MAYO CLINIC
FAMILY HEALTH BOOK

Other Mayo Clinic Titles

Published by

William Morrow and Company, Inc., New York

Mayo Clinic Complete Book of Pregnancy & Baby's First Year

Robert V. Johnson, M.D., Editor-in-Chief, 1994

Mayo Clinic Heart Book

Michael D. McGoon, M.D., Editor-in-Chief, 1993

Mayo Clinic Interactive CD-ROM Discs

Published by IVI Publishing, Eden Prairie, MN

Mayo Clinic Family Health CD-ROM, 1996

Mayo Clinic Family Pharmacist CD-ROM, 1996

AnnaTommy, Mayo Clinic Learning Series CD-ROM, 1994

Safety Monkey, Mayo Clinic Learning Series CD-ROM, 1994

Mayo Clinic Sports Health and Fitness CD-ROM, 1995

Mayo Clinic—The Total Heart CD-ROM, 1995

MAYO CLINIC
FAMILY HEALTH BOOK

David E. Larson, M.D.

Editor-in-Chief

Second Edition

William Morrow and Company, Inc.

New York

Mayo Clinic Family Health Book provides comprehensive health information in a single, authoritative source. *Mayo Clinic Health Letter*, our monthly, eight-page newsletter, offers the same kind of easy-to-understand, practical, reliable information, with a special focus on timely topics. For information on how this award-winning, widely circulated newsletter can be delivered to your doorstep every month, call 1-800-333-9037.

Mayo Clinic Family Health Book provides reliable, practical, comprehensive, easy-to-understand information on issues relating to good health. Much of its information comes directly from the experience of Mayo's 1,600 physicians and research scientists. This book supplements the advice of your personal physician, whom you should consult for individual medical problems. *Mayo Clinic Family Health Book* does not endorse any company or product.

Library of Congress Cataloging-in-Publication Data

Mayo Clinic family health book / David E. Larson, editor-in-chief.—2nd ed.
     p.   cm.
    Includes index.
    ISBN 0-688-14478-0
    1. Medicine, Popular. I. Larson, David E., 1947-   . II. Mayo Clinic.
    [DNLM: 1. Medicine—encyclopedias—popular works. WB 120 M473
    1996]
    RC81.M473 1996
    613—dc20
    DNLM/DLC
    for Library of Congress   96-23661
                                           CIP

Printed in the United States of America

Second Edition

1 2 3 4 5 6 7 8 9 10

Foreword

All of us at Mayo are pleased and proud to recommend the book you are holding. This second edition of our *Mayo Clinic Family Health Book* contains the latest, most reliable health information available. The text has been completely reviewed, revised, and updated. More than 400 Mayo physicians, scientists, nurses, health educators, and other allied health professionals worked closely with Mayo editors skilled at making complex information easy to understand and enjoyable to read.

As in our first edition, this book addresses a broad range of common and rare health conditions and diseases, but we've added many practical, new preventive medicine recommendations. Access to the information you need is improved. The book has been reorganized and redesigned to make it easier to use. You'll also find new self-help tips throughout and a new 8-page color section focusing on the diagnosis and treatment of common disorders such as back pain, high blood pressure, coronary artery disease, breast lumps, and prostate gland problems.

On behalf of the more than 20,000 physicians, scientists, nurses and other health care providers, educators, and support personnel actively engaged at Mayo Medical Center facilities in Rochester, Minnesota; Scottsdale, Arizona; and Jacksonville, Florida, and on behalf of our expanding network of community-based health care partners at each of these locations—thank you for your vote of confidence in selecting our book.

Robert R. Waller, M.D.
President and Chief Executive Officer
Mayo Foundation

Editorial Staff

Preface and Acknowledgments

Six years have passed since this book first appeared in print. In the fast-paced world of modern health care, that's a very long time. Advancements have occurred in many areas, and our health care system has undergone fundamental change. Because of all that has happened, the decision to publish this second edition was easy.

Our first edition was successful. Shortly after the book became available, *U.S. News & World Report* ranked it number one of its kind. *The New York Times* said it "deserves a place on the shelf next to the dictionary and encyclopedia." We are pleased by these votes of confidence.

More than 700,000 copies of the first edition are in print in the English, Dutch, and Chinese languages. We distributed more than 3 million copies in the CD-ROM format, making it a leading source of reliable electronic health information.

How do you go about revising and updating an 800,000-word book?

We began by distributing each chapter to two key groups of Mayo reviewers, one comprised of physicians and scientists, many of whom helped prepare the first edition, and the other of health educators and registered nurses who are members of our Mayo Patient and Health Education Center.

As with our first edition, all physician reviewers are Mayo clinicians. Our Mayo scientific reviewers are engaged in active and varied programs in clinical and basic research. Our patient educators assist Mayo patients with their health information needs on a daily basis.

Despite heavy responsibilities and workloads, all reviewers somehow found time to provide the careful review on which the reliability of health information you'll find in this book is based. As chapter after chapter was returned, marked up with edits and notes and occasionally attachments (such as the latest in Mayo patient education literature), it became apparent that the second edition would be substantially improved in content.

We rewrote several chapters completely. We crafted many new sentences and paragraphs, and we removed information that is now obsolete. We added new information on how to stay well, new facts on self-help, a new "Color Guide to the Diagnosis and Treatment of Common Disorders," and a new listing of organizations that offer health information. We reorganized the content, improved access, and redesigned the book to make it easier and more enjoyable to use. I could go on, but the point is—this is a different, much improved book.

There are many people to thank. Our Assistant Editors top the list. You'll find their names on the preceding page. Our patient educators read chapters and responded to hundreds of editorial queries. Our Section of Publications prepared preliminary page layouts and provided complete manuscript preparation services, including editing, typing, cross-referencing, and proofreading. LeAnn M. Stee again served as an editor while managing with skill, perseverence, and a consistently positive attitude the massive effort required in Publications.

Working with computers that seemed to run perpetually, Margery J. Lovejoy prepared page proofs, distributed them to reviewers, and maintained our production records to help keep the project on track. She was assisted in this effort by Mary K. Horsman. Roberta J. Schwartz coordinated the production process, ensuring that editing, keyboarding, and proofreading tasks were synchronized. Mary L. Schwager again was our chief proofreader and cross-referencer.

Members of our Section of Visual Information Services prepared all line and color medical illustrations and coordinated graphic design. The book was redesigned by our art director, Karen E. Barrie, who developed the attractive new format and selected a new typeface. She also supervised page layout, coordinated the book's conversion to electronic (desktop) publishing, and provided sage advice on a host of issues relating to her specialty. Karen was assisted by graphic designer Kathryn K. Shepel. Working together they solved many design problems while improving the appearance of each page.

Nancy A. Moltaji, visual information librarian, delivered existing line art and photos for scanning by Thomas F. Flood, who processed hundreds of illustrations and photographs with skill and persistence. Graphic design supervisor Ronald R. Ward was a project consultant and helped maintain a smooth work flow.

We were again fortunate to have the services of medical illustrator John V. Hagen, who rendered color and line drawings for the first edition. John updated some of the existing drawings, then worked with Michael A. King to produce the wonderful illustrations you'll find in our new 8-page Color Guide to the Diagnosis and Treatment of Common Disorders. John prepared sketches and Mike rendered them on a state-of-the-art computer. Both are recipients of numerous awards for the consistently outstanding medical art they've produced for many Mayo publications. Dr. J. William Charboneau obtained the radiographic images from Mayo archives to complement this artistic and informative effort.

Photo librarians Jayne H. Feind, Sharon S. Puhl, Lori K. Rehbein, Karlene M. Schulz, and Erica R. Smith, of our Department of Dermatology, helped us find replacements for several images in our Photographic Guide to Common Skin Disorders section, improving the clarity and usefulness of this important visual information.

Once again our publisher is William Morrow of New York City. Senior Editor Toni Sciarra somehow found time to personally review and edit each chapter while coordinating a large publishing team with whom we were in frequent touch throughout the project. We are grateful for the considerable help of Richard Aquan, Michael Beacom, Katharine Cluverius, Michele Corallo, Kaylee Davis, Judy DeGrottole, Jacqueline Deval, Ken Lang, Barbara Levine, Al Marchioni, Michael Murphy, Tom Nau, Tom Oborski, Lisa Queen, Carolyn Robson, Sharyn Rosenblum, Staci Shands, Carol Steuer, Will Schwalbe, Deborah Weiss Geline, Ann Cahn, the Morrow copyediting department, and William Wright. The index was done by Sydney Wolfe Cohen. The book was printed by Kingsport Press/Quebecor.

Special thanks go to my friends and colleagues in the Health

Information Division of Mayo Medical Ventures, including Dr. Richard F. Brubaker, Rick F. Colvin, Marne J. M. Gade, Sara C. Gilliland, Gary E. Peterson, James H. Hale, Christie L. Herman, M. Lillian Haapala, Vicki L. Moore, Kristina L. Randall, Cheryl A. Nelson, Jeanne G. Paulios, Jeanne A. Schmidt, David E. Swanson, and Dr. Kenneth G. Berge, whose decades of experience as a leading Mayo clinician were invaluable in responding to literally hundreds of medical queries. (He also happens to be an outstanding editor.) Suzanne J. Leaf-Brock, of our Division of Communications, coordinated public relations. Special thanks to Arthur Klebanoff, of the Scott Meredith Literary Agency, for energy, creativity, and good advice.

Finally, an extra special thank you to my wife Julie and children Kirstin, Benjamin, and Jonathan, who again supported me with enthusiasm and patience throughout the extra hours required to complete this project.

The following is a list of many of the more than 400 original and new contributors to this second edition:

Administration
Richard C. Edwards
Bruce M. Kelly
Diane E. Quackenbush, R.N.
Alan R. Schilmoeller
David H. Senjem
Richard C. Spavin
David J. Sperling
Stephen Q. Sponsel
Sharon A. Tennis, R.N.

Allergy
Virginia A. Gosselin, R.N.
Lowell L. Henderson, M.D.
James T. Li, M.D.
Richard G. Van Dellen, M.D.

Anatomy
Stephen W. Carmichael, Ph.D.

Anesthesiology
Bradly J. Narr, M.D.

Biochemistry & Molecular Biology
Andrea H. Lauber, Ph.D.
Nita J. Maihle, Ph.D.
Thomas C. Spelsberg, Ph.D.

Breast Clinic
Cindy M. Boyum, R.N.
Jennifer H. Hazelton, R.N.

Cardiovascular Diseases
William T. Bardsley, M.D.
Robert O. Brandenburg, M.D.
John F. Bresnahan, M.D.
Alice M. Flood, R.N.
Gerald T. Gau, M.D.
Raymond J. Gibbons, M.D.
Stephen C. Hammill, M.D.
David R. Holmes, Jr., M.D.
Stephen L. Kopecky, M.D.
Thomas E. Kottke, M.D.
Michael D. McGoon, M.D.
Fletcher A. Miller, M.D.
Sharon A. Neubauer, R.N.
Rick A. Nishimura, M.D.
Jae K. Oh, M.D.
Richard J. Rodeheffer, M.D.
Clarence Shub, M.D.
Lois A. Thorkelson, R.N.
Douglas L. Wood, M.D.

Cardiovascular Health Clinic
Thomas Allison, Ph.D.

Chaplain Services
Warren D. Anderson, M. Div.
Clyde J. Burmeister, M. Div.

Communications
Suzanne J. Leaf-Brock

Dental Specialties
Ronald P. Desjardins, D.M.D.
Joseph A. Gibilisco, D.D.S.
Victoria L. Zook
Bruce A. Lund, D.D.S.
A. Howard Sather, D.D.S.
Phillip J. Sheridan, D.D.S.

Dermatology
David G. Brodland, M.D.
Charles H. Dicken, M.D.
Sigfrid A. Muller, M.D.
Henry W. Randle, M.D.
Randall K. Roenigk, M.D.

Dermatology Photographic Library
Jayne H. Feind
Sharon S. Puhl
Lori K. Rehbein
Karlene M. Schulz
Erica R. Smith
Donna M. Whipple

Education & Professional Development
Katherine J. Flippin, R.N.

Emergency Services
Thomas D. Meloy, M.D.

Endocrinology
Michael D. Brennan, M.D.
Paul C. Carpenter, M.D.
Ian D. Hay, M.D.
Sundeep Khosla, M.D.
Edward G. Lufkin, M.D.
Roger L. Nelson, M.D.
Todd B. Nippoldt, M.D.
P. J. Palumbo, M.D.
Donald A. Scholz, M.D.
Suzanne L. Woolman, R.N.

Family Medicine
John W. Bachman, M.D.

Gastroenterology
David A. Ahlquist, M.D.
Alan J. Cameron, M.D.
Peter W. Carryer, M.D.
Albert J. Czaja, M.D.
Eugene P. DiMagno, M.D.
Willard S. Gamble, M.D.
Christopher J. Gostout, M.D.
Kenneth A. Huizenga, M.D.
Mark V. Larson, M.D.
Edward V. Loftus, Jr., M.D.
Barbara J. Nelson
Albert D. Newcomer, M.D.
Jean Perrault, M.D.
Michael K. Porayko, M.D.
Charlene M. Prather, M.D.
Alfred J. Schei, M.D.
Kenneth W. Schroeder, M.D.
Johnson L. Thistle, M.D.
William J. Tremaine, M.D.
Russell H. Wiesner, M.D.

Hematology
Edwin D. Bayrd, M.D.
Dennis A. Gastineau, M.D.
Morie A. Gertz, M.D.
H. Clark Hoagland, M.D.
C. Christopher Hook, M.D.
Chin-Yang Li, M.D.
William L. Nichols, M.D.
Robert L. Phyliky, M.D.

Hypertension
Gary L. Schwartz, M.D.

Immunology
Paul J. Leibson, M.D.

Infectious Diseases
Juanita D. Heikes, R.N.

Internal Medicine
Darryl S. Chutka, M.D.
Joanne H. Heathman, R.N.
Janet Vittone, M.D.

Laboratory Medicine & Pathology
Curtis L. Bakken, M.D.
Paul G. Belau, M.D.
Keith E. Holley, M.D.
Jurgen Ludwig, M.D.
S. Breanndan Moore, M.D.
Jeffrey L. Myers, M.D.

Legal Counsel
Jill A. Beed, J.D.
Ann E. Decker, J.D.
Francis Helminski, J.D.
Benjamin R. Hippe, J.D.
Kathleen A. Meyerle, J.D.

Library
Dottie M. Hawthorne
Karen E. Larsen
Jean M. McDowall

Mayo Medical Ventures
Ann M. Allen
Richard F. Brubaker, M.D.
Michael A. Casey
Rick F. Colvin, J.D.
Jo Ann Fox
Marne J. M. Gade
Sara C. Gilliland
M. Lillian Haapala
Jody M. Hagan
James H. Hale
Christie L. Herman
Kenneth L. Kurth
Vicki L. Moore
Daniel M. Newton
Jeanne G. Paulios
Judy W. Payne, R.N.
Gary E. Peterson
Kristina L. Randall
Mary L. Rysavy
Jeanne A. Schmidt
Joanne M. Souhrada
Cheryl A. Nelson
Steven P. Van Nurden

Medical Genetics
Gordon W. Dewald, Ph.D.
Noralane M. Lindor, M.D.
Virginia Michels, M.D.

Nephrology
Nancy L. Driscoll, R.N.

Neurologic Surgery
Dudley H. Davis, M.D.
Michael J. Ebersold, M.D.
David G. Piepgras, M.D.

Neurology
Andrea C. Adams, M.D.
J. Eric Ahlskog, M.D.
Allen J. Aksamit, M.D.
Robert D. Brown, Jr., M.D.
J. Keith Campbell, M.D.
Gregory D. Cascino, M.D.
Terrence L. Cascino, M.D.
Bruce A. Evans, M.D.
Gilbert R. Gonzales, M.D.
Frank M. Howard, Jr., M.D.
William J. Litchy, M.D.
Kathleen M. McEvoy, M.D.
James F. Mellinger, M.D.
John H. Noseworthy, M.D.
Ronald C. Petersen, M.D.

Nicotine Dependence Center
Kay M. Eberman

Nutrition/Dietetics
Margaret R. Baker, R.D.
Margaret M. Gall, R.D.
Diane M. Huse, R.D.
Therese K. Liffrig, R.D.
Kathleen A. Lipari, R.D.
Karen E. Moxness, R.D.
Diane L. Olson, R.D.
Rose J. Prissel, R.D.
Charla K. Schultz, R.D.
Jacalyn A. See, R.D.
N. Nicole Spelhaug, R.D.
Susan P. Starkson, R.D.

Obstetrics & Gynecology
Arla J. Bernard, R.N.
Robert J. Breckle
Virginia M. Caspersen, R.N.
Mary E. Cook, R.N.
Lisa D. Erickson, M.D.
Roger W. Harms, M.D.
Edward O. Jorgensen, M.D.
Thomas M. Kastner, M.D.
Linda K. Letts, R.N.
George D. Malkasian, Jr., M.D.
Tammy A. Mulholland
Steven J. Ory, M.D.
Robert G. Rosenquist
Richard E. Symmonds, M.D.
Ann E. Teske, R.N.

Oncology
David L. Ahmann, M.D.
Ann L. Bartlett, R.N.
Donna L. Betcher, R.N.
Edward T. Creagan, M.D.
M. Margaret Gillard, R.N.
Harry J. Long, M.D.
Michael J. O'Connell, M.D.
Paula J. Schomberg, M.D.
Kay M. B. Thiemann

Ophthalmology
Keith H. Baratz, M.D.
George B. Bartley, M.D.
Paul G. Belau, M.D.
Richard F. Brubaker, M.D.
George G. Hohberger, M.D.
Thomas P. Link
Jay A. Rostvold

Orthopedics
Peter C. Amadio, M.D.
Donald C. Campbell II, M.D.
Sherwin Goldman, M.D.
James L. Graham, D.P.M.
Bernard F. Morrey, M.D.
Hamlet A. Peterson, M.D.
William J. Shaughnessy, M.D.
Thomas C. Shives, M.D.
Michael J. Stuart, M.D.

Otorhinolaryngology
Christopher D. Bauch, Ph.D.
George W. Facer, M.D.
Ray O. Gustafson, M.D.
Thomas J. McDonald, M.D.
Cynthia R. McHugh
Anna Mary Peterson
Colleen M. Possehl
Martin S. Robinette, Ph.D.

Patient Health & Education
Susan L. Ahlquist, R.N.
A. Renee Bergstrom
Jeanne M. Ferguson
Eve M. Gehling, R.D.
Margaret C. Harmon, R.N.
Marie A. Ivnik, R.N.
Margo E. Kroshus, R.N.
Diane K. Linbo
Carol J. Mathison
Debra K. McCauley, R.N.
Beverly R. Osmundson, R.N.
Daylene P. Petersen
Deanna M. Radtke
Jane L. Satre, R.N.
Marilyn J. Smith, R.N.
Laurie Jo Vlasak, R.N.
Donna M. Wohlhuter, R.N.

Pediatric Allergy
Edward J. O'Connell, M.D.
Martin I. Sachs, D.O.
John W. Yunginger, M.D.

Pediatric Cardiology
David J. Driscoll, M.D.
William H. Weidman, M.D.

Pediatric Hematology & Oncology
Carola A. S. Arndt, M.D.
Gerald S. Gilchrist, M.D.

Pediatric Neonatology
Fredric Kleinberg, M.D.

Pediatrics
Daniel D. Broughton, M.D.
Edmund C. Burke, M.D.
Roy F. House, Jr., M.D.
Richard D. Olsen, M.D.
K. Hable Rhodes, M.D.
Julia A. Rosekrans, M.D.
Patricia S. Simmons, M.D.
Helen E. Walker, R.N.

Pharmacy Services
James E. Glaser, R.Ph.
Todd M. Johnson, Pharm.D.
Joseph P. Kostick, R.Ph.

Physical Medicine & Rehabilitation
Robert W. DePompolo, M.D.
Tom R. Garrett
Timothy J. Madson
Mehrsheed Sinaki, M.D.
Jack E. Thomas
Jeffrey M. Thompson, M.D.
Gudni Thorsteinsson, M.D.
Lloyd T. Wood, M.D.

Preventive Medicine
Melvin A. Amundsen, M.D.
Richard A. Owen, M.D.
Donald R. Nichols, M.D.

Psychiatry
Nanci A. Bernard
Richard E. Finlayson, M.D.
John E. Huxsahl, M.D.
Ted R. Laska
Ellen J. Lichty
Linda M. Minor, R.N.
Pat M. Oja, R.N.
Lloyd A. Wells, M.D.

Psychology
Donald Eugene Williams, Ph.D.

Publications
Mary K. Horsman
Margery J. Lovejoy
Mary L. Schwager
Roberta J. Schwartz
LeAnn M. Stee

Radiation Safety
Joel E. Gray, Ph.D.
Richard J. Vetter, Ph.D.

Radiology
Thomas H. Berquist, M.D.
Harley C. Carlson, M.D.
Richard L. Ehman, M.D.
Lee A. Forstrom, M.D.
John J. Gisvold, M.D.
E. Meredith James, M.D.
Michael J. Kiely, M.D.
George H. Klann
Andrew J. LeRoy, M.D.
Gary M. Miller, M.D.
Kristie J. Nelson
LeeAnna J. Tomasek
Steven L. Williams
Gregory A. Wiseman, M.D.

Rheumatology
Thomas W. Bunch, M.D.
Sherine E. Gabriel, M.D.
W. Leroy Griffing, M.D.
Thomas G. Mason, M.D.
John G. Mayne, M.D.
Charles H. McKenna, M.D.
Audrey M. Nelson, M.D.
John W. Worthington, M.D.

Speech Pathology
Arnold E. Aronson, Ph.D.
Joseph R. Duffy, Ph.D.
Robert L. Keith
Jack E. Thomas

Social Services
Mary E. Ely

Surgery
Philip E. Bernatz, M.D.
Richard M. Devine, M.D.
John H. Donohue, M.D.
Clive S. Grant, M.D.
Melissa J. Lushinsky
Christopher G.A. McGregor, M.D.
Thomas A. Orszulak, M.D.
Robert J. Spencer, M.D.
C. Robert Stanhope, M.D.
Geoffrey B. Thompson, M.D.
Jonathan A. van Heerden, M.B.,Ch.B.
John E. Woods, M.D.

Thoracic Diseases
Howard A. Andersen, M.D.
W. Mark Brutinel, M.D.
Kathryn A. Cummings
Eric S. Edell, M.D.
Peter J. Hauri, Ph.D.
Ashokakumar M. Patel, M.D.
Udaya B. S. Prakash, M.D.
Jay H. Ryu, M.D.
Paul D. Scanlon, M.D.
Bruce A. Staats, M.D.
Robert W. Viggiano, M.D.

Urology
David M. Barrett, M.D.
Michael L. Blute, M.D.
Karen M. Hyland, R.N.
Stephen A. Kramer, M.D.
Renee E. Kromrey, R.N.
Frank J. Leary, M.D.
Ronald W. Lewis, M.D.
Michael M. Lieber, M.D.
Robert P. Myers, M.D.
David E. Patterson, M.D.
Joseph W. Segura, M.D.

Visual Information
James G. Bambenek
Karen E. Barrie
Robert C. Benassi
Vincent P. Destro
Thomas F. Flood
Mary T. Frantz
John V. Hagen
Elman A. Hanken
Joseph M. Kane
Michael A. King
Nancy A. Moltaji
Kristi Lee Ostrom
Kathryn K. Shepel
Carol J. Sparrow
Ronald R. Ward
Randy J. Ziegler

Writers
Susie Blackmun
Felicia Busch, R.D.
Terry Jopke
Lynn Madsen
Beverly K. Parker
Deborah J. Shuman
Cathy Stroebel
Ruth Taswell
Robin E. S. Taylor
Beth A. Watkins

To one and all, within and outside Mayo Medical Center, my sincere thanks for a job exceptionally well done.

David E. Larson, M.D.
Editor-in-Chief

Contents

Foreword v
Preface and Acknowledgments vii

How to Use This Book xiii

Here you will find practical information about the book's organization, the content and purpose of each division, tips on how you can quickly and easily locate the information you need, and how to interpret your signs and symptoms.

Color Atlas of Human Anatomy xvi

Part I: Your Health Through the Years 1

From your entrance into the world to your later years, your physical and emotional needs change. These introductory chapters review human growth and development and address many of the common health problems you and those you care about may face during the course of your lives.

1   Newborn: The First Month of Life 3
2   Infancy: Ages 1 Month to 1 Year 59
3   Preschool Years: Ages 1 Through 5 81
4   School-Age Child: Ages 6 Through 12 115
5   Teenage Years: Ages 13 Through 19 137
6   Young Adulthood: Ages 20 Through 39 161
7   Middle Years: Ages 40 Through 65 219
8   Later Years: After Age 65 231

Part II: Staying Well 249

Maintaining or improving your health means eating right, exercising regularly, caring for your body, avoiding harmful habits and substance abuse, and practicing other preventive strategies. All of these measures are addressed here. You'll also find tips on safety within and outside your home, dealing with the challenges of our environment, and guarding your health when traveling outside the United States.

9   Nutrition and Health 251
10   Exercise and Fitness 289
11   Controlling Stress 307
12   Tobacco 315
13   Alcohol Abuse and Alcoholism 325
14   Medications and Drug Abuse 335
15   Safety 349
16   Tooth Care 363
17   The World Around Us 371
18   Traveling Abroad 379

Part III: First Aid and Emergency Care 387

How can you best deal with a deep laceration, a high fever, a seizure, or chest pain? In this special section you'll find easy-to-understand, practical information on common health problems, ranging from a nosebleed or sunburn to life-threatening challenges such as an airway obstruction or a heart attack. To find this section quickly and easily, look for pages with blue edges.

Part IV: Human Diseases and Disorders **455**

If you are ill, or if someone you care about is faced with a health problem, look here to find detailed descriptions of signs and symptoms, causes, diagnoses, severity, and treatments for more than 1,000 ailments, from the common to the rare.

19   Your Brain and Nervous System 457

Color Guide to the Diagnosis and Treatment of Common Disorders **512**

20   Your Eyes 519
21   Your Ears, Nose, and Throat 567
22   Dental and Oral Disorders 601
23   Your Heart and Blood Vessels 631
24   Your Lungs and Respiratory System 699
25   Your Digestive System 737
26   Your Kidneys and Urinary Tract 825
27   Your Bones, Joints, and Muscles 859
28   Your Endocrine System 923
29   Your Blood 953
30   Your Skin 983

Photographic Guide to Common Skin Disorders **1008**

31   Allergies 1025
32   Infectious Diseases 1055
33   Mental Health 1093
34   Women's Health 1139
35   Men's Health 1195
36   Health Issues of Partners 1213

Part V: Modern Medical Care **1235**

Here is your introduction to the complexities of modern medical practice. Also, there are chapters on understanding and coping with cancer, and on dealing with death. Look for specific tips in understanding and using the numerous and sometimes perplexing health care options available today.

37   Understanding and Using the Health Care System 1237
38   The Modern Pharmacy 1271
39   Understanding Your Medications 1281
40   Cancer 1289
41   Dealing With Death 1309
42   Home Care and Elder Care 1319
43   Medical Tests 1329

Appendices **1349**

I   Conversion Tables (Weights and Measures) 1351
II   Understanding Medical Terms 1355
III   Where to Go for More Information 1373
IV   How to Prepare an Advance Directive 1381

Index **1390**

> *"The object of all health education is to change the conduct of individual men, women and children by teaching them to care for their bodies well."*
>
> —C. H. Mayo, 1932

How to Use This Book

This book is about answers: *Mayo Clinic Family Health Book* is designed to provide you with the kind of authoritative, comprehensive, practical, easy-to-understand, reliable information you need to live a healthier life.

The Organization

The book consists of five divisions. Parts I, II, and III address normal human growth and development, the changes you can expect as you age, strategies for avoiding illness, and dealing with habits or emergencies that can threaten your health. Parts IV and V mainly concern disease, its diagnosis, treatment, and modern medical care.

To use the book efficiently, you may find it helpful to understand in more detail how the divisions and chapters are arranged. The organization is as follows:

Part I: Your Health Through the Years

If you are about to become a parent, or you want to understand more about normal changes or health problems you might encounter in your children, your parents, or yourself, Part I is the place to look.

Starting with the newborn, separate chapters address each stage of life, including newborn, infancy, the preschool years, school-age children, the teenage years, young adulthood, and the middle and later years.

You'll also find a 16-page Color Atlas of Human Anatomy.

Part II: Staying Well

Good habits are keys to healthful living. This section is filled with practical guidance on nutrition, exercise, how to control the inevitable stresses in your life, tobacco, alcohol, and medications. We also address safety, tooth care, the challenges of our environment, and foreign travel.

Part III: First Aid and Emergency Care

No one is immune to medical emergencies. This lengthy, special section offers comprehensive, easy-to-find information on most of the minor and major challenges you may face any day of the year.

Part IV: Human Diseases and Disorders

For decades, Mayo Clinic has been a storehouse of the latest and best information on human diseases and disorders. In this lengthy division we discuss, individually, most of the common and many rare health problems. It is here that you can find detailed information about a specific ailment.

Each entry begins with a review of signs and symptoms. This is followed by a description of the disease and a discussion on how your physician might make a diagnosis. We often include reviews of the real or potential seriousness of the problem. We discuss treatments including medications or surgery or, when appropriate, self-help.

We address mental health, women's health, men's health, and health issues of partners. Part IV includes an 8-page Color Guide to the Diagnosis and Treatment of Common Disorders and a 16-page Photographic Guide to Common Skin Disorders.

Part V: Modern Medical Care

The goal of Part V is to demystify the increasingly complex world of modern medicine, with chapters devoted to understanding and using the health care system, the modern pharmacy, and medications. There is a chapter that can help you avoid, understand, or cope with cancer. We include a sensitively written chapter that offers guidance on how you or a loved one might deal with death. There's advice on how to select home or elder care. We conclude with brief descriptions of common medical tests.

Appendices

At the close of the book are appendices in which you'll find conversion tables for weights and measures, a comprehensive glossary of medical, anatomic, and health care terms, a helpful listing of organizations offering all kinds of health information, and useful information on how to go about preparing advance directives such as a living will or durable power of attorney for health care.

Finding the Facts You Need

For speedy access to specific information, you will find on the page that introduces each major division a complete listing of chapter titles included in that division. On the opening page of each chapter is a table of contents for that chapter. Throughout the book are numerous cross-references, and we end the book with a detailed index. But beyond these tools is an underlying rationale for the organization of this book.

Using Your Symptoms

You know when you are well: life's activities give you pleasure, whether in your work or play, the meal before you, or the joy of family and friends. There are no pains to distract you from life's satisfactions.

Equally, you know when you are ailing.

Yet, identifying the signs and symptoms of an illness, whether minor or major, is the very essence of caring for your health. For that matter, it is also at the heart of modern medical practice and of this book. A nagging ache, a regular cough, a minor or more significant change in your body's day-to-day messages to you—all are signs and symptoms, potentially meaningful pieces of information for you or your physician.

This book is not intended to teach you to perform independent self-diagnosis. No book can be a substitute for your physician's years of medical school, clinical training, and practical experience. However, you can use this book to help you better understand your body and mind and to help you become a more active partner in your health care.

The fact is you know a great deal about your personal signs and symptoms. You live with them. If symptoms change, your physician isn't the first to know—you are. Therefore, we organized *Mayo Clinic Family Health Book* to help you use signs and symptoms to recognize problems and to better understand your health.

Because it deals with your personal health, this may be one of the most practical and valuable books in your home. We hope you will use it often, and we hope that the reliable information in this book, complemented by the advice of your personal physician, will help you and your loved ones lead a healthier, more fulfilling life.

The Organization of an Entry

For quick and easy reference, most entries pertaining to human diseases and disorders are organized in the format shown on the opposite page:

Name of disease

Aortic Aneurysm

Key indications

Signs and Symptoms
- Often, none
- Pulsating sensation in the abdomen

Basic description of the disease

An aneurysm is an abnormal widening of an artery. A weakened wall of an artery is stretched as the blood is pumped through it, often creating an egg-shaped ballooning.

An aneurysm can occur in any blood vessel, including major ones in the brain (see Stroke, page 461) and minor ones anywhere in the body, but it is most likely to occur in the aorta, the main blood vessel that carries blood from the heart. A common site for an aortic aneurysm is immediately below the kidneys but above the junction of the abdominal aorta and arteries to the legs.

Abdominal aneurysms are thought to be largely the result of atherosclerosis. Complicating factors such as high blood pressure (hypertension) may contribute to the development of an aneurysm.

In addition to the expansion of the arterial wall, an aneurysm also characteristically has an accumulation of cholesterol, calcium, and even small blood clots. The weakened muscle fibers of the artery wall become fragmented and are replaced by scar tissue. Despite all these changes, the size of the artery's central channel may remain roughly normal.

Abdominal aortic aneurysms most often strike people over age 60, and men are more commonly affected than women.

In some people, the layers of tissue that compose the wall of the aorta separate (dissect). Immediate treatment is required for this disorder; often surgical removal of the affected artery is necessary.

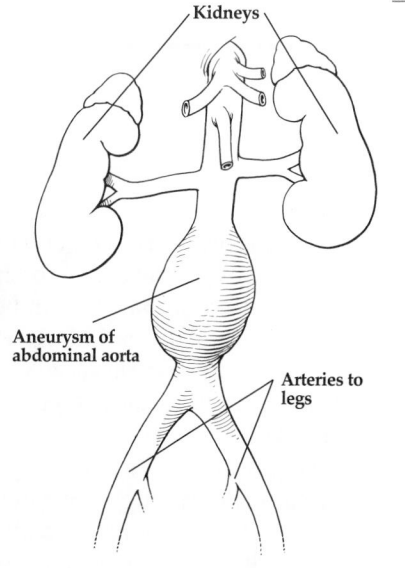

Informative illustration

An aneurysm, an abnormal widening of an artery, can occur in any location, but commonly occurs in the abdominal aorta just below the kidneys. The weakened wall of the aorta balloons out over time, usually growing at a rate of ⅛ to ¼ inch a year.

How the disorder is identified

Diagnosis
Often there are no symptoms. However, in advanced cases, pain may be present in the abdomen and lower back. Aneurysms tend to grow at a rate of about ⅛ to ¼ inch a year and often do not cause symptoms until blood begins to leak from the ballooning wall of the artery. If the aneurysm ruptures, shock, loss of consciousness, and death may be the catastrophic result.

Your physician may feel the pulsating vessel on routine examination of your abdomen. In some cases, an X-ray taken for another reason will reveal an aneurysm. Its presence is usually confirmed with an ultrasound examination or a CT scan (see page 1334).

Potential consequences

How Serious Is an Aneurysm?
An abdominal aortic aneurysm can be life-threatening; all too often, the ailment is discovered during autopsy. Like heart disease, abdominal aortic aneurysm can be considered a silent killer. However, if discovered in time, there is a highly effective surgical procedure available to treat this disorder.

Treatment
Drugs are not of value in treating an abdominal aortic aneurysm. If the aneurysm is small and no symptoms are apparent at the time it is discovered, your physician may recommend a watch-and-wait approach. No changes will be required in your physical activities, but periodic ultrasound examinations or CT scans will be done to determine if the aneurysm is expanding.

Surgery
In an emergency or as a preventive measure, your physician may recommend an operation to replace the diseased portion of aorta with an artificial artery made of synthetic material.

The risk of the aneurysm rupturing—a potentially life-threatening event—increases as the aneurysm grows. The operation is relatively safe when performed prior to rupture, but less than half of those operated on after rupture survive.

Latest information on treatment and prevention

Color Atlas of Human Anatomy

Your body never really sleeps. Day and night it is busy constructing new cells, warding off illness, processing nutrients, and orchestrating a host of physical and biochemical actions, all of which contribute to your health and sense of well-being.

Within this Color Atlas of Human Anatomy you will find easy-to-understand drawings of the human body in all its wondrous grace and complexity. From your skin (your first line of defense against disease), to muscles, bones, and organs (which control movement and bodily functions), to your immune system (where substances too small to be seen wage never-ending war against illness), the drawings in this atlas focus on normal human anatomy. Supporting the drawings are insets offering unique views of various common ailments as revealed by state-of-the-art imaging technology. In recent years, this remarkable equipment has significantly advanced the ability of physicians to diagnose illness at an early stage, when treatment often is most effective.

Contents

Your Skin. A-1

Your Muscles A-2

Your Bones A-4

Your Organs A-6

Your Digestive System A-7

Your Blood Vessels, Heart, and Lungs. A-8

Your Brain and Nerves. A-10

Your Endocrine Glands. A-11

Your Reproductive Organs and Urinary Tract. A-12

Your Senses. A-14

Your Immune System A-16

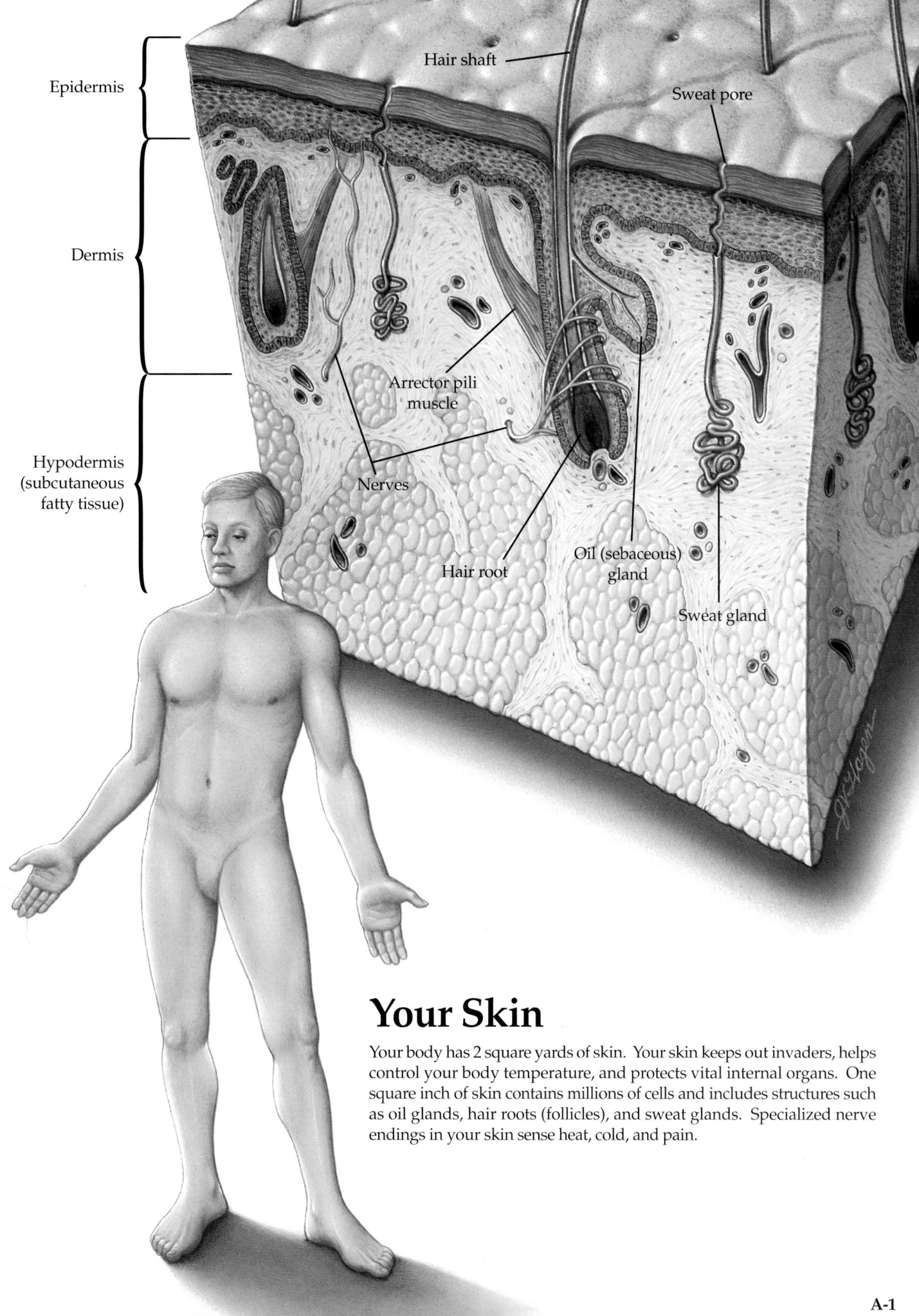

Epidermis

Dermis

Hypodermis
(subcutaneous
fatty tissue)

Hair shaft

Sweat pore

Arrector pili
muscle

Nerves

Hair root

Oil (sebaceous)
gland

Sweat gland

Your Skin

Your body has 2 square yards of skin. Your skin keeps out invaders, helps
control your body temperature, and protects vital internal organs. One
square inch of skin contains millions of cells and includes structures such
as oil glands, hair roots (follicles), and sweat glands. Specialized nerve
endings in your skin sense heat, cold, and pain.

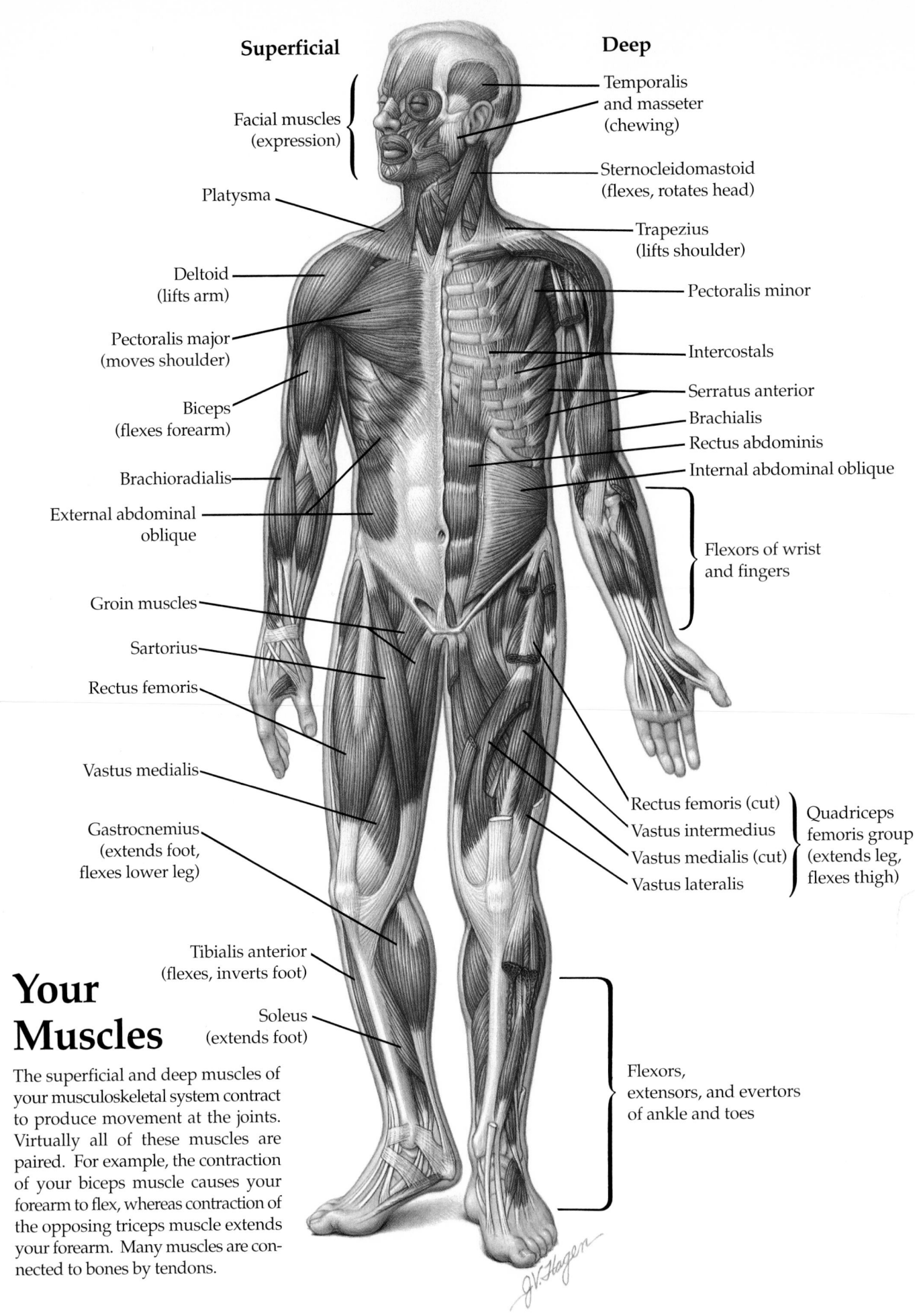

Superficial **Deep**

Temporalis
and masseter
(chewing)

Facial muscles
(expression)

Sternocleidomastoid
(flexes, rotates head)

Platysma

Trapezius
(lifts shoulder)

Deltoid
(lifts arm)

Pectoralis minor

Pectoralis major
(moves shoulder)

Intercostals

Serratus anterior

Biceps
(flexes forearm)

Brachialis

Rectus abdominis

Brachioradialis

Internal abdominal oblique

External abdominal
oblique

Flexors of wrist
and fingers

Groin muscles

Sartorius

Rectus femoris

Vastus medialis

Rectus femoris (cut)

Quadriceps
femoris group
(extends leg,
flexes thigh)

Vastus intermedius

Vastus medialis (cut)

Gastrocnemius
(extends foot,
flexes lower leg)

Vastus lateralis

Tibialis anterior
(flexes, inverts foot)

Your
Muscles

Soleus
(extends foot)

Flexors,
extensors, and evertors
of ankle and toes

The superficial and deep muscles of
your musculoskeletal system contract
to produce movement at the joints.
Virtually all of these muscles are
paired. For example, the contraction
of your biceps muscle causes your
forearm to flex, whereas contraction of
the opposing triceps muscle extends
your forearm. Many muscles are connected to bones by tendons.

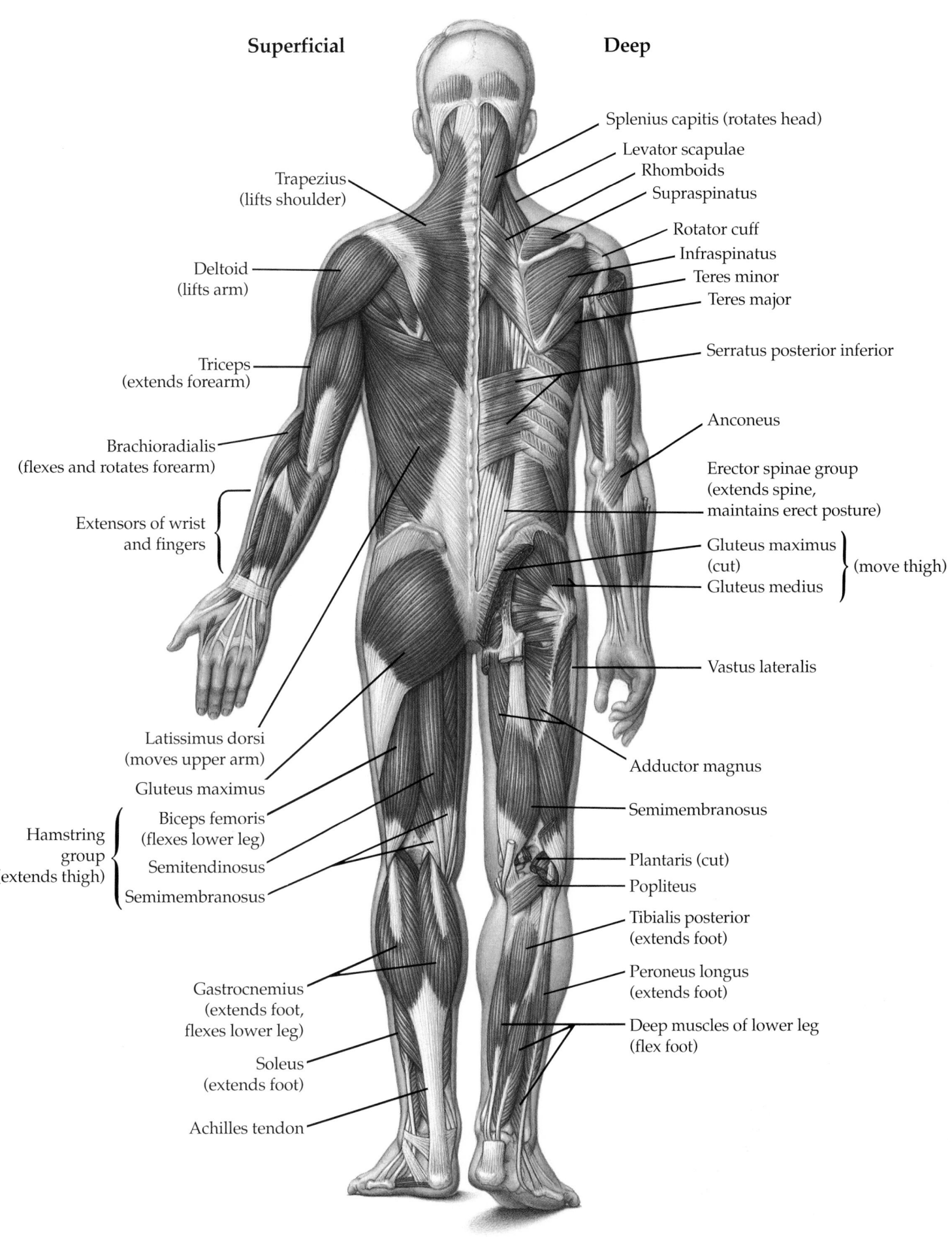

Superficial

Deep

Trapezius
(lifts shoulder)

Deltoid
(lifts arm)

Triceps
(extends forearm)

Brachioradialis
(flexes and rotates forearm)

Extensors of wrist
and fingers

Latissimus dorsi
(moves upper arm)

Gluteus maximus

Biceps femoris
(flexes lower leg)

Semitendinosus

Semimembranosus

Hamstring
group
(extends thigh)

Gastrocnemius
(extends foot,
flexes lower leg)

Soleus
(extends foot)

Achilles tendon

Splenius capitis (rotates head)

Levator scapulae

Rhomboids

Supraspinatus

Rotator cuff

Infraspinatus

Teres minor

Teres major

Serratus posterior inferior

Anconeus

Erector spinae group
(extends spine,
maintains erect posture)

Gluteus maximus
(cut)

Gluteus medius

(move thigh)

Vastus lateralis

Adductor magnus

Semimembranosus

Plantaris (cut)

Popliteus

Tibialis posterior
(extends foot)

Peroneus longus
(extends foot)

Deep muscles of lower leg
(flex foot)

A-3

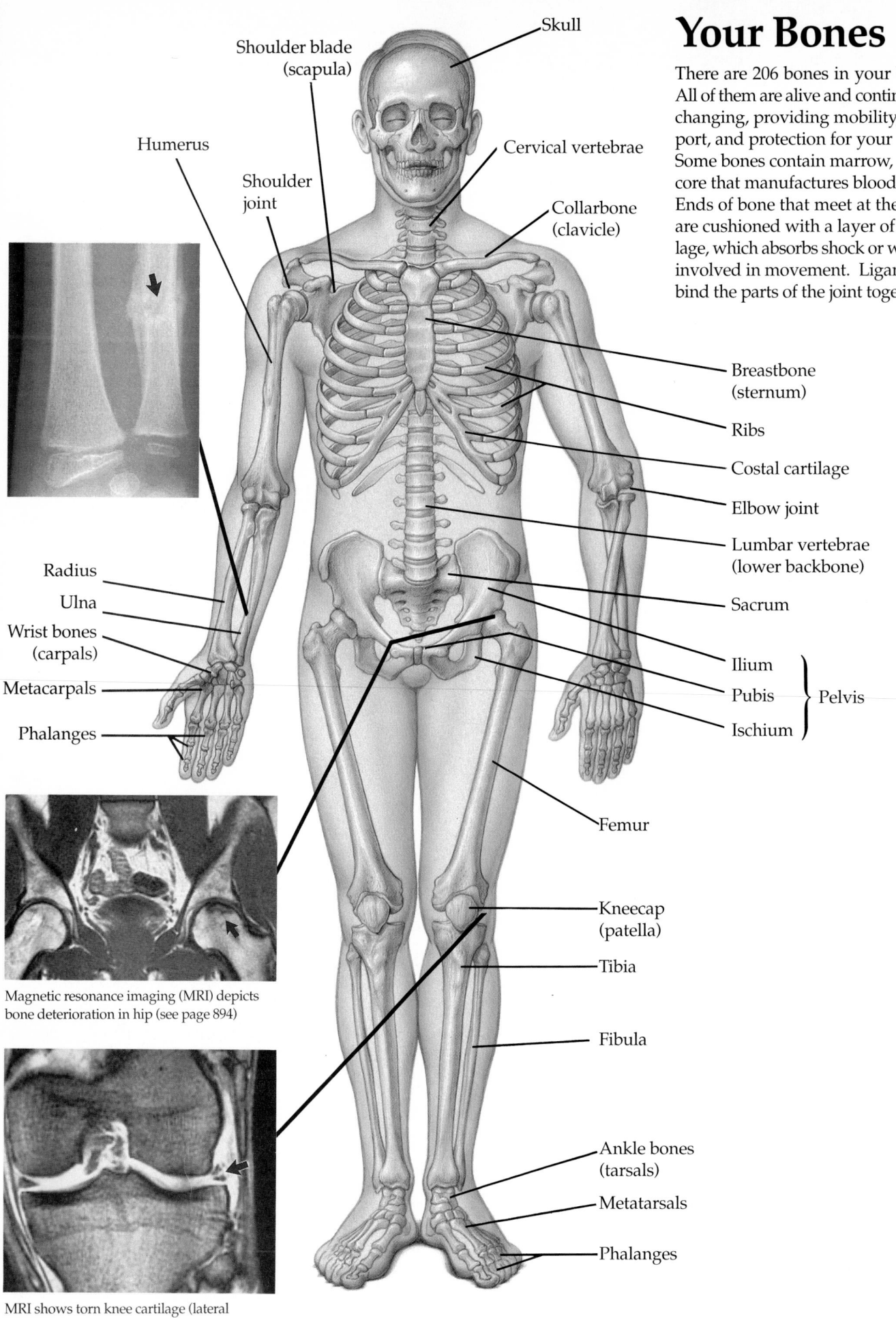

Your Bones

There are 206 bones in your body. All of them are alive and continually changing, providing mobility, support, and protection for your body. Some bones contain marrow, a soft core that manufactures blood cells. Ends of bone that meet at the joint are cushioned with a layer of cartilage, which absorbs shock or weight involved in movement. Ligaments bind the parts of the joint together.

Skull

Shoulder blade (scapula)

Humerus

Shoulder joint

Cervical vertebrae

Collarbone (clavicle)

Breastbone (sternum)

Ribs

Costal cartilage

Elbow joint

Lumbar vertebrae (lower backbone)

Sacrum

Ilium

Pubis

Ischium

Pelvis

Radius

Ulna

Wrist bones (carpals)

Metacarpals

Phalanges

Femur

Kneecap (patella)

Tibia

Fibula

Ankle bones (tarsals)

Metatarsals

Phalanges

Magnetic resonance imaging (MRI) depicts bone deterioration in hip (see page 894)

MRI shows torn knee cartilage (lateral meniscus) (see page 907)

Skull and Vertebrae

Your skull and vertebrae protect your brain and spinal cord. In between the vertebrae are spongy cushions called discs. The vertebrae and discs are held together by a network of muscles and ligaments.

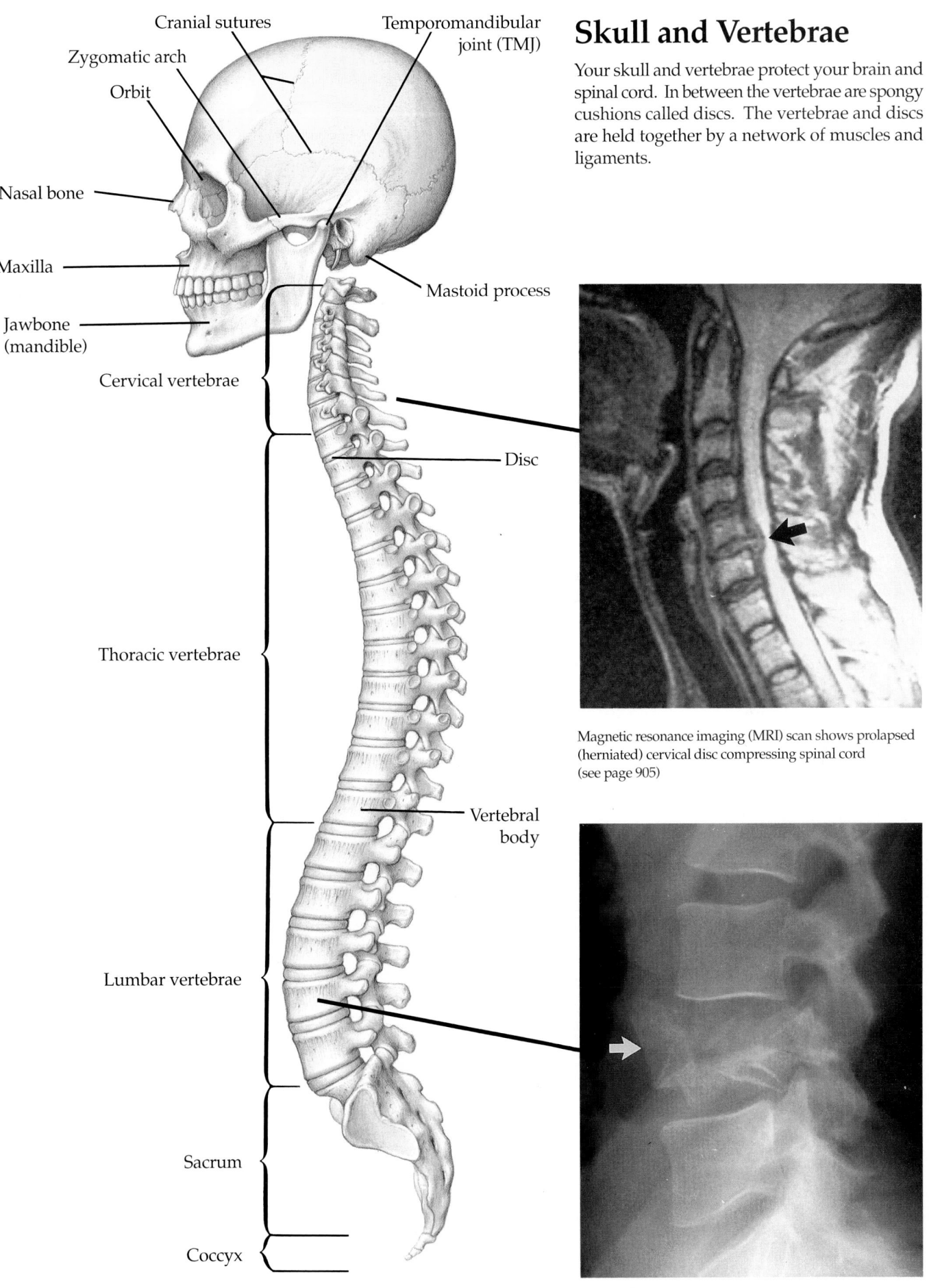

Cranial sutures

Zygomatic arch

Orbit

Temporomandibular joint (TMJ)

Nasal bone

Maxilla

Jawbone (mandible)

Mastoid process

Cervical vertebrae

Disc

Thoracic vertebrae

Vertebral body

Lumbar vertebrae

Sacrum

Coccyx

Magnetic resonance imaging (MRI) scan shows prolapsed (herniated) cervical disc compressing spinal cord (see page 905)

X-ray reveals severe fracture of a low back (lumbar) vertebra

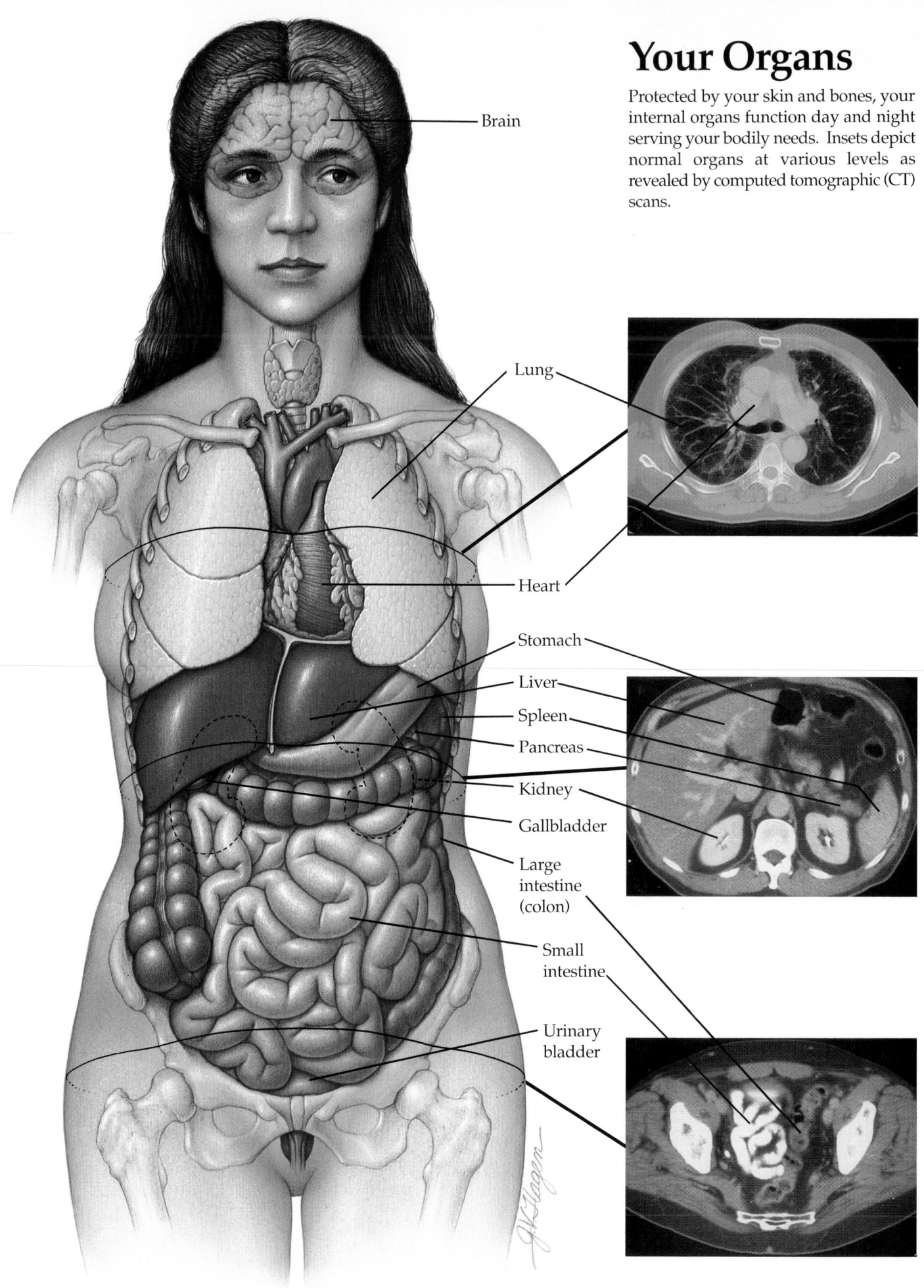

Your Organs

Protected by your skin and bones, your internal organs function day and night serving your bodily needs. Insets depict normal organs at various levels as revealed by computed tomographic (CT) scans.

Brain

Lung

Heart

Stomach

Liver

Spleen

Pancreas

Kidney

Gallbladder

Large intestine (colon)

Small intestine

Urinary bladder

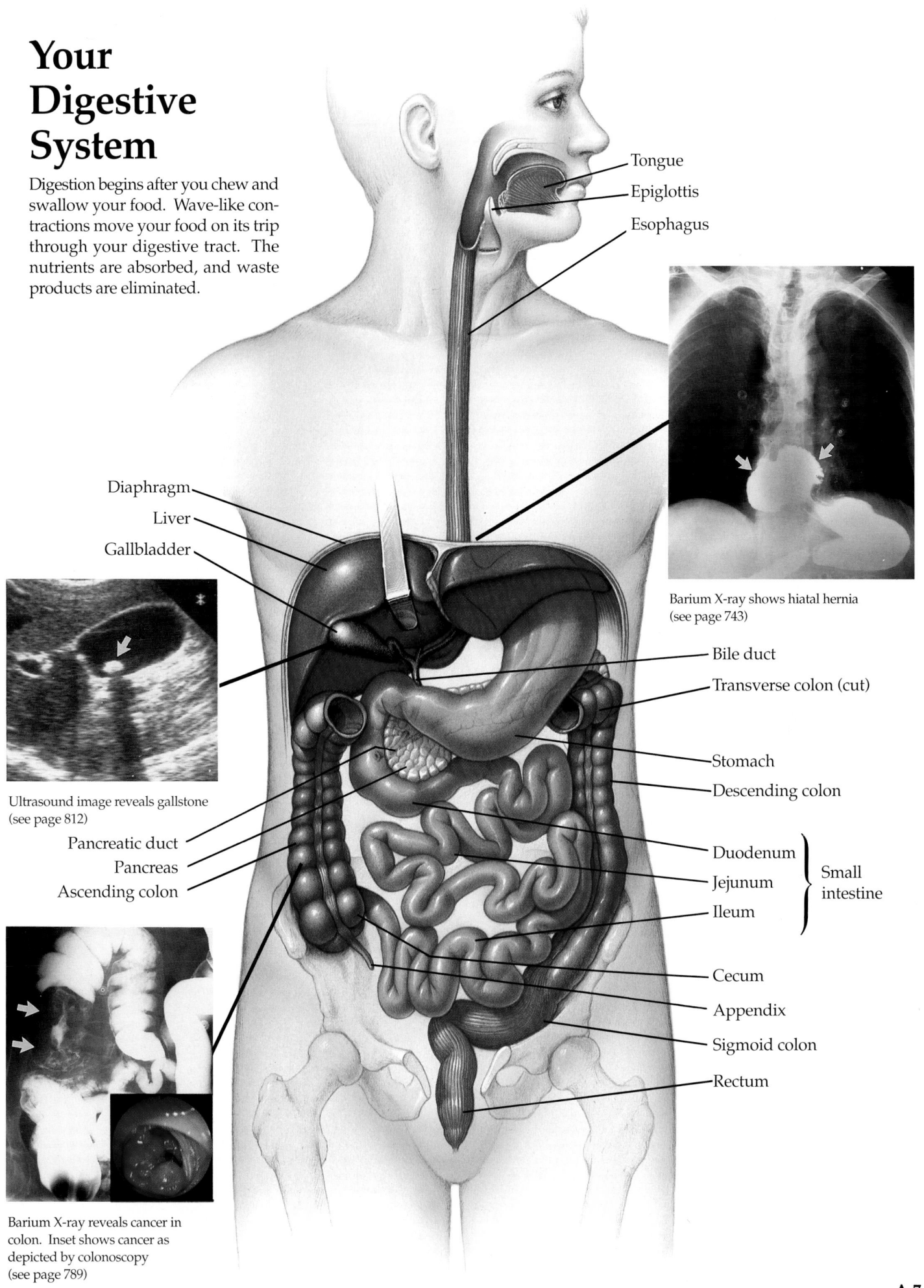

Your Digestive System

Digestion begins after you chew and swallow your food. Wave-like contractions move your food on its trip through your digestive tract. The nutrients are absorbed, and waste products are eliminated.

Tongue

Epiglottis

Esophagus

Barium X-ray shows hiatal hernia (see page 743)

Diaphragm

Liver

Gallbladder

Ultrasound image reveals gallstone (see page 812)

Pancreatic duct

Pancreas

Ascending colon

Bile duct

Transverse colon (cut)

Stomach

Descending colon

Duodenum

Jejunum

Small intestine

Ileum

Cecum

Appendix

Sigmoid colon

Rectum

Barium X-ray reveals cancer in colon. Inset shows cancer as depicted by colonoscopy (see page 789)

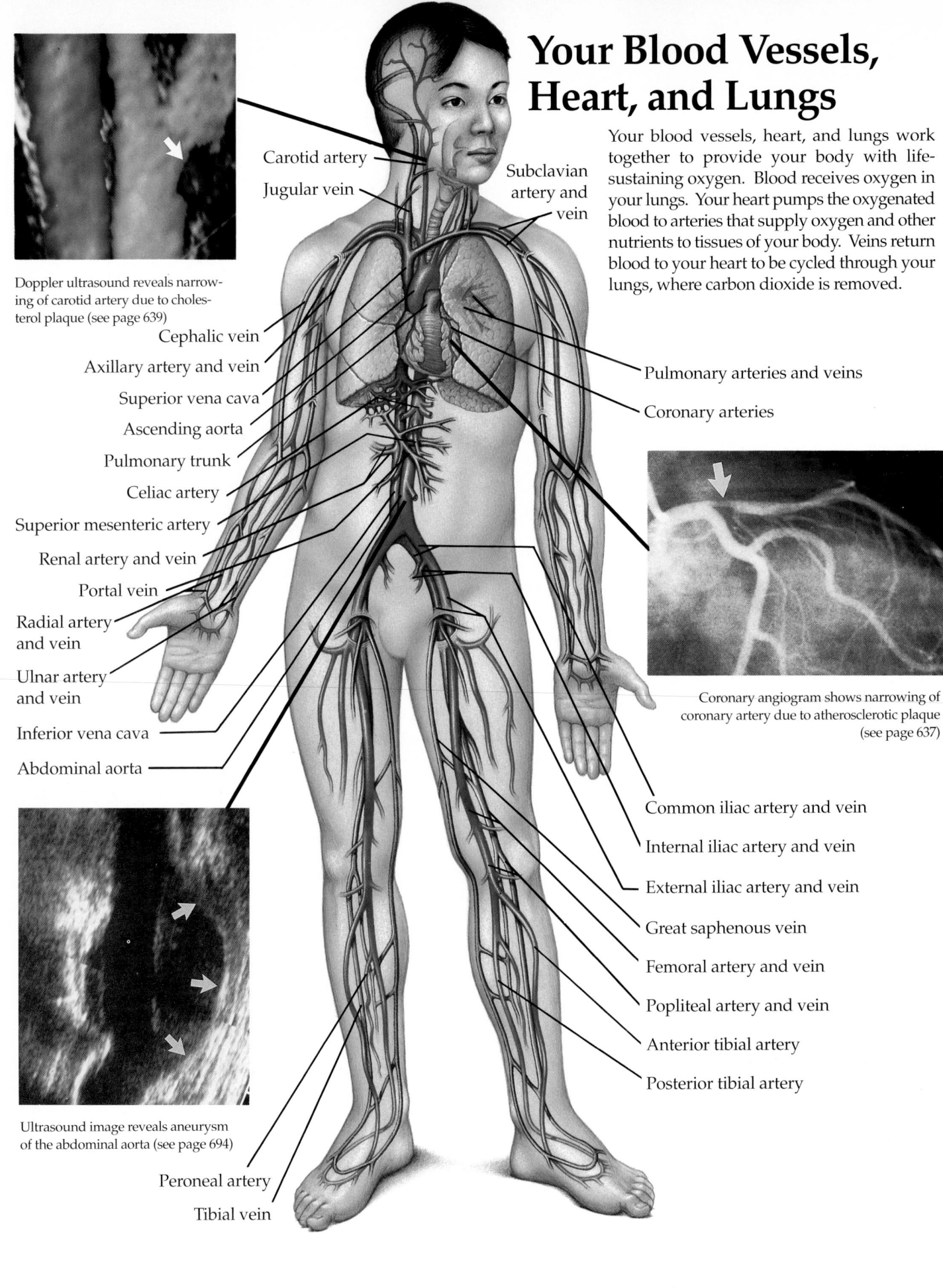

Your Blood Vessels, Heart, and Lungs

Your blood vessels, heart, and lungs work together to provide your body with life-sustaining oxygen. Blood receives oxygen in your lungs. Your heart pumps the oxygenated blood to arteries that supply oxygen and other nutrients to tissues of your body. Veins return blood to your heart to be cycled through your lungs, where carbon dioxide is removed.

Doppler ultrasound reveals narrowing of carotid artery due to cholesterol plaque (see page 639)

Carotid artery

Jugular vein

Subclavian artery and vein

Cephalic vein

Axillary artery and vein

Superior vena cava

Ascending aorta

Pulmonary trunk

Celiac artery

Superior mesenteric artery

Renal artery and vein

Portal vein

Radial artery and vein

Ulnar artery and vein

Inferior vena cava

Abdominal aorta

Pulmonary arteries and veins

Coronary arteries

Coronary angiogram shows narrowing of coronary artery due to atherosclerotic plaque (see page 637)

Common iliac artery and vein

Internal iliac artery and vein

External iliac artery and vein

Great saphenous vein

Femoral artery and vein

Popliteal artery and vein

Anterior tibial artery

Posterior tibial artery

Ultrasound image reveals aneurysm of the abdominal aorta (see page 694)

Peroneal artery

Tibial vein

Heart

Your heart is a muscular pump containing four chambers connected by valves. Venous blood from your body flows through the superior and inferior vena cava into the right atrium, then through the tricuspid valve into your right ventricle. The right ventricle pumps blood through the pulmonary valve, via the pulmonary arteries, into your lungs. From the lungs, blood enters the left atrium via the pulmonary veins and flows through the mitral valve into the left ventricle. The powerful left ventricle pumps oxygen-enriched blood through the aortic valve into the aorta for delivery to your body's tissues.

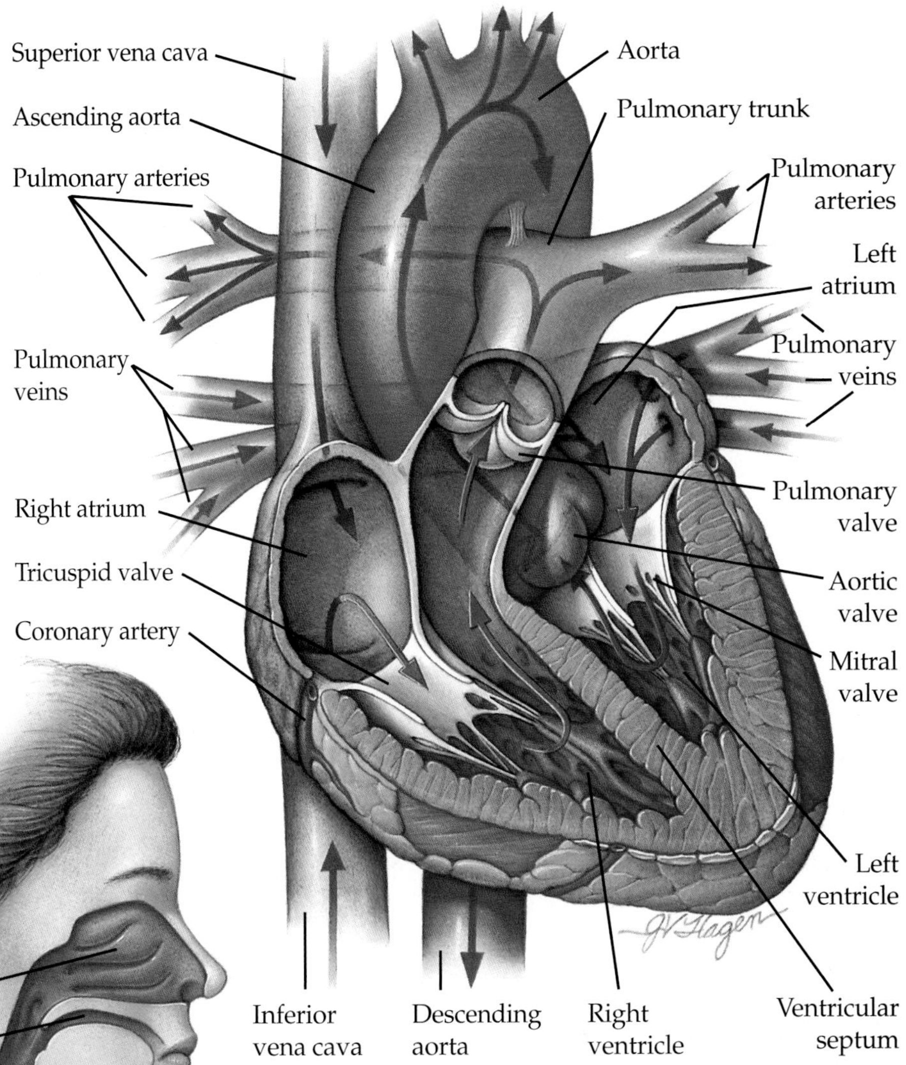

Lungs

Your lungs supply oxygen to your blood and remove carbon dioxide from it. The exchange takes place in tiny air sacs called alveoli.

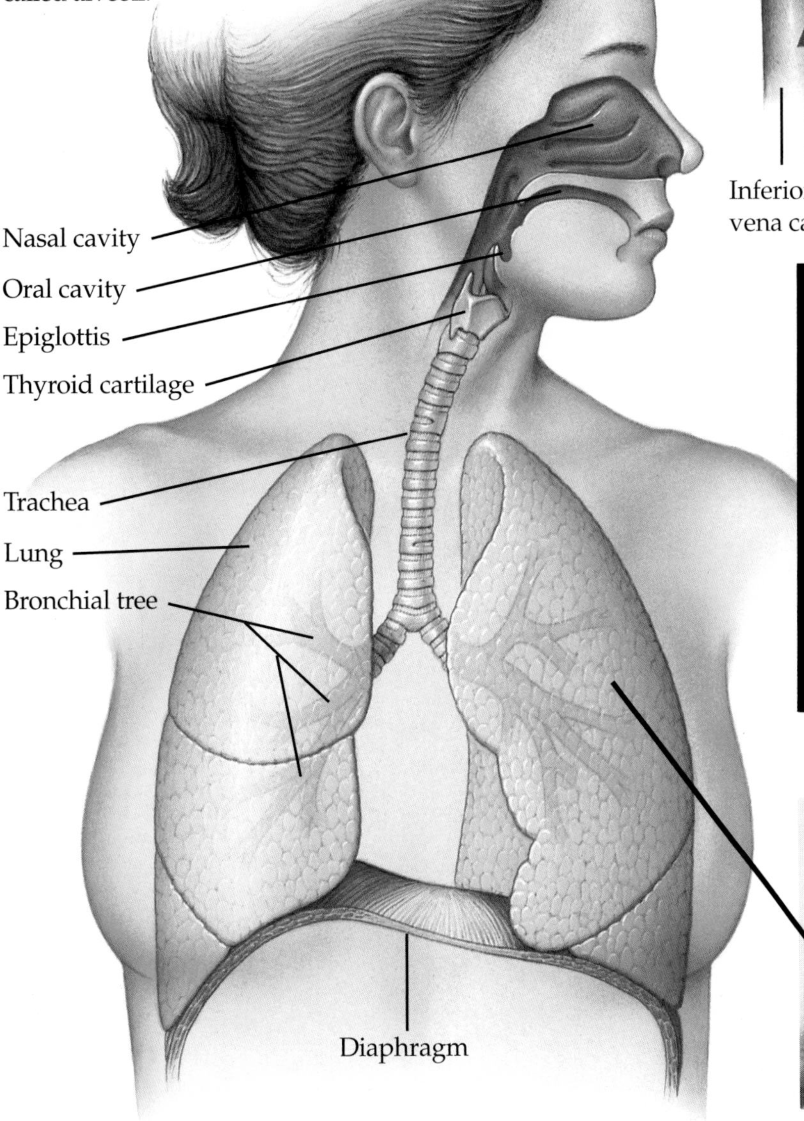

Superior vena cava

Ascending aorta

Pulmonary arteries

Pulmonary veins

Right atrium

Tricuspid valve

Coronary artery

Aorta

Pulmonary trunk

Pulmonary arteries

Left atrium

Pulmonary veins

Pulmonary valve

Aortic valve

Mitral valve

Left ventricle

Inferior vena cava

Descending aorta

Right ventricle

Ventricular septum

Nasal cavity

Oral cavity

Epiglottis

Thyroid cartilage

Trachea

Lung

Bronchial tree

Diaphragm

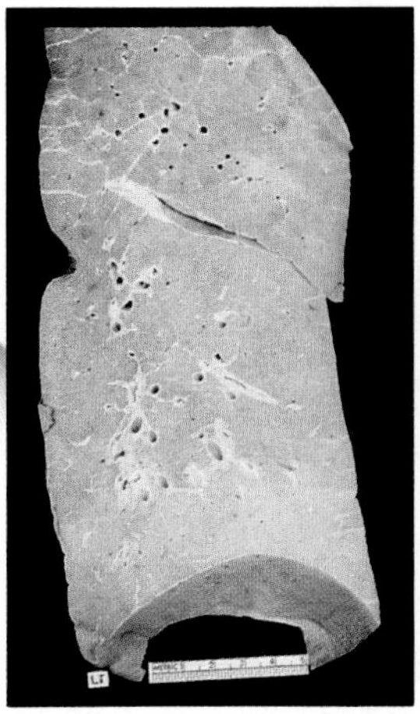

Normal lung tissue

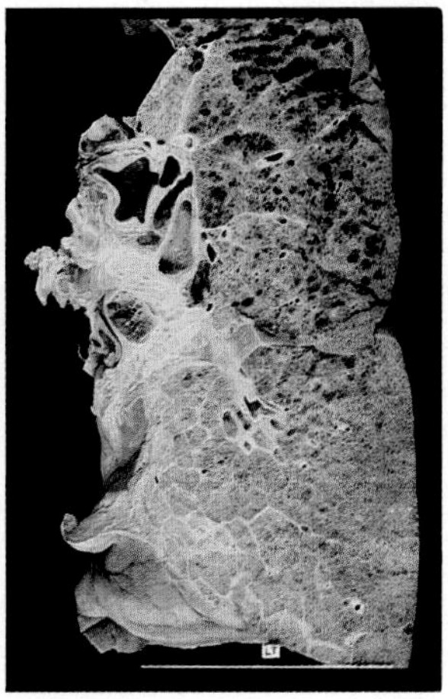

Diseased lung tissue (emphysema) (see page 715)

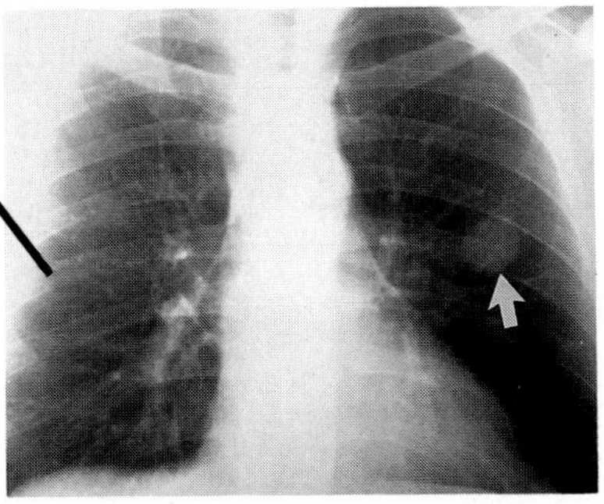

Chest X-ray reveals cancer in left lung (see page 724)

A-9

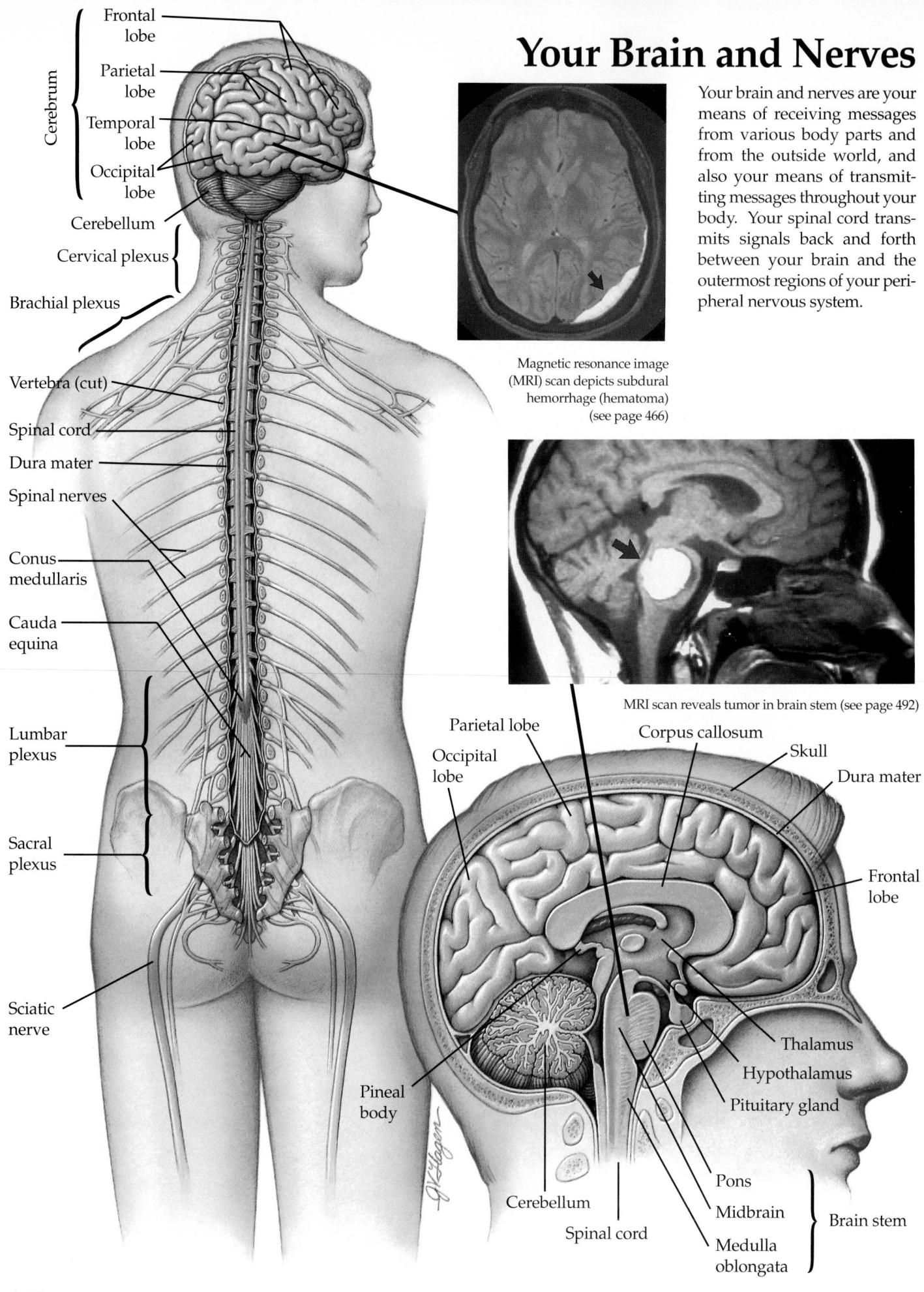

Your Brain and Nerves

Your brain and nerves are your means of receiving messages from various body parts and from the outside world, and also your means of transmitting messages throughout your body. Your spinal cord transmits signals back and forth between your brain and the outermost regions of your peripheral nervous system.

Magnetic resonance image (MRI) scan depicts subdural hemorrhage (hematoma) (see page 466)

MRI scan reveals tumor in brain stem (see page 492)

Frontal lobe
Parietal lobe
Temporal lobe
Occipital lobe
Cerebrum
Cerebellum
Cervical plexus
Brachial plexus
Vertebra (cut)
Spinal cord
Dura mater
Spinal nerves
Conus medullaris
Cauda equina
Lumbar plexus
Sacral plexus
Sciatic nerve

Parietal lobe
Occipital lobe
Corpus callosum
Skull
Dura mater
Frontal lobe
Thalamus
Hypothalamus
Pituitary gland
Pons
Midbrain
Medulla oblongata
Brain stem
Spinal cord
Cerebellum
Pineal body

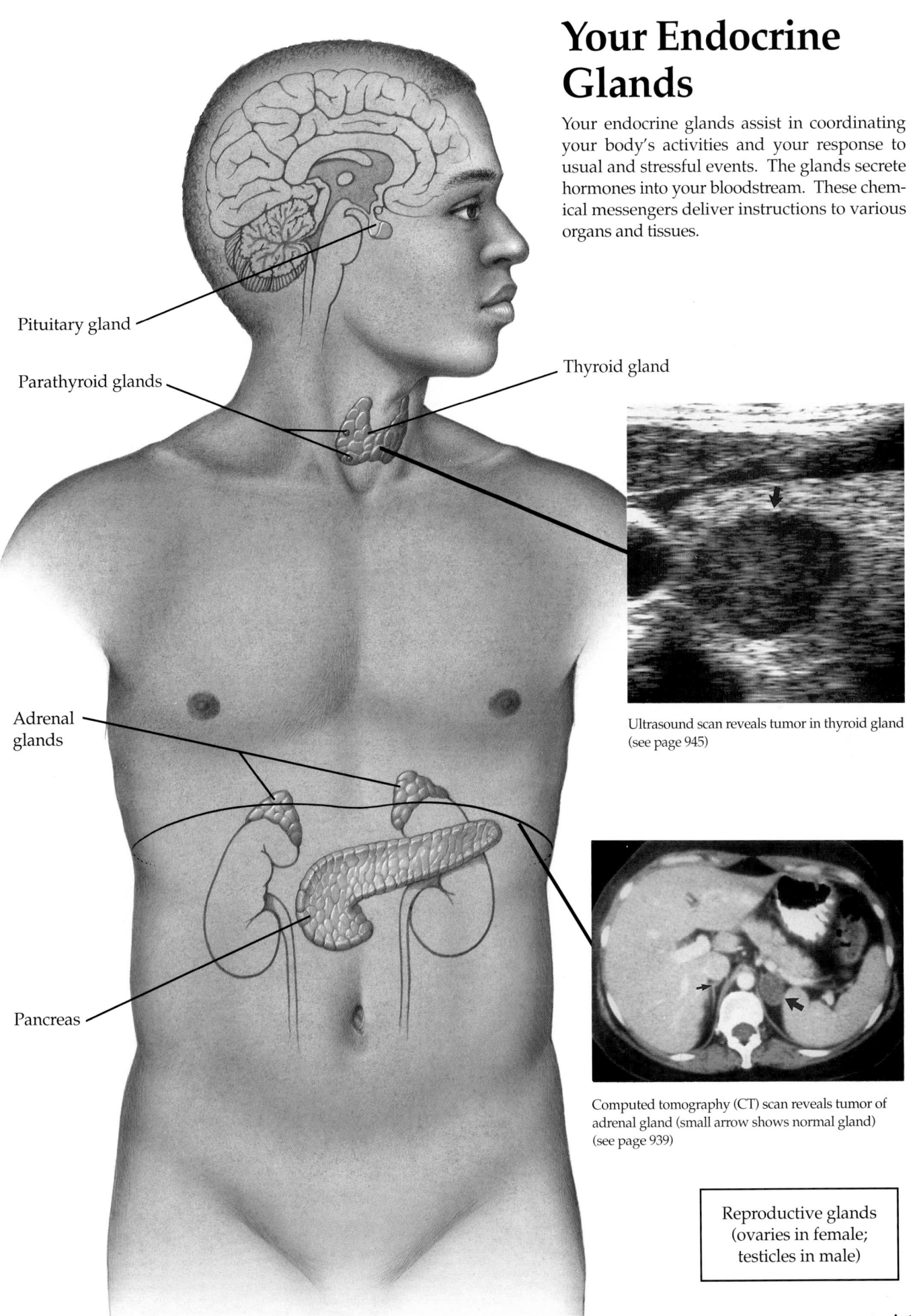

Your Endocrine Glands

Your endocrine glands assist in coordinating your body's activities and your response to usual and stressful events. The glands secrete hormones into your bloodstream. These chemical messengers deliver instructions to various organs and tissues.

Pituitary gland

Parathyroid glands

Thyroid gland

Adrenal glands

Pancreas

Ultrasound scan reveals tumor in thyroid gland (see page 945)

Computed tomography (CT) scan reveals tumor of adrenal gland (small arrow shows normal gland) (see page 939)

Reproductive glands (ovaries in female; testicles in male)

Your Reproductive Organs and Urinary Tract

Reproductive organs of the female include the ovaries, which release an egg at ovulation; the fallopian tubes, where the egg may be fertilized; and the uterus, where the fertilized egg implants itself and grows into a fetus. Reproductive organs of the male (opposite page) include the testicles, where sperm are produced, and the epididymis, which transports sperm for storage in the seminal vesicles. Fluids from the seminal vesicles and prostate are mixed with the sperm and ejaculated as semen through the urethra.

Your kidneys cleanse blood of excess fluid and waste products and pass urine through your ureters to your bladder, where it is stored and then expelled through your urethra.

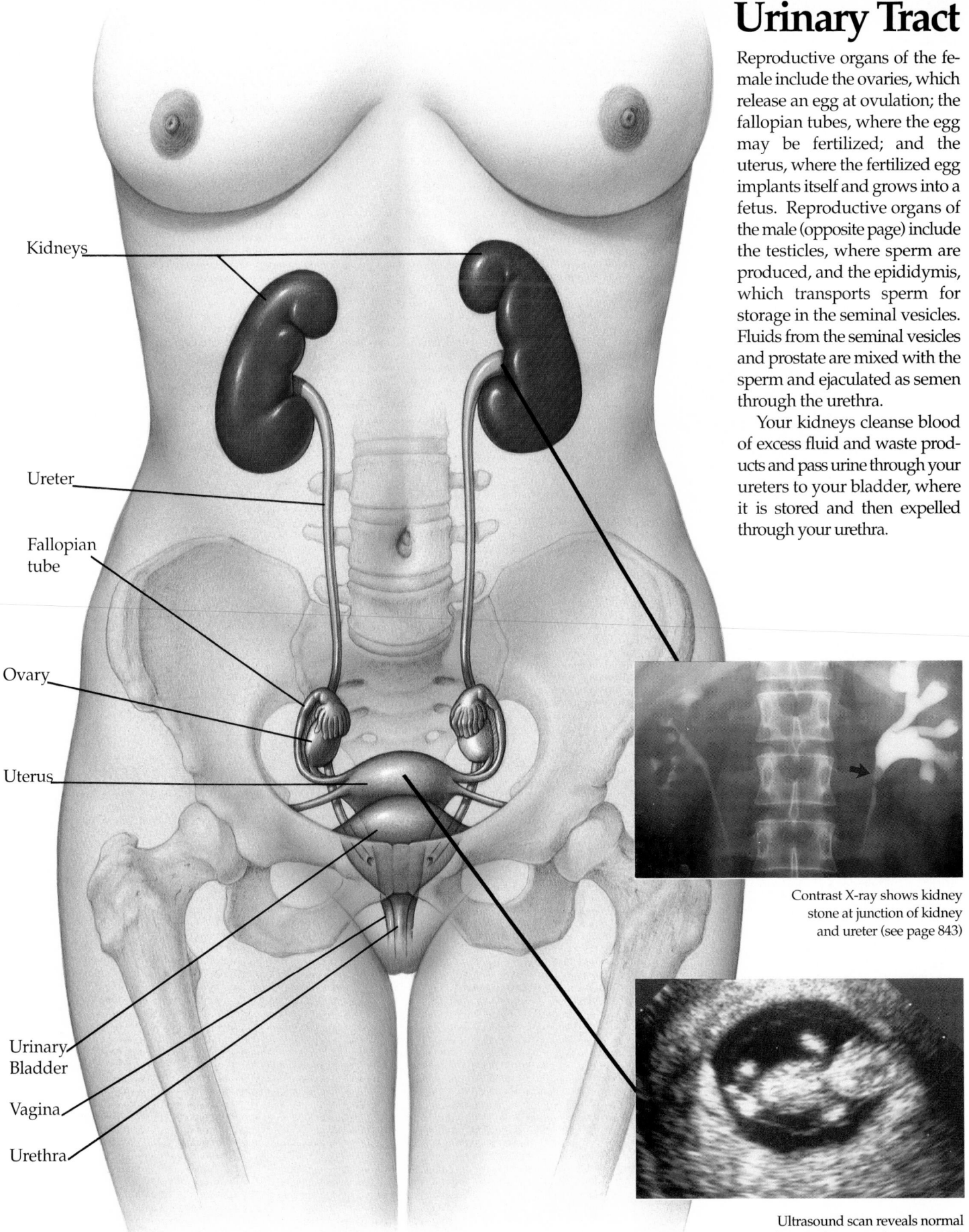

Kidneys

Ureter

Fallopian tube

Ovary

Uterus

Urinary Bladder

Vagina

Urethra

Contrast X-ray shows kidney stone at junction of kidney and ureter (see page 843)

Ultrasound scan reveals normal fetus in the uterus (see page 180)

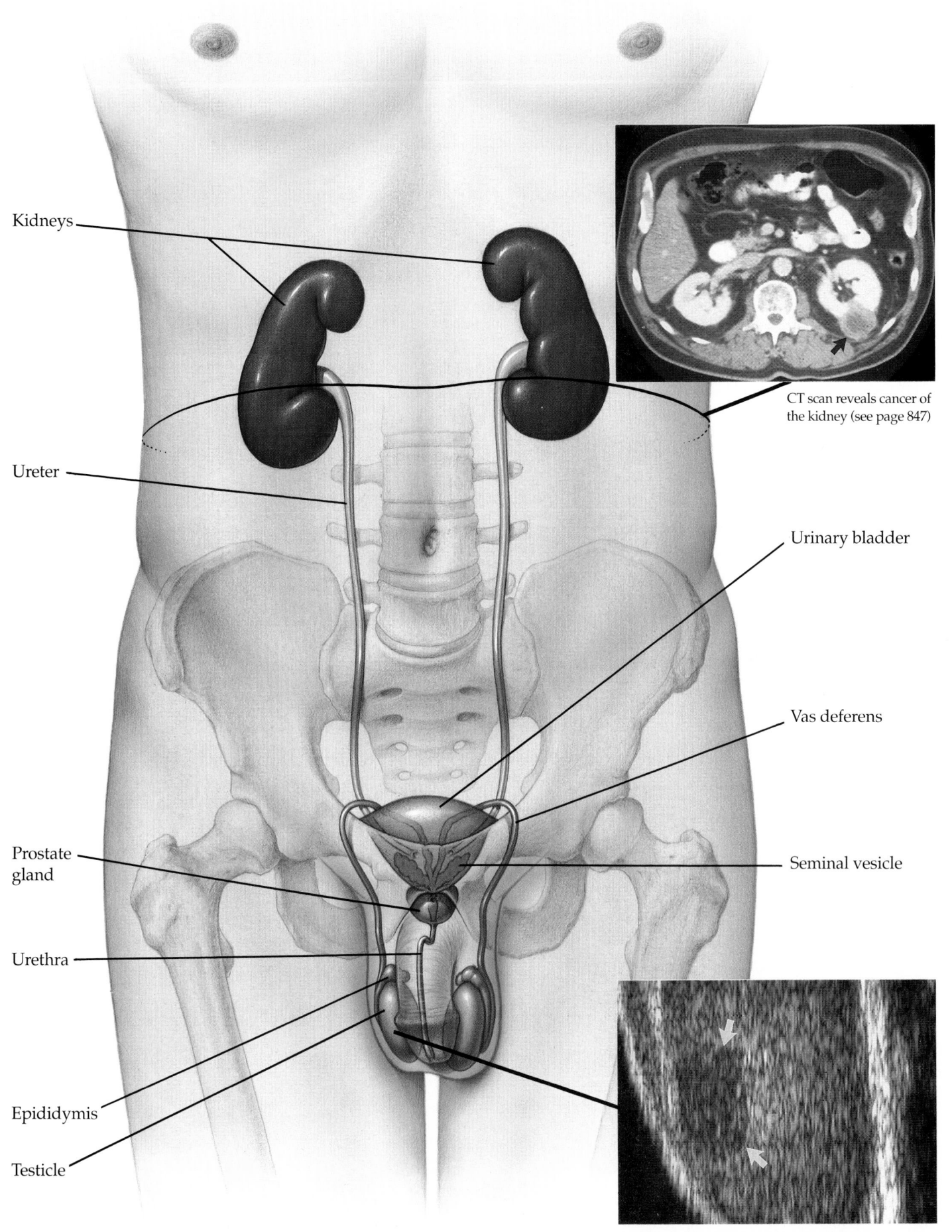

Kidneys

Ureter

Prostate
gland

Urethra

Epididymis

Testicle

CT scan reveals cancer of
the kidney (see page 847)

Urinary bladder

Vas deferens

Seminal vesicle

Ultrasound scan reveals cancer within a testicle
(see page 1202)

A-13

Your Senses

Your five senses—sight, sound, smell, taste, and touch—allow you to perceive the world around you.

Sight

Images first pass through the opening at the front of your eye, the pupil, to the lens, which inverts the image and projects it onto the retina. Your retina processes the image and delivers it to your optic nerve, which carries nerve impulses to your brain.

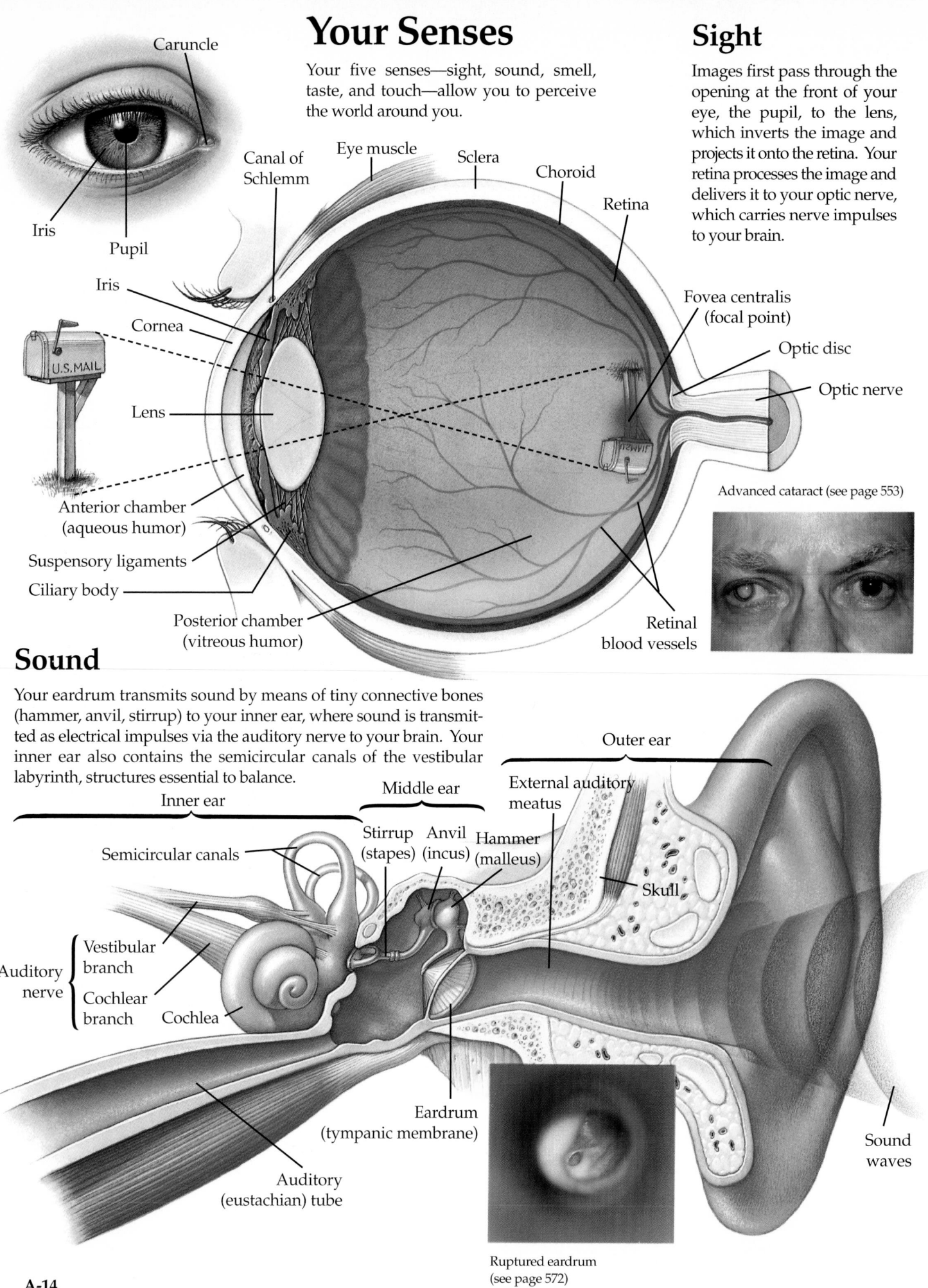

Caruncle

Iris

Pupil

Iris

Cornea

Lens

Anterior chamber (aqueous humor)

Suspensory ligaments

Ciliary body

Posterior chamber (vitreous humor)

Canal of Schlemm

Eye muscle

Sclera

Choroid

Retina

Fovea centralis (focal point)

Optic disc

Optic nerve

Retinal blood vessels

Advanced cataract (see page 553)

Sound

Your eardrum transmits sound by means of tiny connective bones (hammer, anvil, stirrup) to your inner ear, where sound is transmitted as electrical impulses via the auditory nerve to your brain. Your inner ear also contains the semicircular canals of the vestibular labyrinth, structures essential to balance.

Inner ear

Middle ear

Outer ear

Semicircular canals

Stirrup (stapes) Anvil (incus)

Hammer (malleus)

External auditory meatus

Skull

Auditory nerve { Vestibular branch Cochlear branch }

Cochlea

Eardrum (tympanic membrane)

Auditory (eustachian) tube

Ruptured eardrum (see page 572)

Sound waves

A-14

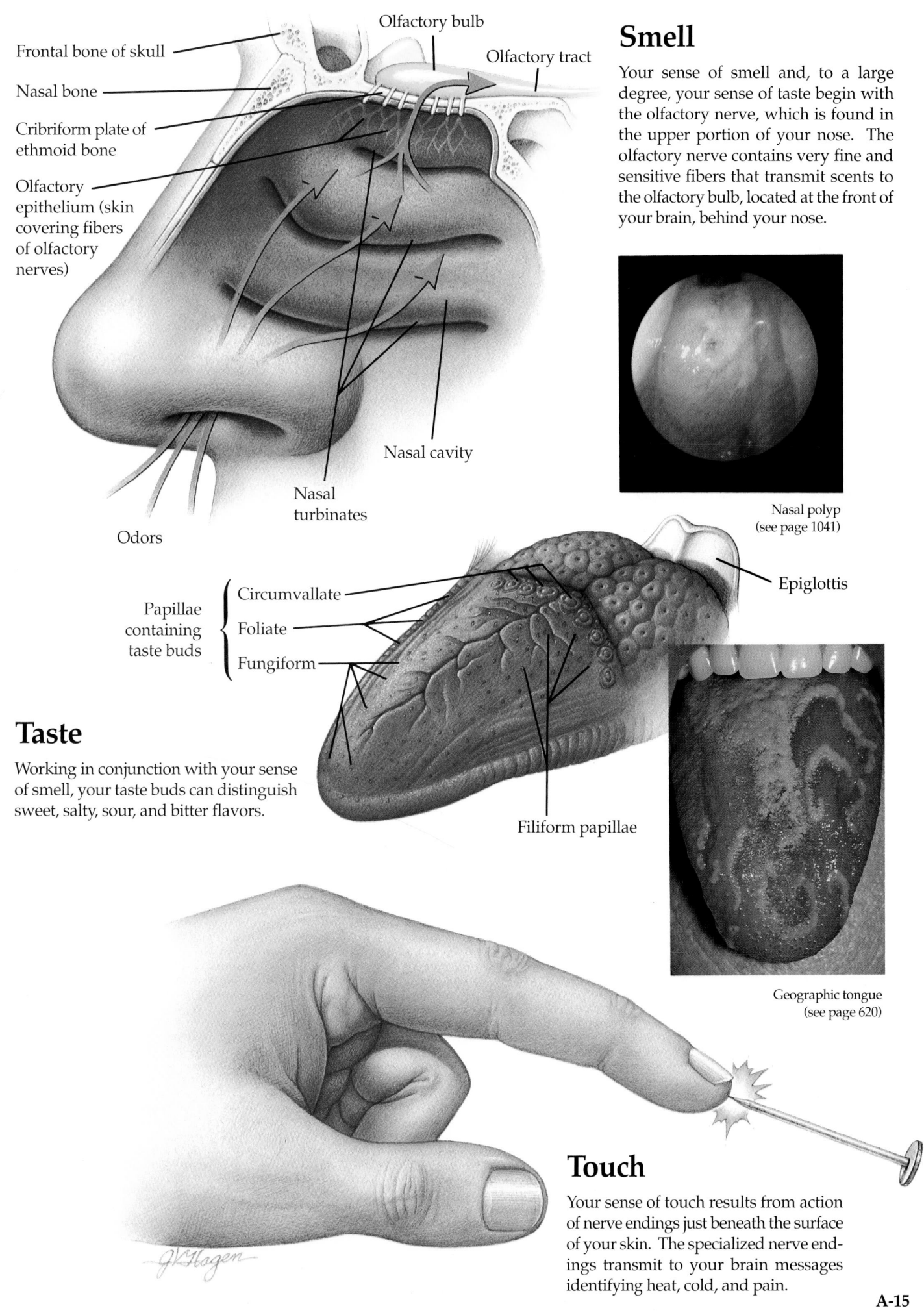

Frontal bone of skull

Nasal bone

Cribriform plate of ethmoid bone

Olfactory epithelium (skin covering fibers of olfactory nerves)

Olfactory bulb

Olfactory tract

Nasal cavity

Nasal turbinates

Odors

Smell

Your sense of smell and, to a large degree, your sense of taste begin with the olfactory nerve, which is found in the upper portion of your nose. The olfactory nerve contains very fine and sensitive fibers that transmit scents to the olfactory bulb, located at the front of your brain, behind your nose.

Nasal polyp
(see page 1041)

Epiglottis

Papillae containing taste buds
- Circumvallate
- Foliate
- Fungiform

Filiform papillae

Taste

Working in conjunction with your sense of smell, your taste buds can distinguish sweet, salty, sour, and bitter flavors.

Geographic tongue
(see page 620)

Touch

Your sense of touch results from action of nerve endings just beneath the surface of your skin. The specialized nerve endings transmit to your brain messages identifying heat, cold, and pain.

JVHagen

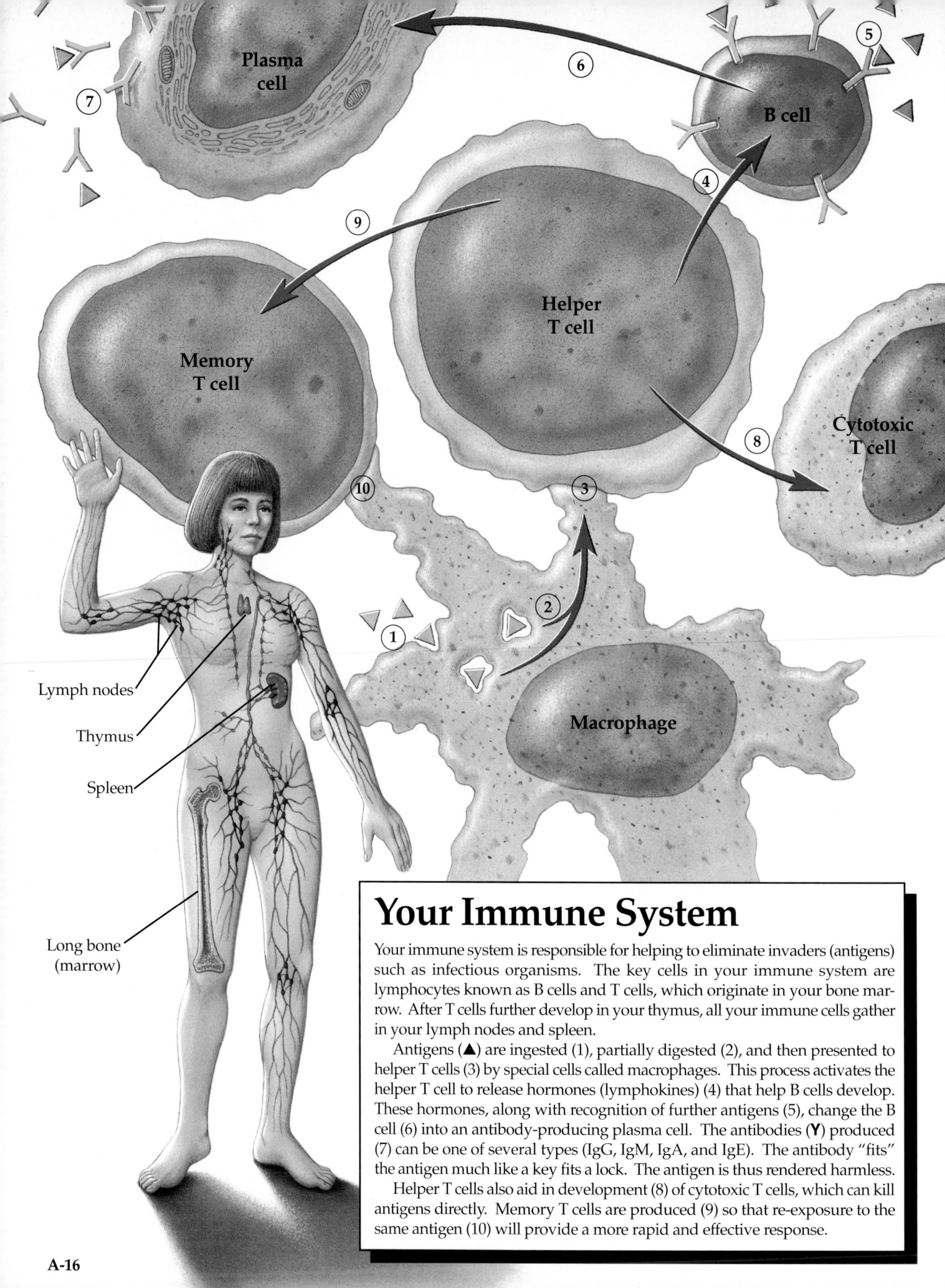

Plasma cell

B cell

Helper T cell

Memory T cell

Cytotoxic T cell

Macrophage

Lymph nodes

Thymus

Spleen

Long bone (marrow)

Your Immune System

Your immune system is responsible for helping to eliminate invaders (antigens) such as infectious organisms. The key cells in your immune system are lymphocytes known as B cells and T cells, which originate in your bone marrow. After T cells further develop in your thymus, all your immune cells gather in your lymph nodes and spleen.

Antigens (▲) are ingested (1), partially digested (2), and then presented to helper T cells (3) by special cells called macrophages. This process activates the helper T cell to release hormones (lymphokines) (4) that help B cells develop. These hormones, along with recognition of further antigens (5), change the B cell (6) into an antibody-producing plasma cell. The antibodies (Y) produced (7) can be one of several types (IgG, IgM, IgA, and IgE). The antibody "fits" the antigen much like a key fits a lock. The antigen is thus rendered harmless.

Helper T cells also aid in development (8) of cytotoxic T cells, which can kill antigens directly. Memory T cells are produced (9) so that re-exposure to the same antigen (10) will provide a more rapid and effective response.

Part I

Your Health Through the Years

We focus on human development and common health concerns in these first eight chapters. Each chapter addresses a specific time of life and reviews, often in detail, medical, behavioral, developmental, and other health issues with which you and those closest to you may have to deal during your lifetimes.

Contents

1 Newborn: The First Month of Life.....................3
2 Infancy: Ages 1 Month to 1 Year......................59
3 Preschool Years: Ages 1 Through 5....................81
4 School-Age Child: Ages 6 Through 12................115
5 Teenage Years: Ages 13 Through 19..................137
6 Young Adulthood: Ages 20 Through 39..............161
7 Middle Years: Ages 40 Through 65..................219
8 Later Years: After Age 65...........................231

Chapter 1

Newborn: The First Month of Life

Contents

The First Month of Life, 4

The Healthy Baby, 5
The Apgar Score, 6
Growth and Development, 6
Weight, 6
Posture and Motor Capabilities, 7
Circumcision, 7
Required Screening Tests, 8

Common Concerns, 9
Signs and Symptoms of Illness, 9
Fever, 10
Crying, 11
Excessive Crying (Colic), 11
Vomiting and Spitting Up, 12
Loose Stools, 13
Constipation, 13
Neonatal Jaundice, 13
Failure to Gain Weight, 14
Diaper Rash, 14
Cradle Cap, 14
Infantile Eczema, 14
Milia, 15
Birthmarks, 15
Erythema Toxicum, 16
Thrush, 16
Innocent Heart Murmurs, 16
Umbilical Hernia, 17

Special Concerns, 17
Premature Babies, 17
Newborn Intensive Care Units, 18
Respiratory Difficulty, 19
Bronchopulmonary Dysplasia
(BPD), 20
Pneumothorax, 20
Babies of Mothers
With Diabetes, 21
Birth Injuries, 21
Drug Withdrawal, 22

General Care, 22
Clothing, 23

When Is Your Baby Warm
Enough? 23
Car Seats, 23
Infant Carriers, 24
Pacifiers, 24
Exposure to Sun and Wind, 24
Care of the Eyes and Ears, 25
Care of the Skin, 25
Trimming Nails, 25
Fontanelle, 26
Appropriate Toys, 26
Bathing, 27
Selecting a Crib, 28
Don't Leave Your Baby Alone, 28
Diapers, 28
Prevention of Disease, 29
Care of the Umbilicus, 30

Personality and Behavior, 30
Healthy Development, 30
Bonding, 31
Infant Reflexes and Responses, 32
Twins, 33
Hearing, 34
Vision, 35
Sleeping, 36
Infant Behavior, 36
Sleeping Issues and Concerns, 37

Your Newborn's Nutrition, 38
Common Feeding Practices, 39
Breastfeeding Versus Bottle-
Feeding, 40
Feeding Concerns, 40
Bottle Care, 41

Genetics and Genetic
Disorders, 42
The Family History, 43
Down Syndrome, 44
Changes in the Hands and Feet, 44
Congenital Disorders of the
Skeleton, 46
Pectus Excavatum, 46

Conditions Affecting the
Genitals, 47
Ambiguous Genitals, 49
Supernumerary Nipples, 49
Enlarged Breasts in the
Newborn, 50
Epstein Pearls, 50
Supernumerary Teeth, 50
Congenital Obstruction of the
Nasolacrimal Duct, 50
Cleft Lip and Cleft Palate, 51

Congenital Heart
Disorders, 51
Ventricular Septal Defect (VSD), 52
Atrial Septal Defect (ASD), 52
Patent Ductus Arteriosus, 52
Coarctation of the Aorta, 52
Tetralogy of Fallot, 53
Pulmonary Stenosis, 53
Aortic Stenosis, 53
Transposition of
the Great Vessels, 53

Central Nervous System
Disorders, 53
Spina Bifida Occulta, 53
Hydrocephalus, 54
Cerebral Palsy, 54

Congenital Disorders of the
Gastrointestinal and
Respiratory Tracts, 55
Pyloric Stenosis, 55
Esophageal Atresia, 56
Biliary Atresia, 56
Intestinal Atresia, 57
Hirschsprung's Disease, 57
Imperforate Anus, 57
Diaphragmatic Hernia, 57
Omphalocele and Gastroschisis, 58
Congenital Lobar Emphysema, 58

The First Month of Life

Few things are as exciting as the birth of a baby. After 9 months of wondering—Will my baby be a boy or girl? Whom will he or she look like? Will he or she be healthy?—the questions suddenly have answers.

Despite the elation that comes with knowing they have a healthy newborn, first-time parents in particular may find themselves a bit overwhelmed—suddenly there is a little person who completely depends on them for his or her very survival.

The newborn period—the first month of life—is an exciting and challenging time for even the most experienced parents because every baby is different. Maybe you have given birth to three children, all of whom nursed well from the beginning, did not cry unless they were hungry, wet, or tired, and slept a good part of the day. Then comes the fourth child. This baby may feed erratically some of the time. He or she may spend 3 hours crying every night for no apparent reason, and may take no more than 1-hour catnaps.

You might feel as though you are at the end of your rope. And you secretly wonder whether something is wrong with the child. Most likely, nothing is wrong. The first month of life is a period of adjustment and challenge for both baby and parents.

How then can you best handle your baby's first month? Physicians and health care givers who specialize in the care of children offer this bit of advice: relax. If a baby naps, a mother should too. Let a few dust balls accumulate. Forget about preparing gourmet meals. Do not feel duty-bound to entertain all visitors who come for a peek at the baby.

As you and your baby begin to adjust to being home together, you may find that life gets easier.

Most newborns (not all) spend a good part of the day sleeping and are alert only a small portion of the time they appear to be awake. You will discover how social the baby is during these brief but important moments. Holding and cuddling, cooing, establishing eye contact, and talking to your baby are all crucial to building a close relationship between the two of you.

Do not underestimate your newborn. Even at 1 month, the infant knows family and recognizes their voices, particularly mother's.

A baby's abilities are amazing and perhaps greater than you might expect. Healthy babies are born with all the basic senses. He or she can see, hear, smell, and communicate by crying or using eye contact and simple body language. The baby also has ways to defend itself to some degree, thanks to certain protective reflexes.

For several days after birth, the gag reflex allows the infant to clear its airway of mucus to breathe. The eyes are protected from bright light by a strong blink reflex. Your newborn will try to avoid pain by drawing away from the source and batting with both arms or legs.

If one part of the infant's body becomes cold, the whole body changes color and temperature; the baby pulls its limbs toward the trunk to reduce the exposure and begins to shiver to generate heat.

Most new parents have many questions during their baby's first month. Your baby's health care provider is an excellent source of information. Although new parents may be

Since the beginning of time, when the discomfort of delivery is past, the arrival of a new person is an especially joyous occasion for mother.

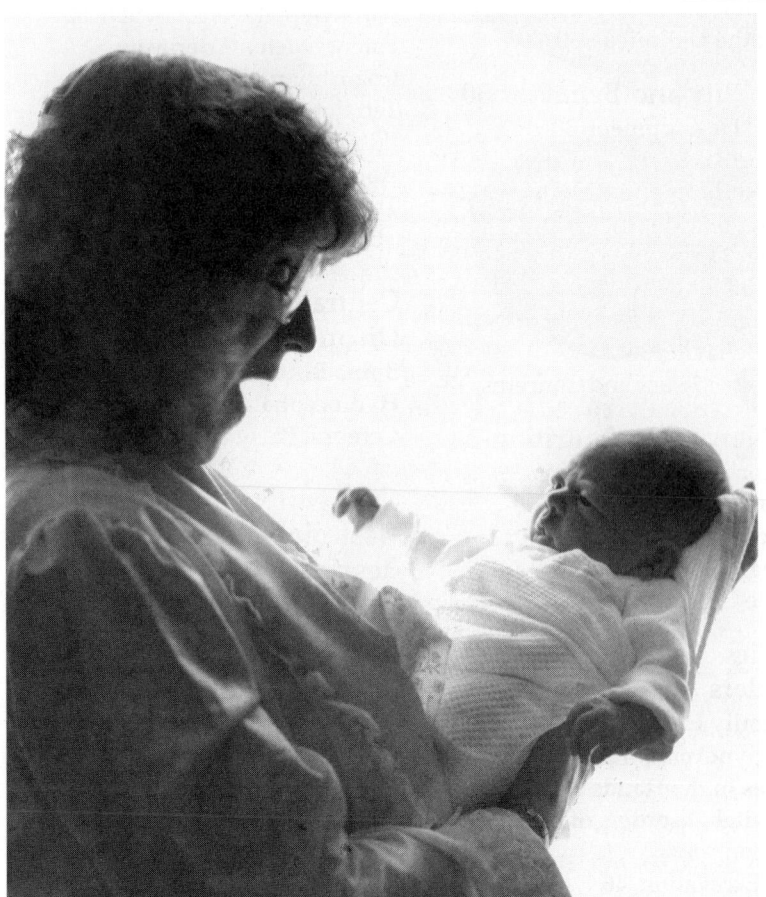

reluctant to "bother" them, most are accustomed to fielding questions over the telephone. Many have pediatric nurse practitioners or other experienced nurses or health professionals who also can be of help.

If you suspect your infant may be ill, call your baby's physician immediately. Your baby is particularly vulnerable during the first month of life. When in doubt, do not be afraid to ask.

The purpose of this chapter is to provide a guide for parents with a newborn. Topics include growth and development, bonding between parents and child, signs of illness, nutrition, care of the newborn, and congenital disorders.

The Healthy Baby

For most expectant parents, the image of their baby begins to crystallize soon after they learn that the results of a pregnancy test were positive. More often than not, the picture that emerges resembles the chubby, smiling 3- or 4-month-old that adorns disposable diaper boxes and baby food jars.

The reality is that the newborn you are handed in the delivery room may be very different from that image. Wrinkled and often with a head that is molded from the trip down the birth canal, this baby may not be the beauty depicted in baby books.

The time from conception to birth may seem an eternity to prospective parents, although the process is completed in about 40 weeks. Babies born anywhere from 38 to 42 weeks after the last menstrual period are considered full-term.

Sometime within that 4-week period, most women go into labor, the climax of which is the delivery of an infant. The average full-term newborn weighs 5.5 to 10 pounds. Boys weigh slightly more than girls. Most full-term babies are between 18 and 22 inches in length.

Immediately after delivery, your baby's mouth and nose are suctioned to remove mucus and blood that could interfere with breathing. The umbilical cord, the former lifeline between mother and child, is clamped and baby is on his or her own!

Your baby receives its first examination in the delivery room to ensure that there are no serious problems. What does a healthy baby look like? The infant may be quiet, or it may be crying at the top of its lungs and actively moving its arms and legs. Immediately after birth, the baby's skin may be mottled and the color may be dusky blue. This is the normal color for a baby before birth. During the first few minutes after birth, the normal increase in oxygen causes babies of all races to become increasingly pinkish, especially the palms and soles of the feet. Some infants have wrinkled and loose skin. Others look rather chubby. Many babies are born covered with vernix, a moist white material that protects the skin while in the womb.

Your baby may be totally bald or have a full head of hair, much of which will fall out by the fourth or fifth month. Fine, dark body hair (lanugo) may cover the infant's back, shoulders, and even parts of its face.

African-American babies have eyes that appear dark brown. Most white babies are born with dark blue eyes. Permanent eye color usually becomes discernible by 2 to 3 months of age, with perhaps some slight change in hue by the end of baby's first year.

You may notice that your newborn's eyes are slightly swollen. This is normal and is due to the erythromycin or tetracycline ointment or solution that is routinely placed in the infant's eyes to protect them from infection.

The baby's head usually looks large in relation to the body and often appears pointed or swollen shortly after birth. This shape is called "molding" and occurs as the head adjusts to the size and shape of the birth canal. The newborn's skull bones are soft and made to overlap so the head can pass through the mother's pelvis without injury. Molding does not result in any head or brain injury, and the infant's head returns to its normal shape in a few days. The top of the newborn's head has a soft spot where the bones of the skull meet, which will remain until between 9 and 18 months.

By the time your baby is 1 minute old, the infant will have been evaluated with the Apgar score, which is an assessment of the baby's apparent health. This score is repeated after 5 minutes. Babies with low Apgar scores may require intervention (see The Apgar Score, this page).

An injection of vitamin K, which helps prevent bleeding, is given to all babies shortly after birth.

If the baby is breathing well and appears healthy, and you are able, the baby will be given to you right away. You should be given an opportunity to nurse your baby immediately. Even though your body has not yet begun to produce mature milk, your breasts do contain early milk (colostrum), a rich liquid that provides nutrients and antibodies that are beneficial to your baby. The act of nursing itself helps develop closeness between you and your child.

Much has been written about bonding between parents and child. Simply put, bonding is the creation of emotional ties between the parents and their infant. By the time the infant is born, some bonding already has taken place. The parents, especially after going through childbirth, have an emotional attachment to their child. From the moment the parents first hold their child, the infant begins to form a bond that will last the rest of his or her life (see Bonding, page 31).

For the first hour or two after birth, your baby is likely to be awake, alert, and quiet.

This is a perfect time to observe and begin to get to know your baby. Babies can hear before they are born. After birth, parents may observe the startle or jerk when the infant hears a loud noise. Newborns also can see and are able to focus on objects within 8 to 12 inches. Parents often are surprised to observe the infant staring intently at an object or face.

Birth is hard work, and the newborn's response may be to settle into a quiet sleep for much of the next day or so. The newborn will have short periods of wakefulness to discover the wonders of these new surroundings, but also needs sleep to regain energy from the tiring birth process. The infant usually will have a variable interest in the breast or bottle in these first few days, but will soon develop more sustained interest in feedings. A newborn usually loses weight in the first few days of life and regains the birth weight by 1 to 2 weeks of age.

Growth and Development

An amazing story is unfolding before your eyes. One day your infant is safe within the womb, and the next it has to breathe for itself, digest food, maintain its own body temperature, and stabilize a host of other functions that it must perform. Despite all of these requirements, your baby adapts and begins the long journey to independence.

It takes time to get to know your newborn and what cues he or she is telling you about discomfort, hunger, boredom, and emotion. Be patient with yourself—you're gaining experience and expertise every moment.

Any parent with more than one child knows that there is no standard approach to caring for an infant. The following guide outlines what to expect of your child during the first month of life. Keep in mind that there are normal variations.

Weight

The average newborn weighs between 5.5 and 10 pounds and is between 18 and 22 inches in length. Within the first few days after birth, a baby will lose from 6 to 10 percent of its birth weight because of normal fluid loss and adaptation to life outside the uterus. At the end of the first month, the average baby weighs 2 pounds more than it did at birth.

The Apgar Score

The Apgar score is used to evaluate the general health of the newborn at 1 minute and again at 5 minutes after birth. The Apgar score aids in determining which measures need to be taken to assist the infant after birth.

The following areas are assessed: heart rate, respiratory effort, muscle tone, response to stimulation, and color.

A score of 8 to 10 indicates that a baby is in excellent condition. The heart rate is more than 100 beats per minute and the baby is breathing well and crying, is active, coughs or sneezes when the nose is suctioned, and appears the appropriate color.

If the score is 0 to 4, the baby has a slow or inaudible heartbeat and is pale or even blue. The reflex response may be absent or depressed.

Most infants have a score of 7 to 9 and require nothing more than having the mucus suctioned from the airway.

Infants with a score of 4 or less at 1 minute after delivery require immediate assistance with their breathing.

Posture and Motor Capabilities

The posture of the newborn simulates the fetal position. At birth, when placed on a firm surface, the baby can move its head from side to side. When held on an adult's shoulder, the infant can lift its head. When on its stomach, it lies in a frog-like position or rolled in a ball. When the baby is pulled to a sitting position, its head falls backward or forward. Fingers are balled into a fist.

At 1 month, the baby's head still needs support but he or she may hold the head steady for longer periods. The baby can roll partway to its side from its back. When the baby's fingers are pried open, it can grasp a rattle but drops it right away.

Vision

Newborns can see. From the moment of birth, your newborn is capable of focusing on objects within 8 to 12 inches of its face.

At 1 month, your newborn will follow objects but will not reach for them. Intermittent eye-crossing is normal until age 2 months. Newborns prefer black and white patterns over color, and they enjoy faces. The baby makes eye contact and is particularly interested in focusing on its mother's face.

Hearing

Babies are born with the sense of hearing and can distinguish volume. A sharp noise may startle the baby, whereas a soft voice may cause the baby to quiet or become more alert.

At 1 month, you may see your infant distinguish between parents' voices.

Language

The language of the newborn is the cry. Some babies cry more than others. By 1 month, the infant's repertoire expands to include soft, throaty, and gurgling sounds.

Feeding

The newborn is hungry at irregular intervals. It is not uncommon for a baby to show little interest in feeding, particularly during the first couple of days after birth. By the end of the first week, most infants eat every 2 to 5 hours.

Feeding is still somewhat disorganized at 1 month. Babies may eat as often as every 2 to 3 hours during the day and have one or more night feedings. Gradually, over the course of the first month, the number of feed-

Circumcision

Circumcision is a procedure in which the foreskin—the sheath of tissue covering the head of the penis—is removed. The practice has been performed since ancient times, and many parents today still have their sons circumcised for religious or other reasons, including concerns about health and hygiene.

Researchers have attempted to learn more about whether circumcision may prevent infection and certain types of cancer, but more studies need to be done to answer some of these questions.

An uncircumcised penis requires no special care beyond regular hygiene.

Like any minor surgery, circumcision poses some risk to the newborn. Local anesthesia may be used to lessen the pain for the baby. If you choose circumcision, it usually will be done a few days after birth.

ings may be reduced from 8 or 10 over a 24-hour period to 6 or 8.

The length of feedings also is erratic. On one day a breastfed infant might want to nurse for 40 minutes at each breast, and the next day it may nurse for only 10 minutes at each.

By 2 weeks of age, your newborn may take in about 18 ounces of milk per day. At 1 month, the infant may increase the amount to about 25 ounces each day. However, each baby's needs for growth are different so it is best to follow your baby's cues and changes in demand to determine feeding frequency and volume.

Bowel Movements

The baby has the first bowel movement usually within 24 hours after birth. Called a meconium stool, it is composed of intestinal secretions and amniotic fluid and is dark green. After the baby begins to drink breast milk or formula, the meconium stool changes to transitional stools, usually on the third or fourth day of life. These stools are usually greenish brown and may contain milk curds. After the passage of transitional stools, the stool resembles the bowel movement of an older infant.

By the end of the first week, most babies pass between three and five stools a day, although it is not uncommon for a baby, especially one that is breastfed, to have more bowel movements each day. However, if your newborn goes for a day without having a bowel movement, do not worry. This does not mean that the baby is constipated.

The stool of the breastfed baby is odorless and mushy. The stool of a formula-fed baby has a characteristic fecal smell and is usually more formed.

By 1 month, most babies have three or four bowel movements a day, often after a feeding. However, some infants, especially some nursing babies, occasionally may not have one for 1 to 10 days. This is normal and not a cause for concern if baby is acting well otherwise.

Sleeping

The newborn often has an alert period immediately after birth. After this hour or two of alertness, the baby sinks into a quiet sleep. During the next several days most newborns sleep anywhere from 14 to 18 hours a day and are alert for only 30 minutes out of every 4 hours.

A 1-month-old baby spends most of the time sleeping, usually at least 14 hours a day. Generally, toward the end of the first month, parents observe that the 7 or 8 daily sleep periods are reduced to 3 or 4 daily naps and a 5- or 6-hour block of sleep at night. Sleep patterns, however, are highly variable.

No matter how much or how little your infant sleeps, he or she is an active sleeper. Hence, even though the baby is asleep, you may see it grimace, cry out, startle, and move about—all without waking up.

Crying

Crying is one of your baby's first methods of communication. The amount a newborn cries, like many other aspects of development, varies. Some babies cry only when hungry or wet; others cry more often.

One day your newborn may cry many times a day, for example, before a feeding, falling asleep, or having a bowel movement. On another day the crying may be infrequent.

Psychosocial Development and Personality

These important areas of development are discussed on pages 30 through 36.

Required Screening Tests

Although the majority of babies are born healthy, most states require routine screening for certain disorders that are not immediately apparent at birth. Some rare but serious defects in the metabolism of various substances can be treated effectively if they are diagnosed during an infant's first weeks after birth. If left untreated, however, these disorders can cause various problems, including mental retardation, poor physical growth, and cataracts.

Many states require that newborns be tested for certain conditions to ensure that proper treatment is initiated immediately to enhance the chance of a normal life. Your infant's health care provider or the nursing staff at the hospital where you give birth will inform you of any screening tests required in your particular state.

Some states test for certain disorders of red blood cell formation such as sickle cell anemia (see page 960) and thalassemia (see page 962). A few states have also begun testing for Maple Syrup Urine Disease, MSUD, which is another inborn error of metabolism like PKU. The following are four metabolic disorders for which newborns are commonly tested:

Phenylketonuria

Phenylketonuria (PKU) is a congenital deficiency of a specific enzyme. Infants born with PKU are often normal at birth. The condition disrupts normal metabolism and may cause developmental delays and IQ loss if diet is not carefully regulated beginning in early infancy. One out of every 10,000 babies born in the United States has PKU.

To test for PKU, only a few drops of the baby's blood are needed. Although PKU can be detected as early as 4 hours after birth, most testing is done after the baby is 24 hours old because the test's accuracy depends on the baby having eaten an adequate amount of protein.

If your baby has PKU, a special diet will be prescribed. With early detection and treatment, normal development is optimized.

Galactosemia

This enzyme deficiency affects the body's ability to metabolize galactose, one of the sugars normally present in milk. One in 40,000 to 50,000 children is born with this inherited disorder which, if left untreated, can cause brain damage, cataracts, and kidney and liver problems.

Galactosemia can cause symptoms such as convulsions, marked lethargy, persistent jaundice, feeding difficulties, or hypoglycemia. Treatment involves a diet restricted in galactose content. When the diagnosis is made early, medical problems can be avoided.

Hypothyroidism

This is an inherited deficiency in the production of thyroid hormone, which is essential for mental and physical growth and development.

Hypothyroidism occurs in about 1 in every 4,000 births and is twice as common in females as males. Before screening became available, this disorder often went unrecognized. Symptoms initially may be absent or mild and then progress slowly, and might include sluggishness, constipation, and poor growth.

If left untreated, these children are usually developmentally disabled and have short stature. Early treatment with thyroid hormone is effective for ensuring normal growth and development. Studies have shown that infants who begin treatment during the first month of life have normal IQs in the first grade. Further studies are needed to assess later school performance (see Hyperthyroidism, page 947).

Congenital Adrenal Hyperplasia (CAH)

This disorder blocks normal metabolism in many ways, resulting in a range of problems for approximately 1 in every 5,000 newborns. Symptoms may include vomiting, diarrhea, failure to gain weight after birth, and ambiguous genitals (the genitals of a girl may be formed in such a way that she appears to be male). Additional problems might include severely low sodium and seriously high potassium levels in the blood.

A blood test in the first days of life can identify many of these infants before serious symptoms develop. Treatment is very effective and usually consists of giving cortisone-type medications and sometimes surgery.

Common Concerns

It is sometimes difficult to determine whether a newborn is indeed sick or simply is having a bad day.

In time, you will become accustomed to your child's moods and patterns. Even before the child is old enough to communicate, you often can sense that something is not right by, for example, a change in your infant's eating or sleeping habits. In short, some behavior change triggers your suspicions. But the newborn and parents are just getting to know each other. What is "normal" behavior for this child has not yet been established. So how can a parent tell whether something is wrong?

Signs and Symptoms of Illness

Illness can be indicated in many ways. Some signs or symptoms always indicate that the baby is ill. Others, such as excessive crying, may or may not be indicative of illness. For easy reference, the most common ones are discussed below in brief. In the pages that follow, most are discussed in detail.

Fever in the newborn is defined as a rectal temperature of more than 101 degrees Fahrenheit (38.4 degrees centigrade). Fever is the body's response to infection. Keep in mind, however, that in the first few months of life, particularly in premature infants, an infection may not cause a fever. The key is how your baby acts. If he or she is more listless than normal or if a fever is present, contact your health care provider.

Excessive crying also may indicate illness, especially if there are other symptoms. Some babies cry more than others—sometimes even for 2 or 3 hours—without being ill. Some babies have colic (severe, often regular, episodes of crying during which the baby's legs are drawn up to its chest, and its abdomen becomes firm). Burping, rocking, or walking your baby often helps a colicky child (see Excessive Crying [Colic], page 11). If nothing seems to work and the crying continues for several hours, the baby may be crying because of illness.

Breathing difficulty is a sign of illness. If the baby is congested, wheezing, or having difficulty breathing, there may be a respiratory problem. Sneezing in an infant is common and normal.

Diarrhea can become a serious condition. If untreated, it can lead to dehydration. Babies' stools are normally loose. As a rule, a baby with diarrhea has an increase in the number of stools, and the consistency changes. A breastfed baby's normal stool is mushy, contains curds, and does not have a foul odor. If the curds disappear, and the stool becomes watery and foul, the baby probably has diarrhea. A baby with diarrhea also looks sick (see page 66).

Vomiting is not the gentle spitting up after eating that occurs in most newborns. Rather, true vomiting is when the contents of the stomach are propelled forcefully from the baby's mouth. Although occasional vomiting usually is not cause for alarm, if it becomes frequent or contains green bile or blood, call your health care provider (see page 67).

Lethargy may be a worrisome sign. If your child is suddenly uninterested, limp, and sleeping more than usual, an infection or illness could be present.

Lack of appetite occurs in most sick newborns. A baby who has been eating well but suddenly refuses the bottle or breast may be sick.

Jaundice (yellowing of the skin) is common beginning the second or third day of life and continuing for the first week. If jaundice is present at birth, appears within the first 24 hours, or develops or persists after two weeks, a serious infection or other disorder may be present.

Failure to move an extremity may be a sign of a fracture, dislocation, or nerve injury.

If your baby has any of the above symp-

toms or signs or is more irritable or lethargic than you think is warranted, and you do not feel comfortable with your concern, call your baby's health care provider immediately.

Fever

A fever is usually the body's response to infection. In the case of the newborn, it also may be the result of dehydration or overexposure in hot climates.

Regardless, a rectal temperature of more than 101 degrees Fahrenheit (38.4 degrees centigrade) warrants a call to your baby's physician. Any fever in a newborn is considered potentially serious and should be investigated.

When should you take your baby's temperature? Does the baby feel warm to the touch? Does the forehead feel warmer than your lips when you kiss it? Is the infant unusually fussy or unusually quiet? Have its sleep patterns abruptly changed? Is the baby vomiting or having diarrhea? Does its chest sound congested? Has the baby stopped wetting its diapers? If the answer to any of these questions is "yes" or if your instincts tell you that something is not right, take the infant's temperature.

In the first 2 months of life, an infant's temperature is most accurately taken with a special rectal thermometer—one with a rounded bulb. You also will need some petroleum jelly to lubricate the tip of the thermometer so that it will slide in more easily.

Insert the thermometer into the rectum about an inch and hold it there for a couple of minutes. Never let go of the thermometer while it is inside the baby because one squirm may push it deeper into the rectum and cause an injury.

An infant's temperature varies. It is often lower in the morning and increases in the afternoon or evening. As long as it is below 101 degrees Fahrenheit, the baby does not have a fever.

If, however, it is more than 101 degrees Fahrenheit, call your health care provider, even if the child has no other symptoms. Your provider may want to examine the baby. It may be nothing more than a harmless virus, but because as many as 10 percent of infants develop infections during their first month, the physician may want to eliminate more serious possibilities.

When you are taking a newborn's temperature with a rectal thermometer, insert the lubricated thermometer approximately 1 inch and hold it there for 3 minutes. Never let go of the thermometer while it is in your child.

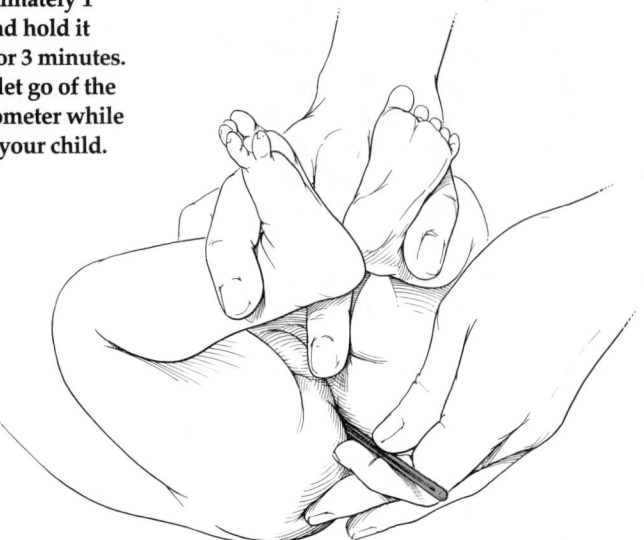

Many physicians recommend acetaminophen (not aspirin) for reducing fever. Do not, however, give your newborn any medicine unless instructed to do so by your physician.

Crying

A baby's cry is one of the major ways of communicating. Most newborns cry easily and frequently. The infant with a sensitive temperament cries more than one less sensitive.

In cultures where parents are in constant physical contact with their newborns, crying is less common than in countries such as the United States, where baby swings, cribs, and infant seats often replace physical contact.

A certain amount of crying each day is a predictable part of a baby's cycle of rest and activity. Although the infant will develop more sophisticated methods, few methods will be any more effective for obtaining a response from the parent.

What is excessive crying during the first month of life? There is no easy answer to that question because every baby and every day are different. All babies cry, some more than others.

On some days your baby may cry for 20 or 30 minutes for 4 or 5 times—typically before eating, sleeping, and having a bowel movement. On another day, the infant may cry for hours. Crying during the newborn period peaks at approximately 6 weeks of age and tapers off by about 3 or 4 months of age.

Trying to figure out what your baby is signaling with his or her cries is like being a detective. "On the job training" by trying different things and seeing what works and what doesn't is the only way to learn. With time and familiarity, your understanding of your baby's needs will increase. At each stage of development, it helps to have a general idea of what's considered normal behavior so you won't expect too much from your baby or miss something worrisome.

Nature would have you cuddling your baby a lot in the early months. Babies come equipped with reflexes to ensure this contact. The grasping and startle reflexes result in clinging motions of the arms, fingers, and feet. Both reflexes occur when the baby is alarmed by a noise or sudden movement. The act of breastfeeding and the composition of human milk support this natural phenomenon.

Mother's milk will let down in response to her infant's cry. The composition of human milk necessitates frequent feedings in the early months. Its low-fat, low-protein, high-sugar content is similar to the milk of mammals who carry their offspring along and feed them often. The milk of mammals who hide their young between feedings while they are out for hours foraging is, by contrast, very high in fat and protein. Interestingly, the grasp and startle reflexes fade as the baby gains maturity, as does the need for frequent feedings.

During infancy, many parents have unrealistic expectations about normal behavior. They don't know what to expect. Although some babies sleep between regular feedings, the vast majority do not. Most babies cry easily and frequently and can only be comforted when they are held.

Feedings are often not predictable. Predictability comes with maturity. Inexperienced parents often are surprised by their baby's erratic feeding needs.

Babies lack experience in reacting to the many new and confusing situations outside the womb. Although some make the transition easily, most need lots of cuddling and human contact day and night in those important few months. As the baby grows and matures, different cries for different needs will emerge.

Can you spoil your newborn by too much love and attention? No. Responding to your baby's cry will not spoil him or her.

Follow your instinct to respond to your baby's cries. Infants who are responded to consistently and quickly during the first 6 to 8 months of life cry less in later months than those left to cry. It seems that an important task for your infant to learn is that others will respond in a caring and predictable way. This helps your baby develop a strong trust in others and in self.

Excessive Crying (Colic)

The colicky baby is one who is healthy and well-fed but has predictable periods of crying (usually at about the same time each day, and most often in the evening) that may last for minutes or may continue for 2 or more hours. While there are many theories as to the cause of colic, the reasons for it are still not understood. Colicky spells usually begin within a few weeks of birth but usually disappear in the baby's third or fourth month. The baby cannot be consoled for more than a few moments by any method. The crying has an effect on the parent-child interaction and is a potential source of major family disruption. These irritable babies are at greater risk for child abuse. Parents express feelings of frustration, anger, guilt, self-doubt, depression, isolation, and being overwhelmed.

Colic occurs with equal frequency in male and female babies, firstborns or subsequent babies, and bottle-fed or breastfed babies. The crying may occur at any time of the day or night, but often seems to have a pattern.

If your baby has colic, the months of crying can seem like an eternity. When you can't end the crying episodes by the usual consoling methods, you'll need to shift your tactics and concentrate on finding ways to survive the colicky weeks. Here are some suggestions:

- Rock your baby back and forth in a hammock motion.
- Try white noise. For example, turn on the sound of a vacuum cleaner, a hair dryer, radio static, or any similar sound while rocking your baby.
- Go for a car ride.
- Put your crying baby in a sling or stroller and go for brisk walks.
- Leave your baby with a supportive caregiver for an hour or two so you can take a nap or get out of the house.
- If no one is available, lay the baby down for 5 or 10 minutes and do some on-the-spot stretching or vigorous exercises to re-energize yourself.

If you are worried at any time that your baby is sick, or if you or others caring for your baby are starting to feel out of control with anger because of the excessive crying, bring your baby to the physician's office or a hospital emergency room.

Though your attempts to console your baby may be unsuccessful, he or she still needs the reassurance of your presence. Also, the support of your partner, family, and friends is essential.

Vomiting and Spitting Up

Newborns and even older infants often spit up after a feeding.

Spitting up is the gentle spilling of what is typically a small amount of milk from the baby's mouth. This should not be confused with vomiting, during which the contents of the baby's stomach are ejected forcefully from its mouth.

One newborn may spit up after every feeding, and another may spit up only infrequently. Spitting up is messy for the parents (some have learned never to hold their baby unless a cloth is on their shoulder), but it rarely signifies a serious problem. Usually, the problem gradually resolves itself by the time the child is between 6 months and 1 year old.

The reason babies spit up is not completely understood, but it probably is related to their immature digestive systems. Unlike the older child or adult, the young baby's muscle between the esophagus and the upper part of the stomach is not yet adept at holding down the stomach's contents. Thus, any movement, even something as gentle as laying down the baby or the act of digestion itself, can cause the milk to be regurgitated.

Often the milk that spills from your baby's mouth smells slightly sour and may be curdled. This is nothing to be concerned about; the milk was undergoing digestion when it was regurgitated.

What should you do if your baby spits up? Sometimes a baby spits up because of air in its stomach. Thus, burping after each feeding is important. Even though it may take a while, try to get the baby to burp after every feeding. Some babies do better sitting upright in an infant seat after eating—others may spit up less when placed on their sides. Try to see if there is a position that works best for your child.

If your baby is a spitter, the problem probably will continue no matter what you do. As long as the baby seems healthy and is gaining weight, there is little cause for concern.

Vomiting, however, may need to be investigated.

A newborn may vomit mucus, often streaked with blood, a few hours after birth. This is often blood from the mother that the infant swallowed during delivery and is normal. Usually this vomiting subsides after a few feedings. If it continues, however, it can signify an obstruction in the esophagus or intestines that will need further evaluation.

Vomiting also can be the result of milk intolerance or an initial sign of another illness.

What should you do if your baby vomits?

Notify your baby's health care provider, but, again, as long as the baby seems healthy and is gaining weight, there is probably no reason to be alarmed.

If there is blood or green bile in the vomit, the baby should be examined immediately because this may suggest a serious illness.

Loose Stools

The stool of a breastfed newborn is naturally a mushy consistency. If your baby does have diarrhea during the first month, it may be caused by an infection. The stool is apt to be greenish, the frequency will increase, the stools will become watery, the curds contained in the normal stool of a breastfed newborn will be absent, and there may be an unpleasant odor.

If you suspect your newborn has persistent diarrhea, call your baby's health care provider. If he or she determines that the baby has only a mild case of diarrhea, you may be advised to change the frequency or amount of your baby's feedings. Let your nursing baby continue to nurse, but do not be surprised if the baby wants less than usual. Occasionally, a prepared fluid solution like Pedialyte may be suggested for a short time. If your physician thinks the diarrhea is more severe or thinks the baby is becoming dehydrated, your baby may need care in the hospital.

Constipation

Constipation, rare in the newborn, refers to the consistency of the stool and not to the frequency. Some breastfed babies have a bowel movement after every feeding, and some newborns have only one a day or one every few days. The baby who has one only once a day or even less frequently is not necessarily constipated.

The breastfed baby passes mushy stools. Sometimes the baby may appear to be straining, and yet the stool that passes is soft. The formula-fed newborn sometimes may have difficulty having a bowel movement. The stools may be hard. True constipation is the difficult passage of hard, dry stools.

Chronic constipation can occasionally indicate a congenital problem and should be discussed with your baby's health care provider.

Neonatal Jaundice

Approximately 60 percent of all full-term newborns develop jaundice during their first week, and the proportion increases to 80 percent in premature infants.

Jaundice (yellowing of the skin) is not a disease itself but rather is the result of the inability of the immature liver of an infant to metabolize bilirubin. Thus, the bilirubin accumulates in the skin and gives it a yellowish tint.

Some babies are jaundiced at birth, and others develop jaundice later, depending on the condition responsible for the jaundice.

Jaundice that is present at birth or appears within the first 24 hours may be the result of several problems, including hemorrhage, sepsis (an infection in the blood), and a blood incompatibility between the baby and mother. If your physician is concerned about these possibilities, special blood tests may be done.

Typically, most jaundiced infants become so during the second or third day of life. This is called physiologic jaundice and is due to the breakdown of fetal red blood cells in combination with the inability of the immature liver to excrete bilirubin. It is common for jaundice to continue through the first week or two, especially in babies receiving breast milk.

If jaundice develops or persists after the second week of life, it may be due to a liver malfunction, severe infection, enzyme deficiency, or abnormality of red blood cells.

Your health care provider will watch your newborn carefully for signs of jaundice. If your baby is getting progressively more jaundiced, your health care provider may order periodic blood tests to measure the bilirubin concentration.

Most infants with physiologic jaundice require little more than observation. Generally the condition is gone within a week or two. However, the severity of physiologic jaundice is influenced by race or ethnic background; Chinese, Japanese, Korean, and American Indian newborns are affected more severely.

If your infant has a significantly increased amount of bilirubin, he or she may be placed under a high-intensity light (phototherapy). Bilirubin absorbs light and is then converted into a form that can be excreted in the bile and urine. This treatment is applied continuously until the amount of bilirubin has been reduced to a level considered safe for the infant.

Side effects of phototherapy can include loose stools, rash, and dehydration.

Failure to Gain Weight

Babies in the first days and months of life undergo dramatic growth. The most common reason for slow weight gain is due to insufficient intake. If you are breastfeeding, your baby's health care provider or a lactation consultant may be able to suggest helpful changes in breastfeeding techniques or patterns. If you are bottle feeding, sometimes a change in formula or an increase in the number of feedings will resolve the problem.

Occasionally the failure to gain weight is a sign of medical problems that would need further investigation. Infrequently, treatment may involve hospitalization. In the hospital, the infant usually is given unlimited feedings to determine whether weight gain will result. Tests and X-rays also can be done if a physical abnormality is suspected.

Diaper Rash

Signs and Symptoms—A rash in the region covered by the diaper

Most infants develop a diaper rash at some time or another; some even arrive home from the hospital with a slight rash. A diaper rash does not necessarily mean that an infant is receiving poor care. It only means that the baby has sensitive skin.

Diaper rash (see color photograph, page C-2) can have many causes. The typical diaper rash is the reaction of the newborn's sensitive skin to contact with moisture and irritants. This rash often goes away with lots of airing and frequent diaper changes.

Babies commonly develop a type of diaper rash that is caused by a yeast infection. The infection may appear on the buttocks and genitals as bright red spots that come together to form a solid red area with a scalloped border. This common rash can be treated with anti-yeast cream or ointment and lots of airing.

Treatment
If your baby has a diaper rash, the first step may be simply changing the diaper more often and gently washing the skin every time the diaper is changed. If you have been using plastic pants to help keep the baby dry, stop using them until the rash has disappeared. Petroleum jelly, a zinc oxide paste, or a lubricating cream can be applied to the rash several times a day. If the rash is particularly persistent and severe, a 0.5 to 1 percent hydrocortisone cream can be used for a limited time (generally a few days).

For persistent diaper rash, many physicians recommend taking the baby's diaper off and exposing the affected area to air as frequently as conveniently possible.

Cradle Cap

Signs and Symptoms—Dry, scaly skin on the scalp

Cradle cap (seborrheic eczema) is a common problem that can occur at any age, but it is most common during infancy and adolescence. Cradle cap often begins during the infant's first month of life and may continue to be a problem throughout the first year. Its cause is unknown.

If your infant has cradle cap (see color photograph, page C-2), you probably first will notice dry, scaly patches on the scalp that give it a dirty appearance. A thick, yellow crust may form over the scales. You may notice some scaly patches around the hairline, eyebrows, eyelids, nose, and ears. Sometimes the rash is so extensive that the entire body is affected.

Treatment
Cradle cap usually has a shorter course than many other rashes, and it responds to treatment. Avoid daily washing with soap and water. Lubricate the affected area with a cream that does not contain a dye or perfume. Avoid clothing that is rough, scratchy, woolen, or too tight.

If the condition does not improve, your baby's physician may recommend a medication to apply to the affected area.

Cradle cap usually is not a problem after the first few months of life.

Infantile Eczema

Signs and Symptoms—Rough, red patches of dry skin

Infantile eczema (atopic dermatitis) is a

rough, red, patchy rash (see color photograph, page C-2) that usually is associated with extremely dry skin. The rash may be a reaction to an irritant, such as food, clothing, baby powder, or urine.

Eczema is more likely to occur in infants whose relatives have allergies. These infants also have a tendency to have asthma and seasonal allergies later in their lives.

If your infant has eczema, you may first notice light red or tannish pink patches of rough, scaly skin. The patches later become red. The baby may seem restless or irritable due to itching. Occasionally, the rash begins to ooze and crust. Infection may follow.

The most common areas for eczema are the cheeks and forehead. The problem may spread to the ears and neck.

Treatment

If you suspect your infant has eczema, see your baby's health care provider. In some infants, the rash can be traced to diet or a change in formula. Sometimes the offender may be a laundry detergent, a fabric such as wool, or excessive perspiration during hot weather. Rarely, eczema is a symptom of a serious disease. Often the cause is hard to identify.

The main complication of eczema is infection of the lesions with a virus or bacteria. Infants with eczema should not be exposed to persons with cold sores (herpes simplex). To decrease the chances of more bacteria being introduced into the open skin, keep your baby's nails clipped as short as possible. If your baby will tolerate them, a pair of cotton mittens, worn especially during sleep when most of the scratching is done, helps prevent further skin damage and infection.

Treatment is geared toward avoiding the source of irritation (if one has been determined). Avoid extremes of temperature. Most babies with eczema do better in a warm climate with moderate humidity because sweating seems to aggravate the rash. Dress the baby in cotton clothing. Avoid wool. A baby with eczema should not even lie on wool carpeting.

Keep baths to a minimum, perhaps once a week, and use bath oil to lubricate the dry skin.

If the eczema is particularly severe, your baby's health care provider may recommend that you apply dressings soaked in a special solution to ease the redness and itching. Corticosteroid lotions and creams can be applied after the dressing is removed. Anti-histamines such as diphenhydramine and hydroxyzine are often effective for controlling the itching. If your baby's lesions become infected, oral or topical antibiotics may be necessary.

Infantile eczema may wax and wane, but most children outgrow it by 3 to 5 years of age.

Milia

Milia are small white bumps or cysts on the newborn's face that resemble whiteheads. More than half of newborns have these little spots (see color photograph, page C-2). They are harmless and disappear without treatment.

Birthmarks

Birthmarks are common among all newborns. Generally, they are of no concern and no therapy is required.

The following are some of the more common birthmarks that occur in newborns:

Salmon Patches. Often called stork bites, salmon patches are small, light pink, flat spots that appear on 30 to 50 percent of newborns. They are collections of small blood vessels (capillaries) close to the skin. Occurring most frequently on the eyelids, the upper lip, the area between the eyebrows, and the back of the neck, salmon patches become more noticeable during crying bouts or when the temperature changes. Salmon patches often seem brighter in the first few months, and then variably fade by 1 year of age. Those on the back of the neck often persist but are usually not noticeable once the infant's hair grows.

Hemangiomas. These markings are benign (noncancerous) tumors made of newly formed blood vessels. Characteristically, hemangiomas are bright red, protruding, sharply demarcated lesions that may appear anywhere on the body.

Strawberry Hemangioma. This type of hemangioma usually appears on the face, scalp, back, or chest, but it may be anywhere on the body. More common in girls, strawberry hemangiomas are seldom present at birth, but usually appear within the first 2 months of life.

Most strawberry hemangiomas grow rapidly, remain at a fixed size, and then begin to disappear. Usually no treatment is recommended. In 60 percent of cases, these lesions disappear by the time the child is 5 years old, and in 90 to 95 percent of cases, they disappear by the time the child is 9. Approximately 10 percent of children with this birthmark have some discoloration or a slight puckering of the skin after the mark is gone (see color photograph, page C-2).

Cavernous Hemangioma. This hemangioma is more deeply situated in the skin layer than a strawberry hemangioma. It is typically a red-blue spongy mass made up of tissue filled with blood.

The outcome of this lesion is hard to predict. Some lesions disappear on their own. Depending on the location and size, sometimes steroid medication or laser treatment is helpful for treating the lesion.

Port-Wine Stain. The port-wine stain is a flat hemangioma (see color photograph, page C-2) that consists of dilated capillaries. The face is the most common site. The size of the hemangioma varies. Occasionally, half the body surface may be affected. This is a permanent condition. Laser therapy has become the treatment of choice, but it is most successful on adolescents and adults.

Erythema Toxicum

Signs and Symptoms—A rash characterized by white pimples or pustules on a red background

An estimated 50 percent of full-term newborns (less in premature infants) develop erythema toxicum 1 to 3 days after birth. It generally appears on the face, trunk, and limbs.

The cause is unknown. The rash is harmless, does not cause the infant discomfort, is not infectious, and requires no treatment. It generally disappears in a few days.

Thrush

Signs and Symptoms—A thin layer of milky matter on, in, and around the baby's mouth

Thrush is a mild yeast infection of the mouth that looks like whitish patches stuck to the inside of the cheeks and on the tongue and the roof of the mouth (see color photograph, page C-10). If the white patches do not come off when gently rubbed with a cotton swab, the baby may have thrush. Some babies will also get persistent diaper rash from the yeast infection, which looks like raised, bright red bumps on the skin and in the skin folds. Breastfeeding mothers may get the infection in their breasts, resulting in red, sore nipples and sometimes a burning pain in the breast. If you suspect that you or your infant may have thrush, consult your baby's health care provider.

Treatment

Thrush in healthy newborns generally resolves on its own, but treatment with an anti-yeast agent called nystatin 4 times a day will hasten the process, particularly if the thrush is extensive. The mother may also need treatment. An anti-yeast cream may be necessary to treat the diaper rash. Because yeast grows well on warm, moist skin, exposing infected areas to air will benefit both babies and mothers with thrush.

Innocent Heart Murmurs

At one time or another, most children have an innocent heart murmur. It is found frequently in newborns or after a child has had a fever, been anxious, or engaged in increased physical activity.

Most parents worry that a heart murmur indicates a serious heart problem. Although some heart murmurs are the result of congenital heart defects, an innocent heart murmur does not cause problems. Most children outgrow the murmur by the time they reach adolescence.

Innocent heart murmurs usually are discovered during routine examinations. Using a stethoscope, the infant's physician can hear the sounds made when the heart's ventricles contract and the heart valves open and close. If your child has a murmur, the physician hears an additional sound. There are several types of murmurs. Each type creates its own sound, and the sounds vary in intensity.

If your baby's health care provider diagnoses an innocent murmur, do not be alarmed. Treatment or special precautions are not necessary.

Umbilical Hernia

An infant with an umbilical hernia has a soft bulge of tissue around the navel that may protrude when the baby cries, coughs, or strains.

The problem is failure of the ring around the navel to close. As a result, a portion of the small intestine slips through the umbilicus.

Umbilical hernia is more apt to occur in black infants and in those with a low birth weight.

Unlike other hernias, there is little danger associated with an umbilical hernia. Most that appear before the age of 6 months disappear by the time the baby is 1 year old. Surgery is rarely necessary unless the hernia becomes progressively larger, fails to heal by the time the child is 5 years old, or causes an obstruction.

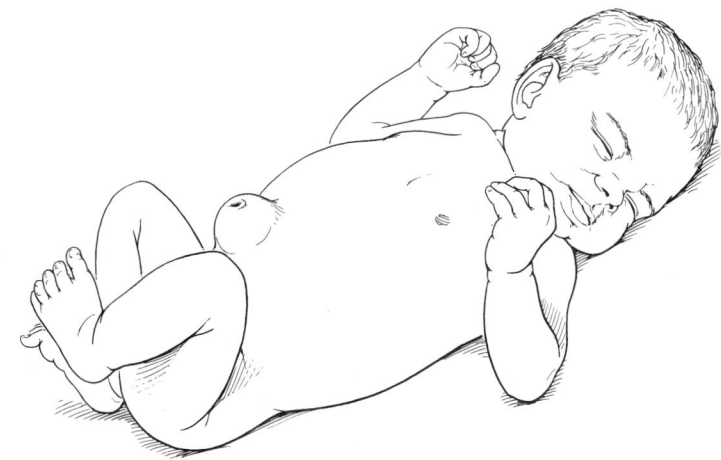

An umbilical hernia is caused by a failure of the ring around the navel to close. This results in a soft swelling that may protrude farther during coughing, straining, and crying.

Special Concerns

Most infants are born fully developed, healthy, and soon ready to be taken home.

Unfortunately, a few babies do not follow this pattern. For various reasons, some babies are born prematurely. These tiny infants, with lungs and other organs that are not yet developed enough to function properly, require special care, often for weeks or even months.

The birth of a seriously ill or premature baby can be a frightening experience. But today, the outlook for these infants is often hopeful. The care provided in specialized neonatal units for these fragile newborns has been a dramatic force in improving their chances of survival.

The following section discusses infants who require specialized care, such as those born prematurely, babies with diabetic mothers, babies with birth injuries or breathing difficulties, and babies born to drug-dependent mothers.

Premature Babies

A premature baby is commonly defined as one born before 37 weeks of gestation.

The word "premature" upsets many expectant parents, and it is true that not long ago the survival rates for premature infants were much lower than those for full-term babies. However, recent advances in the care of low-weight, premature infants have greatly improved their chances of survival.

Many factors contribute to prematurity. Women who are undernourished, are anemic, or have had little or no prenatal care are more likely to give birth prematurely. A history of infertility, stillbirth, abortion, and other premature births can increase the chance of premature birth, as can teenage pregnancy and smoking.

Often the stimulus for early labor comes from other factors. Premature separation of the placenta, uterine abnormalities, and a cervix that is too weak to bear the weight of the developing fetus are all associated with early delivery (see pages 202, 203, and 205). In addition, urinary tract infections in the mother may lead to a premature delivery.

To reduce the likelihood of premature delivery, seek early and regular prenatal care. If problems occur during pregnancy, contact your physician immediately.

If you go into premature labor, decisions

Newborn Intensive Care Units

Babies born prematurely or who have a serious infection, a respiratory problem, or a major birth defect may require care in a newborn intensive care unit (NICU).

Any birthing place must be prepared to assist the newborn with problems at birth. If your hospital or birthing place does not have an NICU and you are at risk of going into premature labor, your doctor will need to make arrangements well in advance in case the need for transfer to such a unit arises.

Some hospitals have units equipped and staffed to handle all but the most serious cases. Often one hospital in a particular area is designated as being the facility to which the sickest babies may be transported. The purpose of the NICU is to provide maximal care and monitoring of patients with life-threatening problems.

In the United States, the neonatal death rate has decreased substantially during the past 40 years, mainly as a result of vastly improved care for sick newborns.

The main elements of an NICU are:

- The staff—neonatologists (pediatricians with specialized training in the care of premature infants), neonatal intensive care nurses, and other health care professionals
- Monitoring and alarm systems so that every vital sign of every baby can be checked
- Respiratory therapy and resuscitation equipment and medications
- Access to physicians in every pediatric specialty, including surgery and anesthesiology
- 24-hour laboratory service

If your newborn requires intensive care, the experience may seem overwhelming at first. Your infant will be placed in an incubator to conserve body heat and reduce the chance of infection from the environment. The baby will be connected to monitors that provide the nurses and physicians with information about heart rate, blood pressure, body temperature, and rate of respiration.

Depending on whether respira-tory distress is present, the infant may be attached to a ventilator so that he or she can breathe through a tube inserted into the windpipe (trachea). The newborn may have a feeding tube through the nose or connected to a needle in a vein to provide liquid nutrition from a special container.

Important factors in the successful care of premature and ill infants are the skill and experience of the nurses and the number of nurses who care for these children. The nursing staff provides most of the baby's care and informs the physician when something goes wrong. A typical NICU is crowded with nurses, and it is not uncommon to see two nurses caring for one particularly sick baby.

Parents usually are encouraged to spend as much time as possible in the unit. Even though you may not be able to hold your baby, eye contact, touch, and any other stimulation you can provide can be beneficial for both you and your newborn.

---

involved in trying to stop your labor are complex. Your physician will assess your health, the health of your baby, how your placenta and cervix are functioning, risks of infection, and how far along you are in your pregnancy. After taking these factors into consideration, your physician will evaluate whether an attempt should be made to stop preterm labor and what these efforts should be.

Interventions may include bed rest, intravenous fluids, and medications to help you stop preterm labor. You may also be given antibiotics to prevent the risk of infection in both mother and baby (see Premature Labor, page 201).

If your membranes have ruptured, a sample of amniotic fluid can predict the maturity of your baby's lungs and also indicate whether there is infection in the amniotic fluid. If the membranes have not ruptured, amniotic fluid can be collected by an amniocentesis test. (For a description of amniocentesis, see page 181.)

If your baby's lungs are not mature enough, you may be given steroids to enhance the maturation of the baby's lungs before birth.

A baby born too soon has not had time for adequate development of body systems that are essential to life. Thus, it is the role of the physician—often a neonatologist (a physician trained to care for premature infants)—and the nursing staff of the newborn intensive care unit to allow the baby time to develop further in a protected environment.

As a rule, the longer the baby is in the womb, the better equipped it is to live outside, the fewer the complications, and the better the chances of not only surviving but also surviving with no long-term disabilities.

Premature babies are at an increased risk of Sudden Infant Death Syndrome (see page 69). Babies born after 23 weeks of gestation have a good chance of surviving with the help of newborn intensive care.

Usually, although not always, the size of the baby is indicative of its age. For example, a baby born at 26 weeks of gestation is apt to be much smaller than one born at 32 weeks.

Although size is important, the older the gestational age of the infant at birth, the greater the chances of survival. Moreover, the younger the gestational age at birth and the lower the birth weight, the more likely the baby is to have a neurologic or developmental handicap such as cerebral palsy, learning difficulties, or vision or hearing problems.

One of the biggest problems of premature birth is underdeveloped lungs. If your baby has breathing difficulty, he or she may require breathing assistance from a ventilator through a tube placed down the windpipe (trachea). The goal is to maintain adequate oxygen exchange, blood circulation, and nutrition while allowing the baby's lungs to develop (see Respiratory Distress Syndrome, this page).

Other problems associated with premature birth include heart problems, pneumonia, low blood sugar concentration (hypoglycemia), anemia, and infection.

The combination of very little body fat and immature skin prevents the premature infant from maintaining body heat. Babies born prematurely are taken to special units (see Newborn Intensive Care Units, page 18), where they are placed under warmers or in incubators to help conserve their body heat.

Premature newborns often receive their initial nutrition intravenously. This is called total parenteral nutrition (TPN), which is used until the newborn is more stable and ready to start breast milk or formula feedings.

Many premature infants have not yet developed the sucking reflex or are too weak to suck. These infants are fed through a tube inserted through their mouth into their stomach. After these early feedings are well established, these infants usually can be fed by breastfeeding or with a bottle. The antibodies in breast milk are important to these premature babies.

The trend today in neonatal nurseries is toward greater parental involvement. Parents are encouraged to spend time with their infants and to touch and caress them even when tubes, wires, and other equipment make cuddling difficult. Whenever practical, parents are encouraged to feed the child and to change a diaper. Some parents bring books and read to their babies, play music, or put family pictures in the incubator.

Finally, one day your baby will be ready to come home. By now the baby may be weeks or even months old. This is an exciting moment, but one that is often mixed with fear and anxiety.

Like countless other parents who have done it, you can too. You can be sure that your infant would not be discharged from the hospital unless the physicians thought it was time. Moreover, you will be instructed fully on any special care your baby will require, and if you have any questions, help is only a telephone call away.

Try to relax. You have come through a difficult time. Now it is time to enjoy the rewards of parenthood.

Respiratory Difficulty

At birth, a newborn must rapidly fill its lungs with air while at the same time clearing them of fluid. Simultaneously, the infant must also increase the circulation of blood through its lungs.

The newborn must breathe without the lungs collapsing every time they are expanded. Most full-term infants are able to accomplish this because the lungs have had adequate time to develop fully. Many premature infants and even some full-term babies, however, have problems breathing.

Two common types of breathing problems occur in newborns: respiratory distress syndrome, which typically affects premature infants, and transient tachypnea (rapid, shallow breathing), which occurs in both premature and full-term babies.

Respiratory Distress Syndrome (RDS)

Respiratory distress syndrome (RDS) is characterized by harsh, irregular breathing; grunting; nasal flaring; difficulty breathing; and a dusky blue skin color.

RDS is a specific diagnosis that refers to a lack of certain agents in the lungs called surfactants. Surfactants help reduce surface tension and prevent collapse of the lungs' small air spaces every time a breath is drawn. Thus, in these infants, greater pressure is needed to expand the lungs. RDS can often be prevented or lessened in severity.

The severity of RDS correlates with the infant's gestational age and birth weight. Thus, the smaller and more premature the infant, the greater the chance the baby will have RDS. This disorder is rarely found in infants born at term. Boys have this condition more often than girls, and white babies are affected more often than African-American babies.

RDS generally is recognized within minutes after birth. In some babies, the distress at birth is so severe that resuscitation is necessary. An X-ray of the lung and blood tests can establish the diagnosis.

If your child is born with RDS, he or she will need to be in a newborn intensive care unit (see page 18), where vital signs will be monitored constantly. The baby will be placed in an incubator that is filled with warmed, humidified air. Nutrition and fluids may be given intravenously.

Many infants with this condition require help in breathing. In such a case, a breathing tube may be inserted into the baby's trachea to provide supplemental oxygen.

Because RDS is due to an insufficiency of surfactant, infants with severe RDS may be given doses of surfactant preparation directly into their lungs. Other medications frequently used in babies with RDS include diuretics (to increase urine output and rid the body of extra water), dexamethasone (to reduce inflammation in the lung), bronchodilators (to reduce wheezing), and theophylline or caffeine (to minimize pauses in breathing).

The goal in caring for infants with respiratory distress syndrome is to keep them complication-free until the lungs have had time to develop adequately. With the advent of special neonatal units and highly trained physicians and nurses, the mortality rate for these infants has declined steadily.

Transient Tachypnea

This form of respiratory distress can occur after an uneventful vaginal delivery or cesarean section and in premature or full-term infants.

Infants born with this form of respiratory distress often have no signs of trouble other than rapid, shallow breathing (tachypnea). In some babies, the skin may have a bluish tinge, which can be alleviated with small amounts of oxygen.

Unlike infants with RDS, these infants rarely appear severely ill. Most of them recover within 3 days.

Treatment often involves postponing feeding to avoid the aspiration of fluid into the lungs. Occasionally, intravenous feedings are necessary if the baby is breathing too fast to be fed orally. Usually no other treatment is necessary.

Bronchopulmonary Dysplasia (BPD)

The lung problems of premature babies generally improve within several days to several weeks. Babies who still require assistance with ventilation or supplemental oxygen a month after birth are often described as having bronchopulmonary dysplasia (BPD).

Symptoms include rapid breathing, wheezing, coughing, cyanosis (in which the lips and the fingernail beds turn blue), and difficulty breathing. BPD often is suspected in infants with RDS who do not recover quickly. It is diagnosed from a chest X-ray.

Babies with BPD continue to need supplemental oxygen for an extended period and medications such as theophylline or caffeine. Most infants recover slowly over several months. However, their lungs are somewhat fragile, and care should be taken to keep them warm and free of infection. Immunization against influenza might be suggested to parents and siblings of an infant with BPD.

Pneumothorax

Every infant is born with collapsed lungs. One of the miracles of birth is that, within a few breaths, the lungs inflate and the baby begins breathing. However, considerable pressure changes occur to inflate the lungs that first time. Occasionally, the lungs do not immediately inflate all the way, and the pressure changes can cause small ruptures in the alveoli (air sacs) of the tiny lungs. These ruptures allow air to leak out into the spaces between the thin membranes (called pleurae) lining the lungs and the inner wall of the chest. If a large amount of air leaks into this area (called the pleural space), the lungs may collapse (pneumothorax) and breathing becomes difficult.

Diagnosis

If a small amount of air leaks, the infant will have shortness of breath, rapid or grunting breathing, and may have cyanosis (bluish lips and fingernail beds). However, if a large amount of air leaks, the infant may suddenly develop severe breathing difficulty. Your physician may take a chest X-ray to try to find out why the breathing difficulty has developed.

How Serious Is Pneumothorax?

Pneumothorax can be very serious if a lung collapses suddenly, but in most cases the leakage of air is small and the air is reabsorbed on its own.

Treatment

Sometimes no specific treatment is necessary. Occasionally, the pneumothorax can be corrected by giving the infant extra oxygen to breathe for 1 to 2 hours. In the case of a large pneumothorax, the air that has leaked into the chest may need to be removed as an emergency procedure. This is accomplished by inserting a tube into the space between the ribs (chest wall) and the lung itself.

Babies of Mothers With Diabetes

Before the availability of insulin, many women with diabetes were too ill to conceive. Today, with improved maternal and prenatal care, more women with diabetes than ever before are able to have babies.

Even so, if you have diabetes, your child is at greater risk than one whose mother does not have diabetes. Newborns whose mothers had diabetes before pregnancy or whose diabetes developed during pregnancy (gestational diabetes) have a slightly higher mortality rate than do those whose mothers do not have diabetes. In addition, these babies are more apt to be born with problems such as respiratory distress and metabolic problems such as low blood sugar (hypoglycemia).

If you have diabetes, seek the care of a specialist. Optimal care begins before conception. It is important for the diabetes to be well controlled, both before and during pregnancy, to minimize the risk of birth defects or other problems in the baby.

The degree to which the mother's diabetes is controlled correlates closely with the infant's outcome. With close monitoring by a physician, the medical problems of infants born to mothers with diabetes are less common than in the past.

All babies of mothers with diabetes need careful monitoring. Blood sugar tests may be done within 1 hour after birth and then frequently thereafter.

In some infants, glucose will have to be given intravenously if the blood sugar value is too low after birth and feedings aren't possible. These changes in blood sugar value are temporary, and normal regulation is established within hours to several days (see Diabetes Mellitus, page 925).

Birth Injuries

Between 2 and 7 of every 1,000 newborns have a birth injury. A birth injury is defined as trauma incurred by the infant during labor and delivery. Most often, the birth injury occurs despite excellent obstetric care.

Certain conditions make the possibility of a birth injury more likely. Prematurity, breech birth, prolonged pregnancy, an abnormally large fetus, an abnormal fetal position, and a small maternal pelvis are conditions that predispose infants to birth trauma.

Forceps sometimes are involved in birth injuries. Forceps are used to assist some difficult vaginal births. Forceps injuries generally are minor, involving facial or scalp abrasions. Often, forceps delivery is the safest way to end a labor that may threaten the life or health of the mother or child.

Another technique used to assist in difficult deliveries is vacuum extraction. In this method, a rubber or plastic cap is placed on the head of the baby while it is in the birth canal. The doctor applies suction with a pump and then gently pulls on the instrument to help ease the baby down the birth canal. Newer methods that prevent too much suction from being applied help protect the baby from injury.

The following are the most common birth injuries:

Caput Succedaneum. This injury involves swelling of the tissues of the scalp. It occurs because of pressure of the head against the birth canal. This swelling usually disappears after a few days, and the baby's head assumes a normal shape.

Cephalhematoma. Caused by slow bleeding, cephalhematoma is a bruise under the scalp. The swelling usually is not visible until several hours after birth. Most cephalhematomas resolve within 2 weeks to 3 months. Treatment is rarely required.

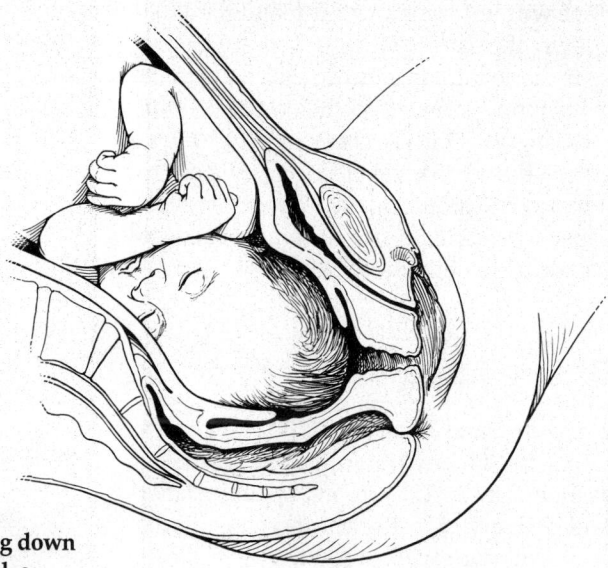

After traveling down the birth canal, a newborn commonly develops swelling of the scalp. Called caput succedaneum, this swelling is not harmful and usually disappears in a few days when the baby's head assumes its normal shape.

Fractured Collarbone. A fracture of the collarbone (clavicle) is the most frequent bone injury during labor and delivery, particularly when there is difficulty in delivering the shoulder. An infant with this injury is reluctant to move the arm on the affected side. The collarbone heals quickly in a young infant. Usually the only treatment required consists of simple measures for pain relief.

Dislocation of the Nasal Septum. Dislocation of the nasal septum (cartilage) can occasionally occur. When this happens, the infant may have difficulty nursing and some problems breathing through its nose. The nose appears asymmetric and flattened. Most nasal flattening resolves spontaneously. More severe flattening may require a minor procedure to fix the dislocated septum.

Facial Nerve Palsy. Weak to absent movement of facial muscles usually results from pressure over the facial nerve during labor or birth. It may involve an entire side of the infant's face.

When the infant cries, the affected side of the face does not move and the mouth is drawn to one side. The eye on the weak side cannot close, and the corner of the mouth droops. In most cases, improvement is rapid and complete.

Drug Withdrawal

The infant of a mother who took drugs frequently during her pregnancy may go through withdrawal at birth. Drugs that may cause withdrawal in infants include narcotics (heroin, morphine, methadone), barbiturates (especially phenobarbital), analgesics (prescription pain medications), tranquilizers and sedatives, alcohol, amphetamines, and phencyclidine (PCP).

The infant whose mother was addicted to narcotics may develop irritability, a high-pitched cry, sleeping and feeding problems, diarrhea, vomiting, and, rarely, convulsions. If the mother was addicted to barbiturates, withdrawal symptoms in the infant may not appear until 7 to 10 days after birth.

After birth, treatment may be required for the drug withdrawal syndrome. The infant is also at increased risk for problems resulting from poor growth while within the uterus and from prematurity. The infant may need oxygen if it has difficulty breathing or if its breathing is depressed. If withdrawal symptoms are mild, they are treated simply by providing a quiet, comforting environment, with swaddling, gentle handling, and frequent feedings.

If symptoms are severe, medications may be required. The smallest dose possible to relieve the symptoms is given. After the newborn has had no symptoms for several days, the physician will begin to decrease the dose until the child is no longer receiving any medication and the symptoms have disappeared.

General Care

Many mothers discover that taking care of their healthy, happy newborn is quite natural. Somehow, as if by instinct, they know what the proper approach should be for a given situation. Others are at a loss, afraid to make a mistake and afraid that they might endanger the well-being of the baby. Regardless of how confident you are with your newborn, you should be aware of some everyday issues.

Clothing

Comfort and convenience should be the important features of any newborn's wardrobe. Keep in mind that it is not economical to buy too many of one item. You will be surprised at how quickly your newborn will grow. Thus, as a rule, try to stay away from newborn and layette sizes. There is no reason why a full-term newborn cannot wear clothing designated for babies 3 to 6 months old. Fit does not have to be perfect.

The following should give you an idea of the types of clothes you may want on hand when your newborn comes home. Of course, there are seasonal variations.

Nightgowns are an essential part of the newborn's wardrobe. These often have a drawstring at the bottom and mittens on the end of the sleeves that keep the baby from scratching himself or herself. Usually, three or four of these are adequate.

Stretch suits are comfortable for the newborn and can be worn day or night. Usually made of polyester, terry cloth, or cotton, they have snaps down one or both legs to make changing diapers easier.

Undershirts come in two styles: those that pull over the head and those that snap down the front. The latter often are preferred because they are easier to put on the newborn. Unless the weather is extremely cold, a short-sleeved, medium-weight undershirt usually is adequate.

Layers of cotton or acrylic tops or shirts, sweaters, or sweatshirts are useful in cool weather or to add extra warmth when the baby is out of bed. If you dress your baby in a sweater, make sure there is adequate room at the neck and that the buttons are sewn on securely.

A snowsuit, jacket, or a bunting is important if your infant will be taken out in cold weather. A bunting is a warm zippered bag in which the baby is encased up to its shoulders. A snowsuit is shaped like a pair of overalls and encloses the feet. These suits are usually made of warm, quilted, water-repellent material. A snowsuit is easier to use with a car seat than is a bunting.

If the baby will be outside in cold weather, a warm hat is necessary. In the summer, a sun hat with a chin strap is needed if the baby will be in the sun any length of time.

Shoes are not recommended for newborns.

Booties and socks are useful for keeping the baby's feet warm in cold weather.

When Is Your Baby Warm Enough?

How can you tell whether your baby needs an extra sweater? The hands are not a good indicator of how warm a baby is because they tend to be cool even when the body is warm. The legs, arms, and neck are better indicators—and the baby's face can also be a guide. If the infant is cold, the cheeks will lose all color. A cold baby also is very likely to be fussy.

Bedding should include fitted crib sheets (probably three to six), a mattress pad for protection, and two or three crib blankets, usually made of a combination of cotton and polyester. Cotton receiving blankets are not particularly warm as a covering but are good for swaddling the infant to keep the baby from kicking off the covers and for security.

The current recommendation is to avoid putting your baby to sleep on sheepskin, waterbeds, or thick layers of quilts and bedding. Studies have found that the incidence of SIDS (Sudden Infant Death Syndrome) goes down when these types of bedding practices are discontinued (see page 69).

Most parents are more likely to put too many clothes on their newborn than too few. Too many clothes can be detrimental because the baby may become overly warm.

Car Seats

Not so long ago, parents assumed that the safest place for their baby during a ride in the car was in someone's arms.

Today, we know that a baby held in someone's arms can be killed or severely injured should an accident occur. Even if the vehicle is traveling at only 30 miles per hour, a newborn would be ripped from your arms with a force comparable to that of falling from a three-story building. If you are not wearing a seat belt, the baby may be crushed between you and the windshield.

All 50 states and the District of Columbia have laws requiring children to be in a specially designed safety seat. A safety seat will be one of your most important purchases. Your baby should not leave the hospital without a car seat. In fact, most hospitals will not allow a parent to take an infant home unless they have a safety seat installed in the car. Many hospitals or civic groups either rent or lend safety seats for newborns.

A safety seat is designed to diffuse the forces of a crash over the child's entire body and to keep the child from being thrown out of the car or from striking anything inside the car. Although no one can predict the outcome of an accident, experts do know that an infant's chance of surviving even a serious accident is improved greatly when a safety seat is used properly.

Two types of safety seats are suitable for a newborn:

One is the infant safety seat designed for a baby weighing less than 20 pounds. It is installed so the baby faces the rear of the car when placed in the seat. This position is crucial because during a crash, the back—the strongest part of the baby's body—absorbs the shock. The safest placement for the seat usually is in the middle of the back seat of your car. Read both the owner's manual for your car and the safety seat manufacturer's instructions to determine the best placement. Do not put an infant seat in the front when the car has air bags.

The other type of safety seat is a convertible car seat that can be used from birth until the child weighs approximately 40 pounds. This seat can be converted from the reclining, back-facing position to an upright and forward-facing position when the child is about 1 year old or weighs about 20 pounds.

When you begin shopping for a safety seat, make sure you buy one that conforms to current Federal Motor Vehicle Safety Standards. Seats manufactured before 1981 may not meet current standards.

Whatever seat you choose, make sure you understand the instructions and then follow them. If the seat is not installed properly and is not used correctly, the baby does not have the benefit of its full protection.

Infant Carriers

Infant carriers are inclined plastic seats and are useful for carrying the infant from place to place. The seat also is a good place to put your awake baby when your arms are full. If you decide to use an infant carrier, however, make sure you always strap the infant into it. Keep the seat on the floor or a low table. Just a few slight rocking motions from the infant are enough to move the carrier off the edge of a countertop and bring baby crashing to the floor. Make sure that any seat you buy has a large enough base so that it will not tip easily once your baby becomes more active. Some car seats do convert to serve as infant carriers, but not all infant carriers meet car safety standards.

Pacifiers

Should you give your infant a pacifier?

The answer to that question is somewhat controversial. Some health care providers are adamantly against the use of pacifiers. Others believe that when used in moderation they can be helpful for some babies, who need the pleasure of sucking more than others. Some babies will suck on their fists, fingers or thumb, and so find a pacifier soothing.

Pacifiers should not be introduced to breastfeeding newborns until their nursing routine is well established.

If you decide to try a pacifier, the most important thing is to use it properly. Do not pop it into your baby's mouth every time it opens. Do not let your baby or yourself become dependent on the pacifier. Encourage your baby to go to sleep without the pacifier. Find other methods for calming your crying baby other than the pacifier alone. And take it away as soon as your baby's need for extra sucking is gone, usually between 12 and 15 months of age.

Exposure to Sun and Wind

Parents often ask their baby's health care provider whether they can take their new-

For all automobile rides, secure your newborn in an infant car seat that is fastened to the seat of your car.

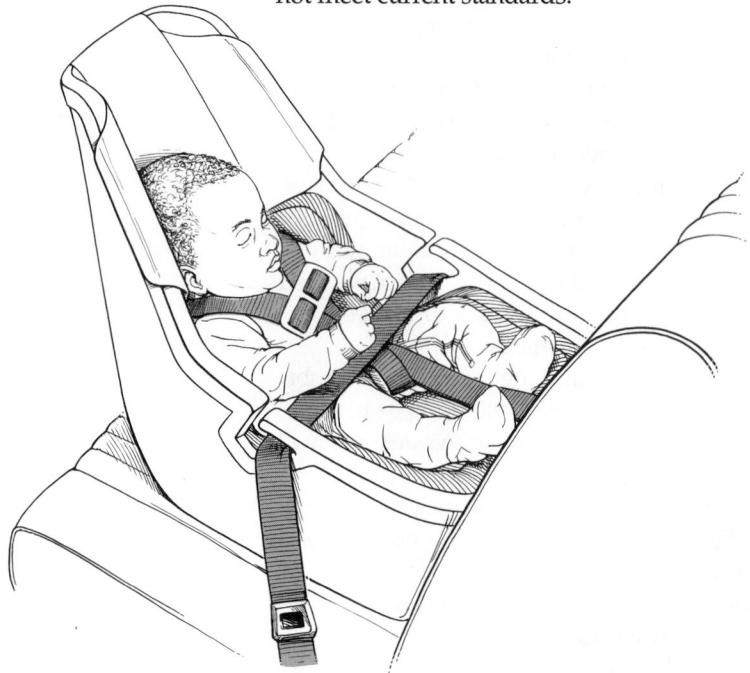

born outside. The answer is a qualified yes.

Babies love the motion of a ride in the stroller or carriage. You need not let winter keep you indoors as long as you dress the baby warmly.

Your baby can and should be exposed to some sunlight, but only in moderation. Direct sunlight contains ultraviolet rays, which create vitamin D in the skin, a vitamin necessary for growth of bones and teeth.

The main danger of sun exposure is sunburn. If a baby is left asleep in a carriage or stroller outside in the sun for even a few minutes, the result may be a sunburn and overheating. The sunburn is not only extremely painful but also damaging to the baby's delicate skin.

Take into account the season and whether the area where the carriage is parked is partially shaded. An infant can take more sun on a cold winter day, when the rays are not so strong, than during the summer. Consider these factors before exposing your infant to the sun.

Most babies should not be out in the summer sun for more than 30 or 40 minutes. At the beach, where the sun is more intense, the infant should be in the shade whenever possible. Put a sun hat on your baby to protect its face. Although sunblock lotions are highly recommended for children and adults, they should not be used on infants younger than 6 months.

Your baby may become overheated in a short time. Generally, young infants don't sweat. Panting may be the first sign of overheating. A flushed skin is a late sign that your infant is too hot.

Care of the Eyes and Ears

The newborn's eyes are bathed constantly by tears secreted by the tear ducts. However, many newborns develop a slight inflammation of the eyes a few days after birth. This requires no treatment. If your baby's eyes are very red or pink, there may be an infection, and you should call the baby's physician. Some newborns have a clear or white discharge from one or both eyes. Typically, the infant awakens with the affected eye "glued" shut. Usually, the eye drains tears down through the nose by the nasolacrimal duct. In infants this duct is easily blocked, causing overflow of fluid or matter from the eye. This blockage usually resolves in the first few months. Treatment is only to clean with plain water and a cotton ball or, infrequently, your baby's health care provider may prescribe antibiotics. If the problem continues to 1 year of age, which is rare, an evaluation by an opthalmologist is recommended.

Routine care of your baby's eyes and ears can be accomplished during the baby's bath. You can wash around your infant's eyes with a soft washcloth or cotton ball and plain water. Do not use soap or any other cleanser because it will irritate the baby's delicate eyes.

Your baby's ears also are easy to care for. The outer ear is the only part you need be concerned with during the baby's bath. Simply wash the ear with a soft cloth and mild soap. Do not be concerned about any wax in the ear canal. Wax is formed by the ears for protection. Caregivers should never attempt to remove the wax, nor should anything be inserted into the ear for cleaning purposes. If an excessive amount of ear wax makes it impossible for your health care provider to examine the child's ears, he or she will remove the wax with a special instrument.

Any blood or discharge from your infant's ears should be reported to the physician.

Care of the Skin

In the first month of life, a baby's skin is not yet self-lubricating. Many newborns have dry, peeling skin, especially on the hands and feet. If lotions are needed, look for nonscented (nonirritating) brands. Use nonscented soaps as well. For baby care, simpler products are usually better.

Trimming Nails

Trimming an infant's nails—especially for the first time—can be a bit of an adventure.

Select a good pair of scissors. Ideally, the scissors should have blunt ends to prevent injury to a squirming baby. Small manicure scissors work well. Some parents prefer nail clippers.

Trimming a baby's nails while he or she is asleep is probably the preferred way because the infant is still. Alternatively, enlist help and make this a two-person job. Have someone hold the baby's hand steady while you do the trimming.

Fontanelle

Every baby is born with a soft spot (fontanelle) on the top of its head.

During birth it is necessary for the baby's relatively large head to move down a narrower birth canal. To do so, the head must adapt itself to this smaller space. A completely formed skull could not do this. Thus, babies have a spot on the top part of the skull where four pieces of bone have not yet come together.

The size of the fontanelle varies. Generally, the larger the soft spot, the longer it takes to close. In some babies the bones come together by 9 months after birth; in others the process may take 2 years. The average is between 12 and 18 months.

New parents often are particularly concerned about this soft spot. Some mothers are afraid to shampoo the infant's hair for fear they will harm its brain. In fact, the baby's brain is well protected from normal handling by a tough, protective membrane over the soft spot. Parents should not be afraid of inflicting damage by simply touching the top of the baby's head.

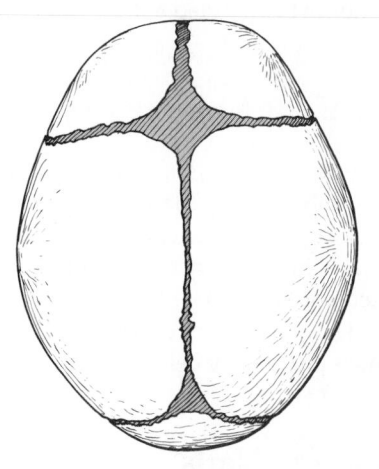

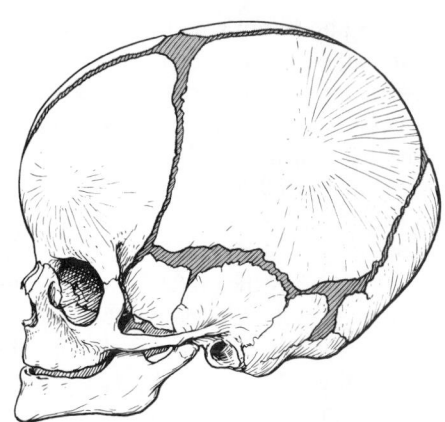

Your child's tiny skull consists of not one but several separate bones. Over the first year or two of life, these bones fuse to form a single protective bone mass. Until then, there will be a soft spot (fontanelle) at the main juncture of the bones.

You may sometimes see the soft spot pulsing. This is nothing to be concerned about. However, if you ever observe marked bulging or if the spot appears to sink, especially if the baby is acting differently than usual, notify your health care provider at once.

Appropriate Toys

A newborn infant does not need a room filled with toys. Parents themselves are the best "toy" for infants because they provide the most desirable interaction of touching and talking. Does this mean, then, that your newborn does not need toys? No. A newborn placed in an empty crib with nothing to look at is going to be bored. The key is finding toys that are appropriate for the newborn's abilities.

The word "toy" may not accurately describe what a newborn needs in that it implies a certain physical interaction that the newborn is not yet capable of. The baby cannot shake a rattle, cuddle a teddy bear, or spin the dials or pull the levers on a busy box attached to the crib. A cluttered crib may hinder the baby's movements.

The newborn has amazing abilities. Your baby has been born with the abilities to see, hear, touch, smell, and taste. In selecting toys, keep this in mind and find objects that will stimulate some of those senses. Even though the baby is not capable of shaking a colorful rattle, he or she can hear the interesting sound it makes when you shake it. Your baby also can appreciate the color and pattern of a mobile hanging over the crib or the soft feel of a teddy bear's fur when you rub it against your baby's cheek.

Because your newborn spends a large portion of the day in bed, every effort should be made to make that environment as pleasant and as interesting as possible. Newborns prefer busy patterns (especially in black and white) to plain solid colors, and they are fascinated by faces. Keeping that in mind, you can buy patterned sheets and bumper pad covers that give your baby something interesting to look at. Bedding with pictures of animals, colorful balloons, or geometric shapes is always preferable to plain-colored bedding.

Many parents buy a mobile to hang over the crib. Mobiles come in various styles. When choosing one, keep in mind the baby's perspective. Some mobiles may look great to parents who are seeing them at eye level, but there may not be much to see from baby's position in the crib. The most useful mobiles are designed so that the baby sees the mobile at its best. Some hang stationary, and others rotate and even play lullabies when you push a button. It is important to position the mobile out of the reach of your child and secure it well. Be sure to take it down when your baby begins to pull up.

A baby can appreciate music. Your newborn can enjoy a small music box in the nursery, a musical mobile, or even a radio playing soft music.

Several toys are designed to hang over infant seats or even car seats. Choose black and white patterns for your newborn, bright colors for an older baby. The newborn cannot reach up to grab these objects, but he or she can enjoy looking at them.

Walking into a toy store for the first time can be puzzling for the new parent. With thousands of toys to choose from, how does one make a decision? Most of the major toy companies indicate on the packages the age for which a particular toy was designed.

When you choose toys from a major company that are age-appropriate for your newborn, you can feel relatively confident that the toy is safe. However, you still should examine the toy to make sure there is nothing sharp or loose that could hurt the baby and nothing on which your infant might choke.

Bathing

Bathing your infant can become one of the most rewarding routines of early parenthood. Your baby thrives on attention, touch, and, eventually, the opportunity to play with you. Although not all infants will love the water from the first encounter, bathing can be a fun and special time for both of you.

Most hospitals give bath demonstrations in the newborn nursery. If not, ask your mother, another relative, or an experienced friend for advice.

Placing a tiny, slippery baby in an adult-sized bathtub can be awkward and uncomfortable for parents. Thus, many parents buy a baby bathtub that can be placed in the kitchen sink or in the tub. Large bowls or washbasins also can be used. If you do not feel comfortable with even the small tub, you can give the baby sponge baths initially. Many health care providers recommend sponge baths until the baby's navel is healed (see page 30).

Never leave the baby unattended in the tub for even a few seconds. The bathtub can be an extremely dangerous place if a baby is left alone, even if it contains only a small amount of water. Let the telephone or doorbell ring. Do not allow anything to take your attention away from your infant. Hence, planning is important. Before you begin the bath, assemble everything you might need: soap, baby shampoo, washcloth, towel, cotton balls, clean diaper, undershirt, and sleeper or nightgown.

After you have run the water in the tub (fill it to a depth of only an inch or two), touch the water with your elbow or wrist to make sure it is comfortably warm but not hot.

Undress the baby. Support the head with your wrist and place the fingers of that hand in its armpit. Then place the baby in the tub. First, wash the face with a soft, wet cloth but no soap. Use a cotton ball soaked in plain water to wipe around the baby's eyes. A shampoo is necessary only once or twice a week. Use a shampoo that is specially designed for infants. Wipe the suds off the scalp with a damp cloth. Do not pour water over the baby's face.

After the face is washed, soap the rest of the body. Most parents find it easier to soap the skin with their hand rather than a washcloth because the other hand is holding the baby. Wash the diaper area last. Remember that infants get chilly fast, and try to keep bath time short.

When the soap has been rinsed away, hold your baby with both hands and move it

While bathing your newborn, support the baby's head and torso with your wrist and hand, to provide your baby both safety and a sense of security. Never leave your child unattended in the bath, even for a moment.

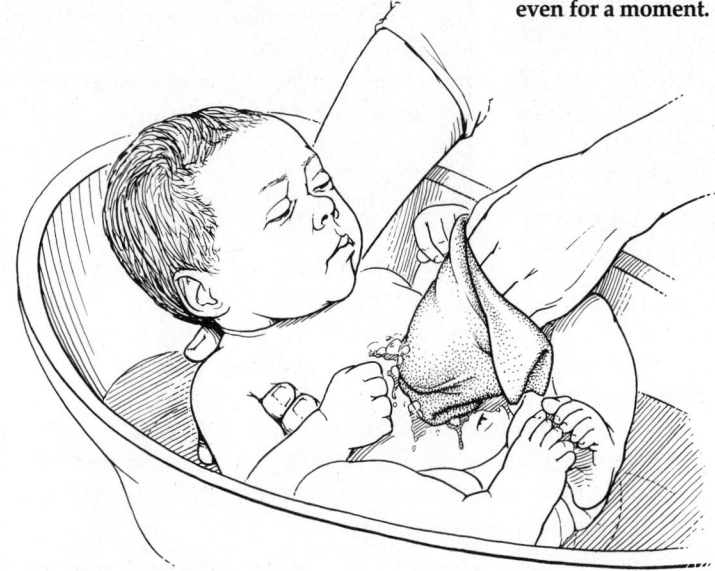

to a soft bath towel. If the navel is still not healed, your baby's health care provider may want you to swab it with a cotton ball soaked in plain water.

Neither lotion nor powder are necessary most of the time. The simplest treatment is usually best for babies' delicate skin, and the agents that make lotions and powders smell good often irritate sensitive skin. If your baby's skin is dry, choose unscented lotion. If you choose to use powder, never dust it directly on the baby because the particles can irritate the baby's lungs. Instead, apply some to your hand (away from the baby) and gently pat it on thinly.

When should you bathe your baby and how often? Each baby is different. Pick a bathing time that works best for everyone involved. As long as the baby's diaper area and the face are thoroughly cleansed daily, infants probably only need to be bathed with soap once a week. If you wish to bathe your baby more often than that, use plain water. Excess bathing can tend to dry out a baby's skin in the winter.

Selecting a Crib

While many parents like to use a bassinet in the early months, your infant will soon outgrow it and need a crib. The crib you choose should have slats that are less than 2⅜ inches apart, a mattress that fits snugly, a locking mechanism that keeps the sides up, and no sharp edges. There should be at least 20 inches from the top of the rail to the mattress surface. The lowered crib side should be at least 9 inches above the mattress surface. Most cribs on the market today meet these specifications. However, if someone has given you an older crib, measure the slats; if they are more than 2⅜ inches apart, the crib

can be dangerous, especially if the mattress does not fit perfectly. Babies have been known to strangle as a result of getting their heads stuck between the slats. Another potential danger of an old crib (one built before 1974) is that it may have been painted with a lead-based paint. Make sure this is not the case. Infants sometimes chew the slats of their cribs, and lead-based paint, when consumed, can be harmful (see Lead Poisoning, page 71).

Bumper pads should be used in the crib to prevent the baby from banging against the sides. A pillow is unnecessary and should not be used. Avoid placing baby on waterbeds, sheep skin, or layers of thick quilts, all of which can pose a potential hazard from suffocation.

Place your newborn on his or her side or back to sleep. A rolled-up blanket can serve as a wedge to keep the baby on his or her side while sleeping.

Diapers

The two basic types of diapers are disposable and cloth.

Disposable diapers are the choice of many parents because of their convenience; the diaper is worn and then thrown away. Disposable diapers come in various sizes and thicknesses. A disposable diaper is easy for even the most inexperienced parent to put on a baby because it is prefolded and secured around the baby with adhesive tape rather than pins. Parents who use these diapers do not have the age-old worry of sticking their newborn with a pin.

Despite their convenience, however, disposable diapers are expensive. Another disadvantage is that they fill up your garbage can and pose an environmental problem as well. In the United States, disposable diapers account for approximately 2 percent of our landfill space, where they decompose slowly. Some argue that the water, energy, and resources used to make, wash, and dry cloth diapers make them no more "environmentally friendly."

If you choose to use cloth diapers, buy the largest size. Cloth diapers are made of several materials, including cotton, gauze, and flannel.

You can launder them or you can hire a diaper service. Those who choose to wash the diapers themselves—the most economi-

---

Don't Leave Your Baby Alone

Leaving your baby alone, in the house or outside, is an invitation to trouble. An infant, or any young child, should never be left alone in the house. If you cannot find a trusted baby-sitter, take the baby with you. Infant carriers and baby slings make taking the baby along easy and fun.

Do not leave the baby unattended on a changing table. Your baby may be capable of flipping over or pulling up before you are aware of this new muscular development, and may put himself or herself at risk of serious injury.

cal method—should buy at least 2 dozen, more if you do not want to be tied to the washing machine every day. You will need a covered diaper pail, partially filled with water, to put used diapers in. Empty bowel movements into the toilet and rinse the diaper before putting it into the pail. Diapers should be machine washed with a mild soap or detergent and rinsed two or three times. Rinsing is important. A diaper with soap residue on it may irritate your baby's skin.

If you hire a diaper service, the service will deliver sterilized diapers to your door and pick up the used ones (stored in a container). You may wish to compare the cost of a diaper service with the cost of disposable diapers—differences may be slight. However, if your baby will be cared for in a child care center, check to see if they allow cloth diapers.

In general, neither cloth nor disposable diapers have been found to cause a higher incidence of diaper rash. Each baby is different, and yours may respond better to one type than the other.

If you use cloth diapers, you can buy disposable diaper liners that help wick moisture away from the baby and make it easier to dispose of the solid waste before washing the diapers. You can also find waterproof nylon shells with convenient Velcro-type closures to hold the diaper in place. If you use diaper pins, slip two fingers between the baby and the diaper to avoid sticking the infant. Sometimes, it helps to soap the pin so that it slides through the diaper more easily.

Some parents change their infants at least once and often twice during a feeding—usu-ally at the beginning and at the end. This frequent changing is not really necessary unless the baby has had a bowel movement. Changing the infant after a feeding is usually adequate.

When changing a baby who has had a bowel movement, use a disposable wipe or a washcloth with soap and water to clean the area thoroughly. A girl should be wiped from front to back to avoid getting stool bacteria into the urethra.

Prevention of Disease

Most of the medical care a newborn infant receives is geared toward the prevention of disease.

Occasionally, bacteria in the birth canal cause serious eye infections in a newborn. Therefore, immediately after birth, every newborn's eyes are protected with erythromycin ointment or tetracycline solution.

An injection of vitamin K is given in the hospital to prevent potential bleeding problems. Babies also should receive the hepatitis B vaccine to protect them from any possible contact with hepatitis B, a viral infection that affects the liver. (Two additional hepatitis B vaccinations will be given in your baby's first year.) Several days after birth, routine screening tests will be performed for congenital problems such as PKU (phenylketonuria), galactosemia, hypothyroidism, congenital adrenal hyperplasia, and possibly others (see Required Screening Tests, page 8).

It may be wise to continue to limit your

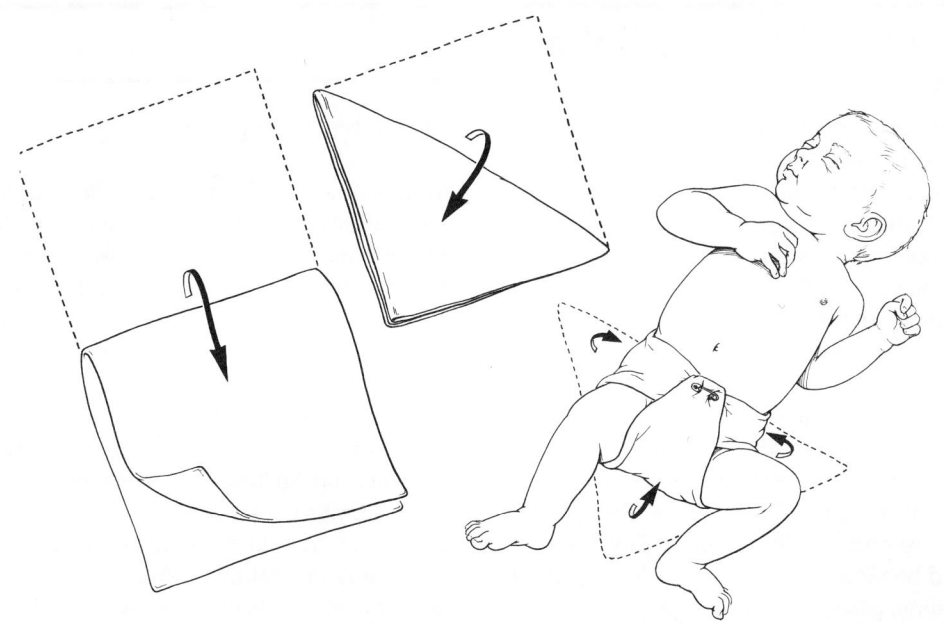

There is no mystery to changing a cloth diaper. First, fold the diaper approximately in half. Second, fold it again, this time on the diagonal, into a triangle. Third, position your baby on the diaper and pin the corners together carefully.

newborn's exposure to outsiders for a while after you leave the hospital. In particular, avoid crowds. Remember, fever and other illnesses that may be considered minor in the older baby may be cause for concern during the first month of life.

It is important for all infants to be seen by a health care provider on a regular basis. Before you go home from the hospital, your health care provider will discuss this schedule with you. Depending on your infant's age at discharge, the first follow-up visit occurs when the baby is 1 to 2 weeks old. Some pediatricians or family physicians recommend monthly visits during the first year of life; others want to see the baby every 2 months, provided everything is going well.

Care of the Umbilicus

The fetus's lifeline to its mother is the umbilical cord. During its 9 months in the uterus, the baby receives its nourishment through the blood vessels of the cord. At birth, however, that connection is severed because it is no longer needed.

All that remains of the cord is a small stump, about an inch long. The cord begins to wither and separate, the raw area becomes covered by a thin layer of skin, scar tissue forms, and, in most babies, the cord drops off within 12 to 15 days after birth.

Most of the time the care of the umbilicus is relatively easy. Many physicians advise parents not to cover the area because this may impede healing. The cord should be kept dry. When diapering the newborn, fold over the top of the diaper so it does not cover the navel. This will allow it to stay dry.

Some physicians recommend sponge baths until the cord has dropped off. Your baby's health care provider may advise you to clean the area with a cotton ball dipped in plain water. Gently swab around the base of the navel to keep the area clean and discourage infection.

A few days of crusted discharge or dried blood is normal until the cord falls off. Until the cord completely heals, infection is possible (although rare) because bacteria can enter the body through the opening. If your infant's navel area looks reddened or there is any discharge, call your baby's health care provider.

Some babies develop small growths in this area, called umbilical granulomas. If your infant has a granuloma, the healing process is delayed. You will notice that the cord area looks dull red or pink and moist and there may be an unpleasant-smelling discharge.

Initially, the physician may recommend cleaning the area several times a day with alcohol. If the granuloma persists, your physician can cauterize or seal the cord with silver nitrate.

Personality and Behavior

A newborn does not arrive as a "blank slate," as was once believed. Rather, from the moment of its birth, your newborn is unlike any other person ever born.

Some babies are quiet, some are noisy. Some stay awake for as long as 90 minutes after birth; others fall asleep within 15 minutes. Some suck better than others. One baby prefers visual stimulation; the newborn in the next bassinet may prefer sounds.

From one healthy baby to the next, the variations are enormous. Part of the wonder of parenting is watching, recognizing, and reinforcing the changes, development, and behaviors as your infant's personality emerges.

Healthy Development

Your baby starts life with traits inherited from generations of your family. The events during pregnancy and birth can also be important for shaping the infant. Did the mother eat well? Did she refrain from smoking, consuming alcohol, and taking drugs? Were labor and childbirth normal, or were there complications? These and other factors influence the person your baby is and will become.

A crucial factor in the development of your infant's personality is the relationship between parent and child. Love and affection are as critical to the infant's emotional survival as food is to the body's well-being.

An infant deprived of human love and attention will wither emotionally and also often physically (see Bonding, this page).

Your infant is a social being from the beginning. Research has found that newborns prefer looking at figures that resemble human faces rather than at other pictures. Some scientists believe that a baby has an inborn tendency to perceive the human face as a source of potential reward. In addition, a newborn infant seems to prefer a high-pitched voice.

During the first month, your infant probably will show a preference for familiar persons. Babies also tend to respond based on the kind of stimulation they prefer. For instance, if your baby loves action, the aunt who rocks him or her may get more response from the child than does the aunt who sings.

Do not be surprised to see your infant smile. Initially, the infant's smile is usually in response to something internal and is seen when the baby is sleeping or drowsy. Between the third and fifth weeks of life, however, most babies have their first social smile, typically in response to a face or voice. This is an exciting moment for most parents.

Your baby is a born mimic. Stick your tongue out, and the newborn can repeat the action. By the time most babies are 4 weeks old, they begin to make small throaty noises—their first attempt at conversation.

Your newborn responds positively to comfort. A crying baby often will quiet when picked up by familiar hands. The baby searches out its mother's face, makes eye contact, and then stops crying. The baby cries when wet or hungry and quiets when the diaper is changed or the breast or bottle is given.

Sometime during the newborn period, you will notice that your baby is expressing a new emotion: enjoyment. For many babies, this is first seen in the bath. A crying infant may stop when put in the bath, relax, smile, and then begin crying (out of disappointment) when the bath is over.

Excitement is another emotion that emerges during the first month. Usually the source is a person or toy. Your baby may move its arms and legs, pant, coo, and even smile at you or at a particularly interesting object.

A newborn does not yet distinguish between actions and their results. By the time your baby is 1 month old, however, you will notice the infant begin to repeat actions for its own pleasure. Your baby may thrust out its legs, like the way that feels, and do it again.

A 1-month-old infant is beginning to take a little control over its environment. For example, your baby may discover that thumb sucking is comforting. During a crying spell, you may see the baby pop his or her fist into its mouth. A moment later, things are quiet.

Many of these areas of development may be inconsistent or variable in the first month or so. At certain times, your infant may be ready to play and react, but at other times may tune out your attempts at interaction. That is perfectly normal. As you become more aware of your baby's cues, these times will be even more rewarding for both of you.

An infant's early weeks are consumed by learning to adapt to his or her new environment. In the first few days of life, the infant begins to communicate and interact through signals. The baby is hungry, the baby cries, and then mother appears with food. The baby is wet, the baby cries, and the diaper is changed. It is through these and similar exchanges that the attachments between parent and child are formed. The infant learns that its needs will be met by someone who cares.

Thus, it is impossible to overemphasize the importance of security and consistency to the newborn. For normal emotional development, the infant must learn to trust, and trust can be learned only when a parent or caregiver responds to the baby's needs in a prompt and loving manner.

Bonding

The bonding (formation of an attachment) between parent and child begins long before the baby is born (or adopted).

When parents-to-be first learn that they are expecting a child (or an adoption placement), they may begin to look through books for a name for their child. They furnish a nursery. They hear their baby's heartbeat on a visit to the obstetrician or receive a photograph of the child they will be adopting. They plan and dream, worry and hope. And finally they are rewarded with the arrival of the baby.

Bonding is the complex array of emotional ties and commitments that characterize the parent-child relationship. By the time a baby arrives, there is already a strong emotional link on the parents' part, a link that is stronger for some than for others. Over the

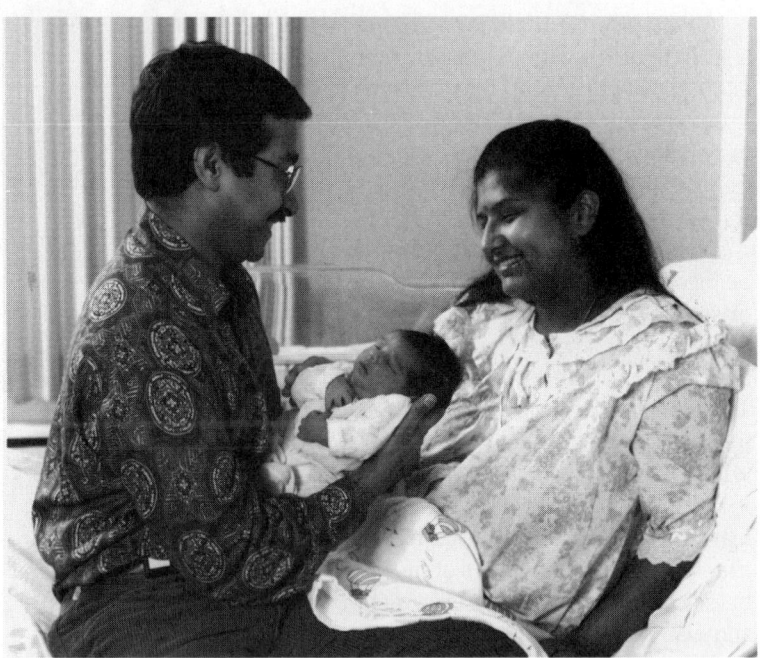

Most hospitals encourage new parents to spend time with their newborn.

course of the next few months, the infant begins to develop an attachment to the person or persons with whom he or she learns to associate protection, love, and guidance.

If your baby is healthy, bonding begins immediately. Most babies have an alert period for an hour or two after the delivery, making it a particularly good time for the parents and infant to begin to know one another. It is not known whether the bonding between humans has a critical period. However, the key is not when it happens but that it does. It is most important that the bonding eventually take place.

How does a parent go about bonding with an infant? There is no easy recipe for bonding, just as there is no way to tell someone how to love. Bonding occurs during the day-to-day exchange of affectionate actions between parent and child.

A mother gently touches her infant, and that touch is pleasurable to the new baby. When the baby's cheek is touched, the infant turns toward the mother's face or toward the breast and begins to nuzzle and lick the nipple. This not only stimulates the production of milk but also is a powerful emotional stimulant. The baby gazes into the mother's eyes during breast- or bottle-feeding. The infant cries and the parent picks the baby up, strokes its cheek, and speaks in a soft and soothing voice.

The importance of bonding is well recognized by hospitals and health professionals. Thus, most hospitals encourage new parents to spend time with their newborn, and adoptive parents will want to do the same.

If, however, your infant is born prematurely or is seriously ill, the situation may be different. Your baby will probably be placed in an incubator and connected to machines that monitor its vital signs. Intravenous and feeding tubes may be present. You may not be able to hold or even feed your infant initially. However, you will still be encouraged to spend as much time as possible with your newborn. You can stroke the baby's skin, hold its tiny fist, and soothe its cries with your voice. Even this limited contact is important and beneficial for both you and your baby and your ultimate relationship.

Once you bring your baby home from the hospital, the bonding process continues. Whether breast- or bottle-feeding, you are feeding the infant frequently, during which time you are cuddling, stroking, and providing comfort as well as nourishment. The infant may cry when picked up by someone other than you. You may notice after a few weeks that your infant recognizes your voice and quiets in response to it. The colicky baby cries, you spend hours walking the floor, and the baby learns that someone cares. These all are ways in which, over the course of the first few months, you and your baby form the lifelong bonds that are the basis for the loving parent-child relationship.

It is not uncommon for parents to wonder before the baby arrives whether they will be able to love this new person who is about to enter and change their lives. Even after birth or adoption, many a parent has looked at the new baby expecting to feel a rush of love and, instead, felt nothing or, worse, disappointment or even dislike.

Do not be too hard on yourself if you do not immediately fall in love with your infant. Parenting is never easy, and at times it can be downright trying. Love for your baby sometimes comes gradually. Again, as you bond with the child, as you get to know each other, as you see the baby's eyes light up when you come into the room, or when the infant smiles at you for the first time, you soon will find yourself loving your baby.

Infant Reflexes and Responses

Your newborn's movements are governed by reflexes. Stroke its cheek and the baby will root and try to suck. Prick the soles of its feet, and the knees and feet flex. Make a sudden noise, and your baby may startle.

Twins

"Twinship" is the closest of all human relationships. Twins need very little encouragement to remain close. As parents, the best gift you can give your twins is a sense of identity. Use their names frequently. Take pictures individually. Spend time alone with each child. These are just a few ways to strengthen their sense of uniqueness.

Caring for two or more babies can be physically and emotionally overwhelming for both new and experienced parents. Here are tips that may help ease your daily responsibilities and help preserve the quality of family life.

Attend to Your Own Needs

Give yourself adequate rest and good nutrition. Keep meals simple, and take naps often. This will help give you the energy you need to meet the high demands of caring for twins.

Share the Workload

Cooperative parenting lightens the load for both parents. Working parents sometimes can shorten workdays during initial weeks to help out at home.

Accept Help

If ever there was a time for a baby-sitter or parent's helper, this is it. Grandparents, neighbors, student nurses, and even school-aged helpers may enjoy the opportunity to share in this special experience. Call on them. Their help allows you some relief and personal time, and it is essential as routine activities such as grocery shopping and going to the post office become much more difficult tasks.

It is easy to be so involved in the daily demands of these two infants that you may overlook people, organizations, or professionals that can offer assistance or advice. Other parents of twins are a natural source of practical advice. Some communities offer support groups for parents of twins. Pediatricians, psychologists, psychiatrists, and social workers often have special interests in, and valuable advice concerning, the more specific problems of nurturing twins.

All healthy babies are born with predictable reflexes that disappear in a predictable order as the voluntary motor functions take control. However, the absence of reflexes and responses may indicate a possible neurologic problem. Part of your newborn's examination in the hospital includes attempts to elicit various reflexes and responses.

The reflexes and responses found in the newborn at birth are described here. All healthy newborns can exhibit these responses, although they may be more subdued in a sleepy or recently fed baby.

Moro Reflex

This is one of the most frequent and dramatic newborn responses. It occurs when your infant hears a loud noise, has an abrupt change in position, or is handled roughly. The infant startles, arches its back, and throws its head back. At the same time, it throws out its arms and legs and then brings them abruptly back toward its body. The infant cries, then startles, and then cries because of the startle. The Moro reflex gradually disappears by the third month of life.

Grasp Reflex

Stroking your infant sets off several responses. Your baby will grasp your finger when you stroke the palm of its hand (palmar grasp). Stroke the sole of your baby's foot and you'll see the toes turn downward, as if trying to grasp (plantar reflex). The more premature the infant, the more reluctant it is to let go. The palmar grasp disappears at about age 6 months. The plantar reflex continues until 10 months of age.

Rooting and Sucking

These are two of your infant's important reflexes. Stroking the baby's cheek or lips produces the rooting reflex. The baby turns toward the stroking object and begins to root for the nipple. The sucking reflex is initiated once the nipple is taken into the baby's mouth. Sucking and rooting reflexes usually stop by the time the infant is 4 months old. However, these reflexes can be produced in a sleeping infant until the seventh month.

Tonic Neck Reflex

This reflex is seen when your baby is on its back and its head is turned to the side. The infant arches its body away from the face side, the arm on the face side extends while the other arm flexes, and the legs are drawn up.

Although present in newborns, this reflex is more prominent in the 2-month-old infant. It usually disappears by the sixth month.

Orienting Response

The orienting response of your newborn is a response to a change in the environment. If, for example, the infant hears or sees something new, it becomes more alert and less active. Its head may turn toward the stimulus and its heartbeat changes. If the infant is adapting to a familiar stimulus, the heartbeat slows. When the stimulus is unfamiliar, the heartbeat accelerates.

Gag Reflex and Blink Reflex

An infant is able to protect itself because of several responses and reflexes. Because of a strong gag reflex, your newborn infant is able to spit up mucus to help clear its windpipe. If a part of the infant's body is exposed to cold air, its entire body changes color and temperature, its limbs are pulled in close to its body to reduce the exposed surface, and it begins to shiver and cry in an attempt to stay warm. In addition, a strong blink reflex protects the newborn's eyes from glaring light.

Your newborn does not like pain any more than you do and will do whatever possible to avoid it. If the baby's leg is hurt, for instance, he or she will pull the leg away. If that does not work, the other foot will attempt to push you away.

Even though your newborn's reflexes will disappear—most of them during the first year of life—their usefulness seems to be more than short-term. Studies indicate that your baby's brain stores information learned from these early reflexes. For example, when infants try to right themselves, this act, even though unsuccessful, probably contributes to their development of the concept of space. Similarly, the strong tonic neck reflex helps a baby learn to use both sides of its body separately and to use its hands voluntarily rather than instinctively.

Hearing

Babies are born with a good sense of hearing. The healthy newborn will blink and startle in response to sound and can distinguish differences in volume. Soft noises may produce something akin to a smile, whereas harsh or loud sounds may cause the infant to cry. Moreover, your newborn already has developed sound preferences, favoring a high-pitched voice such as its mother's over lower pitches.

Hearing is essential in the acquisition of speech and language. Even a minor hearing loss can have a major impact on your infant's ability to understand and later to communicate with language.

Some newborns are in a high-risk group for hearing loss. They include infants whose 5-minute Apgar scores are 6 or less (see page 6); those born with infections such as rubella, cytomegalovirus, syphilis, and herpes; those who have head or neck injuries, severe jaundice, or a family history of hearing loss during childhood; and those who are born very prematurely. The incidence of severe hearing loss in both ears among newborns with any of these conditions ranges between 2 and 5 percent.

It is important that even a minor hearing loss be detected in infancy so that the proper steps can be initiated to avoid problems the loss can cause. If your newborn is thought to be at high risk for hearing loss, hearing tests should be done while the baby is still in the hospital or arranged for in follow-up evaluations. Two tests currently are used: 1) observation of the infant's response to sound and 2) special tests (auditory brain stem-evoked response or oto-acoustic emissions that can check for loss in one ear).

However, none of the current hearing tests routinely used on newborns can detect slight hearing loss or minimal loss that will progress as the child grows. Thus, if any hearing loss is suspected, your infant should have a follow-up hearing test between the ages of 3 and 6 months (see page 64).

Certain types of hearing loss can be corrected. When the loss is due to ear infection (see Acute Ear Infection, page 574), for example, antibiotics can eradicate the infection and the ear can function normally. Surgery sometimes corrects congenital malformations of the ear.

Programs that help parents communicate with their deaf or hearing-impaired infants also are available in many communities. Parents are taught how to make the most of any hearing the child has and to acquaint the child with visual language through signing or lip reading.

The four types of hearing loss found in infants and children are described below.

Conductive Hearing Loss

This type of loss involves some type of interference with the external ear's ability to receive sound or with the transmission of sound from the external ear to the inner ear. The most common causes of this type of hearing loss are congenital abnormalities of the ear and ear infections. This type of hearing loss often can be treated with medication or surgery.

Sensorineural Hearing Loss

This loss results from abnormalities of the cochlear hair cells within the ear or the auditory nerve. More than 50 percent of severe sensorineural hearing loss is hereditary. Other causes include severe jaundice, infection while in the uterus, and medications. Sensorineural hearing loss is usually permanent.

Mixed Hearing Loss

This loss occurs when a child has both conductive and sensorineural hearing loss. This type of loss may be severe. Medication or surgery or both may help restore a portion of the child's hearing loss.

Central Auditory Disorders

These disorders result from a problem in the central auditory nervous system, the ear's nerve linkage with the brain. Children with these disorders can hear sound but only as a jumble of noise.

Vision

At birth, your infant's eyes are about three-fourths the size of what they will be at adulthood. The white part of the eye (sclera) has a bluish tinge, and the colored part (iris) is usually a nondescript blue in whites and dark in other races. The pupils in the newborn are small and may not constrict readily in response to light. The eyes do not always appear to move together.

Your baby probably will keep its eyes shut much of the time. This does not mean the infant cannot see. In fact, physicians now know that babies see immediately after birth, although not clearly. Your newborn will try to focus on objects held in front of its face. If the object is farther than 8 to 12 inches away, the image is hazy and the baby's eyes may wander, each in a different direction.

The newborn is attracted to patterns more than to colors. Most interesting of all to the newborn is the human face.

Most infants are slightly farsighted, although some babies, particularly those born prematurely, are born nearsighted (unable to see objects far away clearly). As healthy infants grow, their eyes change and become able to see both near and far objects more clearly.

Some infants are born with partial or total loss of vision. Common causes include developmental malformations, damage to the eyes due to infection, birth trauma, a significant loss of oxygen (hypoxia), and genetic diseases that affect the eye itself or the nerves to the brain's vision center.

Until the mid-1950s, the leading cause of blindness in infants was retrolental fibroplasia (now referred to as retinopathy of prematurity). This occurred when small or premature infants were given high concentrations of oxygen in incubators to help them survive. In some, this resulted in partial or total blindness.

Retinopathy of prematurity sometimes occurs today in very premature infants with low birth weight who survive because of advances in technology and neonatal care. Fortunately, blindness is less frequent as new understanding of this problem is gained and better treatments evolve.

Occasionally, a physician doing a newborn examination may suspect that the infant is partially or completely blind. There may be dense cataracts, the eyes may be abnormally small (microphthalmia), or the cornea may be opaque. Sometimes, however, the defect lies not in the eye or optic nerve but in the brain itself, requiring neurologic evaluation and studies such as computed tomography or magnetic resonance imaging (see page 494).

Treatment for partial or complete congenital blindness depends on the cause. Sometimes a defect can be corrected surgically. Cataracts, for example, can be removed. Whether or not vision is restored depends on whether the infant has other vision problems and whether they also can be corrected.

Sometimes blindness is permanent. If your child is born blind, your pediatrician or family physician can direct you to social and community agencies that may be able to offer information and help in rearing a child with a visual impairment.

If a severe problem is not apparent in the infant's early days in the hospital, how does a parent know that something is wrong with the baby's vision? The first clue may be what is called nystagmus—the rapid movement of the baby's eyes. The baby's eyes suddenly may begin to move up and down, side to side, in a rotation, or a combination of all three movements. Another common sign is the baby's inability to develop skill in properly aligning both eyes on an object. One eye fixes on an object, and the other deviates. The baby might squint and appear to be cross-eyed. As the baby grows, you might notice that he or she appears to be timid about crawling or seems unusually clumsy. If you have any concerns about your baby's eyes, see your baby's health care provider.

Sleeping

The average newborn spends more time sleeping than any other activity. Some babies sleep as little as 10 hours daily while others may sleep up to 20 hours.

Newborns are light sleepers. They "cat-nap" throughout the day and night. Studies of infant brain waves during sleep have shown that a newborn spends at least half of its sleep time in restless sleep and 20 to 30 percent in deep sleep. Once babies are 8 months old, they spend less time in restless sleep and more time in deep sleep, when they are often seemingly unarousable. Infants have a great knack for tuning the world out during sleep, and the routine noises of your busy household will not wake them.

Newborns require frequent, small feedings due to their rapid early growth rate and tiny stomachs. As they grow and mature, sleep periods will lengthen.

By 6 months, some babies are taking one or more daytime naps and may sleep 6 to 8 night-time hours at a time. Brief awakenings throughout the night are normal.

The older infant is able to "sleep through" the night only when he or she no longer needs night feedings and has learned how to get back to sleep without help.

Infant Behavior

Your baby's sleeping, crying, and eating patterns define your infant's behavior. A baby that sleeps easily, cries very little, and eats predictably is easy to parent. The irritable, fretful baby who feeds irregularly and sleeps little requires more attention. Normal infant behavior covers a wide range of patterns.

Many parents ask: "How do I know what I'm doing is right? Can I spoil my new baby?"

Your baby's behavior will influence how you parent. Initially, the newborn behaves in response to his or her immediate physical needs. However, a newborn's emotional needs are equally important. Newborns need comforting and holding; they need the sound of your voice and the sight of your smile.

Not long ago the prevailing wisdom was that a newborn could easily be spoiled. Babies were put on strict schedules and handled only when necessary. If a newborn cried for any reason other than hunger or a diaper change, the wails often were ignored. Experts now know that responsiveness is a better approach.

During pregnancy, a baby's needs are instantly met. The womb provides an environment of constant security and comfort, and babies seek security and comfort outside the womb as well.

Most newborns cry easily and need frequent cuddling and reassurance. The research of Mary B. Ainsworth and Sylvia Bell shows that the longer a parent takes to answer a baby's cry, the longer it takes to soothe the baby. Babies whose cries are answered quickly in the early months of their development may cry less often and for shorter periods in later months. Instead of becoming clingy toddlers, these babies are more likely to demonstrate healthy independence.

Rigid schedules have been cast aside in favor of flexible schedules that consider the needs of each baby and family. Parents are encouraged to cuddle their child. Health care providers advise parents to meet the immediate needs of their newborn, whether it be for food or comfort. In essence, enjoy your baby.

By observing what works and learning from what doesn't, you will discover many things about your baby's behavior over time. What does your baby enjoy? How much stimulation can your baby tolerate? How can you help your baby quiet down? Human contact works best in the first few months.

Parents often underestimate their baby's ability to "calm down" without any help from mom or dad. Examples of such skills include sucking a finger or knuckle, listening to a repetitive noise, or watching an interesting object. As your baby starts to demon-

Sleeping Issues and Concerns

Sleep patterns, like many activities of the newborn, are unpredictable and disorganized in the early months. One major factor at the root of most concerns about an infant's sleep patterns is unrealistic expectations on the part of the parents.

Don't expect to make sense of your newborn's sleep/wake periods in the beginning. Your infant's first priority is to adjust to life outside the security of the womb. Falling asleep at times convenient to mom or dad is simply not a priority.

Lots of cuddling can help smooth the transition. Meanwhile, be prepared for your infant to fall asleep and be awake at the wrong times. Learn to nap when your baby does, even if it's not a time you prefer. Sometimes, napping while cuddling your baby is the only way either of you will get much sleep. Eventually, with added maturity and subtle persuasion, your baby will adjust and assume a more conventional sleep pattern.

Drooping eyelids, rubbing the eyes, and inconsolable fussiness are usual signs of fatigue in a baby. Many babies cry when they are put down for sleep, but if left alone, most will eventually quiet themselves. It often takes 20 minutes of restlessness for a baby to fall asleep.

If it's bedtime and your baby is not wet, hungry, or ill, try to be patient with the crying and encourage self-settling. Provide your baby with a quiet atmosphere.

Sleeping through the night doesn't happen early for most newborns. It will come with time. Be patient and enjoy the early weeks with your newborn, even the night feedings.

Begin by finding ways to calm your baby: a certain position or a specific object to look at or listen to may help. After a while you'll know how your baby likes to be wrapped and rocked, and what helps him or her to settle down to sleep.

Any of the following steps may help your baby learn how to fall asleep and how to get back to sleep:

- Put your baby to bed drowsy but awake. A baby who falls asleep in someone's arms may wake up in the night and not be able to fall asleep without being held.

- When your baby needs care or feeding in the night, use a soft voice and subtle body language to let the baby know it's nighttime, not playtime. Be business-like and boring. Let your baby know this is not the time for fun activities such as walking, rocking, and playing.

- Think about your own sleep habits. When you awaken in the night, it takes a couple of minutes to find a comfortable position, settle in, and fall back asleep. The same is true of your baby. Unlike you, however, one of the only comforting mechanisms your baby has is crying. Expect some crying as your baby tries to fall back to sleep.

- Make sure your baby is comfortable and safe. If you've made sure the crib and area around it are safe, you won't immediately become concerned about your baby's safety if you hear cries.

- Establish a bedtime routine, a winding down of the day's activities. Perhaps you will want to turn off the TV and have a quiet time 30 minutes before you put your baby to bed.

strate these skills, it's important to know when to intervene during a fussy spell and when to let your baby try to calm himself or herself down.

Interpreting the meaning behind a cry takes educated trial and error. To narrow the possible causes, evaluate the circumstances. When, for example, was the last feeding, the last nap, the last diaper change? Is there too much noise or activity?

Rocking soothes a multitude of needs and will almost always calm a crying baby, unless the baby is hungry. Try to understand the specific needs of your baby and intervene as best you can.

As you and your baby become better acquainted, you can begin to establish a schedule that is mutually acceptable. Nap time, for example, can be determined not only by your baby's need for sleep but also by your need for rest and free time. With growing maturity on the part of your baby, scheduling will become easier and needn't be as loose and flexible as in the early months.

A crying baby can be unnerving, but you must never handle an infant roughly. Shaking or any other rough behavior can cause irreparable damage and even death. It might be best to ask for "time out" and take a break for a short time while the baby is under the care of someone you trust. Let your baby's health care provider know if you feel that your baby's crying is becoming unmanageable.

Your Newborn's Nutrition

Your goal in feeding your newborn is to help the baby grow and to include nutrients that will enhance your baby's health.

Unlike the older baby, the newborn does not have a varied diet. If you are breastfeeding, your baby will be nourished by breast milk. If you are bottle feeding, your infant will be given formula, usually a combination of specially processed cow's milk, vitamins, and minerals mixed with water.

Parents often want to know how they can tell whether their infant is eating enough. The best rule is to personalize your baby's feeding schedule and trust your baby. He or she knows how much food is needed. When you offer the breast or bottle, your baby will eat as much as is needed, regardless of how much is left. When it is time to eat again, the baby will usually let you know.

If a baby does not get enough to eat, you will soon know it. He or she cries until you offer more food. An infant who needs more food than is being given will awaken more at night and will decrease rather than increase the time between feedings. Moreover, these infants finish their milk to the last drop and still do not seem satisfied. You may even observe the baby chewing his or her fist more than usual.

The best indication that your baby is receiving the necessary nourishment is weight gain. Some babies gain weight slowly, and others gain rapidly. Sometimes slow weight gain can be attributed to illness, which might require more visits to the baby's health care provider to make sure nothing is amiss.

As a rule, the average baby gains 2 pounds a month during the first 3 months of life. Most babies who weigh about 7 pounds at birth (the average weight of a newborn) have doubled their weight by the fourth to sixth month of age.

Although it is helpful for a parent to understand the basics of nutrition, the newborn's diet is simple. If you are breastfeeding your infant, the baby is getting the most complete food known. If you opt to feed your infant formula, your health care provider will recommend one that will provide the nutritional ingredients needed. Supplemental vitamins may be prescribed. Regardless of whether the source is mother's milk or formula, the following are the components of the basic diet of the newborn:

A calorie is a measurement of the energy content of food. Everything we eat and much of what we drink contains calories. The distribution of calories in human milk and standard formula is 20 to 30 calories per ounce: between 9 and 15 percent of the calories come from protein, 45 to 55 percent from carbohydrates, and 35 to 45 percent from fat.

Protein is essential for growth and for the repair of cells. Most of the major body organs are composed mainly of protein. If the body does not receive an adequate amount of protein, it begins to break down its muscles to supply protein to the brain and to make enzymes. An infant, or anyone else, deprived of protein for a long enough period will develop lethargy, a distended abdomen, and swelling.

Carbohydrates supply most of the body's energy needs. If the body has an inadequate carbohydrate intake, it improvises by using protein and fat for energy. Carbohydrates are stored in the liver and muscles. The infant's reserve is a fraction of that of the adult. Carbohydrates are necessary for your infant's health, even when he or she is ill.

Fats are a concentrated source of energy. They help protect body organs, vessels, and nerves, provide insulation against changes in temperature, act as a vehicle for the absorption of some vitamins, and delay the time it takes for the stomach to empty, thus giving one a "full" sensation. Although it is important for adults to limit their fat intake, infants and young children should not be on a fat-restricted or low-fat diet.

Water is absolutely essential for human life. Water accounts for 70 to 75 percent of your newborn's body weight, compared with only 60 to 65 percent of an adult's body weight. To remain healthy, an infant must take in larger amounts of water per unit of body weight than an adult. The daily amount of water required is between 10 and 15 percent of the infant's body weight, whereas in an adult the requirement is between 2 and 4 percent.

Fortunately, the water content of both breast milk and formula is very high. Some formula-fed babies like to have water from a bottle between feedings, although water itself is seldom needed unless the baby has a fever or diarrhea or the environmental temperature is high. If the infant is feeding well, the amount of water in the milk or formula is adequate.

Minerals are important to the structure and workings of virtually every part of the body. For example, calcium and fluoride are necessary for the formation of strong bones and teeth, copper and iron are required for the production of red blood cells, and sodium is needed to maintain the water balance in the body.

Vitamins are substances required by the body in minute amounts if every organ is to work properly. Some of the necessary vitamins include vitamin A, which is needed for the eyes and to keep the linings of the bronchial, urinary, and intestinal tracts healthy; vitamin C, which is needed for the development of bones, teeth, blood vessels, and other tissues; and vitamin D, which is also needed for the development of bones and teeth.

Common Feeding Practices

A generation ago, breastfeeding was not the norm for many American women. Today, it is proved to be the ideal feeding method because of its nutritional and immunologic advantages and its emotional benefits (see page 40).

Even so, some women who decide to breastfeed need more flexibility than that method normally allows. Thus, they also introduce the infant to the bottle. If you want to supplement one or more breastfeedings a day with a bottle, you can pump your breasts and store the milk, which can be given later. Have your health care provider or lactation consultant demonstrate the proper procedure for pumping your breasts. Highly efficient breast pumps are now available to enable you to provide breast milk for your baby regardless of your circumstances or lifestyle.

Many parents prefer, and health care providers recommend, that the newborn be allowed to determine the schedule of feedings—at least to some degree. This method considers the differences in babies. Many newborns are content to be fed every 4 hours, whereas other infants may demand a feeding more frequently.

Even if your infant has been on a 3-hour feeding routine, the rules may suddenly change; he or she may shorten the time between feedings. A parent should be prepared for some changes and unpredictability at feeding time during the first months of life.

Most breastfed infants are offered an opportunity to nurse for the first time shortly after birth. The breasts don't produce mature milk until the third day after birth. Closeness between mother and child is facilitated by breastfeeding, and the infant also gets the health benefits of the mother's colostrum, a rich lemon-colored breast liquid that is highly beneficial in protecting the baby against some diseases. In breastfeeding, frequent non-scheduled lengthy feeding sessions are important factors in establishing a good milk supply.

If you choose to breastfeed your infant, you should know that breast milk is easily and efficiently digested. Do not be surprised if initially you are feeding the baby quite often.

It is important for a nursing mother to feel at ease while breastfeeding. Make sure you are comfortable, either lying down or sitting in a comfortable chair, preferably one with an armrest. Support the baby with its face held close to your breast with one arm while the other hand supports the breast so the nipple is easily accessible to the infant's mouth.

Nursing time varies with babies. Most health care professionals recommend that you allow your baby to set the length and frequency of feedings. Most babies need 8 to 10 feedings daily in the first couple of months. Some babies may want to feed hourly. Allow your baby to finish feeding on one breast before you offer the other. There may also be periods of cluster ("bunch") feedings during which your baby may feed hourly for several hours.

Initially, a nursing mother may have tender nipples. Keep your nipples as dry as possible. Position your baby comfortably at your breast to prevent cracked nipples. If soreness persists, call your health care provider or lactation consultant.

Your diet is important to your general health and sense of well-being. While you breastfeed, you can expect to lose approximately 1 to 4 pounds monthly. Be wary of taking any medication unless approved by a physician. Avoid smoking, and consume only a minimal amount of alcohol, if any.

Most bottle-fed babies have their first feeding within 6 hours after delivery. A bottle-fed baby probably will need between six and nine feedings in a 24-hour period by the end of the first week of life.

The setting for bottle feeding is similar to that for breastfeeding. A bottle should never

Breastfeeding Versus Bottle-Feeding

Organizations concerned with children's health the world over agree—breastfeeding, whenever possible, is the preferred form of infant feeding. Science is proving more and more conclusively that breast milk promotes optimal health for babies. Breast milk provides the best nutrition for the baby's physical and intellectual growth. It reduces the risk of serious illness, upper respiratory infection, ear infection, diarrheal illness, and allergies. It also may offer protection from juvenile-onset diabetes, tooth decay, and high cholesterol.

If you breastfeed, offer your baby only breast milk for the first 4 to 6 months after birth. It's best to continue breastfeeding throughout the first year, if possible. If you cannot or choose not to breastfeed, your baby can be well nourished with bottle-feeding.

Breastfeeding offers some hidden emotional benefits: Hormones released during breastfeeding create a calming sensation for mother and baby alike. Breastfeeding continues the nurturing and comforting your body provided during pregnancy. In addition, there are health benefits for mom. The risk of breast cancer decreases. Breastfeeding may also offer protection against osteoporosis and premenopausal ovarian cancer.

Breastfeeding is cost-free and convenient, but information, guidance, support, and reassurance are essential at the start. New and improved breast pumps make going back to work or getting out convenient while continuing to provide mother's milk in your absence.

Although there are some clear advantages to breastfeeding, it is not an option for some women for medical reasons. Others choose not to breastfeed. In these cases, processed infant formula is an acceptable alternative to breast milk. Infrequently, health care providers may suggest a multivitamin preparation supplement that includes vitamin D, vitamin E, and fluoride for breastfeeding infants. Most formulas are prepared with adequate amounts of these nutrients.

As with breastfeeding, bottle-feeding requires guidance and support for the experience to be successful.

You may feel pressure to choose one or the other method of feeding your infant. Check your local public library for information and discuss any concerns you may have about either feeding method with your nurse, midwife, or physician. It is crucial that you feel confident in your decision so you may enlist the much-needed support of family and friends.

Feeding is an important experience for your baby, and fathers can play a significant role with either method you choose. If you are breastfeeding, your partner can show his support by bringing you water to drink while you are nursing, making sure you are comfortable, and reminding you that you are doing what is best for the baby. He can participate in burping or rocking the baby after the feeding. If you are bottle-feeding, he can take turns giving baby the bottle himself.

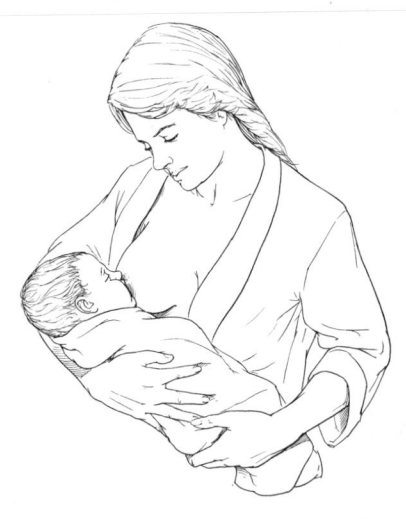

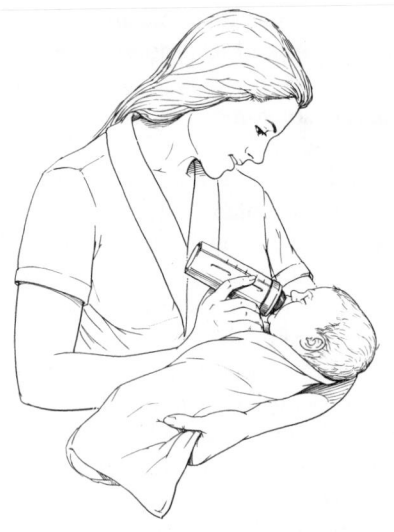

be propped up against the infant. Rather, the parent should take the time to hold the child closely during the feeding.

The formula should be warmed to body temperature, and the temperature tested by dropping a bit on your wrist. A word of caution: do not warm the bottle in a microwave oven. The formula can become very hot and severely burn your infant. A bottle-feeding may last from 5 to 25 minutes, depending on the eagerness and sucking ability of the infant.

Both bottle-fed and breastfed babies should be burped after a feeding.

Feeding Concerns

The newborn period can be challenging in terms of feeding your infant. Maybe your infant simply will not eat—or at least not as much as you want him or her to. Perhaps the baby falls asleep in the middle of a feeding and then wakes up an hour later crying to be fed. Sometimes the baby may savor a feeding and at other times he or she may rapidly finish.

Some common feeding problems are described here.

An Infant Who Does Not Seem to Eat Enough

Your baby may, in fact, be eating plenty. The average 2-week-old newborn takes between 2 and 3 ounces per feeding. By 3 or 4 weeks, your baby usually has increased the amount to between 4 and 5 ounces. Although nursing mothers cannot measure the amount their babies are consuming, they can follow their babies' cues as to when to feed. If a baby seems content, he or she is probably feeding adequately.

Do not expect your infant to eat the same amount every day at every feeding. Babies are like everyone else. They are hungrier on some days than others. You can usually trust your infant to know how much to eat. Do not force food on the infant, or feeding problems may result later.

If your infant is gaining weight, most likely he or she is eating enough. (If you notice a loss of weight or a lack of weight gain, see Failure to Gain Weight, page 14.)

An Infant Who Falls Asleep During a Feeding and Wakes Up Crying Before It Is Time for the Next Feeding

Your baby may be hungry or simply need to be burped. If your baby's intake was just a little under the usual amount, the problem is probably not hunger but an abdominal upset. Many physicians advise trying to let the baby go back to sleep without an additional feeding. If that does not work, offer the breast or bottle again.

An Infant Who Is Underfed

If underfed, your baby may be restless and unhappy, cry a lot, be constipated and unable to sleep, or fail to gain weight. This infant may be emptying the bottle or breast and still may not be getting enough.

The problem may be solved by simply increasing the number of feedings per day, enlarging the size of the nipple holes in the bottle so the infant gets more milk with every suck, or trying a different type of nipple.

Bottle Care

Remember the stories of your mother boiling all the utensils that a baby would use? Today, that is thought unnecessary.

The tap water in most communities is safe and bacteria-free. Bottles, nipples, caps, and baby's other feeding equipment can be washed with soap and hot tap water, rinsed in hot water, and allowed to air dry. They also can be run through a dishwasher.

Once milk is in a nursing bottle, it should not be stored for more than a few hours, and then only in the refrigerator. Discard milk in half-empty bottles.

Breastfed babies who are not gaining weight adequately need to be offered more frequent feedings. Also, be sure your baby is positioned properly and sucking effectively. Allow your baby to remain at your breast long enough to obtain the high fat content of the milk near the end of each feeding.

An Infant Who Is Overfed

When overfed, your baby may spit up or seem uncomfortable. Generally, following baby's cues will avoid overfeeding. Sometimes, however, an infant will respond to a well-intentioned parent's efforts to encourage eating by taking in more than he or she needs.

An Infant Who Spits Up After a Feeding

Many babies spit up or even vomit after a feeding. Spitting up is normal, but vomiting is not and may indicate a serious problem (see Vomiting and Spitting Up, page 12). Spitting up can be reduced by burping the infant after every feeding or noting which positions seem to help your baby keep his or her milk down after a feeding.

Loose Stools

Loose stools are the norm for breastfed infants. If the mother uses laxatives or eats food with laxative properties, the baby's stools may become even looser. Bottle-fed babies generally have firmer stools than do breastfed babies.

Diarrhea will generally not be a problem for breastfed babies who thoroughly finish feeding on one breast before they are offered the other breast.

Constipation

You should not be concerned if your baby misses a bowel movement or even goes for days without having one. The consistency of the stool indicates constipation, not the frequency of bowel movements. A baby who passes hard, pellet-like stools is constipated.

If your infant becomes constipated, it may be due to an inadequate food or fluid intake. Constipation rarely occurs in breastfed infants but if it does, try giving more frequent feedings. For bottle-fed infants, increasing the amount of sugar or fluid in the formula should alleviate the problem (see page 215). Iron in your infant's formula does not cause constipation.

If the constipation is present from birth, your baby's health care provider will want to examine the infant's rectum to make sure there is no obstruction or congenital abnormality.

An Infant Who Fails to Gain Weight

Failure of your baby to gain weight is cause for concern. The average baby gains 2 pounds a month. Your infant may gain more or less. If your infant is not gaining weight at all or is losing weight, your pediatrician or family physician may want to try another formula if you are bottle-feeding. If you are breastfeeding, your health care provider or lactation consultant can assess a feeding session and recommend appropriate measures.

Your infant's rate of growth may simply be slower than average. However, if the baby seems hungry all the time, slow growth may be an indication that your infant is not getting enough to eat and some feeding modifications should be made.

Genetics and Genetic Disorders

Will it be a boy or a girl? Will the child be healthy or have a birth defect or genetic disorder? Will the child have blue or brown eyes, be short or tall, be chubby or thin?

The answers to these questions are determined by the interaction of the genes (the biologic units of heredity) with the social and physical environments in which the child develops.

Genetics is the study of heredity. It is concerned primarily with the study of the origin of the characteristics of the individual and their transmission to offspring. Medical genetics is the branch of human genetics concerned with the relationship between heredity and diseases.

At conception, the mother's egg (ovum) is joined with the father's sperm. The ovum and sperm, called germ cells, each contain 23 chromosomes. During the process of fertilization, the union of sperm and egg produces an individual with 46 chromosomes. This means that, normally, an individual has two copies of each gene, one from the mother and one from the father.

Each chromosome contains many genes. The genes determine many of your offspring's characteristics, which are passed from one generation to another. Usually this occurs uneventfully. Sometimes, however, unexpected changes, or genetic defects, occur. Although most causes of genetic disorders in humans are largely unknown, various environmental agents, such as radiation, viruses, and chemicals, are among the factors that have been identified.

The three basic categories of genetic disorders are the single mutant gene, abnormalities of the chromosomes, and multifactorial disorders:

A single mutant gene is one discrete unit of genetic material that is altered. A disorder caused by the transmission of a single altered gene shows one of three simple patterns of inheritance: 1) autosomal dominant, 2) autosomal recessive, or 3) X-linked.

The term autosomal is applied to a gene that is present in any chromosome other than a sex chromosome, and the term dominant applies to a gene that produces a recognizable condition if passed to the offspring from one parent. The risk of passing an autosomal dominant altered gene to an offspring is 50 percent. The term recessive refers to a gene that does not produce a clinical effect unless both members of the gene pair are altered. Thus, a disease with autosomal recessive inheritance occurs only if an altered gene is received from both parents, who are "silent" carriers of one abnormal gene. The risk of passing an autosomal recessive altered gene to an offspring is 25 percent. Conditions such as cystic fibrosis, sickle-cell anemia, phenylketonuria, and color blindness are caused by alterations of single genes.

The genes responsible for X-linked disorders are located on the X chromosome. The female has two X chromosomes, and the male has only one X chromosome. An important feature of all X-linked inheritance is the absence of transmission of the trait from male to male (that is, father to son). An X-linked trait cannot be transmitted from father to son because the father's Y chromosome, and never the X chromosome, is transmitted to his son. Alternatively, the male's X chromosome always is passed to a daughter.

Chromosome abnormalities result from the lack, excess, or abnormal arrangement of one or more chromosomes, which may produce either an excess or a deficiency in genetic material. Birth defects caused by abnormalities of the chromosomes occur in about 1 in 250 newborns. Moreover, in about 50 to 60 percent of early miscarriages, the fetus has a chromosome abnormality.

Multifactorial inheritance is the process whereby genes interact with environmental factors to produce a congenital defect or disorder. No one knows how many genes are involved. Some researchers believe that the genes are harmless under normal circumstances. However, in combination with certain environmental factors, these genes can cause abnormalities in the developing baby. Some of these environmental factors include drugs ingested by the mother during pregnancy, alcohol, and maternal diseases such as diabetes. In most cases, the external agents are not known.

Many of the common chronic diseases of adults (such as essential hypertension, coronary artery disease, diabetes mellitus, peptic ulcer disease, and schizophrenia) and many of the common birth defects (such as cleft lip and palate, spina bifida, and congenital heart disease) long have been known to run in families. These fit best into the category of multifactorial diseases.

Most of the common birth defects usually have a relatively small risk of recurrence— about 3 to 5 percent. However, in some families the risk could be much higher. Disorders caused by single mutant genes tend to have a much higher risk of recurrence—25 to 50 percent—but in some cases the risk could be almost 0. After carefully analyzing the family history and the nature of the birth defect or genetic disease, a medical geneticist usually can give the parents a fairly precise estimate of the risk of recurrence. A medical geneticist is a specialist in genetic or inherited disorders. Laboratory tests might be used to determine whether a parent is a carrier of an abnormal gene or chromosome.

Sometimes the mother of a child born with a birth defect may wonder, for example, whether medication she took during pregnancy was responsible. Some medicines are known to cause defects; others are thought to be safe. In general, it is best to avoid any unnecessary drugs during pregnancy, particularly during the first 3 months. Sometimes, however, the medicine is necessary because, if untreated, the mother's illness itself would be more harmful to the developing baby than the medication prescribed.

In most cases, birth defects are not the result of something you did or didn't do in pregnancy. If you find yourself feeling guilty about your baby's condition, professional counseling can help you to deal with your concerns.

The Family History

A genetic evaluation can be very helpful if your child is born with a birth defect or inherited condition. The goal of such an evaluation would be to define a diagnosis so that accurate information can be provided on the child's medical needs and prognosis.

Genetic evaluations also are useful for family planning, especially for couples who already have had a child with a birth defect or genetic disorder or who have a family history of these conditions. Such couples often are unsure whether they should have a baby. Sometimes the couple has no family history of birth defects but, because of the relatively advanced age of one or both of them, they might seek information about diagnostic tests that are available for the detection of possible defects in unborn babies. This is important because some genetic disorders can be treated.

A complete family medical history will be taken of a child born with a genetic condition, or of a couple who is concerned about future children. Information will be obtained on all members of the immediate family including siblings, parents, aunts, uncles, cousins, and grandparents. This information includes the given name, surname, maiden name, birth date or current age, age at death, cause of death, and name or description of any disease, birth defect, or medical condition. Questions may include the following:

1. Does any relative have an identical or similar trait to the person being evaluated?

2. Does anyone in the extended family have a different birth defect, trait, or medical condition that is not seen in the person being evaluated? Answers to these questions give the medical geneticist knowledge about the possible pattern of signs and symptoms of a given condition within a family.

3. Does any relative have a condition that is recognized to be inherited?

4. Does any relative have an unusual condition or trait, or has any relative died of a rare condition?

5. Are any blood relatives married to each other?

6. What is the ethnic or national origin of the family? Persons of certain ethnic origins have increased chances of specific genetic diseases, such as sickle-cell disease in African-Americans, cystic fibrosis in persons of northern European descent, and Tay-Sachs disease in Ashkenazi Jews.

Establishing a cause for a genetic condition can be a long process. Sometimes additional information, testing, and medical records may be required. In the case of a preconception genetics evaluation, once you have information about the medical condition and its chances of being transmitted to your child, you can decide whether to attempt pregnancy. If the genetics evaluation was performed after your child was born with an inherited condition, you will be able to learn more about available treatment.

The following pages discuss several genetic disorders.

Down Syndrome

Down syndrome is a condition caused by the presence of extra genetic material from the number 21 chromosome (usually three chromosomes instead of two). An estimated 1 in 600 to 800 infants is born with Down syndrome.

A woman's chances of giving birth to a child with Down syndrome increase with age. For example, the chance of having a baby with this syndrome is 1 in 1,250 for a 25-year-old woman but is 1 in 378 at age 35 and 1 in 30 at age 45.

An infant born with Down syndrome may or may not have a number of distinctive characteristics such as a small head, short neck, transverse palmar crease on the hands, and epicanthal folds (folds of skin over the inner corner of the eyes that sometimes give the eyes a slanted appearance).

Infants born with Down syndrome may be of average size, but typically they grow slowly and remain small. They have developmental delays that range from mild to severe and an increased risk of congenital heart defects and gastrointestinal problems.

The mortality rate during the first year is higher than that for other babies. Babies with Down syndrome may be at increased risk for development of respiratory infections, vision impairment, cardiac problems, or leukemia.

There is no treatment for Down syndrome. Heart or other associated conditions often can be repaired successfully with surgery. Many children with Down syndrome are happy, affectionate, and easygoing. Many live with loving families, go to school, learn to read and write, perform at various levels of jobs as adults, and can live independent or semi-independent lives.

Changes in the Hands and Feet

Hands

Congenital Absence of a Part or All of the Upper Extremities
This condition is more common than absence of a part of the lower extremities. A child may be born with only part of one finger missing, or an entire arm may be absent.

A newborn with only one hand should be examined by a physician who is skilled in the care of this condition. Once the baby is able to sit, a prosthesis, usually a simple paddle, can be fitted to allow the child to develop balanced ability to use both arms. If a prosthesis is not fitted early, the child develops one-handed patterns that are nearly impossible to break.

Polydactyly

Polydactyly is the presence of an extra finger or fingers, most commonly a fifth finger or extra thumb. This defect is more common in African-American newborns. Frequently, the extra digit consists of skin and soft tissue and can be removed easily. However, if the extra finger contains bone or cartilage, removal may require surgery on adjacent structures, which can best be performed after the infant is a few months old.

Syndactyly of the Fingers

Syndactyly (webbing) of the fingers is best treated surgically. Because the bones in the fingers are of various lengths, the joints of the fused fingers do not line up and the fingers are difficult to use. If surgery is not performed, the child will probably not acquire significant use of the fingers.

Camptodactyly

Camptodactyly is the permanent flexion of one or more fingers. This is usually congenital and most often affects the little finger.

Clubhand

Clubhand is the rare absence of the radius (the bone on the thumb side of the forearm) or the ulna (the larger bone, on the opposite side of the forearm). Treatment includes stretching the soft tissues of the arm during infancy. An operation is then necessary to reposition the bone. However, retaining the new position is a problem. Several operations during childhood may be necessary.

Children with this condition often have a higher incidence of cardiac disease and blood problems.

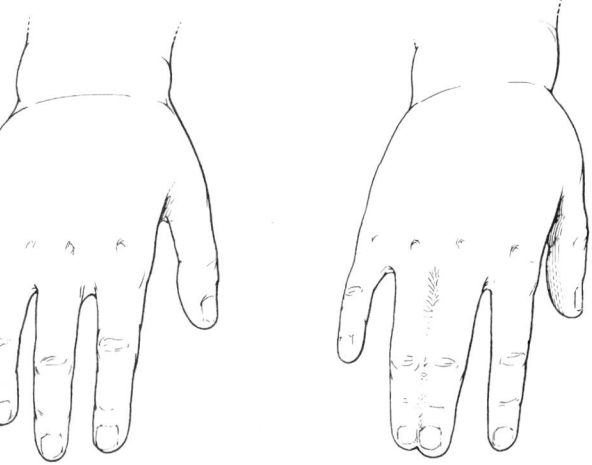

Feet

The newborn's feet are proportionately longer and thinner than those of the older child, and the joints of the ankle and foot are extremely flexible. Although the feet often may appear to be in abnormal positions, there is rarely cause for concern because these minor problems resolve in time.

In-Toeing and Out-Toeing

These are common problems in which the foot or leg turns inward or outward. The condition is aggravated when the infant sleeps face down. They are usually positional or postural deformities that correct spontaneously with growth and development. They rarely require treatment.

Syndactyly of the Toes

Webbing of the toes is rarely more than a cosmetic problem. The scars and distortions of

Both polydactyly (a congenital deformity of the hand in which the newborn has an extra finger) and syndactyly (webbing of the fingers) can be effectively treated surgically.

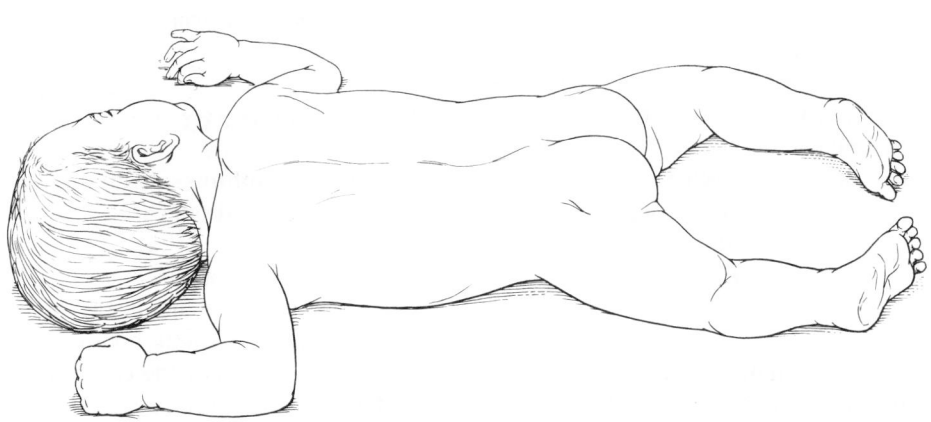

Your baby's feet may occasionally seem to be in an abnormal position, perhaps in-toeing, as shown here. This common, minor concern rarely requires treatment.

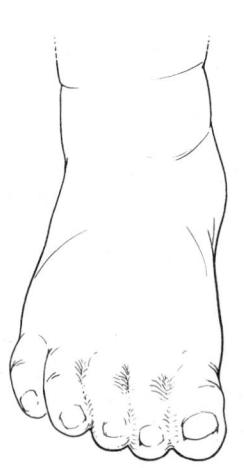 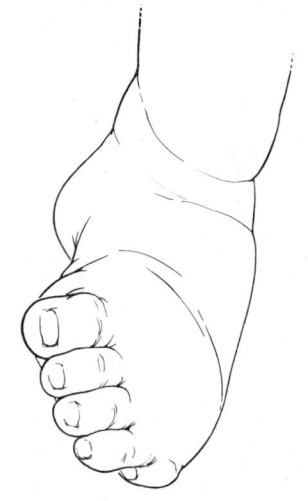

Syndactyly (webbing of the toes) is rarely more than a cosmetic problem, requiring no treatment. In contrast, clubfoot (in which the foot is twisted out of shape or position) requires therapy soon after birth.

surgery may be more unsightly than the webbed toes. In contrast to webbed fingers, webbed toes usually function normally.

Clubfoot

Clubfoot occurs in 1 of every 1,000 births. The term is used to describe several congenital foot abnormalities in which the foot is twisted out of shape or position. This condition is not caused by the position of the fetus inside the uterus. In about 95 percent of cases of clubfoot, the forefoot is twisted downward and inward, the arch is increased, and the heel is turned inward.

Early treatment is essential and is initiated soon after birth. The feet are manipulated to the normal position and then held there by casts or adhesive tape. This process is typically repeated every few days during the first 2 weeks of treatment and then at 1- to 2-week intervals. If this method is successful, corrective shoes may then maintain this position. If this method does not correct the problem, an operation, usually between 4 and 18 months of age, may be necessary.

Although the position of the corrected clubfoot may look relatively correct, the foot will never have completely normal contours, and the calf on the affected leg is often thinner than that on the normal leg. Orthopedic care throughout childhood is necessary for children born with clubfoot.

Extra Toes

Extra toes can make it difficult to fit shoes and thus they often are surgically removed. However, the operation should not be performed until the structures are large enough to be easily operated on, yet it should be done before the child begins to walk and wear shoes.

Congenital Disorders of the Skeleton

Developmental Dysplasia of the Hip (Congenital Hip Dislocation)

This disorder is the result of hampered development of the hip joint. The problem may be detected during the initial examination at birth or later.

The newborn with developmental dysplasia of the hip is fitted with a brace or splint-like device to position the head of the thighbone (femur) in the hip socket (acetabulum). This treatment is often successful within 6 to 8 weeks. Most developmental dysplasias of the hip that are diagnosed during the newborn period can be treated adequately in this manner.

Dwarfism (Dysplasia)

Dwarfism indicates several skeletal abnormalities, most of which have disproportionate lengths of limbs and trunk. Usually, the child's limbs are short initially. As the child grows, the trunk is also disproportionately short. Most dysplasias are not detected during the newborn period. These children may have other congenital problems such as hearing impairment, kidney problems, and immune deficiencies. There is no cure for the actual skeletal disorder, but many of the accompanying problems can be treated.

Treatment involves a combination of orthopedic techniques to maximize the child's mobility and function and to correct malformations of the limbs and spine. Emotional support and psychological and genetic counseling are often beneficial.

Pectus Excavatum

Signs and Symptoms—An indentation of the sternum (breastbone)

Pectus excavatum, also referred to as funnel chest, is a major indentation of the sternum. The lower part of the bone is depressed toward the spine, and the chest has a funneled or hollow appearance.

This is usually a congenital problem, although rarely it is caused by rickets or a chronic airway obstruction. In the latter case,

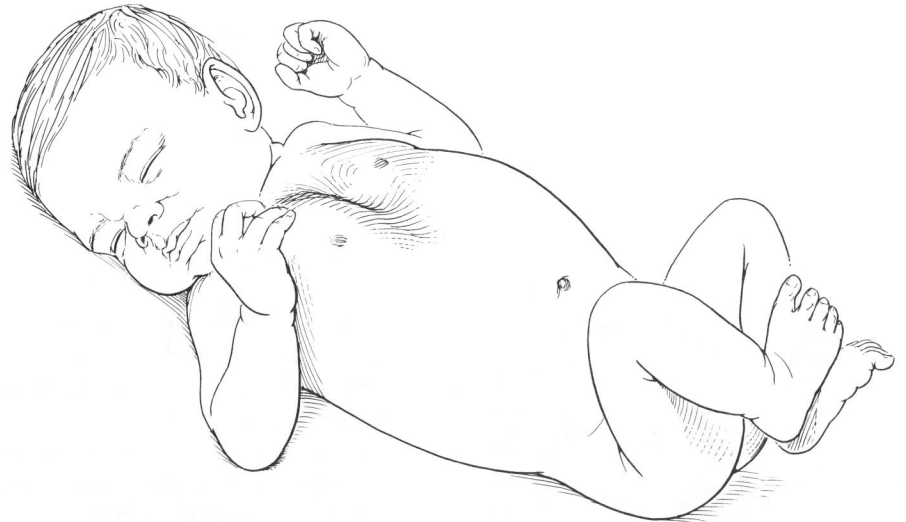

Pectus excavatum, a congenital indentation of the chest, usually will not interfere with breathing.

successful treatment of the obstruction sometimes results in the disappearance of the indentation.

Babies and children with pectus excavatum usually have normal respiratory function. Only rarely is heart function adversely affected. Some inherited muscle diseases also are associated with the finding. This condition tends to run in families.

Treatment
Surgery is usually not recommended for most children with pectus excavatum. However, in severe cases, an operation may be performed later in childhood or adolescence for cosmetic reasons.

Conditions Affecting the Genitals

Boys
The scrotum in the newborn boy is relatively large. The size can be increased by the trauma of a breech birth. In addition, an African-American newborn's scrotum usually is dark before the rest of the skin attains its dark color.

It is common for a newborn boy to have erections. If you cannot fully pull back the foreskin of your newborn's penis, do not be concerned. The skin is normally attached to the end of the penis in a newborn and should never be forced back.

None of these characteristics is cause for alarm. However, disorders of the male genitals are not uncommon, and some require treatment.

Phimosis
Phimosis is a tightness of the foreskin that results in the inability to pull back the fold of skin that covers the uncircumcised penis. It can be congenital or the result of inflammation. Sometimes this requires circumcision.

Paraphimosis
Paraphimosis occurs when the foreskin of the uncircumcised penis is retracted too much and cannot be brought back over the end. This can cause severe and painful swelling. When discovered early, the condition can be treated by gentle but firm pressure applied to the end of the penis to reduce the swelling and to allow the foreskin to be brought back. Sometimes circumcision is required.

Undescended Testicle
Undescended testicle is the absence at birth of one or both testicles from the scrotum. The testicle may be misplaced within the abdomen

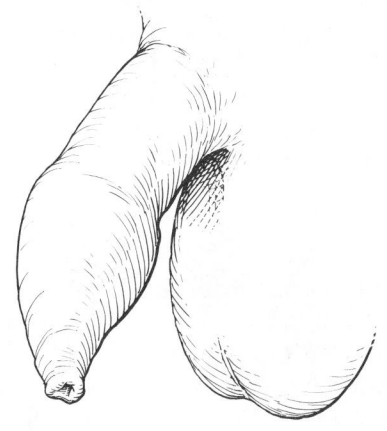

Phimosis is a tightness of the foreskin resulting in an inability to pull back the fold of skin that covers the tip of the uncircumcised penis.

If one or both testicles fail to travel from the abdomen to the scrotum, the condition is termed "undescended testicle" and may require surgery.

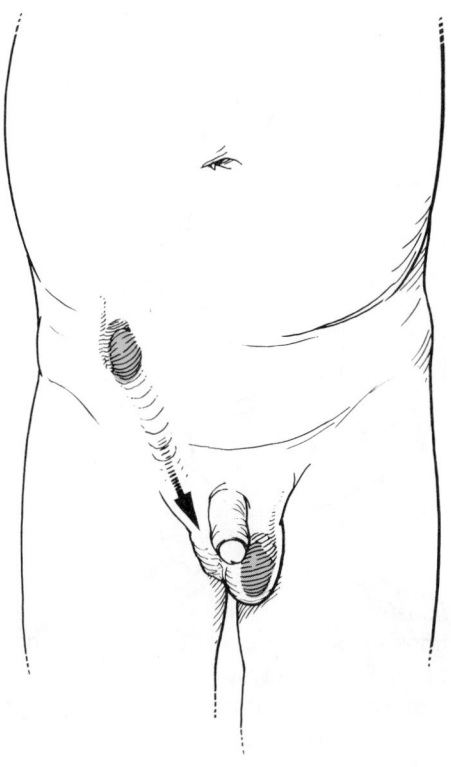

or be absent altogether. The latter condition is rare and usually occurs in a child born with ambiguous sex characteristics (see Ambiguous Genitals, page 49).

Two months before birth, the testicles normally descend from an area near the kidney through a small opening in the abdominal muscles into their normal position in the scrotum. In about 1 of 30 full-term newborns, they do not descend. The incidence of undescended testicles is up to 17 percent in premature infants and up to 100 percent in infants weighing less than 2 pounds, because

Hypospadias is a condition in which the urethral opening is not located at its normal position at the end of the penis. Surgery can correct this congenital defect.

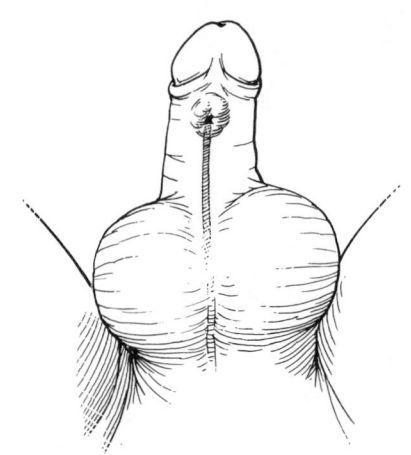

the testicles do not descend until after the seventh month of gestation.

In up to 30 percent of cases, both testicles are affected.

Sometimes hormones are given to bring the undescended testicle into place. If it has not descended by the child's first birthday, however, it will not do so spontaneously, and the condition should be treated surgically at 12 to 15 months of age. Surgery also is important because often the boy with an undescended testicle also has a hernia due to the failure of the opening in the abdominal muscles to close properly. In such cases, the intestines may slip through the muscle opening and become trapped. The operation can be done on an outpatient basis. Occasionally a testicle has shrunk or atrophied so severely that removal is indicated.

When left untreated, undescended testicles may lead to infertility in adulthood.

A boy born with an undescended testicle has a risk of testicular cancer, generally when he is in his 20s or 30s. Correction does not reduce the risk, but it does allow for better examination and earlier detection should a tumor develop (see Undescended Testicle, page 1202).

Hypospadias
Hypospadias occurs in approximately 1 of 500 newborns. In this congenital defect, the urethral opening is not in its normal position at the end of the penis. In its mildest form, the opening is just on the underside of the glans. In its most severe form, it may be as far away as the scrotum. Ten percent of boys born with hypospadias also have undescended testicles.

The more severe the degree of hypospadias, the more curved the penis. This curving of the penis is called chordee.

Hypospadias is treated surgically. Circumcision should not be done because the foreskin is needed for the surgical repair. If the case is mild, the main reason for surgery is cosmetic. The more severe the condition, the greater the need for surgery because of urination problems—the child will not be able to stand to urinate—and inability to function sexually later. The psychological consequences of having malformed genitals also are a factor in the consideration of surgery.

When should the operation be performed? The current thinking is the earlier, the better. Many pediatric urologists believe the ideal age is during the first year, certainly before the child is toilet-trained.

A single surgical procedure is generally all that is necessary to bring the opening closer to the tip of the penis and also to straighten the penis.

Hydrocele

A hydrocele is the accumulation of fluid in a structure of the testicle called the tunica vaginalis. This problem is common in newborn boys. If the testicle can be examined easily and the amount of fluid remains constant, treatment is unnecessary. Small hydroceles usually disappear during the first year. However, if the sac changes size during the day, it may mean there is direct contact with the abdominal cavity. This is a hernia and requires surgery.

Girls

Hormonal changes in the mother before birth often may cause changes in the breasts and genitals of her newborn daughter (described below). Although these changes may be disturbing to the new parent, they are normal and temporary and require no treatment.

Enlarged Clitoris

The clitoris of the newborn girl is often enlarged, especially in premature babies, as a result of hormonal changes that affect the genital area. The size decreases shortly after birth. If the clitoris seems unusually large, tests may be indicated to confirm the child's sex (see Ambiguous Genitals, this page).

Vaginal Discharge

Vaginal discharge sometimes occurs in the newborn. During the first 3 weeks, many mothers notice a thick, white discharge from the baby's vagina. The discharge is the result of normal hormonal changes that took place in the mother before she gave birth. Treatment is unnecessary.

Vaginal Bleeding

Vaginal bleeding is sometimes the newborn girl's response to the absence of the maternal hormone estrogen after birth. This manifests as a few drops of blood shed from the vagina. Parents understandably are shocked to find blood in the diaper. Again, this is a temporary condition. The baby is not hemorrhaging or starting to menstruate, as some anxious parents at first suspect.

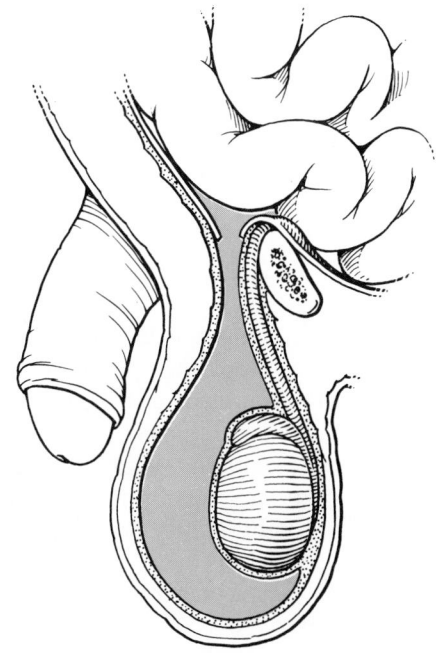

A common problem in newborns is an accumulation of fluid near the testicles, called a hydrocele.

Ambiguous Genitals

Ambiguous genitals refer to the uncertain appearance of the baby's external sexual features. Sometimes a female who has been exposed to an excess of male hormones in the womb is born with ovaries but male-like genitals (female pseudohermaphroditism). A male may be born with testicles but with ambiguous or completely female genitals (male pseudohermaphroditism). Some newborns have both ovaries and testicles and ambiguous genitals (true hermaphroditism).

The numerous causes of ambiguous genitals include tumors, chromosome abnormalities, and hormone excesses or deficiencies.

Treatment

When a newborn's sex is in question, a specialist in hormonal problems of infancy should be consulted promptly. Only after thorough testing and evaluation can a correct diagnosis be established and the correct assignment of sex be made. This is a serious problem with a significant impact on future life and emotional health. Hormones may be given to males to increase the size of the penis. Reconstructive procedures can also be done.

Supernumerary Nipples

Rarely, an infant is born with one or more extra nipples. The nipples may occur with or without breast tissue. Sometimes the nipple

Enlarged Breasts in the Newborn

Enlarged breasts sometimes occur in girls or boys during the first 2 weeks of life because of the large amounts of circulating hormones that reach the baby through the umbilical cord. Breast enlargement usually disappears in the first few months and is no cause for alarm.

does not have an areola (the darker pigment that surrounds a nipple). Supernumerary nipples usually are located in the breast area.

An estimated 1 to 2 percent of North Americans have supernumerary nipples. The condition occurs equally in men and women. The condition may be associated with urinary problems.

If your newborn has supernumerary nipples, they can be removed for cosmetic purposes. The nipples rarely present a medical problem, although they can respond to hormonal changes that occur during puberty, menstruation, and pregnancy. When this happens, the supernumerary nipple may enlarge and become painful. The presence of a third breast also can be emotionally traumatic. Moreover, a supernumerary nipple is at the same risk as a normal nipple of developing breast disorders such as mastitis, abscesses, and cancer.

An infant also can be born with absence of a breast or nipple. Sometimes the muscle underlying the breast also has failed to develop. When this occurs, nothing should be done during infancy or early childhood.

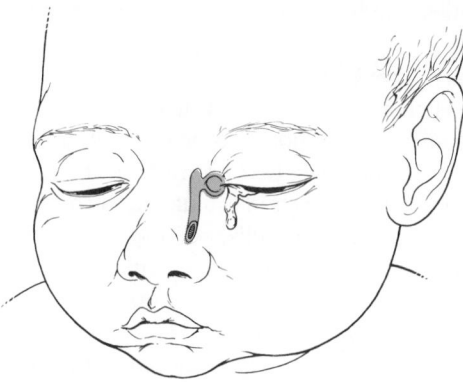

Persisting tears or a white or yellow discharge on the cheek of your infant may indicate an obstruction of the nasolacrimal duct. This can persist for several months. Your physician might prescribe an antibiotic to help prevent infection. Most often, cleansing your infant's eyelid with warm water and massaging the area will suffice.

However, an operation can be performed for cosmetic reasons when the child reaches puberty.

Epstein Pearls

Eighty percent of newborns have Epstein pearls, which are small white cysts on the palate. These cysts are cells that were trapped during the formation of the palate. Similar cysts also may form on the gums, leading parents to suspect the child has a tooth. Epstein pearls are painless, require no treatment, and disappear within a few weeks.

Supernumerary Teeth

Most infants are born toothless. Sometimes, however, a tooth can be observed in the newborn's mouth, usually in the lower front gum. It generally falls out before the infant starts teething. If they persist, supernumerary teeth can interfere with the position and eruption of adjacent teeth.

An X-ray should be obtained to determine that the tooth is supernumerary and not a natal tooth, which is a prematurely erupted primary (baby) tooth.

Congenital Obstruction of the Nasolacrimal Duct

Congenital obstruction of the nasolacrimal duct results from incomplete development of the tear drainage system.

Normally, tears and secretions from the eye drain from the tear ducts, which lead from two small openings at the inner corner of the eyelids, first toward the nose and then down into the nasal cavity. If this drainage system is partially or completely obstructed, the tears are not drained from the eyes.

This problem usually becomes apparent within the first days or weeks after birth. A cold or exposure to wind or low temperature often aggravates the problem. The first sign a parent typically notices is the presence of tears in the baby's eyes. This can range from what appears to be a pool of tears to tears spilling onto the baby's cheeks. There also may be some white or yellow discharge in the corners of the eyes and some crusting that glues the eyes shut during the baby's sleep periods.

Sometimes infants with nasolacrimal duct obstruction develop inflammation in the duct area. The area under the eye may become swollen, red, and tender. The baby also may have a fever and be irritable.

This is a fairly common condition and rarely harms the eye, even when it persists for several months. The main treatment involves cleansing the infant's lids with warm water and massaging the area between the infant's nose and the affected eye two or three times a day. Antibacterial drops or ointment are sometimes used to prevent infection.

In most cases, this is the only treatment that is needed, and the problem usually resolves in the first few months. Occasionally, it persists throughout the first year, and the physician may need to surgically dilate the duct. Rarely, insertion of tubes or a reconstructive operation is necessary.

Cleft Lip and Cleft Palate

Cleft lip and cleft palate are separate birth defects that may occur together. The incidence of cleft lip with or without cleft palate is 1 per 1,000 births; the incidence of cleft palate alone is 1 in 2,500 births. Genetics seem to be more of a factor in cleft lip with or without cleft palate than in cleft palate alone.

An infant born with a cleft malformation, especially if it is a cleft palate alone, has a higher incidence of other problems, including hearing impairment.

An infant born with a cleft lip has a fissure or elongated opening where the upper lip failed to fuse. This can vary from a small notch at the top of the lip to a complete separation extending to the nose. If the palate is also cleft, the roof of the baby's mouth has failed to close.

If your infant is born with either or both conditions, the most immediate problem is feeding. Soon after birth, a specially designed obturator (prosthesis) can be fitted over the palate so that the baby can be fed. However,

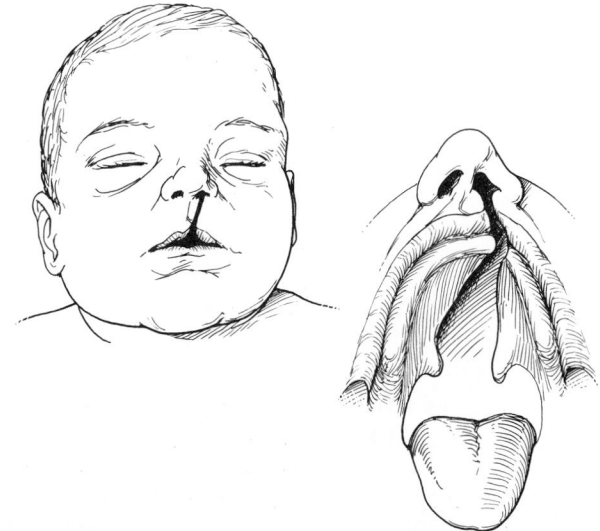

because the infant will be growing rapidly, this will have to be replaced every few weeks.

A baby with a cleft lip typically has an operation to close the lip at 1 or 2 months of age. Frequently, nasal widening is associated with cleft lip deformities. Closure of the cleft lip helps to narrow the nasal base. A definitive nasal operation, however, usually is deferred until the child has reached adolescence. The cosmetic results depend on the severity of the malformation, the absence of infection, and the surgeon's skill.

A cleft palate generally is closed within the first year of life to enhance normal speech development. The goals of surgery are to make it possible for the child to speak in a normal voice and to reduce nasal regurgitation. If a child does not have the operation by age 3 years, a prosthesis may be used to help the child develop intelligible speech.

Complications of cleft lip or palate include recurring ear infections, hearing loss, an excessive number of dental cavities, and displacement of the teeth, which requires orthodontic correction. Some children continue to have speech defects even after surgery because of muscle problems in the palate. Speech therapy often is required (see page 132).

Failure of the lip to fuse together results in a condition called cleft lip. When the roof of the mouth also has failed to close, this is termed a cleft palate. These conditions require surgical correction.

Congenital Heart Disorders

Approximately 1 of every 125 newborns has a congenital heart disorder. These defects range from mild to severe. One of every 500 babies shows the first signs of a heart disorder during the first year of life.

The precise cause of a congenital heart disorder is rarely found, although a combination of genetic and environmental factors (multifactorial inheritance) usually seems to be responsible (see page 43). Some chromosome abnormalities, such as the one that causes Down syndrome, also are associated with heart defects. Infections such as German measles, contracted by the mother during the first 2 months of pregnancy, also increase the risk of congenital heart defects.

With recent advances in heart surgery, many of these heart disorders can be treated successfully. Some of the common congenital heart disorders are described.

Ventricular Septal Defect (VSD)

Ventricular septal defect (VSD) is the most common heart malformation, accounting for 25 percent of the cases of congenital heart disease. The infant born with this condition has an opening between the lower chambers (ventricles) of its heart so that there is an increased blood flow under high pressure to the lungs.

The symptoms of VSD vary depending on the size of the defect. The problem may be discovered during a routine physical examination when the physician may detect a slight murmur. Babies born with large defects develop pulmonary hypertension, feeding difficulties, profuse perspiration, poor growth rates, recurrent pulmonary infections, and cardiac failure in early infancy.

Treatment depends on the size of the defect. Approximately 30 to 50 percent of small defects close spontaneously during the first year of life. Many children have no symptoms and no apparent heart damage.

Treatment for infants with symptoms of VSD is aimed at controlling the heart failure with medications. If this is unsuccessful, an operation to close the defect should be done before the baby is 1 year old.

Atrial Septal Defect (ASD)

Atrial septal defect (ASD) is an opening high in the heart between the upper chambers (atria), which produces abnormal blood flow. ASD is more common in female infants than in males, and it often occurs in children with Down syndrome.

The affected children frequently have no symptoms.

Surgical closure is the recommended treatment, usually at around 4 years of age.

Patent Ductus Arteriosus

The ductus arteriosus is a vessel that leads from the pulmonary artery to the aorta. Normally, this closes immediately after birth. When it does not, blood flows between the pulmonary artery and the aorta. This condition is called patent ductus arteriosus.

In babies who are born prematurely, the ductus is less apt to close spontaneously. In a full-term infant, failure to close is a congenital malformation.

Patent ductus arteriosus occurs more often in female infants, in babies born at high altitude, and in the offspring of women who had German measles (rubella) during the first 3 months of pregnancy.

If the ductus is small, there are often no symptoms. A large ductus will produce a heart murmur, pulmonary hypertension, and growth retardation.

In the premature infant, the ductus often closes spontaneously within weeks or months. In the full-term infant or the premature infant whose ductus fails to close, surgery is necessary, usually between the first and second years of life.

Coarctation of the Aorta

Coarctation (constriction) of the aorta results in increased blood pressure above the obstruction. There are no symptoms initially. However, heart failure may develop because of other associated heart abnormalities.

In the absence of symptoms, significant obstructions should be surgically relieved before 6 years of age to help prevent future complications.

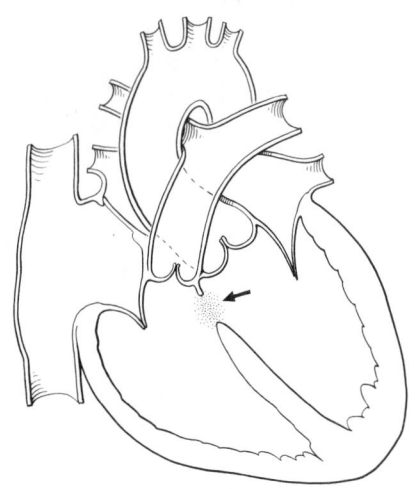

An unwanted opening between two of the chambers of the heart—ventricular septal defect (arrow)—allows blood to flow under high pressure to the lungs. In many cases, the defect resolves itself, but in some instances, surgical correction is required.

Tetralogy of Fallot

Tetralogy of Fallot consists of a large ventricular septal defect (see page 52), obstruction of blood flow from the heart's right ventricle to the lung (pulmonary) arteries, and a shift of the aorta to the right side of the heart. The right ventricle also is enlarged. The result is decreased blood flow to the lungs.

The main symptom of this disorder is a bluish cast to the skin (cyanosis), although this may not always be present at birth.

The symptoms of tetralogy of Fallot often begin slowly during the first year of life. Sometimes, however, the problem is apparent at birth.

Treatment is geared toward providing an immediate increase in pulmonary blood flow. A heart operation is the usual treatment once your child is past infancy. However, occasionally an operation is performed during infancy to improve blood flow to the lung and to decrease cyanosis.

Pulmonary Stenosis

Pulmonary stenosis is an obstruction of blood flow from the heart to the pulmonary artery.

With mild or moderate obstruction, there are often no symptoms. The newborn with a severe obstruction has a bluish cast to the skin and shows signs of heart failure.

Congestive heart failure (see page 659) occurs in severe cases during the first month of life.

Children with mild to moderate stenosis can lead a healthy life, but they should be under the regular care of a physician. Those with more severe stenosis require a procedure to open the valve.

Aortic Stenosis

Aortic stenosis is a narrowing of the valve through which blood leaves the heart to enter the aorta. Aortic stenosis is more common in male infants and accounts for 5 percent of heart malformations.

Severe stenosis generally is detected in early infancy. However, most children have no symptoms, and the problem is found during a routine examination when the physician hears a heart murmur.

Surgery is needed to treat severe stenosis. Children with mild or moderate obstruction should remain under medical care because of the possibility of the obstruction increasing in severity.

Transposition of the Great Vessels

Transposition of the great vessels is a complex condition in which the two arteries arising from the heart are reversed. Blood returning to the heart from the body is pumped back to the body without passage through the lungs.

Infants with transposition are blue (severely cyanotic) and must have immediate medical care. Several surgical procedures are available to relieve the problem.

Central Nervous System Disorders

The central nervous system is the portion of the nervous system consisting of the brain and spinal cord. The most common congenital disorders of the central nervous system are described here.

Spina Bifida Occulta

Spina bifida occulta is a defect in the formation of a portion of the backbone (vertebrae) and surrounding tissues. This can occur in any vertebra but is most common at the base of the back or lower spine.

The clue to the presence of this condition is an abnormal tuft of hair, a collection of fat, or tiny vessels on the skin overlying the defect. Generally, this condition is an insignificant finding on an X-ray or ultrasound and is not associated with any underlying neurologic defect because there is no involvement of the spinal nerves.

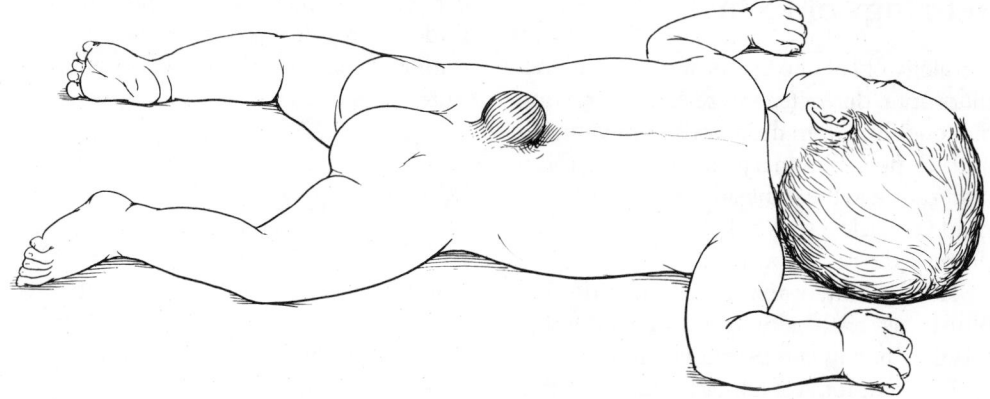

An outpouching of membranes covering the spinal cord (myelomeningocele) occurs in some infants with spina bifida. This may result in neurologic disturbances of the lower legs, bladder, or bowel.

Babies born with spina bifida occulta should receive a thorough neurologic examination because a small percentage of them will have a myelomeningocele (see page 514). This may result in a neurologic disturbance of the lower legs, bladder, or bowel.

Hydrocephalus

A child born with hydrocephalus has an imbalance between the brain's production of cerebrospinal fluid and its ability to absorb it. This accumulation of cerebrospinal fluid in the skull of an infant produces an extremely large head.

The incidence of this condition varies in different populations, but on the average it is 1 per 1,000 births.

The most obvious symptom of congenital hydrocephalus is an abnormally large head. Occasionally, the head of the fetus grows so large that a normal delivery is impossible. In less extreme cases, the head may seem normal at birth but grows at an abnormally rapid rate.

A CT scan and an MRI scan (see page 494) are useful for differentiating hydrocephalus from other disorders and for looking for the cause of the hydrocephalus.

The goal of treatment is to establish equilibrium between the production and absorption of cerebrospinal fluid. Sometimes medication is effective, but generally the best treatment is the surgical insertion of a shunt in the skull to drain the fluid. Shunting is permanent and should be removed only in the event of infection or malfunction of the device itself.

The long-term outlook for children born with hydrocephalus has improved greatly as a result of shunt placement. If left untreated, more than half of infants born with this disorder die. With proper medical management, an estimated 70 percent of infants with hydrocephalus live beyond infancy. Of this group, 40 percent will have normal intelligence, and 60 percent (mainly those with other central nervous system disorders) will have severe intellectual and motor impairment.

Cerebral Palsy

Cerebral palsy is one of the most common handicapping conditions of childhood. It is a result of damage to the motor function areas of the central nervous system before, during, or after birth.

There are many causes of cerebral palsy. One possible cause is the absence of adequate oxygen in the brain tissue (anoxia). Studies also have shown that one-third of infants born with cerebral palsy weigh less than 5 pounds.

Injury to the brain during labor and delivery also is a cause, as are infection (for example, bacterial meningitis) and hemorrhage. Often, however, there is no obvious explanation.

The outlook for a child with cerebral palsy depends largely on whether the child also has intellectual handicaps. Even when a child has severe motor difficulties that necessitate use of a wheelchair, adjustments are easier if the child is capable of going to school. The family's attitude toward the child's condition has an impact on whether the child develops a positive self-image.

There is no cure for cerebral palsy. However, in special cases, surgery is helpful in reducing spasticity. Treatment involves early stretching exercises to help the muscles stay loose and to prevent contractures, the use of aids such as wheelchairs and walkers to improve the child's mobility, and special educational methods to help compensate for the child's motor difficulties and any learning disabilities.

There are four types of cerebral palsy: spastic cerebral palsy, extrapyramidal (athetotic) cerebral palsy, atonic cerebral palsy, and mixed types.

Spastic Cerebral Palsy

Spastic cerebral palsy is the most common type. An infant with spastic cerebral palsy has an abnormal persistence of some newborn reflexes. A hyperactive grasp reflex leaves the infant's hands in a tight fist. As the infant grows, the limbs become more spastic and rigid.

All four limbs may be involved (spastic quadriplegia). When this occurs, there is often some degree of mental retardation as well. Convulsions are common.

If all four limbs are affected but the arms are affected to a lesser degree, the condition is called diplegia. Children with diplegia may have good use of their hands. Their intelligence is often normal or near normal, but they may have some difficulties learning to draw and write letters.

One-third of all children with cerebral palsy have spastic hemiplegia (paralysis on one side of the body only). Children with spastic hemiplegia tend to have intelligence in the low-normal range, although some have average or even above-average intelligence.

Extrapyramidal (Athetotic) Cerebral Palsy

This type of cerebral palsy manifests initially as weakness and floppiness of a baby's muscles. It generally is not diagnosed until the infant is 6 months old. An early sign is abnormal positioning of the hands when the baby attempts to reach for something.

Atonic Cerebral Palsy

Atonic cerebral palsy has two forms: atonic diplegia and congenital cerebellar ataxia. The former is associated with severe mental retardation. Spasticity often develops later in childhood. Congenital cerebellar ataxia is a rare form of cerebral palsy, which may be accompanied by mild mental retardation.

Congenital Disorders of the Gastrointestinal and Respiratory Tracts

There are many congenital disorders of the gastrointestinal tract, some of which are responsible for partial or complete obstruction of the passage of food or stool. The most common obstructions involve the duodenum (the first section of the small intestine) or the rectum and anus at the lower end of the gastrointestinal tract. The most frequent gastrointestinal abnormalities in infancy are described.

Pyloric Stenosis

Pyloric stenosis is a narrowing of the pylorus, the part of the stomach through which food and other stomach contents pass to enter the small intestine. Pyloric stenosis affects approximately 1 out of every 150 male newborns and 1 out of every 750 female infants. About 15 percent of those born with this condition have a family history of the pyloric stenosis, but the precise cause is not known.

If your infant is born with pyloric stenosis, the symptoms usually begin during its second or third week of life. The initial symptom may be regurgitation and possibly vomiting, although not necessarily forceful or projectile vomiting. After the symptoms have been apparent for a week or so, the infant generally begins to vomit more forcefully (projectile vomiting). Rarely, the vomit will contain blood. Vomiting typically occurs during or shortly after a feeding, but it may be delayed for hours. After vomiting, the baby is hungry and wants another feeding.

An infant with pyloric stenosis has very small stools because little food is reaching the intestines. Soon the baby begins to lose weight and may become dehydrated. The infant's eyes may appear sunken and the cheeks wrinkled. The newborn with pyloric

A narrowing of the outlet of the stomach (pylorus) through which stomach contents pass into the small intestine is called pyloric stenosis. This condition requires prompt surgical treatment.

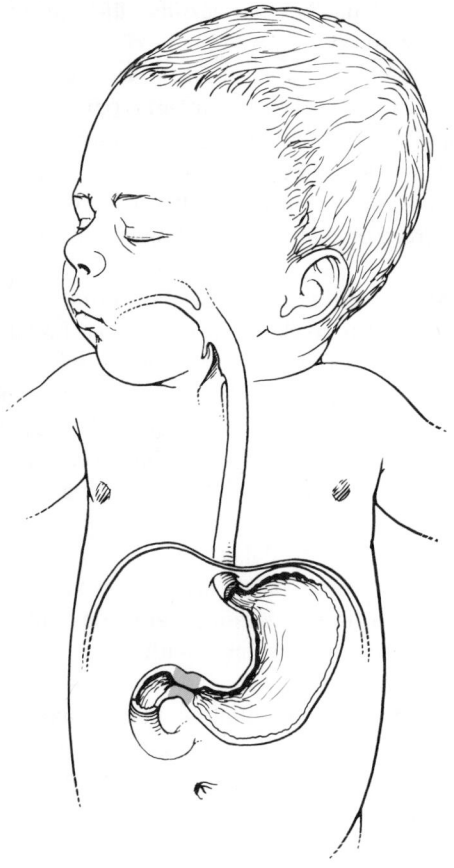

throat to the stomach) that has not fully developed. An estimated 1 in 3,000 to 4,500 infants is born with this malformation.

One-third of babies with esophageal atresia are premature. This condition often is accompanied by other disorders, usually of the trachea (the tube from the larynx into the lungs). Moreover, at least 30 percent of infants with esophageal atresia have other life-threatening birth defects such as heart, urinary tract, and central nervous system problems.

The symptoms of esophageal atresia often are detected in the delivery room. The infant may have an unusually large amount of secretions coming from its mouth or may choke, cough, or turn blue when attempting to feed. If the physician cannot pass a tube through the baby's mouth into the stomach, the infant probably has esophageal atresia.

Infants with this condition require surgery. If the underdeveloped esophageal segment is short, repair can be attempted immediately. If the segment is long, the surgeon might decide to permit growth of the esophagus before attempting repair. In this event, a tube is placed through the abdominal wall into the stomach to permit feeding.

stenosis may appear uncomfortable but does not seem to be in great pain.

Pyloric stenosis usually can be diagnosed from a physical examination, the child's feeding history, and the identification of a pyloric mass on examination of the abdomen. If the mass cannot be felt, an ultrasound examination (see page 1335) is sometimes done.

An infant born with pyloric stenosis requires an operation following rehydration with intravenous fluids. More recently, a nonsurgical approach with endoscopic balloon dilatation has also shown some success.

Within 6 hours after the operation, your baby will begin to receive oral feedings. The amount of the feeding is increased gradually. Most infants can go home 2 days after the operation.

The prognosis for an infant with pyloric stenosis is very good, depending on how early the diagnosis is made and on the overall condition of the infant.

Esophageal Atresia

An infant born with esophageal atresia has an esophagus (the tube leading from the

Biliary Atresia

Biliary atresia (obstruction of the bile ducts) is an uncommon congenital defect, affecting an estimated 1 in 50,000 to 75,000 newborns.

It is often difficult to differentiate hepatitis from bile duct atresia in an infant. If the results of hepatitis tests are normal, a liver biopsy might be done to confirm the diagnosis.

Infants with bile duct atresia have persistent jaundice and an increased incidence of other abdominal abnormalities. The stools are very pale to white, and the liver may be of abnormal size.

If your infant has biliary atresia, your physician may recommend an exploratory operation to determine the precise site. Rarely, the obstruction can be corrected surgically. However, drainage of bile can sometimes be achieved by surgically creating a connection to the intestine. It is important that the operation be performed during the first 3 months of life to ensure success.

Children with biliary atresia often have persistent inflammation of the liver even after surgery. Some may ultimately require liver transplantation.

Intestinal Atresia

Obstruction of the intestine occurs in about 1 of 1,500 births. The obstruction can occur anywhere in the intestines.

If the obstruction is "high," it is located just beyond the outlet of the stomach or in the upper small intestine. The infant's predominant symptom is vomiting, which tends to be persistent even when feedings have been discontinued. An infant with a "low" obstruction has an obstruction in the lower small intestine or colon and has a distended abdomen initially, although vomiting occurs later. Vomiting of bile (yellow-green material) should always be investigated by your health care provider.

An infant with an intestinal obstruction generally does not have a bowel movement, although meconium stools (see page 7) may be passed during the first days of life if the obstruction is high in the small intestine. An obstruction may be complete or partial. When the baby has a partial obstruction, the symptoms may not be apparent immediately.

If your physician suspects that your infant has an intestinal obstruction, an X-ray of the abdomen will be taken.

Treatment depends on the type of obstruction. A complete obstruction requires prompt surgery to prevent severe complications. An operation often is needed for a partial obstruction. Some minor obstructions may not require surgery. When the diagnosis is made promptly and the proper treatment is initiated, most infants tolerate the operation well and recover completely.

Hirschsprung's Disease

An infant born with Hirschsprung's disease (also called congenital megacolon) gradually develops an abnormally large or dilated colon. This condition is due to a failure of the lower rectum to propel stool through the anus. Rare in premature infants, Hirschsprung's disease accounts for about 33 percent of all neonatal obstructions in the colon.

Early signs in the newborn may include the failure to pass meconium stool, vomiting, abdominal distention, and the failure to have a bowel movement. After a rectal examination, the baby often has an explosive bowel movement. Sometimes a newborn even vomits fecal material. Dehydra-

tion and weight loss are common. Many infants have alternating constipation and diarrhea.

The best method of diagnosing megacolon in the newborn is by rectal biopsy.

The treatment for Hirschsprung's disease is an operation during which an opening on the outside of the abdomen is created so that the stool can pass into a disposable pouch. This is a temporary measure. The opening is closed during another operation, typically when the child is between 12 and 18 months old. The treatment is highly successful, although continued bouts of diarrhea are sometimes a problem.

Imperforate Anus

If your infant is born with an imperforate anus, the anal opening is obstructed. Consequently, there is no passage of stool. Congenital disorders of the anus and rectum are fairly common, with minor abnormalities occurring in 1 out of 500 births and major ones in 1 out of 5,000 births.

Children born with anal and rectal problems have a higher incidence of other birth defects such as urinary tract disorders.

Imperforate anus is suspected when a baby fails to pass a meconium stool. X-ray and ultrasound studies can be done to establish whether the obstruction is high or low in the rectum.

Treatment depends on the location of the obstruction. If the anal opening is simply narrowed, an instrument can be used to dilate the opening. In other types of imperforate anus, surgery is required. The higher the obstruction, the more major the surgical procedure. Some children require complete reconstruction of the anus. Others need a temporary colostomy for the first 6 to 12 months of life (see Hirschsprung's Disease, this page).

Children with low anal obstruction generally do well after surgery and develop bowel control. When the obstruction is higher, there may be some fecal incontinence.

Diaphragmatic Hernia

A diaphragmatic hernia occurs when an abnormal opening in the diaphragm enables part of the abdominal contents to poke through into the chest cavity. In severe cases, the stomach and a large part of the intestines displace the heart and lungs.

This condition will probably be evident immediately after birth. It is then a life-threatening situation and requires emergency surgery.

Later-appearing symptoms of diaphragmatic hernia include vomiting, severe colicky pain, discomfort after eating, and constipation. Rarely, there are no symptoms and the problem is discovered on routine X-rays.

If your physician suspects that your infant has diaphragmatic hernia, X-rays will be taken to confirm the diagnosis.

Omphalocele and Gastroschisis

During normal fetal development, the abdominal organs start developing outside the abdominal cavity before returning to the abdomen in an orderly fashion. In both omphalocele and gastroschisis, the abdominal organs (intestines, stomach, and even liver and spleen) are not in the abdomen at birth. When these organs are contained in a protective envelope of tissue, and protrude through the umbilicus, it is called an omphalocele. When they protrude through an opening to the right (or, rarely, to the left) of the umbilicus, it is called gastroschisis. In this instance, the organs are not protected by an envelope, and serious damage to these organs, especially the intestines, may have

occurred. Surgery must be done immediately, but recovery can take a long time.

Congenital Lobar Emphysema

Signs and Symptoms
- Persistent shortness of breath
- Wheezing
- Bluish tinge to the lips and fingernail beds (cyanosis)

Congenital lobar emphysema, also known as infantile lobar emphysema, occurs when air enters an infant's lungs but has trouble leaving. The lungs become overinflated, and air leaks out into the space around the lungs. In most cases, only one lobe is affected, usually an upper one.

Congenital lobar emphysema is almost always identified during the first 2 weeks of life. In most cases, no cause can be identified. The infant's lungs may not have developed completely or something may be obstructing the airway.

A chest X-ray shows the overinflation of the involved lobe of the lung and may reveal a blockage of the air passage.

Treatment
In infants with no or only mild and intermittent symptoms, no specific treatment is necessary. However, surgical removal of the affected lobe may be necessary in some cases.

Chapter 2

Infancy:
Ages 1 Month to 1 Year

Contents

The First Year, 60

Normal Growth and Development, 60
The Milestones, 60

Common Concerns During Infancy, 62
Signs of Illness, 62
Failure to Gain Weight, 63
Concerns About Hearing, 64
    Your Child's Hearing Development, 65
Concerns About Vision, 65
    How to Determine Whether
        Your Infant Sees Properly, 66
Diarrhea, 66
Constipation, 67
Vomiting and Regurgitation, 67
Rashes, 68
Febrile Seizures, 69
Sudden Infant Death Syndrome (SIDS), 69
    What to Do If Your Infant Has a Seizure, 70

General Infant Care and Hygiene, 71
Safety, 71
    Lead Poisoning, 71
Car Seats, 72
Safe Toys, 73
Swings, Jumpers, and Walkers, 73
Comfortable Clothing, 73
Diaper Care, 74
Preventing the Spread of Disease, 74

Development of Personality and
Behavior, 75
Normal Developmental Milestones, 75
Sleep Concerns, 77
Sibling Relationships, 77

Your Infant's Nutrition, 78
Feeding Recommendations, 78
Feeding Problems, 79
    Vitamin and Mineral Supplements
        for Infants, 80

The First Year

The second month of life is the point at which you and your baby have begun to adjust to each other. Mothers usually begin to recover some of their strength by the second month, and the relationship between parents and infant grows.

If you have found yourself adjusting to caring for your baby, think of the phenomenal transformation he or she has experienced in just a few short weeks. The physical changes in appearance from birth to 1 month are dramatic. Your 1-month-old baby also is beginning to fall into a somewhat predictable schedule of eating, sleeping, and eliminating. This is not to say that the schedule will not change. It will—frequently—during the first year of life. But between the changes there is a newfound sense of predictability in what to expect from your baby during a given day.

The first year of life is a time of continuous and rapid change. During this first year your baby will go from a diet of mother's milk or formula to feeding himself or herself table food and even drinking from a cup. The young baby who spends a good part of each day sleeping becomes the 11-month-old who is active the whole day except for an afternoon nap. The baby will progress from being able to sit up on his or her own to creeping and then to walking, which generally occurs between ages 9 and 16 months.

You will watch your infant evolve from a being who communicates only by crying to one who coos and squeals with pleasure when you walk into the room and then to one who can say mama and dada and wave bye-bye.

This chapter is devoted to the infant ages 1 through 12 months. Within its pages we explore the developmental—both physical and psychological—milestones that you can expect during these important months. Common concerns such as diarrhea, rashes, and vomiting will be covered. We will emphasize general care, nutrition, feeding problems, and ways in which you can help keep your curious infant safe in your home.

Normal Growth and Development

How much weight gain is normal? How does a breastfeeding mother know whether her baby is getting enough to eat? How many hours a day should my infant be sleeping?

These are all common questions asked by parents, particularly those with a first child.

It is natural to worry whether your baby is developing normally, even though serious abnormalities are uncommon.

From the standpoint of reducing parental anxiety, it would be easier if your health care provider could tell you with absolute confidence that your baby will gain a specified amount of weight each month, turn over at a definite time, and begin to walk at some exact age. Easier, perhaps, but not realistic.

What this chapter and your health care provider can offer you, however, are guidelines. There is a range within which development occurs in most infants. For example, a child may walk as early as 9 months or as late as 16 months and still be considered to be normal. Just because your baby walks at 15 months does not mean he or she is slow. On the contrary, your infant may have been directing energies toward language and as a result may be more verbally advanced than his or her peers.

Even if your baby fails to reach a developmental milestone within the normal time frame, this still does not necessarily mean that anything is wrong. However, you should discuss your concerns with your health care provider.

The Milestones

The precise timetable is not fixed, yet human development does occur in a predictable sequence of events. An infant simply does not suddenly begin to walk; instead, he or she begins in the first weeks of life to lift his or her head and later to roll over, sit alone, crawl, stand, and then finally walk.

Although the steps involved in the mastery of a skill such as walking are the same for all children, the rate at which the steps occur varies considerably. This variation often leads to concern. For instance, parents remember that their first child walked at 9 months and then become anxious when the second still is not walking at 14 months.

In this section we give you some guidelines for growth and development. Keep in mind, however, that these are only averages.

Growth

By the time your infant is 1 month old, he or she probably has gained 1 to 3 pounds over his or her birth weight and has grown 1 or 2 inches in length. The baby will probably double his or her birth weight by the age of 4 to 5 months and triple it by the first birthday. Your infant's height will increase about 10 to 12 inches over the course of the year. The circumference of the baby's head will increase about 4 or 5 inches during the first year of life.

Your baby will likely develop a first tooth between 5 and 9 months. Most children have between six and eight teeth by the time they are 1 year.

Sleep Patterns

In the first months of life, babies spend most of their time sleeping. They wake up when they are hungry, they eat, play, or fuss for a while, and then go back to sleep. The average 1-month-old may be awake a total of 10 hours out of every 24. Some babies sleep more, others less.

Most 4- to 6-month-old babies sleep 6 or 7 hours nightly.

As a rule, the older the infant, the less he or she sleeps. By the end of the first year, most infants' naps are limited to 1 or 2 hours in the morning or afternoon or both.

Motor Development

The 1-month-old infant's movements seem clumsy and uncoordinated. Unsupported, the baby's head will flop forward or backward. The infant may grasp an object such as a rattle, but lets go quickly. The baby may stare at an object but does not try to reach for it.

Most 2-month-old infants can move their arms and legs smoothly, hold their heads up at a 45-degree angle for a few minutes, and grasp an object briefly.

The 3-month-old can sit supported with minimal head bobbing. At this age, the baby may begin to swipe at objects, but often misses. The body now is less floppy.

A 4-month-old infant can sit with assistance and maintain good control of the head. When on his or her stomach, your baby may rock, rolling from side to side. Some infants at this age can roll from their stomach or side to the back, or transfer an object from one hand to the other.

The 5-month-old can put its feet up to his or her mouth and suck on the toes. The baby can now roll from stomach to back. When on the stomach, he or she can push with the hands and bring up the knees. When pulled to stand, the baby can move his or her body up and down and push down on one foot and then the other, as though walking. The baby may be able to swap objects from hand to hand, and can reach with accuracy.

A 6-month-old rolls from back to stomach. Some babies of this age can get up on their hands and knees and creep. The baby can sit in a chair and bounce and can play with his or her hands by touching them together.

At 7 months, your infant's ability to sit has improved and he or she may even be able to sit unsupported. The baby can use thumb and finger to grasp a block and bang together two objects.

The 8-month-old infant is trying to crawl. Some babies of this age can stand when leaning against something. The baby can hold a rattle for several minutes and tries to pick up small objects.

Many 9-month-old babies can crawl while grasping a toy in one hand. The baby may be able to stand alone for brief periods and can grasp small objects between the thumb and forefinger.

The 10-month-old infant may be holding on to your furniture to walk around the room. Most infants can walk at 10 months provided you hold on to both hands. Your child can climb up and down from chairs and carry two small objects in one hand.

The 11-month-old may be able to stand alone and wave, climb stairs, and squat and stoop. The child may be able to grasp a spoon and bring it to his or her mouth, make marks with a crayon, and pull off his or her shoes.

By the time many children have their first birthday, they are walking, although crawling still may be the preferred method of getting around. The child may be capable of climbing stairs and going down stairs and may be able to climb out of the crib. The child can point with the index finger and can take the covers off containers.

Verbal Development

The 1-month-old baby, besides crying, begins to make small throaty sounds. At 2 months, these sounds begin to sound like coos. The 3-month-old baby's verbal repertoire is expanded with squeals, chuckles, whimpers, and vowel-like sounds such as ooh, ah, and ae. Considerable cooing and gurgling take place during this time. Language comprehension is limited to responses to loud noises and familiar voices.

Between 4 and 6 months is the babbling stage—complete with sighing, grunting, gurgling, laughing, and crying differently for pain and hunger. Your child vocalizes for pleasure and displeasure.

Between 7 and 9 months your child repeats syllables, babbles in a singsong manner, and may produce as many as 12 different sounds, particularly the p, b, and m

sounds. He or she may use different vowels. Your infant may use sounds as a means of play and may repeat the word mama. Toward the end of this period, actual imitation of intonation and speech sounds made by others can be heard. Your child will search for sources of sound, listen intently to speech and non-speech sounds, and recognize dada, mama, and bye-bye. Your child may recognize his or her own name and is able to differentiate friendliness or anger from the tone of people's voices.

Between 10 and 12 months, the babbling may take on some of the melody of actual speech. Your child enjoys repeating sounds made by others. Considerable vocalization is used during play. Almost all of the consonant and vowel sounds are used. In some children, the first words emerge during this period. Your child's comprehension also is improved by this time, and he or she can respond to names and simple requests and recognizes the names of common objects and family members.

Common Concerns During Infancy

As the parent of an infant, you may find yourself frequently wondering whether your baby is well. Is he or she gaining enough weight? Can he or she see and hear normally? Are the infant's difficulties with bowel movements cause for alarm? How do you know whether your fussy baby is really ill or simply having a bad day? In this section we will provide you with information that will help you answer some of these questions.

Signs of Illness

Illness in an infant may be difficult to detect initially. Unlike the older child, the 1-month-old infant cannot tell you that his or her head hurts. Your baby may cry more, but if he or she is a fussy baby anyway, the crying may not arouse your suspicions. Or, the child may—like most of us when we are sick—sleep more.

Trust your instincts! Remember, the most important factor is how the baby is acting. If your infant's eating and sleeping patterns

abruptly change, it is reasonable to suspect that the baby may not be feeling well. Taking the baby's temperature is a good first step, although a baby might not have a fever when ill.

A baby who has a normal temperature but is limp, lethargic, and refusing food or liquids is more likely to be ill than the bright-eyed, into-everything 8-month-old baby with a temperature of 103 degrees Fahrenheit.

Some signs that may indicate illness are described below.

Fever

A rectal temperature of more than 100.4 degrees Fahrenheit is considered a fever, the body's response to infection. Fevers are common during childhood and usually are due to a viral infection. Most fevers less than 102 degrees Fahrenheit do not cause symptoms, and contrary to popular belief, the seriousness of an illness is usually not related to the degree of fever. Again, always ask yourself, "How is my baby acting?"

If a baby younger than 2 months develops

a fever of more than 100.4 degrees Fahrenheit, call your health care provider. A fever of more than 102 degrees Fahrenheit in a child older than 2 months also warrants a call to your health care provider, as does one that has been present for 3 days or more.

Constant Crying

Babies, particularly those younger than 3 months, frequently cry for long periods. Although constant crying during early infancy usually is attributable to colic (see Excessive Crying [Colic], page 11), it also may be an indication that the child is ill. If your baby cries for a long period (2 or 3 hours) or is inconsolable, or if the cry sounds strange (unusually high-pitched or a weak moan), call your health care provider. If you are worried that your baby is sick, do not be embarrassed to call your infant's health care provider or to bring your child in to be examined.

Breathing Problems

Your baby may catch a cold that interferes with his or her breathing. Removing mucus from the nose with a special rubber bulb (available at your local pharmacy) often enables your baby to breathe freely and may be all the treatment required. However, if your baby develops a raspy, harsh-sounding cough, begins to wheeze, has difficulty breathing, or turns bluish around the lips and mouth, call your infant's health care provider or seek immediate emergency care (see Common and Recurrent Colds, page 86).

Soft Spot (Fontanelle)

For the first year and a half of life, your baby has a soft spot on the top front part of the skull where the bones have yet to grow together. Normally, this area is flat or may be slightly depressed. If, however, your baby is sick and the soft spot bulges or if it appears sunken, call your health care provider immediately. Note that the soft spot bulges out naturally with respiration or crying.

Vomiting

Most healthy babies spit up; some do it more than others. Spitting up is the effortless regurgitation of food or milk, and vomiting is the forceful exit of the stomach's contents. If vomiting continues for more than 12 hours or if there is blood in the vomitus, call your health care provider (see Vomiting and Spitting Up, page 12).

Diarrhea

The best indicators of the severity of diarrhea are its frequency and how sick your baby is acting. If the stool is green, it indicates the rapid passage of food through the intestines. This is normal.

If your infant passes more than eight diarrhea stools in 8 hours, is also vomiting, or has blood in the stool, call your health care provider.

Dehydration

The main danger of vomiting and diarrhea is a depletion of the body's fluids. Dehydration is potentially life-threatening and can occur in infancy after only a few hours of illness. Signs to look for include an absence of tears during crying, a dry mouth, the failure to produce a wet diaper after 8 hours, and a sunken soft spot. If your child has any symptoms of dehydration, call your health care provider immediately. You may need to bring your baby in for an examination.

Failure to Gain Weight

The vast majority of babies grow normally. There are differences, of course, from one child to the next in the achievement of specific weights and lengths—after all, some babies are born several pounds lighter or heavier than others.

In rare instances, an infant stops growing or grows unusually slowly. The most evident symptom of a child who is failing to thrive is a lack of weight gain or even weight loss. Moreover, many babies who fail to thrive show signs of developmental retardation and physical and emotional deprivation. They may be apathetic, unwilling to make eye contact, and withdrawn. Some may have gastrointestinal problems such as vomiting, diarrhea, and regurgitation.

Although failure to thrive can occur at any time during childhood, it is most common during infancy. Babies who are mentally retarded or autistic or who have cerebral palsy are much more likely to display a failure to thrive.

The basic cause of failure to thrive falls into one of two categories: organic, which means there is a physical problem responsible for the infant's poor weight gain; and nonorganic, an indication that the cause is psychosocial or environmental factors such as feeding errors, the absence of care, or the lack of a nurturing emotional environment.

Many physical problems can cause failure to thrive. Malabsorption disorders of the small intestine, liver disease, kidney disorders, chronic heart failure, malignancies, central nervous system abnormalities, cleft palate, and endocrine disorders are some of the ailments that can interfere with weight gain. When a specific physical cause is found, treatment of that disorder generally remedies the failure to thrive.

Sometimes parents make feeding errors that result in the baby not consuming enough calories. An inexperienced parent may, for instance, dilute the baby's formula. Or, the parent may not feed the baby often enough, or the feedings themselves may be too small.

Babies who have failure to thrive because of neglect usually wear the signs of their neglect. They often have severe diaper rash, uncut fingernails, untreated rashes, and dirty clothes.

In addition to withholding food, the parents may withhold love and affection. Babies who are treated in this way usually have not been kissed, cuddled, or played with. When the baby is held, it is often done in a rough manner.

What should you do if your infant fails to gain weight? Consult your baby's health care provider. During your infant's first year of life, he or she should be seeing a health care provider every month or two. At each checkup, the baby is weighed and measured and the weight and height are recorded. If your baby is not gaining properly or is losing weight, your health care provider will evaluate your baby's feedings and appetite and ask whether he or she has had any vomiting or diarrhea.

Hospitalization may be necessary. During this time, your infant will be given unlimited feedings and his or her growth will be monitored. If evaluation points toward an organic cause, tests will be done to confirm the diagnosis. For cases in which the cause of failure to thrive is neglect or improper feeding, the infant, ravenous, usually responds with rapid weight gain during a week in the hospital.

The outlook varies for babies who have nonorganic failure to thrive. These families typically require help, including precise feeding instructions and visits from a public health nurse or representative of some form of community service.

A small percentage of affected babies are not treated until it is too late to save them. Although poor weight gain and growth attributable to malnutrition can be reversed, an infant malnourished for more than 6 months may never achieve a normal-sized brain. Moreover, many of these children go on to have reading and language problems and exhibit antisocial behavior in later years.

Concerns About Hearing

In order to develop normal speech and language abilities, a baby must be able to hear.

Normally, babies are born with the ability to hear. But sometimes events that occur in or out of the womb can impair to varying degrees a baby's ability to hear out of one or both ears.

Infants at high risk for hearing impairment include those with severe birth asphyxia (oxygen deprivation) or bacterial meningitis, those who have infections in the womb or in early infancy, some head or neck defects, or severe jaundice requiring exchange transfusions, or those who are born prematurely. It is also important to evaluate hearing if there is a history of hearing impairment in the family.

Hearing loss is an insidious problem and one that might go undetected until the child is 18 to 24 months of age, when concerned parents become aware that he or she is not developing normal speech. All newborns, including well babies, should be screened for hearing loss.

Four types of hearing loss are found in infants.

Conductive hearing loss occurs when something interferes with the reception of sound by the external ear or with the transmission of sound from the external to the inner ear. The most common causes of conductive hearing loss are structural abnormalities of the ear and chronic ear infections. This type of hearing loss often can be treated successfully.

Sensorineural hearing loss stems from abnormalities of the cochlear hair cells or the auditory nerve. More than half of the cases of sensorineural hearing loss are congenital, and the remainder are due to conditions such as birth trauma, intrauterine infections, certain medications, and other factors. Generally, sensorineural hearing loss cannot be reversed.

Mixed hearing loss occurs when the child has both a conductive and a sensorineural hearing loss. The hearing loss is often severe.

Central auditory disorders are a result of a problem with the central auditory nervous system. These problems can occur during pregnancy, birth, or early life.

Early detection of a hearing loss is critical for determining effects on the development of language and speech. Many children with hearing problems can be helped with medical or surgical treatments and hearing aids. Specific testing may be arranged for infants at risk for hearing problems and those with speech difficulties.

Moreover, if your baby is found to have a hearing loss, your health care provider or a specialist in hearing assessment (audiologist) may recommend a parent-infant program that will help you to make the most of your child's hearing abilities.

Concerns About Vision

Although your newborn probably keeps his or her eyes closed much of the time, the baby was born with the ability to see, although not too clearly. Your baby's vision responses and the interior of the eye (retina) are checked shortly after birth by your infant's health care provider.

In most infants, the ability to see things clearly rapidly progresses, and by the time most children are 3 years old or even younger, they have 20/30 or 20/20 vision.

Many normal babies may have difficulty coordinating their eye movements during the initial months. Hence, at times your baby may seem cross-eyed. In most cases, however, this appearance should not persist beyond the first few months.

Sometimes—for various reasons—a vision problem surfaces during infancy. As is so often the case, the earlier the diagnosis, the better the chances that treatment will be successful. For this reason, an eye examination should be a part of even the young child's routine examinations.

Some of the vision problems that may occur during infancy are described below.

Amblyopia

This term describes subnormal vision in one or both eyes. There are numerous causes, including trauma to the eye, diseases of the eye, and disorders of vision such as the failure of the eyes to focus or align properly (lazy eye).

The most important factor in the treatment of amblyopia is early detection and

---

Your Child's Hearing Development

As a parent, there are certain developmental signs that you can watch to determine whether your baby's hearing is within the normal range.

A hearing problem that is not detected shortly after birth is usually not discovered until well into the child's second year, when it becomes apparent that his or her speech is delayed. By this time, a crucial point in language development has been missed.

Under normal circumstances, an infant is born hearing and may even have sound preferences. The 1-month-old often stops moving and appears to listen to a sudden sound. By 2 months, the child should appear to be listening to his or her mother or father. At 3 months, the baby should coo and gurgle in response to speech and look in the direction of the speaker. The child should startle to a clap within 3 feet.

The 4-month-old infant responds differently to angry and pleasant voices, the 5-month-old baby should begin to mimic sounds and respond to his or her own name, and the 6-month-old should be able to protest loudly and squeal with delight. The child should search (turn his or her eyes and head) in an attempt to find the source of sounds or speech.

Most babies at 7 months begin to make some word-like sounds and respond with gestures to simple words such as "bye-bye." At 8 months your baby may stop activity when you call his or her name, at 9 months he or she stops an activity when you say "no," and he or she may begin to speak at 10 months. The 1-year-old baby should be able to answer simple questions (such as, Where is your nose? Where is your hair?) by pointing to the named object.

There is some normal variation in the development of hearing from one child to the next—but if you suspect that your baby's development is abnormally slow, consult your health care provider.

---

prompt treatment. Typically, a child is most susceptible to amblyopia during the first 3 years of life.

Treatment involves providing the clearest vision possible and may include eyedrops, glasses to correct a refraction error, or even surgery. Another crucial component of treatment is forcing the use of the amblyopic eye. This is usually done by putting a patch over the better eye to force the child to use the weaker eye. In some infants, amblyopia can be reversed within weeks of treatment.

Strabismus

Strabismus describes the inability of the eyes to align properly. When this occurs, a person is unable to integrate what he or she sees from both eyes into a single visual image, which is essential to develop normal depth perception.

In one form of strabismus, the eyes malalign only when the child is tired, under stress, or ill.

A child who has alternating strabismus learns to see out of one eye at a time. While one eye is being used to see with, the other one wanders. Because both eyes are used (at different times), vision develops in both, whereas a child who uses one eye exclusively may develop amblyopia in the other eye because it is used improperly.

Another type of strabismus is accommodative esotropia. This form of strabismus usually occurs when a child is between 2 and 3 years, but in some cases it surfaces during infancy. These children are typically far-sighted (unable to see clearly objects close at hand) and cross-eyed. The crossed eyes may be most apparent when the child is looking at something close.

If your infant has strabismus, the first goal of treatment is to establish the best achievable vision and, when possible, equal vision in both eyes. Surgery is often necessary in children born with strabismus, and it should be done as soon as possible so that the infant will be able to develop normal vision. Sometimes several operations are necessary, but in most children with strabismus, one or possibly two operations are usually sufficient. Total correction, however, is not always possible (see Strabismus and Amblyopia, page 534).

Diarrhea

Diarrhea—the frequent passage of abnormally loose or liquid stools—is one of the most common reasons for seeking consultation with a health care provider. During the first 3 years of your baby's life, he or she probably will have from one to three severe episodes of diarrhea.

In infants, diarrhea usually is caused by a viral infection. Occasionally, the offender may be a bacterium or toxin that invades the intestinal tract. Diarrhea also can be due to diet; loose stools often are noted with the introduction of new foods. Finally, diarrhea can be a symptom of chronic gastrointestinal diseases, anatomical defects, and congenital disorders.

Breastfed babies normally have soft, mushy stools. Often, the stools of a healthy baby may be green. As for frequency, many infants have a bowel movement after each feeding, whereas others have only 1 a week.

So how do you know whether your breastfed infant has diarrhea? One clue is the presence of blood, mucus, or a bad odor (stools of a baby nourished exclusively at the breast do not have an offensive odor). An abrupt increase in frequency is another sign to watch for. When in doubt, ask yourself, how is the baby acting? Is he or she feeding poorly, acting sick, or feverish?

In the formula-fed infant, the stools increase in frequency and go from formed to being mushy or watery, in some cases turning green.

If your baby has diarrhea, what should you do? If the baby is acting normally and the diarrhea is mild, continue the usual form of nutrition.

If you are breastfeeding your baby, continue feeding as always. Simply offer your breast more often. More frequent breastfeeding is usually all that is needed.

If your baby has mild diarrhea and is already eating solids, continue the solids. Avoid any foods that usually cause softer stools. If in doubt as to what to feed, consult your physician.

How to Determine Whether Your Infant Sees Properly

Although an important part of a newborn's initial physical examination includes a check for any apparent vision or hearing defects, it is not uncommon for some sensory problems to go undetected during early infancy. Often the problem is later discovered by the parents when the infant fails to develop speech or seems unusually clumsy.

As a parent, there are certain developmental signs that you can watch for to determine whether your baby's vision is indeed within the normal range.

When your infant is between 4 and 6 weeks old, try the following test. Bring your face within 20 inches of your baby's. This should elicit a smile. By the time your infant is 3 months, the baby should be able to visually follow a toy that is dangled in front of his or her face. The infant also should attempt to reach for a toy or rattle. A baby this age also can see objects at least several feet away.

By the time your infant is 4 months old, his or her vision capabilities—the ability of the eye to distinguish color, adjust itself to various distances, see one image instead of two, perceive depth, and orient itself to moving images—are on the way to reaching those of an adult.

Although there is some normal variation in development, if you suspect that your baby's development is abnormally slow, consult your health care provider.

When diarrhea in a formula-fed infant is watery or frequent, your health care provider may suggest giving your baby an oral electrolyte solution for a short time to help replace electrolytes lost in the diarrhea. Drinking fluids is important to prevent dehydration (depletion of the body's fluids). So encourage your baby to drink.

When you begin feeding formula again, your health care provider might suggest trying a soy formula, which is less likely to cause diarrhea than one made with cow's milk, until stools return to their normal pattern.

Anyone caring for a child with diarrhea should be reminded that diarrhea caused by a virus or bacteria is contagious. Be especially diligent about hand-washing after diaper changes.

Most cases of diarrhea are over within 72 hours and require no more than an increased fluid intake and occasionally a brief change in diet. The key again is how your child is acting. Severe diarrhea—particularly in infants and young children—can be dangerous because of the possibility of dehydration. Babies who are dehydrated may require hospitalization, during which replacement fluids are infused into the child's body through a vein.

If your infant has diarrhea, watch carefully for the following signs and symptoms:

- No wet diaper for 8 hours or more
- Crying that produces no tears
- A dry mouth
- Depressed soft spot on baby's head
- More than eight diarrhea stools in 8 hours
- Blood in the stool
- Persistent vomiting of clear fluids, three or more times, with diarrhea
- Actions that indicate the baby is very sick

If your baby has any of these symptoms, call your health care provider immediately.

Constipation

Many parents assume that if their infant does not have a daily bowel movement, the baby is constipated. Constipation, however, is not marked by the frequency of bowel movements but by the consistency and effort required to pass the stool.

Constipation is uncommon in breastfed babies. Typically, breastfed infants have several loose bowel movements a day, often after each feeding; yet sometimes your baby may go several days without having a stool. The infant may grunt and push until he or she is red in the face. Yet when the movement is passed, it is not the hard stool associated with constipation. The seemingly difficult passage of this loose stool may be due to the fact that the baby's intestines are not yet smoothly coordinating intestinal contractions with relaxation of the anus, which is normal and will improve with time.

Some infants who are formula-fed do have constipation. Sometimes an increase in the amount of fluids or other diet changes will alleviate the problem. If the infant is more than 4 months old, adding water, diluted juices, or foods such as fruits or vegetables may help.

Consult your baby's health care provider for further specific advice on foods or before giving a suppository or enema. Some congenital disorders can cause chronic constipation, as can small cracks (fissures) around the anus, which make having a bowel movement painful for the infant.

If the constipation does not improve with these measures, check with your health care provider.

Vomiting and Regurgitation

Vomiting is the forceful ejection of a large amount of food from the stomach, occurring usually when your infant is sick. Vomiting is most often caused by a virus, although it can be the result of more serious problems. Regurgitation is the effortless spitting up of food or milk that frequently occurs in most healthy babies, usually after a feeding.

One or two episodes of vomiting in a baby who otherwise appears healthy is not cause for alarm. However, if the vomiting continues in a sick infant, call your health care provider.

If your breastfed baby is vomiting, your health care provider may suggest shorter, more frequent breastfeedings, or give your bottle-fed baby an oral electrolyte solution available without prescription at any pharmacy. Use small amounts at first, perhaps a tablespoon every 5 to 10 minutes. The solution will help replace electrolytes that are being lost in vomiting. Cautiously increase the quantity and frequency until the vomiting ceases. Then, if the baby is eating solids, try easily digested foods such as bananas, applesauce, and rice cereal.

A baby who vomits repeatedly—especially if diarrhea is also present—is at risk for dehydration, the depletion of the body's fluids. Signs that should alert you to the possibility of dehydration include the absence of wet diapers for more than 8 hours, a sunken soft spot on the baby's head, tearless crying, and a dry mouth. If the baby vomits clear fluids three or more times, call your health care provider immediately.

In contrast to vomiting, regurgitation—seen in more than half of all infants—is the gentle spitting up of small amounts of food or milk, usually shortly after eating. Regurgitation, also called gastroesophageal reflux, occurs because the upper end of the stomach has allowed food to travel back up the esophagus.

Regurgitation, especially for the first 6 months of life, is normal and nothing to be concerned about unless there is blood in the material or the infant is not gaining weight properly. In most infants, regurgitation improves as the child grows older and is upright for longer periods and as solids are added to the diet.

Although nothing will completely stop a baby from spitting up, there are things you can do to improve the problem.

Because overfeeding worsens the problem, start giving the baby less per feeding. Limit the feeding time to less than 20 minutes, and wait longer between feedings.

Be diligent about burping. During pauses in the feeding, try to get the baby to burp so that he or she has several burps during a feeding.

After meals, do not immediately lay the baby down. Try to keep him or her upright in a backpack or frontpack.

Avoid putting tight clothing on the baby or bouncing him or her after a meal.

Rashes

Rashes are common in infancy. The vast majority of rashes are not dangerous and often can be treated at home, but a rash also can be a symptom of an infectious disease (chickenpox or measles, for example) or of a serious disease such as allergic purpura (see Henoch-Schönlein Purpura, page 837).

As a general rule, if your baby suddenly develops a purple or blood-colored rash, develops a rash that looks like a burn, or seems to be acting sick and develops a rash, call your infant's health care provider immediately.

Common rashes that occur during infancy are described here.

Diaper Rash

This rash is the result of prolonged contact with wetness, bacteria, and other waste products from the digestive tract. The diaper area of a child with a diaper rash is covered with red, spotty sores. (See color photograph of diaper rash, page C-2.)

To treat a diaper rash, leave your infant's bottom exposed to air as much as possible. Avoid plastic pants and, if possible, switch to cloth diapers or at least a disposable diaper that keeps wetness away from your baby's skin.

To clean the baby's bottom, use plain water, which is less irritating than baby wipes. Mild rashes do not require ointment unless the skin is dry and cracked. Baby powder such as cornstarch or talcum powder is generally to be avoided because of concerns that it can lead to coughing or choking if inhaled by your infant.

Most diaper rashes respond within 3 days of drying efforts. If your baby's rash does not improve, it could mean the child has a yeast infection, which may require medicated cream. If the rash is so severe that it interferes with the child's sleep, if it is a solid, bright red, if it causes fever, or if the bottom develops blisters, boils, or drains pus, call your child's health care provider.

Cradle Cap

If your baby has yellow, oily scales and crusts on the scalp, he or she has cradle cap (seborrheic eczema). Without treatment, cradle cap will go away over a period of a few months. However, if you want to treat a particularly bothersome case, it may improve within a few weeks.

For cradle cap, avoid the tendency to wash your baby's hair with baby shampoo once a day. Once a week is often enough. After lathering, massage the scaly scalp with a soft toothbrush for a few minutes. If the scalp is very crusty, you can rub in mineral or baby oil an hour before you shampoo. If the rash is red and irritated, you can apply a 0.5 percent hydrocortisone cream, available without a prescription, once a week. Use of an antidandruff shampoo also may provide relief. A particularly stubborn case should be evaluated by your infant's health care provider. (See color photograph of cradle cap, page C-2.)

Infant Acne

About a third of all infants develop acne, usually after the third week of life. The cause appears to be related to maternal hormones that cross the placenta before birth.

The presence of acne can be disturbing, but parents should know that it is only temporary. In some infants, the acne disappears within weeks; in others, it may persist for up to 6 months.

We recommend no treatment other than washing your baby's face daily with plain water and once or twice weekly with a mild soap.

Drool Rash

Many infants develop a rash on their cheeks and chin. The rash, which is caused by contact with food and stomach contents (regurgitation), comes and goes. The only treatment generally required is cleansing the skin after a feeding. Placing a diaper under your infant's face during naps to absorb the drool or regurgitated material also may help.

Milia

These are small white bumps that are found on the faces of 40 percent of all newborns. These blocked skin pores generally open up and disappear by the time the infant is 2 months old. Treatment is not needed. (See color photograph of milia, page C-2.)

Heat Rash

This rash of tiny pink bumps is usually found on the back of the neck and on the upper back and is the result of blocked sweat glands. Typically, the rash occurs during hot, humid weather, although an infant who is overdressed or who has a fever may develop a heat rash at any time.

Treatment involves cooling the skin. Let the skin dry on its own, and dress your infant in as few clothes as possible. Use a fan while the child is sleeping. Cool rinses sometimes help. (For more information about rashes, see Your Skin, page 983.)

Febrile Seizures

A seizure (convulsion) occurs as a result of abnormal activity in the brain's nerve cells. Typically, the infant having a seizure suddenly becomes unconscious, with the arms and legs held rigid. After a few seconds, the limbs and face may begin to twitch rhythmically.

The majority of childhood seizures are related to fevers. When seizures are recurrent and not related to fever, a child is said to have a seizure disorder (see Seizures, page 495).

A febrile seizure is triggered by a fever. Typically, a seizure occurs in a child between 6 months and 5 years of age who develops a sudden fever. The height of temperature does not necessarily correlate with the development of a febrile seizure. Sometimes a febrile seizure is the first indication that a child is ill. Between 4 and 5 percent of all children have at least one febrile convulsion; 50 percent have no recurrence after the initial episode.

Febrile seizures tend to be short—usually less than 5 minutes. Although it was once believed that a child who had a febrile seizure risked brain damage, this is rare. In febrile seizures, the cause of the illness is more important than the extent of the seizure. For example, meningitis is far more serious than a simple febrile seizure (see Febrile Seizure, page 497).

Sudden Infant Death Syndrome (SIDS)

Sudden Infant Death Syndrome (SIDS) is the sudden and unexplained death of an apparently healthy infant.

Typically, the parents go to the baby's crib in the morning and find their baby dead. Sometimes the infant has had a slight cold but, more often than not, nothing seemed amiss when the parents put their baby to bed the night before. In most cases, an autopsy fails to establish the cause of death.

SIDS rarely occurs before 2 weeks or after 6 months of age, and the peak incidence is between the second and third months of life. The incidence in the United States is about 1 in 500 live births. Males are more likely to die of SIDS than females, and the syndrome strikes more often during cold weather.

The parents of a child who dies of SIDS are often torn with grief and guilt. Common thoughts are, If only I had checked the baby during the night. . . . I should have known something was wrong. . . . I am responsible because the baby must have smothered under too many blankets.

Researchers are studying this perplexing syndrome and discovering that many of these children were not really as healthy as they appeared to be. Some evidence now suggests that infants with SIDS may have had subtle abnormalities of the central nervous system.

Although the cause remains elusive, physicians now know that certain infants may be at greater risk than others, although infants who are not in this high-risk group also die of this syndrome. Premature or low-birth-weight babies, the babies of smokers or drug users, babies who have had a sibling die of SIDS, babies who have stopped breathing and then have been resuscitated, and babies with low Apgar scores (see The Apgar Score, page 6) are at higher risk.

Lowering the Risk

Some conditions associated with a higher risk of SIDS, such as premature birth, are beyond your control. SIDS can't be predicted or prevented, but the following recommendations may help reduce the risk of SIDS:

Sleep Position. For the first 6 months, put your baby to sleep resting on his or her side or back and not on the stomach. The back is the best position. If you put your baby to sleep on his or her side, pull the lower arm forward so your baby is less likely to roll forward.

At the age when babies begin to move about the crib while they sleep, parents sometimes become concerned about maintaining a back- or side-sleeping position. However, by the time your baby has learned to roll over (back to front or front to back) the risk of SIDS has decreased.

Some babies have medical conditions that require sleeping on their stomachs. If your baby's health care provider recommends this position, it's probably best to follow that advice. Remember that sleeping tummy-down has not been shown to cause SIDS; it is only one of the factors that may increase the risk of SIDS.

Bedding. Babies should sleep on a firm mattress, not a beanbag or water bed. Avoid thick, fluffy padding under the baby, such as lambskin or quilts. Soft bedding materials may cause your baby to sink in and have difficulty breathing.

Diet. Breastfeeding may reduce the risk of SIDS.

Secondhand Smoke. Provide a smoke-free environment for your baby. This measure is as important during your baby's first year of life as it was during pregnancy.

Room Temperature. Your baby doesn't need a warmer environment than you do. If the temperature in the house is comfortable for you, it should be comfortable for your baby.

What to Do If Your Infant Has a Seizure

Seizures can be frightening for a parent. You are bound to feel helpless, especially the first time.

Remember, in the vast majority of cases, the child is fine after the seizure. The instructions given here can help you deal with a seizure.

Febrile Seizure

If the infant with a fever has a seizure, the most important thing to remember is that the seizure usually stops by itself within several minutes. However, take steps to gradually bring down your baby's fever. Remove your baby's clothes and apply tepid cloths to the infant's head and chest. Sponge the torso with tepid water. Never sponge with alcohol. Do not put the infant in the bathtub during the seizure, because this can be dangerous.

If your baby begins to vomit during the seizure, place the child on his or her stomach or side, never on the back. If the child's breathing becomes labored, gently pull the jaw and chin forward by placing two fingers behind the corner of the jaw on each side. Don't reach inside the mouth.

After the seizure is over and your baby is awake, notify your physician, who will probably want to see the baby right away. If you are unable to contact your infant's health care provider, take your baby to a clinic or emergency room for examination.

Seizure Without Fever

The rules for handling this type of seizure are similar to those for a febrile seizure except that you do not have to worry about bringing down your baby's fever.

Do not try to move the baby or restrain any movements. Although the infant's breathing may stop for a moment, do not begin resuscitation; the child will begin breathing on his or her own. People are often concerned that someone in the midst of a seizure will somehow swallow or bite off his or her tongue. Although occasionally a child will bite the tongue, there is no way he or she will swallow it or inflict a severe injury. Keep your hands and other objects out of the baby's mouth.

Again, after the seizure has passed, call your baby's health care provider.

Electronic Monitoring. Electronic monitoring of heart rate and breathing may be useful in dealing with some infants at high risk for SIDS. It is still uncertain whether electronic monitoring has any protective value. Babies have died suddenly and unexpectedly even while being monitored. Monitoring cannot resuscitate your baby.

If you opt for electronic monitoring, special training will be required.

General Infant Care and Hygiene

Caring for your baby is certainly time-consuming, but it is not difficult.

One of the most important aspects of care falls under the realm of safety. Your infant—especially after he or she begins to crawl—is particularly susceptible to injury in the home. Thus, it is up to you to make certain that the child's environment is as safe as possible. This means childproofing your home and making sure that your infant's toys are both safe and appropriate for his or her stage of development. It also includes being diligent about the use of a car seat.

In this section, in addition to safety, we discuss diaper care and what steps you can take to minimize the spread of disease.

Safety

Making your home as safe as possible for your infant is imperative during these early months when your baby has no sense of danger.

How can you make your baby's environment safe?

First, start with the baby's bed. Since 1974, the federal government has required that the spaces between crib bars be no more than 2⅜ inches. This precaution is important because it prevents an infant from getting his or her head stuck between the bars. If you are using an old crib, make certain that the bars are spaced in accordance with these specifications. Moreover, make certain that the mattress fits the crib snugly, because babies have been known to get their heads caught in the space between the crib and the mattress. In either situation, a baby's breathing may be obstructed and he or she may die.

Make sure that any toys in the crib are soft, with no sharp edges that could hurt your baby. Remember to check stuffed animals for any loose buttons or parts that could find their way into a baby's mouth and cause choking.

As your baby grows older and begins to pull up on crib rails, be sure the rails are positioned at their full height and the mattress is

---

Lead Poisoning

For generations, lead was used in plumbing pipes and paint. It was also used in typesetting, in soldering, for sash weights in windows, and in numerous other products. Many older homes were painted with lead-based paint.

Today, we know that lead is poisonous. When ingested—whether in lead paint chips by children, in water supplies tainted by lead pipes, or in the air from auto emissions—lead can accumulate in the bone marrow, nerves, and kidneys.

In many cases, there are no symptoms of lead poisoning. However, such signs as irritability, weight loss, and sluggishness may occur, perhaps accompanied by vomiting, constipation, or stomach pain.

If you suspect lead poisoning in your child, consult your physician, who may recommend a change in your child's environment or diet or prescribe a medication to treat the lead poisoning.

Prevention

The best approach to prevention is to inspect your home for potential sources of lead—and to eliminate them. If you live in an older home and the paint is flaking off as dust, consult your local health department and have the paint dust tested. Older homes should also be checked to determine whether any of the pipes are lead. Look for the main line where the water pipe enters your house: if there is a swelling at one of the joints, gently tap it with a hammer. If it dents easily, it is made of lead and you should have your water tested to determine whether it contains lead.

Beware of old lead toys or jewelry and fishing or curtain weights—do not let your children play with them. Do not store juices in earthenware jars because the glazes may be lead-based.

at its lowest position. The top of the rail should extend at least to the height of your baby's chest. Also, remove bumper pads on which your baby might stand and topple over a rail. To prevent strangling, don't string toys of any kind across the top of crib rails.

Many parents have no qualms about putting a very young baby in the middle of a bed to nap. This practice can be dangerous because some infants will manage to roll off. If a crib is not available, put a blanket on the floor. The baby will be comfortable there. But select a location well away from stairs or adult "traffic."

An important safety rule is to never leave your infant unattended on a bed or table or in the bath. When bathing the baby, do not allow yourself to be distracted by the doorbell or telephone. Let it ring. All it takes is a second alone for a baby's head to become submerged under water.

Another rule applies to infant seats: do not put your baby in a seat perched on a table or counter. One slight move is often all it takes to tip the carrier and the infant off the table or counter.

As your infant becomes more mobile, your childproofing efforts will have to increase. If you have stairs in your home, make sure you have gates at the top and bottom of the stairway. Babies love to poke and prod, and electrical outlets are often a source of curiosity, so cover your unused outlets. You can purchase protective covers at many drugstores and at hardware and grocery stores that carry infant-related items.

An infant is forever mouthing anything he or she comes into contact with. Although it is impossible to keep the occasional bug or bit of dirt out of your baby's grasp, you must keep your child away from substances that can potentially cause harm. Make sure that all cleaning solutions, insecticides, and medications are stored well out of your infant's reach. If you do not have a high shelf or cupboard, you can buy locks that make it difficult for a child to open a cabinet.

Keep your baby well away from plastic bags. The soft material can quickly smother a baby.

Avoid scalds by lowering the temperature of the water heater in your dwelling. Check to be sure your baby's bathwater is not too hot. Don't drink hot beverages or foods, such as soup or coffee, while nursing your baby. Always check the temperature of any liquid you intend to give to your baby.

Equip your home with smoke and fire alarms in suitable locations, with fresh batteries or backup batteries if the devices are wired into your home's electrical system.

Check your houseplants. Be familiar with the toxic plants in and around your home, and make sure that they are well out of reach of your baby (see Garden-Variety Poisonous Plants, page 440).

Car Seats

Install a car seat in your car before your baby has his or her first ride home from the hospital. Read the instructions to know how to install and use the seat properly. In many hospitals, an infant will not be released to the parents unless they have a safety seat in their car. In all 50 states, the parent who does not strap a young child into a car seat is breaking the law.

If this rule seems extreme, consider the statistics. The major killer and crippler of young children in the United States is automobile accidents. Yet an estimated 80 percent of these deaths and serious injuries are thought to be avoidable if safety seats are correctly used.

When shopping for your car seat, make sure it meets government standards. Since 1981, all manufacturers have been required to meet stringent specifications set down by the federal government. Somewhere on the seat you should see an indication that the seat has met Federal Motor Vehicle Safety Standard 213, which includes crash testing.

Two types of car seats are suitable for infants.

An infant safety seat can only be installed so that the baby faces the rear of the car. This seat can be used until the child is about 1 year old or about 20 pounds.

Most parents find a convertible safety seat more practical because it can be used until the child weighs 40 pounds. During early infancy, the convertible seat is installed so that the baby faces the rear; later, when the infant is 1 year old or about 20 pounds, it can be turned around so that the infant faces the front of the car.

No matter what type of seat you purchase, it will not provide optimal protection unless it is used properly.

Here are tips on proper use of car seats:

- Install the seat in the back seat of the car, preferably in the middle.

- Make sure the seat belt is fastened securely around the car seat.
- Adjust the harness straps so that they fit snugly, and fasten all parts of the harness.
- If the seat has a top anchor strap, make sure it is installed.
- Don't install the car seat on a seat equipped with an air bag.

Always use the car seat. Even if you are just going a block down the road, do not assume your baby will be safe unless he or she is securely fastened in the seat. For more information about car seats, see page 23.

Safe Toys

Like the older child, your infant needs toys to keep him or her amused and stimulated and to learn. The key is finding appropriate toys—your 5-year-old's marbles and jacks could have disastrous consequences in the hands of a 6-month-old.

Always be on the lookout for toys that could be hazardous. Do not give an infant toys that contain small pieces that can easily be swallowed. Keep anything made of a material that can be broken, such as glass, away from your baby. Avoid toys with sharp edges or loose buttons. Discard objects painted with a lead-based paint, because an infant gnawing on the toy can ingest enough lead to cause lead poisoning.

During the first 3 months, your baby needs toys that can be looked at (he or she is not yet adept at grasping). Babies prefer patterns over solids and bright colors over pastels. Buy a colorful mobile, one whose full impact is seen from the baby's position and not from the parent's upright view. Interesting pictures on the wall can capture a baby's attention. A mirror attached to the side of the crib, a music box or tape recorder playing a soothing lullaby, colorful plastic shapes hung on strings suspended between the crib rails, rattles your baby can shake, furry stuffed animals with which you can stroke the baby—these are all good toys for the young infant. They serve to stimulate your infant and promote interaction.

By the end of the fourth month, most babies have mastered the ability to grasp and can swipe at objects, although they often miss. At this age, your baby can appreciate rattles, clacking disks, and stuffed animals.

At 6 months, a baby's greatest pleasure is putting things in his or her mouth. Teething rings, cloth dolls, squeeze toys, and kitchen objects such as measuring spoons, plastic cups, and bowls are good toys. For the older infant, a riding toy such as a small car is often a source of enjoyment, as are balls, blocks, and toy telephones.

When buying toys, read the description on the box to determine whether a toy is appropriate. Most major toy manufacturers indicate on the packaging the age range for which the toy is intended.

Swings, Jumpers, and Walkers

These devices were all designed to give a baby increased mobility while freeing the parent to tend to other tasks. However, they don't live up to their original intention. All of these "toys" need direct and attentive supervision because they can be dangerous.

By 4 months, your baby is probably outgrowing an infant swing. A baby who can wiggle, scoot, and shift can possibly topple out of a swing.

Jumpers that hang on a doorway should always be positioned so the baby's toes barely touch the floor. The baby's heels should not touch the floor. A baby in a jumper should always be supervised. Injuries can occur if the jumper falls or the baby pinches fingers between the jumper and door frame.

Walkers have caused countless injuries and should not be used. Although parents often believe that using a walking will speed a baby's walking abilities, this simply isn't true. In fact, the use of a walker often robs the baby of time to crawl and walk alone.

Walker injuries include pinches and falls. And walkers are especially dangerous because their use can result in a severe accident, such as a fall down a flight of stairs. Although many parents use child gates to help prevent such falls, gates can unintentionally be left unlatched in the midst of a busy day. A walker is one piece of baby gear you don't need.

Comfortable Clothing

When buying clothes for your infant, remember that what is important to your baby is comfort. In general, your newborn needs about one layer more of clothing than you have on.

Is the material soft? Does it feel good to the touch? Is it loose enough for the baby to move about in without feeling constrained? Does your baby appear to be comfortable? For your convenience and the baby's, is it easy to put on and take off?

In planning your infant's wardrobe, remember to buy larger sizes than your baby's age suggests. For example, most newborns can easily wear clothes made for a 3-month-old. And many 6-month-olds may be large enough to wear 9-month or even 12-month sizes. In the same vein, do not stock up on one particular size. Babies grow at an astonishing rate during the first year, and parents who buy too many clothes often end up with a drawer full of unopened packages.

The following are some basic guidelines for dressing your infant:

Knitted Nightgowns and Stretchies. In the first 2 or 3 months it is often easier to dress your baby the same during the day as you do at night. Knitted nightgowns and stretchies (which are usually made of a soft terry cloth material or cotton) are perfect for sleep and wakeful periods. Because many babies virtually live in these clothes, you should have several of each.

Underclothes. There are two styles of undershirts: shirts that are pulled over the baby's head and shirts with a snap closing, which are usually easier to use on a very young baby. Buy three or four in at least a 6-month size for the young infant.

Socks. Buy several pairs. Booties, while cute, are not needed and often do not stay on. Shoes are not necessary until the infant begins to walk.

Sweaters. During cool weather, you may find that your baby needs a sweater for extra warmth over the stretchie. Usually made of acrylic, a sweater should fit loosely around the neck.

Outerwear. If you are taking your baby out in cold weather, he or she will need some type of snowsuit or bunting. A bunting—a zippered bag in which the baby is encased up to the shoulders—is fine for the very young baby. However, once the infant is several months old, he or she will prefer the freedom of a snowsuit. The baby also will need a cap that fits snugly over the ears. If the baby is going to be in the sun, a sun hat is great for protecting his or her skin.

Bibs. Once your infant begins to eat solids, make sure you buy several bibs. Forget the dainty little round bibs. You need bibs large enough to cover the entire front of your infant. Bibs made of plastic are good because they can be rinsed off.

Other Clothes. Once your infant begins to move around, you will probably want to begin dressing him or her more for play and less for sleep. Jeans, cotton overalls with snaps along the legs and crotch, and knit pants and shirts are good choices. When the weather is warm, sunsuits, shorts, and T-shirts are appropriate clothing.

Diaper Care

Stringent care of the diaper area will help prevent diaper rash, a problem affecting most babies at least once during their diaper-wearing years. Follow the key preventive steps given below.

Check your infant's diaper frequently and change it if it is wet or soiled. In a 1-month-old infant, this sometimes means changing the baby before and after feeding. In the 10-month-old baby, it may entail checking every 2 or 3 hours.

After you remove a wet diaper, rinse the baby's bottom with a wet washcloth or an unscented diaper wipe. When changing a soiled diaper, make certain you clean the area thoroughly. On a boy, pay particular attention to the scrotum; on a girl, gently wipe from front to back.

Disposable diapers currently are used widely and are convenient in our mobile society. There is, however, increasing discussion of the fact that disposable diapers are not biodegradable and contribute significantly to the growing problems with managing solid waste and other garbage. As a result, we are beginning to see a renaissance in the use of cloth diapers.

The choice is up to you. In deciding on cloth versus disposable diapers, consider factors such as the cost, convenience, and impact on the environment.

Preventing the Spread of Disease

Once one member of the family contracts an infectious disease such as a cold, preventing others in the household from catching the infection is often difficult.

The following simple measures could reduce the spread of some infectious diseases in your home:

- Hand washing is the most important thing you can do to help reduce the spread of disease. After changing your infant's diaper, using the bathroom yourself, or blowing your nose or wiping your baby's nose, make sure you thoroughly wash your hands with soap and water.

- Avoid touching your mouth and nose.
- Never smoke at home. (Children who breathe tobacco smoke have a higher incidence of respiratory infection.)
- Use a disinfectant in the kitchen, bathroom, family room, and nursery and on your infant's playthings (see Child Care Centers, page 101).

Development of Personality and Behavior

During the first 12 months of life, your baby works harder than at any other stage of his or her existence. In the course of this incredible first year, your infant goes from being totally dependent to walking, feeding himself or herself, and even speaking a few words. Bonds are formed, a routine is established, and, at some point early in the year, the parent notices a distinct personality emerging.

In this section, we examine normal development and we review milestones to look for. We also offer advice on handling sleeping problems that may arise.

Normal Developmental Milestones

A momentous occasion during the early weeks of life is your baby's first smile. Although you often will see a smile on your newborn, an infant generally does not have what is called a social smile until after the first month, usually by the eighth week.

By the time your infant is 6 weeks old, he or she may be showing a clear preference for family members over strangers. Smile at your infant and he or she may smile back. Watch your infant gaze at you intently while he or she is eating.

The infant at 2 months smiles with his or her entire body. Watch your baby when you walk into his or her room. Your baby begins flailing both arms and legs in excitement. He or she gurgles and coos.

Your response to your infant's smiles during these early weeks is important. When you cuddle your infant, smile, coo, or attend to his or her needs, you encourage the smiles.

By the second month of life, your baby can differentiate people from objects, with the former eliciting a much more immediate response. Your infant is beginning to recognize your voice. Thus, you may find that the baby who screams when with a babysitter calms immediately when a parent enters the room and talks in a soothing voice.

The infant at 3 months can play for perhaps 10 or 15 minutes at a time, with minimal parental involvement. The infant at this age is more easily distracted and will even interrupt nursing to look at or listen to something that catches his or her attention. The baby will spend time staring at things—a picture, a mobile, or his or her own hand.

You may notice that your baby's memory seems to improve with each passing day. At this point, the infant may associate certain acts with rewards—for example, the sound of the refrigerator door closing and your footsteps with feeding. The baby may wait patiently for a moment or two anticipating your arrival. Should that arrival be delayed by a ringing telephone, he or she may erupt in a howl.

At 4 months your infant may be less interested in feeding than in the world around him or her. Hence, do not be surprised if it takes longer than usual to finish a feeding.

A milestone during this period—usually at around 20 weeks—is your baby's behavior in front of a mirror. Hold him or her in front of the mirror and watch the infant smile. When the image smiles back, the baby will get really excited and begin to babble. It will puzzle him or her to see two of you and he or she will repeatedly look back at you and then at the mirror.

At 5 months your baby definitely knows the difference between his or her parents and strangers. For the first time, you may notice a real fear of strangers.

At this age, your infant has learned to identify and find objects. For example, if a toy drops to the floor, your infant will try to find it. Similarly, he or she will play with a stuffed animal, lay it down, and later come back to it.

A 6-month-old infant is alert for half of his or her waking hours.

If you are bottle-feeding, your baby may insist on trying to hold the bottle. That's OK, but don't simply "prop" the bottle in his or her mouth. Some babies at this age are ready to start using a cup in conjunction with a bottle.

By this age, solid foods may be a part of the diet. Gone are the days when your baby was content to have you do the feeding. Now that the infant's dexterity is improved, he or she wants to pick up pieces of food and put them in his or her own mouth and anywhere else mood dictates.

Increased motor skills give the infant of 7 months a taste of freedom. At the same time that your baby longs to test his or her wings, however, the infant only wants to do it within sight of your reassuring presence. Do not be surprised if every time you leave the room your baby cries. The infant who has been content up until now to spend time in a playpen may suddenly rebel unless you are in the same room.

The infant of this age loves to mouth things. Chewing on fingers, sucking a thumb, and nibbling toes are very satisfying activities. During feedings, the baby may be able to grasp a spoon.

The 8-month-old baby is clearly attached to the parent providing most of his or her care—generally the mother. Separation anxiety often occurs at this age, and you may find that you cannot leave the room without sending your baby into a panic. The baby who previously was not bothered by strangers suddenly may fear the next-door neighbor or even a grandparent. Or, the infant may cry uncontrollably when the babysitter arrives, even when the caregiver is someone the baby knows. This reaction is a normal part of development and is nothing to be concerned about. Cuddle your child and reassure him or her that you will return soon. Build trust.

Don't sneak out; always tell your infant you're leaving and will return.

The infant at 9 months is sophisticated enough to be bored. This is because his or her memory is more developed. Thus, the infant is constantly searching for new stimulation, and the nightly game that has amused him or her for the past month suddenly has become uninteresting.

Another stage to expect around this time is insecurity and even fears. Every time you turn on the vacuum cleaner your baby begins to cry. Or one day the beloved bath is shunned out of fear. With a little patience and understanding on your part, these fears usually are conquered within a month or so.

The 10-month-old is capable of carrying two small objects in one hand.

During this time your baby's sense of identity within your family is emerging. His or her moods become more apparent. Scold your baby, and he or she looks sad; praise your infant, and he or she beams. Watch your child smack his or her lips after a good meal or light up when your spouse comes in the door after work.

Your baby may begin to say "no" at this age. Your child also is developing a sense of possession and may for the first time distinguish between baby's toys and those belonging to a sibling.

You also will notice how imitation plays a role in your infant's learning. During a meal, the baby may offer you bits of food; afterward he or she may attempt to wash your face and hands.

Although not always cooperative, your 11-month-old baby seeks your approval and will try to avoid your disapproval. Still, the infant cannot avoid trying to test your authority. After you have put your son or daughter to bed, he or she may summon you every 5 minutes. At the same time, your every request is apt to be met with a resounding "no." At this age, "no" sometimes means "yes."

This negativism increases in the 12-month-old baby. Some infants at this age begin to have tantrums; you should expect refusals (see Tantrums and Breath Holding, page 92). Appetite naturally begins to decrease, so do not be surprised when your eager eater suddenly becomes picky. This refusal also may extend to bedtime. Sleep problems are common at this age.

If you are concerned that your infant is not achieving these developmental milestones, see your child's physician.

Sleep Concerns

Parents often find their babies' sleeping habits confusing. Like adults, babies vary in their sleep needs: some get by on very little, while others need more. Babies do not get their sleep in long blocks of time. Newborns frequently sleep for short periods followed by fussing and crying. This goes on day and night. They do not know the difference between night and day. Many new parents do not realize the impact sleep disruption will have on their lives.

Sleep is divided into active and quiet sleep. REM (so named because of rapid eye movements) is the sleep when dreaming takes place and is the lighter sleep. In the REM phase, the baby can easily be awakened. During this lighter sleep, babies may toss and turn, suck, and gurgle in their sleep. This is normal in the early months because newborns have more of this lighter sleep than the quiet, deep sleep. Deeper sleep or quiet sleep is referred to as non-REM sleep. As babies mature, they begin to have more quiet sleep like adults have.

Parents are frequently asked, "Is your baby sleeping through the night yet?" They begin to suspect something is wrong with their baby because he or she is not. Because of the baby's small stomach, you can expect at least two night feedings during the first few months. Try not to be impatient for the baby to reach this milestone of sleeping throughout the night. Sleeping through the night is defined as a 5- to 6-hour stretch somewhere from midnight to 6 a.m. The time that this is accomplished varies from baby to baby but may begin at about 3 months of age. Through the entire first few years, there will be many nights of interrupted sleep from teething, illness, or bad dreams.

Place your newborn infant on his or her back or side. Lying on the stomach is a risk factor for sudden infant death syndrome (see Sudden Infant Death Syndrome, page 69).

Other parental concerns about sleep focus on getting the baby to sleep. Early on it is helpful to establish nighttime routines or rituals. Some ways to get your baby to sleep or calm him or her at the end of the day are as follows:

- Limit stimulation at the end of the day and make sure your baby has had enough stimulation during the day. Start to tone down about an hour before bedtime.
- Talking softly, singing, or reading are nice bedtime rituals to establish early on.
- Some babies settle down after a bath, but others are overstimulated by this activity.
- Rocking and gently swaying are very helpful in calming a baby. Babies like to be rocked in a side-to-side, hammock motion, not a swinging motion.
- Your baby will welcome soothing sounds such as background music, tapes of womb sounds, nature sounds, or lullabies.
- A night-light in the room may help relax your baby.
- Some newborns like to be swaddled, but others do not.
- Some babies sleep better in the family bed. It seems to help newborns organize their sleep patterns.

As a new parent, you need to identify and understand all the issues that may influence your newborn's sleep patterns. It will take time and patience to achieve a balance between meeting your newborn's needs and your own requirements for restful sleep.

Sibling Relationships

If your infant has a brother or sister, he or she is indeed fortunate. Much attention has been devoted to sibling rivalry—the hostilities and insecurities aroused in the older child by the birth of a baby (see page 105). But what about the infant and its relationship with big brother or sister?

Granted, life is not always cozy for the infant with a sibling. This baby is apt to be poked and jabbed more than once, especially as he or she becomes more mobile. On the positive side, watch your 5-month-old's delight when he or she is included in a game with an older sibling. Play with a sibling is so rewarding for the baby that he or she is willing to put up with even a little roughness. Of course, you have to monitor the play and make sure your infant is not endangered.

Besides the simple enjoyment of having a brother or sister to play with, the baby develops mentally and socially from this exposure to an older child. The infant learns self-protection, cooperation, imagination, and how to get along with others. Moreover, the bond between your children is developed and they grow to love each other.

Do not feel guilty that your second and subsequent children do not get undivided attention as did your first child. Remember, your first child did not reap the benefits of an older brother or sister. There will be times when your baby actually prefers a brother or sister over you, or when a sibling's request that baby eat his or her cereal is immediately granted—whereas your efforts were met with resolute rejection.

Look for creative ways to involve older brothers or sisters in caring for the baby. Make a special effort to give your older children individual attention, too. They need to understand that you care about them as much as you care about the baby.

Be prepared for the "low point" in family relationships. It often occurs about 2 months after the baby's arrival. The novelty of a new baby is gone, and so have your helpers. You and your partner may be entertaining second thoughts about the responsibilities and com-

mitments that accompany the arrival of yet another family member. Siblings may have tired of tolerating changes in their lifestyles. You may find it increasingly difficult to plan anything.

Discuss these common emotions with your partner, then persevere. More predictable sleep patterns are on the horizon and things will begin to fall into place again soon.

This is not to imply that relationships will always be smooth. At around 9 months, some babies have trouble getting along with a sibling who only weeks before was an object of admiration. Babies this age are intent on battling their own insecurities and fears. An older sibling who loves to tease or assert authority is just too much sometimes. If this happens to your infant, do not worry. The stage will pass.

Your Infant's Nutrition

One of the important decisions you will be making during your baby's first year regards nutrition. Which is preferable—bottle-feeding or breastfeeding? When should I wean the baby? When is the best time to introduce solids? These are questions on every parent's mind.

Feeding Recommendations

During your infant's first year of life, his or her birthweight may triple. It should come as no surprise, then, that eating will be an important part of your baby's day.

In the first few months of life, your baby's nutrition consists solely of breast milk or formula. Evaporated milk or cow's milk should not be substituted for formula because cow's milk does not provide proper nutrition for young babies. Do not give your baby cow's milk until the infant is 12 months old, unless directed by your physician.

In hot weather, you might offer your baby more frequent feedings to satisfy thirst. Usually babies don't need extra vitamins or water; if in doubt ask your health care provider.

The frequency of feedings depends on your baby's needs and the method of feeding.

A baby between 1 and 3 months old probably will want between five and six feedings a day, eventually eating every 3 hours, except for a longer stretch at night. As the baby grows, the number of feedings is reduced. Typically, a 5-month-old is down to four or five feedings, and by 9 months the child has only three milk feedings. Remember, each infant is a distinct individual. Accept differences in feeding behavior.

Breastfed infants may require more frequent feedings because breast milk is so efficiently digested. Also, more frequent nursing stimulates the availability of breast milk. During the first 3 months some infants want to nurse for comfort as well as for nutrition.

Parents always ask when they should offer their baby solids. This is a difficult question and one that has no shortage of opinions. From a nutritional standpoint, your baby gets everything he or she needs from breast milk or formula for the first 6 months. Yet many health care providers recommend starting babies, particularly formula-fed babies, on solids after 4 months. Moreover, if your infant is nursing more often rather than less, your health care provider may recommend an early introduction to solids.

Before you introduce your baby to solids, consult your health care provider. He or she will be able to tell you whether the child is developmentally ready to handle solid foods. For example, for several months the neuro-muscular development of infants is geared only toward sucking and swallowing liquids. Until the child has the ability to recognize a spoon and his or her tongue and swallowing mechanisms can respond to solid food—usually around 6 months—the infant is not ready to expand his or her diet.

Before 4 to 6 months, your baby's gastrointestinal system may be unable to absorb solids efficiently. Also, your baby may be unable to sit up or hold his or her head erect for feedings.

Once the decision to start solids is made, what foods should you introduce? Many health care providers recommend starting the baby on a cereal. Precooked rice cereal (found in the baby food section of the supermarket) is often used as baby's first solid food because it is easy to digest. Mix a small amount (1 tablespoon) of cereal with 4 or 5 tablespoons of formula or breast milk. Initially, babies generally respond better to solids if the solid foods are thin rather than thick. Put some food on the tip of a small spoon and place it in your baby's mouth. Do not be surprised if it comes back out. Many babies take time to adjust to this new taste and consistency. Be patient. Do not put solids in a bottle or a syringe-type feeder; the former can encourage your baby to overeat, and the latter can cause choking.

You have two options in feeding your baby: buy commercial baby food or prepare your own. Commercial food may be more convenient, but it is more expensive and may contain fillers or sugars, which add empty calories.

Making your own baby food is not difficult if you have a blender or food grinder. Cook meats, vegetables, and fruits (bananas do not need to be cooked) in a small amount of water. Remove fat, skin, and seeds and then puree the mixture in the blender until it is a suitable consistency. A little water aids in the blending process. Fresh fruits and vegetables are best. If you cannot obtain them, select frozen produce. Don't add sugar or salt to your baby's foods.

After your baby is acquainted with cereal, your next step might be a fruit, such as pureed bananas, or a vegetable.

At 8 months, most infants are ready to try pureed meats, but breast milk or formula continues to provide ample amounts of protein. After 8 months most babies are able to eat small pieces of table food. Toast, bits of cheese, pieces of scrambled egg, dry cereals, crackers, mashed potato, and well-cooked pasta are good finger foods.

Avoid foods that could choke your baby. These include hot dogs, grapes, popcorn, nuts, raisins, and raw carrots.

Some general rules are these:

- Introduce new foods as tolerated.
- Avoid seasoning, especially salt, and desserts.
- Do not force your baby to eat. Spitting the food out, putting a hand over his or her mouth, turning his or her head, or fussing are all indications that your infant's appetite has been satisfied.

How much food should your baby be eating? By the time the infant is between 6 and 8 months old, he or she should be eating 3 to 4 ounces of solids at each of the three meals, or between 5 and 8 tablespoons of food per meal. A good diet for an infant of this age would be, for example, cereal and fruit for breakfast, cereal or fruit and vegetable for lunch, and cereal, fruit, and vegetable for supper. Although patterns vary widely, many babies eating this diet reduce their milk consumption to about 16 ounces a day. Many babies also need a mid-morning and mid-afternoon snack, which should be something nutritious such as a fruit or yogurt.

In your baby's second 6 months, you may need to increase feedings with cereal to meet his or her needs for an adequate supply of iron. Sometimes a baby's diet needs to be supplemented with vitamins and minerals (see table, page 80). Consult your health care provider.

Once your child reaches his or her first birthday, the infant probably will be eating table food exclusively.

A note of caution: never allow your infant to have food away from your supervision.

Feeding Problems

Several feeding problems can be encountered during the first year of life. If your baby is not growing adequately or seems to be gaining an excessive amount of weight, is colicky,

Vitamin and Mineral Supplements for Infants

Type of Feeding	Iron	Vitamin D	Fluoride	Other
Breast	Additional iron from a supplement or an iron-fortified infant cereal is needed after 6 months of age	Supplementation may be recommended if the infant has little exposure to sunlight	Supplementation may be recommended based on the fluoride content of the water supply	None
Formula	Supplementation is needed by 4 months of age if the formula does not contain iron	No supplementation needed	Supplementation is recommended for infants receiving ready-to-feed formulas, and it may be recommended for powdered formulas, based on the fluoride content of the water supply	None
Cow's milk plus solid food (after 1 year of age)	Additional iron from a supplement or from an iron-fortified infant cereal is needed	No supplementation needed	Supplementation may be recommended	None

From *Mayo Clinic Diet Manual*, seventh edition, 1994. By permission of Mayo Foundation.

is constipated, or has frequent diarrhea, consult your physician. A change in formula or in the amount the baby is fed may be all that is necessary to eliminate the problem.

Common feeding problems are described here.

Underfeeding

A baby who is not getting enough to eat does not gain weight on schedule, is frequently restless, and cries often. The baby also may be constipated and have wrinkled, dry skin as a result of the loss of fat (see Failure to Gain Weight, page 63).

Although the vast majority of women can successfully breastfeed, sometimes the infant may not nurse well enough to be satisfied. This problem is often temporary, and most women are encouraged to continue breastfeeding. Check with your lactation consultant or health care provider for help with breastfeeding assessment and recommendations.

For bottle-fed infants who do not eat enough, sometimes the problem is solved by enlarging the holes in the bottle nipple. You also can try increasing the number of feedings.

If these measures fail, your health care provider will want to determine whether an underlying disease may be causing the problem.

Overfeeding

A baby who eats too much or too often may have excessive regurgitation or even vomiting. Excessive weight gain, irritability, restlessness, abdominal pain, and bloating are other symptoms of overfeeding.

Unlike adults, most babies stop eating when they have had enough. However, a parent who offers the bottle every time the infant cries, is overzealous in pushing solids, or rewards an older baby with food may contribute to overeating.

Chapter 3

Preschool Years:
Ages 1 Through 5

Contents

A Time of Rapid Change, 82

Growth and Development, 82
Your 1-Year-Old, 82
Your 2-Year-Old, 83
Your 3-Year-Old, 83
    Growth Disorders, 83
Your 4-Year-Old, 84
Your 5-Year-Old, 84

Common Concerns During the Preschool
Years, 84
Signs of Illness, 84
    Warning Signs of Serious Illness, 86
Common and Recurrent Colds, 86
Constipation and Diarrhea, 87
Toilet Training, 88
Teething Problems, 89
Swallowing Objects, 90
Eye Problems, 90
Sleep Problems, 90
Fears and Phobias, 91
Tantrums and Breath Holding, 92
Walking and Falling, 92
Speech and Language Development, 92
    Stuttering, 93
Urinary Tract Infections, 94
Orthopedic Concerns, 95

General Care, 97
Disease Prevention, 98
Diaper Care, 98
Safety at Home and Play, 99

Car Safety, 100
Caring for Your Child's Teeth, 101
Child Care Centers, 101

Psychosocial Development of Personality
and Behavior, 102
Behavioral Development, 103
Negativism, 104
Imagination, 105
Sibling Problems, 105
Thumb and Finger Sucking, 106
Delayed Psychomotor Development, 106
Learning Problems, 106
    Infantile Autism, 108
Mental Retardation, 108
Sexuality in Your Preschool Child, 109
Sexual Abuse, 109
    Child Abuse, 110

Care of Your Handicapped Child, 110
Treat All Your Children Alike, 111
Be Aware of Your Attitude, 111
Do Not Neglect Your Other Children, 111
Accept Your Child's Individuality, 111
Do Not Isolate Your Child, 111
Address Special Needs, 111
You Are Not Alone, 111

Nutrition, 112
Nutrition in Your Preschool Child, 112
    The Balanced Diet for Your Preschool Child, 113
Obesity, 113

A Time of Rapid Change

It may seem like only yesterday that you held your baby for the first time. After 9 long months, the waiting was over when your physician handed you a bundle of energy, tiny and helpless and giving little hint of what he or she would become.

With each passing day a bit of the mystery was revealed—perhaps dark hair from the father's side or the mother's eyes or maybe a preference for rice cereal over oat cereal or for fruits instead of vegetables. Little by little, step by step, you became acquainted.

Now, having celebrated your baby's first birthday, you have a better idea of who this little person is. Although it has been only 365 days—barely enough time to alter your appearance at all—the changes in your baby have been phenomenal. Even so, most of the story of the development of your child has yet to be written. This chapter discusses changes you will see in your child from ages 1 through 5 years.

If you are the parent of a preschooler, you occasionally may have entertained thoughts of taking a permanent vacation. These years can be trying. Preschoolers are demanding and can consume your energy. Caught between wanting to "do it myself" yet longing for the safety net that only a parent can provide, preschoolers are often at odds with themselves and with everything that gets in their way.

Negativism, anxieties over monsters hiding under beds, temper tantrums, toilet training, and discovering the genitals are among the issues during ages 1 through 5.

Helping to offset these often difficult issues are the amazing developmental changes that occur during this time. Your 12-month-old who knows a handful of words grows into the 2-year-old who proudly recites the ABCs and then becomes the 3-year-old capable of carrying on a conversation. This virtual explosion of language is indeed exciting for a parent, as is the determination with which many children this age approach a new task. Watch your child struggle to master a new toy or task. Even a temperamental 2-year-old will usually give it a good try before, out of frustration and disappointment, he or she bursts into a tantrum.

In this chapter we look at common problems such as toilet training, recurring colds and infections, and general care. We devote a large segment to the psychosocial development of children in this age group. Elsewhere in this book (primarily in Part IV, Human Diseases and Disorders) you will find discussions of most of the disorders that commonly occur in this age group.

If the theme of this chapter can be boiled down into a single thought, it should be "enjoy these years." They are special. Although some days may seem endless when your life appears to revolve around temper tantrums and getting your child to the bathroom before an accident occurs, the time will pass quickly. Ask any parent whose children have moved beyond this stage. These are years to be savored.

Growth and Development

Your 1-Year-Old

The rapid weight gain of the first year levels off during the second, with an average gain of 5 to 6 pounds. Your child's physical changes involve a transition from the plumpness of babyhood to the leaner and more muscular body of a toddler.

This is an exciting time for you and your baby. Your 1-year-old begins to walk and talk. These skills, combined with a will of his

or her own and a tentative sense of independence, produce a determined explorer.

Even though your 1-year-old does not have a large vocabulary, he or she develops an increasing ability to understand language. This so-called passive language lays the groundwork for the virtual explosion of language that occurs between ages 2 and 3. The average 18-month-old probably uses only about 10 words, but within a year he or she has a significant vocabulary and can speak in simple sentences. A child of this age is constantly exploring by touching, holding, climbing, and mouthing. Your 1-year-old will leave no wastebasket unturned nor drawer unemptied. Every corner is investigated. Safety becomes vitally important; you must baby-proof your 1-year-old's world (see page 99).

playing side by side with children their age. As your child approaches age 3, he or she will become more interested in socializing.

Your 2-year-old child is a great imitator. If you rake the lawn, your 2-year-old may want to follow behind with a toy rake. Or, your child will insist on his or her own broom and dustpan when you are cleaning house.

Your 2-Year-Old

At 2 years most children begin to communicate verbally. At some point after reaching 2 years, most children can tell you their name and the names of common objects. They can speak in three- to four-word sentences and even carry on brief conversations.

Two-year-olds are most famous for negative behavior. Temper tantrums—often out of frustration—are common (see Tantrums and Breath Holding, page 92).

Most 2-year-olds do not actively play with other children. Rather, they enjoy

Your 3-Year-Old

Your 3-year-old is more coordinated than he or she was at age 2. By age 3, most children can climb stairs with alternating feet, although most cannot descend in the same manner until age 4. A 3-year-old also can stand briefly on one foot.

Your 3-year-old's vocabulary and pronunciation continue to expand. A 3-year-old can tell you his or her age and sex, and crudely imitate simple drawings.

Emotionally, your 3-year-old loves his or her parents and wants to be just like them.

Growth Disorders

Children vary widely in height and weight during their preschool years. If you look at a growth chart, your child may fall in the bottom range for his or her age, in the middle, or near the top. Your child's size generally depends on heredity; large parents are more likely to have a large child, and small parents typically have small children. Most children fall somewhere within the normal range (5th to 95th percentile) for weight and height (see height and weight charts, page 117).

So how do you know whether your child is "abnormal"? If your child is either substantially below or substantially above the range, there may be a problem.

There are many types of growth disorders, the most common of which we discuss here.

Nutritional Deficiencies

The most common nutritional disorder in children in the United States is obesity (see page 113). Malnutrition, although less common, also occurs frequently, especially among lower socioeconomic groups. Malnutrition can be the result of diseases such as cystic fibrosis (see page 720) and celiac disease (see Malabsorption Problems, page 770).

Hormonal Disorders

Sometimes the pituitary or thyroid gland produces an insufficient or an excess amount of hormones, the result of which can be a growth disorder. These rare disorders include gigantism and dwarfism (see Pituitary Gland Disorders, page 941) and hypothyroidism (see page 948).

Chronic Disease

Children with diseases such as congenital heart disorders (see page 51), chronic kidney failure (see page 854), and anemia (see Anemias, page 956) also may have impaired growth.

What to Do

If you suspect a growth disorder, take your child to the physician. Depending on the physical findings, your physician may need to do diagnostic tests, including blood tests and X-ray studies.

Again, treatment depends on the specific problem. An obese child may be placed on a diet, whereas one who is malnourished may need high-calorie supplements and even hospitalization. Injections of the deficient hormone may help children with growth disorders due to a hormone deficiency.

Identification with these powerful role models is important in laying the foundation for your child's character.

Your 4-Year-Old

A child of 4 speaks well enough for strangers to understand him or her, and sentences become increasingly complex.

The imagination of a child this age is vivid, and the line between what is real and what is imaginary often becomes indistinct.

Some children at this age or even younger develop fears. Common fears of the 4-year-old include the fear of death, animals, and the dark.

Your 5-Year-Old

A child of 5 is generally able to hop on one foot and even skip, can accurately copy figures such as a triangle, and continues to develop language skills.

Children this age have the coordination required to write, and many have learned to do so. Moreover, it is not uncommon for 5-year-olds to begin reading before starting school.

Your 5-year-old is a social person. Unlike the younger child, when given a choice between spending time with his or her parents or the afternoon with a friend, a 5-year-old child will almost invariably choose the friend.

Common Concerns During the Preschool Years

How do you know whether your fussy 1-year-old is sick or is simply having a bad day? Is it normal for a preschooler to have repeated colds? What is the best way to toilet train your resistant 3-year-old? How should you handle your 2-year-old's daily temper tantrums?

These are just a few of the common concerns expressed by parents of young children.

We consider a wide range of these concerns in this section.

Signs of Illness

As many parents can attest, preschoolers do get sick with amazing frequency. Some months you seem to be caught in a revolving door between home and your physician's office. No sooner is an ear infection cleared up than your child develops a cold. Before you know it, you are back to see your physician.

Most parents are understandably concerned when their young child seems to fall prey to every virus that hits the block. In the back of your mind, you may wonder whether there is something wrong—a serious underlying illness—that is interfering with your child's ability to fight these infections.

Almost always, these fears are groundless. If your child is active and gaining weight,

there is probably nothing wrong with his or her health. It is a simple fact that young children are particularly susceptible to colds, ear infections, and gastrointestinal viruses. Your child's immune system must be exposed to many viruses before it fully develops its own resistance. Moreover, your child's habits, alone and with others, ensure this exposure. The way young children play and relate is not geared toward avoiding germs. A 2-year-old with a runny nose does not worry about germs before handing a toy to a friend. A cold will not stop a 4-year-old from offering a bite of his or her cookie to a friend.

It is no wonder that the average preschooler has seven or eight colds a year and two or three bouts of intestinal flu. These illnesses may also provide means for our bodies to learn to recognize and fight infections. Many illnesses are actually better tolerated by a young child than by an adult. For example, chickenpox is a common and usually well-tolerated illness of childhood, whereas an adult who develops chickenpox may have a more serious illness. So, some of these illnesses not only may be common but also are an important, normal part of growing up.

In addition to the frequency of minor illness, another common concern is how to tell whether your child is ill. Unlike an older child, a 1-year-old does not have the verbal abilities to communicate distress beyond a cry or crankiness. And even though your 5-year-old can certainly tell you whether he or she is sick, your child may not be able to articulate anything more specific.

Keep in mind that certain common ailments tend to be seasonal in children, as in adults. Thus, if your child seems ill in late winter, the cause may be the flu (see Influenza, page 1065). By the same token, chickenpox is most likely to strike in the spring; colds, ear infections, and croup in the winter; and certain viral infections, including meningitis, in the late summer or fall.

Some signs that will help you to determine whether your child is ill are described below. Keep in mind, however, that there is often no substitute for a parent's intuition. Many parents simply sense that something is wrong with their child even before the child develops a fever or other symptoms. In the absence of obvious symptoms, trust your instincts. You will be surprised how frequently you are on target.

Fever

A fever is a rectal temperature of more than 101 degrees Fahrenheit or an oral temperature of more than 100 degrees Fahrenheit (see How to Take a Temperature and How to Read a Thermometer, page 1072). A fever is one of the body's ways of fighting infection. It is not automatically a cause for alarm, nor does it necessarily need to be lowered.

Children tolerate fever better than adults. If your child is responsive, continues to drink fluids, and wants to play, there probably is nothing to worry about. If you think your child will be more comfortable with a lower fever, you can use acetaminophen to help reduce it.

Extra fluids, minimal clothing, and, perhaps, a sponge bath with tepid water also may help. Do not use aspirin to lower the fever of a viral illness in children, because aspirin has been possibly linked to Reye's syndrome, a potentially life-threatening illness (see Reye's Syndrome, page 484). Some medical experts believe that aggressively lowering all fevers actually will blunt the body's immune response and possibly prolong some illnesses.

Decreased Appetite

Your sick child often will not feel like eating. This is a normal response and nothing to worry about. However, even though it is not important that your child eat normal meals during an illness, an adequate fluid intake is important (although the risk of dehydration is very low in most minor illnesses). Do not insist that your child eat, but do try to coax him or her to drink liquids, whether in the form of water, juices, ice pops, or clear soups.

Increased Sleep

Another sign of illness may be that your child seems to be sleeping more than usual. This too is one way your child's body fights infection and speeds recovery. If, however, it becomes difficult to arouse your child or if your child appears to be confused and drowsy when awake, call your physician.

Lethargy

Surprisingly, even children with high fevers can have much energy. However, if your child is lethargic, does not respond to you, or is limp and uninterested in playing or anything else, this is cause for concern. Call your physician.

Breathing Changes

Noisy breathing and coughing are common with an upper respiratory tract infection. If your child has difficulty breathing, breathes rapidly, or is wheezing, call your physician.

Diarrhea

Diarrhea is a frequent gastrointestinal disturbance. Mild diarrhea is the passage of a few mushy stools, whereas with moderate or severe diarrhea the frequency increases and the stools become more watery. Dehydration is the main danger, because the body can lose so much fluid in the stools.

If your child does not urinate for about 8 hours and has a dry mouth and tearless crying, call your physician immediately. He or she may have severe dehydration. Blood or pus in the stool, severe abdominal pain, the passage of frequent diarrhea stools, or the combination of watery diarrhea and frequent vomiting also warrants a call to your physician.

Vomiting

Vomiting may or may not be associated with diarrhea. If your child is vomiting, avoid feeding solid foods for about 8 hours. Your child may try to drink small amounts of clear liquids or suck on ice pops. If there is no vomiting for about 8 hours, you can try such

Warning Signs of Serious Illness

The following signs and symptoms may suggest a serious illness. If your child has any of these, call your physician immediately:

- Fever higher than 105 degrees Fahrenheit
- Fever that lasts longer than 24 hours without any obvious cause (such as a cold or gastrointestinal symptoms)
- Fever that lasts more than 72 hours
- Lethargy or no drinking of fluids
- Stiff or painful neck
- Such severe pain that he or she does not want to be touched
- Sudden inability to walk
- Breathing difficulty
- Difficulty being awakened
- Painful urination
- A convulsion
- Pain in the groin (boys)
- Blue lips
- Profuse drooling
- Purple or deep red spots on the skin

foods as soda crackers, white bread, or chicken soup. If you see blood in the vomitus or note that your child has severe abdominal pain or a swollen abdomen, if your child is delirious or is difficult to awaken, or if your child has signs of dehydration (no saliva or tears, absence of urination), call your physician immediately.

Common and Recurrent Colds

The common cold is one of the most frequent illnesses of childhood. Preschoolers, in fact, have an average of five to eight infections each year, often during the peak times for colds of early September, late January, and late April.

If your child constantly has a congested head, is sneezing, and even has a fever and a sore throat, there are several possible causes.

The most common cause of a constantly runny nose is simply a recurring cold. Children older than 6 months often have recurring viral upper respiratory tract infections. A young child with a cold is generally sicker than are older children or adults.

Fever in your child under 3 is an early symptom. Irritability, restlessness, and sneezing usually follow. A few hours later a clear liquid begins to drip from the nose, which gradually changes to a thick mucus that makes it difficult to breathe through the nose. The virus irritates your child's throat and windpipe, causing a sore throat and cough. Other symptoms may include headache, lack of appetite, and muscle aches.

What can you do for a cold? In general, there is little anyone can do to make your child better rapidly. Usually, your child's temperature will return to normal in 1 to 3 days. All nose and throat symptoms will disappear within a week; however, the cough may persist for 2 to 3 weeks. Over-the-counter drugs only relieve symptoms. They do not shorten the duration of the illness or prevent complications. Antibiotics are of no benefit for colds caused by viruses.

There is no magic potion for a cold, but there are some things you can do to make your child more comfortable:

1. If your child is too young to blow his or her nose, use a soft rubber suction bulb to remove mucus.

2. If your child's nose is stuffed, try administering nose drops 15 to 20 minutes before meals and at bedtime. You can use saline nose drops, which are available without a prescription. If your child is too young to blow his or her nose, place three drops in each nostril. After waiting 1 minute, use a suction bulb to remove the loosened mucus. For your older child, put three drops in each nostril while he or she is lying face-up on the bed with his or her head over the side. After a moment, have your child blow his or her nose. This can be repeated several times in a row until the nose is cleared.

3. When saline drops do not work, you can buy nonprescription nose drops that will shrink the mucous membranes, allowing your child to breathe easier.

(Do not give nose drops for more than a few days. Prolonged use of these nose drops causes a rebound reaction and actually makes the congestion worse instead of clearing it up. Simply stopping use of the nose drops should clear up the problem; see Beware: Nose-Drop Addiction, page 587. Discuss this with your child's physician. Many physicians recommend use of nose drops only in certain specific circumstances.)

4. If your child has aches or a fever of more than 102 degrees Fahrenheit, you can give acetaminophen. DO NOT give aspirin, which has been possibly linked with Reye's

syndrome, a life-threatening condition (see Reye's Syndrome, page 484).

In addition to an increased frequency of colds, your preschooler is more apt than older children to have complications from colds. The most common complication is an acute ear infection (otitis media) (see page 574). This occurs when bacteria infiltrate the space behind the eardrum.

Symptoms may include an earache (children too young to verbalize their pain may simply cry or pull on the infected ear). You may see a yellow or green discharge from the nose. Drainage from the ear means that your child's eardrum has ruptured. The rupture may relieve the pressure and the pain. See your child's physician. Another symptom may be a return of fever after the initial fever of the cold has already gone down.

Unlike a cold, an ear infection must be treated with antibiotics to clear the infection and to help prevent damage to the middle and inner ear and resulting hearing loss (see Disorders of the Ear, page 570).

Other Possible Causes

Another cause of nasal congestion in some children is environmental respiratory irritants. Air pollution, tobacco smoke, or sudden changes in the air temperature may cause a prolonged stuffy nose and sneezing.

Finally, your child may suffer from hay fever (allergic rhinitis). Usually, it takes several years before your child has been exposed to enough allergic substances to have a reaction to them; therefore, hay fever seldom occurs in children younger than 2 years. Your child will have symptoms that include a constantly runny nose, with large amounts of clear, watery discharge, frequent sneezing, and an itchy nose. Antihistamines may relieve these symptoms. If not, your child's physician may want to obtain a consultation from a pediatric allergist (see Common Viral Colds, page 1071; Respiratory Allergies, page 1040; and Disease Prevention, page 98).

Constipation and Diarrhea

Parents of young children are often overly concerned about their child's bowel movements. If your child skips a day, you may incorrectly assume he or she is constipated. Or, if the consistency of the stool is mushy, you may incorrectly assume your child has diarrhea.

The characteristics of constipation and diarrhea are detailed below.

Constipation

Just because your son or daughter does not have a bowel movement every day does not mean your child is constipated. Although many people do have a daily bowel movement, others may have one only every second or third day.

The symptoms of constipation are the painful passage of the stool; the inability to pass a stool, even though the urge to defecate is strong; going more than 3 days without having a bowel movement; or passing a large, hard stool that may even plug the toilet.

If your child has the symptoms of constipation, they are probably the result of not getting enough fiber or fluid in the diet. Moreover, children may hold back their stool because it is inconvenient to go when the urge hits or as a response to toilet training (see Toilet Training, page 88). Some children hold in the stool because a previous passage of a hard stool created a tear (fissure) in the anal opening. It hurts when they try to have a bowel movement, so they try to avoid the pain (see Anal Fissures and Fistulas, page 796).

Treatment for constipation is generally dietary, including lots of fruits and vegetables, foods high in fiber such as wheat breads, legumes, and whole-grain cereals, and an increased intake of water and other fluids. Encourage your child to have bowel movements at regular intervals, perhaps after breakfast or supper. If this does not resolve the constipation, check with your child's physician.

Diarrhea

A child with diarrhea has a sudden increase in the frequency and looseness of bowel movements. If diarrhea is mild, the stools may only be loose; when it is moderate or severe, they may be watery, green, and very frequent. If your child has only a couple of diarrhea stools, it may be the result of something he or she ate. Diarrhea usually is caused by a virus or, less commonly, by bacteria or parasites.

Some young children develop "toddler's diarrhea." Typically, your child with toddler's diarrhea has several days of loose stools that are malodorous and runny. Some of these children are incredibly thirsty during this time. Despite the diarrhea, a child with toddler's diarrhea usually is very active, appears healthy, and does not have a fever. If the stool is tested for organisms, it almost always is normal. In the case of toddler's diarrhea, dietary restrictions usually do not make much difference.

If your child has diarrhea, take steps to avoid dehydration by increasing your child's fluid intake. Water, juices, ice pops, and broth are good choices. Do not use diet soda or diet juices. In addition, commercially available oral electrolyte replacement solutions, such as Pedialyte or Lytren, provide excellent replacement of what the body loses with diarrhea. They also help slow down the amount of fluid loss.

If your child is not hungry, there is a good reason, so do not force food. If he or she wants to eat, offer a general diet and a lot of fluids. Foods that contain bulk such as cereal, fruits, and vegetables are good, because they usually make the stool firmer.

Diarrhea may last up to a week.

Although it is unnecessary to call your physician every time your child has a bout of diarrhea, consult your child's physician if any of the following symptoms occur:

- Signs of dehydration (no wet diapers or urination for 8 hours, tearless crying, no saliva in the mouth)
- Bowel movement every hour for more than 8 hours
- Blood, pus, or mucus in the stool
- Abdominal pain lasting more than 12 hours
- Diarrhea that does not improve within 48 hours of dietary changes
- Mild diarrhea lasting more than a week

Toilet Training

The toilet training of your toddler can be a difficult time in the lives of you and your child. Or, when handled properly, it can be simply one in a series of many milestones.

The first question most parents ask is, "When is the right time to attempt toilet training?"

That is not an easy question to answer, because every child is different. Your first child may have been day-trained within 24 hours at 24 months, whereas the second one may still be balking near the third birthday. The readiness of one child for toilet training may be different from that of another.

Generally, most physicians advise never trying to train a child before 18 months, and many believe that even this is too early except in rare cases. Unless a child appears extremely interested in being trained, most physicians today usually advise waiting until between 2 and 2½ years.

Control at night comes later. Most children continue to wear a diaper at night for several months after they are day-trained, which usually is accomplished by the time they turn 3. Even so, 40 percent of 3-year-olds wet the bed at least once a month.

There are signs that you as a parent can look for to determine whether the time is right to attempt training. Remember, no rule says that training has to be successful immediately. Try it for a few days, and if your child is clearly not interested or protests, put the plan off for a few weeks. Next time it may work. Signs of readiness include the following:

1. Your child has a vocabulary of bathroom words such as "potty," "pee pee," or "poo poo."

2. Your child has watched others use the toilet.

3. Your child indicates when he or she is wet or dirty and wants to be changed.

4. Your child can briefly control his or her bowel and bladder; in other words, he or she can delay having a bowel movement or urinating until it is convenient.

Once you determine that the time may be right, you will need some supplies:

1. A small potty chair that sits on the floor. There are children's toilet seats designed to fit on a regular toilet, but many children prefer the floor type. This type not only allows the child to get on and off at will but also enables the child to push better because his or her feet are on the floor. Purchase the potty a few weeks before you are ready to begin training so that your child can become familiar with it.

2. Training pants, which are heavy, absorbent underwear.

3. Favorite treats and stars or stickers if you want to use tangible rewards in addition to your praise.

Now, you are ready to begin. Tell your child he or she is now going to wear underpants like the big boys and girls. Save the diapers for nap and bedtime.

There are various ways to go about toilet training. No matter which one you ultimately choose, make sure that you do not turn the bathroom into a battleground.

Many physicians suggest allowing the child to become trained according to his or her own free will. This means no coercion whatsoever. Ask your child if he or she wants to sit on the potty. If the answer is no, do not pressure the child. If your child sits a minute but does not do anything, let him or her get off the potty when ready. If your child urinates or has a bowel movement, be free with your praise. But when there is an "accident" (and there undoubtedly will be), do not scold or shame your toddler.

Other methods use similar principles but require more parental involvement. You take your child to the potty at appropriate intervals and ask him or her to "pee pee." If your child is reluctant to cooperate, you can try entertaining your toddler with books or games. If your child does not go within 5 minutes, take him or her off and try later. When your child does go, offer praise. You can even try rewards such as nutritious snacks, stars, or stickers.

Several months after day-control is achieved, you can try putting your child to bed without a diaper. Although not necessary, taking your child to the bathroom just before he or she goes to bed may hasten night training.

For some children, bowel and bladder control occur simultaneously, whereas others achieve one before the other. In most cases, toilet training can be accomplished within 2 months. If not, it may be an indication that your child is too young, and you should probably try again in a few weeks or months.

If, however, your child is older than 2½ years and still is not trained after 2 months, he or she is resisting toilet training. The most common cause of this resistance is too much parental pressure. Often, these children have been reminded too much; some have been forced to sit for long periods on the potty. Hence, control of one's urine and bowels has become a political issue in the child's mind.

In trying to train your resistant child, shift the responsibility to him or her. Tell your child that you are not going to remind him or her to go to the bathroom and that he or she must decide when to go. Use positive reinforcement and incentives to reward your toddler for a day without wet or dirty pants. Try a reward system such as buying your child a calendar and awarding a star every time the toilet is successfully used. If your child has an accident, change him or her and then involve the toddler in cleaning up the mess. Again, do not punish or criticize. Above all, try to be patient, however difficult that may be.

Encopresis and Enuresis

The involuntary passage of feces far beyond an age at which most other children are toilet trained is called encopresis. It is not a disease, but it may be a symptom of constipation or emotional difficulties (there is rarely a physical cause) (see Encopresis, page 1098).

Bedwetting (enuresis) is also a common problem in preschool children (see Enuresis, page 1098).

Teething Problems

Many babies breeze through teething, the process during which the teeth erupt through the gums. Their only symptoms are increased drooling and an insatiable need to chew on things.

For others, however, the process is fraught with discomfort, daytime restlessness, and crankiness. Your child may take to thumb sucking as never before, rub his or her gums, and temporarily lose his or her appetite.

Teething generally does not cause fever, diarrhea, sleep problems, seizures, bronchitis, or diaper rash. Seek appropriate care for such problems if they are sufficiently severe to be worrisome. Do not assume that they are part of the normal teething process.

If your baby is among those with discomfort, there are some things you can do:

1. If your child allows, massage the swollen gum for a couple of minutes with or without a piece of ice. Some children, however, voluntarily or involuntarily tend to bite your fingers trying to relieve their discomfort.

2. A cold teething ring may help. You also may want to give your child some ice, an ice pop, or a slice of frozen banana to gnaw on. Never, however, tie a teething ring around your child's neck—this could cause strangulation.

3. Do not use lotions or ointments designed to reduce teething pain. These not only are unnecessary but also may contain benzocaine, an agent that could numb the throat and cause your baby to choke. Many of these products also have a bitter taste and your child may refuse to take them.

4. You may use acetaminophen for a few days if your child is uncomfortable.

Swallowing Objects

Young children are naturally curious and are not averse to putting coins, safety pins, buttons, fruit pits, and other things into their mouths. Keep these and other small objects out of reach.

Large chunks of food such as hot dogs occasionally lodge in a child's throat; to minimize this risk, do not allow your preschooler to eat while walking or playing.

In addition to a penchant for small objects, some children chronically ingest non-nutrient substances such as dirt, plaster, clay, paint, and ashes. This eating disorder, called pica, may occur during the first 2 years, when your child's natural curiosity compels him or her to sample everything. However, if your child persists with this practice, inform your physician.

A watchful parent may be able to retrieve an object before it is swallowed. When your child swallows an object, it usually passes through the digestive system uneventfully. A good rule is that if a swallowed object passes into your child's stomach, it will usually pass the rest of the way through the intestines.

However, objects can lodge in the esophagus. If your child has difficulty with swallowing, or if he or she is spitting up saliva, you might suspect that a swallowed object has become stuck in the esophagus. If this occurs, or if your child develops chest or abdominal pain or vomiting, call your physician. Another exception is if your child swallows a button-sized battery such as those found in watches, pocket calculators, cameras, and hearing aids. If this occurs, contact your physician at once even if no symptoms are present (see Children and Button Batteries, page 427).

The most frightening possibility is that an object might become lodged in the windpipe, preventing your child from breathing, crying, or speaking. This is an emergency. If the obstruction is not relieved within a few minutes, your child will become unconscious and may convulse because of a lack of oxygen. Death could follow.

If your preschooler stops breathing because of an obstruction, try the Heimlich maneuver and seek emergency help (see Choking, Breathing Emergencies, and Resuscitation, page 406).

Eye Problems

The preschool years, particularly between ages 3 and 4, are crucial for the detection and successful treatment of many eye problems, including those described below.

Strabismus and Amblyopia

Strabismus occurs when the eyes are malaligned. Cross-eyes is a type of strabismus, for example. In some cases, one eye deviates only when your child is tired; in another form of the problem, both eyes alternate deviating. Treatment may require an operation. The earlier the condition is discovered, the better the chances of substantial improvement.

Amblyopia is subnormal vision in one or both eyes. It can be caused by many vision defects. Susceptibility to amblyopia is greatest within the first 3 years. Amblyopia can be treated. The most important factor in its successful treatment is early detection. Amblyopia, often called "lazy eye," frequently is a consequence of strabismus.

Although examination of the eyes should be a part of your child's regular checkups, a more thorough examination by your eye specialist ideally should occur when your child is 4 years old (see Strabismus and Amblyopia, page 534).

Sleep Problems

Crying uncontrollably at bedtime, waking up frequently during the night, and getting out of bed and attempting to crawl in with the parents are common sleep problems in the preschool age group.

If your child has a sleep problem, you are not alone. This is a frequent complaint of parents. Whether the problem is temporary or intermittent or has been occurring for months, a child who is awakening at night creates tired parents, not to mention a cranky child.

Causes vary, often depending on the age of your child.

If your child is between 12 and 24 months old and has always had problems sleeping through the night, you may have been too responsive to his or her night cries. Most babies older than 4 months awaken several times during the night but can put themselves back to sleep. However, if your baby has learned that Mom or Dad will come rushing every time he or she cries, your child becomes dependent on a parent to get back to sleep. Your child, in essence, becomes trained to cry at night.

To assist your child in improving sleep patterns, avoid the following: nursing your child to sleep or giving him or her a bottle to take to bed, sleeping in the same room, rocking your child to sleep, entertaining him or her at night, letting your child nap more than 3 hours a day, or changing his or her diaper at night.

Then, try the following, whether your child protests going to bed or wakes up at night. Although this approach may leave you wide awake for a while, it will ultimately (usually within 2 weeks) improve the situation:

1. Put your child to bed awake, say good-night, and leave the room despite protests.

2. Do not go in immediately when your baby begins crying. Wait 15 or 20 minutes before checking on your child. Then, stay in the room for less than a minute. Do not turn on the light or pick up your child; simply reassure him or her that everything is all right and that it is time for sleep.

The first night your baby may cry for an hour, but generally the crying time will decrease each night when you use this method.

Some children have not been trained to cry at night but, because of a fear, they resist going to bed or awaken terrified.

If your young toddler's cries sound fearful rather than simply angry, go to him or her immediately. Seeing your face should calm your child, although after you reassure your toddler you may have to sit by the crib awhile. Do not play or talk. You do not want your child to think this is play time.

Older preschoolers also often develop nighttime fears that impede sleep. Again, be reassuring. Do not make fun of your child, be impatient, or try to argue him or her out of a fear. Leaving the door open or using a night-light can work wonders.

If you find your child crawling into bed with you at night, gently but firmly take him or her back to his or her bed. In the long run, this is better for you and your child.

Fears and Phobias

As your child grows, he or she inevitably will have certain fears, which will change with age. Such fears are normal and may even be necessary for psychological development.

Fear—the perception of a threat, whether actual or simply a possibility—is necessary for survival. For example, fear of a barking, snarling dog is normal. Your child perceives a real threat, and it is correct to be frightened and to try to avoid the danger. However, the child who continues to be terrified of the friendly, tail-wagging cocker spaniel who lives next door has an irrational fear or phobia.

Fears vary from child to child, but some appear more commonly in certain age groups. For example, children between 1 and 2 years are commonly afraid of the bath. Often children this age are afraid of slipping under the water or of getting soap in their eyes. Toddlers this age also tend to be fearful of strangers. Fear of separation from parents is another common fear if your child is 2 or younger.

Fears in 3-, 4-, and 5-year-old children often revolve around the dark, animals, monsters, and death.

If your child is going through a fearful time, try to be supportive and encouraging. Do not force your child to confront the object of the fear. A parent who tries to make a child who is afraid of animals pet a dog will only complicate the situation.

Your reassurance in the form of a hug or kiss can be powerful medicine for the 2-year-old who is afraid of the dark. A night-light is often helpful. Be creative in your quest for a solution. One mother whose 3-year-old girl was terrified that there were monsters lurking in her dark room initiated a nightly "monster check." At bedtime every night they would scour the room together in search of a monster. Reassured, the little girl went to bed and immediately fell asleep. Within a few weeks she stopped asking for the monster check.

When your child conquers even a tiny part of his or her fear, do not forget the praise.

Most fears resolve themselves in time. Those that do not or that incapacitate your child or family may require some psychiatric counseling.

Tantrums and Breath Holding

Few children exit their toddler years without demonstrating temper tantrums.

Between the ages of 18 months and 3 years, negativism reigns. "No" (sometimes even when it means "yes") seems to be your child's favorite word. Sometimes everything you do, no matter how innocuous, seems to provoke your child. This stubborn, oppositional, and defiant behavior is simply a natural part of moving from total dependence to a taste of independence.

This time is not called the "terrible twos" without reason. Nothing is more exasperating than when your child decides to throw a temper tantrum. Any parent who has been through one knows that it does not take much to drive a toddler to uncontrollable kicking, screaming, head banging, and even breath holding. Often, in fact, the temper tantrum has nothing to do with you, but is your child's response to frustration.

When a child reaches this point, he or she is out of control and beyond reason. You talk or try to placate to no avail. Generally, a temper tantrum, once started, has to run its course.

What Should You Do?
Giving in is not the answer. If, for example, your 2-year-old has a tantrum because you deny a second cookie, you will be sending the wrong message if you suddenly reverse your decision. Once the tantrum starts, giving your child a "time out" is most helpful. Leave the room. Try to ignore what is going on (it will be difficult). Even if your child holds his or her breath, do not worry, because this is not harmful. As for any head banging, children hate pain as much as adults; when things get too uncomfortable, they know it's time to quit.

When to return to your child is variable. Some parents find that their child finishes the tantrum on his or her own; other children may need to be held for a moment before they can stop crying.

Although ignoring a tantrum is effective in most cases, sometimes you must take other measures. Obviously, the child who decides to throw a tantrum in the middle of the supermarket cannot be left there to kick and flail, nor should a child who is physically aggressive toward someone else or toward property be allowed to continue unchecked. Take the child to his or her room or separate your child from others until your child regains his or her composure.

Walking and Falling

A frequent question is, "When will my baby walk?"

No one can answer this with precision. One child may walk as early as 9 months and another may be content to crawl until 14 months or later.

Your new walker is amusing to watch. On plump feet that look flat because of baby fat, your child will toddle about with the toes turned out. Many babies also may be bow-legged or knock-kneed. Virtually all these characteristics are normal and disappear on their own (see Flatfeet, page 95; Knock-Knees, page 96; and Bowlegs, page 97).

Do not expect your new walker to be graceful. One minute your 1-year-old will be making his or her way across the room and the next he or she will be lying in a heap on the floor. Falls can be frequent at first and usually are no real deterrent to the determined baby. Falls are part of learning to walk.

For the parent, however, they should serve as a signal of things to come. Your child who only weeks before had limited mobility now has discovered the ability to go where he or she wants to. By the time your "explorer" is 18 months old, he or she may be able to climb the stairs while holding your hand; at 20 months, your child can walk down the stairs while holding a hand. By 24 months, it's difficult to stop most children from traversing a steep stairwell; but a safety-conscious parent will install a safety gate at the top and bottom of all staircases in the home.

Speech and Language Development

Your child's speech and language development begins almost immediately on entering the world and is not complete until age 6 or

7. Such development takes place in stages. Be aware that there are considerable developmental variations from child to child, even within the same family. Therefore, the following are general guidelines:

During the first 3 months of life, beginning with what is called the "undifferentiated birth cry," your infant will experiment with making sounds, producing several consonants and vowels that have no meaning. Considerable cooing and gurgling take place during this time. Language comprehension is limited to responses to loud noises and familiar voices.

Between 4 and 6 months, your baby moves into the babbling stage, which is accompanied by sighing, grunting, gurgling, laughing, and crying differently in response to pain and hunger. Your child vocalizes for pleasure and displeasure.

Between 7 and 9 months, your child repeats syllables, babbles in a sing-song manner, may produce as many as 12 different sounds, particularly the p, b, and m sounds, uses different vowels, uses sounds as a means of play, and may repeat the word "mama." You may hear your child utter sounds that mimic the letters m, n, t, d, p, b, and z.

Toward the end of this period, your child begins imitating intonation and speech sounds others make. During this period your child searches for sources of sound, listens intently to speech and nonspeech sounds, recognizes "dada," "mama," and "bye-bye," recognizes his or her name, and is able to differentiate friendliness or anger from the tone of other people's voices.

At 10 to 12 months, the babbling may take on some of the melody of actual speech. Your child enjoys repeating sounds others make and uses considerable vocalization during play. Your child now uses almost all of the consonant and vowel sounds. In some children, the first true words can emerge during this period. By now your child's comprehension is improved. He or she responds to names and simple requests and recognizes the names of common objects and family members.

Between 13 and 18 months, your child uses sentence-like intonations, continues repeating sounds made by others, and uses all the vowels and consonants. However, his or her language is basically unintelligible except for a few words such as "mama" and "dada." During this time your child makes genuine efforts to name objects. Your child comprehends a few simple words, phrases, and commands, shakes his or her head appropriately in response to simple yes-or-no questions, and shows an interest in simple rhymes and songs.

Between the ages of 1½ and 2 years, your child produces words that are more understandable. Jargon usually disappears by age 2. During this period your child may begin to use two-word phrases such as "more milk" and has a vocabulary of 10 to 20 words. Your child may still use jargon that sounds like sentences. He or she uses single words to express larger ideas, such as "wawa" for "I want water" or "Look at the water." When your child is about 2 years old, you should understand about two-thirds of what he or she says. Your child can comprehend well enough to bring objects on command, to point to some body parts, to understand simple questions, and to recognize pictures, although he or she may be unable to name them.

Stuttering

Typically, stuttering begins between ages 2 and 5, while your child is mastering the basics of speech. In some children it first appears between ages 6 and 8, when school lessons include reading aloud and recitation. Occasionally older children develop the problem. Stuttering occurs in 1 to 2 percent of grade-school children but often disappears by adolescence.

We only partially understand what causes stuttering. Several factors may promote tension of the muscles involved with speech and lead to stuttering. Stuttering can run in families. Common stuttering is not linked to intelligence or any measurable brain abnormality.

Occasional lack of fluency is common among children. These episodes usually disappear as speech and language develop and do not require attention.

Professional and Home Treatment

Seek professional evaluation if your child becomes apprehensive about speaking, speaks with a struggle or facial grimace, or begins to avoid sounds, words, or speech altogether.

A speech pathologist can help your child minimize his or her stuttering by reducing tension in his or her lips, tongue, and jaw. A speech pathologist also provides training skills to eliminate unnecessary, undesirable speech patterns.

Never label your child a stutterer. Never interrupt, show impatience, or finish your child's sentence. Build your child's self-confidence by arranging quiet, one-on-one conversation and reading times.

Between 2 and 2½ years, your child uses two- or three-word phrases, has a vocabulary of 50 or more words, begins to use words such as "me," "you," and "mine," and shows considerable substitution and omission of final consonant sounds. You can now understand about 70 percent of what he or she says. Your child ought to be able to point to body parts by this age, understand many complex sentences, and follow three directions in succession.

Between 2½ and 3 years, your child still has many consonant omissions and substitutions, but you should be able to understand most of what he or she says. Your child is able to use three- or four-word sentences, may repeat words when excited or anxious, and comprehends most of what is said.

Between the ages of 3½ and 4 years, your child is able to give his or her full name and age, can use the present and past tenses of verbs, and uses more complicated sentences. You can understand virtually all of what your child says. Your child may begin to use the plural forms of words. People outside your family understand most of what your child says. Your child often will talk to himself or herself. He or she begins to ask "what?" questions. Your child can understand a simple story, recognizes several colors, and can put foods and animals into their proper groups. Your child can understand the concept of time by this age.

Between the ages of 4 and 5 years, your child is able to count to five, uses complete sentences, asks "why?" and "who?", uses four- or five-word sentences, uses 75 percent of all speech sounds correctly, enjoys naming objects, knows most colors, and understands the concept of the past, present, and future forms of verbs and the difference between single and plural nouns. Most of the time you can understand what your child says.

By now your child has a 2,500-word vocabulary and uses most consonant sounds consistently and accurately, although not in all words.

At ages 5 to 6 years, a stranger can understand what your child says. Your child uses words such as "and" and "but," asks many questions, and uses five- or six-word sentences and grammatically different types of sentences. He or she is able to carry on a conversation and can define and explain words. Your child understands most of what he or she hears and can follow three or more directions given at the same time. By age 6, your child may have a vocabulary comprehension of about 13,000 words and understands such concepts as yesterday, tomorrow, more, less, some, many, several, few, most, and least.

By age 6 to 7 years, your child should master all of the consonants and vowels. You should be able to understand everything your child says. With a vocabulary comprehension of 20,000 words, your child understands time intervals and seasons of the year, can print the alphabet and write one-syllable words, can read approximately 10 printed words, and can count to 100.

If you think that your child's speech is not developing at an appropriate rate or if you are having trouble understanding your child's words, see your physician.

Urinary Tract Infections

Urinary tract infection occurs when bacteria enter your child's bladder via the urethra (the channel leading from the bladder to the outside of the body). Under normal circumstances these bacteria are rinsed out of the body during urination. Urine itself has properties that inhibit the growth of bacteria. However, factors such as the virulence of the particular bacteria and anatomic abnormalities in the urinary system can increase the chance of a urinary tract infection.

Urinary tract infections are common in young children, particularly girls. Usually the infection is confined to the bladder and is called cystitis (see page 842). In this situation, your child may seem as though she constantly has to go to the bathroom and complains of pain with urination. The urine may be foul-smelling; bed-wetting may occur in a child who had previously been night-trained. Fever, vomiting, and chills also may occur. In some cases a child has no symptoms.

Sometimes, however, the infection can travel from the bladder up the ureter to a kidney. Symptoms then may include a fever, chills, back pain, and vomiting. When this occurs, your child may have an acute infection of the kidney called acute pyelonephritis (see page 841). Unlike cystitis, a kidney infection may require hospitalization.

If your child has the symptoms of a urinary tract infection, your physician may collect a urine specimen to determine whether there are bacteria in the urine. If a microscopic examination reveals bacteria, the urine may be cultured to determine the type of bacteria. Although this test reveals whether there is infection, it is no indication of whether the infection is confined to your child's bladder or has invaded the kidney. For this, your physician must rely on an accurate description of your child's symptoms, your child's appearance, and a physical examination. A child with a kidney infection will appear more ill than one with a simple bladder infection.

If your child is having recurrent infections, your physician may want special X-rays such as a kidney X-ray after dye injection (IVP) (see page 829) and a voiding cystourethrogram (see page 829) to determine whether there is an abnormality and whether there has been kidney damage as a result of repeated infections.

Most urinary tract infections respond promptly to antibiotic treatment. When properly treated, acute pyelonephritis rarely progresses to chronic renal disease. You should not ignore urinary tract infections. Untreated bladder infection (cystitis) can involve the kidney, and a kidney infection that is not totally eradicated can recur, which may damage the kidney. Moreover, recurrent urinary tract infections can be a symptom of other diseases. One problem frequently associated with recurrent kidney infection is vesicoureteral reflux (see page 830), an abnormality in the ureter that allows urine to reflux back into the kidney. Thus, when your child's urine is invaded by bacteria and urine automatically flows up to the kidney, the result is a kidney infection (see page 841).

If your child has cystitis, he or she will be treated with antibiotics. For acute pyelonephritis, your child may need an intravenous infusion of antibiotics.

Some children who have recurrent urinary tract infections need daily doses of an antibiotic for months or even years to keep their urine sterile. It may be best in these children to use showers or sponge baths rather than baths. Some children should have urine cultures performed at regular intervals (even if they have no symptoms) to ensure that the urinary tract is free of bacteria.

When an abnormality such as reflux is responsible for the infections, your physician may consider surgery if there is concern about kidney damage.

Orthopedic Concerns

Beyond breaking a bone from time to time or pulling a muscle, most children do not have serious problems of their muscles, bones, and joints.

Yet a wide range of growth patterns can occur in the preschool-age child. Flatfeet or pigeon-toes, bowlegs, and knock-knees are all stages through which most children pass during the normal pattern of leg and foot development. For example, your infant's toes tend to bend inward and the feet appear flat because of the abundance of baby fat. As the child slims down, however, arches gradually become visible by the age of 5.

Likewise, legs are ordinarily slightly bowed from birth until about 2 years of age. Then your toddler's legs often overcorrect in the opposite direction, giving a knock-kneed appearance by age 3. Normally legs straighten by 7 years of age.

Even when these variations continue through the school-age years, they seldom require treatment. Only rarely is disease the cause.

Flatfeet

Your child's feet are flat if arches are not apparent. There is no reason to be concerned about flatfeet in infants, whose baby fat always makes their feet look flat. However, if the arches do not become discernible by age 5 years, your child may have flatfeet that are either flexible or fixed.

Flexible flatfeet look flat only when your child stands up. When he or she stands on tiptoe or the foot bears no weight, the arch is restored. Flexible flatfeet tend to run in families and are more common in Jewish and

Flatfeet are feet that have little or no arch. Below at left (top and bottom) is a normal foot and footprint. If your child's foot and footprint more nearly resemble the illustrations at right, then he or she has flatfeet.

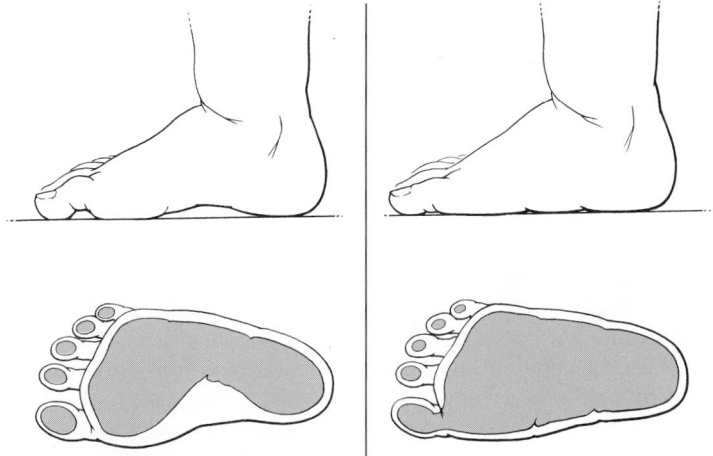

black people. The feet are mobile and painless and have excellent muscle strength.

Usually, flexible flatfeet do not require treatment. However, if the feet are extremely flat, your child's physician may prescribe an arch support in a firm shoe. Although this will not correct the foot, it can permit long walks without foot strain.

Fixed or rigid flatfeet are cause for more concern because they may occur with congenital bone malformations. Your child's physician will take X-rays to determine whether this is the case. An operation may be appropriate if the condition is not relieved by special footwear.

Pigeon Toe

In pigeon toe, the toes turn inward. Most newborns are pigeon-toed as a holdover from their fetal position in the womb. They usually sleep with their toes pointed inward. Then, as they start to walk, their feet often turn inward to keep their balance and make up for such conditions as flatfeet, bowlegs, and knock-knees.

The condition usually resolves spontaneously by age 5. If it persists, your physician will watch your child standing and walking and also may take X-rays. He or she will check for the presence of diseases that can cause pigeon toe, such as congenital bone malformations in which the bones of the

thigh, shin, ankle, or foot turn inward.

Malposition, such as sitting or sleeping on the in-turned feet, does not cause further deformity but may perpetuate the problem. If your infant's foot is flexible, your physician may advise stretching exercises. If the foot is fixed, your child may need special shoes or a cast.

Encourage your child to sit and to walk with his or her toes straight ahead or turned slightly outward. Have your child sit cross-legged rather than with his or her knees together and the lower legs flat on the floor and pointing outward.

An underlying structural malformation can be treated by putting the feet in casts and then in orthopedic shoes. If these measures do not work, an operation may be necessary, but your physician usually will not perform it before your child is 9.

Knock-Knees

When a child with knock-knees stands up, the knees touch each other but the ankles do not. Knock-knees are more common in girls than in boys, partly because their pelvis is wider. They also occur more frequently in overweight children whose developing bones and joints are hard put to support their weight.

A knock-kneed appearance can persist after age 4, but most children's legs straighten by age 7. If the legs do not straighten or if the condition develops after your child is of school age, your physician may rule out diseases of the knee joint that can cause knock-knees, such as juvenile rheumatoid arthritis, rickets, and infections. An unrecognized injury or developmental problem can cause asymmetrical knock-knees. Your physician measures the distance between your child's ankles when the knees are touching each other and takes X-rays to determine the severity of the condition.

Knock-knees are common, especially when they run in your child's family. In most cases the legs tend to straighten as your child grows, so treatment is seldom required.

Children with severe knock-knees often have flatfeet, because the weight falls on the inner edge of the foot and ankle. If your child is overweight, this condition may strain the feet and require an arch support to relieve foot fatigue and to prevent the inner border of the shoe from wearing. Your physician may treat severe knock-knees with braces your child wears at night. Occasionally, an operation is needed, but it should not be

Newborns commonly arrive with pigeon toe, a condition in which the toes turn inward. Most often the condition resolves itself spontaneously by age 5.

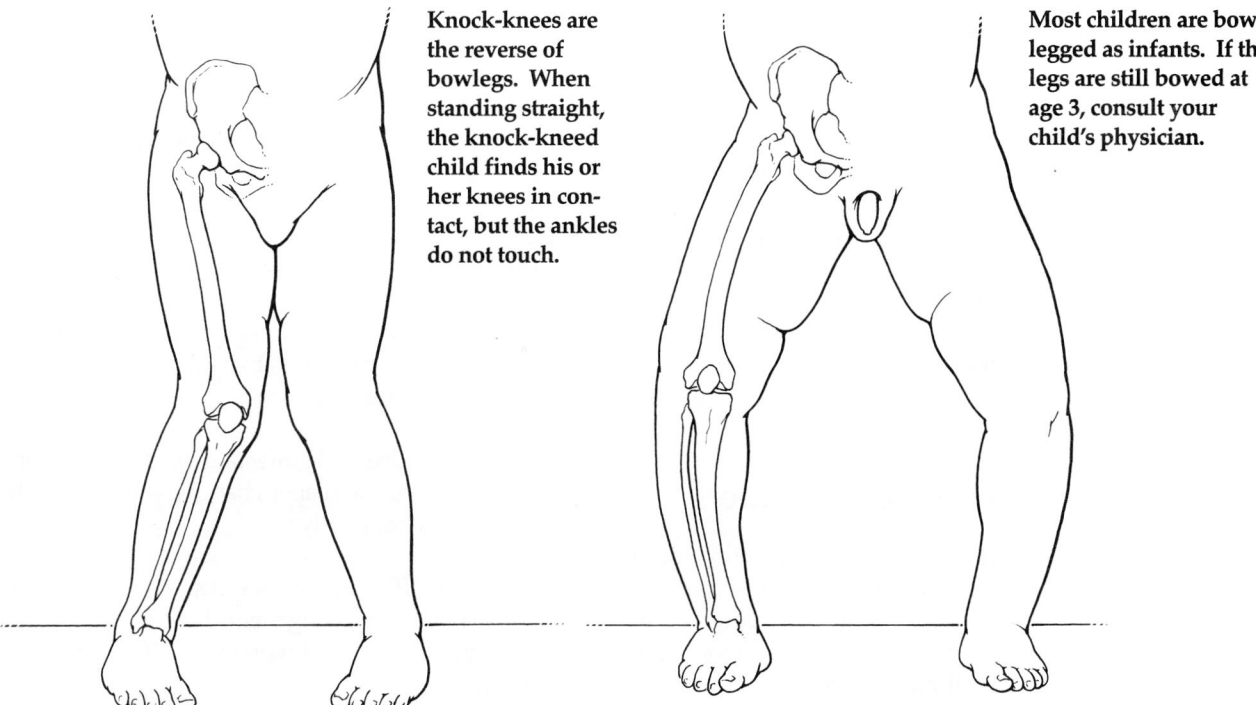

Knock-knees are the reverse of bowlegs. When standing straight, the knock-kneed child finds his or her knees in contact, but the ankles do not touch.

Most children are bow-legged as infants. If the legs are still bowed at age 3, consult your child's physician.

performed until the knees have been given a chance to straighten on their own—after age 10 for girls and 12 for boys, but before growth is complete.

Bowlegs

Legs are considered to be bowed if, when the ankles touch each other, the unbent knees do not. Legs are normally bowed at birth because of the way the fetus's legs are folded over each other in the cramped space of the womb. Legs often stay bowed for up to 2 years. If bowed legs persist or worsen after age 3, they should be examined by your child's physician.

Your physician measures the distance between your child's knees when the ankles touch each other and takes X-rays to determine the severity of the bowing. Sometimes the legs merely appear bowed because of the distribution of the fat on your child's legs. When one leg is more bowed than the other, it may be the result of an injury or a growth problem. Persistently bowed legs usually straighten without treatment by age 8. Occasionally physicians prescribe night braces. Surgical correction is a possibility if conservative measures fail.

In rare cases, bowlegs are caused by disorders such as rickets (see Osteomalacia and Rickets, page 896) or Blount's disease. In Blount's disease, the shin bone curves out below the knee and is not securely inserted into the knee. Severe problems of the knee joint may develop. This disease tends to occur more often in children who are overweight or short or who walked at an early age. It is more common in girls than in boys. An operation on the upper part of the shinbone can correct it.

General Care

Taking care of a preschooler is a full-time job. This section discusses some basic hygiene concerns. When should your child begin regular visits to the dentist? How can you help prevent diaper rash? You can also learn about ways to minimize the spread of infectious disease in your household and how to prevent your child from bringing home every infection to which he or she is exposed.

This section also examines safety. These

early years can be dangerous for your young child if you are not conscious of the safety risks. Young children are curious about everything. They have no qualms about tasting something—anything—they find in a container under your sink, popping beads or other objects into their mouths, or jumping off the edge of the pool. How can you make your home a safe place in which to live and play?

Many times both parents work out of the home; thus, we also offer tips on what to look for in a child care center (see page 101).

Disease Prevention

If you have a young child, you may notice that you also have more colds and viral illnesses. Given the frequency with which young children contract these ailments and their high degree of contagiousness, this is not a surprise.

Infections that typically afflict the American family spread in various ways.

We spread respiratory infections such as colds most often through contact with secretions from the nose, mouth, or eyes of an infected person. Toddlers are great at spreading colds because of their habit of touching and mouthing everything they come across.

Your child's sneeze releases a stream of potentially infectious agents into the atmosphere. Although we less commonly spread colds in this manner, the infectious particles contained in a sneeze or cough can travel up to 6 feet.

Contact with the infected person's feces, which are most often found on the hands of the infected person or on an object touched by the infected person, can spread infections such as diarrhea and hepatitis A.

Finally, sharing combs, brushes, and hats can contribute to the spread of lice, ringworm, and impetigo.

Although it is impossible to totally halt the spread of contagious disease within a family, you can take measures to reduce the chances. These measures are more successful in keeping gastrointestinal illnesses from making the rounds in your family, although they also may lower your incidence of colds somewhat:

1. Wash your hands. This is particularly important after using the bathroom, blowing your nose, or changing a diaper.

2. Do not smoke around your children. Passive smoking increases both the frequency and the severity of your children's colds.

3. Discourage your child from touching his or her mouth or nose.

4. After an illness, throw out the toothbrush. It may contain bacteria that can cause reinfection.

5. Use a disinfectant in the bathroom, kitchen, and diaper-changing area. Clean the areas frequently.

6. If you have pets, discourage your children from kissing them. Pets, especially puppies, can spread worms and other parasites.

7. To help prevent salmonellosis, a form of food poisoning, cook eggs and poultry thoroughly. And be sure that you carefully wash your hands and any object that comes into contact with uncooked food.

Diaper Care

Almost all children who wear diapers have diaper rash at some time. It develops when the skin is in prolonged contact with wetness, ammonia, digestive enzymes, and bacteria.

The following measures can minimize the chance of your child developing a diaper rash:

1. Check frequently for wetness. If a diaper is wet or dirty, change it as soon as you can. Prolonged exposure to feces is particularly conducive to diaper rash.

2. Avoid use of plastic pants.

3. Cleanse your child's bottom with warm water and a mild soap after a bowel movement, and dry it thoroughly before putting another diaper on.

4. If you use cloth diapers, wash them with a mild detergent during the first cycle, then use a cup of bleach during the second cycle. This kills the bacteria. (See color photograph of diaper rash, page C-2.)

Safety at Home and Play

The leading cause of death in young children is accidents. Preschoolers, especially those between 2 and 3 years old, are particularly vulnerable to accidents in the home, some of which can be fatal.

Even though you must take certain precautions to ensure the safety of your young baby (see pages 71 and 352), safety should move to the forefront of your mind once your baby becomes mobile.

By the time your baby is 1 year old, your home should be childproofed. By age 1, most children are beginning to walk. Add to that the immense curiosity that often compels them to explore and their inability to comprehend the dangers of most actions and you have a potentially hazardous situation.

As preschoolers grow up, they will be able to understand why they should not stick their fingers in an electrical socket, put buttons in their mouths, or play with matches. Even so, 4- and 5-year-olds at times do things that they know could hurt them. So even with the older preschooler, never take chances with safety.

Some of the more common accidents in the home or during play and tips on how to prevent them are discussed below.

Burns

In young children, burns are the leading cause of accidental death in the home. Here are some tips for minimizing the chances that your child will be a burn victim:

1. Install smoke detectors on each floor of your home and test them periodically.

2. Have a fire extinguisher in your kitchen.

3. Never leave your child alone in your house.

4. Keep matches out of your child's reach.

5. When cooking, turn pot handles toward the back of the stove.

6. Do not use cloths or mats that your child can pull off the table.

7. Never drink hot beverages with a child on your lap or leave a cup of hot coffee near the edge of a table where your child might easily pull it off.

8. Place electric outlet covers on all unused outlets.

9. Turn down the thermostat on your water heater to between 120 and 125 degrees Fahrenheit. A child can be scalded in less than a second at 160 degrees Fahrenheit.

For procedures to deal with burn emergencies, see page 403.

Drowning

After burns, drowning is the second most common cause of accidental death of young children in the home. Drowning is more common in hot climates, where people are more apt to have outdoor pools. To decrease the chance of drowning, follow these measures:

1. Never leave a preschooler alone in the bathtub.

2. If you have an outdoor pool, install a childproof fence around it.

3. Teach your child to swim.

4. Teach your child never to swim without adult supervision.

5. When boating or around water, always have your child wear a life preserver, and set a good example by wearing your life preserver when boating.

For procedures to deal with drowning emergencies, see page 418.

Poisoning

Another common cause of accidents at home is poisoning; a fifth of all accidental poisonings occur during the second year of a child's life.

1. Keep all medicine in a high or locked cabinet.

2. Keep cleaning solutions out of reach of children. If you must keep them in a low cupboard, install fixtures that make it impossible for your child to open the cupboard door.

3. Do not store anything in the wrong container. For example, if you store paint thinner in a juice bottle, your child may take a drink, thinking it is juice.

4. Look around your garage for toxic chemicals that may be accessible to your wandering child.

5. Many common houseplants are poisonous if eaten. You can obtain a list of these plants from your local Poison Control Center. If you choose to have one of these plants in your home, keep it out of reach of your child. (See Garden-Variety Poisonous Plants, page 440.)

6. Keep the number of the Poison Control Center next to your telephone and call the center immediately if you think your child has taken a poison.

7. Keep a bottle of syrup of ipecac on hand to induce vomiting in case your child ingests something harmful. However, NEVER induce vomiting until you have been advised to do so by a Poison Control Center or your physician. Some substances can cause more damage as they come back up the esophagus.

For procedures in dealing with poisoning emergencies, see page 437.

Falls
Falls also are common during the preschool years. To protect your child from dangerous falls, follow these measures:

1. Keep the side rails up on the crib.

2. Install gates at the tops and bottoms of the staircases in your home.

3. Install a safety net or guard on outdoor decks or staircase openings where a young child could squeeze through.

4. Never let your child use a walker near a staircase.

5. Make sure your windows are locked or have window guards.

6. Do not put a child younger than 6 in the top bunk of a bunk bed.

7. Make sure your child is securely fastened in his or her stroller or carriage.

8. Always supervise outdoor activity.

9. Forbid use of home trampolines; these can result in serious injury even when a parent is supervising.

10. Serious accidents can occur at playgrounds. Before you let your child use play equipment, make sure it is adequately maintained, with no rust, sharp edges or protrusions, or loose nuts and bolts. The surface beneath swings or other playground equipment your child may climb on should not be concrete, asphalt, or packed dirt, but rather should be an energy-absorbing material such as loose sand or wood chips to lessen the chance of injury should your child fall.

Choking
Young preschoolers will put anything into their mouths. This can lead to choking.

1. Select toys appropriate for your child's age. A 1-year-old should not have a toy with small pieces that he or she could accidentally swallow.

2. Make sure your preschooler's toys do not have loose buttons or sharp edges.

3. Avoid giving your child food that could get stuck in his or her throat. Such foods include, for example, whole hot dogs (cut them lengthwise and then into small pieces), popcorn, nuts, hard candy, and raw carrots.

4. Do not allow food to be in your baby's hand away from the table.

See Swallowing Objects, page 90. For procedures in dealing with a choking emergency, see Choking, Breathing Emergencies, and Resuscitation, page 406.

Car Safety

When riding in a car, your preschooler must be strapped into a proper child car seat. After your child grows out of the seat (usually at about 40 pounds), he or she should always wear a seat belt.

Caring for Your Child's Teeth

A combination of measures that include water fluoridation, sealants, brushing and flossing, good nutrition, and regular visits to the dentist can prevent 80 to 90 percent of dental cavities (caries).

Some parents assume that a child has to be a certain age before dental hygiene becomes necessary. In fact, once your baby has a single tooth, you need to begin a daily program of care. Many babies younger than a year will not stand for having a brush in their mouth, but you can at least wipe the tooth with a wet cloth after meals.

The components of a sound oral hygiene program are discussed here.

Fluoride

From the time your child is 2 weeks old until he or she is 12 years old, fluoride is an important deterrent to tooth decay. Fluoride, which helps make your child's tooth enamel cavity resistant, can reduce caries up to 25 percent. Typically, your child consumes fluoride either in drinking water or in a vitamin supplement. If you live in an area where fluoride is added to the water supply, your child must drink at least 1 pint of water daily to reap its full benefits. If your city water supply contains no fluoride or if you have a well, ask your child's physician or dentist to prescribe a supplement. Some children also may benefit from the application of fluoride to the surface of their teeth.

Diet

Never put your baby to bed with a bottle. Sleeping with a bottle containing milk, juice, or anything other than water can cause severe decay, particularly in your child's front teeth. As for sugar, it is virtually impossible to keep children away from it altogether. Avoid sugary foods that stick to teeth or stay in your child's mouth. These include, for example, hard candy and caramels.

Try to limit sugary treats to mealtime, and then insist that your child brush his or her teeth immediately after the meal. Some parents limit sugary treats to being an "award" at one certain time during the day, such as after lunch, followed immediately by toothbrushing. "Smart snacks," such as vegetables and fruits, not only help minimize caries but also are nutritionally better for your child.

Brushing Teeth

Before your child is 1 year old, buy him or her a soft-bristled toothbrush. Although it is fine to let the preschooler attempt to brush his or her own teeth, you will need to do it also to ensure proper cleaning. If your child is negative about brushing, make a game of it. Let your child brush your teeth while you brush his or hers. When possible, brush your child's teeth after every meal. Even rinsing with water or drinking a glass of water after eating is helpful. (See Proper Flossing and Brushing Techniques, page 366.)

The Dentist

Your child should begin to visit a dentist by age 3 years—sooner if the teeth appear abnormal or if he or she complains of toothache.

Child Care Centers

Few issues are as important to working parents as that of child care. Today, more than 50 percent of mothers with preschool children work outside the home. The need for child care centers that provide a nurturing and educational environment has never been so great.

Child care in the United States has become a multimillion dollar business. Still, there are not enough centers that provide high-quality care. Many families, especially those in the lower-income brackets, must accept less-than-ideal conditions for their preschoolers. Many of the truly fine centers have such limited space that parents may put their unborn child's name on a waiting list in anticipation of the need a year down the road.

If you are about to begin the search for a high-quality child care center, here are things to look for:

1. Make sure the center has been licensed by your state. This means that the center meets certain standards and must comply with various health regulations. Family child care centers (those operated out of a private home) are often less expensive but may not be licensed by the state. This means that they may not be monitored by state authorities, as are licensed child care operations.

2. Visit several centers before you make

your choice. A center should be open to parents at all times. You should be suspicious of any center that requires a parent to call ahead before visiting.

3. Once you think you have decided on a center, visit it again, preferably at a different time of day. Are the children happy and busy? Are there lots of things to do, or do the children appear to be at loose ends? Are the teachers warm, encouraging, and willing to hug a crying child? Are there adequate sinks and toilets for the children? Make sure there is a safe playground, with proper fences and equipment that is in good condition.

4. Interview the director of the center and the teacher who would be in charge of your child. Ideally, the staff-to-student ratio should be between 1:4 and 1:6, depending on the preschooler's age (the younger the children, the more staff required). What is staff turnover? What education does the center require of its teachers? Is there a television set and how often are children allowed to watch it? (Television viewing should be minimal and selective, if allowed at all.)

Once you find the center that is right for your child, spend some time helping your child adjust to it. If your child is younger than 2½ years, being apart from you can be painful and tearful, so plan to spend most of the first day with your child at the center. This may be unnecessary for the 4- or 5-year-old, particularly if your child is outgoing and has spent time in the homes of friends.

For the first week or until your child adjusts, avoid rushing off in the morning. Linger for 5 or 10 minutes, until your child begins to interact with someone else. Then, do not sneak away while his or her back is turned. Say "good-bye" and leave. You may find it helpful to let your child bring something from home such as a favorite blanket or a stuffed toy.

Every parent who has a child in child care should expect the child to pick up his or her share of colds and viruses. All young children get sick from time to time, but the chances are that your child will have more bouts of illness during his or her time in child care. In part, this increase is because these common illnesses are so contagious. In addition, children are often contagious before the outbreak of any symptoms, so a seemingly healthy child can infect an entire class. Thus, epidemics of childhood ailments in some centers are commonplace.

What can you do to help prevent the spread of infection in your child's child care center? No practical measures can eliminate the spread of infection, but teachers or assistants can help by making sure they wash their hands thoroughly after changing diapers and before handling food.

As a parent, you can help by not sending your ill child to child care. When is a child too sick to go? Each center generally has its own rules but, as a guideline, most centers do not want your child to attend if he or she has a fever of more than 100 degrees Fahrenheit, is vomiting, or has diarrhea.

As to when your child can return to child care, it usually depends on how well he or she feels and whether the illness is contagious. Many cold symptoms persist for a week or more. Once the temperature is normal for 24 hours, your child probably can return to child care even though he or she still has a slight runny nose and cough.

The following is a guide to when a child with a contagious disease is no longer contagious:

Chickenpox: after all sores are crusted, usually 7 days.
Strep throat: 24 hours after treatment begins.
Conjunctivitis: 24 hours after treatment begins.
Head lice: after one treatment.
Diarrhea: after stools form again.

Psychosocial Development of Personality and Behavior

The development of your child's personality is as important as his or her physical development. During the preschool years, problems may emerge that can affect the way your child behaves around you and other people.

Some of these problems, such as mental retardation and autism, are severe. Others, such as negativism and sibling rivalry, are common.

This section discusses average behavioral development during the preschool years, including the development of imagination and sexual curiosity. We also explore problems that can cause development that is not typical, such as learning disabilities and sexual abuse.

Behavioral Development

During the 5 years that constitute the preschool period, your child goes through many developmental changes. In the course of these few years, your child's vocabulary goes from a few words to hundreds. Your child at 1 year may be barely able to walk but at 5 years may be skipping rope. The 1-year-old who hides behind you when a stranger comes grows into the kindergartner who waves at you nonchalantly from the school bus.

The following are some examples of development that occur typically during these years. Keep in mind that your child's behavioral development does not adhere to a strict schedule. Every child is different and develops according to his or her own schedule. Thus, these are only general guidelines of what to expect. If you think there is a problem with your child's development, consult your physician.

Your 1-Year-Old

Your 1-year-old will hand you a toy when you ask for it. He or she can understand your gestures, obey your commands, and respond to his or her own name. Your child has learned to indicate a need or want in ways other than crying.

He or she is a bit of a "ham," never happier than when there is an audience. Your child sings, plays pat-a-cake, and loves to hide from you, although he or she always wants to keep mom or dad in sight. Although he or she still may fear strangers, your toddler is beginning to adjust to having a baby-sitter from time to time. He or she will hug or kiss either parent spontaneously or when requested and is beginning to show affection to stuffed toys or other objects.

A 1-year-old child loves to drop small objects into a container, dump them out, and then put them back in. He or she will combine objects with other objects to invent new ways of doing things, can retrieve a hidden toy, and is beginning to understand the concept of "up" and "down."

Your 1-year-old probably will insist on feeding himself or herself, can hold a cup with a little help, tries to use a spoon, may fight sleep, and cooperates when being dressed.

Your 2-Year-Old

A 2-year-old child can be bossy. He or she has yet to learn to share, although on rare occasions can put someone else's wishes above his or her own. He or she is able to communicate feelings, desires, and interests to others by using words or gestures.

By this time, most children have a vocabulary of 50 words or more, but they understand much more. Your 2-year-old is beginning to discover that everything has a name, can respond to commands such as "Point to your nose" or "Point to a dog in the book," and can locate items around the house. The child of this age likes to watch television and may be able to identify some cartoon characters.

By the second birthday, most children become more negative. They begin to become more aggressive and may take out their aggression on siblings or playmates. They become more possessive of their toys and more self-sufficient and are more likely to challenge parents' authority.

At play, a 2-year-old mimics parents' behavior, plays better with older children than with those of the same age, and is beginning to pretend.

Your 2-year-old wants to do everything without help. He or she can verbalize toilet needs, although most children are not trained at age 2.

Your 3-Year-Old

A 3-year-old is madly in love with his or her parents and wants to be just like them. Much of the hostility and negative behavior of the 2-year-old recedes into the background.

Your 2-year-old may have picked up his or her mop every time you mopped the floor, but the focus was on the mop. However, your 3-year-old who engages in this imitative behavior is actually trying to be like you. The child this age loves pretend games. After a visit to your physician, your 3-year-old gets out the toy "doctor kit" and examines his or her sick teddy bear or sits in the car and pretends to be daddy driving. Dressing up in your old clothing is a favorite game. At this age, children become more interested in their peers and begin to interact, although side-by-side play is still common.

A 3-year-old can conduct a conversation and uses relatively complex sentences. Many children can recognize several numbers and letters.

At this age, many children develop sleep problems, often as a result of fears.

Most 3-year-old children are toilet-trained and are capable of helping you dress them.

Your 4-Year-Old

Four-year-olds are extremely social creatures, capable of playing with several children at the same time. A 4-year-old has a vivid imagination, and frequent make-believe play reflects that.

Whereas 3-year-olds tend to be quite agreeable, some 4-year-olds are assertive, cocky, and loud.

Your 4-year-old is capable of telling a story. He or she now has the ability to think about language, and his or her speech is intelligible even to strangers. A child this age can accurately count four pennies, pedal a tricycle, play games that require taking turns and following rules, can copy a cross and a square, and can draw a person with as many as four parts besides the head. Some children this age begin writing the letters of the alphabet.

Your 5-Year-Old

Even more so than a 4-year-old, a 5-year-old delights in having other children around. Given a choice between doing something with a friend or with parents, the 5-year-old usually chooses the former.

A 5-year-old can get dressed alone (buttoning some buttons and perhaps even tying shoes). Your child probably also wants to choose what to wear. Your 5-year-old is extremely conscious of the differences between boys and girls. Children at this age often assert that they have a boyfriend or girlfriend whom they plan to marry.

Many children at 5 have been in nursery school for a year or two; some do not begin school until kindergarten. Depending on how much stimulation and exposure a child has had, it is not unusual for a 5-year-old to begin reading and writing and even to have some rudimentary skills in arithmetic.

Negativism

Between the ages of 18 months and 3 years, children go through a period when "No" is their favorite word. It doesn't matter what you say to the child; most of the time it will be met by an emphatic "No."

"Do you want to stay in the bathtub?" you ask your young daughter. "No," she answers. "Well, then, do you want to get out of the bathtub?" "No."

Negativism (along with tantrums) is a normal part of the so-called terrible twos. Although it may seem as though your child is purposely trying to provoke you, he or she is not. This is simply one step down the long road toward independence.

Getting through this sometimes difficult phase of development requires lots of patience and a good sense of humor. If you are the parent of a child in the thick of the terrible twos, remember that every parent goes through this and lives to laugh about it later.

The following are some guidelines that may help make the road a little less bumpy:

1. Do not take your child's negativism too seriously.

2. Don't punish your child for saying "No."

3. Give your child choices: "Do you want to wear the red pants or the green pants?" Letting him or her choose between acceptable choices will give your child a sense of freedom and control and make him or her more likely to cooperate. (Be careful about asking a question when there is only one answer. For example, at bedtime, do not offer your child a choice between staying up and going to bed if you have no intention of letting him or her stay up.)

4. Give your child a transition time between activities. If, for example, your child is having fun but it is time to leave the playground, give him or her adequate time. "You can go down the slide three more times and then we have to go home."

5. Go easy on rules. Children this age are not likely to follow a long list of house rules. Avoid arguing about unimportant things such as whether your child should eat all the carrots on his or her plate. Make

sure that your daily interactions with your child are weighted toward the positive, not the negative.

6. Try to avoid saying "No" yourself. You want the child to see you as an agreeable person, someone he or she can imitate.

Imagination

Preschoolers live part of their lives in a rich, imaginary world where anything is possible. Play during these years often revolves around pretending. Sometimes it is difficult for a child to know where pretend stops and reality starts. Hence, you have the 3-year-old who explains to you that he or she was not the one who broke your bottle of perfume but that it was a little green man with a yellow hat. Your child is not lying, not in the true sense of the word. And you should not punish your child or make him or her feel guilty for making up stories like this from time to time.

However, some children seem to live in their imaginations most of the day. If your child seems to be spending too much time with an imaginary friend whom he or she truly believes in, you might ask yourself whether your youngster's real life is sufficiently interesting. A child who lives in his or her own private dream world may need to spend more time with friends or may not be getting enough attention from parents.

Sibling Problems

Few things are as exasperating to parents as constant bickering among their children.

Problems between siblings can range from rivalry between the young toddler and the newborn to physical aggression to incessant quarreling.

Although these fights can make even easygoing parents wish they were rearing an only child, you should know that fighting and rivalry between siblings are normal. Although at times your children may seem to reside in enemy camps, on other days they may be the best of friends.

The following paragraphs describe some common problems between siblings and offer suggestions that may make them easier to live with.

Sibling Rivalry

Children can be jealous of a sibling at any age. One of the most common situations of sibling rivalry is the jealousy that older siblings feel toward a new baby in your family. The worst age for this rivalry is between 12 and 36 months.

A child who is jealous of a new brother or sister typically demands attention, may show aggression toward the infant, and often regresses (for example, he or she returns to thumb-sucking or wants to wear a diaper even though he or she is toilet trained).

Although you cannot totally eliminate these natural feelings, you can help prepare your child for the new baby by talking about the baby during pregnancy. Let your child help you get ready for the baby. If you need your child's crib, move him or her to a bed long before the baby is due. Praise your child for mature behavior.

At the very least, call your child each day that you are in the hospital. Preferably, your child should be allowed to visit and meet his or her new brother or sister.

When you get home, hand the baby to someone else and spend time alone with your older child.

Fighting

Children must be taught that they cannot kick, punch, or bite each other. When your children physically fight, separate them immediately. Send them to separate rooms for a few minutes.

Quarrels

Make it clear that children have to settle their own arguments. Then, when they do argue, try to ignore it, even if you have to go into another room. Try to stay out of the argument. If they do bring it to you, help them clarify the problem—but let them find the solution. When they do settle it, praise them. Avoid showing favoritism.

Refusal to Share Toys

Some 3-year-olds will share toys, but many do not start sharing until months later. You cannot make your child share with a sibling. Do not punish your child for refusing to share. However, encourage sharing and praise the child when this occurs.

In the same vein, many young children frequently grab toys away from a sibling playing nearby. When this happens, take the toy away from the child and return it to the child who was using it. Always praise the child for asking to use a toy and for returning it on request (see Difficulties With Sibling and Peer Relationships, page 126).

Thumb and Finger Sucking

Thumb and finger sucking is common in infants. Only 6 percent of thumb- or finger-sucking babies continue doing so beyond their first birthday, and only 3 percent do it beyond their second birthday.

By the time most thumb or finger suckers are 4, they have given up the practice, except when the issue has become a power struggle between parent and child or when it has become a deeply ingrained habit.

Thumb sucking is not a serious problem. However, it makes your child appear baby-ish, which may subject him or her to ridicule from peers. Moreover, prolonged thumb or finger sucking can interfere with the normal alignment of the teeth, making orthodontic treatment necessary in later years.

If your child is younger than 4 and sucks his or her thumb, try to ignore or distract the child. Never punish, scold, or pull your child's hand out of his or her mouth. These methods can make the problem worse.

In the older preschooler, you can appeal to vanity. Show your child how his or her teeth are beginning to protrude and the wrinkled skin of the thumb. Remind your child gently when you catch him or her in the act, and lavish praise when you notice he or she is not sucking the thumb.

Because thumb sucking during sleep is involuntary, it ceases when your child's sleep deepens.

Delayed Psychomotor Development

In most cases the development of gross and fine motor control proceeds smoothly. Sometimes, however, a child falls way behind his or her peers. For example, most children walk between 12 and 15 months. But what about the child who is not walking at 20 months? Is there something wrong?

There are several different types of delayed development in either fine (muscles used for hand dexterity) or gross (larger muscles used for walking, jumping, and skipping) motor function.

Some types of fine motor dysfunction may make it difficult for a preschooler to draw or color or may delay him or her in learning to tie shoes. Some children show impairments in hand-eye coordination. Some children with fine motor dysfunction cannot hold a crayon properly. Because of their problems with fine motor skills, these children often have difficulty when they enter school.

Children who are clumsy or who have delayed gross motor skills, such as the inability to skip or jump, often feel self-conscious and humiliated. These are the children who are always the last ones picked to be on the athletic team. Often they develop a poor self-image as a result.

The cause for delayed psychomotor development is generally unknown, although it may run in families.

If you suspect that your child may have a delay in psychomotor development, discuss your concerns with your physician. Tests can determine whether there is a problem.

If there is a developmental delay in your child's motor skills, he or she may lose an important area from which to draw for building self-esteem. As a parent you need to preserve your child's sense of self-esteem by being understanding and patient with his or her progress. If you are impatient, even though your child ultimately will "catch up," your child's self-esteem may suffer.

Learning Problems

Speech, hearing, and vision problems can affect a child's ability to learn. We can treat many of these successfully, or at least make them less severe. Often, the key factor is early detection. A sensory problem you discover during your child's preschool years often can be resolved before it irreparably affects your child's intellectual development.

Thus, it is important that your young child's periodic examinations include vision and hearing tests. Even children with no history or indication of eye problems should see an ophthalmologist by age 4.

The sensory defects that can cause learning problems are discussed below.

Hearing Disorders
In order to develop speech and language, a person must hear. Therefore, even a mild

loss of hearing or hearing loss in one ear during childhood can interfere with your child's language acquisition. The more severe the hearing loss, the greater the learning problem.

An estimated 4 percent of children younger than 5 have some hearing loss in both ears, and as many as 10 percent have a loss in one ear.

We find four types of hearing loss in young children. Conductive hearing loss involves interference with the reception of sound from the external to the internal ear. Sensorineural hearing loss is the result of abnormalities of the cochlear hair cells or the auditory nerve. Mixed hearing loss occurs when both a conductive and a sensorineural hearing loss are present. Central auditory disorders are the result of a dysfunction of the auditory center in the central nervous system.

If your child was born totally deaf, you might suspect it within the first 6 months of life. If deafness is partial, however, it likely will not be diagnosed until your child is between 12 and 24 months old or later. At this point, your child has already missed critical stages for language development and learning. For these reasons, physicians test many infants thought to be at high risk for hearing loss (those with neonatal asphyxia, bacterial meningitis, congenital or perinatal infections, a family history of deafness, or birth defects of the head or neck or those who were very premature) within the first 6 months of life (see Your Child's Hearing Development, page 65).

The extent to which a hearing loss influences your child's ability to learn depends on the severity of the loss and the range of frequencies affected. Moreover, the outcome for your child's language development, learning, and future educational achievements depends on the age at which the loss occurs, how soon it is discovered, and when treatment begins.

Physicians can treat some hearing losses with medication, others surgically. A hearing aid amplifies the hearing your child has and is considered the single most important tool toward allowing your child to function normally.

Your child will probably require some form of special education, even when the hearing loss is mild. This may be restricted to speech and language therapy if the loss is slight; in more severe cases, your child may require special education programs throughout his or her school career.

Finally, you should know that your active involvement is a vital aspect of your child's future academic success. You will need to learn how to make the most of whatever hearing your young child has. Techniques such as lip-reading and sign language can help. A class to learn such techniques may be available in your community.

Speech and Language Disorders

Certain illnesses can interfere with the normal development of articulation of words and sentences as well as with understanding language in your preschool child. The following paragraphs describe problems that can significantly delay development by a mild to a marked degree.

Severely delayed speech and language development that are part of your child's overall developmental retardation can play a part in a broader slowdown in your child reaching other developmental milestones such as sitting, standing, walking, and toilet training.

Hearing loss, resulting from nerve deafness at birth or from middle ear infections during infancy and early childhood, can be a cause of speech and language disorders.

Neurologic disorders involving a lack of muscle strength or coordination, either present at birth or acquired during early infancy or childhood, along with damage to language areas of the brain, also can cause impairment of your child's speech and language.

In addition, environmental deprivation of language and emotional stimulation due to parental conflict, separation, or child abuse may contribute to your child's speech and language disorders.

If you are concerned about an apparent failure of normal articulation, language development, stuttering, or other deviations in your child's speech or comprehension, consult your pediatrician or family physician and a speech-language specialist for proper diagnosis and, particularly, therapy. This step can be important and profitable in many cases of childhood speech and language disorders (see Speech and Language Development, page 92).

Vision Problems

The preschool years are crucial for the detection and treatment of many vision disorders,

Infantile Autism

Infantile autism (now called pervasive developmental disorder) is a severe mental illness of childhood. An autistic child is extremely unresponsive to other people. He or she communicates poorly, does not cuddle, and may even seem repulsed by physical contact. Autistic children fail to seek comfort when distressed, do not imitate adults normally (for example, don't "wave bye-bye"), and have virtually no social interaction.

An autistic child may exhibit stereotyped body movements (hand-flicking or -twisting, spinning, head-banging); is fascinated by parts of objects (say, spinning the wheels on a toy car); gets very upset over even the slightest change in his or her environment (movement of a chair or small objects, for example); and is unreasonably insistent on routines.

Autism usually appears before a child is 30 months old. An autistic child may not speak or may mimic sounds made by others. She or he may have difficulty naming objects and may make bizarre facial expressions and gestures. Occasionally, an autistic child will have an extraordinary talent, similar to the case of the adult "idiot savant." (For more information on Infantile Autism, see page 1100.)

some serious and some, such as myopia, serious only in their ability to create a learning difficulty.

Children with abnormalities of refraction (conditions that require eyeglasses) may show a lack of interest in learning. The child who is farsighted may not want to look at books, and the one who is nearsighted may seem uninterested in any activity more than a few feet away. Squinting, eye rubbing, fatigue, and headaches are common manifestations.

These problems are easily corrected with prescription glasses. When detected in the preschool years, simple vision problems do not have an adverse effect on a child's learning (see Refraction Problems, page 522, and Strabismus and Amblyopia, page 534).

Mental Retardation

Mental retardation, or developmental disability, can range from a slight slowness that makes school a struggle to profound retardation requiring constant supervision. If your child is developmentally disabled, he or she is slow in acquiring motor skills and language. Your child lacks the social skills and emotional maturity appropriate to his or her age.

Your otherwise typical child may lag behind in one or another of these areas of development. This may represent a developmental lag in a child who will eventually catch up. Others have emotional or social immaturities that may indicate a disturbance (see Mental Health, page 1093). However, children with mental retardation are behind in all of these areas and will not catch up with their peers.

Mild forms of retardation may not become evident until your child begins school. Children with mild retardation are able to learn academic skills but do so more slowly than the average child. They are identified as educationally mentally handicapped.

Children with moderate mental retardation may learn self-care skills such as dressing and toileting. They have limited ability to benefit from academic school programs but can attend day activity centers and eventually learn certain simple jobs in sheltered workshops.

Children who are severely or profoundly retarded can learn minimal self-care skills and may become toilet trained but require almost total supervision and care. They have limited communication skills.

In the past, most developmentally disabled children, even those with mild retardation, were institutionalized. Today most of these children live at home or in small group homes in their communities. All school districts offer special education programs for slow learners, and many resources are available in communities to provide social and recreational opportunities for more severely retarded children.

Even when there are some early signs, in many children mild retardation is not actually diagnosed until they begin school, because it is then that we compare them with large numbers of peers and their developmental differences become more apparent.

If your child is developmentally disabled, the goal of treatment is to help your child reach his or her potential, whatever it may be, and to enable him or her to cope as well as possible with limitations.

When a diagnosis is made in infancy, you and your baby frequently can enroll in an infant stimulation program. Such a program offers multisensory stimulation in an attempt to facilitate emotional, intellectual, and physical development. It also helps you to understand more about your child's strengths and weaknesses and offers you support during what is usually a very difficult time emotionally.

Federal legislation has guaranteed an education to all developmentally disabled children in the United States, regardless of the severity of their handicap. Regular community schools teach special education classes. Some children with disabilities may spend part of the day in a class with other children like themselves, and then attend a class or two with children who are not disabled.

Every child needs friends. Despite the mixing (mainstreaming) of developmentally disabled children with other children in schools, classmates do not always accept these children as friends. Thus, you as a parent must often take it upon yourself to plan social and recreational activities for your child. Organizations for developmentally disabled children offer various activities, including summer camps. These programs help your child both to become more comfortable in social situations and to increase his or her independence (see page 1373, Appendix III).

Finally, caring for a child with a developmental disability can leave little time for the rest of the family. However devoted, parents need a break. Because of the child's handicap, though, many parents who would leave an average child with a baby-sitter are reluctant to do so with a child that has special needs. Many communities have recognized this need and opened respite centers where parents can temporarily leave their disabled child with a caregiver experienced in the needs of these children. If you are lucky enough to live in a community with this option, take advantage of it.

Sexuality in Your Preschool Child

Your preschool child has a natural sexual curiosity that manifests itself in various ways.

From birth, boys are capable of having erections, and the vagina of a newborn girl can become lubricated. By the first birthday, one-third of all children have been observed stimulating their genitals; boys typically pull at their penises, and girls rub their external genitalia. Between the ages of 2 and 5, one-half of all boys and one-third of all girls masturbate.

Occasional masturbation is normal and nothing to worry about. The child stimulates himself or herself simply because it feels good. Some children masturbate because they are unhappy or are reacting to punish-

ment to stop the practice.

If your child masturbates, try not to get upset. Masturbation does not mean your child will grow up to be promiscuous or sexually deviant. It is not physically harmful, nor does it cause emotional problems, unless a parent overreacts and sends the message that sex is dirty and frightening.

Because it is difficult to stop a child from masturbating, it is best to simply accept it. However, you need to explain to your child that, although it is all right to masturbate in the privacy of the bedroom, other areas are off limits. If your child suddenly starts masturbating in the middle of a play group, try to distract him or her. If that fails, take your child aside and remind him or her that this is done only in the privacy of the bedroom or bathroom.

In addition to self-stimulation, many preschoolers are curious about their parents' bodies. A young child may want to touch the mother's breasts or father's penis. Another child may be found half undressed, playing "doctor" with the child next door.

These behaviors are normal. Avoid showing shock or anger. Instead, stress that some activities are private and, although it is okay for your child to touch himself or herself, it is not okay for others, even friends, to touch them that way except in special circumstances, such as an examination by a physician. Then point out that this is true for adults as well as for children.

Sexual Abuse

The sexual abuse of children has, in recent years, emerged from the proverbial closet. The problem certainly is not new—but our understanding of the extent of the problem surely is: as many as 1 in 5 girls and 1 in 10 boys will be victims of sexual abuse before reaching the age of 18.

Recognize the Signs
Be alert for the following possible signs of sexual abuse in a child:

1. Sexually provocative behavior in a preschooler

2. Withdrawal from friends, family, or school activities

3. Unusually hostile or aggressive behavior

Child Abuse

Children of all ages can be abused. Most often the abuser is related to the child and is involved in caring for the child. Parents who abuse their offspring come from all walks of life. Some are high-salaried professionals; others are unemployed. Abuse crosses all educational backgrounds, from high school dropouts to people with advanced degrees. Child abusers are rich and poor, white and black, Hispanic and Asian, and of all faiths, economic strata, and political beliefs.

Abusive parents often tend to be lonely, angry, and very unhappy people who often are under stress with which they cannot cope. Many of them were physically abused when they were children. Still, there's never a valid excuse for child abuse.

In dealing with child abuse, protection of the child is the most important objective. The goal of comprehensive treatment of the entire family is for 80 to 90 percent of these families to remain intact and safe for the child, with the parents providing adequate care. Abused children who are returned home without intervention run a significant risk of serious injury or even death.

If our society is going to deal with child abuse, everyone must help by reporting instances of suspected abuse. You can file a report by contacting people who are trained in dealing with suspected abuse, such as local social service and law enforcement agencies. You may obtain further information and assistance by talking to physicians, counselors, clergy, school professionals, or others who deal with child abuse or families with problems.

We encourage parents who fear they have abused or may abuse their children to contact these groups as well. In addition, many communities offer self-help groups such as Parents Anonymous.

There may be no physical signs of abuse, but a physician may identify evidence of trauma to the genital area or the presence of sexually transmitted infections (see page 1087). However, the absence of all of these signs is not necessarily proof that no abuse has occurred.

Why a Child Is Susceptible

Children need affection; depriving a child of healthy physical contact (such as hugging), in fact, is to risk significant problems in a youngster's psychological development.

Children often seek some sexual contact with their peers. This usually is normal curiosity and experimentation. If your child describes an experience in which he or she was touched by a much older child or by an adult in an inappropriate way, take it seriously.

What to Do

If you suspect that your child has been sexually abused, contact your physician or an official in your local child-protection system (child welfare worker, local public attorney, police, or sheriff). If you are tempted to keep the abuse a private or family matter, keep in mind that most perpetrators are involved with many children. Seldom is the abuser a complete stranger to the child. The welfare or even the life of your child may be at stake.

Care of Your Handicapped Child

The care of a handicapped child involves a combination of family support, social and academic adaptation, adjustments in the physical environment to accommodate the child's disability, and, often, special medical care.

Permanent disabilities in children can include severe mental retardation, conspicu-

ous physical deformities such as the absence of a limb, or sensory defects such as blindness or deafness.

Whatever a child's limitations, it does not take him or her long to realize that he or she is different. Helping your handicapped child develop a sense of self-worth and an ability to get along in the world despite this difference is fundamental to the successful rearing of your child. You can achieve this, in part, by helping your child become as self-sufficient as possible and by creating an environment in which your child can develop to his or her full potential.

Few things are as traumatic as the birth of a child with a major disability. Some parents initially try to deny the reality of the situation, especially if the disability is not physically apparent. It's normal to feel guilt, anger, accusation, and fear about your ability to cope with a disabled child, as well as anxiety over your child's future.

If your child's handicap is severe, you may need to address placement into a supervised living service early. It used to be common to place severely retarded infants in institutions. Today, physicians know that infants and young children do better developmentally if they have a consistent parent figure in a nurturing home environment. Still, parents of children with disabilities often come to the realization that they alone cannot care for their child; thus the child may enter a facility equipped for special needs. Even so, you may want to attempt home care before you consider placing your child in an alternate environment.

If you are attempting to rear a child with disabilities at home, there are things you can do to make your child as happy and well adjusted as possible.

Treat All Your Children Alike

Some parents relax household rules for the disabled child, which only makes the child feel more different than he or she is. Rules should apply equally to everyone in the family. Like his or her siblings, your handicapped child should have certain responsibilities around the house and should be punished for breaking the rules (when he or she is capable of understanding the rules), just as any other child would.

Be Aware of Your Attitude

Children are amazingly deft at compensating for a defect. For example, a child born without one hand becomes very proficient with the other hand and, having known nothing else, does not miss the absent hand. However, if you are embarrassed about the defor-mity, your child will sense these feelings and probably become self-conscious.

Do Not Neglect Your Other Children

The care of a child with special needs can be so time-consuming that you ignore other family members. Answer your other children's questions about their brother or sister honestly. Try to set aside time each week to be alone with each child.

Accept Your Child's Individuality

All children have strengths and weaknesses. When your child with special needs accomplishes something, no matter how small, praise him or her. Make your child feel special.

Do Not Isolate Your Child

All children need friends. It is normal to want to protect your child from contagious illness and the potential cruelty of some children, but do not do it at the expense of your child's socialization.

Schools now provide an education for all children within the community. Previously, children with special needs went to one school together. Today, however, by law, most public schools must provide special education classes for children with disabilities. And, in many cases, the children take classes with children in the mainstream student population. Mixing children with disabilities with the rest of the students can benefit everyone in the class.

Address Special Needs

A child's needs may range from a specially designed house and van to home care provided by a trained nurse or weekly visits to a medical facility.

You Are Not Alone

Many community resources can help you meet the needs of your son or daughter. Some agencies offer financial help for qualifying parents who cannot provide for their child's medical needs. Others offer services such as transportation, counseling, psychological evaluation, baby-sitting, child care, and play activities (see page 1373, Appendix III).

Your child's physician can be an excellent source of information about available community resources. Public health nurses and social workers know of local resources and are often a very useful source of information and support. In addition, parent organizations offer help. These groups give parents a chance to express their common concerns and share information. In recent years, these groups have organized and have become a force in influencing legislation that has expanded and improved opportunities for children with disabilities.

Nutrition

Some days it may seem as if your preschooler does not eat enough to keep an ant alive, and other days you cannot keep him or her away from the refrigerator. Such is the preschooler's appetite.

Unlike an infant, who triples his or her weight during the first year and eats well, the 1-year-old child's rate of growth slows considerably, as does his or her appetite. Some preschoolers are reluctant to try new foods or expand their food repertoire beyond three or four old favorites.

If you have a preschooler with a finicky appetite, you may be worried about whether your child is being adequately nourished. Or, your child may be eating too much and is overweight.

This section addresses these and other common nutritional issues.

Nutrition in Your Preschool Child

By the time your child enters the second year of life, he or she should be eating a variety of foods from each of the food groups of the food pyramid (see page 261). These include milk products; meat, poultry, fish, dried beans, and eggs; bread, cereal, rice, and pasta; and fruits and vegetables. The chart on page 113 suggests the approximate serving size and mix of foods that are appropriate for filling your preschooler's nutritional needs.

Keep in mind, however, that every child's energy needs are different. Your child is not growing at the same rate he or she was as an infant, so it will not seem as if your child lives for the next meal. Your child does not need or want the quantities of food that he or she consumed with relish only a few months ago.

You may fail to recognize this important fact and become concerned when your child is uninterested and picks at food. You may attempt to force your child into eating, which can create long-term feeding problems and make mealtime an unpleasant experience for the entire family.

While your preschooler advances to the point where he or she can start to assume the same pattern of eating as that of older siblings or parents—that is, a three-meals-a-day pattern—keep in mind that snacking is acceptable. As parents, your role is to offer a variety of nutritious foods and set a good example.

Do not think that the dietary model has to be followed slavishly every day: a child does not have to eat two servings of vegetables 7 days a week. More to the point, your child, despite occasional daily slips in amounts and choices, should be getting an overall good selection of foods.

Allow your child to help design his or her own eating style. Although the basic three-meals-a-day approach is best, snacks are often appropriate for children. In fact, we recommend them, especially for smaller preschoolers, who cannot eat enough to satisfy their energy needs all at once. Small amounts of a variety of foods eaten frequently over the course of the day as a snack are healthful and normal. However, completely uncontrolled snacking can diminish your child's appetite for meals.

Remember that a balanced diet may also include desserts and fats such as butter, margarine, mayonnaise, and oils. Until age 2, fat should not be limited in your child's diet. Dietary fat and cholesterol are important for

The Balanced Diet for Your Preschool Child

The following foods should form the foundation of your child's diet:

Milk Products. Milk, cheese, cottage cheese, and yogurt are excellent sources of calcium, which is necessary for building strong bones and teeth. We recommend four servings a day. For the 1-year-old child, a serving is ½ cup, and for older preschoolers the serving size may be as large as ¾ cup.

Meat and Eggs. This group includes beef, poultry, lamb, fish, pork, liver, eggs, cottage cheese, dried peas and beans, and peanut butter. These foods are excellent sources of protein, which is necessary for the growth and repair of tissue cells. Your preschooler needs three or more servings a day.

Fruits and Vegetables. Your child should have at least four servings a day from this food group. To obtain an adequate amount of vitamin C, one or more servings should be citrus fruit, berries, tomato, cabbage, or cantaloupe. The child needs at least one serving of a green or yellow fruit or vegetable, which are excellent sources of vitamin A.

Grains. This food group includes whole-grain cereals, crackers, breads, rice, and pasta. We recommend four or more daily servings. The serving size for the 1-year-old is one-half slice of bread, one-half ounce of ready-to-eat cereal, or one-fourth cup of pasta. For the 5-year-old, one and one-half slices of bread, one ounce of ready-to-eat cereal, or one-half cup of pasta constitutes a serving.

These are the food groups necessary for a nutritionally balanced diet; but do not expect your preschooler to eat a completely balanced diet every day. When allowed to choose from a selection of nutritionally sound foods, most children tend to select diets that, over several days, offer the necessary balance. This may mean that one day your child might be eating a lot of peanut butter sandwiches, oranges, and milk and the next day the menu is hamburgers, french fries, and carrots.

In essence, the overall nutrition picture is more important than what he or she eats on any given day.

---

your infant's growth. Fats should be consumed in moderation after your child's second birthday.

In recent years, Americans have become much more conscious of their diets. The excessive consumption of fat may contribute to later health problems—so excess fat should be trimmed from your preschooler's diet, too. However, the intake of fat or calories should not necessarily be limited. Instead, discourage excessive amounts of foods high in fat.

Testing your child's blood cholesterol level is necessary only if your family has a history of premature heart disease or high blood fat levels. If there is a family history and your physician finds an elevated value, take steps to reduce the cholesterol and fat content of your child's diet. Consult your physician.

You needn't do anything radical. Just follow these guidelines when buying food and planning menus:

1. Buy 2 percent milk rather than whole milk for children older than 2.

2. Trim the fat off meats.

3. Serve more fish, poultry, and lean meats.

4. Offer low-fat cheeses, frozen yogurt, or ice milk.

5. Serve cookies that are lower in fats, such as homemade oatmeal cookies, animal crackers, ginger snaps, vanilla wafers, or fig newtons; use skim milk to make pudding.

6. Limit eggs to three or four a week.

7. Replace butter with margarine.

Obesity

Some disorders can cause obesity, but if your child is overweight it is probably because he or she consumes more calories than necessary for growth and activity. However, obesity is more common during the first year of life, after age 5 or 6 years, and during adolescence than it is during the preschool years.

Not all children who are overweight are considered obese. Some children have larger-than-average body frames. These children tend to be stocky and look big, but they are not truly fat.

The obese child looks fat to the casual observer. The obese child is, in fact, more than 20 percent over what is considered his or her healthy weight.

Obesity is generally caused by a combination of factors. Heredity appears to play a role. If one or both parents are obese, their offspring is more likely to be overweight than is the child of thin parents. In addition, overeating may be more common in households whose members are overweight than in those whose members maintain a normal weight. Lack of exercise also may be a factor.

If your preschooler is obese, now is the time to do something, while you still have some control over what your child eats and how active he or she is. Once your child gets older and is more independent, modifying eating and exercise patterns will be much more difficult.

Consult a physician or dietitian if you feel your child needs to change his or her food intake. Consider your child's nutritional needs and growth when making these changes. Do not use fad diets. They can be dangerous.

Of course, prevention is the best treatment. The time to be alert to obesity (especially if there is a family history) is when your child's eating and exercise habits are forming.

Infant obesity has poor or little correlation with adult obesity, but family eating habits may persist into adolescence and adulthood (see Obesity, page 1099).

Chapter 4

School-Age Child: Ages 6 Through 12

Contents

Beginning the School Years, 116

Normal Growth and Development, 116

Common Concerns During the School-Age Years, 118
General Care, 118
Growing Pains, 119
Recurrent Headaches, 120
Recurrent Abdominal Aches, 120
Caring for Sick Children, 120
Nutrition, 121
How Much and What Kind of Food Does Your School-Age Child Need? 122
School Lunch Programs: Do They Make the Nutritional Grade? 123
Memorandum: To Parents and School Officials, 123
Obesity, 123

Psychological and Social Development, 124
Normal Psychosocial Development, 124

Difficulties With Sibling and Peer Relationships, 126
Sexuality in Your School-Age Child, 126
Sexual Abuse, 127
Dealing With Physical Illness and Hospitalization, 128

Learning Disorders, 129
Learning Disabilities, 130
Specific Reading Disability (Dyslexia), 131
Speech Disorder, 132
Attention Deficit Disorder, 132
Hyperactivity, 133
School Phobias, 133

Sexual Development and Gynecologic Disorders, 134
Breast Abnormalities, 134
Vaginal Bleeding, 134
Adrenarche, 135
Premature Puberty, 135
Sexual Precocity, 135
Genital Infections in Young Girls, 136

Beginning the School Years

During the school-age years (ages 6 through 12), your child will gradually become a citizen of a larger world. In particular, peers and teachers become ever more influential as your child develops greater independence from the family. More relationships will be formed outside the home.

Age 6 usually marks the start of your child's formal education. Most 6-year-olds will already have attended kindergarten, and many will have gone to nursery school or child care. These programs, however, tend to have less structured and more flexible settings. First grade is different.

Your child is required to adhere to the rules of an external authority and to devote almost all of his or her time to the work of learning. Suddenly your child has less time to play or to enjoy the informal learning that occurs throughout the preschool years. At school, your child is required to follow a rather fixed schedule. These new rules extend the limit-setting that you started in your child's preschool years.

As with younger children, school-age children are generally healthy, active, and enthusiastic. Not surprisingly, it is often hard for them to control their energy and exuberance enough to conform to rules of good behavior at home and at school. When children enter a more structured environment, such as school, deficits in vision and learning may become more apparent.

Witnessing your child's achievements and successful integration into this wider world can be a great source of pride. At the same time, your child's broad new horizons may provoke anxiety. As your child moves in directions that are new or unfamiliar or of which you do not approve, you may be frustrated by your waning control over him or her. Be assured that you still have a crucial role to play in guiding your child through these years of tremendous physical and psychosocial development.

The increasing independence of your school-age child may stand in welcome contrast to the continual demands of your preschooler. Although it may be easy to allow your increasingly independent child to occupy himself or herself, an open and trusting relationship must be nurtured if it is to be maintained during the turbulent adolescent years.

Seek your child's company. Discuss his or her interests; participate in activities, however mundane, together. The lines of communication you keep open during these critical formative years may prove invaluable in the future.

This chapter is designed to help you identify and play a significant role in your child's development as he or she moves through the school-age years to adolescence. It also outlines the normal growth and development of school-age children. Unlike the changes of puberty, the school-age child's physical, psychological, and social growth move forward in gradual and steady increments. Nonetheless, this is all previously uncharted territory. School, peers, and early puberty all present fresh challenges.

Normal Growth and Development

Growth and development are slow and steady in the early school-age years, in sharp contrast with the rapid changes that occurred during the preschool years and those to follow during adolescence.

Your school-age child will gain about 7 pounds a year, and his or her height will increase by approximately 2.5 inches a year. The growth of your child's head also will slow down. This is the time when your child's brain has almost reached its adult size.

Your child's motor skills also will be refined between the ages of 6 and 12. During this period, running, jumping, and throwing show steady improvement. To enhance this important process, continue to encourage your child to be physically active.

You and your child may enjoy tracking his or her progress on a growth chart at home. Your child's physician may also keep watch of your child's height and weight. Growth charts can provide an opportunity to suspect serious diseases. For instance, when children develop chronic illnesses their weight often stays the same or even decreases and their height does not increase at the expected rate.

During the period of rapid growth toward the end of the school-age years, children suddenly grow at dramatically different rates. If you think your child seems unusually short or tall, you can ask his or her physician about it. The physician may obtain an X-ray of the hand. By reviewing this X-ray with a standardized set of tables, your physician can determine whether the bone age correlates with your child's actual age.

School-age girls and boys have distinctly different growth patterns. There is a period during the late school-age years when girls are taller and heavier than boys because their growth spurt comes first (before the age of about 9½ years, average height is similar for both sexes). By the age of 13½ years, most boys have grown taller than girls. Girls tend to weigh less than boys until almost age 9 and after age 14, but they are heavier than boys between those two ages.

Toward the end of the school-age years, children begin to grow at a dramatic but highly variable rate. This preadolescent growth spurt is a part of puberty, which is a sequence of events that transforms a child into a young adult. Early puberty generally begins at about age 10 in girls and age 12 in boys. For a discussion of normal growth and development in the teenage years, see page 139.

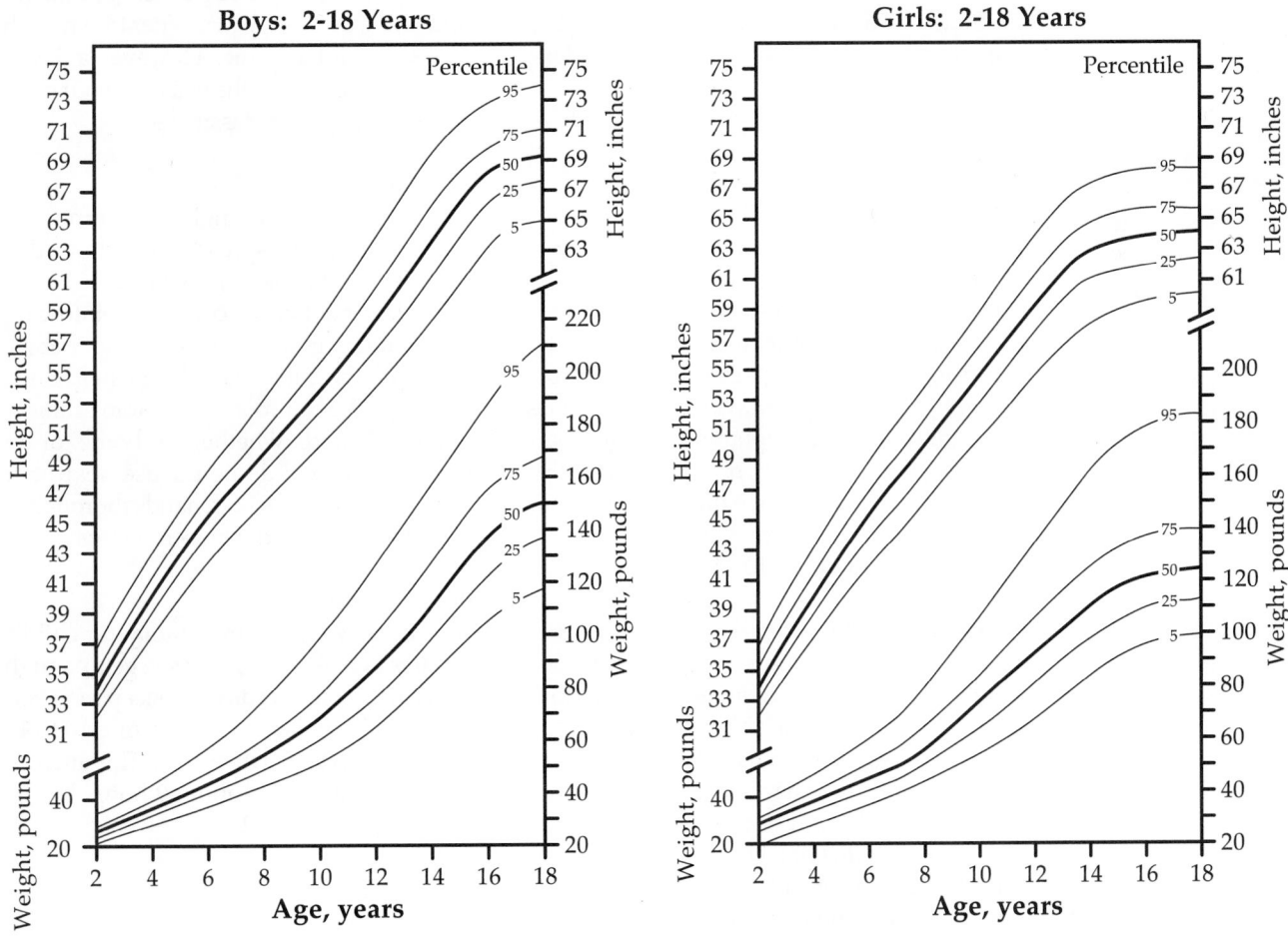

Your physician may use charts like these to assess your child's growth over a period of time.

Common Concerns During the School-Age Years

In this section we give guidelines for general care and nutrition. We also discuss the effects common diseases can have on your child. We emphasize features of these disorders that are unique to children of school age.

School-age children gradually become less prone to the common respiratory infections of the preschooler, including colds (see Common Viral Colds, page 1071) and flu (see Influenza, page 1065). Many school-age children commonly complain of recurrent stomachache or headache and growing pains. In the following pages we will review each of these concerns.

We cover many of the disorders that occur commonly in school-age children elsewhere in this book, specifically in Part IV, Human Diseases and Disorders. Most disorders of school-age children do not have serious consequences. At this age children are extraordinarily resilient, and their young bodies easily recover from most common disorders.

General Care

Immunizations
By age 6, your child should have completed the recommended schedule of childhood immunizations. Most states require that children have a documented, completed series before entering kindergarten. Thus, unless contraindicated, your child may be immunized against diphtheria, tetanus, pertussis, measles, mumps, rubella, *Haemophilus influenzae*, varicella, hepatitis B, and polio before admission to kindergarten (see Immunizations, page 1079).

Regular Checkups
In most schools, children are screened routinely for problems with hearing, vision, height, weight, and spine curvature (see Scoliosis, page 906). If the school health staff detects a disorder, they will tell you and urge you to consult a physician.

However, do not rely solely on the school to address all of your child's health care needs. In addition, schedule occasional visits to your child's physician when your child is well. The physician will check your child's growth and development and blood pressure, among other things, as well as give you an opportunity to discuss any concerns you may have.

Infectious Diseases
At school, your child will come in contact with large numbers of other children. As in child care centers, contagious diseases can spread easily to other children. To help curb this spread, keep your child home from school whenever he or she has a communicable disease. Common examples include colds (see Common Viral Colds, page 1071), flu (see Influenza, page 1065), strep throat (see page 592), and chickenpox (see page 1076).

If you are not sure whether to keep your child home, check with his or her physician, nurse practitioner, or school nurse about whether the disease is communicable—and if so, for how long. It may be difficult if you must rearrange your schedule, get time off from work, or arrange for a sitter to stay with your sick child at home. However, a day at home may be best for the health of your child as well as his or her classmates.

Hygiene
Hand washing is the single most important way to prevent the spread of infectious diseases, including colds. As you started to do in the preschool years, continue reinforcing your child's good hand-washing habits. Insist that the child wash his or her hands after using the bathroom and before eating or preparing food, whether at home or in school. Your child should use soap and warm water to wash both hands thoroughly, including palms and between fingers.

Sleep Requirements
Another way to help maintain your child's health is to make sure he or she gets enough sleep. Your child needs more sleep than you do. At age 6, children may require 10 to 12 hours of sleep to feel their best. This amount declines gradually to about 9 hours by the time they reach age 12.

Dental Care
One by one, your child's permanent teeth will erupt during the school-age years. They replace the primary (baby) teeth at a rate of about four a year. Because the permanent

teeth will have to last a lifetime, it is imperative to care for them well. As you began to do in the preschool years, continue teaching your child to brush his or her teeth after each meal. It is also a good time to start demonstrating how to floss at bedtime (see Proper Flossing and Brushing Techniques, page 366). Schedule visits to your child's dentist about twice a year.

As soon as the permanent back teeth have broken through, your child's dentist may cover them with a brush-on sealant. This will help protect them against tooth decay.

You can do your part to decrease the risks of tooth decay by limiting your child's consumption of sweets. If your water does not contain fluoride, your child's physician or dentist may prescribe fluoride as a supplement. If the teeth need straightening, orthodontic treatment is often started at this age (for a detailed discussion of dental care, see Tooth Care, page 363).

Accident and Injury

Normal behavioral and physical development increase the school-age child's susceptibility to accidental injury. The risk of these accidents is raised by the school-age child's natural inclination to experiment with adventurous behavior. You can minimize your child's risk by diligently taking precautions.

Car accidents are the most common cause of death in school-age children. It is extremely important to require that your child wear a seat belt for the entire duration of each automobile trip, regardless of how far you travel. Set a good example by wearing your seat belt, too.

You can also help by stressing the traffic rules that apply to bicyclists (see Basic Bicycling Safety, page 357).

Peers play an increasingly important role in the life of a school-age child. More and more, your child will enjoy playing with a group and will develop steadfast loyalty to its members. In unsupervised situations he or she may follow the group's lead, no matter how dangerous. The influence of the child's peers tends to increase during the school-age years. Eventually, the peer group may demand that children of late school age (especially boys) perform daring, often hazardous, feats, simply to be accepted.

No parent can supervise every minute of his or her child's life. Yet it is possible—really essential—to instill in your child an idea of what is safe and unsafe. A certain amount of daredevil behavior is normal in the late school-age years. However, you may be able to minimize the danger to your child by promoting a positive self-image so he or she will not feel so much pressure to do what the group says.

Other basic precautions to be taken are ensuring that your child swims in safe, supervised settings, that guns in the house, if any, are kept under lock and key, and that your child follows the rules of pedestrian safety.

It is also important to find the safest possible facilities for your child to use for supervised recreation. Backyards, playgrounds, parks, and community centers are examples. Otherwise, children may choose to play in hazardous or poorly supervised places where the risk of injury is greater and the availability of help is less if an accident does occur. Organized activities such as youth baseball and soccer, under adult supervision, which emphasize the teaching of skills and the discipline of playing on a team rather than winning, are excellent activities for school-age boys and girls.

Healthful Lifestyles

School-age children can take increasing personal responsibility for their own health and can learn the foundations of a healthful lifestyle. This is the time to teach them about hygiene, nutrition, dental care, substance abuse, and accident prevention.

Provide guidance for your child in development and socialization issues, such as discipline, school progress, and relationships with peers. Encourage your child's sense of personal responsibility for chores at home, for schoolwork, and for his or her own behavior.

Growing Pains

Many school-age children, particularly during the later years of this period, experience relatively severe, recurrent limb pain. These pains may come on at any time, but they seem to occur most frequently in the evening, particularly after a day of strenuous activity.

Usually these pains are located in the thighs or calves, and the pains stop after an hour or two. The children are otherwise healthy, and the results of physical examination as well as laboratory tests and X-rays, if needed, are always normal. Although these pains are probably not directly related to physical growth, the symptoms often are labeled "growing pains."

So-called growing pains have no known explanation and disappear over time without any lasting ill effects. Unless other associated symptoms develop, the best treatment for growing pains is sympathy and understanding and offering reassurance that the symptoms do not represent a health problem and will disappear with time.

Recurrent Headaches

Recurrent headaches are common during late childhood and adolescence. They rarely represent any serious problem.

Headache is associated with many viral illnesses. However, if your child frequently complains of headache, even during times when he or she is otherwise well, consult your physician.

Migraine headaches may occur in children and may be suspected if there is a family history of migraine. In children, this type of headache often is accompanied by vomiting, light sensitivity, and sleep. Recovery follows within a few hours (see Migraine Headaches, page 502).

Recurrent Abdominal Aches

Stomachaches are common in children. Typically, the pains are nothing more than the result of eating something that does not agree with them or the beginning of a bout with a gastrointestinal virus.

Sometimes, however, a child complains of intermittent or chronic diarrhea or abdominal pain. These symptoms may relate to some type of stress or fear, such as a school activity.

The prognosis varies. In many children the symptoms disappear, whereas others have recurrent bouts of pain over many years.

Consult your child's physician if vomiting, fever, or loss of weight occurs or if your child refuses to participate in usual day-to-day activities because of such discomforts.

Caring for Sick Children

Although the symptoms of a child's illness can be dramatic—high fevers, for example—recovery is usually easier and quicker than for adults. However, children need a great deal more reassurance and companionship during illness than do adults, so although the nursing experience is likely to be shorter, it can be more demanding.

Giving Medicine
Many children resist taking medication. To sidestep such resistance, approach this task in a natural, matter-of-fact way. Apprehension on your part or the expectation of resistance can become a self-fulfilling prophecy.

It's generally best to avoid mixing medications with foods or drinks. If your child doesn't eat or drink the entire mixture, you won't know how much of the medication was taken.

Do not try to get your child to take medication by promising a treat or, worse, telling him or her that the medication is candy. Children must learn to make a clear distinction between medicine and candy and to take all medications while supervised by an adult.

It is important to give medications exactly as prescribed—in the correct dose and at the correct interval. Give medications at evenly spaced intervals throughout the day. When your child begins to show signs of improvement, do not stop giving the medication unless specifically instructed to do so. Do not give remnants of old prescriptions.

Fevers
Sudden occurrence of fever usually means that an infection has developed. Viral infections, strep throat (see page 592), and ear infections (see Acute Ear Infection, page 574) are the most common causes of fever in children. More serious illnesses can cause fever, but fortunately they are not common.

A temperature of more than 99.5 degrees Fahrenheit (37.5 degrees centigrade) by mouth is considered a fever. The only difference in thermometers is the tip; always use a round-bulb thermometer for taking a rectal temperature (see How to Take a Temperature and How to Read a Thermometer, page 1072).

Although children tolerate most fevers quite well, high temperatures often provoke a great deal of anxiety for parents. A common concern is that there is some critical level of fever that can cause convulsions (see Febrile Seizures, page 69) or brain damage. This is not the case. Febrile seizures are more closely related to how rapidly the fever increases than to any critical level. Children rarely have long-term ill effects from febrile seizures, and high fever by itself does not cause brain damage. Less than 5 percent of all children are prone to febrile seizures.

Contact your child's physician if the fever is accompanied by considerable listlessness, irritability, severe headache, or persistent vomiting or stomachache. Also call if there is a high fever that does not respond to acetaminophen.

Be guided more by how your child acts than by any particular temperature. A high fever is not necessarily cause for alarm, but the absence of a high fever doesn't mean a sick child won't require medical care.

If your child has a fever, the following suggestions may be helpful:

1. Let heat escape. Do not bundle your child up.

2. Provide plenty of liquids to drink.

3. Give acetaminophen in the recommended dosage. This is available in liquid, chewable, and suppository forms. Physicians no longer recommend routine use of aspirin for treating fever in children because of the risk of Reye's syndrome (see page 484).

What to Feed Your Child

Follow your physician's instructions, which will vary depending on the illness. If the symptoms include fever, vomiting, or diarrhea, provide plenty of liquids. Relax household rules about drinking soda pop if making it available helps get sufficient liquid into your child. When vomiting or diarrhea is present, restrict the diet as instructed by your child's physician. If the physician doesn't specify a particular diet, relaxing usual dietary restrictions may encourage your child to eat.

Getting Up

When your child feels well enough, allow him or her to get out of bed. Only in rare cases will physicians instruct otherwise. During the convalescent period, your child may be out of bed part of the time and back in bed when tired. Children are often better than adults at letting their physical condition guide them in how much they can manage.

Long-Term Convalescence

Long-term care of a child with a disease or injury involves keeping him or her busy and occupied (with toys, reading, and suitable television programs). This can require considerable effort on the part of the caregiver.

Unless your child has a contagious disease, you may want to arrange for occasional visits from other children for prescribed periods that suit your child's energy level, interests, and attention span. Encourage your child to participate in the normal activities of the home as much as possible.

Nutrition

By the time your child is of school age, his or her habits are well on the way to being established. The school-age years are a good time to continue the establishment of healthful eating habits that were initiated during the preschool years. Equally important, promote regular physical activity to help maintain normal weight.

In general, the nutritional guidelines are similar for children and adults. Have your school-age child eat a variety of foods that are lower in fat and higher in complex carbohydrate and fiber. Consult the chart on page 122 for an approximate guide to serving sizes and food varieties for your school-age child (see Nutrition and Health, page 251).

At home, you can practice healthful eating patterns to guide what your child learns about food choices. However, no matter how good and consistent your example, your child will be receiving conflicting messages from television, other media, the lunch program at school (see School Lunch Programs, page 123), and his or her friends. These outside influences become even stronger as your child matures. However, so too does your child's ability to make his or her own choices.

Help your child learn that breakfast is an important meal. It is worth getting the whole family up early enough to enjoy this meal together. After school, your child may need a snack. However, the amount and type of this snack should be controlled so that it tides your child over until supper but does not dull his or her appetite for the meal. A good choice is a piece of fruit, a whole-grain muffin, or some low-fat yogurt.

The most common nutritional problem in school-age children is iron-deficiency anemia (see page 957). However, your child will get enough iron, zinc, and other essential minerals if he or she eats lean meats, whole

How Much and What Kind of Food Does Your School-Age Child Need?

Food Group	Servings/Day	Average Size of Serving for Child's Age		
		5-6 Years	7-10 Years	11-Teen
Milk	4			
Milk (whole, skim, * dry, evaporated, buttermilk)		¾ cup	¾-1 cup	1 cup
Yogurt		¾ cup	¾-1 cup	1 cup
Cheese		1 oz	1 oz	1½ oz
Meat	3 or more			
Egg		1	1	1
Lean meat, fish, poultry		¾ oz (3 tbsp)	1½-2 oz	2-3 oz
Peanut butter		2 tbsp	2-3 tbsp	2-3 tbsp
Legumes (dried peas and beans)		½-¾ cup	½-¾ cup	½-¾ cup
Cottage cheese		6 tbsp	½ cup	½ cup
Fruits and vegetables	4 or more			
Fruits		¼ cup	⅓ cup	½ cup
Vegetables		¼ cup	⅓ cup	½ cup
Juice		⅓ cup	½ cup	½ cup
Breads and cereals	4 or more			
Whole-grain breads		1½ slices	1-2 slices	1-2 slices
Ready-to-eat cereals		1 oz	1 oz	1 oz
Cooked cereals		½ cup	½ cup	½ cup
Spaghetti, macaroni, noodles, rice		½ cup	½ cup	½ cup
Crackers		3-4	4-6	4-6
Fats and oils[†]	To meet energy needs			
Margarine, butter, oil, mayonnaise, salad dressing		1 tsp	1 tbsp	2 tbsp
Desserts and sweets[†]	To meet energy needs			
Pudding or ice cream		½ cup	¾ cup	1 cup
Cake		¾ piece	1 piece	1 piece
Cookies		2	2-3	2-3
Pie		½ piece	1 piece	1 piece
Jelly, jam, honey, sugar, syrup		2 tsp	1 tbsp	1 tbsp

*Do not use skim milk before 2 years of age.

[†]Amounts of foods such as fats, oils, desserts, and sweets should be determined by individual caloric needs.

From *Mayo Clinic Diet Manual*, seventh edition, 1994. By permission of Mayo Foundation.

grains, dried beans, fruits, and vegetables.

If your child is involved in vigorous physical activity, he or she will need more calories. If heart disease or high cholesterol runs in your family, discuss this with your child's physician, who will determine whether the child's blood cholesterol should be measured. If this value is high, your child's physician may recommend a diet that controls dietary fat and cholesterol.

However, if your child's cholesterol value is normal, it is important not to overdo a low-fat diet. Your school-age child is still growing and needs a balanced diet and adequate calories to grow to his or her full potential. For this reason, it is inadvisable to impose such dietary restrictions on your child.

It is important that you do not use food as a means of controlling your child's behavior or as discipline, reward, or your primary form of affection.

As in the preschool years, feed your child

School Lunch Programs: Do They Make the Nutritional Grade?

The United States National School Lunch Program now serves many of the nation's children breakfast as well as lunch. The program supplies meals free or at a reduced rate to children. Menus and minimal portion sizes are revised periodically.

But are these programs adequate? A 1995 study of school foods found excess fat in these meals. This finding is of concern because lifetime dietary habits of eating too much fat, sodium, and calories contribute to increased risks of heart disease, high blood pressure, and obesity.

In general, a school lunch—whether homemade or produced at the school—should offer at least five items: meat or other protein, fruit, vegetable, bread or some other form of starch, and low-fat milk. Each meal should provide about a third of a school-age child's recommended daily allowance (RDA) of various nutrients.

Recently, school lunch programs have made some improvements. Many schools have reduced the amount of fat, salt, and sugar and have increased fiber in the foods they serve. Some schools have expanded their offerings, providing children with more options.

Future changes will be limited by conflicting pressures on the school lunch program. One factor is economic: schools save money by getting about a fifth of their food from commodities provided by the federal government. When the agricultural surplus is heavy on processed cheese, ice cream, butter, and ground beef, these items will find their way into school lunches.

Ideally, the food offered in school should complement what your child is taught in school about good dietary practices. Health, social studies, and science programs can reinforce healthful eating habits.

in response to hunger or at mealtimes. When your child feels restless, encourage him or her to be active rather than giving more food. Remember, the best way to teach your child about good nutrition is by setting a good example in your own eating habits.

Obesity

An increasing number of American children are overweight. Being overweight can have various effects on a child. Social or emotional stresses may result from peers making fun of the child's excess weight. There are also potential adult health problems, including an increased risk of diabetes, high blood pressure, and elevated blood cholesterol level.

Physical Inactivity
Weight control at any age is largely a matter of balancing the intake of calories from food with the amount of energy used in everyday activities. If more calories are eaten than are used, the pounds will add up. The cycle is more complicated than it may seem, however, because it is often difficult to determine whether low activity levels are the cause or the result of overeating, or both.

Memorandum:
To Parents and School Officials

Here are some steps for a healthier school lunch:

Reduce Fat
Use nonfat dry or low-fat milk. Serve ice milk, frozen low-fat yogurt, or sherbet rather than ice cream. Limit whipped toppings. Replace butter with margarine.

Use lower-fat (15 percent) ground beef and low-fat ham. Bake or broil rather than fry foods. Rinse ground meat to reduce fat content.

Increase Fiber
Use whole-wheat flour when baking. Add low-fat granola, bran, rolled oats, and cornmeal to quick breads. Offer fresh fruits and vegetables regularly.

Reduce Sodium
Reduce salt in recipes. Use fresh garlic or onion, or garlic or onion powders, instead of onion or garlic salts. Remove salt-shakers from tables in the school cafeteria. Serve soups that are lower in sodium.

Reduce Calories and Sugar
Use less sugar in recipes. Serve unsweetened fruit juice; serve fresh fruit whenever possible. Serve smaller portions of baked desserts.

Heredity

Studies of adopted children reveal that these children take on the weight characteristics of their biological parents and not of their adoptive parents. This occurred even though most of the children had been adopted before their first birthdays. Clearly, heredity is an important factor in obesity.

Controlling Your Child's Weight

Never put your child on a diet without consulting your child's physician or dietitian. Any diet must take into account your child's nutritional needs. Fad diets are dangerous. Stay away from them.

Even an overweight child should not be put on a weight-loss diet. The goal is to slow the rate of weight gain and allow height (growth) to catch up.

Overweight children have the same nutritional needs as other children. Do not restrict meeting these essential needs. Do not give your overweight child special meals; rather, give less total food.

Increase Activity Levels

Encourage physical activity. Plan family activities.

Never Criticize

Support your child: insensitive jokes, especially from parents and loved ones, can be devastating to children. Be patient: do not attempt to solve the problem overnight. Achieving a healthier weight takes time.

Psychological and Social Development

In contrast to your school-age child's relatively slow physical growth, his or her psychological and social development proceed at a rapid clip. Your child is busy mastering a host of psychosocial tasks. Impressive changes take place in his or her ability to reason, learn, act in a moral fashion, follow rules intelligently, and interact with adults and other children. Many of these changes may seem surprising or even shocking to you as a parent, so it is best to have some understanding of the normal course of events.

Normal Psychosocial Development

Starting first grade can be frightening, but most children proudly accept their new status. The school places social and learning expectations on the child, and it can be quite a challenge to meet them.

At the advent of the school-age years, most children have just become able to think logically about concrete things that they experience directly in everyday life. Between ages 6 and 12, children's ways of thinking and remembering become much more sophisticated. They become better at classifying bits of knowledge, and their memories improve. Enhanced memory lets them keep several related ideas in mind while they solve more complex problems.

During the school-age years, most children also progress in their ability to take account of other people's perspectives. They learn to tailor their approach to the viewpoints of others and not to assume that everyone shares their knowledge and interests. For the first time, they understand that mom and dad have other things in life that demand their time. This realization, in turn, hones their powers of persuasion. School-age children become more adept at drawing inferences from incomplete information. They also discover how to coordinate two different but related meanings—an important element in understanding jokes, metaphors, and certain grammatical rules.

Learning to read is the most important part of schoolwork, opening the door to the discovery of all other knowledge. Reading to your child may inspire him or her to want to read. Learning to read starts with reading aloud. Your child must discriminate the letters of the alphabet, then decode them into speech sounds and master how to pronounce common groupings of letters. Eventually, your child can skip these steps and read silently by processing sounds, words, and meanings simultaneously.

You can motivate your child by stimulating his or her desire to learn. Simply showing an interest in your child's performance in school or other activities and spending plenty of time actively involved with your child can help encourage him or her to try harder to learn or acquire skills.

Schoolchildren also tend to shift, gradually, from an impulsive learning style to a reflective one. The 6-year-old is more likely to blurt out a careless answer, whereas the 12-year-old may think about a question longer before answering.

Through the school-age years, children also learn about moral behavior—how to distinguish between what is right and wrong. Your child must learn how to balance his or her needs and wants with the requirements of the family, school, and society.

You can help your child develop a sense of duty, responsibility, and realistic accomplishment. Encourage your child to assume a helpful role in the family. It may help to assign reasonable household chores such as setting the table. As your child accomplishes tasks you set, he or she will develop confidence in his or her abilities and a sense of responsibility regarding the tasks. This will also reinforce that he or she is an important part of the family.

Setting an example of moral behavior is also important. In addition, it is a good idea to limit and monitor your child's television watching and to keep to a minimum his or her exposure to violence and inappropriate sexual behavior.

If you consistently specify what behavior you are rewarding or punishing, and explain why you are doing so, your child will be more likely to develop internal control of moral actions (that is, a conscience). Less desirable are external controls, which influence behavior through fear of being caught or of displeasing parents.

Children who believe securely in their own worth tend to be more industrious, creative, and successful at school. They are also better at resisting pressure to conform to their peers, which is especially important when peers demand that they join in self-destructive behavior.

To help your child develop high self-esteem, it is necessary to show your child that you truly care for him or her. Your child generally wants to do well and will practice hard to do so. Your child will measure his or her performance by the response given by peers and "important" adults. Success at this stage is enabling your child to realize that he or she has strong points and some areas that need work—and that that is okay.

In contrast, low self-esteem often occurs when parents are rejecting, overbearing, or distant. The child may feel inferior to others of the same age or may feel that he or she must be good at everything to be okay.

Set clearly defined limits for your child's behavior, and enforce those limits consistently. Parents who are too permissive may also convey that they do not care for their child. Your school-age son or daughter is becoming increasingly independent but still needs firm guidance and consistent boundaries within which to grow.

During the preschool years, children tend not to conform. Social rules may be confusing to them. The early school-age years mark a decided change in behavior. Children enjoy identifying with their peers and begin to be able to understand social situations. They often show a rigid conformity that makes them embrace each new social norm that they come to comprehend. You may have noticed that your child relishes some strict compulsion, such as never stepping on a crack in the sidewalk. This is one form of the child's temporary infatuation with arbitrary rules.

Toward the end of the school-age years, most children become more flexible about social roles and norms. They gradually learn to reconcile conflicting value systems, such as the ones at home and those at school. They come to recognize that compromise is not necessarily a sign of weakness.

However, the later years of the school-age period are characterized by some degree of rigidity. Eleven- and 12-year-olds are often extremely concerned about acting and dressing like their peers and not being out of the mainstream.

At times, your child may have difficulty with learning at school, interrelationships with peers, or acquiring common exercise-related skills. Sometimes the difficulties arise from a child's unrecognized problems with vision or hearing. At other times, unrecognized learning disabilities or attention-deficit disorders may be contributing to your child's inability to keep up with his or her peers. Emotional problems can also be both a cause and a consequence of learning difficulties.

Even if they are quite intelligent, children who are upset by family troubles can find it difficult to pay attention in school. Sometimes this takes the form of a school phobia, which may prevent your child from taking full advantage of his or her school environment. We discuss these disorders in the following section.

Difficulties With Sibling and Peer Relationships

Peers and siblings play important roles in the integration of your child into society. From their peers and siblings, school-age children learn a great deal about competition and cooperation as well as about conformity and independence.

The influence of other children can rival or even overtake that of adults. Part of the reason is that children play together as equals. It is easy for them to understand each other. Another child's perspective often provides an alternative to the prevailing wisdom that the child has been accustomed to hearing from his or her parents.

Conflicting behaviors may develop. Parents and siblings within the family may advocate different approaches than do teachers and peers at school. This conflict can pose problems for school-age children, who yearn to be liked and accepted by everyone they meet, including adults and other children. However, when sibling and peer norms conflict with those of adults, school-age children are often more inclined to follow their siblings and peers.

Elementary school is the first social world that most children have to deal with without direct help from the family. As school-age children become part of a peer group, new social traits become important to them, such as popularity and leadership. At this age, children are eager to be popular. They are concerned about being left out in the fringes of the group.

In addition to being peers, brothers and sisters may be rivals. A certain amount of rivalry between siblings is normal, and it even helps them learn how to interact with other people. There is not necessarily any reason for concern if your children compete, roughhouse, and bicker with each other. Despite the friction between them, most older siblings do contribute greatly to the education, socialization, and support of younger ones. Frequently, overt rivalry gives way to closeness by the end of the school-age years.

However, sometimes the discord between siblings is severe. If so, you may want to seek family counseling to identify how the trouble started and how it can be stopped. The underlying cause of sibling antagonism may be a family problem such as marital strain. Without realizing it, parents can cast a child in a role that enmeshes him or her in a conflict between the mother and father, and the other siblings react according to their sympathies.

The birth of a sibling can make a school-age child feel that his or her place in the family has been upset. Compared with the preschooler, the school-age child is usually better equipped to control his or her jealousy of a newborn sibling. Still, your school-age child may protest a decline in the amount of your attention that he or she receives by regressing to younger behavior. It helps if you are sensitive to the school-age child's needs and reserve some time just for the two of you. School-age children often enjoy playing with and caring for "their" new baby. (See Sibling Problems of the Preschool Years, page 105.)

If concerns about your school-age child persist, see your child's physician.

Sexuality in Your School-Age Child

Through the school-age years, your child will continue to define his or her sexuality. This process is a vital part of your child's larger task of discovering and deciding whom he or she is. Your child may also make his or her first attempts to explore sexual activity before this period is over. As a result, this is a good age for sex education, if you have not already started it.

Most school-age children are already well on their way to reflecting the divergent sex roles that our society considers appropriate to men and women.

Perhaps you would prefer your child to feel free to express all aspects of his or her personality, including masculine and feminine ones. However, you may notice how often your efforts are thwarted by the startling array of overt and subtle sex-stereotyping pressures from other relatives, peers, teachers, television and other media, and society at large.

Regardless of your own attitudes, your school-age child may choose not to embrace

Sexual Abuse

Sexual abuse of children involves an adult, usually a man, forcing or persuading a child, frequently a girl, to participate in a sexual act.

Recognizing the Signs

Be alert for the following possible signs of sexual abuse in a child:

- Provocative or promiscuous sexual behavior
- Withdrawal from friends, family, or school activities
- Unusually hostile or aggressive behavior

There may be no physical signs of abuse, but your physician may identify evidence of trauma to the genital area or the presence of sexually transmitted infections (see page 1087). However, the absence of all of these signs is not necessarily proof that no abuse has occurred.

Why a Child Is Susceptible

Young people need affection. Depriving a child of healthy physical contact (such as hugging), in fact, is to risk significant problems in a youngster's psychological development. While young children often seek physical contact with adults, their need for affection should not be mistaken for adult sexuality. Adults may inappropriately respond to this by exploiting children for their own sexual gratification.

Children often seek some sexual contact with their peers. This usually is normal curiosity and experimentation. However, if your child describes an experience in which he or she was touched by a much older child or by an adult in an inappropriate way, take it seriously.

What to Do

If you suspect that your child has been sexually abused, contact your physician or an official in your local child-protection system (child welfare worker, local public attorney, police, or sheriff).

If the sexual abuse involved rape, handle it as a specific type of aggression against the child. This will help to minimize the sexual significance of the trauma and to prevent lasting psychological effects. It is best for you and the child's physician not to dwell on the sexual nature of the assault. If you do, your child may become insecure and anxious, without clearly understanding what is going on.

Make sure that your child is safe from further harm. Report the attack to the police. As soon as possible, take your child to an emergency room at a hospital, preferably one that offers emergency and follow-up psychological support. The child will be checked and treated for any internal and external injuries. Later on, the child may be tested for sexually transmitted diseases (see Sexual Assault and Sexual Abuse, page 428).

Have your child talk with a sensitive professional who is experienced at counseling victims of child abuse. This counseling is particularly important if it was a family member or friend, not a stranger, who perpetrated the attack.

Do not keep the abuse a private or family matter. Most perpetrators are involved with several children. Seldom is the abuser a complete stranger to the child. The welfare or even the life of your child may be at stake.

---

the role assigned to his or her sex. The girl may be called a tomboy and the boy, a sissy. Society and the family may tend to put more pressure on boys than on girls to conform strictly to a narrow sex role. Tomboys are often tolerated, whereas sissies are frequently rejected.

If you are concerned that your school-age son is showing too much interest in playing with dolls or dressing up in girls' clothes, it is best to discourage him gently and not to show your anxiety. This type of behavior does not lead to homosexuality. Be reassured that a great many boys are taunted by their peers at some time or other for their lack of masculinity. It is also important to recognize that sexuality and sex roles are not static. They continue to evolve throughout childhood, adolescence, and even adulthood.

Most school-age children devote most of their attention to peers of the same sex. Many even develop "crushes" on their same-sex peers. However, it is also normal for them to explore the opposite sex tentatively. Curiosity and lack of understanding of social taboos are usually the reasons for their "playing doctor."

During the school-age years, most school-age children continue to play occasionally with their own sex organs, as they did in infancy and the preschool years. Masturbation generally should not be a cause for concern.

The onset of puberty provides a good opportunity to educate your child about sexual development, whether or not you have already done so. You can help prepare your child for the cascade of changes that his or her body will go through during the next few years. The goal is for the child to welcome these changes without shame or anxiety that they are occurring too quickly or too slowly.

Unfortunately, events often conspire against this goal. In the late school-age years, children are most eager to conform. Yet this obsession with "normality" coincides with the time when their bodies are diverging most in their development. Even children who are right in the middle of the spectrum of physical maturity often feel they are developing too fast or too slowly. You can help by reassuring your child that he or she fits well within the wide range of normal developmental timetables.

Do not worry if your child's puberty starts a little earlier or later than that of his or her peers. This is not a serious medical problem. However, your child may feel awkward and self-conscious about diverging from the average schedule. Be sensitive to these feelings. At the same time, reassure your child that he or she is fine. It may help to stress that every child, including your child and each of his or her peers, is traveling along the same road toward adulthood and that everyone takes a different amount of time to arrive (see Sexual Precocity, page 135).

Dealing With Physical Illness and Hospitalization

The school-age years are a good time to instill attitudes of wellness and to promote a positive body image in your child. Of course, whenever your child becomes ill, you will want to make him or her as comfortable as possible. However, avoid rewarding your child for being sick, lest he or she gets to like being sick.

An acute illness can have psychological effects on both you and your child. If your child is in the early school-age years, he or she may respond to a mild acute illness with restlessness and hyperactivity. This behavior may frustrate you if you are trying to encourage your child to rest. It is usually best not to insist too strenuously on bed rest because for many disorders rest is not necessarily helpful.

If your child develops a severe acute illness, do not be surprised if he or she becomes listless and irritable. Disturbances in your child's sleeping and eating habits can appear and, if not deftly handled, they may persist long after recovery. Together with

your child's physician, do your best to comfort and inform your child.

A chronic illness is even more likely than an acute one to alter your child's psychosocial development. His or her mood can easily be depressed by the social isolation of extended absences from school and spending much of the day indoors. This is particularly true in the event of a permanent disability. Your child can feel helpless and may start regressing to younger behavior. This can slow and change the evolution of your child's personality and role in the family and in school.

Chronic childhood illnesses, if not handled adeptly, can sometimes foster the development of problems with school. For instance, if the family treats a sick child like a fragile flower, he or she is more likely to cling to the home and even suffer from school phobia (see page 133).

Some chronically ill school-age children become extremely dependent, anxious, passive, and withdrawn. Others tend to deny their illness and act too independently too soon. The best adjustment occurs between these two extremes in children who are able to accept their limitations realistically while finding other ways to achieve competence and self-confidence.

You can help your child find this middle road. However, this task may be too much to shoulder on your own. Accept support from your relatives and friends. Psychological counseling from health-care professionals may, at times, be helpful.

Your school-age child, unlike a preschooler, has the ability to understand disease. With this comprehension comes the opportunity to lessen the psychological burden of the disorder. You can help your child a great deal simply by answering questions in ways he or she can grasp. Your child may fear that the illness is a punishment for bad behavior, even if he or she does not state this fear. You can help by verbalizing such fears and reassuring your child that they are baseless.

Together with your child's physician, encourage your chronically ill school-age child to have an active role in gaining control over the disease. For instance, children with asthma can learn to recognize their symptoms (see Asthma, page 1044). This allows treatment early in an asthma episode, before it becomes serious. Such an approach to a chronic illness can help set the stage for good control of the disease later on in adolescence, when refusal to cooperate with treatment is more often a problem.

If your child has a chronic disease, it is natural for you to be tempted to overprotect your child, to indulge him or her, and to stop setting limits. You may also find it hard to resist seeking out unproven "cures," which can raise false hopes and then dash them. Resist these temptations and encourage your child to live the most full, normal, active life possible.

Do not unnecessarily shelter your child from any activity, including school attendance and physical exercise. Talk with your child's teacher and school nurse to ensure that the child is included in all of the activities in which he or she wants and is able to participate.

In most cases, there is no justification for banishing your child to study hall while his or her peers enjoy themselves in the gym or on the playing field. It is not only the exercise that is missed. Your child also needs the social activity involved. If the group activities are too strenuous for your child, the gym teacher should be flexible enough to propose an individualized program for him or her. Even if your child does special exercises while the rest of the class pursues another activity, at least he or she will not feel so excluded.

Your child may have to spend some time in the hospital. You can help it seem like a less scary place. Beforehand, prepare your child for this new experience by discussing it thoroughly. Many children's hospitals offer pre-admission programs, orientation programs, and tours. Once your child is in the hospital, you can make the stay less threatening by bringing in a favorite toy, book, or picture. It is particularly important to stay with your child as much as you can.

If the treatment involves surgery, try to allay your child's fears. It is good for your child to get a chance to ask the surgeon and anesthesiologist questions in advance (see Your Hospital Stay, page 1258).

As with adults, confronting and fighting an illness are more likely to be successful if the person with the ailment is a partner in his or her care. Even young children instinctively know when secrets are being kept from them. You do not need to discuss every medical detail. Still, your child is more likely to develop normally and to work harder toward recovery if he or she has some degree of control over decisions made about his or her care.

Learning Disorders

Your child's ability to learn depends on the mental processes that make learning possible and on his or her emotional comfort and overall health.

The following pages consider factors within the child that interfere with learning, but many other factors must be considered also. Illness interferes with learning when it leaves a child tired and listless; emotions interfere when a child is depressed or worried about himself or herself or about problems at home. Such worries or daydreaming in school distracts the child from schoolwork. Finally, a motivation to learn is necessary in order for the child to use his or her capacities.

Vision, hearing, and general health are evaluated by your child's physician. Intelligence is evaluated by psychological testing within or outside the school. When your physician suspects an emotional problem, he or she may refer your child to a child psychiatrist or psychologist.

Cognitive learning disorders are more difficult to diagnose than vision or hearing disorders and require specialists such as child psychiatrists and educational psychologists. These disorders of mental processing include problems with remembering, grasping patterns, focusing attention, writing, speaking, and interpreting written words. Sometimes they are caused by birth injuries. More commonly, however, they occur in children with normal health and intelligence.

If your child has a learning disorder, he or she may need help in learning how to learn. The following sections discuss the various cognitive problems and the kinds of special education needed to overcome them.

Learning Disabilities

Signs and Symptoms

- Significant problems in speaking, writing, spelling, or arithmetic
- Inability to listen, read, or organize thoughts
- Chronic impulsiveness, restlessness, or distractibility
- Poor memory

Children can have normal or high intelligence and still be unable to learn. Specific learning disabilities are not disorders of seeing, hearing, emotions, or mental capacity. They are mental process disorders in acquiring or expressing knowledge (cognition).

Your child may be unable to grasp overall patterns, remember what was said, write legibly, copy a drawing, relate printed text to spoken words, interpret written words (see Specific Reading Disability [Dyslexia], page 131), or speak coherently (see Speech Disorder, page 132). These mental process disorders relate to your child's use or comprehension of language and symbols. There are other reasons for some of these signs, such as impulsiveness and restlessness; therefore, the signs do not necessarily indicate the presence of a learning disability.

Another type of learning disability occurs when your child cannot pay attention for more than a minute or two (see Attention Deficit Disorder, page 132) or cannot exercise self-control over certain physical activities (see Hyperactivity, page 133). These conditions may be due to disorders in the normal process of ignoring distractions and focusing attention in a deliberate way.

Various causes have been cited for learning disabilities. In some cases, they may be genetic. Boys are affected 4 to 5 times more frequently than girls, and these disabilities can run in families. In other cases, there is evidence of a disorder in the way the brain functions, although no evidence of brain damage can be found.

Frequently, however, no specific cause for a child's learning disorder is found. Some experts in the field believe it may be due to developmental delays or immaturity.

Learning disorders are thought to occur in 5 to 20 percent of school-age children in the United States. This range is wide because many definitions are used and because no large-scale study has been done to determine the extent of the problem.

Diagnosis

You may not become aware of your child's learning disorder until school failures start in the third or fourth grade. A complete diagnosis is essential for determining the specific disorder and ways to improve your child's education as soon as possible.

The basic diagnosis will require several types of examinations to evaluate your child's mental capacity, educational performance, eyesight, hearing, emotional status, and general neurologic functions. Further testing may be necessary to identify particular disorders in reading, writing, listening, speaking, or understanding mathematics.

Various tests for the processes involved in learning have been developed in recent years, and it is now possible to obtain a very detailed diagnosis. Your child may need to visit a child psychiatrist, child neurologist, psychologist, or educational evaluation clinic for this testing.

How Serious Are Learning Disabilities?

Your child's learning disability can lead to chronic academic failure and to major social and emotional problems. Although children sometimes outgrow their disability, this may occur too late to prevent a severe limitation in future achievements and self-esteem.

The damage often is minimized by early diagnosis and treatment. Many children can overcome their disability and perform much closer to their potential with special education and tutoring. Your child can achieve most academic and occupational goals if the appropriate teaching method and motivation are found.

Treatment

The primary treatment may be a special education program tailored to your child's needs. Many methods are available, including techniques to help your child develop sound-symbol relationships, number concepts, eye-hand coordination, phonetic articulation, sense of time, and pattern recognition. The special education team in your school system or a private clinic may work with you and your child in using diagnostic results to select appropriate methods.

The educational objective is to help your child acquire the missing abilities and to apply them; in other words, your child must learn how to learn. Attendance in a separate class or school may be needed for a while or your child may go to special education facilities during part of the school day. Additional tutoring and practice at home often are needed.

Counseling by a mental health professional may be necessary to help your child cope more effectively with his or her disability and to improve self-esteem. Your physician may prescribe medication if distractibility, poor attention, and hyperactivity interfere with your child's learning.

Specific Reading Disability (Dyslexia)

Signs and Symptoms
- Inability to recognize letters and words on the printed page
- Reading ability much below the expected level for the age of the child

Specific reading disability is often referred to as dyslexia. It is the most common learning disability, and it occurs in children with normal vision and normal intelligence. The child is unable to interpret written language, and reading is therefore difficult. Children with dyslexia usually have normal speech, but often have difficulty with spoken language and with writing. The disorder is an impairment of the brain's ability to translate images received from the eyes into meaningful language.

The reading problem is characterized by a delay in the age at which a child begins to read. Most children are ready to learn this skill by age 6 years, but children with reading disability cannot grasp the basics of reading in first or even second grade. Reversal of letters ("b" for "d") and a reversal of words ("saw" for "was") are common among children with this problem. In normal children younger than 6 years of age, such reversals should not be of concern. With reading disability, however, the reversals persist.

The condition may also manifest itself by your child's trying to read from right to left, failure to see (and occasionally to hear) similarities or differences in letters or words, and inability to sound out the pronunciation of an unfamiliar word.

If you have a child with reading disability, you may find that his or her inability to read does not affect achievement in other school subjects, such as arithmetic. However, because reading is a skill basic to most other school subjects, a child with reading disabil-

ity is at a great disadvantage in most classes.

Although the basis of reading disability is unknown, there is evidence that it is caused by a malfunction of certain areas of the brain concerned with language. A family history of language disorders also is frequently found. Reading disability affects boys more often than girls. Approximately 10 to 15 percent of school-age children have the disorder.

Diagnosis
Reading achievement significantly below that expected for age is the key symptom of dyslexia. An evaluation of medical, cognitive, sensory processing, educational, and psychological factors will be required to plan treatment and follow your child's progress. Thorough vision, hearing, and neurologic examinations are needed to verify that your child's poor reading ability is not due to another disorder.

A battery of educational tests, such as the Wechsler Intelligence Scale for Children (WISC), and academic achievement tests will be performed to help diagnose the problem. More importantly, an expert will analyze the process and quality of your child's reading skills.

How Serious Is Specific Reading Disability?
Inability to read affects most aspects of school learning. If untreated, the disorder may lead to low self-esteem, behavioral problems, delinquency, aggression, and withdrawal or alienation from friends, parents, and teachers.

Reading disability varies in severity. Some children have a relatively mild form of the disorder, whereas some have a severe form.

Treatment
Treatment is by remedial education because there is no known way to correct the underlying brain malfunction that causes reading disability. Psychological testing will help your child's educators to design a suitable remedial teaching program. Techniques emphasizing many of the senses including hearing, vision, and touch are used to improve reading. Most important is frequent instruction by a reading specialist who uses both visual and phonic methods of teaching. It is important to provide emotional support and opportunities for achievement in areas other than reading.

If the reading disability is severe, effective tutoring for remedial reading usually requires several individual or small-group sessions each week. Progress is likely to be slow and laborious. Children with milder forms eventually learn to read well enough to get through school and to be able to read newspapers. Those with severe forms will never be able to read well and may need training for vocations that do not require good reading skills.

Speech Disorder

Signs and Symptoms
- Failure to use speech sounds correctly
- Speech that is hard to understand or scrambled
- Slow speech development
- Stuttering

The critical period for your child's speech and language development is between ages 6 and 24 months, but occasional mispronunciations are normal up to age 7 years as long as your child's conversational speech is understood readily.

Some speech problems, such as a speech impediment (difficulty in articulation), stuttered speech, and voice problems, have no physical cause. Using one letter for another and leaving off the beginnings and endings of words are typical articulation problems. Stuttering is difficulty in getting the words out in a smooth flow. Voice problems include too soft a voice, a nasal voice, or a loud, booming voice.

Other speech disorders may have a recognizable cause such as cerebral palsy (see page 54), cleft palate or lip (see page 51), hearing loss or deafness (see page 578), mental retardation (see page 108), brain damage, or autism (see page 108).

Your child may be normal physically, emotionally, and intellectually, but may have a speech disorder due to mental processing problems with spoken language. These speech problems are associated with learning disabilities (see page 128).

Your child may have difficulty receiving information and making sense of it. Sentences may come out scrambled or with one word substituted for another. The correct ordering of sounds may be impaired. Your child might be unable to tell the difference between two sounds or might have problems focusing on one specific sound or conversation while ignoring background noise.

Speech disorder is common. It occurs in about 10 percent of children younger than 8 years of age and in 5 percent of those 8 years and older.

Diagnosis
Talk to your child's teacher or to your physician if you suspect that your child has a speech disorder. You probably need to seek help from a speech and language clinic. Most school systems offer these services. A speech pathologist will test your child's speech. A game with earphones may be used to check for hearing loss or deafness, and a complete physical and neurologic examination may be needed.

How Serious Is Speech Disorder?
Many children acquire vastly improved speech with proper professional therapy and help from you at home, but the disorder is likely to cause your child frustration. The social penalty can be costly if your child is taunted or rejected by other children at school. Early diagnosis and treatment are desirable before deep frustration and low self-esteem become part of the pattern.

Treatment
Children with speech disorders require speech therapy. This usually entails at least two sessions a week with a speech professional. Your child's speech therapist can explain what you should do at home.

Attention Deficit Disorder

Signs and Symptoms
- Habitual failure to pay attention
- Excessive distractibility
- Inability to organize
- Impulsiveness
- Restlessness and hyperactivity

Your child's ability to learn depends on paying attention and remembering previous lessons. Many sights, sounds, memories, and other stimulating things compete for your child's attention. Sometimes they can cause any child trouble in paying attention. Most school-age children, however, have developed the ability to focus their attention and to ignore distractions.

Attention deficit disorder is the habitual inability to pay attention for more than a minute or two despite repeated requests or even punishment. As a result of attention deficit disorder, your child may have problems with learning, following directions, and remembering information.

This disorder can have different causes. It has been attributed to heredity and to brain injuries during pregnancy, at birth, or after birth. Attention deficit disorder may not noticeably affect your child's intelligence or early development. It may become apparent only later as your child has increasing difficulty with learning after the second or third grade, when sitting still in class and paying attention become more important.

Diagnosis

Your physician will need to observe your child's behavior and get a detailed history of early development. Early symptoms may appear during infancy, including problems with feeding, sleeping, and restlessness. Physical and neurologic examinations are used to identify any sensory or neurologic disorders. Your physician also may refer you to specialists for EEG (see page 1344), psychological, and educational testing.

How Serious Is Attention Deficit Disorder?

Attention deficit disorder is a chronic problem that can continue through childhood and adolescence and into adulthood. It can damage your child's self-esteem and confidence, generate rejection and ridicule by other children, and cause academic failure. Treatment can help the child with learning, behavior control, and self-esteem.

Treatment

Your child may need a special education program (see Learning Disabilities, page 130). Children with attention deficit disorder often have behavior problems that require specialized counseling for the child and parents. This often is provided by child psychiatrists and psychologists.

Behavior modification techniques and restructuring home and school routines, avoiding overstimulation, and providing consistency may be effective for decreasing unacceptable behavior and rewarding good behavior.

Your physician may prescribe medications to help focus your child's attention and to reduce overactivity. The most common medications for this purpose are dextroamphetamine (Dexedrine), methylphenidate (Ritalin), and pemoline (Cylert). When taken

Hyperactivity

Hyperactivity, or extreme overactivity, is not a diagnosis and not a separate disorder. Rather it is a behavior that often accompanies the other symptoms of attention deficit disorder. Contrary to some opinions, sugar alone will not cause or aggravate hyperactivity.

Children normally vary in their level of physical activity. Some youngsters are naturally much more active than others, and boys tend to be more active than girls. In general, young children usually are very active. These variations in activity are not abnormal.

However, a small percentage of children, more often boys than girls, are excessively active. Some seem to be in constant motion; others are erratically active. These children are not necessarily less coordinated or less intelligent than other children. The difference lies in how organized or purposeful the activity is and whether it can be stopped on request.

Hyperactive children tend to act without consideration for results, punishment, or other people's reactions. They cannot direct their activity, and it is difficult for you or the teachers to do so.

by adults, most of these medications have a stimulating effect; they have the opposite effect on hyperactive children, and they improve attention. When the medication is carefully prescribed and when the child's progress is followed closely by your physician, it may be taken safely for as long as it is needed, even for years.

School Phobias

Signs and Symptoms

- Refusal to go to school
- Stomach pain and sometimes fever beginning the day before or the morning school begins
- Illness continues or worsens rather than disappearing after a day or two
- No physical cause for the pain can be found

School phobia or school refusal is distinguished by a cycle of physical symptoms and anxiety that gets worse instead of better. It is not the occasional stomachache or headache that disappears as soon as the school bus pulls away. In school phobia, no physical cause is found to explain the child's complaint.

School phobia actually is not a fear of school but a fear of separation from parents. Your child may be unwilling to sleep over at a friend's house. An older child is more likely to be afraid of something specific at school—a bully or a new class or getting picked on in the bathroom. These fears, unlike school phobia, are rational.

School phobia is a way of responding to overwhelming stress by substituting an acceptable and predictable pain for a situation the child is unable to control. Sometimes the disorder is triggered by the death or illness of a parent, a divorce, or entering junior high or middle school (where students have a variety of teachers, choices, and classmates). The disorder seems to run in families and is most common in the early school grades. It affects boys and girls equally.

Treatment

Sympathy or nurturing the child for missing school is only likely to reinforce the physical symptoms. However, if the parent becomes angry, the child's anxiety is likely to increase, raising the stress level and worsening the physical symptoms.

In children in kindergarten and first grade, the problem can usually be resolved easily by firmly expecting school attendance and providing emotional support for the child. Close cooperation between the parents and school personnel is essential. If the problem persists in an older child, evaluation and treatment by a mental health professional often are necessary.

Sexual Development and Gynecologic Disorders

The onset of puberty occurs in both boys and girls in the later stages of the school-age years. The age at onset may be over a wide range of years. In general, puberty is thought to be premature if it occurs before age 8 in girls and before age 8 to 9 in boys.

In girls, the first sign of puberty is generally the development of the breast bud (thelarche). The onset of menses (menarche) then follows within several years.

In boys, enlargement or growth of the testicles and penis is generally the first sign of puberty, to be followed by the appearance of pubic hair.

Several potential disorders concerning sexual development may occur during the school-age years, especially in girls. Premature puberty is far more common in girls than boys. We discuss this condition, along with other gynecologic problems in school-age girls, in the following section.

Breast Abnormalities

The start of breast development in girls is known as thelarche. Thelarche signals the onset of puberty. Breast development may be the only indication of puberty for 6 months or so; it is not unusual for one breast to develop first and remain larger for months.

When the breasts commence budding in girls younger than 8 years, this sign of early sexual maturation is called premature thelarche. Most often, premature thelarche occurs between the ages of 1 and 3 years. If it is not followed by the other signs of sexual maturity (such as hair growth in the genital area), the girl's puberty is considered to be premature and incomplete.

The budded breasts often flatten within a year, but they may persist until the normal onset of puberty. The condition is harmless and seldom affects the girl's growth. Supportive counseling is usually all that is necessary to help her cope with her temporary difference from other girls.

Consult your physician for a full evaluation to differentiate premature thelarche from premature puberty (see Premature Puberty, page 135).

Vaginal Bleeding

Some school-age girls may have bleeding from the vagina before the expected age of menstruation. Consult your daughter's physician if this occurs.

The physician will first ascertain the source of the bleeding. Often the cause is not the commencement of menstruation but another cause such as vulvovaginitis (an inflammation of the genital and vaginal areas), genital tumor, trauma, or a foreign body lodged in the vagina.

In some cases, however, the cause is premature menstruation due to precocious puberty (see Premature Puberty, this page).

Adrenarche

Adrenarche refers to activity in the adrenal glands. Premature adrenarche occurs most often in girls between ages 5 and 8 years. It is often accompanied by rapid short-term growth. The armpits may sweat and have hair. Pubic hair can develop (pubarche).

The physician may perform tests to determine whether the girl has a tumor or other abnormality of the adrenal glands, which can cause premature adrenarche in rare cases.

Premature Puberty

Premature (precocious) puberty is rare. It is much more common in girls than in boys. In girls it can start at any time before 8 years of age. The events of puberty may proceed as usual but start earlier than normal. In normal puberty (and usually in premature puberty), the breast buds appear first, then pubic hair appears, and later menstruation begins, often with irregular cycles. Ovulation is uncommon but can occur.

Usually no underlying cause can be determined. However, the condition is known to involve early maturation of the ovaries, pituitary, or hypothalamus, which are hormone-producing glands.

Rarely, premature puberty results from a tumor of the brain or ovaries, so the child's physician may initiate studies to rule out these possibilities. The physician may also ask whether the girl has used any face creams or medications containing estrogens, which can also induce the disorder.

A potential long-term consequence of premature puberty is shorter height. It is usually associated with rapid short-term growth that stops earlier than normal.

Treatment may include psychological counseling for the girl and the family to deal with an appearance different from that of her peers. This problem should not be minimized. However, it is reassuring that by about age 10 most of the girl's peers will have caught up with her in sexual maturity, and she should not feel different anymore.

If your daughter undergoes puberty prematurely, it is important not to respond to her according to her physical appearance or to deny her hugs. Keep treating her like the little girl she is. Advise her teachers to do the same.

It is also imperative to guard the girl against sexual abuse and especially to prevent pregnancy. When puberty occurs very early, medication may be considered, but it has drawbacks. A progesterone-like drug can stop menstruation and reverse breast development. However, it does not prevent growth spurts or increase the height eventually attained, and it can cause undesirable side effects.

In boys, the onset, before age 9, of enlargement of the testicles and penis, appearance of pubic hair, deepening of the voice, and accelerated growth may be signs of premature puberty. If your child develops these signs of advanced sexual development at an early age, see your physician. Studies may be done to rule out a tumor of the brain and nervous system, adrenal gland, or gonads. Approximately half of the time an identifiable cause is found.

Newer and better treatments such as luteinizing hormone (LH) analog therapy are being made available for premature puberty. If you are concerned about premature puberty in your child, consult his or her physician for a full evaluation.

Sexual Precocity

Like puberty, sexual behavior has been starting earlier in many school-age children in recent years. It is particularly important to bolster your child's self-esteem and give him or her the strength to resist any pressure from peers or older people to engage in sexual behavior before he or she is ready for it.

Premature puberty (see this page) and sexual precocity are different problems. Precocious sexual knowledge and behavior, and preoccupation with sexual matters, can sometimes be signs that the child has been a victim of sexual abuse (see Sexual Abuse, page 127).

Genital Infections in Young Girls

Genital infections (vulvovaginitis) can occur in girls not only after puberty but also before. The usual cause is inadequate bathing and toilet habits. A young girl may not wash her genitals adequately. Or she may wipe herself from back to front after bowel movements, inadvertently picking up microbes that normally live harmlessly in the intestines and spreading them to the genitals.

Agents that can cause vaginal infections include yeast, parasites, bacteria, and irritants found in soaps and other toiletries. Yeast infections occur more commonly among girls who have diabetes or who have been taking antibiotics. Another possible cause is the insertion of foreign bodies into the vagina.

When sexual abuse has occurred, a sexually transmitted disease may also be the cause. Excessive masturbation or manipulation can also irritate the genital area.

Your daughter's physician will ask whether she has had any vaginal discharge, itching of the anus or vagina, other infections, or bedwetting. The physician will examine the area and may take a sample of vaginal discharge to examine for microbes. Pinworm, which commonly infects the rectums of school-age children, can also contaminate the vagina. Gonorrhea and other sexually transmitted diseases can cause vaginal infections in young girls. If the girl has one of these diseases, she may have acquired it through sexual abuse (see page 109).

Many of these infections can be prevented—and treated—by teaching your daughter about her genital area and showing her how to wipe from front to back. When she bathes, encourage her to wash her genital area well and use no bubble bath preparations. Her toilet paper and underpants should be white, not colored, because dyes can irritate the skin. Her underpants should also be all cotton and changed once a day. Discourage wearing clothing that increases moisture in the area, including such attire as tight-fitting jeans, nylon panties, and panties while sleeping.

Specific treatment for certain problems may involve taking oral antibiotics or applying an antibacterial or antifungal cream to the vagina or the genital area.

Chapter 5

Teenage Years: Ages 13 Through 19

Contents

On Being a Teenager, 138

Physical Growth, 138
Normal Growth and Development, 139
Sexual Changes in Boys, 139
Sexual Changes in Girls, 140

Nutrition During the Teenage Years, 140
The Competitive Edge and Your Diet, 141

Intellectual Growth and Development, 142

Psychosocial Growth and Development of Personality and Behavior, 143
Psychological Changes, 144
Development of Standards, 144

Teenage Sexuality, 145
The Role of Parents, 146
Initial Sexuality, 146
Sexual Activity, 147
Teenage Pregnancy, 147
Contraception, 148
Homosexuality, 149
Sexual Fantasies, 149
Masturbation, 149

Psychological and Behavioral Concerns, 149
Teenage Rebellion, 150
Bizarre Behavior, 150
School Problems, 151
Anxiety and Panic Attacks, 151
Eating Disorders, 152
Use of Tobacco, 152
Drug Abuse and Addiction, 152
Use of Alcohol, 153
Sexual Abuse, 153
Depression and Suicide, 154
Causes of Death in Teenagers, 155

Common Medical Concerns, 155
Keep Up With Immunizations, 156
Routine Examination, 156
Sexually Transmitted Diseases, 157
Acne, 158
Infectious Mononucleosis, 158
Urinary Tract Infections, 159
Iron-Deficiency Anemia, 159
Dysmenorrhea, 159
Migraine Headaches, 159
Scoliosis, 159
Epiphysitis, 159
Injuries, 160
Vision Problems, 160
Hearing Disorders, 160

On Being a Teenager

In chronologic terms, the teenage years extend from ages 13 through 19. During this time a child evolves into an adult. In biologic terms, the time starts with puberty, the phase when sexual reproduction first becomes a physical possibility, and continues through the attainment of mental and social adulthood.

The growth during these years is perhaps most apparent in a physical sense. The teenage boy or girl becomes a taller and heavier person with a recognizably adult shape. Yet equally significant is the broadening of intellectual growth, providing new insights and abilities to understand more and more complex matters. In tandem, the child's psychological development helps integrate the multitude of changes into a better understanding of his or her physical and intellectual self.

Often, the physical, intellectual, and psychological developments occur at different rates; in fact, the differences can lead to anxiety, insecurity, conflict, and other emotional hurdles. For example, in recent generations puberty has been starting earlier, whereas, ironically, graduation from adolescence, signaled by independence, seems to be attained later and later. The result is that the transitional period we call adolescence has been lengthening. In today's world, with drug use and sexual behaviors commencing earlier and earlier, the challenges of these years seem to grow continually.

Adolescence is the time when the ongoing tug-of-war between parents and children begins to be resolved. This struggle, which starts in infancy and continues through childhood and sometimes even into early adulthood, concerns the normal tension between the child's dependence on his or her parents and the growing independence from them.

Just as children are distinct from adults, so too are adolescents, and they are best understood as such. A teenage boy or girl is not an overgrown child or a miniature or immature adult. In the early teenage years, the adolescent begins forging an identity that is separate from that of his or her parents.

As this time of life gives way to young adulthood, perhaps at age 18, 19, or even later, the tension between parents and their children most often is resolved, with both generations learning to accept the new adult's independence. The teenage child continually strives to coordinate his or her physical, intellectual, and psychological growth and to develop a fully formed ego identity and sense of self.

During adolescence, the relationship between parents and children is challenged, stressed, and gradually redefined. To ensure that a good relationship is maintained, it is crucial for both generations to communicate with each other as openly as possible. In part, this chapter is devoted to furthering this communication.

Teenagers are profoundly influenced by the unique physical and mental changes of adolescence. In contrast with younger age groups, adolescents start to take responsibility for their own lives, including their own health care.

The pages that follow speak directly to teenagers and parents. Our goal is to provide you—whether teen or adult—with the information you need to best cope with these uniquely challenging years.

Physical Growth

As an adolescent, your body grows and develops faster than at any other time except for the first year of life.

This growth occurs unevenly. Changes may occur relatively slowly during some of your teenage years and rapidly during the so-called growth spurt, which starts about 2 years earlier in girls than in boys.

It is not the actual stage of your physical growth that is of greatest importance at any one time. More important is how you feel about your body and how you are reacting to the changes you are experiencing.

You may expect or desire an ideal body, perhaps one like that of a much-admired peer or performer or even a parent or teacher. Rarely, however, is this idealized image achieved. More important, in fact, is that you accept and grow accustomed to the changes you are experiencing. At times you may feel as if things are happening to your body that are literally out of your control, especially during the growth spurt. You cannot expect to control the transformation, but you can attempt to understand, enjoy, and accept your body.

Normal Growth and Development

On average, the growth spurt begins at about age 10 in girls and 12 in boys, tending to reach its peak about 2 years later in both sexes. At the peak of this spurt, you grow between 3 and 4 inches a year. Most boys grow faster than girls. When the growth spurt ends, you have nearly attained your adult height. If you have not started a conspicuous increase in growth by age 15, consult your physician.

If you grow and develop either slower or faster than average, you are not alone; it is also normal to feel somewhat insecure about yourself at this time. It is important to remember that there is no standard timetable for growth and development during adolescence. Entirely normal teenagers mature at such widely varying rates that even those whose growth rate falls in the middle may feel that they are the only ones going through such changes at that particular time. Your parents can help by providing love and reassurance, neither minimizing nor overdramatizing your concerns.

The external changes caused by the growth spurt are obvious: your body grows taller and heavier, and its shape changes. Your bones grow too; even the facial bones change, sharpening your features and transforming your face into that of an adult.

Height is not the only physical attribute that is changing. As the spurt starts, fat collects on the buttocks and around the abdomen in both boys and girls. During the course of the spurt, boys accumulate mostly lean tissue (muscle and bone), and girls add more fat, particularly on their hips and breasts. The result is that fat makes up 25 percent of the total body weight in girls and between 15 and 20 percent in boys.

By the time of a girl's first menstrual period or the end of a boy's growth spurt, adult proportions have been reached, with the distinctly different contours of men and women. The respective male and female sex hormones, along with family traits, account for most of this difference. These hormones are also responsible for the secondary sex changes, which usually begin about 1 year after the start of the adolescent growth spurt in boys and girls.

For a chart illustrating growth patterns and rates for teenagers, see page 117.

Sexual Changes in Boys

During the teen years, the child's body gains sexual maturity. Male changes include the appearance of coarse hair in the pubic area, under the arms, and on the face, as well as deepening of the voice.

Your body prepares for sexual maturity by producing more male hormones. These hormones, made mainly by your testicles, cause the physical changes of puberty.

The first male change you are likely to notice is the appearance of sparse, lightly pigmented pubic hair on the skin surrounding the base of your penis. Your scrotum enlarges and darkens. These changes are likely to be well under way before your growth spurt reaches its peak. Do not be worried if you happen to develop some breast tissue about this time. Only rarely is this change (called gynecomastia) due to any hormonal problem. The development usually disappears within a few months.

Your penis has been able to become erect since you were an infant. However, it is usually not until about 2 years after the start of puberty and 1 year after your penis starts to lengthen that you become capable of ejaculating semen for the first time. This may occur while you masturbate, spontaneously while you enjoy a sexual fantasy, or at night during a nocturnal ejaculation (commonly referred to as a "wet dream"; see Masturbation, page 149, and Sexual Fantasies, page 149).

Later, hair begins to appear under your arms and on your face. As your larynx (voice box) develops, your Adam's apple becomes more prominent. Your voice also starts to change, taking on a deeper tone. Occasionally, your higher, younger voice may still be heard, though fleetingly, when your voice "cracks."

Throughout this period of sexual maturation, which usually lasts 4 or 5 years, your testicles continue to enlarge and your penis gets longer and thicker. By the end of this period, your penis, testicles, and pubic hair are fully developed, and your mustache and beard hair have started to appear.

The period of sexual maturation usually starts a couple of years later in boys than in girls. Sexual changes in boys start anytime between ages 9 and 14. If puberty starts outside that age range, it is considered either delayed or premature (see Premature Puberty, page 135).

Sexual Changes in Girls

Female changes include the development of breasts and the appearance of hair in the pubic area and under the arms.

The first visible change is either breast budding—the beginning of breast development—or the appearance of sparse, lightly pigmented pubic hair. The activity of your sweat glands also increases. Do not worry if one breast happens to start developing before the other, even if the difference in size persists for many months.

About 1 year after your breasts begin to develop, your growth rate is likely to reach its peak. Within the year after the peak of your growth spurt, you will probably experience menarche—your first menstrual period (see The Normal Menstrual Cycle, page 1144).

The advent of your first menstrual period means that it is now physically possible for you to become pregnant and bear a child. You can even get pregnant before then if you happen to ovulate (produce an egg) before your first period. If you are sexually active, find out about the various methods to prevent bearing a child as a result of sexual intercourse (see Contraception, page 148).

You may notice an intermittent increase in either white or yellow vaginal discharge during the months before menstruation starts. It is also normal for your first few menstrual periods to occur irregularly. However, within about a year they will start to appear more nearly on schedule. You will experience a 3- to 7-day period about every 24 to 34 days.

Most girls start out using disposable sanitary pads to absorb their menstrual blood. However, because the hymen does not completely cover the vaginal opening, most girls can use tampons, given a little practice in insertion. If you choose to use tampons, use the kind with a plastic or cardboard inserter. Wash your hands before inserting the tampon and do not leave it in place more than 3 or 4 hours. Most physicians recommend that teenagers not use tampons while sleeping and not use the super-absorbent varieties. This helps reduce the risk of toxic shock syndrome (see page 1145).

Painful menstruation (dysmenorrhea) is unusual during the first few menstrual periods but may occur in later adolescence (see Dysmenorrhea, page 159).

As you experience your first menstrual periods, you continue to grow taller. Your breasts will also grow larger. More and more of your pubic and underarm hair appears. Your voice deepens, though not as much as that of a boy who is experiencing puberty. It usually takes 4 or 5 years for puberty to reach completion, resulting in full body development.

There is a wide range of normal ages for you to begin sexual maturation. When a girl's sexual maturation starts before age 8, it is considered premature (see Premature Puberty, page 135). If it begins after age 13, it is deemed delayed.

There is a link between the timing of your puberty and your nutrition. Improvements in nutrition in recent decades explain why the onset of puberty occurs at younger ages in successive generations of young females in industrialized nations such as the United States. In addition, puberty tends to start earlier in girls who have more body fat and later in those who are thin. Participating in some sports may slightly delay puberty (see Sports and Menses, page 1150).

Nutrition During the Teenage Years

Newly acquired independence and decision-making result in teens spending more time outside the home, thus making independent food choices. By trying to understand your teenager's ideas about food and food choices, you can better support the positive aspects of your teen's eating habits.

Adolescence is a period of alteration in lifestyle and self-concept, as well as a time of rapid physical growth and development that has profound nutritional implications. Requirements for energy and all nutrients increase. The typical teen is involved in a busy school schedule, extracurricular activities, and part-time employment. Tight schedules may lead to omitting some meals, especially breakfast, or to eating more frequently. Many teens eat a greater number of meals away from home, especially from fast-food restaurants and vending machines. Altered body image may cause stress and lead to abnormal eating habits such as overeating or restricting intake, making teens more vulnerable to eating disorders.

Greater independence from the family and the desire to be accepted by peers often influence eating practices such as vegetarianism, changing the diet in hopes of improving athletic performance, fad dieting, and indulging in alcohol. All of these factors put the adolescent at greater risk for suboptimal nutrition. The nutritional status of teens as a group has been described as generally good. However, some studies have observed low dietary intakes and marginal deficiencies of iron, calcium, riboflavin, and vitamins A and C.

Iron, for example, is a key ingredient during teenage years. Ample iron is essential because of the expanding volume of blood in the body and increase in muscle mass that teens experience as they grow. Teenage girls are at particular risk for a shortage of iron because of significant iron loss through menstruation.

To ensure an adequate supply of dietary iron, teenagers need to regularly eat meats (especially liver), fish, poultry, eggs, legumes (peas and beans), potatoes, and rice.

Parents: you have a crucial role to play in setting a good example and taking time to prepare and serve wholesome family meals. Get the entire family involved in meal preparation. If family meals are not possible because of differing schedules, stock your kitchen with healthy, convenient snacks such as fresh fruits and vegetables, yogurt, milk, whole-grain bread, and popcorn.

Do not be too critical of your teenager. There is a place in the American diet for hamburgers and pizza. In fact, both of these foods have significant nutritional value. The key is moderation and informed judgment. Adults are no different from teenagers when it comes to making wise food choices. If we want to operate at peak efficiency, we need to make wise choices and exercise a reasonable amount of self-discipline. Some general tips for you and your teenager are described in the following paragraphs.

As at any age, nutritional status as a teenager does not depend on each food choice, but rather the combination of food choices over several days and weeks. All foods, even fast foods and desserts, can be included in a healthful diet if you regularly eat a variety of foods.

Variety means choices from the food pyramid (see page 261). These include protein (meat, fish, poultry, dried beans, and eggs), dairy products (milk, cheese, yogurt), fruits, vegetables, and complex carbohydrates (cereals, grains, potatoes, and rice). Like a health-conscious adult, you may want to make a special effort to eat foods with adequate fiber. Also, go easy on the extra salt and limit fat (especially saturated fat).

As busy as you are, do not skip meals. Complete meals help you control overindulging when you get too hungry. Growth and development require various nutrients and a certain number of calories. Calorie needs depend on height, weight, age, sex, and level of activity.

The Competitive Edge and Your Diet

If you are an athlete (male or female), a balanced diet is especially important for good performance, but this is not to say that you should "load up" on any particular type of food, drink, or supplement. In particular, skip highly publicized vitamin supplements. They will not give you a competitive edge and may even be harmful.

It is important that you have an adequate intake of fluid, especially when you are perspiring heavily. Your best choice is the one that is most readily available and least expensive: water. Drink plenty of it before, during, and after competing.

To offset losses in sodium, some athletes take salt tablets. We do not recommend salt tablets except in unusual circumstances. The salt in your food should be sufficient. In fact, swallowing too many salt tablets can cause an upset stomach and can further enhance dehydration.

For optimal performance, iron plays an important role. It is an essential component of your blood's hemoglobin, which is necessary for transporting oxygen throughout your body. An inadequate supply of iron can significantly reduce your endurance and ability to compete. Be sure to get an adequate supply of meats and grains. Also, you may want to discuss your potential need for an iron supplement with your team physician.

Remember that as physical training increases, your body expends more energy. Therefore, you will need more food than you would under normal circumstances. The key to peak performance is a balanced diet with an adequate supply of foods and fluids. (See Nutrition and the Athlete, page 274.)

Intellectual Growth and Development

During adolescence, your thinking process undergoes a transformation from childhood into adulthood, just as surely as your body does. It is important to realize, however, that your physical growth and intellectual growth may not be synchronized but may develop at distinctly different rates.

At the start of the teenage years, you are thinking like a child; by the end, your thought processes are those of an adult. Until about age 12, your learning primarily concerns understanding the logic of "concrete things," objects that can be seen and felt. The next step in your intellectual development is the achievement of abstract thought.

Throughout adolescence, you become increasingly adept at considering intangible ideas, including concepts that involve the past and the future. Your newfound abilities allow your thoughts to take wing, traveling through time, perhaps even speculating about what you and the world around you might become.

Along the way, the sudden expansion in your powers of thought may blur the boundaries between you and the world around you. As a young teenager, you may feel that you are at the center of the universe and that your power knows no limits. You may assume that others are thinking about you—positively or negatively—more than they really are. This feeling of being onstage also may make you feel self-conscious, essentially powerless, or lost.

You may go through periods when at one moment you believe that everyone thinks as you do, and the next second you may feel with great intensity that no one else in the world can understand your thoughts or feelings. Eventually, you will begin to realize that your thoughts are both distinct from and yet similar to those of others. This realization is accompanied by the knowledge that you are not the focus of everyone's attention.

Ultimately, your abstract reasoning becomes mature and comprehensive. You start to be capable of judging whether the relationships between two or more propositions are logical. You can solve increasingly complex problems. You become able to think like a scientist, conceiving of hypotheses and of ways to test them. In addition, you can also think reflectively, which means that you can think about thinking. For example, you can frame an argument for a discussion or debate and simultaneously make judgments about that argument's strengths or weaknesses.

The advances in your intellectual development change the way you think about the world and how you behave in response to it (see Development of Standards, page 144). You become able to discern much more clearly how past actions have affected what is happening now. You also become capable of predicting more accurately what implications your current actions or those of others will have for the future, even in the long term.

An important aspect of this concerns your health: you begin to appreciate the cause-and-effect relationship between destructive behaviors (such as drug and alcohol abuse) and poor health. Also, the health benefits of good nutrition and ample physical activity may begin to make sense to you. Your actions in these areas affect your future, and you may decide to act on this new understanding.

For the first time, you may be interested in discussing various serious subjects with your friends, family, and teachers. Topics may involve love, morality, work, politics, religion, and philosophy. By the time you complete adolescence, you, like most teenagers, probably will spend a great deal of time wrestling with such major questions as the purpose of life.

Your advancing intellectual development gives you the flexibility of formal thought that you will need to cope with change as you take your place in the world. This will help you make decisions that will affect the rest of your life. Although you will probably still be guided by your parents, teachers, and other adults, your decisions can now be truly your own. For instance, you will decide whether to work or go to trade school or college after high school. You will choose which school to attend or which job to take.

In addition, you will make your choices among various possible career directions, religions, and political parties (see Psychosocial Growth and Development of Personality and Behavior, page 143).

Psychosocial Growth and Development of Personality and Behavior

Much of your psychosocial development as an adolescent involves coping with the profound physical changes that your body is undergoing. You need to come to terms with your sexual development and the emotions that go with it. At the same time, you are developing an identity distinct from that of your parents and becoming independent of them.

Psychosocial development of adolescents is usually divided into three phases: early, starting at about 13 or younger; middle, at around 15 to 17; and late, extending to 19 or often well into the 20s or even 30s in some individuals. In early adolescence, the mental focus starts to shift from the family to peers. The middle phase may involve outright conflicts over independence. By the end of late adolescence, independence is virtually secured, parental advice can be taken or not, and body image and gender role definition are established.

These stages are not easy. The diverse aspects of your physical, psychological, and social development are not synchronized, and the progress is not smooth and easy. You may find yourself alternating between childish and adult behaviors.

Do not blame yourself for having a difficult time with your psychosocial development. You are not alone. When you face challenging situations, you may feel the need for adult guidance and support. For this purpose, many adolescents find themselves turning to an adult outside their family, such as a teacher or counselor. This compromise offers them needed guidance without falling back on parental influences.

Part of your maturation process is developing and accepting a realistic image of your body. Difficulty with this image may manifest itself in eating disorders (see Anorexia Nervosa, page 1102, and Bulimia Nervosa, page 1102), particularly in girls. Because your body changes quickly during adolescence, you might start feeling uncomfortable with your physical self. You may be deeply concerned about whether your developing body is attractive or adequate. Your fears that you are physically imperfect may cause severe anxiety.

You may find yourself measuring your body against that of your peers. If you mature later or earlier than average—and many adolescents do—you may encounter trouble with your peers and your own image of your body. Often it helps to talk about these concerns with an understanding adult. Whether it is your physician, parent, or a trusted teacher, this person can reassure you that your body is normal.

During the teenage years, you also will do a great deal of thinking about what kind of person you are and who you will become. You will muse, and then think seriously, about what you will do when you grow up. In early adolescence, you may set career goals that are idealistic, or unrealistically beyond your given talents and abilities. Later in adolescence, you may set your sights more practically, considering vocations that more immediately suit your abilities and interests. The merging of idle musings with practical planning is yet another part of the maturation process.

Because your psychosocial status is in flux, your role in society is extremely ambiguous. This presents complicated questions such as whether contraceptives should be prescribed for a teenager without parental consent. Generally, professionals in medicine, psychology, and social work will encourage you to involve your parents in your psychosocial concerns; however, they will not reveal your confidences, unless they perceive a serious danger to you.

The gradual changes of this time will enable you to develop a sense of who you are and to understand the nature of personal responsibility, both for yourself and for your actions. You begin to appreciate how what you do—what you eat and the activities you involve yourself in (playing on sports teams at school or pursuing risk-taking leisure-time activities such as illicit drug, alcohol, or tobacco use)—has a major impact on your entire life.

During these years you begin to take an active role in making countless decisions about what you do—and what you elect not to do. Good decisions can have a significant impact on your present and future health.

Psychological Changes

In early adolescence you may start to experiment with new ways of behaving and dressing at home. You may be seeking some approval from your family before you try anything out on the outside world. You may make a few tentative motions toward asserting your independence. You may become less interested in family activities and less willing to accept advice or criticism from your parents. You may find more social comfort in a close relationship with a best friend of the same sex.

As you start to break away from your family's influence, you begin paying more attention to your peers. For some time, they may even dominate your thinking and behavior. Your chosen peer group may be a club, team, gang, or other group of adolescents of about your age. At first, your peer group is likely to be restricted to members of your own sex. During adolescence, it usually shifts to a mixed group.

Your peer group may provide you with social status and a comforting sense of security: you have a place within the group, and you feel a sense of belonging there. In return, however, teenage cliques often demand conformity of behavior, attitudes, and dress.

Privacy becomes increasingly important to you. At home, you may ask for a room, or a part of one, to be yours alone. You may start keeping a journal or diary to record your private thoughts. This secrecy is important to you, and it deserves to be respected.

Your struggle for independence is often most overt in middle adolescence. You may start testing your parents' controls and discipline. You may decide that your parents' standards are unfair. You may develop your own value system, or adopt that of your peer group, and challenge your parents' and teachers' authority.

You and your peers may delight in playing pranks and practical jokes. Your peer group's behavior may involve rebellion (see Teenage Rebellion, page 150). You may feel intense peer pressure to take risks that pose dangers to you and others—for instance, experimenting with drugs, sex, or vandalism. Some teenagers carry this activity even further into negative behavior (see Bizarre Behavior, page 150). If you take it too far, your rebellion can get you into lasting trouble at home, at school, and even with the law.

By late adolescence or early adulthood, you have evolved a new way of thinking about your family. In your mind, you have become a separate entity from your family, even if you still live at home. Either you are financially independent, earning money to support yourself, or you will be soon. As you have become more comfortable with your own identity, you have started to break free of the values of your peer group.

Achieving independence does not mean that you cut yourself off from others. Rather, you have enough resources from your education, family, and community to allow you to start supporting yourself financially, emotionally, and socially. Part of this mature functioning is knowing when and how to use others for support when needed. You may even be able to appreciate your parents' values enough to seek their advice when you need it. Now that you are more your own person, you may no longer feel threatened that your parents are trying to control you or make you a child again.

Parents often have a difficult time coping with the psychological changes in their adolescent children. However, it is possible for your parents to ease your transition to independence. They can achieve a delicate, ever-shifting balance between their often-conflicting responsibilities: providing support and understanding while setting standards and limiting dangerous or harmful behavior.

When your parents disagree with what you are doing, they should seek to be firm without being harshly punitive. They should respect your sincere efforts to achieve independence. Gradually, they should let go of the control that they have exerted over you throughout childhood and trust that you will be guided by the self-control that they have helped to instill in you.

It is important to realize that parents are trying to make an adjustment from being providers and protectors to a less controlling role. The challenge that parents face is to relinquish involvement gracefully rather than abdicate their role.

Development of Standards

Along with the psychosocial development of adolescence comes the evolution of standards. As you move from childhood to adulthood, your moral standards may progress in more-or-less distinct phases. At each stage, a different type of moral reasoning predominates.

As a child and young teenager, you may evaluate situations in a self-centered or opportunistic manner. When you judge whether an action is moral, the sole basis for your decision may be whether that action will help or hurt you. You may be concerned primarily with avoiding punishment and gaining rewards. Thus, most of the definition of your standards comes from outside yourself, not inside.

In middle adolescence, you may become more interested in conforming to legal standards. You start to realize that laws apply to everyone, including yourself. Accordingly, you may judge actions based on whether they are legal or illegal—not just on whether there is a risk of punishment.

However, teenagers do not always obey the law. Indeed, many adolescents go through a phase of rebelling, testing the limits of authority and sometimes even breaking the law. In a way, they may be asking to be disciplined, to experience tangible proof of the reality of the law. Ultimately, however, most teenagers progress beyond this testing phase. They decide that they should follow the law even if they are not likely to be punished for not doing so.

By late adolescence or adulthood, you start caring more about how your actions affect others. Your moral concerns may now extend to rules of human behavior beyond the letter of the law. You may follow standards based on broad ethical principles that in some cases may be even more restrictive than the law. You start to view real-life moral conflicts in abstract terms. You can recognize everyday examples of justice, equality, honesty, responsibility, cooperation, and reciprocity—and their opposites.

Eventually, your standards should evolve so that you become fully responsible for the morality of your own actions. Ideally, you develop your own detailed, individualized definitions of what your society deems as right and wrong. You follow this internalized personal moral code relatively independently of the endorsement or disapproval of others. If you ever violate your principles, you feel guilty and condemn yourself. You do not feel gleeful that you have gotten away without punishment. Unfortunately, standards are not always fully developed by the end of adolescence.

The evolution of standards is intertwined with social interactions and intellectual development. Teenagers who participate in social activities have more opportunities to observe interactions. This experience may help them to form more mature moral judgments. An advanced level of abstract thinking may be needed to decipher the moral concepts that underlie everyday situations. Mature thinking also may aid in developing sensitivity to the roles, perceptions, and feelings of others. However, neither social nor intellectual maturity necessarily guarantees the development of high moral standards.

Your parents can encourage your development of standards by the example they set. Teenagers tend to develop more self-controlled behavior and make more mature moral judgments when their parents have followed a certain style of child-rearing. This style includes the following: consistent disciplining that involves reasoning and explanation; discussing how others feel about actions taken; and promoting democratic family discussions, in which even the young children can have their say.

Teenage Sexuality

In the early teenage years, your closest relationship is usually with a best friend of the same sex. By the mid-teens, you may be most concerned with a larger group of peers, a group within which a natural process of social experimentation is occurring: in some sense, you all learn from and with each other.

Even if you choose a special friend of the opposite sex at this age, your choice is likely to be made with your peer group's accep-tance uppermost in your mind. In the late teenage years, however, you may be ready to establish an intimate relationship with another person. Compared with your earlier relationships, this one demands a different type of sharing and commitment.

Base your relationship with another person on mutual understanding and enjoyment rather than on the opinion of your peers. It is a mistake to get involved in such a serious relationship merely to impress your peers—or to annoy your parents.

The Role of Parents

Parents often feel perplexed and even threatened by their teenager's emerging sexuality. If you are the parent of a teenager, it is best for everyone if you can come to terms with your child's sexuality, show your trust, and give him or her any help needed.

Your child may receive education about sex, family life, and sexually transmitted diseases at school. However, do not rely on the school to explain all of the complexities of sexual relationships that you want your child to know. No matter how awkward it may be for you, you have a responsibility to know what your child learns about the facts of life. If you are unsure how to present the facts, it may help to consult a book or suggest one to your child to read. You can also ask your physician or other trusted persons for help.

If you are like most parents, you want your child to delay the start of sexual activity until after he or she has reached an adequate level of emotional maturity. This is a sensible goal. Unfortunately, however, it is not always achieved (see Sexual Activity, page 147). If your adolescent becomes sexually active, denying or ignoring the fact will not resolve the conflict you have with the situation and with your son or daughter.

Well before your child starts sexual activity, he or she needs your support and assistance in understanding sexual feelings, defining sexual behavior, and learning to respect himself or herself as well as others. Ideally, your instruction about sex and family life should start when your child is a preschooler or even a toddler. Respond honestly and in a straightforward manner to your child's spontaneous questions, including where babies come from. If your child never asks any sex-related questions, do not assume that he or she is not interested. Bring up the subject if the opportunity presents itself.

All along the way, make an effort to gear your advice on sexual matters to your child's current phase of intellectual, psychosocial, and moral development. The younger your child is, the simpler the advice should be.

Do not use only scare tactics in discussing sexual behavior with your teenager. By doing this, you put your child at risk of having insufficient knowledge about sexual situations. A purely negative approach may be less likely to discourage a teenager from embarking on a sexual relationship than providing a basic understanding and perspective from which to make sensible and responsible decisions in sexual matters. In addition, scare tactics may cut off the parent as a source of information for the teenager.

Discuss contraception and sexually transmitted diseases frankly. Be sure your child understands your feelings and works to form his or her own attitudes on abortion, contraception, and teenage pregnancy (see Teenage Pregnancy, page 147).

Teach your child about the dangers of acquiring sexually transmitted diseases, including AIDS (acquired immunodeficiency syndrome). The risk factors for these diseases include sexual activity (especially promiscuity and male homosexual activity) and sharing needles or syringes to inject drugs (see Sexually Transmitted Diseases, page 157, and AIDS, page 1060). If your adolescent is already sexually active, stress the risk of sexual exposure to people known or suspected to be infected with the virus (HIV) that causes AIDS. Explain that the risk of infection is increased by sexual contact with many partners or with a person who has had multiple partners. The use of drugs and alcohol can also interfere with your child's sexuality (see Drug Abuse and Addiction, page 152).

To protect your adolescent from AIDS, other sexually transmitted diseases, and pregnancy, it makes sense to discourage your adolescent from becoming sexually active until he or she is more mature. At the same time, however, it is important to emphasize that sex can be a joyous experience. Stress that when your child does start sexual activity, the regular use of condoms can reduce the risks of infection with the AIDS virus and other sexually transmitted diseases as well as help prevent pregnancy. Concurrent use of spermicidal foam may provide added contraceptive protection.

Initial Sexuality

As an adolescent, your sexual development has started. Along with it, your sexual feelings and fantasies increase. You may find it difficult to deal with these feelings, particularly if they seem to conflict with the attitudes that you have been taught about sex.

At first you may retreat from your emergence as a sexual being into the safety of friendships with members of the same sex. At the same time, you may find yourself intrigued by sexual matters and frequently seeking information about sex. Sometimes the emergence of sexual feelings in early adolescence is relieved through telling dirty jokes.

When your body first becomes capable of sexual intercourse and, if you are a female, of having a child, you are probably years away from being emotionally prepared for either event. However, you have likely started masturbating, or privately fondling your own sex organs for pleasure. This enjoyable and harmless activity may involve reaching an orgasm or climax (see Masturbation, page 149).

In middle adolescence, you start feeling more aware of yourself as male or female. You become more interested in forming relationships with members of the opposite sex. Dating may start, as well as some sexual experimentation. This may involve kissing, fondling your partner, mutual masturbation, or even intercourse.

You may feel strong pressure from your peers to lose your virginity. Some teenagers react to this pressure, and to their own curiosity, by starting to have sexual intercourse at a very young age. Having a series of sexual partners may reflect emotional immaturity.

It is best to wait to have sexual intercourse until you have reasons other than peer acceptance and curiosity. Ideally, sexual intercourse is a joyous union of two people who love each other. Depending on your own moral and religious beliefs—and those of the adults you respect, including your parents—you may want to wait until you are married.

In the meantime, there are many other ways to express your affection. You may enjoy intimate talks, long walks while holding hands, listening to music, and dancing together. Many adolescents give each other great pleasure through kisses and caresses.

By late adolescence, you become more secure about your sexual identity. You may then feel that you are emotionally ready to have sexual intercourse with someone you care about deeply. But you are unlikely to be prepared to become a parent. Therefore, whenever you start having sexual intercourse, use methods to prevent pregnancy and sexually transmitted diseases; a condom (rubber) helps protect you from both (see Contraception, page 148; Sexually Transmitted Diseases, page 157; and HIV Infection and AIDS, page 1060).

You might feel awkward about discussing the subject of contraception with your prospective partner. However, if the two of you are intimate enough to be thinking about making love with each other, you both should feel free to discuss these issues. If your prospective partner does not seem to care about the possibility of pregnancy or sexually transmitted disease, you may want to reevaluate your relationship.

Sexual Activity

If you have had sexual intercourse at least once, you are considered sexually active.

Male and female adolescents tend to report different reactions to their first experience of sexual intercourse. Girls more often say they were scared, guilty, worried, embarrassed, and curious. Boys, on the other hand, usually report feeling excited, thrilled, satisfied, happy, and grown-up.

The reality is that a wide range of experiences is normal. You may not date at all in junior high or high school, or you may have a sole high school sweetheart. The most common pattern, though, is two or three close emotional commitments as a teenager, one after the other. During the course of each relationship, you and your partner will stay monogamous and, if sexual activity is part of the relationship, there will be no other sexual partners.

About 1 in 10 teenagers experiments with many sexual partners, including more than one at a time. These individuals are more likely to have psychological and physical health problems. They raise their risk of acquiring sexually transmitted diseases—including the fatal illness AIDS (see Sexually Transmitted Diseases, page 157, and HIV Infection and AIDS, page 1060).

Teenage Pregnancy

The United States has the highest rate of teenage pregnancy of any Western industrialized nation. More than 1 million American teenage girls become pregnant each year. More than a third of American girls become pregnant at least once during adolescence. Most of those who become pregnant carry their pregnancies to term. One-third of adolescent mothers get pregnant again before the end of their teenage years. Adolescent pregnancy and childbirth are a virtual epidemic in many inner-city communities.

Most of these pregnancies are neither planned nor wanted. They are a direct result of widespread ignorance about birth control along with denial of the risks of becoming pregnant. Two-thirds of the sexually active teenagers in the United States do not regularly use any form of contraception. Among the main reasons teens give for not using contraception are the following: they think it is the wrong time of the month to conceive; they do not know when to expect sexual intercourse; they think they are too young to become pregnant; they think contraception is wrong or dangerous; they do not have access to information about contraception; or they think they have intercourse too infrequently to become pregnant. In fact, having sexual intercourse just once can result in pregnancy. One-half of teenage pregnancies occur within 6 months of becoming sexually active.

If you are thinking about becoming sexually active, find out about contraception. As soon as your sexual activity starts—including the first time you have sexual intercourse—use contraception (see Contraception, this page). Otherwise, you are likely to have an unwanted pregnancy.

If you have missed a menstrual period and you think you or your partner may be pregnant, tell your parents or another trusted adult immediately. The pregnant girl should see her physician as soon as possible. The sooner she seeks medical help, the more options are available.

Terminating the pregnancy may be a legal option. The earlier in pregnancy that abortion is performed, the safer it is (see Pregnancy Termination: Medical Problems and Personal Choices, page 199). If this route is chosen, the abortion should be done by a licensed physician in a hospital or clinic.

For many people, abortion is not a personal or practical option. The prospective mother may choose to carry the pregnancy to term, deciding either to place her child for adoption or to raise it herself. Appropriate prenatal medical care is important to ensure the good health of the mother and the child (see Prenatal Care, page 178).

Raising a child is a serious responsibility that can last 2 decades. Most teenagers are not yet equipped, emotionally or financially, to make the necessary commitment. Some school districts have special programs that help pregnant adolescents continue their education, but having a baby could put an end to your education, employment, and school friendships. It may force you into a strained, short-lived marriage.

It takes two to make a baby. The father bears just as much of the responsibility as the mother does. Just like adults, teenage fathers should participate in caring for their children and supporting them. Often, however, a teenage mother ends up having to raise her child under difficult circumstances, without any help from the child's father. There are not enough hours in the day for the mother to support herself and to care for her child alone. Children in such situations often face an uncertain future.

Despite these drawbacks, most pregnant teenagers carry their pregnancy to term and keep their babies to raise. Unfortunately, teenagers usually receive less medical care during pregnancy than more mature women do; however, they actually need more. Special considerations need to be taken to ensure a healthy mother and child when the mother-to-be is an adolescent who is still growing herself (see Concerns During Pregnancy, page 175).

Contraception

If you are considering sexual intercourse, arrange in advance some method of contraception. If you are already sexually active, contraception is even more crucial.

Consult your physician or a reputable family planning clinic about contraception. Some schools have clinics that offer a range of health care, including counseling about contraception options.

Various methods of contraception are available, and they are discussed elsewhere in this book (see Prevention of Pregnancy, page 170). Your choice of method may be affected by how motivated you are to avoid pregnancy and by how often you have intercourse.

However, it is important to remember that any contraception is better than none. Aside from the intrauterine device, all the contraceptive methods discussed, including birth control pills, are considered safe for teenagers. Your physician or family planning worker can help you decide what is best for you. Certain forms of birth control, such as oral contraceptives (the pill), do not offer any protection against sexually transmitted diseases (see page 1087).

Homosexuality

Some teenagers seek out members of their own sex. They may later become heterosexual adults or choose bisexuality, in which sexual intimacies are shared with members of both sexes. However, if their sexual identity is well defined in adolescence—or even in childhood—they may remain homosexual throughout adulthood.

If you are an openly homosexual teenager, you may face rejection by some of your peers, teachers, and family. If you are having difficulty adjusting to your sexual orientation, or to others' reactions to it, psychotherapy may prove helpful.

If you are a male homosexual, your risk of contracting certain infectious diseases is increased. You are at even higher risk if you have experimented with several sexual partners. The potential infective agents include *Giardia*, *Chlamydia*, hepatitis B, and AIDS (see pages 768, 1088, 801, and 1060). Tell your physician about your sexual orientation. Then, he or she can help you detect these illnesses early.

As a member of an acknowledged risk group for AIDS, be tested for the presence of antibodies to HIV, the virus that causes AIDS. Because AIDS is fatal, you might save your life by using a condom every time you have oral or anal intercourse.

Sexual Fantasies

Daydreaming is an important part of adolescence, providing an outlet for your actively expanding imagination.

Do not be concerned if many of your daydreams have some sexual content. You also may have sexual fantasies at night. Sometimes you may conjure up hypothetical sexual experiences—or remember actual ones—while you masturbate alone. It is normal to have sexual fantasies. They may even be useful in the development of your sexual identity because they allow you to explore sexual situations that would be unsuitable for you to act out in reality.

Masturbation

Masturbation, or stimulation of the genitals for sensual pleasure, is a normal activity. Some teenagers feel guilty about masturbating because of old, unfounded myths. No, masturbation will not cause you to go blind or to develop genital warts—there is no reason for fear.

There is nothing wrong with masturbating during your teenage years and beyond. You may even have started doing so in your school-age years or before. Masturbation provides a way for you to release sexual tension, give yourself pleasure, savor sexual fantasies, and even curb your impulses to engage in inappropriate sexual activity with others. As long as you do not masturbate publicly, there is nothing at all unusual, harmful, or unacceptable about the practice.

Psychological and Behavioral Concerns

Adolescence is often regarded as the worst of times—but it also can be the best of times. It is true that teenagers have to cope with dramatic physical and psychological changes. They sometimes feel confused, moody, or angry as they wrestle with the conflicts that seem to be heightened by the rapidity of all of these changes. However, it is important to remember that all of life, from birth to death, is a process of change.

Difficulties in adjusting to the changes of the teenage years occur in virtually all communities. No matter what their socioeco-

nomic status, teenagers seem to encounter turbulent times, although children who grow up under deprived conditions and in single-parent families seem to be at greater risk. These children are more likely to fall victim to the three leading causes of death in adolescents: accidents, murder, and suicide. They may not receive the positive feedback needed to keep the psychological and behavioral problems of adolescence in check.

All these negatives should be balanced by positives. Developmental studies now show that most teenagers do not go through the turmoil and rebellion that we used to think was the norm. Most teenagers enjoy their new skills, activities, friends, and opportunities.

Teenage Rebellion

A child who previously has been obedient and calm may become moody, inconsistent, unpredictable, and even rebellious in adolescence. Your adolescent may bicker with you about a range of issues, large and small. They can include everything from what to wear and when to take out the garbage to when to come home at night and whether to engage in sexual activity.

A certain amount of teenage rebellion, risk-taking, and testing of authority is normal. Indeed, it may be an essential stage in the adolescent's process of separating from parents and developing an identity. However, most teenagers do not rebel greatly. A lack of rebellion does not suggest that unresolved problems may surface in later years.

Rebellion can be seen as part of the process by which adolescents define their identities. They may take an action merely to see what reactions it provokes in the people around them. This is why you should not just give up on your rebellious teenager. Explain when behavior exceeds the limits you have set. Eventually, the teen will learn from the consequences of the behavior and work toward the establishment of his or her own boundaries.

Mild rebellion is common and even normal in early and middle adolescence. By late adolescence, most teenagers are on their way to developing a sense of perspective. They have become better able to delay gratification, compromise on conflicting demands, and set limits. However, if rebellious behavior becomes more self-destructive or lingers into late adolescence, you should be concerned. Family problems may be causing or worsening the rebellion. Psychotherapy involving the whole family may help alleviate these problems.

If your teenage child is rebellious, hold your ground. Keep stating your concerns and setting reasonable limits. Do not threaten punishments that you will not carry out. In most cases, with your firm handling, your teenager will outgrow this rebellious phase without doing any lasting damage to himself or herself or others.

Even if your teenager has been rebellious, beliefs and behaviors usually change by the time he or she grows up and starts a family. Your child is likely to return to the viewpoints learned from you during childhood. With this in mind, try to prevent rifts during your child's adolescence that will stand in the way of later reunion.

As a parent, you remain the greatest influence on your teenager's beliefs and behavior, even more than his or her peers. Even when your child appears to be disagreeing with everything you say, he or she needs you to hold and defend your own reasonable and consistent view of the world.

Bizarre Behavior

Sometimes rebellion becomes so marked that teenagers lose control over their impulses. They may feel all-powerful and immortal. Together, these characteristics can result in dangerous risk-taking behavior.

The teenager may alternate between self-consciousness and defiance. He or she may relish being dirty, messy, or even totally rejecting society. When teenage rebellion gets out of control, it can appear as bizarre (odd) behavior. Truly bizarre behavior may indicate mental illness, although many people term "bizarre" any behavior that is out of the ordinary.

Almost overnight your polite child who impresses all your friends and neighbors may seem to become a stubborn irritant in your life. Your adolescent's new way of acting may appall you; in fact, it may well be calculated to do so. However, you should recognize that definitions of "odd" and "bizarre" often vary from one person to another. If your child "acts out" by dyeing his or her hair purple, you may be shocked, whereas your child's peer group (and perhaps even his or her teachers) may consider it normal. However, if a teenager is acting violently hostile, this behavior should be regarded as a serious problem by parents and peers alike.

The consequences of exaggerated teenage rebellion can be severe. It may contribute to the high rates of accidents, suicides, drug use, pregnancy, and sexually transmitted diseases in this age group.

Rebellion that is extreme may be seen in highly impulsive adolescents or when there is severe family conflict. Its causes are not always evident, but whatever its cause, bizarre behavior usually subsides with time. Decide which aspects of your child's behavior really matter and try to intervene only in those chosen areas. Individual and family psychotherapy may be needed.

Dropping out of social and sports activities, isolation from peers, and deterioration of schoolwork may be signs of drug or alcohol use (see Coping With Teenage Drinking, page 332).

School Problems

School problems during the teenage years include school phobia, truancy, school failure, learning disabilities, and, occasionally, consequences of chronic illness. School problems can also result from rebellion, bizarre behavior, drug abuse, sexual abuse, depression, anxiety disorders, or alcohol use.

School phobia is an irrational, persistent fear of attending school. The child actually fears leaving home rather than fearing school. This condition most often appears when a student first begins school. Less often, it may accompany entry into junior high or high school or transfer to an unfamiliar school. School phobia can respond to treatment (see School Phobias, page 131).

Truancy involves not going to school. Unlike the teenager with school phobia, the truant is not afraid of school but does not want to attend school and is not fearful of leaving home. Truancy can start with cutting an occasional class and then escalate into prolonged absences. It can result from conflicts within the family, parental expectations that are too high or low, and peer pressure to drop out. Truants are often rebellious teenagers who are in trouble not only at school but also at home and elsewhere.

Sometimes truancy can be reversed with an educational plan that emphasizes behavior management and involves the family, school, and medical personnel. Individual and family psychotherapy also may help. If the teenager still does not start attending school regularly, it may be possible to work out an educational alternative. Examples include early graduation and special programs such as work-study and independent study.

School failure can result from truancy. It is difficult for your child to know what is going on in class if he or she does not attend.

Some schools have policies that automatically drop students who have been absent more than a certain amount of time. A host of other problems may be involved in school failure among adolescents. High school dropouts face a bleak employment future, so it is important to prevent school failure.

Failure in school can be caused by problems with peers or behavior, not only by an inability to achieve academically. For instance, sometimes a young adolescent starts to separate from the family without succeeding in finding an alternative support group of peers. This can create a social void that results in problems at school. In addition, underachievement can result from problems with an overdemanding teacher, parent, or school.

Alternatively, the cause can be the student's failure to perform up to his or her potential. This does not necessarily spring from lack of intelligence or hard work. Learning disabilities and attention deficits can cause teenagers to perform below average in school, regardless of intelligence (see Learning Disorders, page 127). Undetected problems with hearing and vision also can interfere with learning at school.

If your teenager has had a chronic illness through childhood and adolescence, such as asthma or cystic fibrosis, he or she may often have had to stay home from school during acute episodes of the disease. Too often, these absences pave the way for school failure. Your child may need extra encouragement and support to enable him or her to make up the missed schoolwork. As parents, do not support frequent school absences for minor physical complaints. Work with your child's physician, teachers, and school nurse. Together, you can help your child to keep achieving in junior high and high school.

Anxiety and Panic Attacks

Anxiety can be a helpful cue to alert us to danger. However, if it becomes overwhelming and incapacitating, it is considered a disorder. Anxiety disorders can involve fears (phobias), obsessive-compulsive behavior, posttraumatic stress disorder, and panic attacks. Panic attacks are episodes of extreme fear and anxiety. Treatment involves medications and psychotherapy (see Anxiety Disorders, page 1118).

Eating Disorders

Anorexia nervosa is severe food restriction, and bulimia is binge eating, with or without alternating cycles of purging (by self-induced vomiting, fasting, or abuse of laxatives, diet pills, or diuretics). Anorexia nervosa and bulimia are now regarded as different poles in the spectrum of many different eating disorders that occur most often in teenage girls and young women under age 25. Most individuals with eating disorders recover with treatment. Rarely, the disorders prove fatal (see Anorexia Nervosa, page 1102, and Bulimia Nervosa, page 1102).

One hallmark of anorexia nervosa is that the girl perceives her body as fat, even if she is emaciated. Often lacking body fat, girls with anorexia nervosa do not have much development of breasts, thighs, or waistline, and maintain the appearance of small children. Menstrual cycles may be irregular or absent.

Many individuals with anorexia indulge in compulsive, excessive exercising. It is often impossible for these individuals to confront—or even recognize—their conditions.

If your daughter's growth chart shows that she is failing to gain weight, or even starting to lose it, her physician may suspect anorexia nervosa. Unfortunately, bulimia does not send such clear-cut signals. Depending on the frequency and timing of the binges and purges, some girls with bulimia maintain their normal weight, whereas others lose or even gain weight. But one telltale sign of bulimia—not seen in every case—is weight that fluctuates wildly.

Use of Tobacco

Tobacco use can be an expensive, long-term, potentially life-threatening addiction that often is extremely difficult to overcome. Despite widespread public information about the health hazards of smoking, cigarette smoking among teenagers has not decreased. In addition, male adolescents seem to be using more smokeless tobacco (chewing tobacco and snuff). It is not a safe alternative to cigarette smoking, however; smokeless tobacco can cause mouth cancer, throat cancer, and gum disease (see Tobacco, page 315).

Drug Abuse and Addiction

In the 1960s and 1970s, abuse of illegal drugs increased sharply among American teenagers. Drug abuse became a rite of passage in adolescence. Since then, the explosion of drug abuse has subsided somewhat. For instance, fewer adolescents smoke marijuana every day (see Medications and Drug Abuse, page 335).

In some ways, however, the problem has worsened. The age of first experimentation with marijuana has continually grown younger. Today, two-thirds of all teenagers have tried marijuana at least once before finishing high school, some of them during grade school. Also, the marijuana now on the market has higher levels of marijuana's active ingredient, tetrahydrocannabinol (THC). In addition, the "crack" form of cocaine is widely available at prices low enough for an adolescent to afford.

Alcohol also is a drug. Because it is legal for adults, it is easily accessible to teenagers. For most adolescents, experimentation with drugs starts with an alcoholic drink. Next usually comes smoking a marijuana cigarette (joint). Fortunately, relatively few teenagers "graduate" to trying harder drugs or using marijuana heavily or regularly over prolonged periods (see Marijuana, page 342, and Street Drugs, page 342).

Some drugs, such as heroin, are physically addicting. Others, such as marijuana, can cause psychological dependence that is strong enough to approach a form of addiction. Adolescents are at high risk of psychological dependence on drugs because they are so vulnerable to peer pressure.

The teenage years should involve the evolution of independence, increasingly serious scholarship, and the formation of a sexual identity, among other processes. All this may be daunting enough when your adolescent child is clear-eyed. He or she may be tempted to use drugs as an escape from the difficult task of being a teenager. However, if your child is habitually drugged or drunk, the challenges of adolescence can be nearly impossible to meet.

Problems at school make teenagers more likely to abuse drugs. Conversely, drug abuse can dampen the adolescent's motivation to do well in school. Drugs can impair the learning process, causing memory loss and shortening the attention span. Drug-abusing teenagers compromise their future outside school also. They may get into legal trouble for abusing illegal drugs, peddling them, or stealing to get enough money to buy them.

Drugs can disrupt the process by which your teenager develops a secure sexual identity. They can cause sexual anxiety. They can also mar judgment and self-control. They release inhibitions and can make it easier for your child to do things that he or she would not normally consider doing.

Some of these actions can have lasting effects. For instance, drugs might prevent your child from resisting sexual advances or from remembering to use contraception. An unwanted pregnancy could result. The adverse effects of maternal abuse of drugs—particularly alcohol—are well documented (see Risk Factors and Pregnancy, page 194).

Just like an adult who takes a drink to feel more comfortable at a party, an adolescent may take a drug to relax and join the crowd. For adults and teenagers alike, this is a counterproductive strategy. Social interactions are more successful when one is really one's self, rather than some other personality induced by a drug. Drugged or drunk people often withdraw socially and become depressed (see Myths About Alcoholism, page 329). Likewise, depressed adolescents may abuse more drugs in a vain effort to improve their mood.

Most seriously, drug abuse raises the risk of death during adolescence. The three leading killers of teenagers—accidents, murder, and suicide—are more prevalent among drug abusers.

The senses are distorted by drugs. This effect interferes with motor coordination and raises the risk of accidents. It is dangerous to operate machinery or even play sports while under the influence of drugs. Advise your child against the use of drugs. Insist that your child not drive a car while drugged (or drunk).

When adolescents share needles and syringes used to "shoot up" drugs intravenously, they are at high risk of getting AIDS. If they engage in this high-risk behavior, they should be tested for the virus that causes this fatal disease.

The most effective way to discourage your teenage child from abusing drugs—or alcohol or tobacco—is to gear your message to his or her level of intellectual and moral development (see Intellectual Growth and

Use of Alcohol

Most young people try at least one alcoholic drink during their teenage years. Alcohol is widely available, and many adolescents start unfortunate patterns of excessive drinking (see Alcohol Abuse and Alcoholism, page 325).

Alcohol is a potentially addicting drug—and an illegal one for most teenagers. Many of the issues that pertain to drug abuse apply to alcohol use also. Most important, alcohol plays major roles in depression and in the leading causes of death among teenagers—accidents, murder, and suicide (see Depression and Suicide, page 154, and Causes of Death in Teenagers, page 155).

Development, page 142, and Development of Standards, page 144). Particularly in early and middle adolescence, your child may be less impressed by the long-term health effects of these substances than by their immediate social consequences.

Even more important than delivering an anti-drug message is to set a good example. Addictive behavior often repeats itself in successive generations of a family. If your child is abusing drugs and others in your family have struggled with alcoholism or drug addiction, family therapy can help break this cycle. Striving to build your child's self-confidence so that he or she can better resist peer pressure to abuse drugs and alcohol is also helpful (see Teenagers and Drugs, page 338).

Sexual Abuse

Sexual abuse can occur in adolescence or even earlier in childhood (see Sexual Abuse in the Preschool and School-Age Years, pages 109 and 127). It can include incest and rape.

Rape usually involves force or the threat of force. However, rape also includes situations in which the victim is unable to give consent because of being drunk, drugged, mentally ill, or developmentally disabled. Almost half of reported rape victims are adolescents. Most sexual abuse of teenagers involves girls, but the rate of assaults on boys may be increasing.

Incest is sexual contact between close relatives. It can occur between a teenager—or a younger child—and a member of the family. The perpetrator can be anyone perceived to be a family member, even if that person is not related to the adolescent by blood or marriage. Examples may include the boyfriend of an adolescent's mother or a foster parent. Even when it does not involve blood relatives or any threat of force, incest is a betrayal of trust.

Rape and incest are devastating, hostile, and dehumanizing events. Sexual abuse often leaves extensive psychological trauma that has lasting effects on the victim's self-worth and identity. This is especially true for adolescents, who are still figuring out who they are, including their sexual identity. If rape is a teenager's first sexual experience, future sexual adjustment can be threatened.

After being raped, the victim may go through rapid mood swings, feeling alternately degraded, angry, guilty, and helpless. The victim may be plagued for a long time by fears, nightmares, and disturbed sleep. The victim's relationships with peers and consensual sexual partners may suffer. Fearing retaliation from the attacker, the victim may act withdrawn and develop ritualistic behavior as a defense.

Counseling can help the victim and family to cope with long-term effects of the sexual abuse. You may want to seek professional guidance from an established rape crisis center. Unfortunately, some parents reject their children who have become victims, while others overprotect them. You can help your child come to terms with the sexual abuse and then proceed with life by neither denying nor overreacting to the sexual abuse.

The psychological ramifications of incest can be even more complex than those of rape. Fearing that reporting the incest will disrupt the structure of the family, the victim may be too frightened to tell anyone about it. Thus, the incest may occur repeatedly. The incestuous relative may invoke family authority to keep the victim from reporting the abuse. As the incest continues unreported, the victim may feel increasingly helpless, ashamed, guilty, and even responsible.

More cases of incest are thought to be kept secret than disclosed. Serious consequences can occur when adolescents do not have the opportunity to disclose incest, end it, and learn to cope with its aftereffects. They are at high risk of drug abuse, promiscuity, running away, or even suicide. In contrast, professional treatment can deal with incest. Sometimes the abusive relative is rehabilitated. However, temporary or permanent breakup of the family and foster placement may be necessary.

When adolescents are victims of rape or incest, they are sometimes blamed for provoking the sexual abuse. Teenagers experiment with provocative modes of dressing and behavior. However, these experiments are just steps along the road to the creation of a personal sexual identity. In most cases, to say that an adolescent asked for sexual abuse is to perpetuate a cruel myth (see Sexual Assault and Sexual Abuse, page 428).

Depression and Suicide

Transient moodiness in response to a difficult situation is normal in adolescence, even more so than at other times of life. However, prolonged periods of profound unhappiness indicate depression, which can often be treated.

Once it was thought that only adults got depressed. Now, depression is being recognized increasingly in teenagers and even in younger children.

Symptoms of depression may include complaints of insomnia, fatigue, headache, stomachache, weakness, and dizziness. Your child may "act out" with unusual behavior, find it difficult to concentrate, and feel isolated from his or her family and friends. Your child may feel hopeless, expressing inner turmoil, chaos, and worthlessness. He or she may start abusing drugs or alcohol, trying in vain to feel better. Each bout of depression can last longer than 2 weeks. Often, the episode of depression is accompanied by a lack of interest in food and resulting weight loss or failure to gain.

If you think your child may be depressed, seek professional help. Professional treatment can help the depressed adolescent regain hope. He or she can realize that things will get better and problems will be overcome. Treatment involves individual psychotherapy or family therapy, sometimes with antidepressant medication. Hospitalization may be appropriate for a particularly long and severe bout of depression.

If your child has mentioned suicidal thoughts, do not take it lightly. Do not try to treat or manage his or her depression yourself. However, you do have an important role to play at home. Because depressed adolescents often feel that their families do not understand them, make a special effort to bridge this communication gap. Your hopes for your child's happiness, strength, and success should not stand in the way of your accepting his or her revelations of depression.

Ask your child how he or she feels—and listen. Check how long the mood lasts and how intense it is. You can help by offering your support and concern. You can also remind your child that he or she will not feel so bad indefinitely. Each episode of depression ends eventually. However, a teenager who is feeling deep depression for the first time may not recognize this.

Sometimes, depressed teenagers' lives become so painful that they feel they have nothing to live for. They may try to take their own lives. Most adolescents who attempt suicide are depressed. However, others may be motivated by other triggers, such as the breakup of a relationship, the death of a friend or family member, psychological problems within the family, chronic physical illness, drug abuse, or physical or sexual abuse. There are many reasons why teenagers attempt suicide. Sometimes they give no warning, and the attempt cannot be predicted.

The rate of suicide among teenagers, young adults, and even young children is rising rapidly. An estimated 500,000 teenagers survive suicide attempts each year in the United States. Suicide is now the third leading cause of death among American adolescents. In young adults, suicide is the second leading cause of death. The suicide rate may be even higher because many suicides are likely reported as accidents.

Causes of Death in Teenagers

Largely because of violent deaths, adolescents are the only group in the United States whose death rate is actually increasing. The three major causes of death in teenagers are accidents, murder, and suicide. Together, these account for three-quarters of the deaths that occur in adolescents.

Most of the accidental injuries that kill adolescents occur in car crashes. Many of these deaths could be prevented if teenagers wore seat belts and did not drive after drinking alcohol or abusing drugs. Other commonly fatal accidents include drowning (frequently with alcohol involvement), poisoning, burns, falls, and guns going off unexpectedly.

Many of these accidents do not occur randomly. Factors that raise the risk of death in adolescents include poverty, stressful family situations, and risk-taking behavior.

When male adolescents attempt suicide, they are more likely to use guns and to succeed in killing themselves. In contrast, female teenagers more often use drugs, which are not as reliably lethal.

If your child confides that he or she has considered suicide, take this admission seriously and seek counseling for him or her immediately. Even if it does not mean your child is really going to kill himself or herself, it is a cry for help that deserves to be heeded.

For further information, see Adolescent Depression (page 1101), Teenage Suicide (page 1101), Warning Signs of Potential Suicide (page 1125), and Depression and Mood Disorders (page 1122).

Common Medical Concerns

Adolescence has the reputation of being the healthiest of times, and most teenagers appear healthy and robust. However, many adolescents do have significant health problems. Some diseases are more likely to appear during the teenage years. Because it is normal for teenagers to rebel and question authority to some extent, they may find it difficult to comply with treatment for health problems. They may resent any diagnosis that sets them apart from their peers—and any treatment that makes them feel dependent.

Teenagers are bombarded by temptations to experiment with risk-taking behaviors that pose grave threats to their health, including abusing drugs and alcohol and engaging in sexual activity. Therefore, adolescence is a key time for preventive care.

It is a matter of concern that this age group receives the least medical attention. The childhood illnesses have passed and the health problems of the adult may not have yet developed. The annual rate of visits to a physician is less for teenagers than for all other ages. In fact, adolescence is no time to skimp on checkups. Routine visits should be scheduled at least every few years.

Routine examinations allow teenagers to seek professional guidance regarding their health-related concerns. The promotion of good health habits and healthful lifestyle behaviors should be a major focus of these

Keep Up With Immunizations

Adult-type combined tetanus and diphtheria toxoids should be given at age 14 to 16 and again every 10 years after that (see Immunizations, page 1079). A second measles-mumps-rubella vaccine is given at junior high or middle school entry unless it was given at grade school entry. Hepatitis B vaccination, a series of shots over 6 months, is also recommended for adolescents.

medical visits. In addition, school-based health education and health-care programs, with the active participation of physicians and other health-care professionals, should be actively encouraged. This is a critical time for teenagers to begin taking responsibility for their health and health-care decisions.

The teenage years are a time for identifying risk factors for cardiovascular disease, such as hypertension and elevated serum cholesterol (see page 640). Diabetes mellitus often is identified during adolescence.

Your physician or other health-care professionals can counsel you if you smoke or use alcohol or street drugs. Because motor vehicle accidents are a concern, use seat belts regularly and do not use alcohol or drugs while driving. In addition, this is the time to receive counseling regarding sexual activity, preventing sexually transmitted diseases (see page 157), using nonprescription and prescription birth control devices, and postponing sexual activity.

If you have questions about the cause and spread of AIDS (see page 1060) or other sexually transmitted diseases, ask your physician about this. If you are sexually active, you need to protect yourself against exposure to these infections.

Routine Examination

As the years pass and you mature, you will become increasingly independent from your parents and ready to assume increased responsibility for your health. Ideally, your physician should see you alone at each office visit. Privacy is important because your concerns are not always the same as those of your parents.

Many teenagers are reluctant to discuss the health-related problems that concern them most—problems such as acne, contraception, depression, drugs, being overweight, sexual practices, sexually transmitted

diseases, and getting along with parents and other adults. This reluctance can prompt a teenager to make an appointment ostensibly for a sore throat when the true problem centers, for example, on how to cope with depression. Physicians understand this reluctance. Often, it takes time, privacy, and special skill for a physician to draw out the teenager about his or her true concerns.

In the interest of effective communication, try to understand any tendency you may have to be reluctant and avoid it. Be direct and honest when discussing health problems with your physician. You may want to involve your parents, whose support can be a great help. But if you don't, your physician will respect your right to confidentiality unless suicide or some other potentially fatal emergency is threatened.

Your physician will appreciate an opportunity to discuss the issue of confidentiality with you. In most cases, physicians will seek your permission before communicating with parents, schools, other institutions, or previous physicians concerning your personal medical history.

Strive to achieve a comfortable relationship with your physician. You should know each other well. Sometimes teenagers continue consulting the pediatrician they have visited throughout childhood. Other adolescents prefer an internist or a family practitioner. Either way, select a physician in whom you can place your confidence, one who will respect your desire to be treated seriously and confidentially. In late adolescence, some young women consult an obstetrician/gynecologist for all or part of their health concerns. Teenagers with chronic acne may select a dermatologist for this purpose.

As in other age groups, the routine physical examination you will receive involves a review of your skin, head, eyes, ears, nose, mouth, glands, chest, lungs, abdomen, musculoskeletal system, neurologic system, external genitals, growth, and puberty development. A good physician is gentle and sensitive when examining all patients, and you should expect no less. If you would prefer to have a parent in the room, your physician should not object to this. Also, your physician should explain the goals of the examination and provide you with a clean gown and ample time to disrobe privately.

Checkups for teenagers offer an opportunity for early detection of chronic conditions that could stand in the way of health now or in adulthood. For example, your physician will measure your blood pressure at each routine visit. As you grow, your blood pressure will increase. This is normal. Because teenagers grow at varying rates, height tends to be a better determinant than age for deciding whether blood pressure is normal. But if you do have high blood pressure, early identification is important. Your physician can intervene and perhaps prevent consequences of high blood pressure. This is also a good opportunity for screening for scoliosis (see Scoliosis, page 906).

Adolescent girls generally start having pelvic examinations and Pap smears by at least age 18. Your physician can answer any questions you may have about your menstrual cycle (see Normal Menstrual Cycle, page 1144). If you are sexually active and need contraception, if you have symptoms that suggest a possible problem in your urinary tract or reproductive organs, or if you just want reassurance that your anatomy is normal, request a pelvic examination even if you are younger than age 18 (see Pelvic Examination, page 1141). Again, you can expect your physician to be gentle and thorough in explaining what is happening.

If you are an adolescent male, your physician can answer questions about the changes in your body that you are experiencing. Your physician may also instruct you in testicular self-examination (see Self-Examination of the Testicles, page 1200).

As part of your examination, your physician may ask about family practices and attitudes that could lead to health problems. For example, do your parents use alcohol? What are their views toward use of recreational drugs? Is there a history of physical or sexual abuse in your family?

Your physician should know about any diseases that run in your family. For example, has a parent or grandparent had a heart attack or cancer? To answer these questions, you may need help from your parents.

If you have a chronic disease such as diabetes or asthma, take on as much responsibility for managing your personal health problem as you can handle. Learn everything you can about your ailment and how it is to be managed. You may want to keep a journal of chronic symptoms and treatment methods to help determine what treatment works best.

By accepting any potential disability realistically and by taking charge of your ailment, you will come to feel that you have, to the best of your ability, mastered your unique circumstances. Over the long term, this can enhance the effectiveness of treatment and the outcome of your disease.

Sexually Transmitted Diseases

Signs and Symptoms
- Sores, lumps, bumps, or warts on or around the genitals
- Genital or anal itching
- Discharge from the vagina, penis, or anus
- Burning during urination
- Sore throat
- Swollen lymph glands
- Pain in the upper thigh (groin) or lower abdomen
- Rashes, especially on the soles of the feet or palms of the hands
- No apparent symptoms

Sexually transmitted diseases are spread from one person to another during sexual contact. Usually that contact is sexual intercourse, but sometimes it is oral or anal sex or some other sexual activity. These diseases are called STDs for short. An older term is venereal disease (VD). Each type of STD is caused by a different infectious agent. The most common STDs are gonorrhea, chlamydiosis, trichomoniasis, genital herpes, and human papilloma virus. In addition, AIDS is becoming more widespread.

STDs occur most commonly among teenagers and young adults. This age group is more likely to have more than one partner, have a partner who has been sexually active with others, and not consistently use condoms. There may also be biologic differences that make it easier for a teenager exposed to an STD to get infected. Unfortunately, most adolescents' decision-making and communication skills are still developing and may not keep pace with their sexual activity. Lack of adequate sex education may also play a role.

If you are sexually active, you are at risk of contracting an STD. The more sexual partners you have, the higher your risk of catching one of these diseases.

Diagnosis
It is important to note that symptoms do not always accompany STDs. When no symptoms are present, you and your partner

have no reason to believe that anything is wrong, and the infection can easily be passed on. Because of this, if you are a sexually active teenager you should be tested and examined regularly for the common STDs. This step can be part of your routine checkups.

To determine whether you have an STD, your physician first will perform a physical examination, including a pelvic examination and Pap smear if you are female (see pages 1141 and 1181). The next step may be taking samples of your blood, urine, or genital discharge, which can be tested for the presence of either an STD-causing infectious agent or antibodies to such a microbe.

Abstain from sexual contact if your sexual partner tells you that he or she has an STD. If you think you have one, abstain from sexual contact until your STD is cured. Consult a physician immediately. You can visit your own physician, a clinic that specializes in STDs or birth control, or a hospital emergency room. Teenagers, like adults, are entitled to confidentiality regarding the diagnosis and treatment of STDs. That means parents and others are not notified without your permission. In the uncommon situation of a life-threatening STD or the need for hospitalization, your parents would likely need to know. Also, physicians are required by law to report many STDs to state health authorities.

Whenever an STD is diagnosed, it is important for all sexual partners to be examined and treated. Do not feel guilty for revealing the identities of your partner or partners to your physician. Again, this information will be kept confidential.

How Serious Are Sexually Transmitted Diseases?

Most STDs can be cured with medications. AIDS, which leads to death, is the exception (see HIV Infection and AIDS, page 1060). Others, such as herpes or human papilloma virus (HPV), may recur in spite of being treated.

The longer you delay treatment, the more difficult your STD will be to control. Sometimes, STDs are left untreated for so long that they lead to lasting complications. For instance, repeated bouts of pelvic inflammatory disease (see page 1187) can leave a young woman infertile (incapable of having a baby). Teenage girls tend to be at extra risk for such complications of STDs.

Treatment

Various antibiotics are available to cure STDs and kill the bacteria that cause them.

You can avoid contracting an STD by abstaining from sexual activity. If you are sexually active, you can minimize your risk of STDs by being selective about your sexual partners and using a condom. Condoms are relatively effective—although not foolproof—at blocking the spread of infectious agents, including AIDS. Such precautions allow what is termed "safer sex." When used together with a condom, contraceptive foam offers added protection against the spread of STDs (see Sexually Transmitted Diseases, page 1087).

Acne

Signs and Symptoms—Numerous pimples, which come and go, appearing as red lumps, whiteheads, or blackheads

Pimples result from inflammation of the follicles from which your body hair grows. This inflammation is usually caused by overproduction of oil (sebum) by the sebaceous gland in each hair follicle. The oil can block the follicle and predispose it to bacterial infection and inflammation. When a pimple is plugged with white pus, it is called a whitehead. If this plug extends to the skin surface and is exposed to air, it turns black and is called a blackhead.

Acne is so common in adolescence that almost all teenagers have it to some degree. Acne usually starts around puberty and disappears by the end of the teenage years. It is somewhat more common in boys than in girls. When girls have acne, it tends to worsen around the time of their menstrual periods. In both boys and girls, it may be triggered by normal elevations of androgen hormones, which make the sebaceous glands produce extra oil (see Acne, page 990).

Infectious Mononucleosis

Infectious mononucleosis is caused by the Epstein-Barr virus. Even though it is nicknamed the "kissing disease," the virus can be transmitted by coughing and sneezing as well as by kissing, but it is not highly contagious. Many children between 4 and

15 become infected with the virus. However, their initial infection usually results in only mild symptoms—short-term fever and fatigue. Later in adolescence and young adulthood the virus may be a cause of a prolonged, exhausting illness. Symptoms of infectious mononucleosis include long-term fever, swollen glands, sore throat, and fatigue. Rest and adequate fluid intake are the main treatments (see Infectious Mononucleosis, page 1064).

Urinary Tract Infections

The most common infection caused by bacteria multiplying in the urinary tract is cystitis, which is inflammation of the bladder. Cystitis occurs often among teenage girls.

It usually results when traces of stool contaminate the urethra, the canal that transports urine from the bladder out of the body. It can be worsened by sexual intercourse, which can irritate the urethra. The symptoms can include urination that is frequent, urgent, and painful, as well as foul-smelling urine and fever (see Cystitis, page 842).

Iron-Deficiency Anemia

Iron-deficiency anemia is most common in young children between 6 months and 3 years old. Its prevalence increases again in the teens.

Iron deficiency tends to be more common in males than in females during adolescence, unlike in other age groups, because the male teenager has higher iron and hemoglobin needs as a result of his increase in muscle mass. However, girls may lose enough blood with periods (menses) to develop iron deficiency. You can help prevent iron deficiency by eating plenty of meats (especially liver), fish, poultry, eggs, legumes (peas and beans), potatoes, and rice (see Iron-Deficiency Anemia, page 957).

Dysmenorrhea

Dysmenorrhea, or painful menstruation, tends to be most common in adolescence. As a woman matures—and particularly after pregnancy—the problem usually subsides. At some time, more than half of all teenage girls and young women experience dysmenorrhea (see Painful Menses, page 1148).

Migraine Headaches

Migraine headaches are repeated attacks of intense, throbbing head pain lasting at least an hour each. They are often accompanied by nausea, vomiting, loss of appetite, and sensitivity to light. They usually occur for the first time in early adolescence, although they can also appear in young children and in adults. They are more common in girls than in boys, and they tend to run in families (see Migraine Headaches, page 502).

Scoliosis

Scoliosis is a lateral (sideways) curvature of the spine. It is most commonly detected in girls who are 10 to 14 years old. Screening for scoliosis is performed routinely at many schools. Some cases of scoliosis are too slight to need treatment. In other cases treatment is needed with special braces or surgery. If untreated, the scoliosis may worsen rapidly and become permanently disabling (see Scoliosis, page 906).

Epiphysitis

Epiphysitis is inflammation of an epiphysis, the wide end of a long bone such as the shinbone (tibia), thighbone (femur), or upper arm bone (humerus). The epiphysis is considered distinct from the shaft of the bone. Rapid growth, as occurs during adolescence, can place extra stresses on the epiphyses and predispose them to epiphysitis.

The most common type of epiphysitis is Osgood-Schlatter disease, a painful inflammation of the epiphysis of the shin bone. It is caused by overuse in activities that place repeated stress on the top of the shin bone, where the tendon of the kneecap inserts. The major symptom is knee pain, which is worsened by activity and relieved by rest. Treatment involves resting and avoiding activities that place prolonged stress on the flexed knee. These activities include bicycle riding and playing basketball. When growth of the affected bone ends, the pain usually subsides on its own.

Injuries

Among American adolescents, injury is a major public health problem. For teenagers 15 through 19, injuries are responsible for more than three-fourths of all deaths. Automobile accidents are the most common cause. Half of fatal accidents occur during evening hours, even though teenagers do only about 20 percent of their driving at night. Alcohol is often a factor. Seat belts could spare some lives and injuries, but in spite of driver education programs and state laws requiring their use, adolescents often fail to buckle up.

Athletic activities are leading causes of nonfatal injuries. Football is among the most hazardous. Knees and ankles are sites commonly injured, but head and neck injuries occur as well, despite advances in equipment. Although less hazardous, participation in sports such as track and field, baseball, and basketball can lead to injury, especially among boys. For girls, gymnastics poses the highest risk. For both, even sports such as cross-country running, swimming, and tennis carry some risk.

Bicycles can be lethal. Each year 70 percent of bike deaths occur in children younger than age 15. Most of these accidents involve cars and result in head injuries. In-line skating, rollerskating, and skateboarding also can be hazardous to your health. Of these popular forms of recreation, in-line skating is the safest, but all three can lead to head, wrist, elbow, ankle, and other injuries.

What can you do to improve your safety? Buckle up. Don't drink and drive. Minimize your risk of injury by wearing the protective equipment designed for each sport you play and by appropriate physical conditioning.

Accidental injuries and deaths can be avoided.

Vision Problems

The rapid growth of adolescence involves the whole body, including the eyes. Sometimes a teenager's eyes change their shape as well as their size. As a result, problems with vision acuity often develop during adolescence. The most common problem is the development of or worsening of nearsightedness (myopia), which can be corrected by prescription glasses or contact lenses (see Refraction Problems, page 522).

Teenagers are also prone to injury-related vision problems. Most of these problems can be prevented by wearing protective goggles, masks, or other headgear during sports (see Protecting Your Eyes, page 532).

At school, you may be screened for vision problems and hearing disorders. At routine visits, your physician will also check your eyes and ears. If you notice any difficulty seeing or hearing, tell your parents and your physician.

Hearing Disorders

Sometimes teenagers develop a permanent high-frequency hearing loss—that is, it becomes more difficult for them to hear sounds that are higher than 4,000 hertz. You can help prevent this hearing disorder by avoiding extended exposure to loud noises such as the sound of loud amplified music, subway trains, and heavy machinery. Such loud sounds can damage your inner ears (see How to Protect Your Ears, page 573).

Chapter 6

Young Adulthood: Ages 20 Through 39

Contents

The Transition Years, 162

Becoming a Parent, 162

The Male Reproductive System, 163
Reproductive Organs, 163
Sexual Function, 164
Prevention of Pregnancy, 165
Vasectomy, 166
  Reversing a Vasectomy: The Vasovasectomy, 166

The Woman of Childbearing Age, 167
The Reproductive System, 167
Sexual and Reproductive Health, 168
Sexual Function and Dysfunction, 169
Prevention of Pregnancy, 170
Tubal Ligation, 174
  Reversing a Tubal Ligation, 174
Preparation for Pregnancy, 175

Concerns During Pregnancy, 175
Fertilization, 176
Prenatal Development, 177
  Bleeding During Pregnancy, 178
Prenatal Care, 178
Prenatal Tests, 179
  Intrauterine Growth Retardation, 179
Nutrition During Pregnancy, 182
  Where You'll Gain the Weight, 183
  Key Nutrients in Pregnancy, 184
  Smart Snacking, 185
Therapeutic Drugs in Pregnancy, 185
  Caffeine Content of Common Foods, 186
Common Discomforts During Pregnancy, 186
Medical Problems of Pregnancy, 189
Infectious Diseases During Pregnancy, 191
  Rhesus (Rh) Compatibility, 192
Risk Factors and Pregnancy, 194
Exercise During Pregnancy, 195
Travel During Pregnancy, 196

Early Pregnancy: The First Trimester, 196
How Do You Know If You Are Pregnant? 197
Miscarriage, 197
  Pregnancy Tests, 198
  Pregnancy Termination: Medical Problems and
    Personal Choices, 199
Ectopic (Tubal) Pregnancy, 199

Mid-Pregnancy: The Second Trimester, 200
Premature Labor, 201
Hydramnios, 202
Incompetent Cervix, 203

Late Pregnancy: The Third Trimester, 203
Preeclampsia and Eclampsia, 204
Antepartum Hemorrhage, 205
Premature Rupture of Membranes, 205
Placenta Previa, 205
Intrauterine Death, 206
Postmaturity (Prolonged Pregnancy), 206

Labor and Delivery, 207
How Will I Know When Labor Begins? 207
How Long Will Labor Be? 207
  What Is False Labor? 208
Abnormal Fetal Positions, 209
Labor and Delivery Procedures, 210
Pain Relief, 211
Cesarean Delivery, 212
  Twins and Multiple Pregnancies, 213
Postpartum Hemorrhage, 214
Retained Placenta, 214

After Pregnancy, 214
Breastfeeding, 215
Breast Problems, 216
Postpartum Depression and Stress, 216
  Sex After Birth, 217
Contraception, 218

The Transition Years

Becoming an adult is one of life's greatest transitions. The fundamental change from dependence on one's parents—in financial, emotional, and other terms—to independence usually occurs shortly before or after the age of 20.

Part of this change involves the switch from being a student. The world of the student is defined by expanding horizons and new worlds to investigate. Alternatively, having a job implies a wide range of new disciplines and responsibilities.

Working should, of course, offer stimulating challenges and the opportunity for accomplishments. Yet an ex-student who starts work suddenly may face specified hours, the need to master teamwork skills, and a boss whose role is unlike that of any parent or teacher.

For most young Americans, career choices are made in their third decade of life, but that is only one of several major adjustments. Many young adults also come to grips with their sexuality during this period. Relationships are established, and some are cemented. For some, this may be a time of experimentation and risk with numerous sexual partners, alcohol, or drugs.

For the most part, these years are a time of good health: our bodies change relatively little during the third and fourth decades, and concerns of aging seem some distance in the future. Nevertheless, it is a time to develop good habits: healthful exercise patterns and a good nutritional regimen can help make the passage to middle and later years healthier and happier (see Exercise and Fitness, page 289).

Becoming a Parent

Today, many couples delay until the late 20s or 30s the inevitable question of whether to have children. (For some, of course, the question is answered earlier.) An increasing number of women and men are asking another question: whether to end the childbearing years with permanent sterilization.

How does a man or woman maintain sexual and reproductive health? The time to begin is before damage has been done. Be aware of sexually transmitted diseases that could impair your ability to have children (see page 1087). Take the time to practice self-examination, whether it be breast examination by women (see page 1160) or testicle examination by men (see page 1200). The earlier a cancer is found, the better the chance of cure. Also, have medical checkups regularly (see How Often Should I Consult My Physician? page 1250). For a woman in her childbearing years, a Papanicolaou smear (Pap test) (see page 1181) should be a part of the regular examination.

Prevention of pregnancy is a major concern of many young adults. You can minimize the chances of that happening to you by avoiding intercourse or by practicing birth control. Today, couples have more birth control options than ever before, some of which are more effective for preventing pregnancy than others. This chapter explains the options, risks, and benefits of birth control. It also discusses permanent sterilization techniques for both men and women.

Today, more and more often, couples postpone pregnancy. People marry later. More women than ever before are working, many in fulfilling and demanding careers. Inevitably, though, couples must acknowledge the biologic clock. Those in their 30s must realize that if they are to have a child, the years of postponement are nearing an end.

When is the best time in the menstrual cycle to plan intercourse to achieve pregnancy? What happens when the egg and sperm meet? What are the symptoms of pregnancy? These and other concerns are covered in the following pages.

Unfortunately, drug and alcohol abuse are major health and social problems. Some women continue to drink excessively or to use drugs even after they learn they are pregnant, and their infants often pay a price. A section in the chapter discusses the use of alcohol, drugs, and cigarettes during pregnancy.

Although most women are not drug users or alcoholics, many do take prescription drugs even during pregnancy. Is this safe? In some cases these drugs can harm the developing baby. Never take a medication unless your physician recommends it. (Make sure any physician you consult knows you are pregnant.) A list of some prescription medications known to cause birth defects or other medical problems is included in the chapter.

Most pregnancies are medically uneventful. Only a small percentage of women have complications. Complications such as diabetes, preeclampsia, hypertension, and hemorrhage are discussed in this chapter. Factors that increase the risk of problems for either you or your baby also are discussed; these include poor diet, advanced age, and the use of alcohol and cigarettes.

Many women wonder what is involved in, and to some extent fear, labor and birth. What are the signs of true labor and false labor? What are your pain relief options? What are the indications for a cesarean section and what should you expect if your physician deems it necessary? You will get answers to these questions in the pages that follow.

Finally, the chapter discusses concerns during the postpartum period. These can be trying weeks. A husband who is used to his wife's undivided attention may feel resentful when her energies become consumed by the new family member. The wife may be exhausted and suffering from postpartum depression, a not uncommon affliction. To worsen the situation, the couple must avoid intercourse, so both may feel some sexual frustration. Although time usually resolves these problems, this chapter offers advice on getting through the often difficult postpartum period.

The childbearing decades can be packed full of life. In this chapter you will find much guidance about your overall and reproductive health—and also about the new-life process, from conception to birth.

The Male Reproductive System

Unlike the female, whose reproductive abilities usually come to a halt in mid-life, the male is capable of fathering a child well into old age.

A man's sperm is produced constantly. Each time a man ejaculates, millions of microscopic spermatozoa are propelled in a pool of semen. Whether or not one will fertilize an egg depends on several factors, including how well the male reproductive system is working.

Reproductive Organs

The following is a description of the male reproductive organs and their components.

Testicles (Testes)

The testicles function as a sperm and hormone production center. Each testicle contains coiled tubes, called seminiferous tubules, in which sperm are made. Normally, a male child is born with two testicles. While the fetus is in the uterus, the testicles are located near its kidneys, but they gradually work

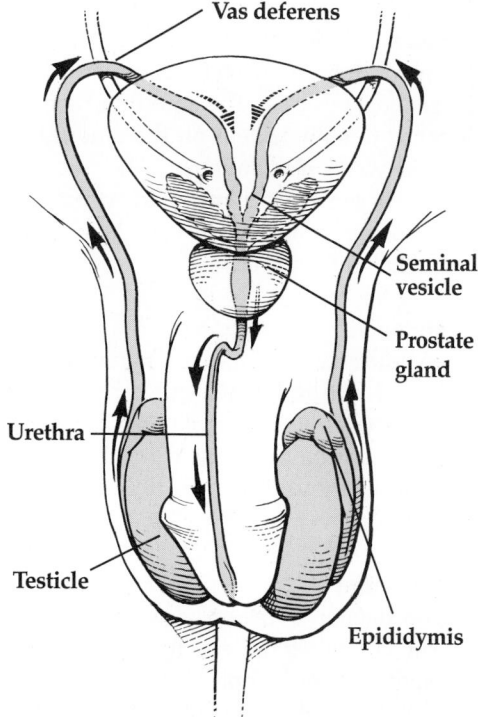

From the testicles, sperm are moved by contractions through the epididymis and the vas deferens. Fluids are added by the seminal vesicles and prostate gland. Semen is comprised of these fluids and sperm. Following sexual stimulation, the semen is ejaculated at orgasm through the urethra.

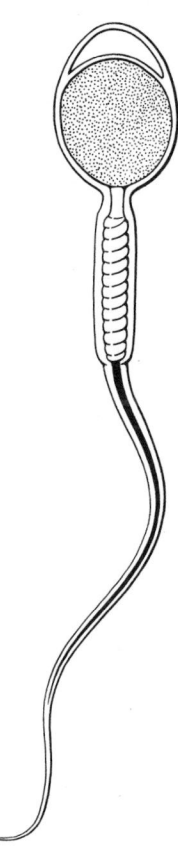

About 1/600th of an inch long, the human sperm is made up of a head, containing the nucleus or center of the cell, a body, and a tail that propels it.

their way down into the scrotum, the sack-like structure below the penis. Premature infants sometimes are born with an empty scrotum because the testicles have not had time to descend. Full-term infants also may have undescended testicles, and treatment with hormones or even an operation may be needed (see Undescended Testicle, page 47).

Within the testicles, the cells whose job it is to make sperm are extremely sensitive to heat. Thus, exposure to excessive heat can interrupt production of sperm.

Scrotum
The scrotum protects the testicles. It is a highly efficient air conditioner, maintaining the temperature of the testicles about 6 degrees below the normal body temperature. When the weather is cold, the scrotum shrinks to maintain heat; in hot weather, it becomes larger and flaccid to expose a larger area for heat loss.

Sperm
A single human sperm is made up of a head, containing the nucleus (center) of the cell, a body, and a tail. A sperm is about 1/600th of an inch long. The mechanism that propels the sperm is in the tail. Depending on whether a woman's vaginal mucus is watery or thick, a sperm can swim an inch in 4 to 16 minutes in the vagina.

Semen
Semen is the ejaculated fluid that contains the sperm. It is produced by the prostate and the seminal vesicles. The amount of semen depends to some extent on the amount of time between ejaculations. The average amount of semen ejaculated varies from ½ to 1½ teaspoons. The average ejaculation contains a half billion sperm.

Epididymis
The epididymis is a long, coiled tube above each testicle through which sperm is propelled by contractions on its way to the vas deferens, a tube that runs from the upper scrotum to the urethra at the base of the prostate.

Vas Deferens
The vas deferens is the body's warehouse for sperm as well as the conduit that carries the sperm from the epididymis to the urethra. Millions of sperm enter the vas deferens daily.

Penis
The penis is the organ through which sperm are released into the vagina. Normally, the penis is soft and flexible. However, when a man is sexually aroused, the spongy tissue of the penis becomes engorged with blood because the exit valves of the penile veins close. The result is an erection. The penis becomes firm, expanding in length and circumference.

Prostate
The prostate is a gland surrounding the urethra, the tube through which urine passes from the bladder. The prostate and the seminal vesicles are sources of the semen.

Hormones
Hormones are chemical messengers produced in various parts of the body. Testosterone, the important masculinizing hormone, is produced within the testicles. It influences body shape, voice, body hair, sexual drive, and the ability to have an erection.

The first step in reproduction is sexual desire (libido), which is regulated by a combination of psychological factors and sexual hormones. When a man is sexually stimulated, an erection occurs. During intercourse, the sexual excitement intensifies to the point of orgasm. It is during orgasm that ejaculation occurs. It begins at the base of the bladder and in the prostate and seminal vesicles. The muscles go through a series of involuntary contractions, resulting in the sudden propulsion of semen through the urethra. This fluid traverses the length of the penis and is released into the vagina.

The vagina is flooded with millions of sperm, swimming in all directions in search of an egg. Most never reach the cervical canal but die within the vagina. Of those that make it to the 1-inch cervical canal, most get side-tracked and never go farther. A few reach the uterus and successfully make the 2-inch journey to the openings of the fallopian tubes.

Out of an average of 400 million sperm, only a few reach the fertilization point—midway down the fallopian tube that contains an egg. The sperm that ultimately fertilizes the egg has overcome enormous odds.

Sexual Function

In men, the ability to function sexually depends on psychological, hormonal, neurologic, and vascular (blood vessel) factors.

The sexual sequence in the male involves five steps: stimulation, erection, ejaculation, orgasm, and detumescence (loss of erection).

Sexual desire (libido) is governed by hormones and psychological factors. The ability to have an erection is controlled by both the nervous system and the vascular system. Ejaculation is controlled by a part of the nervous system. Orgasm is purely a psychological phenomenon that includes the sensation caused by the ejaculation. Detumescence probably is under the control of the vascular system.

Sometimes problems occur that impair male sexual function (see Health Issues of Partners, page 1213). Some neurologic disorders and diseases of the urogenital system directly interfere with sexual performance (see Sexual Problems of Men, page 1212). Many chronic diseases impede a man's ability to perform sexually because of their debilitating effect on overall health. The use of alcohol or other drugs also may impair sexual function.

Many diseases of the male genitals—cancer being the most serious—have an excellent cure rate when detected early. All men should examine their genitals routinely for any suspicious changes (see Self-Examination of the Testicles, page 1200).

Prevention of Pregnancy

Throughout history, men and women have attempted—not always successfully—to prevent pregnancy.

More than 1,500 years ago, the Talmud recommended that couples drink a "cup of roots" to prevent pregnancy. The American Indians brewed a special tea for those who wished to avoid conception. As early as the 16th century, Arabs were inserting crude versions of today's intrauterine device inside their camels to prevent an increase in the herd.

Today, most couples in the United States use some form of birth control.

Two methods of temporary contraception depend primarily on the man: condoms and coitus interruptus. A condom is both more effective and more sexually satisfying.

Condoms
Condoms are used by approximately 10 to 15 percent of all couples practicing birth control. The condom is a thin rubber sheath that the man places over his erect penis just before intercourse. When the man ejaculates, the semen remains inside the condom and is not released into the vagina.

When used correctly, condoms are about 96 percent effective for preventing pregnancy. Moreover, if they are intact and properly used, condoms help to protect an uninfected partner from sexually transmitted diseases (see HIV Infection and AIDS, page 1060, and Sexually Transmitted Diseases, page 1087).

One reason for the popularity of condoms is that they are easy to obtain. Condoms are available without prescription in drugstores and can be purchased from vending machines in some men's restrooms. They are available in various materials, ranging from rubber to animal skin, come with or without a lubricant, and are packaged in small and large quantities. Packaged condoms are good for at least 2 to 5 years when kept in a cool, dry environment. Latex condoms offer the best protection from sexually transmitted diseases.

If you decide to use a condom, make sure that as you unroll the condom down over the penis, you leave room at the tip for semen to collect. If you are uncircumcised, make sure the foreskin is pulled back before you put on the condom. After intercourse, the penis should be withdrawn from the vagina, and then the condom is removed and disposed of.

Condom "accidents" can occur during intercourse, usually as a result of rupture. The chance of an accident can be lessened by always allowing extra room at the tip for semen and by using a water-based lubricant on the condom, especially if your partner's vagina seems dry. (A petroleum-based lubricant may compromise the condom's effectiveness.) Finally, the risk of pregnancy when using a condom is reduced further when a spermicide is inserted into the woman's vagina before intercourse.

The most common complaints associated with condoms are not that they are ineffective but that they dull sensation for the man, thus diminishing sexual pleasure. Some couples also complain that spontaneity is lost.

Coitus Interruptus
Coitus interruptus is the withdrawal of the penis from the vagina before orgasm. It is probably the oldest method of birth control, and it is used throughout the world more extensively than any other form of contra-

Reversing a Vasectomy: The Vasovasectomy

Always consider a vasectomy as permanent sterilization.

However, circumstances do change. Maybe your financial situation suddenly has taken a turn for the better, and you and your partner decide you want another child. Or perhaps you have remarried after being widowed or divorced and you and your spouse want a child.

It is possible to reattach the vas deferens once it has been severed. Unlike the initial operation, however, the vasovasectomy requires the skill of a surgeon trained to work under the magnification of a powerful microscope. Moreover, this is not an office procedure but requires 1 to 2 days in the hospital.

Approximately 80 to 90 percent of men who have their vasectomies reversed do ejaculate sperm. However, only 30 to 40 percent are able to father children after the reversal. The reason for this discrepancy may be that as a result of vasectomy many men develop antibodies that fight their sperm.

Consult your family physician or urologist for referral to a surgeon experienced in this procedure.

ception. In the United States, however, fewer than 3 percent of adults use it as their primary method of contraception.

Although some couples have used coitus interruptus effectively, the overall failure rate is relatively high, and most physicians do not recommend it. Aside from being frustrating for both partners, coitus interruptus requires that the man maintain stringent control. Even a small leak of semen into the vagina can result in pregnancy.

In performing a vasectomy, the surgeon cuts the vas deferens, thus closing off the path taken by sperm to the outside.

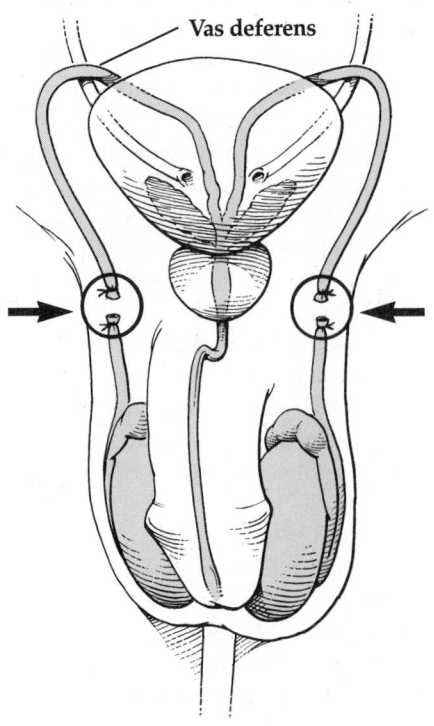

Vas deferens

Male Birth Control Pill

A male birth control pill has been talked about for years. In fact, some hormonal treatments have been tested which do render the male temporarily infertile. Unfortunately, they also take away sexual drive and the ability to maintain an erection. Thus, at this time, there is no male birth control pill on the market.

Vasectomy

At some point, many couples decide that they do not want any more children. For these couples, permanent sterilization may be the answer.

Many couples opt for male sterilization simply because the procedure is less physically traumatic, is less expensive, and involves less time away from work and home than does the counterpart for women, tubal ligation (see page 174). Vasectomy is a relatively simple operation that can be done in a physician's office or in an outpatient surgical setting.

Vasectomy involves cutting and sealing the vas deferens, the tubes that carry sperm. The procedure in no way interferes with a man's ability to maintain an erection or reach orgasm. Nor does it impede the production of male hormones or of sperm in the testicles. The only change is that the sperm's link to the outside has been severed permanently. After a vasectomy, you continue to ejaculate about the same amount of semen because sperm account for only a small part of the ejaculate.

If you have a vasectomy, you will be given an injection of anesthetic in the scrotum to numb the area so you will not feel pain. After your physician has located the vas deferens, a pair of small cuts are made in the skin of the scrotum. Each vas deferens is then pulled through the opening until it forms a loop. Approximately a half inch is cut out of each vas deferens and removed. The two ends of each vas deferens are closed by stitches or cauterization, or both, and are placed back in the scrotum. The incisions are closed with stitches.

The operation takes approximately 20 minutes, after which you will be asked to stay for a short period of observation. After a vasectomy, refrain from any strenuous activity for at least 48 hours. However, if your work does not involve hard physical labor, you can return to your job as soon as you feel like it. The stitches generally are of a type that dissolves in 7 to 10 days.

You may notice some swelling and minor discomfort in the scrotum for several weeks. However, if the pain becomes severe or if fever develops, call your physician.

The failure rate for a vasectomy is less than 1 percent. But your vasectomy is no immediate guarantee against pregnancy because of the sperm stored above the point where the vas deferens was tied. Thus, your physician will want to test your ejaculate for sperm. Generally, in most men the semen becomes sperm-free after 8 to 10 ejaculations following the vasectomy. Until your physician has determined that your ejaculate does not contain sperm, you should continue to use contraception.

The Woman of Childbearing Age

If you are a woman between the ages of 20 and 39, many of your health concerns are related to sexual and reproductive health. Questions that often are asked concerning reproductive health include the following: How often should I have a pelvic examination? What is the correct way to perform a self-examination of my breasts? How safe is the birth control pill if I smoke and am over 35 years old? What are the risks of permanent sterilization? If I do not have orgasms, do I have a sexual problem?

The following section addresses some of these concerns, including ways in which you can spot potential health problems, the benefits of exercise for every woman, common breast problems, and family planning.

The Reproductive System

The organs of the female reproductive system are the two ovaries, the fallopian tubes, and the uterus. The vagina is a tubular structure that extends from the lower portion of the uterus (the cervix) to the external genitals.

Ovaries
The ovaries are situated in the lower part of the abdomen and produce and store eggs and also feminizing hormones. While it is still in the uterus, the female fetus contains hundreds of thousands of eggs, many of which disappear before birth. Later, some of the eggs are surrounded by cells that begin to form a capsule (follicle) around individual eggs. As a girl reaches puberty, a substance called follicle-stimulating hormone (FSH) is secreted by the pituitary gland. As a result, fluid develops within some follicles. Some grow fat and bulge; others shrivel and die. Every month after puberty, one or sometimes two of these fluid-filled follicles (graafian follicles) grow larger until another pituitary substance called luteinizing hormone (LH) stimulates the follicle to release an egg, which then bursts through the surface of the ovary into the pelvic cavity and eventually enters the fallopian tube. This process is called ovulation.

Every month, one of the eggs present at birth in the ovary is released during ovulation. The egg travels down the fallopian tube, where fertilization may occur. The fertilized egg implants itself in the lining of the uterus. If fertilization does not occur, the egg, along with the lining of the uterus, is shed during menstruation.

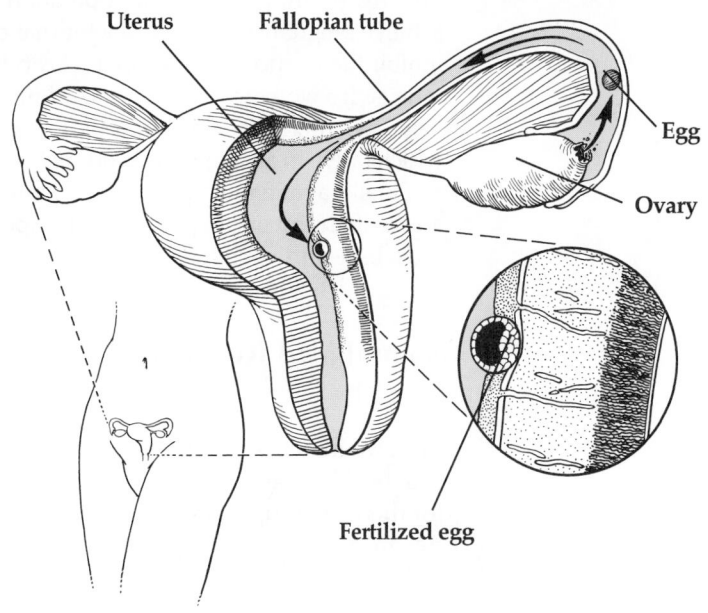

Uterus   Fallopian tube

Egg

Ovary

Fertilized egg

Fallopian Tubes

The fallopian tubes are two thin, 5-inch-long tubes that lead from near the ovaries to the uterus. It is within a fallopian tube that fertilization occurs. In any given cycle, ovulation occurs from only one ovary.

Uterus

The uterus is a pear-shaped, muscular organ. The uterus receives the egg after its journey down the fallopian tube. If the egg has been fertilized, it implants itself within the wall of the uterus and begins to grow into a baby. If it is not fertilized, the egg and the lining of the uterus are shed, the result of which is menstruation.

Reproduction depends on several factors. Timing is critical. To result in pregnancy, intercourse must take place within the 72 hours before the egg enters the fallopian tube or within the 24 hours after it enters the fallopian tube. A sperm cell is capable of fertilizing an egg for only 2 to 3 hours after ejaculation, and an unfertilized egg survives for only about 24 hours after its release from the ovary. Your best chance of becoming pregnant is on the 13th or 14th day preceding the onset of your period.

Even perfect timing, however, does not guarantee a pregnancy. Healthy male and female reproductive systems are necessary. In a woman, irregular ovulation patterns hinder the chance of fertilization. Moreover, the fallopian tubes must be open and receptive to the egg and sperm. Women whose tubes contain scar tissue from a previous infection or surgery may require an operation to achieve pregnancy. Another factor that can inhibit the chance of pregnancy is cervical mucus. If a woman's mucus is too acidic, the vaginal environment may be hostile to sperm, which thrive in alkaline surroundings.

Finally, a man must produce not only an adequate number of sperm but the sperm must be healthy (see Infertility, page 1215).

Sexual and Reproductive Health

Most women ages 20 through 39 are basically healthy. Thus, the major thrust of health care for this age group is prevention rather than treatment.

You can play an active role in helping to ensure your future sexual and reproductive health. This is not to imply that serious diseases of the reproductive organs do not occur in women who take good care of themselves. Unfortunately, they do. However, you can reduce the likelihood of a serious problem or at least discover the problem in its early stages, when it is more easily treated, by following a few simple rules.

Pelvic Examination

Beginning at age 18 years, every woman should have a yearly pelvic examination (see page 1141). For sexually active teenagers, annual pelvic examinations should start earlier. The examination may be part of a routine examination by your internist, family physician, or gynecologist (see Selecting a Gynecologist, page 1142).

The pelvic examination is important in that any abnormalities, such as cysts, tumors, and infections, or problems, such as muscle weakness that causes the uterus or vagina to sag, can be detected. If you have a suspicious discharge, your physician can obtain a sample of the material to be analyzed to identify the cause (see Pelvic Examination, page 1141).

Pap Test

An important part of the pelvic examination is the Papanicolaou (Pap) smear. This simple and painless test is done by removing a few cells from your cervix with a spatula, brush, or swab. The Pap test is used to detect cervical cancer, a disease that occurs more often in women older than 40 years. It is also useful for detecting precancerous conditions.

Starting at age 18 years (earlier if the teenager is sexually active), every woman should have a Pap test at least every 1 to 3 years at the advice of her physicion (see Pap Smear, page 1181).

Pelvic Inflammatory Disease

A frequent cause of female infertility is pelvic inflammatory disease, a condition that ultimately can scar the fallopian tubes. This disease usually occurs when bacteria—often those that cause gonorrhea—are introduced into the vagina during intercourse. It occasionally may occur after abortion, miscarriage, or insertion of an intrauterine device.

This disease most often is found in young, sexually active women. Thus, particularly if you have multiple sex partners, be aware of the risks.

The use of an intact condom is usually

effective for preventing pelvic inflammatory disease and sexually transmitted diseases such as herpes, syphilis, gonorrhea, and AIDS because bacteria or viruses are prevented from passing from one partner to the other.

If you have pelvic pain, tenderness in your lower abdomen, fever, or an unpleasant-smelling vaginal discharge, you may have pelvic inflammatory disease. See your physician immediately. Early treatment with antibiotics is necessary to minimize damage to your fallopian tubes (see Pelvic Inflammatory Disease, page 1187, and Toxic Shock Syndrome, page 1145).

Breast Self-Examination

Unlike your internal organs, you have access to your breasts. You can see them, feel them, and notice change. The female breasts are often the site of various disorders, ranging from annoying to fatal (see Problems of the Breast, page 1157). Thus, the importance of monthly self-examination cannot be emphasized enough.

Until puberty, the female breasts are basically the same as the breasts of a boy. At some point, usually between the ages of 9 and 13, female hormones are released in response to the hypothalamus, pituitary, ovaries, and adrenal glands, in increasing amounts, the result of which is increased female hormone concentration and the beginning of breast development. Often, this is the first concrete sign that a girl is approaching puberty.

A woman's breast is made up of as many as 20 groups of milk-producing glands housed in fatty tissue. Each gland group contains a milk duct that runs to the nipple. Surrounding the nipple is a dark area (areola).

In young adulthood, a woman's breasts are firm and dense. Self-examination (see page 1160) helps you become familiar with your breasts and develop a routine that you will practice the rest of your life.

Examine your breasts monthly, 1 week after the start of your period. After menopause, any day will do as long as it's the same day each month. This enables you to become acquainted with the topography of each breast so that you will be able to detect any change, lump, bump, or thickening.

Remember, the sooner breast cancer is discovered, the better your chance of cure. Ninety percent of breast masses are found by women, either accidentally or during self-examination (see Breast Self-Examination, page 1160). The vast majority of breast lumps are noncancerous (benign).

Mammography

Mammography is an X-ray study of the breasts that can detect tumors long before they are large enough to be felt. There is debate over who should have mammography. In general, women older than 50 years who have no symptoms should have it annually. For women thought to be at high risk of developing breast cancer (those with prior breast cancer or whose mother or sister had the disease), annual mammography is recommended after age 40 years. If you are between the ages of 40 and 50 years and have no family history of breast cancer, have mammography every 2 years (see Mammograms, page 1165).

Sexual Function and Dysfunction

When a woman is sexually aroused, the glands in the vagina secrete a lubricant to facilitate entry of the penis. For this to take place, your vaginal tissues must be functioning properly and there must be adequate sexual stimuli.

The next stage of sexual response is known as orgasm. This is a series of involuntary contractions of the muscles of the pelvis and is controlled by a specific part of your nervous system. For orgasm to occur, the clitoris generally must be stimulated, either directly or indirectly.

Sexual dysfunction can occur at any point during intercourse. If you find sexual intercourse either painful or uncomfortable, if you do not become sexually aroused even when your partner is patient and loving, or if you cannot achieve orgasm, you may have a sexual dysfunction (see also Health Issues of Partners, page 1213).

Sexual dysfunction is not uncommon among either sex. Do not feel embarrassed or ashamed to seek professional help.

The cause of a woman's inability to respond sexually may be organic—that is, there is a physical reason for the dysfunction. For example, diseases such as diabetes and multiple sclerosis cause nerve damage, which may prevent you from becoming sexually aroused. Similarly, pelvic infections or endometriosis (see pages 1185 and 1187) can make intercourse painful. Lack of a sexual response can occur after a disease or as a result of medications.

The more common cause of sexual dysfunction, however, is psychological. Traumatic events such as rape or incest, the perception that sex is "dirty" and not to be enjoyed, guilt over sexual enjoyment or inner conflict over sexuality, fear, anxiety, shame, a poor self-image after a hysterectomy or mastectomy, depression, and chronic fatigue all can cause sexual problems. A selfish and unresponsive partner, a faltering marriage, or other stressful situations may also affect your sexual response.

Often the cause for a lack of sexual response is unknown. If you are concerned about being sexually unresponsive, seek help. If you are in a loving relationship with a caring partner who takes the time to stimulate the sensitive areas of your body before intercourse and you still cannot respond, you may want to explore emotional or psychological factors. Often a combination of psychotherapy with a psychiatrist or psychologist and sex therapy can alleviate the problem (see Desire Disorders in Women, page 1222).

The following are the types of sexual dysfunction that can occur in women.

Painful Intercourse

Painful intercourse (dyspareunia) can be due to psychological or physical causes (see Vaginal Pain, page 1175). The causes of painful intercourse described below are treatable. When the medical problem is eliminated, so is the pain during intercourse (see Sensation Disorders in Women, page 1222).

Vaginismus

A rare cause of painful intercourse is vaginismus. If you have vaginismus, the natural lubrication of your vagina is not activated when you are sexually aroused. At the same time, the muscles surrounding the entrance to the vagina contract, making intercourse difficult if not impossible.

The cause of vaginismus may be psychological, perhaps as a response to a traumatic sexual experience. If you have vaginismus, consult a physician or therapist trained in treating sexual disorders.

Treatment often combines counseling with progressive vaginal enlargement (dilation). Your physician or therapist will prescribe several tubes or dilators of various sizes. You begin by inserting the smallest tube into your vagina. Once you can tolerate that one without pain, you insert the next size, and so on until you can insert a penis-size dilator without pain.

Infection

Infections of the vagina and vulva can make intercourse painful. Genital herpes, cysts, rashes, or allergic reactions make the vulva extremely tender and unable to tolerate the friction during intercourse. A bladder infection (cystitis) or an infection in your urethra (urethritis) also can make intercourse uncomfortable (see page 842).

Disease

Diseases of the reproductive organs such as pelvic inflammatory disease (see page 1187) or endometriosis (see page 1185) can make intercourse painful, especially when your partner thrusts deeply. Occasionally, you may notice blood after intercourse (postcoital bleeding). This can result from a lack of lubrication in your vagina. See your physician to eliminate other causes.

Failure to Reach Orgasm

Failure to reach orgasm differs from a lack of sexual responsiveness in that a woman remains sexually responsive. The vagina is lubricated and ready for intercourse, and lovemaking is enjoyable.

Sometimes a woman's failure to achieve orgasm can be resolved by a frank discussion with her partner. More foreplay, a change in position during intercourse, or direct physical stimulation of the clitoris may help.

Occasionally, however, the problem requires therapy. Your physician may suggest sexual exercises that can be done at home with your partner. These, together with psychotherapy, can be beneficial (see Orgasm Disorders in Women, page 1223).

Prevention of Pregnancy

A healthy woman who becomes sexually active in her teens and uses no birth control whatsoever may have 30 to 35 years of reproductive life. Today, thanks to several effective contraceptive methods, women can choose whether they want to become mothers and, if so, when. Popular birth control methods that depend primarily on the woman are described on pages 171 through 174.

Natural Family Planning

Natural family planning encompasses several methods that rely on a woman's menstrual cycle to determine what days are safe for intercourse. They are variations of the so-called rhythm method.

Each of the approaches in natural family planning involves a conscientious awareness of when you can become pregnant, which is but a brief span approximately in the middle of each menstrual cycle—from about 72 hours before ovulation to about 24 hours after ovulation. The key is to determine when these days are and then to avoid having intercourse during that time.

Overall, these methods are less than 80 percent effective for preventing pregnancy. Predicting ovulation is difficult because a woman's cycle may vary. If you decide to try natural family planning, keep records for several months to establish a pattern for your cycle. There are four ways to calculate the time of ovulation: the temperature method, the calendar method, the mucus inspection method, and the mucothermal method.

The temperature method involves determining when you have ovulated. Most women have a slight rise in basal body temperature just after ovulation. To detect a temperature change, take your temperature every day when you wake up. You'll need to use a basal thermometer to detect these small changes. Basal thermometers are available in most pharmacies. Once you have determined your time of ovulation, refrain from intercourse for 3 days before ovulation and 3 days after to avoid pregnancy.

For the calendar method, you need to keep a record of your cycle for a year. Subtract 18 days from the number of days in the shortest cycle (14 days from ovulation to the first day of your period, and 4 days for the average life of sperm) and 10 days from the longest cycle (14 days from ovulation to the first day of your period, minus 1 day for the lifespan of an egg, and minus 3 days for a margin of error). The numbers you calculate are the first and last days of your cycle during which you can become pregnant.

For example, if your shortest cycle is 24 days and the longest is 35 days, then the time during which you can become pregnant is between 24 days minus 18 days (or the 6th day) and 35 days minus 10 days (or the 25th day). Thus, in this example, during the 6th through the 25th days of each cycle you could become pregnant.

The cervical mucus inspection method depends on the fact that about 4 days before the release of an egg, your vaginal mucus becomes thin, clear, runnier, and profuse. To prevent pregnancy, avoid intercourse from the time the mucus appears until 4 days after it becomes thicker and drier.

The mucothermal method is a combination of the temperature method and mucus inspection. It is the most reliable natural method.

Birth Control Pills

Birth control pills are used by one out of every four American women younger than 45 years. The pill is the most effective method of contraception. If used correctly, only 1 out of 1,000 women on the pill should become pregnant per year.

The most commonly prescribed pill, and the most effective, is a combination of synthetic estrogen and progestin; its actions are the same as the two naturally occurring hormones produced by the body. Some women take the so-called mini-pill, which contains only progestin. Although less effective than the combination pill, it is believed to be marginally safer for women older than 35 years and for those with problems such as hypertension and diabetes.

Birth control pills work by preventing the hypothalamus (a structure in the brain) from instructing the pituitary gland to mobilize follicle-stimulating hormone and luteinizing hormone. If these hormones are suppressed, you simply do not release an egg.

Moreover, the pill also prevents the cervical mucus from becoming watery, as it normally does during ovulation. Instead, the mucus for the entire cycle is scant, making it difficult for sperm to reach the fallopian tubes.

The pill does not suppress menstruation, but the flow is generally not as heavy and does not last for as many days as normal menstruation. (In some women, the flow may be so light they wonder whether they are even having a period.) Most women on the pill do not experience cramps before and during the menses.

If you want to begin taking the pill, you will need a prescription and instructions from your physician. Get in the habit of taking your pill at the same time every day to keep the dosage constant and to lessen the chance that you will forget to take your pill. A common method is to begin taking the pill on the Sunday after the start of your period.

You continue to take a pill for 21 days, after which you do not take one for 7 days. About 3 days after you take the last pill, your period will start. (Note, however, that some prescriptions come in packages with 21 pills that contain hormones and 7 pills that have no active ingredient; thus, the daily pattern of taking a pill is not interrupted. You simply finish one package and start another the following day.)

Sometimes a woman will not have a period. If this happens to you, simply begin your new pills 1 week after you finish the previous pack. If you miss a second period, consult your physician.

Even though birth control pills are effective and easy to use, they have some side effects, most of which are minor. Weight gain, nausea, vomiting, and a sense of tenderness or fullness in the breasts and pelvis may occur. Some women also have spotting or breakthrough bleeding.

The most serious side effect is a tendency to develop blood clots in the veins, which can be fatal if they dislodge and travel to the lungs. The incidence of blood clots is slightly higher in women who take the pill than in those who do not. Those who take pills high in estrogen seem to be at the most risk.

In addition, a small percentage of women who take the pill develop significantly high blood pressure. Strokes and heart attacks that are due to the pill are rare, as are gallbladder problems.

Smoking increases the risk of many of these side effects, especially for women older than 35 years.

The pill does not seem to increase the incidence of cancer in the reproductive organs. In fact, there is good evidence that oral contraceptives may decrease the risk of ovarian and endometrial cancer. In addition, the pill is beneficial for reducing the risk of ovarian and breast cysts, the anemia that results from excessive menstrual flow, and the incidence of rheumatoid arthritis and pelvic infections.

How do you know whether the pill is safe for you? It probably is safe if you are younger than 40 and a nonsmoker. If you smoke, you probably should not use the pill after age 35 years. If you are older than 40 and otherwise healthy and on a "low-dose" estrogen pill, your physician may elect to continue this form of birth control. Women who have had certain forms of blood vessel disease, heart problems, or some types of cancer should find another method of birth control. If you have migraine headaches, hypertension, sickle cell anemia, or diabetes, or if you are about to undergo an operation, the pill may increase your risk of complications. You and your physician must weigh the risks. In general, the risks of the pill are significantly less than the risks of pregnancy itself.

Intrauterine Devices

Intrauterine devices (IUDs) are 95 to 98 percent effective for preventing pregnancy.

The IUD is a small piece of plastic inserted into your uterus by your physician, usually during your menstrual period when the cervix is more open. The device has a small string hanging from it. The string makes it easy for the physician to remove the device. Also, the wearer can use the string to make sure the IUD is in place.

The IUD prevents pregnancy by creating changes in the lining of the uterus that make it difficult for a fertilized egg to implant and grow.

The most common side effects of an IUD are increased bleeding during your period and increased menstrual pain. Sometimes the device can be expelled during a menstrual period, so it is important that you periodically check the string to make sure the device is still in place.

The most serious side effects are pelvic infection and ectopic or tubal pregnancy (see page 199). Severe pelvic infection can render a woman sterile, but this result is rare.

Barrier Methods

Barrier methods of contraception block the sperm from access to the egg. There are both physical barriers, such as the diaphragm, vaginal sponge, and cervical cap, and chemical barriers (spermicides), in the form of creams, gels, foams, and suppositories. The 80- to 90-percent effectiveness of these methods is enhanced when a physical barrier is used with a spermicide.

Diaphragm

The diaphragm is the most effective barrier method for women and has a high success rate of 98.5 percent when used consistently and correctly. The diaphragm always should be used in conjunction with a spermicide.

Developed more than 100 years ago, the diaphragm is a rubber cap that is inserted into the vagina to cover the cervix. If you want to use a diaphragm, you must see your physician to be fitted for one. Proper fit is essential because the diaphragm must cover the entire cervical opening to be effective. If you gain or lose a large amount of weight or deliver a baby, you may require a diaphragm of a different size.

Before intercourse, insert your diaphragm with about a teaspoon of spermicidal cream or jelly, spread around the edge and in the center of the device. After intercourse, wait at least 6 hours to remove the diaphragm. If you have intercourse again within the 6 hours, you must apply more spermicide without removing the diaphragm.

Clean your diaphragm with soap and water. Periodically check for holes or thinning; if either occurs, you need a new diaphragm.

There are no side effects unless you are allergic to spermicide. The most common complaint is that having to interrupt sex to insert a diaphragm interferes with enjoyment.

Vaginal Sponge

Unlike the diaphragm, the vaginal sponge is available without a prescription and does not require a special fitting. It is less effective than the diaphragm, however.

The sponge is inserted deep into the vagina, much like the diaphragm. The significant difference is that the sponge contains spermicide that is released continually for 24 hours. During that time, you can have repeated intercourse without worrying about adding more spermicide. After intercourse, the sponge must remain in the vagina for 6 hours before removal.

Cervical Cap

The cervical cap, a plastic cap designed to fit snugly over the cervix, is similar to the diaphragm in that it must be fitted by a physician. Unlike the diaphragm, however, the cap is difficult for many women to insert because it needs to be placed deeply within the vagina. Thus, the tendency is to leave the cap in for extended periods. Many physicians, however, recommend against this because it can become a breeding ground for toxin-producing bacteria.

The cervical cap is about 85 percent effective for preventing pregnancy, a rate far below that with the diaphragm.

Female Condom

This new form of condom, worn by the woman, comes in several forms. Many are made of thicker latex than typical male condoms. All extend to the outside of the vagina,

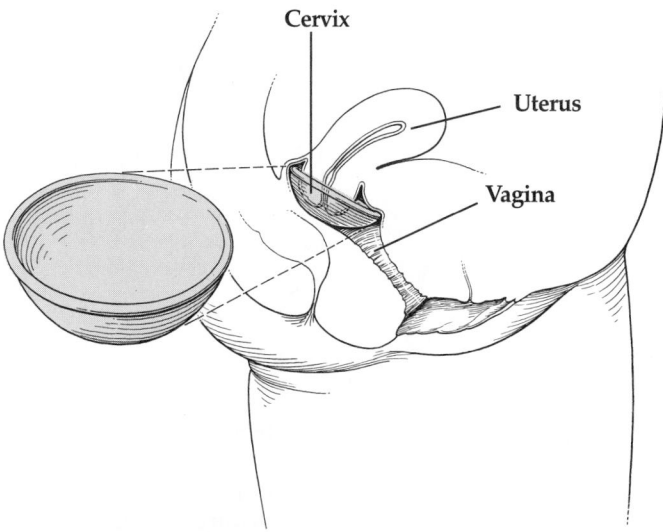

and several have a diaphragm-like end that fits on the cervix. Insertion methods vary. Breakage rate is generally less than half that of male condoms.

Contraceptive Implants

These are similar to progestin-only birth control pills in that they contain hormones that impair fertilization and prevent ovulation. Your physician can implant these small, match-sized hormone sticks under the skin of your upper arm. They will last for 5 years, and there's no need to remember to do anything.

Contraceptive implants may have the same side effects as oral contraceptives, except that they also may cause some irregularity in your menstrual cycle or spotting, and they may adversely affect glucose control if you have diabetes. This method is somewhat expensive initially. Fewer than 5 percent of women who use the implants will become pregnant.

If you opt for implants, be careful to select a physician well trained and experienced in placing and removing implants.

Birth Control Shots

Similar to contraceptive implants, birth control shots contain progestin. You will need to have a birth control shot in the arm or buttock every 2 to 3 months to maintain protection. This method is safe immediately after childbirth and while you are breastfeeding. You may experience irregular monthly periods and spotting, but chances are good you will stop having periods entirely after 6 months. When you stop getting the shots, return to fertility may be delayed.

This method is highly effective in pre-

The contraceptive device known as a diaphragm is a rubber cap that is inserted into the vagina to cover the cervix, which is the opening to the uterus.

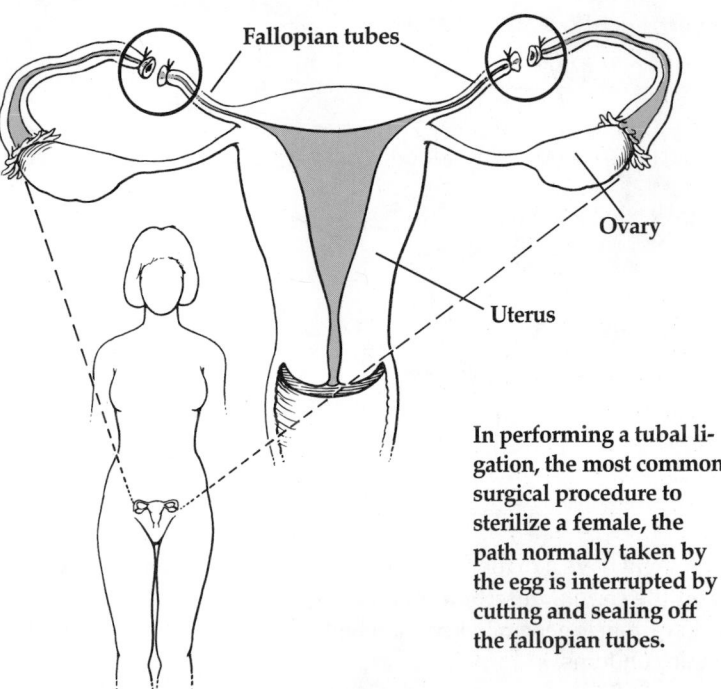

Fallopian tubes

Ovary

Uterus

In performing a tubal ligation, the most common surgical procedure to sterilize a female, the path normally taken by the egg is interrupted by cutting and sealing off the fallopian tubes.

venting pregnancy. There is a slightly higher rate of pregnancy among women who weigh more than 160 pounds. If you exceed this weight, your physician may need to adjust the amount of medication you receive.

Tubal Ligation

Tubal ligation—female sterilization—is accomplished by interrupting the fallopian tubes so that the egg cannot travel down the tubes and the sperm cannot move upward. Hence, contact between egg and sperm is avoided. Tubal ligation is the most common method of female sterilization.

Hysterectomy—the removal of the uterus—should not be done for the sole purpose of sterilization. It is too risky to justify doing unless there are medical conditions that warrant it (see page 1184).

Many women opt to be sterilized immediately or shortly after giving birth. This is

a good time for a tubal ligation because the abdominal wall is relaxed and the top of the uterus is near the navel, the entry point of operation. Minimal anesthesia is usually all that is necessary, and the procedure does not alter the duration of the postpartum hospital stay. When the abdomen is open for a cesarean birth, a tubal ligation can be performed in a matter of minutes.

If you are pregnant and considering sterilization, discuss the options with your physician. Some physicians perform the tubal ligation immediately after childbirth, but most prefer to wait at least 12 hours. There are two reasons. First, the likelihood of a postpartum hemorrhage is reduced greatly after this period. Second, if your infant has a life-threatening condition that could jeopardize survival—and that could change your mind about sterilization—it probably has been detected by this time.

Tubal ligation can be done in a hospital or an outpatient clinic, with a general anesthetic (which means you will be asleep) or a local anesthetic injected into the operative site. If you choose to have a local anesthetic, you will be given medications to relax you, but you will remain awake.

A common method in the woman who recently has had a vaginal delivery is to make a small incision below the navel. The tubes are found easily. A "knuckle "of tube is raised and the base is tied and cut off, and the two separated ends are tied.

Generally, this technique is effective for preventing pregnancy. One in 350 women who have it soon after childbirth eventually will become pregnant. For some unknown reason, the failure rate is slightly higher when the procedure is done immediately after a cesarean section.

Another method of sterilization uses a laparoscope. This is a thin instrument that is inserted through a small incision below the navel after the abdomen has been inflated with gas. The instrument has a viewing scope through which the physician can see the reproductive organs. Using operating instruments through either the same incision or a second one, the physician locates the tubes and either cauterizes them or attaches plastic clips or rings to them.

As with any operation, tubal ligation is not without risk. About 1 in 1,000 women will have a problem from the procedure. Complications include reactions to the anesthetic, pelvic infection, accidental injury to blood ves-

Reversing a Tubal Ligation

Some women who have been sterilized later decide they want to become pregnant. An operation to reverse the tubal ligation can be done. Following the operation, 60 to 80 percent of women eventually conceive. However, the risk of an ectopic (tubal) pregnancy is increased (see page 199). For these reasons, physicians stress that before you undergo sterilization be very sure that you do not want to become pregnant.

sels in the abdomen, bowel injuries, and burns (when the tubes are cauterized). Most women, however, have no major complications.

After a tubal ligation, you may be given pain medication for your sore abdomen. Dizziness, fatigue, nausea, and bloating are not uncommon. Within 8 hours, most women can walk around, eat a regular diet, and care for their infants. Most women go home either the same day or the next day and resume their normal schedules within a few days.

Preparation for Pregnancy

Before attempting to become pregnant, see your physician for a thorough physical examination. This is important because many conditions that are initially without symptoms can complicate pregnancy. Diabetes, high blood pressure, pelvic tumors, and anemia are just a few common conditions that can be detected easily during a comprehensive general examination.

If your physician discovers a health problem, in most cases it does not mean you cannot have a child. But you will want to have the disease under control before attempting pregnancy. Some pregnant women with chronic diseases such as diabetes may be best cared for by an obstetrician who specializes in high-risk pregnancies.

A particular disease or genetic abnormality may run in your family. Or you may be older than 35 years, considering a first pregnancy, and worried about the possibility of having a child with Down syndrome or another birth defect. This is a good time to inquire about genetic counseling. A frank discussion with an expert can provide helpful information about your chances of having a healthy baby (see page 42).

If you have been pregnant before and had a problem such as miscarriage, preterm birth, or abnormal fetal development, then a discussion of possible recurrence, consultation with an obstetrician, and possible therapy are in order. Women who are at high risk (prior history) for having a baby with a neural tube defect should take folic acid from at least 1 month preconception through the first 3 months of pregnancy. For women at low risk, some physicians recommend folic acid in a lower dose.

Once your physician determines you are healthy, you may want to examine your lifestyle before giving up contraception. If you are overweight and want to reduce, do it before you become pregnant. Pregnancy is not the time to begin a diet.

Moreover, if you are a cigarette smoker, quit smoking (for help, see page 321). Women who smoke during pregnancy tend to have babies of lower birth weight than nonsmokers, and these babies may have developmental problems. In addition, smokers have a higher incidence of miscarriages and stillbirths.

If you take medications, prescription or over-the-counter, check with your physician about whether or not to continue using them before you try to become pregnant. He or she will know whether the medication could be harmful and if there is a safer drug that can be substituted.

Don't use alcohol during pregnancy.

If you are unable to become pregnant after 1 year of sexual intercourse without using any contraception, you, your partner, or both of you may have a fertility problem (see Infertility, page 1215).

Concerns During Pregnancy

Pregnancy is a natural condition; most women come through pregnancy and birth uneventfully. Occasionally, however, there are complications.

This section discusses many of these problems. Some are concerns such as morning sickness, heartburn, and backache that make you uncomfortable but generally do not threaten your or your developing baby's health. Problems such as diabetes and hemorrhage are more serious and can have dire consequences for mother or child.

Also covered in this section are ways in which you can help ensure that you and your baby are healthy during pregnancy, the most important being regular visits to your physician, a proper diet, and the elimination of potentially harmful substances such as cigarettes, alcohol, and drugs.

Today, most obstetricians or family physicians who deliver babies will think something is wrong if you do not ask questions—lots of them. You and your partner are expected to be active participants in your pregnancy and the birth of your baby.

Fertilization

The process of fertilization begins with the penetration of the female egg by a single male sperm, one of the hundreds of millions that traveled up the female reproductive system.

It is not completely understood how the minute sperm penetrates the firm capsule (zona pellucida) of the egg. Swimming in an indirect path, the sperm attacks the egg with the side of its head. Several sperm may begin to enter the outer egg capsule, but ultimately only one will enter the egg itself. Approximately 266 days later, a baby will be born.

The egg and the sperm each bring to the union 23 chromosomes containing thousands of genes. This produces a new individual with 46 chromosomes, the correct number for a human being. It is this genetic material that determines sex, physical characteristics such as eye, hair, and skin color, body size and type, facial features, creativity, and, to a large extent, intellectual capabilities and even personality. After the sperm penetrates to the center of the egg, sperm and egg merge to become a one-cell embryo (zygote), and fertilization is complete.

Multiple births result either from the fertilization of two or more eggs or from a single egg being fertilized and then splitting to form two or more embryos.

The next step in the process is cell division. Within 12 hours, the new cell has divided into two cells, each of which then becomes two cells, and so on, with the number of cells doubling every 12 hours.

The new egg continues to make its way slowly down the fallopian tube to the uterus, regularly doubling its cell number and becoming not larger but more complex. Within 4 to 5 days after fertilization, the egg, by this time made up of 500 cells, reaches its destination inside the uterus.

By the time the egg reaches the uterus, it has changed considerably from a solid mass of cells to a group of cells arranged around a fluid-filled cavity. This is called a blastocyst. One section of the blastocyst contains a compact mass of cells that will ultimately produce an embryo. The outer layer of cells, called the trophoblast, will produce the placenta, which provides nourishment.

While all this has been taking place, the rest of the female reproductive system has not been idle. The ovaries have been secreting the hormone progesterone into the bloodstream. The result of this hormonal surge is a uterine lining that is swollen with blood, the perfect environment for implantation to take place.

Initially the egg does not dig deeply into the uterus. It clings to the surface of the uterus for a few days. Then the egg releases an enzyme that eats away at the lining of the uterus, allowing the egg to drop deeper into the lining, where it is surrounded by a pool of the mother's blood. Eight days have passed since fertilization took place. By the 12th day, the egg will be firmly embedded in its new home.

At this point, you are pregnant, although it is too early for you to have missed a period or to have any other symptoms of pregnancy. In the initial days and weeks after fertilization, miscarriage is common, often before a woman knows she was pregnant. In fact, an estimated 50 percent of fertilizations end in miscarriage.

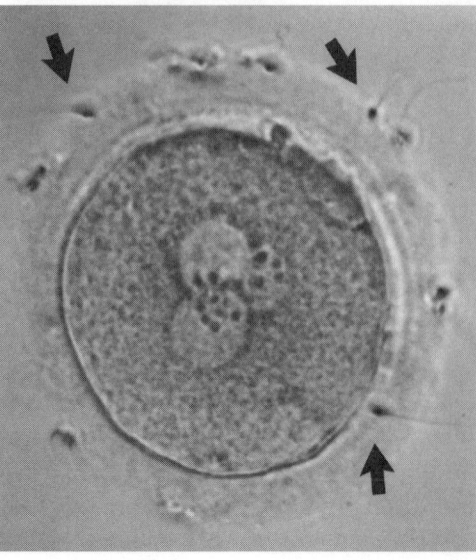

Recently fertilized ovum in early stages of cell division. Arrows point to sperm that entered the capsule but did not penetrate the egg.

Prenatal Development

The average time from fertilization to the birth of a baby is 266 days. Compared with the duration of gestation in most other species, that might seem an incredibly long time. When you consider the magnitude of this creation, it is a wonder it does not take longer.

It is difficult to comprehend how something as complex as a human being can emerge from a single cell. What is equally perplexing is the seemingly effortless development of this microscopic speck. Every aspect of this process, from the creation of the smallest fingernail to the brain itself, is set into an exquisitely scripted timetable that rarely falters. If it does, the result can be a miscarriage or a birth defect.

The following is an overview of the development process during the three trimesters of pregnancy. The two methods used to measure the duration of pregnancy are gestational age and fertilization age.

Gestational age is measured from the first day of your last menstrual period, which is about 2 weeks before actual fertilization. Thus, a pregnancy calculated by this method is about 280 days (9.3 months).

Fertilization age is measured from the time of fertilization. Thus, the duration of pregnancy calculated with this method is 2 weeks shorter than with the other method.

Usually, obstetricians or family physicians calculate the duration of your pregnancy on the basis of gestational age, so this section will also.

First Trimester

The first 3 months of fetal development are in many ways the most important. During this time, all the major organs in the body are formed. By the end of this period your baby is not more than 3 inches long and weighs little more than 1 ounce.

The time from fertilization of the sperm and egg to implantation in the uterus is about 5 to 7 days. After burrowing deep within the uterus, the egg begins to grow, doubling in size every day. By now, the placenta has begun to form. In another week, the rudiments of a spinal cord are evident and, within days, five to eight vertebrae are in place. In addition, the eyes and heart have begun to form.

It is during the third week after fertilization that the embryonic period begins. Before this, the products of conception are referred to as an ovum. This is about the time that an expected period does not happen. If you have a pregnancy test, the results probably will be positive.

Over the next few weeks the components of a human being develop, although at first the human baby is similar in appearance to the developing babies of some other mammals. The head begins to form, as does the intestinal tract.

At the end of the sixth week the brain becomes more noticeable, and arm and leg buds begin to appear. Cells that will later become either an ovary or a testicle have appeared.

By the seventh week, the chest and abdomen are fully formed and the lungs are beginning to develop. The embryo measures slightly more than one-half inch and weighs a fraction of an ounce.

Your baby's face and features are forming in the eighth gestational week. Fingers and toes are beginning to develop, as are the ovaries or testicles. If the embryo is a male, his penis begins to appear at this time.

At the end of the second month of pregnancy, your baby looks like a human infant, albeit in miniature.

By the tenth week, your baby's face, with the exception of the jaws, is well developed. The heart has four chambers and beats at 120 to 160 beats per minute. At this point, the embryo is considered a fetus.

By the end of the first trimester, the fetus has a head that is disproportionately large compared with the rest of its body.

Second Trimester

During the second trimester the fetus grows and the organs that formed during the previous weeks mature.

At 13½ weeks the fetus has tiny fingernails. The genitals are fully formed, and the sex can be determined with certain prenatal tests (see page 179). The fetus can kick and move its toes. The mouth can open and close, and the fetus is capable of bending its arms and of making a fist.

By the end of the fourth month, the heartbeat can be detected with a stethoscope (other specialized instruments can detect a heartbeat much earlier). You are also likely to feel the first signs of life in your abdomen. The fetus's skin at this point is slightly pink and less transparent than it was previously. Fine hair covers the entire body. The first eyelashes and eyebrows begin to appear.

One month later, the fetus may have hair on its head. Fat deposits begin to appear beneath the wrinkly skin. The fetus is now 12 inches long and weighs about 1 pound. If it is born at this time, it will attempt to breathe but probably will not be able to survive.

Third Trimester

The fetus takes on most of its weight during its last 13 weeks of development. At the beginning of this last phase of development, the fetus weighs slightly more than a pound. The average baby is born 3 months later weighing 7½ pounds.

When you are 28 weeks pregnant, your baby is covered with a thick white protective coating called vernix. The infant's eyes are open, and a baby born at this time can cry weakly and move its limbs. Although an infant at this stage weighs only 2 pounds and may experience significant medical problems, two out of three babies born at this stage survive because of recent advances in the care of premature and ill newborns.

One month later the male infant's testicles descend into the scrotum. The infant now weighs 3 pounds 12 ounces. The vast majority of these infants are also capable of surviving with proper care.

The infant born at term, 40 weeks after the mother's last menstrual period, has a more rounded body and is less wrinkly than babies born earlier. The skin may or may not still be covered with vernix. Most of the body hair is gone, although the shoulders and arms may still have a light covering. The fingernails and toenails may extend beyond the fingers and toes.

Prenatal Care

One of the most important things you can do for yourself—and your baby—is to seek prenatal care as soon as you suspect you may be pregnant.

By the time many women call for an appointment with an obstetrician or other physician who provides prenatal care, they already know they are pregnant. They have all the symptoms, and a pregnancy test that they performed at home was positive for pregnancy (see Pregnancy Tests, page 198). If your pregnancy has not been confirmed by a test, you can have one done at your physician's office.

Most physicians advise that as soon as you have missed a period, especially when you are trying to conceive, seek prenatal care. At the very latest, wait no longer than two missed periods.

During your first visit, you may be asked to fill out a detailed health form. Your physician will also ask you questions about your family history and overall health to determine whether there are any preexisting conditions that may cause problems or that call for special measures during the pregnancy.

It is important to determine when you conceived, so the physician will ask you about your menstrual history to try to pinpoint when the baby will be born. This is only an approximation, however. Most babies are not born on the precise date they are expected. It is perfectly normal for a baby to be born anywhere from 2 weeks before to 2 weeks after the due date.

After taking your medical history, your physician will perform a physical examination and a pelvic examination (see Pelvic Examination, page 1141). Typically, after this

---

Bleeding During Pregnancy

Bleeding from the vagina during pregnancy often is an indication that something is wrong. Notify your physician immediately.

In the first 20 weeks of pregnancy, bleeding may be associated with miscarriage (see page 197), ectopic pregnancy (see page 199), or other conditions such as a cervical lesion. Bleeding during a miscarriage may be slight or heavy. There may be no warning, or you may first notice some brownish discharge.

During the first days of pregnancy when the egg is implanting itself within the uterus, you may have some spotting. Moreover, approximately 20 percent of all pregnant women have some bleeding in early pregnancy that does not result in miscarriage. So do not necessarily assume the worst, but do check with your physician.

After the 20th week of pregnancy, bleeding is called antepartum bleeding. This is much less common than early pregnancy bleeding, affecting less than 2 percent of all women. There are many causes of antepartum bleeding, including placenta previa (see page 205), the onset of premature labor (see page 201), miscarriage (see page 205).

Most often the bleeding is mild. However, a severe hemorrhage can endanger your life and your baby's. If you begin bleeding after the first months of pregnancy, see your physician immediately. You may require hospitalization and tests such as ultrasonography (see Prenatal Tests, page 179) to determine the cause of your bleeding. If the hemorrhage is severe, blood transfusions may be necessary. Sometimes labor is induced or a cesarean section is performed.

first visit a pelvic examination usually is not done again until the last weeks of pregnancy, and then it is done to determine whether labor is imminent. Blood and urine tests are done during the first visit.

The visit usually concludes with the physician discussing pregnancy with you, advising you on nutrition, weight gain, and exercise, and alerting you to potential complications such as vaginal bleeding.

Most physicians see their pregnant patients every 4 to 6 weeks for the first 7 months, once or twice during the eighth month, and then weekly.

After the initial visit, your regular visits usually begin with your weight and blood pressure being determined, and you also will be asked to submit a urine sample for testing. Your physician also will want to know whether you are having any problems such as headache, altered vision, abdominal pain, nausea, vomiting, swelling of the legs or feet, or vaginal bleeding. Write down any questions that have occurred to you during the past month so that you remember to ask your physician.

After about 10 to 12 weeks' gestation, an exciting part of the visit is listening to your baby's heartbeat, which can be detected with a Doppler instrument (see Office Doppler, this page).

Your physician will also feel your abdomen to determine whether the baby is growing properly. Sometimes there is a discrepancy between when you thought conception occurred and the size of the fetus. When fetal age is in question, your physician may request that an ultrasound examination (see Ultrasound, page 180) be done to determine whether the fetus is indeed older than believed.

Prenatal Tests

Recent years have seen a virtual revolution in the field of obstetrics. Today, physicians have better technology to examine your baby in the womb. Tests to determine if the fetus has any congenital defect are becoming increasingly common, particularly for women older than 35 years, an age at which genetic abnormalities are more likely. A few years ago, these women had to wait 9 months to know whether their child had an abnormality. Now, women 35 years or older, as well as those with a family history of certain abnormalities, can know earlier in the pregnancy

---

Intrauterine Growth Retardation

An infant who is born extremely small for its gestational age, usually below the 10th percentile, is considered to be growth retarded. Intrauterine growth retardation occurs when the fetus does not get adequate nourishment from the mother via the placenta.

An infant born growth retarded does not have the amount of body fat that a normal-size newborn does. Thus, the infant has difficulty maintaining a normal body temperature and blood sugar level. Moreover, many growth-retarded infants grow slowly throughout at least early childhood. There also may be some delayed intellectual development.

Many conditions and lifestyle characteristics can produce intrauterine growth retardation. A woman who smokes, uses illegal drugs, or drinks large amounts of alcohol is more likely to produce a small infant. A mother who is malnourished or fails to gain adequate weight also is in danger of giving birth to a small infant. Certain chronic diseases also place you at risk.

Conditions related to pregnancy can cause growth retardation. These include abnormalities of the placenta and cord, fetal infections or malformations, and the presence of more than one fetus.

If your physician suspects intrauterine growth retardation, he or she probably will ask you to have an ultrasound examination. When the fetus is not growing at a proper rate because you are smoking, drinking, using drugs, or not eating properly, sometimes a change to a healthier lifestyle can help. Often, however, labor must be induced or a cesarean section performed. If the fetus is still far from term, the risk of such early delivery must be weighed against the risk of leaving it in the womb and allowing further malnutrition.

---

whether the fetus they are carrying has a birth defect. Today, any woman can find out her baby's sex before he or she is born.

In addition, physicians can determine other medical problems. Life in the uterus is not without risk. Sometimes, for various reasons, there is cause to suspect that your baby may be in danger. Perhaps a previously active baby suddenly ceases to move, or blood tests reveal that an Rh-negative mother is developing antibodies against her Rh-positive fetus. Whatever the reason, if your physician suspects something is wrong, several techniques can be used to evaluate fetal health, the goal being to find any sign of distress before irreparable damage has been done.

Office Doppler

The "Doppler" ultrasound can be used to detect the action of the fetal heart. This device can detect a heartbeat and confirm a viable pregnancy.

Ultrasound

The advent of ultrasound examination, also called ultrasonography (see page 1335), has made it possible to visualize the embryo as early as 6 to 7 weeks after your last menstrual period. This noninvasive and painless diagnostic tool uses high-frequency sound waves to record a picture of your baby. Safe for both mother and baby, it has proved invaluable in many cases, although some physicians believe that the ultrasound examination has become too commonplace.

In addition to its use in determining fetal age, ultrasound can show whether you are carrying more than one baby. It also allows your physician to monitor your baby's rate of growth to determine whether it is normal for gestational age or if there is any indication of intrauterine growth retardation (see Intrauterine Growth Retardation, page 179).

With ultrasound, it may be possible to tell whether the fetus has kidney disease, an intestinal obstruction, or is missing an arm or leg. The tiny fetal brain can also be examined for a few abnormalities using ultrasound.

The position of the placenta, particularly if placenta previa (see page 205) is suspected, and your baby's position in the womb can be determined using ultrasound. This diagnostic tool can also detect hydramnios (too much amniotic fluid, see page 202).

In some cases, ultrasound can also reveal the sex of your baby. An examination at 18 to 20 weeks of your pregnancy is an opportune time to obtain this information.

When there is a question about whether the fetus has died in the uterus, ultrasound examination usually can provide the answer.

Not only can problems be diagnosed in the womb but also a few can be treated. Using ultrasonography to visualize the fetus, physicians can perform surgery through the womb to alleviate problems such as urinary obstruction and hydrocephalus (the accumulation of cerebrospinal fluid in the head). This type of intervention can sometimes prevent irreparable damage.

Alpha-Fetoprotein Test

The alpha-fetoprotein analysis is a noninvasive blood test of the mother that is useful for detecting defects in the fetus's nervous system (for example, a neural tube defect) and, to a limited extent, for detecting Down syndrome. Because the test carries no risk to mother or baby, many physicians recommend that all their pregnant patients undergo the test for alpha-fetoprotein at approximately 16 weeks' gestation (see page 179).

Alpha-fetoprotein is a protein made by every fetus. Normally, a small amount crosses the placenta and can be detected in the mother's blood. When it is found in higher than normal amounts, however, the fetus may have a neurologic defect such as spina bifida (open spine, see page 53) because large amounts of alpha-fetoprotein are allowed to leak into the amniotic fluid. These defects are rare, occurring in an estimated 1 or 2 babies out of 1,000.

Your physician will draw blood from your arm for this test. If the test results are within normal limits, the chances are that your baby does not have an open neurologic defect, although a closed neural tube defect could still occur.

Approximately 50 women out of 1,000 have a positive result. If this should happen to you, do not assume the worst. This finding may mean the fetus is simply older than was thought, that you are carrying twins, or that something else increased the alpha-fetoprotein level in your blood. A second blood test is warranted.

When two blood tests are positive, an ultrasound examination usually is done. If this test fails to find a defect, amniocentesis is the next step. Of 50 women with positive test

Ultrasound examination painlessly reveals the shape of the fetus within the uterus. Fetal age can be determined by measuring the width of the skull.

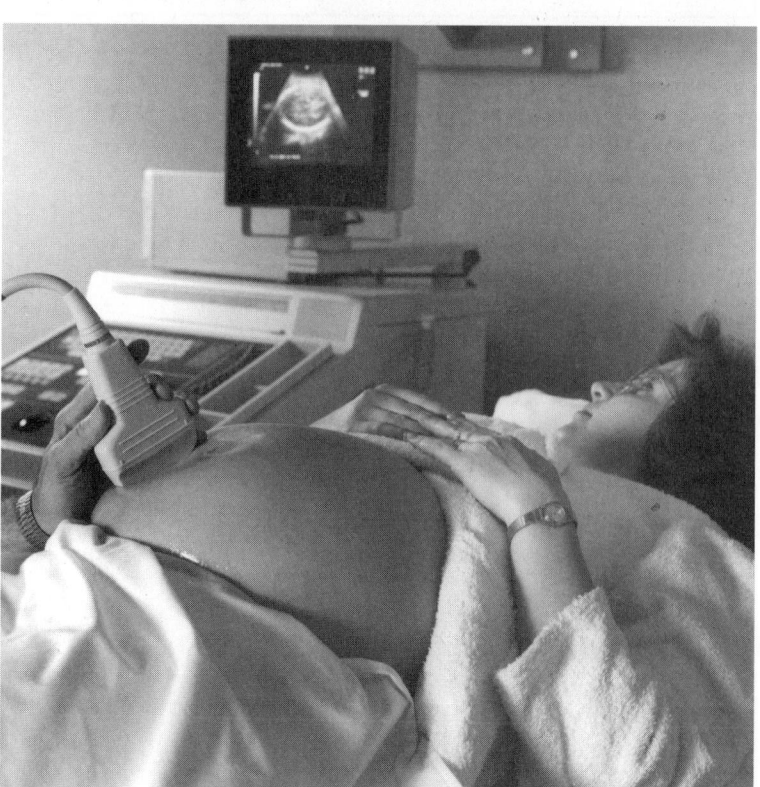

results, only 1 or 2 will be carrying a child with a defect of this kind.

Genetic Amniocentesis

Genetic amniocentesis is performed early in the second trimester of pregnancy, usually between 12 and 16 weeks' gestation. It may be recommended for women 35 or older, those who have a family history of congenital abnormalities such as Down syndrome or spina bifida, those who have previously given birth to an abnormal child, and those with an abnormal level of alpha-fetoprotein.

During amniocentesis, your abdomen is anesthetized with a local anesthetic, and the physician, guided by ultrasonography, inserts a long, thin needle through it into your uterus. This punctures the amniotic sac in which the fetus floats. A small amount of amniotic fluid is drawn into the needle, which is then removed and sent to the laboratory for tests. There is a 1 in 200 risk of losing the pregnancy as a result of the procedure.

This fluid contains valuable genetic information about your growing baby. After a few weeks in a culture medium, the cells can be studied for chromosome distribution.

The presence of Down syndrome, indicated by the presence of an extra chromosome, can be successfully diagnosed with amniocentesis. In addition, other defects such as neurologic problems, kidney diseases, and metabolic disorders may be diagnosed. Your baby's sex also can be determined, which can be helpful if there is a risk of a sex-linked disorder.

Amniocentesis also can be used later in pregnancy to monitor Rh disease (see Rhesus [Rh] Compatibility, page 192) or to ascertain whether the lungs are developed enough to withstand an early delivery.

Amniocentesis is usually safe for mother and child, but there is a slightly increased risk of miscarriage after the procedure.

Chorionic Villus Sampling

Chorionic villus sampling is similar to amniocentesis in that it is an invasive technique that can detect many genetic abnormalities, including Down syndrome. A big advantage is that it can be done between 9 and 11 weeks of gestation. Thus, if a defect is found, you have the option of terminating the pregnancy in its early stages.

During chorionic villus sampling, a small piece of the placenta supporting the embryo is removed. Using ultrasonography, the physician inserts a catheter or small tube into your cervix. A suction procedure is used to suck the tissue into the catheter. You may feel slight discomfort but little more than is normally felt during a pelvic examination.

The removed tissue contains the same chromosomes as your developing baby. After an analysis of the tissue, your physician can determine whether your child has Down syndrome or other chromosome diseases. The test also can determine sex. Chorionic villus sampling is not as effective as amniocentesis for detecting some disorders, however. Sometimes amniocentesis is used after chorionic villus sampling, especially when it becomes important to rule out one of these defects.

Like amniocentesis, chorionic villus sampling slightly increases the risk of miscarriage. Moreover, the risk of intrauterine infection is greater than that associated with amniocentesis.

Percutaneous Umbilical Cord Sampling

This technique tests fetal blood from the umbilical cord for the prenatal diagnosis of some genetic disorders. It is done most easily in the third trimester. Percutaneous umbilical cord sampling also can be used to determine oxygen and carbon dioxide levels in the blood, which may help diagnose growth retardation.

Fetal Activity

You can document fetal movement each day

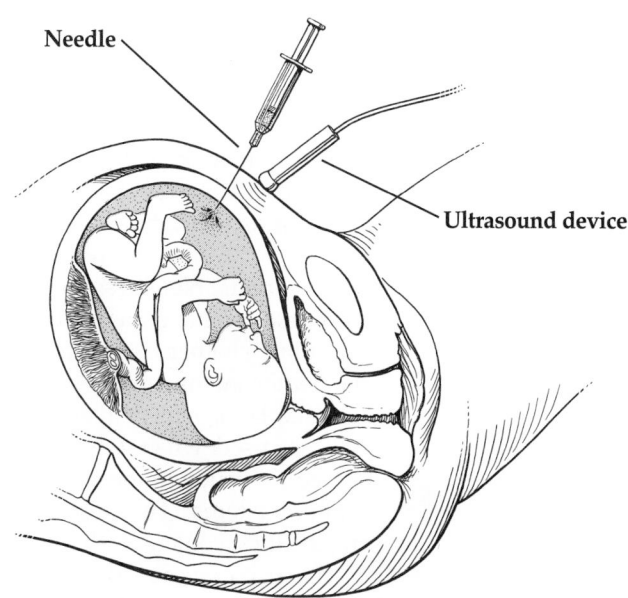

Amniocentesis involves removal of a small amount of amniotic fluid from the sac containing the fetus. Guided by an ultrasound image, your physician inserts a long, thin needle to withdraw fluid. Laboratory analysis of the fluid can reveal such things as your baby's sex, development, and overall health.

Needle

Ultrasound device

by noting at least four movements in an hour during a time of day when the fetus is usually active. Fetal activity is generally felt more often after meals or at night when there are fewer external distractions. In addition, remember that the fetus will have sleep cycles up to 1 hour throughout the day or night, during which time it will not move.

Electronic Fetal Nonstress and Stress Tests

These tests evaluate the fetal heart rate to determine whether there is a problem and whether the infant will be able to withstand a normal labor and delivery. These tests often are used when a woman notices a marked reduction in the amount of movement of the fetus. They also often are prescribed for women with symptoms of preeclampsia (see page 204), a history of stillbirth, or diabetes mellitus and for women whose babies' growth rate seems to be abnormally slow.

Nonstress Test

The first step is often the nonstress test. During this test, you lie on your back and a recording device connected to an electronic monitor is attached to your abdomen. Fetal heart rate, uterine contractions, and fetal movements are recorded.

Stress Test

Contraction stress testing is done when the results of the nonstress test are abnormal. If your physician prescribes this test, you will be given a drug that stimulates contractions. The effect of the contractions on the fetus is then monitored. This test can help your physician determine whether your infant is in fetal distress. If so, a decision to induce labor may be made if the fetus is old enough to survive. The test also can help the physician determine whether the infant is able to withstand a normal labor and vaginal delivery or whether a cesarean section should be done.

Nutrition During Pregnancy

The best time to start thinking about good nutrition is before you plan to become pregnant. Then you can be sure that your baby will have all the essential nutrients from the moment of conception. In fact, the improvements you make in your own diet now can spark a healthful change for the family.

Nutrition Risk Factors

If you have a history of good eating habits, you begin your pregnancy with optimal amounts of all nutrients needed for your baby's tremendous growth and development. However, a background that includes chronic dieting, skipping meals or fasting, or eating a limited variety of foods can put you both at nutritional risk. Other factors that put you at increased risk for poor nutrition include using cigarettes, alcohol, or street drugs; carrying more than one baby; and being significantly underweight or overweight at the time of conception.

Extremely poor eating habits before or during pregnancy can harm both you and your baby. If you eat too few calories or nutrients, cell development can be less than ideal and your baby may be underweight at birth. Low-birth-weight babies have a greater chance for short- and long-term health problems.

In the first weeks of your pregnancy, perhaps before you know you're going to have a baby, most of your fetus's major organs will be forming. That is why it is so critical to make nutritious eating habits a part of your decision to begin a new life.

Weight Gain

Pregnancy is the one time in your life when you're encouraged to gain weight. But weight gain in pregnancy doesn't mean getting fat. Your size increases for various physical reasons, including the weight of the baby you will deliver.

Over the years, the recommended amount of weight to gain during pregnancy has varied dramatically. Twenty or 30 years ago, a minimal weight gain was thought to be best for mother and baby. Now, research has proven that women who are normal weight at the time of conception have the healthiest pregnancies and babies if they gain 25 to 35 pounds.

Your caregiver will estimate the right amount of weight for you to gain. Individual recommendations will vary based on factors that include your pre-pregnancy weight, your medical history, your health, and the health of your developing baby.

How much weight you gain during your pregnancy partly determines your baby's weight, and a normal birth weight is important for good health. A desirable weight for a full-term newborn is between 6½ and 9 pounds. Babies born at these healthy weights have:

- A lower rate of infant death
- Fewer mental and physical handicaps
- Fewer serious childhood illnesses
- A head start, physically and mentally, over smaller babies

Strive for a slow and steady increase in your weight, but keep in mind that individual women gain at different rates. Here are some general guides to weight gain:

- First trimester: 1 to 1½ pounds a month
- Second trimester: ½ to ¾ pound a week
- Third trimester: ¾ to 1 pound a week

Where You'll Gain the Weight

Your baby	6½ to 9 pounds
Placenta	1½ pounds
Amniotic fluid	2 pounds
Breast enlargement	1 to 3 pounds
Uterus enlargement	2 pounds
Fat stores and muscle development	4 to 8 pounds
Increased blood volume	3 to 4 pounds
Increased fluid volume	2 to 3 pounds
Total	22 to 32½ pounds

Calorie Needs

Early in pregnancy, your developing fetus is almost exclusively dependent on the calories you provide through eating and drinking. This need does not mean that you have to eat excessively, but you may need to eat more often. In fact, some of the discomforts of early pregnancy—feelings of hunger, nausea, or vomiting—are often relieved by intermittent snacking. If you feel more comfortable snacking, eat smaller meals to avoid excessive weight gain.

As the placenta develops in the second trimester, hormones are produced that begin to ensure a more steady supply of nourishment for the fetus, and frequent snacking becomes less necessary. By this time, you'll probably be feeling better and eating regular meals.

During your first trimester, an extra 200 calories a day over your normal intake will provide for the recommended 1 to 1½ pounds of weight you should gain each month. It's important that these calories are from foods that offer the most nutrition for you and your unborn baby. For example, a slice of whole-grain bread, a glass of skim milk, and 1 ounce of lean meat will add about 200 calories.

In your second and third trimesters, you'll need a total of 300 to 500 extra calories a day beyond your normal diet. The more active you are, the more calories you will need.

Your health care provider will monitor your weight gain at each prenatal visit.

Food Choices

There are lots of ways to keep track of your food intake. The key is finding a system that works for you. No, you don't have to keep a food diary or analyze your meals and snacks—but you do need to pay attention to some basic guidelines.

The Food Guide Pyramid, developed by the U.S. Department of Agriculture and endorsed by the U.S. Department of Health and Human Services, is a good model for healthful daily eating. This graphic pyramid (see page 261) replaces the old basic 4 food groups and is designed to help you plan a nutritious diet.

The steps of the pyramid show how to make the best food choices for you and your baby. Each of the food groups provides some, but not all, of the nutrients required for a healthful diet. Because foods in one group can't replace those in another, you can't skip or eliminate any category of food if you want to eat right. No single food group is more important than another—for good health and a healthy baby, you need them all.

Eat at least the minimal recommended servings from each level of the pyramid. If you're having trouble gaining enough weight, add extra servings from the bread and cereal group. If you are gaining weight too rapidly, cut back on toppings such as salad dressings, butter, margarine, and oils. If weight is still a problem or if you have special nutritional concerns, seek help from a registered dietitian or your physician.

Vitamin and Mineral Supplements

Pregnant women need more of almost every vitamin and mineral than do women who are not pregnant. Guidelines from the National Research Council advise that pregnant women who eat a well-balanced diet don't need supplements, but most pregnant women cannot eat enough foods high in iron and folic acid to meet recommendations. Some women can't or won't eat enough high-calcium foods to meet the increased need for this mineral, while research shows that multivitamins taken early in pregnancy may help prevent birth defects.

Key Nutrients in Pregnancy

More than 50 nutrients are essential for good health when you're pregnant. Here's a summary of those most critical for you and your baby.

Nutrient	Why You and Your Baby Need It	Best Sources
Protein	The main building block for your baby's cells; provides reserves you'll need for labor and delivery	Eggs, lean meats, poultry, fish, cheese, milk, dried peas, beans
Carbohydrate	Provides energy for you and your baby; allows protein to be used for tissue growth	Whole-grain and fortified breads and and cereals, fruits, vegetables, rice, pasta, potatoes
Fat	Provides long-term energy for growth; critical for the development of your baby's brain	Lean meat, fish, poultry, eggs, nuts, seeds, peanut butter, oils, margarine, butter
Fluid	Helps increase fluid volume; prevent constipation and dry skin; needed for amniotic fluid	Tap and bottled water, soup
Vitamin A	Promotes healthy skin, eyesight, and bone growth	Sweet potatoes, carrots, dark leafy greens, cantaloupe, apricots
Vitamin C	Forms healthy gums, teeth, and bones for your baby; keeps your tissues in top shape; improves iron absorption	Citrus fruits, broccoli, tomatoes, peppers, berries, melons, potatoes with skin
Folic acid	Helps blood cell and hemoglobin formation; early in pregnancy, it may prevent neural tube defects	Dark leafy greens, dried peas and beans, whole-grain breads and cereals, citrus fruits, bananas, cantaloupe, tomatoes
Calcium	Helps form strong bones and teeth	Milk, cheese, yogurt, collard greens, kale, sardines and canned salmon (with bones), broccoli, dried beans
Iron	Develops red blood cells needed to deliver oxygen to your baby; prevents fatigue	Lean red meat, spinach, tofu, dried fruits, whole-grain and fortified breads and cereals

For these reasons, many physicians prescribe a prenatal vitamin specially formulated to provide various essential nutrients. Nevertheless, it's important to eat a balanced diet. Most registered dietitians agree that a bad diet supplemented with vitamins is still a bad diet. Taking supplements will not make up for poor eating habits.

Remember that more is not necessarily better; large doses of vitamin or mineral supplements, especially vitamin A, actually can harm your baby. Take only the supplements recommended by your physician.

Vegetarian Diets

If you are a vegetarian, you can continue your vegetarian diet throughout your pregnancy and still have a healthy baby, but you will need to pay additional attention to meal planning. Make time to review your food intake regularly. If you include fish, milk, and eggs in your diet, it will be easier to balance your nutritional intake. It is no longer necessary to combine complementary proteins at each meal. Simply eat a wide variety of foods each day (see the Food Guide Pyramid, page 261) and include one or two extra servings of plant foods high in iron.

Snacks

Healthful snacking is the perfect way to add the extra calories and nutrients essential during pregnancy. Well-planned snacks are also helpful for the times when you can't eat a full meal. In the early part of your pregnancy, frequent small meals and snacks can help control nausea. In the last weeks the pressure of your baby may limit the amount of food you can comfortably eat at one time. Snacking assures a steady stream of nutrition for your baby to grow on.

Salt

In the past, pregnant women were encouraged to limit their sodium intake. New research suggests that it is better not to. During the last few weeks of pregnancy, almost all women have some swelling in their ankles, legs, fingers, or face. This is a normal response to the high levels of estrogen circulating in your body. Cutting back significantly on salt to reduce this swelling will cause your body to conserve sodium and water, actually making the swelling worse.

If you have high blood pressure or develop complications later in your pregnancy, your physician may suggest you limit your intake of foods high in sodium and table salt. Otherwise, don't make drastic changes.

Artificial Sweeteners

More than 1,500 artificially sweetened foods line the shelves of your local grocery store. They include chewing gum, soft drinks, pudding, gelatin, drink mixes, yogurt, and candy. The National Academy of Sciences' landmark report titled *Diet and Health* suggests that although there is no recommendation either for or against the use of artificial sweeteners, pregnant women might want to consider limiting the amount in their diet. We suggest you keep your use down to no more than two or three products a day.

Caffeine

Caffeine is a drug that has been part of the human diet for thousands of years. It occurs naturally in coffee, tea, chocolate, and cocoa. Caffeine is frequently added to soft drinks and over-the-counter drugs, including headache and cold tablets, stay-awake medications, and allergy remedies. An abundance of research indicates that moderate consumption of caffeine (200 milligrams daily) has no

---

Smart Snacking

Crunchy
Raw vegetables
Whole-grain crackers

Sweet
Fresh fruit
Dried fruit
Low-fat yogurt
Low-fat muffin

Thirst quenchers
Ice water or sparkling bottled water
Fruit juice fizz (½ juice and ½ sparkling water)
Fruit shake made with skim milk
Vegetable juice

Hearty
Fruit muffins or breads
Cereal with low-fat yogurt
Vegetable soup
Tuna sandwich

---

negative effects during pregnancy. Consumed in high amounts (500 milligrams or more daily), caffeine increases the amount of time a fetus spends in an active, awake state and may cause a decrease in your baby's birth weight and head circumference.

Coffee is the most common source of caffeine. Drinking more than 2 or 3 cups of coffee a day is not recommended.

Because little is known about herbs and their effect on pregnancy, avoid herbal teas. Don't take anything that contains comfrey; this herb can cause serious liver disease.

The best advice is to avoid caffeine-containing foods and drugs whenever possible. If you can't give up caffeine during pregnancy, keep your intake below 200 milligrams daily (see Caffeine Content of Common Foods, page 186).

Therapeutic Drugs in Pregnancy

Almost any drug you take during pregnancy affects your baby too. Even a seemingly innocent over-the-counter drug such as aspirin travels through the placenta to your baby. Thus, avoid taking medication unless it is approved by your physician.

Caffeine Content of Common Foods

	Milligrams of Caffeine	
	Average	Range
Coffee, 5 ounces		
Brewed, percolator	115	60-180
Brewed, drip method	80	40-170
Instant	65	30-120
Tea, 5 ounces		
Brewed, imported	60	25-110
Brewed, U.S. brands	40	20-90
Instant	30	25-50
Iced (12 ounces)	70	67-76
Soft drinks, 12 ounces	36	30-50
Cocoa, 5 ounces	4	2-20
Chocolate milk, 8 ounces	5	2-7
Semi-sweet chocolate, 1 ounce	20	5-35
Milk chocolate, 1 ounce	6	1-15
Chocolate syrup, 1 ounce	4	4-5

Sometimes drugs cannot be avoided during pregnancy. If you have a condition for which medication is necessary, your physician will select a drug that will help your problem without jeopardizing your baby unnecessarily.

Some women have chronic diseases such as diabetes or hypertension that necessitate medication. Many pregnant women develop urinary infections that require antibiotics. And often physicians recommend that their pregnant patients with a high fever due to a viral illness take acetaminophen because a prolonged high fever is potentially dangerous to the fetus.

Sometimes the effects of exposure of the fetus to a drug do not appear for many years. Such is the case with the female offspring of women who took diethylstilbestrol (DES). This drug commonly was prescribed for women who were thought to be in danger of miscarriage or who had a history of miscarriage. In the 1970s, many adolescent girls and young women were found to have unusual vaginal, cervical, and uterine changes. The one thing they had in common was that their mothers had taken DES while pregnant.

Drugs that are known to affect the fetus adversely are called teratogens. In general, the most dangerous time to take medication is during the first trimester of pregnancy, because that is when most fetal development occurs and when the fetus is most vulnerable to injury. However, some drugs, such as aspirin, are more dangerous when taken later in pregnancy.

The following are some drugs that are known to cause or are suspected of causing birth defects. This is not a complete list. Always check with your obstetrician before taking any medication.

- Isotretinoin (Accutane) is a drug used for acne. It can cause heart disease and severe facial and ear abnormalities.
- The antibiotic streptomycin can cause deafness when used by a pregnant woman for a long time; tetracycline can lead to retarded bone growth and damage to tooth pigmentation.
- Dicumarol is an anticoagulant sometimes taken by people with heart disease or excessive blood clotting. Abnormal facial features and mental retardation are associated with its use.
- Dilantin, an anticonvulsant used for seizure disorders (epilepsy), can cause tumors, retarded growth, and other abnormalities.
- Diuretics, used when water retention is a problem, can interfere with fetal nutrition if used in excess.
- Methyltestosterone can cause masculinization of the female fetus.
- Tranquilizers may produce tremors that continue for months after birth.
- Valium may cause depression.

In a few cases a drug helps rather than hurts the fetus. Some abnormalities in fetal heart rate can be treated with cardiac drugs through the mother, even though she does not have a heart abnormality. Similarly, if your physician anticipates that labor will have to be induced before 32 weeks of gestation because of a medical problem, the infant can be given corticosteroid medications before labor that may enable the infant to breathe better after birth.

Common Discomforts During Pregnancy

Although most women have pregnancies uncomplicated by serious medical problems or emergencies, few escape without at least some discomfort. Some problems, such as morning sickness, are more common during the early weeks of pregnancy and usually subside by the end of the third month. Others, such as hemorrhoids, may worsen as your pregnancy advances.

Morning Sickness

Morning sickness is the term used to describe the queasiness, nausea, or vomiting that about half of all pregnant women have during the first 12 weeks of pregnancy. Although morning sickness tends to be worse in the morning, some women complain of bouts of nausea throughout the day.

It is not understood why some women have nausea and vomiting. Hormonal changes may be responsible. Although morning sickness is certainly unpleasant, it is rarely dangerous.

If you have morning sickness, there are certain things you can do to minimize your nausea and vomiting, although nothing is 100 percent effective. Many women find that the nausea is worse when their stomachs are empty. Thus, they make it a point to eat several small meals a day. Some keep crackers next to their bedside and find that they feel better when they nibble a few before rising in the morning.

You may find the smell of certain foods brings on the nausea. If this happens, avoid that particular food. If you feel nauseated, stick to a bland diet, avoiding spicy, rich, and fried foods.

Drink lots of fluid, especially if you are vomiting. If plain water upsets your stomach, try crushed ice, fruit juice, or Popsicles.

Some drugs may be effective for eliminating the problem. However, many physicians are reluctant to prescribe a medication for nausea unless the problem is severe. Occasionally, vomiting may be serious enough that a pregnant woman becomes dehydrated. This condition usually requires hospitalization, during which anti-vomiting drugs are administered and lost body fluid is replaced intravenously.

Constipation

Constipation is a common problem during pregnancy. If you usually are constipated, you may find the problem worsens during your pregnancy. It probably occurs because of decreased intestinal contractions and diminished ability of the bowel to expel its contents because of the pressure from the enlarged uterus.

To alleviate the problem, drink plenty of fluids, exercise daily, and make sure your diet contains several servings of fruits (prunes are particularly good), vegetables, and grains such as whole wheat and bran. Bulk formers that contain psyllium (available without a prescription) are often helpful.

Do not take a laxative unless you check with your physician.

Heartburn

Heartburn has nothing to do with your heart. Rather, the burning sensation in the middle of your chest and the sometimes bad taste in your mouth are the result of stomach acid flowing upward into your lower esophagus (see page 742).

This problem occurs in about half of all pregnant women when the muscle that closes off the stomach from the esophagus becomes lax, allowing stomach juices to flow back up and irritate the esophagus. It often worsens with advancing pregnancy because the stomach is moved out of position by the expanding uterus, which delays the emptying of its contents.

If you have heartburn, try eating smaller meals at more frequent intervals, which will keep food in your stomach to soak up the excess acid. Eat slowly and avoid greasy foods. Both regular and decaffeinated coffee may aggravate heartburn. Because heartburn is often worse when you lie flat, your physician may suggest sleeping with the head of your bed on 4- to 6-inch blocks. Also, avoid eating during the 2 or 3 hours immediately preceding bedtime.

If these practices do not help, consult your physician, who may recommend an antacid.

Backache

Backache is common during pregnancy. Often it occurs when you are tired or have been bending, lifting, or walking too much.

When you are pregnant, your ligaments are more elastic, which allows your pelvis to expand during the birth of your baby. Although this is necessary, its negative effect is that your joints are more prone to strain and injury. During pregnancy, as your center of balance changes, so does your posture, inflicting more strain than ever on your already vulnerable back.

Usually the pain is in the lower back. Some women get sciatica (pain that radiates down the legs). Most women also have pain in the abdomen because of the stretching of abdominal ligaments by the expanding uterus. Called round ligament pain, it is generally worse during the second trimester.

Try not to gain more weight than is recommended because weight places stress on your back. Backache usually can be relieved by eliminating as much strain as possible. Sometimes a maternity girdle can help. Your physician also may recommend exercises to relieve the pain. If the pain is severe, your physician may recommend an orthopedic examination to determine whether there is an underlying problem.

Varicose Veins

Varicose veins usually become worse in later pregnancy and are more pronounced in women who stand for long periods and older mothers. Heredity also may play a role in whether you get varicose veins.

As many as 20 percent of all pregnant women have varicose veins. The condition tends to appear earlier and is more pronounced with each pregnancy.

When you are pregnant, your blood vessels must accommodate an increased blood volume to supply the needs of your baby. Your uterus enlarges and the flow of blood from your leg veins to your pelvis decreases. This combination causes the veins in your legs to become swollen and uncomfortable or even very painful.

If you have varicose veins, keep off your feet (and elevate them) as much as possible. Do not wear clothing that is tight around the legs or waist. Support hose can help relieve the pain and swelling. Many physicians recommend that you put on your support hose first thing in the morning and not take them off until just before you go to bed.

Surgery to treat varicose veins generally is not recommended during pregnancy. Rarely is the problem so severe that it becomes necessary.

Hemorrhoids

Hemorrhoids occur when the veins at the anal opening become enlarged due to pressure. When you strain during a bowel movement, the veins may protrude through the anus and cause pain and itching. Generally, they become worse during pregnancy and often occur in conjunction with constipation.

Prevention is the best treatment. Avoid becoming constipated and straining at stool (see Constipation, page 187).

If you notice pain during a bowel movement and feel a swollen mass near your rectum, you probably have a hemorrhoid. To ease the discomfort, take frequent warm water baths. A cotton pad soaked with cold witch hazel cream applied to the hemorrhoidal area also may help.

Sleeping Problems

Sleeping problems often occur during the later months of pregnancy. The frequent urge to urinate contributes to lack of sleep. The movement of your baby also may keep you awake. Some women simply have so much on their minds that sleep eludes them. What should you do if you find yourself staring at the ceiling half the night?

Avoid coffee, tea, or cola drinks because they contain caffeine, which can keep you awake. Also, do not eat a huge meal just before bedtime. Some physicians recommend exercising a little more so you will be more tired and more apt to fall asleep. For some pregnant women, a warm bath helps. If nothing seems to work, get up—read a book, pay some bills, or catch up on household tasks. Try sleeping later.

If the lack of sleep becomes significant, consult your physician. Some physicians will prescribe sleeping pills when a woman is exhausted from lack of sleep. Do not, however, take any medications unless recommended by your physician.

Anemia

Anemia occurs when your hemoglobin—a protein in blood that carries oxygen throughout the body—falls below an adequate amount. A small decrease in hemoglobin is normal during pregnancy. Usually, anemia in pregnancy is due to an iron deficiency or an inadequate supply of folic acid.

If you have mild anemia, you may have no symptoms, and the condition may be discovered accidentally during a routine blood test. With more severe anemia, symptoms include fatigue, breathlessness, fainting, palpitations, and pallor.

Unlike other conditions discussed in this section, anemia can be risky for both mother and child. Should hemorrhaging occur, the anemic pregnant woman is less able to cope with blood loss than a pregnant woman with adequate hemoglobin.

Most physicians prescribe iron and folic acid supplements to prevent anemia. You also can help prevent anemia by eating a diet rich in iron, which is found in foods such as liver, eggs, dried fruit, whole grains, and beef. Green vegetables are a good source of folic acid.

If you do develop anemia, your physician will determine what type of anemia is present and prescribe appropriate treatment. Most often, this will include iron and folic acid supplements (see Anemias, page 956).

Edema

Edema (swelling) is common during pregnancy because of accumulated fluid in body tissues. Approximately one-quarter of your weight gain during pregnancy is fluid, which tends to congregate in various parts of your body, including the lower legs, feet, and hands. You may notice swelling in your legs, ankles, and feet after you have been standing for long periods. The problem usually is worse at the end of the day and in warm weather. After a night of rest, the legs and feet return to their normal size in most women.

The fingers also are a common site for swelling. You may wake up in the morning with your fingers so stiff that you cannot button your clothing. Your fingers also may be puffy. Cold water compresses help relieve the swelling.

Some women notice facial swelling. If your face becomes extremely swollen, especially around the eyes, this may be a sign of preeclampsia, a serious medical condition (see page 204). See your physician immediately.

Use diuretics only at your physician's direction. Often a low-salt diet will prove helpful. Lying down and elevating your legs for an hour in midafternoon also may reduce the swelling in your legs.

Medical Problems of Pregnancy

Most women go through pregnancy without any major complications. For a small percentage of women, however, this 9-month experience is not without problems. You may have a chronic disease such as diabetes or hypertension, or develop disease over the course of the 9 months. Pregnancy does not make a healthy woman immune to disease. This section explores some of the more common medical problems that complicate pregnancy.

Diabetes Mellitus

Diabetes does not preclude a woman from becoming pregnant. Today, if you have diabetes you have an excellent chance of having a healthy baby.

Prior to conception and during pregnancy, keep your blood sugar concentration under control through careful measurements of its value and appropriate adjustment of insulin injections (see page 933). A satisfactory glucose level decreases your baby's risks for birth defects.

If you do not stringently keep your blood sugar under control, the excess blood sugar will travel through the placenta and cause an increase in the fetus's blood sugar concentration. This, in turn, activates the fetal pancreas to produce insulin, which acts as a growth hormone. Babies born to mothers whose diabetes is out of control often are extremely large, a characteristic that complicates labor and delivery. They tend to have more congenital defects and are predisposed to diabetes. Moreover, some of these babies die before birth because of metabolic problems.

For the mother with diabetes, the risks associated with the disease include infection, postpartum hemorrhage, heart and lung problems, and a 4-fold greater risk of preeclampsia than in mothers who don't have diabetes (see Preeclampsia and Eclampsia, page 204).

The pregnant woman with diabetes must adhere to a strict diet to keep her blood sugar under control. If this is not effective, insulin shots are required. Blood tests now available allow your physician to determine how well your diet and blood sugar are being controlled. With strict control of your diabetes, the infant is more likely to be nearly normal in size. Sometimes an early delivery by cesarean section is necessary because of the infant's large size or because the environment of the womb is becoming detrimental to the baby (see Cesarean Section, page 212, and Diabetes Mellitus, page 925). If you have diabetes, seek the care of an obstetrician who specializes in high-risk pregnancy.

Sometimes women who don't have diabetes develop a condition called gestational diabetes during pregnancy. This form of diabetes also requires careful control but may not require insulin injection; it usually goes away after the baby is born. Your physician may order a screening test during the middle of your pregnancy to check for gestational diabetes.

Hypertension

Hypertension (high blood pressure) is a common and potentially dangerous problem during pregnancy. Hypertensive mothers tend to have small placentas and their infants tend to be small at birth. The incidence of fetal death also is higher than in the general population.

Some women have preexisting hypertension. In others, the pregnancy is responsible for an elevation in blood pressure. You may have hypertension but no symptoms. The condition is detected easily during the routine blood pressure check that is a part of every prenatal visit.

Some women with mild hypertension have no major problems during pregnancy. In others, the blood pressure continues to increase, fluid begins to accumulate in their bodies, and protein is detected in their urine. This is called preeclampsia and usually occurs after the 20th week of pregnancy. Convulsions (eclampsia) can follow (see Preeclampsia and Eclampsia, page 204). This is an extreme emergency and can result in death for the mother and child.

Thus, it is important that your hypertension be controlled. This means frequent examinations, blood and urine tests to determine whether your kidneys are functioning properly, and possibly repeat ultrasound examinations to ascertain whether your baby is growing properly.

Sometimes bed rest is advised. If your blood pressure is extremely high, medication may be prescribed (see High Blood Pressure, page 647).

Asthma

Asthma is a chronic respiratory disease that afflicts about 3 percent of adults. The course of asthma during pregnancy is difficult to predict. In some women the disease worsens with pregnancy; in others it improves or remains the same.

If you have asthma, you may be more prone to respiratory infections during pregnancy. The emotional stress of pregnancy may make your attacks more intense. However, most asthmatic women can carry a baby to term safely.

Many women with asthma require medication. Most asthma medication is safe to use during pregnancy.

Heart Disorders

About 1 percent of all pregnant women have a preexisting heart disorder. Although potentially serious, many women with heart disorders have successful pregnancies and healthy babies.

Pregnancy makes your heart and other organs work extra hard. Thus, if you already have a heart disorder, this extra load can cause heart failure. If you have a heart problem, particularly one involving your valves (see Disorders of the Heart Valves, page 677), make sure you discuss the risks of pregnancy with your physician before you become pregnant.

Generally, if you are in good health otherwise and have no evidence of heart failure, you probably will have a successful pregnancy and a healthy baby.

Excessive weight gain, abnormal retention of fluid, and anemia can be particularly dangerous for a woman with a heart disorder, and every effort should be made to avoid these problems. In some cases, bed rest for part of the pregnancy may be recommended.

Seizure Disorders

Seizure disorders (for example, epilepsy), if controlled with medication, generally do not affect pregnancy. However, severe nausea and vomiting during early pregnancy may interfere with your ability to take your anticonvulsant medication. This can increase the risk of seizures.

Rarely, medications to control seizures can cause birth defects and increase the risk of prematurity, low birth weight, and infant death. Some drugs are more apt to cause problems than others, so if you have a seizure disorder and are contemplating pregnancy, make sure you consult a physician who has experience in treating such disorders.

Skin Problems

Skin problems, while a nuisance, usually do not pose a risk during pregnancy. Pruritus (itching), which is more likely to appear in first pregnancies, generally occurs all over the body. One form of pruritus appears as small red patches that usually are found around the abdomen and then spread to the buttocks, hips, thighs, and upper arms.

If you have pruritus, avoid scratching, which may cause infection. Wash the area with a mild soap. If your symptoms are severe, your physician may recommend a cortisone cream (see Itching, page 995).

Pigmentation changes often occur during pregnancy. You may notice brownish spots on your face or on other parts of your body. The discoloration on your face is sometimes called the mask of pregnancy. These spots of pigment usually, but not always, disappear after the baby is born.

Infectious Diseases During Pregnancy

Some common diseases that seem to do little more than make a pregnant woman miserable can, in fact, do irreparable damage to the fetus, depending on when in fetal development they strike.

German Measles

German measles (rubella) is usually a mild disease that causes a mild, itchy rash (see color photograph, page C-1) and fever. If contracted during the first 10 weeks of pregnancy, however, the virus can cross the placenta and infect the fetus. More than half of the infants born to women who have rubella during early pregnancy have congenital malformations such as cataracts, deafness, hernias, heart defects, and defects of the central nervous system.

When contracted in later pregnancy, rubella does not cause congenital defects, but the infant is born with the virus, which can cause serious illness. Many of these babies later develop diabetes.

Your best defense against rubella is immunization. If you have not had German measles, ask your physician about immunization before you become pregnant (see page 1074).

Chickenpox

If you have never had chickenpox, consider receiving a newly available chickenpox vaccine before you become pregnant. Chickenpox (varicella) may be a serious disease in pregnant women. It sometimes can be dangerous for the infant as well. If you have chickenpox (see color photograph, page C-1) during pregnancy, the virus may also infect your developing infant either while it is in the uterus or during delivery. The infant in the uterus may actually develop pockmarks. If there is sufficient time before delivery, the pockmarks generally heal and the infant is born without skin blemishes.

The greatest risk seems to be exposure to the virus just before delivery. If the infant is delivered before receiving your antibodies against the virus, he or she may develop the disease. Unless the infant immediately is given a shot of zoster immune globulin, the baby may die from complications of the virus (see page 1076).

Toxoplasmosis

Toxoplasmosis is a disease due to contact with the parasite *Toxoplasma gondii*. It is contracted by eating infected undercooked meat or through contact with infected cat feces, or it can be passed from an infected pregnant mother to her baby. If you are pregnant, do not handle cats or empty their litter boxes.

As many as 25 to 45 percent of American women of reproductive age carry the organism, although they may not have symptoms. It is estimated that one fetus in every 800 to 1,400 pregnancies acquires toxoplasmosis.

The symptoms of toxoplasmosis are fatigue and muscle pain. You may feel like you have the flu. Some women have no symptoms. The disease cannot be confirmed unless you had a test for toxoplasmosis early in pregnancy and did not carry the antibodies. The infection in the mother can be treated with medication.

If you contract the infection early in pregnancy, you may have a miscarriage.

Most infants born with toxoplasmosis do not immediately show evidence of having been infected, but many physicians advise treatment anyway. In addition, most infants are not infected despite maternal infection. Of those who are, most have only minor symptoms. A few, however, eventually develop neurologic problems and partial blindness. A small percentage of these infants die from the disease.

Genital Herpes

Genital herpes is a sexually transmitted disease that appears as painful blisters on the genitals. The cervix or upper vagina also may have blisters, which may not produce symptoms. In the newborn, herpes can cause serious damage to the eyes and central nervous system or death.

There is no cure for genital herpes. After one attack, it may be a month or years before the next attack. Some women carry the virus but never have symptoms. If you have confirmed herpes or suspect you have the virus, tell your physician. There are tests that can be done to determine whether you have any active lesions.

The danger to the baby is generally thought to be exposure to the virus as it travels down the birth canal. Thus, if an examination, tests, or both confirm that you have active herpes near your delivery time, your physician may want to deliver the baby by cesarean section (see page 1090).

Rhesus (Rh) Compatibility

During childbirth, some of your baby's blood can escape into your bloodstream. If your blood and that of your child are compatible, this is not a problem. However, if they are incompatible, you can develop antibodies that could be a threat to subsequent pregnancies.

Blood groups are determined by whether or not a person has certain protein molecules on the surface of his or her blood cells. The Rh factor is one of these blood groups. Eighty-five percent of Caucasians are Rh positive, which means they have the Rh component in their blood cells. Among African-Americans, the percentage is slightly higher, and virtually all American Indians and Asians are Rh positive.

About 15 percent of Caucasians and 7 percent of African-Americans are Rh negative. If you are Rh negative, you do not have a potential problem unless the father of your baby is Rh positive. If the baby has inherited the father's Rh-positive blood, the blood of the baby is incompatible with your blood (see Blood Groups, page 980).

In most cases, the first child is not at risk even if it is Rh positive because your Rh-negative blood has not had prior exposure to Rh-positive blood. Thus, you have not been sensitized, meaning your body has not yet begun to develop the antibodies that would attack the fetus. However, if you become pregnant again and the fetus is Rh positive, these antibodies can pass through the placenta and harm the developing baby. The risk increases with each Rh-incompatible pregnancy.

Rh disease is not the problem it once was because of more thorough screening techniques, use of a serum that prevents the Rh-negative woman from developing antibodies, and more effective therapy for infants who are affected.

If you are pregnant, your physician will order a blood test that will determine whether you are Rh negative or Rh positive. If you are negative, the baby's father may be tested also (unless you already know his Rh status).

If the father's blood is Rh positive, regular blood tests will be required throughout your pregnancy to check for development of antibodies. Although unlikely to occur during a first pregnancy, this is not unheard of. If you have ever had an abortion or a miscarriage, it is possible that some of the fetus's blood cells entered your body and triggered the development of antibodies. Moreover, there is always the possibility of small leaks of fetal blood during pregnancy.

Physicians now give all their pregnant Rh-negative patients a shot of Rho immune globulin at 28 weeks of gestation to prevent sensitization should there be some early leakage of fetal blood. This serum destroys any fetal red blood cells that have entered your circulation before your body has time to marshal its forces against them.

After the birth of your baby, you may discover that this precaution was unnecessary if your baby is Rh negative. But because there is no risk from the shot itself and because of the possibility of injury to the baby without it, the choice seems clear.

When you deliver an Rh-positive infant, you will be given another dose of Rho immune globulin within 72 hours after the delivery. This will enable you to enter the next pregnancy without having been sensitized.

If you have been sensitized and your baby is being affected, an early delivery may be necessary. Some infants die in the uterus because of severe anemia as a result of this blood incompatibility. The infant may be given a blood transfusion while still in the womb. This is done to "buy time" until the baby's lungs are developed enough so that he or she can withstand an early delivery.

After birth, a baby who has Rh disease is severely anemic and jaundiced. Exchange transfusions will be necessary. These involve slowly removing the infant's anemic Rh-positive blood and replacing it with Rh-negative blood. The outlook for these infants has improved markedly in recent years.

Hepatitis B

Hepatitis B is a liver infection caused by the hepatitis B virus (see page 801). This virus is transmitted in much the same manner as the AIDS virus (see page 1060). If you have the hepatitis B virus, it can be transmitted to your fetus through the placenta. Also, your newborn baby can become infected by the virus from contact with you.

This virus can cause liver failure. The risk of premature birth also is higher among women who have hepatitis B.

If your physician suspects that you have hepatitis B, he or she will test your blood for the presence of antibodies to the virus. If you have hepatitis B, your infant will be given an injection of antibodies against the virus after delivery.

Because the hepatitis virus also may be found in breast milk, a mother with hepatitis B should not breastfeed.

Group B Streptococci

Group B streptococci are bacteria that can be transmitted to the fetus during childbirth. As many as 40 percent of pregnant women tested in the last trimester of pregnancy asymptomatically harbor these bacteria in their vagina. You will be treated during labor if these bacteria are identified.

Many infants are born with this bacteria, but infection develops in only 2 or 3 per 1,000. An infant with group B streptococcal infection usually shows symptoms within 48 hours after delivery. The symptoms include breathing problems and shock. Occasionally, an infant will be a week old before there are symptoms, which then usually appear as meningitis. Immediate treatment with antibiotics is necessary for infants with this infection. Even so, the mortality rate is high.

Syphilis

Syphilis is a serious sexually transmitted disease that can be passed from a pregnant mother to her baby. If you have syphilis, you may see one or more lesions, called chancres, on your genitals, although sometimes they may go unnoticed. They occur 10 to 90 days after exposure. About 6 weeks later you may notice a rash.

During your first prenatal visit you will be tested for syphilis, as required by law. The disease can be treated easily with penicillin.

At birth, your infant will be tested. If the baby has syphilis, treatment will be initiated immediately (see page 1089).

Gonorrhea

Gonorrhea is another sexually transmitted (so-called venereal) disease. It can be treated effectively with antibiotics. However, if you have gonorrhea, your baby will be exposed to the infection during the birth process.

Infection with gonorrhea may result in damage to your baby's eyes. For this reason, all newborns receive preventive treatment immediately after birth. This consists of an antibiotic ointment applied under the baby's eyelids.

A discharge of pus from the baby's eyes may be a sign that the infant has gonorrhea. If you have gonorrhea, your infant will be treated with penicillin (see page 1087).

Chlamydial Infection

Chlamydial infection, another sexually transmitted disease, can cause an eye infection called conjunctivitis (see page 1088) in the newborn. This usually appears during the second week of life. When treated with antibiotics, it does not have any long-term adverse effects.

Cytomegalovirus

Cytomegalovirus is the most common virus affecting the fetus. An estimated 2,500 to 7,500 babies are born infected by this virus each year. It can cause death during the newborn period or numerous birth defects such as blindness, seizures, anemia, and neurologic disorders. Some women carry the virus in their urine or cervix during pregnancy, but few pass the disease to their infants. There is no effective treatment.

Papilloma

Papilloma appears as warts on the skin. The warts usually found on the genitals are called condylomata or venereal warts. These are highly infectious, sexually transmitted, and often painful. The warts tend to grow faster during pregnancy. Usually, treatment during pregnancy is not effective. Sometimes the warts grow so large that they interfere with the baby's passage down the birth canal, necessitating a cesarean section (see page 1092).

AIDS

AIDS (acquired immunodeficiency syndrome) is a fatal disease for which there is no cure (see page 1060). A pregnant woman can be infected by the AIDS virus through sexual intercourse with an infected man, by blood transfusion, or by injecting drugs with dirty needles (as drug addicts often do), or through artificial insemination with semen containing the virus.

If you have AIDS, you can pass the disease to the baby you are carrying. Transmission of AIDS from mother to baby occurs in about one-fifth to one-fourth of cases, but may be reduced to as low as 8 percent by treatment during and after pregnancy with a medication called AZT. Therefore, prenatal screening for AIDS is recommended for everyone.

There is no cure for AIDS. Babies born with the disease usually do not live more than a few years. Therefore, if you have the AIDS virus, do not become pregnant.

Risk Factors and Pregnancy

There are never any guarantees, but the vast majority of pregnant women deliver healthy, normal babies at or near term. Some factors, however, tend to increase your chances of complications such as miscarriage, stillbirth, intrauterine growth retardation, and premature birth. Some of these factors, such as age, are to a large extent beyond your control. Others, including smoking and the use of alcohol and illegal drugs, are dangerous practices that you should avoid (see also Exercise During Pregnancy, page 195, and Travel During Pregnancy, page 196).

Age

Age is especially worthy of some attention today because so many women are delaying pregnancy until their 30s and even 40s. How safe is this? Again, the vast majority of healthy women older than 35 years tend to have uneventful pregnancies. Because many of these women have planned their pregnancies, they are often highly motivated and take especially good care of themselves. There is, however, an increased risk for mother and child.

Women older than 35 tend to develop gestational diabetes and hypertension more frequently than younger women. The rate of miscarriage and stillbirth also is slightly higher. Placenta previa, an uncommon condition requiring premature delivery, is more common among older mothers (see page 205). Labor also tends to be slightly longer in older first-time mothers.

Teenagers also are at higher risk for complications of pregnancy. The risk may not be so much age-related as the result of the youthful mother being uninterested in taking care of herself. These young girls may have inadequate diets and little or no prenatal care, which may result in a higher frequency of preeclampsia and eclampsia—often called toxemia (see page 204)—a potentially fatal condition. Pregnant teenagers also have higher rates of miscarriage, intrauterine growth retardation, stillbirths, and premature births than women a few years older.

Congenital Defects

Congenital defects occur in about 2 to 3 percent of all newborns. Some defects correlate with the age of the mother. For example, if you are 30 years old, your chance of having a baby with Down syndrome is 1 in more than 900, but if you are older than 40 the incidence is about 1 in 100 births.

The risk of congenital defects is known to be increased by some drugs taken by the pregnant mother (see Therapeutic Drugs in Pregnancy, page 185), diseases such as diabetes (see Medical Problems of Pregnancy, page 189), intrauterine infections, and alcoholism (see Pregnancy and Alcohol, page 328).

Inadequate Diet

An inadequate diet increases your risk of giving birth to a low-birth-weight infant, which makes the infant more vulnerable to infection, disease, and death. Failure to gain an adequate amount of weight can affect your baby adversely (see Nutrition During Pregnancy, page 182). If you have been poorly nourished most of your life, the effects may be felt by your baby despite improved nutrition during pregnancy.

Caffeine

Caffeine is a stimulant found in coffee, tea, chocolate, and cola. Women who consume an excessive amount of caffeine tend to have babies who are slightly smaller than average. However, because these women also often smoke, it is not known whether caffeine is responsible for the low weight (see page 273).

Radiation

Radiation from X-rays can damage the fetus. Therefore, avoid X-rays directed at the abdomen if at all possible.

Physicians now are clearly aware of the potential risks of cumulative radiation to a fetus. Moreover, equipment has improved so that less radiation is needed. These factors combine to make X-ray examinations relatively safe when a pregnant woman has a medical condition that requires them.

If you are pregnant, it is safe to have an X-ray of your teeth, head, or extremities. Modern techniques protect your abdomen, and the only part of your body exposed to radiation is the area on which the X-ray is focused.

Smoking

Smoking is a difficult habit to break, but it is not impossible, as millions of Americans can attest. Why should you stop smoking if you are pregnant or contemplating pregnancy?

Studies show that mothers who smoke a pack or more of cigarettes a day consistently produce smaller babies than do nonsmokers. A small baby is generally weaker and more vulnerable to illness than one of average size. Moreover, smokers are more apt to have their pregnancy end in miscarriage or still-birth. (For help in stopping smoking, see page 321.)

Alcohol

Alcohol is a dangerous drug when used during pregnancy. Alcohol use during pregnancy is the leading preventable cause of mental retardation. There is no known safe level of alcohol use during pregnancy, so your physician probably will advise you not to drink at all during your pregnancy.

If you drink heavily, your infant may be born with fetal alcohol syndrome. This syndrome, found in 1 or 2 infants out of every 1,000, is characterized by prenatal and postnatal growth retardation, facial abnormalities, heart defects, joint and limb problems, and intellectual handicaps.

The more alcohol you drink, the greater the chances of producing a child with fetal alcohol syndrome or at least some congenital defects. For example, up to 33 percent of infants whose mothers are heavy drinkers have some congenital abnormality, whereas fewer than 5 percent whose mothers did not drink during pregnancy have a congenital abnormality.

The question that most women ask their physicians is whether it is safe to drink socially during pregnancy. The answer is "no."

Illegal Drugs

Illegal drug use is becoming more common, with the result that more infants are being born with both drug addiction and severe health problems. If you are using heroin or another addictive drug such as cocaine, amphetamines, or barbiturates, your infant is 2 to 6 times more likely to be born prematurely or to be retarded in growth than a baby whose mother does not use drugs. Moreover, your pregnancy is apt to be complicated by hypertension and hemorrhage.

Approximately half of the infants born to addicted mothers also are addicted. Generally, within the first day of life the heroin-addicted infant becomes irritable and has convulsions, congestion, vomiting, diarrhea, and fever. Sedatives such as phenobarbital frequently are given to the baby and then slowly withdrawn. The withdrawal must be slow or the infant may experience convulsions.

Because of the ease with which cocaine or crack (cocaine that is smoked) can be obtained, in some areas of the country mothers of as many as one in four new babies are users (see page 1132). A significant percentage of their infants are born prematurely or with brain damage.

Hot Tubs

Avoid saunas, steambaths, or immersion above your hips in a hot tub (hot bath or hot shower is fine) because of a possible association of increased core body temperature with developmental abnormality or premature labor or both.

Exercise During Pregnancy

Today, an increasing number of health-conscious women are exercising throughout their pregnancies. This is not to say that pregnancy is the time to embark on a vigorous fitness regimen, especially if you have never done as much as a knee bend in your life. However, if you have been exercising regularly before pregnancy, you probably can continue unless your physician advises against it. Many physicians even recommend that previously sedentary patients slowly begin some form of mild exercise during pregnancy.

The long-term benefits of a regular exercise program for men and women are well known. What impact, however, does exercising by an expectant mother have on the fetus? Studies have shown that exercise probably does not have any impact, negative or positive, on the developing fetus. However, it may increase maternal stamina.

The result of this increased stamina may be a shorter and easier labor. Some speculate that this effect may be due to increased cardiorespiratory fitness and better endurance. The latter characteristic of the physically fit mother is particularly valuable when she is to push the baby out during delivery. Women who exercise regularly often can push for longer periods without succumbing to fatigue.

Although the possibility of an easier and shorter labor may entice you to try exercising, proceed with caution. Because of physical and hormonal changes in your body, you are more vulnerable to injury. Your joints are more unstable and easily injured because your connective tissues now stretch more easily. Moreover, as you become larger, your center of gravity shifts and you may find yourself losing your balance.

After about the fourth month of pregnancy, avoid exercises that require you to lie on your back because of the possibility of interrupting blood flow to the fetus.

Avoid overly strenuous and potentially dangerous activities such as horseback riding, mountain climbing, scuba diving, and water skiing. Restrict downhill skiing to your level of absolute safety and stay below 10,000 feet elevation. Pregnancy is not the time to take up marathon running, although some long-distance runners have completed marathons during pregnancy with no adverse consequences to themselves or their babies.

Despite these few exercise restrictions, there are many sports and exercises that are suitable for a pregnant woman. One of the best exercises during pregnancy is swimming. It provides a good cardiovascular workout; there is no risk of injury to your joints because of the water's buoyancy.

Low-impact aerobics are fine, and in many communities there are low-impact aerobic classes geared for expectant mothers. Jogging and cycling also are good if you took part in these activities before conception. You may need to decrease your activity level if you find yourself becoming more fatigued than usual. Walking during pregnancy is often recommended, and it is usually the first exercise advised for the previously inactive pregnant woman who wants to begin exercising.

No matter what exercise you choose, check with your physician before you begin. Although it is safe for most women to exercise during pregnancy, some pregnant women have medical problems such as hypertension that make exertion dangerous.

Never exercise to the point of exhaustion. Drink plenty of fluids to prevent dehydration during a workout. If the weather is hot and humid, delay your run or walk until a cooler day.

Travel During Pregnancy

Travel does not induce labor, miscarriage, or any other pregnancy complication. Thus, there is no medical reason why you cannot travel during your pregnancy unless your physician advises against it.

Before you contemplate a cross-country car trip or a 2-week cruise, however, consider how you are going to feel. Many women, particularly during the first 3 months of pregnancy, have frequent bouts of nausea or morning sickness. (This is a misnomer because the nausea can occur morning, noon, or night.) Travel during this period may make the nausea worse.

A potential risk of traveling while pregnant is lower-extremity thrombophlebitis, blood clots that result from sitting for long periods of time. While traveling, get up and walk around for a few minutes every couple of hours to activate your leg muscles and increase blood flow (see page 694).

Another consideration is the proximity to your due date. Most physicians advise against traveling during the last weeks of pregnancy, particularly if you have a history of any problems. Many airlines will not allow you to fly if you are close to your due date.

If you are feeling well, have plenty of time before the baby is due, and feel like taking an airline trip, go ahead. Make sure, however, that you get up from your seat every 2 hours and walk around.

When traveling by car, remember to always wear your seat belt. A lap belt should be fastened below your uterus, and a shoulder harness should be adjusted between your breasts and to the side of your abdomen.

You may find it is helpful to put a pillow in the small of your back to prevent low-back pain. Also, stop periodically (every couple of hours) to get out and walk.

Early Pregnancy: The First Trimester

The first trimester of pregnancy can be difficult for an expectant mother and is without doubt the time when a developing embryo is most vulnerable. Virtually every organ in your baby's body is being formed during the first 3 months of pregnancy. Thus, the embryo is particularly sensitive to assaults from the outside. If you take drugs, prescription or oth-

erwise, drink alcohol, or are exposed to toxins or improper use of X-rays, this development can go awry—the result can be birth defects. Miscarriage also is more likely to occur during this critical first trimester. Often this is nature's way of dealing with an abnormal embryo that could not have lived a normal life had the pregnancy been brought to term.

For you, the first 3 months of your pregnancy can be like riding a roller coaster. You are delighted and yet have some fears. If the pregnancy was unplanned, you may be losing sleep considering your options (see Pregnancy Termination: Medical Problems and Personal Choices, page 199). Physically, you may feel drained and find yourself napping whenever you get the opportunity. Rest assured that these weeks will pass quickly and so will most of the symptoms.

How Do You Know If You Are Pregnant?

The first sign for most women is a missed menstrual period. If your periods are usually regular and suddenly you are a week late and you have had intercourse during your cycle, take a pregnancy test. Sometimes a woman will have what appears to be a period even though she is pregnant; however, this bleeding usually is scant.

Many pregnant women complain of breast tenderness. Your breasts may seem fuller and tingle. The nipples are often extremely sensitive. Sometimes the breasts actually hurt.

Many newly pregnant women experience morning sickness—the queasiness, nausea, and vomiting that are common during the first trimester. These problems, which often do not confine themselves to the morning, range from a slightly upset stomach to incessant vomiting. This often begins a few days after a missed period.

Fatigue is common during early pregnancy. If you are home during the day, you probably find yourself lying down for a nap. Women who work outside the home often arrive home so tired that they cannot wait to get into bed.

Frequent urination is another sign of pregnancy. This occurs initially because of the hormonal effects on the bladder and later because of the growing uterus exerting pressure on the bladder. As the size of your uterus begins to increase in your abdomen, this symptom will diminish. However, in the final weeks of pregnancy it returns, and many women find themselves unable to sleep through the night because of the urge to go to the bathroom.

If you have missed a period and have some of these other symptoms, see your physician. He or she will confirm your pregnancy with a pregnancy test (see Pregnancy Tests, page 198). Most women receive prenatal care from an obstetrician, a physician specially trained in the care of pregnant women and the delivery of babies. Some family physicians, especially in small towns, also offer this service to their patients. In some communities, licensed certified nurse midwives also provide maternity care.

Miscarriage

Aside from the initial discomfort of pregnancy, the greatest threat in the first trimester is miscarriage (also known as a spontaneous abortion). Miscarriage and abortion refer to the termination of a pregnancy before the time the fetus can survive even for a few minutes outside the womb. This generally occurs before the 20th week after conception. (Any fetus born dead after the 20th week is termed stillborn.)

About 50 percent of all fertilized eggs spontaneously abort, most of them before a woman has any idea she is pregnant. The percentage of miscarriages in women who know they are pregnant is about 10 percent. Three-quarters of these miscarriages occur in the first trimester, most between the 9th and 11th weeks of gestation. Factors associated with miscarriage include age (women older than 35 years), difficulty in becoming pregnant, and a history of miscarriage.

In the first trimester, miscarriage almost always occurs after the death of the embryo or fetus. Why does an embryo die in the uterus? The most common cause of miscarriage, an estimated 60 percent, is an abnormality in development, usually as a result of extra chromosomes. Other possible causes include chronic infections, unrecognized diabetes in the mother, and defects in the uterus.

Women who suffer a miscarriage tend to blame themselves: "I exercised too hard"; "The stress at work caused it"; "The fall off my bike caused me to lose my baby." It is natural to seek an explanation when a miscarriage occurs, but try not to blame yourself—rarely is miscarriage the result of stress or trauma.

The first symptom of a potential miscarriage is usually vaginal bleeding with or without cramping. An estimated one in five women have some vaginal bleeding or bloody discharge during the first trimester, and more than half of these women do not lose their babies. However, if you have any bleeding, call your physician immediately. Special precautions such as curtailing exer-

Pregnancy Tests

The earliest way to know for sure whether you are pregnant is to have a pregnancy test.

The fertilized egg at 4 days of age begins to secrete a hormone called human chorionic gonadotropin (hCG). This hormone spreads into the body's tissues. Initially it can be detected in the blood, and shortly thereafter it is detected in the urine.

Most pregnancy tests are conducted with a sample of urine, which is obtained more easily than a sample of blood. Many types of urine tests are used to detect the presence of hCG. Most depend on a reaction between the hCG and an anti-hCG antibody. A second reaction is then needed to determine whether the first reaction has taken place. Often that is a color change.

Some women use home pregnancy tests. These testing kits can be purchased at most drugstores and other retail outlets. Most contain a solution that is mixed with urine in a test tube. After a specified amount of time—anywhere from a few minutes to a couple of hours, depending on the test—a dark ring forms if you are pregnant. In some brands, a color change indicates pregnancy.

If you decide to use a home pregnancy test, follow the instructions precisely. Moreover, any pregnancy test, whether done at home or in the physician's office, is more accurate if you use your first urine of the day.

How accurate are urine tests? Their accuracy depends on how closely you follow the instructions, which can be complicated. First-time users or inexperienced users are less likely to get an accurate test result, and no test is foolproof. Also, pregnancy tests, particularly when done in the early days of pregnancy, may indicate you are not pregnant when in fact you are. This is because early in pregnancy the levels of hCG are low and may go undetected. For this reason, negative results from any pregnancy test are less reliable than a positive result.

Home pregnancy tests should be considered screening tests. If your test result is negative but you have the symptoms and signs of pregnancy (see How Do You Know If You Are Pregnant? page 197), consult your physician. If the result is positive, see your physician for confirmation and prenatal care.

About three-fourths of the time, results of a urine test done in a clinic or at your physician's office will be positive if you are pregnant and your period is 4 to 7 days late. When your period is 2 weeks late, the accuracy is close to 100 percent. The results of home pregnancy tests are about 95 percent accurate 10 days after a missed period.

Urine pregnancy tests are the most frequently used, but in some cases a blood test may be indicated because it is more accurate and can detect pregnancy earlier. In the case of an ectopic pregnancy (the egg begins to grow in the fallopian tube or someplace other than the uterus), a woman may have all the signs of pregnancy, despite negative results of urine pregnancy tests (see Ectopic [Tubal] Pregnancy, page 199). This occurs because hCG levels are not high when the egg is not in the uterus. The blood test, however, is more sensitive and could detect the pregnancy. Because ectopic pregnancy is a potentially life-threatening condition, this information could ultimately help save the mother's life.

---

cise, staying off your feet as much as possible, and avoiding intercourse may be necessary for several weeks.

When the embryo or fetus dies, miscarriage is inevitable. An inevitable miscarriage usually is accompanied by pain in the lower abdomen or back. The pain may be dull and relentless or sharp and intermittent. Bleeding may be heavy. Some clot-like material may emerge from your vagina. This is the embryo and placenta. If possible, save it and give it to your physician, who can examine it to try to determine the cause of death.

Sometimes only some of the products of conception are expelled. When this occurs, it is called an incomplete abortion, and the pain and bleeding can continue for several days.

If neither the fetus nor the placenta is expelled but the fetus has died, it is termed a missed abortion. You may not have any bleeding or pain during a missed abortion, but the symptoms of pregnancy will disappear soon. Your physician may suspect miscarriage when your uterus fails to grow.

Little can be done to prevent an inevitable, incomplete, or missed abortion. Usually a surgical procedure called a dilatation and curettage (see page 1151) or a vacuum suction procedure is done to empty the uterus of any fetal remains. This is usually done in the hospital.

Most physicians recommend waiting a few months before trying to conceive again.

Pregnancy Termination: Medical Problems and Personal Choices

Therapeutic and elective abortions present an intensely politicized and personal dilemma in our nation. Since 1973, when the Supreme Court ruled in the landmark Roe v. Wade decision that abortions were legal up to the 24th week, speeches, demonstrations, and even violence have been associated with the issue.

Elective Abortion

Resolution of the moral and ethical issues concerning abortion is an intensely personal decision among you, your physician, the father of the baby, and perhaps other counselors. At this time, however, if you do not want to continue your pregnancy, abortion is a legal means of terminating your pregnancy.

In most states, the decision is solely yours until the 12th week of pregnancy; some states have laws that affect the decision after that time. The choice to abort also may be made on the basis of information discovered through prenatal testing about the health of the fetus—for example, finding that the fetus has Down syndrome or spina bifida.

Therapeutic Abortion

Abortions are performed not only as a matter of choice but also for medical reasons. For reasons of the mother's health, either physical or mental, a physician may recommend an abortion. Termed "therapeutic abortion," it is done when the physician believes the mother's life is endangered by the pregnancy, and the mother agrees.

Procedures

There are different procedural options for terminating pregnancy. One, called vacuum suction, involves inserting into the cervix a tube attached to a suction device that removes the fetal tissue. New drugs, such as RU486, are being studied as a medical alternative to surgical termination in early pregnancy.

In second trimester abortions, uterine contractions may be stimulated by intravenous oxytocin or intravaginal prostaglandins or both to expel the uterine contents.

If you are considering abortion, get all the information you need as quickly as possible. The earlier a pregnancy is terminated, the less risk there is of having complications. Although the federal limit for performing abortions is 24 weeks, regulations vary from state to state, and finding a physician who will terminate a pregnancy beyond 20 weeks may be difficult. Your physician or genetic counselor can help you explore your options.

Ectopic (Tubal) Pregnancy

Signs and Symptoms
- Scanty dark brown vaginal bleeding
- Abdominal pain
- Internal bleeding
- Severe cramping
- Sudden urge to urinate or have a bowel movement
- Dizziness and fainting

Ectopic (tubal) pregnancy occurs when the fertilized egg implants itself anywhere other than in the lining of the uterus. The fertilized egg may become implanted on the ovary or in the abdominal cavity, but in 95 percent of all ectopic pregnancies the egg is implanted in the fallopian tube. Thus, an ectopic pregnancy is sometimes called a tubal pregnancy.

The frequency of ectopic pregnancy has increased in recent years. It now occurs in about 1 out of every 100 pregnancies.

Cause
The interior of the fallopian tube is not unlike a maze, with twists and turns and folds. Sometimes, for various reasons, the fertilized egg becomes stuck and implants in this unsuitable environment.

This growing egg immediately begins to produce human chorionic gonadotropin (hCG), a hormone associated with pregnancy (see Pregnancy Tests, page 198). The growing embryo then begins to secrete other hormones, which cause an increase in the tube's blood supply. As the embryo continues to burrow into the tube, vessels begin to bleed. Unlike the uterus, the tube was not made for pregnancy. As the embryo grows, the tube becomes stretched beyond its capacity. Hemorrhage often occurs. If the pregnancy continues long enough, the tube will rupture, a potentially life-threatening situation.

No one is certain why ectopic pregnancy has become more common. Some speculate that an increase in the incidence of pelvic inflammatory disease may be at least partially responsible. It is known, however, that some medical conditions tend to be associated with a higher risk of ectopic pregnancy. These include abnormalities of the tube, tubal adhesions caused by infection, appendicitis, endometriosis, and the absence of one ovary.

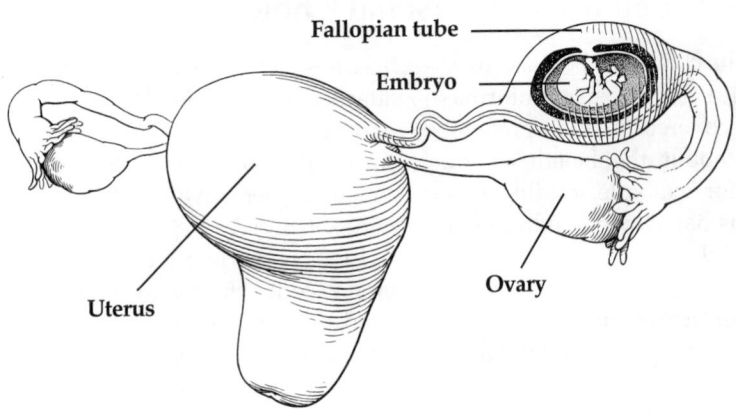

Fallopian tube

Embryo

Ovary

Uterus

Potentially life-threatening, an ectopic (tubal) pregnancy occurs when a fertilized egg implants itself in the fallopian tube rather than the uterus. As the embryo develops, it causes the tube to expand beyond its capacity, producing hemorrhage and potentially serious medical consequences.

Diagnosis

If you have an ectopic pregnancy, initially you may not know that anything is wrong. Despite a missed menstrual period, results of a urine pregnancy test may be negative. This occurs because hCG (a hormone found in pregnant women's urine) is present in much higher amounts when the pregnancy is uterine. Thus, if you have the symptoms of pregnancy but the pregnancy test is negative, your physician will probably order a blood test, which can detect hCG at lower levels.

If you are experiencing any other symptoms listed above, report them to your physician immediately. If your physician suspects an ectopic pregnancy, he or she will first do a pelvic examination to detect any abnormalities. An ultrasound examination (see page 1335) or laparoscopy (see page 1346) may be done to confirm the presence of a mass.

How Serious Is an Ectopic Pregnancy?

An ectopic pregnancy is an extremely dangerous condition—if not detected early, it can have dire consequences. It is a leading cause of pregnancy-related death.

Treatment

There is no chance you can carry this pregnancy to term or to a point at which the fetus has a good chance of surviving. Ectopic fetuses seldom develop beyond 3 months.

Surgery

The treatment may be an immediate operation. If the embryo is still small and the fallopian tube has not been ruptured, the embryo may be squeezed out without further injury to the tube. Some physicians favor removing the injured part of the tube and rejoining the ends.

When there has been massive hemorrhage, blood transfusion may be necessary. In such a case, the physician will have to stop the internal bleeding by clamping off blood vessels. Often the removal of a tube and even of an ovary is necessary.

Medications

Another therapy consists of using a powerful drug called methotrexate, which causes embryo cells to stop growing and eventually disappear. In most cases, this replaces the need for surgery.

Prognosis for Future Pregnancies

If you have had an ectopic pregnancy, what are your chances of having a normal pregnancy later? In women who have had an initial ectopic pregnancy, about 10 percent of subsequent pregnancies will be ectopic pregnancies. Once you have had two ectopic pregnancies, your chances are less than 50 percent of ever having a normal pregnancy. If the ectopic pregnancies have significantly injured both fallopian tubes, in vitro fertilization (see page 1219) may be the only option left if you still want to become pregnant.

Mid-Pregnancy: The Second Trimester

For most women the second trimester of pregnancy is less eventful than the first trimester. The fatigue is lessened. The nausea and vomiting decrease or are absent. And you no longer have frequent urination.

Your abdomen is growing slowly, and you'll probably need to start to wear maternity clothes. Your body is becoming rounder around the middle and probably at the hips, too, but it is not yet unwieldy. For most women, the 4th, 5th, and 6th months of pregnancy are uneventful and even enjoyable.

At this stage, you are still seeing your physician once a month, unless you have a medical condition that warrants more frequent visits. You are taking an iron and folic acid supplement, and you should be making an effort to eat a balanced diet containing several servings each day of protein-rich foods including milk products, fruits, vegetables, and grains (see Nutrition During Pregnancy, page 182).

If you have been contemplating travel, now is probably the best time during pregnancy to take a trip (see Travel During Pregnancy, page 196). Most women feel better during the second trimester than during the earlier months, and as your due date approaches your increased size will tax your energies and you're better off staying close to home.

Although the second trimester is the easiest part of pregnancy for most women, it is not without risks. Miscarriage is not the risk that it was during the first 3 months, but some women begin labor during the second trimester. A fetus delivered this early is not yet mature enough to survive. Although premature labor most often occurs later (third trimester), defects of the uterus can lead to this early labor during mid-pregnancy. This section explores some of the medical complications of this normally uneventful part of pregnancy.

Premature Labor

Signs and Symptoms
- Rupture of your membranes involving a gush of fluid escaping from your vagina
- Mild to severe abdominal contractions

Normally, labor occurs about 40 weeks (280 days) after the first day of your last period. If your baby is born between 38 and 42 weeks, delivery is considered at term. Sometimes, labor—the signal that your baby is about to be born—begins before term. (In some cases, however, your physician may induce labor early if the uterine environment appears to be increasingly harmful to your baby and its chances of survival are better outside the womb.)

Cause
Most often the precise cause of mid-pregnancy labor is never determined. However, the following conditions are associated with premature or preterm labor: spontaneous rupture of membranes (see page 205), cervical infection, incompetent cervix (see page 203), abnormal uterus, hydramnios (see page 202), abnormal fetus or placenta, placenta previa (see page 205), retained intrauterine contraceptive device, preeclampsia and eclampsia (see page 204), death of the fetus, history of premature delivery, multiple fetuses, cigarette smoking, hemorrhage, serious maternal disease, and age—teenagers and women older than 40 are more likely to have premature labor.

Diagnosis
Rupture of your membranes usually occurs when labor is in progress, but occasionally it is the first step. Generally, if you have contractions that last for at least 30 seconds and occur every 10 minutes, you are probably in labor.

How Serious Is Premature Labor?
Premature labor can be an ominous sign. The less time your infant has had in your womb, the less its chances of survival. In recent years, however, major advances have been made in the care of seriously ill or premature infants. Babies as small as 1 pound now have a chance of survival when they are cared for in specialized neonatal units. A reasonable chance for survival of the baby is now being realized as early as 24 weeks after gestation.

Treatment
The treatment for premature labor varies, depending on the age of the fetus. Initially, many physicians prescribe bed rest and hydration. This precaution alone is sometimes successful for stopping contractions. Cultures from the cervix and prophylactic antibiotics may also be considered.

Medications
Thus far there is no specific drug that is always successful for stopping premature labor. However, several therapies have had some degree of success.

Magnesium sulfate may be effective for stopping labor. If your physician prescribes this drug, you will be carefully monitored in the hospital because magnesium sulfate can cause breathing problems. Moreover, the drug passes through to the placenta and may affect your newborn's respiratory movements.

Another group of drugs that has had some success in arresting labor are the beta-mimetics. These drugs, which must be given in the hospital where you can be monitored closely, mimic the effects of epinephrine, the hormone the body secretes in response to danger. (It is well known that fright can delay or halt labor.) These drugs will temporarily stop labor and relax the uterus. If you are given one of these drugs, your heart will beat faster, you may feel shaky and anxious, and your blood pressure and blood sugar concentration will increase. Other possible side effects include fluid in the lungs and chest pain. Like magnesium sulfate, the beta-mimetics cross the placenta, and as a result your baby experiences similar symptoms.

Under certain circumstances, newer drugs such as indomethacin and calcium channel blockers are used either alone or in combination with the drugs mentioned above. However, there can be greater risk of problems. Therefore, these medications are used only when your physician thinks it may do the most good.

Surgery
If your premature labor is determined to be the result of a defect in your uterus, some-

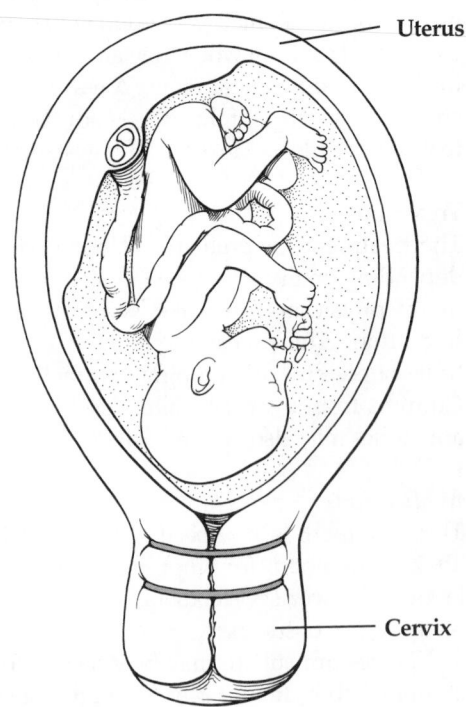

If the lower portion of your uterus, your cervix, opens during pregnancy, a surgical procedure may be done to prevent premature delivery of your baby. Called cerclage, this involves stitching the cervix closed to prevent expulsion of the fetus from the uterus.

times an operation can be done to forestall labor. One procedure, called cerclage, involves placing surgical stitches (sutures) around the cervix so the infant can stay in the womb until term (see Incompetent Cervix, page 203).

Hydramnios

Signs and Symptoms
- Breathlessness
- Indigestion or nausea
- Abdominal distention and accompanying intense pain
- Premature labor (see page 201)

Hydramnios refers to a condition in which there is an excessive amount of amniotic fluid around the baby.

Cause
Normally, the fetus begins to urinate and to swallow amniotic fluid in the second trimester of pregnancy. Later in the pregnancy these functions may help control the amount of fluid in the womb. Hydramnios often is associated with birth defects, particularly with malformations of the central nervous system and gastrointestinal tract. Some of these defects prevent the fetus from swallowing amniotic fluid, and others may cause it to excrete an excessive amount of urine. When hydramnios occurs in a woman who is carrying twins, one fetus perhaps takes over most of the circulation meant for both babies. The result is an increased urine output for this twin.

Diagnosis
If your physician suspects hydramnios, he or she probably will want you to have an immediate ultrasound examination.

How Serious Is Hydramnios?
In most cases the swelling is slight and harmless. In about 1 out of 1,000 pregnancies, however, the condition is severe enough to cause symptoms that can lead to premature labor. Diabetic women and those carrying multiple fetuses have a higher incidence of hydramnios than other pregnant women.

Treatment
If the hydramnios is not severe, no treatment other than resting a little more than usual may be prescribed. If the pain is severe, hos-

pitalization and sedation may be necessary. You may be given drugs to relax your uterus to reduce the chance of premature labor. Sometimes amniocentesis is used to release some of the excess fluid. Although this relieves pain, it must be repeated often, and it can initiate premature labor.

Incompetent Cervix

If you have an incompetent cervix, the mouth (lower portion) of your uterus opens during the second trimester or early part of the third trimester. The result is a miscarriage or premature delivery.

A woman with an incompetent cervix usually has a history of miscarriage, typically in the second trimester of pregnancy. The cervix usually does not open before the fourth month of pregnancy because the fetus is not sufficiently large to dilate it.

The cause of incompetent cervix is unknown, but the condition often is associated with trauma to the cervix after procedures such as dilatation and curettage and with abnormal development of the cervix (such as occurs with exposure to the synthetic estrogen hormone diethylstilbestrol, see page 186).

If your medical history indicates a possible incompetent cervix, surgery can be done to close your cervix during pregnancy. Called cerclage, the procedure is performed while you are under a general anesthetic, usually after the first trimester. Using strong thread, your physician will actually stitch around your cervix to close it to prevent you from expelling the fetus. After the operation you will be given drugs to reduce the chance that the procedure could have stimulated premature labor.

Cerclage is successful in 85 to 90 percent of cases. The thread is cut in your 9th month of pregnancy.

Late Pregnancy: The Third Trimester

During the third trimester of pregnancy, what seemed so far off just a few months ago is now within reach—almost.

No matter how well you have felt, this is probably the point when you ask, "When will it be over?" Your maternity clothes are getting tight. Your walk has given way to the pregnant waddle. You may notice stretch marks on your breasts and abdomen. Your feet and ankles may be so swollen that your shoes do not fit.

You may be exhausted. Somehow you cannot seem to get comfortable at night, and when you do the baby starts kicking. Finally, the kicking stops and you sleep an hour or two and then wake up with the uncontrollable urge to urinate. You awake the next morning, looking as though you have been up all night. But it is hard to find time to sleep. The easy days of middle pregnancy are over.

Many couples attend classes in preparation for childbirth during the last trimester of pregnancy. There you are taught about the birth process, given exercises to strengthen your pelvic muscles and to enable you to push more effectively, and taught relaxation and breathing techniques that may help to relieve some of the pain during labor. Many physicians recommend these classes even for women who know they want to use an anesthetic during labor and delivery.

Many women, particularly those who have previously miscarried in early pregnancy, understandably are relieved to reach the late stage of pregnancy. With proper treatment in a specialized neonatal unit, babies born after 30 weeks have a good chance of survival. However, barring any maternal disease that can make the environment of the womb harmful, there is no substitute for a full 9-month pregnancy. Thus, one of your physician's goals is to prevent premature labor whenever possible.

Your visits to the physician will be more frequent during the final trimester. Up until now, you probably have been seeing the physician every 4 to 6 weeks, unless you have a medical problem that warrants more frequent visits. After the 30th gestational week, your physician may want to see you every 2 weeks until the 36th week, when you will begin weekly visits. Toward the end of your pregnancy, your physician may perform a pelvic examination to see whether your cervix is beginning to dilate in preparation for labor.

The vast majority of women deliver near term and have no major complications. The problem of premature labor may occur in the third trimester as well as in the second (see page 201), but the later in pregnancy it occurs, the better the outlook for the infant.

However, there are some serious conditions associated with late pregnancy. Preeclampsia and eclampsia are dangerous conditions that, when not detected early, can cause both fetal and maternal death (see below). Other problems that your physician will be watching for include hemorrhage (see page 205), placenta previa (see page 205), premature rupture of membranes (see page 205), intrauterine death (see page 206), and intrauterine growth retardation (see page 179).

Preeclampsia and Eclampsia

Signs and Symptoms
- High blood pressure
- Protein in the urine
- Fluid retention that causes puffiness of the hands and face, particularly around the eyes
- Sudden and excessive weight gain
- Pain in the upper right side of the abdomen
- Severe headaches
- Severe convulsions
- Vision disturbances, including seeing flashing lights
- Unconsciousness

Preeclampsia can be a serious disease of late pregnancy. Eclampsia (seizures) is the next stage of the disease, occurring when the symptoms of preeclampsia (the first four listed above) are not brought under control.

These conditions are not as common as they once were, presumably because of improved prenatal care. Preeclampsia occurs in about 5 percent of all pregnancies, and the overall incidence of eclampsia is about 1 in 1,500 pregnancies.

Cause
Preeclampsia and eclampsia are called the toxemias of pregnancy, although thus far no one has been able to identify a toxic substance in a pregnant woman's blood that can cause these conditions. Hence, the cause remains unknown. As a result, there is no treatment that is universally effective. Physicians do know, however, how to diagnose the conditions and that some women appear to be at higher risk.

Diagnosis
If preeclampsia develops, you may not know it. Initially you may feel normal because hypertension and protein in the urine usually do not cause pain. (This is one of the reasons why it is so important to keep your prenatal appointments.) However, as the preeclampsia progresses, the other symptoms will occur.

How Serious Is Eclampsia?
Eclampsia is one of the most dangerous conditions of pregnancy. It can lead to hemorrhage in the brain, liver, or kidney, and it can be fatal for both the mother and her baby. Teenage mothers, women older than 40 years, women in their first pregnancy, women with a history of high blood pressure, and women who are carrying twins all are at higher risk for preeclampsia and eclampsia.

Treatment
If you have very mild preeclampsia, your physician may instruct you to eat a low-salt diet and tell you to rest in bed, lying on your left side as much as possible to take the weight of the uterus off your major blood vessels. These precautions will improve blood flow to your kidneys. Sometimes this is all the treatment that is necessary.

However, you may require hospitalization, during which you may be given medications for your hypertension and to avoid seizures. The goal in treating preeclampsia is to keep it from progressing in severity to eclampsia.

The best treatment for severe preeclampsia is delivery of the baby. If you are near term, your physician may induce labor or perform a cesarean section. If the fetus does not have a good chance of surviving at this stage in its gestation, many physicians will try to forestall labor if the preeclampsia is not too severe. You and your baby will both be monitored continuously to make sure neither of you is in distress.

After delivery, the symptoms of preeclampsia usually become less severe, although in some women eclampsia can still develop during the first 24 hours after delivery or, although rare, later.

Eclampsia is not the problem it once was. However, if eclampsia does occur, your physician will want you to deliver at once. Because of the availability of improved prenatal care, the vast majority of women with preeclampsia never progress to eclampsia.

Antepartum Hemorrhage

Signs and Symptoms—Vaginal bleeding after the fifth month of pregnancy

Cause

Many conditions can cause antepartum (pre-birth) hemorrhage in middle or late pregnancy, including placenta previa (see this page), cervical damage, or separation of the placenta from the uterine wall.

Diagnosis

Report any bleeding during pregnancy to your physician immediately. Your physician will want to determine the cause of the problem. You may need to be hospitalized and have an ultrasound examination and blood tests.

How Serious Is Antepartum Hemorrhage?

Most often, antepartum bleeding is mild and no damage is done. However, when this bleeding becomes heavy, it can be dangerous for both you and your baby.

Treatment

When there is substantial blood loss, blood transfusion is often necessary. Sometimes, when the hemorrhage poses a threat, early delivery of the infant, either by inducing labor or by cesarean section, is warranted.

Premature Rupture of Membranes

Signs and Symptoms—A gush or a constant dribble of fluid from the vagina

Normally, the membranes that surround the fetus rupture either just before labor or during labor. Occasionally, however, these membranes rupture weeks or months before the anticipated delivery date.

Cause

The cause of ruptured membranes usually remains a mystery.

Diagnosis

If your membranes rupture, call your physician immediately. You probably will be hospitalized. Amniocentesis (see page 181) may be done to determine whether your infant's lungs are mature enough for it to survive an early delivery.

How Serious Is Premature Rupture of the Membranes?

When premature rupture of your membranes occurs, there is a high risk that your labor will also begin within a few days—this is a dangerous prospect if you are in the middle of your pregnancy. Moreover, there is a risk of infection once the membranes have ruptured.

Treatment

If your baby's lungs are mature, your physician may give you drugs to induce labor.

If your baby is too immature to have a good chance of survival outside the womb, your physician may give you drugs to help stimulate fetal lung maturity and to relax the uterine muscles to decrease the chance of early delivery. This can be successful, but the risk of serious infection remains, so your condition must be monitored closely.

Placenta Previa

Signs and Symptoms—Painless bleeding from the vagina, usually at the end of the second trimester or later; often first occurs at night when you are asleep and usually stops on its own

Approximately 1 in 200 pregnancies that go beyond the seventh month have placenta previa. Uncommon in first pregnancies, placenta previa is more likely to occur with each subsequent pregnancy. Older mothers tend to be more at risk, as are women who have had cesarean sections.

Cause

In placenta previa, the placenta is not implanted high in the uterus but is located partially or completely over the cervix. Late in pregnancy as the uterus prepares for labor, the cervix expands and any placenta near it is torn loose. The result is a raw area that bleeds.

Diagnosis

If your physician suspects placenta previa, he or she will ask you to have an ultrasound examination.

How Serious Is Placenta Previa?

Bleeding from the placenta can cause fetal brain damage or even death.

Treatment

If you are close to your delivery date, your physician may want you to undergo a cesarean section to prevent further bleeding from the placenta. Blood transfusions may be necessary if the hemorrhage is severe.

Intrauterine Death

Most fetal deaths occur as miscarriages in the first weeks of pregnancy. Occasionally, however, a fetus will die after the fifth month of gestation.

Several conditions are responsible for intrauterine death, including preeclampsia and eclampsia (see page 204), maternal diabetes (see page 189), antepartum hemorrhage (see page 205), postmaturity (see this page), Rh disease (see page 192), and severe congenital abnormalities.

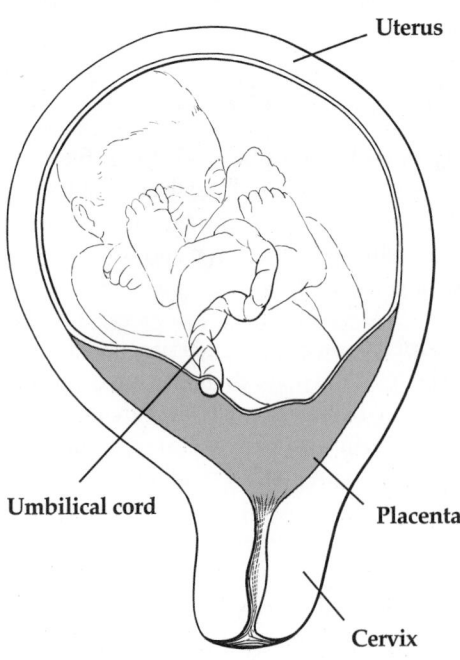

If the placenta is located over the cervix (placenta previa), painless hemorrhage may occur. If this happens, see your physician immediately.

Usually the death of a fetus is silent. One day you may notice that you do not feel the baby move like you used to. When the physician fails to detect a heartbeat, he or she will use monitoring techniques to determine whether the fetus is still alive (see page 210).

Most often, labor begins within 2 weeks after fetal death, although it may be longer in middle pregnancy. If your labor does not begin on its own, you will be given drugs to induce it. There is concern that if your labor is too overdue, you may develop blood clotting abnormalities that can set the stage for a life-threatening hemorrhage.

In most cases, the outlook for future pregnancies is the same as for first pregnancies. The biggest hurdle is the grief that every couple must work through after an intrauterine death (see Grief Responses, page 1109).

Postmaturity (Prolonged Pregnancy)

Signs and Symptoms—Labor and delivery that fail to occur by 42 weeks of pregnancy

The average pregnancy lasts 40 weeks from the onset of the last menstrual period. "Postmaturity" describes a pregnancy that is prolonged beyond 42 weeks.

How Serious Is Postmaturity?

As with prematurity, postmaturity can be dangerous. The overdue infant is living with an aging placenta that often fails to provide adequate oxygen. Moreover, the infant may be getting larger than a newborn is supposed to be, which may make delivery extremely difficult. Or fetal growth may be halted altogether by the increasingly harmful womb environment, and the infant may be literally starving to death. As a result, the stillbirth rate of these babies is twice that of those born after a pregnancy of normal length.

Treatment

If your pregnancy continues after 42 weeks, your physician probably will induce labor, provided he or she is sure that the baby is indeed overdue and there has not been a mistake in calculating the time of conception. If the baby is very large, mechanical assistance may be needed during the delivery or a cesarean section may be performed.

Labor and Delivery

How Will I Know When Labor Begins?

That is sometimes a difficult question because each woman and each pregnancy are different. Maybe this is your first child, and you are confused by friends and relatives who tell you that labor will be the toughest hours of your life or that it will not be so bad. Perhaps you have already borne a child and you expect this labor to be similar to your previous one. Whatever you expect, expect the unexpected.

Every labor is slightly different. But there are some good indicators that labor is beginning or about ready to begin.

1. A few days or hours before labor actually begins, you may have what is called "bloody show." This is the discharge of a small amount of blood-tinged mucus. Actually, it is the mucus plug that formed the barrier between your uterus and your vagina during your pregnancy.

2. The membranes that surround the amniotic fluid may rupture at the beginning of labor or as the labor progresses. If the membranes fail to rupture during labor, the physician ruptures them. When your membranes (sometimes called "bag of waters") rupture, you may feel a gush of fluid from your vagina or simply a slow trickle.

3. Contractions may or may not be a sign that you are in labor. Throughout pregnancy, you may have noticed your uterus contracting. These are called Braxton Hicks contractions, and they usually do not cause discomfort until the last weeks of pregnancy. Many women then have these contractions and believe they are in labor. It is often difficult for pregnant women to distinguish between these Braxton Hicks contractions (false labor) and those of real labor.

As a rule, the contractions of real labor occur at regular intervals. The period between contractions slowly begins to get shorter, and the contractions become longer and more intense. The pain usually begins high in the uterus and then radiates down the abdomen and to the lower back.

If you have any of these signs, notify your physician. Your physician may want to examine you to see whether your cervix is dilating and thinning (effacing), signs that the baby is getting ready to be born. If your membranes rupture, your physician probably will want you to go to the hospital immediately.

How Long Will Labor Be?

That is a common question and one that is impossible to predict with any accuracy until your physician can determine how quickly your cervix is readying itself.

As a rule, labor usually is longer with first babies. The uterus and birth canal of a first-time mother are less flexible, and as such it takes longer for labor and birth. A first-time mother generally can expect about 13 hours to pass between the time she goes into active labor and the birth of her baby. Some women, however, are in labor much longer.

For a woman who has previously given birth, the average time is between 4 and 8 hours.

The three stages of labor are described here.

First Stage
During the first stage your cervix opens so that the baby can pass into the birth canal. Think of the uterus as a large, upside-down, elastic bottle. When labor begins, the cervix is about ½ inch in diameter and almost closed. It would be impossible for a baby to pass through such a small opening, so somehow the cervix has to open.

Contractions cause the cervix to open (dilate) by creating pressure within the uterus. This force is tremendous and is directed against the uterus in two ways. During a contraction, the infant is subjected to an intense pressure that forces it against the cervix. These repeated attempts eventually will stretch the cervix open. The cervix is said to be fully dilated when it is open to a diameter of 4 inches. At the same time, the contractions cause the cervix to become thinned (effaced) or to merge with the uterine walls.

During the first stage of labor, your contractions will become more frequent and last longer. You may be attached to a machine that monitors your infant's heart rate and charts the onset and cessation of each contraction. Your physician or a nurse periodically will do a pelvic examination to determine how you are progressing. When the contractions are not forceful enough to open the cervix, a drug may be given to make your uterus contract.

Some women go through the entire labor with no pain medication. These women usually have taken classes in prepared childbirth and learned breathing techniques. Many women find that they need some pain relief, however, particularly as they get closer to full dilation. If you need something for the pain, do not be afraid to ask your physician.

Prolonged Labor

Sometimes labor drags on without much progress. When this occurs, it is usually because the contractions are poorly coordinated, the contractions are not strong enough, or there is some obstruction.

If the cause is inadequate contractions, the uterus can be stimulated to contract by the intravenous infusion of a medication. This is successful in most cases. In some cases, a cesarean section is necessary.

Conditions that obstruct delivery include a head that is too large to pass down the birth canal or a fetal head position that makes delivery difficult. In these cases, either a cesarean section or a vaginal delivery with forceps usually is done.

What Is False Labor?

Many women have one or more bouts of false labor before real labor begins. False labor is more likely to occur in the final weeks of pregnancy and in women who have already borne a child.

How can you distinguish false labor from true labor? With false labor you will have contractions, but they will be irregular and will not increase in frequency and intensity, as true contractions do. Moreover, the pain will be in the lower abdomen and groin, whereas true labor pains begin higher in the uterus and then radiate throughout the abdomen and lower back. When your labor is false, walking may stop the contractions, whereas with true labor, walking generally has no effect.

If you suspect you are in labor, call your physician. A pelvic examination can ascertain whether your cervix is beginning to dilate, a sign of true labor.

Above all, do not dismiss your symptoms without seeking medical advice. Many pregnant women have postponed going to the hospital, convinced it was only a false alarm, only to end up giving birth before reaching the hospital.

Second Stage

The second stage of labor is when your baby is born. Your cervix is now fully dilated and effaced. This is the baby's signal to start the 5-inch journey down the birth canal. Now that the cervix offers no resistance, each contraction serves to propel the infant downward. You may feel a tremendous urge to push, almost as though you want to have a bowel movement. You must wait, however, until instructed to do so by your physician or nurse. Sometimes this urge to push comes before the cervix is fully dilated.

Push only when you are having a contraction. In this way two forces—that of the contraction and your pushing—combine to move the baby, which conserves your energy.

Both the first and the second stages of labor are longer for first-time mothers. On the average it takes about 1 to 2 hours to push a first baby out, whereas women who have previously given birth usually complete the second stage in anywhere from 15 to 40 minutes.

As you push and the baby begins to move, the vaginal opening becomes more and more dilated and begins to bulge. At this point you might be moved from the labor room to the delivery room. In some hospitals, all stages of labor and delivery occur in specially equipped rooms called birthing rooms. If the vaginal opening does not provide adequate room for the baby to be born and it appears that your tissues may tear, your physician may give you a local anesthetic and then make an incision (an episiotomy) at the opening of the vagina. This will create a larger opening for delivery of the infant (see Labor and Delivery Procedures, page 210).

After you have pushed the baby's head out, you will be instructed to stop pushing for a moment while your physician clears the baby's airway. A few more pushes and your baby is born.

The umbilical cord that connects the baby to the placenta is cut and your baby is examined, weighed, and cleaned.

Third Stage

The third stage of labor is delivery of the placenta. Your uterus will continue to contract to expel it, but you should not feel any great pain.

Abnormal Fetal Positions

Most babies are born head first, with the face toward the mother's back. This position is called occiput anterior. It allows for the easiest passage through the birth canal.

An estimated 4 percent of babies, however, enter the world in other positions, some of which are potentially dangerous and warrant special measures during labor and delivery.

Breech

Breech presentation is the most common of the abnormal positions. If your baby is breech, it is positioned with its buttocks near your cervix. Thus, either the buttocks or feet emerge first instead of the head.

Breech births are particularly common in premature infants because many babies do not assume the correct position until the last few weeks or even days of pregnancy. Other factors that predispose some women to breech birth include multiple fetuses, uterine abnormalities, tumors, hydramnios (see page 202), and placenta previa (see page 205).

If your infant is in the breech position in the last weeks of pregnancy, your physician may attempt to turn the baby externally. If the baby does not turn before labor, most physicians perform a cesarean section, which usually results in a healthier infant but offers a slight increase in risk to the mother.

Transverse

Transverse presentation occurs when the long axis of the infant's body is at right angles to the long axis of the mother's body, usually with the shoulder over the birth canal.

This presentation is more common in women who have had four or more children. Prematurity and placenta previa are other conditions associated with the transverse presentation.

Vaginal delivery is impossible when a live infant is in the transverse position. There is a real danger that the umbilical cord will become obstructed and cut off the infant's oxygen supply. Moreover, an infant in this position cannot move through the birth canal.

Cesarean section should be performed either before active labor begins or just after. If a woman is allowed to labor too long, both she and her baby are at increased risk because of uterine rupture and the chance of cord damage.

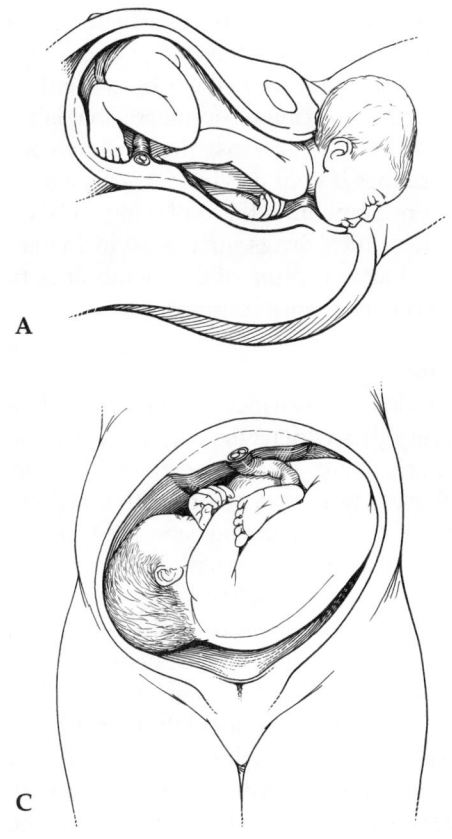

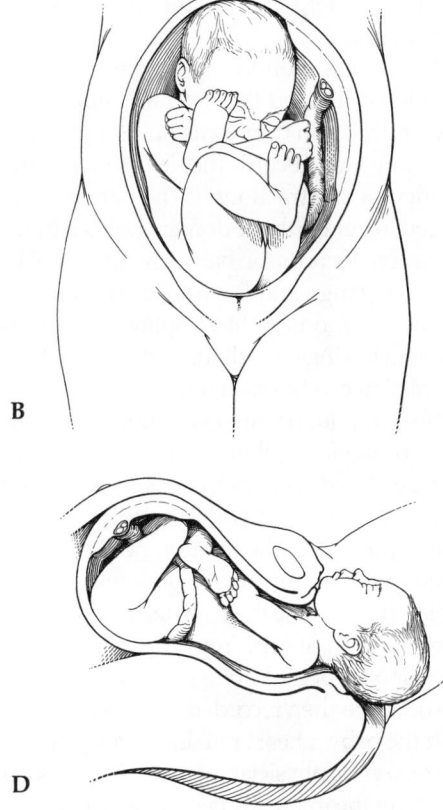

A

B

C

D

At the time of delivery, the normal position for the unborn baby is head first (A), with the face toward the mother's back. This position is called occiput anterior. Other presentations include breech (B), transverse (C), and occiput posterior (D).

Occiput Posterior

Occiput posterior position is when the infant's head is positioned near the cervix but its face is toward the mother's front. This presentation makes it difficult for the infant to travel down the birth canal.

This position can delay labor, especially if the infant is large. Forceps often are used for an occiput posterior presentation. Sometimes a cesarean section is necessary.

Labor and Delivery Procedures

Electronic Fetal Monitoring

Electronic fetal monitoring is commonly used to continuously record the unborn baby's heartbeat during labor.

Fetal monitoring also may be done before labor when the mother has a medical problem that may jeopardize the fetus (see page 179).

As the uterus contracts during labor, there is a temporary reduction in the flow of blood through the placenta. Most fetuses tolerate this without problem, but if the fetus is otherwise compromised and in danger, its heart rate will drop. Thus, many physicians use fetal monitoring during all labors as a precaution to help ensure the safety of the unborn infant.

In external monitoring, two wide straps are placed around the mother's abdomen. The one high on the uterus holds a gauge to measure and record the length and frequency of contractions. The other strap, placed lower on the abdomen, holds a transducer that records the baby's heart rate. The pressure gauge and the transducer are connected to a monitor that displays and prints out both tracings simultaneously so that their interaction can be observed.

If during labor there is a concern for the labor or the fetus, then an internal monitor may be placed. An electrode will be inserted through your vagina onto the baby's scalp. This is done after the membranes have ruptured. At the same time, a pressure catheter is placed alongside the fetal head into the top portion of the uterus. Your contractions and the response of the baby's heart to these contractions are then recorded.

If the baby's heart rate indicates possible distress, your physician may decide it is safer to deliver the infant immediately by cesarean section.

Fetal Blood Sampling

Another method of helping to identify a fetus in distress during labor is by extracting a sample of fetal blood and measuring its alkaline or acid content (pH). If your physician suspects your baby is getting an inadequate amount of oxygen, he or she may perform this test.

A tube called an endoscope will be inserted through your dilated cervix to the baby's skin, usually the scalp. A couple of incisions are then made in the skin and a small amount of blood is drawn into a tube. The pH of the blood is measured. If the pH is lower than normal, you may need an immediate cesarean section.

Induction of Labor

Sometimes it is necessary to start (induce) labor. Although there are cases in which labor is induced because of convenience—either the physician's or the mother's—this is not recommended. Most labor inductions occur because the mother, baby, or both are in danger if the pregnancy continues.

The most common medical reasons for inducing labor include preeclampsia and eclampsia (see page 204) and premature rupture of the membranes, which makes infection a risk (see page 205). Labor also may be induced when the fetus is in distress as a result of its mother's preeclampsia, eclampsia, or diabetes or when the baby is overdue.

If your physician recommends that labor be induced, he or she may first rupture your membranes if your cervix shows no sign of dilation. Sometimes this will bring on labor. At other times, drugs such as oxytocin may be used after rupture of the membranes to bring on or enhance contractions.

Episiotomy

An episiotomy is an incision made just before delivery that widens the vagina so that the mother's tissues are not damaged. This surgical procedure is often done with first pregnancies, during premature labor, and when a forceps delivery is necessary.

If your physician believes your vagina will be torn during delivery, he or she will inject a local anesthetic into the area between your vagina and rectum. An incision is then made just before the emergence of the baby's head.

After the delivery, the incision is sutured with stitches that will dissolve. You may have some pain for a while. The pain can be relieved with hot baths or ice packs, pain medication, and sprays that contain a local anesthetic.

Forceps

Forceps are two blunt blades that resemble a pair of tongs. They are used to pull the baby out of the vagina when the delivery is not progressing as it should or when there are signs of fetal distress.

Reasons for using forceps include an umbilical cord that has preceded the baby down the birth canal, an infant who is too large to pass through the birth canal unaided, a breech birth, or signs of asphyxia (oxygen deprivation). Sometimes use of forceps may be necessary when a woman does not have the strength to push the baby out.

If a forceps delivery is necessary, you will have an episiotomy. You also will be given an anesthetic.

Complications from forceps deliveries are relatively rare. Occasionally, temporary bruises to an infant's face and nerve damage occur. However, when used by a skilled obstetrician or family physician, forceps have saved the lives of many babies.

Vacuum Extraction

The vacuum extractor was designed as an alternative method to replace forceps.

A metal or silicone cup is fitted over the baby's head. A pump is used to attach the vacuum extractor to the baby's head. Grasping the handle on the cup, the physician can then move the baby's head to a better position and pull the baby out of the birth canal. Occasionally there is some bruising under the infant's scalp; this resolves in several days.

Pain Relief

The vast majority of women—80 to 90 percent—choose to use some type of pain medication during the birthing process. What you decide to use, if anything, depends on your informed preferences, your physician's recommendations, what is available at the medical facility you have chosen, and the specific character of your labor. Learn about the different options ahead of time so you can make knowledgeable choices regarding pain medication. Be sure to remain flexible, however, because you may need to change your mind if things don't go as intended.

All medications involve some risk. The risks must be weighed against the desire to relieve pain.

Narcotics

Narcotics offer reasonable pain relief, do not interfere with your ability to push, and can be given as an injection or intravenously. However, they have a sedative effect and often are not as effective as expected. They also can cause nausea and vomiting, dizziness, itching, and occasionally respiratory problems. Because narcotics can slow the baby's respirations at birth, they aren't given too close to the time of delivery. Should the baby be affected by narcotics, however, medications to counter their effect can be given immediately after birth.

Local Anesthetics

A "local" is a medication that is injected directly into tissues, much as a dentist numbs your mouth before drilling. The simplest local used during the birthing process is one that numbs you before an episiotomy is made or repaired. A local anesthetic before an episiotomy has no effect on the baby, nor does it provide pain relief for labor. Injections at other sites have more widespread effects.

Paracervical Block

A paracervical block is an injection into the tissues around the cervix that relieves the pain of uterine contractions and cervical stretching during early labor. Today, because of the increased use of epidural or spinal anesthetics (see below), paracervical blocks are not often used.

Pudendal Block

A pudendal block is injected into the vaginal wall and the ligaments supporting the pelvic floor. Because it affects just the vagina and rectum, and gives no pain relief to the uterus or cervix, it is used only for the later part of labor and for episiotomy.

Epidural and Spinal Blocks

In these increasingly popular procedures, the anesthetic is injected into the space surrounding the spinal nerves, temporarily blocking pain from the chest level down. These blocks are used for labor as well as for episiotomy and cesarean birth. Their use, however, requires the services of an anesthesiologist.

Epidural and spinal anesthesia are the most effective forms of anesthesia for childbirth. You can receive almost total pain relief but still be awake, alert, and able to enjoy your baby's birth. However, you must remain in bed with an IV and a fetal monitor in place. Any regional anesthetic can be an additional expense.

Cesarean Delivery

A cesarean delivery is birth by a surgical procedure that involves incisions through the abdomen and into the uterus. The infant is then lifted out.

Shakespeare was familiar with cesarean delivery: it was basic to the plot of the play Macbeth. Macbeth had been told by an apparition that "none of woman born shall harm Macbeth"—but he later learned that Macduff had been "from his mother's womb untimely ripp'd." Thus, he became Macbeth's slayer.

Although for many centuries cesarean delivery was an accepted procedure for attempting to save the baby after the mother's death, it was not until anesthesia and aseptic surgery were developed in the 19th century that the procedure became feasible as a means of saving both the baby and the mother in a difficult childbirth. In fact, although childbirth through cesarean delivery was once an operation of last resort, today it accounts for more than 20 percent of all births in the United States. Even though many critics think the pendulum has swung too far, there is no doubt that many women and babies are alive today because this alternative to vaginal delivery was available.

When Is a Cesarean Delivery Necessary?

Many conditions call for a cesarean delivery. Some premature infants tend to have a better chance of survival when delivered in this way. Infants in breech or other abnormal positions (see page 209) more often than not are delivered by cesarean delivery. When the infant is too large or the mother's birth canal is unusually small, a cesarean delivery is the only safe way to deliver. Sometimes abnormalities of the uterus or vagina obstruct the birth canal and necessitate this operation. If a mother has preeclampsia, diabetes, genital herpes, or hypertension and the fetus is having trouble, a cesarean delivery may be indi-

cated. Placental abnormalities such as placenta previa often require cesarean delivery. In the event of twins or multiple fetuses, many physicians advise this procedure. When labor is prolonged because of insufficient uterine contractions, many physicians believe a cesarean delivery is better for both the mother and the baby.

Some believe that the procedure is done too often and that physicians do a cesarean delivery whenever they are faced with the possibility of a difficult birth, just to make sure that all precautions have been taken. Some of this so-called defensive medicine is practiced, but the threat of a lawsuit is not the reason for most cesarean births.

Improved fetal monitoring techniques now provide vital information about the health of the fetus and its ability to withstand labor and delivery. If it appears that the fetus may be jeopardized, most physicians are quick to perform a cesarean delivery. At the same time, improvements in the operation itself, in anesthesia, and in antibiotics make the procedure safer for the mother than it once was.

In addition, more women are postponing pregnancy until later in life. These women and their infants are at higher risk of medical complications than their younger counterparts. Hence, cesarean births in this group are more common.

The need for a cesarean section with a subsequent pregnancy will depend upon the type of uterine incision (how high the incision extends into the top of the uterus) and whether the circumstances that led to the first cesarean section recur.

Procedure

If you need a cesarean delivery, you will be given an anesthetic. Unless the procedure is being done because of an emergency—in which case you will be put to sleep with a general anesthetic—you will have either epidural or spinal anesthesia (see page 211), which allows you to remain awake without feeling pain. Many hospitals now allow your partner to be in the operating room, unless you are having an emergency cesarean.

It takes a little less than an hour to perform a cesarean delivery. Two types of incisions into the abdomen can be used. One is the so-called bikini cut, which is a horizontal incision near the pubic hair line. The other is a vertical cut from the navel to the pubis.

Once the incision reaches the uterus, one of two commonly used incisions can be made. The most common method is a horizontal incision in the lower part of the uterus, called a lower uterine transverse incision. This incision heals better and is associated with less chance of uterine rupture at a subsequent pregnancy. On occasion, the physician will use a vertical incision to open the uterus. This incision allows more access to your uterus and is used, for example, when an infant is large or when an infant is known to have an abnormally large head (see Hydrocephalus, page 54).

After the uterus is opened, the baby is delivered from the womb. The placenta is then removed, and the uterus and incision are stitched closed.

Complications

Although cesarean delivery is safer than it used to be and most women recover well, there can be complications. It is a major operation and, as with any other one, there is a risk of infection at the surgical site as well as bladder and kidney infections. Hemorrhage is rare, but when it does occur it can be severe.

The death rate for women who have a cesarean delivery is 2 to 4 times higher than that for women who have a vaginal delivery. Many of the women who die, however, were ill before the operation.

Recovery

From an emotional standpoint, a cesarean delivery can be difficult because it can impede bonding with your new baby. Initially you will feel groggy and be in pain, and so you are less likely to want to spend time with the baby.

After the procedure, you will be encouraged to try to move around your room on the same day. You can eat a regular diet when you have an appetite. You can hold your baby and begin breastfeeding just as you would if you had delivered your baby vaginally.

The average hospital stay after a cesarean delivery is between 4 and 5 days.

Future Pregnancies

Women who have had a cesarean naturally wonder about the next pregnancy. Formerly, once you had a cesarean, you always had one for subsequent births. This was done because of the risk of the uterine scar rupturing during labor, which occurred in about 2 out of 100 births.

Twins and Multiple Pregnancies

What are the chances that you are expecting twins? If you are Asian, you are much less likely to have a multiple birth than if you are African-American. A teenager has a 1 in 167 chance of having twins, and the rate for a 40-year-old woman is 1 in 55. The more children you have, the greater your likelihood of producing twins. Finally, fraternal twins simply run in some families.

Twin pregnancies account for 1 in 90 births in the United States; triplets occur in 1 of 8,000 pregnancies.

A multiple pregnancy occurs when either more than one egg is fertilized or the one egg splits after fertilization. Seven of 10 pairs of twins are fraternal, meaning they came from two eggs and two sperm.

In about 7 of 10 cases, your physician will discover you are carrying multiple fetuses before labor. Abnormal weight gain or size, an excessive amount of movement, and the detection of two heartbeats are common clues. If your physician suspects twins, he or she will order an ultrasound examination.

If you are expecting twins, you need to take especially good care of yourself. Try to increase the amount of rest you get, take in more calories, and be diligent about your prenatal visits; adherence to your prenatal checkup schedule is especially important because the incidence of preeclampsia and eclampsia (see page 204), placenta previa (see page 205), and hemorrhage is higher when you are carrying multiple fetuses.

Multiple pregnancies tend to be shorter, an average of 21 days shorter for women delivering twins. Unless there is a medical reason to indicate cesarean delivery, twins can be delivered vaginally. And a woman who wants to breastfeed can do so.

Now, however, as many as 60 percent of women who have had a previous cesarean delivery may be able to have a vaginal delivery subsequently. This depends on the initial reason for the operation and on whether the condition is still present. For example, if the cesarean section was done because of fetal distress, your next baby may be able to withstand labor and a vaginal delivery. Alternatively, if your pelvis is unusually small, all your future deliveries probably will have to be cesarean.

The other factors that determine whether you can try a vaginal delivery are the type of uterine incision that was made and whether the postoperative course for the first cesarean delivery was free of infection. If your uterine scar is the horizontal type (lower uterine transverse incision), you may be a candidate for vaginal delivery.

Postpartum Hemorrhage

Signs and Symptoms—Continued heavy vaginal bleeding after delivery

Postpartum hemorrhage is the excessive loss of blood after delivery. This is the most common type of serious obstetrical hemorrhage.

Cause

One of the most common causes of postpartum hemorrhage is the inability of the uterus to contract firmly enough to control the bleeding that occurs when the placenta separates from the uterus. This inability often is the result of uterine muscles being exhausted or weak.

Other causes of postpartum hemorrhage include trauma to the vaginal wall from an episiotomy or lacerations, uterine rupture, and retention of part of the placenta. The risk of postpartum hemorrhage increases with the delivery of an excessively large baby or more than one infant, a forceps delivery, vaginal delivery after a previous cesarean section, several previous deliveries, labor that has been induced with drugs, and hydramnios (see page 202).

How Serious Is Postpartum Hemorrhage?

If you have postpartum hemorrhage, the bleeding may be massive or just a steady seepage over a period of hours. Sometimes the blood does not escape through the vagina but collects inside the uterus, causing the uterus to become distended.

Treatment

Postpartum hemorrhage usually can be controlled with drugs that make the uterus contract. If this treatment does not stop the bleeding, your physician will do a pelvic examination. Any torn tissues will be repaired after a local anesthetic is administered.

When the bleeding cannot be brought under control, the body's ability to form clots may be jeopardized. You may be given medications that help your blood clot.

Surgery

An abdominal operation may be necessary if no cause can be found. The first step is tying off the major blood vessels that feed your uterus. If this is successful, the bleeding will stop and your ability to have more children will not be hampered.

If the hemorrhage continues, the uterus must be removed.

Retained Placenta

Signs and Symptoms—A placenta that does not emerge from the birth canal within 30 minutes of the delivery of the baby

Normally, the placenta is delivered after the baby. The physician presses on your abdomen and pulls on the umbilical cord to expel the placenta. A retained placenta is one that is trapped in the uterus after delivery, often because it has not separated completely from the uterine wall.

Treatment

Sometimes the physician has to peel the placenta from the uterine wall manually. You may need extra anesthesia during this procedure.

After any delivery, it is important that the uterus remain contracted because of the possibility of hemorrhage. Techniques such as uterine massage through the abdomen and breastfeeding help the uterus contract. When these measures are insufficient, certain drugs help stimulate uterine contractions.

After Pregnancy

No doubt you will feel a great sense of relief after giving birth to a healthy baby. Accompanying that relief, however, is a whole new set of responsibilities and worries. There are decisions to make and no doubt more than a few problems and hurdles to deal with during the ensuing months.

In the chapter titled Newborn: The First Month of Life, many of the health matters concerning your baby are discussed in detail (see page 3). However, you also may confront a few matters pertaining largely to your health. You may experience postpartum depression, you may still be unsure about whether to breastfeed or bottle-feed, and you may have questions about sexual activity after birth. These and other matters are discussed in the following pages.

Breastfeeding

The feeding of your newborn baby occupies a considerable portion of your time. The first chapter of this book, Newborn: The First Month of Life (see page 3), discusses breastfeeding and bottle-feeding. The section that follows here discusses what you will experience when you nurse.

The vast majority of women are physically capable of breastfeeding. Some small-breasted women automatically assume they will not be able to produce enough milk for a baby. This is not true, because breastfeeding has nothing to do with breast size.

During pregnancy your breasts are preparing to produce milk. The hormones estrogen and progesterone are produced by the placenta and promote the growth of special breast tissue designed to produce milk. At the same time, these hormones suppress the release of prolactin, a hormone produced by the pituitary gland. Your breasts will slowly increase in size, and the nipples will change, becoming thinner, darker, and more prominent.

After the delivery of the placenta, release of the hormone prolactin is triggered. The result of this surge is the production of colostrum, a thin, sticky fluid that fills the breasts.

Besides being a wonderful way to begin bonding with your baby, breastfeeding has several other advantages. The colostrum contains antibodies to resist viruses and bacteria. By nursing, your infant gets the benefits of your body's immune system.

After your baby is born, you probably will be able to breastfeed immediately. The baby's suckling stimulates production of the pituitary hormone oxytocin, which helps contract the uterus. The result is that your uterus returns to its normal size more quickly than usual. Nursing also can help prevent postpartum hemorrhage of the uterus.

The oxytocin also stimulates contraction of the muscles that surround the milk ducts, and this contraction releases the milk into storage areas behind the nipples. This is called the "let-down" reflex.

About 1 or 2 days after delivery, your breasts may feel engorged and uncomfortable. They will be much larger than usual, tender, and firm. You may notice prominent veins appearing. These are normal changes caused by increased fluid to the breast, an increased blood flow, and a greater volume of milk. The best cure for this discomfort is a hungry baby.

As your baby nurses more and empties your breasts, your discomfort will diminish.

For the discomfort of excessive swelling (engorgement), put ice packs on your breasts between feedings. You also can use mild pain relievers. A bra that fits properly will provide support and comfort.

The initial days and weeks of breastfeeding can be trying under the best of circumstances. Relaxing with your baby may be difficult. Take advantage of the soothing effect breastfeeding has on you and your baby. Learn to pay attention to your body's cues. If you feel sleepy, take a nap or nurse your baby while lying comfortably. If you're thirsty, get something to drink. If you're hungry, eat nutritious foods. If your baby cries, recognize that your first instinct is to feed your baby. Follow that instinct.

It is not uncommon for a new mother to wonder whether she is producing enough milk for her baby. You probably are. If your baby is gaining weight and has at least six wet diapers and two or more stools during a 24-hour period, you can assume that the amount is adequate.

Nutrition and Lactation
Adequate milk production can be maintained over a wide range of the mother's eating practices. Whether or not you have gained an appropriate amount of weight during the pregnancy or your baby's birth weight is normal, the chances for successful lactation are excellent.

Dietary Guidelines
Lactation is a physiologic completion of the reproductive cycle. During pregnancy, your body prepares for breastfeeding by storing additional nutrients and energy. After your baby arrives, you will notice an increase in appetite and thirst and a change in dietary preferences.

The need to follow special dietary rules to breastfeed is unfounded. Eat a variety of foods and nutritious snacks between meals. Drink fluids to satisfy your thirst.

You cannot increase your milk volume by drinking additional fluids. You do not need to drink milk to make milk, but you do need to consume 1,200 mg of calcium daily from some source. A few babies may react to dairy products consumed by their mothers or to foods to which a member of their immediate family is intolerant.

Your physician may recommend that you continue taking your prenatal vitamins during lactation. Avoid crash diets to lose weight. A gradual weight loss of 1 to 4 pounds monthly is safe and healthy.

Weaning

Weaning may be mother- or baby-led. Ideally it is a joint decision. Gradual weaning is best both physically and emotionally for both mother and baby. Start by eliminating one feeding. When your breasts have reduced production, eliminate the next feeding and so on until the weaning process is complete. Abrupt weaning can result in engorged breasts.

Breast Problems

During the postpartum period you may have problems with your breasts. These are some that you may encounter.

Engorgement

Early, frequent, and lengthy nursing helps prevent engorgement. Some engorgement is normal. However, increased fluid and accumulation of milk in the breasts can lead to severe engorgement. Hard, swollen, painful breasts result. If your breasts are only moderately engorged, position your baby carefully and increase feedings. For severe engorgement, warm soaks and hand expression may soften your breast and help to get your baby attached for feeding. Cold packs between feeds can help reduce swelling. For unmanageable engorgement, call your lactation consultant or other health care provider.

Cracked Nipples

Cracked nipples most often occur from poor position of the baby at the breast. Correcting the position problem is the first step for healing. Applying expressed breast milk to the damaged areas will aid healing and provide antibacterial protection. It is not clear whether creams aid in the healing process. Softening scabs with warm soaks may also help.

Blocked Milk Duct

A blocked milk duct appears as a small, hard lump in your breast. Sometimes the lump will disappear on its own, or you can use hot water compresses, massage your breast, and extend the length of breastfeeding sessions on the affected side.

Infectious Mastitis

Infectious mastitis occurs when a bacterium, most commonly *Staphylococcus aureus*, enters the breast. Part of the breast becomes red and is hard and hot. You may feel unusually tired and have joint pains, chills, and a high fever.

If you have infectious mastitis, you will be given antibiotics. Continue nursing and increase fluids and rest. You may be more comfortable nursing your baby more often. The antibiotics you are taking will not hurt your infant, although you may notice a change in the color of the baby's stool.

With treatment, mastitis usually clears up within a few days. If it is untreated, an abscess may form, which will require surgical drainage (see Breast Infections, page 1160).

Postpartum Depression and Stress

The "Blues"

Having a baby is a powerful, exciting, frightening, joyous, and awe-inspiring event. In the days that follow, you may be surprised and confused about the many and varied emotions you experience. Having easily handled family and work responsibilities, as a new parent you may feel incompetent and overwhelmed with new responsibilities. Be patient with yourself as you make this transition and give yourself credit for how well you are doing.

Common to 80 percent of new mothers (no statistics for new fathers) is a mild depression called "baby blues." This mild form of distress usually occurs a few days to weeks after birth. It is self-limiting, resolving spontaneously in a few weeks. During this time you may have feelings of sadness, anger, anxiety, irritability, and incompetence. New moms often experience uncontrollable teariness for no identifiable reason. Lack of energy and inability to sleep may cause you to re-identify priorities. Some mothers are surprised by occasional negative throughts they may have about their baby and may interpret this as being a "bad" mother. It can be comforting to know that the baby blues are normal.

In addition to accepting mild depression as a normal part of birth, taking care of yourself by getting adequate rest, eating a nutritious diet, exercising in moderation, and having a social support system will help you toward resolution. Listen and respond to your body's cues for rest. Adequate rest has a significant impact on your emotional, as well as physical, well-being. Try sleeping during the day, when your baby sleeps, to synchronize rest periods. Babies need well-rested parents to care for them. You will know you need more rest when things that didn't bother you before are now perceived as insurmountable events. Accepting assistance from others is sometimes difficult, but it may be just what you need for maintaining a positive and realistic emotional perspective.

Good nutrition provides nutrients your body needs for recovery from childbirth. A few small meals a day may be more comfortable for you than three large meals. Choose fruits and vegetables for snacking to assist with weight control.

Light exercise can be helpful. Take a brisk, 30-minute walk 3 times each week. Your walking should slightly elevate your heart rate. You may enjoy your walk more if you take your baby with you in a baby carrier. Stretching and flexing as you play and talk to your baby will help tone your muscles. Your mind will feel better when your body feels good.

As with pregnancy and delivery, a strong social support system will continue to be valuable. The fatigue, emotional upheaval, and interruptions a new baby brings can strain the best of relationships. With the birth of your baby, your husband may feel left out as you focus your energy on caring for your baby. Crying babies evoke a protective and "fix it" response in the father toward the baby and the mother. However, for the mother, biologic changes take place that elicit an urge to comfort the baby and increase blood flow to the breasts. Fathers who keep this in mind as the mother takes full control of bundling, rocking, and soothing the baby, or repeats what the father has just done, will not perceive her behavior as thinking he is incompetent.

Another normal part of the recovery process is to relive the birth process by sharing your childbirth experience with others.

Sex After Birth

Most couples want to know when they can resume sexual intercourse after the birth of a baby. There is some variation, but most physicians recommend not resuming intercourse too soon. The vagina of a woman who has just given birth has been through some trauma. It has been stretched, cut, and possibly torn. Under the best of circumstances, it is bound to be tender.

Thus, many physicians recommend waiting 3 or 4 weeks before having intercourse. Some ask their patients to wait until after their postnatal examination, which generally occurs 6 weeks after birth. During this time you and your physician can discuss contraceptive methods so that you are not faced with an untimely pregnancy.

Having family and friends who truly listen and accept your feelings can greatly lessen your depressive symptoms.

Postpartum Depression

A more severe form of the blues, called postpartum depression, occurs in approximately 10 to 20 percent of new mothers. Symptoms are more intense and longer lasting than those of the blues and can occur any time within the first year. Additional symptoms could include constant fatigue, lack of joy in life, a sense of numbness, withdrawal from family and friends, lack of concern for self or baby, severe insomnia, overconcern for the baby, loss of sexual responsiveness, strong sense of failure and inadequacy, and severe mood swings. You may have high expectations and be overdemanding, have difficulty making sense of things, or feel trapped.

Inform your health care provider early if even a few of these symptoms are identified by you or other caring family members or friends. Early intervention may result in a more rapid recovery. Treatment varies according to individual needs, but it may include counseling, antidepressant medication, hormone therapy, and vitamin B. Ask about a support group in your area.

Postpartum Psychosis

Another form of depression is postpartum psychosis. This relatively rare disorders calls for immediate consultation with your health care provider.

Again, emotional changes may begin days or weeks after childbirth. You may become severely depressed and may experience any of the following: acute anxiety, racing thoughts or conversation, fear of harming yourself or your baby, hallucinations, irrational thoughts or statements, paranoia, or hysteria. You may need to rely on others to recognize your need for intervention.

The goal of treatment is to keep you and your baby safe and to preserve your sense of competence as a parent while you recover.

Posttraumatic Stress Disorder

Posttraumatic stress disorder can occur in the postpartum period. It is a response to a real or perceived traumatic childbirth or unresolved past trauma—usually sexual in nature—which was triggered during childbirth. Symptoms are similar to those of postpartum depression, but the underlying cause is trauma-related. When sought early, counseling, sometimes in combination with medication and education in stress reduction, generally leads to recovery.

Summary

No single cause for these forms of depression has been identified. Contributing factors may include hormone changes, a perceived unsatisfactory birth experience, a sense of loss in no longer being pregnant, level of marital satisfaction, a baby with a high level of needs, lack of social support, exhaustion, and a family history of postpartum depression.

The transition to parenthood can be difficult at times, and experiencing depression, whether mild or severe, does not mean you have failed as a person or parent. Expect to recover as you learn new ways to balance your daily life and responsibilities. The process of defining your new identity as a parent and what that means for you can also bring with it an enrichment to your life you may never have thought possible.

Contraception

Some new mothers, particularly those who breastfeed, think they are somehow protected from pregnancy. Do not make this mistake.

Breastfeeding does temporarily impair fertility to some degree, and many breastfeeding mothers do not menstruate for several months or even until the baby is weaned. Still, you should not rely on breastfeeding to prevent pregnancy. Use some form of contraception.

The options for contraception are basically the same after delivery as they were before pregnancy (see Prevention of Pregnancy, page 170). However, factors such as nursing, irregular periods, and a change in vaginal size may necessitate a change in your method of contraception. One purpose of your postpartum examination (usually done about 6 weeks after delivery) is to discuss your contraceptive options and preferences.

If you have used a diaphragm and want to continue, do not assume your old one will do. Many women require a slightly larger diaphragm after giving birth. Take your pre-pregnancy diaphragm with you to your postpartum examination. Your physician can check whether it still fits and, if not, refit you.

Although the popularity of the intrauterine device has diminished because of serious side effects, which have led most manufacturers to cease production, many physicians will still fit former wearers with the device. If you want to use this method again, wait at least a month after the birth of your baby to have one inserted. If it is inserted before the uterus is firm, it may fall out.

Many women want to resume taking birth control pills, the most effective contraceptive available. Is it safe for a nursing mother? There is no doubt that the use of some pills, most often the combination of estrogen and progestin pills, will somewhat reduce the milk supply in as many as a third of women who use this method. The reduction, however, is usually only temporary, and it is not thought to be a major deterrent to using the pill. Moreover, if you take the pill, your baby also is getting some of these hormones. Again, the amount is thought to be insignificant. The low-dose pills do not tend to reduce the milk supply. However, they are not as effective a contraceptive as the combination pills. If you are nursing but want to take the pill, ask your physician about this. If you have no medical problems that increase the risk of complications, most physicians will prescribe the pill.

There are several natural methods of contraception that depend in part on a regular menstrual cycle. Even if you were using these methods before you became pregnant, you should use another method for the first few postpartum months because your cycle may be irregular for a while. Consult your physician if your periods fail to return 3 to 4 months after delivery of your baby.

Chapter 7

Middle Years: Ages 40 Through 65

Contents

Why Call Them Middle Years? 220

Life in the Middle Years, 220
Family Life, 220
    Drug and Alcohol Abuse, 221
Work, 222
Planning for Retirement, 222
Depression, 223
    Suicide, 223
Midlife Crisis, 224

Physical Aging, 224
Cardiovascular System, 225
Digestive System, 225
    Preventing Disease With Vaccines, 226
Bones and Joints, 226
Hair, 227
Skin, 227
    Cosmetic Surgery, 228
Sexuality, 228
    Sex and Illness, 230

Why Call Them Middle Years?

To some people, the term "middle age" has a negative meaning. In our youth-oriented culture, a middle-aged person occasionally is viewed as someone past his or her prime years.

This impression, of course, is not true. For most people, the midlife period is the most productive and fruitful time. In fact, in the United States, people of this age group are the mainstream—demographically, culturally, economically, and in a host of other ways.

We deliberately chose not to use the term "middle age" in the title of this chapter because, apart from its negative associations, it means different things to different people. For some, middle age begins in the 50s, for others in the 40s. Or maybe the 40th birthday is the landmark. To the healthy 60-year-old at the height of his or her career, however, the notion of middle age may seem laughable. To make matters more complicated, the changes and events we describe in this chapter can occur earlier or later, sometimes even well beyond what people sometimes refer to as middle age.

For our purposes, the term "middle years" means ages 40 through 65, the years that lie approximately in the middle of the adult lifespan.

During this time, some people barely notice changes in their bodies. Most, however, start to realize they are getting older. Some need to modify their lifestyles or to correct minor problems before they develop into more serious ones that can affect life after the middle years.

For convenience, this chapter groups the problems and challenges of the middle years into two broad categories: those that concern issues of life and lifestyle and those that are manifested by health changes.

Life in the Middle Years

In the middle of our lives, several transitions occur. Children grow up and leave home. Spouses may enter or reenter the workforce. Some people change jobs, whereas others begin to think of retirement or actually do retire. Divorce is as common during the middle years as during other times. Some people experience a midlife crisis. Such changes can present great challenges and opportunities.

Family Life

The middle years are a time of change for your family. They often are referred to as the sandwich years because two key responsibilities dominate them. The first involves your children, on whom you've focused for so many years. They may be preparing to leave home for further schooling or to start life on their own, causing substantial financial, emotional, or logistical adjustments for you. The second involves your parents, who may require your help and care as they face illness, an end to independent living, or death.

Although not unique to this period, changes in your relationship with your spouse occur more frequently and require adjustments in your life. You may have more time to focus on each other as you begin to plan for your "golden years." You might face the dissolution of your marriage if the children, now gone, were the only tie that held you together. One spouse may die, leaving the other to carry on alone.

Parenting
At times it can seem that children are the whole point of marriage or of your life. You spend much time, energy, financial resources, and love on them. But during the middle years, children leave home.

In some people, this change triggers a depression that has become known as "empty nest syndrome." It can occur in both men and women, but it is primarily experienced by women who have had few interests outside the home and so find themselves without a focus in life after the children have left. Try, if you can, to become involved in other things well before the children leave.

Most parents experience a sense of relief when the day-to-day responsibility for children ends. Privacy, freedom, time for yourself, and time to spend together can bring back the mood of early marriage. Everything is easier—shopping, housework, going out, taking trips. You have time for activities you didn't have time for previously and for discovering new ones.

Divorce

Divorce is frequent during all periods of adult life, including the middle years. Going through a divorce and adjusting to the new circumstances that follow the separation and legal proceedings can be among the most stressful events that take place during a person's lifetime. In most divorces, both members experience a decline in financial resources, resulting in adjustments in lifestyle.

Many people are reluctant to visit marriage counselors, but professionals can sometimes prevent a breakup by helping couples work through their conflicts. With something as important as a marriage at stake, it is certainly worth a try. Should all efforts at reconciliation fail, though, you'll have to plan for the events of your future life. These may include entering or reentering the workforce, moving, redefining social relationships, and perhaps starting to date again.

One change almost always begets others. Too much change too fast can be stressful, so try to pace yourself.

Aging and Death of Parents

If you are in your middle years, your parents, if they are still alive, are in their later years. Where they once guided you, now you might have to guide them.

They may be experiencing major health problems. You may have to coax or even coerce them into handing over the car keys. It might be time for them to give up independent living. Should they move in with your family? Choose a retirement community? Enter a nursing home? (See Later Years: After Age 65, page 231, for more information on these choices.) These decisions add to the other stresses you might be experiencing at this time in your life.

The death of a parent can trigger depression over the loss (see page 223) or a midlife crisis (see page 224) brought on by the realization that you, too, are facing mortality.

The death of a parent is a major loss, no matter what your age; even at 60 you can feel

Drug and Alcohol Abuse

The abuse of drugs, including alcohol, is not limited to any particular age group. The stresses of the middle years, however, can cause infrequent substance abuse to progress, developing into a pattern leading to a life that is out of control.

For example, if you rely on tranquilizers to get through difficult periods, you may become addicted to them if the going gets even more difficult during your middle years. If you enjoy a drink before dinner, this method of "relaxing" may, after time, become the only way you can relax and a habit that begins to snowball.

The abuse of prescription or nonprescription drugs, alcohol, or controlled substances will not solve the personal or physical problems associated with the middle years; it can only aggravate them. If you suspect you have an addiction problem, see your physician or call an alcohol or drug abuse hotline for referral to an appropriate support group (see Alcohol Abuse and Alcoholism, page 325, and Medications and Drug Abuse, page 335).

"orphaned," unable to imagine life without a person who has been a strong influence on you. Grieving is the way to work through and accept such a loss. However, if grief gets you down for too long, or if you get stuck in one stage of grief and can't get out, seek help (see Grief Responses, page 1109).

Loss of Spouse

In your younger years, accidents were the primary cause of death among persons your age. In the middle years, "natural causes" take over. Cancer, heart disease, and stroke are the primary killers of people older than 45. You attend more funerals. You no longer feel invincible, but begin to get a sense of your own mortality.

Loss of a spouse can be devastating. You grieve on many levels: you've lost your best friend, the parent of your children, the person around whom your life was structured, the mate you thought you'd grow old with. You must work through a period of grieving before you can get your life in order (see Grief Responses, page 1109). If your grief seems prolonged or destructive, if you cannot eventually proceed to other things, get professional help.

After losing a spouse you'll have to do things yourself that your spouse formerly did with you or for you, adjust to a different financial level, develop new routines, and fill the void in your life with new social bonds. In other words, you'll have to restructure your entire lifestyle.

More women go through this than men, because three out of every four wives outlive their husbands. Women who haven't been working outside the home may face economic hardship. One solution is to reenter the workforce, intimidating as it may be. You can get counseling regarding job choices, and most communities offer courses that can help you regain old skills or learn new ones. Once you begin, you'll meet people, make new friends, and develop a better sense of self-worth as you once again feel needed.

If you're financially comfortable and don't need to work, think about volunteering. You'll fill up empty hours, add structure to your life, and achieve a sense of accomplishment. Museums, schools, hospitals, libraries, and social agencies are some of the places where your experience and help will be welcome.

Work

For some people, the middle years are a time to go back to working outside the home. For others, they afford an opportunity for career shifts or realignment. You may feel that your occupation no longer offers the satisfaction or rewards it once did. Although it may be unrealistic to do a complete about-face, it is appropriate to evaluate exactly where you are and compare what you see with what you would like to see.

Being laid off or phased out of a job makes such an assessment mandatory. It can take on a real urgency if you're concerned that potential employers might want a younger person. How do you go about appraising your skills and needs?

Reassess your financial needs. If your mortgage is paid off or your children grown, you may need less money than before. However, if you need to put children through college, pay for the care of a parent, or support yourself after a divorce, your financial needs may be greater than they were before.

Evaluate your strengths and experience; typically, you have more than you realize. If self-assessment doesn't work for you, seek help from an established career counselor. The important thing is to deal openly with change rather than be intimidated by its prospects.

Match your needs and your strengths with a specific job or career objective. Entering or reentering the job market, or changing careers, is made easier by some of the flexible work arrangements now available. Many jobs offer schedules that don't require strict adherence to a five-day-a-week, 9-to-5 schedule. Part-time work, shift work, temporary assignments, and job-sharing are other possibilities. With the prevalence of home computers, faxes, and modems, many people now work out of the home.

Night Jobs

Some jobs entail working night shifts on a regular basis. Others rotate shifts: for example, you might work 3 p.m. to 11 p.m. one week, 11 p.m. to 7 a.m. the next, and 7 a.m. to 3 p.m. the one after that.

To remain healthy, you need a sound diet, adequate exercise, and enough sleep. When you were younger you could get away with temporarily shortchanging yourself on these healthful habits— subsisting on coffee and doughnuts for an entire day or skipping sleep to finish a project. During the middle years, your body is not as forgiving as it once was. Mistreatment ultimately results in decreased energy and poor health.

Even assuming that you get enough sleep, working shifts that change from week to week becomes increasingly hard on your body. You get accustomed to a particular rhythm of waking and sleeping. Changing this rhythm requires a period of adjustment while your body experiences something akin to jet lag. As you get older, your body has more difficulty readjusting than it did during your younger years. This opens the way for health problems.

Planning for Retirement

The middle years often seem to creep up unnoticed. Nowhere is this truer than in regard to retirement.

Retirement can be a stressful adjustment for which you are unprepared. Or it can be as rewarding and fulfilling as the preceding years. Which way it goes is, to a certain extent, up to you.

Factors to Consider

From about age 40 to 60 is a time to take stock of yourself and prepare for the time when you'll change your focus. "People who think about and prepare for retirement adjust better," says Virginia Richardson, social work professor at Ohio State University. She identifies three factors that usually determine adjustment, described here.

Financial Security

Save and invest wisely now, even though it requires discipline and risk. Attending pre-retirement classes can help you estimate your retirement income and ascertain whether it will be enough for the lifestyle you envision. Starting early gives you time to make changes if the figures don't add up.

Health

Controlling your weight with regular exercise and a healthful diet, plus getting preventive medical care, can pay off later with continued good health and vitality. You want to be able to enjoy your retirement.

Positive Attitude

Optimism about the future is a tonic for a satisfying retirement. Think of retirement as an opportunity for continued growth and enrichment. Explore new ways to achieve a sense of accomplishment, structure, and status.

Control the Process

Will you retire early? How and where do you want to live? The more control you have over these decisions, the better you'll adjust to not working. To exercise control:

Rehearse for Retirement

Plan what you'd like to do with your free time and try it out on weekends and vacations. Gradually reduce your work hours or responsibilities. If your spouse has died, investigate activities for singles.

Reassess Marriage Roles

If you're a homemaker, will having your spouse around hinder or help your daily routine? If you've had a career, how can you become more comfortable at home during the day? If both you and your spouse work, how will your routines change if one of you retires and the other doesn't?

Even the best-planned retirement can have emotional bumps. Feelings of loss, grief, anger, restlessness, anxiety, mild depression, or preoccupation with the past are common during the first 6 months. Acknowledge these feelings as normal. If the feelings seem overwhelming, or if you don't feel better at the end of the first year, get help.

Depression

Signs and Symptoms
- Generalized sad or numb feeling
- Lack of interest or enjoyment in activities
- Loss of appetite
- Difficulty sleeping
- Physical signs such as dizziness, headaches, or impotence
- Irritability, crying for no evident reason
- Difficulty making decisions
- Social withdrawal
- Loss of interest in sex

Everyone feels down from time to time. The feeling may be sadness caused by an event or turn of circumstances, or just a general out-of-sorts mood for no reason in particular. Usually it passes on its own. Sometimes it does not. Physicians refer to this situation as depression. Events that are common in the middle years—such as loss of a loved one, work problems, or a perceived failure to reach a particular goal—can trigger depression. So can physical illness. At other times, depression just appears.

Depression is not a normal state of mind or something you just have to work through

---

Suicide

The events that trigger depression cause some people to consider suicide. Adolescence, the middle years, and old age are times when life is full of transitional events, some of which seem overwhelming.

During the middle years a person may lose a spouse or a parent, watch the children leave home, or be diagnosed with a chronic disease. Any of these events can be all-consuming and provoke a serious depression. If several occur at once, coping becomes even more difficult. Depression also can occur without an identifiable cause. Whatever the reason, life doesn't seem to be worth living.

Thoughts about suicide are not normal; if you are having them, you need help. As impossible as it may seem, just talking about your problems to an understanding listener, such as a spouse or friend, can make you feel better. If not, seek professional help.

If someone you know mentions suicide, even casually, take it seriously. Contact the family, the family physician, a clergyperson, a suicide hotline, or a psychologist or psychiatrist.

Most suicide attempts are a cry for help. Help comes in the form of professional counseling, drug therapy, and, occasionally, temporary hospitalization.

For more discussion, see Warning Signs of Potential Suicide, page 1125.

yourself. With so much help available in the form of counseling or medication, there's no reason to suffer needlessly. But because even persons who are close to you might misinterpret your behavior, you may well have to reach out.

For more on depression and therapy, see Depression in the Elderly, page 1103; Psychotherapy, page 1107; and Depression and Mood Disorders, page 1122.

Midlife Crisis

What constitutes a midlife crisis? Does everyone have one? Is it possible to emerge unscathed, or even better off?

Childhood is a period of preparation for adulthood. As a young adult you start making your own way through life, exploring alternatives and striving to reach your goals. By your middle years, you've constructed a life of stability, comfort, and familiarity and have adequate personal and financial resources. This is a productive period, during which many people achieve their greatest accomplishments.

Where, then, is the crisis? Stability, comfort, and success are not words that describe a crisis.

But a lot happens during the middle years. You may have faced changes in work, marriage, and parenting. You may have dealt with drug or alcohol abuse, depression, divorce, or the loss of a parent, spouse, or other loved one. Changes in your body make it clear that you are no longer as young as you once were. Retirement and old age don't seem all that far away. If you haven't reached all your goals or learned to modify them along the way, you might consider yourself a failure. You may think you made a wrong career choice and that it's too late to change.

In short, it takes considerable personal stability to cope with the full array of problems and changes that the middle years can bring.

However, the word "crisis" probably applies to only the most problematic situations. A crisis occurs when you feel unable to cope with change, to shift directions, to set new priorities and goals. A crisis also occurs when you react to a situation in unproductive or harmful ways: becoming mired in self-doubt, making sudden job changes, becoming obsessed with aging and mortality, or having extramarital affairs.

Not everyone goes through a midlife crisis, but if you experience one, you can emerge from it better off—more aware of yourself as an individual and better able to direct your life under new and challenging circumstances. Taking stock of where you're headed is a positive thing to do at any age. It might be time to make changes in your priorities, to lighten up, or to develop interests apart from your career.

If it's your spouse who is going through these changes, how do you cope? Do you "go with the flow" or remain a rock of stability? Only you can ascertain what will work best to keep your marriage on track.

If you get bogged down in the challenges of the middle years rather than coming to terms with them, seek help from a family member or friend, a clergyperson, a marriage counselor, your family physician, or a professional counselor.

Physical Aging

Human beings have a finite lifespan. The upper limit is around 100 years; only a few people live a century or a little longer.

For years, scientists have wondered why aging occurs. Some postulate the existence of a biologic clock that runs down with time. Others believe that subtle damage to cells impairs their efficiency.

One of the first changes most people notice is with vision. During the middle years, the lens of the eye becomes less elastic. It takes longer to accommodate from distance focus to close up, and eventually you can't focus on close-up work at all. The person who doesn't eventually need reading glasses is a rarity.

Another change is with memory. You might have a harder time learning telephone numbers or remembering everything you have to do. Many people become reliant on lists during this period. It's easy to become worried that you're developing early senility or Alzheimer's disease, but overloaded memory banks are most likely the problem. With decades of information stored in your brain, you have a harder time locating some of the older material and filing the newer.

As you age, changes take place in your organ systems and in your appearance. Some occur without being visible to others, and some you barely notice yourself. During your later years (the topic of Chapter 8), the cumulative effects are more noticeable.

Good health, sound nutrition, and regular exercise tend to delay and minimize some of the changes associated with aging. Conversely, poor nutrition, stress, and an inactive lifestyle accelerate the changes and hamper your ability to fight disease or recover from injury.

This section groups the normal physical effects of aging into those affecting the cardiovascular system, digestive system, bones and joints, hair, skin, and sexuality.

Cardiovascular System

The heart and blood vessels change with age, even in the absence of any disease process. The muscle of the heart becomes less elastic and a less efficient pump, working harder to do the same job. The heart may atrophy with age and therefore weigh less than it did when you were young. There also may be some loss of the pacemaker cells that control the heart's activities.

The blood vessels also become less elastic with age. Atherosclerosis—accumulations of fatty deposits on and in the walls of the arteries—may make the passageway through the vessels narrower (see page 636).

The loss of elasticity in the walls of the arteries, in combination with atherosclerosis, makes the heart work harder to pump blood through a more resistant network of vessels. This effect can cause high blood pressure, which makes the heart work even harder. With age, a mild increase in blood pressure is normal. Blood pressures beyond this, however, are cause for concern. Prolonged high blood pressure (hypertension) can damage the blood vessels, kidneys, heart, or brain. It can cause death.

Such changes in the cardiovascular system occur gradually rather than overnight. By the middle years, the process already may be well along, particularly in men, who have more heart and blood pressure problems than women. Despite such age-related deterioration in your cardiovascular system, your heart is strong enough to meet the normal needs of your body. However, it has less reserve capacity for overcoming injury or handling the sudden demands placed on it by stress or illness. Heart attacks kill as many people as cancer, AIDS, and all other diseases combined.

Activity level and diet play significant roles in keeping your cardiovascular system healthy. An aerobic exercise, such as vigorous walking or running for at least half an hour at least 3 days a week, places demands on your cardiovascular system that sitting at a desk does not. Your body responds to the demands of exercise by increasing its capacity to pump blood. This increased capacity is healthful, becomes a characteristic of your body, and stays with you while you are not exercising (provided, of course, that you keep up the exercise program).

Exercise programs should be phased in gradually to avoid injury. If you have been inactive, contact a physician before embarking on an exercise program (see Cardiovascular Fitness, page 644).

Atherosclerosis occurs in nearly everyone, narrowing the openings in the blood vessels and thereby increasing the resistance to the heart's pumping action. Exercise, in combination with a low-fat low-cholesterol diet, will slow the process. You cannot stop the effects of aging altogether, but you can greatly minimize them.

For more discussion, see Atherosclerosis: What Is It? page 636; High Blood Pressure, page 647; Controllable Risk Factors, page 638; Coronary Artery Disease, page 654; and Heart Attack, page 661.

Digestive System

With age, several changes take place in your digestive system. They are so subtle that you may not notice them until you are past the middle years.

The swallowing motions of the esophagus become somewhat slower. Similarly, the motions that automatically move digested food through the intestine slow down. The amount of surface area within the intestine diminishes slightly because of changes in the shape of the ridges of the intestine. The flow of secretions from the stomach, liver, pan-

Preventing Disease With Vaccines

The middle years are a time to review your immunization history in order to maintain and maximize your health. As you age, you actually become more susceptible to certain infectious diseases, some of which are preventable with vaccines. In addition, the middle years frequently are a time when international travel becomes feasible, adding even more importance to this issue. Get yourself up to date on the following vaccines:

Influenza. Older people and those with underlying medical conditions are at increased risk for complicated illness, hospitalization, and even death from influenza infection. All adults age 65 or older should receive this vaccine on an annual basis, as should younger adults with chronic cardiopulmonary disorders, diabetes, renal disease, liver disease, blood diseases, cancers, HIV infection, or diseases (or taking drugs) that suppress immunity. Healthy adults living in a household with someone who has one of these disorders also should receive the vaccine.

Pneumococcal Vaccine. The indications for this vaccine are the same as those for influenza vaccine, with the addition of alcoholism and surgical removal of the spleen. Adults with these underlying medical conditions should begin receiving pneumococcal vaccine by age 50. Completely healthy adults can wait until age 65.

Tetanus-Diphtheria (Td). Because children receive three primary doses of Td, tetanus and diphtheria in the United States are now predominantly diseases of adults. In the past, adults were advised to get a booster dose every 10 years. Now a single booster at age 50 is recommended.

Certain lifestyles, occupations, hobbies, and foreign travel plans may make other immunizations advisable. Ask your physician for advice.

creas, and small intestine may decrease. These changes generally are inconsequential and do not disrupt the digestive process. Adding vitamin or mineral supplements is not necessary unless your physician finds a specific deficiency.

Constipation may occur more often. Often this is related to a lack of water intake rather than to problems with the intestine itself. Increasing your daily consumption of water and adding fiber to your diet are helpful approaches. Avoid long-term use of laxatives (see Laxative Abuse, page 785).

Older people have more illnesses of the digestive system than do younger people. If you see evidence of blood in your stool, experience abdominal pain or unexplained weight loss, or your bowel habits undergo a dramatic change, consult your physician immediately. If the problem is serious, the earlier it is treated, the better.

Bones and Joints

Although you might think of bones as hard, rigid, and unchanging, living bones constantly undergo renewal and respond to the demands placed on them. For example, a person who does a lot of heavy work using his or her arms not only will develop larger and more powerful arm muscles than someone who does not but also will develop stronger bones in the arms.

Your bones reach their maximal mass between ages 25 and 35. During subsequent years they decline slightly in size and density. One consequence is that during the middle years or after, your height may decrease. Another is that your bones become more brittle, making you more vulnerable to fractures.

Osteoporosis

One of the most serious health hazards that the elderly face is osteoporosis, when the bones become demineralized (see Osteoporosis, page 894). Sometimes they become so porous that even a slight fall or injury can break a hip, wrist, vertebra, or other bone.

Osteoporosis also makes bones more susceptible to being distorted under the pull or weight of the muscles, which can lead to a severely stooped back. This disorder especially affects women after menopause. Men also lose bone density, becoming more vulnerable to hip and other fractures; but because men lose it at a lesser rate, and because they start with a larger bone mass, they are less likely to have difficulty from osteoporosis.

The best treatment of osteoporosis is prevention, which should start well before the middle years. Eating foods that are high in calcium, taking calcium supplements, and getting plenty of weight-bearing exercise will maximize bone mass before depletion begins. After menopause, these measures become even more important. Estrogen replacement therapy, should your physician recommend it, slows bone density loss (see page 1154).

Arthritis

Aging eventually makes your joints a little stiffer and your movements a little slower, changes that may not show up until after the middle years. In addition to the normal stiffening, however, there is arthritis, a familiar problem with joints which often begins during the middle years (see Osteoarthritis, page 907).

Most arthritis is simple deterioration of a joint. Heredity, diet, and previous injuries and diseases in your joints are possible causative factors, but everyday use also is a factor. (This is the reason arthritis is known as the "wear-and-tear disease.")

Arthritis usually starts in the spine or large joints—the hips and knees, which bear the weight of your body. It also can show up elsewhere, such as in the knuckles. During the middle years, most people have arthritis in at least one joint. The symptoms are intermittent pain, stiffness, and occasional swelling in the joint. Sometimes there are no symptoms.

Pain, if present, is usually a minor discomfort, although it can be severe. Because your natural response to a painful joint is to move it less, you use the muscles in the area less frequently, so they start to shrink and lose strength. This process produces a destructive cycle that increases the degree of disability. Arthritis in the hips and knees can substantially affect how you walk.

Arthritis is a process that does not go away, but it can be treated effectively. Describe your symptoms to your physician. He or she can diagnose arthritis easily, although sometimes an X-ray and other tests are needed. If you are overweight, losing weight (so that less is carried by those joints) can help. Exercise and physical therapy are beneficial, and your physician can suggest appropriate pain-relieving drugs.

As with all of the physical changes associated with the middle years, you may experience less change and fewer associated problems if you follow a regular exercise program and avoid joint-damaging activities.

Hair

Hair changes with age, although individual variations are great. On average, half of us are about 50 percent gray by age 50. Graying usually begins at the temples and slowly works its way up the scalp. The new hair is often different in texture. Underarm hair and pubic hair may or may not turn gray.

Graying is considered attractive by some and unattractive by others. How you view it is largely a matter of your personal preference, your cultural background, and current fashion. If you don't like your gray hair, you can change it with rinses or dyes.

Hair also thins with age, in both women and men, and sometimes in places other than the head. Baldness is genetically determined and affects about 60 percent of men by age 50. Several treatment options are available. Medications can stimulate growth of hair on bald patches. Hair follicles can be surgically transplanted from other parts of the head. Toupees and weaves are other options.

With the hormone alterations that occur after menopause, the facial hair in some women coarsens and starts to grow. It can be bleached, or it can be removed by plucking, waxing, or electrolysis or with hair remover. Removal does not stimulate further growth.

For more detailed discussions of hair and baldness, see page 1017.

Skin

As you get older, your body's largest organ, the skin, loses some of its elasticity and begins to droop a bit. You can keep the underlying muscles firm and taut—avoiding a spare tire around your stomach, for example—but in some places (such as your face), the skin will sag anyway. Your skin becomes a little thinner, so that veins or discolorations beneath the surface show through more clearly than they used to. You begin to lose your youthful color and glow. Decreased production of natural oils makes your skin drier. Also, you perspire less.

How fast your skin ages depends on many factors. The most significant is how much unprotected exposure to the sun you have had over the years. The more sun, the more damage (see Senile Skin, page 1000).

Nutrition and fitness also play a part. The skin, like other organs, benefits from a good blood supply provided by a healthful diet and regular exercise.

Although you may enter this period of life with virtually no wrinkles, by the end of the middle years you can expect to have a fair number. This is a natural consequence of aging which can be postponed but not reversed, although some people use cosmetic surgery to improve their looks.

Age Spots
Also called liver spots, these are flat patches of increased pigmentation that range from the size of a freckle to a few inches across (see Liver Spots, page 1003, and page C-4 for color photograph). Although age spots are not dangerous, see your physician whenever

anything new appears on your skin, just to be sure that it is not skin cancer (see Skin Cancers, page 1004, and page C-6 for color photographs).

Sexuality

The middle years do not spell an end to sexual desire or performance for men and women. Such an expectation is detrimental because it can become self-fulfilling. In reality, sex can be more rewarding during the middle years than it was during the frantic pace of your younger years. Biology finally puts sex in sync: for men, setting and mood take on more importance; touch and extended foreplay may become as enjoyable as release. Women may feel more relaxed, less inhibited, and more confident to assert their sexual desires.

Sexual Changes in Women

Menopause is the end of menstruation in women. With it, the possibility of bearing a child ends.

There are many common misconceptions about menopause: it marks the end of interest in sex, it triggers depression, it brings on emotional and mood instability. What are the facts?

Cosmetic Surgery

Some of the common questions about cosmetic surgery are listed here:

What Can It Do? The classic facelift operation tightens and smooths the skin, eliminating coarser wrinkles and sags. Eyelid surgery removes puffiness and bags under the eyes and redundant skin above the eyes (see Cosmetic Surgery of the Eyelid, page 541). Noses can be reshaped and receding chins augmented.

How Is It Done? The surgeon makes incisions in the area of the sideburns, just in front of the ears, and behind the ears in the hairline, then pulls the skin up and back and trims away the excess. Subcutaneous fat in the area of the chin often is removed. Visible scarring is minimal.

Is It Dangerous? Like all operations, it is subject to complications such as excessive swelling and bruising, infection, and injury to nerves. If general anesthesia is used, the anesthesia itself has risks (see General Anesthesia, page 1261).

How Long Must I Hide? Bruising and swelling from a facelift largely disappear after 2 to 3 weeks.

How Long Do the Results Last? The results last from a few to many years. After that, the procedure may have to be repeated.

If you were interested in sex and enjoyed it as a younger woman, you probably will feel the same way after menopause. Yet menopause does bring changes, as described here.

Desire

Sexual desire is the most variable of your responses. Although your sex drive is largely determined by emotional and social factors, hormones such as estrogen and testosterone do play a role. Estrogen is made in your ovaries, and testosterone is made in your adrenal glands. Surprisingly, sexual desire is affected mainly by testosterone, not estrogen. At menopause, your ovaries stop producing estrogen, but most women produce enough testosterone to preserve their interest in sex. And remember: the most important sex organ is the brain. Candlelight, music, food, conversation, books, and thoughts can help create a mood for sex.

Vaginal Changes

After menopause, estrogen deficiency may lead to changes in the appearance of your genitals and how you respond sexually. The folds of skin that cover your genital region (labia) shrink and become thinner, exposing more of the clitoris. This increased exposure sometimes reduces your sensitivity or causes an unpleasant tingling or prickling sensation when you are touched. The opening to your vagina becomes narrower, particularly if you are not sexually active. Natural swelling and lubrication of your vagina occur more slowly during arousal. Even when you feel excited, your vagina may stay somewhat tight and dry. These factors can lead to difficult or painful intercourse (dyspareunia).

Longer foreplay sometimes helps stimulate your natural lubrication, or you can use a water-soluble lubricant such as K-Y jelly. (Do not use Vaseline or other petroleum-based jellies.) Talk to your physician about estrogen cream for your genital area or estrogen replacement therapy. And have intercourse regularly—this is one area where the "use it or lose it" maxim holds true. Women who are sexually active after menopause have better lubrication and elasticity of vaginal tissues.

Orgasm

Because sexual arousal begins in your brain, you can have orgasms throughout your life. It may take longer as you age, but you can still get there.

Emotional Changes

Menopausal women have traditionally been expected to be depressed, moody, fatigued, tense, anxious, and irritable. Yet study after study shows little connection between mood and menopause. Emotional reactions seem, instead, to be a result of whatever is going on in your life. The same stresses that throw some men into a midlife crisis can cause some women to react emotionally. The culprit probably is not menopause, except in one area: women who experience extreme hot flashes and night sweats might become sleep-deprived and irritable.

Your expectations about menopause seem to influence how you experience the "change of life." If you think it will be difficult, it will; if you expect to breeze through it, that's probably what you'll do.

For more discussion of Menopause, see page 1153.

Sexual Changes in Men

Menopause has no functional counterpart in the male. With aging, the production of testosterone, a male hormone, gradually lessens but does not cease. Yet physical changes in a middle-aged man's sexual response parallel those in a postmenopausal woman.

Desire

Many men experience a gradual lessening of sexual desire. Some might call this a focus on quality rather than quantity.

Excitement

You may require more stimulation to get and maintain an erection, and the erection will be less firm. You may need more partner involvement.

Orgasm

During ejaculation, you may expel less semen, and with less force, than previously. After a climax, it will take increasingly longer before you can be stimulated to another. Whereas at 17 you could have a subsequent climax within minutes, by the age of 70 it could take as much as 48 hours.

Impotence

The inability to have an erection when desire and opportunity are present can affect men at any age, although it becomes more common during the middle years. Nearly 20 percent of men are impotent at age 60. Impotence is not an inevitable consequence of aging. Common causes are alcohol abuse, medications that affect sexual desire, and medical problems. Stress, which can be plentiful during the middle years, also ranks high on the list of possible causes.

Don't interpret an episode or two of impotence as a signal that your sex life is about to end. If you experience impotence that is not confined to an occasional episode, however, discuss the problem with your physician. The chances are excellent that, regardless of the cause, it can be cured (see Impotence, page 1225).

Changes Due to Illness or Disability

Whether you're healthy, ill, or disabled, you have your own sexual identity and desires for sexual expression. Yet illness or disability can interfere with how you respond sexually to another person. Some medical problems that can affect sexual expression are discussed below.

Heart Attack

Chest pain, shortness of breath, or the fear of a recurring heart attack can have an impact on your sexual behavior. But if you were sexually active before your heart attack, you can probably be again. If you have symptoms of angina, your physician may recommend that you take nitroglycerin before intercourse.

Even though pulse rates, respiratory rates, and blood pressure increase during intercourse, after intercourse they return to normal within minutes. Sudden death during sex is rare.

Prostate Surgery

For a benign condition, such as an enlarged prostate, surgery rarely causes impotence. Prostate surgery for cancer may cause impotence, but advances in surgical techniques have reduced this risk in recent years. Also, new treatments for impotence are available (see Impotence, page 1225).

Hysterectomy

In this surgical procedure, the uterus and cervix are removed, and in some cases the fallopian tubes, ovaries, and lymph nodes are also removed. A hysterectomy, by itself, doesn't interfere with your physical ability to have intercourse or experience orgasm.

Sex and Illness

Changes in your body due to illness or surgery can affect your physical response to sex. They also can affect your self-image and ultimately limit your interest in sex. Here are tips to help you maintain confidence in your sexuality:

Know What to Expect. Talk to your physician about the usual effects your treatment has on sexual function.

Talk About Sex. If you feel weak or tired and want your partner to take a more active role, say so. If some part of your body is sore, guide your mate's caresses to create pleasure and avoid pain.

Plan for Sex. Find a time when you're rested and relaxed. Taking a warm bath first or having sex in the morning may help. If you take a pain reliever, such as for arthritis, time the dose so that its effect will occur during sexual activity.

Prepare With Exercise. If you have arthritis or another disability, ask your physician or therapist for range-of-motion exercises to help relax your joints before sex.

Find Pleasure in Touch. It's a good alternative to sexual intercourse. Touching can simply mean holding each other. Men and women can sometimes reach orgasm with the right kind of touching. If you have no partner, touching yourself for sexual pleasure may help you reaffirm your own sexuality. It can also help you make the transition to intercourse after an illness or surgery.

Removing the ovaries, however, creates an instant menopause and accelerates the physical and emotional aspects of the natural condition.

When cancer is not involved, be sure you understand why you need a hysterectomy and how it will help your symptoms. Ask your physician what you can expect after the operation. Reassure yourself that a hysterectomy generally doesn't affect sexual pleasure and that hormone therapy should prevent physical and emotional changes from interfering.

Drugs

Some commonly used medications can interfere with sexual function. Drugs that control high blood pressure, such as thiazide diuretics and beta blockers, can reduce desire and impair erection in men and lubrication in women. In contrast, calcium channel blockers and angiotensin-converting enzyme (ACE) inhibitors have little known effect on sexual function.

Other drugs that can affect sexual function include antihistamines, drugs used to treat depression, and drugs that block secre-

tion of stomach acid. If you take one of these drugs and are experiencing side effects, ask your physician for an alternative medication. Alcohol also may adversely affect sexual function.

Hardening of the Arteries and Heart Disease

About half of all impotence in men older than 50 years is caused by damage of nerves or blood vessels to the penis. Hardening of the arteries (atherosclerosis) can damage small vessels and restrict blood flow to the genitals. This can interfere with erection in men and swelling of vaginal tissues in women.

Diabetes

Diabetes can increase the collection of fatty deposits (plaque) in blood vessels. Such deposits restrict the flow of blood to the penis. About half of men with diabetes become impotent. Their risk of impotence increases with age. Men who have had diabetes for many years and who also have nerve damage are more likely to become impotent.

If you are a woman with diabetes, you may suffer dryness and painful intercourse that reduce the frequency of orgasm. You may have more frequent vaginal and urinary tract infections.

Arthritis

Although arthritis does not affect your sex organs, the pain and stiffness of osteoarthritis or rheumatoid arthritis can make sex difficult to enjoy. If you have arthritis, discuss your capabilities and your desires openly with your partner. As long as you and your partner keep communication open, you can have a satisfying sexual relationship.

Cancer

Cancer can cause anemia, loss of appetite, muscle wasting, or neurologic impairment that leads to weakness. Surgery can alter your appearance. These problems can decrease your sexual desire or pleasure.

Cancer may also cause direct damage to your sexual organs or to their nerve and blood supplies; treatment can produce side effects that may interfere with sexual function, desire, or pleasure. Discuss possible effects of your treatment with your physician. If cancer has disrupted your usual sexual activity, seek other ways of expression. Sometimes cuddling or self-stimulation can be enough.

Chapter 8

Later Years: After Age 65

Contents

Healthful Aging, 232

The Aging Process, 232
Statistics About Aging, 232
Physical Changes, 233
    Changing Sleep Patterns, 233
Loss of Independence, 234
    Elder Abuse, 234
Aging Successfully, 235
Exercise, 236

Special Problems of the Elderly, 237
Forgetfulness, 237
    Sharpening Your Memory, 238
Changes in Eyesight, 238
    Problems With Night Vision, 239
Impaired Mobility, 239
    How to Avoid Falls, 240
Incontinence, 240

Constipation, 241
    Special Nutritional Concerns, 241
Changes in Sexuality, 242
Hearing Loss, 242
Voice Changes, 243
Depression, 243
Skin Problems, 244
Support of Pelvic Organs in Women, 244
Problems Related to Too Many Medications, 244

Community Services, 245
Retirement Communities, 246
Home Health Care, 246
Adult Day Care, 246
Respite Care Programs, 246
Day Respite Care Programs, 246
Foster Care Homes, 247
Nutrition Services, 247
Nursing Homes, 247

Healthful Aging

Much material written about aging focuses on loss. Although the older adult sometimes experiences physical, mental, or psychosocial losses, continued growth and creative expression mark the lives of many elderly. They are signs of healthful aging. Older adults are taking college courses and are involved in Elderhostel. They make contributions through tutoring, teaching, counseling (such as peer counseling), and advocating for political and social action.

Some experts believe that there is a creative peak at age 65. Sometimes older adults just need someone to encourage them to pursue latent interests or rediscover forgotten talents that were set aside when family and job occupied much of the day. Increased knowledge of resources available within the community will sometimes stimulate interests and encourage new avenues of self-expression.

The Aging Process

The aging process begins the moment you are born, and it never ceases. By age 65, however, people vary a great deal in how old their bodies appear and how much they have changed. There are 65-year-olds who look like 45-year-olds and 65-year-olds who look like 85-year-olds.

These differences occur because people differ greatly in their genetic makeup, in their health history, and in their environments, including personal nutritional and exercise habits and patterns of stress.

It is not possible to predict what will happen to you in your 60s, 70s, and 80s because you are different from your spouse, your parents, your neighbors, and everyone else. However, we can develop a description of the typical human lifespan by examining statistics concerning older people. The next few pages discuss these statistics and characterize the physical changes that are to be expected during this period. Finally, we take a look at independence and consider how it can be maintained for maximal health of mind and body.

Statistics About Aging

There always have been elderly people. We know this from ancient writings as well as from skeletal remains. Until fairly recently, however, people did not live through what we call the middle years (40 to 65), let alone beyond age 65.

Disease was rampant, medicine was primitive, and nutrition was poor. A woman born in 1841 could expect to live to age 42; for a man born the same year, the life expectancy was 41. A woman born today can expect about 78 years of life, and a man can expect 73. These are average numbers that include deaths in infancy, young adulthood, the middle years, and the elderly years.

The maximal human lifespan seems to be about 100 years; a few exceptional cases have been recorded, and a lifespan exceeding 120 years has been verified. A woman who is 65 today can expect about 18 more years of life; a 65-year-old man can expect about 13 more years.

On average, women live longer than men. If a woman is age 75 today, she can expect to live about 12 more years; a man at age 75 can expect to live about 9 more years. This difference seems to be due to a combination of biologic, genetic, and environmental factors that are not fully understood. Because women tend to live longer, the proportion of women among people 65 or older is greater than it is in younger population groups.

Many people now reach the later years and continue to thrive. In the United States, each day about 5,000 people reach age 65 and about 3,600 people age 65 or older die. The net increase of 1,400 people a day is changing the makeup of our society.

In the United States, 26 million people are now age 65 or older—1 person in 10. This segment of the population is increasing twice as fast as the rest of the population. Today, we have one-fourth more people age 65 or older than we had as recently as the 1970s and twice as many as in 1950.

The United States has neither the highest nor the lowest proportion of older people in the world. Europe has a larger proportion of the elderly, while Japan has a slightly lower proportion. Developing countries have far lower proportions; in Egypt, for example, only about 6 percent of the population is age 60 or older; in Nigeria, the figure is only 2 percent. A little more than a century ago, the proportion was 2 percent in the United States.

In industrialized societies, we can expect the increase in the proportion of elderly to continue. Even if we assume that medicine will make no advances in prolonging the lives of this age group (an unlikely assumption), a large segment of the existing population is about to reach their later years. In 2011, the postwar "baby boomers" will start turning 65. In that year, and for each of the 20 years that follow, we can expect our elderly population to increase by about 1 million people annually.

By the year 2000, the number of Americans older than age 85 is expected to triple. At that time we should have 100,000 people 100 years of age or older.

In other words, you could say that it is "in" to be 65 or older. If you are older than 65, you are a member of a growing group, and you will have more company than ever before in history. Society also shows some signs of gearing up to accommodate the greater numbers of elderly.

With the increasing proportion of our population in their later years and the greater frequency of illness in this group than in younger age groups, medicine (except for pediatrics and obstetrics) is dealing with older persons. Your physician has become accustomed to dealing with the problems of the elderly and is helped by a large and growing body of scientific research that almost daily is discovering more about the aging process and how to go about living a longer, healthier life.

Physical Changes

The old saying that "you are as young as you feel" has a great deal of truth to it. In the absence of serious diseases or other crushing problems, as people age they "feel" just about like they did when they were young. The essence of a person does not change; the body does.

The degree to which the body changes varies enormously. Some men and women in their 60s and early 70s participate regularly in vigorous exercise. Conditioned older athletes have hearts, lungs, and muscles that are in better shape than those of many younger people. Moreover, they have a lot more vigor than someone years younger who has let his or her body get badly out of condition.

In the later years, healthful living with regular exercise, weight control, adequate rest, a balanced diet, avoidance of tobacco, and moderation in consumption of alcoholic beverages can produce a feeling of well-being and vigor that surpasses that of an overweight, sedentary, 30-year-old smoker. Good health also helps ensure a satisfying sex life in the later years.

What are the general body changes you will face? The changes that started during the middle years (described in Chapter 7) continue. Your heart, lungs, stomach, and other internal organs become somewhat less efficient. Regardless of conditioning, even the best of athletes lose some of the physical abilities they enjoyed in earlier years. Your muscles lose tissue and strength, and your bones get a little lighter and smaller. Bones that are less dense break more easily, and recovery from illness and injury takes longer. You may move more slowly.

Changing Sleep Patterns

Your need for sleep remains about the same most of your life. If you need about 6 hours nightly now, chances are you'll need that amount—give or take a half-hour—10 years from now.

However, aging can cause you to sleep less soundly. After age 70, it's common to spend more time in bed but less time asleep. That's because delta sleep, which is the deepest, most restorative sleep, decreases with age. Delta sleep occurs soon after you fall asleep.

If you think you're sleeping less, remember to count afternoon naps. Many older people who rest during the day find that the combination of naps and nighttime sleep totals just about the same hours of rest they had when they were younger.

Your hair may turn gray and become thin, and your skin—which has protected you from the environment for decades—shows the effects of this battle, with more wrinkling and a bit of sagging as elastic tissue is lost. Eyesight and hearing often begin to fail, and illness is more common. Prostate problems in men, weakening of muscles supporting pelvic organs in women, and incontinence with involuntary loss of urine in both sexes are common concerns that must be dealt with.

Elder Abuse

In this context, abuse means anything from a consistent pattern of harsh words and marked unfriendliness to slapping, pushing, hitting, and sexual molestation, at times by the people on whom these victims are dependent.

According to the American Medical Association, about 10 percent of people age 65 or older suffer some kind of chronic abuse. Frequently, the pattern emerges gradually, beginning with verbal abuse and progressing to physical abuse. Since 1981, there has been an increase in cases reported each year, to about 100,000 a year. In other words, abuse of the elderly is a common problem that is only beginning to be recognized.

Who Is Most Likely to Be a Victim?
Those who are age 75 or older and who are dependent on others for basic care such as bathing, dressing, and eating are the ones most likely to be abused. Abuse is three times more likely among the elderly who live with someone. Although men are more often the victims, abused women suffer more physical harm. Abuse seems to occur in all economic and ethnic groups.

Who Are the Abusers?
In about half of the cases, they are the children or other younger relatives of the victims. About 40 percent of the time the victim's spouse is the abuser. In institutions, professional caregivers also may be abusers. The abusers may be reacting to stress and exhaustion. They may have psychological or drug abuse problems. Some were abused themselves as children.

What Can Be Done?
If you are being abused, first realize that this kind of treatment is not acceptable. Your dependence on another person does not give that person the right to mistreat you. Call the police or ask a visiting nurse to assess the situation and contact the authorities. Your local senior citizens center can provide help. Physicians and social workers also can help. Most cities and counties, according to state law, protect the vulnerable adult from elder abuse through their welfare and social service agencies.

Remember that to get help from someone, you have to ask for it. Talking with the abuser about the problem is not likely to help.

Loss of Independence

One of the toughest adjustments to make in the later years is the loss of independence that some people experience. However, most do not lose it or do not lose all of it.

Moving into a nursing home has come to symbolize loss of independence. More than 1 million Americans who are 65 or older live in nursing homes. This is only about 5 percent, or 1 out of every 20, of those in this age group. Even among people age 85 or older, only about 1 in 5 lives in a nursing home.

When you find that you need a little help doing things or that your living arrangements do not quite work, you have a lot of choices. Here is just a partial list:

1. Move to a smaller place, all on one floor, if possible.

2. Outfit your home with special equipment to help prevent falls and make life easier.

3. Use home health services, including housekeeping, visiting nurses, and Meals on Wheels.

4. Move to a retirement community with congregated dining and convenient services.

5. Arrange for a companion to live with you and help you do things.

6. Move to special housing for the elderly which offers temporary or permanent nursing care, depending on need. These apartment communities often have arrangements from complete independence to skilled nursing care, all in one location.

7. Use the services of home health care, adult day care, or a respite care program (all are described later in this chapter).

8. Move in with your family, or have them join you.

9. Hire help.

10. Join forces with another older person or share your home with a younger person. Placement services are now available at many senior citizens centers throughout the country.

These are not all the possibilities. Situations vary just as needs vary. For one person, being independent means having time to read and a ready supply of good books. To another, it means the chance to play golf several times a week. To another, it means not having to take orders from anyone. To most, it means the freedom to get up, move about, do things, have friends in, make telephone calls, go places, and pursue activities they deem to be important.

Before you make changes in your living situation, think about what the word "independence" means to you. You may be able to adapt your current way of life, perhaps with just a little change, to accommodate your aging.

However, if you require a lot of nursing help, especially constant care, then someone does have to provide it. Living in a nursing home may limit your independence, but it may be the only wise thing to do.

In the past, admission to a nursing home was regarded as the "last stop." Today, physicians often recommend a stay in a nursing home during recovery from a stroke, hip fracture, or other mishap; 25 percent of persons who are in a nursing home for these reasons are able to leave after they complete their rehabilitation.

In the past several years, there has been a rapid increase in the number of nursing homes that specialize in the care of patients who no longer need hospitalization but still require specialized and skilled care. Examples include the care of patients who require intravenous medication or intensive rehabilitation. The average length of stay in these homes is 7 to 21 days.

Nursing homes vary in the amount of independence they provide. If one is in your future, temporarily or permanently, try to pick a facility that suits your expectations, your personality, and your budget (see the information on nursing homes later in this chapter). If you cannot actually visit the different nursing homes yourself, have someone else go and ask your questions for you.

Another threat to your independence is the possibility of no longer being able to drive. As you grow older, your reflexes become slower. Even more important, you lose the ability to deal quickly with two or more problems that occur simultaneously—to handle the most urgent first and the less urgent later. As a result, you become less able to react to traffic situations. This may be coupled with decreased visual acuity and problems with night vision (see Problems With Night Vision, page 239).

First you stop driving at night, then you stop driving on the highway, and finally you even give up driving around your neighborhood. Senior safety programs are an excellent way to relearn defensive driving and may restore your confidence behind the wheel.

The American Association of Retired Persons (AARP) has a "55 Alive" course that offers tips on safe driving and avoidance of common accident situations. All states provide the course and give elders who complete the course a 10 to 15 percent reduction on their auto insurance.

At some point, however, your enemy on the road may become yourself. For many people, turning in the car keys seems like giving up on life altogether; but if your skills have eroded to the point that you pose a danger, doing so may avoid a lawsuit or a tragic traffic death.

Aging Successfully

Who fares best when it comes to aging? That question has never been more important, because never in history have so many people lived so long. By the year 2000, one-fourth of America's population will be age 65 or older. And the fastest-growing segment of elderly people consists of those age 85 or older.

Aging isn't about retirement or even reaching a particular chronologic age, such as 65. It's a lifelong process. The people who do best are the ones who've successfully passed through each stage of life. Successful aging involves many factors within your control: your attitudes, activities, and relationships.

Advice for succeeding at the business of growing older is provided on the following pages.

Anticipate and Accommodate

Many people plan for retirement. Successful aging means making plans for after you retire as well. Consider the "big picture." Do you want to start a part-time consulting business? Live near a year-round golf course? Also consider details. How will you spend your days?

Structure your time with specific plans, such as working out three mornings each week or visiting the library regularly. Setting priorities helps you avoid stress. It gives you a sense of excitement about the future and a feeling of success when you attain your goals. It means taking charge and making choices.

Have Diverse Interests

Balance solitary activities with group activities. You can enjoy swimming or water exercises in a class or by yourself. Think about adapting rather than about giving up favorite pastimes. If arthritis keeps you from playing the piano, attend concerts or check out music from your local library. When you can no longer play singles in tennis, switch to doubles. Expand your horizons. If you've always loved reading, consider joining a book discussion group.

Accept Limitations

Do your grandchildren live out of state? Stay in touch by exchanging "letters" on cassette tape. Share favorite memories, tell them about your interests and activities when you were their age, or make a special album of old family photos.

Establish Financial Security

You don't have to be rich to be happy, but try to budget for activities and a lifestyle that you value. Financial planning is as important now as when you were starting out.

Seek qualified, professional advice as you consider your insurance needs, charitable goals, providing for your loved ones, managing assets from your pension, or the sale of your home or business. Financial planning also could mean moving into a smaller home with less upkeep.

Draw on the Kinship of Others

Turn to family and friends for support and encouragement. To make new friends, attend activities for people with similar interests, such as woodworking or astronomy classes at a local college.

Maintain Your Faith

Participating in religious services brings you into contact with people of other ages and walks of life. Your faith can provide a sense of continuity amid the changes you face and can offer peace of mind.

Cultivate a Positive Outlook

No matter how cloudy your disposition may be, remember that the sun will shine again, flowers will grow, and things probably will improve. Don't dwell on clouds unless you enjoy overcast weather.

Be Engaged in the World Around You

You could be a volunteer grandparent at a local child care center or deliver for Meals on Wheels. One woman didn't like the view from her new apartment—she looked onto the loading dock of a factory. But rather than get depressed about it, she visited the factory to learn what people did there, and now she follows their activities with interest.

Be Flexible

You've already seen a lot of change in your life. Change will continue. An ability to roll with the punches and a sense of humor are tools that can help you cope.

Practice Good Health Habits

This doesn't have to be an unpleasant regimen of dull dos and don'ts. Look for ways to incorporate regular exercise, such as walking, into your daily routine. Also, eat a balanced diet and get adequate rest.

Exercise

Don't believe that life after 65 is a time of disability. Aches and pains are inevitable, but your later years can be some of the most pleasant and productive years of your life. Strive to live life to the fullest by maintaining a reasonable level of fitness. Modest, regular exercise can help you live better and longer and can reduce the period of disease or disability that may precede death.

The new approach to exercise is called functional fitness, a broad term that involves the four components described here.

Aerobic Capacity

This is a measure of the ability of your heart, lungs, and blood vessels to deliver oxygen to your muscles—and of your muscles, in turn, to use that oxygen efficiently. Exercises that develop aerobic capacity require your large muscles (arms or legs, for example) to work continuously for 20 to 40 minutes.

Regular aerobic exercise slows your resting pulse rate and increases the volume of blood your heart pumps with each contraction. Also, your muscle cells develop increased capacity to use the oxygen they receive. This capacity leads to a more efficient exchange of oxygen for carbon dioxide.

The net effect? More vim and vigor.

Regular physical exercise can increase the aerobic capacity of a sedentary adult by at least 20 percent. Thus, you may be able to perform at a level of physical activity comparable to that of an inactive person 10 to 20 years younger.

Muscle Strength and Endurance

When is the last time you asked for help with a stubborn jar lid? Have you declined to swing your grandchild overhead because you can't easily lift 30 pounds? Your ability to perform such tasks is a measure of your muscle strength. Strength allows you to lift an ax to chop wood. Endurance determines how many times you can swing the ax before tiring.

Nine nursing home residents, ranging in age from 86 to 96, enrolled in a program of lifting and lowering leg weights. At the end of 8 weeks, five of them could walk faster and two gave up their canes. Of three residents who needed to use their arms in rising from a chair before the program, one could get up without support after the program.

Flexibility

Can you easily tie your shoes? Is it difficult to stretch to reach items on an overhead shelf? Physical therapists talk about flexibility in terms of "range of motion," the range to which you can bend and stretch joints, muscles, and ligaments.

If you have arthritis, appropriate exercise helps you move joints more easily. If you find it difficult or impossible to exercise on weight-bearing joints, consider swimming or water exercises.

Coordination and Balance

Strong muscles and your brain are key components in a complex system involving coordinated movement and balance. To prevent a stumble from becoming a fall, for example, your brain first receives the signal that you've lost your balance. Then it triggers your muscles to compensate. If your reaction is quick and your muscles are strong, your muscles pull you back and keep you upright. Regular activity conditions this integrated pattern of movement, keeping it coordinated and finely tuned.

The payoff on relatively small investments of time and energy can be long-lasting. From armchair exercise, if you use a wheelchair, to marathon competition, there's an exercise suitable for you.

It's never too late to become more active. But before you begin an exercise program that is more vigorous than walking, get a medical evaluation from your physician. Then plan activities that you enjoy, because if exercise is drudgery, you won't do it for long.

Special Problems of the Elderly

Although health problems can occur at any age, some are more common among older people. This section covers problems with memory, mood, eyesight, hearing, and mobility. For women, support of pelvic organs is discussed. Also covered are incontinence, constipation, changes in sexuality, voice changes, and skin problems.

This is not a list of things that will happen to everyone. Aging is a time when the body reveals its wear and tear, but the odds are high that you will avoid some of these problems. And often, those that occur are easily managed and not disabling.

Forgetfulness

Do you frequently misplace the car keys, or forget what time you agreed to meet your friends for golf? Have lists become an essential component of daily living?

Memory falls into three categories:

Short-term—looking up a phone number and remembering it long enough to dial

Long-term (recent)—what you ate for breakfast today or the outfit you wore a few days ago

Long-term (remote)—events from the distant past, such as incidents in high school

Aging doesn't generally affect short- or long-term (remote) memory, but long-term (recent) memory often declines. To store and retrieve information, your brain performs a complex chain of chemical and electrical functions involving nerve cells. As you age, some of these cells may deteriorate and function less efficiently.

Your brain, however, compensates in remarkable ways. Even though you might not have the same number of brain cells as a 19-year-old, consider how much more wisdom and judgment you have. These qualities are difficult to measure, but they reflect the ability to make sound decisions based on a lifetime of experience.

Memory can decline for various reasons, including depression, medical illness, and side effects of drugs. A progressive loss of memory that affects your daily activities could indicate a more serious problem, such as Alzheimer's disease. If you don't recall where you put your glasses, that's forgetfulness. If you can't remember that you wear glasses, that's a serious concern. Contact your physician if you notice these warning signs:

- Memory lapses that become more frequent and severe
- Severe difficulty in learning new facts or skills
- Regularly forgetting things you learned recently

- Losing awareness of daily events
- Repeating phrases or anecdotes in the same conversation
- Losing interest in daily activities and physical appearance

(For detailed discussions of Alzheimer's disease and other degenerative brain disorders, see page 469.)

Changes in Eyesight

Signs and Symptoms
- Difficulty in focusing on objects
- Blurring of the central portion of the field of vision
- Clouding of vision in one or both eyes
- Double vision
- Difficulty driving at night because of glare from oncoming headlights

Like the rest of your body, your eyes age. As a result, they become less "elastic." This change most often affects the lens, resulting in difficulty in focusing on nearby objects (see Presbyopia, page 526). If you do not need glasses at least some of the time after age 65, you are the exception.

When changes in vision become more pronounced, something other than normal aging is frequently at work. Glaucoma, the buildup of fluid within the eyeball to an abnormally high pressure, narrows the field of vision and can lead to blindness if not diagnosed and treated appropriately. Most people have no symptoms, although occasionally patients with glaucoma have pain or redness of the eyes and see colorful halos around lights. About 3 percent of people older than 65 have glaucoma. Cataracts (clouding of the lens) blur the field of vision, may cause double vision, and typically create problems in night driving. Macular degeneration, possibly caused by a diminished blood supply to the macula (the center of vision), can affect reading acuity and visual sharpness.

These illnesses can affect one or both eyes. Because they generally come on gradually and are usually painless, they often are mistaken for the normal effects of aging on the eyes.

Diagnosis
It is important to visit an ophthalmologist promptly when a vision problem occurs. In particular, seek prompt medical attention if

---

Sharpening Your Memory

These tips may help enhance your memory:

Get Organized. Manage daily activities with a routine. Wind the grandfather clock every Sunday after breakfast.

Use Lists. Don't bother to memorize things you can list on paper (for example, grocery lists and birthdays).

Nudge the Numbers. Find ways to cue your memory. If your wedding anniversary is September 5, think, "We didn't have 5 minutes alone until our honeymoon."

Make Associations. When driving, look for landmarks and repeat, "Clark's house, Central School." Next time, you'll remember to turn there to reach your friend's house.

Practice. Practice paying attention. When you're introduced to someone, listen carefully and repeat the person's name: "How do you do, Anne?" Repeat the name in the ensuing conversation. At parties, take an inventory of people you see. Rehearse names in your mind.

Try Not to Worry. Fretting about memory can lead to more forgetfulness, especially if you're tired or under stress.

you develop a painful, red eye or if you lose full or partial vision in an eye. If left untreated, some eye disorders can cause you to lose a substantial part of your eyesight or even to go totally blind. The tests that an ophthalmologist performs are generally painless.

How Serious Is Failing Eyesight?

The moderate degree of eyesight failure that is normal to aging is not serious and can be corrected with eyeglasses. Cataracts and diseases of the eyes are serious because they have the potential for significant loss of vision.

Cataracts and glaucoma usually can be treated. Macular degeneration is sometimes treated with laser therapy, although the results often are disappointing.

What Can Be Done?

Many low-vision aids are available. Finding one that's right for you can take some trial and error, so be patient. Here is a list of just some of the devices that are available:

Good Lighting. As you grow older, you need more light, whether you have vision problems or not. A flexible light, such as a gooseneck lamp, can direct illumination onto your reading or work area.

Special Eyeglasses. Bifocal or trifocal glasses that are stronger than normal may help. Also, high-power, prismatic "half-eye" reading glasses are available.

Magnifiers. Magnification devices come in many styles. They can be hand-held, free-standing, mounted on a headband or your eyeglasses, or even worn around your neck. Many models have a built-in light or incorporate various magnification powers.

Easy-to-See, Practical Items. Everything from magnifiers to items such as clocks, telephones, playing cards that have extra-large letters or numbers, and large-size game boards is available from mail-order catalogs. To order a catalog, contact the American Foundation for the Blind Product Center, 3342 Melrose Ave. N.W., Roanoke, VA 24017; telephone number (800) 829-0500.

Telescopes. Miniature telescopes and binoculars, some of them worn like eyeglasses, can help you with distance viewing.

High-Tech Systems. If you have severely poor eyesight, consider a video system. This equipment, although expensive, allows you to adjust the magnification up to 60 times.

Problems With Night Vision

Night vision refers to how well you see in poor light or in the dark. With age, healthy eyes become a little less adept at night vision. A common and potentially dangerous consequence is difficulty in driving at night. For example, your eyes may not be able to recover as rapidly from the momentary blinding caused by the glare of oncoming headlights.

There are other causes of diminished night vision. Vitamin A is vital to night vision; a diet marginal in vitamin A or a disease process that results in a vitamin A deficiency can all but eliminate night vision. Today, though, vitamin A deficiency severe enough to impair vision is rare.

In addition, other problems with the eyes, such as cataracts and glaucoma, can cause difficulty with night vision (see pages 553 and 550).

If you have a night vision problem, consult your eye specialist. Never assume that a vision problem is simply something you have to put up with as you age. It could be that you have an easily treatable condition or, conversely, that a delay in seeking help could jeopardize your sight.

Finally, if night driving bothers you, reexamine your need to drive after dark. For safety's sake it may be wise to avoid such trips.

(For detailed discussions, see Cataracts, page 553; Glaucoma, page 550; and Macular Degeneration, page 556.)

Impaired Mobility

There is a saying that "once you're over the hill, you start to pick up speed." Unfortunately, at least when it comes to physical mobility, this is seldom true. Muscles, tendons, and joints generally lose a certain amount of their strength and flexibility, and the metabolic "power plant" that provides the energy for your body burns a little slower. You do not move as fast as you once did.

If you have had an active life, by age 60 your muscles will have lost little or none of the strength they had in your youth. However, you will have less flexibility, your reflexes will be slower, and your coordination will be poorer. With advancing age, and especially with lack of regular strenuous physical activity, muscles may lose some of their strength.

If you have a disease that saps your energy or an ailment that affects a body part involved in locomotion—such as hip, knee, ankle, or back—then you experience greater impairment. Arthritic changes in

How to Avoid Falls

Losing your independence is one of the biggest fears you may have about aging. Falling is one of the most common causes. Half of all people older than 65 who are hospitalized for a fall never regain their former level of independence. The checklist provided here will help you prevent a fall.

Your Health

Have your vision and hearing checked regularly. If they are impaired, you lose important cues that help you maintain your balance.

Exercise regularly. Exercise improves your strength, muscle tone, and coordination. These results not only help prevent falls but also reduce the severity of injury if you do fall. Walking is a good form of exercise.

Ask your physician about the drugs you take. Some drugs, or combinations of drugs, used to treat high blood pressure, angina, and depression may affect balance and coordination.

Avoid alcohol. Even a little alcohol can cause falls, especially if your balance and reflexes already are impaired.

Get up slowly. A momentary decrease in blood pressure, due to drugs or aging, can cause dizziness if you stand up too quickly.

Maintain balance and footing. If you sometimes feel dizzy, use a cane or walker to help you keep your balance on uneven ground or slippery surfaces. Wear sturdy, low-heeled shoes with wide, nonslip soles.

Your Home

All rooms. Remove raised doorway thresholds. Rearrange furniture, if necessary, to keep electrical cords and furniture out of walking paths. Fasten area carpets to the floor with tape or tacks, and don't use throw rugs.

Stairways. Be sure stairs are well-lighted and have sturdy handrails. If you have a vision problem, apply bright tape to the first and last steps.

Bathrooms. Install grab handles and nonskid mats inside and just outside your shower and tub and near the toilet. Shower chairs and bath benches minimize the risk of falling. Elevated toilet seats, which can be purchased at a medical supply store, can be a significant help for persons who have a problem getting off the seat.

Kitchens. Don't use difficult-to-reach shelves. Never stand on a chair. Use nonskid floor wax, and wipe up spills immediately.

Bedrooms. Put a light switch by the door and by your bed so you don't have to walk across the room to turn on a light. Plug night-lights into electrical outlets in bedrooms, halls, and bathrooms.

---

joints slow the movements of millions of Americans. Occasionally, medications have the same effect.

What Can Be Done?

If you have a disease that affects your movements, it should be treated. But what about the usual slowing down that comes with age or with deterioration of a joint?

First, take a little more time to get where you have to go. In particular, avoid falls. The possibility of a fall is a special danger. As you age, your bones become more brittle (especially in postmenopausal women who may have some degree of osteoporosis; see page 894). A fall that you would have easily walked away from as a younger person may cause a fracture. And certain fractures, such as those of the hip, may end your independence or even your life. However, surgical procedures now available may provide good recovery of joint function if you are in good health (see Joint Replacement, page 911).

Do not live your life in fear of falling. The best single strategy to avoid this and many other problems of aging is to keep yourself in good general health. This requires regular exercise—especially walking. Weight training in people older than 65 can increase muscle strength and improve walking ability. Among the elderly who have accidents, those who are in good physical condition before the accident recover the most quickly and completely. Stay active, but be sensible. Think prevention.

Incontinence

At any age, and whether it involves urine or stool or both, incontinence usually is caused by an underlying illness or ailment. Elderly people are more vulnerable to incontinence than are younger people. As you age, the muscles and ligaments that control urination and defecation become somewhat less efficient and thus are more readily disturbed by a physical ailment. However, incontinence is not an inevitable part of getting older.

(For detailed discussions of urinary incontinence in women, see Urine Incontinence and Other Urine Loss Problems, page 1193; in men, see Urinary Incontinence, page 1207. For a discussion of Fecal Incontinence, see page 799.)

Constipation

Signs and Symptoms
- Hard and occasionally painful bowel movements
- Diminished frequency of bowel movements
- Difficulty in evacuating stool

Many people define constipation as not having at least one stool per day. This definition simply is not accurate. The range of normal stool patterns varies widely from individual to individual. For one, it may be a bowel movement one to three times a day, and for another it may be only once every 2 or 3 days. Constipation means a decrease in the frequency of your normal bowel habits. In addition, with constipation, stools often tend to be harder in composition and the act of defecating occasionally may be painful. Evacuating stool can be difficult, or there is a sense of incomplete emptying of stool from the rectum.

Constipation can be caused by an improper diet, changes in diet, dehydration, medications, or inactivity. Sometimes it is a symptom of an underlying disease such as cancer of the colon, hypothyroidism, or depression. You are not necessarily constipated more frequently as you age.

What Can Be Done?
The vast majority of cases of constipation are not serious. If the signs and symptoms described above are of recent onset, see your physician. He or she will review your medications and dietary habits to see whether they are the cause. Your physician may perform an examination, obtain appropriate laboratory tests, and probably recommend examination of your colon (see pages 784 and 788).

If these studies do not reveal any signifi-cant abnormality, minor dietary modifications may be helpful. These include increased consumption of water or other fluids and the addition of fresh fruits and vegetables to supply fiber in your diet. Your physician's recommendations might also include the use of bran in your breakfast cereal or a bulk former that contains psyllium. Psyllium is nothing more than a vegetable fiber ground into a powder. You mix it thoroughly with water or other liquids and drink it once or twice a day.

Continue to be as active as you can. When you feel the urge to go to the bathroom, don't delay; holding a bowel movement can foster constipation. Avoid commercial laxatives because, over time, they can aggravate your constipation.

(For a detailed discussion of constipation, see page 784.)

Special Nutritional Concerns

Is there a single "old-age" diet that can help all elderly people live longer, healthier lives? No. But we can offer some nutrition strategies.

The maladies you accumulate as you age are unique to you. If you have hypertension, you will be advised to avoid salt. People with diabetes are told to avoid simple sugars.

Although there is little evidence that your need for vitamins changes as you age, other nutritional needs do change. For example, there is reason to believe that your requirements for protein increase. At the same time, your need for energy may decrease. Thus, if you do not reduce the calories in your diet, you probably will gain weight. Obesity, in turn, puts you at risk for many ailments such as diabetes. So it is important to work at maintaining proper weight, especially as you age.

Nutrition Strategies
Variety and moderation are the keys to a healthful diet—at any age. A balanced diet ensures proper intake of vitamins, minerals, proteins, carbohydrates, and other food elements. Moderation controls calories and is especially important with regard to consumption of alcohol.

Drink plenty of water. Insufficient intake of water is a common cause of constipation.

If you have specific ailments, your physician or a registered dietitian will provide dietary advice tailored to your needs. Follow it. Sometimes these recommendations require changes in lifelong habits or food preferences. Be assured that the self-discipline required is well worth the effort. It may enhance your health and even add years to your life.

Changes in Sexuality

Signs and Symptoms
- Diminished sexual desire
- Absence of sexual desire
- Problems in sexual performance (such as impotence or painful intercourse)

It takes determination to resist the "over-the-hill" mentality espoused by society today. The widespread perception is that older people are not sexually active. The reality is that many older people enjoy an active sex life that often is better than their sex life in early adulthood.

Age brings changes at 70 just as it does at 17, but you never outgrow your need for intimate love and affection. Whether you seek intimacy through nonsexual touching and companionship or through sexual activity, you and your partner can overcome most obstacles that aging or illness brings. The keys are caring, adapting, and communicating.

Your brain is an important sex organ. Sexual arousal begins with external stimulation of your senses—touch, sight, smell, and hearing. Because of this you can have orgasms throughout your life, although your response may be diminished or slower.

Changes in Women
Sexual desire is the most variable of your sexual responses. Although your sex drive is largely determined by emotional and social factors, hormones such as estrogen and testosterone do play a role. Estrogen is made in your ovaries, testosterone in your adrenal glands. Surprisingly, sexual desire is affected mainly by testosterone, not estrogen. At menopause, your ovaries stopped producing estrogen, but most women produce enough testosterone to preserve their interest in sex.

If you experience decreased desire, mood enhancers (candlelight, music, romantic thoughts) often help. Medical interventions include hormone replacement therapy, treatment for depression, and behavioral counseling.

After menopause, estrogen deficiency may have slowed the natural swelling and lubrication of your vagina during arousal. Even when you feel excited, your vagina may stay somewhat tight and dry. The result can be dyspareunia—difficult or painful intercourse. Try a lubricant such as K-Y jelly, or talk to your physician about estrogen cream for your genital area or about estrogen replacement therapy. Even regular intercourse can help—women who are sexually active after menopause have better vaginal lubrication and elasticity of vaginal tissues.

Women in their 60s and 70s have a greater incidence of painful uterine contractions during orgasm.

Changes in Men
Sex, something you may have taken for granted most of your life, may become "iffy" in your later years. Physical changes in a man's sexual response parallel those in women.

Although feelings of desire originate in your brain, you need a minimal amount of the hormone testosterone to put these feelings into action. The great majority of aging men produce well above the minimal amount needed to maintain interest in sex, but they may require more physical and mental stimulation to get an erection, and the erection will be less firm and will not last as long. Accept changes in erections as a normal part of aging, and use a position that makes it easy to insert the penis into the vagina. To enhance stimulation, don't use a condom unless necessary to prevent disease transmission.

Aging increases the time between possible ejaculations from just a few minutes at the age of 17 to as much as 48 hours by age 70. Emphasize quality, not quantity. Have intercourse less frequently. Alternatively, engage in sexual activities that don't require an erection.

If you have problems reaching orgasm, talk to your physician. Counseling, medications, vacuum devices, and vascular surgery are some of the treatments possible. For information on penile implants, see page 1227.

(For detailed discussions, see Loss of Sexual Desire in Women, page 1225, and Loss of Sexual Desire in Men, page 1229.)

Hearing Loss

Signs and Symptoms
- Increasing difficulty in hearing well
- Difficulty in hearing a conversation when surrounded by other noises

Although some people retain perfect hearing throughout their lives, most lose some hearing sensitivity gradually, starting in the 20s. This normal hearing loss begins with the higher frequencies and, by age 65, generally has started to affect the lower frequencies also.

Hearing impairment associated with aging is caused by changes that occur within the inner ear or in nerves attached to it. Wax in the ears, ear injuries caused by excessive exposure to noise, and various diseases also can impair hearing.

How Serious Is Hearing Loss?

Hearing loss can be serious in that it can interfere with your safety as well as your social life.

Treatment

Hearing Aids

Many types of hearing impairment can be treated by wearing a hearing aid. A good one costs from $500 to $2,000, but it is worth the money if it helps you hear better and improves your quality of life. Yet, people often aren't fully satisfied with their hearing aids. Complaints range from improper fit to poor repair service to lack of hearing improvement. Dissatisfaction can be caused by unrealistic expectations and by the lack of skill and training of some hearing-aid salespeople.

Technical improvements during the past decade have made hearing aids better than ever, but to take advantage you have to be an informed consumer. Before you buy a hearing aid, be examined by a physician, preferably an ear, nose, and throat specialist (otorhinolaryngologist). Also, have an audiologist give you a hearing test. The results will help a dispenser select the aid that best compensates for your particular hearing loss. Buy from a reputable company, be alert to misleading claims, and ask about a trial period. Get another hearing test while wearing the aid, and return it if it doesn't improve your hearing.

Personal Assistive Listening Devices

These are relatively inexpensive amplifiers that work like a headset. They often are available at church services and other activities.

Surgery

Some types of hearing impairment and loss are treatable by surgery (see Hearing Loss and Hearing Aids, page 580).

Voice Changes

The characteristic sound of a person's voice can change. Three causes of voice changes are throat infection, stroke, and cancer.

Throat infections sometimes cause hoarseness. Most often, treatment is not required. If the hoarseness is severe, medications are available.

Stroke sometimes affects the voice. Speech may become slurred and slow. After a stroke, the voice usually recovers on its own. If not, many physicians recommend speech therapy (see Stroke, page 461).

Hoarseness can be a symptom of cancer of the larynx. With early detection and prompt, appropriate treatment, this potentially fatal illness often can be controlled or even cured. Cancer of the larynx is associated with smoking and excessive use of alcohol. It affects men more often than women (see Cancers of the Throat, page 599).

Hoarseness can also be caused by an underactive thyroid gland or by anxiety.

If you experience rapid or chronic changes in the quality or loudness of your voice, consult your physician.

Depression

Signs and Symptoms

- Loss of interest or pleasure in usual activities
- Feeling sad or "blue"
- Poor appetite
- Sleep disturbance
- Fatigue, loss of energy

Sometimes people become depressed over specific events, such as the loss of a spouse or friend or the course an illness has taken. Or they just may have a general "out-of-sorts" mood for no reason in particular. This second type of depression generally passes on its own.

When the feeling does not pass, physicians describe the condition by the term "major depression." It is common among people of all ages. Among the elderly, it is sometimes mistaken for Alzheimer's disease, which can have the same symptoms of withdrawal and apathy. However, there is no connection between the two.

One feature of depression in the elderly is an obsession with mortality. Depressed people often think they are about to die, or they dwell on the inevitable approach of death. Some consider suicide (see Warning Signs of Potential Suicide, page 1125).

(For a detailed discussion, see Depression in the Elderly, page 1103.)

Skin Problems

Age brings changes in your skin. It becomes more wrinkled, thinner (so that the veins are more apparent), and less supple than it was in youth. Blotches and spots are common. You probably perspire less.

Some of these changes are caused in part by skin dryness, which can be minimized by good skin care throughout life (see Proper Skin Care, page 986). Your skin also will benefit from sustained, sound nutrition. Avoid excessive exposure to the ultraviolet rays of sunlight (see page 996).

If you are white, age spots (also known as liver spots) probably will appear. These small, flat patches look like freckles. Their color ranges from light brown to black. Their cause is unknown. They may be cosmetically troublesome but are medically insignificant. In particular, they have nothing to do with the liver and never become cancerous. Most people do not seek treatment for liver spots (see page 1003).

Tiny blood vessels just below the surface of the skin may become fragile, break, and bleed. This causes superficial bruising, a condition called senile purpura. It occurs mainly on the forearms.

Another skin condition that sometimes occurs is asteatosis. This is characterized by intense itching on your back, lower legs, hands, or elsewhere. It is caused by a loss of natural skin oils, and it produces scaly skin that, in some cases, cracks deeply. Asteatosis is often treated by commonsense measures such as restricting the frequency of baths, not wearing wool, increasing the humidity of dry rooms in winter, and applying oils to the skin. See your physician about itchy skin, though, because it can be caused by some other underlying condition (see page 995 for other skin conditions).

Skin cancer, which can appear as various types of spots or growths, usually can be cured if found early. The appearance of any sore that does not heal is a good reason to consult your physician (see Skin Cancers, page 1004).

Support of Pelvic Organs in Women

As women age, muscles supporting the organs in their pelvic area may weaken. This condition is more likely to develop in women who have borne children. Childbirth, particularly repeated childbirths, can stretch the supporting muscles and ligaments of the abdomen, and the results of this stretching show up later in life. In addition, the aging process itself sometimes weakens these tissues.

The conditions that occur include cystocele, rectocele, enterocele, uterine prolapse, and urinary incontinence. Although such problems are not an inevitable consequence of aging, you should be aware of them so that you can recognize their symptoms and know the treatment options.

(For detailed discussions of these problems, see Women's Health, page 1139.)

Problems Related to Too Many Medications

In your later years, you may be at risk for problems with the medicines you take. Older Americans take a disproportionately high percentage of the prescription drugs sold; the average number of prescriptions per person is seven. Because older adults tend to have more than one health problem, they often find themselves taking several different medicines at various times of the day or night. This situation can be risky.

It is easy to forget a dose or mistakenly take an extra dose or two. In addition, aging alters the ways your body absorbs, metabolizes, and excretes medications.

The Risks

Many medicines can cause sedation or confusion. Many can cause stomach distress or other gastrointestinal problems. Some combinations of drugs can interfere with the action of your heart or other organs.

For many medicines, an occasional skipped dose or a double dose makes little difference. With some, however, precise dosage and timing are of great importance. To organize your schedule for taking medications, use a pill box with multiple compartments. If you miss a dose, the omission will be apparent. For example, if you think you forgot to take the pills scheduled at your previous meal, the empty compartment will indicate that you actually did take the medicine at the proper time.

Drug Interactions

The action of one drug can sometimes be altered by the action of another drug. The effects of anticoagulant medications, for example, can be influenced by over-the-counter drugs such as aspirin. Non-prescription drugs can be potent. Some cause serious reactions when mixed with prescription medications.

Today, "going to the doctor" often means going from one specialist to another. Ideally, all of your medications should be under the control of one physician. Bring along your medicines, in their original containers, when you visit the physician. List any over-the-counter drugs you take, such as aspirin, laxatives, and hay fever products. Ask your physician to determine the proper dosage of the over-the-counter drugs, because the amounts recommended on the package may be too great for older people or when mixed with prescription medications.

Then, follow your physician's instructions carefully and inform him or her of any side effects. If you take many medications, your physician might arrange a medicine calendar for you. This is a compilation of your drugs with directions for what and how much you should take throughout the day or night (see page 1278).

It is essential to notify any physician you see if you have conditions such as heart disease, high blood pressure, or glaucoma or if you are allergic to certain drugs. In such cases, a standard prescription could threaten your life.

Aging Brings Change

As you age, the way your body handles medications can change, as follows:

Distribution. Some drugs concentrate in body fat. Others concentrate in other tissues. As you age, body fat makes up a greater percentage of your weight. If you take a drug that concentrates in fat, its effects may be delayed and prolonged.

Metabolism. With age, your organs lose some of their effectiveness. For example, the flow of blood through your liver may be only 40 to 50 percent that of a younger person. This means you don't process drugs as quickly; therefore, their effects may be delayed or exaggerated.

Elimination. The ability of your kidneys to clear drugs from your system decreases.

To offset these differences, your physician considers your age when prescribing a medication and deciding on its dosage and frequency.

Curbing Costs

Many pharmacies will offer 5 to 15 percent discounts for senior citizens, so comparison shop. Ask your physician whether a generic form is available or suitable. Not all medications are, but if so they often cost 30 to 50 percent less than the brand name. Check with your insurance, too; some plans cover the costs of only generic drugs. If you'll be taking a drug for a long time, ask your physician if it's appropriate to order a bulk supply, which costs less than small refills.

Community Services

If you, or a relative or friend, need a little help getting through the day, what can you do? If you require periodic or around-the-clock nursing attention, where can you best get it?

To find out what is available in your area, ask physicians, nurses, social workers, clergy, and friends. Check the Yellow Pages, which in many cities have a community information section that includes numbers for information and referral centers, seniors help lines and hot lines, and the area agency on aging.

The U.S. Administration on Aging runs a public service called the Elder Care Locator. If you call 1-800-677-1116, they will put you in touch with someone who can advise you of what's available in your community.

Today, only a minority of people in their later years live in nursing homes because so many other options are available. Some make it possible for you to remain at home.

Retirement Communities

Continuing-care retirement communities (CCRCs) meet the needs of many older adults. These offer both residential and health care facilities that can effectively serve all your needs. Nearly 250,000 people now live in CCRCs, and the number of facilities is expected to double to about 1,500 within the next decade.

At a CCRC, you purchase a contract for care. You pay an entry fee, which may be refundable, and a monthly fee for services. These services include the following:

Housing. You typically choose from apartments of different sizes. In some communities, penthouses, townhouses, and detached houses also are available. The retirement community takes care of security and maintenance.

Meals. You might have the option of cooking in your unit, eating in the communal dining room, or having meals delivered.

Amenities. Most facilities provide transportation, housekeeping, laundry service, a library, religious services, a beauty salon, and recreation and cultural activities.

In-Home Care. At extra cost, some CCRCs help with bathing, dressing, and taking medications.

Health Care. An on-site nursing home offers temporary or permanent care.

Most CCRCs have similar services, but their financial terms—especially for health care—differ sharply. Shop carefully to find the place that best meets your needs.

Home Health Care

Many hospitals or other health agencies offer home health services. A nurse or nurse's aide will come to your home and provide services such as giving injections, changing bandages, or helping with speech or physical therapy. Or someone will help you bathe, dress, and even cook meals. Depending on the service and arrangements, care is provided for a portion of every day or for several days a week. Medicare, Medicaid, private insurance, and other programs sometimes pay for some or all of such care, even for extended periods. Home health care and other types of community facilities can be especially helpful if you live alone.

Adult Day Care

Adult day care is available in some communities. In this service, an older person who cannot function independently is looked after in a supervised setting during the day. Transportation to the day care center usually can be arranged and, depending on the program, people can attend for part of a day, a day or two each week, or even daily. This type of program often is appropriate for people mildly incapacitated by a stroke or for those who have physical or mental handicaps.

A midday meal often is served. Contact with others is possible and, in some cases, organized activities are arranged. The services provided generally are limited, although some programs do provide medical and nursing attention.

Respite Care Programs

People who need limited nursing or medical care often can check into a hospital or nursing home for a limited time during which they receive specific services. The help commonly offered includes rehabilitation programs such as physical or speech therapy after a stroke. After the service is provided, the patient returns home. This may occur within a week or two or after a month or more. Repeat or regular visits can be arranged.

To find out whether these services are available, check with your local hospital or nursing home.

Day Respite Care Programs

These are similar to the respite programs described above but the services are more limited. Again, you can visit the facility (a hospital or nursing home) on an as-needed basis for some particular medical procedure, nursing care, or therapy. Generally the visit is limited to several hours or perhaps once or twice a week.

Foster Care Homes

In some communities, foster care homes are available. Another option is home sharing, in which an elderly person can stay at home and rent a room to someone who helps out with simple work around the house. Ask your physician or social service worker for advice.

Nutrition Services

The Meals on Wheels program has changed life for elderly Americans. It delivers hot meals, generally one meal a day, to older people in their homes, sparing them the chore of cooking for themselves or the unhealthful option of skipping meals altogether.

The program receives some public funding, making the cost charged for meals nominal. Programs similar to Meals on Wheels also are offered by volunteer groups and churches, particularly in larger cities.

Congregate dining (dining with others) is commonplace at senior citizens centers and at housing designed specifically for older people. The meal and the social gathering can become the high point of your day. More meals can be served with greater economy to senior citizens this way than by home delivery programs.

Nursing Homes

More than 1 million Americans age 65 or older now reside in nursing homes. This is about 5 percent, or 1 out of every 20 people in this age range. Among people age 85 or older, approximately 20 percent live in nursing homes. About three-fourths of all nursing home residents are women.

In the past, admission to a nursing home was considered to be the "last stop." This is not necessarily the case today. Many physicians recommend a stay in a nursing home to recover from a stroke, a hip fracture, or some other mishap. Once rehabilitated, nursing home residents often return to independent living.

Among the common problems that lead to nursing home admission are incontinence, thinking disorders, stroke, a bone fracture, walking disabilities, general debility, loss of spouse or caregiver, and terminal illness.

When Is a Nursing Home Appropriate?

It is not a matter of course that everyone who is old or who has a chronic illness has to enter a nursing home. Individual circumstances vary considerably. In addition, admission to a nursing home is getting more difficult.

The single most important reason for entering a nursing home probably is the need for intensive care. Nursing home residents receive help with many of the routine activities of daily life. Eighty-five percent need help bathing, 70 percent need help dressing, more than 50 percent need help going to the bathroom, and more than 30 percent need help eating. The average nursing home resident also has several chronic illnesses that require medical attention. More than half have Alzheimer's disease or some other mental impairment.

Families often care for elderly family members who cannot live alone. How much care a family can offer depends on many factors. If a household consists of two working parents and children in school, no one is around during the day to provide care to an elderly person. Some mentally disoriented people can pose a hazard to themselves and to others when left unsupervised.

If you have an elderly family member in your home, you must balance his or her care needs against the well-being of the rest of your family. Someone who needs long-term help in eating, dressing, bathing, and going to the bathroom can wear an entire family down. Families sometimes recruit temporary help for part of the day or for relief in order to shop, take a vacation, or pursue their own interests. Care provided at home should be shared by family members so that it does not all fall to one person, and it should lie within the limits of a family's physical, emotional, and financial resources.

When care at home is not feasible or threatens to destroy the fabric of a family, a nursing home should be considered. If the elderly person is physically able to visit prospective nursing homes and psychologically fit enough to help make the decision, then he or she should participate in the selection process.

Selecting a Good Home

In selecting a nursing home, the first person to turn to for advice is a social worker or hospital dismissal planner. These experts are excellent sources of information on nursing homes and are familiar with entry criteria and options for different levels of care.

Service agencies funded by your county or the United Way are another source of help, or ask a member of the clergy, a friend, or your physician. Nursing homes are listed in the Yellow Pages of your telephone directory. Your state or county social services agency, health department, or county medical society also can provide a list of nursing homes. They also may have information on how best to evaluate and select a home.

Most nursing homes now are termed skilled-care homes; so-called intermediate-care homes are being phased out in most areas. In a skilled-care home, you get 24-hour nursing service as well as restorative, physical, occupational, and other therapy. If you are deciding between skilled-care and intermediate-care homes, consider your future as well as your current health needs.

To select a nursing home, visit several. Before you go, however, prepare yourself for the visits. Write down the things you want to find out. Here are four suggestions:

Atmosphere. Are the staff members qualified? Friendly? Caring? How about the residents? Ask some residents what they think about the home. Also consider the facilities. Luxury is not necessary, but basic hygiene is. Notice odors. A pervasive urine smell suggests neglect or bad ventilation. Find out how hair care and personal laundry are handled.

Food. Ask the residents how they rate the food. Look at a menu. If you have special dietary needs, ask if the home can accommodate them. Do residents get help in eating if they need it? If possible, time your visit so you arrive at mealtime.

Activities. Ask about the home's activity program. A skilled-care nursing home must post its activity program; take a look at it. Is there anything going on that interests you? Can you pursue your own hobbies and interests there? Can you leave the home to go out and shop or just take a walk? Is it easy to get to a telephone? Can you have a say in choosing roommates?

Medical Care. Usually your physician will continue to take care of you after you enter a nursing home. However, see what medical care the home itself offers. Can it meet your needs for physical or occupational therapy or other specialized needs?

Paying the Bill

The cost of nursing home care can be high. However, financial assistance is available from Medicare, Medicaid, private health insurance policies, the Veterans Administration, trade unions, and fraternal organizations. Federal, state, and local governments pay for more than half of the nursing home care provided in the United States. Individuals and their families fund a little under half. Private insurance pays for less than 5 percent.

Reimbursements change and vary widely from state to state, so check current state and federal programs locally. A hospital social worker can help you.

Other Alternatives

During the past 20 years, the United States has seen the development of group homes for children and adults with mental disabilities. As the population ages, more group homes are becoming available for seniors with specific medical problems such as Alzheimer's disease (see page 470).

Part II

Staying Well

The chapters in this section are devoted to helping you maintain and even improve your health by establishing and maintaining a healthful lifestyle. You'll find practical tips on topics such as eating right, exercising, controlling stress, avoiding harmful habits, and traveling overseas. You'll also find useful information on safety within and outside your home, and on steps you can take to help protect the environment.

Contents

 9 Nutrition and Health 251
10 Exercise and Fitness 289
11 Controlling Stress 307
12 Tobacco 315
13 Alcohol Abuse and Alcoholism 325
14 Medications and Drug Abuse 335
15 Safety 349
16 Tooth Care 363
17 The World Around Us 371
18 Traveling Abroad 379

Chapter 9

Nutrition and Health

Contents

What Is a Healthful Diet? 252
Is There an Ideal Diet? 252
Butter vs. Margarine, 254
Importance of Vitamin D, 255
"Healthy" Weight, 258
How Much Should You Weigh? 259
Prudent Diet, 259
A New Guide to Healthful Eating, 260
Preventing Excess Gas, 260
Nutritional Advice for the Stages of Life, 261
The Food Guide Pyramid, 261
What Counts as a Serving? 262
How Many Servings Do I Need? 262
Food Labeling, 263
Understanding Food Labels, 263
Nutrient Claims on Food Labels, 264
Vitamin and Mineral Supplements, 264
Selecting a Breakfast Cereal, 265
Antioxidant Nutrients, 265
Do You Need an Antioxidant Supplement? 266
Calcium and Osteoporosis, 266
What If I Don't Drink Milk? 266
Foods Rich in Calcium, 267
Food Safety, 267
Pesticides, 268
Food Safety at Picnics, 269
Food Safety in Your Home, 270

Food Processing, 271
Food Scares, 272
Proper Handling of Food, 272
Caffeine and Your Health, 273
Approximate Caffeine Content of Foods, 273
Nutrition and the Athlete, 274
Vegetarian Diets, 276
Weight Control, 277
Curbing Your Appetite, 278
Role of Exercise in Weight Control, 278
How Many Calories Are in My Drink? 279

Diet and Disease, 280
Avoiding Heart Disease, 280
Nutrition and Cancer Protection, 280
Nutrition and the Cancer Patient, 281
Salt and Hypertension, 283
Salt in Drinking Water, 283
Diabetes Diet, 284
Controlling Your Blood Sugar, 285
Specialized Diets for Chronic Diseases, 285
Dietary Risks of Alcoholism, 286
Food Fads, 286
Food Myths, 288

What Is a Healthful Diet?

Not many subjects are of consuming interest to virtually all of us—but food is certainly one of them. It is a principal pleasure of life and also a life-giving essential.

Without the continual replacement of nutrients in our bodies, we would die. Food is so important that from time immemorial it has formed the basis for rituals in every society. One measure of the success of a society is the abundance and quality (or lack thereof) of its food.

As recently as 50 years ago, the focus of nutrition research was to fight malnutrition and diseases caused by a lack of basic nutrients. Today, the pendulum has swung, and overconsumption has replaced deficiency as America's leading nutrition problem.

Dr. C. Everett Koop, Surgeon General under President Ronald Reagan, in a report on the nation's health, placed nutrition high on the nation's health agenda, along with reducing the spread of AIDS and eliminating smoking.

Recommendations on how Americans should eat have been made by several government and private agencies and are discussed in this chapter. Remember that these guidelines are for the general public. You are an individual and, depending on your family background and your own health findings, your physician or dietitian may recommend more stringent dietary restrictions, or possibly a more relaxed approach. It is reasonable to expect that as scientific knowledge advances, changes will be made in these guidelines from time to time.

This chapter also includes basic information on how your body uses food, weight control, and how to eat well when faced with disease.

If you need specific advice about a nutrition question beyond what is offered in these pages, talk to a registered dietitian. The letters R.D. (for Registered Dietitian) after a person's name show that he or she is registered with the American Dietetic Association. To obtain this credential, a person must earn an undergraduate degree in a 4-year program in food science and nutrition at an accredited college or university, complete 6 to 12 months of accredited or approved training in practical aspects of dietetics, and pass a national examination. In addition, registered dietitians must complete 75 hours of professional education every 5 years.

Some states have licensing procedures, and a dietitian may also be a licensed dietitian under the regulations of the state health department. Your local health department or physician can refer you to a competent dietitian.

Other people may also be helpful in examining or improving your nutritional status. Some physicians have a particular interest in nutrition. Home economists are often a good source of information on meal planning, food preservation, and food preparation, but they are less qualified than a registered dietitian for advising about the nutritional needs of a specific person.

The term "nutritionist" is not specifically defined and, unfortunately, it is sometimes used by people who have no credible nutritional training and who seek to sell dietary supplements or weight-loss schemes. Some may even display a diploma or certificate that may mean very little.

You can verify whether a school listed on a diploma is a bona fide educational institution by asking your local librarian to check whether the school is accredited by an agency recognized by the U.S. Department of Education or the Council on Post-Secondary Accreditation. The nutrition staff at your local hospital may also be of help for evaluating qualifications.

Is There an Ideal Diet?

In this day of intense interest in diet and health, many people yearn and often search for the perfect diet—one that will produce super health and above-normal vigor, strength, and resistance to disease, one that will delay aging, and one that will keep them slim. So pervasive is this interest that thousands of people spend vast quantities of time and money searching for the perfect answer.

Does or can such a diet exist? In all likelihood, the answer is no. Our nutritional needs differ at each stage of our lives from infancy through childhood, maturity, pregnancy, and old age and in states of disease. We also vary in our genetic tendencies toward diseases, including hypertension, some cancers, and heart and other vascular diseases, so food components such as salts or fats pose different risks to different people.

The human body needs various substances from the environment in order to grow, reproduce, and survive. We breathe air to acquire the oxygen our cells need to survive, we drink water to replenish vital supplies of liquid, and we eat to provide us with all-important energy sources, because energy is provided by the body's use of ingested protein, fat, and carbohydrates. Other components are also needed, although in much smaller amounts. These include essential amino acids, fatty acids, minerals, trace minerals, and vitamins.

All the foods we eat provide some level of nutrition. There may be no one perfect diet for all of us or even for one of us at all times, but there are some general principles for food selection that apply to most of us (see Dietary Guidelines for Americans, page 259).

Basic Components of Food

Our food is made up of many components that, when combined in appropriate proportions, provide a complete diet. The major groupings of nutrients include water, carbohydrates, proteins, and fats. Other groups are trace nutrients, known as vitamins and minerals, needed in smaller amounts. Each category has a different function in the regulation, growth, and repair of the body.

Water

Water seems so ordinary that you may forget how vital it is to good health. Water plays an important role in nearly every major function of your body. Water regulates body temperature, carries nutrients and oxygen to cells, and removes wastes. It also cushions joints and helps protect organs and tissues.

Drinking eight 8-ounce servings of water daily will help meet your body's need for proper hydration. Your individual need for water can increase for various reasons. Exposure to extreme hot or cold weather, eating a high-fiber diet, being pregnant, breast-feeding a baby, and vigorous exercise may all increase your need for water.

You can meet part of your water requirement through other fluids such as milk, juice, and soup. Keep in mind that beverages containing caffeine or alcohol have a dehydrating effect and do not count toward your daily water intake.

Some tips for increasing your water intake include the following:

- Taking water breaks instead of coffee breaks
- Having a glass of water before meals and snacks
- Substituting sparkling waters for alcoholic drinks at parties and social gatherings
- Bringing a supply of bottled water when traveling

Carbohydrates

Carbohydrates are starches or sugars and are found primarily in breads and cereals and in fruits and vegetables. The starches are referred to as complex carbohydrates, and sugars (found in fruits and in refined sugars) are called simple carbohydrates. Surprisingly, some of the complex carbohydrates may be digested, broken down into sugars, and appear in the blood as sugars, almost as rapidly as simple sugars themselves. Cane or beet sugar, known technically as sucrose, and corn syrup, which contains the sugar known as fructose, make up a considerable portion of the average American diet.

Proteins

Proteins are composed of building blocks called amino acids. Some of these amino acids can be produced by your body; others cannot. Those that must be obtained from the diet are called essential amino acids.

The essential amino acids in meat, eggs, milk, and cheese are very efficiently used. Proteins found in vegetables, cereals (such as wheat, rice, or corn), peas, and beans (except for soybeans) do not provide an optimal ratio of essential amino acids. Thus, more protein of plant origin is needed to meet your body's requirements than protein of animal origin. Vegetarian diets, when properly planned, can readily meet one's needs for protein (see page 276).

Fats

Fats are found in various foods and in various forms. Fats are found in foods of animal origin, such as meat, poultry, and fish, and in foods of vegetable origin. Some fats, such as cooking oils and salad oils, are liquid, whereas others, such as butter, margarine, vegetable shortening, and trimmed meat fat, are solid at room temperature.

Chemists classify fats according to the structure of their building blocks, the fatty acids. Fatty acids are saturated or unsaturated. Unsaturated fats are further classified as

Butter vs. Margarine

Not only the type of fat but also the amount of fat influences the level of cholesterol in your blood. Your goal is to limit total fat. Instead of worrying about the difference between margarine and butter, see how little of either spread you can use.

Nutritional comparisons:

- Margarine has 100 calories and an average of 11 grams of fat per tablespoon—virtually the same as butter
- Butter contains cholesterol; some margarines do too
- Margarine averages only 2 grams of saturated fat and 2 grams of trans fatty acids per tablespoon. Butter has almost 8 grams of saturated fat in the same serving size
- Stick, tub, and squeeze margarines are about equal in calories and total fat. But stick margarine has slightly more saturated fat
- Diet margarine has an average of 50 calories per tablespoon and about half the fat and saturated fat of regular margarine

monounsaturated (*mono* means "one") and polyunsaturated (*poly* means "many").

The chemical structure of saturated fatty acids is different from that of unsaturated ones, and this structure determines the characteristics of each type of fat. Saturated fats usually are solid at room temperature, and unsaturated fats are liquid at room temperature. Saturated fats are less likely to turn rancid, which is why they are used in many processed foods that must withstand long storage times.

Unsaturated fats can be made into saturated fats through a process called hydrogenation. This makes them more solid. Hydrogenated fats are common ingredients in commercial baked goods and other processed foods.

No food contains just one type of fatty acid. All foods contain a mixture of fats in various proportions. For example, olive oil is termed a monounsaturated fat, although it contains small proportions of saturated and polyunsaturated fatty acids.

Various fatty acids have different effects on blood cholesterol levels, which have been shown to have a relationship to heart disease. Saturated fats tend to raise your total blood cholesterol level by increasing both low-density lipoprotein (LDL, "bad" cholesterol) and high-density lipoprotein (HDL, "good" cholesterol). Monounsaturated fats tend to raise HDLs without raising total blood cholesterol. Polyunsaturated fats tend to reduce your total blood cholesterol level, but at the expense of the protective HDLs.

During the process of hydrogenation, a portion of the unsaturated fatty acids is converted to the saturated form and another portion remains unsaturated but changes into a "trans" form. Trans fatty acids have adverse effects on blood fats, increasing the "bad" LDL cholesterol and decreasing the "good" HDL cholesterol. The amounts of trans fatty acids are not shown on current nutrition labels. As a practical matter, avoid or minimize the use of foods identified as containing partially hydrogenated fats.

In addition, there are several different fatty acids within the categories of fat. Each of these may have somewhat different properties from those of its group as a whole. One group of polyunsaturated fatty acids found in fish is known as omega-3 fatty acids. These modify normal blood clotting mechanisms and have a mixed effect on blood fats. There is some suggestion that fish in the diet may have a protective effect against heart disease, but supplemental fish oil is generally not recommended.

While monounsaturated and polyunsaturated fats have few or almost no adverse effects on blood fats, many persons seek to reduce the fat in their diet as much as possible. Actually, certain polyunsaturated fatty acids (like vitamins) are necessary for health and life and are called essential fatty acids.

A very low-fat diet is difficult for some people to follow over any length of time, but it will have a favorable effect on blood fats and presumably on the process of atherosclerosis (a deposition of cholesterol in the lining of the arteries). Because foods low in fats such as grains and vegetables supply only a small amount of calories for their bulk, you might have difficulty eating enough to maintain your weight. Conversely, foods high in fat contain a large amount of calories for their volume and it is easy to consume enough to gain weight. Furthermore, fatty foods are often tasty and appealing. Almost any diet plan that greatly restricts choices of foods is also likely to reduce one's consumption of calories and lead to weight loss. (For more about fats and your health, see What Do Measurements of Blood Fats Mean? page 640).

Vitamins

Vitamins are substances that are essential in certain chemical transformations in your body and need to be present in your diet only in very small amounts. They help the body process proteins, carbohydrates, and fats. Certain vitamins also contribute to the production of blood cells, hormones, genetic material, and chemicals of your nervous system. Our bodies are unable to synthesize adequate amounts of most vitamins, so we must get them from the foods we eat.

The essential vitamins (there are 13 in all) are divided into two categories: fat-soluble and water-soluble.

The fat-soluble vitamins are A, D, E, and K. Vitamins A and D are stored in the liver, and reserve supplies may be sufficient for as long as 6 months. Reserves of vitamin K, however, may be sufficient for only a few days, and the supply of vitamin E is somewhere in between.

Both vitamins A and D can produce toxic effects when taken in excessive amounts. Toxic effects from taking large amounts of vitamin E have not been clearly demonstrated, but it does accumulate in the body's fatty tissues. Vitamin K is scarcely stored at all, and toxic effects from taking large amounts have been found only rarely.

The water-soluble vitamins include vitamin C (ascorbic acid) and the B vitamins. They are stored to a lesser extent than fat-soluble vitamins. Although it is popularly believed that the water-soluble vitamins are harmless when taken in large amounts, this is not always true.

Some of the water-soluble vitamins may have strong medicinal effects—good and bad—when taken in large amounts. Large amounts of niacin, for instance, are sometimes used to reduce high levels of fats in the blood; however, they also can cause abnormal liver function and an increase in blood sugar levels. Ascorbic acid in high amounts can increase oxalate excretion in the urine and may promote oxalate kidney stones (see page 843). In large doses, pyridoxine (a B vitamin) can cause nerve damage. In short, taking megadoses of vitamins is rarely warranted—and often it is potentially hazardous.

Minerals

Minerals such as calcium, magnesium, phosphorus, potassium, and sodium are also essential parts of the diet. Known as macrominerals, they are needed in relatively large amounts in the diet (those we need less of, termed "microminerals," are discussed below). Calcium, phosphorus, and magnesium are important in the development and

---

Importance of Vitamin D

Calcium is essential for strong bones, but to enhance the amount of calcium that ultimately reaches your bones you also need vitamin D.

Your body makes vitamin D from two sources—sunlight and food. Most of the vitamin D your body makes starts with the sun. When you're exposed to ultraviolet (UV) light rays, a chemical in your skin is changed into an inactive form of vitamin D.

Butter, eggs, and fatty fish such as herring, mackerel, and salmon naturally contain vitamin D. Other food sources are foods fortified with vitamin D such as milk, margarine, and some breakfast cereals.

Your liver and kidneys work to change vitamin D into the active form your body can use. Despite the availability of the sun and vitamin D-rich foods, several factors can interfere with obtaining enough of this essential nutrient:

Age. As you get older, your body turns UV rays into vitamin D less efficiently. If you spend limited time outdoors exposed to the sun and don't drink 2 or more cups of milk a day, you may want to consider a supplement. Don't take more than 400 IU of vitamin D a day unless prescribed by your physician.

Illness. Kidney or liver disease reduces your ability to change vitamin D into its usable form. Medications such as phenytoin, prescribed for seizure disorders, can also lead to vitamin D deficiency.

Vitamin D is like no other nutrient in that one of the best ways to obtain it has nothing to do with food. Although excessive sun exposure isn't healthful for your skin, a little bit of sun is good for your bones.

---

health of bones and teeth. Potassium is a major component of our muscles. Sodium helps regulate the fluids of the body.

The microminerals (trace minerals) are found in much smaller amounts in our food. Essential trace elements are minerals that, like vitamins, are needed in only small amounts. They include iron, iodine, zinc, copper, fluoride, selenium, and manganese, among others. They are all necessary for normal growth and health.

Calories

A calorie is a measure of energy. When carbohydrates, proteins, or fats are metabolized (burned) in the body, they produce energy, which is measured in a unit known as the kilocalorie. The kilocalorie is a common "calorie" used in expressing the energy content of foods and energy expenditures. It is defined as the amount of energy required to raise the temperature of 1 kilogram (2.2

pounds) of water by 1 degree Celsius (1.8 degrees Fahrenheit).

We all need energy, but our needs vary considerably. A small, elderly, sedentary woman may need only about 1,000 calories per day, but a large, young, physically active man may need as many as 4,000 calories daily.

Dietitians use food composition tables to calculate the nutrient content of various diets. The tables give the calorie, protein, carbohydrate, and fat content of various foods. When such food composition tables are used, the portion of food must be measured accurately, preferably by weighing it.

The term "empty calories" applies to sugars and to alcohol. These foods contribute energy (calories) but no other essential food elements such as vitamins or trace elements. Sugars include cane and beet sugar, fructose, glucose, and lactose. Some of these sugars, such as fructose and lactose, are an inherent part of some of the foods we eat (fruit and milk, respectively). Consuming sugar and even alcohol in moderation should not affect your health adversely, as long as you eat a variety of other foods to provide a good pattern of essential nutrients.

However, if you derive too many of your daily calories from sugars and alcohol, nutritional deficiencies can develop.

Fiber

Fiber is an important part of our diet. It is a complex mixture of chemicals derived from plant food that cannot be digested. There are two categories of fiber: soluble and insoluble. Fiber-rich foods usually contain more of one than the other. Examples of soluble fiber-rich foods are citrus fruits (not juice), strawberries, apples, legumes, oatmeal, and oat bran. Insoluble fiber is found in wheat bran, cereals, apples, vegetables, and root vegetables. (Note that apples are in both categories.) Soluble fiber has a favorable but usually not a major beneficial effect on blood cholesterol, and diets high in insoluble fiber appear to have a protective effect against cancer of the colon. Psyllium seed is used in the manufacture of many fiber supplements and provides a form of soluble fiber. You should seek to obtain the necessary fiber from foods, but fiber supplements may be used also, particularly for regulating stool habits (see page 784). Your physician can advise you whether fiber supplements are appropriate for your needs.

Currently, there is no Recommended Daily Allowance (RDA) for fiber, but many authorities recommend that we consume 20 to 25 grams per day.

Your Body Composition

Understanding the principles of nutrition involves more than a basic understanding of the various kinds of food we eat. The next step requires some comprehension of the makeup of our bodies. The fact is that water, protein, fat, and carbohydrate are primary ingredients of the human body. Water is a major component of the protein structures and carbohydrate stores, but there is only a small amount of water in our deposits of fat. Water makes up about 40 percent of body weight for the very obese to 70 percent of body weight for the very lean. In fact, measurements of the amount of water in the body can be used as a means of estimating how much fat one is carrying.

Protein structures make up about 30 to 60 percent of body weight. These tissues (muscle and vital organs such as the liver) function as the machinery of your body.

Your body does not store extra protein. If you eat more protein than your body needs, your muscle mass will not increase, nor will you have protein on reserve should you need it. Rather, extra protein is converted to fat. In a state approaching starvation, your body will tear down protein tissues in order to use the amino acids as fuel for energy processes. Death by starvation occurs when the body uses up between a quarter and a third of its protein structures.

Carbohydrate exists in the liver and muscles of the body as glycogen stores. Carbohydrate in the form of glycogen makes up about 1 to 5 percent of your body weight.

If your diet is high in carbohydrates and you are eating your full complement of needed calories each day, your glycogen stores, found largely in the liver, will be maximized. This store of fuel can be quickly called upon. For example, marathon runners may eat a diet rich in carbohydrates before a race. Glycogen, after conversion to glucose, is used as a fuel for the brain during brief fasts—such as during an overnight sleep (see Nutrition and the Athlete, page 274).

Conversely, if you eat a diet low in carbohydrates or if you are on a restricted-calorie diet, your glycogen stores will be rapidly depleted. If you switch from a normal diet to a very low-calorie or a very low-carbohydrate diet, you may lose 3 or 4 pounds within a day or two of the change. Such weight loss, however, will be in the form of glycogen and not fat.

Another "ingredient" of your body is fat. Fat is unlike protein and carbohydrates in that it is an extremely concentrated form of reserve energy and is associated with very little water. Body fat represents nearly 10 times as much energy for its weight as protein or carbohydrate tissues, about 3,500 calories per pound. In a normal person, 15 to 20 percent of body weight is from fat, although extremely obese people may have as much as 50 percent of their body weight in the form of fat.

These discrepancies in stored fats are the result of the way our bodies work. If you eat larger amounts of food than your body can burn, whether in the form of protein, fat, or carbohydrate, your body will store the extra energy as fatty tissue. However, because fat in our diet is so high in calories, indiscretion in fat intake can supply more calories than if protein or carbohydrates were eaten. Conversely, if we eat less food than our bodies need, our fuel reserves are mobilized to meet the daily energy deficit, and fatty tissues diminish—but relatively slowly because of the caloric richness of the fatty tissue.

The primary function of body fat is as a reserve of fuel, but it also constitutes a form of padding and insulation. Have you ever noticed that overweight people can sit longer and more comfortably on an unpadded bench or chair than can lean people, or that lean people become chilled more easily in cold surroundings?

Body fat also contributes to the regulation of certain hormones in women. Women whose body fat stores become very scant tend not to have menstrual periods. This is often the case with young women who have anorexia nervosa or some other form of starvation, and it can be a problem among lean women athletes.

Estimating degrees of personal fatness is difficult. Skinfold measuring is one method, but it requires a trained professional using skinfold calipers with considerable skill and accuracy. Even then, the results should be regarded as only approximate. Other methods, such as measurements of total body water and body density, used in research projects have a greater degree of accuracy.

Perhaps the easiest methods to assess body composition are with weight and height tables (see How Much Should You Weigh? page 259). Keep in mind, however, that the weight assigned to your sex and height does not consider your individual makeup and such factors as skeletal structure (are you big-boned?) and the amount of muscle (are you unusually muscular?). These are useful averages, but they are not to be taken as the final word in establishing your place on the slimness-to-heaviness scale.

One final word on the subject of fat. Physicians and scientists often debate whether having a very small amount of body fat is a hedge against some degenerative diseases, such as coronary artery disease (see Atherosclerosis: What Is It? page 636).

Alternatively, having only a small reserve of calories in the form of minimal body fat may lessen your chances of survival in the event of serious injury, infection, or disease with prolonged stress and convalescence. Obesity can under no circumstances be termed healthful, but being underweight may offer other health risks.

Changing Body Composition

The composition of the adult body changes during the course of a lifetime. Muscle mass tends to decrease slowly after the age of 30 or 35 and more rapidly after the age of 55. Translated into what your scale tells you, that means that if at age 65 you weigh 10 pounds more than you did at 30, you may actually be 15 to 20 pounds "fatter."

We seem to be equipped genetically for a certain distribution of fat. Women tend to carry more of their fat around the hips and thighs. Men often carry excess weight around their abdomens.

The distribution of fat is also related to age. As we get older, our subcutaneous fat tends to shift from the periphery (face, arms, legs, and neck) to the center of our bodies (trunk and abdomen). Furthermore, as we age, fat seems to shift from the subcutaneous depots to accumulations within the body cavity and around the kidneys. This is one reason why older people often have thin faces and extremities. At the same time, they may have protruding stomachs but little "pinchable" subcutaneous fat over the abdomen.

Excess fat about the abdomen and upper part of the body is considered to be a greater health risk than excess fat around the hips and thighs.

Metabolism

The processing undergone by the carbohydrates, proteins, fats, and other food substances we eat is termed "metabolism." It is the extremely complex process by which the food we eat is converted into energy. The process produces heat, carbon dioxide, water, and waste products. The energy created is used to carry out essential chemical transformations in the body and for muscular activity, and the heat helps maintain body temperature.

The rate of metabolism can be determined by measuring how much oxygen is used and how much carbon dioxide is given off. This rate, measured shortly after waking and before eating, is called the basal metabolic rate (BMR). Physicians have formulas to calculate average BMR or resting calorie expenditure based on metabolic rate standards, but you can get a very rough idea of your daily calorie expenditure with normal activity by multiplying your weight in pounds by 12.

The rate of metabolism, and therefore production of body heat, increases for an hour or two after meals. The rate of metabolism also increases with physical exertion. When you exert yourself, fat and glycogen (stored starch) are used up at an increased rate (see Exercise and Fitness, page 289).

We have discussed the basic components of food: fat, protein, carbohydrate, vitamins, and minerals. We have reviewed the process by which your body metabolizes fuel to keep you healthy and active. Now it is time to translate that knowledge into action and to identify what, for you, is a healthful weight and a prudent, healthful diet.

"Healthy" Weight

How much do you weigh? How much would you like to weigh? How much should you weigh?

In the best of all worlds, the answers would be the same. In reality, they aren't.

Ever since the Metropolitan Life Insurance Company issued height-weight tables in the 1940s, consumers and health experts alike have struggled with the concept of acceptable weights.

The latest version of recommended weight for height comes from the 1990 edition of Dietary Guidelines for Americans, published by the U.S. Department of Agriculture.

Height-weight tables are controversial. We can't settle the debate, but we can offer insight into what the latest height-weight table means to your health.

What Is a "Healthy" Weight?

The Dietary Guidelines for Americans recommend that you maintain a healthy weight. Figuring healthy weight should be based on three factors: a height-weight table, your body shape, and your health status.

Height-Weight Table

Depending on your age and height, the latest table lists broad ranges of recommended weights.

For example, if you're a 60-year-old man or woman who stands 5 feet 8 inches, you can weigh from 138 to 178 pounds. Higher weights generally apply to men; lower weights to women. This allows for differences in muscle and bone.

Don't focus on the numbers alone. The table is helpful only as a guide.

"Apple" vs. "Pear" Shape

How excess fat is distributed on your body can be a health risk. Extra weight that settles about your waist (apple-shaped body) puts you at a higher risk for heart disease, high blood pressure, stroke, and diabetes.

However, additional fat on your hips and thighs (pear-shaped body) means you probably don't have any greater health risks than people who aren't overweight at all.

Take a good look at yourself in the mirror. Does your shape resemble that of an apple or a pear? One way to determine whether you have the "apple" or "pear" silhouette is to determine your waist-to-hip ratio. Measure around your waist near the navel while standing relaxed, not pulling in your stomach. Measure around your hips over the buttocks where they are the largest. Divide the waist measurement by the hip measurement. If you are a woman and this number is greater than 0.80 or if you are a man and the figure is greater than 0.95, you have the "apple" silhouette and may be at greater risk for several health problems such as hypertension and heart disease. The distribution of your body fat stores is determined largely by heredity, although the amount is determined by how you eat and exercise.

Work at attaining and maintaining a lower body weight to reduce weight-related health risks due to storage of body fat.

Health Status

Some medical conditions such as diabetes, high blood pressure, heart disease, and stroke are related to weight.

If losing extra pounds may improve your health, then a lower weight in your height-weight range may be healthier and thus more important for you than it is for someone who does not have a medical problem.

What's the Right Weight for You?
Health experts agree that there's no exact answer to the question, "What's a healthy weight for me?" Researchers need to gather more data on obesity and its relation to disease and death. However, using tables with suggested weight-for-height-and-age and measuring waist-to-hip ratios are popular methods of estimating fat distribution and body weight.

Review Your Health Condition
Despite what tables say, you may not have to lose weight if you are in generally good health and have a sense of vigor and normal values for blood sugar, blood pressure, and triglyceride and cholesterol levels.

In the end, the weight that's most healthful for you may be one that you can comfortably attain and maintain through sensible eating habits.

Practice a healthful lifestyle, and chances are you'll keep your weight at a healthy level.

Prudent Diet

Except for people who are in need of a therapeutic diet to deal with a specific health problem, the best approach is to adhere to the principles of food selection advised by the government agencies concerned with health and nutrition. These recommendations incorporate the best judgment of nutritionists based on current knowledge.

Dietary Guidelines for Americans
The latest revision of Dietary Guidelines for Americans is intended for healthy persons older than 2 years. The following paragraphs summarize the guidelines.

Eat a Variety of Foods
Your body needs more than 40 nutrients for good health. These nutrients should come from many different foods, not from a few highly fortified foods or supplements.

Maintain a Healthy Weight
A "healthy" body weight depends on the percentage of body weight as fat, the location

How Much Should You Weigh?

The 1990 edition of Dietary Guidelines for Americans includes this height-weight table. Your weight may be healthy 1) if it falls within the range shown for your height and age, 2) if your pattern of fat distribution doesn't place you at risk for certain diseases, and 3) if you have no medical problem for which your physician advises you to gain or lose weight.

U.S. Department of Agriculture, U.S. Department of Health and Human Services Acceptable Weights for Adults

Height*	Weight in Pounds, by Age[†‡] 19 to 34 Years	35 Years or Older
5'0"	97-128	108-138
5'1"	101-132	111-143
5'2"	104-137	115-148
5'3"	107-141	119-152
5'4"	111-146	122-157
5'5"	114-150	126-162
5'6"	118-155	130-167
5'7"	121-160	134-172
5'8"	125-164	138-178
5'9"	129-169	142-183
5'10"	132-174	146-188
5'11"	136-179	151-194
6'0"	140-184	155-199
6'1"	144-189	159-205
6'2"	148-195	164-210
6'3"	152-200	168-216
6'4"	156-205	173-222
6'5"	160-211	177-228
6'6"	164-216	182-234

*Without shoes.

[†]Without clothes.

[‡]The higher weights in the ranges generally apply to men, who tend to have more muscle and bone; the lower weights more often apply to women, who have less muscle and bone.

From The Human Nutrition Information Service. The U.S. Department of Agriculture. Report of the Dietary Guidelines Advisory Committee on the Dietary Guidelines for Americans—1990. Hyattsville, MD: U.S. Government Printing Office, June 1990: 8.

A New Guide to Healthful Eating

Many people think that choosing a healthful diet requires making drastic changes in what they eat. Often, that's not the case at all. For most people, a few small, gradual changes can make a big difference in the long run. To select a healthful diet:

Try Something New. No single food supplies all the nutrients you need. Increase the variety of foods you eat by trying new fruits and vegetables, whole-grain breads and cereals, and dried peas and beans.

Balance Your Choices Over Time. Your food choices over several days should average out to the right balance of nutrients. Not every food or meal you eat has to be perfect. If you eat some foods high in fat, salt, or sugar, select other foods that are low in these ingredients.

Moderate Your Intake. If you eat reasonable portion sizes, it's easier to include all the foods you enjoy and still have a healthful diet. See the Food Guide Pyramid (page 261) to determine the right amount of food for your individual needs.

of the fat deposition, and the existence of any weight-related medical problems. (See What's the Right Weight for You? page 259.)

Choose a Diet Low in Fat, Saturated Fat, and Cholesterol

Fat intake should be limited to 30 percent of calories, with less than 10 percent of calories from saturated fat. Most people can keep their blood cholesterol at a desirable level by eating plenty of vegetables, fruits, and grain products; choosing lean meats, fish, poultry without the skin, and low-fat dairy products; and using fats and oils sparingly. Persons interested in assessing their diets for fat content should be encouraged to seek more information from their physicians, registered dietitians, or other health care professionals.

Choose a Diet With Plenty of Vegetables, Fruits, and Grain Products

Consuming more vegetables, fruits, and grain products is emphasized, especially for their complex carbohydrates, dietary fiber, and other components linked to good health. It is stressed that some of the benefits from a high-fiber diet may be from the food that provides the fiber, not from fiber alone, so fiber from foods is recommended over fiber obtained from supplements.

Use Sugars Only in Moderation

Sugars should be used in moderate amounts and sparingly if calorie needs are low. Because sugars can contribute to tooth decay, excessive snacking should be avoided and teeth should be brushed and flossed regularly.

Use Salt and Sodium Only in Moderation

Most Americans consume much more salt and sodium than they actually need. A reduction in salt and sodium intake will benefit people whose blood pressure increases with salt intake.

If You Drink Alcoholic Beverages, Do So in Moderation

Drinking alcoholic beverages has few health benefits and is linked to many health problems and accidents. Therefore, persons who drink alcoholic beverages are advised to use moderation. Moderate drinking is defined as no more than one drink per day for women and two drinks per day for men. One drink may be 12 ounces of beer, 5 ounces of wine, or 1½ ounces of distilled 80 proof spirits. (Avoid alcohol if you are trying to become pregnant. Don't drink alcohol if you are pregnant.)

For More Information

For more on how to put the dietary guidelines into practice, contact the Human Nutrition Information Service, USDA, Room 325-A, 6505 Belcrest Road, Hyattsville, MD 20782, or a registered dietitian in your area.

Some nutrition professionals suggest more stringent nutrition goals, with greater restrictions of dietary fat and salt and

Preventing Excess Gas

Too much gas is typically caused by the incomplete absorption of certain starches and sugars. Bacteria then ferment the sugars and gas forms. To prevent excess gas:

Avoid or Limit Gassy Foods. The worst gas-formers are beans and other legumes, wheat and wheat bran, cabbage, onions, Brussels sprouts, sauerkraut, apricots, bananas, and prunes. Milk and other dairy products can also cause gas if you have reduced amounts of lactase, the enzyme needed to digest lactose, the main sugar in milk.

Limit Sugar Substitutes. Up to half of healthy people poorly absorb sorbitol and mannitol contained in some sugar-free foods such as candies and gums. The amount of sorbitol contained in five sticks of sugar-free gum can cause gas and diarrhea.

Don't Rely on Antacids. Antacids neutralize stomach acid to relieve heartburn, but they don't reduce gas.

Do Try Some Anti-Gas Products. Adding Beano (a trade name of a food enzyme) to high-fiber foods reduces the amount of gas these foods make. Lactaid and Dairy Ease reduce excess gas caused by lactase deficiency.

greater consumption of fiber. One goal that is realistic would be to have less than 25 percent of calories as fat and more than 25 grams of dietary fiber daily.

The Food Guide Pyramid

Gone are the days of the basic four food groups. Now health and nutrition experts suggest planning your diet based on the shape of a pyramid. The Food Guide Pyramid is an outline of what to eat each day by incorporating the Dietary Guidelines for Americans.

The Food Guide Pyramid lists a range for number of servings in each of five food groups based on age, sex, and level of activity. Serving sizes are also specifically defined. Use the pyramid as an outline of what to eat each day.

The small tip of the pyramid includes fats, oils, and sweets. These are foods such as salad dressing and cooking oils, butter and margarine, sugar, soft drinks, candy, and most dessert foods. Foods in this section of the pyramid provide calories but have very little nutritional value. Use them sparingly.

The next level of the pyramid contains two food groups that are predominantly animal products. Included in this section are milk, yogurt, cheese, meat, poultry, fish, dry beans, eggs, nuts, and nut butters. These foods are important for the protein, calcium,

Nutritional Advice for the Stages of Life

See Your Newborn's Nutrition, page 38
See Your Infant's Nutrition, page 78
See Nutrition in Your Preschool Child, page 112
See Nutrition in Your School-Age Child, page 121
See Nutrition During the Teenage Years, page 140
See Nutrition During Pregnancy, page 182
See Nutrition and Lactation, page 215
See Special Nutritional Concerns After Age 65, page 241

iron, and zinc they contribute to your diet. Choose skim or low-fat dairy products whenever possible. Select lean cuts of meat and poultry without skin and prepare them without added fat. Nuts, seeds, and nut butters are high in fat, so eat them in moderation. Vegetarians need to pay particular attention to eating a wide variety of non-animal protein foods to ensure a healthful diet.

The third level of the pyramid includes fruits and vegetables. Most people need to eat more of these foods for the abundance of vitamins, minerals, and fiber they supply. Plain varieties of frozen fruits and vegetables offer nutrition similar to that of fresh produce. Avoid canned or frozen fruits in heavy syrups or vegetables in cream sauce unless you can afford the extra fat and calories they provide.

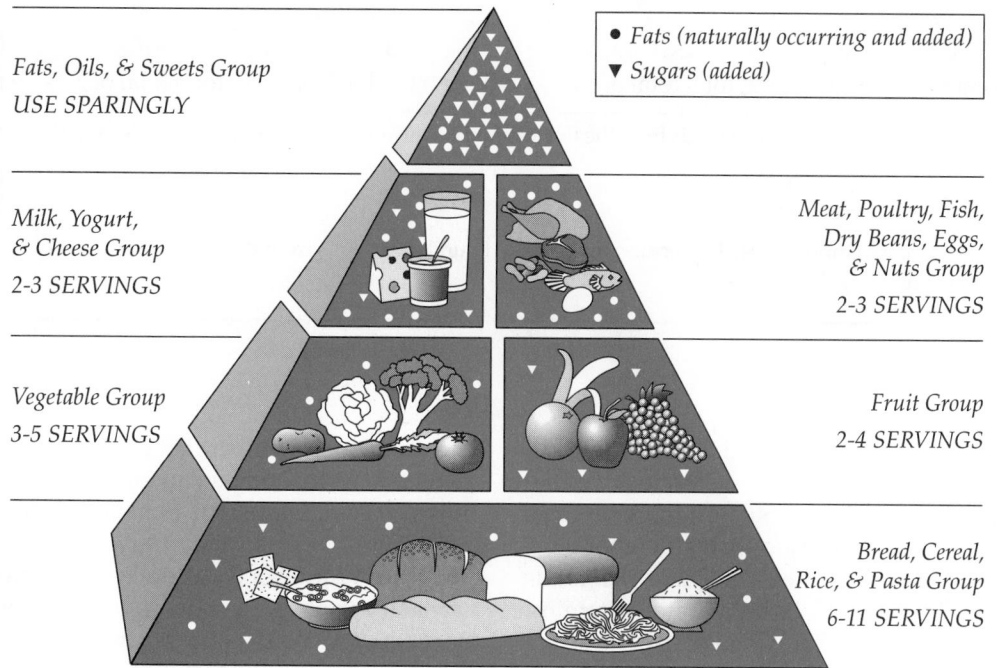

The Food Guide Pyramid provides a guide to your daily food choices.

What Counts as a Serving?

Food Groups

Bread, Cereal Rice, and Pasta	Vegetable	Fruit	Milk, Yogurt, and Cheese	Meat, Poultry, Fish, Dry Beans, Eggs, and Nuts
1 slice bread	¾ cup vegetable juice	¾ cup fruit juice	1 cup milk or yogurt	½ cup cooked dry beans
1 oz ready-to-eat cereal	1 cup raw leafy vegetables	1 medium apple, banana, or orange	1½ oz natural cheese	2-3 oz cooked lean meat, poultry, or fish
½ cup cooked cereal, rice, or pasta	½ cup other vegetables, cooked or chopped raw	½ cup chopped, cooked, or canned fruit	2 oz processed cheese	1 egg or 2 tbsp peanut butter counts as 1 oz of lean meat

How Many Servings Do I Need?

	Women and Some Older Adults	Children, Teenage Girls, Active Women, Most Men	Teenage Boys and Active Men	Pregnant and Breastfeeding Women
Calorie level*	About 1,600	About 2,200	About 2,800	About 1,800-2,800
Bread group	6	9	11	9
Vegetable group	3	4	5	4
Fruit group	2	3	4	3
Milk group	2-3†	2-3†	2-3†	3
Meat group	2, for a total of 5 oz	2, for a total of 6 oz	3, for a total of 7 oz	3, for a total of 7 oz

*These are the calorie levels if you choose low-fat, lean foods from the five major food groups and sparingly use foods from the fats, oils, and sweets group.

†Teenagers and young adults to age 24 years need 3 servings.

From *Mayo Clinic Diet Manual*, seventh edition, 1994. By permission of Mayo Foundation. Also from the U.S. Department of Agriculture Food Guide Pyramid.

The base of the pyramid includes breads, cereals, rice, and pasta—all foods from the grain group. You should eat more servings from the grain group than any other level of the pyramid. These nutrient-rich foods provide complex carbohydrates, vitamins, minerals, and fiber. Choose at least several servings each day of whole-grain breads and cereals. Remember that starchy foods aren't fattening—unless you top them with butter, cream, cheese, or rich sauces and gravies.

Copies of the Food Guide Pyramid are available from The Superintendent of Documents, Consumer Information Center, Department 159-Y, Pueblo CO 81009.

Food Labeling

Food labels can serve as an important guide to better nutrition. "Nutrition Facts" on food labels help you make good decisions about food choices which may help reduce your risk for heart disease, high blood pressure, obesity, diabetes, and some cancers.

Almost all foods in the supermarket are required to carry the Nutrition Facts panel. Voluntary information for the 20 most com-monly eaten raw fruits, vegetables, and seafood should be available in your local store. This information may be provided in the form of a brochure, pamphlet, sign, or poster.

Nutrition labeling is also voluntary for single-ingredient raw meat and poultry products. Ground beef and chicken parts, for example, are not required to have a nutrition label. However, processed products such as corned beef, hot dogs, and frozen entrees with meat must have nutrition labeling on each package.

Understanding Food Labels

At first glance, a food label may look intimidating. But as you become familiar with the format, you'll see how the label can help you compare products for nutritional quality.

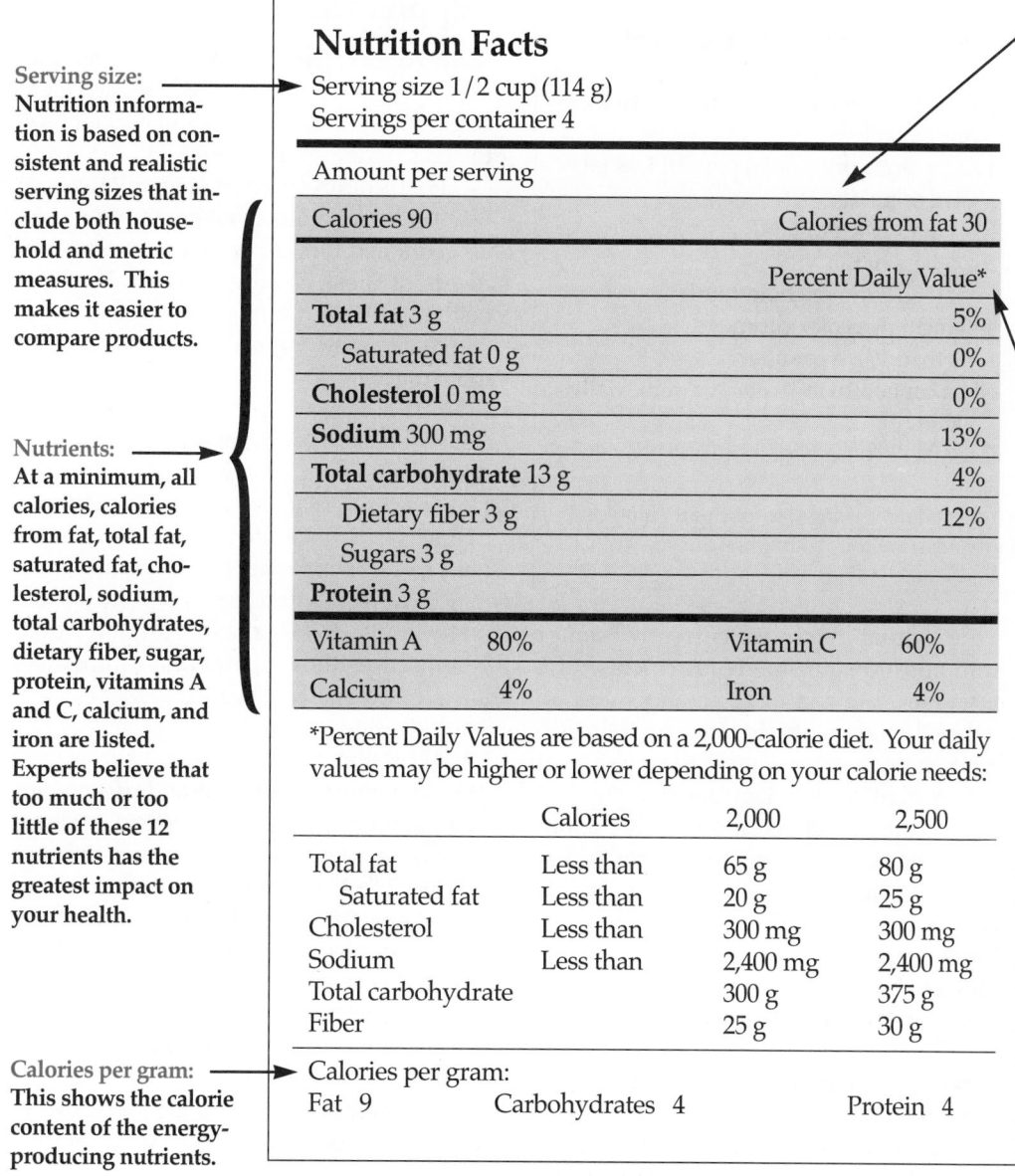

Serving size:
Nutrition information is based on consistent and realistic serving sizes that include both household and metric measures. This makes it easier to compare products.

Nutrients:
At a minimum, all calories, calories from fat, total fat, saturated fat, cholesterol, sodium, total carbohydrates, dietary fiber, sugar, protein, vitamins A and C, calcium, and iron are listed. Experts believe that too much or too little of these 12 nutrients has the greatest impact on your health.

Calories per gram:
This shows the calorie content of the energy-producing nutrients.

Calories from fat:
This information underscores the fat content per serving of foods to help you meet the recommendation of no more than 30 percent of calories from fat. Remember, it's your total fat intake over time, and not the amount in one food or meal, that's important.

Percent daily value:
The percent daily values show the percentage of a nutrient that is provided by this product serving, based on a 2,000- or a 2,500-calorie diet. Use the percent daily value figures to easily compare products and to tell whether a food is high or low in nutrients.

Nutrition Facts

Serving size 1/2 cup (114 g)
Servings per container 4

Amount per serving

Calories 90	Calories from fat 30

	Percent Daily Value*
Total fat 3 g	5%
Saturated fat 0 g	0%
Cholesterol 0 mg	0%
Sodium 300 mg	13%
Total carbohydrate 13 g	4%
Dietary fiber 3 g	12%
Sugars 3 g	
Protein 3 g	

Vitamin A	80%	Vitamin C	60%
Calcium	4%	Iron	4%

*Percent Daily Values are based on a 2,000-calorie diet. Your daily values may be higher or lower depending on your calorie needs:

	Calories	2,000	2,500
Total fat	Less than	65 g	80 g
Saturated fat	Less than	20 g	25 g
Cholesterol	Less than	300 mg	300 mg
Sodium	Less than	2,400 mg	2,400 mg
Total carbohydrate		300 g	375 g
Fiber		25 g	30 g

Calories per gram:
Fat 9   Carbohydrates 4   Protein 4

From Food & Drug Administration, 1992.

Nutrient Claims on Food Labels

Three basic types of nutrient claims are permitted on food labels:

Absolute Claims. Products making absolute claims such as "low sodium" or "fat free" must meet specified government-defined restrictions.

Relative or Comparative Claims. Products that compare the amount of a specific nutrient with the amount of the same nutrient in a comparable food (reduced calorie, light).

Implied Claims. Products making implied claims lead you to believe a nutrient is present or absent in a food. A product that claims "high in bran" implies it is high in fiber and must meet the corresponding nutrient claim.

Products making absolute claims such as "low sodium" or "fat free" must meet specified government-defined restrictions.

Here are some of the federal definitions for common nutrient claims:

Nutrient Claim	Definition per Reference Amount*
Low calorie	40 calories or less
Reduced calorie	At least a 25 percent reduction from the original
Light or lite	1/3 fewer calories or 50 percent less fat than original
Fat free	Less than 1/2 g of fat
Low fat	3 g or less of fat
Cholesterol free	Less than 2 mg of cholesterol
Low sodium	140 mg or less of sodium
Sugar free	Less than 1/2 g of sugar
Good source of. . .	Must contain 10 to 19 percent of the daily value
High or rich in. . .	Contains 20 percent or more of daily value

*The reference amount is the standard serving size for a particular food as determined by the Nationwide Food Consumption Survey.

Restaurant menus are currently exempt from nutrition labeling requirements. If a restaurant, cafeteria, or deli makes nutrition or health claims off the menu (advertisements, posters, or brochures), then they must meet current labeling regulations.

Seven health claims are currently permitted on the packaging of food products that meet the requirements for certain nutrients such as fat, fiber, sodium, and cholesterol. These claims link foods or food components with reducing the risk of certain chronic diseases. They are as follows:

- Eating enough calcium may help prevent osteoporosis (thin, fragile bones)
- Limiting the amount of sodium you eat may help prevent hypertension (high blood pressure)
- Eating fruits, vegetables, and grain products that contain fiber may help prevent heart disease
- Limiting the amount of saturated fat and cholesterol in your diet may reduce your risk of heart disease
- Limiting the amount of total fat you eat may help reduce your risk for cancer
- Eating fiber-containing grain products, fruits, and vegetables may help prevent cancer
- Eating fruits and vegetables that are "low in fat" and "good sources" of dietary fiber, vitamin A, or vitamin C may help prevent cancer

Vitamin and Mineral Supplements

Many American adults take vitamin supplements regularly. Some people regard them as essential food replacements; others see them as harmless "insurance."

The recommended dietary allowances (RDAs) are amounts of vitamins and minerals estimated to meet or exceed the requirements of most healthy people. They are neither minimal nor required amounts.

A daily multivitamin and mineral supplement that supplies close to 100 percent of the RDAs is not harmful, and it could be beneficial if you eat a very limited diet—one that does not contain a wide variety of foods. However, true vitamin or mineral deficiencies in the United States are rare, and few people need to take supplements of any kind.

There is also a danger: those who decide, on their own, to take megadoses (more than 10 times the RDA) of vitamins or minerals are taking significant health risks.

Food Is Better

The unglamorous but tried-and-true recommendation of eating at least 6 to 11 servings of breads and cereals, 3 to 5 servings of vegetables, 2 to 4 servings of fruits, 2 to 3 servings of low-fat milk and dairy products, and 2 to 3 servings of lean meat or meat substitutes a day is still the best way to ensure adequate nutrition. Food contains many components that work together to maximize your absorption of nutrients.

Although a nutritionally balanced diet is ideal, it may be unrealistic for some people. If you routinely eat less than 1,200 calories a day, a balanced diet will be difficult to achieve. Regardless of how many calories you eat, if your diet regularly falls short in one or more of the groups from the Food Guide Pyramid, a daily multivitamin and mineral supplement may be a reasonable precaution.

Here is what to look for when choosing a supplement:

Avoid Gimmicks. Disregard labels that suggest the product is specially formulated for certain groups of people—such as women, athletes, or the elderly—or for a specific purpose—such as "stress formula."

Maintain Balance. Read the label for the amount of vitamins and minerals or the percentage of the USRDAs (simplified RDAs) per dose. Choose a supplement that supplies close to 100 percent of all the vitamins and minerals instead of one that supplies, for instance, 500 percent of one vitamin and only 20 percent of another.

The exception to this approach is calcium. Multivitamin and mineral supplements do not contain 100 percent of the RDA for calcium because the tablets would be too large to swallow.

Organic Versus Synthetic. There is no advantage to taking "organic" or "natural" vitamins instead of synthetic ones. Your body does not know the difference and uses them in the same way.

Brand Name Versus Generic Name. Nationally advertised brands are not necessarily better than generic or store brands. Compare the list of ingredients and the percentages of the RDAs. The nationally advertised brands may cost more without offering any real advantage.

Special Needs. Physicians often prescribe specific supplements for persons with special needs. For example, women with heavy menstrual flows may need iron supplements. Women who are pregnant or breastfeeding need additional amounts of iron, folic acid, and calcium. Some vegetarians, especially those who eat no animal products, may not receive enough vitamin B_{12}, vitamin D, calcium, and iron in their diets; thus, a vitamin supplement may be essential.

Before taking any supplement other than a standard multivitamin and mineral supplement, check with your physician or a registered dietitian. As little as 5 to 10 times the RDA for vitamin A, for example, taken over an extended period, can harm your health.

Again, as is so often the case in matters of nutrition, moderation is the best strategy.

Selecting a Breakfast Cereal

At least 100 new cereals debut on supermarket shelves each year. That can make choosing confusing. Most breakfast cereals have only modest amounts of fat and salt. Here are three keys to selecting a nutritious cereal:

Look for Fiber First. Choose products that contain at least 3 grams of fiber per serving. If you don't normally eat high-fiber foods, consider a cereal that provides as many as 15 grams of fiber in a serving.

Scan for Sugar. To prevent sweeteners from crowding out nutrients and fiber, look for cereals with no more than 5 grams of sugar in a serving.

Don't Be Fooled by Fortification. Fortified cereals may appear superior, but there's little justification for adding huge amounts of vitamins to breakfast foods. Any cereal that provides 10 to 25 percent of the daily values for several nutrients is a good choice.

Aside from supplements your physician prescribes (perhaps because of the action of a drug you are taking), we do not recommend mineral or vitamin supplementation that goes beyond 100 percent of the USRDA, and then only if your diet is significantly limited in one way or another.

Antioxidant Nutrients

Can eating a diet rich in the antioxidant vitamins beta carotene, vitamin C, and vitamin E reduce your risk of cancer, cardiovascular disease, or cataracts? Some scientists say "yes."

Oxygen damage (oxidation) to your cells may be partly responsible for the effects of aging and certain diseases. Researchers are studying how antioxidants in your food may protect against this damage.

But how does this new research translate into your daily diet? Is eating lots of fruits and vegetables enough? Do you need to take a vitamin supplement? The answers are not yet available.

How Do Antioxidants Work?

As a part of their normal function, cells make toxic molecules called free radicals. A free radical is a damaged molecule—one that's missing an electron.

Because the free radical molecule "wants" its full complement of electrons, it reacts with any molecule from which it can take an electron. By taking an electron from certain key components in the cell, such as fat, protein,

Do You Need an Antioxidant Supplement?

Despite the support for the health benefits of vitamin C, vitamin E, and beta carotene, there are good reasons for not taking large supplemental doses:

No Proof of Benefit. The evidence for using antioxidant vitamins to lower your risk of chronic disease is preliminary. It has not yet been proved in clinical trials.

No One Knows the Right Dose. Researchers don't know which antioxidant, or combination of antioxidants, offers the greatest potential to prevent disease. Further, they don't know the amount of antioxidants you may need.

No One Knows the Long-Term Risk. Vitamin C, vitamin E, and beta carotene generally aren't toxic. Yet controlled studies in people typically last less than 6 months. There's no proof that a daily supplement of 500 or 1,000 IU of vitamin E, for example, carries no risk over 5 years—or a lifetime.

or DNA molecules, free radicals damage cells.

Antioxidants that occur naturally in your body and certain foods may block some of this damage by donating electrons to stabilize and neutralize the harmful effects of the free radicals.

Even though most free radical damage is repaired, a fraction still may remain. The environment also is a source of free radicals caused by ultraviolet radiation or airborne pollutants such as cigarette smoke.

Eventually, free radical damage may overwhelm your body's natural defenses. As cell damage accumulates, it may contribute to aging and certain diseases. More antioxidant vitamins from your diet may help counter some of the damage.

What If I Don't Drink Milk?

Two cups of skim or low-fat milk as part of a varied diet will help most people meet the recommended dietary allowance (RDA) for calcium for adult men and women 25 years or older. If you can't or won't drink milk, try these suggestions:

Buy Treated Milk or Milk Products. If you have an intolerance to lactose, try milk treated with Lactaid. Lactaid and Dairy Ease are also available as chewable tablets that you take with a meal that contains lactose.

Choose Foods Rich in Calcium. It takes a concerted effort to get enough calcium from non-dairy foods (see page 267).

Consider a Calcium Supplement. Calcium carbonate is the preferred supplement because the rate of calcium absorption is comparable to that of milk.

How Antioxidants May Delay Disease

Research designed to study free radicals and how antioxidants may protect against their damage has led to these associations:

Cardiovascular Disease. Scientists theorize that low-density lipoprotein (LDL) cholesterol damages the lining of your arteries when it becomes oxidized. Vitamin C, vitamin E, and beta carotene may help protect against the oxidation of LDL cholesterol by neutralizing free radicals.

Cancer. Evidence from more than a hundred studies suggests that eating fruits and vegetables rich in vitamin C or beta carotene is linked with a reduced risk of virtually all cancers.

Cataracts. A cataract is a clouding of the normally clear lens of your eye. Scientists suspect cataracts develop partly as a result of oxidation of proteins in the lens of your eye. Vitamin C, vitamin E, and beta carotene, acting as antioxidants, may help prevent some lens clouding.

Calcium and Osteoporosis

If you are a woman, you have one chance in four of developing osteoporosis after menopause. In osteoporosis, bones become thin, fragile, and prone to fracture. A stooped posture and fractures of the spine, wrist, and hip are common. For some older people, complications arising from such fractures can prove fatal (see Osteoporosis, page 894).

The cause of osteoporosis remains unclear. We do know that one factor seems to be the amount of dietary calcium you consume during your lifetime. Therefore, your diet should include adequate amounts of calcium.

The recommended dietary allowance (RDA) of calcium for men and women is 1,200 to 1,500 milligrams a day from ages 11 to 24 years and 1,000 milligrams a day from age 25 years on, although most experts now recommend 1,000 to 1,500 milligrams a day. However, many women consume barely half the RDA for calcium. Dairy products, such as milk, cheese, and yogurt, are particularly rich in calcium. Many women avoid dairy products on the assumption that they are fattening. If this is your concern, consider this—dairy products made from skim milk supply as much or slightly more calcium than do higher-calorie products made with whole milk.

Other sources of calcium include canned salmon and sardines (with the bones), dark green vegetables such as broccoli, kale, spinach, and bok choy, and beans such as kidney, navy, pinto, soy, and black-eyed peas. Because of differences in absorption, the calcium in fiber-rich vegetables is probably less available to your body. Thus, if you consume a high-fiber diet, be careful to include other food sources that are high in calcium. (Note: If you take a bulk-forming agent containing psyllium, take it at times other than mealtime.)

Some brands of yogurt, orange juice, and milk are calcium-enhanced. They usually command a premium price, but they may be worth it if your intake of calcium from other sources is low.

What about supplements? In general, it is better to get as much calcium as you can from your diet. However, if you cannot attain your RDA of calcium from food, supplements can help make up the difference. The most common recommended dosage for a supplement to prevent osteoporosis is 1,000 to 1,500 milligrams a day. Discuss taking a dietary supplement with your physician, particularly if you are already through menopause.

Food Safety

Our food and water supplies generally are remarkably safe. However, the food you eat and the water you drink can make you sick. In the following pages, we review these risks and offer tips on how you can avoid trouble. The risks include food poisoning from bacteria or other organisms, natural toxins, and possible contamination from pesticides.

Federal and local health departments monitor our food supply, but their resources are limited. There has been, and probably will continue to be, controversy regarding how much funding should be provided to these agencies and how their resources should be allocated. Should monitoring be done widely, or should more intense scrutiny be given to certain target areas where the probability of difficulties is greater? How valid are assumptions based on observations made on test animals given large amounts of a substance that humans consume in very small amounts? These and other food safety issues may be better understood in the next several years so that our food supply perhaps can be made even safer.

Foods Rich in Calcium

The following foods contain approximately 300 milligrams of calcium:

Milk
⅓ cup dry milk powder
1 cup milk (skim, 2%, whole)

Cheese
1½ oz cheddar-type cheese
2½ oz American (processed) cheese
1¾ oz mozzarella (part skim milk) cheese

Other dairy products
1¾ cups ice cream or ice milk
1 cup pudding
6 oz low-fat plain yogurt
1 cup low-fat fruited yogurt

Fish
5 oz salmon, with bone
7 sardines, with bone

Vegetables
2½ cups Great Northern beans (dried, cooked)
1¼ cups spinach (fresh, cooked)
2 cups collards (fresh, cooked)

Miscellaneous
1½ cups macaroni and cheese
1¼ cups tofu (soybean curd)

From *Mayo Clinic Diet Manual,* seventh edition, 1994. By permission of Mayo Foundation.

Infectious Food Poisoning

Food poisoning is a gastrointestinal infection caused by eating contaminated food. Common symptoms are loss of appetite, nausea, vomiting, diarrhea, and stomachache. In most people, the discomforts of food poisoning pass within a few hours (see Infections of the Gastrointestinal Tract, page 766).

Bacterial contamination of food can occur if food is handled improperly. Thus, cleanliness in the kitchen is of paramount importance. Wash your hands before you handle food. Wash dishes in hot, soapy water. Cook foods at temperatures that minimize the number of bacteria. Cool and refrigerate foods adequately and rapidly (see Proper Handling of Food, page 272).

The recent popularity of salad bars in restaurants and grocery stores poses a potential new risk. Observe how well the items

Pesticides

Pesticides protect crops from harmful insects. Yet the protection provided by pesticides raises questions about the safety of long-term chemical exposure to humans. Here are ways you can reduce your exposure to pesticide residue on foods at home:

- Scrub and rinse thoroughly all fresh produce before you handle or eat it
- Don't use soap to wash produce; you may be adding chemicals back to your food. Just use plenty of clear, plain water
- Remove and discard the outer leaves of leafy vegetables such as lettuce and cabbage. These outer surfaces tend to have the most exposure to sprayed pesticides

are chilled and how well they are protected from the inevitable sneezes and coughs of the public before buying from them.

Many of our common foods carry large numbers of bacteria. Raw vegetables, salads, and milk products, in particular, contain or carry bacteria. Ordinarily, these bacteria pose no risk because the body is capable of destroying them. However, people with suppressed immune function, such as those with AIDS, those receiving chemotherapy, or organ transplant recipients, may become vulnerable to infections from uncooked everyday foods.

Unfortunately, particularly virulent strains of usually harmless bacteria can arise from time to time. Recently, a "new" strain of *Escherichia coli* found in ground meat was identified as being responsible for several cases of serious illness and death. This virulent strain was apparently in the intestinal tract of the animals and small amounts contaminated the meat during the process of butchering. When meat is in the form of steaks or roasts, bacteria on the surface are killed during cooking and there is no danger. When contaminated meat is ground, however, some of the bacteria are distributed through the meat patties, and the interior of the patties are a good environment for their multiplication. When patties, or any ground meat, are cooked at too low a temperature to kill the bacteria in their centers (the centers are pink), you can ingest a large dose of the bacteria and become seriously ill.

Food inspection practices are being improved by doing bacterial studies in addition to the traditional visual inspection of the carcasses, but it is probably impossible to keep our food supply completely free of potentially dangerous bacteria. For this reason, your procedures for handling and cooking food in your home must be the final line of defense against potential bacterial hazards.

Staphylococcus aureus

The most common bacterium that causes food poisoning is *Staphylococcus aureus*. Outbreaks can occur among large numbers of people. Sometimes these infections are traced to an open wound on the hand of a food preparer. Bacteria from the wound are passed to the food, where they can multiply rapidly if the food is left at room temperature.

Foods with mayonnaise or cream bases make particularly good environments for growth of bacteria. Within 3 to 6 hours after eating, people experience nausea, vomiting, and diarrhea, which persist for about 12 hours.

Clostridium perfringens

A form of infectious diarrhea is caused by *Clostridium perfringens*. This can result from allowing cooked meat to cool slowly to room temperature over a period of 12 to 24 hours. Symptoms of abdominal pain and diarrhea begin within 6 to 12 hours after eating the contaminated meat and last about 24 hours.

Salmonella

These bacteria are responsible for another common and potentially fatal form of food poisoning. The bacteria are found most commonly in poultry, eggs, and meat. Symptoms (which may last less than a day) usually appear 12 to 48 hours after you eat contaminated foods. In addition to gastrointestinal discomforts, you may run a fever. Infants or older people are especially at risk from this infection.

An epidemic due to *Salmonella* was traced to the transport of ice cream mix in a tanker truck that had previously been used to carry raw eggs and had not been adequately cleaned between loads. This epidemic extended across much of the country because of the wide distribution of the ice cream. Precautions against the recurrence of such an epidemic include designating tanker trucks solely for carrying either the eggs or the ice cream mix.

Botulism

This is a particularly dangerous form of food

poisoning. Fortunately, it is rare because of modern canning techniques. Unlike most other bacteria that cause food poisoning, *Clostridium botulinum* organisms grow in the absence of oxygen. Botulism can occur when sealed foods are not processed at high enough temperatures to kill the organism. Also, cooking this canned food after you remove it from the container will not destroy the toxin. If you are about to open a canned food, be sure that the can is not swollen or that the safety button in the center of the lid has not popped up. If you see either, throw the food away.

Botulism can be fatal. It requires prompt treatment with a substance called antiserum. Symptoms include muscle weakness in addition to nausea, vomiting, cramps, headache, and double vision. (For more information on Botulism, see page 488.)

Traveler's Diarrhea

Another common bacterial food hazard is traveler's diarrhea. This form of poisoning results from eating strains of the common intestinal bacterium *Escherichia coli* (known as *E. coli*), which produces toxins. These toxins can cause a severe diarrhea that lasts several days. You are most likely to be exposed to this bacterium, to which you may have little immunity, when you travel abroad. In many countries it is common in the water supply and on foods prepared in a less-than-hygienic manner. Outbreaks of this form of food poisoning can occur among large groups of people.

When traveling in developing countries, shun untreated water and ice, salads, raw fruits and vegetables that you cannot peel, and uncooked milk products (see Traveler's Diarrhea, page 383).

Contamination from *E. coli* bacteria also can occur from eating meat that has been handled, such as ground meat, and then not thoroughly cooked. Regardless of where you are in the world, avoid hamburgers that are pink in the middle.

Hepatitis A

Hepatitis A can be caused by eating raw shellfish harvested from sewage-contaminated waters. Even though federal regulations and posting of contaminated waters offer some protection, there is a risk to eating raw shellfish. The wisest course is to consume them in the cooked state (see Acute Viral Hepatitis, page 801).

Contaminated Fish

Other forms of food poisoning can occur from eating fish that have ingested certain one-cell organisms. Such infections occur occasionally from eating fish such as snapper, sea bass, barracuda, and amberjack caught off Florida or the West Indies or puffer fish from the Pacific Ocean. In addition to the gastrointestinal symptoms common to food poisoning, symptoms include a rash, numbness in the hands and feet, headache, muscle ache, tingling of the lips and tongue, and face pain. In some cases, the debilitating symptoms can last for months.

Another form of food poisoning results from eating certain kinds of fish that are not fresh. Bacterial decomposition of tuna, mackerel, bonito, mahi mahi, or bluefish can cause immediate gastrointestinal distress as well as a rash and pain around the abdomen. Symptoms usually last only a day or so.

Sushi, the popular Japanese dish made of raw fish, can be responsible for a form of gastrointestinal distress characterized by abdominal pain in addition to nausea and vomiting. Its cause is not a bacterium but a parasitic worm, anisakiasis, which infests small crustaceans upon which many kinds of fish feed.

One final note on food poisoning from seafood: environmental toxins such as PCBs

Food Safety at Picnics

When going on a picnic, follow these tips for food safety:

Pack Right From the Refrigerator. Keep food cold or frozen before putting it in your cooler or cold vacuum bottle (Thermos).

Use an Insulated Cooler. Put ice or a frozen gel-pack on top, with foods to be kept the coldest on the bottom.

Wrap All Foods Separately in Plastic. Don't place foods directly on ice that's not of drinking quality. Keep raw meat, poultry, or fish well wrapped so that drippings don't contaminate other foods.

Don't Put Your Cooler in a Hot Trunk. Keep it in the shade at your picnic or campsite. Keep the lid on.

Keep Food and Utensils Covered Until Serving Time. Flies, other insects, and household pets can carry Salmonella.

Keep Hot Foods Hot and Cold Foods Cold. Use a vacuum bottle or insulated dish for serving.

Clean Your Hands. Take along disposable premoistened hand towels to use before and after working with food.

Remember the 2-Hour Rule. Return leftovers to your cooler as quickly as possible. Two hours is the maximal time food should be left unrefrigerated—1 hour if the temperature is 85 degrees Fahrenheit or higher.

Food Safety in Your Home

The bacteria that cause food-borne illness are almost everywhere. They occur in soil, on plants, in animal wastes, meats, and fish, and even on your own skin. Basic to food safety are three simple rules:

Keep Hot Foods Hot. Avoid letting food sit out on the table after meals. When serving large quantities of food, bring out small batches at a time. Throw out any leftovers that have been at room temperature more than 2 hours.

Keep Cold Foods Cold. Purchase eggs, dairy products, meat, poultry, and fish last at the grocery store. Avoid making stops on the way home, and immediately refrigerate all cold items. Keep eggs in their original carton on a shelf in your refrigerator—the door compartment is not cool enough.

Keep Everything Clean. Wash your hands in hot soapy water before preparing foods. Keep all kitchen surfaces, especially cutting boards, meticulously clean.

Symptoms of food-borne illness include diarrhea, nausea, vomiting, fever, or cramps. You may begin to feel sick anywhere from 30 minutes to 2 weeks after eating contaminated food. If you develop food-borne illness, rest and drink plenty of liquids. If your symptoms are severe, or if you are elderly, pregnant, or already ill, contact your physician immediately.

(For more information on food safety, see Proper Handling of Food, page 272.)

(polychlorinated biphenyls) and methyl mercury are potential problems with fresh and saltwater fish. Read and heed the warnings from your state's department of natural resources. Most fishing licenses come with a booklet that flags unsafe waters and dubious fish species. Generally, water near industrial complexes, sewer plants, and runoff areas poses the greatest hazard. Young, small fish will have accumulated fewer contaminants than large or predator fish.

Naturally Occurring Food Toxins

Certain foods contain toxins that can cause serious or even fatal gastrointestinal ailments. For example, certain forms of mushrooms, most commonly those of the *Amanita* family, can produce poisons that cause severe intestinal distress as well as tearing of the eyes, salivation, sweating, dizziness, mental confusion, and coma. If not treated within a few hours, you can die.

Amanita mushrooms are not cultivated, so they can be gathered only in the wild. To be safe, never eat mushrooms you find outdoors unless you are positive of their identity (see Poisonous Plants, page 440).

We all know the benefits of the potato. Not everyone knows, however, that potatoes can develop a toxin. This toxin can produce intestinal distress. Do not eat potato sprouts or potato eyes. If you prepare green potatoes, be sure to peel away all portions that have any tint of green.

Peanuts, another ordinarily healthful food, can develop an unhealthful mold when not stored properly. Do not eat moldy or shriveled peanuts.

Safe Drinking Water

Even though a mountain stream may look, smell, and taste "pure," animal waste is a common contaminant that can make you ill. Conversely, chemicals used to purify water supplies may add unpleasant tastes or odors, but they're safe if used properly.

Under the Safe Drinking Water Act of 1974 and its amendments, the Environmental Protection Agency (EPA) regulates 83 contaminants in drinking water, enforces compliance by public suppliers, and promotes protection of groundwater sources. Yet water sometimes can be unsafe to drink.

In April 1993, health officials advised residents of some areas of Milwaukee, Wisconsin, not to drink tap water. They warned of contamination with a water-borne parasite called *Cryptosporidium* that causes diarrhea and nausea. Other outbreaks of *Cryptosporidium* have hit additional municipal water supplies.

In May 1993, the EPA reported that the drinking water in 819 cities, supplying water to about 30 million people, contained unhealthful levels of lead.

Even though America's drinking water is among the safest in the world, some states may lack funding for adequate enforcement of regulations. And, as with any complicated mechanical process, water-treatment equipment sometimes can break down temporarily.

The EPA requires public suppliers to notify you if your water doesn't meet safety standards or if required monitoring isn't being done.

In addition, here are some general precautions:

Don't Drink Water of Unknown Safety. Water from streams or lakes near campsites or hiking trails can be contaminated. Carry your own bottled water or boil on-site water for about 10 minutes before using for drinking or cooking.

Put Your Water to the Test. Ask your county health department about potential contaminants. The most common ones are bacteria, nitrates, and lead. The health department can also help you find certified testing laboratories and then help you interpret results. Costs for tests range from $25 to $50.

If your water supply comes from a private well or groundwater source such as a lake or stream, you're responsible for ensuring that your water is safe. Have your water tested annually or anytime you notice a change in color or odor.

If you are unsure whether lead is in your plumbing or water service line, use only cold water for cooking or drinking. Also, let your cold water run for a few minutes after it has sat in pipes for 2 or more hours.

If your drinking water meets EPA standards, you generally don't need a home water filter. If you decide to buy a unit, choose one that's specifically suited to your water problem. And be sure to follow suggested maintenance.

If your water is safe, but you don't like the taste, bottled water is an acceptable substitute. Be sure you select water and not a water beverage that also contains sugar and calories.

If you have children and drink bottled water exclusively or have a private water system, contact your child's dentist to see whether fluoride supplements are indicated.

For more information about your drinking water, call the EPA Safe Drinking Water Hotline, (800) 426-4791.

Other Contaminants

The possibility of contamination of foods with pesticides and other substances is a continuing cause for concern. Always wash fruits and vegetables carefully. Pesticides and most other contaminants are likely to be on the surface.

One of the problems presented by such substances is largely psychological. Today's techniques for measuring such substances allow detection of exceedingly small amounts. Even if the quantities are thought to be harmless, our anxieties may be sustained simply by the knowledge that toxins are present. Unless they reach a level determined to be harmful, these substances in our food supply do not seem to pose a significant risk. Still, alertness and monitoring programs conducted by our public health departments continue to be important.

Food Processing

Many people are concerned about the effects of food processing. "Processing" covers anything done to a food to prepare it for market. Processing efforts may range from simple washing to creation of a nearly new synthetic food.

For instance, soybean proteins can be prepared in a highly purified form and then used as a constituent in foods meant to resemble meats of various sorts. Such foods may contain substances for preservation, flavoring, and texture.

Some people focus their concerns on food preservatives. Chemical preservatives and antioxidants are present in many of the foods and beverages most of us consume each day. For several decades, sulfur dioxide and similar compounds have been used to preserve flavor and color. Commonly known as sulfites, these chemicals generally are useful and appropriate for human consumption. Sulfites are used by stores and wholesalers on fresh fruits and vegetables and by restaurants to keep certain foods fresh. Many processed foods also contain sulfites. By preventing spoilage, they help to keep food wholesome, palatable, and safe from molds and other decay.

Some people, however, have a sensitivity to sulfites and experience unpleasant symptoms shortly after eating or drinking foods or beverages containing sulfites. If you have this problem, avoid foods containing sulfites (see Food Allergies, page 1048).

One concern about processed foods is whether the nutritional value is lost during processing. In commercial canning and freezing operations, small losses of vitamins and minerals may occur. Ingredients such as sugar, salt, and fat—which sometimes are added in considerable quantities—can make these processed foods less nutritionally sound than those you prepare yourself.

Food Irradiation

Several years ago, alarming reports about *Salmonella* contamination in chicken made headlines. In 1990, the Food and Drug Administration (FDA) approved a process that could virtually eliminate this disease-causing bacteria from poultry.

The process is called food irradiation. Yet, despite its safety, fears may keep commercial use of food irradiation from becoming a success.

When foods are irradiated, exposure to a high dose of gamma radiation kills insects, parasites, and microorganisms that cause gastrointestinal diseases and spoilage. Another benefit is that irradiation delays spoilage in fresh produce. For example, strawberries that usually develop mold within a few days stay fresh for up to 2 weeks when irradiated.

Worldwide Acceptance

Food irradiation isn't new. In 1963, the FDA approved use of food irradiation in wheat. Since then, the FDA has approved the process for potatoes, spices, pork, fruits, vegetables, and poultry.

The World Health Organization (WHO) also endorses food irradiation. In its "10 Golden Rules for Safe Food Preparation," WHO states as its first rule: "Choose foods processed for safety... if you have the choice, select fresh or frozen poultry treated with ionizing radiation." Still, U.S. companies have shied away from food irradiation because of unfounded consumer fears that it leaves radioactive residue in foods and produces cancer-causing substances. Health experts agree that radioactivity fears are groundless. Radiation is not left in the food. In fact, cooking changes the chemical structure of food more significantly than does radiation.

Food irradiation is an FDA-approved process designed to enhance the safety and extend the shelf life of food.

Food Scares

Our food and water supplies are the safest they have ever been and are among the safest in the world. Although continuing vigilance over the safety of the foods we eat and the water we drink is important to our individual and collective health, perhaps it is our overconcern that sometimes allows unnecessary food scares to develop.

We should not ignore possible risks to health from chemical agents in our food and water. However, we do need to keep the focus on more important, ongoing risks (such as smoking, use of alcohol, and lack of use of auto seat belts) and not be swept away by momentary panics. We need to be careful—but we have to realize that we can never make our lives absolutely free of risk.

Proper Handling of Food

Foods that present the greatest risk for contamination during storage, preparation, cooking, and serving are meat, poultry, and eggs. The principles of proper handling are as follows:

Wash Your Hands. To avoid contamination by Salmonella bacteria or other organisms when preparing any food—especially poultry and meat—wash your hands thoroughly with soap and water before and after handling the food. Then wash your utensils (or cutting board) with hot soapy water before allowing them to come into contact with any other food.

You can wash an acrylic board in your dishwasher, where high temperatures kill organisms. After use, disinfect a wooden cutting board with a solution of 2 teaspoons of household bleach mixed with 1 quart of water. Flush the board thoroughly after applying the bleach. To minimize contact with other foods, reserve a separate cutting board for poultry and meat.

Do Not Thaw Meat at Room Temperature. Thaw meat or poultry in a microwave oven or in your refrigerator, then cook the meat immediately.

Do Not Consume Uncooked Marinades. If you marinate meat or poultry, do not serve the marinade unless it has been cooked at a rolling boil for several minutes. (Also, serve poultry and meat on a clean plate with a clean utensil, so as not to contaminate the cooked food with its raw juices.)

Cook Poultry, Pork, and All Ground Meats Thoroughly. Use a meat thermometer. Place it in the thickest portion of the pork or the poultry thigh (not in contact with a bone or fat). Before the meat is done cooking, the thermometer should register 180 to 185 degrees Fahrenheit for poultry and 137 degrees Fahrenheit for pork. Juices should run clear when the meat is pierced.

Do not cook poultry such as turkey at a low temperature over a long time. Cook all ground meats thoroughly, eliminating centers that are pink.

Refrigerate Leftovers Promptly. Cool poultry and meat quickly when refrigerating it. In particular, do not let stuffed fowl stand for long periods before refrigerating it. Better yet, remove the stuffing promptly after cooking and before refrigerating.

Never Use Cracked Eggs. Salmonella bacteria can enter cracked eggs and contaminate them; therefore, it's safest to check eggs for cracks before you use them—and discard any questionable eggs.

Cook Eggs Thoroughly. Even an uncracked egg may contain bacteria, but Salmonella bacteria are destroyed by heat, so cook eggs thoroughly. Avoid dishes that use raw eggs such as Caesar salad dressing, hollandaise sauce, homemade eggnog, and high-energy drinks that use raw eggs. To keep eggs fresh longer, refrigerate them in their original cartons. Resist the temptation to sample raw cookie dough or other batters that contain uncooked egg.

Do Not Eat Moldy Foods. Generally, it is best to throw out foods that are moldy, such as leftovers. Cheese is an exception—just trim off the mold before serving the cheese.

Caffeine and Your Health

You hear a great deal these days about caffeine. Can it harm you? How much is too much? We cannot know because the research is incomplete.

Most of us tend to associate caffeine exclusively with coffee. Coffee certainly is a large source of caffeine. Half the world's coffee supply is consumed within the United States. But coffee is not the only source of caffeine. Tea, carbonated beverages such as colas, cocoa, and chocolate all contain caffeine.

Certain medications, particularly nonprescription drugs for colds and allergies, use caffeine to counteract the sleep-inducing effects of antihistamines. Nonprescription stimulants such as NoDoz and Vivarin rely on caffeine as their main component—usually about twice the amount of caffeine per dose as a cup of coffee.

Benefits
For all its recent bad press, caffeine does have benefits. Its most obvious effect is its ability to stimulate.

Caffeine has certain medical applications. It constricts blood vessels in the brain; thus, it is used to treat certain types of migraine headaches and to counteract certain drugs that depress the central nervous system. It is used to treat hyperactive children, on whom it seems to have a calming effect.

Drawbacks
Caffeine's disadvantages include potentially undesirable effects on health. People who drink large quantities of coffee run the risk of developing irregular or rapid heartbeats, insomnia, upset stomach, increased blood pressure, anxiety reactions, and increased body temperature. Caffeine also can interfere with fine muscle coordination and timing. It may have a small adverse effect on blood fats.

The Food and Drug Administration (FDA) warns pregnant women not to consume excessive amounts of caffeine because it may harm their fetuses. Some researchers believe there is a link between consumption of caffeine and stillbirth, miscarriage, and birth defects. Although such associations remain unproved, why take a chance? We endorse the FDA recommendation.

What Should You Do?
As with many decisions regarding your diet, moderation is the best approach. For the average person, one or two 6-ounce cups of regular, caffeine-containing coffee or 20 ounces of a caffeinated soft drink per day are considered safe. If you have ulcers, avoid even decaffeinated coffee because of its acid-producing qualities. If you have hypertension, use caffeine with caution because it can increase your blood pressure. If regular coffee keeps you awake at night, switch to decaffeinated.

Coffee Drinks
The strong taste of espresso and cappuccino doesn't mean they have more caffeine or fewer calories than regular "American" coffee.

A standard 2-ounce serving of espresso has about 100 milligrams (mg) of caffeine, and a 6-ounce cup of coffee has about 115 mg. Cappuccino, made from 2 ounces of espresso with milk added, also has about 100 mg of caffeine.

However, the amount of calories and fat whipped into the trendy coffee drinks can be

Approximate Caffeine Content of Foods

6-oz cup brewed coffee	115 mg
6-oz cup instant coffee (one rounded teaspoon)	55-60 mg
6-oz cup decaffeinated coffee	2 mg
6-oz cup tea	35-40 mg
6-oz cup cocoa	5 mg
12 oz cola	40-50 mg
1 oz bittersweet chocolate	20 mg
1 oz baking chocolate	25 mg

different from the amount in regular coffee and espresso, which have practically no fat or calories. Depending on the type of milk used (skim, 2 percent, or whole), an 8-ounce cappuccino or latté drink contains between 50 and 100 calories and 0 to 5 grams of fat.

Cutting Down

To cut down on the amount of caffeine you consume, do so gradually to avoid possible ill effects of sudden withdrawal. (People often report headaches, drowsiness, nausea, and reduced attention span when they abruptly stop using caffeine.) There are several methods:

- Mix decaffeinated coffee in with your regular coffee when it is brewing
- Substitute regular instant coffee because it contains less caffeine per cup than brewed coffee
- Cut your consumption by 1 cup a day over the course of a week or two

You can, of course, do the same with tea or other beverages that contain caffeine. Be careful when switching to herb teas, however. Some types, particularly homemade varieties, can have the same effects as coffee—or worse.

Nutrition and the Athlete

For various reasons, people sometimes follow special dietary strategies. For example, some vegetarians regard avoiding meats as a moral imperative. Athletes may select a special diet in the hope of improving strength or endurance. For healthy, active people, there are alternatives to the rules of a conventional diet.

Many people have a mental image of athletes at the "training table." The vision may be of a team of muscular football players devouring huge slabs of steak before a game, or of runners swallowing mounds of spaghetti before a marathon. In fact, there is no one diet that produces optimal vigor or athletic performance—and there are as many misconceptions about so-called training diets as there are diets.

One myth is that high-protein diets increase strength. Many athletes consume commercially prepared protein or amino acid supplements in an effort to increase their muscle bulk and strength.

If you are an athlete and you eat a nutri-tionally balanced diet, you have no need for extra protein. The protein requirements of athletes are only a little higher than those of nonathletes. However, most athletes already receive this additional protein in their normal diets. The typical American diet is between 50 and 75 percent above the recommended dietary allowance for protein.

If increased muscle mass is your goal, weight lifting and increased calorie intake can help (but select complex carbohydrates instead of, for example, meat or dietary supplements).

Similarly, exercise does not increase your body's vitamin needs. Thus, taking vitamin supplements cannot improve athletic performance.

All of us need fat in our diets. Although our bodies can make most fats from carbohydrates or protein, there are some fatty acids, known as essential fatty acids, that the body must have which can be obtained only by eating foods containing fat. Moreover, athletes, who burn a great many calories in exercise, may need to consume a significant amount of fat if they are to maintain body weight.

For the athlete and nonathlete alike, the need for carbohydrates is greater than the need for protein or fat. In fact, the recommended distribution of dietary calories for athletes is the same as that for healthy adults: 55 to 65 percent of your food should be complex carbohydrates, 25 to 30 percent fat, and only 12 to 15 percent protein. (This recommended nutrient distribution is the same for those wanting to lose, maintain, or gain weight.)

If you participate in athletics, there are certain dietary precautions you should take to ensure good health:

Drink Enough Water. Adequate fluid is vital for the athlete. Proper hydration is the most frequently overlooked aid to athletic performance. For most of us, thirst is a good sign of our need for water; however, it is not a reliable indicator during physical activity. If you are going to engage in vigorous exercise in which you perspire, drink an extra pint of water 2 hours before the competition or workout and 3 to 6 ounces every 10 to 20 minutes during exercise.

To determine how much liquid you lose during a workout, weigh yourself before and after it. Then, over the course of a few hours afterward, drink about a pint of fluid for every pound you have lost.

Drinks containing a high percentage of sugar may delay stomach emptying; thus, avoid them. Instead, select a drink that contains less than 10 percent sugar. (The rate of stomach emptying is similar to that when water is consumed.) Orange juice is 11 percent sugar, and you can mix water with the orange juice in equal amounts to lower the sugar content.

Commercially prepared drinks are available. They contain sugars and electrolytes such as sodium and potassium. These drinks are designed with the intent of preventing undue depletion of body water and electrolytes during exercise. Such drinks ordinarily are unnecessary but may be useful if exercise is unusually intense and prolonged and is performed under hot, humid conditions that cause profuse perspiration.

If you train in a hot environment for several weeks, acclimatization will take place and the loss of electrolytes in your sweat will be reduced. Generally, the amounts of sodium and potassium you lose in your sweat are small enough that they can be replaced by eating ordinary food lightly salted. Also, you do not need salt tablets. They can irritate your stomach and cause nausea.

Eat Foods Rich in Iron. Certain kinds of athletic training can have an effect on your body and on its use of and need for certain nutrients. Blood hemoglobin concentrations tend to decrease in the highly trained athlete and may appear to be evidence of anemia (lack of iron). This decrease in blood hemoglobin level appears to result from a dilution due to an increased amount of fluid in your blood vessels. (Runners who exercise several hours each day actually may lose small amounts of blood in the intestinal tract.)

Athletes should eat foods rich in iron and also consume citrus fruits. Citrus fruits eaten or taken as juice help facilitate your body's absorption of the iron in vegetables, cereals, and other nonmeat sources. These foods can help prevent potential iron-deficiency anemia. But consult your physician before taking iron supplements. Excess iron consumption over a period of time can pose a significant health threat.

Eat Foods Rich in Calcium. Women athletes can be vulnerable to osteoporosis (weakening of bones as a result of loss of calcium). When a woman's body fat content falls below a certain amount, her hormones react so that menstruation ceases. Because many women athletes are involved in sports in which leanness is required for maximal performance, the diminished amount of female hormones in association with the cessation of menses may be a factor that contributes to future development of osteoporosis. A lack of calcium in the diet does not seem to be the major factor in these women, as it seems to be in other women. But if you are an athlete, be particularly careful to eat foods rich in calcium to achieve the recommended dietary allowance of this important mineral (see Calcium and Osteoporosis, page 266). You may need to take supplemental calcium carbonate tablets to reach the goal of about 1,000 to 1,200 milligrams per day (see Osteoporosis, page 894).

Dietary Strategies for Athletes

Carbohydrate seems to be the preferred fuel for working muscles. In general, like everyone else, athletes should rely on bread, grains, cereals, vegetables, and fruits for at least 55 to 60 percent of their daily calorie needs. However, there are specific strategies you can use in advance of a particular event.

Carbohydrate Loading

Carbohydrate loading is a practice sometimes used by long-distance runners. It can only benefit athletes participating in endurance events (90 minutes or more), and it should be done no more frequently than three or four times per year. Two or 3 days before a competition, you eat a diet high in carbohydrates. You do this after consuming a low-carbohydrate, high-fat, high-protein diet in combination with continued exercise for up to a week before the competition.

Carbohydrate loading supplies your muscles with a large amount of glycogen, which is the most readily available fuel during competition. It also tends to increase your body weight by 2 to 3 pounds. The glycogen is stored in your muscles (and your liver), and this contributes to your body weight. Carbohydrate loading will increase your endurance, especially if your diet is not normally high in carbohydrates.

We believe athletes who participate in endurance events such as long-distance running should follow a high-carbohydrate diet throughout training. From the seventh to the fourth day before competition, reduce your consumption of carbohydrates. During that time, you should receive approximately 50 percent of your calories from carbohydrates. (Training activity remains intense on these days.) On the third to the second day before competition, you decrease training and increase carbohydrate intake to approximately

70 percent of daily calories. This modified sequence results in muscle glycogen levels equal to those provided by carbohydrate loading. In addition, most athletes find this new routine easier to follow.

High-Protein Diets

A low-carbohydrate, high-protein diet tends to reduce glycogen stored in your muscles and liver and to impair endurance. Still, this diet often appeals to wrestlers, whose weight is crucial for qualifying to compete in a given weight class. If a wrestler wants to compete in a lower-weight category, a low-carbohydrate diet in the days immediately preceding the event can help keep weight down by several pounds while not greatly impairing strength. It will, however, affect endurance.

Water-Weight Diets

Some wrestlers use sodium-restricted diets and diuretics in an effort to reduce body weight from water. Such practices can encourage faintness and weakness and may cause the loss of potassium, an essential nutrient. Avoid these diets.

Pregame Meal

In the past, much attention was given to the meal eaten before a competition. Often it consisted of meat and other high-protein foods.

Today we know that it is better to eat a meal primarily of carbohydrates, with a moderate amount of protein and a low amount of fat. Such a meal provides glycogen, the most readily available fuel during competition. Eat this meal 3 to 4 hours in advance of competition to ensure that the food has left your stomach (you should not feel full or heavy). Remember, as a general rule, carbohydrates empty from your stomach faster than proteins, and proteins empty faster than fats.

Vegetarian Diets

Vegetarian diets appeal to people for various reasons. For some people, religious and philosophical teachings prompt adherence to a vegetarian regimen. Other people seek health benefits.

There is much to be said for most of us making our food choices in the direction of vegetarian principles, eating less meat and eggs and substituting foods of vegetable origin. Such choices will reduce the amount of fats, particularly the saturated ones, and increase the amount of fiber consumed. Although such choices will reduce the amount of protein we eat, most of us consume more protein than we need.

At the same time, a poorly planned vegetarian diet can put you at risk for disorders such as vitamin B_{12} deficiency, iron-deficiency anemia, growth retardation (in persons who have not yet achieved their full adult growth), and osteoporosis, to name a few. Avoiding these risks means devising a healthful vegetarian diet—that is, one in which all of your body's nutrient needs are met.

Careful planning is the key to such a diet. Because many of the nutrients a human body needs are found most readily in animal products, finding substitutes requires effort.

There are various degrees of food restrictions in vegetarian diets. Total vegetarians, known as vegans, restrict their foods to those of plant origin only. Fruitarians further restrict their foods to only raw or dried fruits and nuts, honey, and olive oil. Lacto-vegetarians eat foods of plant origin plus milk and other dairy products. Lacto-ovovegetarians eat plant foods, milk and other dairy products, and eggs.

Obviously, the question of the nutritional adequacy of a particular vegetarian regimen depends on the extent of food restrictions. Also, children and teenagers, pregnant and lactating women, and people recovering from a serious illness or injury who are vegetarians need to take precautions to ensure that all of their body's needs are met. Such people should follow a vegetarian regimen only with the careful supervision of an experienced, registered dietitian.

Protein is of some concern when planning a strict vegetarian diet. Protein found in foods of plant origin tends to have only small amounts of one or more essential amino acids. (Essential amino acids are those that your body cannot manufacture—you must obtain them from your diet.) Protein from animal sources contains essential amino acids in an optimal proportion.

Grains and cereals with ingredients including wheat, corn, oats, and rice provide some essential amino acids, while legumes such as peas, peanuts, and dry beans provide others. When, during the course of a day, you combine a grain with a legume, or cornmeal with beans, you have a more nearly complete set of essential amino acids.

Another important nutrient in the vegetarian diet is vitamin B_{12}. Vegetarians who consume milk or eggs will get enough of this vitamin. Those who do not can eat foods artificially enriched with vitamin B_{12}. Some commercial foods made from soybeans and other plant proteins are fortified with vitamin B_{12}. A deficiency of this vitamin is a serious medical disorder (see Pernicious Anemia, page 958).

Vegetarians who eat eggs and dairy products also usually receive enough calcium and riboflavin, but the vegan has to devise special dietary strategies. Many foods of plant origin contain calcium, but they may not be as easily used by the body because of the presence of fiber and oxalic acid in the foods. Oxalic acid and fiber may interfere with the body's ability to use the calcium present in the foods. Thus, if you are a strict vegetarian, you may need calcium supplements.

Vitamin D, iron, and zinc are other nutritional elements needing special attention in the vegetarian diet. Most of us obtain vitamin D through fortified milk and exposure of our skin to sunlight. If you do not drink milk, you must rely on sunlight or on a vitamin supplement. However, children and pregnant and lactating women who are vegetarians should not rely solely on sunlight but should take a supplement.

The high fiber content of most vegetarian diets tends to impair the absorption of iron and zinc. Good sources of iron include enriched cereals and grains, legumes, dates, prunes, raisins, and leafy green vegetables. You can enhance absorption of the iron in vegetables by including citrus fruit or juice or other foods high in vitamin C with meals that contain plant sources of iron. Vitamin C helps increase the iron absorption from plant foods. Good sources of zinc include legumes and nuts.

Weight Control

Anyone who has struggled with a weight problem yearns for the ability to become thin immediately. Indeed, each year the market is flooded with the latest in instant weight-reduction plans.

Just remember this: most claims are greatly exaggerated.

Consider this, too: anything that makes you lose weight at a sustained overall rate of more than 2 pounds per week is a possible risk to your health.

The good news is that you need not master complicated formulas or scientific theories to learn about real, healthful weight loss. The concept is simple: your excessive stores of fat can be used up by expending more energy (calories) than you consume.

Daily Calorie Deficit

Let's take a more detailed look. The first step is to reduce your food consumption so that you eat less food than your body needs to perform the physical, mental, and other tasks that you demand of it. The difference between your daily calorie expenditure and calorie intake is called the daily calorie deficit.

The daily calorie expenditure can be calculated approximately by multiplying your weight in pounds by 12. This formula may underestimate your expenditure somewhat if you are younger or male—and overestimate it if you are older or female. The calorie intake of a diet can be estimated from food composition tables, although you must carefully measure amounts and sizes of portions. There may be substantial error in estimating both intake and expenditure of calories. A dietitian can help with such a calculation.

The second step involves the way your body fills the daily calorie deficit. Ideally, to lose weight, your body would use only body fat to provide extra calories. In fact, however, body protein also is used (more is used if the deficit is large and if the dietary protein intake is small and of poor biologic quality). Loss of this body protein increases the rate of weight loss because approximately the same number of calories is contained in a pound of body protein tissues as found in one-eighth to one-tenth of a pound of body fat.

Rate of Weight Loss

If you are considerably overweight and begin a weight-loss program by eating less food, you may notice a rapid loss during the first week or two. This initial weight loss can help give you confidence in your plan. However, be aware that such loss may not be limited to a loss of fat alone. Your weight loss also may be due in part to a loss of fluid and a depletion of glycogen stores in your muscles and liver. Thus, the 2 to 5 pounds you may lose those first few days can make you feel good about the plan, but permanent weight loss (fat loss) is a slower process.

To lose a pound of fat a day requires a deficit of 3,500 calories, a nearly impossible goal—although many quick-weight-loss schemes imply that this is possible. A more reasonable goal is to plan for a deficit of about 500 to 1,000 calories a day. Such a limitation will generally result in a weight loss of body fat of about 1 or 2 pounds a week.

The advantage of the smaller calorie deficit (500 calories) is somewhat greater confidence that the protein tissues of your body are not being lost in the process of weight reduction. The advantage of the greater calorie deficit (1,000 calories) is that a faster rate of weight loss results. Also, minor errors in measuring quantities of food are less likely to negate results of your dietary efforts.

Remember that any program that promises you more than 2 pounds of weight loss weekly may be unhealthful because the additional weight loss will be in the form of water, protein, and glycogen—not just body fat.

You can calculate your approximate weight loss per week over a long term by multiplying your daily calorie deficit by 0.002. For example, if you expend 2,000 calories per day in energy and eat 1,500 calories worth of energy, your deficit will be 500 calories per day. Five hundred calories multiplied by 0.002 yields an expected weight loss of 1 pound per week.

Setbacks

If you binge in the form of a single big dessert generous in calories and carbohydrates, you may well find your weight up 2 or 3 pounds the next day, mainly because of the increase in glycogen stores. This might lead you to the disheartening conclusion that a single meal or dessert can wipe out a week of dieting. Not so.

If you return to your dietary program promptly, most, but not quite all, of that increase in weight will disappear during the next day or two. The weight loss will be behind schedule by the amount of calories in the big dessert, but it usually amounts to wiping out no more than a day or two of previous dieting.

Your physician may want to refer you to a registered dietitian for planning a diet appropriate for your needs. Diets very low in fat and generous in vegetables and fruits are inherently high in fiber. They are filling, and you may find this helpful in following such a plan. Your likes and dislikes can be changed gradually, and following a proper plan may become easier as time goes on.

Half the process of dieting is controlling your intake of calories. The second half involves increasing the number of calories you burn.

Curbing Your Appetite

If the "just-say-no" technique doesn't work, try these tips to help appease an overactive appetite:

Eat Breakfast. Eating regular meals and snacks prevents the "famine-then-feast" syndrome. Make breakfast a high-fiber cereal, whole-grain bread, or fresh fruit, and you're more likely to eat less at lunch.

Eat When You're Hungry. By responding to physical signals to eat, you may be less apt to eat in response to stress or boredom.

Eat Slowly. Savoring each flavor and texture can boost satisfaction. Remember, it takes about 20 minutes for your brain to receive the signal that you're full.

Ride Out the Urge. Cravings generally pass within minutes—maybe even seconds. Busy yourself with an activity unrelated to food until the desire to eat passes.

Start Small. If you always finish what's in front of you, start with half the amount of food you usually eat. You may find smaller servings more satisfying. To make less food seem like more, serve your main course on a salad or dessert plate.

Splurge Now and Then. If you're really committed to eating less, an occasional lapse is OK. It has little impact on a lifetime plan for controlling your appetite.

Role of Exercise in Weight Control

Losing weight and keeping it off are much easier if you combine a food plan with an exercise plan.

Exercising increases your calorie expenditure. When it is combined with a reduction in calorie intake, exercise is a great asset to a weight loss program, and it can help strengthen and tone muscles and increase your vigor and feeling of well-being. Lack of vigor is a common complaint among people who are dieting (see Exercise and Fitness, page 289).

The benefits of exercise are great, but do not expect a rapid loss of weight due simply to a vigorous exercise plan. Loss of weight should be steady and is best achieved by combining good eating habits with regular exercise. Keep in mind, however, that even a little exercise will help burn off fat. It may be too small to be apparent in the day-to-day fluctuation of weight, but every little bit does help. Remember also that with exercise, protein needs may increase.

Before embarking on an exercise and diet plan, visit your physician. If you have a physical disability that prevents even moderate exercise such as slow walking, don't despair. You can lose weight successfully solely by reducing your calorie intake. It just takes longer.

Motivation

One of the problems with exercising is keeping motivated. Many people find that once they reach their weight goals they gradually lose interest in their exercise programs as well as in their careful eating patterns. First they skip a workout or two, then several in a row. After a time they find themselves back in their old sedentary habits.

The only way to keep fit long-term is to incorporate your exercise into your normal routine—like managing your money and keeping in touch with family and friends. The following are some suggestions for creating an exercise plan that becomes part of your normal routine, one that you can use while you lose weight and, just as important, one you will maintain after you reach your goal:

Be Realistic. Few of us will ever have the perfectly shaped bodies that exercise videos and some publications show. Do not be intimidated by them. Do not compare yourself with them.

Instead of trying to carve out the perfect physique, concentrate on toning your muscles and strengthening your heart and lungs. In this way you will be focusing your exercise toward the most important aspect of your program—your increased good health.

Choose Your Activities Carefully. What you do should match your personality. Select an individual sport such as tennis or racquetball if you like to compete on a one-to-one basis. If you like to socialize, choose a team sport or one in an organized group, such as dancing or aerobic exercise classes. If you enjoy solitude, try walking (highly recommended for all ages and many stages of fitness), jogging, bike riding, or cross-country skiing. Whatever you choose, make sure it is something you can do regularly, at least three times each week for 20 minutes or more. Try to schedule the activity for a regular time. This helps you get into a habit of exercise (see What Exercise Is Right for You? page 294).

Set Priorities. Lack of time is the most common excuse for dropping an exercise program. However, studies show that people who exercise have the same amount as or even less leisure time than sedentary people—it is just that they find the time for exercise.

Take charge of your time. If your schedule is in disarray, exercise becomes just one more nuisance. If you make a commitment, 20 minutes to an hour of exercise three to five times each week can be easy to maintain.

Vary Your Routine. If you get bored with a constant pattern of exercise, mix it up. Varying your activities is also a good way to prevent wear and tear on your body. Ride your bike one day, jog the next, dance another—they are all good aerobic exercises. Weight lifting, calisthenics, and swimming all firm muscles.

Do Not Overdo. Some people who finally make a commitment to exercise over-train. They become so enthusiastic about exercise that they set unrealistic goals for themselves.

How Many Calories Are in My Drink?

Are you counting calories? Don't forget to include any alcoholic beverages you may consume.

You burn most of the calories in alcohol as fuel for your body, or it is transformed into body fat.

To determine the calorie content of an alcoholic beverage, read the label first. If the beverage is a distilled liquor such as whiskey or vodka, what is the proof? If it is wine, what is the percentage of alcohol?

A distilled liquor identified as 100 proof is 50 percent alcohol by volume. "Proof" is twice the percentage of alcohol contained. Thus, a liquor that is 80 proof contains 40 percent alcohol. If a wine label states that the alcohol concentration is 10 percent by volume, then it is 20 proof (although wine is not traditionally referred to by its proof).

Although the label on beer only rarely indicates its alcohol content, beer is usually 4 to 5 percent alcohol and is, therefore, about 8 to 10 proof.

The amount of calories contributed by the alcohol portion of various forms of alcohol drinks can be calculated by the following formula: number of ounces x proof x 0.8 = number of calories. For example, a 2-ounce drink of 80 proof gin: 2 x 80 x 0.8 = 128 calories.

Because dry wines and distilled liquors contain essentially no calories beyond those found in the alcohol, this formula can reveal the calorie content with good accuracy. Remember, though, that sugar in a sweet wine contributes additional calories; likewise, the carbohydrates in beer may furnish perhaps a fourth, or half again as many calories, as the alcohol itself. "Lite" beers have smaller amounts of carbohydrates and often lesser amounts of alcohol.

This can lead to injury or frustration when the body does not respond as quickly as desired.

To get started on the right track without overexerting, use a trainer or fitness advisor for the sport you choose. Start your exercise program by investigating local community programs or membership in a health club. Adopt a moderate pace and be sure to get enough rest. If you develop problems, contact a trainer, physician, or specialist in sports medicine promptly.

Make an Investment. Many people feel more committed to an activity if they put money into it. Some people also find that the peer pressure of a class helps keep them involved. Look at such spending as an investment in your health.

But spend wisely. You do not have to sign up for the deluxe membership if all you plan to do is take a few classes. You do not need the very best athletic equipment to pursue an activity. Buying a pair of jogging shoes may help motivate you to start your program, but buying the most expensive pair will not make your body tone up any faster.

Do not worry about how you may appear to others. The class is for your benefit. Forget about how you look in a leotard. Remember that most people in these classes are most concerned about their own appearance—not yours.

Reward Yourself. Just as you may occasionally indulge in a treat while on your eating plan, you may find that moderate self-indulgence in your exercise program helps keep you motivated. Treat yourself occasionally to a new tape to listen to while you walk, or to a new sweatshirt.

Have Fun. "No pain, no gain." "Feel the burn." Unfortunately, such attitudes can make working out such serious business that you really do not look forward to it. And if it seems like a never-ending unpleasant chore, you may well look forward to stopping it. Try to look at exercise as a way to release tension or frustrations, a time for quiet reflection, or something that makes you feel good. That is why it is important to choose an activity that gives you some kind of pleasure.

Diet and Disease

There are many theories regarding preventive nutrition. Claims seem always to be made that preventing or curing countless disorders, ranging from the minor and inconvenient to the debilitating and fatal, is merely a matter of using this or that food or food additive.

Not all diseases and disorders have a nutritional component. However, several ailments do, including heart disease, cancer, hypertension, diabetes, and various chronic gastrointestinal disorders.

In the following pages, we consider the diet-and-disease link for each of these ailments as well as some of the often ineffective therapies associated with various food fads and vitamin and mineral supplementation programs.

Avoiding Heart Disease

Some factors that put you at high risk for heart disease are beyond your control (for example, your heredity). But one risk factor, a high blood cholesterol concentration, may be affected by what you eat.

In short, reduce the amount of fat and cholesterol you consume, particularly if you are susceptible to having a high cholesterol value. For most people, this need not involve a revolution in eating patterns. Moderation is the key. Small changes, consistently followed, can have a significant impact.

For a detailed discussion of preventing heart and blood disease, see Controllable Risk Factors, page 638.

Nutrition and Cancer Protection

These days there is great interest in the effect of diet on cancer risk. Much research is under way to evaluate and clarify the role that diet and nutrition play in the development of cancer. Although no direct cause-and-effect relationship has been proved, statistics do show that some foods may increase or decrease the risk for certain types of cancer.

The American Cancer Society and the National Cancer Institute have developed dietary guidelines to help reduce the risk of developing certain kinds of cancer. These dietary recommendations are consistent with dietary guidelines for Americans put forth by the U.S. Department of Agriculture and the Department of Health and Human Services. They include general recommendations for an overall healthy diet. They are as follows:

Keep a Normal Body Weight. Obesity is linked to increased death rates from some cancers in humans, particularly those of the prostate, pancreas, breast, ovary, colon, gallbladder, and uterus.

Avoid Too Much Fat in Your Diet, Both Saturated and Unsaturated. Evidence from epidemiologic studies suggests a relationship between dietary fat levels and the occurrence of prostate, colorectal, and other cancers. Currently, the reasons for such correlations are unclear.

Recent reports suggest that dietary fat intake may be unrelated to the incidence of breast cancer. No guideline for fat intake has been established, but it seems clear that in general the lower the fat intake, the less the risk of cancer. A prudent guideline for fat intake is 30 percent or less of your total calorie intake. (Do not try to eliminate fat from your diet; it is neither healthful nor possible.)

Eat Foods Rich in Fiber. The National Cancer Institute recommends a fiber intake of 25 to 35 grams each day. Dietary fiber appears to protect the body against some forms of cancer, particularly colorectal. The manner in which specific types of fiber work is unclear. Therefore, eat fiber daily from various dietary sources such as fresh fruits, vegetables, and whole-grain products.

Eat Foods Rich in Vitamins A and C Daily. Examples of these foods include dark green and deep yellow fresh vegetables and fruits, such as carrots, spinach, sweet potatoes, cantaloupe, and apricots, as sources of vitamin A. Oranges, grapefruit, strawberries, and green and red peppers supply vitamin C. Vitamin A may help decrease the incidence of several cancers, including those of the oral cavity, pharynx, larynx, and lung. Also, animal studies have shown that ascorbic acid, commonly known as vitamin C, can inhibit the formation of some carcinogenic compounds that are produced when nitrates are eaten. Still, there is no suggestion that you should consume supplemental amounts of these vitamins (see Do You Need an Antioxidant Supplement? page 266).

Include Vegetables as Part of Your Regular Diet. Broccoli, cabbage, Brussels sprouts, kale, cauliflower, kohlrabi, mustard greens, and Swiss chard are a few recommended examples. Research shows that these foods seem to offer protection from the development of colorectal, stomach, and lung cancers.

Eat Only Moderate Amounts of Salt-Cured, Smoked, and Nitrite-Cured Foods. This group of foods includes smoked and cured meats such as bacon, sausage, ham, and others. The incidence of cancers of the esophagus and of the stomach is higher among populations in which large quantities of these foods are eaten.

Some cooking methods, such as barbecuing or smoking, can produce substances that might cause cancer—thus, be moderate in using these methods.

If You Drink Alcohol, Do So in Moderation. Drinking large quantities of alcohol over a long period of time increases your risk of liver cancer. Combining alcohol consumption with smoking or chewing tobacco increases your risk of cancer of the mouth, larynx, throat, and esophagus. A limit of two or fewer drinks per day is recommended.

These suggestions are reasonable. You can follow them with little alteration in your daily dietary regimen. Still, the degree of protection from cancer that such actions may confer remains uncertain.

Nutrition and the Cancer Patient

Good nutrition is important for everyone. However, it is particularly important for people undergoing treatment for cancer, and proper eating habits can be especially difficult at this time. Treatments such as chemotherapy and radiation often disrupt eating patterns. You may feel nauseated. You may have no appetite or find that medications change your ability to taste accurately. Foods may seem tasteless.

You may find that you are so tired or ill that the last thing you feel able to cope with is eating. Some cancer patients lose their appetite even when they are not undergoing treatment.

Proper eating is important during cancer treatment. People who eat well during treatment maintain their stamina better and thus are more able to withstand potential side effects of chemotherapy and radiation therapy. They also tend to have fewer infections and remain more active during treatment.

Frequently the loss of appetite and other difficulties in eating that result from the cancer treatment lead to loss of weight and depletion of body protein. To obtain adequate amounts of calories and protein, you may need to choose foods such as eggs, ice cream, cheese, or commercial liquid nutritional formulas because alteration in taste sensation is common in advanced cancer, and meat often becomes distasteful. Fruits and vegetables should be tried, but often the amounts that can be consumed provide only limited amounts of protein and calories.

Pay special attention to eating protein-rich foods. They are particularly useful in helping to repair and build body tissues. In general, you need to eat enough food so that your body does not need to call on its stores of protein for energy, thus leaving it less able to repair itself.

Tips for Eating Well During Treatment
How do you go about eating well when you feel ill? Choose foods that are most palatable, then time your eating to take advantage of the times when you feel up to it.

Many people find that some of their favorite foods have scant appeal during therapy. Thus, they end up eating a very limited diet. As more foods seem unappetizing, their dietary choices shrink. To avoid this problem, keep an open mind about the foods you might eat. Something that is unpalatable today might taste better tomorrow or next week.

When you do feel well, make the most of it. Eat as much as you can of various foods. If you are cooking for yourself, prepare meals you can freeze and easily reheat for those times when you feel ill. Frozen dinners and prepared foods can be a help if cooking requires special effort. To make meal preparation easier, combine canned soups and sauces with fresh foods.

Even if you don't feel like it, give meals a pleasant atmosphere. Surroundings can do a great deal to help you forget how poorly you feel. A meal eaten on your lap may not be nearly as appealing, especially if you have no appetite, as one eaten at the table—from attractive china, with flowers on the table.

Perhaps the biggest problem to overcome during treatment is finding foods that are both appealing and nutritious. Many people find that meats do not appeal to them. If this is a problem for you, try poultry, mild-flavored fish, or cheeses. Mild-tasting dairy products such as cottage cheese and tangy yogurt also are good sources of protein. Even ice cream contains some protein. Also, try eating a peanut butter sandwich or peanut butter spread on fruit such as apple slices. Legumes such as kidney beans, chickpeas, and black-eyed peas are good sources of protein, especially when combined with grains such as rice, corn, or bread.

Pack as many calories as possible into the foods you eat. Warm your bread, and spread it with butter, margarine, jam, or honey. Sprinkle foods with chopped nuts. Enrich foods with nonfat dried milk.

Many people report losing interest in foods that are not particularly healthful. Fried foods, candy, potato chips, and alcoholic drinks are often unappealing, as are coffee, tea, or red meat. Some vegetables, such as those that have a tendency to cause gas or bloating (broccoli, cauliflower, corn, and beans), are also often disliked.

Foods that seem to cause fewer problems include fresh fruits and many vegetables and foods that, in general, are easy to eat and digest. Lightly seasoned dishes made with milk products, eggs, poultry, fish, and pasta often are well tolerated.

If you have trouble eating an adequate amount of food at a single sitting, eat smaller amounts more frequently. Chew your food slowly. Drink liquids at other times. Also, make sure that the liquids you drink have nutritional value, such as juices, milk shakes, or milk. If carbonated drinks help calm your stomach, mix fruit juice with sparkling water rather than relying on soda alone. Keep snacks handy so that when you do feel a little hungry you can eat easily. Also, avoid greasy foods and rich, buttery sauces. They may make you feel satiated much faster than other foods.

If the aroma of food being prepared makes you feel ill, avoid these smells. Heat foods in a microwave oven, or choose foods that require little cooking or can be warmed at a low temperature.

Many people report problems of elimination, either constipation or diarrhea, during the course of treatment. These conditions may be due to various factors, including medication that irritates the intestine and causes diarrhea or that slows down action of the bowel and promotes constipation. Radiation to the abdomen also can cause diarrhea. A decrease in activity and in the variety of foods eaten also can cause constipation and bloating from gas. Some people develop an inability to break down the lactose in milk products during treatment and have to refrain from eating them until treatments are completed.

In the case of constipation, eating foods rich in fiber often can help prevent or combat the problem. Such foods include fresh fruits and vegetables, dried fruits, whole-grain cereals and breads, and nuts. Drinking plenty of fluids also helps (see Chronic Constipation, page 784).

Diarrhea can result in a loss of important minerals and fluids. Sometimes a high-fiber diet is effective in treating diarrhea because fiber tends to absorb liquid in the stool and solidify it. Your physician may prescribe an antidiarrheal medication. You may want to avoid dairy products until the diarrhea clears up. If you have cramps, avoid foods that cause gas, such as carbonated drinks of all kinds, cabbage, broccoli, cauliflower, highly spiced foods, and even some forms of chewing gum (those that contain sorbitol). Also, drink liquids between meals (see Nutrition and Cancer, page 1303).

Salt and Hypertension

Too much salt (sodium chloride) in the American diet has been the focus of much study and has been given much attention by the media in recent years.

Findings indicate that people in certain population groups that habitually consume large amounts of salt develop hypertension (high blood pressure) more frequently than do individuals who use less salt. Also, research shows that people with hypertension generally can lower their blood pressure if they follow a low-sodium diet.

Blood pressure refers to the force exerted by the bloodstream on the walls of arteries. When there is more fluid in the bloodstream or when the blood vessels are narrowed, the pressure is greater. Roughly 20 percent of people in the United States are sensitive to the effects of sodium.

The American diet tends to be high in salt. We all should be aware of the amount of salt we eat, but a major effort to restrict salt is necessary only if you have hypertension (or if you are prone to developing hypertension). Even then, reducing the amount of salt in your diet is but one important step in lowering your blood pressure.

Sodium is present in nearly all plants and animal foods we consume. Indeed, our bodies need only a small amount of sodium to function properly (approximately half a gram daily, the equivalent of about a quarter teaspoon). The average American consumes 4 to 6 grams (2 or 3 teaspoons) per day. However, with current publicity about salt in the diet, this amount is decreasing.

If you need to limit your salt intake, begin with the food you prepare. Do not use salt when you cook, or use it only in very small amounts. Remove the saltshaker from your dinner table. If food tastes bland without salt, use herbs instead. Avoid salty foods such as chips and pickled foods. Switch from salted butter and margarine to unsalted.

Be aware that many processed foods contain large amounts of salt. Get in the habit of scrutinizing food labels (see Understanding Food Labels, page 263). Condiments such as ketchup, prepared mustard, and soy sauce are all high in sodium. Prepared foods such as canned soups, stews, and broths and cured foods such as ham, bacon, cold cuts, and hot dogs also are high in salt content.

For a detailed discussion of High Blood Pressure, see page 647.

Sodium

Sodium makes up 39.3 percent of the chemi-

Salt in Drinking Water

If you have heart or kidney disease or if you are on a sodium-restricted diet, softened water may provide too much extra salt.

In the water-softening process, calcium carbonate, a naturally occurring chemical compound that makes water "hard," is exchanged for sodium chloride (salt). This process can increase the sodium content of water to as much as 100 milligrams (mg) per liter (about a quart) after softening.

If you have softened water and are concerned about the water you use for cooking and drinking, you can have it tested. Your local or county health department, a water softener retailer, or a private laboratory can provide this service.

If your water contains more than 40 milligrams of sodium per liter, here's what you can do:

- Readjust your water softener line to bypass the tap used for drinking and cooking
- Buy bottled water with a low sodium content. Check the nutrition facts panel for sodium levels
- Consider a home water purifier
- If your sodium restriction is severe, buy distilled, demineralized, or deionized water for cooking and drinking.

cal compound sodium chloride (salt) and 27.4 percent of sodium bicarbonate (baking soda). Its concentration in the body fluids that bathe the cells is closely regulated. An excess in the body increases the volume of these fluids and thereby causes swelling or edema. Hypertension is more frequent in populations consuming larger amounts of sodium.

Sodium added during processing and manufacturing of foods constitutes about 75 percent of the sodium intake in the United States. An additional 15 percent is added as salt in cooking and at the table. The remaining 10 percent of sodium is contained naturally in food.

As a part of the treatment of hypertension, restriction of sodium to less than 2 or 2.5 grams daily is commonly recommended. This restriction can usually be achieved without great inconvenience. Greater degrees of restriction are used for treatment of persons who have certain forms of kidney disease.

Should everyone attempt to avoid every possible source of sodium in the diet? To do so would create considerable inconvenience, remove much of the enjoyment of eating, and result in benefit mainly to a small proportion of the population. Those who would benefit the most would be those considered "sodium sensitive" and vulnerable to developing hypertension, if they have not already been found to have increased blood pressure. However, those not considered to be sodium sensitive probably would benefit from avoiding excesses of sodium in their diet. A reasonable strategy for most of us would be to avoid salty foods and minimize the use of the saltshaker.

How are we to know who is sodium sensitive? Most of those persons will show some trend toward increased blood pressure. Only about half of those who have definitely increased blood pressure are sodium sensitive and may not require stringent restriction of sodium. Those receiving treatment for hypertension with diuretic agents usually are advised to restrict sodium intake carefully because this precaution will add to the blood-pressure-lowering effect and lessen losses of potassium associated with these agents. The benefits of several other categories of blood pressure medications are also increased by sodium restriction. Your physician can advise you whether a more relaxed approach is sufficient, although there is no simple procedure for distinguishing the sodium-sensitive person.

Diabetes Diet

In the past, if you were diagnosed with diabetes, your physician often handed you a standard preprinted diet sheet. No more. One set of guidelines just doesn't apply to everyone, and newer recommendations stress the need for personalizing your diet.

The American Diabetes Association (ADA) recommends working with a registered dietitian to develop a meal plan based on your food preferences, health concerns such as weight or blood cholesterol level, and insulin therapy.

Other recent changes in diabetic management include:

Reasonable Weight Goals. Being overweight can make it more difficult to control blood sugar. But rather than encouraging you to reach your ideal weight, new guidelines suggest "reasonable" weight goals. Dropping as few as 10 pounds may be enough to improve blood sugar control.

Flexible Fat Levels. If you're at a healthful weight and have a normal blood cholesterol level, new guidelines encourage you to keep fat to no more than 30 percent of total calories. (These are the same guidelines recommended for all Americans.)

However, if you need to lose weight or have a high blood cholesterol level, some experts suggest 20 to 25 percent of calories from fat is healthier. These lower levels correspond to the recommendations of the National Cholesterol Education Program for all people with cardiovascular disease.

But the key is individualization. If you're used to eating about 50 percent of daily calories from fat, lowering to even 40 percent can help you lose weight and improve blood cholesterol levels.

Calculated Use of Sugar. Sugar is no longer forbidden. People with diabetes have long been told that simple carbohydrates—sweets such as table sugar, honey, jelly, fruit juice, and candy—cause a rapid rise in blood sugar.

Complex carbohydrates—starches such as breads, cereals, and potatoes—were believed to cause a moderate increase in blood sugar. But new information shows that table sugar affects blood sugar about the same as bread, rice, and potatoes. It's the total amount of carbohydrate in the diet, rather than the source, that is the critical factor affecting blood sugar levels after meals.

Using modest amounts of sugar may not interfere with blood sugar control—as long as you substitute a sugary food for a starchy food that contains an equal amount of carbohydrate. Meal planning for people with diabetes continues to be a nutritionally balanced, flexible style of eating.

Greater flexibility, however, takes responsibility. More than ever, it's critical that you work with a registered dietitian and the rest of the diabetes team to learn how to enjoy more variety within the limits of your diet.

Specialized Diets for Chronic Diseases

Some chronic diseases require use of specialized diets. Such diseases include a sensitivity to gluten in foods (known as celiac sprue), liver failure, kidney failure, and kidney stones. When used with proper medical programs, appropriate diets can be important in controlling these conditions.

Celiac Sprue and the Gluten-Free Diet

Celiac sprue (also called nontropical sprue) can cause improper absorption of nutrients (see page 770). The disease is caused by the body's intolerance of gluten, a protein found in wheat, rye, oats, and barley. The sensitivity to gluten causes the lining of the intestine to lose its many tiny folds (villi) through which nutrients are absorbed. In addition, necessary digestive enzymes cease to be produced in large enough quantities. Symptoms include foul-smelling diarrhea, weight loss, a bloated abdomen, and anemia. Children fail to grow and may develop rickets; adults may develop a bone disease called osteomalacia (see Osteomalacia and Rickets, page 896).

Strict adherence to a gluten-free diet is the main course of therapy. Such abstinence seems, at first glance, to be fairly easy. However, it is actually difficult. You must avoid all foods containing wheat, barley, oats, and rye. Products made from gluten-containing grains are staples of American and European diets.

For example, many processed foods contain emulsifiers, thickeners, and other additives derived from such grains. These foods include commercial beverages such as chocolate milk, dietary supplements, cold cuts and prepared meats, breaded prepared foods, cheese foods and spreads, commercial souf-

---

Controlling Your Blood Sugar

The American Diabetes Association (ADA) treatment guidelines encourage not only avoiding high blood sugar but also keeping blood sugar as close to normal as possible. The ADA defines the normal range as 80 to 120 mg/dL before meals and 100 to 140 mg/dL at bedtime. Keeping blood sugar in tight control delays the progression of blindness, kidney failure, and nerve degeneration—common complications of diabetes.

You're most likely to be successful with this new approach if you're:

Motivated. You must be willing to test your blood sugar before each meal and at bedtime.

Organized. In view of the potential benefits, are you willing to keep daily records of your blood sugar levels?

Adaptable. You need to give yourself insulin 3 or 4 times each day—either by separate injections or with an insulin pump.

Flexible. Are you comfortable adjusting insulin to accommodate changes in your diet and activity?

Objective. For some people, the structure and intensity of treatment can be overwhelming.

Team-Oriented. By providing guidance and support, your diabetes physician, diabetes educator, and registered dietitian play a critical role in your success.

---

flés, omelets, fondue, and soy protein meat substitutes. Also included are commercial salad dressings and gravies, seasoned rice and potato mixes, vegetable mixes, canned baked beans, commercial soups and broths, and commercial ice creams and sherbets. Wheat breads of all kinds contain gluten, as do most baked goods. Commercially prepared condiments such as ketchup, mustard, soy sauce, meat sauces, vinegar, pickles, and syrups all may contain gluten unless the manufacturer specifically states that the product is free of gluten.

Rice (which does not contain gluten) may become the mainstay of your diet insofar as grains are concerned. Breads and pastries made with rice flour, corn flour, or potato starch are acceptable. Plain meats, fish, fowl, eggs, dairy products, vegetables, and fruits contain no gluten. Beverages including coffee, tea, carbonated drinks, chocolate drinks made with pure cocoa powder, wine, and distilled liquor contain no gluten. If you are on a gluten-free diet, you can also eat such things as soups and desserts thickened with tapioca, cornstarch, arrowroot, or eggs (see Celiac or Nontropical Sprue, page 770).

Kidney Stones

Renal lithiasis, the technical term for kidney stones, is a relatively common disorder. An estimated 5 percent of women and 10 percent of men will have at least one stone by the time they reach 70. For most people it is a very painful experience.

A kidney stone is a hard, mineralized deposit that occurs within the urinary passage. There are many kinds of kidney stones (see page 843). If you have kidney stones, your physician will determine the particular kind of stones you have and may make some dietary recommendations. In general, you will be advised to drink plenty of fluids each day—up to 3 or 4 quarts—to keep your urine diluted, particularly at night.

If you have calcium stones (the most common form), you may be advised to limit your intake of calcium to no more than 600 milligrams per day. Your physician may also ask you to limit your sodium intake to 2 grams per day, to avoid excessive protein, and to eat whole-grain foods.

If you have stones containing calcium oxalate, your physician may recommend first that you limit oxalate-containing foods (such as tea, chocolate, berries, and rhubarb) and second that you avoid supplements of vitamin C.

Kidney Failure

Kidney failure occurs when the kidneys are unable to remove waste products from the blood. It may result from infection, injury, exposure to toxins, or disease.

The two types of kidney failure are acute and chronic; both have nutritional implications. If you have acute kidney failure you will probably be placed on a diet high in carbohydrates and low in protein. If you are on dialysis, you may need more protein and your sodium and potassium intakes may be restricted. (Your physician or dietitian will monitor this carefully.)

Chronic kidney failure has many nutritional implications. Nausea, vomiting, and lack of appetite may be helped by eating a diet low in protein. A diet low in protein may also help preserve kidney function. You may also have to control the amount of water you drink. If you have hypertension associated with the disease, you may need to restrict the amount of liquids you drink as well as the amount of salt you eat. Your physician may limit the amounts of phosphate and potassium you consume (for more information about kidney failure, see page 852).

Liver Disease

Another problem that has nutritional implications is advanced liver disease. If this occurs, it may result in an increased amount of ammonia in your blood. Protein tends to be broken down into ammonia, so your physician may suggest a diet low in protein. Because vegetable and dairy proteins produce less ammonia than animal protein, your physician may also recommend these foods. People with liver ailments often retain fluids. To minimize this, you may need to restrict salt in your diet.

Dietary Risks of Alcoholism

Problems caused by alcoholism are many. They touch virtually every aspect of an alcoholic's life. Not least among them are the nutritional deficiencies and abnormalities that prolonged heavy drinking often will cause.

Alcohol contains only "empty calories"—those that have no nutritional value beyond their energy value. Alcoholics commonly substitute alcohol for food—thus their diets are lacking in essential nutrients.

Eating improperly, of course, is not the only problem alcoholics have. Many important nutrients, particularly thiamine and folic acid, are poorly absorbed by alcoholics. In addition, fat accumulates and is stored in the liver in only partially processed forms. Soon the liver swells, producing a condition called "fatty liver," and its function is impaired.

Excessive use of alcohol may result in a condition known as cirrhosis of the liver (see page 804). Some of the protein metabolized by the damaged (cirrhotic) liver is broken down into ammonia and substances called amines. These substances can build up in the body and can impair consciousness, resulting in a condition called hepatic encephalopathy (see page 808).

Consumption of large quantities of alcohol also may cause gastric bleeding or it can damage the pancreas, resulting in pancreatitis, both of which can be fatal (see page 818).

For a detailed discussion of Alcohol Abuse, see page 325.

Food Fads

Food can be symbolic. From ancient times, humankind has endowed particular foods with various attributes. In some of the early

Near East civilizations, for example, foods were designated as having either hot or cold qualities, and one was advised not to mix these at the same meal. Certain primitive societies believed that eating a tiger's heart enhanced a man's courage.

Even now, the rhinoceros is being hunted to near extinction because of the belief that eating powdered rhinoceros horn will aid sexual potency. The simplistic expectation that the properties of foods are assumed by or passed into the eater with little alteration is exemplified in the modern Western world by the practice of athletes who eat large amounts of protein foods and take protein supplements for the purpose of building muscle.

Adoption of specific eating habits or food boycotts can be a vehicle for expressing one's political views or a means of protest.

There are certainly plenty of unqualified people ready to make nutritional claims. The fads they spawn come and go and are generally characterized by a brief but intense enthusiasm and then a fading away of interest, often to be supplanted by another similarly strong and dwindling interest or hope.

Scientific exploration of various foods we eat and their relationship to health sometimes unwittingly spawns some of the fads we see each year. A few scientific reports about the properties of a specific food are published, sometimes in reputable publications, and soon the machinery of faddism is under way. Before long, newspapers, magazines, and even computer bulletin boards across the country discuss the magical benefits or serious toxicity of certain foods.

An example is the promotion of oat bran. There are undoubted nutritional benefits from the use of fiber in the diet, soluble fiber in particular; but the manner in which oat bran has been promoted and the way in which it has been received by the public justify describing the popularization of oat bran use as a fad.

People consume oat bran believing that this is all they need to do to lower their cholesterol levels. They fail to recognize that other dietary changes are needed for proper control of blood fats. In addition, oat bran and other fibers may combine with calcium in the gut to form a compound your body cannot absorb. Thus, the calcium and the fiber are eliminated from the body before potentially beneficial effects occur. Thus, if your diet is high in fiber, you may need more calcium than usual.

Some of the preparations, such as muffins, used to make oat bran palatable, are high in fat and sugar. Increasing your intake of fiber, in general, is a good idea, but focusing too closely on one specific food is not—especially if eating one muffin for its bran also means consuming quantities of butter, sugar, and other ingredients whose potential for increasing blood cholesterol far outweighs the potential benefits of the oat bran.

A similar fad several years ago involved a largely mythical disease. Hypoglycemia is a condition characterized by an abnormally low blood glucose level. It occurs in people with diabetes who are taking insulin or oral hypoglycemic drugs (see Diabetes Mellitus, page 925) and as a result of certain rare tumors (see page 936). The belief arose, however, that feelings of shakiness and anxiety that might occur within a few hours of eating were the result of a low blood sugar at the time. It is now recognized that many people who experience such symptoms are actually suffering from panic or anxiety attacks.

Other common misconceptions about foods include the extraordinary powers sometimes attributed to vitamins and minerals. Vitamin E seems to be one target for commercial exploitation. One theory holds that large doses of vitamin E will increase sexual performance. Vitamin C also has been touted as helpful in preventing colds. Controlled studies have shown neither of these tales to be true.

Claims often are made that honey has unique nutritional benefits. Not true. Honey has essentially the same nutritional properties as ordinary sugar. Your body does not differentiate the way it processes and uses them.

Much has been made of the supposed higher quality nutrition in foods grown in "organic" conditions. Promoters claim that foods produced by using inorganic (chemically produced and processed) fertilizers are of poorer nutritional quality. However, when studied in a laboratory, foods grown using "organic" manure and those grown using commercial fertilizers show few or no such differences. Organic gardening and farming practices may be desirable from a conservation standpoint (they are friendlier to the environment), but the food produced is not nutritionally superior to conventionally produced food.

For any person who eats a well-balanced diet containing the necessary proteins, fats, carbohydrates, vitamins, and minerals, fad diets promising improved health are less than useless. Because they are misleading, they are potentially harmful. The harsh reality is that additives or special foods cannot cure or prevent disease. The best way to avoid disease by dietary means is to eat a balanced diet (see Prudent Diet, page 259, and Vitamin and Mineral Supplements, page 264).

Food Myths

The more things change, the more they stay the same. This adage holds especially true when it comes to food. Despite advances in understanding the relationship between nutrition and health, some food myths are as prominent today as they were years ago. Here are some of the most common:

Myth: The only way to lose weight is to eat less.

Fact: One of the best ways to lose weight may be to eat more—at least of certain foods. Which seems like more to you—a handful of peanuts or seven cups of light microwaved popcorn? The popcorn, of course. Yet both foods have 150 calories. The difference is in the amount of fat and fiber.

Foods that are low in fat and high in fiber (like popcorn) naturally contain fewer calories than foods higher in fat (like peanuts). Gram for gram, fat has more than twice as many calories as carbohydrate or protein. Fat makes a little food add up to a lot of calories.

Myth: Vitamins provide energy.

Fact: Calories from fat, carbohydrate, and protein provide energy. Vitamins don't have calories, so they can't give you energy. The myth likely stems from the action of B vitamins. They don't actually provide energy. Yet each of the eight B vitamins plays a critical role in the chemical reactions that release energy from foods.

Myth: Fasting flushes out impurities and toxins.

Fact: No evidence supports the claim. Your body was designed to process food. This includes removal of naturally occurring toxins such as ammonia that results from the breakdown of protein.

For most people, one-day fasts are neither healthful nor harmful. But longer fasts threaten your health. Risks include dehydration, dangerously low blood pressure, muscle and organ tissue breakdown, and irregularity of your heartbeat. Never fast if you have heart disease, insulin-dependent diabetes, or kidney or liver problems.

Myth: Wheat bread has more fiber than white bread.

Fact: Only if it's "whole-wheat" bread. Otherwise, wheat and white bread are essentially the same. Both are made from refined wheat flour and have about one-half gram of fiber in a slice.

The only real difference is color. Manufacturers often add caramel coloring or molasses to wheat bread to darken its hue.

To be sure bread is whole-wheat, look for the word "whole" in the first ingredient. The nutrition label should also list the fiber content per slice as about 1.5 grams.

Myth: You were born to be fat.

Fact: Heredity strongly influences your body size and shape. Studies show that the weights of adults who were adopted as children closely resemble the weights of their biologic parents, not their adoptive parents.

But you don't inherit fatness as you do eye color or skin tone. Instead, you may have a genetic predisposition toward obesity.

That means having overweight relatives makes you more vulnerable—but not destined—to obesity. To gain weight, you still have to eat more calories than you burn.

Myth: Spinach is a good source of iron.

Fact: Sorry, Popeye, but it's not so. Spinach contains plenty of iron, but it also contains a lot of oxalic acid. Because oxalic acid binds iron, only 2 to 5 percent of the iron in spinach is actually absorbed by your body.

Spinach does, however, contain beta carotene. One-half cup of cooked spinach has more than half a day's supply of this important antioxidant.

Chapter 10

Exercise and Fitness

Contents

Benefits of Exercise, 290
What Is a Good Exercise Program? 290
  Getting Started: Five Little Rules, 291

Elements of Exercise, 292
Warm-Up, 292
Exercise, 292
Cool-Down, 294

What Exercise Is Right for You? 294
Identifying Your Goals, 294
Recognizing Your Condition, 295
  Perceived Exertion Scale, 295
  Finding Your Target Heart Rate, 296

Common Forms of Exercise, 297
Walking, 297
Jogging, 298
  Starter Jogging Program, 298
Exercise Machines, 299
Cross-Country Cycling, 299
Weight Training, 300
  How Many Calories Does It Use Up? 301

Avoiding Injury, 302
Consult Your Physician, 302
Warm Up Before Exercising, 302
Cool Down After Exercising, 302
Pace Yourself, 302
Select the Right Sport for You, 303
Make It a Habit, 303
Take Care of That Injury, 303
Take Care of Your Back, 303

Exercise in the Heat and Cold, 304
Hot Weather, 304
Cold Weather, 304
  Exercising at High Altitudes, 305

Getting Motivated, 305

Staying Active, 305
Don't Toss Your Tennis Shoes, 306
Does It Really Help? 306

Benefits of Exercise

A century ago, most Americans lived and worked on farms. Just staying warm and well fed involved countless daily tasks, all of which required actual physical labor.

For many of us today, the daily routine involves little or no compulsory exercise. Our service economy and innumerable labor-saving devices have made our lives more pleasurable in many ways but have robbed us of the natural, regular exercise we need to achieve optimal levels of health, performance, and appearance.

Physical inactivity and the aging process can result in a steady decline in your capacity to do physical work. If you withdraw from a physically active existence, activities that require strength and stamina become more difficult, the chances of injury become greater, and your risks of heart disease and other ailments increase.

However, there has been a healthy trend in recent years to "work out." More and more men and women are working out regularly because they like the way it makes them feel as well as its long-term benefits. In some social circles, the after-work cocktail has been replaced by a workout at the health club.

It is not hard to understand why so many people are turning to a healthier lifestyle that includes regular exercise. People like the healthy glow of the skin, the toned muscles, and the extra energy that comes from exercise.

The outward signs of a good exercise program are readily apparent. You can tell when your physical fitness improves: your ability to perform physical and even mental work increases. There may be an accompanying reduction in fatigue, tension, and anxiety.

Your muscles and joints will feel more flexible and seem to function better. You may be able to shed extra pounds, especially if a moderate reduction in food intake accompanies your exercise program. But perhaps the most important benefits cannot be seen.

When you exercise vigorously, your muscles require more oxygen. Thus, you must breathe more deeply to fill your lungs with air. Your body's most important muscle—your heart—must beat harder and faster to pump blood to your muscles. In time, your heart becomes stronger and more resilient.

In addition to a stronger heart, fat and sugar levels in the blood also may be decreased by exercise.

Women who exercise have a better chance of avoiding osteoporosis, a degenerative bone disease that afflicts many women, provided that they do not become so active that menstruation stops (see page 894). An exercise program may even be a factor in helping you quit smoking. Exercise also relieves stress, gives you an overall feeling of well-being, helps you sleep better, and improves concentration.

Just as exercise is important to your health— setting aside time for three 20-minute workouts a week is a sound practice—it is also essential that you match the exercise to your age, physical condition, and temperament.

In the following pages, you will learn about exercise programs. If you establish realistic goals, devise a suitable variety of exercise that fits into your lifestyle, and stay at it, your health will benefit. An important warning to remember, however, is that you should consult your physician before starting a new exercise regimen if you are obese, lead a largely sedentary life, or are older than 40 years and have never exercised; if you have diabetes, heart disease, a kidney disorder, or other serious health problem or had a relative who died of a heart attack before age 50 years; or if you smoke or have high blood pressure. Your physician may conduct an exercise tolerance test (see page 655) to help you establish safe limits for your exercise program.

What Is a Good Exercise Program?

A key distinction among kinds of exercise is whether they are aerobic or anaerobic.

Aerobic exercise involves continuous motion. An aerobic activity is one that requires your heart and lungs to function at an increased rate to supply your cells with more oxygen (literally, aerobic means "exercise with oxygen"). The increased respiration and heartbeat improve the condition of those vital organs and thus improve your overall conditioning and endurance, words that often are used interchangeably with aerobic health (see Cardiovascular Fitness, page 644).

Getting Started: Five Little Rules

First, visit your physician before you begin an exercise program. If you smoke, are overweight, are older than 40 years and have never exercised, or have a chronic condition such as heart disease, diabetes, high blood pressure, or kidney disease, it is particularly important that you check with your physician.

Second, begin gradually. Rome wasn't built in a day, and one doesn't go from strolls around the block to being a decathlete overnight. Do not overdo it. If you have trouble talking to a companion during your workout, you are probably pushing too hard. Slow down a bit.

A body not accustomed to vigorous exercise can be easily injured. Thus, in the beginning, your joints, ligaments, and muscles are vulnerable. Your body is less likely to be injured after it has been conditioned. Use your target heart rate (see Finding Your Target Heart Rate, page 296, and the Perceived Exertion Scale, page 295) to help you establish a suitable pace.

Third, select the exercise that is right for you. It should be something you enjoy—or at least find tolerable. Otherwise, in time you will avoid doing it. Vigorous walking, running, swimming, biking, racket sports, dancing, skiing, and aerobics are a few good forms of exercise.

Fourth, do it regularly. For real benefit, it is important that you have at least three exercise sessions of at least 20 minutes every week. When you exercise, it should be vigorous enough to make you breathe more deeply. Your heart rate will probably increase. However, never exercise to the point of nausea or dizziness.

Fifth, stay with your program. Do not get discouraged. You do not have to be a natural athlete to have a regular exercise program. Nor should you have unrealistic expectations. If you have short, thick legs, do not expect exercise to give you a ballet dancer's body. What you can expect is a better-toned body and more energy.

Walking, bicycling, jogging, aerobic dancing, and swimming are familiar aerobic exercises. They involve continuous activity and will help condition your cardiovascular system. They increase the rate and depth of breathing. Your body becomes warm and, if the exercise is sufficiently long and vigorous, you may also perspire.

Anaerobic exercise can be healthful, too, but does little for the health of your heart. Weight lifting is a classic example: strong muscles may be the result of a weight-lifting program, but lifting heavy barbells a few times offers little challenge to your heart and lungs to deliver oxygen in a sustained fashion to your body's tissues. A workout with light weights that is of sufficient duration may be aerobic.

A personal exercise program is a logical way to incorporate physical activity into your daily routine. It need not be very strenuous exercise to improve your fitness. In fact, a moderate amount of exercise is sufficient and will be more enjoyable for most people.

An exercise program should also be gradual: do not try to whip yourself into shape overnight, or even in a week or two. By gradually increasing the amount of exercise performed and by allowing your body to adapt to the change in activity level, you can improve your fitness in 8 to 12 weeks.

Tailor your fitness program to your needs, abilities, schedule, and other personal factors. Develop a regimen that works for you and your lifestyle because you must do it consistently to benefit. If you make your program so difficult that you rarely find the desire to do it or if the length of your workout is such that you cannot seem to fit your workout into your schedule more than once or twice a week, rethink your fitness program. You need a minimum of three 20- to 30-minute periods of conditioning exercise each week.

For maximal gain and to avoid injury, any exercise program should consist of three distinct elements: the warm-up, the primary exercise or activity itself, and the cool-down.

Elements of Exercise

Warm-Up

The purpose of the warm-up is to prepare your body for exercise. Gentle stretching exercises enhance flexibility, and low-intensity aerobic exercise gradually increases muscle blood flow and temperature. Muscles that have been inactive are "cool"; stretching and other low-intensity exercises gradually increase heart rate (pulse), body temperature, and blood flow to your muscles. Your warm-up regimen can ease you into the principal exercise. It will help you to avoid muscle stiffness, soreness, and even injury.

Stretches
In performing stretching exercises, remember to hold each stretching position for 30 seconds—do not bounce rhythmically. You should experience a definite pulling sensation in the muscles you are stretching, but it should not be painful.

We recommend at least 3 to 5 minutes of stretching at the start (and the end) of every workout. Your selection of stretches should depend on the kind of exercise that is to follow. For example, if you are a runner, emphasize your legs and lower back. Among good candidates for stretches are those shown on page 293.

Exercise

Your principal exercise should be an aerobic exercise. This is any activity that requires continuous rhythmic muscle contraction of the legs and possibly the arms and that increases the rate and depth of breathing. Common aerobic (endurance) activities include walking, cycling, jogging, swimming, cross-country skiing, rowing, rope skipping, dancing, and racket sports. The key is to find an activity that you enjoy.

Your selection of exercise should be made with three characteristics in mind: intensity, duration, and frequency.

Intensity
The right intensity for your exercise will improve your fitness; however, your workout should not be too strenuous. In general, correct intensity of exercise requires you to reach 50 to 80 percent of your "maximal endurance exercise capacity." For most people, the ideal is about 70 percent.

By measuring your heart rate (pulse) you can determine the intensity of a given workout: the more intense your aerobic exercise, the greater your heart rate. When you exercise as hard as you can (your "maximal endurance exercise capacity"), your heart will be beating at its maximal rate. This rate decreases as you age and is affected by heart disease and some heart medications.

Additional benefits from going full-tilt in your workouts are small. That is where your "target heart rate" comes in. You can measure the efficiency of your exercise by determining your target rate (a calculation that factors your age into the equation; see Finding Your Target Heart Rate, page 296). During the conditioning portion of your workout, your heart rate should reach the target rate and remain there for perhaps 20 minutes or more. Exceeding your target rate puts you at increased risk of muscle or joint soreness or injury and adds little fitness benefit.

To use your target heart rate as a guide, you need to take your pulse. With the tips of your index and third fingers, locate the pulsing artery (radial artery) between your wrist bone and tendon on the thumb side of either wrist. Do not press too hard on the blood vessel; you could temporarily obstruct the flow of blood. Count your pulse for 10 seconds, timed by the sweep hand of a watch or clock. Multiply this count by six to obtain your pulse (see page 645).

At rest, the pulse is likely to be about 70 for men and about 80 for women. When you exercise, your rate may more than double (depending on your age and the intensity of your workout).

Frequency
Exercising three times each week on nonconsecutive days is the minimal frequency for aerobic exercise. Exercising more often will increase conditioning and speed weight loss if you are overweight.

Duration
The duration of your conditioning exercise should be at least 20 to 30 minutes; 45 to 60

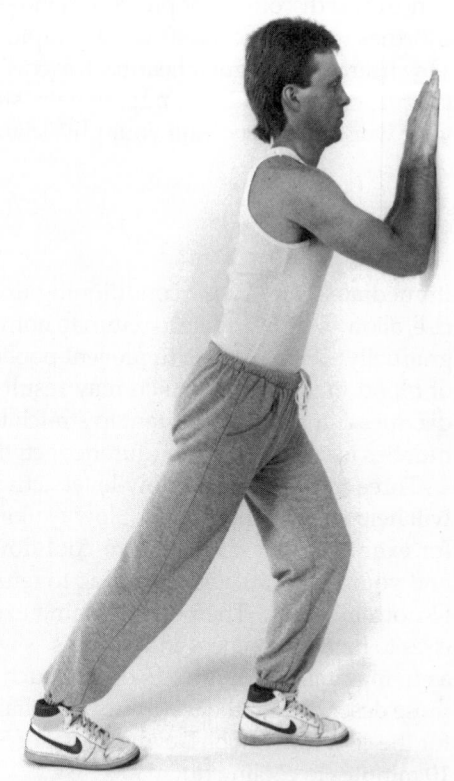

Calf Stretch

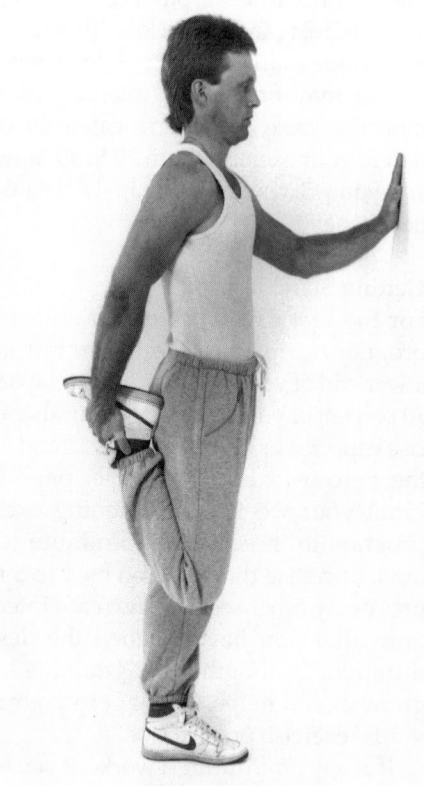

Thigh Stretch

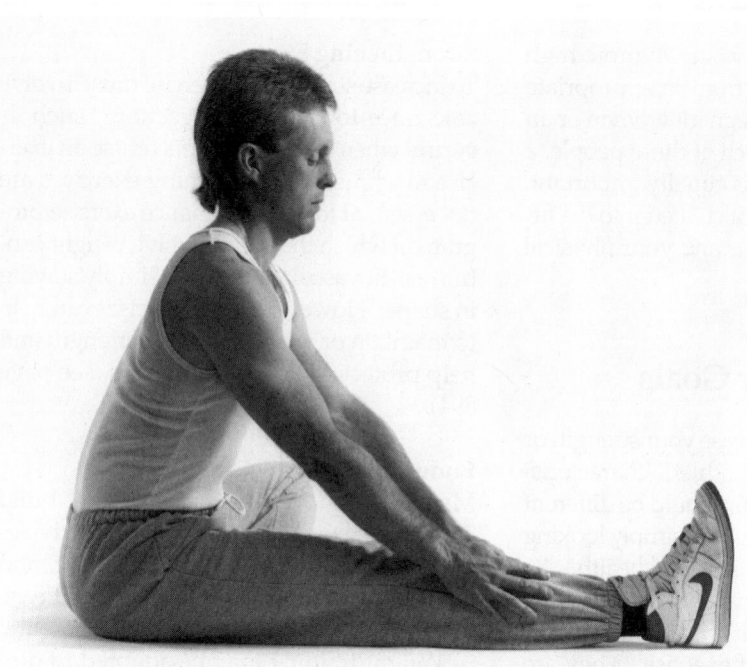

Hamstring Stretch

Calf Stretch
Stand an arm's length away from the wall.
Lean forward, rest your forearms on the wall,
and align your forehead with the backs of
your hands. Bend one leg at the knee and
bring it toward the wall. Keep the other leg
stiff, with the heel on the floor. Move your
hips toward the wall, keeping your back
straight. You will feel a stretch in the calf
muscles. Hold this position for 30 seconds,
and then repeat the stretch with the other leg.

Thigh Stretch
Place your left hand on the wall for balance.
Reach behind you and hold onto your right
foot or ankle with your right hand. Pull the
foot toward your buttocks. Again, you will
feel your muscles stretching, this time in the
front of the thigh. Hold this position for 30
seconds, and then repeat the stretch with the
other leg.

Hamstring Stretch
Sit on the floor and extend your right leg
straight ahead of you. Bend your left leg so
that the bottom of your left foot touches the
inner thigh of your right leg. Bend forward
from your waist and slowly move both hands
down your right leg—you will feel a stretch
in the back thigh muscles (hamstrings). Hold
this position for 30 seconds, and then repeat
the stretch with the other leg.

minutes of exercise will produce faster progress in conditioning and weight loss. These times do not include warm-up and cool-down periods.

You may find lower intensity exercise more enjoyable; if so, then increase the duration of your exercise (from 20 to 40 minutes) and you will continue to reap the desired fitness benefits.

Getting Started

For the first several weeks of an exercise program, keep your target heart rate at the lower end of your target zone (perhaps 50 to 70 percent of your maximal endurance exercise capacity, or between levels 11 and 13 on the Perceived Exertion Scale, page 295). Limit your weekly conditioning exercise program to three 10- or 15-minute workouts. Increase the duration by 1 to 5 minutes every other session. Increase intensity only after you have reached the desired duration. A month-long, graduated program should help you adapt to your individual exercise prescription.

If at any time during a workout you experience chest discomfort or pressure, faintness, shortness of breath, bursts of very rapid or slow heart rate, irregular heartbeat, excessive fatigue, or severe joint or muscle pain, stop your workout and consult your physician.

Cool-Down

Immediately after your conditioning exercise, allow your heart rate to return to normal gradually. Keep moving to prevent pooling of blood in your legs, which may result in dizziness. It also is important to stretch the muscles used during the endurance activity.

Three to 5 minutes of low-level activity will help achieve these ends. Slow walking, for example, will allow you to cool down and your heart rate and breathing to return to normal levels. Then do stretching exercises to prevent soreness and stiffness as well as to maintain flexibility. Exercises such as those described for the warm-up are suitable for the cool-down too. Devote a total of 5 to 10 minutes to cooling down.

What Exercise Is Right for You?

The perfect workout for an Olympic high jumper is very different from an appropriate fitness program for a pregnant woman or an elderly man. Yet, for each of these people, a good exercise program is equally important.

Two factors must be calculated into the fitness equation: your goals and your physical condition.

Identifying Your Goals

If you are looking to increase your strength or quickness or some other athletic characteristic, your exercise program should be different from that of the person who is simply looking to maintain his or her basic good health.

Any exercise program should involve a mix of activities but, for practical purposes, there are three kinds of exercise. They are distinguished by the goals they are intended to help attain.

Strengthening Exercise

To increase strength, an exercise must involve resistance to muscle contractions, such as occurs when you lift weights or use an exercise machine. Strengthening exercises are not essential for a maintenance exercise program in which the goals involve weight control, cardiovascular health, or simply staying in shape. However, these exercises can help to maintain or increase muscle strength and help protect against osteoporosis (see page 894).

Endurance (Aerobic) Exercise

Many other kinds of exercise can build endurance too. In particular, aerobic activities such as running, swimming, walking, and cycling build the endurance of your heart, lungs, and muscles (cardiovascular benefit).

Weight training may be adapted to provide some aerobic benefit by reducing the resistance and increasing the number of repetitions for each exercise to 20 to 40 (circuit weight training).

Endurance (aerobic, cardiovascular) exercise is a form of exercise that requires your heart and lungs to increase the amount of oxygen provided for the working muscles. Three 20-minute aerobic workouts a week should be a part of any basic conditioning program (see Cardiovascular Fitness, page 644).

Flexibility Exercise

Flexibility exercises also are basic. They are less about conditioning and more about avoiding injury and discomfort. Stretching and warm-up exercises get the blood flowing, literally warming up your muscles and getting them ready to work out. At the close of a period of activity, flexibility exercises are also essential to help your muscles cool down and to help prevent muscle tightness.

Recognizing Your Condition

Your physical status is the other key factor—are you overweight, of a certain age, or pregnant? You and the members of your family each will be in one of the categories described here.

Child

For many parents, the idea of having to encourage their children to be more active is absurd. Kids never stop running around. How could they possibly need more exercise?

For some children, however, particularly those who are overweight, an increase in physical activity is very important. Weight control at any age is largely a matter of balancing the intake of calories with the amount of energy expended in everyday activities—when more calories are burned than are consumed, the excess pounds will begin to disappear.

Scheduling regular workouts is a suitable approach for an adult, but it probably is not for a school-age or even teenage child. A better approach is to encourage sports or physical fitness activities at times of the child's choosing. These activities burn calories and may have a beneficial effect on self-esteem and self-image as well.

Healthy Adult

The aging process often makes us realize how important exercise is: our bodies grow

---

Perceived Exertion Scale

Rating of perceived exertion is another tool to help you determine if you are exercising at a satisfactory intensity.

Perceived exertion refers to the total amount of physical effort experienced during a given activity. The scale takes into account all sensations of exertion, physical stress, and fatigue. When using the rating scale, do not become preoccupied with any one factor, such as leg discomfort or labored breathing, but try to concentrate on your total inner feeling of exertion.

A rating of "6" indicates a minimal level of exertion, such as sitting comfortably in a chair. A rating of "20" corresponds to a maximal effort, for example jogging up a very steep hill.

Ratings between "11" and "15" on the scale are generally recommended. A rating of "13" corresponds to 70 percent of maximal exercise capacity and is considered ideal for most people.

6		
7	Very, very light	
8		
9	Very light	
10		
11	Fairly light	
12		Exercise Training Zone
13	Somewhat hard	
14		
15	Hard	
16		
17	Very hard	
18		
19	Very, very hard	
20		

---

less forgiving of our minor excesses and sedentary ways as we grow older. Muscles that are rarely used lose strength, tone, and definition. In particular, if your heart and lungs are unchallenged, you increase your risk of heart attack and other disorders.

The good news is that there are a wide variety of exercise options for a healthy adult. You might consider jogging (see The Starter Jogging Program, page 298), bicycling (see Cross-Country Cycling, page 299), swimming, rowing, or any number of other options.

These are the key considerations: start slowly and work up gradually; eventually work out a minimum of three times a week; and determine your target heart rate (see page 296) and perceived exertion load (see page 295). Maintain exercise at that level for no less than 20 minutes at each workout.

If you are older than 40, overweight, or a smoker, or if you have had a heart attack or have diabetes, consult your physician first. An exercise stress test may be necessary to assess the risks and limitations (see The Exercise Tolerance Test, page 655).

Pregnant Woman

Reasonable exercise programs probably have little or no impact on your unborn child—but they can affect you in numerous ways, including your stamina (perhaps making labor shorter and easier) and even your overall attitude. However, during pregnancy you may be more vulnerable to injury, so take appropriate precautions when planning a program (see Exercise During Pregnancy, page 195).

Obese Adult

Any complete weight-loss program should involve an exercise component: reducing your intake of calories is a key element, but exercise expends calories and can increase your resting metabolic rate and make you feel better. However, if you are overweight and have been largely inactive for several months or more, consult your physician before embarking on an exercise regimen. He or she may give you an exercise stress test to determine the response of your heart to the stresses of exercise (see The Exercise Tolerance Test, page 655). When you begin to exercise, start slowly, perhaps with a walking program.

Heart Attack Survivor

Having had a heart attack, coronary artery bypass surgery, or coronary angioplasty (see pages 665 and 666) does not mean you can no longer exercise. On the contrary, appropriate workouts are an important part of your treatment and recuperation. Your physician can help you plan an exercise program. A local civic organization may even have group workouts for persons who have had a heart attack or heart surgery (see Cardiac Rehabilitation, page 668).

Elderly Person

If you have led a sedentary life, consult your physician before starting a conditioning program. Your physician may conduct an exercise stress test to help you plan the pace of your exercise (see The Exercise Tolerance Test, page 655).

In general, walking is an excellent exercise for elderly people. It delivers cardiovascular benefit yet does not stress the bones and joints, in contrast to some more vigorous forms of exercise. In particular, women beyond menopause are at increased risk of fractures because of bone demineralization (see Osteoporosis, page 894), so avoiding unnecessary stresses is sensible.

If you experience chest pressure or pain, dizziness, shortness of breath, bursts of very rapid or slow heart rate, irregular heartbeat, excessive fatigue, or severe joint or muscle pain, stop your workout and consult your physician.

If You Have a Disability

Exercise is as important to persons with a disability as to those without physical limitations. The health of the heart and lungs is equally crucial to those with disabilities, and cardiovascular conditioning exercises should be sought.

Finding Your Target Heart Rate

Whenever you run, swim, or cycle, your heart beats faster—this is the point of a conditioning exercise. But is your increased heart rate fast enough to provide maximal benefit but not so fast that there is an unnecessary strain on your heart?

In selecting the right exercise for you and in creating your exercise program, look for the right pace: this means identifying your "target heart rate." To do this, subtract your age from 220, and then take 70 percent of this number. For example, if you are 40 years old, 220 minus 40 is 180; 70 percent of 180 is 126, so your target heart rate is about 125 beats per minute. That means that you should aim to reach and maintain that level or slightly above it for the duration of your workout.

However, if you have been inactive for several months or more, have a chronic health problem, or are recovering from an injury, consult your physician before starting a workout regimen. If you have high blood pressure, high cholesterol level, diabetes, or a family history of heart disease or if you are a smoker, your physician may recommend an exercise stress test to help determine the best approach for you (see The Exercise Tolerance Test, page 655).

Your physician may recommend that, rather than the 70 percent factor, a lower value, perhaps 50 percent, is appropriate, at least to start with.

Common Forms of Exercise

Walking

We take walking for granted. We do it every day, taking dozens or even hundreds of little trips to the kitchen, car, bathroom—going just about anywhere involves taking at least a few steps.

Yet, taking a brisk walk can be a safe, effective means of improving your physical fitness. Especially if you lead an inactive life and are a bit out of shape, a program of walking could be just the challenge you need—not too taxing, yet providing fitness benefits.

An appropriate regimen of walking can help you increase the efficiency of your heart and lungs, improve the ability of your body to use oxygen during exertion, and decrease your resting heart rate. It also may decrease your blood pressure.

Walking expends calories—a 175-pound person expends approximately 210 calories by walking 2 miles in an hour, 275 calories at 3 miles in an hour, and 340 calories at 4 miles in an hour. Walking can improve muscle tone, which helps to shape and tone muscles in your legs, hips, buttocks, and abdomen. Walking also can be a valuable part of a weight-loss program.

Walking can be a tonic for the mind as well as the body. Walking can relieve stress, helping you unwind at the end of the day or after a difficult task.

Regular walking also can help you prevent age-related diseases. Walking increases bone density and, according to recent research, may lower the risk of osteoporosis developing (see page 894). For some people, regular exercise can lessen the pain of osteoarthritis.

About 30 million Americans walk today for fitness—in fact, fitness walking is the fastest-growing participant sport in the country. It requires no special skills or instruction. You can vary your route to keep it interesting. Walking is a convenient, inexpensive, and even social workout, if you can get a spouse or a friend to join you. Walkers also are less prone to injury than participants in most other kinds of physical activity.

Decide on your goals before you begin. For aerobic benefit, plan on a minimum of three workouts a week, on alternating days,

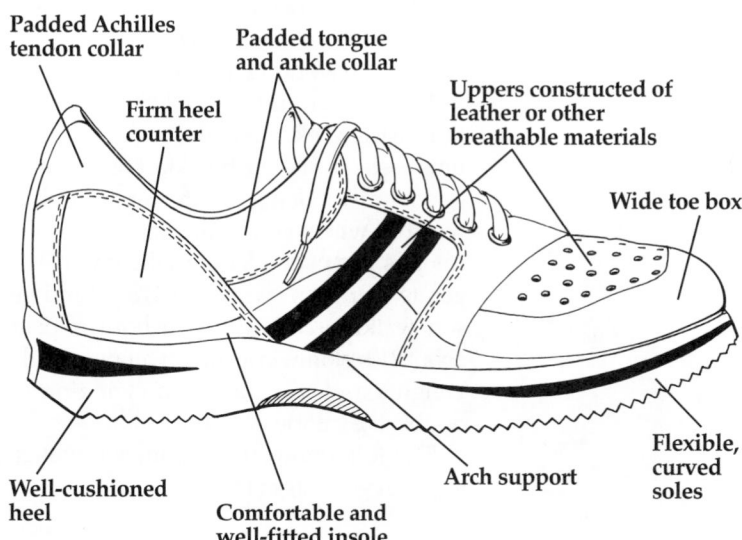

Padded Achilles tendon collar

Firm heel counter

Padded tongue and ankle collar

Uppers constructed of leather or other breathable materials

Wide toe box

Well-cushioned heel

Comfortable and well-fitted insole

Arch support

Flexible, curved soles

A good walking shoe should include these features.

of 20 minutes or more each.

Get yourself a pair of good walking shoes. Such shoes should be lightweight, fit comfortably, and have a slightly elevated heel. They should also provide substantial arch support, plenty of width in the toe area, a firm heel counter (the curved support at the rear of the shoe) to guide your foot through its roll forward, a well-cushioned heel and midsole to absorb shock, and a durable outersole with good traction. The rest of your attire is important, too, especially in an excessively warm or cold condition (see Exercise in the Heat and Cold, page 304).

Do stretching exercises before and after you work out. In fact, a safe, effective workout consists of the same basic components: a warm-up with flexibility and stretching exercises, the conditioning exercise itself (in this case, walking), and a post-exercise cooldown period with more stretching and flexibility exercises.

Stretching should be done for at least 3 to 5 minutes before the walking exercise. This loosens joints and stretches key muscles. Begin by walking slowly for approximately 5 minutes to increase heart rate, muscle blood flow, and muscle temperature. After each walking session, cool down by walking slowly for a few minutes, and then conclude with 3 to 5 minutes of stretches.

Start slowly. If you are just beginning, increase the duration and rate of your workout slowly over a period of 4 to 6 weeks. Begin by walking on flat ground. If walking on flat ground becomes too easy, look for gentle hills to increase the intensity of your program. If you're working so hard you can't talk, you're working too hard.

Establish a routine, and do it at least three times each week. Take your walk at the same time each day; before breakfast or dinner is a good time. Using 1- to 3-pound hand weights when you walk can increase the calories you expend, especially if you exaggerate your arm swings. A 175-pound person walking at 2 miles an hour expends about 210 calories in an hour without weights. Weights and vigorous arm swinging can double the calories you burn.

The following chart outlines a walking regimen you might follow:

Week of Program	Distance, miles	Time, minutes per mile
1-2	1-2	15-30
3-4	2-2.5	12-25
5-6	2.5-3	12-20
7-8	3-4	12-20
9-10	4-5	12-20

Keep your water consumption high. When you exercise, you need the extra water to maintain your normal body temperature and to cool working muscles. Drink water before and after your workout.

Starter Jogging Program

	Exercise Time, minutes		Repetitions, number		Total Time, minutes
Step	Jog	Walk	Jog	Walk	
1	1	1	12	12	24
2	2	1	8	8	24
3	3	1	6	6	24
4	4	1	5	5	25
5	5	1	4	4	24
6	7	1	3	2	23
7	10	1	2	2	22
8	12	1	2	1	25
9	15	1	2	1	31
10	20	—	1	—	20
11	25	—	1	—	25
12	30	—	1	—	30

And listen to your body. It will send warning signals—pain, nausea, dizziness—if something is amiss. Stop and rest. If symptoms persist, consult your physician.

Especially if you have been inactive for several months or more, have a chronic health problem, or are recovering from an injury, consult your physician before beginning walking workouts. If you have high blood pressure, high cholesterol level, diabetes, or a family history of heart disease or are a smoker, your physician may recommend an exercise stress test to help determine the best approach for you (see The Exercise Tolerance Test, page 655).

Jogging

Jogging is not for everybody (if you have a heart or lung ailment, discuss jogging or any proposed exercise program with your physician before beginning it). But many people find that a regular program of jogging suits their exercise needs and can fit into busy schedules.

If you have not been active for several months, do not start with a multi-mile run. Begin by walking. When you are able to walk 2 miles in 30 minutes comfortably, you are ready to try alternating jogging and walking.

Follow the guidelines in the chart on this page. Move from one step to the next every 2 to 7 days—your body will tell you when you have gone too far too fast. To minimize the risk of injury and of muscle and joint discomfort, do not jog more than three or four times a week, and jog on alternate days.

Jog at a comfortable pace, aiming at the lower end of your target heart rate (perhaps 50 percent; see Finding Your Target Heart Rate, page 296). After step 12, you can then gradually increase the intensity of your workout.

Remember the warm-up and cool-down. Do not forget to allow 5 to 10 minutes before and after your jogging for stretching and acclimating your body to the change in pace (see Warm-Up and Cool-Down, pages 292 and 294).

To begin, give your body a break. Do not try to accomplish too much. Step 1: Jog for 1 minute, and then walk for 1 minute. Repeat this sequence 12 times for a 24-minute workout. Exercise three times a week on alternate days. Each week, move up one step in your Starter Jogging Program.

Exercise Machines

There are five basic exercise machines, each with something unique to offer. Some machines exercise only your lower body, and others build strength or aerobic (cardiovascular) capacity. The following devices can build both strength and aerobic capacity:

Stationary Bicycle. Builds leg strength and cardiovascular capacity and is an excellent choice for both beginning and serious exercisers. Some cycles have moving handlebars that provide an upper body workout as well. If you have knee problems, be sure the resistance can be adjusted to a low setting.

Rowing Machine. Offers a good aerobic workout by putting your entire body in action. Helps strengthen your back, shoulders, stomach, legs, and arms. Machines with a flywheel and chain drive generally are easier to operate and are more effective than piston-type rowers, which are less expensive and more compact. Proper technique is important to avoid back strain.

Treadmill. Builds leg strength and aerobic capacity. Some models offer adjustable inclines simulating hills. You can adjust speed for walking or jogging. Higher horsepower models run smoother and are more durable.

Stair-Climber. Helps tone and strengthen hips, buttocks, thighs, hamstrings, calves, and lower back. It provides an effective aerobic workout. Compared with jogging, it reduces wear and tear on ankles and knees. Still, the device can aggravate knee problems.

Cross-Country Ski Machine. Offers a good overall workout, but can be difficult to master, requiring practice in moving arms and legs in rhythmic opposition.

Shopping for a Machine

In general, you'll get what you paid for when you purchase an exercise machine. The low-priced models may do little more than raise your blood pressure once you realize the machine is unstable, uncomfortable, and even unsafe.

Make sure the device is solidly built, with no exposed cables or chains. Avoid spring-operated components, and look for a machine that operates smoothly.

Be sure it's comfortable to operate. A comfortable seat is critical for cycles and rowing machines. Try it out at the dealer, or visit a fitness center. Some vendors allow a home trial. You may need instruction, and some vendors offer it free when you purchase the machine.

Look at the warranty—it's usually a sign of quality. And avoid making a purchase decision based on gizmos to monitor your performance. Many of the machines are laden with such things as calorie counters, timers, computer printouts, and video displays. Don't get talked into something you don't need and won't use.

Cross-Country Cycling

As the old cliché has it, "You never forget how to ride a bicycle." This is more or less true, and a good thing to remember if you are looking for a conditioning exercise.

Cycling is not just for kids. Increasingly, fitness-minded adults are returning to cycling. About 20 million adults get on their bicycles at least once a week; many of them use their bicycles regularly in a pattern of three or more workouts a week for maximal aerobic benefit. However, there are some important considerations in planning for a true workout.

Selecting the Right Bicycle

Some bicycles are designed for smooth surfaces and high speeds; others are suitable for rough terrain. Consider your needs: do you need a racing, mountain, or touring bicycle?

Racing bicycles are lightweight and have narrow tires, low-slung handlebars, and many gear settings, usually between 10 and 18. When riding a racing bicycle, the upper part of your body is parallel to the ground.

Mountain bicycles have sturdier frames and wider tires that have more tread. They are designed for off-the-road riding and often have many gear settings too. The handlebars are more upright. The riding posture is more erect.

Touring bicycles are between mountain and racing bicycles. The posture is more upright. Older models typically had gears for 3 to 5 speeds, but today's touring bicycles often have 10 or 12.

In selecting a bicycle, keep in mind that, when you are seated and have your foot on the pedal lowest to the ground, your leg should be not quite fully extended. You should be able to reach the handlebars and to work the brakes and shift mechanism while

keeping your eyes on the road. When strad-
dling a racing bicycle with your feet on the
ground, there should be 1 to 3 inches of clearance above the crossbar; a mountain or touring bicycle should have 3 to 6 inches of
clearance. Always wear a helmet when riding a bicycle.

Designing Your Exercise Program

As with any form of conditioning exercise,
schedule regular workouts. We recommend
three rides a week (at least) of 30 minutes in
duration or more. Stretch your muscles
before and after you cycle.

Intensity is also a factor. As you become
comfortable with your bicycle and workout
schedule, determine what your target heart
rate and perceived exertion level should be
and work up to maintaining them for the
duration of your workout (see Finding Your
Target Heart Rate, page 296, and Perceived
Exertion Scale, page 295).

If you have been inactive for several
months or more, have a chronic health problem, or are recovering from an injury, consult your physician before starting a
workout regimen. If you have high blood
pressure, high cholesterol level, diabetes, or
a family history of heart disease or are a
smoker, your physician may recommend an
exercise stress test to help determine the
best approach for you (see The Exercise
Tolerance Test, page 655).

Select a time of day that works for you
for your cycling. For example, if managing
stress is a goal, perhaps your ride is best
scheduled when you need a safety valve
from pressure—a ride after work may relax
you for your evening at home.

Do not be tempted to challenge yourself by setting the gears to make pedaling
hard, producing a strain resembling that
of a hard run. This does not work your
heart and lungs effectively, except when
you are ascending a hill. Pedaling more
rapidly at all times—even while going
downhill—will help make your ride an
aerobic activity.

Is the workout challenging enough?
According to the "talk test," you should be
able to carry on a conversation during your
workout but have to time your words with
your breathing pattern. If you cannot talk,
then slow down a bit. But, if you do not
need a shower after your ride, you have
probably not challenged yourself enough.
(See also Basic Bicycling Safety, page 357.)

Weight Training

Weight training is about more than big
biceps. Lifting weights can increase muscle
size, but it also can tone and tighten muscles
and enhance overall conditioning. However,
weight training is of limited aerobic value,
even if you move rapidly from one exercise
to another.

Types of Weight Training

Olympic weight lifting and power lifting are
competitive sports in which the aim is to lift
the greatest amount of weight at a single
time. Bodybuilding is another category in
which participants use weights for conditioning, but the emphasis is on shaping or
"sculpting" and enlarging the muscles for
visual effect.

Weight (resistance) training, in contrast, is
not competitive. It involves lifting moderate
amounts of resistance several times for each
of a series of specific exercises.

Today, more people are likely to incorporate resistance training into their exercise
programs. At its simplest, resistance training
is an overall weight-training approach for the
purpose of conditioning muscles for other
sports.

Resistance training works on the principle
of overload. You exercise certain groups of
muscles, such as in the arms, legs, or chest, to
the point of mild fatigue. Then, after a recovery phase, you exercise them again,
gradually increasing the amount of weight
used (progressive resistance).

Designing Your Program

How much and how often should you lift?
Get advice from a qualified instructor—many
gyms and schools have qualified strength-
and-conditioning professionals. Such an
advisor can help you design a program that
meets your needs and is varied enough to
keep you interested.

The design of a weight-lifting program
depends on your goals. To build strength
quickly, lifting a weight that will exhaust you
after 6 lifts is appropriate; to enhance the size
and contour of your muscles, weight that
fatigues you after 8 to 12 lifts is best; for
endurance (such as for swimming or running), lifting a weight that creates muscle
fatigue after 15 to 20 times is best. It is best to
start with very conservative amounts of
resistance to minimize the risk of injury and
to learn the proper technique of lifting.

How Many Calories Does It Use Up?

Even when you are asleep, you require energy (calories) to fuel your heartbeat, breathing, and other body functions. When you move about slowly, you burn more calories. When you exercise, your expenditure of calories may increase dramatically.

The chart on this page shows the range of energy expended while performing various activities for 1 hour.

Remember that you may expend up to 100 calories just sitting quietly for 1 hour.

From the numbers in the table, it is obvious that calorie expenditure varies widely with different forms of exercise. You can indulge in an activity with a great intensity or with a low degree of intensity or any degree between. In addition, the trained athlete may perform a given activity with greater economy of motion and less expenditure of energy.

Walking at ordinary speeds is the exception. The amount of energy you use for walking depends only on body weight and distance covered. The heavier the person, the greater the calorie expenditure; the greater the distance covered, the greater the calorie expenditure. The athlete has no advantage over the rest of us.

It also is apparent that all forms of activity cost a lean person fewer calories than they cost a heavy person. This is the reason that middle- and long-distance runners strive to be as lean as possible. With less body weight, they need less oxygen and less fuel (calories) to cover the same distance.

Activity	Average Calories Expended in an Hour*	
	120-130 lb Person	170-180 lb Person
Aerobic dancing	290-575	400-800
Backpacking	290-630	400-880
Badminton	230-515	320-720
Basketball		
Game	400-690	560-960
Nongame	170-515	240-720
Bicycling		
Outdoor	170-800	240-1,120
Stationary	85-800	120-1,120
Bowling	115-170	160-240
Canoeing	170-460	240-640
Chopping wood	170-575	240-800
Dancing	115-400	160-560
Gardening	115-400	160-560
Golfing (walking, carrying or pulling bag)	115-400	160-560
Handball	460-690	640-960
Hiking	170-690	240-960
Jogging		
5 mph (12 min/mile)	460	640
6 mph (10 min/mile)	575	800
Racquetball	345-690	480-960
Rope skipping	345-690	480-960
Rowing	170-800	240-1,120
Running		
7 mph (9 min/mile)	690	960
8 mph (7.5 min/mile)	745	1,040
10 mph (6 min/mile)	860	1,200
Scuba diving	290-690	400-800
Skating, ice or roller	230-460	320-640
Skiing		
Cross-country	290-800	400-1,120
Downhill	170-460	240-640
Soccer	290-690	400-960
Squash	345-690	480-960
Stair climbing	230-460	320-640
Swimming	230-690	320-900
Table tennis	170-290	240-400
Tennis	230-515	320-720
Volleyball	170-400	240-560
Walking		
2 mph (30 min/mile)	150	210
3 mph (20 min/mile)	200	275
4 mph (15 min/mile)	250	340

*To adjust for your body weight, multiply calories by your weight (in pounds) and divide by 175.

Types of Weights

There are several varieties of weights that can be used for weight training:

Free Weights. These are what most people think of as traditional weight-lifting equipment. Free weights consist of dumbbells (weights held in one hand) and barbells (requiring a two-handed grip). You lift the weight and control its direction. These are inexpensive, suitable for home use, and effective, but their potential for injury should not be ignored. For safety, work with a training partner.

Machines. Machines can isolate a particular group of muscles and provide variable resistance. Some of these machines look very high-tech and intimidating, but in general they are easier and safer to use than free weights. Machines typically are found in health clubs, but they can be purchased for home use also. Given the expense, however, it makes sense to try weight lifting at a public gym and buy the machine later, after you know that weight training is for you.

Establishing Your Routine

An investment of time and energy is required to benefit from weight training. Typically, increases in strength are noticeable after 6 weeks of programmed lifting; improvement in muscle shape and size takes longer, perhaps 8 to 16 weeks.

Do not try to do it all at once. Using too much weight too soon can result in injury. For the same reasons, incorporate proper warm-up and cool-down periods into every workout.

Listen to what your body tells you: muscle aches are common after workouts, but lingering aches or burning sensations should not be. Take a day or two off; if the discomfort does not go away, consult your physician.

Some Cautions

If you have high blood pressure or heart disease, consult your physician before beginning a weight-training regimen. Lifting can cause your blood pressure to soar.

Be sure to use proper technique. Do not bounce the weight or bend and shift your body while lifting. Breathing correctly is important too—inflate your chest to support your spine during exertion. (A support belt also can be helpful.) Set a regular rhythm, breathing in before the lift, exhaling during the lift. Never hold your breath.

Avoiding Injury

Most injuries that occur during an athletic activity result from unusual demands on bones, muscles, or other tissues. The novice runner who struggles to complete 5 miles the first day on the track will experience aches and pains; the over-40 ex-jock who comes out of retirement for the company softball game is an excellent candidate for a sprain or some other painful injury.

An injury-free life is an unrealistic goal. But there are a few sensible rules to follow that will help you avoid inconvenient, painful, expensive, and, at times, disabling injuries.

Consult Your Physician

If you are older than 40, obese, or a heavy smoker, have had unexplained chest pains, heart problems such as a previous heart attack, irregular heart rhythms or other serious health problem, or lead a largely sedentary life, consult your physician before starting a vigorous exercise regimen. Your physician may suggest a stress test (see The Exercise Tolerance Test, page 655) to evaluate the condition of your heart and lungs and will offer valuable dos and don'ts specific to your physical condition.

Warm Up Before Exercising

To avoid injury, invest at least 3 to 5 minutes in stretching and loosening the muscles that will be used in your activity. Take the first 5 minutes of the particular activity at a modest pace. The increased blood flow of such a warm-up will decrease tension in your muscles, improve their range of motion, and even may improve your performance. Simultaneously, you are significantly decreasing the chance of muscle pulls, strains, and other injuries.

Cool Down After Exercising

After your workout, allow your muscles to cool down. Muscles that have carried you through a workout have contracted, and a session of stretching is critical. Muscles that are not properly stretched are more likely to sustain pulls, strains, and spasms.

Pace Yourself

Sudden and unfamiliar exertion is most likely to cause injuries. If you are bent on improving your performance, do so, but at a sensible pace. Do not double your distance or your duration overnight. Develop a program that allows your body to become conditioned to the activity so that it adjusts over time to the challenges you offer it.

Select the Right Sport for You

If you have back problems or perpetually sore knees, the pounding of jogging is not for you; perhaps a daily swim or riding on a stationary cycle more nearly suits your needs.

Make It a Habit

Working out only once a week, no matter how vigorous the activity, puts you at risk of injury (and fails to provide you with maximal aerobic and conditioning benefits; see Benefits of Exercise, page 290). Try to establish a schedule of a minimum of three 20-minute workouts a week.

Take Care of That Injury

If you sprain an ankle or twist a knee, make sure you get medical advice and then follow it. A key element is almost sure to be what physicians commonly refer to as the "tincture of time." Allow the injury to heal before testing it too vigorously (see Principles of Sports Rehabilitation, page 875).

Take Care of Your Back

Many athletic activities put your back at risk for injury. If a sneeze can produce a twinge of back pain in some people, then lifting weights surely can. Reportedly, four of five Americans complain of back pain at least once in their lives.

As you go about your daily activities and, in particular, if you start a new exercise regimen, it is an excellent idea to keep some commonsense strategies in mind to avoid back discomfort.

Maintain Good Posture
Whether you are walking to the bathroom to brush your teeth or running a marathon, good posture is important. Keep your backbone straight. Hold your shoulders back. Pull in your stomach and buttocks. Trim your profile. Pull in your chin.

Lifting
Whether the object to be picked up is a newspaper or a 100-pound barbell, squat down with your back straight and let your legs do the lifting. Bring tension on your muscles gradually: never jerk or lunge to lift the load.

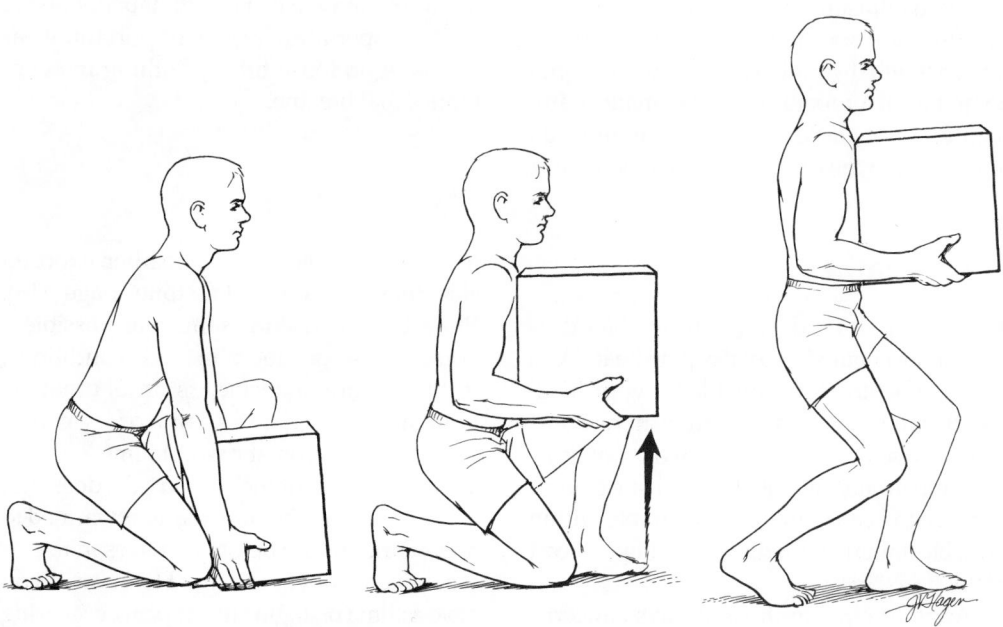

When lifting any object, let your legs do the work. Bend your knees rather than your back. Hold the object close to your body and lift gently. Avoid jerking or lunging upward.

Exercise

If you have had back problems, remember that sports involving sudden jerking motions (stops and starts, twists and turns) put your back at increased risk of stress and strain. Falls and collisions also can endanger the health of your back. Perhaps you should retire from the Saturday afternoon touch-football game and take up swimming, bicycling, walking, or jogging instead.

If the muscles of your back are poorly toned, your chance of injury also is increased. Exercises can be done to stretch and strengthen your back muscles (see a physical medicine specialist for instructions).

Sleeping

Lying down provides relief for backache and also an opportunity for backache prevention. Do not sleep on your stomach unless your abdomen is cushioned by a pillow; sleep on your side with your legs drawn up slightly toward your chest. Pick a firm mattress, one that provides your back with proper support. If the mattress is too soft or sags, place a board of ½-inch plywood between your mattress and springs.

Avoid Stiffness

If you are seated at a desk, standing in one position, or behind the wheel of a car for hours every day, you are at risk of stiffness and muscle fatigue. Make it a point to break the routine at frequent intervals. When standing, shift your weight from one foot to the other periodically; when sitting, get up, even for a few seconds, as often as possible. Take frequent breaks when driving and get out and stretch. A small pillow at the base of your back also can help to support your spine.

Weight Loss

One frequent cause of backache in the United States is being overweight. The extra pounds at your waistline put additional strains and stresses on your back. An appropriate program of weight loss and exercise may help you avoid back pain.

Exercise in the Heat and Cold

The environment in which you work out has a significant effect on your exercise. Extremes of heat or cold and high altitude may require that you adjust not only your attire but also the duration and intensity of your exercise. Listen to what your body advises you about extremes of temperature and climate: maintain your schedule of workouts if you can, but adjust to the conditions when necessary.

Hot Weather

On warm, humid days, more blood is directed to your skin to dissipate heat. As a result, less blood is available for your muscles than on cool days, so your heart rate during exercise will be higher than on cool days. To compensate, decrease the intensity of your exercise to keep your target heart rate within sensible limits (see Finding Your Target Heart Rate, page 296).

Another strategy for hot days concerns scheduling: try exercising indoors or work out during a cooler time of day (morning or evening). Make sure you drink water before and after exercise in warm, humid weather. If you exercise for more than 30 minutes, stop and drink water every 15 to 20 minutes during the exercise (see Heat Exhaustion, page 415). Proper attire also is important: wear lightweight, loose-fitting clothing made of fabrics that breathe.

Cold Weather

In extremely cold, windy weather, exposed skin may freeze (see Frostbite, page 416). Protect exposed skin as much as possible if you exercise outdoors in such conditions; using an indoor facility is an alternative. Walking or jogging in snowy or icy conditions also puts you at risk of falling.

Breathing extremely cold air does not injure your lungs because the air is warmed to body temperature before it arrives in the air sacs (alveoli) of your lungs. However, if you have asthma or angina (heart pain), exercising in cold weather may worsen these symptoms. Try wearing a soft scarf or a cold-air mask over your mouth and nose in extremely cold or windy conditions. You can purchase a cold-air mask at your local drugstore or pharmacy. Also, breathe through your nose because your nose warms, filters, and humidifies the air before it enters your lungs.

When you exercise outdoors, dress for the conditions. Dressing in layers is the best strategy in the cold. This provides added insulation, and you can add or shed layers as appropriate to warm up and cool down. Thick, absorbent socks are important, especially for runners and walkers. A windbreaker will help protect you against excessive heat loss in a strong wind. If you exercise outdoors in the dark, wear reflective material on your clothes, and try to stay in well-lighted areas where traffic is limited.

Exercising at High Altitudes

If you travel to an altitude much higher than that to which you are accustomed, you may experience a decrease in performance during endurance exercise. Less oxygen is available for the blood to transport at high altitudes, but do not allow that to deter you from exercise unless you experience symptoms of acute mountain sickness.

Acute mountain sickness is caused by a shortage of oxygen in the blood (hypoxia) and usually has symptoms such as headache, breathlessness on mild exertion, fatigue, nausea, vomiting, and disturbed sleep. It is much more likely to occur at high elevations (8,000 feet or more) and in people who have ascended rapidly.

Getting Motivated

Motivation is a matter of "skill power." The good news is that anyone can master the skills necessary to break down barriers to regular exercise. A few common barriers and solutions are given here:

1. You're not sure what you can gain from exercise. Talk with your physician about specific goals for your blood pressure, weight, and cholesterol and triglyceride levels.

2. You're afraid of overexerting. Get a baseline health evaluation from your physician.

3. You have trouble allotting time for exercise. Set aside time blocks on your personal calendar for exercise.

4. You argue with yourself about crawling out of a warm bed in the morning for a walk. If you deliberate, you'll probably sleep in. Put your exercise clothes and shoes near the foot of your bed and avoid deliberating.

5. You don't feel like making a long-term commitment to exercise. Take it a week at a time. Select activities you enjoy.

6. You don't have the willpower. Exercise with a friend who is motivated and can help keep you motivated.

7. You really don't see any improvement. Keep track of your progress by logging measures such as time, distance, weight, or feelings of exertion.

Staying Active

The intense workout programs touted for the past 2 decades may have left you with an "all-or-nothing" attitude toward exercise. Recently, experts convened by the Centers for Disease Control and Prevention and the American College of Sports Medicine created new guidelines for exercise. The guides put hope for a healthy body within reach of almost everyone as the emphasis shifts from becoming an athlete to just being active.

Their recommendations center on one idea: choose moderate-intensity activities that burn at least 200 calories daily. If you'd rather count minutes than calories, that translates into about 30 minutes, depending on your weight and the type of activity you choose (see How Many Calories Does It Use Up? page 301).

The best news for busy people is that you can accumulate your activities throughout the day. Ride your bike to the newsstand and back in the morning. Spend a few minutes hoeing your flower bed in preparation for spring planting. Take a brisk walk with your dog after dinner.

Of course, not all daily activities count. Playing croquet or ironing doesn't burn enough calories.

In "moderate activity," you should burn 4 to 7 calories a minute—comparable to the effort you exert during a brisk walk.

Don't Toss Your Tennis Shoes

Do the new recommendations mean you should give up your aerobics dance class or cut back on cross-country skiing? Definitely not.

The emphasis on regular moderate activity is meant to complement—not replace—previous advice to exercise for 20 continuous minutes in higher-intensity activities at least three times a week.

There's nothing wrong with the old recommendations, except that few people follow them.

Only 22 percent of American adults are active enough to meet or exceed the level recommended in the new guidelines. About 54 percent are active but not active enough to meet the guidelines, and 24 percent are sedentary and never exercise. The new guidelines are designed to encourage the people who are not active enough, or are not active at all, to get the health benefits of moderate activity.

Does It Really Help?

If you're striving to build up your muscles or train for sports activity, a program of moderate activity probably isn't enough. Stay with a program based on 20 or 30 continuous minutes of more vigorous exercise.

But if you want to reduce the risk of cardiovascular disease or osteoporosis, enjoy better mental health, and improve your balance, coordination, and agility, the moderate-activity guidelines are for you.

You can have all these health benefits by starting a lifestyle of moderate activity. Remember, it's the total amount of activity, not great exhibits of endurance, that counts.

Chapter 11

Controlling Stress

Contents

Keeping Your Stress Under Control, 308
The "Fight-or-Flight" Response, 308

Recognizing Stress, 309

Dealing With Stress, 309
Interpersonal Conflicts, 310

Methods of Coping With Stress, 311
Keep Things in Perspective, 311
Seek Help If You Cannot Cope, 312
Techniques for Managing Stress, 312
Does How You Think, Feel, and Act Aggravate
Your Medical Problems? 312

Keeping Your Stress Under Control

Most of us know something about stress—the term has become common in our society. In addition, nearly everyone experiences stress on a day-to-day basis.

Stress is an individualized, personal response to situations and circumstances that create pressures. It is a normal and perhaps necessary part of our lives.

Stress is not an outside force; rather, it is our physiologic response to specific stimuli or "stressors." These responses mobilize bodily systems so that they can help us adapt to the constant demands and changes of our lives. For example, athletes frequently perform best in competition rather than in practice. Many people find that goals and deadlines are stimulating and necessary for accomplishment.

Sometimes stress responses may be so mild that they go virtually unnoticed. At other times, they can seem to be an overwhelming burden. One of the greatest current stressors may be the feeling that we should not have the discomfort associated with increased stress. When this discomfort happens, some of us may assume that we are not coping well or that this is a sign of illness.

The assumption that we should feel good all the time, no matter what changes or problems we are facing, can add to the pressures we already feel.

There are two basic types of stressful events. One is intense, an alarm reaction that readies your body for an emergency. The other is less intense and alerts your body to meet a long-term problem that calls for endurance.

In instances when the stimulus is intense, as in a perceived threat, a phenomenon referred to as "fight or flight" occurs. The physical signs of this stress response are almost always conspicuous and may include an increased heart rate, muscle tension, or perspiration.

The effects of stress are not always instantaneous or fleeting. In many people the impact can be deferred for weeks or months. As a result, many illnesses are thought to be affected by accumulated stress, whether the illness has been either brought on or worsened by stress. Simply stated, stress produces or worsens symptoms when demands outweigh personal resources to cope with them.

The "Fight-or-Flight" Response

Since the "fight-or-flight" phenomenon was first described nearly 50 years ago, we have learned much about how the body produces chemicals in preparation for a fight-or-flight response.

Your pituitary, a gland attached to the base of your brain, secretes hormones that regulate many body processes. When you perceive a danger, your pituitary secretes a hormone called adrenocorticotropic hormone (ACTH), which causes your adrenal gland to release other hormones. These hormones—adrenaline (epinephrine) and cortisol—immediately cause your pulse to quicken, your muscles to tense, and your blood pressure to increase. Your body is made ready to fight or flee (see Your Endocrine System at Work, page 924).

The change in blood flow is produced by adrenaline (epinephrine). During an emergency, you need more blood in your large muscles, so your heart beats faster and your blood pressure increases abruptly. Also, blood is directed away from your stomach and skin. Your body releases potential sources of energy into your bloodstream in the form of blood sugars and fat. Your body even secretes certain chemicals that make it easier for your blood to clot in case of an injury.

Your nervous system also is brought into action so that the pupils of your eyes dilate (to permit better vision), your facial muscles become tense (possibly to look more menacing), perspiration increases (to keep your body cool), and respiration accelerates (to increase available oxygen in your blood). All of these changes prepare your body for an emergency, real or imagined.

Recognizing Stress

Many of us are not very good at recognizing the emotional reactions we have and consequently find that first we notice the physical responses to stress.

Stress can produce such symptoms as headache, insomnia, upset stomach, or digestive changes. You may feel physical symptoms or emotional fatigue as the first clues of increased stress. An old nervous habit such as nail-biting may reappear. Because you may not recognize that you are under increased stress, you may interpret the symptoms as those of an illness rather than the manifestation of an adjustment or adaptation process.

The thought that you may have an illness can be frightening and can add to the emotional burden you already have.

The stress experience also may become apparent through psychological changes. The most common change is increased irritability with people who are close to you. You also may feel more cynical, pessimistic, or resentful than usual. Many people report a sense of being victimized, misunderstood, or unappreciated. You may find that things to which you normally look forward seem burdensome. Some people become anxious or reclusive or prone to crying or laughing or to inappropriate aggressive behavior. Occasionally, these changes are so gradual that you or others around you may not recognize them until your health or relationships change.

As with the physical symptoms described earlier, you may not recognize such emotional changes for what they really are—signals of increased stress. Many people find themselves perplexed by the changes and often feel guilty or prone to blaming others. The term "burnout" often is used to describe a combination of physical and psychological responses to stress.

Dealing With Stress

In the course of daily events, we develop various ways of dealing with stressors. We work hard to decrease the newness of the changes we face, we talk about the experience, and we use things that we can count on already in our lives as "safe havens" from the new or adaptive changes.

Much of this we do without really thinking about it. However, some of these changes are monumental, such as switching jobs or moving to another part of the country. Others are routine, such as turning in a report, taking a test, meeting a new client, interviewing a baby-sitter, meeting a new teacher, or dealing with a child's temper tantrum. Mostly, we do pretty well in getting through fairly major as well as minor crises. Sometimes, we could do better.

The first step in learning to manage our stress-related reactions better is to become more aware of the things that may be particularly stressful for us individually. Not everyone responds to the same life event with the same amount of distress. For instance, a so-called workaholic may be thought by others to be working into an early grave, but he or she may have found that taking on extra challenges in a work-related environment helps him or her to feel more in control. For this person, the work itself may be a form of stress management, and unstructured time of a vacation without goals or "relaxation" at home may be a much greater stress.

We must learn to recognize in ourselves those things that cause the most stress. We may not be able to avoid them, but, when we encounter them, it may reassure us to know they are the source of our extra discomfort. Just recognizing such elements helps to make us feel more in control. Understanding the real cause of discomfort also can minimize anxiety about the manifestations of stress we experience.

As a part of our overall strategy to manage stress in our lives, most of us must become more self-tolerant. We need to understand

and accept that we constantly have to adapt to changes, losses, and events in our lives over which we have, at best, only partial control.

Most of us tend to be a great deal more understanding of other people's distress than we are of our own. We tend to think that we should always feel all right. As long as we believe this, we are sure to be disappointed. Accepting the fact that we may experience stress-related discomforts and that they are normal is helpful in managing stress.

Another important step involves actually dealing with the stress. Most of us want to do something when we are distressed so that

we can feel as if we are making an active choice to reassume control in our lives—the very thing we feel we have lost to some degree in facing life's challenges. What we do is largely determined by a method most easily called "trial and success."

Over the years, most of us have found techniques that help us feel more comfortable. These vary from person to person and from personality to personality, so there is no way to provide a list of things everyone should do.

Each person needs several tools, or techniques, at his or her disposal. Some of the tools may include learning and using specific

Interpersonal Conflicts

Difficulties in coping are not always a matter of the individual and his or her circumstances. Often, life's hurdles include dealing with personality conflicts with others. Typically, such conflicts are of three kinds: family, marital, or job-related.

Family Conflicts

All families are a complex network of relationships. Each member has a different relationship with each of the others in the family. These differences may be a reflection of age, birth order, sex, or personality type, or a combination of several factors. Each of these relationships, in turn, affects the rest of the family.

Physicians often recommend family therapy—in which the client is the entire family unit and the sessions include the whole family—when more than one member seems to have serious emotional problems, when a pattern of blame has become entrenched, or when an adolescent is particularly rebellious.

Often, problems within a family may be brought to the attention of a professional therapist when one member is showing signs of a problem—for example, trouble in school, substance abuse, or inappropriate sexual behavior.

Through family therapy, each member can discover his or her role in the problem.

There may be a pattern of behavior that everyone is contributing to and that everyone needs to help change. Rather than focusing on the gripes of individual family members, the therapist will identify specific problems in communication that all can work on. The therapist does not solve problems for the family but shows families how to understand their problems and how to cope with them more effectively.

Marital Conflicts

Marriage counselors frequently observe that one of the greatest problems in the couples they treat is that partners often enter into the relationship with unrealistic expectations. Our culture's romantic view of marriage fosters this tendency. Instead of realizing that they are marrying ordinary human beings with strengths and weaknesses, people tend to idealize their mates and expect nothing short of perfection.

Over the life of a marriage, couples typically face a predictable series of transitions. Consequently,

researchers often speak of "different marriages" within a single marriage. Adjustments to the first child and subsequent children, changes in jobs, loss of a spouse's parents, and changing sexual needs all present challenges. If the marriage is to survive, the couple must communicate and resolve inevitable conflicts effectively.

At a time of conflict in a marriage, a marriage counselor often can help bring such issues to light so that the couple can begin to deal with current problems in a more mature way.

Job-Related Conflicts

Interpersonal conflicts in the workplace can represent a multitude of issues. Competition between co-workers may reflect a genuine lack of the potential for upward mobility; there may simply be too many candidates for promotion. Conflict also can stem from downsizing or from an individual's desire for power and control. Problems often result from a lack of proper communication between co-workers and between management and employees.

If conflicts prove to be a continuing problem, seek counseling.

relaxation techniques—meditation, exercise, hobbies, and such. Others may require interaction with people to decrease the sense of social isolation that they may feel. They may include group sports or hobbies, attending social events, meeting with a group of friends or talking with a particularly valued friend. Finally, more specific treatment by a skilled professional may be necessary. Discuss this with your physician.

Be particularly careful about using drugs, either prescribed or recreational, as a management technique. The so-called happy hour, which many people use as a way to release tensions from their work, functions as a stress reliever for some, not because of the alcohol consumed but rather because of the social setting. The happy hour works because the person has made a choice to be in a setting with friends and with few work expectations.

Drugs, whether tranquilizers, alcohol, or so-called street (recreational) drugs, may increase symptoms of loss of control, depression, and emotional or behavioral impulsiveness. Conscious or regular use of drugs to manage stress can be a manifestation of problems with the substances (for more information about alcohol and substance abuse, see pages 325 and 335).

In summary, experiencing stress is an ongoing and normal part of living. We are constantly called on to adapt to changes within ourselves (such as aging or health problems) or in our surroundings (such as a new job, family structure, or social relationships). The reactions to these stressors may be physical or psychological and usually are unpleasant. The fact that they may be unpleasant does not mean that they are abnormal or that they constitute illness.

You can minimize the effects of stress by learning to recognize when you are experiencing it, by acknowledging and accepting it, and by choosing or learning to use methods for managing it. Some of these tools for managing stress include both physical and psychological approaches using individual and interpersonal skills and techniques.

A caution: Physical or psychological symptoms that affect your ability to work, to play, or to find pleasure in life or hope for the future are unlikely to be merely due to stress. Consult your physician for further evaluation. Stress-management techniques alone are unlikely to provide relief.

Methods of Coping With Stress

Events that cause stress will always be with us. We can do many things to lessen the effects of stress and to relieve the discomfort it causes, but some stress is inevitable. Accept situations that cannot be changed. But remember—you can make acceptance easier. Here are some suggestions to help you.

Keep Things in Perspective

Most of us tend to worry about things over which we have no control. For instance, how many times have you worried about whether the weather will be pleasant for a special event, such as a wedding? Clearly, there is nothing you can do about it except to prepare for the possibility of inclement weather.

When faced with worries and fears, try to look beyond the specific event. Ask yourself a few questions, such as:

What is the worst thing that can happen?

How likely is it that the worst will happen?

Have I done everything I realistically can to influence the outcome of the situation?

Will the outcome change my life substantially, and will I even remember it several years from now?

How would I counsel a friend in a similar situation?

Try giving yourself a little pep talk of reassurance. Do not let feelings of defeat, fear, or disappointment overtake you. The more positively you can approach the situation, the more likely it is that you will be able to face and influence the outcome.

Seek Help If You Cannot Cope

You do not need to handle all of your problems alone. Sometimes the help of a counselor, psychiatrist, psychologist, clergyperson, or friend may be just what you need to help you handle stress. Many people believe that seeking outside help is a sign of weakness, which adds to their sense of despair, hopelessness, or anger. Nothing could be further from the truth. It takes strength to realize that you need help. Ask your physician, local community health organization, or employer for recommendations if you need help in finding appropriate assistance.

Techniques for Managing Stress

Even if you cannot always identify causes of stress, you can relieve some of the discomfort. Just feeling that you can do something often is a help in itself.

Relaxation Techniques

Many of us think of relaxation as simply not working. We tend to think that watching television with our feet up or reading a book or the newspaper is relaxing. Such activities may or may not be. If your teeth are clenched or your muscles tense as you follow the action, or if you relive the irritations and problems of the day while paying only partial attention, you are anything but relaxed. Relaxing involves skills you can learn.

Relaxation techniques can help lessen the discomfort and duration of symptoms of stress such as headaches, anxiety, high blood pressure, trouble falling asleep, Raynaud's syndrome (see page 697) or other causes of cool or cold hands, hyperventilation, and clenching or grinding of teeth, to name a few.

One simple method of relaxation is to remove yourself from the stressful situation. Block the world out and concentrate on your body. Here is how:

1. Sit or lie in a comfortable position and close your eyes. Allow your jaw to drop and your eyelids to be relaxed and heavy but not tightly closed.

2. Mentally scan your body, starting with your toes and working slowly up through your legs, buttocks, torso, arms, hands, fingers, neck, and head. Focus on each part individually. Where you feel tension, imagine it melting away.

3. Tighten the muscles in one area of your body and hold them for a count of 5 or more before relaxing and moving on to the next area. This is a good method for releasing tension. Tighten the muscles of your face, shoulders, arms, legs, and buttocks.

4. Allow thoughts to flow through your mind, but do not focus on any of them. Many people find using autosuggestion to be a great help: suggest to yourself that you are relaxed and calm, that your hands are warm (or cool if you are hot) and heavy, that your heart is beating calmly, or that you feel perfectly at peace.

5. Breathe slowly, regularly, and deeply during the procedure.

6. Once you are relaxed, imagine you are in a favorite place or in a spot of great beauty and stillness.

7. After 5 or 10 minutes, rouse yourself from the state gradually.

Does How You Think, Feel, and Act Aggravate Your Medical Problems?

If you have a medical problem or illness, it certainly can affect the way you think, feel, and act. However, how you think, feel, and act can in turn affect your medical condition. If stress, psychological, or social factors are a part of your illness, your doctor may refer you to a specialist in behavioral medicine. This specialist can help you better understand how such factors affect your illness as well as gain control over your symptoms. Such help often contributes to the successful treatment or management of an illness.

People who have the following medical problems are often referred to a behavioral specialist: high blood pressure, chronic pain, habit problems or tic disorders, headaches, insomnia, irritable bowel syndrome, obesity, Raynaud's phenomenon, sexual dysfunction, infertility problems, or trouble following a medical treatment plan.

Referral to a behavioral specialist rarely means you have a mental illness. However, if your doctor diagnoses a mental illness, he or she may recommend that you visit with a psychiatrist for more treatment options. If you are already seeing a psychiatrist, you may still see a behavior specialist to supplement your treatment.

Relaxed Breathing

Make relaxed breathing a part of your total relaxation program. This type of breathing can be helpful because of its quick, calming effect.

Different methods of breathing involve moving different regions of your torso. Most adults breathe by expanding and contracting their chests (chest breathing). Some lift their shoulders in an attempt to fill their lungs (shoulder breathing). Infants and children, however, usually breathe from the diaphragm, the dome-shaped muscle that separates the chest cavity from the abdominal cavity. This diaphragmatic breathing provides a more efficient exchange of oxygen and carbon dioxide than chest or especially shoulder breathing. Diaphragmatic breathing also takes less effort.

With relaxed diaphragmatic breathing, your shoulders do not move up and your chest does not move out noticeably. Air flows smoothly into and out of your lungs rather than being drawn in and blown out forcefully. Your abdomen rises with each inhalation and lowers with each exhalation. The overall effect is relaxing to your entire body.

With practice, you can breathe in a deep and relaxing manner as a matter of course. At first, practice lying on your back while wearing clothing that is loose around your waist and abdomen. Once you can breathe easily in this position, practice while sitting and then while standing. After a while you will be able to breathe from your diaphragm whenever and wherever you wish.

1. Lie on your back on a bed, a well-padded floor, or a recliner chair.

2. Place your feet slightly apart. Rest one hand comfortably on your abdomen near your navel. Place the other hand on your chest.

3. Inhale through your nose because this allows the air to be filtered and warmed. Exhale through your mouth. If you have trouble breathing through your nose, inhale through your mouth.

4. Concentrate on your breathing for a few minutes and become aware of which hand is rising and falling with each breath.

5. Gently exhale most of the air in your lungs.

6. Inhale while slowly counting to 4, about 1 second per count. As you inhale gently, slightly distend your abdomen, causing it to rise about 1 inch. (You should be able to feel the movement with your hand.) Remember, do not pull your shoulders up or move your chest.

7. As you breathe in, imagine the warm air flowing in. Imagine this warmth flowing to all parts of your body.

8. Pause 1 second after inhaling.

9. Slowly exhale to the count of 4. While you are exhaling, your abdomen will slowly fall as your diaphragm relaxes upward against your lungs.

10. As air flows out, imagine that tension is also flowing out.

11. Pause 1 second after exhaling.

12. If it is difficult to inhale and exhale to a count of 4, shorten the count slightly and later work up to 4. If you experience light-headedness, alter the length or depth of your breathing.

13. Repeat the slow inhaling, pausing, slow exhaling, and pausing 5 to 10 times. Exhale. Inhale slowly: 1, 2, 3, 4. Pause. Exhale slowly: 1, 2, 3, 4. Pause. Inhale: 1, 2, 3, 4. Pause. Exhale: 1, 2, 3, 4. Pause. Continue on your own.

As you practice you may notice that initially not every breath will reach the lower parts of your lungs. This will improve with practice. The idea is to concentrate on slow, even, easy breathing.

If it seems difficult to make your breathing regular, take a slightly deeper breath, hold it for a second or two, and then let it out slowly through pursed lips for about 10 seconds. Repeat this once or twice and return to the other procedure.

Physical Exercise

Another method for coping with stress is physical activity. If you are physically fit, your body can handle stress better, both physically and emotionally.

Exercise also has a calming effect that lasts well after you finish your workout. Activities such as running and swimming, which require repetitive movements, can produce a mental state similar to that of meditation. Aerobic exercise that increases your heart rate for at least 20 minutes is good for cardiovascular fitness (see page 645) and also may decrease feelings of stress. Yoga and other nonaerobic stretching exercises are calming and produce a meditation-like state.

Almost any exercise can be good for you. Jogging, swimming, aerobic exercises, and brisk walking all may help to relieve symptoms of stress. Stretching can relieve tension in certain muscles or all over, and it can be done at almost any time.

Dealing With Tension

Tension is common in the shoulders and neck. To relieve it, roll your shoulders, raising them toward your ears. Then relax your shoulders.

To reduce neck tension, move your head gently in a circle going clockwise and then counterclockwise.

Relieve tension in your torso by reaching toward the ceiling and doing side bends.

To help relieve foot and leg tension, draw circles in the air with your feet while flexing your toes.

To help ease muscular tension throughout your body, stand up and stretch all over.

Chapter 12

Tobacco

Contents

Why Smokers Smoke, 316
How Addictive Is Nicotine? 316

How Hazardous Is Smoking? 317
Common Health Effects, 317
Tobacco Advertising and Your Health, 317
Lesser-Known Health Effects, 318
Smoking and Skin Wrinkles, 318
Low-Tar, Low-Nicotine Cigarettes, 318
Chewing Tobacco, 319

Teenage Smoking, 320
Secondhand Smoke, 320
Smoking and Pregnancy, 320

How to Stop Smoking, 321
Methods of Stopping, 321
If You Light One Up, You Don't Have to
Smoke It, 322
Problems of Stopping, 323
Benefits of Stopping, 324

Why Smokers Smoke

The health care costs of tobacco use in the United States are staggering. It is estimated that the costs of smoking in the United States annually exceed $100 billion for health care expenditures for tobacco-related diseases and lost productivity of workers. Each year, smoking kills more than 400,000 Americans, more than died in battle in World War II and the Vietnam War combined.

The indirect costs of smoking are equally astonishing. Each year, fires started by cigarettes cause more than $400 million in property damage. Higher insurance premiums and taxes needed to fund disability benefits for people who are ill as a result of cigarette smoking are part of the cost also.

Warnings about the hazards of smoking have had an effect on smokers. Today, more than 40 million Americans identify themselves as former smokers. The number of men who smoke has declined substantially, from one-half of the adult men in 1965 to less than one-third today; among women, it has declined slightly but is now very close to the rate of smoking in men.

Yet, in the face of the well-known dangers of cigarette smoking, an estimated 25 percent of the 50 million people over the age of 20 who smoke are still unaware of or do not accept the health risks of their smoking, while 70 percent realize that cigarette smoking is addictive.

Very few people restrict their smoking to a few cigarettes a day. Fifty million American smokers consume 80 million packs of cigarettes each day.

Because tobacco use is legal and for the most part is still socially acceptable in this country, education about the perils of smoking may be the most effective way of providing reasons either to stop or to never start smoking. The following pages explain many of the health hazards of smoking and some of the methods for quitting.

The medical evidence is clear: smoking cigarettes, pipes, or cigars, or using smokeless tobacco, endangers your health. Even the infrequent use of tobacco is unhealthy.

The reasons people start smoking or refuse to quit are rarely simple. Some smokers report that their cigarettes offer them a surge of energy, especially to wake them up in the morning or keep them awake at other times (for example, while driving). Nicotine acts as a stimulant with an adrenaline-like effect. It increases your heart rate and blood pressure while you are smoking.

Some smokers report that when they are under tension, their cigarettes act to calm them. The cigarette gives them something to do with their hands if they are nervous and provides a mild form of distraction or even a feeling of security.

The nicotine in tobacco is an addictive drug. Nicotine can provoke an addictive response in regular smokers that can be relieved only by using tobacco. The degree of addiction depends to some degree on how much and how long the smoker has smoked.

The addiction most smokers experience may be both psychological and physical. For some, the regular use of cigarettes in many life situations may have persuaded them that they could not cope with life without smoking.

How Addictive Is Nicotine?

Nicotine can be as addictive as alcohol or cocaine. You may be dependent if you have regularly used tobacco and experience one or more of the following characteristics:

- You have made a serious but unsuccessful attempt to quit or reduce the amount you use.
- Your attempts to stop have led to physical withdrawal symptoms, such as craving for tobacco, anxiety, irritability, restlessness, difficulty in concentrating, headaches, drowsiness, and stomach upset.
- You continue to use tobacco even when you have a serious physical problem, such as heart or lung disease, that you know is worsened by tobacco.
- You develop a "tolerance" to tobacco. For example, your first few cigarettes may leave you feeling nauseated or light-headed. After smoking a short while, these effects generally subside, but you may notice a certain number of cigarettes daily produce less effect and that you need to increase the number you smoke to achieve a desired sensation.

The central element of addiction is loss of control. The substance controls your behavior by producing temporary alterations in your mood when it is not in your system. You may want to quit but you can't, even when you know nicotine is harmful to your health.

How Hazardous Is Smoking?

Smoking is the single largest preventable cause of premature death and disability in this country. One in five deaths in the United States each year is associated with cigarette smoking. The American Lung Association states that smoking kills more Americans each year than cocaine, heroin, alcohol abuse, auto accidents, homicide, AIDS, and suicide combined.

Although more than 400,000 Americans annually die prematurely from the effects of smoking, millions more live with damaged lungs and hearts. Cigarette smoking accounts for the vast majority of deaths from lung cancer and from chronic obstructive pulmonary disease (see Emphysema, page 715, and Chronic Bronchitis, page 714). For years, lung cancer has been the number 1 cause of cancer death in men; lung cancer has now surpassed breast cancer as the leading cancer killer of women, too.

Smoking contributes substantially to the development of atherosclerosis, which affects the heart and peripheral blood vessels (see Atherosclerosis: What Is It? page 636). Smoking is also implicated as a cause of or is associated with other diseases and types of cancer including cancer of the mouth, throat (pharynx), voice box (larynx), esophagus, urinary bladder, kidney, pancreas, stomach, and cervix.

Common Health Effects

Cigarette smoke contains more than 4,000 chemicals, including trace amounts of such known poisons as cyanide, arsenic, and formaldehyde. There are 43 known cancer-causing chemicals (carcinogens) in tobacco smoke. Carbon monoxide in cigarette smoke displaces oxygen from your red blood cells, thereby robbing your tissues of oxygen.

The delicate tissues of the mouth, throat, and voice box are exposed repetitively to the effects of cigarette smoke. The cancer-causing agents of tobacco smoke are directly responsible for most cancers of the mouth, pharynx, and larynx seen in this country. The profile of someone with oral cancer is a man older than 50 who has been a heavy cigarette smoker most of his life. Pipe and cigar smokers run the same risks of oral and laryn-geal cancer; use of chewing tobacco is linked primarily to cancers of the lip and mouth.

After the smoke passes through your mouth, your lungs retain 70 to 90 percent of the compounds you inhale. A few puffs on a cigarette reduce the effectiveness of the cilia inside your bronchial tubes. Cilia are tiny, hairlike bodies that normally work like brooms to sweep foreign particles out of your lungs. Smoking just one cigarette can slow the sweeping action of the cilia. Regular smoking virtually paralyzes the cilia, leaving your lungs exposed to billions of tiny particles from cigarette smoke. With the cilia largely inactive, tar from the cigarette smoke begins to build up and damage delicate lung tissues. When cooled inside your lungs, the tar forms a brown, sticky layer on the lining of breathing passages. This layer contains the tar and other chemicals that can cause cancer (see Lung Cancer, page 724).

The link between smoking and lung cancer is inescapable. At the turn of the century, lung cancer was relatively rare. But with the widespread practice of cigarette smoking among men after World War I, and then among women 30 years later, lung cancer has become the most common cause of cancer

Tobacco Advertising and Your Health

Cigarettes are the most heavily marketed consumer product in America, with the tobacco industry spending more than 4½ billion dollars a year on advertising and promotion.

Many advertisements show smoking as part of physical, outdoor activities such as backpacking, jogging, and boating. Tobacco companies also sponsor events of high visibility with major crowds of young people, such as rock concerts, automobile and horse racing, and athletic events. In recent years, advertising efforts have been more targeted toward women, minorities, and youth.

To counteract the educational efforts of the medical community, the tobacco industry through its public relations efforts, opinion surveys, and lobbyists persistently challenges the relationship between cigarettes and disease and claims that nicotine is not addictive. Even though the tobacco manufacturers claim that their advertising is meant only to establish brand loyalty among existing smokers, the extravagantly expensive advertising, promotional, and political campaigns of the industry are considered a significant influence on the many young people who start and continue to smoke.

death in this country. The risk of having lung cancer is approximately 10 times greater for cigarette smokers than for nonsmokers. Pipe and cigar smokers as a group have a somewhat smaller risk for developing lung and bladder cancer, probably because they generally do not inhale the smoke as deeply.

Various studies and reports issued by the Surgeon General of the United States clearly document that cigarette smoking is also the major cause of chronic lung diseases such as chronic bronchitis (see Chronic Bronchitis, page 714) and emphysema (see Emphysema, page 715). In addition to paralyzing or destroying the cilia in your lungs, the smoke irrevocably damages or destroys the alveoli, the tiny air sacs in your lungs in which carbon dioxide is exchanged for oxygen. When these air sacs are injured to a critical extent, your body is unable to transport adequate levels of oxygen to your vital organs and, eventually, the chronic bronchitis or emphysema becomes fatal.

Lesser-Known Health Effects

It is well known that smoking is the leading cause of lung cancer and chronic lung diseases. Yet, the single most important health effect of smoking may be in the development of heart attacks: cigarette smoking is the suspected cause of approximately one-fourth of deaths from coronary artery disease. There are many different chemicals and substances in tobacco smoke that injure the cardiovascular system.

The nicotine in tobacco smoke acts on your adrenal glands, causing them to secrete hormones that temporarily increase your blood pressure and your heart rate, which makes your heart work harder. Tobacco smoke also contains carbon monoxide. When inhaled, the carbon monoxide binds to the hemoglobin, taking the place of valuable oxygen. Thus, smoking decreases the amount of oxygen available to your heart.

The result is that every cigarette places a small but unnecessary load on your heart and blood vessels. In addition, the carbon monoxide may have a direct effect on the heart muscle itself, on your blood vessels, and perhaps even on the clotting of your blood.

Smoking probably increases the clumping ability of certain blood cells (platelets). The mechanism is complex, but the result is that smoking is a contributing factor to the deposition of cholesterol in the arteries (see Atherosclerosis: What Is It? page 636). This may be why smoking is also associated with stroke, the nation's third leading cause of death. Smokers may be at a 2 or 3 times greater risk of having a stroke.

Smoking contributes to peripheral obstructive arterial disease (see Circulatory Problems, page 690). This can result in leg or thigh pain with exercise and, ultimately, in gangrene of the foot.

Female smokers who use one type of oral contraceptive (birth control pills that combine estrogen and progestin), especially after age 35, are at risk of serious problems with their heart and blood vessels.

Smoking decreases the senses of smell and taste and so makes eating food less enjoyable. Smoking also can impair the healing of peptic ulcers (see Peptic Ulcer, page 753) and may increase the likelihood of a recurrence.

Low-Tar, Low-Nicotine Cigarettes

The low-yield cigarette is not a magic answer to the problems caused by smoking.

During the past 30 years, the average tar and nicotine yield of American cigarettes has

---

Smoking and Skin Wrinkles

In all of us, skin wrinkles develop with age, but cigarette smoking can accelerate the process. Smokers in the age group from 40 to 49 years frequently have facial wrinkles that are similar to those of nonsmokers who are 20 years older.

Tobacco can affect your cardiovascular system, including blood circulation within your skin. Nicotine constricts small blood vessels and thus may impair your skin's nutrition. Direct exposure to cigarette smoke, which contains hundreds of toxic substances, can dry and irritate your skin and promote wrinkles.

The telltale wrinkles caused by smoking may include:

- Lines or wrinkles spreading from the upper or lower lips, or at right angles from the corners of the eyes (crow's feet).
- Deep lines or numerous shallow lines on the cheeks and lower jaw.
- Slight hollowness of the cheeks, which emphasizes the bony contours of the face and leads to a gaunt appearance; a leathery or worn appearance to the facial skin, which may have a grayish tinge.

declined substantially. On the face of it, the decrease in these substances is good news, and the message from advertisers has been that the low-yield cigarettes may be safer than the older, conventional cigarettes.

The addition of a filter tip that selectively removes tar and nicotine was an important first step in decreasing the levels of these substances in the smoke. Further refinements to decrease tar and nicotine have included expanded, or puffed, tobacco (so that there is less tobacco per cigarette), faster burning times, more porous paper, and ventilated filters that allow dilution of the tobacco smoke with air.

The fact is, however, that the low-yield cigarette contains the same tobacco and nicotine as other cigarettes—it has simply been engineered to make more dilute smoke available to the smoker. In addition, filters do not remove carbon monoxide or other gaseous components from tobacco smoke.

Don't Be Misled

Most smokers smoke because they are addicted to nicotine. When using low-yield cigarettes, smokers tend to change their smoking behavior. They take more frequent puffs, inhale more deeply, and often smoke more cigarettes. After switching to low-yield cigarettes, you may still take in as much, or more, tar, nicotine, and carbon monoxide as with your old brand.

Use of low-yield cigarettes probably does not decrease the risk of cancer, emphysema, or other diseases—even if you do not increase the number of cigarettes you smoke per day.

In addition, there appears to be no difference in the risk of a heart attack between high-yield and low-yield cigarette smokers. However, the risk of a heart attack diminishes within a year after you stop smoking, no matter which type of cigarette you smoked.

Thus, even if you switch to a low-yield cigarette, the chance of decreasing your risks for lung cancer, emphysema, heart attack, or other diseases is nil. To decrease these risks significantly, there is only one clear message: stop smoking. Do not be misled; there is no such thing as a safe cigarette.

Chewing Tobacco

At the turn of the century, smokeless tobacco was the most popular form of tobacco used in this country. Chewing tobacco and snuff remained commonplace until the discovery that tuberculosis was transmitted through spitting, and it became both illegal and socially unacceptable to spit in public places.

Before the early 1970s, smokeless tobacco users were almost all older men. In the 1960s the tobacco industry, to counter a decline in cigarette smoking, decided to retarget marketing of smokeless tobacco, focusing on young males and altering the nicotine delivery of entry-level smokeless products. The effort apparently was successful, because since the early 1970s, there has been an upswing in the use of smokeless tobacco, especially among male adolescents. Surveys have found that in some areas more than one-third of all male high school and college students regularly use smokeless tobacco. Of the 12 million users in this country, an estimated 3 million are younger than 21. Studies have also revealed that children as young as 8 and 9 years old use smokeless tobacco regularly.

Smokeless tobacco is sold in two forms. One is a cured, ground tobacco called snuff, which may be dry, moist, or finely cut. The other form is chewing tobacco, which is sold in loose-leaf, plug, or twisted forms. When you chew tobacco or place a small amount of it between your gum and cheek, the tobacco mixes with your saliva and nicotine is absorbed through the lining of your mouth into your bloodstream.

The use of smokeless tobacco is linked to an increased chance of oral cancer (see Oral Cancer, page 621). The cheek and gum are the locations most often affected. Leukoplakia—white spots or patches on the tongue, lip, or cheek which can become malignant—has been found in a high percentage of people who use smokeless tobacco. Smokeless tobacco has also been associated with cancers of the esophagus, larynx, and pancreas.

Another health problem associated with use of this tobacco is periodontal disease. Smokeless tobacco can cause the gums to become so inflamed that they swell and bleed (see Gingivitis, page 610). In addition, chewing tobacco extract can increase the growth of two types of oral bacteria that are associated with dental cavities.

Treatment for addiction to smokeless tobacco differs from techniques used in treating addiction to cigarettes. It may involve specialized counseling or higher doses of prescription nicotine gum or patches.

Despite marketing claims, smokeless

tobacco is highly addictive and is not a safe alternative to smoking. On the contrary, it is clear that smokeless tobacco poses a serious threat to the health of anyone who uses it.

Teenage Smoking

Most cigarette smokers start early in life. Grade school children were surveyed and asked to identify products associated with various symbols, including the friendly camel that appears on a popular brand of cigarettes and the familiar ears of Mickey Mouse. The children recognized the camel and its cigarette product equally as often as they recognized the ears of Mickey Mouse.

Among smokers born since 1935, more than 80 percent started smoking before age 21 and more than half started before age 18. Today, a million teenagers take up smoking each year. A growing number of them are female. Even though smoking has generally declined since the mid-1960s, an increasing number of teenage girls smoke. This group continues to be a major target for advertising by the tobacco industry.

It has been well documented that a high percentage of teenagers who smoke are from families in which one or both parents smoke. An explanation of this may be that, because more mothers now smoke than in past generations, more of their daughters mimic their mothers' smoking behavior.

Cigarette smoking among teenagers also seems to be connected to peer pressure. In a survey of 3,000 junior high school students, the most likely predictor of whether a boy or girl smoked was having friends who smoked.

Education does not appear to be an effective deterrent to smoking among teenagers. Nine of every 10 teenagers surveyed believed that smoking was harmful to their health and 85 percent of those who smoked said that they did not plan to be smokers for more than 5 years. It is interesting to note that most of the teenagers who took up smoking had been adamantly against smoking in their younger years. But the power of example, good or bad, is often persuasive: parents who continue to smoke with no visible ill effects can have a substantial influence. The teenagers' concerns about smoking diminish, and many take up smoking.

Young women smokers find it harder to quit than men do. One of their fears is that they will gain weight if they quit smoking. Weight gain is a frequent occurrence in people who stop smoking, but the increase is usually only a few pounds. If you stop smoking, your senses of taste and smell tend to return and with this a greater enjoyment of food. Simply being on guard against the temptation to exploit the newly returned enjoyment of the taste of food may prevent undue weight gain. In a national survey, one of four ex-smokers had actually lost weight.

Young people are not exempt from the health risks of smoking. Lung damage can begin at an early age, and atherosclerosis, which can lead to heart attacks and strokes, can have its start early in life, especially among smokers.

Secondhand Smoke

The health threat to the nonsmoker from exposure to tobacco smoke is well documented. As a result of the effects of this secondhand (passive) smoking, most states have enacted laws limiting smoking in public places.

The Environmental Protection Agency (EPA) has classified environmental tobacco smoke as a class A carcinogen responsible for more than 3,800 cases of lung cancer in nonsmokers each year. Other class A carcinogens are asbestos, radon, and benzene.

The inhaling of secondhand smoke causes your heart to beat faster, your blood pressure to increase, and the level of carbon monoxide in your blood to increase. Sidestream smoke from a burning cigarette contains twice as much tar and nicotine as does the inhaled smoke, 3 times as much of a compound called 3,4-benzpyrene (a cancer-causing agent), 5 times as much carbon monoxide, and possibly 50 times as much ammonia. Clearly, people with respiratory or heart conditions, and the elderly in general, are at

---

Smoking and Pregnancy

Many women who smoke during their pregnancies choose to deny that there are unique health hazards both to themselves and to their developing fetuses. The primary risks associated with cigarette smoking during pregnancy or at the time of delivery include an increased chance of miscarriage, a low-birth-weight baby, and increased incidence of fetal or infant death (see Risk Factors and Pregnancy, page 194).

special health risk when exposed to second-hand smoke. Infants are three times more likely to die from sudden infant death syndrome if their mothers smoke during and after pregnancy.

Children younger than 1 who are exposed to smoke have a higher frequency of admissions to hospitals for respiratory illness compared with children of parents who do not smoke. Secondhand (passive) smoke increases a child's risk of getting ear infections, pneumonia, bronchitis, or tonsillitis. Furthermore, children of parents who smoke are at increased health risk because their parents are more apt to have respiratory infections that they pass on to their children.

The health issues regarding environmental smoke are so grave that all parents who smoke should smoke outdoors or quit if for no other reason than the health of their children.

How to Stop Smoking

Most smokers understand that tobacco use, and smoking specifically, is a behavior that is hazardous to their health. What many beginning smokers fail to understand, however, is that smoking is also an addiction that involves chemicals that affect emotions and behavior.

The cigarette user smokes to maintain a certain level of nicotine in his or her blood. After the smoker has not had a cigarette for several hours, this level decreases and the smoker becomes irritable and edgy—he or she "needs a smoke." Smoking a cigarette may then relieve these symptoms of withdrawal. Smoking a cigarette will not relieve nervousness in a nonsmoker. The only kind of nervousness that smoking will relieve is the nervousness that comes from nicotine withdrawal.

Because nicotine is an addictive drug, quitting smoking can be difficult—in fact, most people fail in their first attempt. As difficult as it may be to stop, however, it is not impossible. Each year, a million Americans are successful, although many of them failed on previous attempts. The reasons many people initially fail vary, depending on how long and how much they smoked, their sensitivity to the nicotine, and how well they prepared for their attempt to stop.

Remember, there is no reason to give up trying to quit even after a failed attempt or two or more. If you failed in past efforts to stop smoking, do not be discouraged. Instead, learn from your experiences and set another stop date. Making a commitment to stop and then following through with an attempt to stop can be a most rewarding accomplishment and of great importance to your continued good health and the health of others.

Methods of Stopping

There is no one perfect plan or technique for quitting smoking. What most successful approaches have in common, however, is a commitment on the part of the person to quit, coupled with a realistic expectation that quitting probably will not be easy.

You may experience physical withdrawal symptoms for 3 to 10 days. When these symptoms begin to lessen, you may still have an impulse to smoke at those times you habitually would "light up" in the past (after a meal or when getting behind the wheel of your car).

For some ex-smokers, periodic urges to smoke may come and go for months to years. However, the intensity and duration of these urges invariably grow smaller with the passage of time.

Most relapses occur within four weeks after a person stops. The reason for a relapse depends on many factors, including the strength of the addiction. Occasionally, relapses occur because the smoke-ending program was not thorough enough or individual commitment weakens. A smoking cessation program should include various changes in your routine because it is thought that people revert to smoking during the first 3 months most often because of a lack of new nonsmoking behaviors. Reduced resolve may be due to complacency or the belief that "just one cigarette" won't hurt. Attending a support group can help reinforce commitment.

Consider the strategies listed here in designing your personal stop-smoking regimen.

Do Your Homework First

In organizing your plan for quitting, your physician can be helpful or you can seek a smoking cessation program in your community. Before you start your program, examine the wide range of self-help materials available from the American Lung Association, American Cancer Society, American Heart Association, and your local library.

Set a Stop Date

Pick a date to quit. Then list on paper the reasons you want to stop. Review the points on your list both before you begin your attempt and periodically during the program.

If You Light One Up, You Don't Have to Smoke It

If you start it, you don't have to finish it. And if you finish it, you're not a failure. This is nothing more than a temporary setback. Experts in the field suggest it is important to retain a vision of the day when you no longer smoke and to refer to it when the urge to smoke occurs: no more messy ashtrays, stained yellow teeth, cigarette breath, or burn marks on your furniture, rugs, or clothes. No more breathlessness and lack of stamina.

If you find yourself returning to old patterns of smoking, set a new stop date, develop a plan using your experience to make changes to enhance success, and try again. Remember that most lifelong ex-smokers have succeeded after five or more serious attempts to stop.

If you are unable to stop on your own, there are many organized group and individual programs available to help you succeed in becoming an ex-smoker. The assistance of a trained counselor can help you develop a personalized plan of coping strengths for quitting. Some programs offer weight control and stress management skills training as well. Contact your local hospital, your physician, the American Lung Association, American Cancer Society, or the public health department for information. A few persons will find it extremely difficult to quit, often despite health complications from smoking. If you are one of these persons, consider entering a residential treatment program that keeps you confined and safe while you cope with initial withdrawal and practice behavioral changes that improve your chances of success.

Involve Other People

Do not make your plans to quit a secret merely to avoid talking about a potential failed effort. Tell your family, friends, and colleagues. Give them specifics of when and why you want to stop and ask for their support. Ask your spouse or a friend to quit with you.

Before You Reach Your Stop Date

Make yourself aware of each cigarette you smoke by keeping a log. Make it inconvenient to smoke, and delay lighting up each cigarette until the urge is strong. Buy cigarettes by the pack rather than by the carton. Make other changes in your normal routine, such as using matches instead of a lighter and vice versa. Use only one ashtray and clean it after each use. Invent your own methods of making yourself aware of every cigarette you smoke.

Most heavy smokers can benefit from cutting down slightly before the stop date. However, it is a rare smoker who can actually stop smoking completely by tapering down. Tapering to 10 to 20 cigarettes a day before the stop date can reduce the severity of withdrawal symptoms.

Reduce the number of smoking cues by limiting the places you smoke (for example, smoke in one room only or outdoors, stop smoking in your car, smoke only on breaks, or stop earlier in the evening than usual). This will reduce the behavioral cues to smoke so that when you stop smoking, you can be comfortable in more situations without having a cigarette. Remember, you are changing a behavior that has been a ritualized part of your life, perhaps for years.

Read about stopping smoking. Plan your stop date with places to go that are smoke-free, with methods to cope with cravings and with an easy schedule.

Attend a support group and talk to ex-smokers for tips and increased motivation. You may want to see your physician or a counselor to discuss your plans and seek advice about quitting and support. Medications may help reduce withdrawal symptoms. Discuss this with your doctor.

Take It One Day at a Time

On your stop day, quit completely. Make it your commitment to not smoke today. Focus all of your attention on achieving that goal. Then take care of tomorrow.

Change Your Routine

Avoid or change situations in which you previously smoked. Drink your morning coffee in a different location, or have tea or juice instead of coffee. Leave the table immediately after meals if they formerly ended with a cigarette. Take a walk instead of lighting up. If you smoked while using the telephone, avoid prolonged conversations or change the location of the telephone you use. If you have a chair you favor for smoking, avoid it temporarily. Drive a different route to work.

Before the urge to smoke strikes, start activities that make smoking physically difficult to perform, such as washing the car, weeding the garden, or taking a shower. Almost any kind of physical exercise may help. Your smoking behavior may be very ingrained and seem automatic. Anticipate this automatic behavior and plan alternatives.

Handling Each Urge

Check your watch whenever an urge hits. Most are short. Once this is apparent, you will be better able to resist the urge.

Plan short, distracting activities to use during urges, such as chewing gum, using a toothpick, or doing a crossword puzzle or handicrafts. Reverse the negative "I can't do it" thinking. Take a positive approach. "I can make it another few minutes and then the urge will pass and I will be okay."

Medications to Reduce Withdrawal

Nicotine gum (nicotine polacrilex), popularly known by its trade name Nicorette, may help as an adjunct to a treatment program. This product gradually releases nicotine when it is used properly.

The goal is to use just enough nicotine gum to maintain your nicotine level, thus holding in check any withdrawal symptoms. Bite into the nicotine gum a few times and then "park" it between your cheek and gum in order to maximize its absorption. It can be used daily in decreasing amounts for several weeks while the behavior of reaching for a cigarette is slowly being broken.

Once you feel comfortable in your smoke-free behavior you can taper off within 3 to 6 months after you stop smoking.

Nicotine gum is only an aid and may not be appropriate for everyone. Your physician can help you decide; the gum is currently available only by prescription from a physician, but it may be available as an over-the-counter product in the future. Some people experience side effects such as indigestion or stomachache, but these discomforts usually are mild and are most often caused by improper use (such as chewing rapidly and swallowing the saliva).

Nicotine patches are also available to help people stop smoking. They are designed to provide nicotine to your circulatory system through your skin. They are used daily for 6 to 12 weeks and have been shown to be very effective, but they are not a magic cure. You need to pay attention to all of the other elements of stopping smoking that have been described.

The most common side effect of nicotine patches is skin irritation, which can be minimized by rotating the site where you apply the patch. Apply a cortisone cream to the skin that is irritated. This cream can be purchased without a prescription.

New nicotine delivery systems such as nicotine nasal sprays and nicotine inhalers are being studied alone and in combination with nicotine gum and nicotine patches to help smokers stop smoking. Bupropion (Wellbutrin) also can help reduce withdrawal symptoms and help smokers stop. Other prescription medications may be available in the future.

Problems of Stopping

Immediately after quitting, you may feel more hungry, tired, and short-tempered than usual. You may have strong cravings for a cigarette and find it difficult to concentrate and maintain your focus. You also may have trouble sleeping and there may be an increase in coughing.

Nicotine withdrawal symptoms are the result of your body's clearing itself of the nicotine. Most of the nicotine will be gone within 3 days, but your body's desire for it may continue for several weeks.

You may experience increased hunger or an improvement in your senses of taste and smell. Indirectly, this can result in weight gain. Quitting does not mean that you automatically will gain weight. A modest, temporary weight gain can be addressed after you are secure in your new, nonsmoking status. Here are tips for guarding against a major weight gain:

- Drink a glass of water before every meal.
- Plan well-balanced menus carefully and literally count the calories.
- Arrange beforehand that you will eat only low-fat, low-calorie snacks, including low-calorie beverages.
- If you miss having something in your mouth, chew sugarless gum or snack on foods such as carrots, pickles, or celery.
- If you must have sweets, eat hard candy.
- Weigh yourself weekly.
- Exercise regularly.

If you become constipated during your recovery, add fiber to your diet, such as raw vegetables and whole-grain cereals, and be careful to drink plenty of water (approximately six 6-ounce glasses daily).

Tension and irritability are common withdrawal symptoms. Become familiar with suitable relaxation techniques. Take a walk or a shower, or soak in the bathtub. Breathe deeply and slowly, as though you are inhaling a cigarette, and repeat this procedure several times.

Benefits of Stopping

Within a few days, you will begin to notice some remarkable changes in your body. Your senses of smell and taste may improve. You may breathe easier, and your smoker's cough will begin to disappear, although you may still cough and bring up mucus for a while. You may also notice an improvement in your stamina.

The more lasting and serious benefits of quitting smoking begin almost immediately. Within 24 hours the levels of carbon monoxide and nicotine in your system will decrease rapidly. The effects of smoking on bronchitis will begin to be reversed from the very first day you quit. Although the effects of emphysema are irreversible, breathing is made easier and the progress of the disease is slowed.

By the end of the first nonsmoking year, your risk of a heart attack begins to decrease; by 5 years it is almost the same as for lifetime nonsmokers. The American Cancer Society believes that quitting smoking immediately decreases the chances of esophageal or pancreatic cancer; within 7 years your risk of bladder cancer will drop to that of a nonsmoker, and after 10 to 15 years of not smoking the statistical risk of the ex-smoker getting cancer of the lung, larynx, or mouth approaches that of people who have never smoked.

By stopping smoking you have reassumed control over a very important part of your life. Your self-esteem will improve and you will feel better about yourself and your abilities. In addition, those around you will benefit from not inhaling smoke from your cigarettes. You will also rid yourself of the unpleasantries associated with smoking, such as health risks, bad breath, yellow teeth, and smelly clothing and hair.

Chapter 13

Alcohol Abuse and Alcoholism

Contents

Understanding Alcohol Use, 326
What Is Alcoholism? 326
What Is Alcohol Abuse? 326
How Alcohol Works in Your Body, 326
Alcohol Intoxication, 327
Short- and Long-Term Effects of Excessive Alcohol Use, 327
  Pregnancy and Alcohol, 328
Recognizing the Alcoholic, 329
  Myths About Alcoholism, 329

Self-Administered Alcoholism Screening
  Test (SAAST), 330

Treating Alcoholism and Alcohol Abuse, 331
Acknowledging the Problem, 331
  Coping With Teenage Drinking, 332
Treatment Programs, 332
  Alcoholics Anonymous and Al-Anon, 334

Understanding Alcohol Use

Many people who choose to drink alcohol can limit their consumption to amounts that cause no harmful health or social consequences. Millions of other people, however, use alcohol excessively and suffer adverse consequences. According to the National Institute on Alcohol Abuse and Alcoholism, more than 13 million Americans abuse alcohol.

As a result, alcohol abuse and alcoholism are major social, economic, and public health problems. In the United States alone, the annual cost of lost productivity and health expenses related to alcoholism is estimated to be almost 100 billion dollars.

Treating people who have drinking problems—or their agreeing to get treatment themselves—is particularly complex given the very nature of the problem. Most people with a drinking problem deny there is a problem. It is important to keep in mind, however, that alcoholism is a disease. In fact, alcoholism is the third-largest killer in the United States, ranking behind heart disease and cancer. If traffic fatalities and death certificate diagnoses related to alcohol use were included in the statistics, alcoholism would be recognized as our nation's number one killer.

Controversy persists over what levels of drinking are problematic or unhealthful. The importance of distinguishing between alcoholism and alcohol abuse is chiefly that the treatment approaches and goals may differ considerably.

What Is Alcoholism?

Generally, alcoholism is considered a chronic disease, often progressive and fatal, with genetic, psychosocial, and environmental factors influencing its development. It is characterized by periods of preoccupation with alcohol, distortion in thinking (most notably denial), impaired control over alcohol intake, and repetitive use of alcohol despite adverse consequences. Each of these symptoms may be continuous or periodic. It is the physical dependence (addiction) on alcohol (demonstrated by tolerance and withdrawal symptoms) and compulsive behavior related to alcohol use that usually distinguish alcoholics from other problem drinkers.

What Is Alcohol Abuse?

Drinking problems in people who do not have all the characteristics of alcoholism are often referred to as "alcohol abuse," "harmful use of alcohol," or "problem drinking." Persons who abuse alcohol also engage in repeated excessive drinking that results in health or social problems or both. They may also continue to consume alcohol despite knowing that continued intake poses social problems for them. However, they neither are dependent on alcohol nor have lost control over the use of alcohol.

Although it takes years for an adult to develop alcohol dependence, teenagers can become addicted in just months. Alcohol consumption among high school students overall is decreasing, as it is among adults, but use of alcohol is still high and often increases dramatically during the 10th and 11th grades. Also, more and more adolescent girls are taking up drinking even though drinking continues to affect males predominantly. Each year in the United States, more than 2,000 young people between the ages of 15 and 20 die in alcohol-related automobile accidents, according to the National Highway Traffic Safety Administration. Alcohol is also often implicated in other causes of death in teenagers, including drownings, suicides, and fires.

How Alcohol Works in Your Body

Alcohols are a group of compounds, many of which are ingredients in perfumes, extracts, tinctures, paints, and other products. Alcohols are also essential to many manufacturing processes.

The form of alcohol in the beverages we drink is ethyl alcohol (ethanol), a colorless liquid that in its pure, undiluted form has a biting or burning taste. It is produced by the fermentation of sugars that occur naturally in grains such as barley and in fruits such as grapes.

When you drink alcohol, it depresses your central nervous system by acting as a sedative or tranquilizer. In some people, the initial reaction may be stimulation, but as drinking continues, sedative effects occur. By depressing the controlling centers of your brain, alcohol relaxes you and reduces your inhibitions. The more you drink, the more you are sedated. Initially, alcohol affects areas of thought, emotion, and judgment. In sufficient amounts, alcohol can impair your speech and muscle coordination and produce sleep. Taken in large enough quantities, alcohol is a lethal poison—it can cause life-threatening coma by severely depressing the vital centers of your brain.

The principal site for alcohol absorption is your small intestine, although very small amounts are absorbed in your mouth and esophagus and only slightly more is absorbed in your stomach. The rate at which the alcohol is absorbed depends on several factors.

If your stomach is empty, most of the alcohol is usually quickly absorbed. Food in your stomach or small intestine, especially solid and fatty foods, slows the emptying of your stomach and the absorption of the alcohol into your bloodstream. Once the alcohol has been absorbed, it is quickly transported throughout your body to wherever there is water, including inside individual cells. This distribution accounts for the intoxicating effects of alcohol. Taking a drink on a full stomach spreads the metabolism of that drink over a longer time, and thus the concentration of alcohol attained in your blood is lower.

Nearly all of the alcohol is burned as fuel for your body, although small amounts are lost in your urine and from the lungs. It is the alcohol in the air you exhale that is measured in breath tests to determine the amount of alcohol in your body. The level of alcohol in your exhalations closely parallels the concentration of alcohol in your blood.

Alcohol also dilates your peripheral blood vessels (those nearest your skin) to produce an initial feeling of warmth, although this is only temporary (see page 329). Your pulse rate increases, and you produce more urine because of the increased fluid intake and the action of the alcohol on your kidneys. Alcohol also stimulates your stomach to secrete acid.

Your body uses alcohol just as it uses other food—by metabolizing it in the liver to gain heat and energy. The food value of alcohol is limited because its calories provide no vitamins, minerals, or proteins. Alcoholics often have deficiencies in nutrients. Common deficiencies include thiamine (vitamin B_1), riboflavin (vitamin B_2), niacin, folic acid, pyridoxine (vitamin B_6), magnesium, potassium, and zinc. Physicians once thought that the effect of alcohol on nutritional status was the only cause of the long-term liver damage that alcoholics commonly have (conditions called fatty liver and cirrhosis; see Enlarged Liver, page 809, and Cirrhosis, page 804). Today, it is known that the toxic effect of alcohol can harm the liver directly.

Alcohol Intoxication

How much food you have eaten and how recently you have eaten before drinking are not the only factors that affect how you respond to a given amount of alcohol. Size and body fat also play important roles. Drinking equal amounts of alcohol may have a greater effect on a woman than on a man. Women generally are smaller and have a higher percentage of fat tissue than men. They may also metabolize alcohol less efficiently than men.

The intoxicating effects of alcohol relate to the concentration of alcohol, which, in turn, reflects levels present in your blood and brain. For example, if you are not an alcoholic and your blood alcohol concentration is more than 100 mg/dL (milligrams of alcohol per deciliter of blood), you may become intoxicated and have difficulty speaking, thinking, and moving around. If your blood alcohol concentration increases, mild confusion may give way to stupor and, ultimately, coma.

Most states define legal intoxication as a blood alcohol concentration of at least 70 to 100 mg/dL, or 0.1 percent. Even at concentrations much lower than the legal limit, many people lose some coordination and reaction time. Reaction time is the speed with which you can react to a situation—for example, how rapidly you can apply the brakes while driving a car.

Short- and Long-Term Effects of Excessive Alcohol Use

Excessive drinking of alcohol can produce several harmful effects on your brain and nervous system. If you are an alcoholic, genetic factors may also influence some neurologic complications. Excessive use of alcohol can also damage your liver, pancreas, and cardiovascular system.

Brain and Nervous System

Alcohol abusers and alcoholics, as well as occasional or first-time drinkers, commonly forget all or part of what occurred during the time they were drinking. This temporary loss of memory is referred to as a blackout. Some excessive drinkers can have problems with short-term memory that may persist for several weeks after stopping drinking. However, memory is usually restored with abstinence.

Excessive alcohol use can also leave you exhausted in the morning, even after a full night's sleep. This morning fatigue is partially accounted for by the anesthetic effect of alcohol. It interferes with your brain's ability to produce an adequate amount of dreaming periods of sleep, called rapid-eye-movement (REM) sleep (see Sleep Disorders, page 1112).

If you are an alcoholic and are deficient in nutrients, particularly thiamine, you may be affected by a neurologic disorder called Wernicke-Korsakoff's syndrome. This syndrome consists of two separate disorders that often occur together in alcoholics. The first symptom of Wernicke's syndrome is often a weakness and paralysis of your eye muscles, which may result in double vision. Over time, you may not be able to stand or walk without help. Korsakoff's syndrome involves severe amnesia, particularly loss of recent memory. If you have both syndromes, you may experience episodes in which you forget your identity, become disoriented, and have hallucinations.

Treatment for Wernicke-Korsakoff's syndrome is straightforward: thiamine supplements and abstinence from alcohol. The symptoms of this disorder, however, are usually not completely reversible.

Gastrointestinal Tract

Alcohol can irritate the mucous lining of your stomach and produce gastritis (see page 758). This also may cause vomiting, which, in turn, can cause small tears in the upper part of your stomach and the lower part of your esophagus. These tears, called Mallory-Weiss tears, can bleed. Persistent drinking can interfere with the absorption of the B vitamins, particularly folic acid and thiamine, and other nutrients. Most of these problems will disappear if you stop drinking.

Other alcohol-induced problems, however, such as a fatty or enlarged liver, hepatitis (see page 803), or esophageal varices (dilated veins of the esophagus, see page 750), may require immediate medical attention. Damage caused by alcohol-induced cirrhosis of the liver tends to be progressive.

As the circulating alcohol moves through your liver, enzymes metabolize it. A healthy liver can process alcohol at a rate of about 50 calories an hour. This is equivalent to about 1 ounce of 40 percent alcohol in about an hour. If your liver becomes overwhelmed by large amounts of alcohol, the alcohol will circulate in your body until your liver can process it.

The cause of the common hangover (headache and dry mouth) is not entirely clear. One possibility is that alcohol is a diuretic, causing loss of water through the urine. This can lead to dehydration. The treatment for hangover symptoms is rest, plenty of liquids, and aspirin or other simple analgesics.

In alcoholics, both acute and chronic pancreatitis also may develop (see pages 818 and 819).

Cardiovascular System

An alcoholic drink temporarily reduces blood pressure. But if you consume alcohol excessively, it can increase your blood pressure.

Similarly, although recent reports indicate that moderate daily drinking may prevent one type of heart trouble, the harmful effects of excessive use of alcohol outweigh any potential benefits. One or two alcoholic drinks per day, or up to one ounce of ethyl alcohol, may reduce your risk of developing coronary artery disease. This protective effect may, in part, be due to changes in blood fats. People who regularly consume alcohol have

---

Pregnancy and Alcohol

If you are pregnant, don't drink alcoholic beverages—they pose a major threat to your unborn child's health and development. Many children of mothers who consume excessive amounts of alcohol during pregnancy are born with fetal alcohol syndrome, a pattern of birth defects consisting of a small head, heart defects, a shortening of the eyelids, and various other abnormalities (see page 195). As these children grow older, many are recognized as being developmentally disabled or unable to understand the consequences of their actions.

The means by which alcohol causes this damage is not clearly understood. Nor is it known how much alcohol must be consumed to cause fetal defects or an abnormal infant. The best precaution for your future child's well-being is the warning stated above: don't drink alcoholic beverages if you are pregnant.

increased amounts of a type of fat in their blood known as high-density lipoprotein cholesterol (see page 639). This "good cholesterol" may inhibit hardening of the arteries (atherosclerosis). In excessive alcohol drinkers, however, a condition called cardiomyopathy frequently develops. This is a disease that destroys the heart muscle and produces symptoms that range from arrhythmias (irregular heartbeat) to heart failure (see Cardiomyopathy, page 686). If you are male and you drink excessively, you also may be at greater risk for a stroke.

Sexual Functioning and Menstruation

Alcohol abuse can cause impotence in men. In women, it can interrupt menstruation.

Cancer

After cardiovascular disease, cancer is the next leading cause of death among alcoholics. Alcoholics have a rate of cancer higher than that of the general population, especially cancer of the larynx, esophagus, stomach, and pancreas.

Recognizing the Alcoholic

How can you tell whether you or a friend or loved one is an alcoholic? Anyone with a drinking problem can be an alcoholic. Alcoholism knows no social or economic bounds. Many people with alcoholism are highly regarded and pass for years among friends and associates as healthy and normally functioning people. It strikes the young and old, men and women, rich and poor, and people of all races.

The American Medical Association considers alcoholism to be a disease. Nevertheless, many people in this country have been slow to accept alcoholism as a disease and still believe that an alcoholic is someone who has disgraced himself or herself because of personal weakness. Because of the lingering social stigma that many people place on the disease of alcoholism, many alcoholics see themselves as weak and bad people. Some may rationalize the problems that are brought on by their alcoholism, such as a broken marriage or a lost job, as the consequence of bad luck or something caused by others. This burden of shame and blame is one of the greatest stumbling blocks to an alcoholic's recovery.

The fact is, alcoholism is a treatable disease. A step toward recognizing whether you

---

Myths About Alcoholism

There has never been a shortage of myths about alcoholism. Here are some examples:

Older People Don't Become Alcoholics. Older adults are not immune to alcoholism, although the disease is less prevalent among persons 65 years or older.

A Drink Can Warm You Up. Alcohol dilates your blood vessels and does give you a sensation of warmth—but only very temporarily. Increased heat loss through your skin actually decreases your body temperature when you drink alcohol. Consequently, the risk of serious, even fatal, low temperature (hypothermia and pneumonia) is increased if you drink alcohol excessively in a cold environment.

When Drunk, You Reveal Your True Personality. Although alcohol may permit traits to surface that you suppress when you are sober, excessive drinking can distort your personality. Your true personality is revealed when you are sober.

Strong Black Coffee Can Help You Sober Up. Coffee can neither increase the rate at which your liver processes alcohol nor change your blood alcohol levels. The initial lift that coffee provides may lead you to believe that you are reasonably alert and sober when, in fact, you are not.

If You Admit to Being an Alcoholic, You Can Never Get Another Decent Job. It is illegal to discriminate in hiring on the basis of any medical disability, including alcoholism. Often, recovered alcoholics are admired by potential employers for the commitment that is necessary to treat the disease. Employers are learning that it often is less expensive to support an employee in treatment, usually through a health insurance policy, than it is to replace the employee.

---

or someone you know may have a drinking problem is to evaluate the drinking patterns and ask yourself what drinking habits have caused you or your family problems. Indications of alcoholism are discussed below.

Denial

Persisting in the belief that your problems are caused by factors other than drinking, even when the consequences of drinking behaviors are evident, is a clear sign of alcoholism. Denial acts as a powerful barrier to protect against the truth about drinking. Rather than admit the problem, alcoholics often become angry, blame others, and continue to drink abusively for years without seeking help.

Increased Tolerance

Tolerance to the effects of alcohol is an early symptom of alcohol dependence. If you find you need to drink more than the usual amount of alcohol to feel its effects, you have developed tolerance. Alcoholics may appear sober even after consuming more alcohol than would intoxicate moderate drinkers. This is not an accomplishment. It indicates that your body has become accustomed to alcohol. Long-time drinkers of moderate amounts may also develop tolerance to alcohol.

But beware: no matter how much tolerance you seem to develop, your liver is still unable to metabolize pure alcohol at a rate faster than approximately 1 ounce of 40 percent liquor every hour. If your tolerance begins to decline, your liver may no longer be able to metabolize alcohol at the same rate. Using tolerance as a measure of how much to drink is unsafe because it may damage your liver and lead you to believe that you do not have a drinking problem.

Withdrawal and DTs

If you're dependent on alcohol and then suddenly stop drinking, you are likely to experience physical and psychological withdrawal symptoms. In most alcoholics, these symptoms include hand tremors; increase in pulse, blood pressure, and body temperature; nausea, diarrhea, and other gastrointestinal discomfort; and insomnia. Generally, these symptoms last 3 to 7 days, although some may last for weeks.

With DTs (delirium tremens), more dangerous withdrawal symptoms can occur: delirium, confusion, aggression, vivid hallucinations, severe tremors, paranoid ideas, and seizures. These symptoms often last for 3 to 5 days, sometimes longer, and require urgent medical evaluation and treatment.

Your physician can help you deal with withdrawal symptoms if you have a mild problem with alcohol. If you are an alcoholic and you want to stop drinking, a hospital detoxification program can be helpful and may be necessary.

Impaired Health

Your physician can conduct tests to reveal signs of physical damage caused by alcohol, such as cirrhosis of the liver, alcoholic hepatitis, or cardiomyopathy. However, the diagnosis of alcoholism should be made long before complications develop. Sometimes physical signs are absent.

Preoccupation With Alcohol

Looking forward to the next time you'll be able to drink, selecting social activities based on whether alcohol will be available, associating mainly with others who drink, talking a lot about drinking, and feeling uneasy if your supply of liquor is not available are all signs of alcohol dependency. Keeping alcohol in unlikely places at home, at work, or in your car is also a sign.

Drinking Excessively and Often

Gulping drinks, ordering doubles, becoming intoxicated intentionally to feel good, or

---

Self-Administered Alcoholism Screening Test (SAAST)

Some disorders have symptoms that make a diagnosis easy. Alcoholism, however, defies easy classification: the symptoms vary greatly from one problem drinker to the next.

To cope with this difficulty, Mayo Clinic has developed the Self-Administered Alcoholism Screening Test (SAAST). Based in part on the Michigan Alcoholism Screening Test, the SAAST consists of 37 questions. In use since 1972, the test can identify 95 percent of alcoholics ill enough to be hospitalized.

The test aims to identify behavior patterns, medical symptoms, and consequences of drinking in the alcoholic—not to accuse. Here is a sample of questions from the test:

1. Do you have a drink now and then?

2. Do you feel you are a normal drinker (that is, drink no more than average)?

3. Have you ever awakened the morning after drinking the previous evening and found that you could not remember a part of the evening?

4. Do close relatives ever worry or complain about your drinking?

5. Can you stop drinking without a struggle after one or two drinks?

6. Do you ever feel guilty about your drinking?

7. Do friends or relatives think you are a normal drinker?

8. Are you always able to stop drinking when you want to?

9. Have you ever attended a meeting of Alcoholics Anonymous (AA) because of your drinking?

10. Have you gotten into physical fights when drinking?

These responses suggest you are at risk of alcoholism: 1. Yes; 2. No; 3. Yes; 4. Yes; 5. No; 6. Yes; 7. No; 8. No; 9. Yes; 10. Yes. If your answers to the above-listed questions suggest you might have a drinking problem, you need a professional evaluation.

drinking to feel "normal" are indications of alcohol dependency.

Symptomatic Use
Using alcohol as a medicine to relieve pain, to relax, or to sleep is a frequent behavior of people with alcoholism.

Solitary Drinking
Drinking alone is a part of the dependency pattern. Alcohol is more important to an alcoholic than the company of other people.

Making Excuses for Drinking
Rationalizing drinking behaviors by making excuses for drinking is a sign of alcohol dependency. To an alcoholic, any event or occasion may provide a reason to drink.

Adverse Consequences
Difficulties with relationships, employment, finances, legal problems, and mood disturbances are common in people addicted to alcohol.

Impaired Control
You may be unable to predict or control how much you drink. For example, you may stop for a "quick one" on the way home, stay for the entire evening, and become intoxicated.

Blackouts
Temporary lapses of memory and feelings of anxiety, concern, and guilt over what may have taken place are also a part of the dependency pattern.

Treating Alcoholism and Alcohol Abuse

Acknowledging the Problem

Most alcoholics, and alcohol abusers, who enter treatment do so reluctantly, usually under pressure from their families, employers, or friends, or as a result of health or legal problems. This pressure is often necessary because the denial used by people who have a drinking problem enables them to believe they do not need treatment.

Penetrating the Protective Shell
People who have a drinking problem often build a protective shell by developing strategies, both conscious and unconscious, to avoid being found out. The subconscious denial may be so profound that an alcoholic may genuinely not recognize the extent of the problem. One of the first goals of treatment is to penetrate these personal defenses that have developed over the years and allowed destructive drinking to continue. Most importantly, anyone who has alcoholism or who abuses alcohol needs to admit there is a problem.

Blaming the person with alcoholism for the illness only feeds that person's feeling that no one understands him or her. It is important to understand that an alcoholic is someone who has been made ill by the disease of alcoholism.

Intervention
The pretreatment phase of alcoholism and alcohol abuse is crucial for family members, friends, employers, and other concerned persons involved with someone who has a drinking problem. The chances of recovery are increased if those concerned can constructively confront the person who has a drinking problem with the truth about the negative consequences of his or her drinking.

There is no ideal person or persons to confront an alcoholic or alcohol abuser. Confrontation facilitated by a professional knowledgeable about alcoholism and alcohol abuse can result in sparing family members, including the person with a drinking problem, years of suffering and destruction of relationships. An employer or an authority figure whom the alcoholic or alcohol abuser respects may also be appropriate. Sometimes, the best person to intervene is a recovering alcoholic.

There is also no ideal time or place for a confrontation. However, do not confront an alcoholic or alcohol abuser when the person is drunk or even while drinking. Pick a time when he or she is sober.

In a kind but candid way, tell the alcoholic or alcohol abuser to either get help or be prepared to suffer the consequences—such as being fired, divorced, or expelled from the family. Do not allow the person to deny your concerns about his or her drinking. And do not try to bail him or her out of trouble or offer another chance. An escape from the consequences of drinking is usually interpreted as permission to drink again.

Family Members

Drinking problems can impair relationships. Troubled relationships begin to develop in the family and the workplace. The National Council on Alcoholism estimates that 1 employee in 20 has an alcohol or drug abuse problem that affects work performance, either his or her own or that of a family member.

Family members often overlook their own need for counseling. Unaware of the true nature of alcoholism and alcohol abuse, and of the need for specialized treatment for someone who has a drinking problem, the family continues to become increasingly distraught and traumatized. Families may experience psychological, marital, parental, social, economic, physical, and spiritual problems as the disease of alcoholism progresses. By directing their attention toward the alcoholic or alcohol abuser, families neglect these other problems. Families use denial as a coping mechanism as readily as the person who has a drinking problem. It often becomes the family's major defense mechanism in attempting to deal with the unending series of crises that the alcoholic or alcohol abuser poses, which sap their energies and spirits.

Family members often respond to the havoc in their lives with anger, sarcasm, and emotional outbursts. Although understandable, blame is counterproductive in dealing with alcoholism or alcohol abuse. Family members must become knowledgeable about problems associated with alcoholism and alcohol abuse. They must learn why the person who has a drinking problem behaves as he or she does. With guidance, family members can learn how to abstain from enabling and rescuing the alcoholic or alcohol abuser. Instead they need to react constructively and establish a climate for positive responses from the person who has the drinking problem.

Parents, spouse, children, and other family members need to regain their own emotional health, whether or not the alcoholic or alcohol abuser is helped. Loss of trust and intimacy are common among families of people who have a drinking problem, as are the resentments and fears they develop. By attending to their own needs, family members often directly or indirectly influence the alcoholic or alcohol abuser to get the treatment he or she needs. Countless numbers of people with alcoholism or alcohol abuse are recovering today simply because their families chose to start the process of recovery.

Treatment Programs

Many treatment programs are available to help you if you have a drinking problem. It is important, however, to first determine if you are alcohol-dependent. If you have not lost control over your use of alcohol, your treatment might involve attempting to reduce your drinking. If you are an alcohol abuser, you may be able to modify your drinking. This approach is ineffective and

---

Coping With Teenage Drinking

Of the nearly 20 million adults who abuse alcohol in this country, more than half started drinking excessively as teenagers. For young people, the likelihood of addiction depends on factors such as the influence of parents, peers, and other role models, susceptibility to advertising, how early in life they begin to use alcohol, their psychological need for alcohol, and, perhaps, genetic factors that may predispose them to addiction.

Two of the most important elements in any effort to prevent the abuse of alcohol or cope with it are education and early intervention. Schools are growing increasingly aware of the need for alcohol and drug education. Parents also need to learn more about the appeal that alcohol holds for young people, the signs of abuse, the short- and long-term effects of abuse, how to handle a child who is abusing alcohol, and what type of help to seek.

Self-esteem and communication play vital roles in alcohol abuse. Many young alcoholics report that their parents had little understanding of their personal sense of inadequacy and that it was impossible to communicate with them about sensitive issues. For school-age children, peer pressure is the source of many value judgments, including those regarding alcohol use.

Many child psychologists believe that home life and television are primary factors in establishing the attitudes children below the fifth grade form toward use of alcohol. A history of abstinence or responsible use of alcohol and well-established, trusting communication in the home early in your child's life are crucial to preventing teenage drinking. If you abuse alcohol, the likelihood that your child will abuse alcohol is greater. If your children see you treating alcohol as a drug, the abuse of which is dangerous, they are far more likely to adopt a healthy respect for its use.

inappropriate if you have alcoholism; abstinence must be a part of the treatment goal.

Treating Alcohol Abuse

For people who are not physically dependent on alcohol but are experiencing the adverse effects of drinking, the goal of treatment is prevention of alcoholism by a screening procedure or "brief interventions."

Screening

There are two major types of screening. One is designed for people who seek medical care for problems unrelated to alcohol use, those who participate in random alcohol testing programs, or drivers who are stopped at random for testing of their breath to determine alcohol intake. The other type of screening program involves people who have been identified as possibly having a drinking problem. Hospital-based programs screen patients admitted for traumatic injuries. Court-mandated programs screen adolescents or adults arrested for violent crimes or drivers who have positive results on a breath test. Employee assistance programs screen workers with impaired performance.

Brief Interventions

Brief interventions usually involve alcohol abuse specialists who can establish a specific treatment plan. These interventions may include direct feedback, contracting and goal setting, behavior modification techniques, use of written material such as self-help manuals, counseling, and follow-up care extending over multiple visits to a treatment center.

Treating Alcoholism

The most common approach to residential alcoholism treatment in the United States is based on a program developed in Minnesota. The "Minnesota Model" includes abstinence, individual and group therapy, participation in Alcoholics Anonymous, educational lectures, family involvement, work assignments, activity therapy, and use of recovering lay counselors and multiprofessional staff.

A wide range of other treatments that have claimed success in alcoholism are available, but they often have had only modest trials and incompletely evaluated studies. Some treatment approaches that have serious advocates include acupuncture, electroencephalography, biofeedback, and aversion therapy. This last treatment involves pairing the drinking of alcohol with a strong aversive

response such as nausea or vomiting induced by a medication. After repeated pairing, the alcohol itself causes the aversive response and that decreases the likelihood of relapse. Although often effective, aversion therapy tends to be unappealing to people with alcoholism because it is unpleasant.

Some programs include a comprehensive medical examination, a psychiatric evaluation with treatment for other personality disorders if necessary, and other consultations and treatment as required.

Here is what you might expect from a program based on the "Minnesota Model."

Acceptance of Your Disease

Effective treatment is impossible unless you accept the fact that alcoholism is a disease and admit that you are addicted and unable to control your drinking. If you refuse to see yourself as having the disease of alcoholism, your denial will hamper treatment or even render it useless. The admission of powerlessness over alcohol is an act of letting go of the alibis and excuses that once supported your abuse of alcohol. It is the most important step to recovery.

Detoxification and Withdrawal

Your treatment may begin with a program of detoxification. In a detoxification unit, you will receive medical care and be carefully monitored through the withdrawal process. This usually takes 4 to 7 days.

A physician's guidance may be required if you have withdrawal symptoms (see page 330). Administration of medications (benzodiazepines), also under the supervision of a physician, may be necessary to prevent delirium tremens (DTs) or withdrawal seizures.

Medical Treatments

Medical problems associated with your alcoholism will be treated. Common problems include high blood pressure, increased blood sugar, liver disease, and heart disease. Your physician can give you dietary regimens to correct any nutritional deficiencies you may have.

Abstinence

If you continue to drink, you will have little or no control over your disease. Continuing to drink may prove fatal. For these reasons, most treatment programs for alcoholism require abstinence.

Recovery Programs

Detoxification and medical treatment are only the first steps for most people in a residential treatment program. Education about the disease of alcoholism, the damage it does to the body, the problems it causes, and the experience of recovery is also a critical part of treatment. During this phase of treatment, most programs include daily classes, group therapy, individual counseling, recreational therapy, and an introduction to the principles of Alcoholics Anonymous. Psychological support and additional nursing and medical care, if indicated, may also be provided.

Some of the trained professional staff involved in recovery programs are recovering alcoholics themselves and are able to offer insiders' knowledge of alcoholism and recovery. They also serve as role models.

Psychological Support and Psychiatric Treatment

Group and individual therapy support recovery from the psychological aspects of alcoholism. Sometimes, emotional symptoms of the disease may mimic psychiatric disorders. A psychiatrist may need to evaluate you. If you have a psychiatric illness, such as major depression (see page 1123), you will need specific treatment apart from the recovery program.

Drug Treatments

If you are participating in a long-term recovery program, don't expect to receive tranquilizers or sedatives. Like alcohol, they are subject to abuse. (An exception is the use of medications to treat withdrawal symptoms or a psychiatric illness in addition to alcoholism.)

If you have trouble abstaining from alcohol, an alcohol-sensitizing drug called disulfiram (Antabuse) may be useful. Taken orally, this drug disrupts the metabolism of alcohol in your liver. If you drink alcohol, the drug produces a severe physical reaction that includes flushing, nausea, vomiting, headaches, and abdominal pain. You may also trigger a mild reaction when taking the drug if you use skin creams, mouthwashes, or anything else that contains alcohol.

Disulfiram will not cure your alcoholism, nor can it remove your compulsion to drink. But it can be a strong deterrent.

Naltrexone (ReVia), a drug long used in treating narcotic addiction and newly approved for the treatment of alcoholism, may decrease cravings for alcohol by blocking the intoxicating effects of alcohol. Unlike disulfiram or other medications such as metronidazole and chlorpropamide, naltrexone does not cause violent illness within a few minutes of taking an alcoholic drink. Nevertheless, it can produce harmful side effects if managed improperly. The use of this agent or any medication is effective only in conjunction with a comprehensive chemical dependency treatment program.

Continuing Support

What happens after residential treatment ends is critical to the success of your program. A major focus of aftercare is helping you and your family. A long-standing recommendation is attendance and participation in support systems such as Alcoholics Anonymous and Al-Anon. By maintaining your program, you can focus recovery on living in the present and acquiring healthful, truthful relationships built on self-understanding and growth.

Alcoholics Anonymous and Al-Anon

The Fellowship of Alcoholics Anonymous was formed in 1935. As a self-help group of recovering alcoholics, Alcoholics Anonymous (AA) offers a sober peer group as an effective model of how you can achieve total abstinence.

The AA program is built around Twelve Steps, which are straightforward suggestions for men and women who choose to lead sober lives. The Twelve Steps are not requirements for membership but rather are guides for people who choose to live their lives sober. As guides to recovery, the Twelve Steps help alcoholics accept their powerlessness over alcohol. They stress the necessity for honesty about the past and present.

Recovery in AA is based on accepting the unique experience of each alcoholic. Through listening and sharing stories, alcoholics learn that they are not alone. There are no fees for membership, only a willingness to remain sober.

In the mid-1950s, family members of recovering alcoholics formed a complementary self-help group called Al-Anon. Al-Anon is designed for people who are affected by someone else's alcoholism. In sharing their stories, they gain a greater understanding of how the disease affects the entire family, not just the alcoholic. Al-Anon also accepts the Twelve Steps of AA as the principles by which participants are to conduct their lives. It also emphasizes how members need to learn detachment and forgiveness if they too are to be free of the disease.

In many communities, Alateen groups are also available to provide support for teenage children of alcoholics.

Chapter 14

Medications and Drug Abuse

Contents

Use Versus Abuse, 336
**What Happens When You Take a
Medication? 336**
  Pregnancy and Drug Use, 336
What Is Drug Abuse? 337
**How to Recognize Drug Abuse and
Addiction, 337**
  Teenagers and Drugs, 338

**Abuse and Misuse of Legal
Medications, 339**
Medication Misuse in the Elderly, 340
Addiction to Tranquilizers, 340
Addiction to Analgesics, 341

Street Drugs, 342
Marijuana, 342
Cocaine, 343
Hallucinogens, 343
Phencyclidine (PCP), 344
Inhalants, 344
Opiates, 344
Drugs and Sports Performance, 345

Use Versus Abuse

Medication use is part of modern life in the United States. Annually, American physicians write countless prescriptions, and consumers purchase hundreds of millions of dollars worth of nonprescription medications.

When taken as directed, prescription or nonprescription drugs can effectively treat many illnesses. However, if they are not used as directed or are intentionally abused, health problems can result. In the following pages, we discuss the misuse and abuse of legal and illegal drugs.

What Happens When You Take a Medication?

When you swallow a medication, it travels to your stomach. In your stomach or intestines, the drug is dissolved and absorbed into your blood. Once in your blood, the drug passes through your liver and is distributed throughout your body to muscle, fat, and major organs.

Some drugs are metabolized (chemically altered) as they pass through your liver. This process changes the drug into an active form. Sometimes, other organs play a role in metabolizing medications. And some drugs, including many antibiotics, are active in their original form and are not metabolized at all but are excreted from your body unchanged. Your body eliminates most drugs through your kidneys in your urine. Other drugs are eliminated from the liver in the bile, where they pass into your intestine.

Aging Changes Your Body's Response

As you age, the way your body handles distribution, metabolism, elimination, and response to medications changes. In fact, because of such changes, one age group that is particularly sensitive to the actions of many drugs and more likely to experience adverse reactions is the elderly. Your organs lose some of their effectiveness with age as well. For example, the flow of blood through your liver may be only 40 to 50 percent that of a younger person. This means you don't metabolize or process drugs as quickly. As a result, the effects of a medication may be delayed or exaggerated. Your kidneys' ability to clear drugs from your system also decreases, so the rate at which you can eliminate a medication from your body slows.

As you age, body fat makes up a greater percentage of your weight. If you take a drug that concentrates in fat, its effects not only may be delayed but prolonged.

Changes in your circulatory and nervous systems also may affect your responsiveness to many drugs. And changes in your mental functioning may make taking medications according to instructions more difficult.

To offset these differences in effect, your physician considers your age when prescribing a medication and deciding on its dosage and frequency.

Other Interactive Factors

Besides age, other factors including your body weight and health can affect how you respond to a drug. So can other medications you may be taking as well as what you eat or drink. Whether you take a generic medication or a brand name drug also may make a difference in some instances (see Is It a Generic or a Brand Name Drug? page 1274). Be sure to tell your physician about all your medical conditions, other medications you are using, if you have any allergies, or if you are pregnant or planning to get pregnant.

Pregnancy and Drug Use

Many drugs pass through the placenta and reach the fetus. During the first trimester of pregnancy, the fetus may be the most sensitive to drugs in the mother's body. Therefore, inform your physician if you have been taking any drugs just before becoming pregnant or during pregnancy.

Some drugs are known to cause problems with pregnancy and the reproductive system. Many women who smoke marijuana during their pregnancy deliver premature babies or babies who have low birth weight. If you use tranquilizers and amphetamines while pregnant, your baby may be born with congenital malformations. Taking barbiturates, opiates, and cocaine while pregnant may cause your baby to be addicted (see Risk Factors and Pregnancy, page 194).

Marijuana may also make your menstrual cycle irregular. In addition, it can cause a temporary loss of fertility in both women and men. If you're breastfeeding and use marijuana, it may pass through your breast milk to your baby.

If you take two or more drugs at the same time, they may interact and lead to undesirable effects. For example, some sedatives (barbiturates) will cause blood thinners (anticoagulants) to be less effective. On the other hand, antibiotics can increase the blood-thinning effects of these drugs.

Food delays or reduces the absorption of many drugs. Other drugs are better absorbed or less irritating to your stomach when you take them with food. Unless otherwise directed by your physician, it's best to take medications with a full glass of water at least 1 hour before or 2 hours after a meal.

Drinking alcohol may either enhance or reduce the effect of a drug. For example, drinking alcohol while taking an antihistamine enhances the sedative effects of the antihistamine. Chronic use of alcohol can cause changes in your liver that speed up the metabolism of some drugs, such as anticonvulsants, anticoagulants, and diabetes drugs. The drugs don't work as well because they don't stay in your body long enough.

Side Effects

Along with intended helpful effects, most medications can produce adverse reactions. Most side effects are mild, but some can be serious. For example, morphine or codeine, which can relieve or diminish pain, may also slow your rate of breathing or cause constipation.

Some side effects disappear as your body becomes accustomed to the presence of the medication. Other side effects are more serious and require medical attention.

Learn what side effects are common with the medication you are taking. Know whether the potential side effects may require medical attention. When your physician prescribes a medication for you, he or she should brief you on the potential side effects. He or she should also tell you about signs and symptoms that may alert you to a serious or even dangerous side effect.

Be aware of effects that indicate that you should stop taking the medication and see your physician. Some of the symptoms may be related to an overdose. These symptoms may occur when you take a larger dose or take the medication more frequently than prescribed. If upon taking a new medication you experience worrisome symptoms, consult your physician immediately.

What Is Drug Abuse?

The abuse or misuse of addicting drugs is an increasing public health issue in this country. Drug abuse and dependence is one of the most frequently reported psychiatric disorders for men ages 18 to 65 years and for young women ages 18 to 24.

Abused drugs are not just those substances that are considered illegal or are used inappropriately (that is, without a prescription). Drug abuse occurs if you take any drug for purposes other than for what it was intended or in a manner or quantities other than directed.

Drug abuse also applies to the excessive consumption of drugs such as nicotine (see Tobacco, page 315) and alcohol (see Alcohol Abuse and Alcoholism, page 325). Both nicotine and alcohol have properties that categorize them as addictive drugs. They also may cause dangerous medical problems.

People abuse illegally obtained drugs for various reasons. Mind-altering psychedelics produce effects that alter the way we experience reality. Stimulants such as amphetamines give the sensation of increased energy and lifted spirits. Analgesics reduce the sensation of pain and induce drowsiness. And antianxiety and antidepressant drugs create a feeling of relaxation. To achieve such effects or become intoxicated deliberately is a frequent motivation.

Most of the millions of people who take prescription medications do not abuse them. However, many misuse them, sometimes out of ignorance and carelessness. Others, particularly the elderly, may underuse prescription drugs, often in an attempt to reduce the cost of their medications. It is important to your health that you follow your physician's instructions as to proper medication use, report any persistent side effects to your physician, and never use someone else's medication. At no time should you use medications for any purpose other than the one prescribed.

How to Recognize Drug Abuse and Addiction

Drug abuse occurs if you take any drug other than as directed—whether for a different use or in another manner or quantity. The abuse of drugs may lead to an addiction, often referred to as drug dependence. Drug abuse or drug dependence can cause health problems that range from physical to psychological, mild to severe, and reversible to permanent.

Compulsive use of a drug, or loss of control over its use, suggests an addiction. The state of addiction may include psychological dependence and physical dependence—

there is a need to take the drug again. Psychological dependence occurs when the desire or need grows to a desperate craving for the drug—the drug is required for the abuser to feel better. A person who abuses drugs may develop a tolerance so that he or she needs more and more of the drug to get the same effect. Physical dependence occurs when withdrawal symptoms appear

Teenagers and Drugs

The best time to prevent drug abuse is before it begins. For parents, it is critical that you learn to talk to your children and develop good listening skills.

What they are not telling you, however, may be even more revealing than what they do report. Teenagers who use drugs are often unhappy, lonely, and anxious. Although they are not eager to talk about their problems, they do want their parents' understanding.

Pay attention to what evidence you are offered. Do you know your children's newest friends? The pressure of peers cannot be exaggerated during adolescence. Studies generally indicate that the approval of peers is often decisive in a teenager's decision to use drugs.

How can you know definitely whether your youngster is using drugs? In lieu of an admission or direct evidence of drug use (such as a "high"), there are signs that may indicate abuse. Keep in mind, however, that these clues are not definitive signs but only possible indications that something is troubling your youngster.

School
Many children may grow to dislike school at some point, but the child who suddenly shows an active dislike of school and looks for excuses to stay home may be in trouble. Contact school authorities and especially the child's teachers: Does your son's or daughter's official attendance record match what you

know about his or her sick days? What about missed classes? An unexplained pattern of tardiness at school is also telling.

Another change that is a matter of concern is a student who generally gets A or B grades but suddenly begins to fail courses or receives only minimal passing grades and expresses general indifference toward school performance.

Another example of a sudden change that is most likely a significant sign is a school athlete who stops participating in a favorite sport for no apparent reason.

Physical Health
Most healthy youngsters have sufficient stamina to see them through their busy lives. Many sleep long hours during weekends and vacations. However, listlessness and apathy, possible indications of drug use, are not common characteristics of teenagers.

Appearance
Appearance is extremely important to adolescents, especially keeping up with the varied and changing dress codes of young people. Thus, it can be a significant warning sign if your youngster suddenly shows little interest in clothing and appearance.

Personal Behavior
Teenagers enjoy their privacy and often will go to great lengths to protect it. However, exaggerated efforts to bar you from going into

their bedrooms or knowing where they go with their friends can be a signal. Do not ignore any unexplained and lengthy stays in the bathroom if you've observed other behavioral changes.

Other causes for concern include temper tantrums, unexpected displays of anger over relatively small matters, or the onset of discipline problems. These may occur at home or at school.

Sudden requests from your teenager for more money without a reasonable explanation for its use may also be a sign that he or she is buying drugs.

Keep Communication Lines Open
Adolescents need to feel that there is an open line of communication with their parents in which they can risk sensitive disclosure without the fear of being censured. During adolescence, children may find it difficult to share their concerns with their parents. Many young people choose peers as their only confidants. Even in the face of your child's reluctance to share, continue to express an interest in listening to your child talk about his or her experiences.

Most children want their family relationships to be marked by understanding and forgiveness. Even if they are abusing drugs, your children must believe that you will always be available to help (see Teenage Years: Ages 13 Through 19, page 137).

shortly after discontinuing use of the drug. These may become severe and possibly life-threatening, sometimes requiring immediate medical attention. Examples of these symptoms include agitation, tremors, anxiety, insomnia, depression, convulsions, and hallucinations.

Recognizing the signs of addiction (to legal or illegal drugs) in someone can be difficult. These signs vary from drug to drug and person to person. However, people who are addicted to one or more drugs often exhibit changes in their behavior that may gradually affect personal relationships and work performance.

Their behavior may be erratic and their mood unpredictable, alternating between periods of exhilaration or agitation and exhaustion or lethargy. Some addicted persons find that they no longer sleep well; others "crash" and sleep for long periods. They may lose their interest in eating or experience unexplained loss of weight.

Eyes that are bloodshot or that have a dazed or expressionless appearance can be clues to drug abuse. Persons abusing hallucinogens may appear to be daydreaming and may have to be spoken to several times before responding, or they may gaze at or examine an object without explanation for long periods.

Other drugs may produce excessive sweating or flushed skin. An unexplained rash or an irritated nostril or runny nose may be a sign that someone has been using an opiate. Alternatively, many drug-dependent persons appear normal even to their friends.

Genuine changes in personality, such as spending increasing amounts of time away from home, behaving differently in or missing classes or work, or constantly demanding or needing money, may also suggest a drug dependence. However, as with all medical conditions, the person should get a proper evaluation to assess the true nature of the problem and to rule out disorders that might cause similar behavior.

Abuse and Misuse of Legal Medications

Drug abuse and drug dependence in this country involve more than just the better-known illegal (street) drugs. Millions of Americans abuse prescription and nonprescription medications, sometimes with tragic results.

In fact, these drugs dominate the statistics on drug-related deaths and emergencies. They are associated with most of the deaths attributed to drugs. Hospital emergency rooms report that approximately the same percentage of drug emergencies are due to misuse of legal medications as compared with misuse of illegal drugs. Many people associate drug dependence treatment only with street drugs, but treatment is essential for anyone with a drug dependency, whether it is for prescription or nonprescription drugs (see Drug Dependency, page 1131).

The abuse of prescription drugs, especially painkillers (see Addiction to Analgesics, page 341) and tranquilizers (see Addiction to Tranquilizers, page 340), is widespread. Frequently, a person is able to maintain a dependence by obtaining prescriptions from multiple physicians.

Many people misuse numerous over-the-counter drugs as well, with negative consequences. The misuse of drugs such as laxatives, for example, can have long-term effects. This form of drug misuse is common among people who have chronic constipation or irregularity. The habitual use of certain kinds of laxatives can, over time, damage the muscular action of the large intestine (colon). The result may be, ironically, a worsening of chronic constipation (see Chronic Constipation, page 784).

Nasal sprays are another example of an over-the-counter drug that can produce a dependence. People who have used a nasal spray for an extended period often find that when they stop using the spray their noses become stuffy sooner and they feel even worse (see Beware: Nose-Drop Addiction, page 587).

Aspirin, cough medicines, laxatives, diet pills, nasal sprays, and numerous other medications can be abused or misused, especially if taken in higher dosages or more frequently than recommended. Read the instructions on the package and follow them. If you find your condition fails to improve, or if you are concerned that you are misusing the drug, consult your physician.

Medication Misuse in the Elderly

Because aging may make older people more sensitive to medications, the elderly may require lower doses to achieve the desired effects and to avoid toxicity or other side effects. Estimates indicate, however, that as many as 1 in 4 drugs taken by the elderly in institutions may be ineffective or unneeded. Compounding the problem, many elderly people use nonprescription drugs without the knowledge of their physician, or mix drugs and alcohol. In addition, some elderly people misuse drugs by taking less than the prescribed dosage in a misguided attempt to reduce expenses (see The Modern Pharmacy, page 1271).

Multiple Drug Use

Perhaps the most common form of drug misuse in the elderly is multiple drug use. This involves taking too many drugs or inappropriately taking drugs that interact with each other.

Elderly persons often have numerous symptoms or illnesses. They may visit a physician each time a new symptom occurs, and all too frequently begin taking another new prescription without sufficient regard to the schedule of medications they're already taking. This pattern can lead to taking numerous medicines, some of which may interact harmfully with others.

Do not expect a medicine for every new symptom. Sometimes a symptom can be resolved by reducing the dose of another medicine or reorganizing the schedule of medications. Also, review all your medicines with your physician on every visit (particularly if a medicine is added) to determine whether you can simplify the schedule.

If you're using multiple drugs, it is not uncommon to get confused and take too little or too much of one or more drugs or experience unwanted side effects from drug interactions. Older people often need assistance in organizing their medication schedule, especially if they have multiple diseases

that require taking several medicines at different times of the day. If you are not taking your medications as prescribed, they may be ineffective or interact to cause severe adverse reactions (see Problems Related to Too Many Medications, page 244).

Beware of Mixing Drugs and Alcohol

In an effort to alleviate some of the age-related problems of loneliness and boredom that many elderly people face, some older people use drugs, such as alcohol, prescription drugs, and even illegal (street) drugs. According to a National Institute of Drug Abuse survey, two-thirds of people older than 65 use prescription drugs, and only cardiovascular medications are used more commonly than are sedatives and tranquilizers. More than half of all the people using tranquilizers and sedatives feel they could not perform their daily activities without these drugs.

If you use sedatives or tranquilizers, take special care not to abuse them. Using these medications along with alcohol can cause harmful interactions. The drugs remain in the body for a much longer time in the elderly and can accumulate to hazardous levels. If you are an older person using one of these drugs, your physician may suggest a dosage lower than that used in younger persons.

Addiction to Tranquilizers

Addiction to tranquilizers, or antianxiety medications, is a major drug problem in this country. Although it is not clear how many people are addicted to tranquilizers, as many as 10,000 emergency room visits a year are related to an addiction to tranquilizers, and every year thousands of people enter drug treatment centers for the same reason. Many of the more than 1.5 million people who each year take tranquilizers on a regular basis for 4 months or more may be addicted.

Inappropriate Use

Part of the problem appears to be that tranquilizers, such as diazepam (Valium), alprazolam (Xanax), and chlordiazepoxide (Librium), all part of a family of drugs named benzodiazepines, are appropriately prescribed for a limited time for nervousness or tension caused by the stress of everyday life or for psychosomatic symptoms (physical symptoms that may be caused by a mental or emotional source). However, many people may then use these drugs too long or at too high a dose. As a general rule, physicians do not treat minor stress and tension with drugs; at most, use of drugs for this purpose is limited to a short period of time. Education in managing the stress of daily living is a better option.

Are Tranquilizers Addicting?

Another issue related to the abuse of benzodiazepines is the mistaken belief that they are not addicting. When they first became available, many people used them because barbiturates, another family of tranquilizing drugs, have a higher risk from overdosage and toxicity. Subsequently, benzodiazepines have been found to have strong addictive potential. In fact, virtually all of the drugs in the benzodiazepine group can cause physical and psychological addiction if used in high doses or over a prolonged time. Even relatively low doses may result in an addiction if taken over a sufficient period. Some people who have taken only the prescribed doses for several months have developed signs of dependence.

What Are the Signs of Addiction?

The most serious signs are withdrawal symptoms that appear if you abruptly stop taking the drug and that quickly disappear if you resume using the drug. These symptoms may start anytime from the first day to several days after you stop taking the drug. They can persist, although probably not with the same intensity, for as long as 7 to 10 days. The symptoms usually include anxiety, restlessness, nausea, loss of appetite, sleeping difficulty, blurred vision, tremors, twitching, or muscle pains. In severe cases, delirium or convulsions may occur.

Mixing Medications

It is never a good idea to take several drugs at the same time without your physician's knowledge. In combination with tranquilizers, some otherwise safe drugs may cause adverse symptoms. For example, the action of some medications may slow the elimination of the tranquilizer from your body, thereby increasing the risk of a toxic buildup. Let your physician know you are taking tranquilizers before he or she prescribes other medications.

Alcohol Interactions

Avoid alcohol when taking tranquilizers. If you drink alcohol while taking tranquilizers, it can cause drowsiness, intoxication, impaired memory, or even death. Taken together, these two depressant drugs cause hundreds of fatal drug overdoses each year.

Addiction to Analgesics

The ideal analgesic (painkiller) would be one that furnishes sufficient pain relief, produces a minimum of side effects, acts promptly and over time with a minimal amount of sedation, prevents any tolerance from developing, and is nonaddicting. Unfortunately, there is no such ideal painkiller.

Individual needs determine the suitability and choice of the most appropriate drug, each of which has advantages and disadvantages. Analgesics can be divided into addictive and nonaddictive types. The first group includes the opiates (and opioids) such as morphine (and methadone). The second group includes nonopioids such as aspirin and acetaminophen.

The strongest painkillers, although not always the most effective, are opiates and opioids. Opiates are narcotic drugs derived from opium. Opioids are synthetic narcotic substances with the same properties. Morphine, a frequently used opiate for treating severe pain, is usually prescribed for only short periods because it is addictive. In the case of terminally ill persons who are in chronic, severe pain, there is no reason to be concerned about the addictive property of morphine or other narcotics. The opiate codeine often is used in combination with other nonnarcotic drugs as a pain reliever and cough suppressant.

People who are most likely to develop an addiction to narcotic analgesics are those who have chronic pain. To help people with chronic pain avoid developing a drug dependency, treatment usually includes other therapies (see Chronic Pain Centers, page 1136).

Symptoms of withdrawal from opiates include diarrhea, elevated respiratory rate and blood pressure, dizziness, nausea, sweating, uncoordinated muscle movements, general weakness, body pain, insomnia, and intense drug craving. The withdrawal symptoms may begin within 4 hours after the last dose, which explains why some addicts awaken from sleep in mild withdrawal.

Street Drugs

The term "street drugs" is used to describe drugs sold illegally—often, these drugs are literally sold on the street. Many people abuse these drugs by using them "recreationally" in an attempt to relax, experience euphoria, enhance sexual activity, or heighten the senses. Some street drugs are used by athletes to try to improve performance.

Whatever their intended use, illegal drugs are extremely hazardous to your health not only because of their nature but also because of the unknown potency and risk of contamination with other dangerous substances. Most of these drugs are also highly addictive. If you are dependent on any of the following drugs, treatment is essential (see Drug Dependency, page 1131).

Marijuana

The most popular illegal drug in America is marijuana. A significant percentage of high school seniors have smoked marijuana, and studies indicate that at least a few of these students smoke it every day.

The hemp plant (*Cannabis sativa*), from which marijuana is derived, contains more than 400 chemicals, including tetrahydrocannabinol (THC). The THC in marijuana is what causes the effect on mood and is probably responsible for the hunger many people experience after using marijuana.

Marijuana cigarettes are made from the leaves and tops of the plant. The amount of THC varies from plant to plant and from cigarette to cigarette. Hashish, a more powerful derivative drug prepared from the resin of the hemp plant, contains far greater concentrations of the psychoactive THC.

If you smoke marijuana, THC is quickly absorbed from your lungs into your bloodstream and rapidly distributed to most tissues and organs of your body. To eliminate THC, your liver converts the substance into waste products (metabolites). Most of these metabolites are excreted through the feces and urine. The rate at which they are cleared from your body is slower than that of many other psychoactive drugs. If you smoke marijuana regularly and then stop, THC can be found in your urine for more than 4 weeks after use.

The effects of marijuana are almost immediate, especially if you smoke it. Your pulse quickens by as much as 50 percent, depending on the potency of the marijuana. People with a poor blood supply to the heart may have chest pains.

Most people experience a feeling of relaxation and mild euphoria. Some first-time users undergo an acute panic reaction in which they feel they are losing control. This panic usually subsides within a few hours. Depending on the level of intoxication, some people have trouble remembering events that happened while "high" and experience difficulty in performing functions that require concentration, rapid reactions, and physical coordination. High doses of marijuana may produce many of the same behavioral effects as severe alcohol intoxication. Although the high may subside, many of the negative effects may linger for up to 6 hours after you smoke marijuana.

Chronic marijuana smokers show evidence of decreased lung capacity and chronic bronchial irritation. Marijuana also may contain the fungus *Aspergillus*. Studies suggest that serious lung infections may result from inhaling this organism. Because chronic marijuana smoking may impair your body's immune system, your lungs may be more susceptible to this and other infections.

Regular daily marijuana smokers often inhale the smoke deeply and retain it in their lungs as long as possible to increase their "high." This practice also increases the risk of damage to the lungs.

Marijuana is occasionally contaminated by animal droppings containing *Salmonella* bacteria either at the time of drying or during storage. This organism, which is not destroyed by drying, can cause diarrhea, abdominal pain, and fever (see page 767).

A herbicide called paraquat, widely used by the government to destroy marijuana plants, poses another kind of health hazard. If plants sprayed with paraquat are harvested before exposure to sunlight, unaltered paraquat remains on the leaves. This herbicide is highly toxic to humans and can irreversibly damage your lungs.

Clinical testing suggests that marijuana may negatively affect your reproductive system, possibly causing irregular menstrual cycles in women and a temporary loss of fertility in both men and women. Some studies have suggested that there may be a significant relationship between use of marijuana during pregnancy and premature birth (see Pregnancy and Drug Use, page 336).

Depending on the length of use and the potency of the marijuana you use, you may experience withdrawal symptoms when you discontinue using it. Some of the mild or moderate symptoms include tremors, sweating, nausea, vomiting, diarrhea, irritability, and sleep disturbances. However, these withdrawal symptoms are less severe than those heavy users of opiate or alcohol experience.

Although often misunderstood and misrepresented to the public, marijuana is a drug of dependence. Regular use often results in the same type of drug dependence described for other substances (see page 1134).

Cocaine

Cocaine was once referred to as the champagne of drugs, in part because it was an expensive drug preferred by the well-to-do. Today, it is one of the most widely used illegal drugs in this country. Cocaine is eagerly sought by drug users because it creates a sense of euphoria. These effects are the basis of the profound psychological dependence associated with the drug.

Cocaine dilates your pupils and accelerates your heart and respiratory rates. It also causes a slight rise in body temperature. These effects are mostly short-term. They reach their peak about 15 to 20 minutes after you inhale the drug through your nose (snort it) in the form of a powder, and they dissipate in approximately 1 hour. Unwanted effects of chronic use of cocaine are a persistent restlessness, anxiety, and sleeplessness.

Another problem associated with inhaling cocaine is a mildly stuffy or runny nose. Long-term use can cause ulcers on the mucous membranes of your nose and may even cause a hole (perforation) in your nasal septum. In addition, people who chronically abuse cocaine may develop paranoid hallucinations, called cocaine psychosis, that may involve the sense of smell, taste, touch, or sight.

Smoking (free-basing) cocaine creates a faster and more intense high. In this form, the drug can cause confusion, slurred speech,

and anxiety. Crack cocaine is also smoked and has essentially the same effect as free-base cocaine. Both forms are extremely addictive.

Crack is aptly named because it produces an intense high in a matter of seconds. Within a few minutes, a profound low follows, usually leaving the chronic abuser despondent and desperate for more.

Short-term physical effects of crack are increased heart rate and increased blood pressure. Cocaine can overwork your heart, forcing it to beat too fast and too powerfully. As your heart tires, it becomes susceptible to irregularities in its normal rhythm which can cause it to stop.

Cocaine can also induce coronary artery spasm—a sudden narrowing of the arteries leading to your heart. Such spasms can cause a blood clot to form, even in otherwise normal arteries. If the spasm of clot completely blocks the flow of blood to your heart, it can cause a heart attack, dangerous heartbeat irregularities, or sudden death.

Injecting cocaine by means of shared needles increases the risk of exposure to AIDS and other communicable diseases that are passed by sharing nonsterile needles or solutions that are contaminated (see Central Nervous System Stimulants, page 1132). If you have never tried cocaine, remember—your first "experiment" could be your last!

Hallucinogens

Hallucinogenic drugs were widely used in the 1960s and early 1970s. The popularity of such drugs diminished during the next 20 years. Some observers report that there may be a renewed interest today in the use of hallucinogens, especially lysergic acid diethylamide (LSD).

Hallucinogens were popular because they produced a vivid perception of changes in sensation, depth perception, passage of time, and body image. Some experimenters reported experiencing a mixing of the senses; under the influence of LSD, one could seemingly "hear" colors or "see" sounds.

LSD also can cause powerful negative experiences, referred to as "bad trips," in which there is an overwhelming sense of fear, perhaps of being abandoned, going insane, or dying. In some instances, abusers have had no comprehension of their limitations and have died because they tried to fly out of windows or walk on water.

An effect of hallucinogenic drugs is the production of sustained altered mental states that can last for 8 hours or more. Flashbacks also may occur days or weeks after the conclusion of the initial "trip," in which the user reexperiences previous effects even though he or she has not ingested any more of the drug.

LSD and other psychedelics, such as mescaline, increase heart rate and blood pressure, dilate pupils, and cause loss of appetite, sleeplessness, and tremors. Death from overdose is also possible.

It is not yet known whether all of the symptoms dissipate after LSD is no longer ingested. Heavy long-term use of hallucinogens, however, is known to cause impaired memory, abbreviated attention span, and a difficulty with abstract thinking (see Hallucinogens, page 1134).

Phencyclidine (PCP)

This powerful hallucinogen, sometimes referred to as "angel dust," was once used by veterinarians to sedate large animals. But the drug so disturbed and bewildered the animals before it put them to sleep that veterinarians abandoned its use. From this use, however, came other street names for the drug, such as "hog" and "horse tranquilizer."

In contrast to its effect in animals, PCP taken in very small doses by humans causes a loss of inhibition and induces a state of general euphoria. Other physical symptoms are increased heart rate and blood pressure, sweating, flushing of the skin, and an increase in body temperature. It also may cause some unsteadiness. But what makes the drug so dangerous is its unpredictability.

Almost any dose may result in destructive, violent behavior. When users have turned violent or acted in bizarre ways, they have been known to lose all control. Other symptoms include muscle rigidity, loss of concentration, vision disturbances, speech impairment, convulsions and delirium, fear of isolation, and paranoia. PCP also can lead to heart and lung failure or a stroke. It has been known to induce a toxic psychosis that resembles schizophrenia (see Hallucinogens, page 1134).

Inhalants

Some people inhale various substances that can give them a high, many of which do not require a prescription. One common inhalant that does require a prescription is called amyl nitrite. This drug is a vasodilator that relaxes smooth muscle in small blood vessels, causing them to expand and lower blood pressure. It is usually prescribed for treating angina pectoris (see page 657). But people inhale amyl nitrite, or "poppers" as they are sometimes called, because it produces an intense and immediate high and seems to intensify orgasm during sex. The effects are short-lived, lasting only minutes.

Amyl nitrite is not physically addictive, but it is not free of side effects. Users suffer headaches, dizziness, accelerated heart rate, nasal irritation, and coughing. The headaches seem to be the one side effect that can persist long after use.

Other substances people inhale that do not require a prescription include a category of volatile inhalants, sold as room deodorizers. These generally contain butyl and isobutyl nitrite. Butyl nitrite is also thought to intensify a sexual experience. Other inhalants that some young people use are solvents such as Freon (trichlorofluoromethane), other halogenated hydrocarbons (for example, trichloroethylene), esters (for example, ethyl, amyl, and butyl acetates), and aromatic hydrocarbons (for example, benzene).

The physical risks from inhaling these solvents range from cardiac arrhythmia with use of Freon and trichloroethylene to liver and kidney impairment with use of aromatic hydrocarbons and ethyl acetate.

Opiates

Heroin, methadone, morphine, and opium all are considered opiates. They are derived from the opium poppy. Generally, opiates are prescribed to relieve severe pain, but they are often obtained illegally. Given in low doses over short periods, they are not addictive, but in large doses given over time, these drugs are highly addictive.

Side effects include decreased respiration and drop in blood pressure (in high dosages), dizziness, nausea, sweating, uncoordinated muscle movement, general weakness, and euphoria. Heavy use also will depress your sex drive.

When the drug is injected using a shared needle, users sometimes acquire diseases or disorders such as AIDS, hepatitis, blood poisoning, congested lungs, and pneumonia. When the drug is taken with other sedatives, death can result (see Opioids, page 1133).

Drugs and Sports Performance

When you exercise, your nervous system is naturally aroused. Your stimulated nervous system boosts production of hormones, including adrenaline (epinephrine). These hormones increase the amount of blood your heart pumps, resulting in more blood for muscles and a release of sugar (glucose) from the liver and of fatty acids from body fat to serve as fuel for the muscles.

These effects are important to anyone who is exercising. The increased blood flow ensures that your muscles receive a constant supply of oxygen and nutrients, and potentially toxic waste products produced by the accelerated metabolism are more quickly removed.

Some athletes use drugs obtained illegally solely in an attempt to improve their physical abilities and performance. Such risky practices that may give an athlete an unfair advantage are called "doping." The abuse of anabolic steroids and other drugs by athletes is now often front-page news. The problem is international in scope, involving professional and amateur athletes who participate in a wide range of sports.

This elevated level of awareness of the problem has led to more drug testing. Some athletes who require a drug for a medical disorder are even banned from using that drug during competition, because it may artificially boost performance. The result is that today there are two important reasons for an athlete not to get his or her "competitive edge" from anabolic steroids or other medications. First, these drugs can put your future as an athlete at risk because of the bans and penalties now meted out to offenders. Second, and even more important, these drugs might put your health at risk. The unapproved use of any medications, including those described here, has no place in sports or any activity.

Anabolic Steroids
A group of drugs some athletes use illegally are androgenic-anabolic steroids. The name of this group of drugs comes from three Greek words: *andro* and *gennan*, which mean "male-producing," and *anabol*, which means "to build up." Because these drugs are closely related chemically to natural male hormones, anabolic steroids mimic the effects of the male sex hormone testosterone. Athletes have used these drugs illegally because they stimulate the buildup of muscle tissue.

Anabolic steroids have several legitimate medical uses. They may be used to treat skeletal and growth disorders and certain types of anemia as well as to offset the negative effect of irradiation and chemotherapy.

Whether you take them in large or moderate doses over a prolonged period, anabolic steroids have many potentially serious side effects, especially on the liver, cardiovascular system, and reproductive system.

Liver
An overload of anabolic steroids can cause liver damage to the point of jaundice and even liver failure. Another potential liver problem from anabolic steroid use is peliosis hepatis. In this instance the liver develops blood-filled cysts that can rupture. Liver failure can result. There is also the potential for liver tumors forming as a result of anabolic steroid use.

Cardiovascular System
Use of anabolic steroids has been linked to an increase in several risk factors leading to the development of cardiovascular disease. These include decreased blood concentrations of HDL (the "good" cholesterol; see Atherosclerosis: What Is It? page 636) and an increase in blood pressure. Animal research has shown that use of anabolic steroids also can lead to damage of the heart.

Reproductive System
Anabolic steroids can reduce sperm production, decrease the size of the testicles, and reduce the amount of sex hormones produced, resulting in a diminished sex drive. Among female athletes, these drugs have reduced the production of female sex hormones (both estrogen and progesterone), inhibited development of eggs and ovulation, and disrupted the menstrual cycle. All of these changes are reversible when use of anabolic steroids is discontinued. Female athletes, however, sometimes find that male secondary sex characteristics, such as an increase in facial hair or a deepening of the

voice, remain after they stop using anabolic steroids.

Other undesirable effects associated with abuse of anabolic steroids include a reduction of breast size in women and changes in overall hair growth patterns in both men and women, an increased thinning of hair or hair that falls out, and acne. Another concern is the effect the drug has on behavior, which may result in increased aggressiveness.

Sympathomimetic Amines

Some professional and world-class athletes have admitted using sympathomimetic amines, a class of stimulant drugs that mimic the natural effects of a stimulated sympathetic nervous system. These drugs can increase alertness and physical endurance as well as postpone the onset of fatigue.

This class of drugs includes ephedrine and its derivatives (pseudoephedrine and phenylpropanolamine), which are often present in cold and hay fever preparations as decongestants. Ephedrine is also a common ingredient of asthma medications. Athletes who have asthma and have used ephedrine to prevent asthma during competition have been disqualified. These drugs have been banned by most athletic organizations including the International Olympic Committee.

Psychomotor Stimulant Drugs

Athletes also have been disqualified for using psychomotor stimulant drugs. The drugs in this category that are most often abused are amphetamines (namely, amphetamine, dextroamphetamine, and methamphetamine) and methylphenidate hydrochloride (Ritalin).

Amphetamines have a limited role in medicine, especially in the treatment of hyperactive children (see Hyperactivity, page 133) and of narcolepsy (see page 1114). But their unprescribed use is illegal. The most common street name for these drugs is speed. Other slang names include bennies, dexies, greenies, and pep pills. Amphetamines are usually taken orally, but chronic abusers often prefer to inject the drug because it produces a more immediate and stronger effect.

The effects of psychomotor stimulants are not unlike those of sympathomimetic amines. They increase heart rate, respiration, and blood pressure and generally heighten the activity of the sympathetic nervous system. These drugs also affect the brain so that the athlete feels more alert, confident, and perhaps even euphoric. Consequently, psychomotor stimulants may lead to an improved athletic performance, more through their psychological than their physical effects. However, apart from increasing endurance, the benefits of these stimulants on athletic performance are limited or even negative.

In addition to the dangers of a physical and psychological addiction, these stimulants also generate many adverse physical and psychological reactions such as insomnia, dizziness, tremors, heart palpitations, irregular heartbeat, sexual impotence, and possibly amphetamine psychosis. Deaths have resulted even when normal doses have been used under conditions of maximal physical activity.

Beta$_2$-Agonists

These medications often are used to treat asthma and other respiratory ailments. Like ephedrine, they can have stimulant properties. Currently they are banned in athletic competition when taken orally, but their use is permitted in aerosol or inhalant forms. Examples of these medications include metaproterenol (Alupent and Metaprel), salbutamol or albuterol (Ventolin and Proventil), and terbutaline (Brethaire).

Narcotic Analgesics

Narcotic analgesics (painkillers) may produce a sensation of euphoria or psychological stimulation. They also may increase the pain threshold so that an athlete may fail to recognize injury, leading to more serious damage. These drugs have been banned by the International Olympic Committee.

Nonnarcotic analgesics, however, such as aspirin or the nonsteroidal anti-inflammatory drugs have good analgesic and anti-inflammatory actions and are useful in treating minor injuries. These drugs are not banned. Be careful that you do not use a narcotic such as codeine in combination with another medicine such as aspirin.

Beta Blockers

These are drugs commonly used in cardiovascular disease to lower blood pressure and decrease heart rate. Beta blockers also block stimulatory responses. Thus, athletes have used them in sports such as shooting to steady the trigger finger and to relax the nerves. Use of these drugs is considered doping and is banned.

Growth Hormone

Use of this hormone is considered doping by the U.S. Olympic Committee and is prohibited.

Diuretics

Diuretics increase the elimination of fluid from the body as urine. Athletes sometimes misuse them to reduce weight quickly in sports such as wrestling in which strict weight classifications are involved. Some athletes have also used diuretics to reduce the concentration of drugs in their urine so that illegal drugs are not detected. Using diuretics can affect the balance of such minerals as potassium and sodium in your body and can cause, among other things, heart arrhythmias and even death.

Corticosteroids

The International Olympic Committee also bans the use of corticosteroids if taken by mouth or injected into a muscle or a vein. Athletes can use these drugs topically (in the ear, eye, or skin), in local or intra-articular injections such as for bursitis, or in inhalation therapy for disorders such as asthma (see Corticosteroid Drugs, page 919).

Chapter 15

Safety

Contents

The Safer Way, 350

Home Safe Home, 350
Fire Prevention, 350
    Beware of Fireworks, 351
Preventing Poisonings, 351
    Label All Poisons, 352
Childproofing Your Home, 352
Household Safety: A Checklist, 353
    Microwave Oven Safety, 354
    Herbal Supplements: Natural Doesn't
    Mean Safe, 355
Guns in Your Home, 356

Safety Outside the Home, 356
Safety on the Road, 356
    Basic Bicycling Safety, 357
Hotel Fire Safety, 357
Safety in the Workplace, 358
    VDTs: Sensible Precautions, 359
Safety on the Farm, 359
Safety While Hiking and Camping, 360
Water and Boating Safety, 361
Safety and the Elements, 361

The Safer Way

Today, a great deal of time, money, research, and personal effort are being invested in prevention of disease. Perhaps you, like millions of others, are increasingly conscious of improving your diet, getting proper exercise, and using other methods to help ensure the continued good health of you and your family.

All too often, however, we overlook the more obvious risks that confront us daily. Nearly 1 in every 20 deaths in the United States results from accidents. Accidents are the most common cause of death in persons younger than 35. Half of all childhood deaths are due to accidents. On the highway, in the workplace, and at home, accidents injure or disable tens of millions of Americans annually. Many of these accidents could be avoided.

In the following pages, we offer various safety tips. This information is not comprehensive, but it may alert you to other potentially dangerous circumstances in your everyday life and during leisure activities.

Home Safe Home

Every year, tens of thousands of Americans die of injuries sustained in their own homes. Many of these accidents could be prevented by taking simple measures toward fire prevention, childproofing, firearm safety, and commonsense safety.

Fire Prevention

Fire is a leading cause of death and injury at home, not to mention an expensive cause of property damage. Most fires in homes result from carelessness and can be prevented with a few simple precautions and a little common sense. Here are steps you can take to decrease the risks of personal injury and property damage from fires in your home.

Install Smoke Detectors
Smoke detectors are invaluable safety devices. Every home should be equipped with them. Locate your smoke detectors on the ceiling in the sleeping areas of your home and the areas where fires are most likely to start (the kitchen or garage). Have a detector on each level and in each bedroom area of your home.

Place the smoke detector at least 6 inches from where the wall joins the ceiling (the dead air space in a corner could prevent smoke from reaching the detector immediately). Keep the detector away from shower areas because steam can set off a detector.

Test your smoke detector monthly to make sure the batteries are good. Change batteries annually. If your smoke detectors are wired to your home electrical system, make sure they have backup batteries.

Keep a Fire Extinguisher on Hand
Have a fire extinguisher and fire blanket in the kitchen; if you have a garage, have another set there, too. Be sure family members are familiar with the operation of the extinguishers. Check annually.

Establish Escape Routes
Be sure there are adequate escape routes. If needed, purchase fire ladders or other means of escape from upstairs windows. Rehearse with your family procedures to follow in the event of fire. Designate a family meeting place so you can make sure everyone is accounted for. Keep stairways and halls uncluttered. Never padlock an exit door.

Beware of Wood and Coal Stoves and Other Space Heaters
Be sure that the area around an open-flame space heater in your home is properly fireproofed. Building codes vary, but for most space heaters the walls around them must be a specified distance from the stove or insulated with a fireproof material. The floor beneath and in front also must be insulated with a nonflammable material.

Keep kerosene or other freestanding

heaters out of frequently used traffic paths in your home and away from hallways and stairways in particular. Many fires are started when such heaters are knocked over, spilling fuel and igniting nearby furniture and surfaces.

Maintain Electrical Equipment

Make sure that the wiring in your home is up-to-date and in good order. If it is not, hire a qualified electrician to make the necessary repairs.

Do not overload wall outlets with adapters. Never increase the size of a fuse or circuit breaker as a means to sustain service of a line that is overloaded. If you do not increase the capacity of the wire in the line itself, it could heat up and start an electrical fire in the walls of your home.

Do not run extension cords across floors or under rugs or carpets. You can easily trip over exposed extension cords (especially at night). Over time, the wear and tear on a cord beneath a carpet can damage the insulation and lead to overheating and a fire hazard.

Keep Fireplaces and Chimneys Clean

Use a screen in front of your fireplace to prevent sparks from jumping out of the firebox. Never leave an open fire unattended.

Clean your chimney regularly. If you vent a woodstove into your chimney, clean the chimney twice a year. If a wood fire in your fireplace is only an occasional event, an every-other-year chimney cleaning may be sufficient.

If you use your fireplace or wood-burning stove at all, however, have your chimney inspected for a buildup of creosote (a flammable resin that is a by-product of wood fires). Be sure that the chimney lining is intact. Do not postpone chimney repairs. Keep a chimney fire extinguisher on hand.

Never Smoke in Bed

Careless smoking leads to the greatest number of deaths by fire in the United States. Keep cigarettes, cigars, or pipes out of your bedroom. When disposing of butts and ashes, be sure no embers remain.

Remove Flammable Materials

Dispose of rags or papers contaminated with paint remover or other chemicals immediately; spontaneous combustion can occur, producing dangerous fumes and fire.

Beware of Fireworks

The brilliant illumination and resounding bangs and pops of fireworks provide thrills and excitement for young and old. But to avoid being an injury statistic, take care when using fireworks. Remember, one of every three fire-related injuries is caused by fireworks.

The Risks

When stored in your home, fireworks are a potential fire hazard. When put to use, they are even more dangerous. The potential risks include vision and hearing loss (about 1,000 people annually sustain permanent eye injuries from fireworks). Fingers and hands are often burned by carelessly used fireworks, which ignite at temperatures up to 1,000 degrees Fahrenheit. Hearing loss is a common fireworks-related injury.

Preventing Problems

The most important advice we can give is this: be familiar with and obey laws that govern the purchase and use of fireworks in your state.

Use fireworks outdoors only, and in an open area. Stay a discrete distance from them after they are lit. Locate fireworks on level ground.

Allow no horseplay. These devices are especially dangerous if tossed at a person or pet.

Never relight a dud. Douse it with water and discard it. Do not explode fireworks in a bottle, tin can, or clay pot, and never tamper with or disassemble fireworks.

Have a pail of water or hose on hand to douse the fireworks area when you're finished.

Store newspapers, other paper refuse, and any flammable trash away from heat sources. Locate paints and other household chemicals on a shelf that is both out of reach of children and away from any risk of exposure to sparks or heat. Store matches out of reach of children.

Preventing Poisonings

Small children are at special risk of poisoning: their curiosity is boundless and their bodies are small enough that relatively little poison can be harmful. Also, most small children put whatever they find into their mouths.

Keep Poisons Out of Reach

Seemingly innocent products such as shoe polish, nail polish, and nail polish remover can be hazardous. Make it a rule in your home that all hazardous items are to be kept

Label All Poisons

If you store any poison in a container other than the one in which it was originally packaged, be sure to label the can or bottle clearly. The word "POISON" should be prominently printed. Never use baby food bottles or other familiar food containers to store poisons. Young children are likely to assume they contain food and may help themselves.

in high cupboards, on tall shelves in closets, or in locked cabinets. Designate such an area in your kitchen or utility room for household cleaners, another in your garage for garden or automotive poisons, and another in your bathroom. Garden sheds, cellars, and other areas where such goods are stored require similar precautions.

Household Goods

Here is a sampling of common, potentially dangerous household poisons: alcohol of all kinds; virtually all cleaning products, especially those that contain chlorine bleach, ammonia, and detergents; toilet and drain cleaners (the latter often contain lye); cosmetics; paint and paint products such as turpentine and paint thinner; and furniture and floor polishes.

Garden and Garage Aids

Many of us use chemicals to control pests in or around our homes. Roach powders, rat pellets, rose dust, and other home, yard, and farm chemicals are common and, when used as directed, quite safe. However, when swallowed, virtually all are dangerous poisons, as are fuels and oils (including gasoline and kerosene); weed killers; flower, garden, and shrub sprays; and roach, rat, and other poisons.

Medications

Aspirin, acetaminophen, prescription medications, cough medicine, cold pills, and all other drugs can also pose a danger.

(For more information on preventing or dealing with poisonings, see page 437.)

Childproofing Your Home

Accidents are the leading cause of death among children. Indeed, about one of every two children who die does so because of an accident.

Making your home safe for youngsters is an important priority, whether your child is very young and has no sense of danger or is old enough to experiment deliberately with the hazards of your home.

Protecting Your Baby

Today, beds for babies must meet federal standards. Space between crib bars can be no more than 2⅜ inches. This prevents infants from getting their heads stuck between the bars. If you are using an old crib, make certain that the bars are spaced in accordance with the specifications given here.

The crib should have no sharp edges. A locking mechanism should keep the sides up. The distance from the top of the rail to the mattress should be at least 26 inches when the mattress is at its lowest level. The mattress should fit snugly. Use bumper pads to prevent your baby from banging against the sides. A pillow is unnecessary and should not be used.

Check for lead-based paint. One potential danger of an old crib is that it may be painted with a lead-based paint. Infants sometimes chew the slats of their cribs and, if consumed, lead-based paint is poisonous. Make sure that your crib does not have lead-based paint.

Keep plastic bags away from your infant. Young children can suffocate while playing with such bags.

Select blankets and pajamas that are fireproof.

Fasten mobiles securely. If there is a mobile over the crib, make sure that it is firmly secured and positioned well above the crib. If your child can reach the mobile, remove the mobile.

Select toys carefully. Toys in the crib should be large and soft, with no sharp edges that can hurt your baby. Avoid stuffed animals or other toys with buttons or parts that can be swallowed.

Remember that every moment of the day, you are your child's protector. Be alert for hazards until your child learns safety rules (see Safety, page 71).

When Your Child Begins to Crawl

Before your baby reaches 6 months of age, childproof your home. This gives you a chance to practice safety measures before your child becomes mobile. Protect your infant not only from risks within immediate reach but also from hazards to which your baby might crawl or climb. Remember that almost overnight, your child's universe will expand from a crib, baby seat, and playpen to the entire house (see Safety, page 71).

Place gates at the tops and bottoms of staircases in your home. Make sure to lock or guard windows that may be accessible to your child. If your child is younger than 6, he or she should not be in the top bunk of a bunk bed. Make sure your bunk bed has sturdy safety rails.

Electrical outlets are often a target of curiosity, so cover unused ones; inexpensive plug covers are available at most hardware stores.

Young children are forever experimenting, putting into their mouths whatever comes to hand. Keep substances that can hurt children (such as cleaning solutions, insecticides, and medications) stored well out of their reach. You may need to buy fixtures that make it difficult for a child to open lower cabinets.

Never store toxic substances in the "wrong" container. For example, if you store paint thinner in a juice bottle, your child may take a drink, thinking it is juice.

Identify toxic plants in and around your home. Keep them well out of reach of your baby (see Garden-Variety Poisonous Plants, page 440).

Keep matches out of your child's reach. In the kitchen, keep pot handles pointed toward the back of the stove. Do not use cloths or mats that your child can pull off the kitchen or dining room tables. Never leave a hot beverage near the edge of a table. Your child might pull the beverage off. Do not drink hot beverages with your child on your lap.

Keep the thermostat on your hot-water heater between 120 and 125 degrees Fahrenheit. At 160 degrees Fahrenheit, a child can quickly scald himself or herself.

In the bathroom, keep toilet seats covered. Use no-slip tub mats. Never leave your infant unattended in the bathtub, no matter how little water is present.

At Play

In laying out an outdoor play area for your child, locate it so that you can monitor activities from inside your home. Position equipment on grass, sand, or other soft surfaces to reduce the risk of injury from inevitable falls. Anchor the equipment below the ground to prevent it from tipping.

Make sure that the equipment is safe and in good condition. Plane or sand rough wood to prevent slivers; file metal burrs smooth to avoid scrapes. Discard equipment that is fragile or worn out.

Establish rules: one person on the swing at a time, hold on with both hands, no standing or kneeling allowed.

At the playground—whether it is a public facility or in your backyard—supervise your young child's activity constantly.

Household Safety: A Checklist

There is no such thing as an accident-free home. Accidents happen even to the most conscientious and careful people. However, you can decrease your risk of accident and injury at home. Some suggestions are given here.

Kitchen

Clean up spills promptly. Water, foods, or other substances on a hard-surfaced floor can cause slips, falls, and injury.

Use a step stool to reach high shelves; do not stand on a chair or countertop.

Keep your kitchen knives stored out of the reach of children, perhaps on a wall rack. When using them, hold the food you are cutting with your hand curled, not with your fingers extended.

Position pot and pan handles toward the back of the stove or counter. If they protrude over the front, a careless movement or a curious child could spill hot liquids or foods and cause burns. Always use a potholder or insulated gloves when handling heated pots, pans, trays, or other food containers.

Be careful to keep grease and drippings away from open flames. Keep curtains away from the stove.

In case of a small kitchen fire, use salt or baking soda to extinguish the flames. Do not throw water on them. Keep a fire extinguisher on hand for more serious fires.

Unplug appliances that are not in use—in particular, irons, toasters, and food processors. Before inserting tools into a toaster, be sure it is unplugged. Before washing or cleaning any electrical device, unplug it.

Iron clothes on a well-balanced, sturdy surface covered with a fireproof material. Never leave a hot iron unattended.

Never leave small children alone in your kitchen.

Microwave Oven Safety

Are microwave ovens safe to use in your home? Yes they are, so long as they are well maintained and used properly. The risk from microwave radiation itself is small. But shocks, fires, and burns can result from improper or careless use of your microwave oven.

Electrical shock perhaps is the most common danger. Be sure your oven is properly installed and grounded. Periodically examine the electrical cord to be sure it is in good repair.

Fire can occur when food placed on paper or plastic becomes overheated.

An explosion can occur if you use glass containers not designed for your microwave oven. Be sure that dishes are designed for use in your microwave.

Burns can also occur. If you cover food containers to help hold in moisture (plastic wrap is commonly used for this purpose), beware of steam. During the heating process, steam can build up. When you remove the covering, a gush of steam can leave you with a serious and painful burn. Therefore, for safety's sake, remove such covers carefully with a long-handled wooden spoon.

Microwaves heat your food, but your dishes may remain cool. Nevertheless, use a hot pad to take containers out of your microwave oven. Be careful with the first few bites. You may be lulled into a false sense of confidence by a dish that is not hot to the touch. Also, foods may be heated unevenly.

Baby bottles warmed in a microwave oven present the same danger: always test the milk temperature to prevent burning your baby's mouth.

Finally, there is some risk of microwave radiation if the door, seal, or hinges are damaged. If you suspect any such damage, consult a qualified service person.

Keep matches out of reach.

Store cleaning fluids and other chemicals in a high or locked cabinet.

Make it a habit to keep drawers and cupboards closed.

Be sure that all poisons are safely stored and clearly marked.

Living Room

If you have a fireplace, use a fire screen to prevent sparks from flying into the room.

Make sure no electrical cords cross the room. They can trip you or, if worn, can cause a fire.

If you have a humidifier to moisten the air in your home, wash the water reservoir thoroughly on a regular schedule (at least once every 2 weeks during the heating season and when it is emptied for the summer). Bacteria and fungi can grow in such moist environments and create a health hazard for you and your family. Fungicide tablets are available to help prevent this.

Bathroom

Never turn electrical switches on or off while you are in the bathtub or shower or standing on a damp floor. Do not use electrical appliances such as hair dryers or electric shavers when you are wet or in the shower or bathtub. Electrical shock or death from electrocution can result. Change all conventional bathroom outlets to ground-fault outlets. Building codes in many states require them in new construction.

Use nonslip mats in and adjacent to the shower or bathtub to prevent slips and falls. Grab rails also can prevent falls.

Never leave your baby or young child alone in the tub. He or she can drown in only a small amount of water.

Install a night-light in or adjacent to the bathroom.

Keep all medicines safely out of the reach of children.

Avoid discarding razor blades, hypodermic needles (for insulin or other shots), or other potentially dangerous items into wastebaskets to which your child has access. Flush expired medications down the toilet.

Bedroom

Have a lamp within reach on your bedside table. Keep your glasses at hand, too. A telephone within reach may be useful in an emergency, especially if you have a heart problem or other potentially debilitating chronic ailment. A special communication system also may be appropriate.

If young children visit your home, keep medications securely out of reach. For your own safety, and to avoid confusion, keep no more than one medication at your bedside.

Keep house keys on your bedside table or in an easy-to-reach, familiar place. Shoes and robe, too, should be easily available in the event you must leave quickly (such as in case of fire). This is also good practice when staying in a hotel or motel.

Never smoke in bed. Smoking in bed is particularly hazardous after drinking alcohol or when you are tired.

Unplug heating pads or electric blankets when they are not in use.

Entrance and Stairway

All stairs should be in good repair; replace

broken or cracked stairs outside and within your home.

Fasten carpeting on stairs securely.

Every stairway should have a sturdy railing.

Stairway and entryway lighting is very important: if the light is not bright enough for reading, improve the lighting. Place a switch at the bottom and top of each set of stairs.

To help prevent falls, never leave objects on stairs. Do not wax stairways or stair landings. Falls are of special concern to the elderly (see How to Avoid Falls, page 240).

Basement, Garage, and Utility Room

Proper lighting is essential. Install appropriate lighting fixtures near the washing machine and dryer, workbench, and entrance areas.

Have your washing machine and dryer installed and serviced by a qualified electrician or technician. Follow factory instructions for use. Make sure that your dryer is vented. Both machines should be grounded; the area must not be damp or have standing water.

Keep cleaning fluids, paints and additives, and fuels and oils labeled and well out of the reach of children. Never reuse food containers to store toxic liquids; your child might take a sip out of a pop bottle that now contains paint thinner or some other poison.

If you have a workshop, keep it neat and organized. Wood shavings on the floor are a potential fire hazard. A clutter of tools and materials can result in falling or stumbling, doubly dangerous events in the presence of tools.

Wear proper attire when working. Safety glasses, earplugs, and protective clothing (including work shoes or boots) may help you avoid injury. Never wear a scarf or a shirt with sleeves that can become entangled in power tools.

Do not allow children to handle tools until they are old enough to understand and obey instructions regarding safe use. Limit use of most power tools to people older than 18. Keep tools in good repair with blades sharp, cords intact, and guards in working order.

Place a fire extinguisher in the basement, workshop, or utility room. Check it periodically to make sure it is fully charged. Be familiar with instructions for its use.

Herbal Supplements: Natural Doesn't Mean Safe

Americans spend almost $700 million a year on herbal remedies, yet there's scanty proof they actually help you. Worse, scientists know little about the ingredients in some products.

Many of today's pharmaceuticals originated from plants. Yet, what separates these from herbal supplements sold in health food stores is careful scientific study. Many herbs are sold in drug-like formulas and potencies, but the Food and Drug Administration (FDA) hasn't evaluated them for safety and effectiveness.

Known Hazards

Avoid these supplements, which can have serious side effects:

- Comfrey, Borage, and Coltsfoot. Toxic chemicals in these herbs may cause liver disease.
- Chaparral. Several cases of liver disease have been linked to the use of this medicinal herb. No evidence supports the claims that it cures cancer, slows aging, "cleanses" the blood, or helps treat skin problems.

- Ma huang. Not only is this herb ineffective for helping you lose weight, as claimed, but it can cause a dangerous increase in blood pressure. It's particularly unsafe if you have heart disease, diabetes, or thyroid disease.
- Germanium. This substance has no properties of a food or nutrient, yet it's claimed to promote overall health and neutralize heavy metal toxicity. Long-term use may lead to kidney damage and death.
- Yohimbine. Used to enhance sexual performance, this supplement has side effects that include tremors, anxiety, high blood pressure, and rapid heart rate.

A Game of Russian Roulette

When you take an herbal supplement, you do so at your own risk. At a minimum, use these precautions:

- Don't self-treat serious illnesses such as heart disease, cancer, or arthritis.
- To avoid interactions with other medications, tell your physician about all supplements you take.
- Don't give herbal supplements to children.

Guns in Your Home

If you have a rifle or shotgun for sporting purposes, make sure that it is stored without ammunition and in a locked storage cabinet.

We do not recommend the use of handguns or any other potentially lethal weapons for the purpose of home security. If you decide to keep a weapon for security reasons, be sure it is stored out of the reach of children.

Maintain the weapon carefully. Periodically, remove it from its place of storage and make sure that it is clean and working properly. Reacquaint yourself with the weapon's safety and with loading and unloading procedures.

Safety Outside the Home

More accidents occur in the home than anywhere else; not far behind, however, are accidents in the workplace, on the highway, and during recreation. Consider the following recommendations for safer practices while traveling, at work, and at play.

Safety on the Road

Approximately 50,000 people die on our roads and highways every year. Many more are severely injured. This terrible toll is more often the result of alcohol or carelessness than it is of mechanical failure. To help ensure your safety, follow these suggestions.

Always Wear a Seat Belt

Seat belts save lives. Wear one every time you get into a car, even if you are traveling only a short distance. Make sure your passengers wear seat belts, too. Most accidents occur within a few miles of home.

Car Seats

In most states, children who weigh less than 40 pounds must ride in specially designed car seats. Even if your state does not have this law, buckle up your baby or young child when traveling by car—always.

Infant safety seats are designed for babies weighing less than 20 pounds. This type of seat is installed so that your baby faces the rear of your car. The baby seat can be placed on a back or front seat. Many parents, initially at least, put the seat in front. This enables mom or dad to observe the baby while driving. A convertible seat can be used from birth until the child weighs approximately 40 pounds. This seat can be converted from the reclining, backward position (for an infant) to an upright and forward position (to accommodate a heavier child). Also, do not use the car's shoulder harnesses for children who weigh less than 40 pounds. If worn by small children, shoulder harnesses can be hazardous.

When you begin shopping for a safety seat, look for one that conforms to the Federal Motor Vehicle Safety Standard of 1981 and has been crash tested (see Car Seats, page 72).

Drive Defensively

Driving legally and sensibly is not enough. If other drivers are not capable or careful, they can be the cause of an accident. Never assume that other drivers will drive responsibly. Driving defensively means that you are aware of other cars at all times and are prepared to take evasive action. Try to anticipate what other drivers are going to do. Be prepared to react promptly if another driver suddenly makes an unexpected maneuver.

Do not follow other cars too closely. For every 10 miles per hour of speed, allow one car length between you and the car in front (thus, at 50 mph, five car lengths or about 100 feet should separate you from the car ahead).

Make sure that at all angles your visibility is clear. Do not allow accumulation of toys or other objects to block your rear view. Make sure that your windows and mirrors are clean. Turn your head and use your eyes (in addition to rearview mirrors) to verify the presence or absence of other cars when changing lanes, pulling out from the curb, or turning. Always use turn signals, even when pulling away from the curb.

Pedestrians, bicyclists, animals, runners, and motorcyclists all require special caution. Learn where the "blind spots" are in your car.

Consider the Weather

When it is snowing or raining or if visibility is reduced for any reason, slow down. If conditions become severe, do not travel until they improve.

Be ready for the unexpected. In very cold weather, carry food, blankets, and cold-weather clothing. Keep your gas tank as full as possible. You may need to run your engine and heater in the event your car becomes stalled in a blizzard. Do not leave your car in such an emergency. If your engine is running, roll windows down an inch or two to help avoid a potentially fatal buildup of carbon monoxide fumes.

Driving While Impaired

Do not drive after consuming alcoholic beverages or when you have taken medications that make you drowsy or impair your reaction time. If you feel especially tired or ill, someone else should be behind the wheel.

Avoid Distractions

Control the behavior of children in your car. Do not let them get too animated while you are driving. Also, do not let the radio, an interesting conversation, or a roadside attraction distract you from your driving.

Proper Maintenance

Keep your car properly serviced at the recommended intervals (at least every 6 months or 7,500 miles, whichever comes first). Keep your tires (including your spare) in good condition. Make sure your lights, brakes, windshield wipers, and steering work properly. Have a first aid kit (see page 392), flashlight, and emergency flares in your car. Obeying proper maintenance schedules can help ensure that a mechanical failure will not cause a highway mishap.

Hotel Fire Safety

Most hotels and motels are safe, protected by sprinklers and other precautions required by law in most states. But the unexpected can happen. Thus, take a few simple precautions:

- On arrival, find the two exits nearest your room. Determine where they go and

---

Basic Bicycling Safety

Wear a Helmet

Three of four cyclists killed in cycle-related accidents die of head injuries; the majority of bicyclists' injuries involve the head. So wearing a helmet is a sensible precaution.

Your helmet should have a durable outer shell and a polystyrene liner. Adjustable foam pads should help ensure a proper fit at the front, back, and sides, and the straps should hold it snug. Check for a sticker from the American National Standards Institute or the Snell Memorial Foundation, the two groups that have established voluntary testing standards for bicycling helmets.

Ride With Traffic

Wrong-way riders are much more likely to be involved in accidents with motor vehicles. In addition, all 50 states require cyclists to go with the traffic flow.

Stop at Stop Signs

Stop signs are there for bicycles as well as cars. Look both ways before proceeding.

Check for Traffic Before Turning

Always look back, signal, and check for traffic before turning.

Watch Out for Water

In wet conditions, braking ability is greatly decreased. Watch out for wet leaves in the fall; they can be slippery and hazardous.

Bicycle Defensively

Make eye contact with other riders, drivers, and pedestrians. Watch out for potholes, rubbish, and other hazards. Know your own reaction time and other skills. Ride with care at speeds commensurate with your abilities. Beware of motorists who may be inclined to make a right turn into or in front of you.

---

make sure they are unlocked. Locate the fire alarm nearest your room, too.
- Once inside your room, familiarize yourself with its layout. If it ever were to become smoke-filled, you would not be able to see clearly. Review the hotel's fire safety information (often, it is fastened to the back of the door or is in a special brochure).
- Never smoke in bed.
- Keep your room keys on your bedside table.
- If you smell smoke or see flames, call the fire department directly and activate the hotel fire alarm.
- If the fire alarm sounds, feel your door before you open it. If it is hot, do not open it; telephone for help. If your door is cool,

open it slowly. Be alert for smoke and flames in the hall, and go to the nearest exit. Take your room key with you. If smoke or flames block your exit, you may have to return to your room. Your room may be the safest place.

- If the fire is nearby and you are forced to stay in your room, telephone for help, turn off all air-conditioning and heating systems, and open your window slightly for ventilation. If smoke seeps into your room, soak sheets and towels and stuff them under and around the door to block out heat and smoke. Get as close as you can to the floor (for freshest air) and hold a wet washcloth over your face to keep cool and to filter out smoke particles.
- Do not attempt to run through smoke or flames.
- Never use elevators during a fire.

Safety in the Workplace

In recent years, the Occupational Safety and Health Administration (OSHA) and state and local agencies have made important gains in eliminating hazards in the workplace. Yet many potential dangers remain. Be on the alert for such dangers and protect yourself and others by following these safety rules and commonsense guidelines.

Protective Eye Wear

If your job carries a risk of eye injury, your employer is required by law to provide you with protective glasses, and you are required to wear them. If they interfere with your efficiency, try another design; many safe and practical varieties are available. Wear them whenever you are operating machinery or exposed to fumes or particles in the air that could endanger your eyes (see Protecting Your Eyes, page 532).

Protection From Noise

If your workplace is so noisy that you have to shout to make yourself heard, the noise level may be great enough that it can permanently damage your hearing. Under such conditions, your employer should measure noise levels and see if there is a need to decrease the noise or provide protective devices.

Specially designed earmuffs are available. Some types close out the outside world; others are fitted with earphones and a microphone that enables you to communicate with other workers. Commercially available earplugs made of foam, plastic, or rubber or custom-molded plugs also effectively decrease your exposure to excessive noise. Cotton balls are not adequate and can get stuck deep in your ear canal (see Foreign Objects in Your Ear, page 571). (See Noise and Sound Levels, page 573, and Occupational Hearing Loss, page 572.)

Fumes, Smoke, Dust, and Gas Hazards

A wide variety of respiratory symptoms can result from exposure to toxic fumes, gases, particles, and smoke in the workplace. The exposure may be long-term with low levels of chemicals; accidental exposure also may occur, in which high levels of industrial toxic chemicals are inhaled for a short time.

A sampling of dangerous chemicals includes ammonia, cyanides, formaldehyde, acid fumes, hydrogen sulfide, diazomethane, halides, nitrogen dioxide, isocyanates, ozone, phosgene, phthalic anhydride, and sulfur dioxide. The processing of metals such as cadmium, chromium, nickel, beryllium, copper, magnesium, and zinc can produce dangerous fumes. Dust diseases (pneumoconiosis), including asbestosis (from asbestos), silicosis (from silica), byssinosis (from cotton), and miners' disorders like black-lung disease, also result from long-term inhalation of dust particles (see Occupation-Related Lung Disease, page 728). Workers who use high levels of heat, such as during welding, brazing, smelting, pottery making, and furnace work, also are at risk.

If your job involves any of these potential dangers, be sure to obey safety precautions posted in your workplace. Be especially careful if handling hazardous materials such as asbestos. Read the safety information on the Material Safety Data Sheet (MSDS) for the chemicals you handle. Wear proper clothing, air-filtration masks, eye gear, and other appropriate protection. Be sure ventilation is adequate. Make sure that you are familiar with the hazards of the substances with which you work.

If you are pregnant or are trying to become pregnant, avoid any exposure to hazardous chemicals.

If you suspect that there may be dangerous smoke, fumes, dust, or chemical exposure in your workplace, discuss the matter with your physician. Remember that many permanent respiratory ailments develop slowly as a result of industrial exposure over a period of years. Small exposures that may seem harmless can result in chronic disease. If you think that you or your co-workers are at unnecessary risk (see Occupation- Related Lung Disease, page 728), consult with your employer or company safety officer. For further information, contact OSHA or a state or local agency charged with workplace safety, your employer, or your union.

Medication, Drug, and Alcohol Use

Do not consume alcohol before or during working hours. Never use illegal drugs. Do not operate machinery when you are taking medications that might make you drowsy. Always ask your physician or your company or plant physician, pharmacist, or nurse about the effect a medication may have on you.

Working Shifts

If your job requires that you work night shifts on a regular basis or if you rotate shifts from one week or month to the next, health problems may occur.

Changing your normal rhythm of waking and sleeping, as a result of switching shifts, requires a period of adjustment. If you have ever flown across multiple time zones, you know what can happen when your body's internal clock is disrupted. Insomnia, mental and physical fatigue, indigestion, and an overall feeling of ill health are common side effects. Business people commonly refer to this condition as jet lag.

If your job entails constant changing of shifts, your body will have more difficulty adjusting and readjusting as you get older. Some studies suggest that too frequent shift changes over a lengthy period of time can put you at an increased risk of coronary artery disease or peptic ulcer. Also, fatigue can lead to injury and error in the workplace.

There are no clear-cut solutions to this "occupational jet lag," but there are some strategies you might try:

- Work a shift for 3 weeks rather than rotating to a different schedule every week.
- Change the sequence. Research suggests that a more normal sleep pattern results when the shift sequence is day-evening-night rather than the more usual day-night-evening sequence.
- Tolerance to shift rotation varies widely among people. If you have difficulty making the adjustment, consider chang-

---

VDTs: Sensible Precautions

Video display terminals (VDTs) are the screens that more than 15 million Americans look at for hours each day. Also occurring daily are questions about the potential health risks of these helpful new devices.

Among concerns raised are the potential risks posed by the electrical and magnetic fields and radiation produced by screens of VDTs. To date, however, these risks are discounted by experts as being insignificant. The exposure levels from the screens are well below currently acceptable levels. In addition, no major health risks have been found. However, eye and hand (musculoskeletal) strains have been reported.

Avoidance Strategies

If you work at a VDT daily, try these strategies to minimize eye and hand strain:

- Position the top third of the screen at eye level, between 20 and 26 inches from where you are seated.
- Keep your neck relaxed and your head facing forward.
- Locate the keyboard so that your elbows are bent at approximately 90 degrees; you should not have to bend your wrists to type.
- Pick a chair that offers ample back support, and position it about an arm's length from your terminal. Your feet should rest on the floor or on a footrest so that your thighs are parallel to the floor.

There are no proven long-term health risks from VDTs, but research is continuing. In the meantime, follow the above suggestions. In addition, take a 5-minute stretch break every hour.

---

ing your job. If you experience severe insomnia, your physician may consider prescribing a short-acting sleeping pill that you can take for a few days after each shift change (see Insomnia, page 1112).

Safety on the Farm

Today's farmer works long hours and uses complex, dangerous machinery. However, with proper precautions, the potential for an accident can be reduced or eliminated.

Operate Machinery With Care

Half of all serious farm injuries involve mechanical equipment. Tractors, power take-offs (PTOs, which provide power from tractor shafts to other equipment), hay balers, augers (corkscrew-like devices used to move grain into storage bins), and corn pickers are high-powered devices that, if not used properly, can cause serious injury or death.

Never take your machinery for granted, especially if you use it every day. Never reach into equipment while parts are moving; turn the equipment off before making repairs. Do not remove safety shields or guards. Service the equipment at appropriate intervals.

When at work, never wear baggy clothing (loose shirttails, long sleeves, scarves), loose jewelry, or long hair that is unprotected. These can get caught in moving equipment (such as PTOs) and pull you into the mechanism. Use safety glasses, noise protection, and other precautions including masks when using chemicals and pesticides (see Safety in the Workplace, page 358).

Children on the Farm

Supervise children at all times. Assign them tasks within their level of competence and appropriate to their ages.

Do not allow youngsters to play with farm equipment. Children should never get the impression that tractors and other farm machinery are toys. This equipment is too dangerous to risk a child's misuse when you are not present to supervise. Children should not ride in back of an open pickup truck.

Pesticides, Fuels, and Fire Risks

Store poisons and toxic materials in a safe, secure location. Keep flammable materials in fireproof areas away from barns and fodder storage.

Make sure that wiring is properly maintained. Keep fire extinguishers at hand for use in the event of fire. Enforce "no smoking" rules in areas where flammable goods are stored.

Safety While Hiking and Camping

The outdoors can be a wonderful place for exercise, fun, and experiencing nature firsthand. Without proper consideration of the risks, however, a casual hike in the woods can be a dangerous or even life-threatening activity.

Recognize Your Limits

Suit your outdoor activity to your physical condition. A newborn baby or an elderly person with a heart condition probably does not belong on a trek into the wilderness. Match the recreational activity to the capabilities of the campers.

Plan

If you are visiting an unfamiliar area, map your route in advance. Take the map with you, and locate your position on it from time to time. Know the weather forecast in advance, and monitor changes as you travel (see Safety and the Elements, page 361). Let someone know where you are going and when you plan to arrive and return.

Dress for the Occasion

Sturdy shoes are important for the hiker. If you are hiking up a mountain, be prepared for climate changes. It probably will be cooler or damper on top. Desert areas have unusually wide swings in temperature from midday to nighttime.

Carry Appropriate Equipment

Know your needs. Plan ahead, and be sure that you have what you need for your outdoors adventure. Tents, sleeping bags, food, water, extra clothing, insect repellent, matches, flashlights, and other goods may be required.

Always carry first aid supplies when camping (see Basic First Aid Supplies, page 392).

Watch, Don't Touch, the Animals

Beware of wild animals. If they are acting oddly, rabies may be the cause; check wildlife conditions with the Forest Service before going in. Do not approach a young animal; a protective mother may be nearby. Do not keep food in your tent because it may attract unwanted animals. Instead, hang it from a tree nearby.

Avoid Stings, Bites, and Blisters

Carry insect repellent with you if the area has bees, mosquitoes, flies, ticks, or other insects (see Lyme Disease, page 1067). If there is risk of an allergic response, consult your physician first because an antiallergy kit may be needed (see Anaphylaxis, page 444). Watch out for resinous plants such as poison oak and sumac (see Contact Dermatitis, page 987).

Don't Drink the Water

Never drink the water unless you know it is clean. An important risk is giardiasis, infestation by a tiny parasite that produces diarrhea, abdominal cramps, and bloating. Even if the water looks crystal-clear, it may be contaminated. In fact, rushing mountain streams are more likely to infect you than placid lakes, because the parasites cannot settle to the bottom (see page 768).

Boil any water for a minimum of 3 minutes before drinking it. Adding halazone tablets (which contain iodine) to the water will also kill disease-producing bacteria.

Various types of lightweight, portable filters are available to remove *Giardia* from water, but do not rely on them. Experts disagree on their effectiveness.

Don't Pick the Berries
Do not eat berries, mushrooms, or other plants unless you are positive that they are edible.

Douse Your Campfire
Never risk the safety of other campers and animals by failing to drown your campfire.

Water and Boating Safety

Rule number 1 of water safety is that everyone, young and old, should know how to swim. It is never too late to learn. Classes are readily available in most towns and cities.

Going for a Swim
If you have an outdoor pool, there must be a childproof fence around it. Never let a child play alone at the edge of a pool, pond, or any body of water.

Never swim alone, not even if you are an excellent swimmer. Teach your child that he or she is never to swim without adult supervision.

Do not dive into water without first checking its depth. Also, look beneath the surface of the water for obstructions that may pose a risk.

Know your limits. Do not try to swim too far or in hazardous conditions (such as in areas with a strong undertow).

Teach your child to swim. Check out local classes before you enroll your child to make sure that the instructors are qualified and experienced.

Flotation devices on the arms can be used for toddlers. Avoid flotation vests on toddlers; these actually can cause drowning. Never leave your child unattended. Know the basics of cardiopulmonary resuscitation (see Cardiopulmonary Resuscitation, page 408).

Do not go swimming when:

- You have been consuming alcoholic beverages
- A storm threatens, especially a lightning storm
- Boats or fishermen are operating in the immediate vicinity

Boating Safety
Know and obey the rules when using any boat—rowboat, powerboat, or sailboat. Keep your boat properly equipped and maintained. Never consume alcoholic beverages while boating.

Wear a life jacket (now called PFDs—personal flotation devices). When you are in a boat, have as many life jackets as there are passengers. Adult nonswimmers and all children should wear life jackets at all times; it is a good idea for adult swimmers to wear them, too.

Do not overload your boat. Be sure that the operator of the boat is familiar with its workings and is qualified to drive it. Know the boating rules and obey them. Stay off the water in dangerous weather conditions. If your boat capsizes, stay with it until help arrives. Do not try to swim to shore.

Drowning Emergency
For procedures to deal with drowning emergencies, see Near Drowning, page 418.

Safety and the Elements

In our daily lives, we develop strategies to minimize the impact of weather on our normal activities. Most of us take for granted our ability to deal with rain, snow, or other challenges of climate. A word to the wise: never underestimate climate as a potential hazard to your health.

Lightning
In the event of an electrical storm, take appropriate precautions. Avoid the tallest object in the area, such as an isolated house on a hill or a single tree. Avoid being the tallest object, too. Never carry your golf clubs or fishing rod in an open area during a storm. Go indoors and close windows and doors. Do not use your telephone, bathtub, or shower.

Get away from open water, tractors, or metal equipment (motorcycles, scooters, golf carts, bicycles). Avoid metallic structures (fences, clotheslines, pipes, rails) that can carry electricity to you from a distance. Your car, with windows and doors closed, is a safe place.

Intense Cold
Dress for the cold. Many layers of thin clothing that trap insulating air between them are better than a single, bulky covering. For example, to keep your upper body warm, wear a T-shirt, a long-sleeved shirt, a sweater, and then a parka over everything. Add another layer if you get cold.

Always wear a hat to conserve body heat. Also wear mittens or gloves. Boots should have room for two pairs of warm socks.

Do not drink alcohol or smoke cigarettes before going out in extreme cold. Nicotine decreases circulation to your extremities, the areas most susceptible to cold injury. Alcohol enhances the removal of heat from your body, making you vulnerable to hypothermia. Adequate nutrition is especially important in cold weather. People with diseases that limit the blood supply to their extremities are especially at risk.

If you or a companion experiences frostbite or hypothermia (significant decrease in body temperature), seek immediate emergency treatment (see Frostbite, page 416, and Hypothermia, page 416).

Protection From the Sun
Exposure to the sun can damage your skin. Take precautions, especially if you will be exposed to the sun's rays for long periods or at the hottest part of the day (10 a.m. to 2 p.m.). Wear appropriate sunscreens such as those containing para-aminobenzoic acid (PABA) or benzophenone on your face, lips, and any other exposed skin. A rating of 15 is appropriate for most people (see How to Avoid Sunburn, page 997).

If you are exposed to sun for long periods, especially when there is little breeze and high humidity, heatstroke or heat exhaustion may result. Heatstroke and heat exhaustion are emergencies and require immediate care (see Heat Stress, page 414).

Avoid the risk of heatstroke or heat exhaustion by staying out of the sun for extended periods (see page 414). Do not consume alcoholic beverages on hot, humid days when you are outside. Drink plenty of water. Wear a hat with a wide brim to protect yourself from sun exposure. Wear lightweight, loose-fitting clothing; light-colored clothing will reflect the heat. Frequent cool showers or baths may be helpful. Never leave children or pets unattended in a car in the sun—not even for a few minutes.

Sun Exposure in Children
A very young child should not be exposed to more than 2 minutes of sun on the first day of exposure. Then increase exposure by no more than 2 minutes on successive days. Always use sunscreens and hats.

Chapter 16

Tooth Care

Contents

The Care of Your Teeth, 364
How to Choose a Toothbrush, 365
Sensitive Teeth, 365

Proper Flossing and Brushing Techniques, 366
Flossing, 367
Brushing, 367

Toothpaste, 367
Antiplaque, 367

Tartar Control, 367
Baking Soda, 368
Desensitizing, 368
Extra Whiteners, 368
Natural, 368

Controlling Tartar, 368

Dental X-Rays, 369

Fluoride and Tooth Decay, 370

The Care of Your Teeth

Your teeth are among your most important assets. Attached to jaws driven by powerful muscles, your teeth enable you to chew your food into a form that aids digestion.

Teeth, of course, also have a cosmetic dimension. Frequently, the first thing we notice about other people is their smile.

Clean, healthy-looking teeth seem to be a sign to the world of general good health. In the past, a healthy smile belonged only to the young because, until recently, most people lost their teeth by middle age. Now, however, dental care, improved nutrition, and good dental hygiene make it possible for most of us to keep our teeth for our entire lives.

Essential to maintaining a set of healthy teeth is a lifelong program of good dental hygiene—one that you begin early and practice consistently through the years. This includes modifying your diet to lessen the effects of sugar and carbohydrates.

In most children and adults, tooth decay (cavities or, more formally, caries) is the primary problem. Tooth decay is mainly caused by bacteria and carbohydrates. Bacteria are present in a thin, almost invisible film on your teeth. Enzymes in your saliva change starches into sugar in your mouth. Bacteria convert the sugar to an acid that decays your teeth.

Start your child early on a program of regular brushing and flossing. Decay can begin as soon as your child's baby (primary) teeth begin to erupt.

Never allow your infant to sleep with a bottle of fruit juice or milk. The sugar content of these beverages encourages decay. If your baby seems to require the soothing presence of a bottle at bedtime, fill it with water.

Teach your toddler to brush his or her teeth in the morning and evening. Reinforce the habit by setting a good example. Make sure that all of your children brush with fluoride toothpaste and have regular dental checkups, beginning no later than age 3.

The principal cause of tooth loss in adults is cavities. In addition, advanced periodontal disease can lead to tooth loss (see Dental and Oral Disorders, page 601).

Periodontal disease is an infection of the gums and other tissues that support the teeth. The frequency of gingivitis (a mild form of periodontal disease) is high in all age groups—reportedly more than 80 percent in adults age 45 or older. The frequency of periodontitis (a more serious form) increases with age. Close to 50 percent of adults age 45 or older are thought to be affected.

Advanced periodontitis can lead to loosening and eventual loss of teeth. However, you can prevent gum disease with proper daily care of your teeth.

The principal cause of tooth loss is dental cavities (caries). The accumulation of tartar (calculus) can lead to gingivitis and, eventually, periodontitis—another cause of tooth loss.

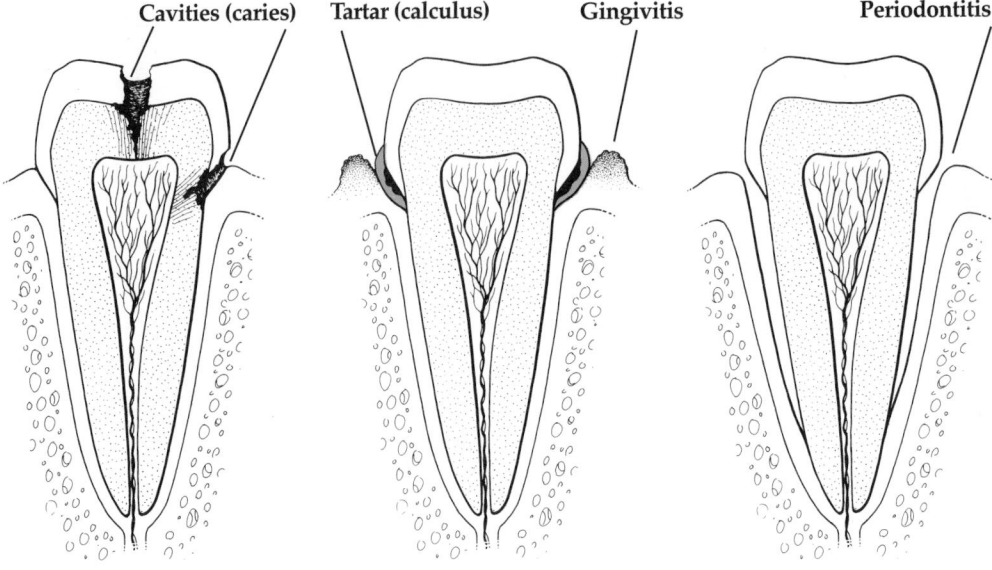

Cavities (caries)   Tartar (calculus)   Gingivitis   Periodontitis

The most frequent sign of gum disease is swollen gums that bleed easily, especially during brushing and flossing. Other symptoms include bad breath, soft or tender gums, pus from the gum line (where the gum forms a collar around the tooth), shrinkage of the gum away from the tooth, a loose tooth, and changes in the tooth position and bite.

Like tooth decay, the cause of periodontal disease is plaque. Plaque consists of an accumulation of bacteria and sugars on the surface of the teeth. Plaque forms constantly in your mouth and collects on the surfaces of your teeth. As plaque accumulates along the gum line, it irritates your gums, making them tender and likely to bleed. This condition is called gingivitis (see Gingivitis, page 610). If you do not remove the plaque daily by brushing and flossing, it continues to accumulate and reacts with minerals in your saliva to form a calcified deposit known as calculus (tartar).

As plaque builds on top of the calculus, the gums slowly separate from the teeth, leaving pockets that fill with bacteria and sometimes pus. When the disease goes untreated, it attacks and destroys bone that supports the teeth. As a result, otherwise healthy, unde-

cayed teeth loosen and can be lost.

The best method for controlling plaque and tartar is to brush thoroughly and regularly (at least twice each day) and to floss at least once a day. As with tooth decay, limit the amount of sugar you eat, particularly between meals (see Prevention of Periodontal Disease, page 613).

How to Choose a Toothbrush

A toothbrush with soft, rounded-end or polished bristles is best for cleaning your teeth and gums. Stiff or hard brushes are more likely to injure gum tissues.

The size and shape of the brush should allow you to reach every tooth. There are brush sizes for children and for adults, and there are various configurations of bristles. Remember that only the tips of the bristles do the cleaning, so there's no need to exert a great deal of pressure.

Replace your toothbrush every 3 to 4 months, or sooner if the bristles become bent. Then you always will be using bristles that are effective in brushing plaque (bacteria and sugars) from the surface of your teeth and gums. Splayed bristles are a sign that it is past time to replace your toothbrush.

If you have doubts about the proper brushes for you and your family, ask your dentist for a recommendation.

Sensitive Teeth

When your teeth become painful to certain stimuli—touch, cold, hot, air, plaque (bacteria), sweet or sour foods—you may have what dentists call "dentin hypersensitivity," or sensitive teeth. This condition is usually caused by enamel erosion or gum recession that exposes the root of the tooth.

If you avoid sensitive areas during brushing, flossing, chewing, or drinking because of discomfort, you need treatment. Failing to clean your teeth thoroughly because of sensitivity may lead to tooth and gum disease.

After determining the cause of your sensitive teeth, your dentist can treat the troubled area and recommend a maintenance program. This may include using a desensitizing toothpaste, applying a prescribed fluoride solution daily at home if sensitivity continues, and having your dentist cover the exposed areas with bonding agents.

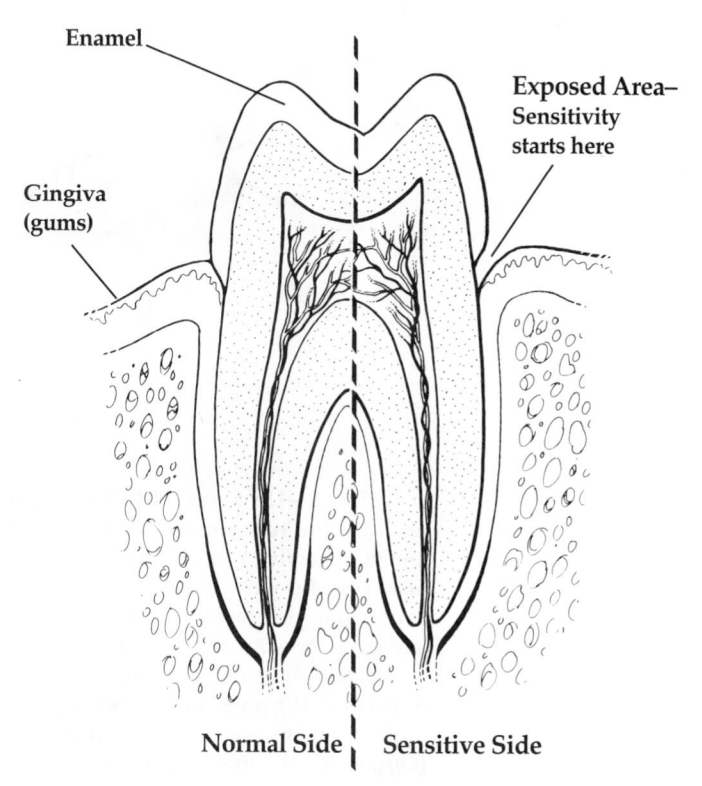

Enamel

Exposed Area–
Sensitivity
starts here

Gingiva
(gums)

Normal Side | Sensitive Side

Proper Flossing and Brushing Techniques

Total mouth care depends more on brushing and flossing techniques than on use of any product. Rather than paying a premium price for a so-called antiplaque or antitartar toothpaste, your best aid is frequent brushing and flossing.

Brushing and flossing are the best ways to remove bacteria and food particles before dental problems begin. Start by flossing your teeth once each day and brushing them at least twice a day (in the morning and before going to bed). Better yet, brush after each meal or snack. A complete cleaning with a fluoride toothpaste, toothbrush, and dental floss (thread that you draw between your teeth) should take 3 to 5 minutes. The proper order for cleaning is floss first, brush second. This order allows you to brush away food particles and bacteria loosened by the flossing.

How to Brush and Floss

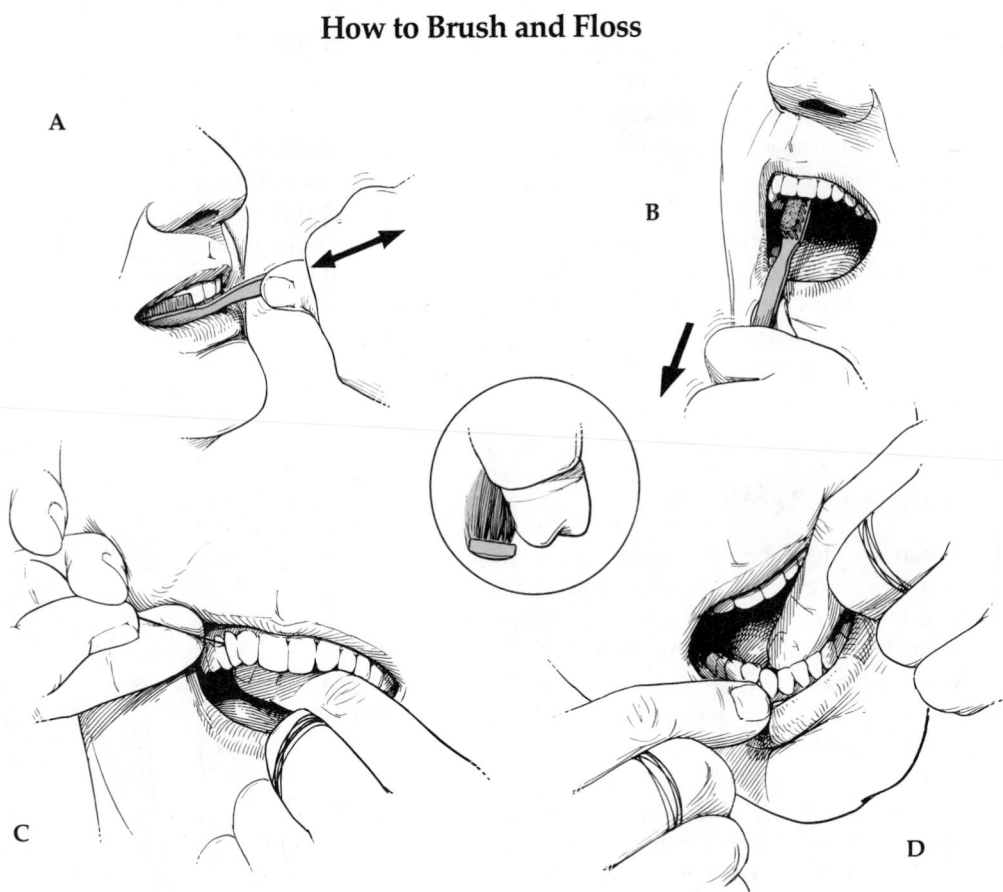

To Brush—Use a soft-bristle brush and minimal pressure. Begin with the outer surfaces of all teeth and the inner surfaces of your back teeth. Position your brush horizontally and brush back and forth gently (A) with short (half-a-tooth-wide) strokes at the gum line. Next, brush vertically away from the gum line. To clean inner surfaces of upper and lower front teeth, brush vertically (B), moving your toothbrush over both teeth and gums. To clean the junction between your teeth and gums, brush at a 45-degree angle (see inset), keeping the bristles angled against the gum line.

To Floss—Wrap waxed or unwaxed dental floss around the middle fingers of both hands. For upper teeth (C), position floss between your thumb and index finger, then insert it between your teeth and gently move it back and forth from the top to the bottom of your teeth. For lower teeth (D), positioning floss between your index fingers works best.

Flossing

Take at least 18 inches of dental floss—unwaxed or waxed, whichever is more comfortable for you—and wind most of it around the middle finger of one hand. Wind a turn or two around the middle finger of the other hand so that you have 2 to 3 inches of floss between these fingers.

For your upper teeth, position the floss over the thumb of one hand and the index finger of the other hand. Guide about an inch of floss into each gap between your teeth. Use a gentle up-and-down motion, holding the floss tightly, to rub the sides of each tooth.

When the floss reaches your gum line, curve it into a "C" shape around your tooth and move the floss up and down, gently scraping the wall of the tooth. Wind the used floss around your middle finger, exposing a fresh section, and repeat the procedure for each tooth.

For the lower teeth, wrap the dental floss around your middle fingers and insert it between your teeth. Use the same motion as described for the upper teeth, and repeat the procedure for each tooth.

Do not be alarmed if your gums bleed the first few times you floss. If the bleeding continues each time you floss, consult your dentist. The problem may be improper flossing. Your dentist can demonstrate the proper method for you (see How to Brush and Floss, page 366).

Brushing

Brush your teeth at least twice daily, especially in the evening. When you brush, position your toothbrush horizontally on your teeth. To effectively clean the top and bottom surfaces of all teeth, move the brush back and forth horizontally and then vertically away from the gum line in a series of short, gentle strokes.

For surfaces adjacent to your gums, move the brush in short back-and-forth strokes or in a rotary motion over both teeth and gums.

Positioning your toothbrush at an angle will help clean the junction between your teeth and gums more effectively. Also, brush chewing surfaces with a gentle scrubbing motion, and brush your tongue to freshen your breath (see How to Brush and Floss, page 366).

Toothpaste

With few exceptions, most toothpastes have enough fluoride to protect your teeth against decay. But a growing awareness of dental health has led to a burgeoning array of specialty products. Gone are the days when a toothpaste promised only to prevent cavities. Now they claim to also fight plaque, control tartar, reduce sensitivity, and more. To clean and protect your teeth, what type of toothpaste do you really need? Here's our analysis of some popular claims.

Antiplaque

Some products claim to remove plaque or kill bacteria that can cause plaque. But all toothpastes remove some plaque if you floss and brush well. Regardless of the product, you can't remove all plaque by brushing alone. Even if you use a plaque-fighting toothpaste, be sure to have regular dental checkups.

Tartar Control

No toothpaste can remove tartar below the gum line. It takes professional cleaning by your dental hygienist to remove any tartar, also called calculus. Tartar is the white or yellowish deposit that plaque hardens into when mixed with minerals in your saliva.

Antitartar pastes can help prevent a buildup of tartar on the teeth. Regular flossing and brushing remove plaque, however, leaving little plaque to harden into tartar.

An antitartar paste may increase your teeth's sensitivity to cold. If so, change to a product without tartar control.

Baking Soda

Baking soda is a mild abrasive and stain remover—but when wet, it loses some of its stain-removing power.

Some pastes contain hydrogen peroxide to help kill bacteria and loosen plaque. However, effective brushing with a fluoride toothpaste serves the same purpose.

Desensitizing

Desensitizing pastes contain chemicals that block the perception of pain in your teeth. Before using such a product, however, check with your dentist. Sometimes sensitive teeth may be a sign of a problem that needs treatment, not cover-up.

Extra Whiteners

Before using any kind of whitening gel or polishing cream, ask your dentist for advice. Whitening toothpastes contain ingredients such as peroxide bleach or papaya enzymes, which may be harsh on delicate gum tissue, especially if you have receding gums. Smokers' pastes also contain strong abrasives that may be harsh on gum tissue.

Natural

If you use a natural toothpaste product—most don't contain artificial ingredients such as a sweetener—be sure it has fluoride. Without it, natural pastes won't effectively fight decay.

Controlling Tartar

Tartar (calculus)

Tartar (your dentist may call it calculus) is an accumulation of minerals and plaque on the surfaces of your teeth. When cleaning your teeth, your dental hygienist will remove the tartar, especially at or below the gum line, because it is a primary cause of gum disease.

Called calculus by your dentist, tartar is a product of minerals in your saliva and plaque. Tartar is a primary cause of gum diseases such as gingivitis and periodontitis. Tartar is most troublesome when it forms below the gum line.

Tartar is chalky, hard, and difficult to remove. Part of a regular dental checkup involves cleaning your teeth and removing tartar. This is often done by scraping the teeth, particularly below the gum line, with instruments known as scalers and curettes. The procedure can be uncomfortable and make your gums bleed. Another method uses a vibrating device that helps remove tartar.

Tartar below the gum line can lead to periodontitis, the gum disease that can result in loss of teeth. Tartar-control toothpastes may have a cosmetic effect and make your teeth easier to clean when you see the dentist, but they are of little use in keeping tartar from building up below the gum line (see Toothpaste, page 367).

Dental X-Rays

Almost all of us have had dental X-rays taken. As in other medical fields, these X-rays are used to aid in diagnosing disease or injury. They often are useful in diagnosing the presence and extent of dental cavities, bone damage from periodontal disease, tooth abscesses, impacted teeth, fractures of the jawbone and teeth, and other abnormalities of the teeth and jaw.

When it comes to cavities, X-rays can show the presence of decay in a tooth even when the enamel looks intact, particularly if the decay is hidden between teeth or under the gum line. If your dentist suspects that something may be wrong, he or she may take an X-ray of your tooth.

The amount of radiation used to make dental X-rays is extremely small, and the process is simple. To detect cavities, dentists use bitewing (BW) X-rays. A small piece of film is placed in your mouth, next to your teeth. You hold the film in place by biting down on the paper that covers the film. The X-ray machine is then aimed at the tooth, and the exposure is made. After developing the film, which takes a few minutes, your dentist can determine an appropriate course of action.

X-rays, particularly a complete set of all the teeth, should not be taken as part of a routine examination but only as a diagnostic tool. No one should have more radiation exposure than absolutely necessary. A set of full-mouth X-rays should not be made more than once every 5 years, unless necessary for a specific purpose. Your dentist will advise you on the proper set of X-rays to obtain.

As a precautionary measure against excess radiation, your dentist should fit you with a lead apron that covers you from chest to lower abdomen. Everyone should wear the apron, but it is particularly important for pregnant women and women of childbearing age.

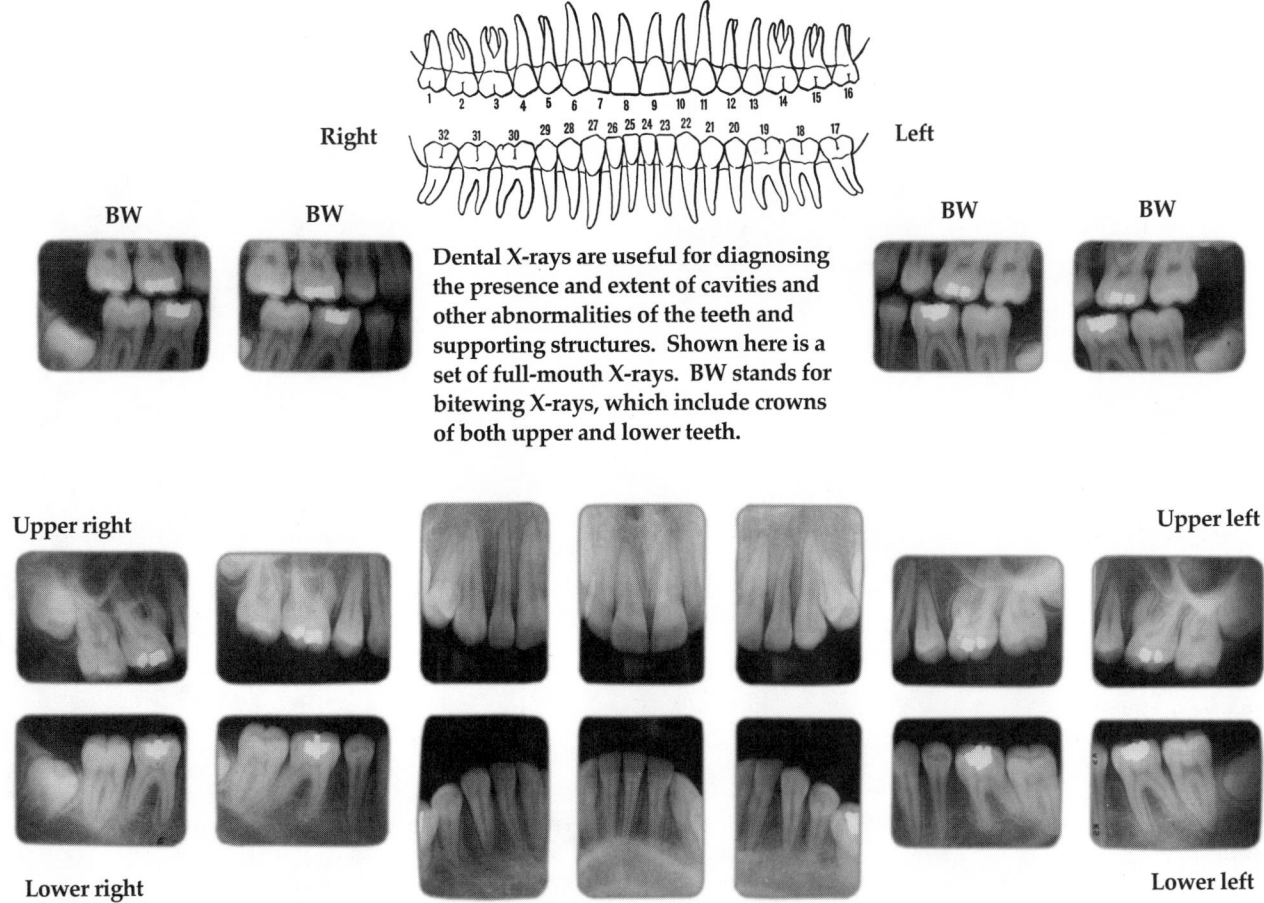

Right   **Left**

BW   BW   BW   BW

Dental X-rays are useful for diagnosing the presence and extent of cavities and other abnormalities of the teeth and supporting structures. Shown here is a set of full-mouth X-rays. BW stands for bitewing X-rays, which include crowns of both upper and lower teeth.

Upper right   **Upper left**

Lower right   **Lower left**

Fluoride and Tooth Decay

Several decades ago, scientists found that adding fluoride to drinking water deficient in fluoride greatly decreased the number of cavities in children and adolescents who drank that water. Today, the scientific evidence is conclusive: the addition of fluoride to drinking water and toothpaste helps to prevent cavities, particularly among children.

Ingestion of fluoride is especially helpful during early childhood, when the teeth are developing. Fluoride is incorporated into the enamel structure of the teeth and provides continuing protection.

You and your family should always brush with a fluoride toothpaste. Many fluoride toothpastes are available, including flavors specially formulated to appeal to children (see Prevention of Tooth Decay, page 608).

The results of fluoride use are so impressive that now not only toothpastes but also many public water supplies contain fluoride. Fluoride is inexpensive, safe, and effective.

Still, only half of our population drinks fluoridated water. If you have children and your municipal water supply is not treated, ask about fluoridation for drinking water in your schools. If you do not have access to fluoridated water, whatever your age, you will benefit from taking supplemental fluoride drops or tablets available by prescription from your dentist or physician.

Older children, adolescents, and senior citizens are most susceptible to tooth decay. For them, fluoride mouth rinses can be useful, as can topical fluoride treatments applied by a dentist.

Chapter 17

The World Around Us

Contents

Drinking Water, 372
Solutions, 372

Cancer Prevention, 373

Air Pollution, 373
20th-Century Syndrome: Fact or Fiction? 374
Indoor Pollution, 374
What to Do, 375

Lawn Chemicals, 375
Recommendations, 375

Carbon Monoxide Poisoning, 376
CO Contamination in the Home and on the Road, 376
Prevention, 376

Radiation and Your Health, 376
What Are X-Rays and What Do They Do? 376
The Radon Risk, 378

In the past quarter century, Americans have made environmental matters a priority. Some rivers that were unswimmable 2 decades ago have regained recreational usefulness. The creation of the Environmental Protection Agency, the passing of the Clean Air Act of 1970, the establishment of a toxic waste "superfund," and various other private and governmental efforts are making a difference in the quality of the air we breathe and of the water we drink.

The job is far from complete. As a member of the general public, you may be concerned that further steps be taken to address continuing and new pollution problems. In your own home, too, there are everyday concerns to be addressed to ensure that you and your family avoid exposure to dangerous and even potentially cancer-causing pollutants. In the following pages we consider some of these concerns.

Drinking Water

In recent years, we have developed a new consciousness of the cleanliness of our water supply. Once, we regarded clean water as automatic because public health programs early in the century had greatly decreased the risks of cholera, typhoid, and other diseases caused by contaminated water.

Today, the risks are different. Infectious disease no longer is our greatest concern. Now the presence of heavy metals, polychlorinated biphenyls (PCBs), pesticides, and other contaminants in drinking water are of greater concern.

Landfills, especially those in which hazardous wastes have been discarded, are potential sources of contamination. Outmoded or improperly maintained tanks at gas stations and fuel oil depots also may contaminate groundwater and wells. Runoff from agricultural lands that have been treated with certain chemical fertilizers and pesticides may contaminate rivers, streams, lakes, and groundwater, as can industrial pollution. Septic tanks for homes in rural and semirural areas may contribute to groundwater pollution.

Among the most serious potential risks are the following:

Trihalomethanes. Chlorine, the chemical responsible for clearing our drinking water of infectious organisms, can undergo chemical reactions in the presence of water pollutants. The resultant chemical compounds, the trihalomethanes (THMs), are potentially cancer-causing (carcinogenic), as demon-strated by tests on experimental animals.

Nitrates. Nitrate contamination as a result of runoff of fertilizer from fields poses a danger. In adults as well as children, ingested nitrates can result in the exposure of your digestive system to nitrosamines, potentially potent carcinogenic compounds.

Asbestos and Heavy Metals. Cadmium (from old galvanized pipes), lead in old homes (from lead-based paint and pipes), and asbestos (from asbestos-cement water pipes and other sources) are potentially dangerous substances (see Asbestosis, page 728).

Solutions

Using bottled water may or may not be the answer. It is expensive, and often the water in these bottles is no better than water from your tap. Boiling water is another option if your water is contaminated with bacteria, but this will not remove lead and cadmium. Commercially available filters may help, although claims made for them sometimes exceed their actual usefulness.

If your water comes from a well, test it every year for pollutants. Find out when the last sanitary testing was done and what was found. You then can take steps to solve any problem.

The Environmental Protection Agency and local and state organizations are responsible for monitoring public water supplies.

Cancer Prevention

The causes of the diverse group of diseases we call cancer remain largely unknown. Medical science continues to add new clues to our understanding of cancer, but much remains to be learned (see The Biology of Cancer, page 1291).

We do know that many cancers occur as a result of exposure to certain substances called carcinogens. These cancer-causing agents can be found in cigarettes, asbestos, certain food substances, and various household and industrial chemicals.

Common sense suggests you should identify carcinogens to which you or members of your family are exposed and then devise strategies to eliminate them. Carcinogenic risk factors include the following:

Passive Smoking. It is not just smokers themselves who are at increased risk of cancer from tobacco smoke—anyone nearby who inhales the smoke also is at risk. In fact, the so-called sidestream smoke from a cigarette (that which curls up from a lighted cigarette in an ashtray) contains 2 times as much tar and nicotine as the inhaled smoke does, 3 times as much of a cancer-causing compound called 3,4-benzpyrene, 5 times as much carbon monoxide, and possibly 50 times as much ammonia.

In addition to quitting smoking yourself, convince other smokers to do the same. Parents who smoke put the health of their children in jeopardy (see How to Stop Smoking, page 321).

Diet and Cancer. The relationship between diet and cancer is under close scrutiny. Recent reports suggest a link between certain foods and some forms of cancer (see Nutrition and Cancer Protection, page 280).

Sun Exposure. Do not get burned by the sun. Chronic exposure to the ultraviolet rays of the sun is the major cause of skin cancer. Use sensible strategies to limit your exposure. Wear long-sleeved, loose-fitting clothes and a hat. Use sunscreen (one with a 15 rating will block out most of the sun's ultraviolet rays). Stay out of the sun at the hottest time of the day, between 10:00 a.m. and 2:00 p.m. (see How to Avoid Sunburn, page 997).

Industrial Exposure. Certain chemicals, the processing of certain metals, and the inhalation of some fibers and dusts have been linked to the occurrence of certain cancers. If you work with hazardous substances, follow instructions about protective clothing or equipment, including goggles, masks, gloves, and overalls (see Safety in the Workplace, page 358).

Air Pollution

The air we breathe often is not clean. Industry, automobiles, and other sources, in combination with weather factors, can decrease air quality to the point that it can be hazardous to your health, especially if you have heart, lung, or other chronic disease.

Key sources of potential outdoor air pollutants include the following:

Motor Vehicle Exhaust. Cars and trucks release a range of pollutants, including carbon monoxide, oxides of nitrogen, and lead.

Industrial and Power Plants. Factories and power plants that burn fuels (such as oil

or coal) that contain sulfur are the principal industrial polluters. They send oxides of sulfur into the air. Oxides of nitrogen (mostly from car exhaust) and oxides of sulfur are the principal causes of acid rain.

Chlorofluorocarbons. Scientists believe that the ozone (an atmospheric layer that protects us from the sun's ultraviolet rays) is gradually being depleted. Chlorofluorocarbons, which are used in refrigeration systems (air conditioners and refrigerators), dry cleaning chemicals, and numerous other products, are thought to be causing this

20th-Century Syndrome:　Fact or Fiction?

In recent years, a concept of illness variously named 20th-century syndrome, total allergy syndrome, or multiple chemical sensitivities has been developed by "clinical ecologists," a group of physicians at the fringe of orthodox medicine.

The working hypothesis is that the health of some people is harmed by exposure to "unnatural elements" in the environment. Unnatural elements can range from synthetic materials to certain foods. People sometimes are told that their immune systems have been damaged. This damage supposedly renders them excessively sensitive to a wide range of naturally occurring and synthetic substances. Various symptoms have been attributed to the supposed disorder, but the symptoms are not those that ordinarily result from an allergy. Symptoms commonly include fatigue, headache, depression, dizziness, anxiety, and mood swings. Furthermore, laboratory tests are never conclusive as to a potential cause for the discomforts these people describe.

There is no clear definition of the disorder. Its potential existence has attracted supporters because of widespread concern about the environment.

This supposed ailment has been examined in depth by the American College of Physicians. The conclusion of this group is that there is no convincing evidence to support the concept of 20th-century syndrome.

Persons for whom this diagnosis has been proposed may indeed have a disorder. Depression is one possible explanation. The physical discomforts commonly described by depressed people are numerous and vague and comparable to the symptoms people with 20th-century syndrome complain of.

The practice of clinical ecology lacks scientific validation. In many situations, the lives of "patients" have been severely constrained because of recommendations made without documentation. In addition, enormous costs are sometimes incurred for ineffective treatment while less costly methods that are potentially helpful are shunned.

change in the atmosphere of the earth. Loss of the ozone layer may be a major risk factor in increasing the incidence of skin cancer.

Other Pollutants. Certain workplaces, including some mines, manufacturing plants, and old buildings, may expose workers to asbestos (see Asbestosis, page 728) and other particulate matter that can produce lung damage and tumors.

Indoor Pollution

The inside of your home also is a potentially polluted place. Especially in homes that are superinsulated (tightly sealed to prevent the loss of heat or cooling), indoor environments can become contaminated with hazardous levels of indoor pollutants.

Prolonged exposure to indoor pollutants can result in symptoms of allergies (including rashes, eye irritation, cough, sore throat, and other cold symptoms). There is also evidence of increased risk of cancer from exposure to certain indoor pollutants.

Among the most common indoor pollutants are the following:

Cigarette Smoke. High in carbon monoxide and particulates such as tar and nicotine, cigarette smoke is a health hazard, even for the nonsmoker who merely shares an interior space with a smoker (see Secondhand Smoke, page 320, and Carbon Monoxide Poisoning, page 376).

Formaldehyde. Various construction products (including particle board and urea-formaldehyde foam insulation), some synthetic carpet and curtain material, fabric softeners, and many cosmetics can release formaldehyde in your home. Although the level of formaldehyde usually is negligible if materials are installed or used properly, an accumulation of high concentrations of formaldehyde may result in chest and lung discomfort. The risk generally is higher in mobile homes because materials that contain formaldehyde sometimes are used in building and decorating these structures.

Household Products. Household cleaning agents, personal care products, paints, hobby products, and solvents can contain harmful substances that contribute to indoor air pollution. Some products release contaminants into the air at the time of use, others do so more gradually.

In particular, be careful when using the following types of household products: pesticides, aerosol sprays, phosphate detergents, chlorine bleach, spot removers and other solvents, furniture and floor polishes, oven cleaner, paints, air fresheners, and glues and epoxy.

The American Lung Association offers these guidelines:

- Use nontoxic alternatives whenever possible.
- Buy only as much of a product as you need.
- Minimize your exposure to these products. Use them only in a well-ventilated area.
- Always read the product label and follow manufacturer instructions. Don't mix chemical products, especially chlorine bleach, with ammonia.
- Store and dispose of hazardous products properly.

Other Pollutants. Gas cookers produce nitrous oxide. Carbon monoxide may come from various indoor heating and cooking devices (see Carbon Monoxide Poisoning, page 376). Asbestos, most often from deteriorating insulation on heating pipes, is an especially dangerous risk (see Asbestosis, page 728). We discuss radon, another indoor pollutant, on page 378.

What to Do

Monitoring the quality of the air outside your home and enforcing the regulations regarding it are the responsibility of the federal Environmental Protection Agency and other such agencies on the state and local levels. In the workplace, the Occupational Safety and Health Administration (OSHA) is charged with monitoring conditions. If you are aware of a source of air pollution in your neighborhood, town, or workplace, report your concerns to one of these agencies.

Make sure that pollution control devices on your car are functioning properly. Your state may require an emissions test as a part of the schedule of inspections.

In your home, be alert to potential airborne poisons. If your house often seems to accumulate smoke, fumes, or other indoor pollution, poor ventilation may be a problem. Have your ventilation checked by a heating/air conditioning specialist. If you live in a house with limited air exchange (a house tightly insulated to hold heat or cool air in), a duct system of air exchangers may be in order.

Make sure that your furnace is installed, maintained, and vented correctly. The same holds true for any other open-flame device you may have in your home (such as a fireplace or cookstove).

Lawn Chemicals

Experts don't agree on the possible long-term health effects of exposure to lawn chemicals such as herbicides, pesticides, and fertilizers.

The hundreds of chemicals used on lawns are registered with the Environmental Protection Agency (EPA). Registration, by itself, however, does not assure safety. Many chemicals registered before the EPA was established were not evaluated for long-term health effects.

Today, two lawn chemical mainstays are receiving scrutiny: diazinon and 2,4-D. Diazinon, an insecticide, was banned by the EPA for use on golf courses and sod farms. The chemical is readily absorbed through skin and is toxic to birds. Yet diazinon remains available for home lawn care.

The herbicide 2,4-D, an ingredient in more than 100 landscaping and agricultural products, has been linked to a higher incidence of a form of cancer (non-Hodgkin's lymphoma) in dogs and possibly in humans.

Recommendations

Be careful when using lawn chemicals. Wear waterproof gloves and shoes, a long-sleeved shirt, a breathing mask, and protective goggles.

Federal law requires you to follow instructions on pesticide labels. Many pesticides are easily absorbed through skin and can be harmful if you inhale them.

In addition, contact your local garden center, nursery, or extension office to learn about low-chemical lawn care techniques.

Carbon Monoxide Poisoning

Carbon monoxide is tasteless, odorless, colorless–and deadly. Often referred to by its chemical formula, CO, this gas is produced by the incomplete combustion of carbon-based fuel. Many cookstoves, lamps, space heaters, furnaces, hot water heaters, and engines produce it.

If the CO level is too high, it takes the place of oxygen in the hemoglobin in your red blood cells, preventing the vital function of this oxygen-carrying molecule.

CO Contamination in the Home and on the Road

The risk of CO poisoning is greatest during cold weather. We seal and weather-strip our homes as tightly as possible to conserve heat, but in so doing we also decrease ventilation and increase the accumulation of indoor pollutants such as CO (see Indoor Pollution, page 374). CO buildup is most likely to occur as a result of defective control valves or pilot lights on cooking or heating units such as portable kerosene space heaters or of inadequately ventilated flame-burning heaters or cookers.

Many recreational vehicles, trailers, and pickup campers have been found to have engine exhaust fumes leaking into them. They may have unvented ovens, stoves, and flame-burning lamps that also produce CO.

The signs and symptoms of CO poisoning are vague. Headache, nausea, vomiting, fatigue, and dizziness may occur but are easily confused with flu-like illnesses that are common in winter months. When the concentration of CO is very high, muscle paralysis and loss of consciousness may occur.

If you suspect CO poisoning, get away from the source immediately. Consult your physician, who will conduct a blood test to identify the amount of CO being carried by your hemoglobin.

Prevention

Make sure wood stoves, space heaters, fireplaces, and flame-burning appliances are properly installed, adjusted, operated, and ventilated. Do not use ovens or gas ranges for heating. Do not operate gas-powered vehicles in confined spaces (such as a garage or basement). Never burn charcoal inside your home, recreational vehicle, or tent.

Radiation and Your Health

When necessary, your physician may schedule you for an X-ray examination to obtain information that will help in diagnosing your problem. The examination itself will be performed by a radiologist or a radiology technician. The results will be interpreted by the radiologist.

What Are X-Rays and What Do They Do?

X-rays are a form of radiation (energy that moves from one place to another). Most radiation is nonpenetrating—it cannot pass through structures. One example of nonpenetrating radiation is visible light. X-rays are one of the few types of radiation (called ionizing radiation) that can penetrate your body.

Because X-rays are able to penetrate your body, they can create a picture of internal body structures on film. This allows your physician to see inside your body without a surgical procedure.

Are X-Rays Safe?

For most X-ray examinations, the amount of radiation you receive is small and the risk of harm is very low. This risk is outweighed by benefits of the examination. In addition, great care is taken to use the lowest dose possible to produce an image for your radiologist to evaluate. No radiation remains in your body after an X-ray examination.

Note: Neither magnetic resonance imaging (MRI) (see page 1334) nor ultrasound examination (see page 1335) involves the use of X-rays; thus, there is no ionizing radiation exposure with these procedures.

Are There Limits on the Number of X-Ray Examinations You Receive?

Because the benefits from these examinations far outweigh the low risk associated with this type of radiation exposure, limits have not been placed on X-ray examinations that are considered medically necessary.

How Is Radiation Measured?

The amount of radiation to which you are exposed is measured in a unit called a roentgen, named after the man who discovered X-rays in 1895, Professor Wilhelm Conrad Röntgen. Other units, the rad and the rem, have technical differences from the roentgen but, for practical purposes, 1 roentgen equals 1 rad or rem. A smaller unit of measurement, the mrad (1/1,000 of a rad), is more useful for measuring exposures to radiation.

What Are the Sources of Radiation Exposure?

Every year, the average person is exposed to approximately 360 mrads of ionizing radiation. This radiation comes from many sources. Natural sources of radiation, which include outer space, rocks, and soil, vary throughout the country. X-rays are an artificial source of radiation. They account for 11 percent of our average yearly exposure to radiation. In recent years, radon has become, in some situations, a significant source of radiation (see page 378).

Should I Have an X-Ray Examination When I Am Pregnant?

The risk of ill effects from exposure of an unborn child to diagnostic X-rays is very low. Nevertheless, because fetal tissues are growing rapidly, they are more sensitive to radiation than the tissues of an adult. Therefore, if you think you might be pregnant, tell your physician. If it is important for you to have an X-ray examination even though you are pregnant, special precautions can be taken to minimize the radiation exposure to your unborn child. For example, in the case of a chest X-ray, a CT scan of your head, or a mammogram, your unborn child can be shielded so there is virtually no exposure.

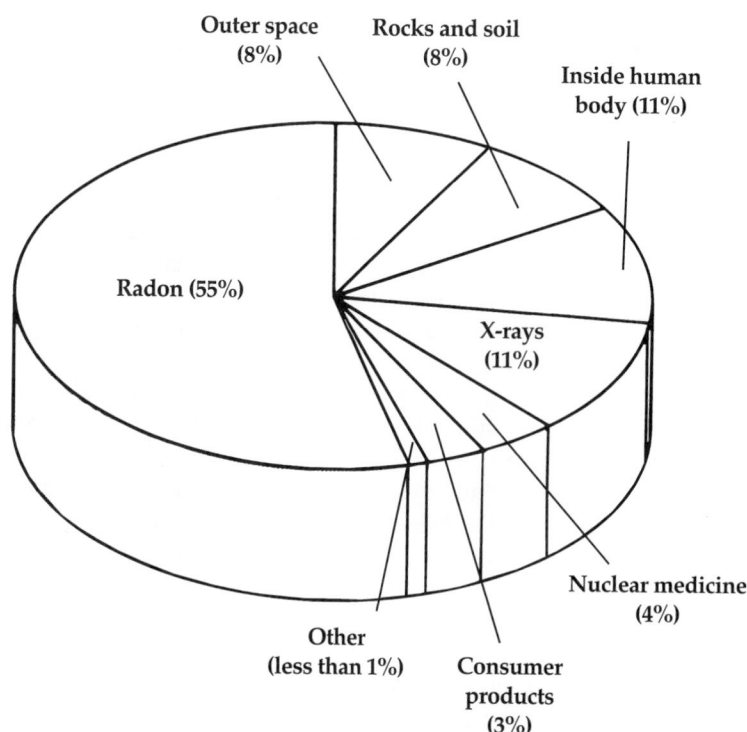

Sources of radiation exposure of United States population. Total is 360 mrads per year. Courtesy: National Council on Radiation Protection and Measurements.

What About Radioactive Iodine?

Occasionally, persons with thyroid problems are given a dose of radioactive iodine to help cure their disease (see Hyperthyroidism, page 947). When this happens, it is important to follow your physician's instructions in order to minimize radiation exposure to members of your family during the first few days after the radioactive iodine treatment. Because radiation exposure decreases rapidly with distance, these instructions usually consist of simple steps such as not holding children on your lap, not sharing eating utensils, and sleeping alone for several days. Such steps decrease radiation exposure of family members to nearly zero.

What About Other Radiation?

There is little you can do about most natural radiation exposure. Radiation is in the air around us, and we cannot avoid it. However, if your occupation or geographic location exposes you to greater than normal amounts of radiation, you might consider lifestyle changes to decrease your exposure. If levels of radon in your home are high, make adjustments to decrease them (see page 378).

The Radon Risk

The element uranium is found in soil and in rocks that contain granite, shale, or phosphate (which means it is also found in masonry building material such as bricks and concrete). As it decays, the uranium releases a gas called radon in such small quantities that it is usually harmless.

Sometimes, however, especially in the interior of some homes, radon can accumulate and the level can become relatively high. Radon decays to radioactive atoms that may attach themselves to dust particles and, when inhaled, may release small bursts of energy that can damage lung tissue and may increase the risk of lung cancer after many years of exposure.

Measuring Radon

A commonly used measure of radioactivity in the United States is the curie. The Environmental Protection Agency urges you to take action if the average annual radon level in your home is 4 or more picocuries per liter of air (a picocurie is one-trillionth of a curie).

The Testing Process

Several tests are available; we recommend use of an alpha track detector in the fall and winter months. Available in hardware stores and supermarkets, this detector measures radon over several months to a year.

Use at least two detectors in your home. Place one in the lowest part used as a living area (such as a family room) and one in an upper area (such as a bedroom). Follow the directions you receive with the testing device, and return the device to the manufacturer as soon as the testing period ends. The manufac-turer will send you the test results, usually within 2 weeks.

Making Changes

If tests conducted over a period of years indicate that average radon levels in your home are more than 4 picocuries per liter of air, minor adjustments to your home may be recommended. Rarely is expensive remodeling required.

Try the following approaches. In the cellar or crawl space, cover large openings to the soil; cover sump pumps and vent them to the outside. Use a high-quality caulk that adheres to concrete to seal cracks and other openings in your basement floors and walls. Insulate the floor above any crawl space and keep vents open on all sides of your home to ventilate the basement or crawl space.

If the radon reading is very high, you might consider installing a small fan that brings in fresh air. Another option is the installation of an air-to-air heat exchanger.

Retest your home after making the changes to determine whether you have decreased the amount of radon in the air.

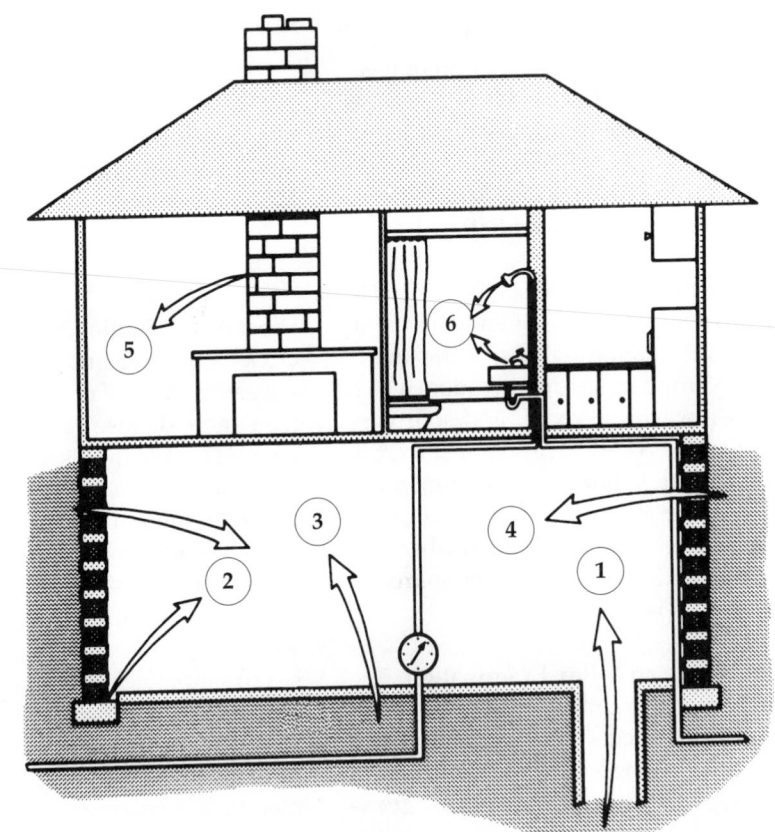

Here, in descending order of frequency, are the six most common routes by which radon can enter your home: (1) open sump pump, (2) gaps between wall-to-wall joints, (3) cracks in foundation floors and mortar joints, (4) pores in concrete blocks, (5) building materials, and (6) water supply.

Chapter 18

Traveling Abroad

Contents

Pre-Travel Planning, 380
Tips for Getting Ready, 380

Immunizations, 380
Your Medical Traveling Packet, 381
Diphtheria, Tetanus, Pertussis, 382
Polio, 382
Influenza, 382
Pneumococcal Pneumonia, 382
Hepatitis A, 382
Hepatitis B, 382
Meningococcal Meningitis, 382

Rabies, 382
Malaria, 382
Cholera, 383
Typhoid, 383
Plague, 383
Yellow Fever, 383
Smallpox, 383

Common Ailments of Travelers, 383
Traveler's Diarrhea, 383
A Drink to Replace Lost Fluids, 384
Jet Lag, 385

Pre-Travel Planning

More than 45 million Americans travel abroad each year. Getting your passport and visa in order and packing appropriate clothes are activities most people take for granted. Getting the proper immunizations before you leave is sometimes overlooked but equally important.

You should also anticipate and plan carefully for minor maladies and major medical emergencies while traveling. About 1 in 4 people experience some type of illness or injury while traveling. One-half million need a physician or require hospitalization.

Tips for Getting Ready

Begin Planning 2 to 3 Months Ahead

As soon as you know your travel destinations, contact your physician to see if there are immunizations you will need. Some immunizations require a series of vaccinations that you should get several weeks to a month before you leave.

Also talk to your physician about what medications or medical supplies you should carry with you for the particular areas to which you will be traveling.

If you have underlying health conditions such as heart disease, high blood pressure, or diabetes, or are handicapped, discuss with your physician any problems you should anticipate and recommendations for dealing with them. You may want to consider staying in larger cities where medical expertise and equipment are more readily available.

Get Names of English-Speaking Physicians

For each area you visit, have a name, address, and telephone number for a physician who speaks English. For a world directory of English-speaking physicians who are available 24 hours a day, write to the nonprofit International Association for Medical Assistance to Travelers (IAMAT), 417 Center St., Lewiston, NY 14092.

The American embassy or consulate can usually provide a list of local English-speaking physicians. If neither resource is available and you need care urgently, go to the nearest university medical center.

Other 24-hour international emergency telephone numbers include the following: U.S. Assist: 800-756-5900; the U.S. State Department's Overseas Citizens' Emergency Center: 202-647-5227; and American Express: 800-554-2639. There may be a charge for these services.

Consider Travel Protection Insurance

Most foreign physicians and hospitals will not bill your American insurance company directly. Rather, they will require cash in advance or at least verification of your ability to pay for services. You must seek reimbursement when you return home. Medicare does not pay for foreign medical services.

Although you should have someone prepared to wire you money from home, this often takes 24 hours or longer. Some travel protection insurance plans offer immediate hospital deposit, emergency travel arrangements, and, if necessary, emergency air evacuation. Ask your travel agent for more information.

Immunizations

Before you leave on a trip out of the country, and especially if you are going to a less-developed country, make sure that you and your children are adequately immunized against any infectious diseases you might encounter.

Every adult and child should have up-to-date immunity against tetanus and polio, whether traveling or not. The other immunizations you need depend on the country you are visiting and perhaps the region of that country. Generally, you are more likely to be exposed to an infectious disease in a rural area than in an urban one (particularly in less-developed countries) because water supply systems and sanitary conditions may not be as up to date in rural areas.

Many countries have immunization requirements that travelers must fulfill before

Your Medical Traveling Packet

When traveling abroad, taking your wallet, passport, and suitcases is a given. But it's also important to include medications, first aid supplies, and medical records.

Medications

Make sure that you have an ample supply of medications you or anyone in your family take regularly. Prescriptions should be up to date. An extra supply also is a good idea because you may stay longer than you anticipated.

If you have allergies that you periodically need to treat, take the necessary medications along as well. A familiar remedy may not be available in a foreign land.

Be sure to include any special medications your physician recommends, such as for motion sickness if you tend to feel nauseated during bumpy travels.

In addition to your regular medications, taking a simple first aid kit is a sensible precaution. Supplies might include alcohol wipes, antiseptic cream, adhesive and gauze bandages, aspirin or acetaminophen, a thermometer, elastic wrap for sprains, insect repellent, sunscreen, lip balm, an antacid, a mild laxative, and a decongestant.

Also include polarizing sunglasses and a second pair of prescription glasses or contact lenses with more wetting and cleaning solutions than you would ordinarily use.

Keep prescription medications in their original pharmacy containers with labels intact. This avoids problems if officials check for illicit drugs.

Transport medications in carry-on luggage. If your checked-in suitcase turns up missing, your medications won't.

Medical Records

In case of illness or an emergency, the physician you consult on your trip will need to know something of your medical history. Carry a brief medical report in your wallet or where it is easily accessible. Make sure other members of your family or traveling group know where it is so they can quickly and easily provide relevant information to any medical professional who may need it. The medical information should include the following:

- Your name, address, telephone number, social security number, and person to notify in case of an emergency.

- Your health status, including any chronic diseases you have— in particular, diabetes, glaucoma, heart disorder, or hypertension—as well as any allergies to drugs, foods, or insect stings. If you have a health problem or allergy, wear a medical bracelet. (To obtain one, call 800-344-3226.)
- Recent test results of any abnormalities on an X-ray or electrocardiogram (especially if you have an implanted pacemaker) for comparison in an emergency.
- A list of your medications and eyeglass or contact lens prescription for easier replacement. For medications, include the generic and brand names (if any) and the doses and frequency at which you take them.
- Your immunization record, including dates. Some countries require certificates of vaccination against diseases such as cholera and yellow fever.
- The names, addresses, and telephone numbers of your primary care physician and your traveling companions' physicians.

entering. These are listed in the booklet *Health Information for International Travel*, written by the Centers for Disease Control (CDC) and published yearly by the U.S. Government Printing Office. For more up-to-date information, you can call the CDC in Atlanta, Georgia. You can also ask your physician, local or state health department, or the consulate or embassy of the country you plan to visit.

If you are going to an area where diseases are prevalent, check with your physician about immunization at least a month before you plan to depart, because some vaccines must be given several weeks before exposure to the infectious agent.

Take immunization records with you when you travel out of the United States. Some countries require certificates of vaccination against diseases such as cholera and yellow fever (see Your Medical Traveling Packet, this page).

Some trip-related illnesses do not become evident until after you return home. When you report symptoms to your physician, be sure to mention any trips you have recently taken.

Some suggestions for basic immunization schedules are given here.

Diphtheria, Tetanus, Pertussis

Diphtheria, tetanus, and pertussis (DTP) immunization usually is given to children as a series of shots and is completed by the time the child enters school. A tetanus/diphtheria booster is given to adults and children every 10 years thereafter. Every child and adult should have up-to-date immunity at all times. If you get a contaminated wound, and it's been more than 5 years since you last received a tetanus booster, you should get a booster dose.

Polio

Poliomyelitis immunization generally is performed by giving a live vaccine orally at ages 2, 4, and 18 months (and 6 months if polio is prevalent in the area) at the same time as the DTP vaccine. All adults and children should be immunized, whether they are traveling or not. A booster may be recommended for travel to some developing areas of the world.

Influenza

Immunization is not recommended for the general population, but certain persons who are at high risk of serious illness should be vaccinated (see page 1066) before leaving the country. Elderly and chronically ill people in particular should be vaccinated.

Pneumococcal Pneumonia

Elderly and chronically ill people who have not received this vaccine previously should be vaccinated once before traveling, several weeks before departure. Once a person has received this vaccine, no further doses should be given. However, individuals without a spleen should get a repeat dose every 6 years.

Hepatitis A

Hepatitis A vaccine is recommended for all travelers to any area of the world where sanitation is poor. You are at risk of contracting hepatitis A from contaminated food or water or from contact with someone infected.

Hepatitis B

If you plan to travel to a country where hepatitis B is prevalent, or if you are at risk of acquiring the disease (see page 801), you should be vaccinated. Persons at increased risk include those handling blood or blood products, homosexuals, illicit drug users, or those staying more than 6 months in a developing country.

Meningococcal Meningitis

If you are traveling to some regions where meningitis is prevalent, you should receive types A, C, W-135, and Y vaccines against this disease. Check with your health care provider.

Rabies

If you plan to stay or live in areas where rabies is common, you may want to acquire immunity to the virus before leaving by obtaining injections of human diploid cell vaccine.

Malaria

There is no vaccine, as yet, against malaria, but effective preventive medications are available. In most countries of the world where malaria exists, resistance has developed to chloroquine. If you will be traveling in such areas, your health care provider may provide you with mefloquine.

You should start taking either of these medicines 1 week before you leave home and continue to take the medicine while you are traveling and for 4 weeks after leaving the malaria area. Discuss with your physician possible adverse reactions to mefloquine. Also be sure to review your past and current medical history for any contraindications to taking the medicine.

Because malaria infection often is initially thought to be a flu-like illness or some other viral disease, be wary if you develop an illness, with fever, within 12 months after traveling to a malaria area. Tell your physician about your trip. A blood test can determine whether you have the disease.

Other preventive measures include avoiding mosquito bites—the *Anopheles* mosquito carries the malaria parasite. Stay in dwellings with screens on exterior doors and windows. Spray rooms with insecticide. Use mosquito repellent on exposed parts of your body and on your pillow at night (effective repellents contain diethylmetatoluamide). Sleep under mosquito netting. Avoid being outside between dusk and dawn. If you must be outside, wear protective clothing, apply repellents to exposed skin, and keep moving.

Cholera

The risk for cholera to tourists in affected areas is considered extremely low. Still, travelers to areas with epidemic cholera need to scrupulously follow precautions for preventing traveler's diarrhea (see this page). The general rule "boil it, cook it, peel it, or forget it" has been proposed for preventing cholera. Travelers to areas with cholera should not consume the following:

1. Unboiled or untreated water and ice made from such water

2. Food and beverages offered by street vendors

3. Raw or partially cooked fish and shellfish, including ceviche

4. Uncooked vegetables

Travelers should eat only foods that are cooked and hot, or fruits you peel yourself. Carbonated bottled water and carbonated soft drinks are usually safe if no ice is added.

Cholera vaccination, which protects approximately 50 percent of vaccinated persons for 3 to 6 months, is not recommended, nor is it a substitute for scrupulously choosing food and drink.

If you develop severe watery diarrhea, or diarrhea and vomiting, during or within 1 week after travel to an area with known cholera, you should seek medical attention immediately.

Typhoid

If you are traveling to a country where typhoid is prevalent, your physician may suggest that you get a weakened live vaccine. Taken orally, it generally is effective for up to 5 years. If you live in that country for an extended period of time, the vaccine should be repeated every 5 years while you are at risk of exposure.

Plague

Vaccination consists of three injections a month or more apart and is given to people traveling to areas where the disease is still prevalent. This vaccine is not currently available in the United States and must be obtained in the country in which you are traveling.

Yellow Fever

If you are traveling to certain areas of Africa and South America where yellow fever is widespread, you should receive a live virus vaccine, available only at certain yellow fever vaccination centers. You must repeat vaccination at least every 10 years.

Smallpox

Smallpox has been eradicated as of 1980—vaccination is unnecessary.

Common Ailments of Travelers

Traveler's Diarrhea

Signs and Symptoms
- Diarrhea
- Abdominal cramps

"Traveler's diarrhea," "turista," "Montezuma's revenge," and "Tut's tummy" are familiar names for a common ailment of travelers. A trip to a foreign country by no means guarantees a bout with gastrointestinal discomfort. But if you travel to a land where the climate, social conditions, or sanitary standards and practices are significantly different from yours at home, particularly developing nations, the risk may be high.

The Causes

Traveler's diarrhea may be attributed to a number of causes, including unaccustomed food and drink, change in the bacteria that naturally live in the bowel, change in living habits, and, sometimes, viral infections. Usually the problem is due to inadequate sanitation. Contaminated food and water contain bacteria that attach themselves to the lining of your small intestine and release a toxin. The toxin causes diarrhea and abdominal cramps.

How Serious Is Traveler's Diarrhea?

Traveler's diarrhea most often begins abruptly while traveling or shortly after you return home. Usually it is mild. Symptoms generally subside in 3 or 4 days, but you may not feel well for several more days.

Sometimes traveler's diarrhea can be more troublesome. If it is caused by organisms other than common bacteria, symptoms may be more severe, long-lasting, and difficult to overcome. Drug therapy is often needed to rid your body of the organism.

Prevention Strategies

Discuss Medications With Your Physician

There are no vaccines that offer protection against traveler's diarrhea. Taking antibiotics or other medications as a preventive measure before and during your trip is not generally recommended by public health experts.

These experts are concerned that the organisms that cause the problem may become resistant to medications. Also, the effective drugs, doxycycline and trimethoprim/sulfamethoxazole, can cause side effects that may spoil your trip.

Taking bismuth subsalicylate (Pepto-Bismol) tablets throughout your trip as a preventive measure can decrease your risk of diarrhea.

Use Proper Water Sources

The first rule for avoiding diarrhea while traveling: do not drink the water—whether it comes from a stream, a well, or a tap—unless it has been sterilized. Bottled water may be safe, if it is factory bottled. In addition, you can purchase from camping stores a water filter pump that removes many microorganisms. Check to see that they have microfilters that prevent passage of viruses.

Iodine tablets or crystals, which you also can purchase at camping stores, will kill most microbes. However, be sure to follow the directions and allow the treatment to continue long enough before drinking the water. (Keep in mind that drinking large amounts of water containing iodine is not always a good idea either.) Water that has been chlorinated or boiled is usually safe.

At some of the newer resort hotels you may be able to drink tap water if the water system is up to date, but do not rely on it.

Often, tourists will conscientiously avoid drinking water from the tap, only to come down with traveler's diarrhea from drinking beverages that contain ice. If the water used to make ice is not free of bacteria, when the ice melts into your drink you will be exposed to foreign bacteria.

Be careful as well of fruit juices because they often are diluted with tap water. Bottled wine, beer, and carbonated sodas (without ice) are safe.

Eat Safe Foods

Cooked foods are usually safe, but do not eat raw foods—especially salads that contain lettuce or raw vegetables. Fruits and vegetables with a rind or skin that can be peeled immediately before you eat them usually are safe after careful washing. Avoid fruit and vegetables already peeled. Eat in restaurants that have a reputation for safety.

Do not eat foods from street vendors, and consume only foods (especially meat products) that are thoroughly cooked. If you

---

A Drink to Replace Lost Fluids

If you experience severe weakness after a bout of traveler's diarrhea, your body may have lost an excessive amount of vital fluids, salts, and minerals. To help correct the problem if professional help is unavailable, prepare this replacement solution.

Mix ½ teaspoon of table salt (sodium chloride), ½ teaspoon of baking soda (sodium bicarbonate), and 4 tablespoons of table sugar (sucrose) in 1 quart of carbonated water. If carbonated water is not available, tap water boiled for 15 minutes is a suitable substitute.

You can prepare this solution in your hotel room. Drink it over the course of the day as a supplement to a clear liquid diet.

cook your own food, keep cold those items that can spoil. Even cooked food can be contaminated. Avoid unpasteurized milk and dairy products.

Treatment

If you do get traveler's diarrhea, drink plenty of safe liquids to replace lost fluids, salts, and minerals. It is important not to get dehydrated. Orange, apple, or other fruit juices are good for replacing lost potassium, but remember to avoid juices that are diluted with tap water. Broths, sweetened tea, and soda are also good for keeping up your strength.

As soon as you feel like eating again, start with nonfat soft foods to avoid irritating your intestinal system. Bananas are a good source of potassium and can help slow diarrhea. Bland cereals, rice, gelatin, jellied consommé, simple puddings, and soft-cooked eggs are other possibilities (see Infections of the Gastrointestinal Tract, page 766).

While some travelers take antibacterial medications as a preventive measure even though public health experts discourage this, other travelers pack them and take them only if symptoms occur during the trip.

Most physicians recommend that you take prescription medicines that offer symptomatic relief rather than powerful antibacterial drugs that attack infectious agents and can cause side effects. Paregoric or codeine and newer synthetic drugs such as loperamide or diphenoxylate often ease cramps and diarrhea and can be taken orally. Although some authorities believe these medications may prolong the diarrhea and cramps, most people are pleased with the prompt relief the drugs offer.

Jet Lag

Symptoms

- Fatigue, drowsiness
- Irritability
- Difficulty in sleeping
- Loss of mental acuity
- Minor coordination problems

If you've ever traveled by air across several time zones, you're probably familiar with what it's like to get jet lag—that dragged-out, out-of-sync feeling that can affect your regular patterns of eating, working, relaxing, and sleeping.

The Cause

The precipitating event that produces jet lag is clear—the sudden readjustment you demand of your body when traveling across time zones.

How Serious Is Jet Lag?

Not all jet lag is the same. Flying eastward—and therefore resetting your body clock forward—is often more difficult than flying westward and adding hours to your day. (Flying north or south does not produce jet lag.)

Most people's bodies adjust at the rate of about 1 hour a day. Thus, after a four-time-zone change, your body will require about 4 days to resynchronize its usual rhythms.

Prevention Strategies

Reset Your Body's Clock

Begin resetting your body's clock several days in advance of your departure by adopting a sleep-wake pattern similar to the day-night cycle at your destination. Or try setting your watch to the time of your destination when you are halfway through the trip so that you start thinking in terms of the new time.

Another strategy is to try to schedule your arrival at your destination at roughly your usual bedtime according to the clocks in the time zone to which you are flying. Or try sleeping on the plane and planning to arrive at the hour you usually start your day. In these ways, you immediately begin to orient your body systems to the new time schedule, a valuable psychological and physiologic advantage.

Getting added sleep before departure may also help to ease the symptoms of jet lag.

Alternatively, if you have an important event or meeting at your destination, get there 2 or 3 days in advance. That way, you will not be disadvantaged by a fresh case of jet lag.

Drink Plenty of Fluids, Eat Lightly

Drink extra liquids during your flight to avoid dehydration, but limit beverages with alcohol and caffeine. They increase dehydration and may disrupt your sleep.

Eat a high-protein, low-calorie diet just before, during, and after your flight. Limit your intake of salty or fatty food. If you have a special diet, be sure to follow it. Many airlines offer special meals (low-sodium, fruit plate, kosher), but you'll need to make arrangements in advance.

Don't Sit Still

During your flight, and especially on lengthy flights, get up frequently to stretch and walk the aisles. Extended sitting can put you at risk for a potentially fatal condition in which a blood clot forms in your leg, breaks loose, and blocks an artery in your lung.

Support hose also can help prevent clots or swelling of your feet and ankles during lengthy flights. But avoid socks or stockings with elasticized tops that constrict your legs and interfere with blood circulation.

Adjust Your Medication Schedule

If you are on a regimen of medications, you may have to make adjustments as to when you take them to account for changes in time zones. Check with your physician before leaving. If you have diabetes and are taking long-acting insulin, you may have to switch to regular insulin until you adjust to the new time, food, and activities.

Part III

First Aid and Emergency Care

This heavily illustrated special section focuses on a wide range of unexpected events, from a severe burn, a deep cut, breathing difficulty, a seizure, or chest pain, to dealing effectively with a nosebleed or a sprained ankle. We begin with basic rules to follow in addressing any emergency medical problem—minor or major.

Contents

Commonsense Medicine 391

Bites and Stings 394

Bleeding Emergencies 399

Burns 403

Choking, Breathing Emergencies, and Resuscitation . . . 406

Environmental Emergencies 414

Faints, Seizures, and Strokes 420

Fever 423

Foreign Bodies 425

Genitourinary Emergencies 428

Intoxication and Behavioral Emergencies 429

Pain Emergencies 432

Poisoning Emergencies 437

Shock 441

Trauma Emergencies 445

Part III

First Aid and Emergency Care

Contents

Commonsense Medicine, 391
  Emergency Warning Signs, 391
  Basic First Aid Supplies, 392
Care of Minor Wounds, 392
  Tetanus Immunization, 393
Care of Minor Illnesses, 393

Bites and Stings, 394
Animal Bites, 394
  The Risk of Rabies, 395
Human Bites, 395
Insect Bites and Stings, 395
Snake Bites, 398
Jellyfish Stings, 398

Bleeding Emergencies, 399
  How to Stop Severe Bleeding, 400
Bleeding From a Wound or Injury, 401
Bleeding From Body Openings, 401
  Detecting Internal Bleeding, 402
Nosebleed, 403

Burns, 403
Burn Classifications, 403
Electrical Burns, 404
Chemical Burns, 404
  Treating Minor Burns at Home, 405
  Treating Major Burns, 405

Choking, Breathing Emergencies, and
Resuscitation, 406
  The Universal Sign, 406
Recognizing an Obstructed Airway, 406
Coughing Versus Choking, 406
Clearing an Obstructed Airway, 406
  The Heimlich Maneuver, 407
Cardiopulmonary Resuscitation, 408
  Performing CPR on an Infant, 412
  Breathing Difficulty Due to Croup, Epiglottitis, or

Bronchitis, 413
Severe Asthma Attack, 413

Environmental Emergencies, 414
Sunburn, 414
Heat Stress, 414
  Skin Emergencies, 415
Hypothermia, 416
Frostbite, 416
Altitude Disorders and Decompression Sickness, 417
Near Drowning, 418
Electrical Injury, 418
Smoke Inhalation, 419
Carbon Monoxide Poisoning, 419

Faints, Seizures, and Strokes, 420
Fainting Spells, 420
Seizures, 421
Strokes, 421
Hypertensive Crises, 422
Diabetic Emergencies, 422

Fever, 423
When Is It an Emergency? 423
What Is a Fever? 423
  Using a Thermometer, 424
What Is a Fever Emergency? 424
  Treatment of Fever in a Child, 425

Foreign Bodies, 425
In the Eye, 425
In the Ear, 426
In the Nose, 427
Inhaled Foreign Objects, 427
Swallowed Foreign Objects, 427
  Children and Button Batteries, 427

Genitourinary Emergencies, 428
  Sexual Assault and Sexual Abuse, 428

Testicular Torsion, 428
Trauma to the External Genitals, 428

Intoxication and Behavioral Emergencies, 429
Alcohol Intoxication, 429
Acute Drug Intoxication, 430
    Sudden Personality Changes, 430
Suicidal Thoughts and Behavior, 431
Hyperventilation, 431

Pain Emergencies, 432
    Abrupt Onset of Severe Pain: When to Be
        Concerned, 432
Head Pain, 432
Chest Pain, 433
    Chest Wall Pain, 434
    Is It a Heart Attack? 434
Abdominal and Pelvic Pain, 435
Pain in the Extremities, 436
    Acute Joint Pain, 437

Poisoning Emergencies, 437
Handling Poisoning Emergencies, 438
    Poison Center Resources, 438
Medications as Poisons, 439
    Acids and Alkalis, 439

Poisonous Plants, 440
    Garden-Variety Poisonous Plants, 440
Food Poisoning, 440
Food Allergies, 441

Shock, 441
Kinds of Shock, 441
Loss of Blood, 441
    Recognizing and Treating Shock, 442
Dehydration, 443
Heart-Related Shock, 443
Septic Shock, 444
Anaphylaxis, 444
Toxic Shock Syndrome, 445

Trauma Emergencies, 445
Fractures, 445
    Types of Fractures, 446
Sprains, 449
Dislocations, 449
Traumatic Amputation, 450
Head Injuries, 451
Eye Emergencies, 452
Tooth Loss (Avulsion), 453

How to Respond

Medical emergencies require immediate action. Be prepared by reviewing the sections listed below:

In the Event of	See
A possible heart attack	Is It a Heart Attack? page 434
Heavy bleeding	Bleeding Emergencies, page 399
A broken bone or severe sprain	Trauma Emergencies, page 445
Inability to breathe	Choking, Breathing Emergencies, and Resuscitation, page 406
A possible stroke	Strokes, page 421
Diabetic emergencies	Diabetic Emergencies, page 422
Poisoning emergencies	Poisoning Emergencies, page 437

Commonsense Medicine

There's been an accident.

Someone—you, a companion, or another person—has been injured or is suddenly very ill. You must do something, but what?

In this special section we will discuss dozens of common emergencies and suggest appropriate procedures for dealing with them. Some commonsense ground rules to follow in addressing an emergency medical problem, whether it's major or minor, are listed below:

Keep Calm. Try not to panic: you may experience an overpowering sense of fear, but keep control. Often, a few deep breaths will help.

Reassure the Victim. If it is another person who has sustained the major injury, reassure the person. A hand on the shoulder or a light, reassuring touch may help.

Do No Harm. Do not move someone who has been injured, who has seemingly lost consciousness, or who complains of neck pain. He or she may have an unstable injury such as a neck fracture.

Be Prepared. Keep the numbers of emergency services posted near your telephone. Although you can find some or all of them printed on the back cover or on one of the opening pages of your telephone book, it is better to have them always in view by or on the telephone.

Take a Class in First Aid. Your local branch of the American Red Cross or YMCA/YWCA or other civic organization offers such a course free or for a nominal fee. Instruction in cardiopulmonary resuscitation (CPR) may be invaluable if someone in your family is at risk of heart attack. CPR courses are also generally available and inexpensive, and they require just a few hours.

If in Doubt, Call for Help. It's human nature to want a problem to be small, even to resolve itself. Sometimes the temptation with a minor injury or illness is to say, "Oh, you'll be okay." That prediction may be so, of course, and lots of unnecessary trips are made annually to the nation's emergency rooms, but, as the cliché says, "It's better to be safe than sorry." (See Emergency Warning Signs, this page.) If in doubt, make the call. In most communities, the emergency call number is 911.

Calling for Help. When you summon emergency assistance, speak clearly. As calmly as you can, give the emergency dispatcher the key information. This includes the victim's location ("He's at 111 Old Farm Road, in the big red barn, just beyond the house"), what the problem is, when it happened, your name, and the victim's name. Do not hang up until the dispatcher has all the required information; he or she will probably also need your telephone number and perhaps directions to the scene. After dark, make sure your house number is clearly illuminated.

In the Emergency Room. Patients are treated in the emergency room according to need: it's not first come, first served; it's a who-needs-help-now priority. A member of the emergency care team will evaluate the extent of the injury or illness.

The examining physician will need to know the circumstances of the injury; the symptoms as they developed; the person's medical history and what medications he or she uses, especially if they bear directly on the situation; and when or if treatment or medication for the emergency has been administered.

Before You Go Home. Make sure when the physician or nurse releases you or the person being treated that any follow-up

Emergency Warning Signs

The following warning signs, compiled by the American College of Emergency Physicians, suggest an immediate trip to your physician's office or emergency room:

- Sudden pain at any location in your body. Chest pain or pressure in the upper abdominal area, for example, can signal a heart attack
- Sudden dizziness, headache, or change in vision
- Weakness or faintness
- Difficulty breathing or shortness of breath
- Severe or persistent vomiting or diarrhea
- Suicidal or homicidal feelings
- Significant bleeding, whether or not accompanied by pain

The presence of one or more of these symptoms suggests that you should seek immediate medical help.

Basic First Aid Supplies

Always keep your medicine chest or first aid kit well stocked—emergencies do not occur on a schedule. Include the following basic supplies:

Adhesive or gauze wrappings or pads in several sizes
Soap
Absorbent cotton
Tweezers
Cotton-tipped swabs
Thermometer
Aspirin or acetaminophen
Antiseptic solution (such as hydrogen peroxide)
Hydrocortisone cream (for bites and stings)

Bandages or surgical tape (Steri-Strips)
Sterile gauze
Adhesive tape
Sharp scissors
Tissues
First aid manual
Syrup of ipecac
Antiseptic cream (such as bacitracin)

If a member of your family reacts severely to bee or insect stings (anaphylaxis, see page 444), have a kit containing a syringe with epinephrine (adrenaline) readily available.

Other medications you may want to have on hand include antihistamine tablets, an antidiarrheal medication, insulin and a simple sugar (for diabetics), and reserve supplies of medications required by your family members.

instructions are clearly understood. You may want to write down follow-up instructions. (Sometimes a stressful situation makes recall difficult.) These may include advice on rest, exercise, medication, or scheduling further medical consultations, perhaps with a specialist or your family physician.

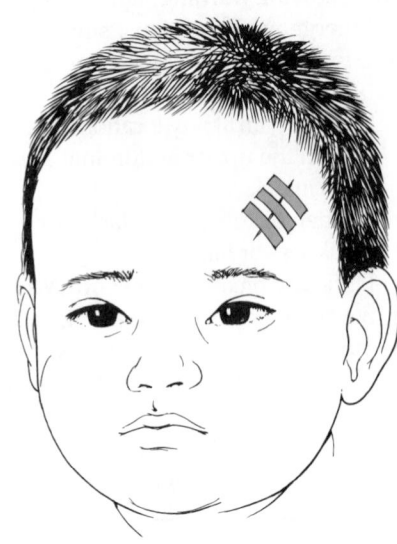

Steri-Strip bandages can be used to effectively close a superficial cut if the cut has edges that can easily be drawn together.

Terms of the Trade. An "emergency" is a general term describing any situation in which immediate care is required. The term "trauma" implies an injury, such as a burn, wound, or broken bone. The terms are often used interchangeably, but the distinction is a useful one.

Care of Minor Wounds

Everyday cuts, scrapes, or wounds often do not require a trip to the emergency room. Yet proper care is essential to avoid infection or other complications. The following guidelines can help you in caring for simple wounds:

Stop the Bleeding. Minor bleeding from a cut or scrape usually will cease spontaneously within a few minutes. If it does not, apply pressure, using a gauze pad or clean cloth.

Emergency Bleeding. If bleeding is persistent—if the blood spurts or continues to flow after pressure has been applied—emergency care is called for. Seek immediate medical assistance (see Bleeding Emergencies, page 399).

Keep the Wound Clean. Wash the area with mild soap and water, being sure to remove any dirt or grit (if dirt or other material is embedded in the wound, consult a physician). Pat the wound dry with a clean cloth. If you want, apply an over-the-counter antibiotic cream. Cover the wound with a protective bandage unless the cut or scrape is on the face; if the wound is facial, leave it unbandaged, but apply a thin layer of antiseptic or antibiotic cream.

Does It Need Stitches? A deep, gaping, or jagged-edged wound may require stitches to hold it together for proper healing. A strip or two of surgical tape (Steri-Strips) may close a minor cut, but if the mouth of the wound is not easily closed, seek a physician's care. Proper closure also will minimize scarring.

Follow-Up Care. Change the dressing at least once a day, taking care to keep the area of the injury clean and dry.

Danger Signs. If any wound becomes inflamed—that is, tender to the touch and reddened—or if it oozes pus or other fluids, consult your physician. There may be an infection that requires additional treatment (see Wound Infections, page 1016).

Tetanus Immunization

A cut, laceration, bite, or other wound, even if minor, can lead to a tetanus infection. The result, days or even weeks later, can be "lockjaw"— literally, a stiffness of the muscles of the jaw and other muscles. This may be followed by a range of other symptoms, possibly culminating in convulsions and an inability to breathe.

Source of Infection

The tetanus bacteria usually are found in the soil but can occur virtually anywhere. If their spores enter a wound beyond the reach of oxygen, they germinate and produce a toxin that interferes with the nerves controlling your muscles.

A tetanus infection is serious and can result in death if you have not been immunized previously (see Tetanus, page 1070).

Treating the Wound

The good news is that tetanus infection is avoidable, given proper preventive steps. Consult your physician immediately if you sustain any cut or puncture wound and have not had a tetanus shot in the past 10 years. If your wound is severe, or if you had a series of tetanus shots many years ago, your physician probably will give you a booster shot of the vaccine. Your body will quickly manufacture the needed antibodies to protect you against tetanus.

If you have not had tetanus shots previously, your physician may administer tetanus immune globulin, which gives immediate protection but only for a few weeks. Your physician may decide to cleanse the wound carefully, cutting away dead tissue and leaving it open without stitches and only a light gauze dressing so that air can reach all parts of the wound. Several antibiotics can help eliminate the tetanus bacterium, but there is no substitute for proper care of the wound and use of a booster shot or the immune globulin (see Care of Minor Wounds, page 392, and Immunizations, page 1079).

Prevention

Active immunization is vital for everyone in advance of any injury. The tetanus vaccine usually is given to children as a DPT shot, in which diphtheria and pertussis (whooping cough) vaccines are given with the tetanus vaccine. Tetanus booster shots should be given every 10 years or at the time of a major injury.

Care of Minor Illnesses

Everybody gets sick from time to time. The problem may be familiar, such as a cold or flu virus, or it may be a seemingly mysterious ailment. Most often, recovery from the common minor illnesses is a matter of time and commonsense treatments. For everyday minor complaints, follow the guidelines given below.

Take It Easy

If you do not feel well, the first rule is to get some rest—or at least slow your usual pace. If you have the flu, bed rest, proper nutrition, and lots of liquids may help you recover more quickly (see Influenza, page 1065). For a cold, patience is the first treatment: it will take a few days to recover. If you feel poorly, stay home and take it easy. However, if you feel up to it, go about your business (see Common Viral Colds, page 1071).

Monitor the Symptoms

Whatever your ailment, pay attention to what your body tells you. The familiar runny nose, minor cough, and stuffed-up head of a cold usually come and go without the help that modern medicine can offer. However, a seemingly trivial ailment that persists for more than a week or two may actually be something more serious.

A few symptoms that normally accompany minor ailments are described below. However, they also can be danger signs to keep in mind when assessing that "minor ailment" from which you are suffering—just in case it is something more serious:

Pain. Acute pain (that is, pain that arrives suddenly) is usually a warning. If you experience a sudden, severe pain you have not had before, consult your physician or seek emergency care.

Fever. Many minor ailments commonly are accompanied by fever. Elevated body temperature is your body's way of fighting infection and certain diseases. A fever also increases fluid loss from the body. Therefore, adequate water intake is important if fever is present.

Although your body temperature normally varies during the day (it is lower in the morning and higher in the afternoon), a low-grade fever (when measured with a thermometer placed beneath the tongue) is usually classified as a temperature between 99.5 and 101.5 degrees Fahrenheit.

Consult your physician if a temperature of 101 degrees Fahrenheit or more persists for more than a day or two, if your temperature is higher than 103 degrees Fahrenheit, if a fever persists for more than 3 days, or if a child 3 months or younger has a temperature of 100.5 degrees Fahrenheit (see What Is a Fever Emergency? page 424). A temperature of more than 103 degrees Fahrenheit can, in an adult, confuse the mental processes.

Cough. A cough due to a cold is normal. However, a cough that persists for more than 2 or 3 weeks or one that produces bloody sputum is reason to consult your physician.

Persistent Diarrhea or Vomiting. The loss of body fluids can, if severe, be life-threatening, especially in children. Consult your physician if you or your child is unable to retain fluids. If watery diarrhea or vomiting persists longer than 2 or 3 days or is associated with a fever, blood in the stool, or a sensation of faintness when standing, see your physician.

Bites and Stings

A dog, a bee in a flowering bush, a spider or a snake, or even another person can deliver potentially dangerous bites or stings. Every such injury must be treated promptly and properly to minimize the risks of infection, allergic reaction, or other complications.

The following pages discuss animal and human bites; bites by spiders, scorpions, and other insects; bee stings; snake bites; and stings by jellyfish.

Animal Bites

Domestic pets are the cause of most animal bites. Dogs are more likely to bite than cats. However, cat bites are more likely to cause infection. For these reasons, the best treatment for an animal bite is prevention.

Teach your child from an early age not to approach strange animals. If you have a dog, obey the leash law in your town, and insist that your neighbors do the same. If an animal bites you or another person without provocation, report it to the local authorities. Animals that habitually bite should be constantly restrained or destroyed.

The vast majority of animal bites are inflicted by household pets, but strays and wild animals such as skunks, raccoons, bats, and others also bite thousands of people each year. Animals living in the wild are especially dangerous because they may carry rabies, but any animal that bites a human should be impounded and checked for rabies.

Emergency Treatment

Minor Bites
Treat a minor bite (one in which the skin is broken but not torn, and bleeding is limited) as you would any minor wound. Wash the wound thoroughly with soap and water, and apply an antibiotic cream to prevent infection (see Care of Minor Wounds, page 392).

Establish whether the person who was bitten has had a tetanus shot within the past 10 years; if not, seek medical care from your physician or local emergency room.

Serious Bites
If the bite results in a deep puncture wound, if the skin in the bitten area is badly torn, or if bleeding persists, apply pressure to stop the bleeding (see How to Stop Severe Bleeding, page 400). Then seek emergency medical assistance. Your physician will examine, wash, and treat the wound; he or she also may give a tetanus shot (see Tetanus Immunization, page 393).

Indications of Infection
Whether the wound is superficial or more serious, watch for any signs of infection in the hours and days after the bite. Swelling, redness, pus draining from the wound, or pain should be reported immediately to your physician.

Certain diseases also can be transmitted through bites and scratches. In addition to swelling or soreness at the site of the wound, accompanying symptoms may include fever,

The Risk of Rabies

Bats, foxes, and other wild animals may carry rabies—but so can the usually friendly pooch next door, especially if it runs wild in the woods from time to time.

Rabies is caused by a virus that affects the brain. Transmitted to humans by saliva from the bite of an infected animal, the rabies virus has an incubation period (the time from a bite until symptoms appear) of between 3 and 7 weeks, although it can be much longer (see Rabies, page 1070).

Symptoms

Once the incubation period is over, a tingling sensation usually develops at the site of the animal bite; a more generalized skin sensitivity may occur and changes in temperature become very uncomfortable. As the virus spreads, foaming at the mouth may occur (a consequence of excess saliva that cannot be swallowed). You may choke when you attempt to swallow even a small quantity of liquid. Uncontrolled irritability and confusion may follow, alternating with periods of calm. Convulsions and paralysis leading almost inevitably to death will result if the rabies virus is untreated. In the later stages, the virus is found in the person's saliva and could infect others.

Observe the Animal

In the event of an unprovoked bite by a domestic dog, cat, or farm animal, the animal should be caught, confined, and observed by a veterinarian for 7 to 10 days. Even a licking from an infected animal can spread the disease if its saliva touches broken skin. If a wild animal has bitten you, the animal should be killed in such a way that the animal's brain is not crushed or damaged. Then notify officials at your local health department. They will be able to assist in testing the animal for rabies. Wild raccoons, skunks, bats, coyotes, and foxes, if not caught, are generally presumed to have rabies.

Treatment

Extensive cleaning of the wound with soap and water followed by a second scrubbing with antiseptics should be carried out as soon as possible after the bite. Your physician must decide whether to treat you for rabies. Treatment consists of a passive antibody, half injected directly into the wound and half injected into the muscle, and a vaccine, usually given in five injections over 28 days.

Consult Your Physician

If circumstances suggest you may have been exposed to rabies, consult your physician or health department immediately.

---

headache, and other flu-like symptoms. Again, consult your physician immediately.

Human Bites

Human bites are of two kinds. The first is what we usually think of as a bite: an injury that results from flesh being caught between the teeth of the upper and lower jaws. The second kind, called a fight bite, occurs when, in the act of striking another person, an assailant cuts his or her knuckles on the opponent's teeth. (See page C-13 for color photograph of a human bite.)

Human bites are the most dangerous of mammalian bites—in part because people frequently delay seeking treatment out of embarrassment or fear of legal action. Human bites are also dangerous because of the considerable risk posed by the bacteria found in the human mouth. Carried by the saliva, the bacteria enter the tissues at the site of the bite and can lead to serious infections. There is also the obvious risk of injury to tendons and joints when the cut extends below the skin.

Emergency Treatment

If you sustain a human bite of either kind, seek emergency medical assistance. Do not treat a human bite yourself. A serious infection could put you at risk of a prolonged hospital stay, permanent joint stiffness, and even amputation if not appropriately treated.

Stop the bleeding by applying pressure, wash the wound thoroughly with soap and water, and bandage the wound. Then visit your physician or an emergency room. In addition to examining and treating the wound, your physician may prescribe antibiotics to prevent the development of infection.

Insect Bites and Stings

The symptoms of an insect bite result from the injection of venom or other agents into your skin. With minor bites, the reaction is temporary and local: a bump rises on your skin at the site of the bite, the area may itch for a few hours, and then over a period of days the skin irritation and discomfort disappear. Typically, the bites of mosquitoes, fleas, flies, bedbugs, ants, and chiggers follow this course.

However, your entire body can be affected if the venom is potent, as is the case with certain spiders and scorpions, or if you are hypersensitive, as some people are, to bee, wasp, and yellow jacket stings.

Spider Bites

The black widow spider (*Latrodectus mactans*) is shiny and black and about a half inch long, usually with an hourglass-shaped splash of red on its stomach. The brown recluse spider (*Loxosceles reclusa*) has long legs, and its body is roughly three-eighths of an inch long. Both the black widow and the brown recluse spiders usually are found in dark places; the black widow likes dampness (stumps and woodpiles provide excellent hiding places), and the brown recluse likes dry environments. Both are most common in the southern United States.

The bite of the black widow spider is little more than a pinprick-like sensation—some victims are not even aware of the bite. At first there may be only slight swelling and faint red marks. Within a few hours, however, intense pain and stiffness begin. Other symptoms may include chills, fever, nausea, and severe abdominal pain. The bite is rarely lethal.

The bite of a brown recluse produces a mild stinging, followed by local redness and intense pain within 8 hours. A fluid-filled blister forms at the site and then sloughs off to leave a deep, growing ulcer. Your body's reactions can vary from a mild fever and rash to nausea and listlessness. In rare cases, death can result. (See page C-14 for color photograph of a brown recluse spider bite.)

Scorpion Stings

Scorpions are found in the southwestern United States. About 3 inches long, they have eight legs and a pair of crab-like pincers. At the end of their narrow tail is the stinger.

Some scorpions have a potentially lethal venom that is injected by a sting. They live in cool, damp places: basements, junk piles, and woodpiles are favored locations. They tend to be nocturnal, and they are most likely to sting in the cool of the evening.

Because it is difficult to distinguish the highly poisonous scorpions (*Centruroides sculpturatus*) from the nonpoisonous scorpions, all scorpion stings are to be treated as medical emergencies.

Bee, Wasp, Hornet, Fire Ant, or Yellow Jacket Stings

Perhaps 1 person in 50 is allergic to the venom injected by insects in the Hymenoptera family. For such sensitive individuals, being stung by a bee or other Hymenoptera insect can be a life-threatening emergency, called an anaphylactic reaction.

Symptoms of such a reaction after a bee sting may include swelling around the eyes, lips, tongue, or throat; difficulty in breathing; coughing or wheezing; and widespread numbness or cramping. Hives may appear on the skin. Speech may be slurred, and anxiety, mental confusion, nausea and vomiting, and unconsciousness may occur. (See Insect Sting Allergies, page 1051, and Anaphylaxis, page 444.)

Tick Bites

Ticks live like fleas in the fur or feathers of many species of birds and animals. The principal risk usually is not from the tick bite itself but from a bacterium carried by the insect which can cause Lyme disease. Lyme disease manifests mainly as a form of arthritis but, in addition, may cause a wide variety of symptoms (see Lyme Disease, page 1067).

If you have a circular skin eruption when you have been in an area where ticks may live (mainly underbrush or tall grass), you may have had a bite by a tick carrying the infectious agent. This may occur even though you may not have seen this very small tick at that time.

(See page C-14 for color photograph of Lyme disease rash.)

Emergency Treatment

Mild Insect Bites and Stings

If the stinger from a bee or other insect remains in your skin, it must be removed carefully. Remove the stinger, particularly the tip of the stinger, so as not to inject more venom. (A plastic credit card can be used in a scraping motion.)

Mild insect bites can be treated with an application of a paste of baking soda, a cold, wet cloth, or ice cubes to reduce pain. You also may apply a hydrocortisone cream (purchased without a prescription) or calamine lotion to reduce itching and inflammation.

If you react more severely to minor bites, consult your physician.

Poisonous Bites and Stings

If bitten by a black widow spider, brown recluse spider, or scorpion, or if you are allergic to insects in the Hymenoptera family (such as bees and wasps), seek immediate emergency medical care.

Before seeking emergency care, however, take the following steps:

1. If the bite is on an arm or leg, snugly bandage the limb above the bite (between it and the heart). This will slow or halt the movement of the venom. The bandage should be tight enough to slow the flow of blood at skin level but not so tight as to halt all circulation in the arm or leg.

2. Remain calm. Excessive excitement or activity increases the flow of venom through your bloodstream.

3. Apply a rag dampened with cold water or lined with ice to the bite.

4. Remove the bandage after 5 minutes, but keep the arm or leg dangling down.

5. Seek emergency medical assistance.

If you know you are sensitive to bee stings, your physician may provide you with a special emergency kit containing a single-dose auto-injector or a hypodermic syringe

Distinctive marks of individual insects are emphasized to simplify identification; however, the insects are not drawn to scale. The deer tick, for example, is in reality only about the size of a sesame seed.

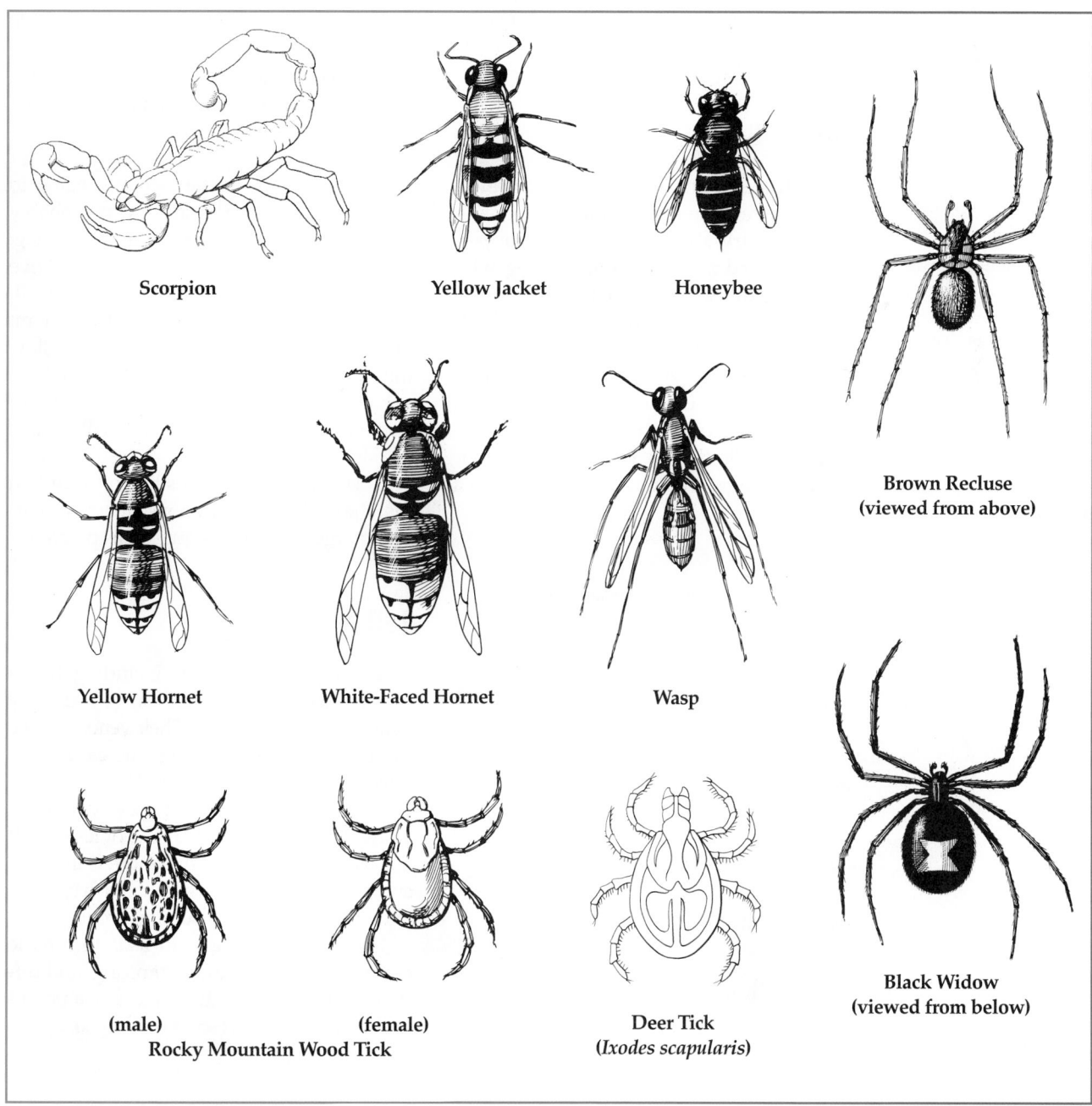

Scorpion

Yellow Jacket

Honeybee

Brown Recluse (viewed from above)

Yellow Hornet

White-Faced Hornet

Wasp

**(male)   (female)
Rocky Mountain Wood Tick**

**Deer Tick
(*Ixodes scapularis*)**

Black Widow (viewed from below)

with epinephrine (adrenaline) and an anti-histamine pill. Keep this kit handy, especially at the time of the year when, or in situations in which, you are at risk of being bitten by an insect in the Hymenoptera family. A person who loses consciousness after a bee sting should be treated for shock (see Anaphylaxis, page 444).

Tick Bites

If you find a tick crawling on your skin, carefully remove it. Do not crush it between your fingers. Wash your hands afterward.

If the tick has already bitten you and is holding on to your skin, do not pull it off. Remove the tick carefully, with tweezers.

After the tick has been removed, wash the area thoroughly. Watch carefully for the next week or two for signs or symptoms of Lyme disease (see page 1067).

Snake Bites

Most snakes are not poisonous. However, because a few are—including rattlesnakes, coral snakes, water moccasins, and copperheads—avoid picking up or playing with any snake unless you have been trained in distinguishing and handling snakes. If you are bitten by a snake, it is important to be able to determine whether the snake is poisonous. Most poisonous snakes (including the rattlesnake, copperhead, and water moccasin) have elliptically shaped (slit-like) eyes. Their heads are triangular in shape, with a depression or "pit" midway between the eyes and nostrils on both sides of the head (thus the collective name for these snakes, pit vipers). Rattlesnakes are also distinguished by a rattling sound made by the rings at the end of the snake's tail.

The water moccasin has a whitish, cottony lining in its mouth, and the coral snake has red, yellow, and black rings along its length.

Emergency Treatment

If the snake was not poisonous, wash the bite thoroughly, cover it with an antibiotic cream, and bandage it. In general, such a snake bite is more scary than dangerous.

If, however, you suspect the snake was poisonous, follow these steps:

1. Remain as quiet and still as possible after the bite. Lie down quietly and, if possible, keep the bitten area lower than the level of the heart. This position will limit circulation of the venom.

2. If the area changes color, begins to swell, or is painful, the snake was probably poisonous. If the bite is on an arm or leg, tightly bandage the limb a few inches above the bite (between it and the heart). This will also help slow the movement of the venom. The bandage should be tight enough to slow the blood flow at skin level but not so tight as to halt all circulation in the arm or leg. Do not remove the band: the physician will do that.

3. Whether you are positive or uncertain that the snake was poisonous, go to the nearest emergency room as quickly as possible.

Jellyfish Stings

Several aquatic organisms, including the jellyfish and the Portuguese man-of-war, carry venom in their tentacles. Their venom can be discharged on contact, in some cases even after they are dead.

Stinging and pain are the key symptoms, along with a red, hive-like line of lesions. If a considerable amount of venom is injected, shortness of breath, nausea, stomach cramps, and emotional upset also may occur.

More severe stings can lead to muscle cramps, fainting, cough, vomiting, and difficulty in breathing. In rare cases, a potentially fatal reaction (see Anaphylaxis, page 444) may occur.

Many poisonous snakes, including the rattlesnake, copperhead, and water moccasin, are known as pit vipers. These snakes have triangularly shaped heads, elliptically shaped (slit-like) eyes, and a depression (pit) midway between the eyes and nostrils.

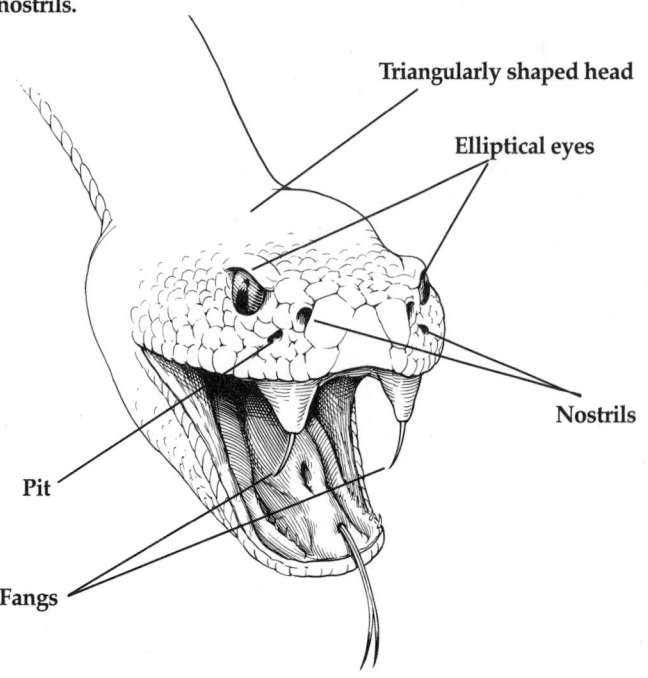

Triangularly shaped head

Elliptical eyes

Nostrils

Pit

Fangs

The Portuguese man-of-war is found in the waters of the Atlantic Ocean, ranging from Canada to the West Indies and the Mediterranean Sea. They also live in the Pacific Ocean near Hawaii and southern Japan.

(See page C-13 for color photograph of a man-of-war skin reaction.)

Emergency Treatment

If you are stung by a jellyfish or Portuguese man-of-war, do the following:

1. Get out of the water: pain and cramps can be disabling and you could drown.

2. Inactivate the stinging: sprinkle the area with meat tenderizer, vinegar, salt, sugar, or even dry sand. Gently rub the material into the wound; this step often offers quick relief.

3. Cleanse the wound: after waiting 15 to 20 minutes, gently wash the area with sea-water. Do not use fresh water and do not rub the skin because either action could trigger discharge of more venom.

4. Remove the stinging tentacles: apply a paste made of seawater and sand (or baking soda, talcum powder, or flour). Scrape the residue with a knife or other sharp object, such as a clamshell. It is best to wear gloves or use a towel when removing the man-of-war debris.

5. Apply 1 percent hydrocortisone cream (available without a prescription) to reduce redness and swelling. A local anesthetic ointment (such as benzocaine) helps relieve pain, and a calamine-type lotion lessens itching. Mild analgesics, such as aspirin and acetaminophen, are often used, but prescription pain killers may be necessary after severe stings.

6. For severe stings and other symptoms, seek emergency care.

Bleeding Emergencies

When an injury results in bleeding (hemorrhage), steps must be taken to stop the loss of blood. If substantial amounts of blood are lost, shock (see page 441), unconsciousness, and death can result.

Most bleeding injuries are not life-threatening, although appropriate care must be taken not only to stop the bleeding but also to avoid infection and other complications. The pages that follow discuss appropriate emergency procedures to accomplish these ends.

It is often useful to distinguish the kind of bleeding that was sustained. The three main classifications are capillary, venous, and arterial:

Capillary Bleeding. The capillaries are the most numerous and the smallest blood vessels in the body. When a minor cut or skin scrape opens some capillaries, the bleeding is usually slow. The body's clotting action is generally sufficient to stop the bleeding in a matter of minutes.

Venous Bleeding. Deep cuts often open veins, releasing blood that is on its way back to the heart. Having delivered its load of oxygen to the cells, the blood is dark red. It flows steadily but slowly. Placing pressure on the wound will usually stop the blood flow.

Arterial Bleeding. The least common but most serious type of bleeding involves the opening of an artery. The blood that is released is bright red and often spews forth in rhythmic spurts that coincide with the contractions of the heart. If a major artery is severed and not treated promptly, it is possible to bleed to death in as little as a minute. In most cases, however, direct, firm pressure on the wound will stop arterial bleeding.

The location and nature of the wound itself also have an impact on the choice of treatment. The following pages discuss wounds to the skin, bleeding from the mouth or other body openings, and bleeding or severe bruising beneath the skin.

How to Stop Severe Bleeding

To stop a serious bleeding injury, follow these steps:

1. Lay the affected person down. If possible, the person's head should be slightly lower than the trunk or the legs should be elevated. This position reduces the chances of fainting by increasing blood flow to the brain. If possible, elevate the site of bleeding; for example, an injured hand can be held up, over the level of the heart, in order to reduce blood flow.

2. Remove any obvious debris or dirt from the wound. Do not remove any objects impaled in the person. Do not probe the wound or attempt to clean it at this point. Your principal concern is to stop the loss of blood.

3. Put pressure directly on the wound with a sterile bandage, clean cloth, or even a piece of clothing. If nothing else is available, use your hand.

4. Maintain pressure until the bleeding stops. When it does, bind the wound dressing tightly with adhesive tape. If none is available, use a piece of clean clothing.

5. If the bleeding continues and seeps through the gauze or other material you are holding on the wound, do not remove it. Rather, add more absorbent material on top of it.

6. If the bleeding does not stop with direct pressure, you may need to apply pressure to the major artery that delivers blood to the area of the wound. In the case of a wound on the hand or lower arm, for example, squeeze the main artery in the upper arm against the bone. Keep your fingers flat; with the other hand, continue to exert pressure on the wound itself.

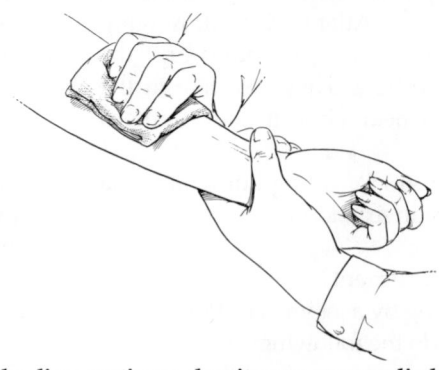

If bleeding continues despite pressure applied directly to the wound, maintain pressure and also apply pressure to the nearest major artery.

7. Immobilize the injured body part once the bleeding has been stopped. Leave the bandages in place, and get the injured person to the emergency room as soon as possible (see Traumatic Amputation, page 450).

Arterial pressure points

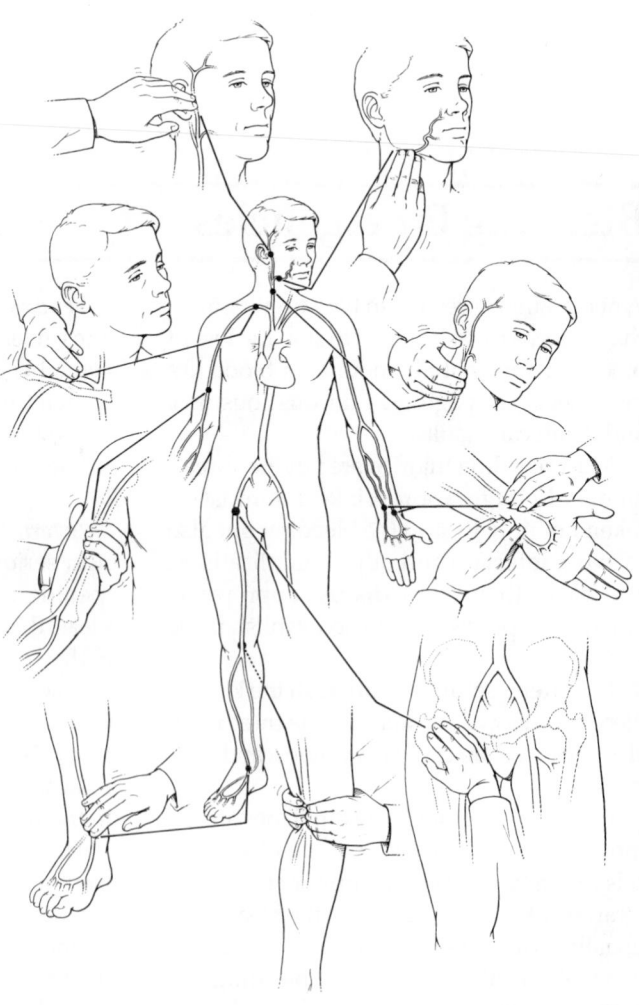

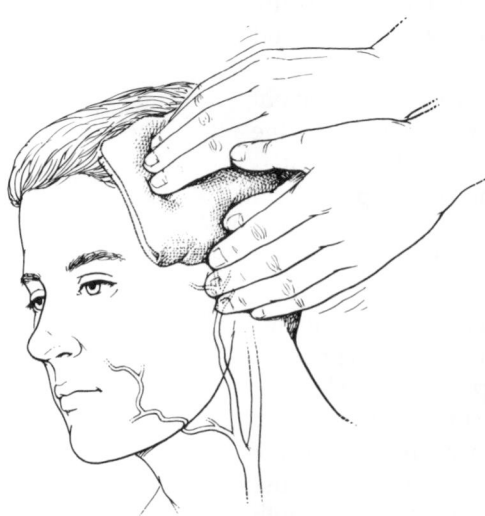

To stop bleeding, apply pressure directly to the wound, using gauze or a clean cloth.

Bleeding From a Wound or Injury

Bleeding from the surface of your body can range from very minor—the prick of a sewing needle can produce a droplet of blood—to major, as with a deep gash in which an artery is severed and blood gushes forth in rhythmic spurts. All wounds, however, require appropriate care and treatment; inadequate care can result in serious infection (see Wound Infections, page 1016). Make sure your tetanus immunizations are up to date (see page 393).

Cuts

If you sustain a small cut that bleeds only slightly, wash the cut thoroughly with mild soap and water. Apply a bandage to keep it clean.

If your cut is more serious—that is, the bleeding does not cease on its own in a short time or the cut is large, deep, or rough on the edges—consult your physician. But first stop the bleeding by applying pressure directly to the injury, using a sterilized gauze pad or clean cloth. Maintain pressure on the wound until the bleeding stops.

For severe bleeding, see How to Stop Severe Bleeding, page 400.

Bruises

Bruises (contusions) usually result from a blow or a fall. Bleeding beneath the skin then occurs, producing an accumulation of blood (hematoma).

When the skin is not broken, a bandage is unnecessary. To reduce discomfort, elevate the injured area and periodically apply ice or cold packs for 30 to 60 minutes several times daily for a day or two after the injury.

Punctures

A puncture wound—stepping on a nail is a common example—does not usually result in excessive bleeding. Often, in fact, little blood will flow and the wound will seem to close almost instantly. These features, however, do not mean that treatment is unnecessary.

Puncture wounds are dangerous because of the risk of infection. The object that caused the wound, especially if it has been exposed to soil, may carry spores of the tetanus or other bacteria. These can result in serious infections (see Tetanus Immunization, page 393). Note: A puncture wound through a shoe is particularly prone to serious infection.

If you sustain a puncture wound, stop the bleeding, if necessary, by applying pressure with a sterile gauze pad or clean cloth. Then seek emergency care for appropriate treatment to prevent tetanus or other infection.

Soft Tissue Injuries

Another kind of injury that may involve considerable bleeding is termed a soft tissue injury. The skin is damaged, as are underlying tissues such as muscle, supporting structures, and blood vessels. Such injuries can occur when an area is struck (contusions), when an area is badly cut (lacerations), when skin is separated from the underlying tissues (degloving injuries), or when areas of skin are forcefully torn away (avulsions). Soft tissue injuries require special treatment once you reach the emergency room, but they are to be given emergency medical care like other bleeding incidents.

Abdominal Wounds

Because of the presence of numerous internal organs, a wound that penetrates the abdominal wall is a potentially serious injury. Seek emergency care immediately by calling the emergency telephone number in your community (911 in many areas) or your local ambulance service if such a wound is sustained.

Before moving someone with an abdominal wound, position the person on his or her back. If no internal organs protrude through the wound, use a gauze pad or sterile cloth and exert pressure on the injury to stop the bleeding. When the flow has stopped, tape the bandage in place.

If organs have been displaced by the wound, do not try to reposition them: cover the injury with a dressing, and do not apply more than very gentle pressure to stop the bleeding.

Bleeding From Body Openings

Internal bleeding may accompany seemingly superficial injuries: for example, a blow to the head that produces minor bleeding from the skin may result in much more dangerous internal bleeding. In some cases, internal injury may produce no signs of external bleeding; in others, the person may vomit blood or have bleeding from the ears, nose, mouth, anus, vagina, or penis.

Internal bleeding, especially in the abdomen, head, or chest, is extremely serious and can be life-threatening. Blood loss can be considerable—even if there is no evident external bleeding.

If the person has sustained a traumatic injury—an injury sustained during a fall, automobile accident, or other event involving an external force or violence—suspect internal bleeding (see Detecting Internal Bleeding, this page).

Vomiting of Blood

Hematemesis is the medical term for the vomiting of blood. This can occur as the result of injury to or disease of the throat, esophagus, stomach, or duodenum (initial portion of the small bowel).

Seek Emergency Assistance

While waiting for help to arrive, keep the person lying down with legs elevated, if possible. The person should not attempt to eat or drink anything, even if he or she complains of being thirsty.

Coughing of Blood

The medical term for the coughing up of blood is hemoptysis. The source of the blood is usually the lungs or windpipe. The blood that appears is usually frothy, is bright red, and has a salty taste. Some possible causes include bronchial or lung infection, blood clot in the lung, blunt injury to the chest, and lung cancer.

Summon emergency assistance immediately if the person coughs up large amounts of blood. While waiting for emergency help to arrive, the person who is coughing up blood should be lying down with his or her head elevated slightly and supported by pillows. Loosen clothing that is tight around the throat and chest. Keep the person warm, quiet, and as comfortable as possible. If the person complains of thirst, small amounts of crushed ice or sips of water may be given.

Detecting Internal Bleeding

In the event of a traumatic injury, such as might be experienced in an automobile crash or a fall, internal bleeding may not be immediately apparent. However, because of the dangers of internal bleeding, consider it if you observe any of the following signs:

- Bleeding from the ears, nose, rectum, or vagina, or the vomiting or coughing up of blood
- Bruising on the neck, chest, or abdomen
- Wounds that have penetrated the skull, chest, or abdomen
- Abdominal tenderness, perhaps accompanied by hardness or spasm of the abdominal muscles
- Fractures

Internal bleeding may produce shock. The volume of blood in the body becomes inadequate and the person may feel weak, thirsty, and anxious. His or her skin may feel cool. Other symptoms of shock that may indicate the presence of internal bleeding include shallow and rapid breathing, a rapid and weak pulse, trembling, and restlessness.

The person may faint and lose consciousness when standing or seated but recovers when allowed to lie down. Elevating the legs may be of additional help.

Emergency Treatment

If you suspect internal bleeding, request immediate emergency assistance by calling the emergency number in your community (often 911) or by summoning your local ambulance. Treat the person for shock (see Recognizing and Treating Shock, page 442). Keep him or her lying quietly and comfortably. Loosen clothing, but do not give the person anything to eat or drink, even if he or she complains of being thirsty. If internal bleeding is in an extremity (as with a fracture or evident bruise on an arm or leg), apply pressure directly to this area or manually compress the major artery above the fracture or bruise to stop the bleeding (see How to Stop Severe Bleeding, page 400).

Rectal Bleeding

Bleeding from the anus can be the result of various causes. Hemorrhoids can produce bleeding, a relatively minor event that produces bright red blood in the toilet bowl or on the toilet paper. Black, tarry stools, maroon stools, or bright red blood in the stool may suggest the presence of considerable bleeding in the gastrointestinal tract. (Note that the use of bismuth or iron-containing preparations also may cause black stools.) If you observe rectal bleeding of unknown cause, consult your physician.

If rectal bleeding occurs in moderate to large amounts, seek immediate emergency care.

Vaginal Bleeding

Vaginal bleeding is a normal part of menstruation; however, bleeding from the vagina also may signal a wide range of medical and gynecologic difficulties. Consult your physician immediately if you experience any unexpected vaginal bleeding, especially if you are pregnant.

Blood in the Urine

Blood in the urine, termed hematuria, may be frightening. A relatively small amount of bright red, fresh blood in the toilet may make the bowl appear to be full of blood. The chances are high that relatively little blood has been lost. Nevertheless, seek your physician's guidance because the cause could be a tumor, infection, stone, kidney disease, or other serious medical problem.

If the blood precedes the flow of urine and is bright red, it probably is coming from the urethra. Blood that seems to have been well mixed with the urine suggests that the source is the bladder or kidneys.

Nosebleed

This common condition involves sudden bleeding from one nostril. It may result from trauma (the most common example being a punch in the nose), from breathing dry air, from allergies, or for no apparent reason.

Most nosebleeds begin from the septum, the cartilage that separates the nasal chambers and is lined with fragile blood vessels. This form of nosebleed is not serious and is usually easy to stop.

In some people, nosebleeds may begin deeper in the nose. These nosebleeds, which are less common, are often harder to stop.

Emergency Treatment

Stop the flow of blood from a common nosebleed using the following steps:

1. First, sit or stand upright. The upright positions slow the flow of blood in the veins of the nose. Do not tip your head back or insert anything in your nostril.

2. Pinch your nose with your thumb and index finger; breathe through your mouth. Do this for 5 or 10 minutes; this should stop the flow of blood.

If you succeed in stopping the flow of blood, there is no need for professional medical assistance. However, if the bleeding proves hard to stop, seek emergency medical assistance (see Nosebleed, page 586).

Burns

Burns can be caused by fire, the sun, chemicals, heated objects or fluids, electricity, or other means. They can be minor medical problems or life-threatening emergencies.

Burn Classifications

Distinguishing a minor burn from a more serious burn involves determining the degree of damage to the tissues of the body. The three classifications physicians use are described here.

First-Degree Burns

The least serious burns are those in which only the outer layer of skin (epidermis) is burned. The skin is usually reddened and there may be swelling and pain. However, the outer layer of skin has not been burned through. Unless such a burn involves substantial portions of the hands, feet, face, groin, buttocks, or a major joint, it is to be treated as a minor burn (see Treating Minor Burns at Home, page 405). If the burn was caused by exposure to the sun, see Sunburn, page 414.

Second-Degree Burns

When the first layer of skin has been burned through and the second layer of skin (dermis) is also burned, the injury is termed a second-degree burn. Blisters develop, and the skin will take on an intensely reddened appearance and become mottled. Severe pain and swelling are accompanying symptoms.

If a second-degree burn is limited to an area no larger than 2 to 3 inches in diameter, see Treating Minor Burns at Home, page 405; if the burned area of skin is larger or if the burn occurred on the hands, feet, face, groin, buttocks, or a major joint, see Treating Major Burns, page 405.

Burns are classified according to the degree of damage to skin and body tissue.

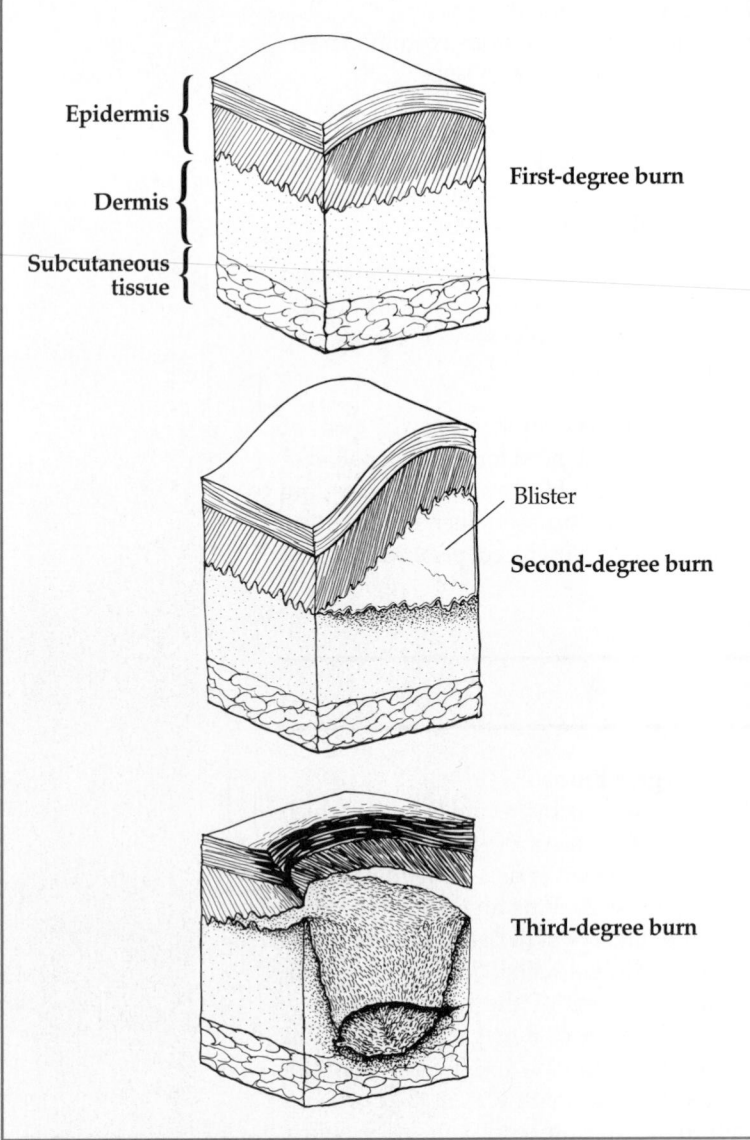

Epidermis

Dermis

Subcutaneous tissue

First-degree burn

Blister

Second-degree burn

Third-degree burn

Third-Degree Burns

The most serious burns involve all layers of skin. Fat, nerves, muscles, and even bones also may be affected. There are usually areas that are charred black or that appear a dry white. There may be severe pain or, if nerve damage is substantial, no pain at all (see Treating Major Burns, page 405).

Electrical Burns

Any electrical burn should be examined by a physician. An electrical burn may appear minor, but the damage can extend deep to the tissues beneath the skin. A heart rhythm disturbance, cardiac arrest, or other internal damage can occur when the amount of electrical current that passed through the body was large.

Sometimes the jolt associated with the electrical injury can cause the person to be thrown or to fall, resulting in fractures or other injuries. For first aid measures to institute before reaching the emergency room, see Treating Major Burns, page 405.

Chemical Burns

To treat chemical burns, follow these steps:

1. Make sure the cause of the burn has been removed. Flush the chemicals off the skin surface using cool running water for 20 minutes or more. (If the burning chemical is a powder-like substance such as lime, brush it off the skin before flushing.)

2. Treat the person for shock if he or she is faint, pale, or breathing in a shallow, hurried fashion (see Recognizing and Treating Shock, page 442).

3. Remove the victim's clothing or jewelry contaminated by the chemical.

4. Wrap the burned area with a dry, sterile dressing (if possible) or clean cloth.

5. If the victim complains of increased burning after you have washed the area, rewash the burn with water for several more minutes.

6. Minor chemical burns will usually heal without further treatment. However, if the

chemical burned through the first layer of skin and the resulting second-degree burn covers an area more than 2 to 3 inches in diameter, or if the chemical burn occurred on the hands, feet, face, groin, buttocks, or a major joint, seek emergency medical assistance.

Chemicals in the Eyes
If chemicals have splashed in the eyes, the eyes should be flushed with water immediately. Any source of clean drinking water will do—it is more important to begin the flushing than it is to find sterile water.

Continue to flush the eyes with running water for at least 20 minutes. After washing the eyes thoroughly, close the eyelids and then cover them with loose, moist dressings. Seek emergency medical assistance.

Treating Minor Burns at Home

To treat minor burns (see Burn Classifications, page 403), follow these tips:

1. Cool the burn by holding it under running water for 15 minutes. If impractical, immerse the burn in cold water or cover it with cold compresses. Don't put ice directly on the burn. Doing so can cause frostbite and further damage.

2. Once the burn is completely cooled, apply a lotion or moisturizer to soothe the area and prevent dryness. Don't apply butter to burned skin. It holds heat in the tissues and can cause more damage and increase the chance of infection.

3. Cover the burn with a sterile gauze bandage. Wrap loosely to avoid putting pressure on the burn. Bandaging keeps air off the burn and reduces pain.

4. Fluid-filled blisters sometimes form to protect against infection. Don't break the blisters. If they break by themselves, wash the area with mild soap and water, and apply an antibiotic ointment and gauze bandage.

5. Aspirin or acetaminophen may help relieve pain and swelling.

Treating Major Burns

In treating major burns (see Burn Classifications, page 403), immediately request emergency assistance. While waiting for medical assistance to arrive, follow these steps:

1. Make sure the cause of the burn has been extinguished or removed. If clothing is on fire, do not let the person run—that will only feed the fire. Put out the flames with water or roll the person in a blanket or coat on the ground. Do not remove burnt clothing, but do ensure that the victim is not in contact with smoldering materials.

2. Make certain the burn victim is breathing; if breathing has stopped or you suspect that the person's airway is blocked, see Choking, Breathing Emergencies, and Resuscitation, page 406.

3. If breathing is not a problem, cover the area of the burn with a dry, sterile bandage (if available) or clean cloth (do not use a blanket or towel; a sheet will do if the burned area is large). Do not apply any ointments. Avoid breaking burn blisters.

4. Await the arrival of emergency medical assistance.

Choking, Breathing Emergencies, and Resuscitation

Choking results from a blockage of the respiratory passage in the throat or windpipe. The flow of air to the lungs is blocked; in turn, the circulation of oxygen to the brain and other cells ceases. If the choking is not dealt with promptly, unconsciousness and death may result.

Choking, heart disease, or other causes may also result in the stoppage of the heart and breathing. In such an emergency, breathing and blood circulation must be restored if the life of the injured person is to be saved. Resuscitation is the process of restoring breathing. Cardiopulmonary resuscitation (CPR) is a technique that combines artificially breathing for the person (mouth-to-mouth resuscitation) and compressing his or her chest to aid circulation.

On the following pages you will learn the basics of determining the nature of the emergency at hand—that is, is your dinner partner having a heart attack or choking on a piece of steak? In addition, you will read about how to react to and deal with the medical emergency, including techniques for dislodging an obstruction in the airway and what is involved in performing CPR. (Effective CPR is a practiced skill. We recommend taking a class in CPR from your local Red Cross or hospital.)

Recognizing an Obstructed Airway

Choking is often the result of inadequately chewed food becoming lodged in the throat (pharynx) or windpipe (trachea). Most often, solid foods such as meats are the cause.

Commonly, persons who are choking have been talking while simultaneously chewing a chunk of meat. False teeth may also set the stage for this problem by interfering with the way food feels in the mouth while it is being chewed. Food cannot be chewed as thoroughly with false teeth as with natural teeth because less chewing pressure is exerted by false teeth.

Panic is an accompanying sensation: the choking victim's face often assumes an expression of fear or terror. At first, he or she may turn purple, the eyes may bulge, and he or she may wheeze or gasp.

Coughing Versus Choking

If a morsel of food "goes down the wrong pipe," often the coughing reflex will resolve the problem. In fact, a person is not choking if he or she is able to cough freely and has normal skin color. However, if the cough is more like a gasp and the person takes on a bluish tinge, the individual is probably choking.

If in doubt, ask the choking person whether he or she can talk. If the person is capable of speech, then the windpipe is not completely blocked and oxygen is reaching the lungs.

Clearing an Obstructed Airway

There are several techniques for opening an obstructed airway. First, determine that the individual is unable to breathe: if so, the person will be unable to speak, and his or her skin, if white, will be taking on a blue, gray, or ashen color.

The Heimlich maneuver is perhaps the best-known technique (see page 407), but there are several other options for certain situations, as described here.

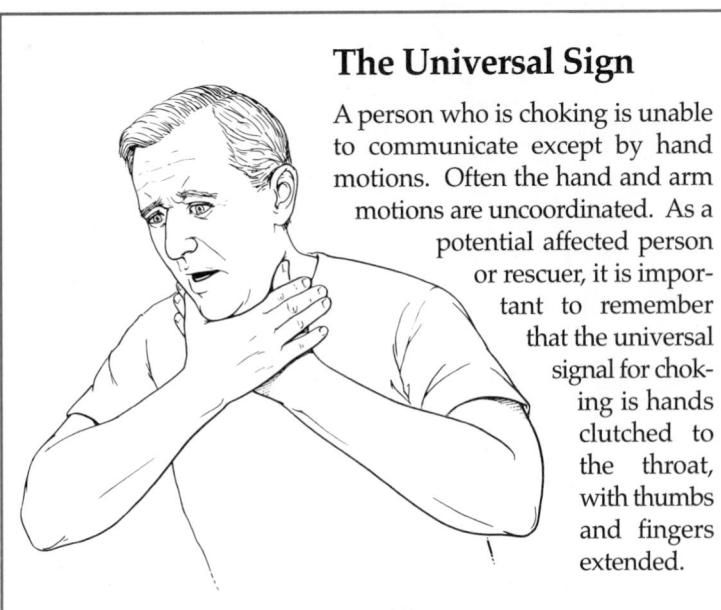

The Universal Sign

A person who is choking is unable to communicate except by hand motions. Often the hand and arm motions are uncoordinated. As a potential affected person or rescuer, it is important to remember that the universal signal for choking is hands clutched to the throat, with thumbs and fingers extended.

Finger Sweep

The simplest method involves reaching a finger into the back of the throat. If you can see into the person's mouth, can you see the cause of the blockage? If so, sweep a finger into the back of the mouth to clear the airway.

This method works only if the blockage is at the very back of the mouth or high in the throat. Be very careful not to push the food or object deeper into the airway. Do not perform a finger sweep in children less than 8 years old unless an object is visible.

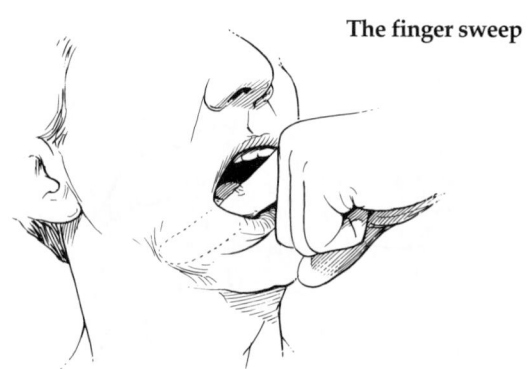

The finger sweep

The Heimlich Maneuver

You have seen it on television and on posters, but do you remember how to do it? Here's how:

1. Stand behind the victim, and wrap your arms around his or her waist. Tip the person forward slightly.

2. Make a fist with one hand and position it slightly above the person's navel.

3. Grasp the fist with the other hand, and press hard into the abdomen. A quick, upward thrust—as if you were trying to lift the person off the ground—works best.

4. Repeat the Heimlich maneuver until the food or other blockage is dislodged.

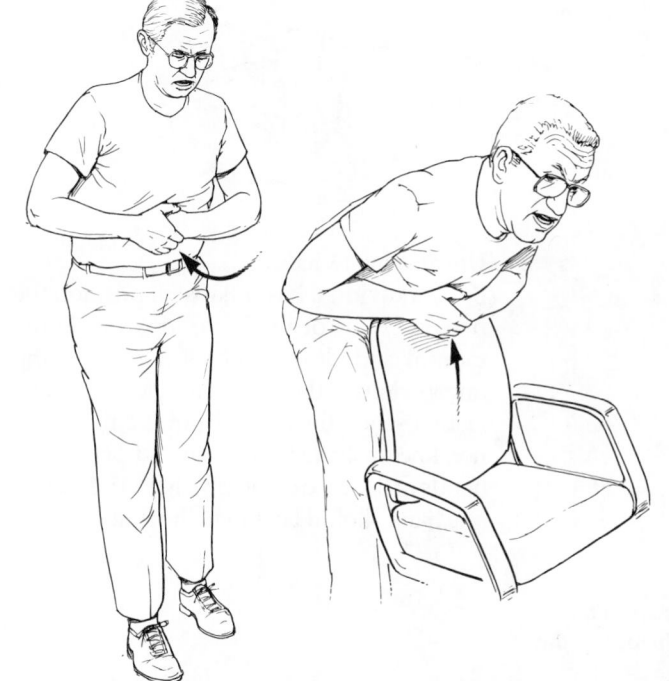

If help is unavailable, you can perform the Heimlich maneuver on yourself. With clenched hands positioned slightly above your navel, thrust your hands upward or drape your body over a chair or rail or some similar object.

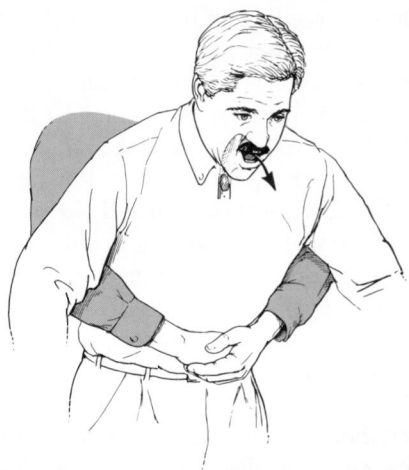

The Heimlich maneuver

Using It on Yourself

You can use a variation of the Heimlich maneuver if you begin to choke. Place a fist above your navel. Grasp your fist with the other hand, and bend over a hard surface (a countertop or chair will do). Shove your fist inward and upward.

For a Pregnant Woman or Obese Person

The abdomen of a pregnant woman or the flabby stomach of a very overweight person can prevent the effective use of an abdominal thrust.

Position your hands at the base of the breastbone, just above the joining of the lowest ribs. Proceed as for the Heimlich maneuver, pressing hard into the chest with a quick thrust. Repeat the maneuver until the food or other blockage is dislodged or the person becomes unconscious (see Unconscious Victim, page 408).

To clear the airway of an unconscious victim lying on his or her back, kneel over the individual and apply upward thrusts to the upper abdomen.

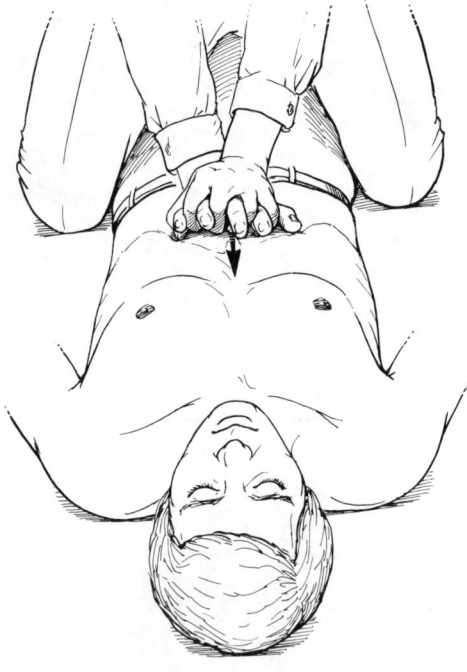

Unconscious Victim

If the individual has collapsed, position the person on his or her back, look inside the mouth, and do a finger sweep. Falling unconscious and relaxing muscles may have just loosened the object from the throat. If not, kneel astride the person and place your hands at the base of the rib cage. The heel of one hand should be down, the fingers of the

A gentle slap on the back can help clear the airway of a choking infant.

upper hand between those of the lower, grasping the palm. Deliver five quick upward thrusts to the abdomen, remembering to be more gentle with a child less than 8 years old.

Choking Infant

Assume a seated position. Hold the infant facedown on your forearm which, in turn, is resting on your thigh. Thump the infant gently five times firmly on the middle of the back using the heel of your hand: the combination of gravity and the blows to the back should release the object blocking the airway.

If the back blows are unsuccessful, hold the infant faceup on your forearm with the head lower than the trunk. Using two fingers placed at the center of the infant's breastbone, give five quick chest compressions. If breathing has not resumed, repeat the back blows and chest thrusts. *Call for help.*

Mouth-to-Mouth Resuscitation

If one of these techniques opens the airway but the infant does not resume breathing, perform mouth-to-mouth resuscitation (part of CPR, described on page 412).

Cardiopulmonary Resuscitation

This lifesaving technique is applicable to a range of emergencies, including cardiac arrest, choking episode, and drowning. Each has key components in common: the person is unconscious and has ceased breathing. Training in cardiopulmonary resuscitation (CPR) will prepare you to handle these life-threatening emergencies effectively.

Before proceeding with resuscitation, you must ascertain that the person is actually unconscious and has stopped breathing. You can actually do harm by performing CPR on somebody who does not need it.

Death comes quickly when the heart stops: the absence of oxygenated blood can cause irreparable brain damage in only a few minutes, and death can occur in 8 to 10 minutes. Time is all-important when you are helping an unconscious person who is not breathing. Thus, the first rule if you are alone is to immediately begin cardiopulmonary resuscitation. After 1 minute activate the emergency medical services (EMS) system by calling 911 or your local ambulance. (If you are not alone, direct someone to call EMS as soon as you determine that the unconscious person is not breathing.)

The American Heart Association, which sets standards for CPR, distinguishes the three parts of the CPR process with the familiar letters ABC: A is for airway, B is for breathing, C is for circulation. These steps are described in order below.

Clear the Airway

"A" is for airway. Many procedures are involved in clearing the victim's airway, beginning with an assessment.

Are You Okay?

The first step in dealing with an unconscious person is to be sure that he or she is not simply resting or sleeping. Firmly shake or tap his or her shoulder and ask, "Are you okay?"

Summon Assistance

If you get no response, immediately shout for help. If you are alone, begin CPR immediately and continue for 1 minute before seeking assistance. If you are not alone, direct someone to call your local emergency number (in many communities the number is 911) or your local ambulance service.

Position the Victim

Lay the person on his or her back. If necessary, roll the person over so that he or she is faceup. Position yourself at a right angle on your knees, perpendicular to the person's neck and shoulders.

Head Tilt/Chin Lift

This is the primary maneuver for opening an airway. Position your palm on the person's forehead and gently push backward, placing the second and third fingers of your other hand along the side of the person's jaw, tilting the head and lifting the chin forward to open the airway.

Modified Jaw Thrust

If you suspect a neck injury, a modified jaw thrust (without the head tilt) may be used. This is done by placing your hands on each side of the person's face, your thumbs on the cheekbones (but not pushing), and pulling the jaw forward with your index fingers.

Examine the mouth to make sure no foreign material is present. If present, use a finger sweep to clear it.

Check for Breathing

Check for breathing, positioning your ear directly over the person's mouth. Look across the person's chest for the rise and fall of breathing. Listen for breath sounds. Feel for air on your face. If no breathing is evident, begin mouth-to-mouth resuscitation immediately.

Breathe for the Person

"B" is for breathing. In the absence of emergency equipment or professional medical help, the restoration of the flow of oxygen to the lungs is best done by mouth-to-mouth resuscitation.

The basis of mouth-to-mouth resuscitation is simple: you are to provide breathing for the victim. You are to expel breath from your lungs into the victim's through that person's nose or mouth.

Deliver Two Slow Breaths

Position yourself at a right angle to the person's shoulder. Use the head tilt/chin lift maneuver and pinch the person's nose closed using your thumb and forefinger.

Take a deep breath. Open your mouth wide, and place it tightly over the victim's mouth. Exhale into the victim. Remove your

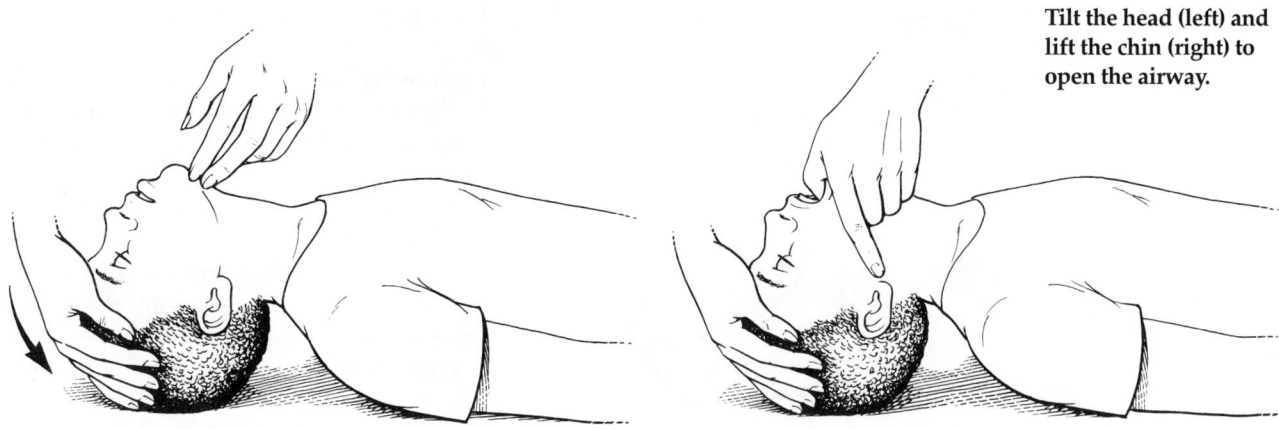

Tilt the head (left) and lift the chin (right) to open the airway.

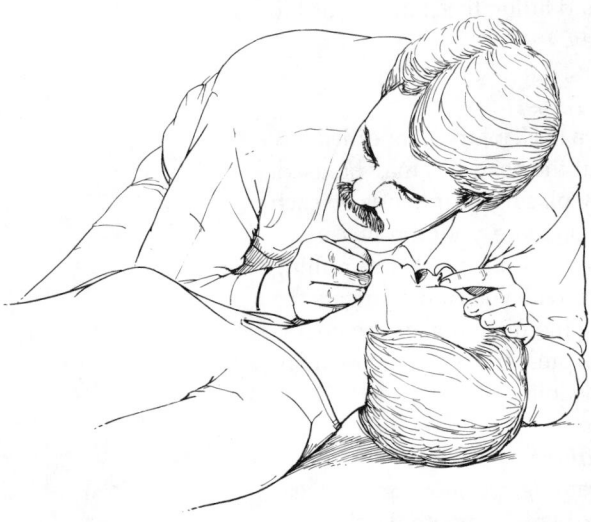
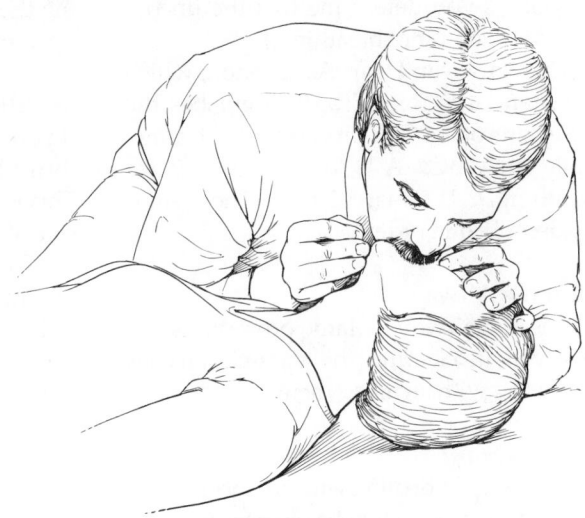

Left: Look, listen, and feel (for air against your cheek) for indications of breathing. Right: Mouth-to-mouth resuscitation.

mouth from the victim's, inhale, and do it again. Deliver two big breaths. Observe the person's chest with each breath to note whether the air you are breathing into the person is actually causing his or her lungs to expand. Make sure you let the person exhale before delivering more breaths. If the victim's stomach bulges excessively, the airway may be blocked, or your breaths may be too full.

Check for a Pulse

After you have delivered two breaths, position two fingers just to the side of the victim's Adam's apple. If the heart is pumping, the carotid artery on either side of the neck should be pulsating. If you do not feel it immediately, move your fingers a fraction of an inch up or down to be sure you are in the right place.

If There Is No Pulse

If there is no pulse, cardiac compressions are necessary to circulate blood to the brain (see below).

Continue Breathing

If the person has a pulse but is not breathing, continue mouth-to-mouth breathing. Using the same technique, blow a big breath into the adult victim every 5 seconds (12 breaths per minute). Take your mouth away between breaths. Listen for signs of breathing and watch chest movement.

If the victim is breathing but the breaths are weak, shallow, or labored, mouth-to-mouth resuscitation may still be appropriate. However, coordinate your breathing assistance with the victim's breathing: deliver a breath when he or she inhales, and allow the person to exhale before you breathe for him or her again.

Call EMS if you haven't already done so. Continue to breathe for the person until he or she breathes on his or her own or until professional medical help arrives.

Restore Circulation

"C" is for circulation: the blood flow must be restored in order to deliver oxygen to the brain. Without oxygen, brain cells will die and, in a matter of minutes, irreversible damage can result.

If you are unable to find a pulse in an unconscious person, heart compressions are necessary to restore circulation. Also called closed heart massage, the heart compressions must be coordinated with mouth-to-mouth resuscitation: the breathing delivers the air

Check for a pulse at the carotid artery on either side of the person's neck.

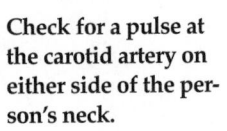
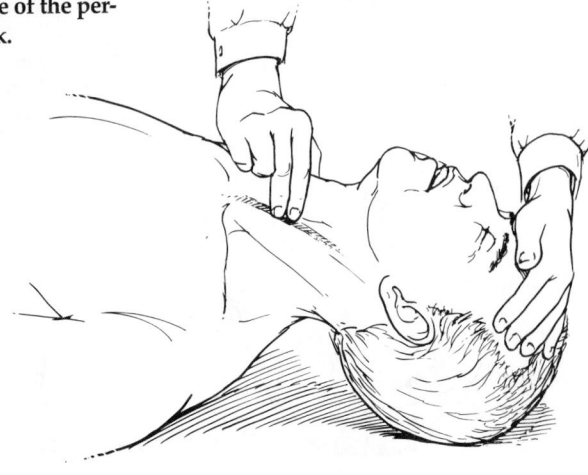

to the lungs, then the heart massage pumps the oxygenated blood to the brain and other parts of the body.

Just as you are to act as a breathing machine for the lungs when you perform mouth-to-mouth resuscitation, performing heart massage means you are artificially pumping the heart muscle.

Position Your Hands

Work from a kneeling position at right angles to the victim's chest. Find the base of the breastbone at the center of the chest where the ribs form a V. Position the heel of one hand on the chest immediately above the V; with the other hand, grasp the first hand from above, intertwining the fingers.

Lock Your Elbows

Shift your weight forward and upward so that your shoulders are over your hands; straighten your arms and lock your elbows.

Pump the Heart

Shift your weight onto your hands to depress the victim's chest (it should fall about 1½ to 2 inches in an adult). Count aloud as you do it, five times in an even rhythm, slightly faster than 1 compression per second (80-100 per minute): one-thousand-one, one-thousand-two, and so on. Repeat the pattern three times for a total of 15 chest compressions.

Breathe for the Victim

You must also give the person oxygen. Use the same technique outlined above for mouth-to-mouth resuscitation. Use the head tilt/chin lift maneuver to open the airway. Pinch the nose closed with the thumb and forefinger. Take a deep breath, then cover the victim's mouth entirely with yours. Exhale into the victim. Give two slow breaths. Repeat.

Alternate Pumping and Breathing

Pump the person's chest 15 times, then breathe for him or her twice. Establish a regular rhythm, counting aloud. Reassess pulse and breathing after 4 cycles. Call EMS if you haven't already done so. Continue until help arrives if physically possible.

Performing CPR on a Child

The procedure is essentially the same. The differences are that you use only one hand and pump the child's chest five times. You then breathe for the child once, and more gently. Reassess every few minutes.

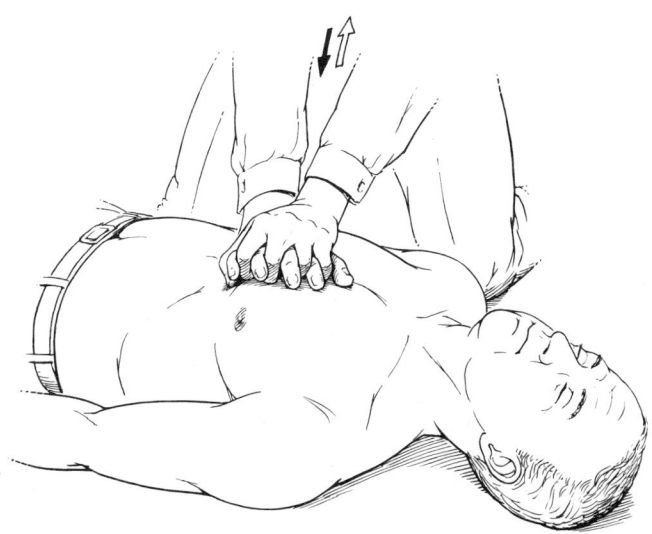

Heart compression (massage) must be coordinated with mouth-to-mouth resuscitation.

Two-Person (Two-Rescuer) CPR

Before beginning, together assess the victim. Then perform one-person CPR while the other rescuer calls 911 for an ambulance. When the other rescuer returns, begin two-person CPR.

Two-person CPR is similar to one-person CPR with the exception that one person provides breathing assistance while the other pumps the heart. Pump the heart at a rate of 80 to 100 times a minute. After each five compressions, a pause in pumping is allowed for a breath to be given by the second rescuer.

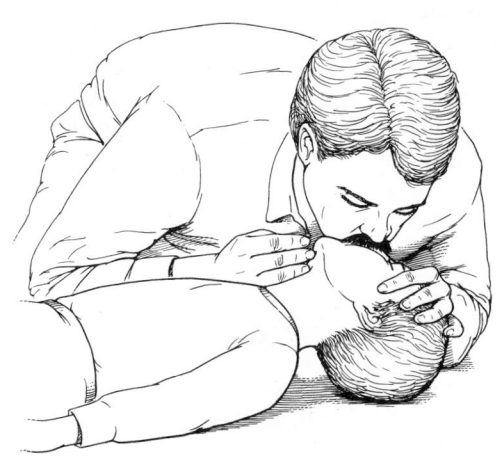

Use mouth-to-nose resuscitation if injury to the mouth or face makes mouth-to-mouth resuscitation difficult. First, hold the victim's mouth closed by lifting the chin. Then, cover his or her entire nose with your mouth and blow into the nose. After breathing, remove your mouth from the area to allow air to escape. Until help arrives, repeat these steps in a steady, rhythmic breathing pattern.

Performing CPR on an Infant

CPR may also be used on infants (babies up to 12 months of age). The techniques are different but the goal is the same as with an older child or an adult victim: you need to restore oxygen and blood flow to the baby's brain.

Does the Baby Need Help?

Be sure that the baby is not simply resting or sleeping. Stroke the child: is there a discernible response? Does breathing seem to have stopped? If you are not alone, direct someone to call 911 or your local ambulance service immediately.

Position the Baby

Put the baby on its back on a table. The floor or ground will do, too. Using the head tilt/chin lift maneuver described on page 409, gently tip the head back. This opens the airway.

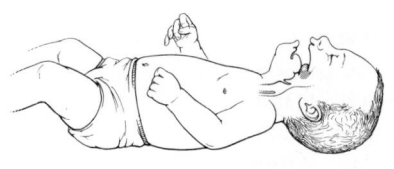

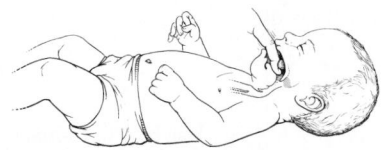

Before giving mouth-to-mouth resuscitation to an infant, tilt the child's head back to open the airway (top). Then, if visual inspection reveals a foreign object in the infant's mouth, remove the object with a sweep of your finger (bottom). Be careful not to push the food or object deeper into the child's airway.

Examine the mouth to make sure no foreign material is in the mouth. Check for breathing: position your ear directly over the baby's mouth and look at the chest

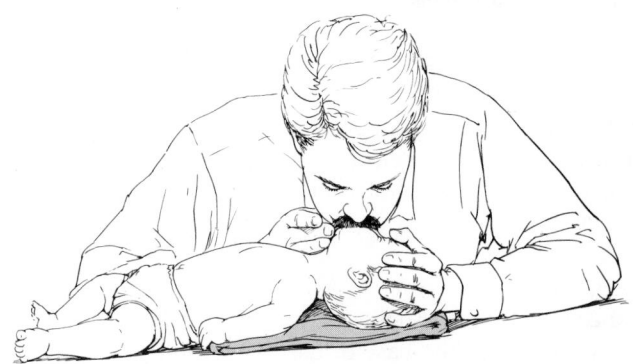

Mouth-to-mouth resuscitation of a baby.

for the rise and fall of breathing. If no breathing is evident, begin mouth-to-mouth resuscitation immediately.

Deliver Two Gentle Breaths

Cover the baby's mouth and nose with your mouth. Using the strength of your cheeks rather than your lungs, breathe two times slowly—the breaths are more like puffs than deep exhalations. (Too much air can result in a distended stomach and vomiting, an unneeded complication.)

Check for a Pulse

After you have delivered two breaths, check for a pulse on the inside of the baby's upper arm. If no pulse is evident, begin chest compressions (see below). If there is a pulse, continue mouth-to-mouth breathing, delivering a breath every 3 seconds.

Call 911 or emergency medical services (EMS) if you haven't already.

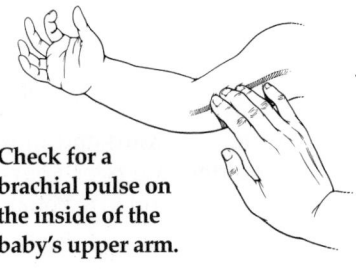

Check for a brachial pulse on the inside of the baby's upper arm.

Continue to breathe for the baby until it breathes on its own or until professional medical help arrives.

Cardiopulmonary Resuscitation

To pump the baby's heart, position your index and middle fingers on the baby's breastbone (between the nipples). Compress the chest (no more than ½ to 1 inch: be gentle).

Count aloud as you pump in a fairly rapid rhythm. You should pump roughly 1½ times a second, or about 100 times a minute. Breathe for the baby gently on every fifth compression.

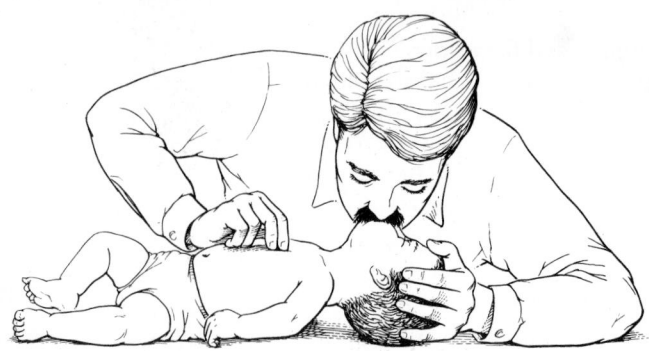

To perform cardiopulmonary resuscitation on an infant, alternate compression of the baby's chest with gentle breaths from your mouth while covering the baby's mouth and nose.

Breathing Difficulty Due to Croup, Epiglottitis, or Bronchitis

Several disorders of the upper respiratory tract can produce difficulty in breathing, especially in children. In most cases, the appropriate treatment is to keep the person with the ailment breathing moistened air, consuming plenty of fluids, and resting in bed.

These illnesses most often are temporary, but occasionally they can lead to extreme swelling in the airway, which produces labored breathing.

Croup

This infection is most likely to affect children 8 years or younger. The symptoms are fever, sore throat, hoarseness, and cough. The cough often sounds distinctly like a bark (see Croup, page 1076).

Epiglottitis

The epiglottis is the lid-like cartilage that covers the windpipe during swallowing. When it becomes inflamed, the condition is termed epiglottitis; its symptoms include sore throat, fever, difficulty swallowing with drooling, and hoarseness (see Epiglottitis, page 594).

Bronchitis

Characterized by a soreness and feeling of constriction in the chest, bronchitis is a common viral infection of the bronchi and the trachea, the principal air passages in the chest. Accompanying symptoms are cough, chills, an overall malaise, and slight fever (see Acute Bronchitis, page 702).

Wheezing, the sound made by air passing through narrowed breathing passages, may be common to all three of these conditions. Wheezing induced by these three conditions may sound similar to the wheezing of asthma. In fact, many individuals with asthma can develop severe asthma attacks with upper respiratory infections or bronchitis.

Emergency Treatment

If your child has any of these ailments, observe his or her breathing carefully. Croup, epiglottitis, and bronchitis, along with asthma, can lead to an obstructed airway because of the swelling of the tissues in the airway.

Exposure to warm, humid air may provide relief. To humidify the air, fill your bathtub with hot water.

Seek immediate emergency assistance if breathing becomes labored. Perform mouth-to-mouth resuscitation if breathing stops (see Cardiopulmonary Resuscitation, page 408).

Severe Asthma Attack

In people with asthma, occasional or even frequent asthma attacks occur. Usually the key symptom is a difficulty in breathing, accompanied by a tightness in the chest and coughing that may bring up excess mucus. Wheezing will be more pronounced when breathing out than when breathing in. Your physician's treatment strategy will be aimed at minimizing or eliminating these breathing difficulties (see Asthma, page 1044).

Occasionally, however, more serious or even life-threatening asthma attacks may occur. Symptoms of a serious asthma attack may include extreme difficulty in breathing, a bluish cast to the face and lips, severe anxiety, an increased pulse rate, and heavy perspiration. Severe asthma attacks also may occur in a non-asthmatic person exposed to something that causes severe difficulty in breathing, such as croup or insecticide sprays.

Emergency Treatment

1. Establish that the problem is not a choking emergency. People with asthma, like the rest of us, choke on food or other foreign objects that block the airway. If the incident occurs during a meal, see Recognizing an Obstructed Airway, page 406.

2. Keep calm and try to reassure the person having the asthma attack.

3. Call the person's physician; if you are unable to reach the physician, call the emergency room at your local hospital.

Before you call, locate any asthma medications being taken by the person. When speaking with the physician, identify the person with the asthma attack by name and age. Describe the symptoms and other details about the person's recent medical history. Tell what medications and what dosages the person has been taking.

Follow the physician's instructions: he or she may suggest you go immediately to the hospital or may send an emergency vehicle. In some cases, the recommendation may be that you stay calm, medicate the person with doses of the drugs on hand, and allow the episode to pass.

Environmental Emergencies

The world around us presents a range of hazards to our health. For example, the sun warms us, but it also can burn our skin or cause our bodies to overheat (see Heat Stress, this page). In a similar way, overexposure to cold and damp can also produce medical emergencies (see Hypothermia, page 416, and Frostbite, page 416).

In the following pages we discuss these environmentally induced emergencies and others as well, including near drowning (see page 418), electrocution (see page 418), smoke inhalation (see page 419), and carbon monoxide poisoning (see page 419).

Sunburn

Prolonged exposure to the sun's ultraviolet rays produces red, tender, swollen skin. The skin also may develop water blisters.

The symptoms of sunburn do not appear until a few hours after exposure, but the painful, hot-to-the-touch quality of sunburned skin is unmistakable. The swelling and redness are due to inflammation of the skin.

The effect of sunburn is like that of any burn, but its development is relatively slow, rather than rapid as from a heat burn. With mild sunburn, there may be only redness and mild pain on touching the sunburned skin. With more severe sunburn, there may be swelling, blisters, severe pain, and an overall sensation of illness.

Emergency Treatment

Mild Sunburn
Most cases of sunburn can be treated adequately at home with a cool bath or shower followed by the application of hydrocortisone cream several times a day. Do not break the water blisters: leaving them intact will speed healing. However, if they break on their own, remove the skin fragments and use an antibacterial ointment on the open areas. Dress them with clean gauze to promote healing.

Aspirin will help alleviate the general discomfort and may reduce swelling.

Severe Sunburn
If you have received a severe sunburn (after

falling asleep in the sun, for example), contact your physician even before the sunburn is fully developed. Your physician may elect to give you an oral corticosteroid and thereby decrease the reaction and prevent some of the symptoms. Once the sunburn develops, treat it as you would a minor burn.

Prevention
Sun exposure in general is discouraged by most dermatologists. Damage to your skin cells from recurrent sunburn is cumulative, and continued overexposure to ultraviolet radiation produces long-term effects. These can include skin discolorations, actinic keratosis (see page 1002), and skin cancer (see page 1004). Chronic sun exposure also prematurely ages your skin and increases wrinkling (see Wrinkled Skin, page 1000).

For detailed strategies to prevent sunburn and protect your skin, see How to Avoid Sunburn, page 997.

Heat Stress

Under normal conditions, a healthy body temperature is maintained by mechanisms involving your skin and perspiration. However, if you are exposed to high temperatures for prolonged periods, particularly where there is little breeze and high humidity, the normal control mechanisms may fail to dissipate the heat. The ability to tolerate high temperatures may be increased somewhat by being in warm surroundings for a few weeks (acclimatization).

Heatstroke
Elderly and obese people are particularly at risk of heatstroke. Other contributing factors can be dehydration, alcohol consumption, heart disease, certain medications, and vigorous exercise.

Adequate hydration and the ability to sweat are your main protections against heatstroke. A few people are born with impaired ability to sweat and are particularly at risk. A few drugs may impair sweating and render you more vulnerable. Examples are medications for motion sickness or depression.

The key indication of heatstroke is a fever of 105 degrees Fahrenheit with hot, dry skin.

Skin Emergencies

Hives and Angioedema

Hives (urticaria) are raised, red, often itchy welts of various sizes that appear and disappear at random on the surface of the skin. They are more common on areas of the body where clothes rub on the skin. Hives tend to occur in batches rather than singly; they may last a few minutes or for several days.

Angioedema consists of large welts below the surface of the skin, particularly around the eyes and lips. Angioedema also may occur on the hands and feet and within the throat.

Both hives and angioedema result from a bodily reaction to foods, drugs, pollen, animal dander, insect bites, infections, illness, cold, heat, light, emotional distress, or other, unclear, factors. In most cases, hives and angioedema are harmless, leave no lasting marks, and sometimes are not even uncomfortable. Taking cool baths or showers, wearing light clothing, and minimizing vigorous activity often will speed recovery. An antihistamine prescribed by your physician also may help relieve itching and assist in your recovery.

Characterized by swelling that does not itch, one rare, hereditary variety of angioedema produces such symptoms as abdominal cramping and diarrhea and can cause fatal obstruction to the breathing passages (see page 1038). When angioedema affects the throat or tongue, causing the air passage to be blocked, it can be life-threatening.

Seek emergency medical assistance if you experience serious angioedema, especially if it makes breathing difficult. If a companion experiences a stoppage of breathing or unconsciousness, resuscitation must be performed (see Cardiopulmonary Resuscitation, page 408).

Severe Contact Dermatitis

The term "dermatitis" simply means an inflammation of the skin. "Contact dermatitis" is the term used to describe such inflammation when redness and itching and, in severe cases, blisters and weeping from the sores occur after contact with a causative agent.

In sensitive individuals, the causes can include poison plants such as poison ivy, oak, or sumac; certain metals found in rings or other jewelry; household products; or certain cosmetics.

(See page C-3 for color photograph of contact dermatitis.)

In contact dermatitis, only the areas of skin contacted by the offending substance will react, and those areas with the greatest exposure will react first.

It is rare for contact dermatitis to be more than a discomfort and an inconvenience. However, if extreme swelling, redness, and inflammation occur, especially around the eyes or in the area of the throat, or if the amount of dermatitis is extensive, consult your physician (see Contact Dermatitis, page 1036).

Contact dermatitis usually can be treated by cleansing the affected area with a mild soap and water and applying 0.5 percent hydrocortisone cream (which can be obtained without a prescription) up to four times daily. An antihistamine, in a dose prescribed by your physician, may relieve the itching.

Other signs include rapid heartbeat, rapid and shallow breathing, and either elevated or lowered blood pressure. Often, the level of consciousness also may be altered, resulting in confusion or delirium. In extreme cases, seizures or even coma and death may occur.

Emergency Treatment

If you suspect heatstroke, get the person out of the sun and into a shady spot. A cool, air-conditioned location is best.

Summon emergency medical assistance immediately. Extreme elevation of temperature is a medical emergency requiring professional treatment to cool the victim, replace lost fluids, and monitor heartbeat and breathing.

While you are waiting for the emergency vehicle to arrive, cool the person by covering him or her with damp sheets or spraying with water. Direct air onto the person, either with an electric fan or by fanning with your hands or a newspaper. If possible, monitor the person's temperature with a thermometer. Stop attempting to cool the person when his or her temperature is normal. If breathing ceases, start cardiopulmonary resuscitation (see page 408).

Heat Exhaustion

Think of heat exhaustion as a failure of your heart and vascular system to respond properly to high external temperatures. It often occurs in elderly people taking diuretics. Heat exhaustion sometimes occurs after excessive perspiration, coupled with inadequate consumption of water or other liquids to replace lost fluids. Symptoms often begin suddenly, and hence the term "heat collapse" is sometimes used. The symptoms resemble those of shock (see page 441), including faintness, rapid heartbeat, low blood pressure, an ashen appearance, cold clammy skin, and nausea.

Emergency Treatment

If you suspect heat exhaustion, get the person out of the sun and into a shady spot. A cool air-conditioned location is best. Once you get the person out of the sun into a cooler, shady location, lay the person down and elevate his or her feet slightly. Loosen or remove most or all of the person's clothing. Give the person cold (not iced) water to drink, but first stir in a teaspoon of salt per quart.

If signs of heatstroke appear—in particular, confusion, delirium, and a temperature of more than 102 degrees Fahrenheit—seek emergency medical assistance.

Heat Cramps

Heat cramps consist of painful spasms of muscles, usually experienced after vigorous exercise, along with profuse perspiration. These do not always occur in very hot surroundings. The muscles most affected are usually the ones you used during the exercise or your abdominal muscles.

Emergency Treatment

Brief rest and ingestion of water with a teaspoon of salt per quart usually will resolve the symptoms. Often salt can be taken more conveniently in the form of a salty food, such as salted nuts. Although salt and fluid replacement are necessary in all forms of heat-related illness, the use of salt tablets is unwise and can prove dangerous.

Massaging the cramped muscles may also help alleviate discomfort.

Hypothermia

Under most conditions, your body is able to maintain a healthy body temperature. However, when exposed for prolonged periods to cold temperatures or a cool, damp environment, particularly if clothing is wet or damp, your body's control mechanisms may fail to keep your body heat normal. When more heat is lost than your body can generate, hypothermia can result.

Falling overboard from a boat into cold water is a common cause of hypothermia. An uncovered head in winter is another frequent source of heat loss.

The key symptom of hypothermia is a body temperature that drops below 94 degrees Fahrenheit. Signs include shivering, slurred speech, an abnormally slow rate of breathing, skin that is cold and pale, a loss of coordination, and feelings of tiredness, lethargy, or apathy.

The onset of symptoms is usually slow; there is likely to be a gradual loss of mental acuity and physical ability. The person experiencing hypothermia, in fact, may be unaware that he or she is in a state requiring emergency medical treatment.

The elderly, the very young, and very lean people are at particular risk of hypothermia. Other conditions that may predispose you to hypothermia are malnutrition, heart disease, and excessive consumption of alcohol or other drugs. Contributing medical factors may include untreated hypothyroidism (see page 948), hypopituitarism (see page 943), and diabetes mellitus (see page 925).

Emergency Treatment

Get the person out of the cold and put warm, dry clothing on him or her. If going indoors is not possible, get the person out of the wind, cover his or her head, and insulate the person from the cold ground. If at all possible, get the person inside to an area at room temperature and cover him or her with warm blankets.

Seek emergency medical assistance.

Monitor the person's breathing and pulse. If either has stopped or seems dangerously slow or shallow, initiate resuscitation immediately (see Cardiopulmonary Resuscitation, page 408).

In extreme cases, hemodialysis given in the same manner as for kidney failure (see page 856) is sometimes used to restore normal body temperature quickly.

Do not give the victim alcohol. Do give the person warm nonalcoholic drinks (unless he or she is vomiting). In most cases of hypothermia, warm baths are helpful for warming the person.

Frostbite

When exposed to very cold temperatures or cold temperatures with a low wind chill factor for a prolonged period, the skin and the underlying tissues may freeze. This condition is called frostbite. The areas most likely to be affected are the hands, feet, nose, and ears. While anyone can get frostbite during extended exposure to cold conditions, people with circulatory problems such as atherosclerosis are at greater risk (see Atherosclerosis: What Is It? page 636).

Frostbite is distinguishable by the hard, pale, and cold quality of the skin that has been exposed to the cold for a length of time. The area is likely to have a definite lack of sensitivity to touch, although there is probably a sharp, aching pain. As the area thaws, the flesh becomes red and painful.

In severe cases, the flow of blood to the affected area actually stops and the blood vessels sustain damage. Immediate treatment is necessary if there is to be a chance of reversing the damage.

Emergency Treatment

A person with frostbite on the extremities may also be subject to hypothermia (lowered body temperature): check for hypothermia and treat those symptoms first (see Hypothermia, page 416).

Warming Process

If your fingers, ears, or other areas are frostbitten, get out of the cold. Warm your hands by tucking them into your armpits; if your nose, ears, or face is frostbitten, warm the area by covering it with dry, gloved hands. If the skin tingles as it warms and there is a burning sensation, the circulation is returning. However, if numbness remains during warming, seek professional medical care immediately.

Do not rub the affected area. If the feet are affected, do not walk on them: allow them to dangle and wait for help to arrive.

If you are unable to get immediate emergency assistance, warm severely frostbitten hands or feet in warm—not hot—water (the water should be between 100 and 105 degrees Fahrenheit). Do not apply other heat sources (such as a heating pad) because the tissue, although desensitized because of the cold, can still be burned by temperatures that are comfortable for you to withstand under normal conditions.

Do not smoke cigarettes (nicotine causes your blood vessels to constrict and may limit circulation).

Prevention

Wear proper clothing when in cold conditions. On arriving in a cold climate from a warmer one, allow your body to adjust. Be sure to protect your hands, feet, nose, and ears, and avoid consuming large amounts of alcohol before and when you are exposed to prolonged cold (see Frostbite, page 416).

Altitude Disorders and Decompression Sickness

Traveling to extremes of depth and altitude can cause serious health problems. Scuba divers who ascend too rapidly or individuals who fly in aircraft soon after diving can experience decompression sickness, commonly referred to as the "bends." Rapid ascent in a poorly pressurized aircraft will cause this same problem.

Decompression sickness can lead to joint pain, chest pain, shortness of breath, and uncontrollable cough. A blotchy, red rash may appear on the trunk, and the person may experience headache, dizziness, and confusion. These symptoms may occur minutes to hours after the ascent takes place. In extreme cases, there can be paralysis, shock, coma, and even death.

High-altitude illness is an entirely different entity and can occur in various forms at altitudes of more than 8,000 feet above sea level. People who reside at lower altitudes and make the transition to a high altitude quickly are at increased risk compared to those who reside at high altitude. Acute mountain sickness results in the development of headache, nausea, fatigue, sleeplessness, shortness of breath, and loss of appetite. It usually develops several hours after arriving at high altitude and may last for several days. Skiers who travel to mountainous slopes from lower elevations are commonly affected. More serious forms of high-altitude sickness involve either the development of severe respiratory distress or severe neurologic illness that can prove fatal if not recognized and treated appropriately.

Emergency Treatment

People who develop decompression sickness require emergency care with intravenous fluids, high-flow oxygen, and prompt transfer to an emergency facility with a recompression (hyperbaric) chamber. Mild altitude sickness can be effectively prevented and treated with high-carbohydrate intake and increased fluid before and during one's stay at high altitude. Certain medications may be prescribed by your physician if he or she is aware of your travel plans. For serious altitude sickness, descent to a lower altitude, oxygen, and rest are effective.

Near Drowning

If the person is still floundering in the water and you believe you are strong enough and sufficiently well trained in swimming and water rescue to get him or her out, do so immediately. However, if you are not a swimmer or are unsure that you can manage the person by yourself, summon help.

Other options include using a throw rope attached to a buoyant object such as a life ring or life jacket. Toss it to the floundering person, then pull him or her to shore. Using a rowboat or canoe to reach the person is another option; the person can then cling to the side of the craft while you row or paddle to shore. Unless there is an access ladder, do not encourage the person to try to climb into the boat, however, because the boat might capsize and force you both into the water.

Emergency Treatment

If the drowning person's breathing has stopped, and you are alone, perform CPR for 1 minute before calling for help. If you are not alone, send someone for help and begin mouth-to-mouth resuscitation as soon as you can safely help the person. This means starting the breathing process even before the person has been positioned on shore: clear the airway and deliver two quick breaths while in shallow water. Continue to breathe for the person every few seconds while moving him or her ashore.

Do not waste time trying to drain the person's lungs of water. Begin immediately to breathe for the person, hard if necessary. The air should still reach the lungs.

For step-by-step instructions on resuscitation, see Cardiopulmonary Resuscitation, page 408.

Summon emergency medical assistance. Near drowning can lead to various medical complications; thus, emergency medical care is required.

Electrical Injury

Most of us experience minor electrical shocks now and again. They are usually more surprising than they are dangerous, because a reflex action almost instantly jerks our hands or other parts away from the source of electricity. For most of us, there is less pain from the stinging sensation than there is fear.

Under certain circumstances, however, even small amounts of electricity can be life-threatening. Electrical current passing through the body can produce unconsciousness, cardiac arrest (see page 443), and a cessation of breathing. Electrical shocks also can produce serious, deep burns and tissue injury, although often even a serious electrical burn appears as only a minor mark on the skin.

Get the Person Away From the Electricity

If you find a person who you think has been electrocuted, look first—do not touch. He or she may still be in contact with the electrical source, and touching him or her may pass the current through you and render you unable to help.

Turn off the power if the fuse box or circuit breakers are nearby; often, simply turning off the appliance itself will not stop the flow of electricity.

Move the source of the electricity away from you and the affected person. Use a nonconducting object: cardboard, plastic objects, or wood (a broom handle, for example) are best. Do not use a metal implement, which will conduct the electricity and also endanger you.

Emergency Treatment

Once the victim is free of the source of electricity, check the breathing and pulse. If either has stopped or seems dangerously slow or shallow, initiate resuscitation immediately (see Cardiopulmonary Resuscitation, page 408).

Summon emergency medical assistance.

Treat for Shock

If the person is faint or pale or shows other signs of shock (see Recognizing and Treating Shock, page 442), lay the person down, with the head slightly lower than the trunk of his or her body and the legs elevated.

Treat any burns (see Treating Major Burns, page 405) and wait for emergency medical assistance to arrive. Remember, have a physician see any person with a significant exposure to an electrical current, even if he or she is not unconscious or lethargic, to verify that no internal injury has occurred.

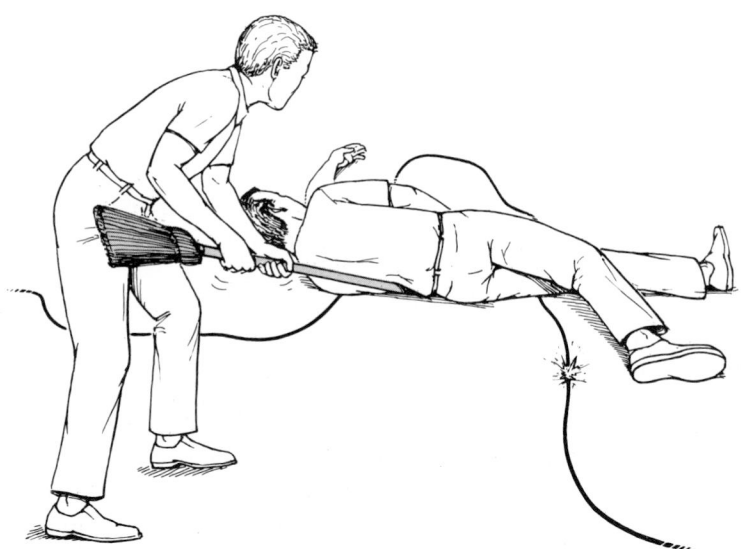

Use a nonconducting object (such as a wooden broom handle) to pull or push a victim of electrical shock away from the live electrical source.

Smoke Inhalation

In addition to the risk of burns, fire presents another deadly danger: smoke inhalation. All combustion produces smoke that contains poisons. When burned, plastics and other synthetics, wood, chemicals, and other flammable materials can produce carbon monoxide and fumes that can irritate the eyes, burn the skin, and result in breathing problems when the lungs and airway are smoke-damaged.

The key symptoms of smoke inhalation usually appear in the victim's eyes and breathing pattern (the victim may gasp for breath). The eyes are likely to be irritated. Treat the eyes as you would if a foreign object were lodged there by flushing with quantities of clean water (see Foreign Bodies in the Eye, page 425). There also may be associated burns, which should be treated appropriately (see Burns, page 403).

Emergency Treatment
Move the victim to a smoke-free area a safe distance from the fire or source of smoke. In doing so, be careful to avoid flames and smoke. Keep as low to the floor as possible (the hot smoke rises, so the air at floor level is less toxic). If the smoke is especially dense, do not enter the area without a proper breathing apparatus, and leave the lifesaving to professional rescue personnel.

Once the person is clear of the smoke, check for breathing and heartbeat; if they are not apparent, begin resuscitation (see Cardiopulmonary Resuscitation, page 408).

If the person is breathing, loosen any tight clothing and make the person as comfortable as possible. Summon emergency medical assistance—even if the person seems recovered.

Finally, treat the person for shock (see Recognizing and Treating Shock, page 442).

Carbon Monoxide Poisoning

A by-product of combustion is carbon monoxide. If inhaled in quantity, the carbon monoxide will take the place of oxygen in your bloodstream and reduce the supply of oxygen to your body's cells.

Typical symptoms of carbon monoxide poisoning are headache, nausea, vomiting, and confusion. Seizures and death may occur when levels of carbon monoxide in the blood become very high.

If you wake up at night with a headache—especially if another member of your family complains of headache and is hard to arouse—get out of the house immediately. Go to a neighbor's home; seek emergency medical care. Inadequately vented furnaces and wood and coal burning stoves, among other things, can result in carbon monoxide accumulation in your home. Carbon monoxide detectors are available for home use and could save your life.

Emergency Treatment
Treat the person with carbon monoxide poisoning as specified for smoke inhalation on this page. Transport the individual to an emergency facility as quickly as possible and administer oxygen.

Faints, Seizures, and Strokes

Sudden loss of consciousness is among the most alarming of medical emergencies. Fainting spells are generally the least serious of such events—some perfectly healthy people faint at the sight of blood, for example, only to recover completely in a matter of minutes. But all faints, seizures, and strokes must be treated as potentially serious medical emergencies. The unconscious individual should receive immediate and appropriate care.

Fainting Spells

The medical term for fainting is syncope. It occurs when the supply of blood to the brain is momentarily inadequate. The person becomes pale as too little blood reaches the skin, and consciousness is temporarily lost.

In syncope, the loss of consciousness is by definition brief. Usually within a minute of lying flat, blood flow is restored and the individual who fainted is again aware of the world around him or her.

Fainting spells can occur as a result of various causes. Several medical disorders, including heart disease, severe coughing spells, and circulatory problems, can produce syncope. Some people, however, faint when they are extremely tired, when they receive news that is emotionally upsetting, or when they simply see blood. The heart slows, the blood vessels dilate, and blood pressure falls.

A fainting episode can have no medical significance or it can be a symptom of a serious disorder. No matter how trivial the cause, however, loss of consciousness is to be treated as a medical emergency until the symptoms are relieved and the cause is known.

Emergency Treatment

If Lying Down

If a fainting spell results in the person slumping to the floor, position the individual on his or her back. Be aware that people who lose consciousness frequently vomit: their airway must be checked carefully.

Check for vital signs. Is the person breathing? Position your ear over the person's mouth to listen for breathing sounds. Can you feel a pulse? It may be weak and slow, so check carefully. If breathing and heartbeat have ceased, the problem is more serious than a fainting spell and CPR must be initiated (see Cardiopulmonary Resuscitation, page 408).

Raise the legs above the level of the head. If the person is breathing, position the individual's legs on a chair or other object. This position allows gravity to increase blood flow to the brain. Loosen belts, collars, or other constrictive clothing. The person should revive quickly.

If Seated

If a companion complains of faintness or dizziness while sitting, have the person lie down. If there is not space to do so, have him or her remain seated but position the head between the knees. This will help increase circulation to the brain. If a person faints, yet remains seated, quickly lay him or her on the floor.

Take It Easy

After a fainting spell, the person's facial color should return to normal. Often, however, the person will continue to feel weak for a short time after fainting, so lying quietly for a few minutes is advisable.

Check for Other Symptoms

Is chest pain present? Does the person complain of head pain? Is there apparent breathing difficulty? Does the person complain of numbness or continuing weakness? These may be signs of underlying medical problems. Seek emergency medical assistance.

Provide First Aid for Injuries

If the person was injured in a fall associated with the faint, treat any bumps, bruises, or cuts appropriately (see Care of Minor Wounds, page 392).

Seek medical assistance immediately if:

- This is the person's first fainting spell
- The symptoms mentioned above are present on awakening
- The person has sustained an injury during the faint

Seizures

Normally, the brain cells produce various coordinated electrical discharges. If, however, the electrical discharges become disorganized, a seizure occurs.

A seizure (also called a convulsion) is an involuntary episode of alternating muscular contractions and relaxations with loss of consciousness. Epileptic seizures are perhaps the most familiar variety of seizures, but several other disorders also can produce them. These include uremia (kidney failure, see page 852); meningitis (see page 481); toxemia of pregnancy (see page 204); withdrawal from benzodiazepines (such as Valium), barbiturates, or alcohol; or intake of certain poisons or street drugs. Rarely, a seizure may be the first manifestation of a brain tumor (see Seizures, page 495).

Emergency Treatment

During the Episode
When a seizure occurs, keep the person from injuring himself or herself. If vomiting occurs, try to turn the head so that the vomitus is expelled and is not aspirated into the lungs or windpipe. Frequently urine or stool will be involuntarily released during a seizure.

To reduce the risk that the individual will injure himself or herself in uncontrolled movements, clear the area around the person of furniture or other objects.

Do not try to limit the movements of a person having a seizure.

Although the person may cease breathing (and occasionally turn blue) for a part of a minute, breathing almost invariably returns without the need for CPR (see Cardiopulmonary Resuscitation, page 408).

If poisoning is suspected, attempt to determine the poison consumed. Call for immediate medical assistance.

In an infant or child, if the seizure seems to be the result of high fever (and your child is awake), lay your child on his or her side and wait until the seizure ends, then cool your child gradually, using a dampened sponge or cool compress and tepid water. An appropriate dose of acetaminophen may be used. Do not, however, immerse your child in a cold bath (see Febrile Seizures, page 69). Seek immediate medical assistance.

After the Episode
If the person has never had a seizure before, if the episode lasts more than a few minutes, or if the seizure recurs, seek professional medical care: call for an ambulance.

Once the seizure is over, position the person on his or her side. This position will allow normal breathing and any vomitus or fluids to drain from the mouth and airway. Frequently, a person will have blood coming from the mouth from biting his or her tongue or cheek.

Confusion may be present for a period of time after the seizure. Watch the affected person until there is complete return of mental function.

If the person injures himself or herself in a fall associated with the seizure, treat any bumps, bruises, or cuts appropriately (see Care of Minor Wounds, page 392).

Record details of the seizure for the physician. Important observations include duration of the seizure, extremities involved, apparent precipitating factors, nature of the seizure, and any other characteristics you noticed.

Strokes

A blockage of blood flow or bleeding (hemorrhage) in the brain can result in a medical condition called a stroke. Symptoms of stroke may include:

- Sudden numbness, weakness, or paralysis of the face, arm, or leg, usually on one side of your body
- Loss of speech, or trouble talking or understanding speech
- Sudden blurred or decreased vision, usually in one eye
- Dizziness, loss of balance, or loss of coordination
- Sudden, severe headache, with no apparent cause
- Difficulty swallowing

A stroke is a brain attack. Seek immediate medical assistance, just as you would for a heart attack. Every minute counts. The longer a stroke goes untreated, the greater the damage. Success of treatment may depend on how soon care is given.

The warning signs may be temporary, lasting from a few minutes to 24 hours, but even symptoms lasting only a short time may indicate a stroke. Treat them seriously.

Emergency Treatment

While waiting for an emergency vehicle to arrive, watch the person suspected of having a stroke. If breathing ceases, CPR is necessary (see Cardiopulmonary Resuscitation, page 408). Minor breathing difficulty may be alleviated by positioning the head and shoulders on a pillow. Watch for vomiting and potential aspiration of vomitus into the lungs. If vomiting occurs, turn the head to the side.

Do not allow the person to eat or drink anything. If paralysis is present, protect the paralyzed parts.

For a detailed discussion of Stroke, see page 461.

Hypertensive Crises

High blood pressure is a common ailment—perhaps one in four Americans has high blood pressure (also known as hypertension). It is a serious but treatable ailment (see High Blood Pressure, page 647). However, a hypertensive crisis is a medical emergency.

Hypertensive crisis is extremely uncommon. It occurs when the blood pressure in your arteries rises to a dangerously high value (more than 140 mm Hg diastolic; see Normal Blood Pressure, page 648). Among the possible causes are stroke (see page 461), toxemia of pregnancy (see page 204), kidney failure (see page 852), and drug interactions. The cause also can be simpler: if a person with hypertension forgets to take his or her medication, blood pressure can become dangerously high.

In addition to a very high blood pressure, the following symptoms may indicate hypertensive crisis:

- Severe headache, accompanied by confusion and blurred vision
- Chest pain
- Nausea and vomiting
- Seizures

Emergency Treatment

If the symptoms listed above occur, seek emergency assistance. While waiting for help to arrive, the person experiencing the symptoms should lie down and be encouraged to rest quietly. No food or fluids should be given.

In the event of seizures, care for the person as outlined in Seizures (page 421).

Diabetic Emergencies

People with diabetes may experience one or more of several different emergencies characteristic of their disorder. Among them are the insulin reaction, coma caused by ketoacidosis, and hyperosmolar coma.

For a detailed discussion of diabetes mellitus, see page 925.

Insulin Reaction

An insulin reaction is sometimes known as insulin shock or hypoglycemia (low blood sugar). An insulin reaction is most likely to occur in a middle-aged or younger person who is taking insulin for his or her diabetes. Some older persons with diabetes also take insulin and are vulnerable to this problem. Rarely, an individual who is not known to have diabetes also may experience an insulin reaction.

An insulin reaction is most likely to occur several hours after eating. Exercise also can cause an insulin reaction unless the person with diabetes takes less insulin or extra food before exercising.

Symptoms vary, but they usually consist of nervousness, feelings of hunger or apprehension, confusion, cold and clammy skin with sometimes profuse perspiration, loss of consciousness, or a seizure. This progression of symptoms may take place rather quickly, usually in less than an hour. The individual may be wearing a bracelet that identifies him or her as a person who takes insulin. It is also possible for the person taking one of the oral hypoglycemic tablets to have a mild reaction, but this is unusual and the symptoms are often less severe.

Once you recognize the problem, give the person some kind of carbohydrate or sugar. He or she may stubbornly resist taking the food because the thinking process has become affected by the low blood sugar. Fruit juices, candy, or sugar-containing carbonated drinks are effective. If the person vomits, wait a few minutes and then give small amounts of the carbohydrate cautiously. If the person is unable to cooperate in swallowing, a teaspoonful of a syrup can be placed in the cheek at intervals of a few minutes. There often will be a period of 15 to 30 minutes from the time the sugar is administered until symptoms abate. Call a physician if recovery is not prompt. Administration of glucose in a vein or glucagon given just under the skin (subcutaneously) may be needed to reverse the symptoms.

Someone responsible should remain with the person for an hour or so after apparent recovery because full mental function sometimes does not promptly return.

Diabetic Ketoacidosis

Diabetic ketoacidosis (diabetic coma) tends to occur in middle-aged or younger persons, but older persons can also be affected. It usually occurs when a person with insulin-dependent diabetes omits an insulin dose, uses too small a dose, or is stricken with a serious illness such as pneumonia. In some cases, diabetic ketoacidosis may be the condition that leads to the identification of previously undiagnosed diabetes.

Symptoms begin more slowly than in an insulin reaction and usually will progress over several hours or days before becoming severe. Nausea, vomiting, weakness, thirst, warm and dry skin, increased rate and depth of breathing, and gradual alteration of consciousness culminating in coma are characteristic symptoms.

Treatment is directed by a physician. If you are uncertain initially whether impaired consciousness in someone with diabetes results from an insulin reaction or from ketoacidosis, give sugar by mouth (treat as an insulin reaction). If there is not an improvement in the person's condition, seek immediate medical assistance.

Hyperosmolar Coma

This condition tends to occur in older persons with diabetes who do not require insulin injections. The most common sequence is an illness, such as gastroenteritis or stroke, that interferes with the person's ability to drink water or perceive thirst. The combination of the stress of the illness and the inability to consume enough water to maintain normal hydration leads to a progressive elevation of blood sugar to very high levels and a gradual loss of consciousness.

Hyperosmolar coma can be prevented by ensuring that older persons with diabetes consume generous quantities of water and by treating the precipitating illness promptly. Once consciousness is altered, this condition requires emergency evaluation.

Fever

Fever is one of the body's reactions to infection. Although the mechanism is incompletely understood, a fever apparently plays a role in the way the body adjusts to and fights off many infectious diseases. Fever also can occur as a result of a reaction to a medication or for no apparent reason.

When Is It an Emergency?

Your body temperature normally traces a definite pattern. Low in the morning, it gradually rises during the course of the day and reaches its maximum during the late afternoon and evening. Ordinarily, body temperature varies 1 or 2 degrees Fahrenheit over the course of the day, and it usually does not exceed 99 degrees Fahrenheit.

Thus, the value of 98.6 degrees Fahrenheit, generally considered normal body temperature, is only a general guide. Values somewhat above this are not necessarily abnormal; elevated body temperature usually does not become dangerous until it goes above 105 to 106 degrees Fahrenheit (see Heat Stress, page 414).

What Is a Fever?

When fever is present, the mechanisms that control body temperature are simply set a few degrees higher. The new set point may be, for example, 102 degrees Fahrenheit instead of the normal 97 to 99 degrees Fahrenheit. As fever begins, the body seeks to elevate its temperature and you feel chilly

Using a Thermometer

There are several ways to take your temperature, all of which require use of a thermometer. Traditional oral and rectal thermometers are glass tubes containing a column of mercury. The mercury expands, moving up the column in response to heat from your body.

Oral thermometers, which have a long, slender bulb at one end that contains mercury, are used for taking temperatures orally or under the armpit (axillary temperature). A rectal thermometer, which has a shorter, stubby bulb of mercury at one end, is used for taking a child's temperature from the rectum.

Electronic and temperature strip thermometers are also available. When you are purchasing a thermometer, look for one that is easy to read and with degrees that are clearly marked.

Before taking a temperature with a glass thermometer, make sure that the mercury is down near the bulb. Holding the thermometer firmly, shake it with several abrupt downward flicks of your wrist. Then wash the thermometer in cold water. To read the thermometer, hold it near the light and rotate it slowly until you see the silver column of mercury.

In adults and in children older than 7, the temperature is usually taken orally. The bulb end of the thermometer is inserted under the tongue and the person closes his or her mouth. After 2 or 3 minutes, you can remove the thermometer and read it.

In children younger than 7, the temperature can be taken by placing an oral thermometer in the armpit and having the child cross his or her arms across the chest. After 3 minutes, remove the thermometer, read the temperature, and add 1 degree Fahrenheit for an accurate measurement. You also can use a rectal thermometer in young children. Insert the bulb end of the thermometer about an inch into the child's rectum, while holding the child down with your arm, if necessary. Never let go of the thermometer while it is inside your baby because one squirm may push it deeper into the rectum and cause an injury. After 2 or 3 minutes, remove the thermometer and subtract 1 degree Fahrenheit.

After taking someone's temperature, rinse the thermometer in cold water or alcohol.

Newer thermometers using digital readouts and those that are able to take temperatures quickly off the eardrum (tympanic membrane) have simplified temperature-taking in the very young and very sick.

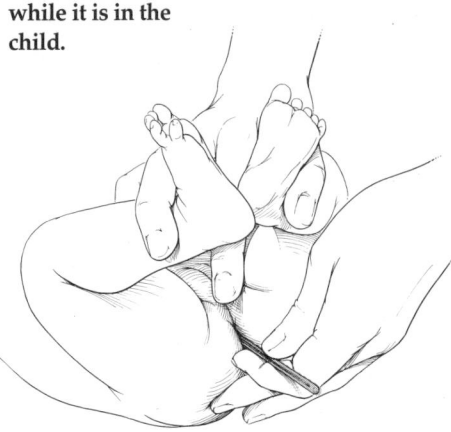

When using a rectal thermometer to take a newborn's temperature, insert the thermometer approximately 1 inch. Never let go of the thermometer while it is in the child.

and may shiver to generate heat. You may be more comfortable wrapped in a blanket and huddled with a heating pad. These methods will help your body gain heat and reach the new set point. Then, when the temperature reaches that new set point (for example, 102 degrees Fahrenheit), you will no longer feel cold and will stop shivering and not need the blanket and heating pad.

If the cause of the fever disappears, or if you take aspirin or acetaminophen or another medication to reduce the fever, the set point will return toward the normal range and you will feel warm. You may seek cooler surroundings and have profuse perspiration, both of which tend to dissipate body heat.

What Is a Fever Emergency?

In the following situations, seek professional medical assistance.

In a Newborn
In babies 3 months or younger, any rectal temperature of 100.5 degrees Fahrenheit is reason to call the baby's physician immediately.

High or Prolonged Fever
A child with a temperature of 103 degrees Fahrenheit or more must be given the emergency treatment discussed below. In an adult, consult your physician if you have a temperature of 101 degrees Fahrenheit that persists for longer than 3 days or if your temperature is 103 degrees Fahrenheit or more.

Severe Headache, Stiff Neck, Severe Swelling of the Throat, or Mental Confusion
If any of these symptoms accompany a fever, consult your physician immediately.

Unexplained Fever
In an adult, call your physician if you have no apparent symptoms except a temperature of 101 degrees Fahrenheit that lasts more than 3 days or a low-grade fever that lasts for several weeks.

Other Symptoms
Fever that accompanies sore throat, the aches and pains of the flu, coughing, and other symptoms suggests the presence of infection. Consult your physician and discuss your symptoms with him or her.

Treatment of Fever in a Child

Dress a child with a fever in light clothing and, at most, cover with a sheet or light blanket. Follow your physician's instructions about giving the child acetaminophen or other medication. Ordinarily, a child does not need acetaminophen for a temperature less than 102 degrees Fahrenheit. A child with a temperature of 102 to 104 degrees Fahrenheit should be given an appropriate dose of acetaminophen. Do not give aspirin to a child with any unidentified or viral illness (such as influenza or chickenpox) because it can increase the risk of Reye's syndrome (see page 484).

A child with a temperature of 104 degrees Fahrenheit or higher should be cooled gradually with a sponge bath of lukewarm water and be given an appropriate dose of acetaminophen. Check the child's temperature every 30 minutes; when the temperature decreases to less than 102 degrees Fahrenheit, stop the sponging. If your child has a temperature of more than 104 degrees Fahrenheit, contact your physician.

If the fever does not moderate or if seizures occur, seek immediate medical assistance (see Febrile Seizure, page 497).

Foreign Bodies

Children and adults alike occasionally get foreign objects in their eyes, ears, nose, or other body orifices. You can take appropriate steps in some cases to remove the object; in other situations, the care of your physician or a visit to an emergency room is required. (If the foreign body is caught in the throat, see Choking, Breathing Emergencies, and Resuscitation, page 406.)

Foreign bodies in the vagina (such as a retained tampon), rectum, and urethra always require the evaluation and treatment of a physician. In such circumstances, seek immediate medical attention.

In the Eye

Often, the eye will clear itself of an airborne object. Involuntary blinking and tearing will wash the particle out. If these natural mechanisms do not remove the foreign body, however, the eye must be treated with prompt and proper care because vision can be threatened by trauma, infection, or exposure to chemicals or particulate matter (such as dense smoke).

Emergency Treatment

Clearing Someone Else's Eye
Follow the emergency steps listed below. (The same procedure applies if you think the object has been removed from the eye but redness and pain persist.)

1. Do not rub the eye. Wash your hands before examining the eye. Seat the person in a well-lighted area.

2. Locate the object in the eye visually. Is it embedded in the eyeball? Examine the eye by gently pulling the lower lid downward

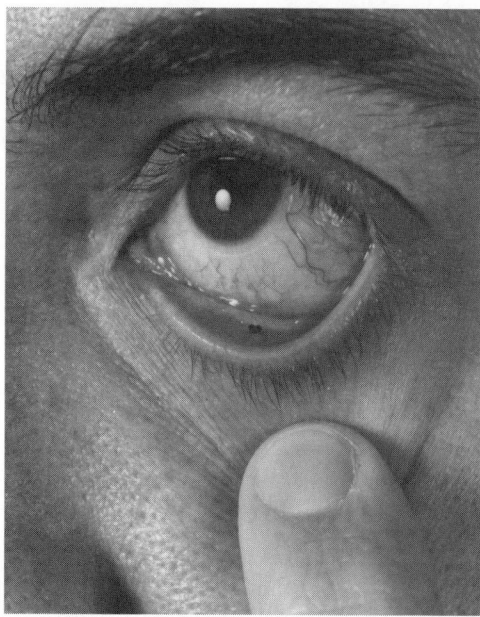

Examine the eye for foreign objects.

and instructing the person to look upward. Reverse the procedure for the upper lid: hold the upper lid and examine the eye while the person looks downward.

If you find that the foreign object is embedded in the eyeball, cover the eye with a sterile pad (if available) or a clean cloth. Do not try to remove the object.

If the object is large and makes closing the eye difficult, cover it with a paper cup and tape the cup to the face and forehead. Seek emergency medical assistance immediately (see Trauma to the Eye, page 531).

3. If the object is floating in the tear film or surface of the eye, you may be able to flush it out or remove it manually. While holding the upper or lower lid open, use a moistened cotton swab or the corner of a clean cloth to remove the object. If you are unable to remove the object easily, cover both eyes with a soft cloth and seek emergency medical assistance.

4. If you do succeed in removing the object, flush the eye with an ophthalmic irrigating solution or with clean, lukewarm water.

5. If pain, redness, or vision problems persist, seek emergency medical care.

Clearing Your Own Eye

The procedures outlined above are very difficult to follow when examining your own eye because involuntary blinking and tearing may make it impossible to see clearly.

If no one is nearby to help you when you get a foreign body in your eye, try to flush the eye clear. Using an eyecup or small juice glass, wash your eye with clean water. Position the glass with its rim resting on the bone at the base of your eye socket and pour the water in, keeping the eye open. If you do not succeed in clearing the eye, seek emergency medical help.

In the Ear

Children often insert objects into their ears; sometimes an insect or an airborne object will accidentally enter the ear.

Emergency Treatment

If an object becomes lodged in the ear, follow these steps:

1. Do not attempt to remove the foreign object by probing with a cotton swab, matchstick, or any other tool. To do so is to risk pushing the object farther into the ear and damaging the fragile structures of the middle ear.

2. If the object is clearly visible, is pliable, and can be easily grasped with tweezers, gently remove it.

3. Try using the pull of gravity: tilt the head to the affected side. Do not strike the victim's head, but shake it gently in the direction of the ground to try to dislodge the object.

4. If the foreign object is an insect, tilt the person's head so that the ear with the offending insect is upward. Try to float the insect out by pouring mineral oil, olive oil, or baby oil into the ear. It should be warm but not hot. As you pour the oil, you can ease the entry of the oil by straightening the ear canal: pull the earlobe gently backward and upward. The insect should suffocate and may float out in the oil bath. Do not use oil to remove any object other than an insect. Do not use this method if there is any suspicion of a perforation in the eardrum.

5. If these methods fail and the person continues to experience pain in the ear,

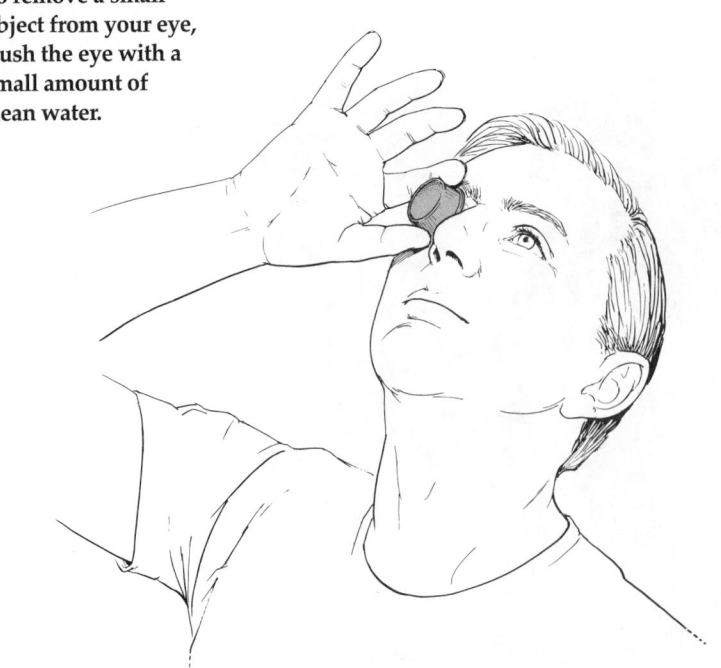

To remove a small object from your eye, flush the eye with a small amount of clean water.

reduced hearing, or a sensation of something lodged in the ear, seek emergency medical assistance (see Foreign Objects in Your Ear, page 571).

In the Nose

Occasionally, an object may become lodged in the nose.

Emergency Treatment
Try the following procedures:

1. Do not probe at the foreign object with a cotton swab, matchstick, or other tool. To do so is to risk pushing the object further into the nose. Do not try to inhale the object by forcefully breathing in. In fact, you or the person with the foreign object lodged in the nose should breathe through the mouth until the object is removed.

2. Try gently blowing your nose to try to free the object. However, avoid blowing the nose hard or repeatedly.

3. If the object is clearly visible, is pliable, and can be easily grasped with tweezers, gently remove it.

4. If these methods fail, seek emergency medical assistance.

Inhaled Foreign Objects

When accidentally inhaled, some objects can lodge in the windpipe (trachea) or lungs (bronchial passages). If an inhaled object causes choking, the Heimlich maneuver and immediate medical intervention may be required (see Choking, Breathing Emergencies, and Resuscitation, page 406).

In some cases, however, the foreign bodies that become lodged in the trachea or a bronchial passage do not inhibit breathing—but they do constitute a hazard to the health of the person involved. If you or your child inhales a foreign object, consult your physician.

Your physician may order an X-ray to establish the presence and location of the object. A procedure involving a bronchoscope (see Bronchoscopy, page 726) may be performed, in which a hollow tube that contains an optical system is introduced through

---

Children and Button Batteries

Increasingly, button-sized batteries are used in portable electronic equipment—cameras, pocket calculators, watches, hearing aids, and other items. To a curious young child, these shiny objects can be most intriguing. They are also most dangerous when swallowed.

These batteries contain dangerous alkali fluids; some also contain potentially life-threatening amounts of mercury. If released into the stomach or intestine, the battery fluid may eat through the lining, producing symptoms such as abdominal pain and tenderness, constipation, vomiting, and fever.

If your child swallows a button-sized battery, seek the care of your child's physician immediately. Surgery may be required.

Prevention
Parents and grandparents should consider this hazard in childproofing a house. Store unused batteries out of the reach of children. When disposing of exhausted batteries, do not toss them into a wastebasket that a toddler can easily explore.

---

the throat into the bronchial airways to find and remove the object from your windpipe or bronchi.

Swallowed Foreign Objects

Occasionally children swallow non-food objects such as coins, pins, buttons, fruit pits, safety pins, and other household objects. These foreign bodies usually pass through the digestive system uneventfully, but some can lodge in the esophagus. In adults, especially those who have esophageal disorders or chewing problems, there is also the risk of esophageal blockage.

If any swallowed object lodges in the throat and blocks the airway, it is a medical emergency requiring immediate intervention. The Heimlich maneuver may dislodge an offending piece of food (see The Heimlich Maneuver, page 407).

If you swallow a non-food object or if your young child seems to have difficulty swallowing, or if he or she is spitting up saliva, especially if abdominal pain or vomiting occurs, call your physician. The object may be blocking the entrance to the stomach and may have to be removed with an endoscope, a hollow tube that contains an optical system. The endoscope may be introduced through the throat and then into the esophagus. It is used to find and remove the object from the esophagus (see Foreign Bodies, page 749).

Genitourinary Emergencies

Medical emergencies involving the genitals and urinary tract may produce intense pain in the groin (as occurs with testicular torsion or trauma to the external genitals), difficulty with urination, or inability to urinate. Sexual, violent, or abusive crimes to the genitals constitute a medical emergency that requires appropriate and immediate care.

Pain in the flank, scrotum, or vulva, especially when accompanied by blood in the urine, may be a consequence of trauma, kidney stones, or a tumor of the genitourinary system. If these symptoms occur, seek emergency medical evaluation.

Sexual Assault and Sexual Abuse

When an act of sexual assault, violence, or abuse occurs, the physical injuries are often less significant than the emotional damage that may have been inflicted. However, if serious physical injury has been sustained, treat the injury with appropriate emergency measures (see Bleeding Emergencies, page 399; Choking, Breathing Emergencies, and Resuscitation, page 406; or Shock, page 441).

The victim of a violent crime, physical abuse, or sexual assault (forced sexual activity in which the person has not consented to the sexual act performed upon him or her) must be approached with care and sensitivity. Make sure the person understands that you are not going to hurt him or her. Do not ask lots of questions. Instead, be a good listener. Try to provide emotional support and reassurance. A child, in particular, may be distracted from the situation by talk of other matters.

Sexual crimes and crimes of abuse and violence, even if the associated physical injuries are minor, require careful evaluation. Many major hospitals have sexual assault treatment centers and are accustomed to dealing with the legal and emotional as well as the medical manifestations of crimes of violence and abuse. Your regular physician is another option.

If you are uncertain where to go, look in the telephone book under "rape," "sexual assault," or "child abuse." There may be a special hot line with trained operators to provide advice and physician referrals as well as other help, including personal support and legal advice.

In the case of sexual assault, call for emergency assistance immediately. Do not wash your body or change clothing before being examined by a physician. Your physician will treat any injuries and provide psychological support. He or she also will be concerned with assembling possible evidence that can be used to prosecute the attacker. (For more information on sexual abuse in the preschool years, school-age years, or teenage years, see pages 109, 127, and 153.)

Painful or burning urination may suggest an infection of the urethra, bladder, or kidney. If these symptoms occur or if you experience a sudden difficulty in urinating, obtain prompt medical evaluation.

Testicular Torsion

A sudden, severe pain in one testicle may be a condition called testicular torsion. This uncommon problem occurs when a testicle twists on its spermatic cord, cutting off the blood supply to the testicle. Testicular torsion sometimes occurs without any apparent cause, even during sleep. It also may follow strenuous physical activity.

Accompanying symptoms may include nausea and vomiting, abdominal pain, faintness, and fever. This condition is more likely to occur in teenagers around the time of puberty, but it may occur in younger and in older males. Epididymitis (see page 1198) is also a frequent cause of a painful testicle.

Emergency Treatment

Consult your physician immediately. Whenever you or a friend or family member experiences pain in the testicles, seek immediate medical help. In cases of testicular torsion, if the testicle is not untwisted and returned to its normal position within a few hours—and often an operation may be required to do so—it will atrophy due to lack of a blood supply and will have to be removed from the scrotum.

Keep the person with testicular torsion as comfortable and still as possible while seeking professional help. For a detailed discussion of this condition, see Testicular Torsion, page 1197.

Trauma to the External Genitals

The male genital organs are not protected by being inside the abdomen, so the penis and testicles are prone to injury. The pelvis and thighs usually prevent injury to the external genitals, but when injury does occur, it can be intensely painful and dangerous.

Emergency Treatment
If the injury involves bleeding, use direct pressure to control it (see How to Stop Severe Bleeding, page 400). After bleeding has been controlled, the entire genital region should be protected with a large, triangular dressing applied like a diaper, and emergency medical assistance should be sought. When the genitals are struck a hard blow but no bleeding results, an ice pack and firm support by a soft athletic supporter may be used to lessen severe pain in the testicles.

If the testicles have been struck by a blunt object or are injured in a fall, and if the pain and swelling of the scrotum lessen within about an hour, there is probably no serious damage.

However, seek emergency medical assistance if the scrotum remains swollen, if it is bruised, if the pain persists, or if the penis or scrotum is seriously cut and bleeding.

If the scrotum is struck and penetrated by a sharp object, immediate emergency care is required.

Intoxication and Behavioral Emergencies

Intoxication, emotional difficulties, and behavioral disorders are common and require professional intervention. In the following pages we will discuss alcohol intoxication, drug intoxication, sudden personality changes, and suicidal thoughts and behavior, the most common signs of emotional and mental distress for which emergency care is appropriate.

Alcohol Intoxication

Alcohol is a drug, a central nervous system depressant with a range of effects depending on the amount consumed and the condition and metabolism of the person drinking the alcohol. Abuse of alcohol can result in short- and long-term illness, unpredictable behavior, and even death.

Recognizing Alcohol Abuse
The signs of acute alcohol intoxication range from slurred speech, uncoordinated movements, and loud and unruly behavior to vomiting, lethargy, and unconsciousness. The person may appear flushed and there may be a noticeable odor of alcohol about the person.

Recognizing Alcohol Withdrawal
When a habitual drinker suddenly ceases to drink, physical symptoms of withdrawal may occur. Delirium tremens (DTs) may result, in which the person hallucinates, acts strangely, is confused or restless, and may have a noticeable shaking of the hands (see Withdrawal and DTs, page 330).

Emergency Treatment
Establish, if possible, whether the cause of the condition is alcohol consumption (or withdrawal). Ask the person about the cause of his or her condition. Do so in a nonthreatening, calm way. You are more likely to get a candid answer to a gentle query than if you appear to be menacing or challenging.

Look for the symptoms cited above, but also ask the person whether any medications have been taken while drinking. Mixing certain drugs, legal and illegal, and alcohol can be lethal, and such an interaction may be the cause of the symptoms.

Monitor breathing and other signs. If vomiting occurs, be sure the person does not inhale (aspirate) vomitus into the lungs. Keep the person leaning over or, if lying down, with the head turned to one side.

If the person has sustained any injuries in falls or other accidents, treat the injury to stop bleeding or immobilize fractures. Ask the person whether he or she has injuries of which you are not aware. (Remember: Alcohol can be a strong painkiller, so the person may not be aware of the severity of an injury.)

Most episodes of alcohol intoxication result in little more than a few hours of nausea and a morning-after headache. However, if you observe any of the following circumstances, seek emergency medical assistance:

- If the person is withdrawing from habitual alcohol use
- If there is no evidence of alcohol consumption but behavior is unusual
- If the person loses consciousness or aspirates vomit

- If there is evidence of both drug and alcohol consumption

(See Drug and Alcohol Abuse, page 1102; Alcohol- or Drug-Induced Psychosis, page 1129; the chapter Alcohol Abuse and Alcoholism, page 325; and Physical Abuse, page 1231.)

Acute Drug Intoxication

Few drugs have no side effects; most can, in certain sensitive individuals, produce dangerous, strong reactions that require emergency medical care. Drug interactions also may produce adverse effects. That is why it is essential that you list for your physician any and all drugs you are taking and whether they were prescribed by a physician or purchased over the counter.

Legal Drugs

If on consumption of a medication you (or a friend or family member) experience severe headache, confusion, emotional instability, anxiety, vision problems, rashes, loss of consciousness, coma, or seizures, immediately stop taking the drug and consult your physician or seek emergency assistance.

Illegal Drugs

The signs of illegal drug use vary according to the type of drug that is used. With a drug such as marijuana, the effects may be minor, and you may observe dilated pupils or redness about the eyes of the user. The person may have speech patterns that are exaggeratedly fast or slow and confused. In acute drug intoxication, however, the symptoms are likely to be more serious (see Hallucinogens, page 1134).

Mind-Altering Drugs

LSD and many other street drugs may produce rapid pulse rate, dilated pupils, and a flushed complexion. The person may talk

---

Sudden Personality Changes

Emotional problems, poisonings, alcohol or drug abuse, head injuries, insulin reactions, high fever, stroke, or other problems can result in various personality changes, ranging from disorientation or delirium to violent or self-destructive behavior. Intense stress can sometimes be overwhelming and result in disorganized and, at times, aggressive outbursts.

Reassure the Person
If you find yourself dealing with a person who is acting or talking in an unpredictable, bizarre, or "crazy" fashion, begin by trying to talk calmly to that person. Try to reassure him or her that you are there to help. Listen and respond gently. With eye contact and a nonthreatening manner, try to establish some kind of interaction with the person.

Safeguard the Person and Yourself
If the person has threatened suicide or harm to others, make certain the person is not armed. Do not try to deal with someone who has a weapon and has threatened to use it. The threat may be very real indeed, a danger to both you and the person. Summon the police or other law enforcement authorities.

Do not try to restrain a person unless you have proper training. Doing this puts you and the person you are trying to help at risk of harm. A person in a disturbed state turned violent can be more dangerous and stronger than you may imagine.

Seek emergency medical assistance if the person is disoriented, incoherent, or agitated or poses a danger to himself or herself or others; also seek assistance if you are unable to communicate with the person.

While you are waiting for help to arrive, continue to try to reassure the person. Do not make jokes: humor may be misconstrued under such circumstances. Do not make threats: ask the person whether he or she is hurt or in pain or whether you can help in any way.

A person who is on a "bad trip"—regardless of whether it is the result of drug use or emotional stress—needs, for his or her own safety, to be isolated in a safe, quiet environment and accompanied by someone who will provide firm reassurance.

For guidance in dealing with these specific emergencies (each of which may be accompanied by strange behavior), see Insulin Reaction (Hypoglycemia), page 927; Alcohol Intoxication, page 429; and Suicidal Thoughts and Behavior, page 431.

incoherently and "see" or "hear" things that you cannot (hallucinations). Some people experience great anxiety and fear. Paranoia, aggressive behavior, or extreme withdrawal also may occur (see pages 343 and 344).

Uppers and Downers

The so-called uppers produce excitement, physically stimulating the body to increase the rates of heartbeat and breathing. Rapid speech, dilated pupils, perspiration, and sleeplessness also may occur. The effects of downers are the opposite, with reduced rates of heartbeat and respiration and stumbling or slurred speech patterns (see Drug Dependency, page 1131).

Narcotics

As with downers, pulse and breathing patterns are likely to be reduced. The skin may be cool, although perspiration may be apparent. Sleepiness and even unconsciousness may result from overdoses (see Street Drugs, page 342).

Emergency Treatment

Seek emergency assistance if you suspect a person has consumed an overdose of drugs. Emergency signs include loss of consciousness, breathing that seems dangerously slow or to have stopped (respiratory arrest), or aggressive, panicky, hostile, delusional, violent, or fearful behavior after use of a street drug.

If you believe that the overdose was taken orally within the past hour, it may be appropriate to induce vomiting (see Handling Poisoning Emergencies, page 438).

Drug Withdrawal

If a person abruptly stops the chronic use of alcohol or certain drugs, drug withdrawal may occur. The chronic alcoholic or drug abuser is in danger of seizures, delirium tremens (DTs), or even death if detoxification is not carried out in a systematic manner. Other complications may occur with cessation of the habitual use of benzodiazepines, barbiturates, heroin, morphine or other opioids, and alcohol.

Proper detoxification often requires a week or more of treatment, ideally in a hospital. Seek emergency medical assistance if you find someone experiencing signs of acute drug withdrawal (see Detoxification, page 1133).

Suicidal Thoughts and Behavior

Conventional wisdom asserts that people who talk about committing suicide do not do it. Do not believe it: that old cliché simply is not true.

Recognizing the Signs

No two suicidal people are alike, but they often manifest similar behavior. Behaviors that may indicate a suicidal state include withdrawal, moodiness, a sudden emotional crisis, a sudden personality change, depression, or aggressive behavior in which respect for his or her own life and for other lives is lacking (see Warning Signs of Potential Suicide, page 1125, and Teenage Suicide, page 1101).

Dealing With a Potential Suicide

If a friend or family member talks of suicide or behaves in a way that leads you to believe suicide is on his or her mind, treat the person with respect and seriousness. It is not unreasonable to ask the person if he or she is contemplating suicide.

Watch the person closely to prevent him or her from finding the opportunity. Seek professional help as soon as possible. Begin by calling your local suicide hot line or local physician, psychiatrist, or emergency room. These sources will be able to suggest where immediate help is most easily available.

Dealing With an Attempted Suicide

If you encounter a person who has attempted suicide, treat the situation as a medical emergency and get help as quickly as possible. If the person has stopped breathing, resuscitation must begin immediately (see Cardiopulmonary Resuscitation, page 408). If the person is bleeding, see How to Stop Severe Bleeding, page 400; if the person has taken an overdose of pills or poison, see Handling Poisoning Emergencies, page 438.

Hyperventilation

Hyperventilation means overbreathing (too many breaths or breathing too deeply). Paradoxically, it leaves you with the sensation of not being able to get enough air.

This condition may be characterized by spasms of the hands in which the fingers are extended while the thumb and fifth finger are drawn together. The feet also have similar spasms. Hyperventilation usually stems from anxiety or panic attacks (see page 1119), but it can occasionally be associated with diseases that cause pain or distress. It is important to establish that a person is not having chest pains or severe headache before being treated for hyperventilation.

Treatment

Treatment of hyperventilation consists of reassuring the person and persuading him or her to breathe more normally. Sometimes breathing into a paper bag, so that the person is rebreathing the air from his or her lungs (the bag should expand and collapse if this is done properly), will be helpful.

Pain Emergencies

The single most common symptom reported to almost every physician is pain. "My head hurts." "It's my left leg." "It comes and goes, especially at night." In an average of one out of two office visits, the principal complaint is pain.

Pain can have many causes; consequently, there are many kinds of pain. Chronic (long-term) pain can be constant or intermittent; acute pain tends to occur suddenly, often as the result of a specific event, and may last minutes to hours. Localized pain occurs in a relatively small, confined area of your body; generalized pain is spread over a larger area.

When describing symptoms to your physician, identify the nature of your pain using these terms. The pain of arthritis, for example, which may endure for decades, is chronic pain; the brief but intense pain of a minor injury such as a burn, scrape, or abrasion is acute, localized pain.

In the following pages, we are concerned with distinguishing pains that signal medical emergencies. Certain chest pains, for example, may signal a life-threatening heart attack; others are the result of indigestion and are no more than a minor gastrointestinal discomfort. Because someone's life may depend on the availability of proper medical assistance in treating heart attack or some other serious medical emergency, distinguishing minor and transient discomforts from serious signs and symptoms is essential.

Head Pain

We have all had a headache at one time or another. Most headaches are minor, passing discomforts that are usually forgotten after the pain has faded—and often a headache disappears almost as quickly as the discomfort arrives.

However, a headache can also be a symptom of a more dangerous and serious medical problem. Discuss with your physician any persistent headache or a headache that you would describe as "my worst ever." Some of the most common causes of head pain are discussed below.

Migraine Headache

An intense head pain, often predominantly on one side of the head and perhaps accom-

---

Abrupt Onset of Severe Pain: When to Be Concerned

Pain is part of your body's warning system. When you experience an intense pain, it usually means some tissues have been irritated or damaged: you may have burned yourself on the stove, or perhaps you sprained your ankle in a fall.

If you experience sudden, severe pain of no known cause that you have not had before, seek your physician's guidance. Infection or internal disease could be the cause, and it may require immediate and appropriate treatment. If the cause is known to you, it may still be appropriate to seek professional help, as is the case with an injury or discomfort after surgery.

Long-term pain from conditions such as arthritis or a back ailment may become a fact of life and something you learn to live with. Your physician may refer you to a chronic pain center for help in dealing with your pain (see Chronic Pain Centers, page 1136). However, if the nature of the pain suddenly changes, seek your primary physician's advice. For your own health and safety, do not try to "tough it out." Disregarding a serious, unfamiliar pain can put you at risk of unnecessary complications and even death. Seek prompt medical assistance.

panied by nausea and vomiting, may be the result of a migraine headache. A migraine headache is often throbbing in character and may last from a few hours to a few days. Another common symptom of migraine headache is sparkling lights or black spots in your field of vision. You may want to avoid bright lights.

Migraine headaches can interfere with your activities and are painful, but they are not life-threatening and there is no indication that they lead to other disorders. However, if you suspect you have migraine, seek your physician's guidance in order to rule out other, more serious ailments. Your physician may devise a program of treatment to prevent migraine headaches or to be used in the event of future episodes (see Migraine Headaches, page 502).

Meningitis
The presence of severe headache accompanied by fever, vomiting, confusion, or drowsiness, and perhaps by a stiff neck, may indicate meningitis. This dangerous disorder is an infection or inflammation in the lining that surrounds your brain tissue.

Because long-term damage may occur if you go untreated, seek emergency care immediately (see Meningitis, page 481).

Cerebral or Subarachnoid Hemorrhage
Bleeding in or around the brain may be signaled by a range of symptoms. These include the following:

- Sudden, severe headaches, frequently accompanied by vomiting
- Deterioration in vision, speech, or sensation over minutes to hours
- Sudden weakness or loss of sensation in one limb or in an arm and a leg, with or without involvement of the face
- Acute onset of double vision, slurred speech, vertigo (the sensation of either you or your surroundings spinning), incoordination, or difficulty swallowing
- Loss of consciousness shortly after onset of headache

Summon emergency assistance immediately (see Stroke and Vascular Disorders, page 461).

Dental Abscess
If you experience persistent throbbing pain in a tooth, find chewing painful, or have sensitivity to liquids or hot or cold foods, you may have an abscessed tooth.

You also may have a slight fever and swollen neck glands and feel generally unwell; a pus-filled boil may develop on the gum near the sore tooth. At some point, this may burst, releasing foul-tasting and foul-smelling pus into your mouth and relieving the pain.

Left untreated, the pain will probably go away over time, but the infection will remain, slowly destroying the bone. If you experience these symptoms, see your dentist immediately.

Acute Ear Pain
If you experience pain in an ear with a sense of fullness and diminished hearing in the ear that is not due to trauma or a foreign object, the cause may be a middle ear infection (otitis media, see page 574).

Ear infections can be intensely painful. In the case of outer ear infections, called external otitis, there may be itching, hearing loss, and an oozing of yellowish and foul-smelling pus.

Infants are likely to cry often when they experience ear infections; they also may tug at their ears.

Consult your physician without delay. Ear infections are relatively easy to treat. In most cases, permanent hearing loss is unlikely. However, consult your physician for appropriate antibiotic or other treatment.

To relieve the pain of an ear infection before seeing your physician, place a warm (not hot), moist cloth over your ear. Taking aspirin or another analgesic may also relieve the discomfort. Do not use ear drops before being evaluated by a physician.

Chest Pain

Pains in the chest are among the most difficult of symptoms to interpret. Simple indigestion can result in chest discomfort, especially when coupled with a growing anxiety that a heart attack might be the cause.

Chest pain can result from excessive sneezing or coughing brought on by allergies. If severe enough, the coughing can actually fracture a rib. The muscles between the ribs can become sore from prolonged coughing. Stress also can produce a tightening in the chest that resembles the pain of a heart attack.

Chest Wall Pain

One of the most common varieties of harmless chest pain is called chest wall pain. One kind of chest wall pain is known as Tietze's syndrome, or costochondritis. It consists of pain and tenderness in and about cartilage that connects your ribs to your sternum (breastbone).

Often, pressure over a few points along the margin of the sternum will demonstrate remarkable tenderness limited to these small areas. If your pain is duplicated by the pressure of the examining finger, you probably can conclude that a serious cause of chest pain, such as a heart attack, is not responsible. This discomfort generally lasts only a few days. Use of aspirin or some other type of analgesic can help alleviate symptoms.

Other causes of chest wall pain include strained chest wall muscles from overuse or excessive coughing and muscle bruising from minor trauma. These pains tend to be worsened by chest wall movement and will usually resolve in several days with rest, heat, and use of aspirin or acetaminophen.

Heart Attack

A heart attack occurs when an artery that supplies oxygen to the heart muscle becomes blocked. The heart attack may be preceded by chest pain (angina pectoris), for days or weeks, during or after exertion or even at rest. Or it may occur in the absence of any previous pain.

During a heart attack, a portion of the heart muscle gradually dies, producing the signs and symptoms listed in Is It a Heart Attack? below.

By definition, a heart attack is a medical emergency. If you think you are having a

Is It a Heart Attack?

A heart attack may be characterized by the following signs and symptoms:

- Intense, prolonged chest pain, often described as a feeling of heavy pressure or heaviness. The pain may extend beyond your chest, radiating to your left shoulder and arm, to both arms, to your back, and even to your teeth, jaw, and neck. At times, the pain may occur in the upper abdomen and be described as akin to severe indigestion. Sometimes the pain occurs suddenly; sometimes it does not
- Nausea, vomiting, shortness of breath, and intense sweating
- Weakness, restlessness, and anxiety
- Occasionally, loss of consciousness is the only sign

If you experience these symptoms, summon emergency medical help immediately.

heart attack or are with someone who is, get immediate medical attention. If your companion's heart attack has caused him or her to cease breathing, resuscitation must be initiated immediately (see Cardiopulmonary Resuscitation, page 408).

Do not delay in seeking medical help: that mistake takes thousands of lives every year. If you experience symptoms that resemble those listed on this page, seek emergency medical assistance—call 911 or call an ambulance. If you think you are having a heart attack, do not try to drive to the hospital yourself.

Pulmonary Embolism

Another medical emergency frequently signaled by chest pains is a pulmonary embolism. An embolus is an accumulation of foreign material (usually a blood clot) that blocks an artery. Tissue death (infarction) occurs when the tissue supplied by the blocked artery is damaged by the sudden loss of blood. When a clot (usually from veins of the pelvis or lower extremity) lodges in the lung, it is termed a pulmonary embolism.

The symptoms of a pulmonary embolism include the following:

- Sudden, sharp chest pain that begins or worsens with a deep breath or a cough (pleurisy), often accompanied by shortness of breath
- Sudden, unexplained shortness of breath without pain
- A cough that may produce blood-streaked sputum
- Rapid heartbeat
- Anxiety and excessive perspiration

As with a suspected heart attack, seek emergency medical help immediately (see Pulmonary Embolism, page 734).

Pneumonia With Pleurisy

The term "pneumonia" actually identifies a wide range of infections, each of which affects tissues of the lungs. A frequent symptom of pneumonia is chest pain (together with chills, fever, and a cough that may bring up bloody or foul-smelling sputum). When pneumonia is accompanied by an inflammation of the membranes that surround the lung (pleurisy), the accompanying chest discomfort upon inhaling or coughing may be considerable.

One sign of pleurisy is that the pain is usually relieved temporarily by holding your breath or putting pressure on the painful area of the chest; the same is not true of heart attack (see Pleurisy and Pleural Effusions, page 711, and Pneumonia, page 704).

Seek your physician's care. If your chest pain is accompanied by a cough and fever or chills, consult your physician. Appropriate antibiotics and other treatment may be required.

Other Causes

Chest pain also may be the result of other causes. For example, a dissecting aneurysm (tearing of an artery due to a weakness in its wall) that occurs in the main artery leaving the heart (the aorta) may produce severe chest pain (see Aortic Aneurysm, page 693). This is a medical emergency requiring immediate treatment.

Heartburn (esophageal pain) tends to occur more frequently when lying down or bending over. Often it is associated with an acid or sour taste in the mouth and generally can be relieved by belching or use of liquid antacids. Sometimes the pain of heartburn is confused with signs and symptoms of a heart attack.

As with other sudden, unexplained pain, all chest pain may be a signal for you to seek medical help.

Abdominal and Pelvic Pain

For purposes of identification, the trunk of your body is divided into three main areas, the chest, abdomen, and pelvis. The chest is defined by the rib cage and contains the heart and lungs; the abdomen and pelvis contain digestive and other organs, including the stomach, large and small intestines, liver, gallbladder, pancreas, spleen, appendix, and some of the reproductive and sexual organs.

Given this number of organs, the potential sources for pain and medical problems are many and varied. If you experience intense, persistent pelvic or abdominal pain, go to the emergency room or seek your physician's guidance. The following medical emergencies may possibly be the cause of acute pains in the abdominal or pelvic area.

Perforated Peptic Ulcer

If a peptic ulcer, usually located in the lower part of the stomach or in the initial portion of the duodenum, erodes completely through the wall, it is said to have perforated.

A perforated peptic ulcer is a potentially life-threatening complication of an ulcer. The symptom is intense pain, generally in the upper abdomen. Leakage of stomach or duodenal material into the abdominal cavity may cause peritonitis (see page 792) and shock (see page 441). Emergency surgery to close the leak is usually required.

Gallstones

An intense and sudden pain on the upper right side of the abdomen that moves up to the right shoulder blade or between the shoulder blades may signal gallbladder or bile duct disease. A small, stone-like accumulation of cholesterol or calcium salts, gallstones result in pain that may last for hours and be followed by general abdominal soreness. Nausea, loss of appetite, and sometimes fever and chills may be accompanying symptoms.

If you develop these symptoms, seek your physician's guidance (see Gallstones, page 812).

Pancreatitis

Intense, constant abdominal pain lasting many hours or even days may signal an attack of pancreatitis. The pain may radiate straight through to the back and chest; it may begin after the consumption of a large quantity of alcoholic beverages. Other symptoms may include fever, bulky stools that float, nausea or vomiting, clammy skin, abdominal distention, and an increase in pain on lying on your back.

Pancreatitis is an inflammation of the pancreas, the gland located behind the stomach. The pancreas secretes enzymes essential to digestion in addition to the hormone insulin.

If you develop these symptoms, seek your physician's guidance (see Acute Pancreatitis, page 818).

Gastroenteritis

Gastroenteritis is a common and uncomfortable ailment. Characteristic signs include nausea or vomiting, diarrhea, abdominal cramps, and bloating. A low-grade fever may accompany the other symptoms.

In an adult, most gastroenteritis will usually last no more than about 36 hours. If the symptoms persist longer than 36 hours, consult your physician (see page 766).

Appendicitis

A small structure attached to the large intestine, the appendix has no known function. However, when the appendix becomes inflamed, it is a medical emergency requiring immediate evaluation. The symptoms are initially a dull pain around the navel, gradually followed by pain and tenderness in the lower right side of the abdomen. Often a fever, lack of appetite, nausea, and occasionally vomiting and constipation accompany the pain.

If you suspect you or your child has appendicitis, seek emergency medical treatment (see Acute Appendicitis, page 772).

Bowel Obstruction

Occasionally, individuals who have developed scar tissue from prior operations will develop a bowel blockage or obstruction (see page 793). Commonly, severe cramps in the mid or lower abdomen are present and often associated with diarrhea and vomiting. Fever does not usually occur. There may be an urge to defecate or pass gas but an inability to do so. Occasionally, individuals without prior abdominal surgery can have a bowel obstruction. Emergency care is usually necessary to further evaluate this condition.

Diverticulitis

A severe, cramping pain, usually more severe on the left side of your abdomen, may indicate the presence of an infection or inflammation in the lower portion of your large intestine (colon).

Seek your physician's guidance if you experience such a discomfort (see Diverticulosis and Diverticulitis, page 781).

Ruptured Ectopic Pregnancy

Ectopic pregnancy (sometimes called tubal pregnancy) occurs when a fertilized egg begins to grow in the fallopian tube or someplace other than the uterus. The result is abdominal pain or cramping and, often, vaginal bleeding. Dizziness and the urge to urinate or have a bowel movement also may occur.

This is a potentially life-threatening condition that requires prompt surgical treatment. Seek your physician's guidance immediately (see Ectopic [Tubal] Pregnancy, page 199).

Ovarian Cysts

Most ovarian cysts are minor problems that present only minor discomfort and difficulty.

In occasional instances, however, sudden, severe pain may occur in the abdomen, accompanied by fever and even vomiting. Consult your physician if such pains and symptoms occur (see Ovarian Cysts and Benign Tumors, page 1189).

Kidney and Ureteral Stones

If you experience flank pain on urination, blood in the urine, or a severe pain that moves downward from the flank to the groin, vulva, or testicle, you may have a stone in your kidney or ureter (the tube that conveys urine from the kidneys to the bladder). This intensely painful kidney condition usually is resolved when the stone is passed into your bladder or out of your body (sometimes there are several stones).

If you develop these symptoms, seek your physician's guidance (see Kidney Stones, page 843).

Cystitis

Painful urination, a frequent need to urinate, blood in the urine, a sensation of not being able to empty your bladder, and lower abdominal pain may indicate cystitis (an inflammation of the bladder). Consult your physician. This problem usually can be treated routinely, but it should be properly diagnosed to be sure that no other underlying cause is present (see Cystitis [Bladder Infection], page 842).

Pyelonephritis

If the symptoms of cystitis are accompanied by pain in the flank and fever, an infection may be present that involves the kidney and ureter as well as the bladder. Symptoms may be accompanied by severe chills, followed by high fever and even shock (see page 441). Severe pyelonephritis often is associated with an extension of the infection from the kidney into the bloodstream (septicemia).

Consult your physician (see Acute Pyelonephritis, page 841). Hospital admission and administration of antibiotics and fluids through a vein may be required.

Pain in the Extremities

Sudden, unexplained pain in the arms, legs, hands, or feet may be indications of medical problems requiring treatment. Among the potential causes are the conditions described here.

Acute Arterial Occlusion

Sudden and severe pain accompanied by paleness and coldness in an arm or leg may indicate the presence of a blocked (occluded) artery.

The blockage commonly is the result of atherosclerosis (see page 636), with a clot (embolism) of fragments of atherosclerotic plaques lodging where a major artery divides into two smaller ones. This most often occurs at the level of the knee.

Because diabetes seems to accelerate the process of atherosclerosis, diabetic persons are more vulnerable. Because of the risk of gangrene (see page 692) and the possible need for amputation, seek emergency care immediately. Protect the leg from both cold and heat. Wrap it in soft cloths or sheeting while getting the affected individual to the hospital.

Thrombophlebitis

When a blood clot occurs in a deep vein in an extremity (usually a leg), there may be tenderness, pain, and swelling in the thigh or calf. Fever also may be present.

Because of the risk of pulmonary embolism (should the clot break loose and travel to the lung) and other complications, seek emergency medical assistance (see Thrombophlebitis, page 694).

Acute Venous Obstruction

Sudden, unexplained swelling of one or both ankles or feet may be caused by an acute venous obstruction in the pelvis or legs. It can occur without pain, especially following incidents such as prolonged bed rest, long auto or plane trips, or surgery. Visit your physician or emergency room promptly.

Acute Joint Pain

Gout

If you experience a sharp, intense pain in a single joint and it is not the result of a blow or other injury, you might have gout. Gout most often strikes the so-called bunion joint at the base of the big toe.

A type of arthritis, gout also produces swelling and redness in the painful joint. Although gout pain usually will disappear of its own accord over a period of days, consult your physician. He or she may prescribe medications to relieve your discomfort and to help prevent future occurrences (see Gout, page 916).

Joint Infections

Pain and stiffness in one joint, typically a knee, shoulder, hip, ankle, elbow, finger, or wrist, accompanied by the warmth and redness of inflammation and perhaps chills, fever, and weakness, may mean a joint infection. This can be the result of a recent wound in which the infecting agent entered your tissues, or there may be no evident cause. Contact your physician or visit your emergency room immediately (see Infectious Arthritis, page 914).

Other Possible Causes

Joint soreness after a period of exercise may result from several causes (see Runner's Knee, page 873; Acute Painful Shoulder, page 917; and Bursitis, page 917), but any intense, continuing pain in a joint is cause for consulting your physician.

Poisoning Emergencies

Any substance that is swallowed, inhaled, injected, or absorbed by the body and that interferes with the body's normal functioning is, by definition, a poison. Some poisons are familiar: pesticides, animal poisons, and cleaning and other household chemicals bearing printed warnings are examples.

In fact, almost any non-food substance is poisonous if taken in large doses. Aspirin is a case in point. This useful medication is found in most homes and is ordinarily safe. Yet each year more children die of aspirin overdoses than from overdoses of more familiar poisons.

Be aware of poisons in and around your home. Take steps to protect young children from toxic substances (see Handling Poisoning Emergencies, page 438). Keep the number of the Poison Control Center near your telephone (see page 438). Know the procedures to follow in case of a poisoning emergency.

Be familiar with plants in your home, yard, and vicinity. Keep your children informed too (see Garden-Variety Poisonous Plants, page 440). If you are concerned that industrial poisons might be polluting nearby land or water, report your concerns to your local health department or to the state or federal Environmental Protection Agency.

Handling Poisoning Emergencies

Recognize the Problem

The poisoning may be obvious. There's no denying the child seated on the floor, surrounded by aspirin tablets, some half-chewed, in his or her mouth. Alternatively, some guesswork may be involved. Look for these signs if you suspect a poisoning emergency:

- Burns or redness around the mouth and lips—they can result from drinking certain poisons
- Breath that smells like chemicals (perhaps gasoline or paint thinner)
- Burns, stains, and odors on the person, his or her clothing, or on the furniture, floor, rugs, or other objects in the area in which the person was playing or working
- Difficulty breathing, vomiting, or other unexpected medical symptoms

Note, however, that many conditions mimic the symptoms of poisoning, including seizures, alcohol intoxication, stroke, and insulin reaction. If you can find no indication of poisoning, do not treat the victim for poisoning. However, summon emergency assistance. Meanwhile, make the person as comfortable as possible. Treat for shock (see Recognizing and Treating Shock, page 442) or begin resuscitation if breathing slows or ceases (see Cardiopulmonary Resuscitation, page 408).

Emergency Treatment

If you conclude that a poison has been consumed, take the following steps:

1. Call your local Poison Control Center. In most communities, the number is listed on the inside cover of the telephone book (see Poison Center Resources, this page), or find the number and write it down near or on your telephone before you need it. (If the number is not readily available or if there is no response, go immediately to the nearest emergency room.)

The person who answers will ask, in brief, the following questions:

What happened? "I came back inside and found Johnny with a bottle of laundry detergent. He had some of the blue fluid on his lips and was crying."

Who are you? "My name is Jane Doe. I'm Johnny's mother."

Where are you? "I'm calling from 555-5555. The address is 111 Anywhere Lane, Middletown."

Who is the victim? "Johnny is my son. He is 4 years old."

Is he conscious? Has he vomited? "He's crying, but he's okay, I think. He's not vomiting or unconscious."

What was the poison? "It was this detergent. Here, I'll read you the label . . . ."

You will be asked other questions too, such as How much was consumed? and What have you done so far? and When did this happen?

2. Do not hang up. After consulting reference materials, the person will tell you what to do.

3. Should you induce vomiting? Certain poisons should be vomited up; others, such as petroleum products, acids, and alkalis, should not (see Acids and Alkalis, page 439). If you do not know the identity of the substance swallowed, do not induce vomiting.

Poison Center Resources

A Poison Control Center is not a hospital or treatment center—it is essentially a library staffed by persons familiar with poisonings. The information it can offer may be crucial to delivering prompt and proper treatment in a poisoning emergency.

In an Emergency

In a poisoning emergency, call the Poison Control Center in your area. The telephone number is usually listed inside the front cover of the white pages of the telephone directory; call the operator if you are unable to find it. Post it on or near the telephone before you have to use it.

Poison Control Centers operate 24 hours a day. They need to know circumstances—who you are, who the poisoned person is, his or her condition, your location, and, most important, exactly what was swallowed.

Have the Substance at Hand

When you call, have the poison that has been consumed at hand. In order to analyze the poison and recommend treatment, the control center will need to know the name of the substance or product and any chemical description found on the label.

Poison Control Centers often are associated with large hospitals or emergency rooms. Each meets the standards for reference material and staff established by the American Association of Poison Control Centers.

If you are told to induce vomiting in the person who has swallowed poison, follow these instructions. Insert a finger into the person's mouth and touch the back of the throat (it may be easier for the poisoned person to do this himself or herself if he or she is old enough). If you have syrup of ipecac at hand (and every household with children should), use it. Ipecac is an emetic (an agent that causes vomiting) that can be used to eliminate poison from the stomach. In both children and adults, use a glass or two of warm water with the ipecac.

Whether vomiting is induced or occurs naturally, make sure that the person does not inhale (aspirate) the vomitus into the lungs. A small child can be held over your knees, facedown. A larger person should bend way over or lie down, hanging the head off the side of a bed. In any case, the chin should be held lower than the level of the hips.

After the person has vomited, give milk or water.

4. Monitor vital signs. Be alert for changes in the person who has been poisoned. If breathing stops, CPR must be performed (see Cardiopulmonary Resuscitation, page 408). Treat for shock (see Recognizing and Treating Shock, page 442).

5. If the poison has spilled on the person's clothing, skin, or eyes, remove the clothing and flush the skin or eyes with water. You may need to hold the person's eyelids open while flushing (see page 425).

6. Go to an emergency room immediately. If you are unable to transport the poisoned person, summon an ambulance. Be sure to take the container or packaging in which the poison was stored with you. If the identity of the poison is unknown, but the person has vomited, take a sample of the vomitus for analysis.

Medications as Poisons

Lifesaving medications also can be killers. Overdoses of seemingly harmless medications such as the common painkillers aspirin and acetaminophen take many lives each year. Numerous other over-the-counter drugs are dangerous if taken in large doses, especially by a child or elderly person. Prominent on the list are sleeping medications, antihistamines, and vitamin supplements.

Acids and Alkalis

Acid and Alkali Poisons
Highly acidic and highly alkaline substances are, when swallowed or exposed to our skin or eyes, poisonous. Acids produce pain and corrosion of the tissues with which they come into contact. Difficulty in swallowing, nausea, intense thirst, shock, difficulty in breathing, and death can result from acid that is taken internally. The effect of alkalis varies, but the symptoms are similar—pain in the mouth, throat, and stomach as the alkalis damage the tissues of the gastrointestinal tract.

Emergency Treatment
Treat acid and alkali poisonings as seriously as you would any poisoning emergency. Call the Poison Control Center for specific instructions. Seek emergency medical care to further evaluate the situation. However, do not induce vomiting.

Follow the Instructions
Children are not the only ones at risk. Anyone who fails to obey dosage instructions is in danger of overdose. Read the label carefully; follow the instructions given there or given by your physician. If you are taking numerous medications daily, extra care and record keeping may be necessary (see Hazards of Multiple-Drug Use, page 1277).

Prevention Is Best
Keep all your prescription and nonprescription drugs stored out of the reach of children. Do not absentmindedly leave them available to a toddler on a kitchen counter, bedside table, or pocketbook. Buy childproof packages. If you have medications that must be refrigerated, put them on a high shelf out of the reach of children. If medications are placed in drawers, lock them or install a latch that only an adult can use.

Drug Allergies
Some people have allergic reactions to medications: even a proper dosage taken at the recommendation of your physician can, in a sensitive person, produce hives, facial swelling, wheezing and difficulty breathing, various rashes, itching, and even shock. These reactions are not common, but consult your physician immediately if you suspect a drug allergy (see Drug Allergies, page 1050).

Emergency Treatment
If a child takes too much of an appropriate or any of an inappropriate medication, call the Poison Control Center or nearest emergency

room (see Handling Poisoning Emergencies, page 438).

Poisonous Plants

Many attractive plants—both cultivated and wild—are potentially poisonous if swallowed. Be aware of plants in your home, garden, and neighborhood. Instruct your children never to eat unfamiliar berries and plants.

Emergency Treatment
If you or your child consumes a poisonous plant, among the symptoms that may occur are a burning pain in the mouth and throat; swelling in the throat that may lead to difficulty in breathing; vomiting, abdominal pain, or other gastrointestinal distress; and hallucinations, seizures, and unconsciousness.

Seek emergency assistance. With a sample of the plant on hand, call your local Poison Control Center for instructions (see Handling Poisoning Emergencies, page 438).

Food Poisoning

Food poisoning can cause various ailments, often distinguishable by the types of poison consumed. Among them are gastroenteritis and botulism.

Gastroenteritis
Unwashed or improperly handled food of almost any sort, raw fish or meats, or contaminated water can lead to food poisoning. A good example is the potato salad left unrefrigerated for too long at a family picnic.

If you become ill after eating such food, your physician probably will call the condi-

---

Garden-Variety Poisonous Plants

Plants are essential sources of food—but many are also poisonous. Did you know that apple seeds, potato vines, and tomato leaves are poisonous?

Do Not Eat Any Unfamiliar Plants
Beware of unidentified berries: they may be poisonous. Some mushrooms are edible and, to some people, great delicacies, but many are deadly. Do not experiment with the unknown in the woods, and do not encourage your children to do so.

Be Careful at Home
Lilies of the valley make lovely borders—but they are poisonous, as are daffodil bulbs in the garden, butter-

cups in the field, the jack-in-the-pulpit on the forest floor, and the holly (berries) and poinsettia in your house at Christmas. Do not eat any plant unless you know it to be safe.

Skin Reactions
Certain poisonous plants, including poison ivy, poison oak, and poison sumac, produce an itchy rash and blisters in sensitive people after contact with the resin of such plants (see Skin Allergies, page 1035).

Common Plants to Avoid

Name	Poisonous parts
Cherry	Pits
English ivy	Entire plant
Holly	Leaves and berries
Jimsonweed (also known as thorn apple)	Entire plant
Lily of the valley	Entire plant
Mistletoe	Berries
Mushrooms (especially amanita)	Entire plant
Potatoes	Sprouts, roots, and vines
Rhododendron	Entire plant
Rhubarb	Leaves

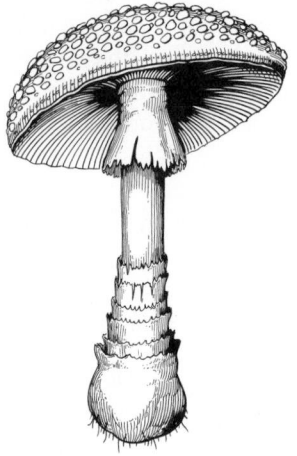

Amanita mushroom

tion gastroenteritis. Typically, within 1 to 6 hours of consuming food or water contaminated with staphylococcal bacteria, abdominal cramps and pain, diarrhea, and vomiting occur. The symptoms usually are gone in about 12 hours (see Infectious Food Poisoning, page 267).

Botulism

Botulism is a potentially fatal food poisoning. It results from the ingestion of a toxin formed by certain spores in food. Botulism toxin is most often found in home-canned foods.

Symptoms usually begin 12 to 36 hours after eating the contaminated food; they may include headache, blurred vision, muscle weakness, and eventually paralysis. Some people also have nausea and vomiting, constipation, urinary retention, and reduced salivation. These symptoms require immediate medical attention; a person with botulism needs to be hospitalized (see Botulism, page 488).

Food Allergies

Some people are allergic to certain foods. After consumption of a food to which the person is allergic, symptoms such as abdominal pain, diarrhea, nausea or vomiting, hives, swelling of the lips, eyes, face, tongue, and throat, and nasal or respiratory congestion may occur.

For most people, food allergies are uncomfortable, often extremely so. Responses vary from minor sniffles and a cough to abdominal cramps, vomiting, and even (rarely) anaphylaxis (see Anaphylaxis, page 444). When a person reacts severely with an anaphylactic response—narrowed air passageways, rapid pulse, drop in blood pressure, cardiovascular collapse, and shock—food allergies can be life-threatening. In such cases, summon emergency assistance immediately (see Food Allergies, page 1048).

Shock

The name itself vaguely suggests the nature of the problem—only rarely does shock result from an electrical current. In fact, a wide range of incidents or problems can cause it. Shock is a common complication of injury, infection, burns, and other conditions. It is not a consequence of emotional stress such as the sudden death of a loved one.

Shock is a condition in which there is a slowing or diminution of the flow of blood around your body (peripheral circulation). This produces a decrease in your blood pressure and an inadequate volume of red blood cells. The result: the supply of oxygen to tissues falls below normal amounts. This decrease may produce various symptoms.

Seek emergency assistance if you recognize the signs of shock. Shock is a medical emergency that requires appropriate and immediate care. You can take certain simple steps to help alleviate the symptoms, but summon professional medical help immediately.

Kinds of Shock

Shock—insufficient blood flow resulting in an oxygen deficiency for normal functioning—can result from serious bleeding

injuries (see Loss of Blood, below), major trauma, or dehydration resulting from loss of fluids due to vomiting or diarrhea. This type is called hypovolemic shock because it results from too little blood volume (*hypo* comes from the Greek word for "below"; thus, below-volume shock).

Cardiogenic shock results when the heart does not pump effectively. Causes may include heart attack or heart arrhythmias (see page 669).

When blood vessel size or tension is affected, vasogenic shock (*vaso* for "blood vessel") can result. Causes include insect and bee stings (see Anaphylaxis, page 444), infection (see Septic Shock, page 444, and Toxic Shock Syndrome, page 445).

Loss of Blood

Excessive loss of blood can produce hypovolemic shock, in which the volume of blood falls below (*hypo*) a healthy amount. A traumatic injury can result in shock, whether the bleeding is external (as with a severe cut) or internal, as with a fractured pelvis or from the rupture of an internal organ or vessel. Bleeding (hemorrhage) due to a lesion in the

Recognizing and Treating Shock

Symptoms

The following signs and symptoms indicate the presence of shock in an ill or injured person:

Skin. It may appear pale or gray, and it is cool and clammy to the touch.

Pulse and Breathing. The heartbeat is weak and rapid and is accompanied by a shallow, hurried breathing pattern. Blood pressure is reduced, perhaps below measurable values.

Eyes. The eyes are lusterless, staring, perhaps with dilated pupils.

Alteration of Consciousness. The shock victim may be unconscious, but even if still awake he or she is likely to be faint, confused, or weak. Sometimes a person in shock becomes anxious and excited. Many persons in shock will complain of being thirsty. Do not give fluids except for small sips of water or ice chips.

The person must be treated for shock immediately. Summon professional emergency assistance: this is a medical emergency.

Treatment

Serious injury, especially one that involves considerable blood loss, is likely to be accompanied by shock. Immediate first aid treatment for shock is essential. Even if a person who has been hurt seems alert and in control, treat him or her for shock.

Get Hospital Care as Soon as Possible

Shock in each of its forms is potentially life-threatening. Care by medical professionals with appropriate equipment is essential. Summon emergency medical assistance immediately.

Get the Person to Lie Down

Lay the person down, face upward, with the head below the level of the feet. This position will help maintain blood flow to the brain and may relieve symptoms of faintness. Elevating the feet on a chair, cushions, or another available prop is usually the easiest means to establish this position. However, if the person has sustained an injury in which raising the legs will cause pain, leave the person flat on his or her back.

Keep movement to a minimum.

Keep the Person Warm and Comfortable

Loosen tight collars, belts, or constricting clothing. Cover the person with a blanket if the air is cold; if the ground is cold, put the blanket beneath the victim. If it is hot outside, position the person in the shade if possible, on top of a blanket or coat or other material.

If the Person Is Vomiting or Bleeding From the Mouth

Position the person on his or her side. This position will help prevent choking or inhaling (aspirating) the vomitus or blood and make the person more comfortable.

Treat Injuries Appropriately

If an injury has occurred, stop any bleeding (see Bleeding Emergencies, page 399), immobilize any fracture (see Fractures, page 445, and Sprains, page 449), or take other appropriate first aid steps. Handle potential spinal injuries with special caution (see page 448). The pain from a fracture that is not immobilized can worsen shock.

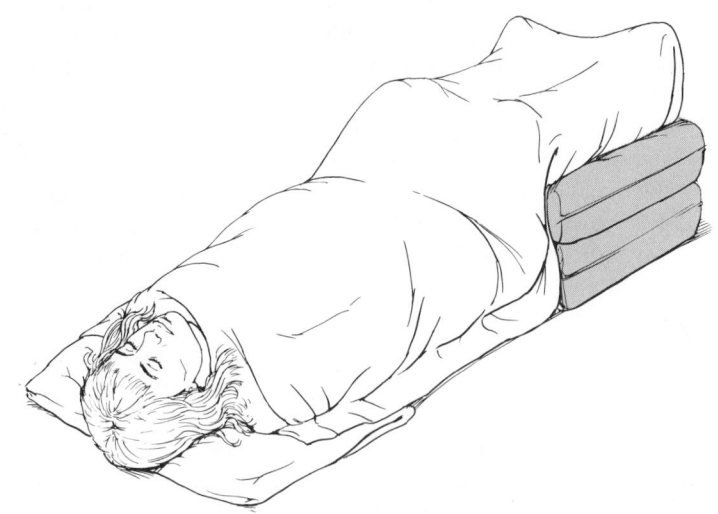

Keep the shock victim warm. Elevate legs and feet above the level of the heart to maximize flow of blood to the head.

gastrointestinal tract or heavy vaginal bleeding also can result in hypovolemic shock.

The symptoms will resemble those for other kinds of shock (see Shock, page 441). The skin will be pale and cool and clammy to the touch. The heartbeat will be weak and rapid, accompanied by a shallow, hurried breathing pattern, and blood pressure may have fallen below a measurable level. The person may be anxious and restless and complain of thirst. The skin at the knees and elbows may be mottled.

Emergency Treatment

Seek immediate emergency care. Hypovolemic shock can be fatal, and emergency medical care must be initiated. Summon help immediately. When the emergency medical team arrives, oxygen may be administered, along with intravenous fluid replacement.

While waiting for help to arrive, reassure the victim and make him or her as comfortable as possible. Treat as for other sorts of shock (see Recognizing and Treating Shock, page 442). If he or she stops breathing, perform resuscitation (see Cardiopulmonary Resuscitation, page 408).

Dehydration

When the body's supply of fluids falls below certain amounts, hypovolemic shock may result. The loss of fluids usually will be known because the person will be aware of persistent vomiting, diarrhea, or loss of fluid through the urine. The other symptoms are similar to those for other kinds of shock (see Recognizing and Treating Shock, page 442).

The skin will be pale and cool and clammy to the touch. The heartbeat is weak and rapid, accompanied by a shallow, hurried breathing pattern, and blood pressure may have fallen below measurable levels. The person may be anxious and restless and complain of thirst. The skin at the knees and elbows may be mottled.

Emergency Treatment

Seek immediate emergency care. Hypovolemic shock can be fatal, and emergency medical care must be initiated. If the person stops breathing, initiate mouth-to-mouth resuscitation (see Cardiopulmonary Resuscitation, page 408).

Potential Causes

Some of the ailments that can result in extreme fluid losses and hypovolemic shock are discussed below.

Gastroenteritis

Gastroenteritis is an infection or inflammation of the gastrointestinal tract. It is frequently called stomach or intestinal flu, and it is usually caused by a virus or bacterium that irritates the lining of the intestine.

These common infections usually last no more than 36 hours. Particularly in children and the elderly, however, the severe loss of fluids that can result from gastroenteritis can produce hypovolemic shock. In such cases, seek your physician's guidance (see Infections of the Gastrointestinal Tract, page 766).

All of the following ailments are to be regarded as medical emergencies. Seek emergency care immediately if you suspect that you or a member of your family suffers from any of them.

Cholera

This acute infection results from the consumption of water or foods contaminated by human wastes infected with the cholera bacterium. Vomiting and severe diarrhea are the major symptoms of cholera and can result in dehydration, hypovolemic shock, and death.

Addisonian Crisis

When the adrenal gland fails to produce the quantities of the steroid hormones your body needs for normal functioning, the disorder is termed Addison's disease. When the shortage of hormones becomes acute, adrenal failure (addisonian crisis) can occur.

There is loss of salt through the urine, and this leads to hypovolemic shock. Fortunately, this syndrome is rare. It may be suspected if the person looks deeply tanned without having been exposed to sunlight (see Addison's Disease, page 938).

Excessive Use of Diuretics

Among the most commonly prescribed drugs, diuretic medications stimulate your body to increase the rate and volume of urination and the loss of salt and potassium in the urine. Used in treating many ailments (including hypertension, certain liver disorders, and heart failure), they are valuable, often lifesaving, medications.

However, you must monitor use of diuretics carefully. Overmedication combined with zealous adherence to a low-salt diet can result in fluid depletion. In extreme cases, shock can result.

Heart-Related Shock

Certain cardiac events and disorders can result in a decrease of blood flow. Heart-related shock occurs when the supply of blood to the tissues falls below certain levels due to inadequate pumping strength of the heart. This condition is also called cardiogenic (or cardiac) shock.

Heart attack (myocardial infarction; see Heart Attack, page 661), heart failure (see page 659), heart arrhythmias (see page 669), or cardiac tamponade (see Pericarditis, page 687) can result in your heart's inability to pump sufficient blood to supply the cells of your body with enough oxygen for normal functioning. Shock can result.

The symptoms will resemble those for other kinds of shock (see Recognizing and Treating Shock, page 442). The skin will be pale and cool and clammy. The heartbeat is weak and rapid and is accompanied by a shallow, hurried breathing pattern, and the blood pressure may have fallen below measurable levels.

Emergency Treatment

Seek immediate emergency care. Cardiac shock is often fatal, so initiate emergency medical care immediately. When the emergency medical team arrives, oxygen may be administered, along with medication to control chest pain, if present.

While waiting for help to arrive, reassure the affected person. Make him or her as comfortable as possible. Treat as for other sorts of shock (see Recognizing and Treating Shock, page 442). If he or she stops breathing, initiate resuscitation (see Cardiopulmonary Resuscitation, page 408).

Septic Shock

If an infection enters the bloodstream and circulates around your body, your body fights back. The unwanted bacteria are killed, but substances called endotoxins are also released.

The presence of endotoxins in your bloodstream can produce symptoms, which may include reddened, flushed skin that is warm to the touch, chills and fever, rapid heartbeat, and shallow breathing. Typically, these symptoms last from 30 minutes to a few hours and then give way to cool, clammy skin, a drop in blood pressure, extreme thirst, shortness of breath, and even respiratory failure. In many cases the person has an infection, such as a kidney infection, before septic shock results. It is the spread of that infection to the bloodstream that produces septic shock.

Emergency Treatment

Septic shock is a life-threatening emergency requiring a range of medical care. Seek immediate emergency help (see Recognizing and Treating Shock, page 442).

Medical professionals may administer oxygen, intravenous fluid therapy, antibiotics, and perhaps other drugs to fight the infection. The blood may be cultured before antibiotics are given so that the nature of the problem can be identified.

Anaphylaxis

Anaphylaxis is a severe allergic reaction. Certain people react more strongly than others to certain allergens, and the introduction of the allergen into their systems can produce anaphylactic shock.

Anaphylaxis most often is experienced by people who have a history of allergies. It is to be suspected if symptoms develop within minutes after the person is bitten or stung by a bee or insect, has ingested a causative food, or begins taking a new medication. There are also other possible causes, but they typically occur while the person is under the immediate care of a physician. In sensitive individuals, these causes include the introduction into the body of certain vaccines, anesthetic agents, or the dyes used in certain diagnostic tests. A blood transfusion occasionally can produce anaphylactic shock.

The usual symptoms of anaphylactic shock are the following:

- The skin is warm to the touch. There is also a notable redness to the skin (erythema), perhaps over much of the body in raised blotches (hives)
- The person usually wheezes and has difficulty breathing
- Accompanying symptoms may include nausea, vomiting, abdominal cramps, increased pulse rate, and a sudden drop in blood pressure
- Without prompt and proper treatment, loss of consciousness and, eventually, death can result

Death from anaphylactic shock is most commonly due to severe breathing difficulty. Swelling of tissues in the throat may result in the airway becoming blocked.

Emergency Treatment

Seek emergency medical assistance immediately or rush the person to an emergency room. If the person stops breathing, perform mouth-to-mouth resuscitation (see Cardiopulmonary Resuscitation, page 408).

If the cause was a bee sting, remove the stinger if it is still attached to the site of the sting. Apply an ice pack or a cold, moist cloth.

Prevention

If you or a member of your family have severe allergic (anaphylactic) reactions to stings, keep a properly equipped emergency kit available. Your family physician can advise you on its contents, but it may include epinephrine (adrenaline) to be administered with a hypodermic needle or a single-dose auto-injector in case of an anaphylactic emergency.

Be careful when bees are around. Wear long-sleeved shirts and trousers. Avoid bright colors. Do not wear perfumes or colognes. If a bee hovers nearby, do not panic. Move away slowly and avoid wildly slapping at the bee or other insect (see Anaphylaxis, page 1053).

Toxic Shock Syndrome

Toxic shock syndrome is a rare but dangerous disorder associated with the use of tampons, especially by women younger than 30. Typical symptoms may include a sudden fever of 102 degrees Fahrenheit or higher; vomiting or diarrhea; dizziness, weakness, fainting, or disorientation; and a rash resembling a sunburn, which may appear even on your palms and the soles of your feet.

Summon emergency help immediately. If you or another female member of your family experiences the preceding symptoms, especially if they occur during menstruation and tampons are being used, summon emergency help. (Even before you call, remove the tampon.) Tell the physician what the symptoms are, how long they have been apparent, and when menstrual bleeding began.

Toxic shock syndrome can cause blood pressure to plummet, resulting in a state of shock (see Recognizing and Treating Shock, page 442, and Toxic Shock Syndrome, page 1145).

Trauma Emergencies

A trauma wound is an injury sustained as a result of external force or violence. A broken bone, a severe blow to the head, a knocked-out tooth—all are trauma emergencies.

Fractures are among the most common trauma emergencies. A fracture is, simply, a broken bone; it results when the forces exerted on the bone are greater than the bone can withstand. The term "sprain" is frequently used to identify a wide range of injuries, but a true sprain involves damage to the ligaments that connect the bones.

Fractures, severe sprains, dislocations, and other serious bone and joint injuries usually require professional medical care. You risk permanent disability, deformity, and, in the case of skull, neck, and spinal injuries, even death if proper care is not given promptly. Likewise, head trauma, eye injuries, and tooth loss (avulsion) must be given appropriate emergency treatment. Each of these emergencies is discussed in the pages that follow.

In the case of blunt trauma to the chest or abdomen (as may occur in an automobile accident), seek emergency medical attention.

Internal injuries can be sustained in such accidents, and even in the absence of apparent bleeding, life-threatening complications can result.

In all instances of trauma emergencies, the principal objective is to seek immediate medical assistance and to get to an emergency medical facility as quickly as possible.

Fractures

A fracture usually occurs as a result of a fall, blow, or other traumatic event. If you suspect a fracture, the proper approach is to protect the affected area from further damage. Do not try to set the broken bone. Reduction (the medical term for the process of setting the bone) is to be left to a physician. Obvious signs of a fracture may include the following:

- Swelling or bruising over a bone
- Deformity of the affected limb
- Localized pain that is intensified when the affected area is moved or pressure is put on it

Types of Fractures

In identifying types of fractures, your physician may use some of the terms explained or illustrated below.

Open fracture: The broken bone protrudes from the skin. This may allow entry of bacteria from the environment, which increases the risk of infection.

Simple fracture: A fracture in which the broken bone does not protrude through the skin.

Complete fracture: Fracture in which the bone snaps into two or more parts.

Incomplete fracture: The break is limited to a crack (the bone is not separated into two parts).

Impacted fracture: One fragment of bone is embedded into another fragment of bone.

Pathologic fracture: A bone break in a person with bones weakened by disease. Bone cancer (see page 899) or a bone disorder such as osteoporosis (see page 894) can result in weakened bones that fracture spontaneously or when only minor stresses are exerted on them. Such breaks are termed pathologic fractures because a principal cause is an underlying disease.

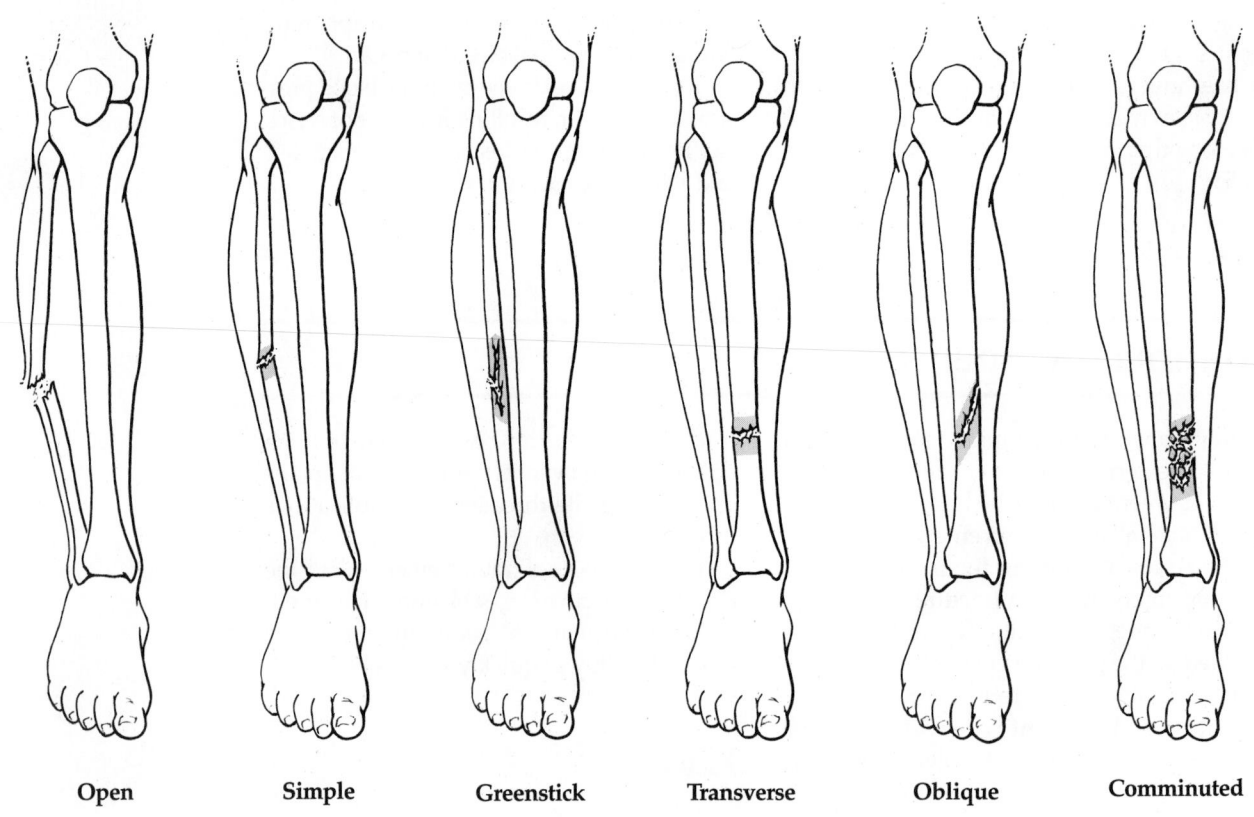

| Open | Simple | Greenstick | Transverse | Oblique | Comminuted |

- Loss of function in the area of the injury
- A broken bone that has poked through adjacent soft tissues and is sticking out of the skin

Emergency Treatment

Immobilize the Area

Before the person with the broken bone is transported to a hospital, the bone should be splinted to prevent movement. Keep joints above and below the fracture immobilized. A splint will stabilize the damaged parts and prevent unwanted movement of the parts that could aggravate tissue damage. Proper splinting may reduce pain.

Splinting depends on the location of the break (see Limb Fractures, page 447; Spinal Injuries, page 448; Hip or Pelvic Fractures, page 448; and Other Broken Bones, page 449).

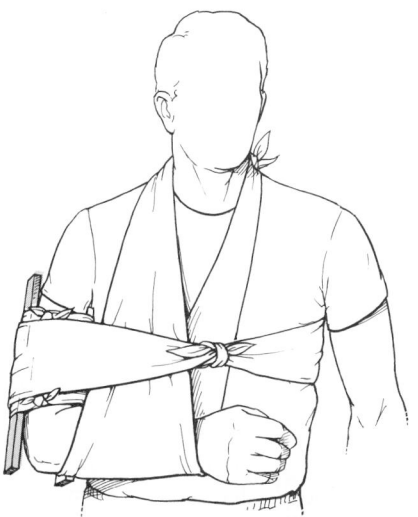

If professional help is unavailable, immobilize an upper arm fracture with splint and sling.

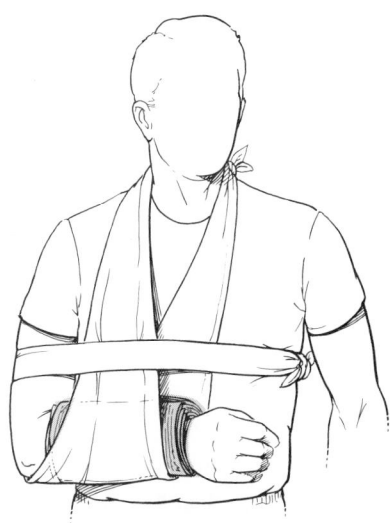

A rolled newspaper or magazine can serve as an effective temporary splint for a fracture of the lower arm.

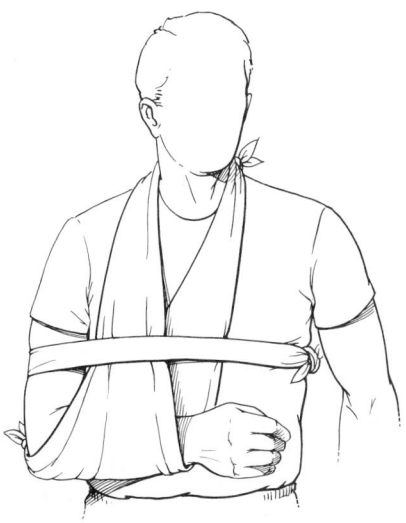

A simple sling can effectively immobilize an injured elbow.

Stop the Bleeding

If the broken bone is an open fracture (that is, the broken bone protrudes through the skin) or there is other bleeding associated with the injury, apply pressure to stop the bleeding.

The site of the fracture should be elevated. (For example, a broken arm can be held up, over the level of the heart, in order to reduce blood flow.)

Put pressure directly on the wound with a sterile bandage, clean cloth, or even a piece of clothing. If nothing else is available, use your hand. Maintain pressure until the bleeding stops (see How to Stop Severe Bleeding, page 400).

Treat for Shock

If the person is faint, pale, or breathing in a notably shallow, hurried fashion, treat the person for shock. Lay the person down, with the head slightly lower than the elevated trunk and legs (see Recognizing and Treating Shock, page 442).

Limb Fractures

If the fracture occurred in the hand, wrist, arm, thigh, or lower leg, a rigid splint should be used. Apply the splint after bleeding (if any) has been stopped, the wound has been bandaged, and the victim has been treated for shock.

Splints can be made of wood, plastic, metal, or other rigid material. Pad the splint with gauze, then apply it to the limb. The splint should be longer than the bone it is

splinting and extend below and above the injury.

Pad the splint wherever possible. Pads make the splint more comfortable and help keep the bones straight.

Fasten the splint to the limb with gauze or strips of cloth, string, or other material. Start wrapping from the extremity and work toward the body. Splint the limb firmly to prevent motions but not so tightly that blood flow is stopped.

Arm Fractures

Rolled magazines or newspapers can be tied around a broken lower arm. A sling over the shoulder and band around the sling can help keep an elbow still.

A leg splint can effectively immobilize a fracture of the lower leg.

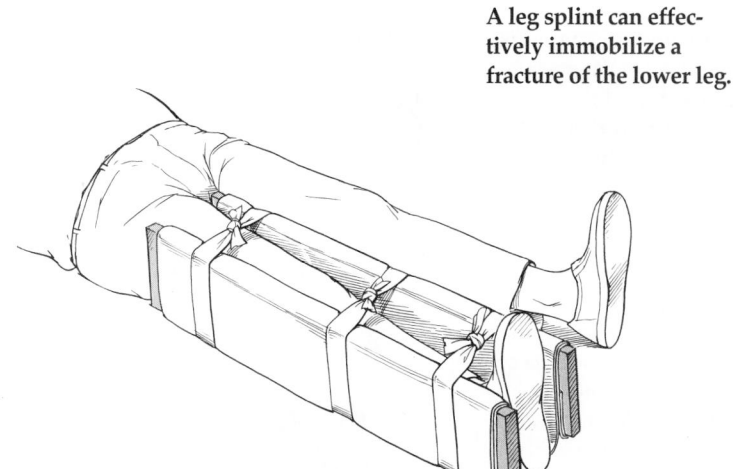

Fracture of a thigh-
bone requires splint-
ing of the trunk and
lower leg.

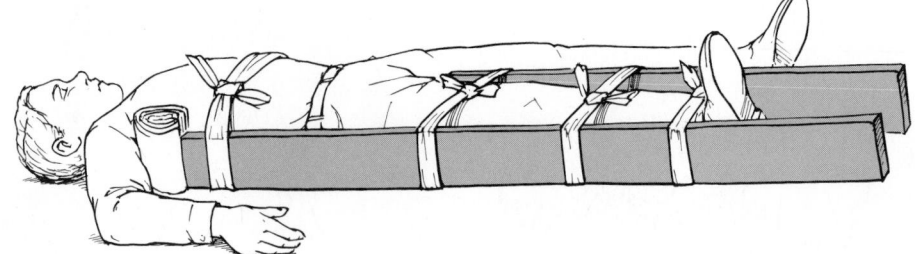

Leg Fractures

If a lower leg is broken, place the entire leg between two splints. If no splints are available, the healthy leg can be used as a splint to limit movement of the broken one.

A broken thighbone requires that the hip joint also be immobilized.

Regardless of type, treat all suspected fractures with proper first aid (see page 446), then consult a physician (see Fractures, page 445), who may obtain an X-ray of the bone to evaluate the extent of the injury.

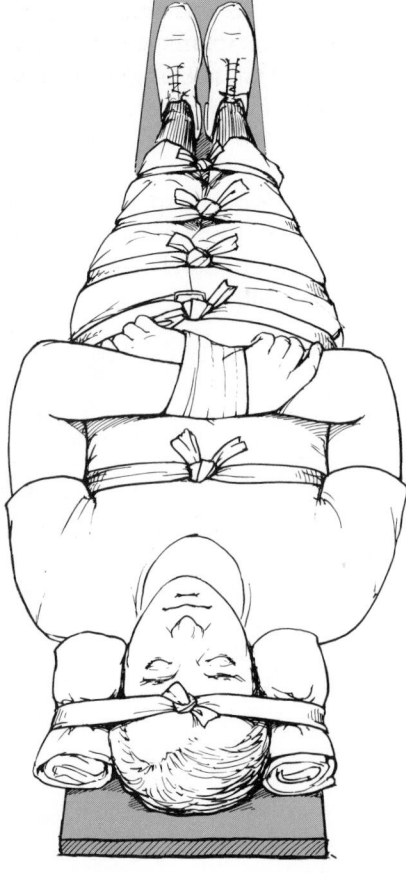

Neck and back injuries
require special precau-
tions. If professional
help is unavailable and
the victim must be
moved, recruit several
people to help. Neck
and back injuries can
lead to permanent
paralysis; therefore,
special precautions are
required. Proper use of
a backboard immobi-
lizes the victim's head,
neck, and spine.

Spinal Injuries

If you suspect a spinal injury (back or neck), do not move the affected person. Permanent paralysis and other serious complications can result from moving a person with a spinal injury.

Assume the person has sustained such an injury if:

- There is evidence of a head injury
- There is severe pain in the neck or back
- An injury exerted substantial force on the back
- The person complains of weakness, numbness, or paralysis or lack of control of the limbs, bladder, or bowel
- The neck or back is twisted or positioned oddly
- The person has been knocked out or is intoxicated and cannot describe his or her pain appropriately

Summon emergency assistance immediately. Keep the victim still. Do not try to move the person unless he or she is choking or in immediate danger.

If the person must be moved, gently reposition him or her on a rigid board (a tabletop or door will do). Get several people to help, and make sure that the person's neck, head, and spine are held firmly in alignment. Make sure the neck is stabilized: use a heavy towel or scarf, pocketbook, or other soft, bulky material to prevent the head from rotating while the person is being moved.

Hip or Pelvic Fractures

Hip or pelvic fractures usually occur as a result of falls or accidents, but in some elderly people whose bones have thinned from osteoporosis (see page 894), such breaks can occur spontaneously.

Suspect a broken pelvis or hip if the person complains of the following:

- Pain in the hip, lower back, or groin area
- Pain in these areas which worsens with movement of the leg

As with a spinal injury, do not try to move the victim. Summon emergency medical assistance immediately.

If the person must be moved, immobilize him or her on a board or tabletop as for a spinal injury (see Spinal Injuries, page 448). Do not attempt to straighten an injured leg or hip that seems oddly positioned.

Other Broken Bones

In the case of broken bones in the fingers, toes, rib cage, or face, splinting is not usually necessary. Stop the bleeding and treat the victim for shock (see Recognizing and Treating Shock, page 442), then seek emergency treatment.

Sprains

A sprain occurs when trauma such as a violent twist or stretch causes the joint to move outside its normal range of movement and ligaments are torn. The usual indications of a sprain are the following:

- Pain and tenderness in the affected area
- Rapid swelling, sometimes accompanied by discoloration of the skin
- Impaired joint function

Emergency Treatment

For most minor sprains, you can probably treat the injury yourself. The combination treatment approach is termed P.R.I.C.E., for protection, rest, ice, compression, and elevation. The steps are described below.

Protection

Immobilize the affected area to encourage healing and to protect it from further injury. Use elastic wraps, slings, splints, crutches, or canes as necessary.

Rest

Avoid activities that cause pain or swelling; rest is essential to promote tissue healing.

Ice

Apply ice immediately to decrease swelling, pain, and muscle spasm. Ice packs, ice massage, or slush baths are all useful applications. Reapply the ice periodically for the first day or two.

Compression

Swelling can result in loss of motion in an injured joint, so compress the injury until the swelling has ceased. Wraps or compressive (Ace) bandages are best.

Elevation

Raise the swollen arm or leg joint above the level of the heart to reduce swelling. This is especially important at night.

Serious Sprains

If an audible popping sound and immediate difficulty in using the joint accompany the injury, seek emergency medical care. If you suspect bone or serious ligament damage in the joint or if the pain and difficulty in moving the joint do not recede within 2 or 3 days, seek professional medical care. Your physician may order an X-ray to look for a fracture (see Sprain, page 869).

Dislocations

A dislocation is an injury in which the ends of bones are forced from their normal positions. In most cases, it is a blow, fall, or other trauma that causes the dislocation, although in some cases an underlying disease such as rheumatoid arthritis, a congenital weakness, or a joint weakened by previous dislocations can be the cause.

The usual signs are as follows:

- An injured joint that is visibly out of position, misshapen, and difficult to move
- Swelling and intense pain

Emergency Treatment

Do not try to return the joint to its proper place unless you have had training in how to do it. Have a physician examine and obtain an X-ray of any suspected dislocation as soon as possible. In the case of a suspected neck or back injury, however, do not move the injured person (see Spinal Injuries, page 448).

The dislocation should be treated as quickly as possible: if it is not treated within half an hour, the swelling and pain are usually such that treatment without an anesthetic is more difficult. Further damage can result from improper attempts at joint manipulation (see page 866).

Splint the affected joint in its fixed position; treat it as you would a fracture (see Limb Fractures, page 447). Seek immediate medical attention.

Traumatic Amputation

An amputation is the removal, usually by operation, of a limb, part of a limb, or even an organ. When an amputation occurs as the result of injury, as when a finger, toe, or larger body part is severed, it is an emergency requiring immediate medical attention. There are various attendant risks, including loss of blood, shock, and the risk of infection.

Seek Emergency Medical Assistance

Have someone call for an ambulance immediately. It is important that the affected person and the severed part reach a hospital, where the finger or limb can potentially be reattached, as soon as possible.

Emergency Treatment

Stop the Bleeding

The first goal of emergency treatment is to stop blood loss. If the amputation involves a small amount of tissue (a fingertip, for example), it may be sufficient to apply pressure on the wound with a sterile bandage, clean cloth, or a piece of clothing. When the bleeding is under control, wrap the wound with additional layers and bandage.

Treat the Victim for Shock

The victim should be lying down, if possible, with his or her head lower than the heart and the area of the severed part elevated slightly (see Recognizing and Treating Shock, page 442).

If the Bleeding Continues

If a hand, foot, leg, or arm has been amputated, the bleeding may be difficult to stop. First, apply pressure to the artery that feeds the area (see How to Stop Severe Bleeding, page 400). If that fails, a tourniquet may be necessary.

Applying a Tourniquet

This is a last resort because tissue damage may result that will make reattaching the amputated part difficult or impossible. Wrap a necktie or other piece of cloth around the tissue immediately above—but not touching—the wound. It must be long enough to wrap around the area twice with enough material left for a knot. Tie a half knot first, then place a screwdriver, stick, dowel, or a similar object on top of the knot and tie the second half. Twist the screwdriver to tighten the tourniquet.

Tighten the cloth only as much as is required to stop the flow of blood. Note the time at which you applied the tourniquet. Tie the tool in place with the cloth once bleeding has stopped.

Treat Other Injuries

Once you have the bleeding at the site of the amputation under control, examine the person for other signs of injury that require emergency treatment. Treat fractures, additional cuts, and other injuries appropriately.

Save the Severed Part

Once the amputation victim is stable and you

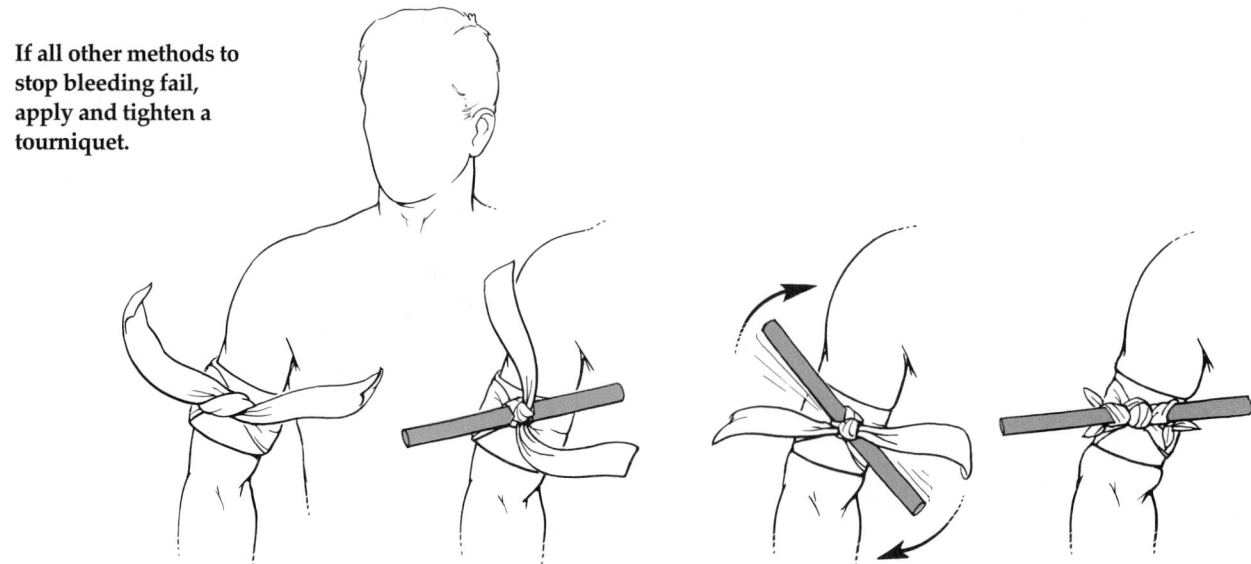

If all other methods to stop bleeding fail, apply and tighten a tourniquet.

have requested emergency assistance, carefully seal the amputated part in a clean plastic bag (if one is not available, wrap it in a clean cloth). If ice is at hand, put the bag with the part in it inside a second bag containing ice. Avoid putting the ice in direct contact with the amputated part. Do not use dry ice. If ice is not available, use very cold water.

Remarkable advances have been made in recent years in reattaching fingers, hands, and even severed limbs. The results depend on many factors, but if you pay proper attention to caring for the severed body part and a qualified surgeon is readily available, the chances are good that a reattachment is possible (see Absence or Loss of a Limb, page 879).

Head Injuries

Most head injuries are minor: the skull provides the brain with considerable protection from injury. Only about 10 percent of all head injuries require hospitalization, and simple cuts and bruises can be treated with basic first aid techniques (see Care of Minor Wounds, page 392). However, seek emergency medical care if any of the following signs or symptoms are apparent:

- Severe head or facial bleeding
- Change in level of consciousness—if the injured person is confused, lethargic, or experiences even temporary loss of consciousness as a result of a head injury. Even if the person regains consciousness quickly, emergency care should be sought
- Cessation of breathing—if the person stops breathing or if no pulse is found, CPR is essential (see Cardiopulmonary Resuscitation, page 408).

In all cases of worrisome head injury, do not move the neck because it may have been injured. Among the potential complications of a head injury are concussion, intracranial hematoma, and a skull fracture.

Concussion
When the head sustains a hard blow as the result of being struck or from a fall or other cause, a concussion may result. The impact creates a sudden movement of the brain within the skull.

Usually a concussion involves a loss of consciousness, either temporary or for a longer time. Amnesia (loss of memory), dizziness, and vomiting also may occur. Partial paralysis and shock are other possible symptoms.

During the 24 hours after the injury, headache, vomiting, increased pulse rate, and anxiety may occur. A concussion requires immediate emergency monitoring and care (see Concussion, page 490).

Intracranial Hematoma
An intracranial hematoma occurs when a blood vessel (either an artery or a vein) ruptures between the skull and the brain. Blood then leaks between the brain and the skull and forms a blood clot (hematoma) that compresses the brain tissue. Symptoms occur from a few hours to several weeks or more after a blow to the head.

Intracranial hemorrhage is caused by injury to the head, often as a result of automobile or motorcycle accidents. There may be no open wound, bruise, or other outward sign.

In intracranial hematoma, pressure on the brain mounts, producing such signs and symptoms as headache, nausea, vomiting, alteration of consciousness, and pupils of unequal size. As more and more blood floods into the narrow space between brain and skull, there is progressive lethargy, unconsciousness, and death if the condition is not treated. Immediate emergency care is required (see Extradural Hemorrhage, page 468, and Subdural Hemorrhage, page 466).

Skull Fracture
When trauma to the head results in skull fracture, the injury may be apparent, as when bleeding or bone fragments are seen. However, if any of the following signs are apparent, there may also be a skull fracture:

- Bruising or discoloration behind the ear or around the eyes
- Blood or clear, watery fluid leaking from the ears or nose
- Unequal size of pupils
- Deformity of the skull, including swelling or depressions

A skull fracture is a medical emergency and must be treated to help avoid potential permanent brain damage and even death.

Emergency Treatment
If a concussion, intracranial hematoma, or

skull fracture is suspected, summon immediate emergency assistance. Keep the person who sustained the injury lying down, with head and shoulders slightly elevated, perhaps on a pillow or blanket.

Observe the person for vital signs. If he or she stops breathing, CPR is essential (see Cardiopulmonary Resuscitation, page 408).

Stop any bleeding with a gauze band or clean cloth (see Bleeding Emergencies, page 399).

Eye Emergencies

There are several common eye injuries and ailments. Described below are those that you are most likely to encounter, and appropriate emergency treatments.

Corneal Abrasions
The cornea is the clear membrane at the center of your eye that functions to refract light from the front of your eye to the retina at the rear of your eye, where visual images are transmitted to your brain. The cornea is easily injured—a speck of sand or even a contact lens worn for too long can scratch (abrade) its fragile tissues. This injury also can result from prolonged exposure to bright light outdoors or in a tanning booth.

Instantaneous pain at the moment of the injury and the persistent pain and redness that follow are the key symptoms of a corneal abrasion (although in occasional cases the pain develops over a period of hours).

If eye pain persists after cleansing the eye to remove any foreign object (see Foreign Bodies in the Eye, page 425), close your eye and cover it with soft gauze or an eye patch. Seek emergency medical care to be sure that the foreign body has been removed and that no serious abrasion requiring surgery or other treatment has occurred.

Blood in the Eye
Blood visible in the front chamber of the eye is a condition called hyphema (see page 533). It can result from a blow to the eye, an injury that perforates the eye, or certain medical conditions.

In most cases, the blood is completely absorbed within a few days. However, a more serious eye injury may be apparent. Seek the care of an ophthalmologist or see your personal physician.

Eyelid Laceration
If the eyelid is cut or damaged, loosely apply clean gauze to the eye. Do not apply pressure. Seek emergency medical care for the person with the injury.

Retinal Detachment
Your retina is a thin, transparent membrane located in the back of your eye. The retina contains cells (rods and cones) that are sensitive to light. It is attached to a layer of tiny blood vessels that provide oxygen and necessary nutrients.

If the retina separates from the layer of blood vessels, the condition is termed "retinal detachment." There is no pain associated with the condition, but symptoms may include sensations of lights flashing and of many tiny floating objects in the eye. Vision may be blurred or double, and there often seems to be a shadow over a portion of your field of vision.

Retinal detachment is a medical emergency requiring immediate treatment in order to avoid permanent vision loss or damage. Seek emergency ophthalmic care. It is unnecessary to cover the affected eye unless the visual disturbance is uncomfortable (see Retinal Detachment, page 557).

Central Retinal Artery Occlusion
When one or more of the blood vessels that serve the retina become blocked, you may experience a sudden blurring or loss of vision in a portion or all of the visual field of one eye only.

If you experience acute blurring of vision or partial blindness, seek emergency medical care. Contact your ophthalmologist or personal physician or go to a local emergency room immediately (see Retinal Vessel Occlusion, page 559).

Acute Glaucoma
The symptoms of acute glaucoma are a red, painful eye, blurred vision, and often the appearance of halos around lights. It occurs when the pressure of the fluids inside the eye becomes too great.

This is a medical emergency requiring immediate medical care. Contact your ophthalmologist immediately (see Glaucoma, page 550).

Orbital Cellulitis
An infection of the eye socket, orbital celluli-

tis may produce pain in the affected eye, decreased vision, fever, swelling of the eyelid, and a general malaise.

If your eye becomes swollen and painful or there is pain with movement of the eye, this is a medical emergency requiring that you seek immediate medical care. Contact your ophthalmologist or personal physician immediately (see Orbital Cellulitis, page 545).

Acute Iritis

An inflammation of the iris, iritis and its associated disorder uveitis can result in redness of the eye, blurred vision, and a sensitivity to light.

Seek emergency medical care (see Uveitis and Iritis, page 544).

Acute Conjunctivitis

Often referred to as pinkeye, conjunctivitis is an inflammation of the transparent membrane (the conjunctiva) that lines the eyelids and the eyeball up to the margin of the cornea. It is usually caused by a virus.

A highly contagious disorder common in children, its symptoms include redness, itching, and a gritty feeling about the eyes. There also may be a discharge in the eye that forms a crust (mattering) during sleep. Blurred vision and sensitivity to light also may result.

In most cases, conjunctivitis is irritating but harmless to your vision. However, because it is extremely infectious, take special steps to prevent conjunctivitis from being spread to others. Avoid sharing eating utensils. Wash your hands thoroughly and often (see Conjunctivitis, page 542).

Emergency Treatment

If you have redness and mattering of your eyes and you suspect pinkeye, irrigate several times daily with artificial tears, which you can purchase without a prescription. This may relieve the symptoms, which generally last less than 5 to 7 days. You can place a cool compress (washcloth) over the closed eyelids to help relieve any itching or swelling.

If your symptoms do not improve or if you have difficulty with vision, seek medical attention. Rarely, conjunctivitis may be due to bacteria, which may respond to specific treatment. If the conjunctivitis occurs in an eye with a contact lens, see an ophthalmologist immediately.

Tooth Loss (Avulsion)

When a tooth is accidentally knocked out (avulsion), it is an event requiring appropriate emergency dental care, whether a child or an adult is involved. Today, permanent teeth that are knocked out sometimes can be reimplanted, but only if you act quickly. A broken tooth, however, cannot be reimplanted.

Emergency Treatment

If a permanent tooth is knocked out, save the tooth and consult your dentist immediately. If it is after office hours, call your dentist at home. If he or she is unavailable, go to the nearest emergency room.

Successful reimplantation depends on several factors: prompt reinsertion (within 30 minutes if possible, no longer than 2 hours after loss), and proper storage and transportation of the tooth. Keeping it moist is essential.

Here is what to do if a tooth is knocked out:

1. Handle the tooth by the crown only.

2. Do not rub it or scrape it to remove dirt.

3. Gently rinse the tooth in tap water, but not under the faucet.

4. Try to replace the tooth in the socket and bite down gently on gauze or a moistened tea bag to help keep it in place.

5. If the tooth cannot be replaced in the socket, immediately place it in milk, your own saliva, or warm, mild, salt water.

Part IV

Human Diseases and Disorders

Most people enjoy reasonably good health most of the time, but all people sooner or later must deal with health problems. Information in the following chapters can help you avoid or manage—sometimes with help from a health care provider—a wide variety of problems. Look for information on prevention and for detailed descriptions of causes, signs and symptoms, diagnosis, severity, and treatments for more than 1,000 common and rare ailments.

Contents

19 **Your Brain and Nervous System** 457
Color Guide to the Diagnosis and Treatment
of Common Disorders. 512
20 **Your Eyes** 519
21 **Your Ears, Nose, and Throat** 567
22 **Dental and Oral Disorders** 601
23 **Your Heart and Blood Vessels** 631
24 **Your Lungs and Respiratory System** 699
25 **Your Digestive System** 737
26 **Your Kidneys and Urinary Tract** 825
27 **Your Bones, Joints, and Muscles** 859
28 **Your Endocrine System** 923
29 **Your Blood** 953
30 **Your Skin** 983
Photographic Guide to Common Skin Disorders. . . 1008
31 **Allergies** 1025
32 **Infectious Diseases** 1055
33 **Mental Health** 1093
34 **Women's Health** 1139
35 **Men's Health** 1195
36 **Health Issues of Partners** 1213

Chapter 19

Your Brain and Nervous System

Contents

How the System Works, 458
The Neurologic Examination, 460

Stroke and Vascular Disorders, 461
Stroke, 461
Transient Ischemic Attack, 463
Cerebral Arteriography, 464
Rehabilitation After a Stroke, 465
Subdural Hemorrhage, 466
Carotid Endartectomy, 467
Extradural Hemorrhage, 468

Chronic Disorders, 469
Alzheimer's Disease, 470
Vascular Dementia, 471
Parkinson's Disease, 472
Tests for Dementia, 473
Tic Disorders, 475
Essential Tremor, 475
Multiple Sclerosis, 475
Amyotrophic Lateral Sclerosis, 477
Huntington's Chorea, 477
Friedreich's Ataxia, 478
Cerebral Palsy, 478
Myasthenia Gravis, 479
Torticollis, 479
Physical Therapy in the Rehabilitation of
Chronic Neurologic Problems, 480

Infections, 481
Meningitis, 481
Encephalitis, 482
Reye's Syndrome, 484
Lumbar Puncture, 485
Poliomyelitis, 485
Epidural Abscess, 486
Post-Polio Syndrome, 487
AIDS and the Nervous System, 488
Botulism, 488

Structural Problems, 489
Hydrocephalus, 489
Concussion, 490
Other Brain Injury, 491
Brain Tumor, 492
Neuroblastoma, 493
Bell's Palsy, 493
CT and MRI Scans, 494

Seizures, 495
Grand Mal Seizure, 496
Petit Mal Seizure, 497
Febrile Seizure, 497
Temporal Lobe Seizure, 498

Headaches, 499
Assessing Your Headaches, 500
Tension-Type Headaches, 501
When Headache Spells Trouble, 502
Migraine Headaches, 502
Muscle Relaxation Techniques, 504
Cluster Headaches, 505

**Problems of the Spine and
Peripheral Nerves, 506**
Spinal Cord Trauma, 506
Spinal Tumor, 508
Rehabilitation in Paraplegia and
Quadriplegia, 508
Cervical Spondylosis, 509
Peripheral Neuropathies, 509
Myelography, 510
Guillain-Barré Syndrome, 513
Charcot-Marie-Tooth Disease, 513
Syringomyelia, 514
Myelomeningocele, 514
Neuralgias, 514
Trigeminal Neuralgia, 515
Spinal Stenosis, 516

How the System Works

The brain and nervous system are your means of receiving input from various body parts and the outside world. The brain works to analyze bits of information before transmitting these messages throughout your body. These messages affect functions such as coordination, learning, memory, emotion, and thought.

The basic unit in the system is the nerve cell (neuron). A neuron consists of a cell body, one major branching fiber (axon), and numerous smaller branching fibers (dendrites). Each neuron is connected to other neurons by contacts (synapses) on the axons and dendrites. A neuron receives chemical signals from other neurons through the synapses. All of these incoming signals are combined as an electrical signal within the neuron, and it may or may not send an outgoing chemical signal down its axon to another set of synapses.

Your brain is composed of approximately 100 billion neurons, their connections, and supporting cells, which add up to roughly 3 pounds of tissue. This dense network of interconnected neurons is organized to convey all the control signals necessary for your activities. The components of this system are the cerebrum, the brain stem, the cerebellum, and the spinal cord.

Your spinal cord is connected to your brain by the brain stem, which is composed of the medulla, the pons, and the midbrain. Your brain stem controls many of your vital functions, such as breathing and circulation of blood. Cranial nerves (nerves connected to your brain) exit from the brain stem to control muscles in your face, eyes, tongue, ears, and throat. They also convey sensations from these parts back to the brain.

In addition to the brain stem, the two other major areas of your brain are the cerebrum and the cerebellum. The cerebrum consists of thick, convoluted masses of nerve tissue. It is divided into two sides (cerebral hemispheres), which are connected in the middle by the corpus callosum.

Conscious functions such as speech, memory, and vision are controlled in the cerebral hemispheres. Specific areas within these hemispheres are known to be responsible for certain functions, such as speech and the control of muscles in particular parts of the body. In general, control of the muscles of the right side of the body resides in the left hemisphere of the brain, and muscles of the left side of the body are controlled by the right hemisphere of the brain. The linking of higher brain functions with cerebral areas is a very active field of research.

The other major portion of the brain, the cerebellum, is tucked beneath the cerebral hemispheres. It helps control your coordination and balance.

At the core of your brain, atop the brain stem, are other key areas, including the hypothalamus and thalamus. The hypothalamus is an endocrine regulatory center that affects sleep, appetite, and sexual desire (see Your Endocrine System, page 923). The thalamus is a collection of nerve cells whose function is the integration and transmission

The nerve cell (neuron) is the basic unit of the brain and nervous system. It consists of the cell body, a major branching fiber (the axon), and numerous smaller branching fibers (dendrites). Each nerve cell is linked to adjacent nerve cells at contact points called synapses.

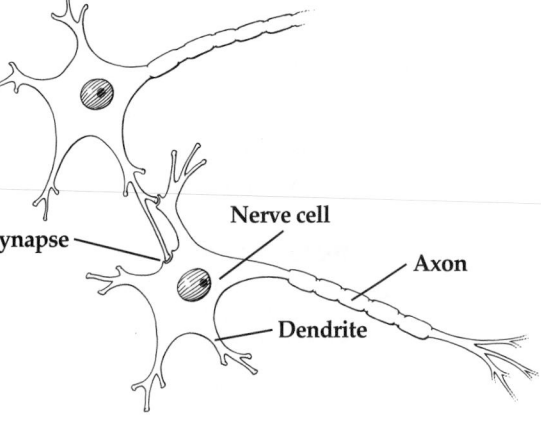

Synapse

Nerve cell

Axon

Dendrite

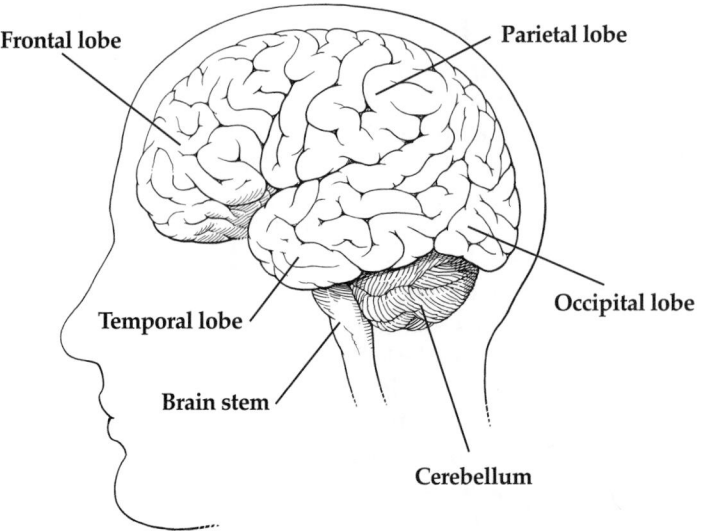

Frontal lobe

Parietal lobe

Temporal lobe

Occipital lobe

Brain stem

Cerebellum

The outer cerebrum is composed of the frontal, parietal, occipital, and temporal lobes. Other major areas of your brain include the brain stem and the cerebellum.

of many of your sensations. In addition, centers under the cortex, such as the basal ganglia, limbic nuclei, and other areas, play critical roles in relaying messages between different areas of the brain. Some disorders, such as Parkinson's disease, involve defects in these areas.

Your brain and spinal cord, collectively called the central nervous system, are encased in bone. The brain is protected by the skull, and the spinal cord is protected by the vertebrae. The brain and spinal cord are sheathed in three layers of membranes (meninges): dura mater (outermost), arachnoid (middle), and pia mater (innermost). These layers provide cushioning for the brain and spinal cord. In addition, a liquid called cerebrospinal fluid, between the arachnoid and pia mater, further protects your brain and spinal cord from injury.

Peripheral nerves run from the spinal cord to all other parts of your body. The parts of this system are named for the four spinal regions from which they branch: neck (cervical), chest (thoracic), lower back (lumbar), and pelvis (sacral). The spinal cord acts as a central communication network to transmit signals back and forth between your brain and the farthest reaches of your peripheral nervous system.

Your autonomic nervous system distributes nerves to smooth muscles in blood vessels (vascular) and internal organs (visceral), to exocrine and endocrine glands, and to function-controlling cells of internal organs. This intricate system controls unconscious but vital activities such as distribution of blood flow, regulation of blood pressure, heartbeat, sweating, and body temperature. Connections between autonomic and other

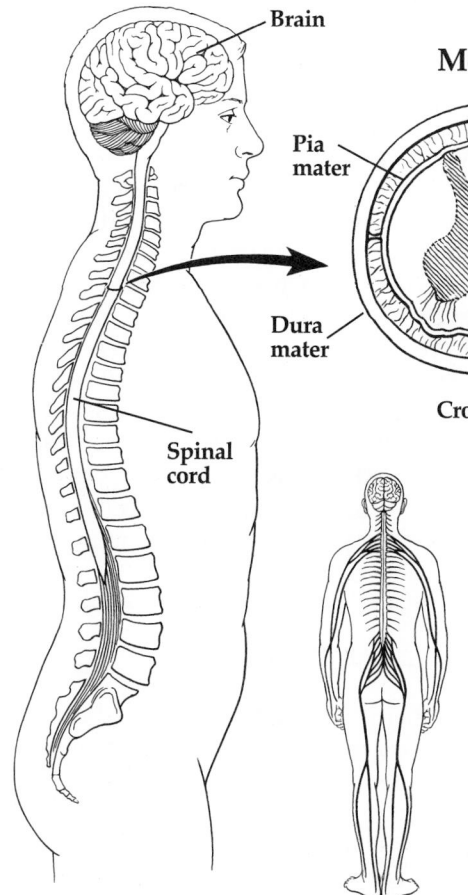

Peripheral Nervous System

Your central nervous system (brain and spinal cord) is protected by your skull and vertebrae and by three layers of membranes: dura mater, arachnoid, and pia mater (collectively known as meninges). Your peripheral nervous system (lower right) extends from your brain and spinal cord to all other parts of your body.

brain functions occur at the brain stem and hypothalamus.

The arterial blood supply, carrying oxygen and nutrients, is critical to the functioning of your brain. Despite its small size and weight, your brain uses 20 percent of the heart's output of blood and 20 percent of the oxygen consumed by your body at rest.

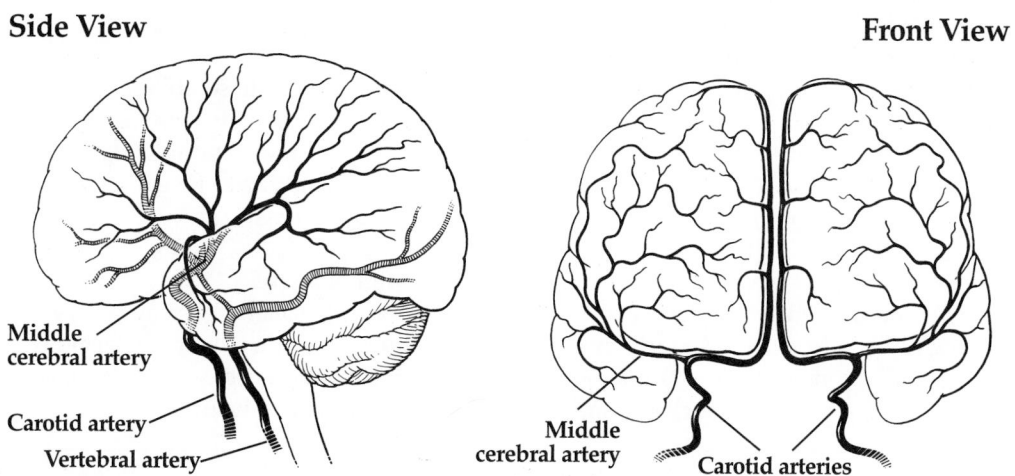

Side View

Middle cerebral artery

Carotid artery

Vertebral artery

Front View

Middle cerebral artery

Carotid arteries

Your brain needs a constant supply of oxygen and nutrients from blood delivered through several key arteries.

Blood is brought to the brain by the vertebral and carotid arteries, which extend up through your neck from your aorta. These large arteries then divide into smaller ones to distribute blood to various regions of your brain.

The central nervous system is vulnerable to a wide variety of insults. Interruption of the blood supply to the brain causes strokes. Degeneration of nerve cells causes illnesses such as Alzheimer's disease, amyotrophic lateral sclerosis, and Parkinson's disease. Inflammatory reaction of the brain to infection causes meningitis and encephalitis. Polio is a viral infection that involves parts of the spinal cord and brain. Head injury or a tumor of the brain may cause structural damage. Problems in mental processing and learning are called cognitive disorders and can result from a variety of conditions affecting certain brain functions. Seizures are caused by abnormal firing of nerve cells. Neuralgias are problems that affect nerves. The following sections describe these and other common nervous system disorders in detail.

Neurologists and neurosurgeons are the medical specialists who treat nervous system disorders. Diagnosis can be difficult because the symptoms and signs are numerous and diverse. Difficulties also may be encountered in distinguishing between neurologic and psychiatric disease. A careful assessment of the character and pattern of symptoms over time, in addition to laboratory tests, may be required to decide among several possible diagnoses.

The Neurologic Examination

The most important element in the diagnosis of a nervous system disorder is a description of your symptoms and how they developed. Headaches, blurred vision, or tingling sensations, for example, can be caused by many disorders. To determine what disorder you might have, your physician may need to ask questions about your symptoms and then conduct a neurologic examination.

The examination systematically tests how well the various parts of your nervous system are functioning. Abnormalities that you may not notice can be detected with simple tests done in your physician's office. The tests are not painful, and no surgical procedure or injections are required. Some of the routine tests for nervous system functions are described here.

Tendon Reflexes

Your tendon reflexes are tested to evaluate motor nerve functions, spinal cord connections, and peripheral nerve conditions. For example, your physician will stimulate your reflexes by tapping your knee or ankle lightly with a special rubber-tipped hammer.

Babinski Reflex

Light stroking of the underside of your foot may produce a certain type of involuntary movement of your big toe, which can suggest an abnormality in the nerve tracts that originate in the brain.

Muscle Strength

Weakness of a muscle or group of muscles can be a manifestation of a neurologic disorder. Therefore, your physician will test your muscle strength as part of your examination.

Muscle Tone

To test your muscle tone, your physician moves your arm or leg to assess the ease and range of movement. For example, both legs may be tested to check for differences between the two sides of your body. Increased tone (spasticity or rigidity) or decreased tone (flaccidity) can indicate particular problems in the nerves that stimulate different muscle groups.

Sensory Function

Sensory tests are important in a neurologic examination because sensations such as pain, heat, touch, and vibration travel through your peripheral nerves to your central nervous system. Your physician evaluates these functions by asking what you feel when your skin is touched lightly by a pinprick, a hot or cold object, a cotton ball, or a tuning fork.

Nervous system disorders also can affect your eyes and senses of taste, smell, and hearing. Eye testing is particularly useful. The size of your pupils, a difference between the sizes of the pupils, range of eye movement, gaze, and field of vision are often useful for diagnosing disturbances that may include the nerves that control your vision.

Gait, Posture, Coordination, and Balance

To evaluate these abilities, your physician may ask you to stand, walk, or move your body in a particular way to reveal possible abnormalities.

Mental Status

Your physician also may ask you questions that help determine whether your thinking, judgment, or memory is disturbed.

Stroke and Vascular Disorders

Your brain requires 20 percent of your heart's output of fresh blood and 20 percent of the blood's oxygen and glucose contents. Two major artery systems extend through your neck to distribute this blood supply throughout your brain.

Any disturbance in blood flow—even for a few seconds—usually produces a dramatic effect on your brain's functions. Depending on what areas of your brain are affected, you can have vision or speech difficulties, paralysis in part of your body, or loss of consciousness.

If this disturbance continues for more than a few minutes, brain cells in the affected area may be destroyed, causing permanent impairment or death. Two important types of blood supply disturbance are described in this section: reduced blood flow (ischemia) and bleeding (hemorrhage).

Stroke

Signs and Symptoms

- Sudden numbness, weakness, or paralysis of the face, arm, or leg, usually on one side of your body
- Loss of speech, or trouble talking or understanding speech
- Sudden blurred or decreased vision, usually in one eye
- Dizziness, loss of balance, or loss of coordination
- Sudden, severe headache, with no apparent cause
- Difficulty swallowing

Stroke is the common name for several disorders that occur within seconds or minutes after the blood supply to the brain is disturbed.

A stroke is a brain attack. Seek immediate medical assistance, just as you would for a heart attack. Every minute counts. The longer a stroke goes untreated, the greater the damage. Success of treatment may depend on how soon care is given.

The warning signs may be temporary, lasting from a few minutes to 24 hours, but even symptoms lasting only a short time may indicate a stroke. Treat them seriously.

Symptoms may progress or fluctuate during the first day or two after onset. This is called stroke in evolution. When no further deterioration occurs, the condition is considered to be a completed stroke. The only warning signal that suggests you may be prone to a stroke is a transient ischemic attack (TIA, see page 463).

The medical term for the cause of stroke is "cerebrovascular disease," which indicates that it originates in the blood vessels (from the Latin *vasa* for "vessels") of your brain (*cerebrum* is Latin for "brain"). Strokes are characterized by the location and type of disturbance. The most common disturbance is a deficient supply of blood through an artery (ischemia). When this happens, the nerve tissue served by that artery rapidly loses its ability to function and may die. The dead tissue is called an infarct.

The most common arterial disease leading to ischemia is atherosclerosis, a condition in which a fatty deposit forms in the inner layer of an artery and results in the formation of plaque (see page 636). A blood clot (thrombus) may then develop at the site in the artery narrowed by the plaque and block the flow. This type of ischemic stroke is a cerebral thrombosis.

Another type of ischemic stroke, cerebral embolism, may occur when either a plaque fragment or a blood clot (the embolus) that is formed elsewhere is carried by the blood until it lodges in one location and blocks the flow. Emboli may arise from another vessel or from the heart.

A less common type of stroke (cerebral hemorrhage) occurs when an artery leaks

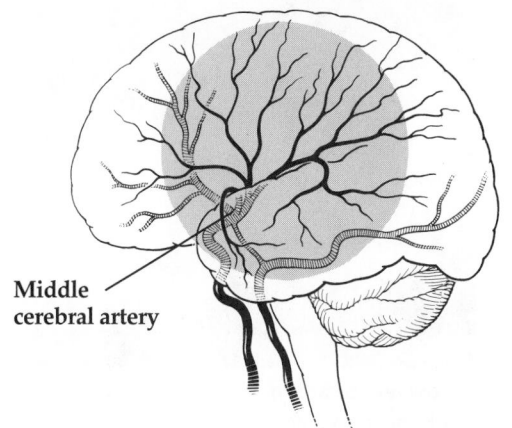

Middle cerebral artery

If blood flow is blocked, brain tissue may die. An obstructed middle cerebral artery will affect the shaded area, producing an ischemic attack or stroke.

blood into the brain, causing compression, displacement, and death of nerve tissue. The initial effect of a hemorrhagic stroke is often more severe than that of an ischemic stroke; the long-term effects, however, are similar in both cases. A severe headache followed by the other signs and symptoms described above is more typical of hemorrhagic than ischemic stroke.

A subarachnoid hemorrhage occurs when there is bleeding between the arachnoid membrane and the surface of the brain. Spontaneous subarachnoid hemorrhage most commonly occurs after the rupture of a saccular aneurysm. A saccular aneurysm is a balloon-like bulge with a narrowed neck that develops in the artery wall. Aneurysmal bleeding sometimes produces bleeding into the substance of the brain (intracerebral hemorrhage).

An arteriovenous malformation is a tangle of abnormal blood vessels. These large, thin-walled vessels usually lead to bleeding into the brain and may cause seizures. Occasionally, arteriovenous malformations run in families.

Stroke is the third leading cause of death in developed countries. Approximately 300,000 Americans suffer a stroke each year. One-fourth of them die, and half the survivors have long-term disabilities. Stroke is more likely to occur as you get older, and the risk doubles each decade after age 35 years. Five percent of the population older than 65

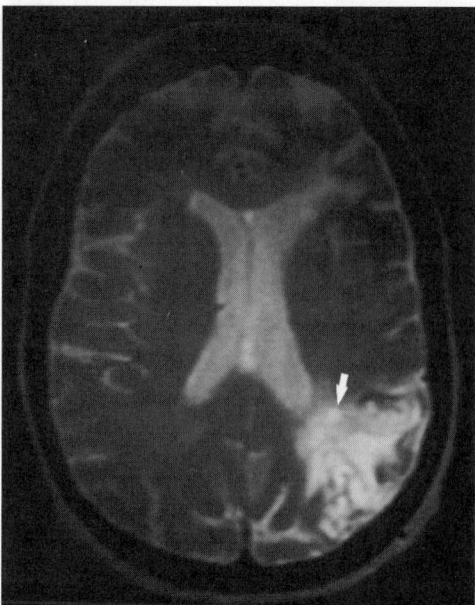

Arrow reveals area of brain tissue affected by stroke as shown on magnetic resonance imaging (MRI) scan.

years has had a stroke.

Several risk factors are associated with stroke. It is estimated that 70 percent of all strokes occur in persons with high blood pressure (see page 647). Some forms of heart disease, such as atrial fibrillation, valvular heart disease, or recent heart attack (see pages 670, 677, and 661), increase the chance of stroke because blood clots from the heart may travel up the major arteries to the brain. Smoking, diabetes, and high blood cholesterol concentration also are thought to be liabilities (see pages 318, 643, and 650). Although young women have a very low risk, their chances may be slightly increased by the use of birth control pills. For women who smoke, chances are greatly increased. Men have a higher risk than women.

Diagnosis

The diagnosis of stroke does not depend on any single symptom, but a rapid development of symptoms is significant. A large blockage such as a clot or a fragment from a cholesterol plaque deposit that is carried in the blood until it blocks flow (embolism) tends to cause a completed stroke within a few minutes. However, even in a completed stroke, early care may decrease the amount of damage.

A blockage that develops in place (thrombus) often occurs more slowly. The presence of symptoms that correspond to specific arterial areas within the brain is further evidence of stroke.

To select a treatment, your physician must decide what type of stroke occurred and its location. In addition, other possible causes of your symptoms, such as tumor, need to be excluded.

One or more of the following diagnostic tests may be used to study your blood vessels: carotid ultrasonography (see page 1335), arteriography (see page 464), computed tomography (CT, see page 494), and magnetic resonance imaging (MRI, see page 494).

How Serious Is Stroke?

Stroke is a very serious illness. A physician's attention is required immediately.

After any kind of stroke, an area of dead nerve tissue (infarct) may remain after the stroke is complete. Recovery depends on whether other nerve tissue can assume the function of that area. A series of strokes can lead to vascular dementia (see page 471).

Stroke is an acute (immediate) event that

most frequently stems from chronic conditions such as high blood pressure, atherosclerosis, or heart disease. If you have one or more of these chronic disorders, you need close medical supervision.

Emergency Treatment

While waiting for an emergency vehicle to arrive, watch the person suspected of having a stroke. If breathing ceases, CPR is necessary (see Cardiopulmonary Resuscitation, page 408). Minor breathing difficulty may be alleviated by positioning the head and shoulders on a pillow. Watch for vomiting and potential aspiration of vomitus into the lungs. If vomiting occurs, turn the head to the side.

Do not allow the person to eat or drink anything. If paralysis is present, secure and protect the paralyzed parts.

Treatment

Intensive care for a comatose stroke victim includes life-support equipment to supply oxygen, nutrients, and medications and catheterization for bladder function. If the ability to swallow is lost, it may return within 1 to 2 weeks or may never return. In the interim, food and water can be supplied intravenously or directly to the stomach after a procedure called a gastrostomy (see page 747). Sometimes a stroke results in much less neurologic damage and requires less care.

Medication
The most important consideration following a stroke is to prevent another, possibly more severe, event. Medications that decrease the blood's tendency to clot may be used. These drugs may include aspirin, ticlopidine, and anticoagulants such as heparin or sodium warfarin.

Anticoagulants are potentially dangerous in persons with high blood pressure and extensive damage to brain tissue because they increase the possibility of hemorrhage. (The term blood thinners is used commonly to describe these medications, which decrease the tendency of the blood to clot but do not actually thin the blood.) New drugs that actually open the passageway or "lyse" the clot, called thrombolytic agents, are currently being evaluated.

For hemorrhagic stroke, pain relievers may be needed to relieve headache. If nausea and vomiting are present, intravenous administration of nutrients and fluid may be required for a few days.

Surgery
Surgical procedures sometimes are used to remove blood that has leaked into the tissues from a cerebral hemorrhage. The decision depends on where the hemorrhage occurred and how far it has progressed. If a subarachnoid hemorrhage has occurred, surgical treatment of the underlying aneurysm or arteriovenous malformation is often needed.

Although surgery is used rarely during ischemic stroke, an operation called carotid endarterectomy (see page 467), which removes arterial plaque deposits, may be used as a preventive measure in some cases. Carotid endarterectomy sometimes is used soon after a minor stroke to prevent a recurrence.

Transient Ischemic Attack

Signs and Symptoms
- Sudden onset of weakness, tingling, or numbness typically involving one limb, or an arm and leg (usually on the same side), with or without involvement of the face
- Incoordination of the limbs
- Vision loss, double vision
- Speech difficulty
- Vertigo and imbalance

A transient ischemic attack (TIA) is caused by a temporary deficiency in the blood supply to the brain. Most episodes last only a few minutes. It has the same origins as ischemic stroke (see page 461).

A TIA most frequently is due to a disease called atherosclerosis, which develops when plaque deposits form inside arteries (see page 636). Plaque forms after the inner lining of an artery is injured. This, then, allows platelets to clump at the area of injury. This, along with the formation of cholesterol at the same site, forms a mass that protrudes into the artery. With further injury, other changes such as ulceration of the plaque and the local formation of a clot (thrombosis) can occur. A plaque fragment can break off and be carried by the blood and lodge at a distant site in the brain. This may cause a TIA.

The major risk factors contributing to TIAs are high blood pressure, some types of heart disease, smoking, diabetes, and advanced age.

Cerebral Arteriography

Cerebral arteriography, also called angiography, is a form of X-ray imaging that permits a physician to see the blood circulating through the brain. This diagnostic procedure is used to locate the specific source of a blood vessel abnormality in the brain or neck so treatment can be prescribed. Cerebral arteriography also is useful to evaluate mass abnormalities such as tumors, especially if surgery is contemplated.

In preparation for the procedure, you will be hospitalized and not given food for several hours before the test. You will receive a mild sedative, but you will remain awake during the procedure because your cooperation is necessary for monitoring your neurologic status.

The test may last 1 to 3 hours. As a precaution, a device will be inserted in a vein in case some form of medication is needed during testing. A long, thin, flexible tube (a catheter) is then inserted through a small incision, usually in your groin. A local anesthetic generally is applied at the point of insertion. The catheter is manipulated up through the major arteries of the trunk and into the carotid or vertebral artery. Once the catheter is in place, dye (contrast medium) is injected through it. The dye outlines arteries not normally seen in X-ray imaging and helps to reveal abnormalities or obstructions.

Cerebral arteriography is a tiring procedure. You may have to lie in awkward positions for short periods. The dye sometimes causes a brief burning sensation in the head. You will probably be discharged from the hospital the same day.

Although arteriography is a wonderful diagnostic tool, it has its drawbacks. The procedure may cause a stroke if the catheter dislodges a blood clot or plaque deposit in an artery. Other risks involve possible allergic reaction to the dye. If you previously have shown a sensitivity to dye, special preparations are required, or this test may be avoided. Much of the risk depends on the training and experience of the team that performs the test. Statistics show that when the procedure is performed in a hospital that does fewer than 100 of these tests a year, the risks are 8 times greater than in a hospital that does at least 400 procedures a year.

As with many medical decisions, you must weigh the risks against the benefits. The risk of a complication with this test is about 0.5 percent.

With the advent of effective CT, MRI, and carotid ultrasound (see pages 494 and 1335), cerebral arteriography increasingly has become a supplementary technique in brain imaging. Cerebral arteriography nevertheless continues to be useful, especially for identifying the site and nature of problems in the brain's blood vessels. These problems include plaque deposits in the arteries, the source of hemorrhages, aneurysms, and blood vessel malformations.

This test may precede the decision for or against a surgical procedure to be done on a blood vessel, such as carotid endarterectomy (see page 467). Arteriography also may be used to establish the location of brain tumors and abscesses.

In cerebral arteriography, a catheter is threaded through the major arteries of the trunk and into the carotid or vertebral artery. Dye (contrast medium) is injected to outline arteries not normally seen on X-ray imaging. This helps reveal abnormalities or obstructions.

Rehabilitation After a Stroke

Some 500,000 Americans survive strokes each year. Half of them live 5 years, and 10 to 15 percent live for 10 years.

An estimated 2.5 million disabled stroke survivors are alive in the United States. Some persons live with only minor disabilities despite having had additional strokes. Four out of 5 long-term survivors will walk again without help, and 2 out of 3 will be able to care for themselves. One-third can return to work. But 2 out of 10 stroke survivors require extended care, some because of the mental or physical disabilities that result, and others because they lack a family member or helper at home.

After a stroke, rehabilitation is crucial for morale and a return to maximal function. Those who return to work are usually white-collar workers younger than 65 who were not totally disabled when they started rehabilitation.

A healthy home environment has a beneficial effect on rehabilitation. Regardless of age, stroke survivors who can go home to a healthy spouse or other companion are more likely to become independent and productive. Encouragement and early treatment are important.

Various adaptive devices and architectural modifications such as ramps, hand bars on the tub and toilet, and walking frames facilitate independence and safety. Contact your physician, local rehabilitation professionals, or independent living center for information and assistance.

Recovery and rehabilitation depend on the area of the brain involved and the amount of tissue damaged. Harm to the right side of the brain may impair sensation and movement on the left side of the body. Damage to brain tissue on the left side may affect movement on the right side and, in right-handed people, may also cause speech and language disorders. Speech disorders may include difficulty in understanding or in expressing words and can be very frustrating for the stroke survivor. Some loss of vision may occur regardless of the area of the brain that is affected. A stroke that occurs in the brain stem can cause disturbances in breathing, swallowing, balance, hearing, and eye and tongue movements. There may be a loss of sensation also. Bladder and bowel function are disturbed in many people.

In addition to the various physical side effects, depression is a common response to stroke. Affected individuals may feel helpless, frustrated, and uninterested in activities they once enjoyed. Diminished sex drive, mood changes, and thoughts of suicide are not unusual.

The way in which a person thinks, interacts with others, or interprets everyday events may be affected. These side effects may be due in part to changes in the production of chemical transmitters within the synapses, and antidepressant drugs may be prescribed.

The professional rehabilitation team normally includes a rehabilitation physician, a nurse, a dietitian, a physical therapist, an occupational therapist, a recreational therapist, a speech therapist, a social worker, a psychologist, and a chaplain. The makeup of the team varies with the needs of the individual. Therapy is focused on maximizing the individual's capabilities. Early and repeated appraisals of status are needed to design the remedial program. This program will emphasize the use of the remaining function for self-care, mobility in the home and community, and reestablishing recreational and vocational pursuits tailored for the individual. Many survivors regain partial use of affected limbs, especially with the help of rehabilitation professionals. Rehabilitation returns $10 for every $1 invested by reducing costs of long-term care, and it improves quality of life.

Some persons recover satisfactorily without specific rehabilitation therapy. In others, damage is so severe that intensive rehabilitation is impractical. Prevention of complicating muscle contractures, skin ulcers, pneumonia, malnutrition, bowel and bladder dysfunction, social isolation, and depression is a minimal objective and should be provided in any living setting. The most important and effective help over the long term may come from family and friends, and it must be given with patience and persistence.

Diagnosis

The most significant symptom of TIA is the speed at which it comes and goes. Rapid onset, brief duration, and then a return to normal is the usual sequence. Recurrence of the same or similar symptoms is also significant. You may be aware of the physical symptoms as a mild loss of function or sensation.

A complete description of your symptoms is helpful for diagnosing TIA. Weakness in only one arm or leg, for example, may point to a disturbance in a branch of the internal carotid artery, whereas weakness in both arms or legs suggests disturbances in the vertebral-basilar artery. Other information that assists in diagnosis includes your eye and arm blood pressure and the noise (bruit) heard with a stethoscope when there is impairment of blood flow in various arteries. Tests might be required to gather complete information. These could include CT or MRI (see page 494) or arteriography (see page 464) to provide images of the arteries for evaluation.

How Serious Is Transient Ischemic Attack?
The signs and symptoms of TIA are similar to those of ischemic stroke, with an important difference—the symptoms disappear completely within 24 hours. A TIA may be repeated in the same day or some time later, and each episode typically lasts only a few minutes. You should regard it as a warning that a stroke may follow. Approximately a third of persons with TIAs will later have a stroke, a third will have more TIAs, and a third will have no further cerebrovascular symptoms.

Arterial plaque deposits are very common, but they do not necessarily cause a TIA. The separate arterial networks in the brain have a built-in safety factor through extensive, small interconnections between them. When blood flow is gradually impeded in one network, these interconnections tend to enlarge so another arterial network can take over the blood supply to that region, a phenomenon called collateral circulation. As a result, a completely blocked artery may be harmless if collateral circulation is sufficient.

An additional safety factor is that the arteries to the brain are large enough to provide an adequate blood supply even when they are narrowed up to 75 percent by a plaque deposit. A TIA, therefore, is a warning that your safety factors are being overwhelmed.

Treatment
The purpose of treatment of TIA is prevention: to improve the arterial blood supply to the brain and avoid stroke.

Medication
If you have high blood pressure and TIAs, your high blood pressure generally is treated first (see page 651). In the absence of high blood pressure, medication may be prescribed to reduce the tendency of the blood to clot. The most common medication used for this purpose is aspirin. (In addition to its pain-relieving ability, aspirin also inhibits the way platelets clump together. The presence of too many platelets at a narrowed site may further compromise the flow of blood to the brain.) Another drug that acts in the same way is ticlopidine. Your physician may prescribe it first as trial therapy. Anticoagulants (such as heparin or sodium warfarin) may be recommended in some situations. Anticoagulants reduce the tendency of the blood to clot. They are sometimes referred to as "blood thinners," although they do not actually thin the blood. Pharmaceutical firms are testing drugs that reduce or eliminate plaque deposits.

Surgery
In carefully selected cases, carotid endarterectomy, a surgical procedure to remove arterial plaque (see page 467) may prevent further TIAs. The ideal candidate for this operation has had a TIA caused by plaque deposits in the neck arteries to the brain, has no further symptoms of stroke, and is thought to be a good surgical candidate.

Subdural Hemorrhage

Signs and Symptoms
- Steady or fluctuating headache, drowsiness, seizures, or confusion after a head injury
- Partial paralysis on one side of the body
- Slowed thinking; changes in personality

Emergency Symptoms
- Convulsions, stupor, or loss of consciousness after a head injury
- Enlarged pupil(s)

Subdural hemorrhage is caused by an injury to the head. It may be the result of a car accident or a seemingly trivial event such as bumping your head. The hemorrhage occurs when blood vessels (usually veins) rupture between the brain and the dura mater, the outermost of three membrane layers that cover the brain. The leaking blood forms a mass (hematoma) that compresses the brain tissue. If the hematoma keeps growing, there is a progressive decline in consciousness that can culminate in death.

The interval between injury and the onset of significant symptoms, such as headache, confusion, paralysis, and loss of consciousness, can vary. The hematoma is considered acute if the interval is less than 48 hours, subacute if it is between 48 hours and 2

Carotid Endarterectomy

Endarterectomy is a surgical procedure that removes the plaque from inside a blood vessel. This plaque can reduce the flow of blood or be the source of particles that break off and flow to the brain. Plaque formation is a common disease. It is also called atherosclerosis (see page 636). It frequently occurs in the neck arteries to the brain, particularly in the carotid artery, where it divides into its internal (to the eye and brain) and external branches.

Plaque at this junction is a common cause for transient ischemic attack (see page 463) or ischemic stroke (see page 461). Carotid endarterectomy usually is done after one or more transient ischemic attacks to prevent their recurrence and subsequent stroke. Occasionally, carotid endarterectomy will be done during the first few hours of an evolving ischemic stroke.

In addition, carotid endarterectomy is effective in reducing the risk of stroke in people who have advanced narrowing of the carotid artery but have not yet experienced any symptoms.

Although it has a high success rate, the procedure has its risks, and your physician will have to weigh several factors when deciding its benefits in your case. If you have symptoms, such as transient ischemic attack, that may be due to plaque in the carotid artery, your physician will check several indicators, including the sound (bruit) made by your blood flowing through a narrowed segment of the carotid artery and the blood pressure in your arms and eyes. If these indications are positive, you may need carotid ultrasonography (see page 1335), MRI scan (see page 494), or arteriography (see page 464) to locate and evaluate the blockage.

Your physician also will assess other factors before recommending this operation, including the possibility of high blood pressure and other cardiovascular disease. Active coronary artery disease may make the risk of this operation too great. Chronic high blood pressure generally must be corrected preoperatively. If there is complete blockage of the artery, endarterectomy is rarely indicated.

In some persons, the combined risk of diagnostic arteriography and this surgical procedure may be greater than nonsurgical therapy, such as medication to control clotting of the blood. The risk is highest for persons with acute stroke or stroke in evolution (see Stroke, page 461) and lowest for those with no stroke symptoms at the time of surgery. For those without stroke symptoms, the rate of mortality and major neurologic complications ranges from 1 to 4 percent at medical centers that have special expertise in the treatment of this condition.

The procedure begins with an incision in the neck to expose the carotid junction. Clamps are inserted to stop blood flow. The artery is opened to remove the plaque. Closure of the artery may require a patch of synthetic material. Restoring the blood flow must be done carefully to prevent clots from entering the flow.

Complications, including stroke, can arise during this operation. To minimize the risk of intraoperative stroke, monitoring of the brain activity by electroencephalography (see page 1344) is helpful. It allows the surgeon to determine if circulation to the brain is adequate while the carotid artery is clamped for repair. If not, steps can be taken to assure adequate blood flow.

As with any surgical procedure, the success rate of carotid endarterectomy depends on the expertise of your physician and surgical team. Blockage may recur after surgery, but this is uncommon. In properly selected persons, the operation is usually successful because it eliminates some risk of further transient ischemic attacks and reduces the chance of a stroke.

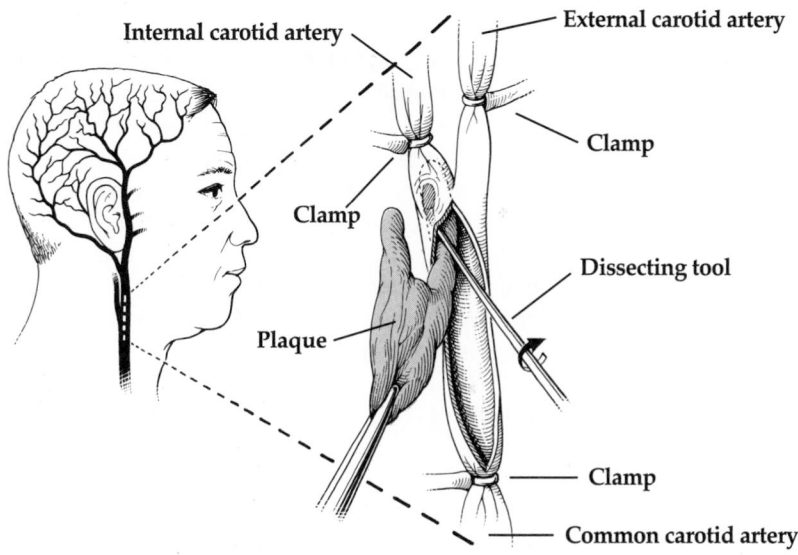

If blood flow to the brain is blocked by an obstruction in the carotid artery, a surgical procedure called an endarterectomy may be done. Clamps are placed on the artery to stop blood flow while the plaque is removed with a dissecting tool.

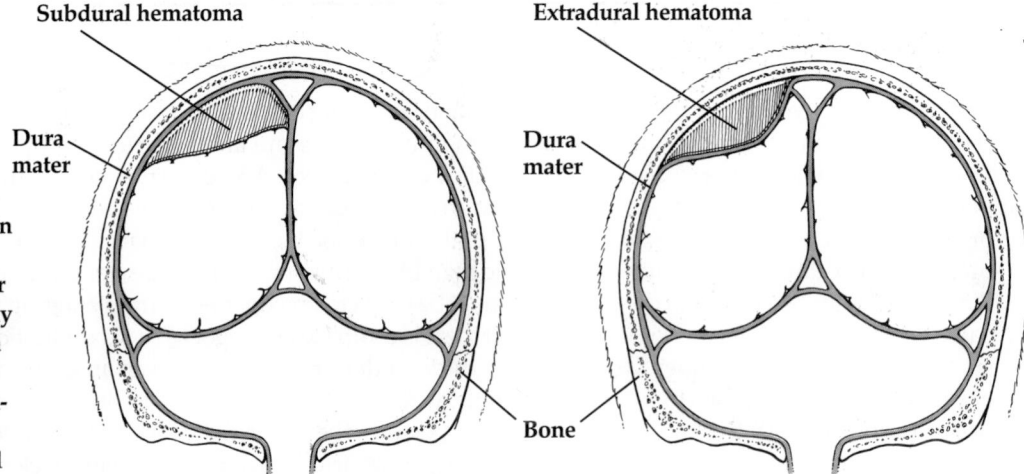

When an injury results in bleeding between the brain and the dura mater (left drawing), blood may accumulate, producing a mass called a subdural hematoma. When bleeding occurs between the dura mater and the skull (right drawing), the accumulation is termed an extradural hematoma. Both of these conditions can put pressure on the brain, potentially causing unconsciousness and requiring immediate treatment.

weeks, and chronic if it is more than 2 weeks. Infants and elderly people are most likely to suffer chronic subdural hematoma, and the injury that caused it may not be remembered.

Diagnosis

Chronic subdural hematoma is hard to diagnose. The progressive loss of consciousness after a head injury, however, generally is presumed to be caused by a hemorrhage inside the head (intracranial) until proved otherwise. The best method to define the position and size of the hematoma is CT (see page 494), if there is time to perform it. In some cases, arteriography may be used instead (see page 464). When there is no time to do these tests, immediate surgery may be required.

How Serious Is Subdural Hemorrhage?

Acute subdural hematoma is often fatal with or without immediate surgery, and death may occur despite prompt medical attention.

The subacute and chronic forms have less risk, but they also require medical attention as soon as symptoms are apparent, or permanent brain damage may result. The risk is greater for persons who use aspirin and anticoagulants on a daily basis.

Treatment

Medication

Intensive care includes various procedures and medications such as corticosteroids and diuretics to control the brain swelling (edema) caused by other fluids accumulating after a head injury. After surgery, anticonvulsant drugs, such as phenytoin, may be prescribed to control or prevent posttrau-

matic seizures. Seizures can begin as late as 24 months after the trauma.

Surgery

Treatment of the hematoma usually requires an operation. If the blood is localized and liquid, the only procedure required may be a perforation (creation of a hole through the skull) and evacuation by suction. Large hematomas or clotted blood may require that a section of skull be opened (craniotomy) to remove the blood. Some subdural hematomas are small and do not cause symptoms or need to be removed.

Convalescence

Amnesia, giddiness, attention difficulties, anxiety, and headache may occur and continue for some time. In adults, most recovery occurs within the first 6 months, and smaller improvements occur over 2 years. Incomplete recovery is due to brain damage. Children fare better; they have superior immediate recovery and small improvements spread over a longer period.

Extradural Hemorrhage

Signs and Symptoms

- Headache, drowsiness, or confusion after a head injury
- Nausea, vomiting, or dizziness
- Enlarged pupil(s)

Extradural (also called epidural) hemorrhage occurs when a blood vessel (usually an artery) ruptures between the outer surface of the dura mater (the outermost of three membrane layers that cover the brain) and the skull. The blood vessel usually is damaged by a skull fracture. Blood then leaks between the dura mater and the skull to form a mass (hematoma) that compresses the brain tissue.

Extradural hemorrhage is caused by injury to the head. It occurs most frequently as a result of automobile or motorcycle accidents. There may be no visible signs, such as an open wound or bruise.

In extradural hematoma, pressure on the brain increases as more and more blood flows into the narrow space between the brain and skull. The signs and symptoms described above may lead to unconsciousness, permanent brain damage, and even death. Immediate diagnosis and treatment are important.

Diagnosis

Symptoms are likely to occur within minutes to hours after injury. Several tests may be required to locate and assess extradural hemorrhaging, such as a skull X-ray and CT scan (see page 494). When there is no time to do these tests, immediate operation may be required.

How Serious Is Extradural Hemorrhage?

Head injuries are common, but only approximately 10 percent require hospitalization. Although only a small percentage of head injuries result in acute extradural hemor-

rhage, the risk of dying is substantial unless prompt treatment is obtained. Up to a third of victims may remain conscious, but most are drowsy or comatose from the moment of trauma.

Treatment

Surgery

If diagnostic tests indicate the presence of extradural hemorrhage, an operation will be necessary to stop the bleeding. The surgical procedure will involve excising a portion of the skull (craniotomy) to remove the blood clot and stop the bleeding. Prompt surgery usually results in complete recovery.

Convalescence

A period of convalescence may be required after an extradural hemorrhage. Headache may occur and continue for some time, along with anxiety, amnesia, and difficulty with concentration. Personality changes and memory deficits may go unnoticed. Speech disorders and paralysis usually disappear. In adults, most recovery occurs within the first 6 months, and smaller adjustments are made over 2 years. Incomplete recovery is due to brain damage. Children fare better; they have superior immediate recovery and small improvements spread over a longer period.

Chronic Disorders

Your brain, spinal cord, and peripheral nerves form an intricate organization consisting of billions of nerve cells. Each of these cells is a complex electrical and chemical transmitter that carries signals to make your muscles move and to relay information throughout your nervous system.

If a few scattered cells die or malfunction, you will not notice any change because surrounding cells then carry the transmissions. When there is progressive deterioration in any

part of your nervous system, however, you gradually will lose some ability to function. This loss can involve mental ability (dementia), muscular movement (paralysis), muscular control (tremor), or impaired coordination.

Compared with many other diseases, the degenerative disorders described in this section are less well understood and their prognosis is often less hopeful. These disorders may be disabling and, in most cases, there is no known cure.

Alzheimer's Disease

Signs and Symptoms
- Gradual loss of memory for recent events and inability to learn new information
- Growing tendency to repeat oneself, misplace objects, become confused, and get lost
- Slow disintegration of personality, judgment, and social graces
- Increasing irritability, anxiety, depression, confusion, and restlessness

Dementia is a syndrome (collection of symptoms) characterized by a decline in intellectual and social abilities to a sufficient degree to affect daily activities. Alzheimer's disease is the most common form of dementia. It is due to a degeneration of brain cells. Some forms of dementia are caused by specific neurologic or medical diseases and may be treatable. The cause of Alzheimer's disease, however, is unknown, and no effective treatment exists. The symptoms of Alzheimer's disease are progressive, but the rate of degeneration varies greatly from person to person.

Alzheimer's disease gradually produces abnormalities in certain areas of the brain. The particular behavioral characteristics of the disease depend on which area of the brain is most affected by the disease process. The brain cells of persons with Alzheimer's disease have characteristic features that were first described in 1907 by Alois Alzheimer. The brain also has chemical abnormalities related to the substances that allow the brain cells to communicate with one another.

Research on the cause and treatment of Alzheimer's disease is progressing. Among the several possible causes that are being explored are genetic factors, toxic exposures, abnormal protein production, viruses, abnormalities in the barrier between the blood and the brain, and neurochemical abnormalities. No particular hypothesis has turned out to be the entire answer thus far, but aging and genetic factors seem to contribute to the disease.

Recently, research has identified a form of protein that carries lipids (fats such as cholesterol) in the blood as a risk factor of Alzheimer's disease. This protein does not provide a diagnostic test for the disease, but it does provide information about the likelihood of developing Alzheimer's disease in the future. The protein is currently the focus of a great deal of research, and its ultimate usefulness is yet to be determined.

Alzheimer's disease accounts for approximately 50 to 60 percent of all cases of dementia. About 4 million persons in the United States have Alzheimer's disease. The disease occurs in approximately 4 percent of persons 65 to 74 years old, 10 percent of those 75 to 84 years, and up to 20 percent or more of those 85 years or older. Alzheimer's disease is extremely rare in young people and uncommon in middle age.

Diagnosis
No single test can be used to diagnose Alzheimer's disease, with the exception of a brain biopsy or an autopsy. Many of the signs and symptoms of Alzheimer's disease, such as memory loss, occur as a normal part of aging or as a part of other diseases such as vitamin B_{12} deficiency, hypothyroidism, depression, an adverse reaction to prescribed medications, or a chronic subdural hematoma (see pages 958, 948, 1122, 340, and 466). Many of these disorders can be treated, and thus it is important for an individual with mental status abnormalities to have a thorough medical and neurologic evaluation.

A person with dementia may lack insight into his or her disability. Consequently, if you know someone who shows signs of changes in mental ability, encourage him or her to be evaluated. The person's family and friends are essential in helping diagnose dementia or Alzheimer's disease and also are needed for ongoing support.

Alzheimer's disease is diagnosed by eliminating other possible causes for the changes in mental status. Initially, the person's history is reviewed in detail, and additional information from family or friends is obtained. The person then has a thorough physical examination and a neurologic examination (see page 460) to determine whether some other disease is present. Hearing is often evaluated. A series of laboratory tests then are used to assess other possible causes for the changes in mental status.

A neuropsychologist may be asked to evaluate the person's cognitive function. In particular, performance on various memory and intelligence tests will be compared with performance by normal persons of the same age. Laboratory tests to rule out other causes of the changes in mental status may include chest X-ray, electrocardiography, blood tests, CT or MRI of the head, electroencephalography, and lumbar puncture (see Tests for Dementia, page 473).

How Serious Is Alzheimer's Disease?

Alzheimer's disease is generally not an acute condition and often does not require emergency treatment. Abrupt changes in mental status may be due to other diseases, and they warrant medical attention. Alzheimer's disease, however, is ultimately fatal. Affected persons eventually may become bedridden and unable to care for themselves. They eventually may die of pneumonia or other infections because of this disability. The course of Alzheimer's disease can run from a few years to as many as 10 to 15 or more years. In the final stages, persons with Alzheimer's disease may be unable to communicate or feed themselves and have bowel and bladder incontinence.

Treatment

During the early stages of the disorder, you can provide care at home for a friend or member of your family who has Alzheimer's disease. It is necessary, however, to care for the person under the direction of a physician. Providing care for an individual with Alzheimer's disease can be difficult and may be stressful to the spouse and family members. Often, those providing care need assistance from support organizations and a network of family and friends. Caring for someone with Alzheimer's disease requires patience and compassion to deal with the frequent repetition of stories and questions and the occasionally offensive behavior. Eventually, the person's condition deteriorates such that additional full-time nursing care is required, and often placement in a nursing home is necessary.

Medication

Currently, tacrine is the only medication approved for the treatment of Alzheimer's disease in the United States. This medication is intended to modify some of the symptoms of the disease, but probably does not alter the overall course. Several experimental drugs are being evaluated for the treatment of Alzheimer's disease. Thus far, none have proved successful for reversing the course of the disease. However, medications can be prescribed to deal with some of the behavior problems that may accompany Alzheimer's disease. Occasionally, mild sedatives, antidepressants, or antipsychotic medications may be necessary to control behavior. These drugs, often used in low doses, can improve the person's quality of life and assist the family in caring for the patient.

Other Therapies

Education can be very important for the caregivers in families. Learning more about the disease process and techniques for dealing with problem behaviors can be very beneficial to the patient and family. These services are often provided by local support groups.

A person with Alzheimer's disease should be encouraged to continue his or her daily routines, physical activities, and social interactions as much as possible. General health maintenance, including proper nutrition and fluid intake, is critical, but generally, special diets and supplements are unnecessary. Exercise is important, and your physician may recommend specific physical therapies. The person should not be restricted from trying new activities, and travel with a supportive companion may be possible if arrangements are not overly complicated.

Avoid dramatic changes in routine, such as moving to a new location, reorganizing furniture, and disrupting daily habits. Avoid dangerous equipment or materials in the living environment, and monitor carefully the person's ability to drive.

Provide practical assistance by using notes as reminders of activities. The living situation can be modified to provide calendars, lists of routine tasks, and directions for daily activities. A medical bracelet may be helpful in case the person becomes disoriented and wanders into unfamiliar settings.

Alzheimer's disease can be a difficult disorder to deal with, but concern and compassion on the part of the persons providing care can make a difference. The assistance of a physician and the services provided by Alzheimer's disease support groups should be sought.

Vascular Dementia

Signs and Symptoms

- Loss of memory or other cognitive functions relatively abruptly
- Cognitive loss usually accompanied by the symptoms of a stroke (paralysis, difficulty with language, visual loss)
- Gait (walking) disturbances, perhaps early
- Loss of control of bowel or bladder, perhaps early
- Sudden involuntary laughing and crying

Emergency Symptoms—Abrupt change in mental state

Vascular dementia is caused by a series of strokes (see page 461) that leave areas of dead brain cells (infarcts). The disorder produces a step-by-step degeneration in mental ability, with each step corresponding to a stroke. Memory, particularly of recent events, usually is affected first.

Approximately 5 to 10 percent of all cases of dementia are classified as vascular, and 10 percent are attributable to a combination of Alzheimer's disease (see page 470) and multiple infarcts. More than 4 million Americans have moderate to severe mental impairment due to dementia.

In the early stages, before too much damage has occurred, the affected person often is aware of impaired ability, and frustration tends to increase the characteristic depression.

Strokes and the resulting vascular dementia are typically the consequences of one or more underlying disorders, including high blood pressure and resultant artery damage (see High Blood Pressure and Atherosclerosis, pages 647 and 636, and Tests for Dementia, page 473).

Treatment

Prevention of stroke is the only potentially effective treatment for this dementia. If you have high blood pressure (see page 647) or transient ischemic attacks (see page 463), or have had a stroke, you will need continuing treatment for these diseases to minimize their recurrence and avoid vascular dementia. Affected persons require care similar to that needed for those with Alzheimer's disease (see page 470).

Parkinson's Disease

Signs and Symptoms
- Shaking at rest (rest tremor)
- Masking or reduction of facial expression
- Slowness of movements
- Shuffling gait
- Stiffness or rigidity of limbs
- Slow, soft, monotone voice
- Difficulty in maintaining balance
- Stooped posture
- Small, illegible handwriting

Parkinson's disease, which years ago was called shaking palsy or paralysis agitans, was first described by Englishman James Parkinson in 1817. It is a progressive degeneration of nerve cells in the part of the brain that controls muscle movements.

This particular group of nerve cells makes a chemical called dopamine. Dopamine is important for transmitting signals from one specific group of cells to another within your brain. In Parkinson's disease, the group of cells that makes the dopamine (called the substantia nigra) is lost, resulting in impairment of walking, arm movement, and facial expression.

Although much research has been done on Parkinson's disease, the cause remains unknown.

Parkinson's disease manifests itself in various ways. These may include only one side of the body or both sides.

If the disease becomes severe, your facial expression may become fixed, your eyes are unblinking, and your mouth may open slightly with an excess of saliva at the corners. Your posture is typically stooped. Your limbs or trunk may be rigid. Some people find it hard to start walking, beginning with hesitant, small steps, but then they have to break into a run to avoid falling forward. Some persons stop their movement in a "frozen" position and are unable to resume movement.

If your symptoms include tremor, it may be aggravated by tension or fatigue. Tremor of the hand may take the form of a continuous rubbing of thumb and forefinger (called pill-rolling tremor). The tremor disappears during sleep.

Parkinson's disease ordinarily starts in middle or late life and develops very slowly. More than 1 million Americans have the disorder.

Diagnosis

The diagnosis is made primarily on the basis of a history and comprehensive neurologic examination. Similar symptoms are caused by certain medications, especially specific drugs used to treat nausea or severe psychiatric disorders. In addition, your physician or neurologist will carefully consider a variety of other degenerative brain conditions that share some of the features of Parkinson's disease but differ in other respects, including a poor response to medicines used to treat Parkinson's disease.

Tremors, although commonly associated with Parkinson's disease, may have many

Tests for Dementia

Dementia is a syndrome characterized by a decline in intellectual and social abilities that affects a person's daily functioning. The symptoms of dementia are a progressive loss of memory and other mental abilities, often accompanied by increasing behavior abnormalities and personality changes. These symptoms are not specific for dementia and may be caused by various other disorders, such as depression, adverse reactions to medication, vitamin B_{12} deficiency, thyroid function abnormalities, alcoholism, drug abuse, or diseases affecting other organs in the body. The purpose of testing an individual for dementia is to identify a possible treatable cause of the changes in mental status. Therefore, an accurate diagnosis is important.

The evaluation of a person with dementia begins with a detailed history of the symptoms and physical and neurologic evaluations (see page 460). The laboratory tests that are then ordered are selected to identify a specific cause of the abnormality in mental status. A mental status examination is often part of the neurologic evaluation. This test is not an evaluation for sanity; rather, it assesses various mental functions such as memory, attention, language, and perception skills. Your physician or a clinical psychologist may ask questions to assess several mental processes. These questions may include an evaluation of insight into the problem (What is your difficulty?), orientation (What is the date, month, and year? Where are you now?), memory (learning a list of words and repeating them later), recall (remembering information learned

at a previous time), abstract reasoning (explanation of a proverb), attention (recite the months of the year forward and backward), language (name objects and demonstrate an ability to read, write, and comprehend the spoken word), general information (Who is the President? How many weeks are there in a year?), and thought content (What are your fears and concerns?).

Memory function may be tested in more detail because impairment of memory is a prominent finding in dementia. Various tests of a person's ability to learn both verbal and nonverbal information and to recall items from the remote past may be used. The ability to construct objects by drawing also may be assessed, and the person may be asked to recall these drawings at a later time.

Cognitive function also may be assessed in more detail by formal neuropsychological testing. This uses standardized tests of intelligence (such as the Wechsler Adult Intelligence Scale—Revised), memory (such as the Wechsler Memory Scale—Revised), language (such as the Boston Diagnostic Aphasia Examination), and prior academic achievements (such as the Wide Range Achievement Test). These tests have been standardized using large groups of people. Typically, an individual's performance score is compared with scores obtained from other persons of the same age. These tests will help to determine whether any changes in mental status performance are within the normal range of aging or whether they may be due to other disease processes. For example,

depression may interfere with some attention and memory tasks in a manner somewhat similar to that found in Alzheimer's disease.

After the clinical examinations, several laboratory tests may be done to identify a specific disease that may be causing the symptoms. These diseases include certain brain disorders, such as strokes, tumors, abscesses, or fluid accumulations, and other general medical disorders that may affect mental status, such as heart and lung disease, liver disease, kidney disease, and infections such as AIDS or syphilis. Because some of these disorders are treatable, a thorough evaluation is essential in newly diagnosed cases of dementia.

Tests that may be ordered to assess the presence of these disorders include CT or MRI of the head (see page 494), electrocardiography (see page 655), chest X-ray (see page 657), blood chemistry and urine tests, and drug screening. Additional neurologic tests that may help in the diagnosis include electroencephalography (see page 1344), lumbar puncture (see page 485), and radioisotope studies (see page 1337).

If no specific cause for the decline in mental status is identified after a thorough medical, neurologic, neuropsychological, and laboratory evaluation, the person may have Alzheimer's disease. In the absence of a brain biopsy or an autopsy, the diagnosis of Alzheimer's disease is based on the exclusion of other causes of the symptoms. The diagnosis of Alzheimer's disease must not be assigned before a thorough evaluation of all other treatable causes has been completed.

other causes, such as essential tremor (see page 475). Many persons with Parkinson's disease have little or no symptomatic tremor.

The onset is not readily apparent, and you may not recognize the early symptoms as a

medical problem for some time. The first symptoms you experience may be a slight dragging of one foot while walking, a sense of stiffness in a limb, or a mild tremor in the fingers of one hand.

Symptoms beyond these early indications become so clear-cut, however, that your physician may be able to diagnose the disorder by a simple examination.

How Serious Is Parkinson's Disease?

Parkinson's disease tends to be progressive—symptoms worsen eventually. The time involved in this process varies greatly, and you may have years of productive living after developing this disease. During the later stages, however, you may need assistance. In its most severe form, you may become helplessly incapacitated by rigidity and tremor. Fortunately, this occurs only in a small minority.

Many individuals with Parkinson's disease have depression. In addition, some degree of mental deterioration occurs in about one-third of those persons with Parkinson's disease. In the later stages, auditory and visual hallucinations may develop. These may be activated by the medication prescribed to lessen other symptoms of the disease.

Treatment

In early stages of the illness, you may not require therapy. Medication normally is introduced at a time when Parkinson's disease interferes with daily activities.

It is critical that you maintain good general health and continue to exercise. Your energy level may go up and down, and you will need to adjust your activities accordingly. Rest periods during the day are needed, and a contented frame of mind is important because fatigue, anxiety, and unhappiness may aggravate your symptoms considerably. You will need emotional support and encouragement to deal with the illness. There are support groups nationwide for this purpose. Ask your physician for information about these groups. Getting involved in physical and occupational therapy programs is stimulating both physically and emotionally. This can help you maintain a positive mental attitude and avoid depression.

Medication

The main goal of treatment is to reverse the problems with walking, movement, and tremors by restoring your brain's supply of dopamine. A medicine called levodopa is used to increase the amount of dopamine in your brain. Levodopa can be dramatically effective for improving the deficits in movement and balance. Physicians typically prescribe levodopa in combination with another medication (carbidopa) that is designed to reduce the side effects of levodopa and make levodopa more potent. Anticholinergic drugs also may be used to decrease tremor, but they have various side effects. Other drugs that might also be prescribed include amantadine, pergolide, or bromocriptine.

Close medical supervision is required during drug therapy. Dosage and the time at which you take the medication must be changed as your symptoms change. You may experience side effects such as involuntary movements, nausea, dizziness, and mental changes. Report these changes to your physician so that medication can be adjusted to your needs. Most people respond, in some degree, to drug therapy. Some are relieved of symptoms almost completely. However, over a period of years, control of symptoms may become less complete, and the response to medication may vary.

Surgery

Several surgical procedures directed at the brain have been used to decrease tremor and sometimes other symptoms of Parkinson's disease. Tissue deep within the brain and in areas called the thalamus and globus pallidus is sometimes surgically destroyed in selected patients. Recently, stimulating electrodes similar to a heart pacemaker have been implanted within the brain and used to control certain symptoms of parkinsonism. Because of computer-assisted technology now available, these procedures are being done much more precisely than in the past.

Several years ago, the transplantation of adrenal gland tissue to precise locations deep in the brain was under investigation. Although early reports on this form of treatment were encouraging, subsequent experience with this type of transplantation was discouraging. Several centers in North America and Europe have investigated transplantation of other types of tissue into the brains of persons with Parkinson's disease in an effort to restore lost brain circuits. For the most part, this has involved the transplantation of fetal brain tissue. This has been partially beneficial but has raised ethical concerns and may not be practical on a large scale. However, genetically engineered cells, which are being developed in laboratories, may eventually circumvent these ethical and practical limitations.

Tic Disorders

Signs and Symptoms—Habitual, repetitive movements or twitches of the face

Tics are semivoluntary mannerisms, usually starting in childhood. Grimaces, eye or mouth twitches, head turning, and shoulder shrugging are examples of common tics. Adolescents sometimes display such tics, which later resolve with age.

Multiple, more prominent tics that develop in youth and include vocalizations (for example, sniffing, grunting, compulsive swearing) characterize Gilles de la Tourette's syndrome. This syndrome is 4 times more frequent in boys than girls and sometimes runs in families. An evaluation is needed to exclude other disorders.

Treatment

Medication

Sometimes no medication is needed. Small dosages of clonidine or clonazepam can be used for mild tics. Neuroleptic drugs control multiple tics more effectively in a considerable number of persons. However, they have significant side effects and are reserved for the more severe disorders.

Essential Tremor

Signs and Symptoms
- Rhythmic, alternating movement of your hands, arms, head, tongue, or larynx
- Arm and head symptoms that worsen with use

Essential tremor is not a serious condition. When there is a family history, it is called familial tremor. Although it is the most common form of tremor, its cause is unknown. The rhythmic tremor may range from a moderate to a rapid frequency (6 to 12 movements per second).

Almost half the cases run in families, appearing at adolescence or later. It most commonly begins in middle to late life and develops slowly. Over time, the tremor may affect your arms, your head, your hands, or your voice. Your voluntary movements, such as holding a coffee cup or a fork, usually make the tremor worse. This is in contrast to Parkinson's disease (see page 472), in which the tremor tends to decrease with movement.

Stress also may increase the tremor. You may notice that it usually appears while you are active. It disappears during sleep.

The diagnosis is usually made on the basis of a history and examination. Only limited laboratory tests are necessary.

Treatment
Often, treatment is unnecessary. The usual medications include propranolol, which reduces the tremor (and also slows heart rate and reduces blood pressure), primidone (an antiseizure drug), or limited tranquilizers.

Stimulants such as caffeine, in excess quantities, may increase the tremor. Consumption of alcohol tends to decrease the tremor but can lead to alcohol abuse.

Multiple Sclerosis

Signs and Symptoms
- Numbness, weakness, or paralysis in one or more limbs
- Impaired vision with pain during movement in one eye
- Tremor, lack of coordination, or unsteady gait
- Rapid, involuntary eye movement

Multiple sclerosis (MS) is a disease of your central nervous system. Its cause is unknown. It generally proceeds in episodes (attacks) that last weeks or months and can be separated by periods in which symptoms diminish or even disappear (remission). Attacks ordinarily recur (relapse), however, and disability may persist and the symptoms may increase in severity. MS is the chief cause of major disability in adults of working age.

Attacks are most frequent 3 to 4 years after they begin. The first attack, sometimes too mild to be remembered, most commonly occurs between the ages of 20 and 40 years.

MS has a wide variety of symptoms because of the way it affects the central nervous system. Each attack is thought to be due to inflammation in an area of your nervous system. This may result in the destruction of the insulating sheath (myelin) that covers nerve fibers, leaving multiple areas of scarring (sclerosis). Muscle coordination, visual sensation, and other signals are slowed or blocked.

The most common general symptoms of MS are movement or coordination problems; sensory problems such as brief pain, tingling,

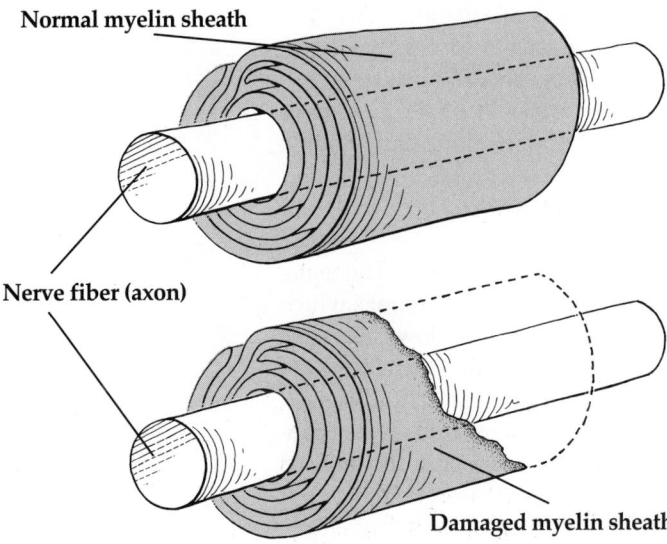

Normal myelin sheath

Nerve fiber (axon)

Damaged myelin sheath

Your nerve fibers are protected by an insulating sheath (myelin). In multiple sclerosis, the sheath is damaged, producing symptoms.

or electric shock sensations; vision problems such as blurred or double vision; and problems with bladder control or mental functions. Lack of energy and fatiguing easily are also common complaints of persons with MS.

Any of these symptoms may be caused by other disorders. One of the early indications that MS may be present is symptoms that appear briefly (usually lasting days to weeks) and then disappear completely or become less noticeable. This pattern corresponds to the attack-and-remission cycle of MS. Symptoms may become more prominent when your body temperature is raised by a hot bath, by being out in the sun, or by a stressful situation.

The cause of MS is not completely understood, but medical research is very active. Preceding the MS symptoms, the concentration of immune cells in your central nervous system is high. These cells are usually beneficial for fighting disease. When you have MS, however, they are thought to destroy the cells that produce the myelin sheath. The presence of a virus, in either immune cells or sheath-producing cells, is one suspected cause.

Your risk for MS is greater if a relative has the disease. An environmental source of the virus or an inherited factor in the immune system genes or a combination of the two may be involved. Your susceptibility to MS probably is acquired before you are 15 years old.

The chances for developing MS also vary with geography; the risk is greater in northern states than in southern states. More than 200,000 Americans have MS. Women have a slightly higher risk than men.

Diagnosis

The neurologic symptoms of MS are varied and difficult to diagnose in the initial stages. However, the sequence of an attack, remission, and yet another attack strongly suggests MS. It is very important to get an accurate diagnosis because all subsequent symptoms may be attributed to MS and the onset of another neurologic disease may be overlooked. If MS is suspected, your physician probably will refer you to a neurologist for a detailed examination.

Criteria for diagnosing MS include a reliable history of at least two attacks and an observable abnormality of the central nervous system such as altered reflexes or sensation. Because the lesions tend to be distributed randomly in the brain and spinal cord, the symptoms can vary considerably.

Laboratory tests may be used to help establish the diagnosis. Recordings may be made of the electrical activity in the brain (electroencephalogram, see page 1344) when your senses are stimulated. You may be given a standard visual stimulus to determine how your brain's nerve cells process this input signal. Other tests may include magnetic resonance imaging (MRI) scan (see page 494). Lumbar puncture (see page 485) also may be used to check the concentration of immune cells and proteins in your cerebrospinal fluid.

How Serious Is Multiple Sclerosis?

The effect of MS is unpredictable. The average life expectancy is more than 35 years after onset of the disease, and it has increased 10 to 15 years in the past few decades as a result of better medical care, particularly in dealing with complications of the disease. Most persons with MS are ambulatory, and many are employed even after having MS for 20 years. An uncommon acute form of MS can be fatal within weeks or months.

Treatment

Currently, there is no cure for MS. Medication varies depending on the symptoms. Baclofen is sometimes useful for suppressing muscle spasticity. For severe attacks, corticosteroid drugs or the hormone ACTH may be prescribed to reduce inflammation and provide temporary relief. Several experimental drugs are being evaluated; most of them are designed to suppress the immune system.

Physical and occupational therapy are important for maintaining a positive mental attitude and avoiding depression. A planned exercise program may be needed.

In 1993, the U.S. Food and Drug Administration licensed a form of interferon for use in ambulatory (still able to walk) persons who have frequent attacks of relapsing/remitting multiple sclerosis. This form of interferon is given as a subcutaneous (under the skin) injection every other day. Research showed that regular use of interferon decreased the frequency of multiple sclerosis attacks and kept more persons free of attacks over a 2-year treatment period. Interferon may be associated with a number of adverse reactions, including inflammation and pain at the injection site, flu-like symptoms, abnormalities of liver function, and, rarely, severe depression, including suicidal depression. Interferon has not been shown conclusively to prevent progression of the disease.

Amyotrophic Lateral Sclerosis

Signs and Symptoms
- Slow loss of strength and coordination in one or more limbs
- Muscle twitches or cramps
- Increasingly stiff, clumsy gait
- Swallowing, speaking, or breathing difficulty

Amyotrophic lateral sclerosis (ALS) is a progressive degeneration of the nerve cells in the brain and spinal cord which control your voluntary muscles. It commonly is called Lou Gehrig's disease after the baseball player who died of ALS in 1939.

The affected nerve cells shrink and disappear with no other signs of abnormality. The muscle tissues then waste away because the nerves that stimulated them are gone.

ALS is not contagious. About 30,000 Americans have ALS, more men than women. It occurs worldwide. A defective gene has been identified as the cause of some cases of inherited ALS.

The onset is gradual. Most often there is increasing weakness in one limb, especially a hand. Later, other limbs may be affected. This may be accompanied by twitching and cramping. Additional muscle areas become affected as ALS progresses, and complete paralysis may result. One in five persons lives longer than 5 years, but death generally occurs within 2 to 10 years after diagnosis.

The disease may be well advanced before you seek medical attention. If so, the diagnosis may be based on your symptoms and signs. Electromyography (see page 1344) to test for nerve damage may be required.

Treatment
There is no cure for ALS. Individually designed therapy is useful for maintaining your muscle function and general health during the early stages. The disease does not affect your mind, and several years of enjoyable life may be possible. A distressing feature is the difficulty in swallowing and the tendency for food and saliva to be inhaled into the windpipe. This complication can be avoided by insertion of a tube through the wall of the abdomen and into the stomach through which liquid feedings can be given (see Gastrostomy, page 747).

The Food and Drug Administration has approved a drug for treating ALS. Riluzole (Rilutek) appears to slow the progression of the disease in some people, slightly prolonging life. Emotional support from family and friends helps encourage positive attitudes. The ALS Society of America can provide information and help.

Huntington's Chorea

Signs and Symptoms
- Wide, prancing gait
- Hesitant speech
- Involuntary, jerky movements in arms, neck, trunk, and face
- Personality changes
- Intellectual deterioration

Emergency Symptoms—Abrupt change in mental state

Huntington's chorea (Huntington's disease) is a progressive degenerative disease stemming from a disorder within the brain which causes certain nerve cells to waste away. The severity of the symptoms is related to the degree of cell loss.

The disorder was first documented in 1872 by American physician George Huntington. Chorea comes from the Greek word for dance and refers to the characteristic incessant, quick, jerky, and involuntary movements.

Onset is usually between ages 35 and 50. Younger patients often have a more severe condition. Rare cases may occur in children.

One or 2 in 20,000 people have the disease.

It is an inherited disease. If one parent has the single faulty gene, the chance that an offspring will have the defect, in some degree, is 50 percent. Because the onset is typically in middle age, some parents may not know they carry the gene until they have already had children, possibly passing on the trait. If your family history includes this disease, it is important to get genetic counseling (see page 42).

The development of the disease is slow. Personality changes, from moodiness to paranoia, may occur first. Involuntary facial movements may begin mildly and develop into grimaces. Other symptoms, including severe chorea and mental impairment (dementia), appear as the disease progresses. Death occurs after many years due to complications of the bedridden stage.

Treatment

Medication
No satisfactory treatment is available. Medication may be prescribed to lessen the chorea symptoms.

Friedreich's Ataxia

Signs and Symptoms
- Difficulty in maintaining balance while walking or standing
- Abnormal speech rhythm or articulation
- Weakness in limbs
- Tremor of hands or arms
- Deformed spine or feet
- Paralysis, particularly of the legs

Friedreich's ataxia, named in 1863 for German physician Nikolaus Friedreich, is a rare, inherited disease. The symptoms, which begin in youth, are due to nerve fiber degeneration in areas of the spinal cord, peripheral nerves, or cerebellum. The diagnosis of this disorder takes into consideration family history and neurologic findings and is confirmed by electrical changes in nerve conduction (see Electromyography, page 1344).

Survival beyond early adulthood is rare. Death is frequently caused by impairment of heart muscle (cardiomyopathy, see page 686).

Treatment
No specific treatment is available. Continued physical activity is recommended for general health.

Cerebral Palsy

Signs and Symptoms
- Full or partial spastic paralysis or weakness in one or more limbs
- Tremor or other involuntary movements
- Vision, speech, or hearing disorders
- Occasionally, mental retardation

Emergency Symptoms—Convulsive seizures (uncommon)

Cerebral palsy refers to a group of disorders caused by injuries to the cerebral area of the brain that occur before or during birth or in the first few months after birth. Damage to the cerebrum may cause paralysis (palsy) in one or more parts of the body. Cerebral palsy is the most common crippling childhood disorder. Although the damage sustained by your child continues throughout adult life, it usually does not get worse.

Cerebral injury can occur in several ways, including inadequate blood or oxygen supply to the fetus, premature birth, birth trauma, diseases in infancy (encephalitis, meningitis, or herpes simplex), intracerebral hemorrhage in premature babies, or blood vessel damage. Any resulting paralysis is classified clinically after the child is 2 years old. There are three main categories, and a fourth category is used to indicate mixed symptoms. The first, spastic cerebral palsy, is the most common and the mildest form, occurring in 50 percent of cases. Your child may have varying degrees of paralysis in paired limbs (paraplegia), one side of the body (hemiplegia), or all four extremities (quadriplegia).

The second classification is dyskinetic or athetoid cerebral palsy; it occurs in 20 percent of cases. Your child may have abnormal involuntary movement such as twisting, twitching, or writhing, or abrupt, jerky movements that may increase with tension and disappear during sleep.

The third classification is ataxic cerebral palsy. It is the least common form, occurring in 10 percent of cases. Your child may have tremor, unsteadiness, incoordination, and choreic movements (see Huntington's chorea, page 477).

Diagnosis
It is difficult to diagnose cerebral palsy in early infancy, although some babies exhibit symptoms after age 6 months. Their symptoms can include a tendency to tuck their

arms into their sides, to cross their legs in a scissors-like fashion, or to toe walk from the ankle. Once the symptoms develop, laboratory tests may be required to exclude other disorders. If your child shows signs of mental retardation, blood tests may be needed to check for abnormalities in amino acid levels and other biochemical abnormalities.

How Serious Is Cerebral Palsy?

Cerebral palsy is a chronic ailment that may require long-term care, but it is not life-threatening. The seriousness of the disorder depends on the amount of cerebral damage and can range from a speech disorder to mental retardation and a physical handicap. With special treatment, many children with cerebral palsy grow up to live long and productive lives.

Treatment

The goal of treatment is to develop your child's maximal level of independence. Regular attendance at school is recommended if the symptoms are not too severe. Physical and occupational therapy may be needed (see page 480). Some children may require an orthopedic operation. Guidelines for treatment should be determined by your child's learning capacity and physical limitations. You will need guidance and help in understanding your child's disorder and future potential.

Medication

Your child's physician may prescribe medications to alleviate some symptoms. These may include muscle relaxants to ease muscle stiffness and anticonvulsants to reduce the seizures that some children experience.

Myasthenia Gravis

Signs and Symptoms

- Facial muscle weakness (including drooping eyelids)
- Double vision
- Difficulty in breathing, talking, chewing, or swallowing
- Muscle weakness in the arms or legs

Emergency Symptoms—Increasing difficulty in breathing or swallowing

Myasthenia gravis is a chronic fluctuating disorder characterized by weakness and

---

> ## Torticollis
>
> Torticollis is an intermittent or continuous spasm of the large muscles of the neck. It is usually more prominent on one side than the other. When the neck is in spasm, this may cause permanent turning or tipping of the head. Often, torticollis is worse when the individual sits, stands, or walks. Generally, this occurs in middle age, and women are affected more often than men.

---

rapid fatigue of your voluntary muscles. Muscle weakness develops gradually and may appear first in your face.

Myasthenia gravis is caused by a problem relating to the immune system. Antibodies that are normally formed to fight infection react instead against normal tissue. Most persons with myasthenia gravis also have abnormalities of the thymus gland, which is an organ that helps program the immune system early in life.

Myasthenia gravis is rare; in the United States, it develops in 1 of 20,000 persons, occurring most frequently in women between the ages of 20 and 40.

Diagnosis

The key symptom that will alert your physician to the possibility of myasthenia gravis is muscle weakness that improves with rest. Tests to confirm the diagnosis may include a neurologic examination (see page 460), electromyography (see page 1344), and a blood analysis for the presence of certain antibodies. After the strength of various muscles is tested, you may be given a drug called edrophonium. Improved muscle strength after taking this drug is suggestive of myasthenia gravis.

How Serious Is Myasthenia Gravis?

There is no cure for myasthenia gravis, but treatment can often lead to a remission. In a crisis phase of the illness, affected persons become so weak they need help breathing, but this effect rarely persists beyond a few weeks. With proper treatment, most can lead productive lives.

Pregnancy is possible for women with myasthenia gravis, although you should stay in close consultation with your physician.

Treatment

Plan activities to take advantage of your

Physical Therapy in the Rehabilitation of Chronic Neurologic Problems

Physical therapy, also called physiotherapy, is used to achieve maximal potential in persons with a disability resulting from multiple sclerosis, stroke, cerebral palsy, muscular dystrophy, traumatic brain injury, and many other disorders. Physical treatments can be valuable for helping to relieve pain, to improve your strength and mobility, and to train you to perform essential tasks so that you can regain as much independence as possible.

Before you begin a program of physical therapy, have a complete medical examination with diagnostic, functional, and psychological testing, as determined by your physician. Your physical therapist, usually at a local hospital or clinic, will consult closely with your physician. Testing and consultation are needed to plan a program that will work best for you and to reevaluate the therapy frequently as you make progress.

Physical testing will include a determination of your joint mobility, muscle strength (any weakness or paralysis), coordination, heart and lung response to exercise, posture, and ability to change position, walk, communicate, follow directions, and perform other essential daily activities.

Your physical therapist, if indicated, will work with you in retraining your bladder and bowel and managing spasticity (muscle rigidity). A therapist may also advise you about ways to rehabilitate or compensate for losses in your cognitive abilities (perception, thought, memory).

Physical therapists are trained and licensed in the use of exercise, water, heat, cold, light, electricity, ultrasound, and other agents that may help relieve symptoms and signs of disease.

Exercise is the most varied and widely used of all physical therapy techniques. Your exercise routine will be designed to overcome the manifestations of your disorder as much as possible, whether it be to increase the degree of joint mobility, muscle strength, or endurance or to retrain your muscles to contract and relax in useful coordination with other muscles.

Exercises may be simple or complex. They are performed actively by you alone or with the help of your therapist or passively as your physical therapist moves your arm or leg through prescribed motions. Active exercises are necessary to improve your muscle function, but passive exercises are helpful when you have muscle contractures or need to relearn certain movements. Exercises against resistance can improve your strength.

Various types of equipment may be used for this therapy, including an exercise table or mat, a stationary bicycle, walking aids, wheelchair, practice stairs, curbs, ramps, parallel bars, and pulleys and weights.

Heat generally is used to stimulate circulation, relax tense muscles, and relieve pain. It is applied with hot-water compresses, infrared lamps, short-wave radiation, high-frequency electrical current, ultrasound, hot paraffin wax, or warm baths. In some cases, cold treatment may be necessary. This is applied with ice packs or cold-water soaking. Alternating hot and cold water immersion of the hands or feet may be used in certain circumstances.

Whirlpool baths can ease the pain from muscle spasm and help guide or strengthen your movements because the water partially supports you and provides resistance to your motion.

Massage is used to aid circulation, help you relax, relieve local pain or muscle spasms, and reduce swelling. It can be done by trained therapists with special equipment or by family members trained in specific techniques.

Electrical currents of very low strength may be applied through your skin to stimulate superficial muscles and make them contract. This helps paralyzed or weakened muscles to respond again. For example, if you have amyotrophic lateral sclerosis (see page 477), such therapy may be used to maintain your muscle function as long as possible. Electrical instruments also are used to test the condition of the nerves supplying your muscles and affecting sensation in your skin. Certain medications can even be supplied through your skin by means of a low-voltage electrical apparatus. Portable electrical current devices (TENS units) frequently are used to control chronic pain.

Your therapy may include learning how to use assistance devices for walking (cane, crutches, walker, braces, or others), mobility aids to substitute for walking (wheelchairs or motorized scooters), or transfer aids for changing position (boards, lifts, and bars). Special equipment that you may be trained to use ranges from simple aids, such as a cane or walker, to sophisticated devices that can make it easier to fasten buttons, hold a fork, dial a telephone, or drive a car.

Many persons are involved in the team approach to rehabilitation. In addition to your physician and physical therapist, other members of your rehabilitation team may include a corrective therapist who uses physical education techniques and an occupational therapist to help you regain the ability to perform routine daily tasks such as grooming and dressing or to help you develop an alternative to compensate for a lost function. Sometimes an orthotist may be needed to construct braces or other devices needed for mobility. Often, a rehabilitation counselor advises you on how, where, and from whom to get the necessary rehabilitation.

energy peaks, and schedule daily rest periods. To relieve double vision, wear an eye patch. Stress also can worsen your condition, and you and your family will need to cooperate in minimizing your level of stress.

Medication

Drugs may be prescribed to increase the amounts of nerve chemicals at the junctions of your nerves and muscles. Arrange to eat meals about 30 minutes after taking your medication to minimize chewing and swallowing difficulty. Medications such as prednisone also may be prescribed.

Other Therapies

Plasmapheresis is a treatment in which the plasma component in your blood is removed and discarded because it contains antibodies that may contribute to your disease. Your blood cells along with other fluids that replace your plasma are returned to your body. This treatment may reduce the immune response and improve muscle strength temporarily.

Surgery

In some cases, removal of the thymus gland may be recommended. This can lead to permanent improvement in symptoms.

Infections

Infections can attack your central nervous system in several ways. They can be direct invasions by a virus or bacteria. They also can attack you indirectly when some minor condition, such as an ear infection or a case of measles, leads to a major infection of the nervous system. You also can be infected by bacterial toxins or certain tick bites.

These infections vary in seriousness. They may result in several days in bed, months of sickness with residual mental and physical impairment, or even death.

Meningitis

Signs and Symptoms
- Fever
- Severe headache
- Vomiting
- Confusion
- Seizures
- Progressive lethargy
- Drowsiness
- Stiff neck

Emergency Symptoms
- Stupor
- Coma
- Convulsions

Acute bacterial meningitis is an infection and inflammation of your central nervous system that attacks the membranes (meninges) and cerebrospinal fluid surrounding your brain and spinal cord. Bacteria usually invade through the bloodstream, but direct spread to the brain or spine can occur.

Bacteria generally enter the blood as a result of infections in other parts of your body. The infection often starts in the respiratory system. Infection of the heart valves, bones, or other areas of the body also can spread to the meninges via the bloodstream. Infection also can occur by direct invasion of bacteria already localized near your central nervous system (for example, from an infected ear, sinus, nose, or even tooth).

Other less frequent causes for acute bacterial meningitis include epidural abscess and medical procedures such as lumbar puncture. Alcoholism, diabetes mellitus, drugs used for organ transplantation, and AIDS may make you more vulnerable to meningitis. In Lyme disease, there can be an inflammation of the lining of the brain from the organism that causes the disease.

The incidence of meningitis is 5 to 10 cases per 100,000 persons annually. About 70 percent of all cases occur in children younger than 5, but the disease can strike at any age.

Like the brain, the spinal cord is protected by several layers of membranes (meninges): dura mater, arachnoid, and pia mater. Cerebrospinal fluid (shown in blue) surrounds your brain and spinal cord. If you have meningitis, your meninges and cerebrospinal fluid are affected.

Meninges

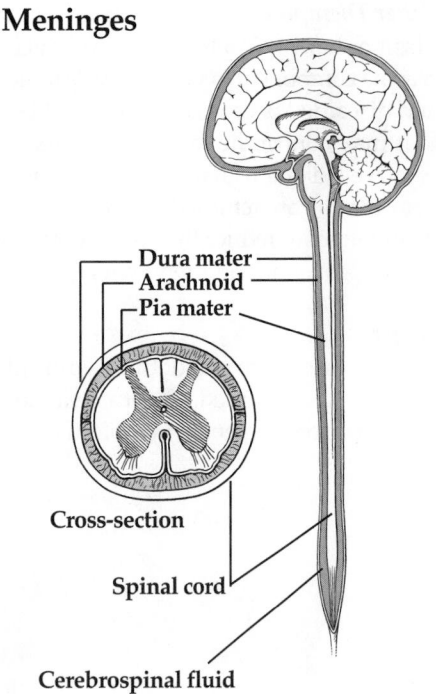

Dura mater
Arachnoid
Pia mater

Cross-section

Spinal cord

Cerebrospinal fluid

Diagnosis

The symptoms of meningitis may not develop early in the course of the infection, but if meningitis is suspected, seek immediate medical consultation. Your physician will examine your head, ears, and skin (especially along the spine) for sources of infection. You may have X-rays taken of your chest, skull, and sinuses. CT (see page 494) may be done to determine whether there is an abscess or deep swelling. The definitive diagnosis, however, will be made by analyzing your cerebrospinal fluid, which is extracted by lumbar puncture (see page 485). One of the signs of the disease is a low glucose level and increased white blood cell count in the fluid. Some of the fluid will be cultured to determine what type of bacteria may be present.

How Serious Is Meningitis?

Acute bacterial meningitis is a medical emergency. The longer you have the disease without diagnosis and treatment, the greater your risk of permanent neurologic damage, such as hearing loss, brain damage, retardation, or loss of vision. Meningitis is most dangerous to infants and elderly persons.

Other, normally less acute, forms of the disease include aseptic, subacute, and recurrent meningitis. Aseptic meningitis is an inflammatory reaction of the meninges that is not caused by bacteria. This disease is most commonly caused by certain viruses but also can be a reaction to certain medications or cells that are not normally present in the cerebrospinal fluid. This form causes many of the same symptoms as a bacterial infection.

Subacute meningitis can be caused by fungal infections, the dissemination of malignant cells, or syphilis. Subacute symptoms evolve over a period of weeks.

Recurrent meningitis may be the result of a channel between the nose and the areas between the brain and one of its protective layers (subarachnoid space). This channel, usually the result of an injury, permits loss of fluid through the nose in certain positions. It also may allow bacteria to travel from the nose or sinuses to the subarachnoid space.

A certain bacterial strain (meningococcus) may cause local epidemics within relatively confined environments, such as boarding schools or military bases. It produces a purplish rash in 50 percent of cases. The disease may be rapidly fatal if not treated promptly with penicillin or another suitable antibiotic. A vaccine will be recommended to those who may have been in contact with affected individuals. In addition, other bacterial strains that cause sporadic cases of meningitis include *Haemophilus influenzae*, *Streptococcus*, and *Staphylococcus*. A *Haemophilus* vaccine is available for children who are at least 18 months of age to prevent *Haemophilus* infections (see page 1079).

Treatment

Medication

After diagnosis of acute bacterial meningitis, antibiotic drug therapy is instituted immediately and will vary, depending on the type of bacteria causing the infection. In some cases, treatment for brain swelling, shock, convulsions, or dehydration may be needed.

Other Therapies

Drainage of infected sinuses or mastoids may be needed. If fluid has accumulated between your brain membrane layers, it may need to be drained or surgically removed.

Encephalitis

Signs and Symptoms

- Drowsiness
- Confusion and disorientation
- Seizures
- Sudden fever

- Severe headache
- Nausea and vomiting
- Tremor
- In infants, bulging in the soft spot of the skull
- Occasionally, a stiff neck

Emergency Symptoms—Altered levels of consciousness

Encephalitis is a rare and acute inflammatory disease of the brain caused by a viral infection. Encephalitis sometimes occurs in a primary form when the disease is due to a direct viral invasion of your central nervous system. Its most common form, however, is secondary (postinfectious) encephalitis, which follows or occurs with a viral infection in some other part of your body such as measles, chickenpox, rubella, or mumps. The cause in some of these secondary cases is believed to be a hypersensitivity reaction.

Secondary encephalitis arises from within your body, but the primary form results from the environment around you. The viruses can be sporadic or epidemic. The most common sporadic form, herpes simplex encephalitis, can be particularly deceptive when it starts as a minor illness with headache and fever. This is followed by neurologic symptoms, which may include difficulty in talking, weakness, confusion, unconsciousness, repeated seizures, and the symptoms described above. Epidemic varieties may be due to arboviruses. These are mosquito-borne and infect you only in warm weather.

Some 1,500 to 2,000 cases of encephalitis are reported annually in the United States.

Diagnosis
In infants, a bulging in the soft spot of the skull (the fontanelle) and a stiff neck are key symptoms. In older children, severe headache and sensitivity to light may be more significant. In adults, mental disturbances, from severe disorientation to coma, may be the most outstanding clinical feature.

After the initial signs, the onset of neurologic symptoms can be variable. You may be severely ill within 24 hours, or a week may pass before the neurologic symptoms are apparent. In the case of secondary viral encephalitis, the disease may develop 5 to 10 days after onset of the initiating viral infection.

Encephalitis usually is diagnosed by analyzing your cerebrospinal fluid, which is extracted by a lumbar puncture (see page 485). Analysis of the fluid reveals a normal glucose level, increased white blood cell count, and failure of culture of the fluid to show the presence of bacteria. Your physician will be able to rule out acute bacterial meningitis (see page 481). When hemorrhages are part of the illness, your cerebrospinal fluid may be slightly bloody. Electroencephalography, MRI, or CT (see pages 1344 and 494) can help to confirm the diagnosis of encephalitis.

Diagnosis of herpes simplex encephalitis is sometimes difficult. Recent advances using sensitive DNA methods have allowed detection of virus in the spinal fluid, confirming the diagnosis. However, if negative, and if symptoms warrant, a biopsy from the brain may be necessary. Because this biopsy involves some risk, treatment with an antiviral agent is initiated early. If no response occurs with antiviral treatment, a brain biopsy may be advised.

How Serious Is Encephalitis?
The course of viral encephalitis is variable. It may be of short duration and benign, or it may strike with great severity and leave significant mental impairment. Such impairment can include loss of memory, the inability to speak coherently, lack of muscle coordination, paralysis, or hearing or vision defects.

The most acute phase of the illness can last from a few days to a week. The duration of the characteristic fever may be 4 to 14 days. Resolution may be gradual or abrupt. Resultant neurologic defects can continue to resolve over weeks or months. Even severely ill persons can have complete recovery.

The mortality rate varies with the source of the virus. Insect-borne sources might cause low mortality one year but severe mortality in the next.

Treatment

Medication
In the case of herpes simplex encephalitis, an antiviral agent such as acyclovir has been used with success in the early stages. For some patients, anticonvulsant medication may be needed.

Other Therapies
Because viruses that cause encephalitis do not respond to antibiotics, basic treatment is supportive and consists of rest, nourishment,

and sufficient fluid intake to let your natural defenses fight the virus. In early convalescence, irritability is common. For persons left with mental impairment, physical and speech therapies may be needed.

Reye's Syndrome

Signs and Symptoms—Persistent nausea and vomiting after a viral infection

Emergency Symptoms
- Drowsiness
- Stupor
- Loss of consciousness or coma
- Delirium, seizures, or convulsions

Reye's syndrome is relatively rare. It was first identified as a distinct disease in 1963. This is a serious disturbance that follows a viral infection in children. It affects the blood, liver, and brain. Characteristics include high levels of ammonia and acidity but a low level of sugar in the blood, fat deposition and swelling in the liver, and brain swelling that produces the emergency symptoms listed above.

The specific cause for Reye's syndrome is unknown, although giving aspirin may trigger it in children. It occurs almost exclusively in children between 2 and 16 years old, soon after a viral infection such as chickenpox or influenza or even an ordinary upper respiratory infection. There is, however, almost never any evidence of a virus in the liver or brain, which are the two areas most affected by Reye's syndrome. Fever is usually not a symptom, although fever occurred with the prior illness.

Diagnosis
Symptoms typically start almost a week after the viral infection. At first there is persistent nausea and vomiting for 1 to 3 days, followed by a progressive decline in your child's mental alertness as the brain swelling increases. This progresses from lethargy and drowsiness to stupor and deepening stages of coma. Episodes of agitation, seizures, or convulsions may occur. These symptoms develop rapidly over a few days, and immediate medical attention is required.

After examining your child, your physician may require further tests to complete the diagnosis. A blood analysis may provide further evidence of Reye's syndrome, but a liver biopsy is the definitive test. Cerebrospinal fluid may be extracted by lumbar puncture (see page 485) to exclude other diseases with similar symptoms, such as meningitis or encephalitis (see pages 481 and 482).

How Serious Is Reye's Syndrome?
Although the severity varies greatly, Reye's syndrome is usually an acute, life-threatening disorder. Emergency treatment is required. The chance for your child's survival depends on how far the disease has progressed and how quickly the body chemistry is stabilized.

Previously, the fatality rate was more than 40 percent. Now, with earlier diagnosis and better treatment, this rate has decreased to about 10 percent. Most children recover completely in 2 to 3 months, but brain damage may persist in a few cases.

Treatment

Prevention
The occurrence of Reye's syndrome is reduced by avoiding the use of aspirin in children younger than 16 years who have a viral infection. Moreover, aspirin is not recommended for children younger than 12 years with any illness. Other, safer alternatives include acetaminophen or ibuprofen.

Medication
Your child may require hospitalization in an intensive care unit while medications are given and vital signs are monitored. Medications usually are given intravenously. Your child's low blood sugar level is increased by giving glucose, the blood chemistry values are corrected with electrolyte solutions containing sodium, potassium, and chloride, and acidity is treated with basic solutions. Small amounts of insulin may be given to increase glucose metabolism. Brain swelling is controlled with a corticosteroid (dexamethasone) to reduce inflammation, and a diuretic (mannitol) is given to increase fluid loss through urination. Other medications may include purgatives, vitamin K_1, and oral nonabsorbable antibiotics (neomycin).

Monitoring of the pressure inside your child's skull may be used to guide the therapy. Arterial catheters commonly are used to monitor blood gases, acidity, and pressure. Other common procedures include the insertion of a tube into your child's airway to aid breathing (mechanical ventilation).

Lumbar Puncture

Lumbar puncture (spinal tap) is the procedure used to measure pressure in your cerebrospinal fluid (CSF) and to remove small samples of CSF for laboratory analysis. It also is used to inject spinal anesthetics, some medications, and substances for diagnostic imaging.

A local anesthetic is used at the puncture site. A thin, hollow needle then is inserted between two vertebrae in your lower back (lumbar region), through the spinal membrane (dura), and into the spinal canal. The vertebrae must be spread apart slightly to provide access, so you will be asked to lie on your side with your knees drawn up to your chest and both arms clasped around your knees. This position flexes the back and spreads the vertebrae. Some conditions, such as a spinal fluid blockage in your middle back, require the puncture to be made between two cervical vertebrae in your neck rather than the lower back.

Once the needle is in place, the fluid pressure is measured, CSF is extracted, and then the pressure is measured again. If a drug or substance is being injected, its volume will equal the volume of CSF that is withdrawn. The substance is at body temperature and injections are made slowly to avoid any shock to the central nervous system. The procedure usually takes about 30 minutes when a CSF sample is being extracted, but more time may be required for an injection. After the procedure, the puncture site is bandaged.

You may have a feeling of pressure during the procedure. Afterward, you may have a headache because of a decrease in CSF pressure if there is a persistent leak of CSF into the tissues. Lying down usually alleviates the headache, and it usually goes away as the pressure returns to normal in a few days.

A sample of your CSF may be required to aid in the diagnosis of various diseases. These include multiple sclerosis, Reye's syndrome, Guillain-Barré syndrome, infections of the central nervous system (meningitis, encephalitis, polio, or AIDS-related diseases), certain kinds of tumors, and subarachnoid hemorrhage that cannot be seen on a CT scan (see page 494). The CSF sample can be tested for protein, sugar, red and white blood cells, and malignant cells. The sample can be cultured to identify bacterial and viral infections.

Lumbar puncture also is used for injecting dye (contrast material) or radioactive substances when they are needed to make diagnostic images of CSF flow (see Myelography, page 510). Medications such as antibiotics and antitumor agents occasionally are injected during this procedure.

There are some risks with lumbar puncture, although they are fewer now than previously. Greater care is used to prevent infection, and the procedure is used more selectively. The availability of CT, for example, reduces the need to use lumbar puncture for diagnosing most types of intracranial hemorrhage when a lumbar puncture may be dangerous. The risks remain for persons with blood coagulation disorders, in which the procedure can cause bleeding where the needle penetrates the spinal membrane, and for persons with increased spinal fluid pressure, which can lead to compression of the brain stem after a sample of CSF is removed.

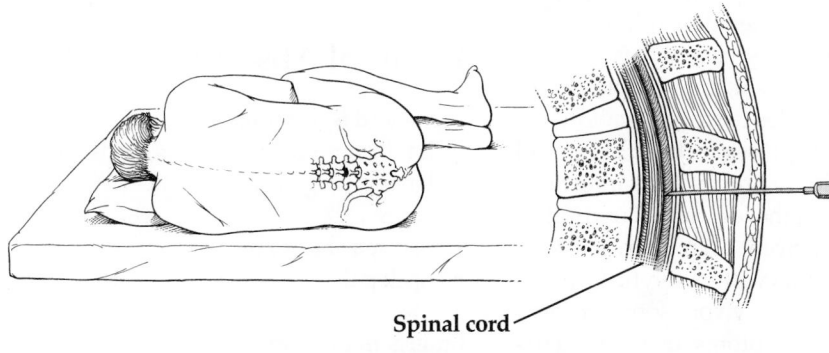

Spinal cord

In a lumbar puncture (spinal tap), you lie on your side, knees pulled to your chest, while a needle is inserted between two vertebrae and a small amount of cerebrospinal fluid is extracted for laboratory testing.

Poliomyelitis

Signs and Symptoms (for the acute paralytic form)
- Fever
- Headache
- Stiff neck and back
- Muscle weakness
- Difficulty in swallowing

Emergency Symptoms
- Weakness or paralysis
- Respiratory failure

Poliomyelitis, also called polio or infantile paralysis, is the result of a viral infection. The virus gains entry through your mouth, invades your body through the throat and digestive system, and spreads throughout the lymphatic system and the bloodstream. The polio virus is contagious and is passed by direct contact with feces or saliva contaminated with the mixture.

The disease may manifest as a minor illness (sore throat, mild upset stomach, and low-grade fever), as aseptic meningitis (see page 482), or as paralytic poliomyelitis. The paralytic form occurs when the virus goes from your bloodstream into your central nervous system and then infects the nerve cells of your brain stem or spinal cord which control muscular activity.

Diagnosis

Paralytic poliomyelitis sometimes is preceded by fever and a brief illness. The incubation period is usually 7 to 14 days and can be up to 35 days.

The key evidence is limb paralysis without loss of sensation. An analysis of your cerebrospinal fluid, extracted by lumbar puncture (see page 485), will show a normal cell count but increased protein level.

How Serious Is Polio?

A minor illness with complete recovery in a few weeks occurs in 90 percent of cases, mostly in children. Paralytic poliomyelitis, however, is an acute disease that occurs both in children and adults, striking adults most severely. It requires prompt medical attention.

The paralysis varies depending on the area of your nervous system that is affected. Brain stem involvement, for example, causes weakness in muscles used for swallowing, talking, facial expression, breathing, and blood circulation. Spinal cord infections cause paralysis of the legs, arms, or trunk.

About 2 to 5 percent of children and 15 to 30 percent of adults with paralytic forms of polio virus die. For survivors, some recovery from paralytic symptoms usually occurs gradually over 6 months. The paralysis that remains after 6 months is likely permanent and may be accompanied by severe pain. Fewer than 1 in 4 people with polio incur permanent disability.

Other possible complications include diseased heart muscles, high blood pressure, fluid in the lungs, shock, and urinary tract infection.

In some people, progressive weakness and atrophy of muscles occur many years after an acute episode of polio. The cause of this is uncertain (see Post-Polio Syndrome, page 487).

Treatment

Prevention

The two forms of vaccine are the Salk vaccine, which is given in a series of intramuscular injections and boosters, and the Sabin vaccine, which is administered orally. The Sabin vaccine is favored in the United States for routine childhood immunization. The Salk vaccine is recommended for those with immunodeficiency. The incidence of polio is low in the United States because of widespread vaccination. If you have never been immunized or are traveling to a developing country, consult your physician (see page 382).

Other Therapies

Mild illness requires bed rest for several days. Persons with paralysis need to be on a firm bed with a footboard to prevent the permanent inability to lift the foot (footdrop). Medications may include bethanechol for urine retention and antibiotics for urinary tract infections. A respirator (mechanical ventilator) may be required if the paralysis affects the respiratory muscles. A surgical incision into your windpipe (tracheotomy) may be needed if your breathing must be supported by a machine for an extended period of time. Physical therapy (see page 480) is important during convalescence.

Epidural Abscess

Signs and Symptoms

- Ear or nose pain with pus discharge
- Unrelenting headache
- Fever
- Nausea and vomiting
- Back pain and tenderness

Emergency Symptoms

- Reduced consciousness
- Growing loss of sensation, weakness, or paralysis in one side of the body or both legs
- Seizures or convulsions
- Speech disturbance

Epidural abscess is usually due to bacterial infection that causes pus to form between the outermost brain membrane (dura mater) and the bones of your spine or skull. Sometimes it invades the bone surface inside the skull or vertebrae. It also can penetrate the membrane layers to become a subdural

Post-Polio Syndrome

The late effects of polio, which some physicians call post-polio syndrome, can resemble arthritis, tendinitis, or amyotrophic lateral sclerosis (ALS, see page 477). Weakness can develop in any muscle, whether or not it was associated with the earlier polio attack. Joint pain and flu-like aching of the muscles are common. The syndrome affects about 25 percent of polio survivors.

Post-polio syndrome does not appear to be the reactivation of a long-dormant virus or a new infection. Because most individuals with post-polio syndrome are in their 30s or 40s, it cannot be attributed to aging. Current research focuses on nerve cells in the spinal cord. Normally, these cells deteriorate over time, but other cells compensate for the change. Polio survivors, however, lost some of their nerve cells during their childhood illness. People who recovered and then led physically active lives may have unknowingly overworked their remaining spinal nerve cells. Also, chronic overuse of undamaged muscles can lead to pain and weakness after many years.

To confirm the diagnosis of post-polio syndrome, physicians look for these criteria:

- Previous exposure to polio—the syndrome usually occurs in persons who were age 10 or older during the initial attack of polio and whose symptoms were often severe.
- Long interval period—the onset of late effects varies widely but typically begins about 30 years after the initial infection.
- Gradual onset—weakness can develop quickly over a few months but tends to be imperceptible until it interferes with daily activities. You may awaken refreshed but feel exhausted by midday, tiring after activities that once were no problem.

It is difficult to forecast the course of symptoms. Fortunately, the progressive weakness in post-polio syndrome commonly occurs only in minor degrees.

Although there is no specific treatment for the syndrome, see your physician if you are a polio survivor experiencing new muscle weakness or pain. Medications, including aspirin and nonsteroidal anti-inflammatory drugs, may relieve some painful symptoms. An occupational or physical therapist can analyze the ways you move during work or leisure and suggest ways to reduce muscle fatigue. Try exercises that are not as strenuous, such as swimming or water aerobics, and avoid overuse of your muscles.

Your attitude also plays an important part in your adjustment. Many communities are developing support groups for polio survivors which offer counseling, self-help tips, and practical advice.

---

abscess, a brain abscess, or meningitis (see page 481).

Epidural abscesses in your head may originate as infections in your sinuses, your ears, or the mastoid bones behind your ears. Head injuries also may allow the infection to penetrate the skull. Occasionally, bacteria will be carried by the blood to the epidural space from an infection elsewhere in the body. Abscesses in the spine can start from a boil on your skin, an infection in your lung or abdomen, or an infection associated with operation.

Epidural and similar abscesses are now relatively rare because the widespread use of antibiotics controls many infections in their early stages. The greatest risk is from chronic sinus or ear infections.

Diagnosis

As with meningitis, epidural abscess can be caused by direct infection or by an infection that is carried to the epidural area by the blood. Progressive headache or back pain with fever and tenderness around the infec- tion site may develop. As the abscess enlarges, it can cause direct pressure on the spinal cord or brain, resulting in pain and the loss of neurologic function.

The diagnosis of epidural abscess is suggested by the presence of an infection and the subsequent development of symptoms. Your physician probably will require an X-ray or MRI or CT scan (see page 494) of your head or spine to complete the diagnosis.

How Serious Is Epidural Abscess?

An epidural abscess can cause serious neurologic damage or even death if it is not treated promptly. Prompt treatment generally results in complete recovery.

Treatment

Medication

You will be given intravenous antibiotic therapy immediately to start controlling the infection. Epidural abscess sometimes is not cured by antibiotics alone, however, and an operation may be needed to drain the infected area. After the operation, antibiotics are usually given for 1 to 2 months.

Surgery

Prompt operation is sometimes required to empty the abscess and remove the pressure (decompression) on your spinal cord or brain. A section of your skull or spine is opened to provide access to the abscess and to facilitate drainage. If the abscess has penetrated any area of your skull or vertebrae, some of the affected area may be removed. Sometimes it is difficult to find and remove all traces of the infection, and your recovery may be complicated by reinfection.

AIDS and the Nervous System

Signs and Symptoms

- Headache
- Stiff neck
- Fever
- Speech difficulty
- Vision impairment
- Loss of memory, concentration, or other mental abilities
- Weakness, loss of sensation, or incoordination

Emergency Symptoms

- Partial paralysis, seizure, or convulsions
- Stupor
- Loss of consciousness or coma

Acquired immunodeficiency syndrome (AIDS) may lead to various nervous system diseases. AIDS is caused by a virus called human immunodeficiency virus (HIV). HIV may directly infect your central nervous system and cause progressive degeneration of nerve cells. The AIDS virus also suppresses your immune system. Thus, other microorganisms have an opportunity to infect you (opportunistic infection), and tumors may invade the nervous system. HIV can infect any level of the nervous system, including the meninges (outer covering of the brain), brain, spinal cord, or peripheral nerves.

Most persons with AIDS develop pneumonia or a rare skin cancer (Kaposi's sarcoma). Approximately a third develop nervous system diseases, which include viral, fungal, or bacterial infections that cause meningitis, encephalitis, or myelitis (inflammation of the spinal cord). Other diseases of the nervous system that occur in association with AIDS include parasitic cysts in the brain, abnormal growth of lymphoid tumors in the nervous system, and a progressive form of dementia. Peripheral nerve disease also has been associated with AIDS.

The occurrence and diagnosis of AIDS are described on page 1060. If symptoms of secondary diseases appear, your physician may obtain an MRI scan (see page 494), lumbar puncture (see page 485), or other laboratory tests for diagnosis.

Treatment

Some AIDS-related diseases of the nervous system are treatable, but the effectiveness of standard treatments (such as antibiotic therapy for bacterial infections) is limited by the state of immunodeficiency. Research on treatment is very active, and new medications are being tested.

Botulism

Signs and Symptoms

- Weak, limp muscles within 12 to 36 hours after consuming contaminated food
- Double vision
- Dry mouth
- Speech and swallowing difficulty
- Vomiting and cramps

Emergency Symptoms

- Rapidly progressive weakness or paralysis
- Breathing difficulty

Botulism is acute poisoning from the toxin produced by a microorganism (*Clostridium botulinum*) commonly found in soil. The organism is similar in many ways to that causing tetanus (see page 1070).

You can be poisoned from canned or home-preserved foods that were not cooked enough to destroy the organism's spores. Your infant may be poisoned by sources, such as raw honey, that do not affect adults. It also can occur from wounds that get contaminated by soil. Usually, but not always, the lids or sides of containers contaminated by this organism will bulge.

The poison blocks nerve signals to the salivary glands of the mouth and to muscles. This effect begins 3 hours to 14 days after consuming the poison. The diagnosis is based on the signs and symptoms and is confirmed by identifying the toxin in blood, food, or feces. Respiratory failure because of weakness of the muscles that control breathing causes death in 10 percent of food botulism cases and in 2 percent of botulism cases in infants. The disorder is now very rare because of careful preparation of food. Heating to boiling for 10 minutes will destroy the toxin.

Treatment

Avoid obviously contaminated or poorly prepared foods. Giving honey to infants is not recommended. Specific treatment consists of administration of antitoxins.

If the person affected with botulism survives the first few days, recovery is usually complete.

Structural Problems

The nerve tissue in your brain is delicate and easily torn, bruised, or damaged by pressure. Under ordinary circumstances, your skull and spinal membranes (meninges) provide protection, but during motor vehicle, industrial, and other accidents, the skull and membranes may prove inadequate. Structural damage to your brain from an accident can range from a mild concussion to permanent disability or death.

Other structural problems described in this section include tumors inside your head. Structural problems from bleeding inside your skull are described under subdural (see page 466) and extradural hemorrhage (see page 468). Structural problems with your spinal cord are described under spinal trauma (see page 506) and spinal tumor (see page 508).

Hydrocephalus

Signs and Symptoms

- Abnormal enlargement of the head (in newborns)
- Mental decline
- Slow and restricted body and eye movements
- Urinary incontinence

Hydrocephalus is caused by interference with the normal circulation of the cerebrospinal fluid (CSF) in the brain. CSF is produced by a membrane in your brain and later is reabsorbed from the subarachnoid spaces above your brain.

Congenital or postnatal hydrocephalus in infants can be due to a blockage in the brain's CSF circulation system or to an inability to reabsorb the fluid. The resulting pressure expands the loosely connected sutures in the skull so that in a newborn or young child, the head is enlarged abnormally in all directions, especially in the frontal area.

Your infant's symptoms may be mild and the progression might stop but then reappear in later childhood. The skull becomes firmly closed by age 5 years, so subsequent symptoms do not include appreciable head enlargement.

Congenital or childhood hydrocephalus due to a blockage in the circulation of CSF in the brain may be caused by various congenital malformations of the brain, a fetal viral infection, birth injury, or tumor. Hydrocephalus due to problems of reabsorption can result from brain malformation, an infection such as bacterial meningitis (see page 481), subarachnoid hemorrhage (see page 433), or spinal cord defects such as syringomyelia (see page 514) and myelomeningocele (see page 514).

In adults, a variation of hydrocephalus may occur in which the CSF pressure is normal (normal-pressure hydrocephalus) but the reabsorption of CSF is defective. The symptoms arise slowly after meningitis, head injury, or subarachnoid hemorrhage. They also may develop for no known reason.

Hydrocephalus in children is relatively uncommon; it occurs in approximately 1 of 1,000 children. In adults, normal-pressure hydrocephalus is also uncommon and occurs most frequently among elderly people.

Diagnosis

Your child's head may be measured at birth. If the circumference of the head exceeds a certain size, hydrocephalus may be suspected and the head will be measured frequently during the first weeks of life.

In later childhood and adulthood, symptoms will lead to further testing. In all cases, the diagnosis may require a skull X-ray or CT or MRI scan (see page 494) and an examination and culture of a CSF specimen obtained by lumbar puncture (see page 485).

How Serious Is Hydrocephalus?

The severity depends on the time of onset and whether the disease is progressive. If the condition is well advanced at birth, major brain damage and physical handicaps are inevitable. Death usually occurs early from an underlying infection. In less severe cases, with proper treatment, 40 percent of the affected persons have a nearly normal life span and intelligence.

Treatment

The goal of treatment is to reestablish the balance between CSF production and reabsorption. In young children with a slowly progressive condition, the drug acetazolamide sometimes diminishes CSF production. When the imbalance is due to a reabsorption problem, treatment may consist of repeated lumbar punctures to relieve pressure.

Surgery

An operation to implant a shunt is effective in many children and adults. The shunt, with tubing or valves (or both), is placed to circumvent the blockage or to divert excess CSF into the bloodstream or abdominal cavity, where it is reabsorbed. A successful shunt procedure will allow an infant's head size to become normal and will relieve symptoms in older children and adults. Shunt tubes may require replacement as a child grows. Successful shunts usually are maintained for life, but shunt infections can be a serious complication. In selected cases with a blockage (obstructive hydrocephalus), a new opening in the brain (ventriculostomy of the third ventricle) can eliminate the need for a shunt.

Concussion

Signs and Symptoms

- Brief loss of consciousness or memory after a head injury
- Headache
- Faintness
- Nausea or vomiting
- Slightly blurred vision
- Difficulty concentrating

Emergency Symptoms

- Persistent confusion or delirium
- Persistent drowsiness
- Progressive lethargy
- Dilation of a pupil
- Speech difficulty
- Partial paralysis
- Stupor
- Coma

Concussion is a brief loss of consciousness after a head injury. The impact creates a sudden movement of the brain within the skull. Such traumatic movement can produce a wide range of injuries, and concussion is the mildest form of these. No evident structural damage to your brain occurs with concussion, although there may be cuts or bruises on the skin outside your skull.

Head injuries usually are caused by traffic or industrial accidents, falls, and physical assaults. Accidents are the leading cause of death for males younger than 35 years, and head injuries are involved in more than 70 percent of these accidents.

The fatality rate due to head injury has been reduced in recent years through the use of motorcycle and sports helmets, hard hats, and seat belts and because of better ambulance services. Nevertheless, head injuries remain a serious problem.

Diagnosis

Get prompt medical attention for any impairment of consciousness or dazed feeling after a head injury. Diagnosis is complicated by the possibility of serious bleeding within the skull, which could require emergency surgery. Serious damage may include epidural or subdural hemorrhage (see pages 468 and 466) or other brain injuries (see page 491).

Symptoms of serious damage may be immediately obvious or they may not appear until hours or days after injury. Your state of alertness and attentiveness provides the key information for how much damage has occurred.

Your physician will examine you for signs of skull fracture and brain damage. Skull X-rays or a CT scan (see page 494) may be required to determine whether serious damage has occurred and whether your injuries are limited to a concussion. An observation period of 24 to 48 hours is recommended in a hospital or at home with your family or friends checking to see whether further symptoms develop.

How Serious Is Concussion?

Concussion is a minor, temporary injury without permanent brain damage. Accidental head injuries, however, cause death or brain damage in one of five cases, and any head injury is potentially serious.

The loss of memory (amnesia) associated with concussion usually involves only your experience just before and during the accident that caused the concussion. It may, however, encompass a few weeks (or rarely months) before the accident. Your recovery of memory commonly progresses from the more distant past to the recent experience.

About a third of all persons with concussion have a combination of symptoms, called postconcussive syndrome or post-traumatic syndrome, for some time after a head injury. In addition to headache and dizziness, these symptoms may include insomnia, irritability, restlessness, inability to concentrate, depression, or personality changes such as moodiness. Precisely why these symptoms occur in some people is unknown.

Treatment

Concussion is generally self-healing and little or no treatment is required. Your physician may prescribe acetaminophen or a stronger painkiller, such as codeine, to relieve your headache. Aspirin should be avoided because it can contribute to bleeding. Rest and relaxation with no activities requiring concentration or vigorous movement usually will facilitate recovery within a few days.

Athletes, such as football players or boxers, who have had a concussion should have a medical evaluation before returning to their sport.

Other Brain Injury

Signs and Symptoms—Headache

Emergency Symptoms
- Persistent confusion, drowsiness, or delirium
- Speech or breathing difficulty
- Difference in size of eye pupils
- Partial paralysis
- Seizures or convulsions
- Stupor
- Coma

Brain injury may result from a blow to the head or from an object that penetrates the head, such as a bullet or piece of industrial equipment. Traffic accidents, falls, industrial accidents, and physical assaults are the major causes of such injuries. Accidents, usually involving head injuries, are the leading cause of death in males younger than 35 years.

Concussion (see page 490) is the mildest form of head injury resulting in loss of consciousness without brain damage. Brain damage does occur, however, in about 20 percent of the 10 million head injuries reported each year.

Moderate to severe brain injuries can be associated with a fracture, torn membranes or nerve tissue, and bruises or hemorrhaging within your brain. There may be brain swelling or leaking of cerebrospinal fluid. Subdural or extradural hemorrhage is possible (see pages 466 and 468). Your symptoms may not appear for several days after the accident.

Diagnosis

Get prompt medical evaluation for any head injury that causes even a brief loss of consciousness or persistent symptoms. After an examination, your physician probably will recommend hospitalization for observation, testing, and treatment if you show any indications of brain injury. A CT scan (see page 494) may be needed.

How Serious Is Brain Injury?

Most persons with moderate head injuries recover in 1 to 6 weeks, although some disability may persist. Continuing convulsive episodes may occur in up to 50 percent of those who experience seizures after injury (see page 495). Severe injuries can be fatal or permanently disabling despite the best medical and surgical treatment.

Treatment

Emergency treatment is required for comatose patients with severe brain injuries. Medications, such as corticosteroids (see page 919), and possibly an operation are sometimes needed to control brain swelling, which can cause death.

Brain Tumor

Signs and Symptoms
- Headaches of recent onset
- Vomiting
- Weakness and lethargy
- Personality change
- Double vision
- Recent incoordination or clumsiness of arm or leg
- Intellectual deterioration

Emergency Symptoms
- Vision, sight, or speech difficulty
- Seizures
- Stupor

A tumor is any mass or growth of abnormal cells. Whether it forms in your brain or elsewhere, it can be benign or malignant. A malignant tumor is cancer. The disorders described here relate to the two major categories of brain tumor: primary and secondary.

Primary brain tumors develop directly in your brain. Their cause is unknown, and occasionally they are congenital or hereditary. Secondary (metastatic) brain tumors originate elsewhere in your body and are more common than primary tumors. They occur in one-fourth of persons with a malignant condition in other parts of the body (systemic cancer). Secondary brain tumors most often come from primary tumors in your lung or breast. Tumor cells from these organs move through the bloodstream (metastasize) to the brain, which is a common target of metastasis.

Both primary and secondary tumors may be located within your brain or in proximity to it, such as in the skull, brain membranes, supportive tissue, cranial nerves, or pituitary or pineal gland. Many types of tumors can originate in these locations, and each has its own symptoms, treatment, and prognosis.

Brain tumors can occur at any age. They may produce no symptoms (asymptomatic), or they can grow very slowly over many years and remain asymptomatic until they become large. Progressive problems then can develop rapidly.

Diagnosis
The symptoms listed above are typical of any expanding tumor because they increase the pressure in your skull and compress brain tissue, cranial nerves, and blood vessels. Emergency symptoms indicate the onset of serious neurologic involvement. Headaches of recent onset may be the key symptom. Neurologic problems then may be evident within days or weeks. Seek medical attention for any new or persistent headache.

A thorough physical examination might establish the suspicion of brain tumor. A CT or MRI scan of the head (see page 494) might be needed to confirm the diagnosis. A chest X-ray to check for possible metastasis from the lung or other tests to evaluate other areas of the body may be needed. Cerebral arteriography (see page 464) may be required if an operation is planned.

How Serious Is a Brain Tumor?
Once a brain tumor has caused neurologic symptoms, it is extremely important to proceed quickly with appropriate treatment. Benign tumors frequently are curable, although sometimes their location makes total removal impossible. If a tumor infiltrates the brain in an area where the tumor tissue cannot be totally excised, recurrence is likely after surgery. Both benign and malignant tumors can produce profound and irreversible neurologic impairment.

Treatment
Your therapy may include surgery, X-ray radiation to kill tumor cells, or anticancer drugs (chemotherapy) to halt the progress of the disease. Corticosteroid drugs to diminish brain swelling, anticonvulsants for seizures, and analgesic painkillers for headaches also may be prescribed. Some benign and malignant tumors can be removed com-

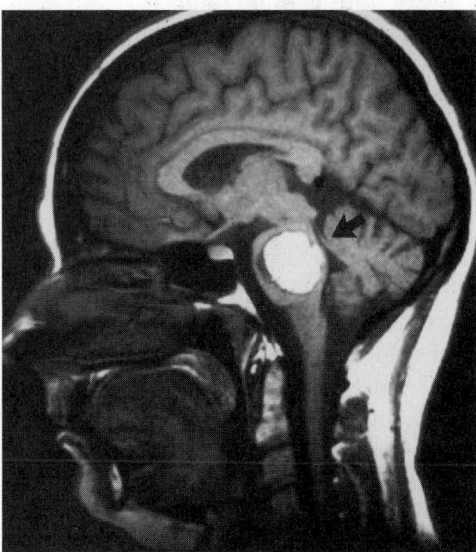

Magnetic resonance imaging (MRI) scan shows a tumor in mid brain (arrow).

pletely at operation. Others can be removed only partially or not at all, and radiation or chemotherapy may be recommended. Advances in computer-assisted surgery (stereotactic surgery) are making it possible to remove some tumors deep within the brain. If widespread cancer is present, the primary consideration is to provide comfort and preserve neurologic function.

Neuroblastoma

Signs and Symptoms

- Pallor
- Hypertension
- Diarrhea
- Abdominal mass, perhaps accompanied by liver enlargement if the tumor has spread to the liver
- Bone pain if tumor has spread to bone
- Respiratory distress if tumor has spread to chest

A neuroblastoma is a malignant tumor made up of neuroblasts, which are embryonic cells from which nerve tissue is formed. Neuroblastomas occur first in the abdomen, often around the adrenal gland, in 70 percent of cases. The disease then may spread to various parts of the body, including the liver, bone marrow, and bones.

Unlike most tumors, neuroblastoma has a high rate of spontaneous regression, although why this occurs is not clear. Neuroblastoma is found in 1 of 100,000 children under the age of 15; 75 percent of cases are diagnosed by the time a child is 5, with 24 months being the median age at time of discovery. The tumor occurs slightly more often in boys.

Diagnosis

The site of the suspected tumor and whether it is believed to have spread will determine what diagnostic studies will be done. If there is an abdominal mass, a CT scan (see page 494) may be done. To determine whether it has spread to bone, a bone scan and bone marrow biopsy may be done.

How Serious Is Neuroblastoma?

The prognosis of this disease depends on the age of the child and how advanced the disease is. The older the child and the more widespread the disease, the more likely that the cancer will not respond to treatment.

Treatment

If the tumor has not spread and is small, surgery alone or with local radiation therapy may offer a cure. In more advanced disease, chemotherapy may be successful. In persons with the most advanced disease, the long-term survival is less than 10 percent. A bone marrow transplantation in these children may achieve a 25 percent survival rate.

Bell's Palsy

Signs and Symptoms

- Sagging muscles and weakness on one side of the face
- Inability to close one eye

Bell's palsy (also known as facial palsy) is a paralysis of the muscles that control expression on one side of your face. Bell's palsy results from damage to the facial nerve, a nerve that runs beneath the ear to the muscles of the face of the same side. This damage results in weakness of these muscles because the electrical impulses directed to them are impaired by the damaged nerve.

The cause of the disorder is unknown, and its development is not well understood. The prevalent theory is that the facial nerve becomes swollen and injured, perhaps by a viral infection such as herpes zoster (see Shingles, page 1011). The nerve then has no room to expand within its bony channel. Bell's palsy is due to this restriction or compression.

Full paralysis on one side will leave you looking expressionless, and you will have virtually no movement of the muscles from the forehead to the mouth on the paralyzed

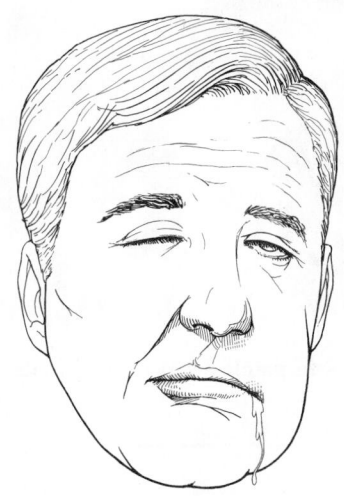

If you have Bell's palsy, one corner of your mouth may droop, and you may have difficulty retaining saliva on that side of your mouth. Most often, this disorder is temporary.

CT and MRI Scans

The computerized scanning equipment introduced during the past 20 years has virtually revolutionized diagnostic neurology and neurosurgery. The two types of procedures most commonly available are computed tomographic (CT) scanning and magnetic resonance imaging (MRI).

Although their computerized scanning techniques are similar, CT and MRI rely on two distinct methods for producing the diagnostic image. CT scanning uses an ultrathin X-ray beam; MRI uses a very strong magnetic field. Both procedures are noninvasive.

During CT scanning, an X-ray beam passes through your body. Various tissues, such as bone or fluid, absorb different amounts of the beam. The intensity of the beam that emerges from your body is then measured by an X-ray detector. Your tissues appear as different shades of gray on the scan. Bone is at one end of this spectrum and appears white on the image; air is at the opposite end of the spectrum and appears black.

When you are in a magnetic field during MRI testing, each hydrogen atom in your body responds to the magnetic field. The degree of hydrogen response depends on the type of tissue or its water content. A magnetic field detector measures the responses of the atoms. You receive no radiation. The magnetic field may affect metallic devices such as a heart pacemaker, inner ear implant, brain aneurysm clip, or embedded shrapnel.

Scanning with CT or MRI is done by taking detector measurements from thousands of angles all around your body while you lie on a special table. These measurements are made automatically by the equipment, and all the data are then processed by computer to create a composite, three-dimensional representation of your body. Any two-dimensional plane, or slice, can be selected electronically from this representation and displayed on a television-type screen for examination. Photographic images can also be produced from the screen for further analysis.

CT and MRI have several advantages over other procedures. CT shows internal structures (soft tissues) much better than conventional X-rays do, and it often reduces the need for higher-risk invasive procedures, such as cerebral arteriography (see page 464) or exploratory surgery. It is particularly useful for clear images of brain disorders, including strokes, hemorrhages, injuries, tumors, abscesses, cysts, swelling, fluid accumulation, and areas of dead brain tissue. CT scanning sometimes can distinguish benign from malignant tumors, because it is sensitive enough to show their different densities.

MRI applications still are undergoing rapid development. It is particularly useful for imaging areas of your head where soft and hard tissue meet, your spinal cord, and areas affected by stroke that cannot be seen well on CT scans. MRI often is used in the diagnosis of nerve fiber disorders, such as multiple sclerosis, because of its high-resolution images of the brain's white and gray matter. CT and MRI also are finding significant applications in the diagnosis of disorders in other parts of the body, including the kidneys, urinary tract, pancreas, and liver.

CT and MRI are safe, painless, simple procedures often done on an outpatient basis. They allow prompt diagnosis and treatment and enable effective follow-up studies.

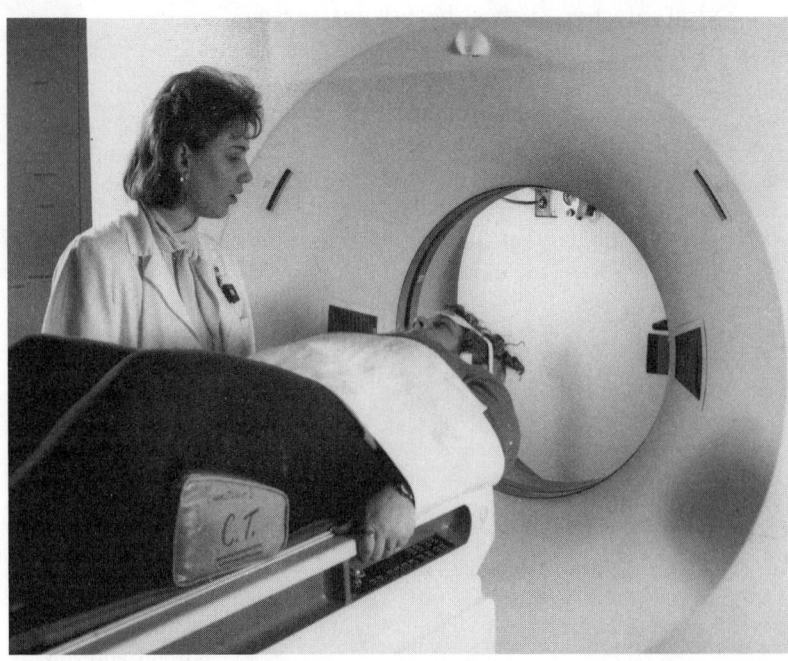

Computed tomography (CT) is a safe, painless way to obtain a detailed image of the brain.

side. The corner of your mouth may droop, and you may have difficulty retaining saliva on that side of your mouth. When you move the muscles of the unaffected side, facial distortions result. The eye on your affected side may close only partially, and tears may leak from that eye. Some persons complain of pain behind the ear, in the jaw, or on the entire side of the face. You may feel that the unaffected side is twisted or contracted, and you may experience changes in salivation and sense of taste, heightened sensitivity to sound, or difficulty in speaking or eating. Extra tearing from your eye on the affected side may result if the lid loses its normal function of moving tears into your tear ducts.

One-sided facial weakness is a common neurologic sign, and Bell's palsy is the most common cause. It occurs at any age, but it is most common between 30 and 60 years. Sometimes it seems to be associated with an infection of the middle ear. Annually, about 40,000 Americans get the disorder (1 person in 60 or 70) during their lifetimes. If it involves both sides of the face, other disorders such as Lyme disease (see page 1067) or sarcoidosis (see page 721) may be the cause.

Diagnosis

The onset is fairly abrupt, and you may notice it when you wake up. Pain behind your ear can precede the palsy by a day or two. Maximal weakness or paralysis may be apparent within 48 hours after onset.

Your physician may be able to make a preliminary diagnosis by looking at your face and asking you to attempt to move your facial muscles. Other conditions, such as a stroke (see page 461), can cause one-sided facial paralysis, and careful evaluation is needed to exclude these disorders. Abrupt onset with no prior symptoms, however, is indicative of Bell's palsy. After several days,

your physician may arrange for you to be tested by electromyography (see page 1344) to determine the severity of your nerve damage.

How Serious Is Bell's Palsy?

Bell's palsy is usually a temporary problem. In 80 percent of cases, recovery begins in 2 to 3 weeks and is complete within a few months. A mild case may be noticeable only when you smile, and it normally disappears in 1 month. A partial resolution of the paralysis by the end of the first week suggests a favorable outcome.

Recovery after total paralysis is variable, and electromyography (see page 1344) may be helpful for determining the possibility of long-term or incomplete regeneration of nerve fibers. If the damage to the facial nerve is unusually severe, the fibers may become irreversibly damaged. Another complication can arise from misdirected regrowth of nerve fibers, which can result in contraction of other muscles during facial movement or "crocodile tears" during salivation.

Treatment

Treatment is controversial. Some physicians believe that recovery, to whatever extent, will occur without treatment. If you cannot close your eye, however, it will need to be protected. Excessive dryness in your eye may lead to a corneal ulcer. A temporary patch or ointment may be recommended for sleeping. Use of moisturizing eyedrops, such as methylcellulose drops, during waking hours will help guard your eye from dust and dryness. Use of eyeglasses also may help.

Physicians sometimes prescribe a corticosteroid medication, such as prednisone, to reduce the suspected swelling of your facial nerve. Physical therapy and facial massage to prevent long-term contracture may be recommended.

Seizures

During normal waking and sleeping, the brain cells produce various electrical patterns that can be recorded and identified with a test called electroencephalography (EEG, see page 1344). If the electrical discharges by the brain cells become disorganized, a convulsion or seizure occurs.

Seizures have many causes. If you have a single episode, it does not necessarily indicate that you have a seizure disorder. When seizures recur, however, the condition is termed a seizure disorder. This designation is now preferred to the older term epilepsy.

Grand Mal Seizure

Signs and Symptoms—Episode of loss of consciousness with convulsions

A grand mal (tonic-clonic) seizure starts with a loss of consciousness and falling down, followed by a 15- to 20-second period with muscle rigidity (tonic phase) and then a 1- to 2-minute period of violent, rhythmic convulsions (clonic phase). The seizure ends with a few minutes of deep, relaxed sleep before consciousness returns with no memory of the seizure. You may experience a headache and drowsiness or confusion afterward. A grand mal seizure also is called a generalized tonic-clonic seizure in reference to its phases.

Grand mal seizures are due to abnormal electrical activity throughout the brain. In most cases, seizures seem to occur randomly, but for some susceptible persons, they are associated with menstruation and, rarely, reactions to a specific stimulation by light, sound, touch, or reading. Sometimes the seizures will involve only a few muscles, such as one side of the face or one extremity. This is called a focal seizure.

Research has shown that seizures can be produced in normal brains by various chemical and electrical stimulants. Sometimes seizures run in families. Other identified causes for recurring seizures include scar tissue from brain disease or injury; brain infection, tumor, abscess, or hemorrhage; alcohol or drug withdrawal; and metabolic disturbances from kidney or liver disease. Nevertheless, the cause frequently is unknown when the disorder starts before age 25. Seizures that start after age 25 may be caused by slowly growing brain tumors.

Up to 2 percent of the population have a seizure disorder, and as many as 10 percent of the population have a single seizure episode. Of these, the vast majority are grand mal seizures, sometimes in combination with other types of seizure.

Diagnosis

Grand mal seizure is recognized easily, but the cause may be difficult to diagnose. Your physician will need a detailed medical history. After physical and neurologic examinations, you will need electroencephalography (see page 1344). Other diagnostic tests may include CT or MRI (see page 494), blood tests, or lumbar puncture (see page 485). Focal seizures are sometimes caused by scarring or tumor in a specific part of the brain. A CT or MRI scan may help confirm such a diagnosis.

How Serious Is Grand Mal Seizure?

A single seizure, with no other signs of abnormality, does not necessarily mean you have a seizure disorder. Recurrence, however, may indicate a serious underlying disorder.

A seizure that produces either loss of awareness or control can be dangerous if you are driving a car or operating other equipment. Therefore, many states have licensing restrictions that are related to how well your seizures are controlled. Seizures also can produce injuries associated with falling.

Treatment

If your seizures are infrequent, you can lead a relatively normal life with the grand mal form. Medication may be very successful in controlling this type of seizure disorder. Discuss antiseizure medication side effects with your physician. Pregnancy may alter your need for medicine. Inform your physician if you are contemplating becoming pregnant. Avoid lack of sleep, forgetting medication, and excess alcohol. Regular and adequate rest is important. Wear a bracelet or necklace stating who should be contacted if a seizure occurs.

Children with a seizure disorder may attend school while taking medication.

Medication

Medication controls or greatly reduces seizures for more than 75 percent of affected persons. Drug selection and dosage require close medical supervision and testing. You may have side effects such as drowsiness, restlessness, upset stomach, or a rash. In some cases, the medication can be discontinued after several years without seizures, but this must be done by a gradual decrease in dosage, not abruptly. If your seizures are due to an underlying condition such as an infection or endocrine disorder, they may be eliminated when the cause is treated.

Gabapentin (Neurontin) is a new medication that improves management of epileptic seizures in 25 percent of people with seizure disorders who don't respond to traditional drug therapy. When taken in combination with other drugs for seizure disorders, gabapentin can prevent seizures that were previously uncontrollable.

Surgery

Seizures caused by a brain tumor, abscess, or hemorrhage may stop after surgical removal of the lesion. Occasionally, for people whose seizures are difficult to control, surgery may be an option. The site of seizure activity can be identified using an electroencephalogram (EEG) and surgically removed.

Petit Mal Seizure

Signs and Symptoms

- Brief, sudden absence of conscious activity
- Decline in a child's learning ability

Petit mal seizure, also called absence seizure, is a form of seizure disorder. Each seizure lasts only seconds or minutes, but hundreds may occur each day. In typical seizures, there may be no movement at all, fluttering eyelids, or a twitching hand during the brief lapse of consciousness. Full recovery takes only seconds, and afterward you will have no confusion. You will not remember the incident.

Atypical petit mal seizures include more noticeable muscle movement such as rhythmic convulsions, rigidity, or falling down. After atypical seizures, there may be a period of confusion, and recovery takes longer than after typical petit mal seizures.

In either case, these seizures almost always begin in children age 6 to 12 and rarely start after age 20. After onset, they may occur for weeks or months before any adult notices them because they usually occur when the child is sitting quietly and seldom during physical activity. Your child may begin to have learning problems before you or a teacher discovers the seizures.

Less than 10 percent of all persons with seizure disorders have petit mal seizures, sometimes in combination with other types of seizure. Usually, no identifiable cause is found for the typical seizures, and your child probably is neurologically normal otherwise. Atypical seizures often are associated with other neurologic disorders that may or may not have identifiable causes, such as congenital malformations in the brain, chemical disturbances from kidney or liver disease, or brain tissue scarring from head or birth injuries.

Diagnosis

No findings on physical or neurologic examination will confirm the diagnosis of petit mal seizures. Your child will need electroencephalography (see page 1344) to test for signs of the distinctive brain electrical pattern associated with these seizures. Your physician also may order blood tests or a CT scan (see page 494) to check for other possible causes for the symptoms.

How Serious Is Petit Mal Seizure?

About 90 percent of all children with petit mal seizures have significantly fewer or no seizures when they take medication. About a third outgrow the seizures, a third continue with only petit mal seizures, and a third continue with petit mal and have occasional grand mal seizures (see page 496).

Treatment

Most children with typical petit mal seizures can live fairly normal lives and should be encouraged to do so. Your physician probably will advise you that your child can participate in physical activities and school with few restrictions. There may be some restrictions with driving or operating dangerous equipment when your child gets older.

Medication

Petit mal seizures are usually very responsive to antiseizure medications. On these medications, most persons are seizure-free. Close medical supervision and testing are required to determine the best drug and dosage for your child. These drugs may cause side effects such as dizziness, upset stomach, or lethargy.

Febrile Seizure

Signs and Symptoms—Brief episode of loss of consciousness and convulsions during fever

Febrile seizure is a type of grand mal seizure (see page 496). It frequently occurs in young children between 3 months and 5 years during an illness with fever. Susceptibility to fever-induced seizures often runs in families, and your child probably will outgrow this reaction to fever.

Approximately 2 to 5 percent of children have seizures at some time in their lives when they get a fever. The cause is unknown, but seizures can occur easily and from many causes.

Diagnosis

If your child has a convulsion while a fever is present, seek medical attention immediately. Often the seizures occur when the temperature is either rising or falling rapidly. Other, more serious diseases such as meningitis (see page 481), encephalitis (see page 482), or poisoning also may first become apparent with this combination of symptoms, and emergency treatment may be required.

Your child's physician will ask about your family medical history and perform physical and neurologic examinations on your child. A lumbar puncture (see page 485) may be required at this time to help rule out the presence of serious infections that may have caused the seizures. If the fever is clearly due to a common childhood illness, only electroencephalography (see page 1344) may be required to test for abnormalities in the electrical activity of the brain. If there is no sign of abnormality, the diagnosis is usually febrile seizure.

When there is any sign of another cause for the fever or the seizure, however, a CT scan or MRI (see page 494), lumbar puncture (if not done earlier), blood tests, and further EEG testing may be required.

How Serious Is Febrile Seizure?

Febrile seizure is not a chronic condition. It happens suddenly and only when your child has a fever. If the seizure causes a loss of consciousness that does not last more than 5 minutes, the chances of mental impairment or a convulsive disorder are minimal.

There is a significant risk of future seizures, however, if your child has a prolonged seizure, local rather than general convulsions, an abnormal electroencephalographic recording, or signs of any neurologic abnormality. Most often, seizures can be controlled or reduced significantly with medication.

Treatment

Your child's febrile seizure should last only a few minutes. Place your child on the ground or lying flat and remove any nearby objects that could be a source of injury. Do not put anything into your child's mouth during a seizure. Roll the child onto his or her side to make sure the tongue does not block breathing. Keep attentive to your child's needs during the entire seizure. Following the episode, report the seizure to your physician. Rapidly cooling the child does not prevent further seizures.

Medication

After your child has a single episode of seizure during a fever, your physician may or may not prescribe medication. When susceptibility to febrile seizure is demonstrated by at least two episodes, your physician may recommend quick and vigorous control of fever during childhood illness as a way to avoid seizures. An alternative procedure is continuing treatment with anticonvulsant medication. In this event, further medical tests and supervision may be required to select the best drug and dosage. Side effects, such as restlessness, may result from some medication.

If no seizures occur after a few years or less and results of electroencephalography and neurologic examinations are normal, your physician may start reducing your child's medication dosage. Many children eventually can stop taking all medication and remain free of seizures.

Temporal Lobe Seizure

Signs and Symptoms

- Sensory or mental aberrations preceding a seizure
- Brief loss of awareness

Temporal lobe seizures frequently are preceded by a peculiar sensation (aura) and are followed by physical movements. These seizures most often originate in the temporal lobe areas of your brain, the portion that extends from your temple to just past your ear. If the seizure is associated with altered consciousness, it may be termed a complex partial seizure. Another name for this disorder is psychomotor seizure. The recurrence of this or any other type of seizure is called a seizure disorder.

Temporal lobe seizures frequently are characterized by 1- to 2-minute episodes of lost awareness or contact with your surroundings. The physical movement can be a simple repetitive act such as lip smacking or picking at your clothes. You may take seconds to hours to recover normal mental activity, and you may not remember the seizure.

Complex partial seizures are due to abnormal electrical activity in the temporal lobe or, less frequently, in another part of the brain. The aura, the first symptom, is caused by an electrical discharge in the area. This is followed by spread of the abnormal firing of the brain's nerve cells, which gives rise to other manifestations of the seizure such as loss of awareness.

The aura, which usually precedes the seizure by seconds or a few minutes, is variously described as hallucinations (sight, sound, or smell), visual illusions (rotating, shrinking, or magnifying), distorted understanding (déjà vu, or recurrent memory), and sudden, intense emotion (anxiety or fear).

Seizures sometimes are caused by a specific disorder in the temporal lobe, such as tiny scars or a tumor, but often there is no identifiable cause. Of the 1 to 5 million persons in the United States with a seizure disorder, about one-half have complex partial seizures.

Diagnosis

Your physician will need an extensive medical history for you and possibly your family. Diagnostic tests usually include electroencephalography (see page 1344), blood tests, and CT scan or MRI (see page 1334).

How Serious Are Temporal Lobe Seizures?

Once they begin, these seizures may become a chronic condition and may not be controllable with medication. Sometimes the source of the abnormality can be removed surgically. The frequency of seizures is reduced significantly in three or four out of five persons who have such an operation. Associated congenital or personality disorders sometimes exist and may not change after operation.

A medical bracelet can be helpful. These bracelets state who should be contacted if a seizure occurs and what medications are to be used.

Treatment

Medication
You will require long-term use of medications to minimize seizures. Medication may not completely control these seizures. Selection of the drug and its dosage requires close medical supervision and testing. These medications may produce side effects such as restlessness or sedation. Complex partial seizures are harder to control with medication than are other seizures. New drugs are being tested for this purpose.

Surgery
When the cause of temporal lobe seizures can be identified as a tumor or can be localized to an area within one lobe, operation may be recommended to remove the source.

Headaches

Almost everyone experiences a headache at one time or another. During a few hours of television viewing, you probably will see several advertisements for painkillers to ease this common complaint. Headaches have many causes, and the site, severity, and frequency with which they occur vary greatly.

Your brain tissue cannot ache. However, there is evidence to suggest that certain pathways within the brain stem and other portions of the brain may contribute to the production of various types of headaches. In fact, pain cannot occur in most of your skull and a large portion of your brain membranes. Observations made during surgery indicate that only certain structures in your head are pain-sensitive. On the outside of the skull, these structures include your skin and the tissues lying just beneath it: muscles, arteries, the skull coating, eyes, ears, and nasal and sinus cavities. The pain-sensitive structures inside your skull include arteries, venous sinuses and their tributary veins, parts of the outer membrane at the base of the brain, and certain cranial and cervical nerves. Pain is practically the only sensation produced by stimulating these structures.

Cranial or cervical nerves send pain sensations from these parts of your head to your central nervous system. Dental and jaw pain, for example, is conveyed by the cranial nerves. Your cervical nerves convey messages about pain in your neck and the base of your head.

Assessing Your Headaches

To help assess your pain, your physician may ask several questions about your headaches, such as the following:

- What is your age?
- What is the circumstance of a headache's onset?
- How frequently do they occur?
- Do they occur at regular intervals, and at what time of day or night?
- Where do you experience the first pain?
- What does the pain feel like? Is it intense?
- Do your headaches begin slowly or rapidly and how fast do your headaches go from beginning to peak?
- How long do your headaches typically last?
- Do other symptoms precede your headache?
- Do symptoms accompany your headache?
- What kinds of things make your headaches go away?
- Is there a history of headaches in your family?
- What are your present and past responses to medication?
- What ideas do you have about your headaches?
- Why are you seeking help now?

Outside your skull, pain is caused by inflammation or tension in muscles, inflammation of scalp arteries, and inflammation in your sinuses, ears, or gums. Inside your skull, enlargement or contraction of arteries, inflammation of brain membranes, and pressure from a tumor or hemorrhage can cause a headache.

Inflammation of your scalp arteries and subsequent stretching of pain-sensitive structures are associated with migraine and cluster headaches. Research suggests that migraine may be due to changes in your brain's blood vessels from disturbances in a chemical called serotonin, which is produced by nerve cells. Cluster headaches are more likely due to an interaction of the nerves and arteries of the head and release of a brain chemical transmitter.

Tension-type headaches (tension or muscular contraction headaches) are of uncertain origin. Some headache specialists feel that they are not completely distinct from migraine, but rather simply a milder form. Other experts see them as a completely different disorder, perhaps in part related to scalp-muscle tension.

Your physician's diagnosis will be based on a medical history and examination. If your headache is of recent onset, occurs in abrupt attacks, is triggered by exertion, is typically present in the morning and accompanied by vomiting, or is associated with other symptoms such as fever, weight loss, or neurologic abnormalities, further testing may be required.

Testing may include a CT scan of your head (see page 494) to look for any structural abnormalities and to examine your sinuses, facial bones, and neck tissue and bones. X-rays of the upper spine may be needed if your headaches began after a head or neck injury. Your physician may require other tests such as MRI (see page 494), a lumbar puncture (see page 485), or cerebral arteriography (see page 464), and also may consult with medical specialists to complete your diagnosis.

Your headache might feel dull, throbbing, or sharp. Your description of the quality of your pain will be helpful in diagnosing what type of headache you have. A throbbing pain is usually a vascular headache. When accompanied by nausea or transient visual disturbances, it is probably a migraine. Sharp, stabbing pain is more likely to be neuralgia (see page 514). Steady, nonthrobbing pain that may feel like a tight band is usually a tension-type headache.

Unrelieved headache pain that continues for 6 months or more as a major and disabling condition is considered chronic. Approximately 42 million Americans have chronic headaches, of which migraine (see page 502) and tension-type (see page 501) headaches are some of the most common forms.

Another common form is sinus infection headache. It usually is felt in your forehead, cheek, eye, or top of your skull. Headaches of this sort may also be caused by a vacuum or suction on the sinus wall. This occurs when air can enter the sinus because of congestion of the nose due to an infection or allergy. The vacuum effect also may be the source of the ear and sinus pain many people experience during the descent of an airplane, especially when they have a cold.

Premenstrual headaches, typically migraine or tension-type headaches, occur in some women during the premenstrual syndrome and usually disappear during the first day of vaginal bleeding. Headaches from high blood pressure tend to occur on awakening in the morning, are uncommon, and occur only with severe hypertension. Migraine headaches frequently occur in the morning. Headache can result from an infection in your nasal cavity, and it can be particularly painful when you bend over. Eyestrain headaches may occur after long periods of reading or driving a car at night. Headaches may occur from overexertion and can last intermittently for weeks or months.

Head pain also can be an indication of many underlying diseases. An acute, severe headache with tingling sensations, nausea, and vision or speech difficulties, for example, may be a symptom of a very serious cerebral hemorrhage. Any persistent headache of recent onset is potentially serious because it may be a symptom of a tumor, hemorrhage, or an aneurysm and also of meningitis, encephalitis, polio, abscess in the brain, or hemorrhage within the head. You need not be concerned by the occasional headache, but if one appears with other less-usual symptoms or if you have one that you might call "the worst ever," seek medical help.

For the common, everyday headache that may be caused by fatigue, stress, or overuse of alcohol or tobacco, your physician may advise you to avoid the offending activity and take a non-narcotic analgesic painkiller such as aspirin or acetaminophen.

Chronic headaches are more of a problem. Non-narcotic analgesics may relieve your pain but not get rid of it completely or prevent it from coming back. Antidepressant drugs may be prescribed. They are believed to work on certain brain chemicals to lessen pain and to modify your perception of it. Narcotic analgesics, such as codeine, may bring relief and can be particularly useful in combination with aspirin or acetaminophen. However, these should be used with caution because of the risk of addiction. The stronger the dose, the worse the side effects of nausea, constipation, and drowsiness. Ergot preparations, sumatriptan or methysergide, may be used to treat severe vascular headaches. These medications are unsafe if you are pregnant or breastfeeding or have high blood pressure or poor blood supply to your brain or legs.

Your physician will have two goals in helping control your chronic pain. First, he or she will try to simplify or minimize your medications to eliminate ineffective drugs. Dosages of your remaining medication will be decreased systematically until you are taking only those drugs that have the most benefit and the fewest side effects. Second, your physician will try to help you develop a better understanding of your pain and the factors that make it worse so that you can avoid them and increase your ability to function. Antidepressant medication may be useful for helping you do whatever is required to cut down your rate of headaches, from practiced relaxation techniques (see page 504) to a serious change in lifestyle.

Tension-Type Headaches

Signs and Symptoms—A dull or pressure-like pain in the scalp, temples, or back of the neck

A tension-type headache (also known as a muscle-contraction headache) is usually felt as diffuse and intense pain over the top of your head or back of your neck. It may feel like fullness or pressure, as if your head were surrounded by a constricting band or vise. The cause for this sensation is thought to be, at least in some cases, a tight, spastic contraction of the cranial and cervical muscles on the outside of your skull. There is some evidence that enlargement of the blood vessels in your scalp also may contribute to the pain.

You may find it difficult to sleep. Some people complain of a superficial stinging or burning sensation on their skin.

These headaches are common. Because they respond well to over-the-counter analgesic painkillers, persons with tension-type headaches usually do not consult their physicians. Tension-type headaches that occur two or more times weekly for a period of months or longer are considered chronic. Some persons report such headaches over a period of years or even decades. The headache pain usually has a waxing and waning quality.

Tension-type headaches are probably the most common cause of head pain. Some of them may be caused by poor posture, working in awkward positions, or a sudden strain. Stress, depression, and anxiety are the most common triggers.

These headaches may strike persons of any age or sex. The chronic form most frequently develops during middle age, and it can last for several years after onset.

Diagnosis
To establish a diagnosis, your physician will exclude other possible sources for your pain. Tests may include a urinalysis, vision tests, sinus X-ray, skull X-ray, or a CT scan (see page 494).

Your physician may want information about how you feel and will look for evidence of anxiety or depression and of whether you have any unusual fears about the state of your health. You may be asked whether there is any particular stress in your job or family situation that is associated with worsening of the headache.

How Serious Are Tension-Type Headaches?

Tension-type headaches are not life-threatening and do not lead to more serious disorders. They may, however, be a sign that you are depressed and anxious or subject to stress. Some persons who have tension-type headaches need treatment for depression.

Treatment

Tension-type headaches respond best to massage, hot and cold showers, practiced relaxation techniques (see Biofeedback, page 1121), and close attention to adequate rest and exercise. Physical therapy may be helpful. Keep a headache diary (see Migraine Headaches, this page) to try to identify the source of your pain. Medication is not a cure.

Moreover, the effectiveness of your painkillers or other drugs may eventually wear off. If tension-type headaches persist, your body may be telling you that serious changes are needed in your lifestyle.

Medication

Simple analgesics such as aspirin, acetaminophen, or ibuprofen are usually effective. Antidepressant drugs may be prescribed for a chronic problem. Avoid tranquilizers.

Migraine Headaches

Signs and Symptoms
- Intense head pain
- Nausea and vomiting
- Sparkling, rainbow-like colors, blank spots in your field of vision, or other auras

Migraines are also known as vascular headaches. The exact cause of migraines is unknown, although evidence suggests involvement of the blood vessels of your head.

A migraine headache usually begins in the early morning or during the day with intense, gripping pain on one side of your head that may gradually spread. The pain begins to throb on one side or over your entire head. It reaches the peak of severity in minutes to an hour or 2 and lasts for hours to 2 days, unless it is treated. It is often terminated by sleep, but you may be listless after waking up. The frequency of attacks can range from daily to one in several months. These attacks can be associated with nausea and, at times, vomiting.

Migraine has several clinical patterns: classic migraine (migraine with typical aura), common migraine (migraine without aura), and complicated migraine.

In migraine with aura (classic migraine), your headache is preceded by warning symptoms. About 20 minutes before the headache, neurologic symptoms often appear, including sparkling flashes of light, dazzling zigzag lines, slowly spreading blind spots, dizziness, or a feeling of numbness on one side of your body. The symptoms preceding the headache are referred to as the aura. Less commonly, aura symptoms include a slowly spreading weakness or numbness of your face, a hand, or a leg; a tingling and numbness in your lips; or difficulty with talking or writing. Rarely, these symp-

---

When Headache Spells Trouble

Headaches that signal a serious medical condition are uncommon, but they can accompany conditions such as a blood clot, a brain tumor, or a weakened blood vessel that could burst (aneurysm).

One rare headache-related condition that almost always begins after age 55 is temporal arteritis. This is an inflammation that affects arteries in your scalp, brain, and eyes. It's treatable, but if ignored, it can lead to blindness or, rarely, a stroke.

Tell your physician about any headache that concerns you. Even if you have a history of headaches, see your physician if the pattern changes or if it feels different.

If you have any of the following warning signs, see your physician or go to the emergency room immediately:

- Abrupt, severe headache, often like a "thunderclap"
- Headache with fever, stiff neck, rash, mental confusion, seizures, double vision, weakness, numbness, or speaking difficulties
- Headache after a recent sore throat or respiratory infection
- Headache after a head injury, even if it's a minor fall or bump, and especially if it gets worse
- Chronic, progressive headache that worsens after coughing, exertion, straining, or a sudden movement
- New headache pain after age 55

toms can be permanent, presumably because of a stroke (infarct).

Migraine without aura (common migraine) has no characteristic warning symptoms. Hours before the headache, you may be elated, full of energy, thirsty, hungry for sweets, drowsy, irritable, or depressed. These are sometimes referred to as premonitory symptoms. The headache usually builds to full intensity over several minutes or longer.

Complicated migraine is associated with prolonged neurologic symptoms that may outlast your head pain.

Less common forms of migraine headache include familial hemiplegic migraine (migraine with aura and paralysis of one side of the body; the affected person has at least one immediate relative who has identical attacks), migraine aura without headache (occurs mostly in elderly persons), ophthalmoplegic migraine (migraine with partial paralysis of the eyes), status migrainous (migraine persisting longer than 72 hours), and migrainous infarction (one or more aura symptoms that persist unabated for longer than 21 days).

Migraines may begin in childhood, adolescence, or early adulthood, and tend to taper off in number and intensity as you grow older. Migraine headaches strike many persons. Women are 3 times more likely to have migraines than men. Migraines may be associated with premenstrual tension. Attacks tend to decrease during pregnancy. There is a family history of migraines in about half of all cases.

The biologic causes of migraine are unknown, but many precipitating factors have been identified. A period of hard work followed by relaxation may lead to a "weekend migraine." Stress, premenstrual changes, alcohol consumption, hunger, or use of oral contraceptives causes migraines in some persons. Certain foods may produce attacks, including red wine, chocolate, aged cheese, milk, chicken livers, meats preserved in nitrates, or anything prepared with monosodium glutamate. Some persons even report that exposure to sunlight or exercise triggers their attacks.

Diagnosis

If you have migraines with characteristic warning symptoms or a family history of these headaches, your physician probably will have little difficulty diagnosing the con-

dition. If you do not have these traits or if the headaches are severe and of recent onset, you may need testing to rule out tumors, aneurysms, or other structural disorders that could cause your pain. You may need to have a lumbar puncture (see page 485) to analyze your cerebrospinal fluid, skull and sinus X-rays, vision tests, and CT scanning (see page 494).

How Serious Are Migraine Headaches?

Migraine is a chronic disorder without cure. The headaches are not life-threatening, and there is no proof that they lead to other disorders. With treatment, you should be able to reduce the number and severity of attacks.

Treatment

For Acute Attacks

Mild analgesics such as aspirin, acetaminophen, ibuprofen, naproxen sodium, or other nonsteroidal anti-inflammatory drugs may provide relief for mild to moderate migraines.

A combination of analgesic and barbiturate agents (such as aspirin, caffeine, and butalbital) helps some patients. The regular use of barbiturate compounds, however, may trigger daily headaches, and therefore they should not be used more than 2 days a week.

Antinauseants, such as metoclopramide, may be prescribed if your headaches cause nausea or vomiting. Some antinauseants can be prescribed in suppository form.

A drug called ergotamine has been used effectively for acute migraine. Sometimes, an analgesic painkiller is used in combination with it. Ergotamine can bring on headaches and other side effects such as nausea, vomiting, cramps, and tingling sensations. It should be used only a few times a week and not at all during pregnancy or breastfeeding.

Isometheptene is a drug related to ergotamine and provides relief for some patients when it is given in combination with an analgesic and a mild sedative (isometheptene, acetaminophen, and dichloralphenazone). Isometheptene may not be as effective as ergotamine, but it is better tolerated and produces fewer side effects.

The medication sumatriptan is a newer drug for the treatment of acute migraine attacks. There is evidence that it works by binding to certain serotonin receptors on cranial blood vessels.

Muscle Relaxation Techniques

When physicians refer to a muscle-tension problem, primarily involving pain, they may be speaking about a habit. People sometimes develop, over years, habitual muscle responses to stress (a tension habit). Muscle relaxation techniques have been developed to deal with pain from muscle tension. These techniques have been useful in disorders such as tension headaches, TMJ syndrome (see page 624), and backaches.

You may set yourself up for your symptoms. After a particularly trying day, you may wonder just when your headache will begin. You need strategy and discipline to break this cycle of tension causing pain causing more tension. Relaxation classes, yoga, walking, and jogging are a few of the many ways people help themselves relieve tension. Practiced relaxation techniques have been successful stress relievers for many individuals.

If you feel anxious, sit in a comfortable chair or lie down. Close your eyes. Begin to breathe slowly and deeply. Keep breathing deeply and rhythmically throughout the session. As you breathe in, let your stomach and chest expand with air. Contract them as you breathe out. In between, hold your breath for a few seconds. After some practice, a few breaths taken this way can calm you down during stressful situations.

Now tense the muscles of your toes and press down your feet. Hold them taut. Feel the tension in your toes and feet. Notice where the tightness is. Keep the muscles tight and concentrate on the tension for about 20 seconds. Then relax your toes and feet. Feel the tension leave your muscles. Feel them grow more and more relaxed, more and more heavy. Feel the warmth circulate through them as the tension drains away. Let all the tension in your toes and feet go. Say the words "calm" and "relax" silently to yourself. Put away all other thoughts. Let yourself feel more and more relaxed, and let that feeling increase.

When your feet and toes feel limp, perhaps in 30 seconds or more, go through the same procedure with another set of nearby muscles, moving very slowly up your body with one group of muscles at a time: your ankles and lower legs, your thighs, your pelvis and buttocks, your stomach, your fists, your arms, and your shoulders. Do not rush. Press your head into the cushion or pillow and tense the muscles in your neck. Clench your jaws. Frown and squint your eyes.

As you relax each section of your neck and head, keep telling yourself "calm" and "relax." Tell yourself how good it feels when you relax that part, and breathe deeply and fully.

When your entire body feels relaxed, keep your eyes closed and feel your heaviness. Press your heaviness into the surface you are on. As you breathe deeply, tell yourself several times that you are feeling very refreshed. Count to 3 and open your eyes (see Controlling Stress, page 307).

After taking medication when the first symptoms appear, some persons respond well to rest in a dark room and sleep, especially during a fully developed attack.

If your migraine is prolonged and associated with continued attacks of vomiting, seek emergency medical treatment to replace lost fluids and to control the pain.

Prevention

If you know that certain foods trigger a migraine, avoid them. It also may help to avoid oversleeping on holidays and weekends. You might consider discontinuing the use of birth control pills if you take them; about 30 percent of women with migraine have increased attacks when they take these.

If you have frequent headaches, keep a diary to give yourself clues about what triggers your attacks. Note the time a headache began, what you ate during the preceding 24 hours, how you felt (and what you were doing) when the headache started, unusual stress, how long the headache lasted, and what made it stop. Relaxation techniques (see this page) help some persons cut down the number of headaches.

If you have more than two migraines a month or your pain is especially prolonged, medications such as beta-adrenergic blockers, calcium entry blockers, nonsteroidal anti-inflammatory drugs, or methysergide maleate may be prescribed for daily use to prevent attacks.

Cluster Headaches

Signs and Symptoms

- Steady, boring pain in and around one eye, occurring in episodes that often begin at the same time of day or night
- Watering and redness of an eye, with nasal stuffiness on the same side of the face

Cluster headaches are characterized by intense burning, boring pain frequently located in or around one eye and temple and occasionally in one cheek or jaw. Your affected eye is bloodshot and teary. The nostril on that side often becomes blocked and may run profusely. Other features can include reduced pupil size on the painful side, a drooping eyelid, and a flushed face.

The pain swiftly intensifies within 5 to 10 minutes to a peak that typically persists for 30 minutes to 2 hours. Affected persons usually do not lie down during an attack because this position worsens the pain.

Cluster headaches have an abrupt onset and can occur at any time, but they most commonly occur 2 to 3 hours after you fall asleep, usually during the phase of deep sleep known as rapid eye movement (REM). Headaches can occur daily for days, weeks, or months before a remission period that lasts weeks or years (episodic attacks), or they can occur for a year or more without remission (chronic attacks). A chronic phase may begin after a period of episodic attacks.

Unlike migraine headaches, which more often affect women, cluster headaches predominantly affect men. The first attack most frequently strikes men during adolescence or their early 20s. Almost all affected persons are heavy smokers. There is usually no family history of similar headaches.

No specific cause has been found for cluster headaches. Some researchers believe these headaches are related to a chemical present in the brain and certain cranial nerves. This chemical causes blood vessels to enlarge and become painful. Consumption of alcohol can trigger cluster attacks if you are predisposed to them. Rarely, some foods may precipitate a cluster headache.

Diagnosis

If your symptoms are typical of cluster headaches, your physician might have little difficulty in diagnosing the condition. Nevertheless, you may need tests to exclude other ailments that can cause similar pain, including an aneurysm of the carotid artery in your head, a tumor made up of newly formed blood vessels, sinusitis, or glaucoma.

How Serious Are Cluster Headaches?

Cluster headaches are a chronic ailment. There is no known cure and little understanding of the periodic pattern of attacks. The headaches can be a lifelong disorder. The pain during an attack can be debilitating, but there is no permanent harm, and the condition does not lead to other disorders.

Treatment

If you have cluster headache attacks, keep a diary of your personal patterns and try to identify a trigger (see Migraine Headaches, page 502).

Cluster headaches are resistant to analgesic painkillers because these drugs take effect too slowly. Inhalation of 100 percent oxygen often provides relief. This may be the most effective treatment for frequent cluster headaches that occur primarily at night.

Ergotamine in suppository, tablet, or aerosol form is an effective pain reliever for some people, but the dosage must be limited to avoid side effects, especially nausea. It also may be prescribed to prevent attacks.

Corticosteroid medications, such as prednisone, may be prescribed if your cluster headaches are of recent onset or you have a pattern of short attack episodes and long remissions. Side effects prohibit long-term use.

About 60 percent of persons with cluster headache respond to methysergide maleate, which acts to relieve and to prevent the attacks. It is used during periods of pain and is tapered off slowly during remission.

Lithium carbonate can be effective during a chronic phase of cluster headaches. Then its dosage is tapered to avoid side effects.

Calcium channel blocking agents such as verapamil are effective for the prevention of cluster headaches in many persons. They often are continued for 3 to 4 weeks after the last headache and then are gradually tapered and discontinued under the direction of your physician. Occasionally, if the headaches are chronic, long-term use is required.

Chronic cluster headaches may require a management program that includes two or more of these medications. Surgery on certain groups of nerve cells near the brain may be recommended if drug management has not worked for you. Operation provides relief for approximately 66 percent of persons with chronic cluster headaches, but residual muscle weakness or sensory loss in certain nerves of the face and head can be a permanent disability.

Problems of the Spine and Peripheral Nerves

Your peripheral nervous system runs from your brain and spinal cord to all other parts of your body. It is the network of nerves that you use for all your movements and sensations. Damage to your spine or peripheral nerves can interfere with communication between your brain and other areas of your body.

Your symptoms can include pain in the affected area, impairment of your ability to move muscles, and numbness or abnormal sensations. The seriousness of damage may range from mild numbness that disappears in a short time to more chronic symptoms or even permanent injury such as paralysis. The following sections discuss many disorders that involve your spine and peripheral nerves.

Spinal Cord Trauma

Emergency Symptoms
- Weakness, incoordination, or paralysis in a part of the body after an accident
- Numbness or loss of sensation
- Loss of bladder or bowel control

Most spinal cord injuries are the result of traffic or industrial accidents, falls, gunshot wounds, and sports injuries, such as from diving or sledding. Sometimes a minor injury can produce severe trauma if you have a predisposing condition such as rheumatoid arthritis.

Various parts of your body can be affected by trauma at different places along your spinal cord because of the way its nerve fibers are organized. Your spinal cord is composed of long nerve fibers (tracts) leading from your brain.

The nerve tracts of the spinal cord feed into nerve roots that emerge between the vertebrae and organize into peripheral nerves that extend to your skin and muscles. If the spinal cord is injured, the nerve tracts passing through the injured region can be affected so that part or all of your corresponding muscles and sensations below that level may be impaired.

Spinal injuries occur most frequently in the lower back (lumbar) and neck (cervical) areas of the spine. A lumbar injury can affect leg and bowel and bladder control and sexual function. A neck injury may affect breathing as well as movements of the upper and lower extremities. Trauma on one side of the spinal cord typically impairs the muscles on the same side and some sensations on the same and opposite sides of your body.

Injury may result from your spinal cord being pulled, compressed, pushed sideways, or cut. It also could result from bleeding or the accidental insertion of a fragment of bone or metal into your spinal cord. Striking your chin on the steering wheel during a traffic accident, for example, may stretch your spinal cord and cause a tear. A bullet or knife wound can cut the cord. Often, injury to the spinal cord in the neck area occurs from a sharp bending of the neck during contact while playing football, from a shallow-water dive, or from a motor vehicle accident. Injury to the lower spine may result in a compression injury of the spine. Again, car and motorcycle accidents are common causes.

Bleeding within the spinal cord can cause some permanent loss of sensation and muscle weakness. When bleeding occurs outside the spinal cord, however, the cord may be compressed. This compression results in weakness or loss of sensation of the limbs and trunk, depending on the site of the bleeding.

Compression also may occur from fluid accumulations and swelling in your spinal cord. The resulting paralysis may continue for several days and then improve dramatically when the swelling subsides or the accumulated fluid is removed surgically, although some impairment may persist.

Most cuts and other severe forms of trauma to the spinal cord will cause permanent disability or paralysis because nerve fibers seldom regenerate. Paralysis below the neck can involve all four extremities (called quadriplegia) or only the legs and lower body (called paraplegia). Approximately 10,000 persons, mostly young and otherwise healthy, become paraplegic or quadriplegic each year in the United States because of spinal cord trauma. About 200,000 persons in the United States have quadriplegia.

Diagnosis

Numbness or paralysis may occur immediately after the injury. These symptoms also might appear gradually as fluid accumulates in or around the spinal cord after an accident. Urgent medical attention is required to minimize the long-term effects of this trauma.

After a physical and neurologic examination, diagnostic tests probably will be needed. These usually include X-rays, CT scanning or MRI (see page 494), or myelography (see page 510). Occasionally, lumbar puncture (see page 485) is also necessary.

How Serious Is Spinal Cord Trauma?

The immediate effect of a spinal cord injury is often paralysis or loss of sensation in part of your body. This can be fatal if a neck injury has paralyzed breathing. The time between injury and treatment is a critical factor that can determine the extent of your recovery.

Recovery of movement or sensation within the first week usually means the eventual recovery of most or all functions. Any impairment remaining after 6 months probably will be permanent. If your bladder control is lost, as is often the case with quadriplegia or paraplegia, you become susceptible to recurring urinary tract infections. You also will be susceptible to injury of any part of your body that has impaired sensation.

Treatment

You will need emergency care, prolonged hospitalization while the injuries heal, and possibly months of specialized therapy for rehabilitation.

Medication

You may be given corticosteroids (dexamethasone or methylprednisolone) to reduce any swelling that compresses your spinal cord. Antibiotics may be required for urinary tract infections.

Surgery

Surgical procedures may be necessary to remove fragments of bone or foreign objects, to fix fractured vertebrae by fusing the bone or inserting metal pins, or to decompress the spinal cord by draining accumulated fluids.

Other Therapies

Traction may reduce some dislocations of your spine and immobilize the back for healing. Sometimes traction is accomplished by placing fixation tongs into the skull to hold it in place. Bed rest is the primary treatment. Further neurologic assessment is used to check for signs that reflexes and sensations are returning.

Injuries will heal in 2 to 4 months, and then the physician can estimate how much

Paraplegia

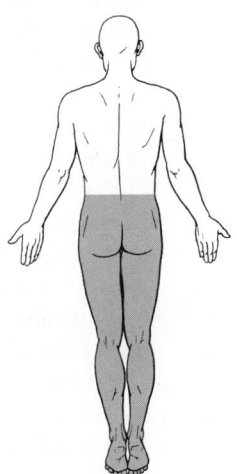

Quadriplegia

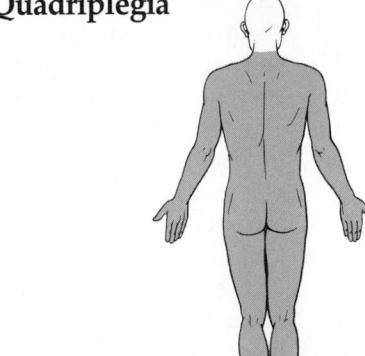

Paralysis of the lower body is called paraplegia. Paralysis below the neck is called quadriplegia.

disability will remain. At that time you may require the services of a special therapy team to obtain the best use from remaining muscle strength and to learn how to move with mechanical assistance.

Spinal Tumor

Signs and Symptoms
- Steadily increasing back pain
- Numbness or cold sensations
- Muscle weakness in one or more limbs

Emergency Symptoms
- Loss of bowel or bladder control
- Progressive loss of lower limb strength or sensation

Spinal tumors are abnormal growths that can occur within your spinal cord, between its covering membranes, or outside the membranes in the spinal canal. These growths are malignant in 40 percent of cases. Spinal cord tumors are similar to brain tumors (see page 492) but are only one-fourth as common.

Sometimes spinal tumors start elsewhere in your body (usually a lung or breast) and move through your bloodstream (metastasize) to the spinal area. More commonly, they originate in the spine itself. The cause is often unknown, although nonmalignant tumors can be congenital or hereditary.

Symptoms appear when the growing tumor presses against the spinal cord. Similar symptoms are caused by other spinal disorders that are not tumors. If a spinal cord tumor is suspected after a physical and neurologic examination, your physician may require X-rays, CT scanning or MRI (see page

Rehabilitation in Paraplegia and Quadriplegia

In the first stages of paraplegia or quadriplegia, your physician will treat the injury or disease that caused the paralysis. Your physician also will watch for possible dangers such as stool or urine retention, respiratory or cardiovascular difficulty, stomach or intestinal ulcers, breakdown of skin, contractures, and phlebitis in the extremities.

After the initial injury or disease has become stable, care will focus on problems that may arise from immobilization, such as deconditioning, muscle contractures, bedsores, urinary infection, and blood clots. Early care will include changing your position frequently, range-of-motion exercises for paralyzed limbs, help with your bladder and bowel functions, applications of skin lotion, and use of soft bed coverings or flotation mattresses. Hospitalization will last from several days to several weeks, depending on the cause of the paralysis and the progress of your therapy.

During this time, a rehabilitation team will be assembled to work with you. Your team may include a physiatrist, a physical therapist, an occupational therapist, a rehabilitation nurse, a rehabilitation psychologist, a medical social worker, a recreation therapist, and any other professionals needed to design an appropriate therapy program for you. Their main goals will be to improve your remaining muscle strength and to give you the greatest possible mobility and independence for living a full and active life.

Therapy (see page 480) will include exercise and various therapeutic agents, such as whirlpool baths, to relieve your pain and relax your muscles. You will be given training on day-to-day tasks and on the devices you need to assist you, such as a wheelchair or equipment that can make it easier to fasten buttons or dial a telephone. This therapy may require several months in a rehabilitation facility.

The rehabilitation team will smooth your transition to living at home through short-term leaves from the hospital. They will acquaint you with support services in your community and share information and expertise for optimal care. The medical services in your community will be directed by your physician. He or she will monitor your health and help you, with the assistance of your family or friends, to adapt to a lifestyle that is healthful and as independent as possible.

Needed equipment and modifications in your home should be determined with your rehabilitation professionals. The goal is optimal independence and efficiency at minimal cost. Transportation needs also are best addressed in collaboration with the rehabilitation team.

Your mental state is extremely important. Sudden disability may be followed by depression. Many people with a disability learn to counter their depression by vigorous rehabilitative activity. It is essential for you to find or rediscover interesting things to do for yourself and for and with others. In addition, there are many support groups and peer counselors to help you.

494), and usually myelography (see page 510) to complete the diagnosis.

If you are diagnosed as having a spinal tumor, proceed with treatment as quickly as possible to minimize the risk of permanent impairment.

Treatment

Corticosteroids (such as dexamethasone) are used to reduce spinal cord swelling. Surgical removal is usually successful for isolated tumors outside the spinal cord. Other tumors may not be completely removable, and radiation therapy may be needed.

Early diagnosis and treatment provide a higher success rate, although neurologic symptoms often may continue after initial treatments. Physical therapy programs often are needed after completion of surgical or radiation therapy.

Cervical Spondylosis

Signs and Symptoms
- Pain or stiffness in the neck
- Pain, numbness, or pins-and-needles sensation in the shoulder or arm
- Numbness or weakness in the legs or arms
- Bladder control problems
- Imbalance or stiffness of the legs

Cervical spondylosis (cervical osteoarthritis) is due to growth of bone spurs on the vertebrae in your neck. This happens slowly, and your neck will become stiff gradually. The bone spurs eventually may press against the peripheral nerve roots leading to your shoulders and arms. This compression causes pain or other sensations in these areas. If the spurs also press against your spinal cord, your leg muscles and bladder and bowel control can be affected.

A neck injury can lead to spondylosis many years later. However, the bone spurs generally are caused by normal aging, and this disorder is common in older people. As the discs of your neck vertebrae become worn and thin, they can prolapse (see page 904) or allow the bone growths of spondylosis, or both. The symptoms are similar, but spondylosis is usually much less acute than a herniated disc.

Diagnosis
A stiff neck is the key symptom, and it may not be very painful. If your symptoms become troublesome, your physician may require a neck X-ray or a CT or MRI scan (see page 494) to diagnose how much the spurs interfere with your nerve roots and spinal cord. When there is pressure on the spinal cord or nerve roots, your physician probably will need a myelogram (see page 510) to determine whether you need an operation.

How Serious Is Cervical Spondylosis?
The symptoms of cervical spondylosis are often mild, and you may never require medical treatment. Your discomfort may be chronic or occur only under certain circumstances, such as sleeping in the wrong position or turning your head suddenly.

Cervical spondylosis causes permanent disability in a few cases when there is pressure on the spinal cord or nerve roots.

Treatment
For a mild case of cervical spondylosis, your physician may recommend exercises, the use of a neck collar, or traction therapy at home. Traction involves using a head halter, carefully selected weights, and a pulley arrangement to stretch your neck for 15 to 30 minutes at a time.

For a more severe case, you may need 1 or 2 weeks of hospitalization, complete bed rest, and neck traction. You may need exercises and medication to loosen your neck muscles and to relieve symptoms.

Medication
Your physician may prescribe analgesic drugs (painkillers) or a muscle relaxant.

Surgery
Surgery may be required to remove the bone growths and to fuse your vertebrae. Fusion of two or more vertebrae may help by stiffening that part of the neck or back. This helps prevent painful movement or neurologic problems related to compression of the spinal cord or nerve roots by the unstable spine.

Peripheral Neuropathies

Signs and Symptoms
- Tingling sensation in the hands or feet
- Numbness in the same areas
- Unsteadiness or lack of coordination
- Weakness and pain of the feet and hands

Myelography

Myelography is a diagnostic examination. It is performed while you are lying face down on an X-ray table that can be tilted. A local anesthetic is injected into the skin over the small of the back. A needle is inserted between two of your lower vertebrae, and a small amount of your cerebrospinal fluid is withdrawn.

Contrast medium then is injected slowly through the lumbar puncture needle. A series of X-rays are then made to show the configuration of the space around the spinal cord and whether it is distorted by the presence of a protruded disc or bony spur. After this injection, your diagnostic team can see the medium in your spinal area on X-rays. The table is tilted up and down to move the medium to the location of the suspected disorder in your spine.

Once the medium is appropriately located, X-rays are taken from different directions until the problem area can be seen clearly. Most contrast agents are absorbed by the bloodstream and excreted in the urine. Therefore, they generally do not have to be removed when myelography has been completed.

You may feel pressure or nausea during the injection, although your preparation beforehand should minimize these effects. Afterward, you may have a headache because of changes in the pressure of your cerebrospinal fluid. Lying down

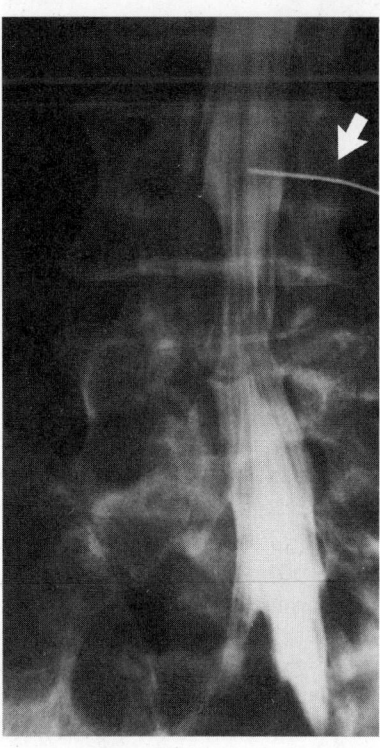

In myelography, a liquid "dye" (contrast medium) is injected through a needle (arrow) into the space around your spinal cord.

will help alleviate your headache, which is usually short-lived.

You probably will be hospitalized for the test, and no food or drink will be allowed for several hours before it. You may be given a sedative. The procedure generally requires 45 to 90 minutes.

There are risks associated with myelography. Some conditions, such as pressure on your spinal cord from a tumor or herniated disc, can be worsened from the change in cerebrospinal fluid pressure, and prompt operation may be required. The risks involved with myelography are well understood, however, and significant complications are rare.

Noninvasive diagnostic tests, such as CT or MRI, provide good resolution and often are used for a general diagnosis of spinal disorders. In many cases, however, myelography continues to be the preferred test because its resolution generally is sharper and fluid obtained from the puncture provides additional diagnostic information. With myelography, your physician can test your cerebrospinal fluid for evidence of infection, inflammation, and cancer cells.

Your peripheral nervous system is the network of nerves used for all of your movements (motor nerves) and sensations (sensory nerves). This network of nerves is connected to your central nervous system at your brain stem and at many points along your spinal cord. It reaches to the remote parts of your body.

Your peripheral nerves provide communication between your brain and your organs, blood vessels, muscles, and skin. Your brain's commands are conveyed by motor nerves, and information is delivered to the brain by your sensory nerves.

Damage to a peripheral nerve can interfere with communication between the area it serves and your brain. This can impair your ability to move muscles or to feel normal sensations in an affected area. It can produce tingling, burning, and even painful sensations in the area of the affected peripheral nerve.

Peripheral neuropathy is the term used to describe damage to your peripheral nerves that does not affect your brain and spinal cord. With minor damage, you may have acute burning pain, whereas major damage can result in imbalance or muscle weakness and even paralysis. You may have damage to a single nerve, as is the case in carpal tunnel syndrome (see page 884), or damage to many nerves at the same time, as in Guillain-Barré syndrome (see page 513).

The causes for peripheral neuropathy are numerous. A partial list includes immediate injury, continuing pressure on a nerve, and nerve destruction from disease or poisoning. The most common causes of peripheral neuropathies are diabetes mellitus, vitamin deficiency, alcoholism associated with poor nutrition, and inherited disorders.

Pressure on a nerve can be due to a tumor, abnormal bone growth, use of a cast or crutches, or prolonged periods in unnatural postures. Rheumatoid arthritis, excessive vibration from power tools, bleeding into a nerve, herniated discs (see page 904), exposure to cold or radiation, and various forms of cancer also cause pressure on nerves. A common peripheral neuropathy, meralgia paresthetica, is characterized by burning sensations, numbness, and sensitivity of the front of the thighs.

Microorganisms can attack your nerves directly and result in peripheral nerve damage. The cause also can be toxic substances, including heavy metals (lead, mercury, arsenic), carbon monoxide, organic solvents, and even some medications.

Your symptoms usually begin gradually over many months but, in certain cases such as arsenic poisoning, the onset may be abrupt. A tingling sensation usually begins in your toes or the balls of your feet and spreads upward. Occasionally, it begins in your hands and extends up your arms. Then numbness may proceed in the same way. Your skin can become sensitive, and even the lightest touch can be painful. In some peripheral neuropathies, weakness may come before or may be more noticeable than the sensory symptoms.

With diabetes mellitus (see page 925), symptoms of a peripheral neuropathy may not appear until you have had the disease for 15 or 20 years. If blood glucose levels are poorly controlled, the symptoms may occur much earlier. Specific symptoms, in addition to those described above, also can include intermittent episodes of sharp pain.

A severe form of vitamin B_{12} deficiency, known as pernicious anemia (see page 958), occurs when your body cannot absorb vitamin B_{12} as it should. Specific symptoms before the onset of peripheral neuropathy include paleness, weakness, fatigue, faintness, or breathlessness. Your skin may turn yellow, and your mouth and tongue may be sore.

Alcoholics may be the most prone to peripheral neuropathies. Their frequently inadequate diet (especially for the vitamin thiamine) contributes to the neuropathy. Pernicious anemia may occur and increase the chances for peripheral neuropathy.

Diagnosis

Because peripheral neuropathies are a complex of symptoms rather than a single disease, the cause for your particular disorder may be difficult or impossible to diagnose. Your physician will conduct a physical and neurologic examination after asking you questions. You will be asked about your symptoms, which symptoms appeared first, medications you are taking, recent viral illnesses, kinds of toxic exposure, your level of alcohol consumption, and if your family or coworkers have similar symptoms. A detailed history of your known medical disorders and past medical problems will also be needed.

Your physician may also request further testing to identify the cause of your peripheral neuropathy. The tests will depend on your answers to the questions and the results of the examinations. These can include blood tests, urinalysis, a chest X-ray, metabolic test, thyroid function studies, electromyography (see page 1344), lumbar puncture (see page 485), and sometimes a nerve biopsy.

How Serious Are Peripheral Neuropathies?

In contrast to the nerve fibers of your central nervous system, peripheral nerve fibers have a good ability to regenerate with proper care. In some disorders, recovery occurs, but the symptoms may recur if the cause is not eliminated.

Treatment

Specific therapy will be directed at the cause of your peripheral neuropathy. This may mean closer control of your underlying disease, such as regular injections of vitamin B_{12} for pernicious anemia, returning your blood glucose level to normal if you have diabetes mellitus, or avoidance of alcohol. Multivitamin therapy may be appropriate.

In severe cases with permanent impairment, physical therapy (see page 480) will be needed to maintain as much muscle strength as possible and to avoid muscle cramping or spasms. Mechanical devices may be needed for mobility. Also, check your skin, especially the skin of your feet, regularly and report any severe bruises or open sores to your physician.

Chapter 19 continued on page 513.

Color Guide to the Diagnosis and Treatment of Common Disorders

Considering the complexity of the human body, it's a wonder that most people enjoy good health most of the time. But problems do occur. In this illustrated section we focus on a wide range of common disorders and diseases—some a nuisance or needless worry and others life-threatening. We provide page references to guide you quickly and easily to a more complete discussion within the text, including information on prevention, treatment options, and self-help tips. The section includes an overview of laparoscopy, a surgical technique increasingly used to reduce pain, recovery time, and health care costs. We end with an illustrated explanation of the role genes play in health and disease.

Contents

Back Pain. B-1
High Blood Pressure (Hypertension) B-2
Coronary Artery Disease B-3
Breast Lumps B-4
Prostate Problems B-5
Joint Trouble. B-6
Laparoscopic Surgery. B-7
Genes and Your Health B-8

Back Pain

It won't kill you, but back pain certainly can make you miserable. People worldwide could save thousands of hours of agony and dollars in health care costs by practicing techniques to avoid the most common cause of back pain—muscle strains and spasms. Other causes are summarized below. (For more information, see page 899.)

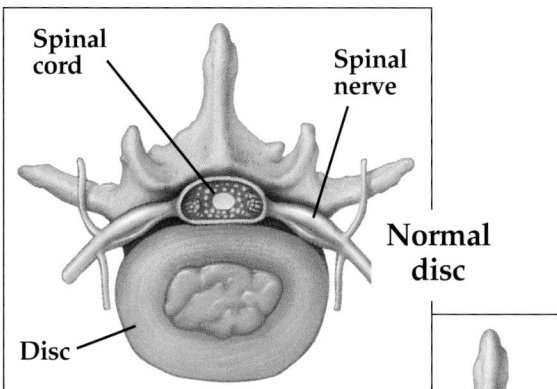

Normal disc — Spinal cord, Spinal nerve, Disc

Herniated disc — Pinched nerve, Disc

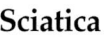

Sciatic nerve

Above: A herniated (slipped) disc places pressure on a spinal nerve, causing pain and, sometimes, loss of sensation or paralysis.

Below: Elastic structures called discs cushion vertebrae in a normal spine, keeping it flexible. In osteoarthritis, discs may narrow and spurs form. Pain and stiffness may occur where bone surfaces rub together. When osteoporosis occurs, vertebrae may become compressed and fractured as a result of weakness in bone structure.

Sciatica

Above: Pain radiating from your back down your buttock to your lower leg may be caused by inflammation or compression of the roots of your sciatic nerve. This is called sciatica (see page 905).

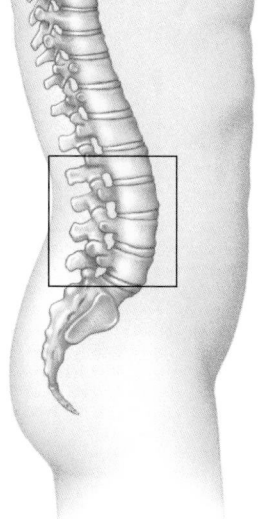

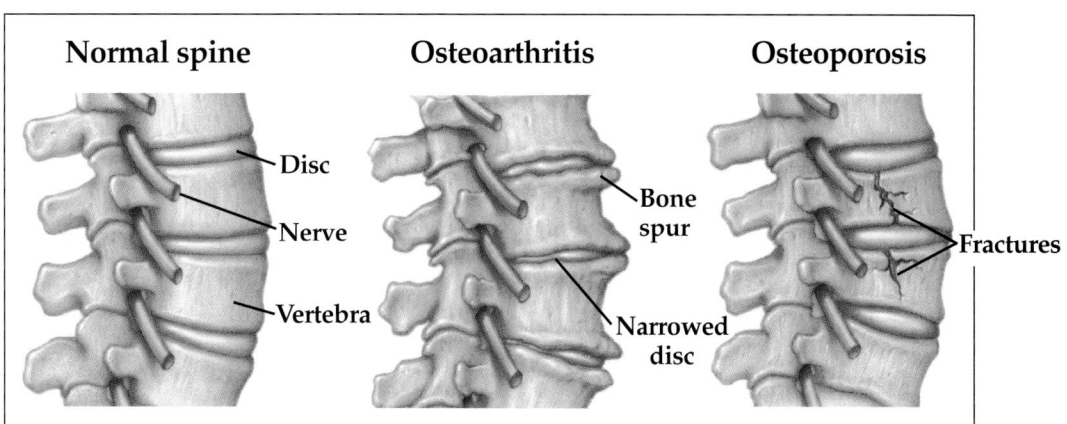

Normal spine — Disc, Nerve, Vertebra

Osteoarthritis — Bone spur, Narrowed disc

Osteoporosis — Fractures

High Blood Pressure (Hypertension)

High blood pressure (hypertension) is a leading chronic adult illness worldwide. Often without symptoms, high blood pressure is associated with heart disease, stroke, and disorders of the kidneys, eyes, and blood vessels. It can be a "silent killer." If your blood pressure is increased, you need professional help. Listed below are health problems often associated with uncontrolled high blood pressure. (For more information, see page 647.)

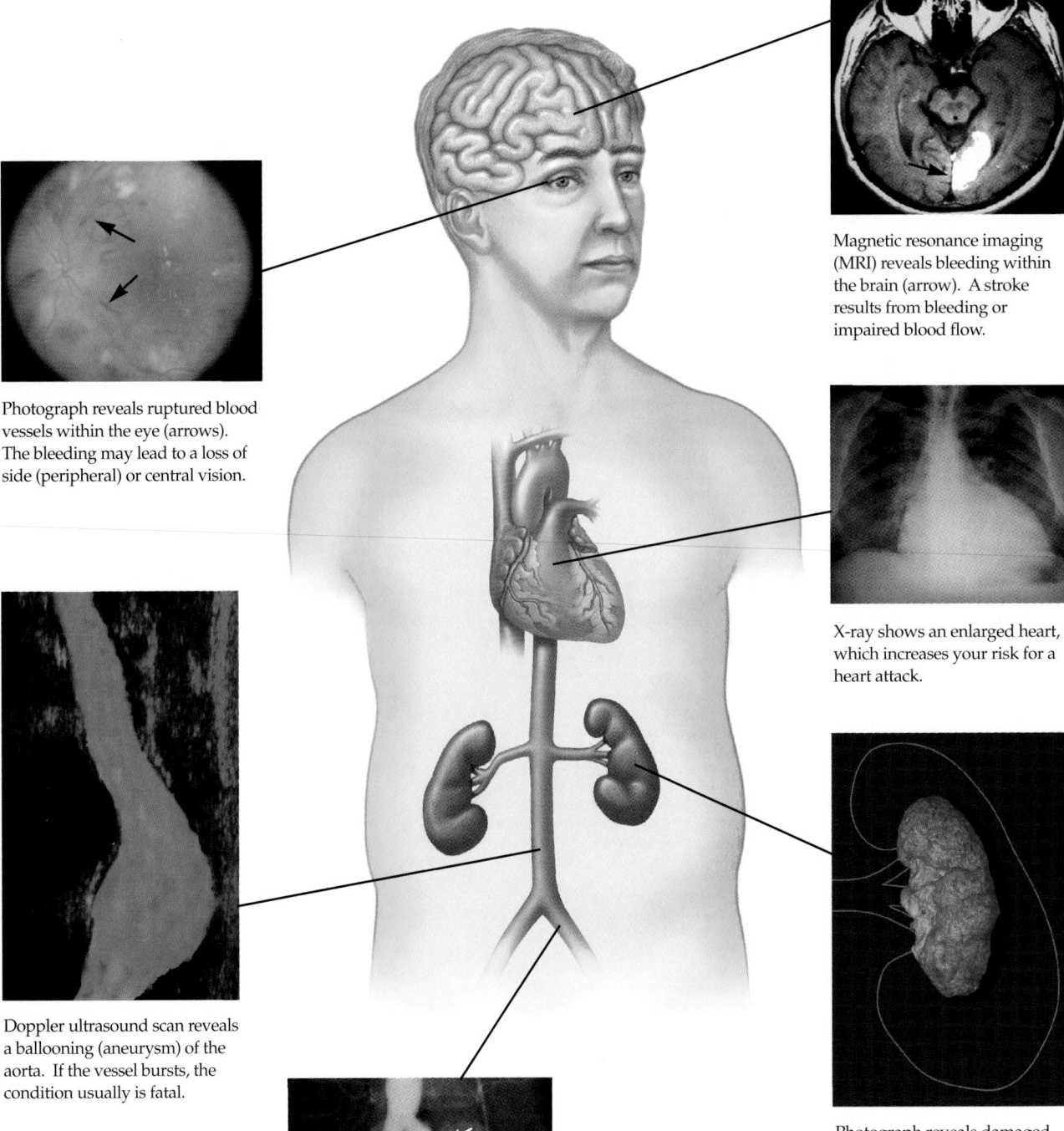

Magnetic resonance imaging (MRI) reveals bleeding within the brain (arrow). A stroke results from bleeding or impaired blood flow.

Photograph reveals ruptured blood vessels within the eye (arrows). The bleeding may lead to a loss of side (peripheral) or central vision.

X-ray shows an enlarged heart, which increases your risk for a heart attack.

Doppler ultrasound scan reveals a ballooning (aneurysm) of the aorta. If the vessel bursts, the condition usually is fatal.

Angiogram reveals a buildup of atherosclerotic plaque (arrow) inside a blood vessel, which can increase your risk for heart attack, stroke, or, in this case, gangrene of the leg or foot.

Photograph reveals damaged, shrunken kidney (nephrosclerosis) due to narrowing or blockage of arteries within the kidney. Dialysis or organ transplantation may be required.

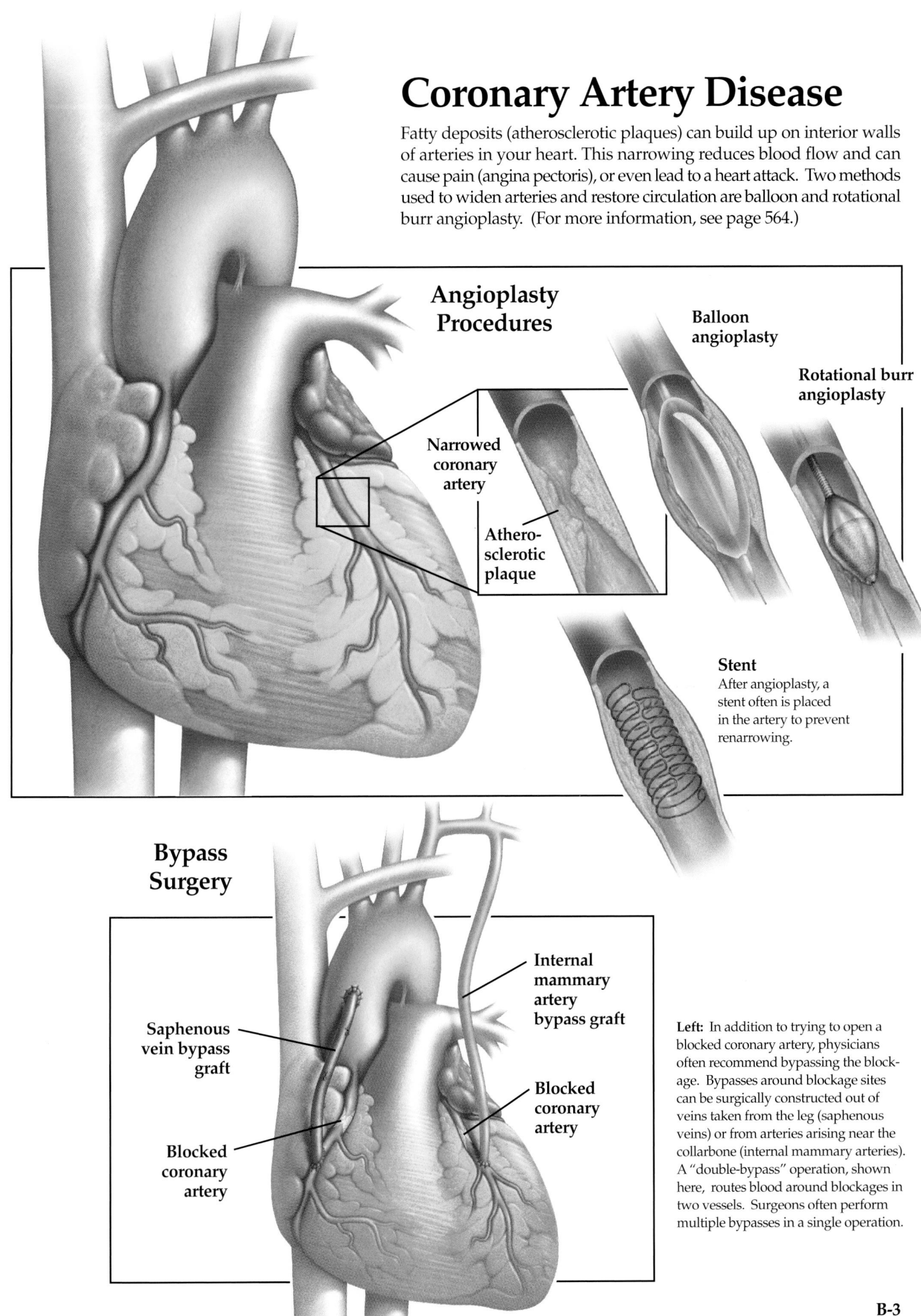

Coronary Artery Disease

Fatty deposits (atherosclerotic plaques) can build up on interior walls of arteries in your heart. This narrowing reduces blood flow and can cause pain (angina pectoris), or even lead to a heart attack. Two methods used to widen arteries and restore circulation are balloon and rotational burr angioplasty. (For more information, see page 564.)

Angioplasty Procedures

Narrowed coronary artery

Athero-sclerotic plaque

Balloon angioplasty

Rotational burr angioplasty

Stent
After angioplasty, a stent often is placed in the artery to prevent renarrowing.

Bypass Surgery

Saphenous vein bypass graft

Blocked coronary artery

Internal mammary artery bypass graft

Blocked coronary artery

Left: In addition to trying to open a blocked coronary artery, physicians often recommend bypassing the blockage. Bypasses around blockage sites can be surgically constructed out of veins taken from the leg (saphenous veins) or from arteries arising near the collarbone (internal mammary arteries). A "double-bypass" operation, shown here, routes blood around blockages in two vessels. Surgeons often perform multiple bypasses in a single operation.

B-3

Breast Lumps

Because a breast lump may represent cancer, it needs to be taken seriously and investigated promptly. But remember the vast majority of these lumps are noncancerous (benign) and may be the result of a woman's monthly hormone cycle. (For more information, see page 1158.)

Monthly breast self-examination is important for women. The most common site for a lump is the upper, outer quadrant, but be sure to examine your entire breast (see page 1160).

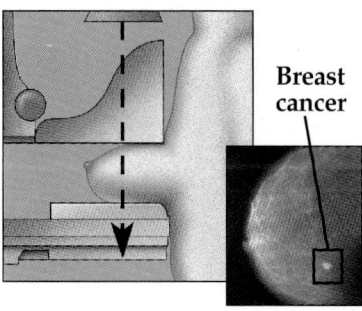

Breast cancer

Mammography and a breast examination done by your physician are the two most effective ways of reducing your risk of dying from breast cancer. Arrow shows path of radiation. Mammogram at right reveals breast cancer.

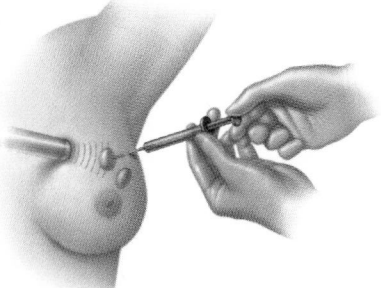

If cysts are suspected, your physician can use a fine needle in an attempt to withdraw fluid for examination. If the lump is solid, a small piece may be removed surgically, or with a larger needle, and tested for cancer. An ultrasound probe can identify the site.

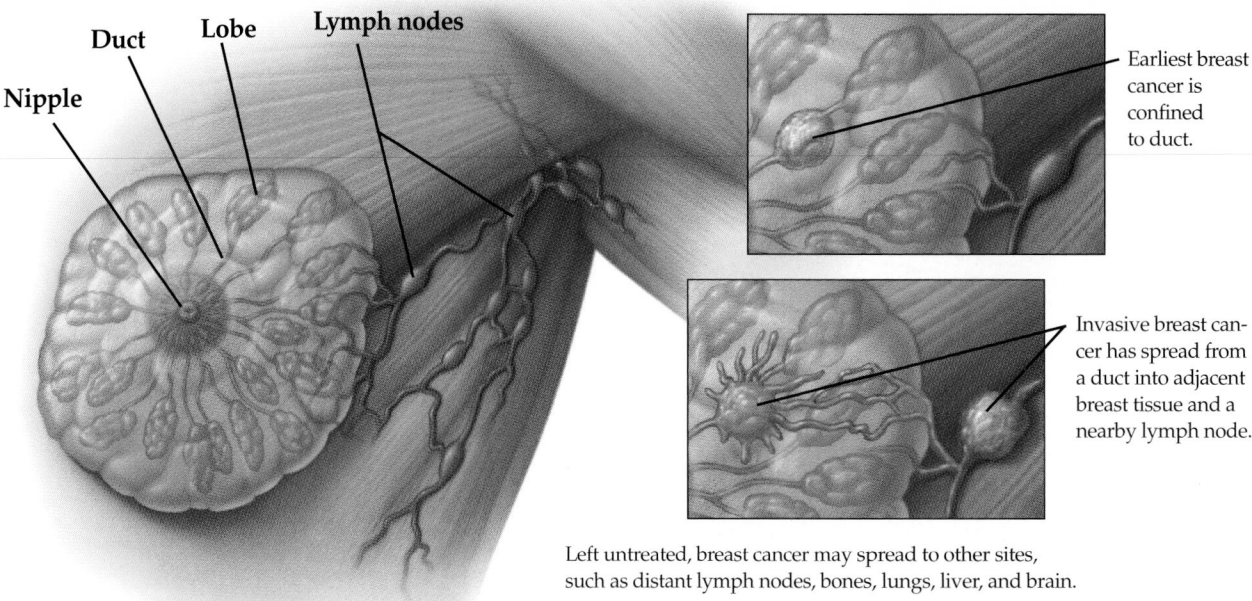

Nipple

Duct **Lobe** **Lymph nodes**

Earliest breast cancer is confined to duct.

Invasive breast cancer has spread from a duct into adjacent breast tissue and a nearby lymph node.

Left untreated, breast cancer may spread to other sites, such as distant lymph nodes, bones, lungs, liver, and brain.

Breast Cancer Treatment Options

The goal is to remove all of the cancer while saving as much of the breast as possible. If the cancer is small and confined to your breast, your physician probably will recommend a lumpectomy. If the cancer has spread, several more invasive surgical options are available. But radical mastectomies, in which the breast, lymph nodes, and chest muscles are all removed, are rarely done today (see page 1166).

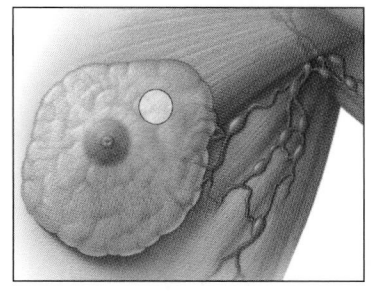

Lumpectomy— The tumor is removed along with some underarm lymph nodes. Radiation therapy follows to kill any remaining cancer cells.

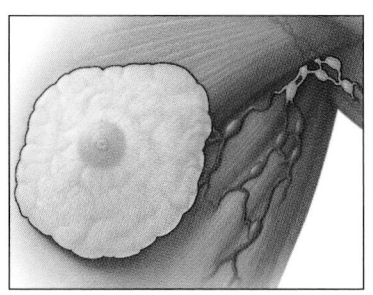

Modified Radical Mastectomy—The breast is removed with some underarm lymph nodes. Chest muscles are left intact.

Prostate Problems

Noncancerous enlargement of the prostate gland, called benign prostatic hyperplasia (BPH), is common as men get older. A more serious disorder is prostate cancer. Several new techniques give men more treatment options to consider for either condition. (For more information, see page 1209.)

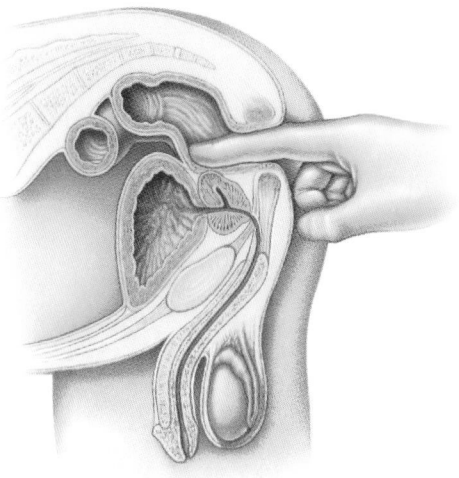

Digital Rectal Examination—Your physician can examine your prostate by inserting a gloved finger into your rectum to determine the size, shape, and texture of your gland.

Prostate-Specific Antigen Test—Your prostate gland secretes a protein called prostate-specific antigen (PSA). If you have an increased level of PSA in your blood, you may have prostate cancer. Additional tests are often required.

Bladder

Prostate gland

Urethra

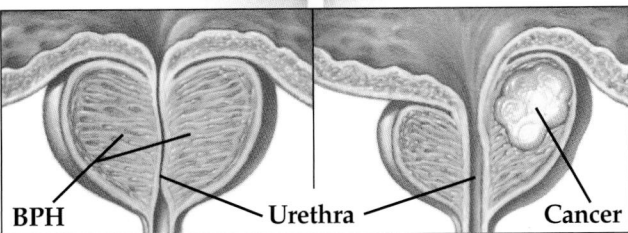

BPH — Urethra — Cancer

Above left: As you age, your prostate gland may enlarge and gradually compress your urethra, slowing the flow of urine. This is called benign prostatic hyperplasia (BPH). **Above right**: Prostate cancer, which may be symptomless.

Prostate Treatment Options

For BPH—Your surgeon can decrease the size of your gland with a procedure called a transurethral resection of the prostate (TURP). The operation is done through a thin tube inserted into your urethra, eliminating the need for an incision. This is the most common surgical treatment. Other techniques are being evaluated, but no single treatment is universally appropriate.

For Prostate Cancer—Removal of the prostate (radical prostatectomy) is a common treatment option for prostate cancer that has not spread

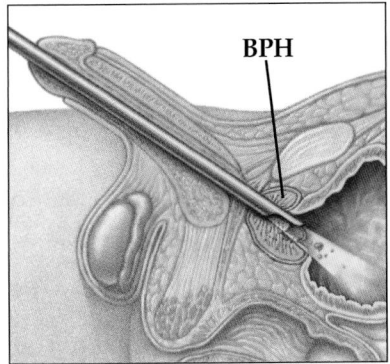

BPH

Transurethral Resection

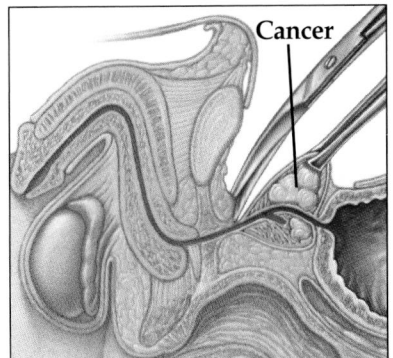

Cancer

Radical Prostatectomy

beyond the gland. Other options might include radiation therapy or "watchful waiting" with no treatment. If spread has occurred

outside the gland, treatments to consider include removal of the testicles (orchiectomy) or hormone therapy.

Joint Trouble

Pain and stiffness in a joint can be caused by arthritis. Of the more than 100 forms of arthritis, osteoarthritis is the most common, affecting nearly everyone older than 60. Hailed as one of this century's best medical developments, joint replacement surgery often restores a near-normal, pain-free lifestyle. Called arthroplasty, this increasingly common procedure has become widely available in recent years for treatment of many joints, including the hip, knee, shoulder, elbow, wrist, and even fingers. (For more information, see page 911.)

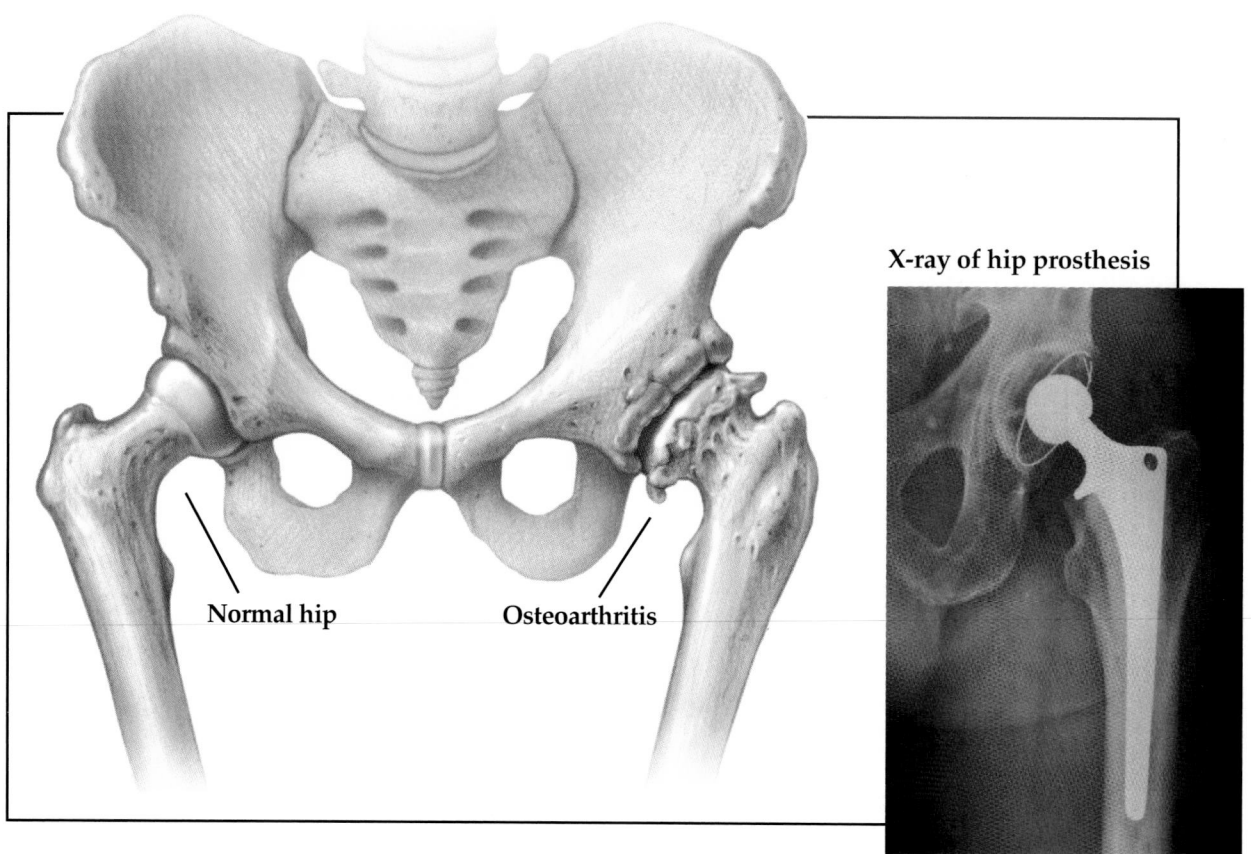

X-ray of hip prosthesis

Normal hip   Osteoarthritis

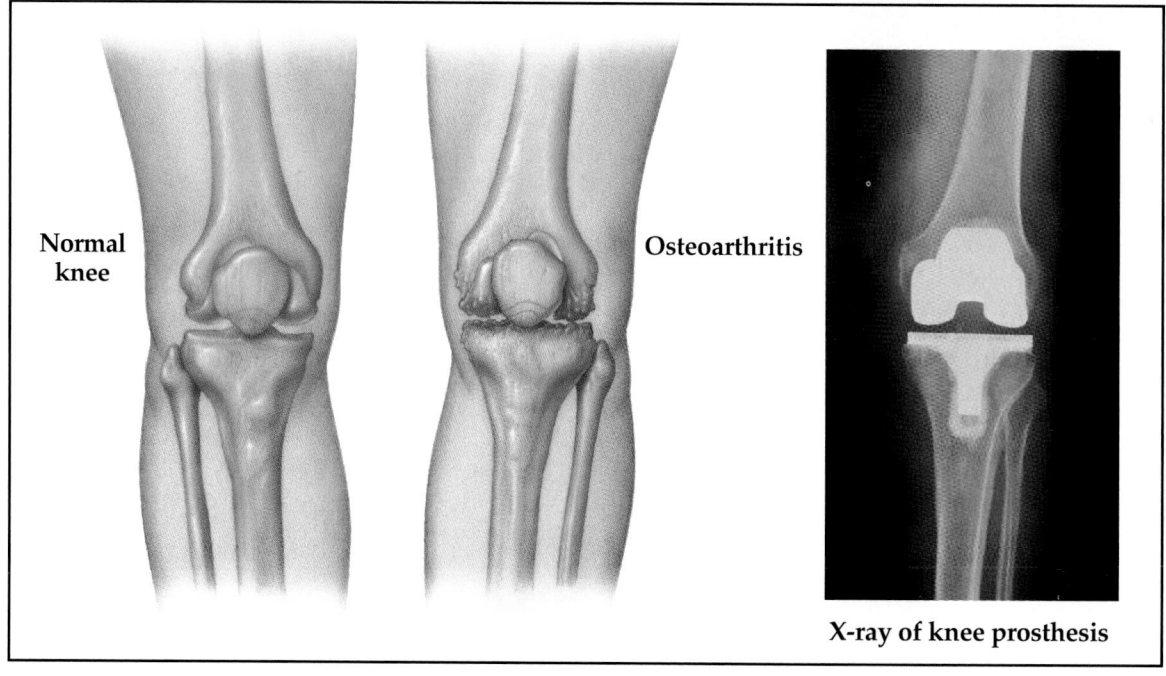

Normal knee   Osteoarthritis

X-ray of knee prosthesis

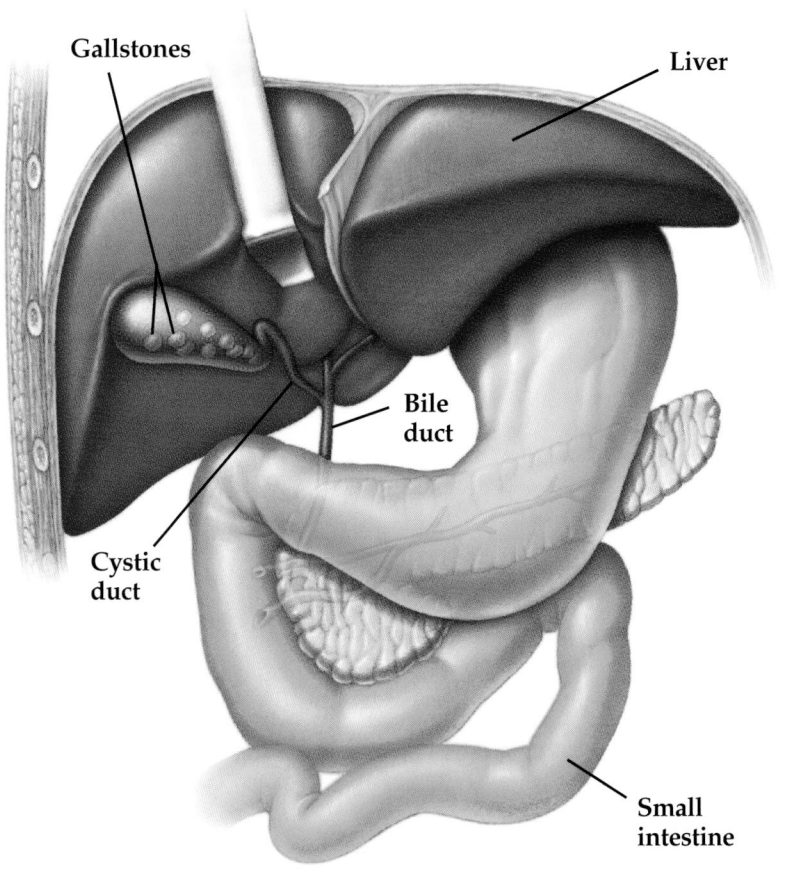

Gallstones

Liver

Bile duct

Cystic duct

Small intestine

Laparoscopic Surgery

Tube-like instruments called endoscopes are indispensable for diagnosing a wide variety of ailments and diseases. These instruments are increasingly being used for surgery because only tiny incisions are required. Endoscopic surgery can often reduce pain, recovery time, and cost.

Not long ago, surgery for gallstones required a 3- to 6-inch incision, a hospital stay of a week, and about 6 weeks of recovery. Now, surgeons often remove the gallbadder with a laparoscope, a special kind of endoscope. The operation, called laparoscopic surgery, or more precisely laparoscopic cholecystectomy, is done through several small incisions, sometimes as an outpatient procedure, generally with a recovery time of less than 1 week. (For more information, see page 817.)

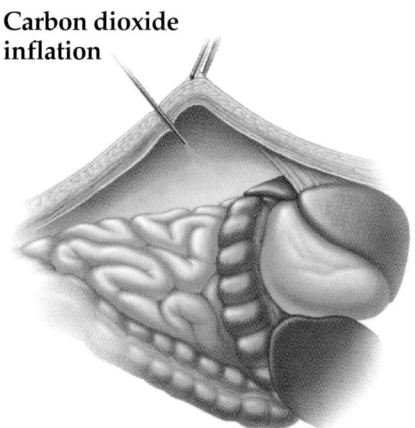

Carbon dioxide inflation

How Is Laparoscopy Done?

To remove the gallbladder with a laparoscope, your surgeon makes small incisions beneath your rib cage. Instruments are inserted through hollow tubes. The surgeon inflates your abdomen with carbon dioxide gas to improve visualization. A video camera and television monitor give your surgeon a clear view of your internal organs. Your surgeon grasps the sac-like gallbladder, cuts it free, and pulls it out through one of the small puncture sites.

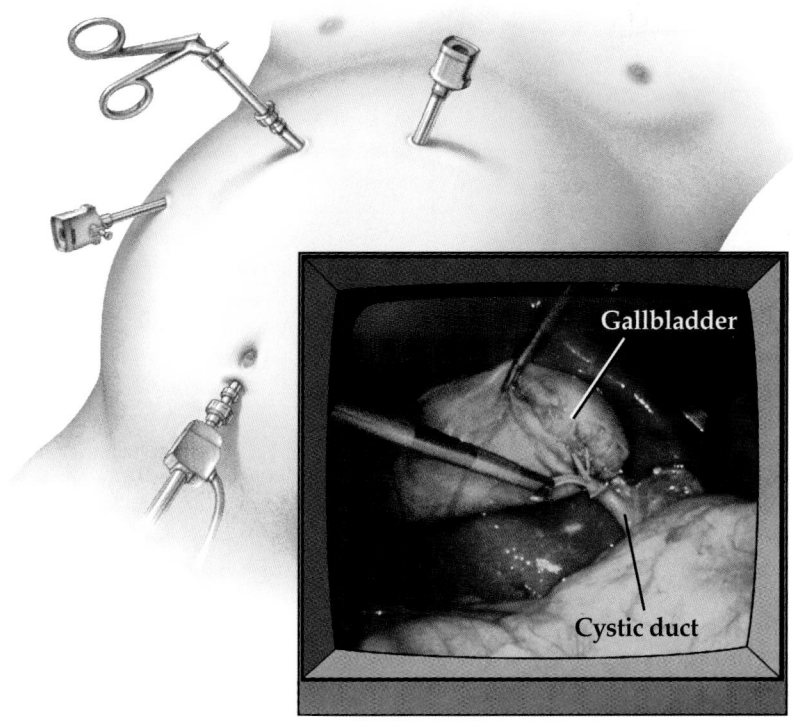

Gallbladder

Cystic duct

Television monitor

Genes and Your Health

Just as your lifestyle and environment can affect your health, so do the genes you inherit. In addition to determining your appearance and other traits, your genes direct your cells to produce proteins essential to the healthy functioning of your body.

The nucleus of each cell in your body contains structures called chromosomes. Chromosomes contain twisted, double strands of material scientists call deoxyribonucleic acid (DNA). You might think of DNA as a twisted ladder.

Your genes are made of portions of these DNA strands. Throughout your life, your genes are telling your cells what proteins they need to make to help keep you healthy. If a gene is missing, incomplete, damaged, or duplicated, this process is altered, which may lead to disease.

Each of your cells contains approximately 100,000 genes. A single abnormal gene may increase your risk of becoming ill. A combination of altered genes and external factors (your diet or a harmful habit such as smoking) can increase your risk of becoming ill.

By pinpointing the location, on the chromosome, of each gene in the human body, and understanding its function, scientists are discovering promising new ways to approach the prediction, prevention, diagnosis, and treatment of disease.

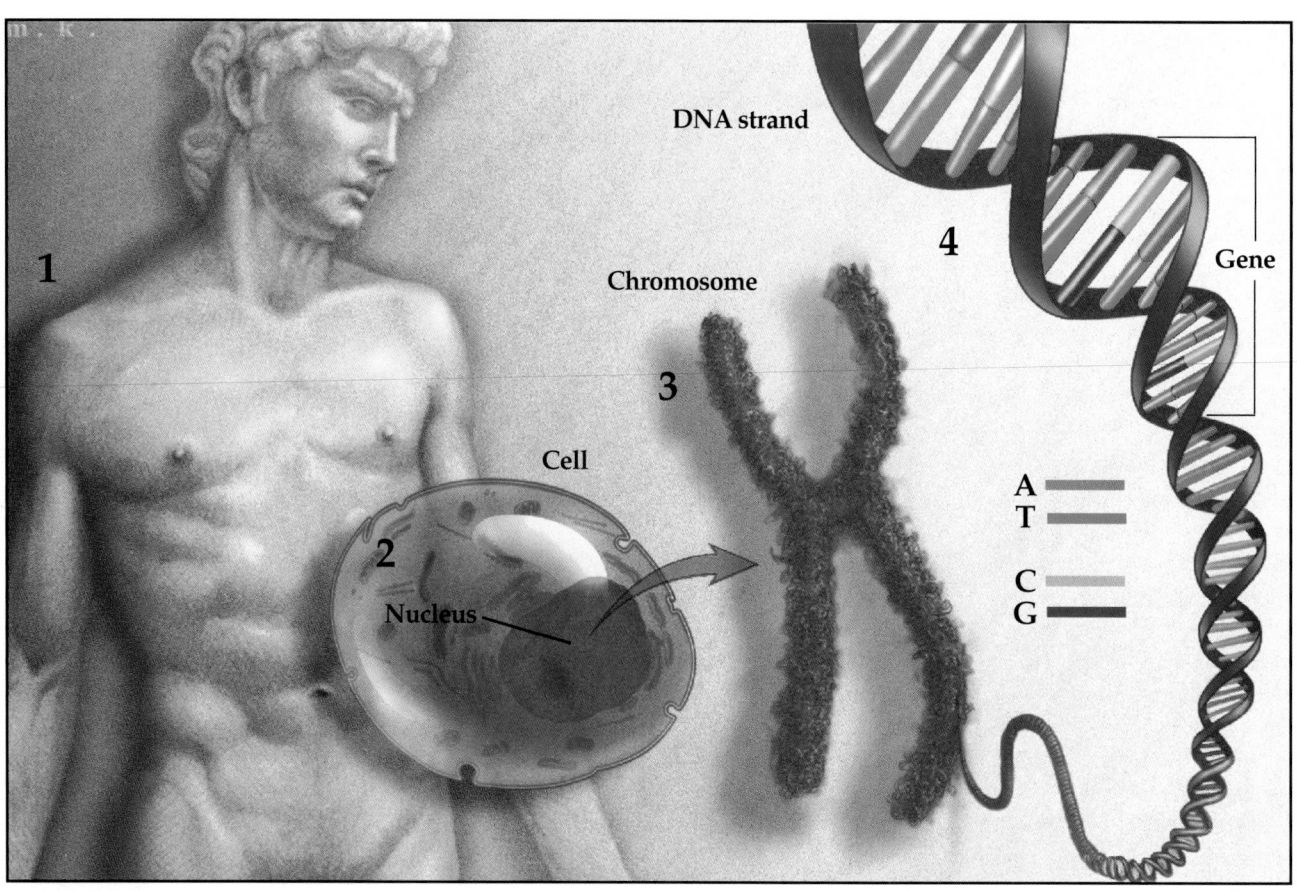

DNA strand

Chromosome

Cell

Nucleus

Gene

1

2

3

4

A
T

C
G

(1) Your body is made up of cells—about 100 trillion of them. Different kinds of cells (for example, skin, muscle, bone, and blood) perform different functions. Each of your cells has a "control center" called the nucleus.

(2) Within the nucleus of each cell are 23 pairs of structures called chromosomes. Half of your chromosomes came from your mother and half from your father.

(3) Each chromosome contains strands that resemble a twisted ladder. The strands, called deoxyribonucleic acid (DNA), are held together by chemical "rungs."

(4) Each gene is comprised of sequences of thousands of pairs of chemicals: adenine (A) and thymine (T), and cytosine (C) and guanine (G). The precise sequence of these chemical pairs (A/T and C/G) in the gene directs the cell to produce another chemical, usually a protein, that has a specific task to do. Think of the sequence of A/T and C/G as a chemical manual, and the protein produced by the cell as the device accomplishing a given task. This is how each gene tells each cell in your body precisely how to act, thereby controlling your appearance and growth and influencing, or directly affecting, the function of your organs and your health.

Guillain-Barré Syndrome

Signs and Symptoms
- Spreading numbness and tingling beginning in the fingers or toes
- Muscle weakness

Emergency Symptoms
- Widespread tingling and numbness
- Difficulty breathing

Guillain-Barré syndrome is acute and frequently causes severe damage to all or part of your peripheral nerves (see also Peripheral Neuropathies, page 509). The illness results from inflammation and destruction of the myelin sheath that covers your nerve fibers.

The cause of Guillain-Barré syndrome is unknown, but in two-thirds of the cases it occurs after a viral infection, either one you know about or one that is found by subsequent blood tests. The viral infection may be a form of herpes, such as Epstein-Barr virus, but it can also follow a bacterial infection such as campylobacteriosis. Flu symptoms, a cold or other minor infections, or other conditions such as Hodgkin's disease (see page 969) may also precede the syndrome.

Guillain-Barré syndrome sometimes is associated with medical procedures. Five to 10 percent of all cases occur after an operation. For a brief period, a vaccine was thought to be a potential cause. Initial concern was raised when many cases of Guillain-Barré syndrome were reported after a major flu vaccination program in 1976 and 1977. Further study revealed that the number of cases was no greater than what would have occurred without the vaccination.

Your symptoms can appear a few days to a week or two after the initial infection or 1 to 4 weeks after operation. Tingling sensations in your fingers and toes may be followed by general muscle weakness. A sensation of weakness usually spreads from your legs to your arms and face. In some cases, the weakness may be severe enough to produce paralysis, and your respiratory muscles also are affected. The muscles responsible for eye movement, facial movements, speaking, chewing, and swallowing also may become weak or paralyzed.

The syndrome occurs at a rate of 3,500 cases annually in the United States and Canada. It can strike any race at any age.

Diagnosis
The diagnosis is based on your symptoms, a physical examination, tests such as electromyography (see page 1344), and analysis of cerebrospinal fluid extracted by lumbar puncture (see page 485).

How Serious Is Guillain-Barré Syndrome?
In its severe form, Guillain-Barré syndrome is a medical emergency and may require intensive care hospitalization. A few persons with Guillain-Barré syndrome need respiratory assistance at some point during the illness.

Most often, recovery occurs over a period of months. If you are severely affected, you will need long-term rehabilitation to regain your independence. Some permanent impairment remains in about 10 percent of cases. The mortality rate is 3 or 4 percent.

Treatment
Guillain-Barré syndrome generally is treated by supportive care. A procedure called plasmapheresis, which removes plasma and damaging antibodies from your blood, is used during the first few weeks of a severe attack. This may improve your chance for full recovery.

Once your condition is stabilized, rehabilitation therapy is initiated. Whirlpool hydrotherapy is used to relieve pain and facilitate retraining of movements. Physical therapy (see page 480) such as passive exercise can be done safely during the acute phase of the illness. After your symptoms subside, your rehabilitation team will prescribe an active exercise routine that will help you regain muscle strength and independence. Training with adaptive devices, such as a wheelchair or braces, may be needed to give you mobility and self-care skills if the recovery period is protracted.

Charcot-Marie-Tooth Disease

Signs and Symptoms
- Weakness in legs and (to a lesser degree) arms
- Absence of muscle stretch reflex
- Foot deformity

Charcot-Marie-Tooth disease is a relatively common example of a group of hereditary disorders caused by degeneration of the insulating sheath (myelin sheath) covering peripheral nerve fibers, or the nerve fibers themselves. Symptoms frequently become obvious between mid-childhood and age 30. The symptoms develop slowly and sometimes appear to stabilize spontaneously.

The diagnosis may require a physical and neurologic examination, electromyography (see page 1344), and sometimes a biopsy of a nerve in the leg. Recent genetic studies have identified abnormalities of chromosomes in this disorder and possibly an option for treatment through gene replacement therapy.

Treatment

Vocational counseling or leg braces may be needed, as may an orthopedic operation or corrective shoes to improve walking. The disorder does not necessarily affect your life span, and you may be active for years.

Syringomyelia

Signs and Symptoms

- Gradual loss of sensation in the nape of the neck, shoulders, and upper arms
- Weakness of the arms or legs

In syringomyelia, a fluid-filled cavity grows within your spinal cord, usually in the neck area. The cavity may expand gradually along your spinal cord, initially reducing your sense of heat or touch and then causing wasting of your muscles. Severe disability can develop. Frequently, the progression of symptoms is very slow.

Syringomyelia can be caused by spinal cord trauma, tumor, or a congenital defect that triggers syringomyelia in adolescence or early adulthood.

Treatment

Surgical therapy to drain the cavity and decompress the spinal cord frequently stops progression of the disorder. About half of the persons with syringomyelia improve significantly after an operation.

Myelomeningocele

Signs and Symptoms

- Sac protruding from the spinal cord on a newborn's back
- Weakness of the lower limbs

Myelomeningocele (open spina bifida) is a congenital defect that leaves your baby's spinal canal open along several vertebrae in the lower or middle back. It is a severe form of spina bifida, a birth defect that occurs on the back.

The spinal cord and membranes protrude shortly after birth. Neurologic impairment below the defect, often including either partial or complete paralysis, is common.

Other congenital malformations often are associated with myelomeningocele, such as syringomyelia (see this page), clubfoot, or hip dislocation. Meningitis (see page 481) can occur with a leaking sac. This defect should be promptly treated with surgery. If there are problems with neurologic control of the bladder, urinary infections are likely to occur as your child gets older.

Treatment

Immediate surgical repair frequently is recommended. With proper care, a long life is possible in some cases, although problems, particularly impaired bladder and bowel function, may persist.

Neuralgias

Signs and Symptoms—Attacks of extremely sharp, stabbing pain, or constant burning pain

Neuralgias consist of severe spasms of pain that extend along the path of one of your nerves. They may be due to injury or irritation of the nerve, but in many cases the cause is unknown.

Your pain may have a background sensation of burning and aching with sharp, stabbing jabs superimposed on it. The pain comes in episodic attacks that might last for seconds or minutes, and the episodes may recur for days or weeks.

During an acute phase of your disorder, you may be hypersensitive to touch and to any slightly painful sensation—you may even perceive that nonpainful sensations cause you pain.

Some neuralgias can occur as a result of a herpes zoster or chickenpox virus infection causing shingles (see page 1011), and occasionally infection by herpes simplex virus. Postherpetic neuralgia, for example, can be a most debilitating complication of herpes zoster virus. It typically produces a constant burning pain that is more prominent than the brief shooting or jabbing component. New attacks are provoked by contact or movement such as sneezing or eating. Your nerve pain can continue for weeks, months, or sometimes years after all signs of the herpes virus have disappeared.

Glossopharyngeal neuralgia is characterized by recurrent attacks of severe pain in the back of your pharynx, tonsils, middle ear, and the base of your tongue. The attacks may be precipitated by movements such as talking or swallowing, and the pain can be intense.

Occipital neuralgia causes pain in the back of your head. Intercostal neuralgia occurs between your ribs. Trigeminal neuralgia, the most common of all forms, is characterized by severe sharp, electric shock-like pain on one side of your face.

Neuralgias usually strike after age 40 and occur most commonly in elderly persons. Fortunately, postherpetic (that is, neuralgias that occur after shingles) and trigeminal neuralgia are the only neuralgias that occur commonly.

Diagnosis

Your physician's diagnosis is determined by your symptoms and by exclusion of other disorders that may be causing your pain. You may need to see a neurologist for a thorough examination. Your dentist also may need to examine your teeth and gums when your face is affected. If you also have swelling as a sign, rheumatic diseases (see page 918), phlebitis (see page 694), and bone fractures will need to be ruled out.

How Serious Are Neuralgias?

Although your pain may be incapacitating, it is not life-threatening. Your attacks may come and go variably, but the time between attacks can grow shorter as you get older.

Treatment

Medication

Treatment will depend on your symptoms, but analgesic drugs (painkillers) commonly are required. For mild neuralgias, your physician may prescribe non-narcotic analgesics such as aspirin, acetaminophen, or ibuprofen. In more severe cases, a narcotic analgesic such as codeine may be temporarily necessary. Carbamazepine, baclofen, and phenytoin are sometimes used for trigeminal neuralgia. Sometimes an antidepressant medication is prescribed to help control your pain. Physical therapy may be useful in the treatment of postherpetic neuralgia.

Trigeminal Neuralgia

Signs and Symptoms—Brief flashes of excruciating pain in the lips, gums, cheek, chin, or, rarely, forehead

Trigeminal neuralgia, also called tic douloureux, is a condition of recurring pain on one side of your face, emanating from one or more of the three branches of the fifth cranial (trigeminal) nerve. The pain may be a tearing, darting, or sharp cutting sensation that occurs in a portion of the face. An attack may last for seconds or a few minutes, and its intensity may make you contract your facial muscles, hence the term tic. Episodes may recur for days or weeks or months. The cause of the disorder usually is considered to be a blood vessel or sometimes even a tumor pressing on the nerve inside the skull.

Often there are trigger zones—spots on the face—or certain movements that precipitate the pain. These may include smiling, talking, chewing, brushing your teeth, or blowing your nose.

The disorder is found almost exclusively in persons older than 50 years and often in those older than 70 years. Women are 3 times more likely to have it than men.

Your physician usually can diagnose the disorder after excluding other disorders that

If you have trigeminal neuralgia, pain may occur in areas supplied by one of the three branches of the trigeminal (fifth cranial) nerve.

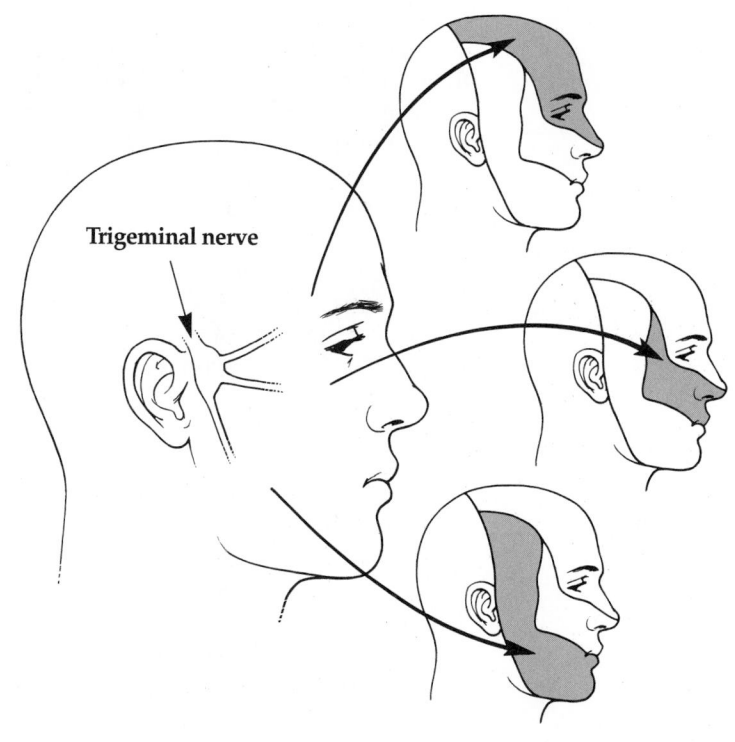

Trigeminal nerve

may cause pain in your head, jaw, teeth, or sinuses. Multiple sclerosis (see page 475) can cause trigeminal neuralgia. Frequently, a delayed diagnosis results in multiple unnecessary dental procedures in an attempt to correct the pain.

Although the pain may be incapacitating, it is not life-threatening. Attacks come and go variably, but periods of remission may grow shorter as you age.

Treatment

In general, attempts to control the pain of trigeminal neuralgia begin with medications such as phenytoin or carbamazepine. If drug treatments fail to control the discomfort, nerve blocks or surgical procedures to reduce the sensitivity of the nerve are an option. An operation to free the nerve from the blood vessel or tumor compressing it also can eliminate the pain permanently. However, this is a major neurosurgical procedure with several potential complications.

Spinal Stenosis

Signs and Symptoms
- An ache in your buttock, thigh, and calf
- Pain radiating from your lower back to your calf
- Progressive numbness or weakness in your leg
- Trouble with bladder and bowel control

You may first notice an ache in your buttock, thigh, and calf when you walk or stand. If you bend forward at your waist or sit for a few minutes, the pain passes. These symptoms suggest spinal stenosis, a source of leg pain caused by narrowing of your spinal canal. Symptoms are often subtle and similar to those associated with other causes of back and leg pain.

Spinal stenosis typically affects adults after age 50. It can develop because of a congenital defect, but it usually results from osteoarthritis (see Osteoarthritis, page 907).

Excessive use, previous injury, or aging can slowly deteriorate the protective tissue (cartilage) covering joint surfaces in your spine. Discs between vertebrae in your spine become worn and spaces between vertebrae narrow. Bony outgrowths called spurs (osteophytes) may also develop. These changes can cause vertebrae and soft tissue to move inward into your spinal canal, compressing nerves.

Pressure may develop on roots of your sciatic nerve. This may cause pain to radiate from your lower back down your buttock to your calf. Numbness or weakness in your legs may eventually develop. Occasionally, nerves to the bladder and bowel become compressed, which leads to incontinence.

Bending forward at your waist or sitting relieves the pain because these positions increase the diameter of your spinal canal, reducing pressure on spinal nerves. In severe cases, the pain persists regardless of activity or position.

Diagnosis

Your physician may first perform tests to exclude other conditions that can cause leg pain or numbness, such as a spinal tumor (see Spinal Tumor, page 508) or a circulatory problem (see Arteriosclerosis of the Extremities, page 690). A herniated (slipped) disc can also cause similar symptoms (see Prolapsed Disc, page 904).

Pain from spinal stenosis tends to be more noticeable when you walk downhill and persists when you stand. (Pain caused by poor circulation is usually worse when you walk uphill and subsides when you stand.)

If after an initial evaluation your physician suspects spinal stenosis, tests may be ordered. CT (see page 494), MRI (see page 494), or myelography (X-ray after injecting a contrast material) can detect narrowing of your spinal canal.

Treatment

For mild to moderate spinal stenosis, bed rest, medication, and physical therapy may be all the treatment you'll need. However, spinal stenosis can be progressive and lead to disabling pain or other symptoms that require surgery.

Bed rest was once the mainstay of treatment. Now it is recommended for only a few days if pain is severe. Prolonged bed rest can reduce muscle strength and lead to further disability.

Medication
Nonsteroidal anti-inflammatory drugs and muscle relaxants prescribed by your physician can relieve chronic pain. Over-the-counter analgesics such as aspirin or acetaminophen also may help. Corticosteroid

medications may be injected for temporary relief, but they don't cure spinal stenosis.

Physical Therapy

For acute pain, applications of heat, cold, or gentle massage performed by a physical therapist may help. Once the pain subsides, your therapist can design an exercise program to improve your flexibility, strengthen your back and abdominal muscles, and improve your posture.

A brace or corset worn around your lower back also can improve your posture. Limit use of back supports to activities that put extra stress on back muscles. Extended use of back supports can lead to muscle weakness in your back and abdomen.

Surgery

Your physician may recommend a surgical procedure if you have disabling pain, progressive weakness in your legs, or reduced control of your bladder or bowel. During the operation, called a laminectomy, your surgeon removes bone and soft tissues that protrude into your spinal canal or put pressure on your spinal nerves. If you have spondylolisthesis, some vertebrae in your lower back may be fused.

Laminectomy often improves or eliminates pain in the buttocks and legs, but it may not relieve low back pain that is caused by underlying conditions such as osteoarthritis.

The average hospital stay for a laminectomy is 4 to 7 days. After 3 months, you will be able to resume most of your daily activities with the exception of heavy physical labor. Your recovery and rehabilitation may take longer if a spinal fusion was required.

Chapter 20

Your Eyes

Contents

How You See, 520
Parts of the Eye, 520
The Mechanism of Sight, 522
Eye Experts, 522

Refraction Problems, 522
Nearsightedness, 523
The Eye Examination, 524
Radial Keratotomy, 525
Farsightedness, 525
Hereditary Disorders of the
Eyes, 526
Presbyopia, 526
Refraction Errors Due to
Changing Blood Sugar
Concentration, 527
Astigmatism, 527

What You Should Know
About Contact Lenses, 528
Who Can Wear Contact
Lenses? 528
How Do They Work? 528
Types of Contact Lenses, 528
Get Them Fitted Properly, 529
Be Alert for Problems, 529
Caring for Your Contacts, 530

Trauma to the Eye, 531
Foreign Bodies, 531
Chemical Burns, 531
Protecting Your Eyes, 532
Black Eye, 533
Hyphema, 533

Strabismus and
Amblyopia, 534
Early Recognition, 534
Corrective Measures, 535
Double Vision, 535

Eyelid Disorders, 536
Sties and Lumps, 536
Problems of Tearing, 537
Eyedrops, 538
Blepharitis, 539
Itchy Eyelid, 539
About That Twitchy
Eyelid, 540
Drooping Eyelid, 540
Cosmetic Surgery of the
Eyelid, 541
Entropion and Ectropion, 541

Disorders of the Eye, 542
Conjunctivitis, 542
Scleritis and Episcleritis, 543
Eye Hemorrhage, 544
Uveitis and Iritis, 544
Orbital Cellulitis, 545
Retinoblastoma, 545
Melanoma of the Eye, 546

Corneal Problems, 546
Corneal Injury, 546
Vitamin A Deficiency, 547
Corneal Ulcers and
Infections, 547
Corneal Transplantation, 548

Disorders of Vision, 548
Color Blindness, 548
Glaucoma, 550
Acute Glaucoma, 550
Chronic Glaucoma, 551
Risk Factors for Chronic
Glaucoma, 551
Tonometry and Your Eyes, 553
Cataracts, 553
When Is Cataract Surgery the
Right Choice? 555
Alternatives to Intraocular
Lens Implant, 556
Vision Problems After
Cataract Surgery, 556
Macular Degeneration, 556
Retinal Detachment, 557
Lasers and Eye Disease, 558
Retinal Vessel Occlusion, 559
Optic Neuritis, 560
Optic Neuropathy, 560
Coloboma, 560
Choroiditis, 560
Retinitis Pigmentosa, 561
Spots and Floaters, 561

The Eye in Systemic
Diseases, 562
The Eye and Diabetes, 562
Third Nerve Palsy, 563
Graves' Disease and Eye
Problems, 563
Hypertension and Vision, 564
The Eye and Warning Signs of
Stroke, 564
Cranial Arteritis and Vision, 565

How You See

Your eyes are singular and unique instruments, able to receive in an instant millions of unrelated pieces of information about the world outside your body. The eye is often compared with a camera, but the comparison is hardly fair to the eye. As with the camera, an image enters your eye by passing through a lens. And the image is in some sense recorded at the back of both devices: on film in the camera and by a communication system that instantaneously transmits the image to your brain. True, the eye is like a camera, but it is more sophisticated than any machine imaginable.

Thousands of times a day, your eyes move and focus on images near and far, picking out objects for interpretation within a vast available field. Instantaneously, your eye records what a dozen cameras could not, providing you with an ever-changing, incredibly detailed chain of three-dimensional pictures of the world around you.

Parts of the Eye

The complex structure of the eye is compact: each of your eyes, lying within protective

Protective Structures of the Eye

sockets formed by the skull and surrounding tissues, measures about 1 inch in diameter. The delicate workings of your eye are protected by the bridge of your nose, your eyebrow, and your cheekbone. The bones and tissues surrounding your eye are known collectively as the orbit.

Your eye is also protected by your eyelids. The eyelids open and shut involuntarily, shielding the eye from intense light, impact, and foreign particles.

Tears serve to lubricate, clean, and nourish your eye. Tears are secreted by glands in your upper eyelids and in the orbit above and to the side of the upper lids. Tears are drained into your nose from two tiny openings located in your upper and lower eyelids, very close to where the lids join adjacent to your nose (inner canthus). The ducts that convey tears from your eyes to your nose are called the nasolacrimal ducts.

When you blink, which happens every few seconds, your eyelids act like windshield wipers complete with fluid, washing away dirt and particles and applying lubricant. During sleep your eyes are protected from drying out by being closed.

The movement of your eye is controlled by six muscles attached to the outside covering (sclera) of the eye. They act in concert to move both eyes up, down, around, and from side to side so that your two eyes will center on exactly the same point. (When the centering mechanisms are impaired, the eyes are said to deviate from one another.)

The eyeball itself is composed of several layers of tissue. The conjunctiva runs along the inside of the eyelid and the outermost portion of the eye. It meets the sclera, the tough white layer that covers most of the eyeball. Both contain tiny blood vessels that nourish the eye.

Inside the conjunctiva at the center of the eye lies the cornea. This layer of clear tissue with its overlying film of tears provides about two-thirds of the focusing power of the eye. The cornea is shaped to refract light as it enters the eye, directing it through the lens and to the retina at the back of the eye.

The pupil and iris lie behind the cornea. The pupil is the opening through which light passes to the back of the eye. Muscles controlling the iris (the colored part of the eye)

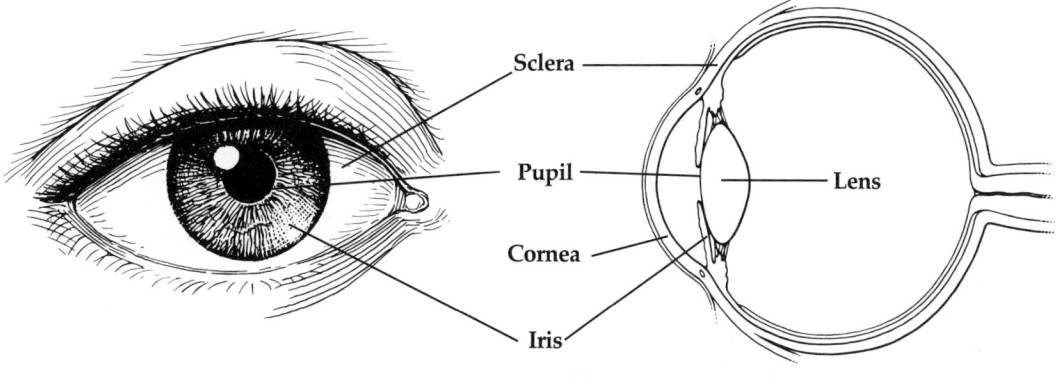

Front View   *Side View*

allow it to change the size of the pupil to adjust to the amount of light. The pupil becomes larger in dim light to allow more light in and smaller in bright light to protect the delicate retina from excessive light. The pupil also opens (dilates) in response to excitement and as a reaction to certain drugs.

Between the cornea and the iris lies the anterior chamber. This space is filled with aqueous humor, a transparent fluid. This fluid is manufactured in the posterior chamber of the eye close to the attachment of the iris. The fluid passes into the anterior chamber through the pupil and then is absorbed into the bloodstream through the canal of Schlemm in the angle where the iris meets the cornea. Your body regulates the pressure of the aqueous humor.

Behind the iris and anterior chamber is the lens. This transparent, colorless tissue is enclosed in a capsule and suspended in the middle of the eye by a net of fibers. The lens can change shape in order to focus light rays on the retina. When an object is nearby, the lens thickens to best perceive the image; when an object is farther away, the lens thins in order to focus the image clearly on the retina. Throughout one's life the lens accumulates more fibers. These added fibers gradually make the lens less elastic, so that generally by middle age you become less able to focus on near objects.

The bulk of the eyeball, which is behind the lens, is formed by the round posterior chamber. It is filled with a colorless, gelatin-like substance known as the vitreous humor. You may notice that occasionally you see spots or what look like tiny bits of string or lint in your vision. Suspended in the vitreous humor, these are known as "floaters" and are usually leftover bits of material from the

growth of the eye before birth. Occasionally they can be a sign of a more serious eye disorder.

Behind the vitreous chamber is the retina. The retina of the eye is equivalent to the film of the camera. Composed of 10 layers, the retina processes the light images projected from the cornea and lens.

Rod cells within the retina perceive light, and cone cells perceive both light and color. Rod cells outnumber cone cells 20 to 1, and they can respond to faint light. Cone cells need more light to function, which is one reason why it is difficult to see colors in the dark. The responsibility of the rods and cones is to transform the light that they perceive into electrical impulses.

Parts of the Eye

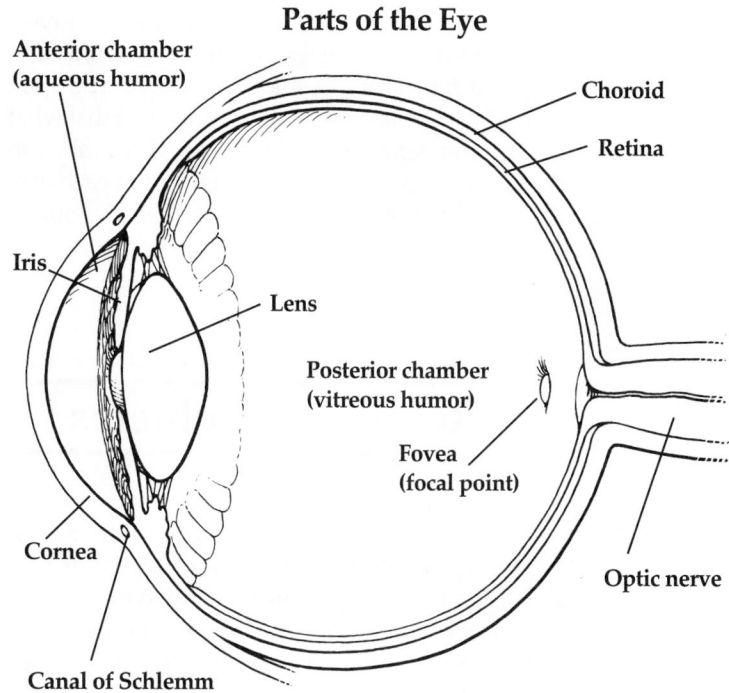

A small depression in the center of the retina, known as the fovea, provides the most acute vision. This section contains only cones and is the most visually sensitive part of the eye. The small area surrounding the fovea is known as the macula lutea, and as a whole it is responsible for central vision.

The retina is nourished primarily by the choroid. This multilayered tissue, which lies between the retina and the sclera, is composed of veins and arteries.

The optic nerve takes the electrical impulses recorded by the retina and transmits them to the brain. The point at which the optic nerve leaves the retina on its way to the brain is known as the optic disc. The optic nerve carries impulses to the visual cortex at the back of the brain. The brain interprets these messages into what we perceive as sight.

The Mechanism of Sight

The listing of all of the eye's parts may make the organ seem complicated indeed. Yet the basic mechanism of sight is relatively simple.

Rays of light project through the cornea, the pupil, and then the lens. The internal eye muscles help adjust the shape of the lens to focus the light rays on the back of the retina. There, the rods and cones turn the light into electrical impulses that are carried by the optic nerve to the brain.

Once the brain receives the electrical impulses, it must interpret them. The image received by the retina is upside down, a characteristic of a simple convex lens. The brain reinterprets the image, however, so that what you perceive is right side up. The brain also must coordinate the images from each eye, which are slightly different. The merging of the two images produces three-dimensional (stereoscopic) vision.

Eye Experts

An ophthalmologist specializes in the treatment of eye diseases and conditions. He or she is a medical doctor (M.D.) who has, in addition to medical school training, at least 4 years of specialized training in the care of the eyes and the diagnosis and treatment of eye ailments. An ophthalmologist can prescribe eyeglasses and contact lenses; complete eye examinations and eye care can be provided by ophthalmologists. An ophthalmologist also treats injuries to the eye and performs various surgical procedures when they are required.

In addition, an ophthalmologist is well trained in the use of specialized instruments to make a correct diagnosis, especially if your eye symptoms are not perfectly obvious. This is crucial in acute eye symptoms when a delay of a few hours may make the difference between good vision and blindness.

An optometrist is a person trained to diagnose refraction errors and to prescribe corrective lenses. Optometrists graduate from a school of optometry and earn a doctor of optometry (O.D.) degree. They can conduct certain tests, and often they detect signs of eye disease or other kinds of disease apparent from examination of the retina. In some states, optometrists are licensed to diagnose and treat eye diseases.

An optician is a technician who fills the prescriptions of ophthalmologists and optometrists. Opticians grind and fit lenses, but they do not examine eyes for disease or refraction problems.

Refraction Problems

The most common eye problems—myopia (nearsightedness), hyperopia (farsightedness), astigmatism (asymmetrical cornea), and presbyopia (the inability to focus on an object at close range as one ages)—are all due to errors of refraction of the lens and cornea of one or both eyes.

If you are to see an object clearly, its well-focused image must reach your retina, the light-sensitive membrane at the back of your eye. As light rays enter your eye, your cornea and lens refract (bend) them to converge on your retina.

For the image to be clear, the focusing power of the lens and cornea must be coordinated with the length of your eyeball. In normal eyesight, the image then appears focused.

When the focusing elements and the eyeball are not properly coordinated, however, the image will not reach the retina in focus, and the light will then be focused in front of or behind the retina. When the shape of the eyeball is such that light is focused in front of the retina, the condition is known as nearsightedness because only objects at near range are focused on the correct part of the retina. Farsightedness is the result of light being focused better on the retina at long range. Astigmatism is a condition in which the cornea is shaped more like a football than a basketball, thereby misdirecting some of the rays of light.

Nearsightedness, farsightedness, and astigmatism may be the result of heredity or other causes. However, another refractive error is a basic part of aging. This is known as presbyopia, and it is the result of changes in the lens of the eye. The lens hardens with age, reducing its ability to change shape and focus light at close range. This hardening results in a difficulty with focusing on near objects.

Most errors of refraction are treated easily with corrective glasses or contact lenses. For most people, a pair of glasses or lenses prescribed and fitted by an ophthalmologist or optometrist provides the necessary correction for them to function easily in daily activities. Also, a new operation may prove useful for people with mild or moderate myopia (see page 525).

Nearsightedness

Signs and Symptoms—Blurred vision of distant objects

Nearsightedness (myopia) is a common vision problem, affecting about 20 percent of the population. If you are nearsighted, your eye is not round. It probably is too long from front to back, so that the light rays that are refracted by the cornea and lens meet in front of (rather than at) the retina. The result is that distant images are blurry.

You may be able to focus on nearby images, although the degree of your myopia determines the focusing ability. If you are severely nearsighted you may be able to see clearly only objects that are a few inches from your eyes; if you are mildly nearsighted, you

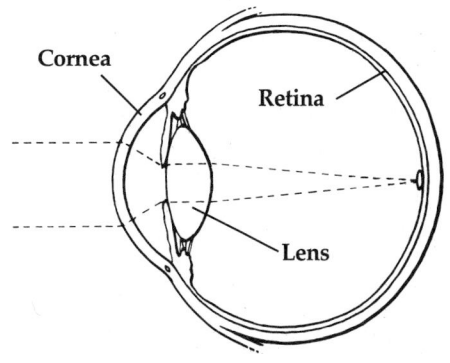

Normal

For clear eyesight, the lens and cornea must be coordinated with the length of your eyeball.

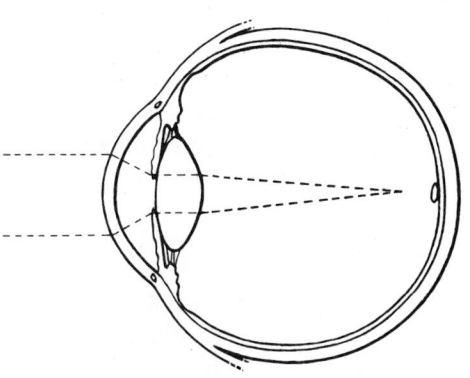

Nearsightedness (myopia)

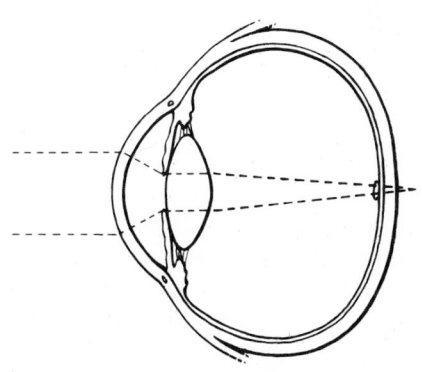

Farsightedness (hyperopia)

may see clearly the objects that are several yards away.

Occasionally, nearsightedness results not from an elongated shape of the eye but from too much focusing power in the lens and cornea. The result is the same in that, again, the light rays focus in front of the retina.

Nearsightedness often is observed during childhood, from the early school years through the late teens; it affects boys and girls equally. It can develop rapidly during this time, requiring new lenses every few months. It tends to stabilize during young

The Eye Examination

How Often Do I Need to Visit the Ophthalmologist?

Everyone should have an eye examination from time to time. If you do not have eye problems, have your eyes examined every 3 to 5 years until about age 50. After 50, have them checked more frequently for signs of glaucoma and other eye disease. If you have refractive or other eye problems, have your eyes checked every 2 years, or as recommended by your eye specialist.

Children should have their first examination at around age 3 or 4, unless you have reason to believe there may be a problem earlier. If you do, tests are available that can be performed on toddlers.

Examination

Your eye specialist may begin by asking a series of questions about your family's medical history and your personal medical history. Then a series of tests will be conducted. One simple test involves passing a light in front of your eyes in a set pattern in order to check the movements of the eyes, both separately and together. Your eye doctor will check peripheral vision by moving an object at the edge of your field of vision.

The Snellen Chart
You will be asked to read letters on a chart known as a Snellen chart. In this test you usually are asked to read the letters on each line of the chart from 20 feet away. If you can read the letters that people with perfect eyesight can read at 20 feet from the chart, you are said to have 20/20 vision. If you read at 20 feet what most people can read 40 feet from the chart, you have 20/40 vision. For children who are too young to recognize letters, another similar test using shapes can be conducted.

The Ophthalmoscope
The back of the eye is examined with an instrument known as the ophthalmoscope. The device has a magnifier and a light that shines through to the back of the eye, allowing the examiner to see clearly the rear (posterior) portions of the eye, particularly the retina.

The back of each eye (known as the fundus) provides many clues to your general health. The region is unique from other portions of your body in that tiny blood vessels and nerve tissue of the retina can be seen directly.

The condition of the retinal vessels often has a tale to tell. For example, if you have hypertension (high blood pressure), the changes in these vessels often indicate the severity of your problem and the urgency with which treatment should be started. Clues to circulatory disturbances in the brain sometimes are provided by the small particles appearing in the blood vessels of the fundus, which indicate the formation of cholesterol-containing plaques or clots of other material. Changes in the blood vessels characteristic of diabetes also can be visible, as can holes or tears in the retina and a host of other problems.

The optic nerve head (optic disc) is also visible with the ophthalmoscope. The optic disc is actually an extension of your brain. If the nerve is swollen it may indicate that you have a disorder, even a problem as serious as a brain tumor, causing increased pressure within your skull.

For the ophthalmoscope examination, a few drops are placed in your eyes to dilate the pupils so that more of the fundus can be seen. The lights of the room are dimmed also so the pupils will widen. Then the bright light of the ophthalmoscope is shone in and each eye is examined.

The use of dilating eyedrops is a routine part of most eye examinations. They can make it temporarily difficult for you to focus on near objects or to tolerate bright light. If you are being checked for signs of cataracts or retinal problems, however, eyedrops are necessary.

People older than 50 should be tested regularly for signs of glaucoma. A simple test to measure the pressure inside the eyeball is done with a device called a tonometer (see Glaucoma, page 550).

adulthood, so that during your 20s and 30s you may not require a change of eyeglasses or contact lenses. At about age 40, however, the normal effects of aging may begin to change your vision. Nearsightedness tends to run in families.

Diagnosis

If you notice that your child persistently squints, sits close to the television, movie screen, or class blackboard, holds books very close while reading, and seems to be unaware of distant objects, have your child's vision tested by an ophthalmologist or optometrist.

The examination will begin with your child reading a chart of letters to determine the vision in each eye (visual acuity). Special charts are available for young children who are unable to read letters (see The Eye Examination, above). Your physician also will perform a series of tests to determine the extent of correction needed.

How Serious Is Nearsightedness?

Nearsightedness in children can be socially, emotionally, and educationally debilitating if not diagnosed early and treated with corrective lenses.

Treatment

Corrective Lenses

Nearsightedness is treated easily with eyeglasses or contact lenses. Your eye specialist will determine a specific prescription to suit your child's needs. This prescription, a specially made concave lens for one or both eyes, can correct vision to normal or nearly normal. The prescription can be made for glasses or contact lenses in various forms, although contact lenses are usually unsuitable for preteen children.

Surgery

Other possible treatments include radial keratotomy (RK) and photorefractive keratectomy (PRK) (see Radial Keratotomy, this page).

Farsightedness

Signs and Symptoms

- Blurred vision at close distance
- Eyestrain, including aching eyes and headache

Farsightedness (hyperopia) is a common refraction problem. In most cases it is the result of the eyeball being too short from front to back. Thus, the rays of light converge on the retina short of the focal length at which they would be in focus. The angle between the iris and the interior surface of the cornea is narrowed in the farsighted individual, making him or her more vulnerable to closed-angle glaucoma later in life (see Chronic Glaucoma, page 551).

Farsightedness also can be caused by a weakness in the ability of the lens and cornea to focus. Whatever the cause, however, close images appear blurry, although distant ones may appear clear.

Farsightedness usually is present at birth and tends to run in families. Young people

---

Radial Keratotomy

Radial keratotomy is a surgical technique to correct mild to moderate nearsightedness. The process seems simple, but it requires careful microsurgical technique.

Procedure

A series of delicate incisions is made in the cornea of each eye in a radial or spoke-like pattern. Each eye is done separately, on different days. The center of the cornea flattens and the outer downward-sloping portion becomes steeper. This changes the way light rays are bent, focusing them more on the retina.

Recovery

The procedure is done on an outpatient basis—it takes only 15 to 30 minutes—and with the person under local anesthesia. The individual may wear a patch or dark glasses for several days. Complete recovery may take weeks to months.

Results

Radial keratotomy in principle seems like a good solution to nearsightedness. A 10-year follow-up study of individuals who have had the procedure suggests that approximately 70 percent were not wearing glasses. Three percent experienced a significant decrease in vision.

Other drawbacks to radial keratotomy include the potential for fluctuating vision—particularly a tendency toward farsightedness, late infections of the cornea, and slightly increased risk of traumatic corneal rupture.

Many eye surgeons remain uncertain of the usefulness of radial keratotomy. At this point it is impossible to know who might have long-term benefits from the procedure. We advise caution when considering it.

More recently, the FDA approved a laser operation called photorefractive keratectomy (PRK) for nearsightedness. This procedure uses a beam of ultraviolet light to flatten the cornea by vaporizing corneal cells. The procedure is irreversible and, although rare, can sometimes lead to vision that is worse, even with glasses. As with radial keratotomy, we recommend caution.

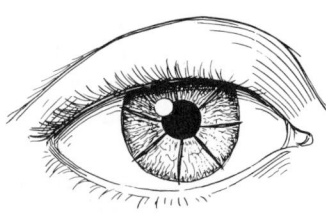

Radial keratotomy uses a series of surgical incisions in the cornea to correct nearsightedness (myopia).

Hereditary Disorders of the Eyes

Conditions and diseases affecting the eyes can be passed from generation to generation. Such conditions range from simple farsightedness (which can be corrected with glasses or contact lenses, see page 525) to more serious eye diseases such as retinoblastoma (see page 545). Certain systemic diseases, including diabetes and hypertension, also can produce eye complications.

Refraction errors such as nearsightedness, farsightedness, and astigmatism are due to the shapes and characteristics of the cornea, lens, and eyeball, and often they are present from birth. The cause of such abnormalities is unknown but, because the deformity often recurs generation after generation, genetics is thought to play a key role. Often, however, only certain members of a family inherit a disorder and others are entirely free of the problem.

Heredity seems to play a part in the incidence of strabismus (habitual squint, see page 534) and amblyopia (poor vision, usually secondary to misalignment of the eyes, see page 534). If your eyes were misaligned as a child, you have a greater chance of having a child with the same problem.

Defects of color vision, commonly and often wrongly termed color blindness, usually are present from birth, having been passed along through the mother, usually to her sons. Most people who have defects of color vision cannot distinguish between reds and greens in dim light; some people cannot separate the colors even in bright light. Only a minority of so-called color-blind people see everything in tones of gray, and only they are truly color-blind. Color vision defects are common. They are caused by a lack of one or more of the light-sensitive substances found in the cones of the retina.

Certain eye diseases also seem to have a genetic factor. People with glaucoma (see page 550) often have a family history of the disease, as do people with cataracts (see page 553). Retinitis pigmentosa is a serious threat to sight, and often there is a pattern of recurrence of the disease within families (see page 561). Retinoblastoma, a cancerous tumor of the eye that occurs in young children, seems to have a genetic component in 30 to 40 percent of cases (see page 545).

Other general disorders that affect the eyes and have a hereditary component include diabetes and hypertension. Diabetes affects eyesight after many years (see Diabetes Mellitus, page 925, and The Eye and Diabetes, page 562). Hypertension (high blood pressure) affects eyesight when the disease is particularly severe, and it can even be diagnosed on the basis of changes seen within the eye (see High Blood Pressure, page 647, and Hypertension and Vision, page 564).

can often overcome mild farsightedness naturally as the eyes accommodate to the condition; the ciliary muscles contract and change the shape of the lens to bring the focal point forward to meet the retina. Thus, they do not need corrective glasses for their hyperopia. However, with age, the ability of the eyes to "correct" the condition is lost, and glasses or contact lenses are required.

Diagnosis

You may not have symptoms for several years, if ever, depending on the severity. You may, however, find it difficult to focus on objects close at hand. You may have headaches or general eye discomfort after doing close tasks such as reading, writing, or drawing.

If you have such problems, consult an eye specialist, who will conduct a series of tests to determine the nature and extent of the problem and who will then prescribe eyeglasses or contact lenses precisely suited to your needs (see The Eye Examination, page 524).

Treatment

Farsightedness is treated easily with eyeglasses or contact lenses made to suit your needs. Your eye specialist will determine the precise prescription needed to correct one or both eyes with convex lenses. The shape of the lens serves to refract the light at an angle that brings the convergence forward to meet the retina. The prescription can be made for glasses, which are appropriate for all ages, or contact lenses, which are best suited to adults and teenagers.

Surgical techniques to treat farsightedness are available but are not in widespread use.

Presbyopia

Signs and Symptoms
- Decreased ability to focus on objects at close range
- Eyestrain that may include a feeling of tired eyes and a headache

When functioning correctly, the lens in your eye changes shape in order to focus on objects: when you are looking at something at close range, the ciliary muscles contract and thicken the lens to bring the object into focus. However, as you age, the lens becomes harder and less elastic, making it more difficult to see nearby objects clearly.

The resulting condition is known as presbyopia. This hardening process is a normal part of life, and it happens to everyone to some degree.

Diagnosis

Many people begin to notice a change in their vision around age 40. Close-up objects that were once easy to see become blurred. The print in newspapers and books begins to seem smaller, and you instinctively hold them farther away from your eyes to read them.

If you are already farsighted you may notice the changes somewhat earlier and will need to have stronger corrective lenses made. Even if you are nearsighted you will experience the effects of presbyopia, and you may find yourself taking off your glasses to read small print. You may find that your eyes seem increasingly tired after reading, or you may experience frequent headaches as a result of eyestrain.

When close work such as sewing and reading becomes difficult to do at a normal distance or if you experience frequent eyestrain and headaches, see your ophthalmologist or optometrist, who will test your eyes and prescribe appropriate lenses (see The Eye Examination, page 524).

Treatment

Presbyopia usually is treated with glasses and only occasionally with contact lenses. Your eye specialist will fit you with a prescription to help adjust the focal point more narrowly. As your own lenses lose the ability to adjust, you may need a new prescription every few years until about age 65. At that point the lenses of your eyes will have lost most of their ability to accommodate, and so changes in your prescription are less frequent.

If you are already nearsighted or astigmatic, you will probably find yourself needing a second pair of glasses to counteract the effects of presbyopia. Some people require a third set for middle distances (2 to 4 feet). You need not constantly shuffle glasses, however, for they can be made with two or

---

Refraction Errors Due to Changing Blood Sugar Concentration

A prolonged increase in the blood sugar concentration (a problem characteristic of poorly controlled diabetes) tends to cause a metabolic change in the lens of the eye, altering its shape.

When diabetes develops, often the blood sugar concentration gradually increases over a period of weeks or months. The subsequent change in the shape of the lens causes a slow change in focus, which often is not noticeable immediately. However, when the diabetes finally is discovered and treatment produces a rapid decrease in the blood sugar concentration, a rapid change in focus toward farsightedness (hyperopia) often occurs, a change that may be alarming.

It is worthwhile to postpone fitting of glasses until your blood sugar concentration has been well controlled for at least a month. Subsequent minor fluctuations in the blood sugar concentration from day to day or week to week are unlikely to cause perceptible changes in vision or the strength of glasses required (see Diabetes Mellitus, page 925).

---

even three lenses. The double lens, which is known as a bifocal, was first introduced by Benjamin Franklin. The top portion of each lens (upper segment) is corrected for distance; the bottom portion (lower segment) is corrected for near objects. Trifocals include a third (middle) lens for focusing at about arm's length.

Some practice is needed to become accustomed to bifocals and trifocals. Be certain that the frames are adjusted to your head: it is important that as you tilt your head up and down, your line of vision will move from one segment to another in both eyes at precisely the same time.

Astigmatism

Signs and Symptoms—Portions of your visual field are blurred, typically vertical, horizontal, or diagonal lines

Astigmatism is a refraction error due to an uneven curvature of the cornea, blurring some of what you see. In a normal eye, the cornea is symmetrically curved, but an astigmatic eye typically has areas of the cornea that are steeper or flatter than normal, a shape that produces the distorted vision. In some instances, astigmatism may result from abnormalities of the lens inside the eye, although the cornea is normal.

Astigmatism is usually present from birth and may occur in combination with nearsightedness or farsightedness. It is a condition that tends to remain constant, neither improving nor deteriorating considerably with age.

Diagnosis

You may notice that your vision is blurred. If you notice that your child seems able to see some things clearly but not others, in a seemingly random pattern, consult your eye doctor for complete testing (see The Eye Examination, page 524).

Treatment

Astigmatism can be treated readily with corrective glasses or contact lenses. After careful examination, your eye specialist will determine your needs. Lenses then can be made to counteract the unevenness of the cornea of one or both eyes or to correct for a combination of astigmatism and nearsightedness or of astigmatism and farsightedness.

What You Should Know About Contact Lenses

Gas-permeable hard lenses, soft lenses, and extended-wear soft lenses are far more comfortable for long-term wear than any previously available. However, with the increase in the types available and their rapidly expanding use, more problems are reported, some of them serious.

Who Can Wear Contact Lenses?

Contact lenses are most useful for people with refraction errors such as nearsightedness, farsightedness, and astigmatism. In addition, certain unusual conditions such as keratoconus (cone-shaped cornea) are better treated with contact lenses than with glasses. Some people who have had artificial lenses implanted during cataract operations find contact lenses preferable to glasses.

In all cases, however, only people who are highly motivated to wear contact lenses should consider them. Learning to wear them requires varying periods of adjustment, during which your eyes may be uncomfortable. You also need a certain amount of manual dexterity to put these tiny lenses in and remove them. Also, most contact lenses require daily care, varying from minimal for some kinds to fairly elaborate for others.

For these reasons, contact lenses are not for everyone. They generally are not suitable for small children or for people with certain diseases that limit mobility of the hands, such as arthritis or Parkinson's disease. In addition, contact lenses are not suitable for people with certain eye diseases and disorders. Your eye specialist can advise you.

How Do They Work?

As its name implies, a contact lens is worn in contact with the eye. The specially shaped plastic disc sits on the cornea of your eye. (The cornea is the transparent window that lies in front of the pupil, like the crystal of a watch.) The lens floats on the tears that bathe the eye when you blink. This liquid also allows necessary oxygen to reach the cornea.

Each contact lens is made according to a prescription to focus light on the retina of your eye, just as each lens for a pair of eyeglasses does. However, in contrast to the situation with eyeglasses, with contact lenses your entire field of vision is corrected because all images reaching the eyes pass through the lenses. The outer and inner surfaces of each lens are ground to correct your particular refraction error and to fit the curvature of your eye.

Types of Contact Lenses

The two basic types of contact lenses are hard (rigid) and soft. Hard lenses are small plastic discs that fit just over the cornea. Soft lenses are made of a thin plastic polymer and fit over a slightly larger portion of the eye.

Hard Contact Lenses

These are the sturdiest contact lenses, but they are the least comfortable. Because they are rigid, they do not scratch or tear easily. They also need less maintenance than the delicate, soft variety. However, the rigid plastic is more water resistant and so it is harder to keep wet and more difficult to keep fixed in position on the eye.

Soft Contact Lenses

Soft contacts are delicate because the polymer can be torn more easily. They are usually much more comfortable to wear than hard lenses because the soft plastic causes less friction on the eyelid than do hard lenses. Soft lenses require more care than hard ones because they must be cleaned and often soaked in special solutions. They tend to stay on the eye better than hard lenses. Daily disposable lenses are available.

Disposable Soft Contact Lenses

These soft contact lenses can be worn for up to 2 weeks and then thrown away. Extended-wear disposable lenses have not been shown to cause infectious ulcers on the cornea any more frequently than standard extended-wear soft contacts. Daily disposable lenses are available.

Other Types

Two other types of lenses are gas-permeable hard lenses and extended-wear soft lenses. One of the problems with all contact lenses is getting enough oxygen to the cornea. Soft lenses have a varying amount of water in them that allows oxygen to pass through the medium. Hard lenses move a little each time you blink, allowing oxygen to reach the cornea. Gas-permeable hard lenses also have pores in the rigid plastic to allow more oxygen to reach the cornea when you blink.

As their name suggests, extended-wear soft lenses can be worn for greater lengths of time because they have sufficient water in them to allow oxygen to pass into the cornea, even while you sleep. They are even thinner than daily-wear soft lenses, a feature that makes them more comfortable but also more fragile.

Tinted soft lenses are a popular choice among fashion-conscious people. These lenses are tinted in the portion of the lens that covers the iris. They come in shades of blue, brown, and green and provide an intense color to the eyes. They are also useful for disguising defects of the iris, corneal scars, and irregularly shaped pupils.

Bifocal Contact Lenses

Bifocal contact lenses are available for people needing corrections for near and far distances. However, because they move with the eye, in some individuals it is difficult for the eye to adjust for near and far vision. Often, a more satisfactory solution is reached by correcting one eye for distant vision and the other for close vision with regular soft lenses.

Combination Contact Lenses

Piggyback contact lenses are designed for people with certain eye disorders. These lenses are a combination of hard and soft lenses. A soft lens with a central excavation is fitted for comfort, and then a hard lens is placed to correct for vision. People with corneal malformations are particularly helped by these lenses.

Get Them Fitted Properly

Good vision, comfort, and the overall health of your eyes depend on properly fitted contact lenses. Whichever form of lens you choose, make sure that you have them custom-fit by a professional who can determine your exact needs.

Be Alert for Problems

If you receive a careful fitting of your lenses and are free of other eye problems, expect good results from your contact lenses. Be aware, however, that on rare occasions potentially sight-threatening problems can develop.

Several of these problems are related to the amount of oxygen your cornea receives. One of the more common of these rare problems is overuse. If you wear contact lenses for too long at a time, your corneas may become starved for oxygen. The symptoms are blurry vision, pain, tearing, redness, and sensitivity to light.

Remove your lenses immediately. If the pain persists, see your eye specialist.

Corneal vascularization is another response of the cornea to inadequate amounts of oxygen. In this condition, tiny blood vessels grow into the clear tissue of the cornea.

Caring for Your Contacts

Proper care of your contact lenses is vital to your comfort and the overall health of your eyes. Each kind of lens has its own requirements, but no matter what variety you wear, the first rule is to keep them clean.

Wash your hands before handling your lenses. Keep your lens case clean and readily available so you can remove and safely store your lenses if your eyes begin to hurt or become red or if your vision blurs.

Hard Lenses

These are the easiest to care for because they are less fragile than other kinds. Use only a commercial contact lens wetting solution to moisten them for insertion (never use saliva). Clean the lenses each day with a commercial cleaning solution.

Gas-Permeable Hard Lenses

These hard lenses have pores in them to allow oxygen to reach the cornea. Wash them each day in a commercial cleaning solution and store them overnight in a conditioner. Clean them each week with an enzyme solution. When rinsing, use distilled water because tap water leaves a residue.

Soft Lenses

These lenses require careful maintenance. They must be cleaned each day with a surface cleaner designed specifically for soft lenses. Disinfect them either daily with a disinfecting solution or every other day with heat (be sure to follow the manufacturer's instructions for temperature and duration).

Do not use a mixture of salt tablets and distilled water for cleaning because it can allow infections to develop. Use a bottled or aerosol saline solution without preservatives. Never use tap water. Apply an enzyme treatment weekly, rinse with saline, and disinfect to neutralize the enzyme.

Extended-Wear Soft Lenses

Remove your lenses most nights and clean them in the same manner as for regular soft lenses.

In extreme cases your vision can become clouded. Should this occur you may need to switch to another type of lens or stop wearing contact lenses altogether.

Corneal warpage is yet another problem of too little oxygen reaching the cornea, and it involves a gradual change in the cornea's shape. The result is uneven or fluctuating vision for hours or days after removing your lenses. The problem is infrequent for wearers of gas-permeable hard lenses or soft contact lenses, but it is more common among those who use standard hard lenses.

Giant papillary conjunctivitis is a relatively common allergic disorder among wearers of soft lenses. It evolves gradually. You may find it increasingly difficult to wear your lenses for long. Your sight may be blurry when you blink (one or both contacts ride up under your eyelids), or one or both eyes may itch and ooze soon after you remove your lenses. The condition is more common among people whose soft contact lenses are fairly old or whose lenses have developed a layer of protein on the surface. See your ophthalmologist; it may be necessary to stop using your lenses until the problems subside. Switching to a newer type of soft lens or a gas-permeable hard lens may be helpful.

Sensitivity to the cleaning solution is another fairly common problem. Some people develop a reaction to chemicals found in contact lens solution, particularly the preservative thimerosal. If you experience discomfort, see your eye specialist. He or she may advise you to switch to another solution that uses different chemicals.

A bacterial or fungal infection of the cornea resulting in a corneal ulcer is rare but serious (see Corneal Ulcers and Infections, page 547). You may notice a loss of vision, and your eye becomes red, very painful, and sensitive to light. Such infections are sometimes the result of improper cleaning of contact lenses. Extended-wear soft lenses are associated with the problem most frequently. If you suspect you have a corneal ulcer, see your ophthalmologist immediately.

Acanthamoeba keratitis is a rare but dangerous infection. The cause is an amoeba organism that lives in stagnant water, certain tap water, and occasionally saliva. It causes a painful, red eye that is difficult to treat. It usually develops as a result of improperly cleaned soft contact lenses and can be avoided by using commercial saline solutions or by heat-sterilizing the lenses.

Finally, if you are a contact-lens wearer, have a pair of glasses available as a backup in case an eye problem develops that requires you to stop wearing your contacts temporarily.

Trauma to the Eye

From time to time, eye injuries of one kind or another happen—whether they result from an errant foul ball at a Little League game, a grain of sand at the beach, a splash of household chemical, or some other cause.

Many such injuries can be avoided by properly protecting the eyes with goggles or glasses when participating in hazardous activities: for example, make it a habit to wear safety glasses when using tools. If an accident occurs and your eye is injured, immediate, careful examination and proper medical care are required (see Eye Emergencies, page 452).

Trauma to the eye can result from objects striking or entering the eyes (see this page) or from chemical burns (see this page). Injury can lead to infections such as orbital cellulitis (see page 545). The following pages also discuss proper eye protection. (For a full discussion of first aid for eye injuries, see Foreign Bodies in the Eye, page 425.)

Foreign Bodies

Signs and Symptoms
- Sudden pain in the eye
- Sudden worsening of vision
- Redness of the eye

Everyone occasionally gets a speck of dust in the eye; usually, all that is required is that you blink until your tears wash the particle away. However, you may find that this does not work or that something more serious has entered your eye.

The injury may be limited to the conjunctiva and cornea (these are the most frequent sites), or it may affect the eyeball. Whenever pain and redness persist, the injury should be treated professionally to ensure that vision is not lost (for emergency treatment, see Foreign Bodies in the Eye, page 425).

Diagnosis
If severe pain develops suddenly in an eye and your vision is suddenly worse, you may have a foreign object in your eye. If the pain is severe, go to a hospital emergency room or arrange to see your ophthalmologist as soon as possible.

Do not try to remove the object yourself.

Your physician will examine your eye under strong light to see whether the cornea has been scratched (abraded) by the foreign object. An injury to the cornea can be very painful. A local anesthetic may be administered to lessen the pain.

If the object has entered the eye itself, an X-ray or a CT scan may be obtained. You will be asked a series of questions to determine the nature of your activities at the time of the accident and thus what substance might have entered the eye.

How Serious Are Foreign Bodies in the Eye?
A foreign body in the eye can be a serious threat to sight, particularly if the object enters the eye itself or damages the cornea or lens. Professional emergency treatment is required.

Treatment
If the object can be seen on the eye surface under strong light, your ophthalmologist may be able to remove it with surgical tweezers. If the object is no longer present but has scratched the cornea, your eye will be treated topically with an antibiotic. Then a patch will be placed over the eye to protect it overnight. Generally, this treatment will allow the cornea to heal itself.

If the object has entered the eye, it must be removed by an ophthalmic surgeon. In the meantime, emergency treatment usually is begun. The pupil may be dilated and antibiotics may be prescribed. A metal shield is placed over the eye to protect it until surgery is performed.

Chemical Burns

Signs and Symptoms
- Pain in the eye
- Decreased vision
- Increased sensitivity to light

Chemical burns of the eye can endanger your vision. If your job entails the use of hazardous chemicals, be aware of the dangers and protect your eyes with goggles. Household cleaning products, particularly those that contain ammonia or bleach, and garden chemicals also can cause serious harm.

Protecting Your Eyes

Myths about care of the eyes abound. For example, the warnings that reading in dim light or watching television while sitting close to the screen will damage your eyes are not true. Reading by flashlight is a harmless activity, too, as are sitting in the front row of a movie theater, doing close work with your eyes, and driving or doing other things in bright sunshine without sunglasses. These activities may make your eyes feel tired or strained, but they do not harm them.

Grease and Chemical Hazards

However, many situations can seriously harm your eyes. Some of the most common injuries are the result of accidents while doing everyday tasks such as cooking, cleaning house, or working in the garden or yard. Spattered grease, splashed household chemicals, or sprayed garden chemicals are common causes of serious eye injuries. The most dangerous substances to the eye are those that contain alkali or lye.

Use Safety Goggles

Protect yourself by wearing safety glasses or goggles. Make sure your children also get in the habit of wearing protective eyeglasses when helping with hazardous housework, cooking, or gardening tasks. Teach children early to wear goggles when using tools.

The Hazards of Makeup

A scratched or abraded cornea can be the result of hastily applying mascara or accidentally squirting hair spray in the eyes. Be careful when using anything near your eyes, from brushes to fingernails. Shield your eyes when applying hair spray.

Sports Risks

Sports carry their share of eye risks. If a hockey puck or racquetball contacts your eye, it easily can cause internal damage. Protective eyeglasses or shields can help prevent such injuries. Basketball players frequently suffer corneal abrasions from finger pokes, and football players sometimes sustain broken bones near the eye. More and more professional athletes now wear protective shields or goggles. You should, too.

Workplace Practices

Anyone whose job carries a risk of eye injury is required by law to have protective glasses provided by the employer and to wear them.

Should I Wear Sunglasses?

There is increasing concern about the effects of ultraviolet radiation from the sun on the eyes. Generally speaking, you do not need to wear sunglasses every time you step outside. However, if you spend a great deal of time in the sun, wear sunglasses designed to screen ultraviolet radiation.

Such sunglasses are available in inexpensive and expensive models. Be sure to wear them if you use an ultraviolet sunlamp. Never look at the sun directly, even through sunglasses or X-ray film, because it can cause permanent damage.

Choose sunglasses that provide maximum protection from ultraviolet A (UVA) and ultraviolet B (UVB) light at a reasonable cost. Long-term exposure to ultraviolet light increases your chance of cataracts. The greater the blockage of ultraviolet light, the lower your risk of damage. Nonprescription sunglasses should carry an American National Standards Institute label telling how much ultraviolet light they block. To minimize ultraviolet light that can enter from the sides, choose sunglasses that fit close to your face or wraparound sunglasses.

Reduce glare with darker lenses that block more visible light. For activities on water, sand, or snow, choose darker lenses than for around-town driving. For reflected glare, choose gray-tinted, polarized lenses. Gray- or green-tinted lenses offer the least color distortion.

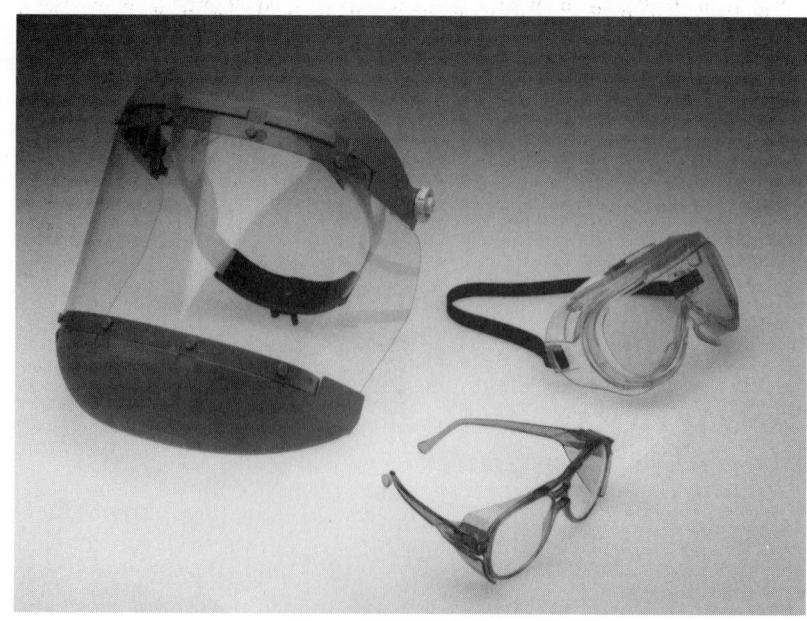

Safety goggles are available in a wide variety of styles.

Direct contact (chemicals splashed in your face, for example) is most hazardous, but concentrated fumes and aerosols also can be dangerous. Wear goggles or protective glasses and try to work in well-ventilated surroundings. Be careful not to splash when mixing and pouring chemicals.

Diagnosis

You probably will know when a chemical is burning your eyes. They hurt and may be more sensitive to light, and your vision may be blurred. If pain is present, seek prompt medical care: chemical burns to the eyes are to be regarded as a medical emergency and should be treated promptly by an ophthalmologist.

Treatment

Before you do anything, flush the eye immediately with water, and continue doing so for 15 to 30 minutes. Hold your head under a water faucet or pour water into your eye from a clean container. Keep your eye open as widely as possible during flushing.

Go to the emergency room of your local hospital or contact your ophthalmologist. The physician examining and treating the eye may use a local anesthetic to lessen the pain. Depending on the extent of injury, the eye may be bandaged, treated with an antibiotic, and left to heal.

Serious damage to the conjunctiva, cornea, or eyelid may require surgical repair at a later date.

Black Eye

Signs and Symptoms

- Bruising around the eye
- Broken blood vessels in the white of the eye
- Swelling of the lid and tissue around the eye

Perhaps you were in an accident and a blunt object hit your eye, or maybe your child encountered the schoolyard bully. Whatever the cause, there is a bruise about the eye—the so-called black eye.

If you sustain such an injury, it may be limited to a small amount of bleeding beneath the skin that gives you the characteristic black-and-blue bruising about the eye.

You might also incur more serious damage to the eye itself. Sometimes a black eye will indicate a more extensive injury, even a skull fracture, particularly if the area around both eyes is bruised. In any case, such an injury should be examined by an ophthalmologist to be sure the eye itself has not been hurt.

Diagnosis

If the area around your eye bleeds under the skin, the lid and nearby tissues also may swell. The eye itself can become red and swollen. The injury may not be serious, but recurrent bleeding within the eye can reduce vision and damage the cornea. In some cases, glaucoma also can result (see page 550).

Treatment

Apply ice to the injured eye, taking care not to press on the eye itself. Your ophthalmologist can determine whether more serious damage has occurred. If so, the eye may be bandaged, bed rest will be prescribed, and you may be sedated to lessen the pain and anxiety. In addition, your physician may prescribe medication to reduce pressure within the eye.

Hyphema

Signs and Symptoms—Bleeding within the front portion (anterior chamber) of the eye

Bleeding into the front portion (anterior chamber) of the eye may follow trauma to the eye. This may occur from either a blunt blow to the eye or a perforating injury. At times, hyphema may occur from severe inflammation of the iris, a blood vessel abnormality, or a cancer within the eye itself. Generally, the blood is absorbed completely within a few days.

Treatment

In some cases of hyphema, an ophthalmologist may recommend hospitalization. Repeat bleeding may occur, and it is a serious complication. Medication may be prescribed to decrease the risk. If the bleeding is severe, your ophthalmologist may elect to evacuate the blood through a small opening in the eye. This drain can be reopened on subsequent days if further bleeding occurs.

Strabismus and Amblyopia

Strabismus and amblyopia are usually first observed during early childhood. Strabismus, from the Greek word for squinting, is the general term for crossed eyes or those that in some other way are misaligned. Amblyopia, often called lazy eye, can be a consequence of strabismus.

Normal vision depends on the eyes focusing together, producing what is known as binocular vision. However, when the eyes do not function in tandem, double vision results. In a young child with strabismus, however, one of the images will be ignored and the development of nerve connections between that eye and the brain will fail to take place normally.

The resulting single vision will lack the depth perception of binocular vision. The affected eye probably will not develop good vision unless it is made to "work"; this is accomplished by surgery (to bring the eyes into alignment) or perhaps by wearing a patch over the unaffected eye.

Amblyopia (literally, dull eye) is a condition in which the vision in the nondominant eye is poor, usually as a result of strabismus. It also can be caused by a greater degree of farsightedness, nearsightedness, or astigmatism in one eye; it can even be caused by the rare occurrence of a childhood cataract. The more-affected eye is then "turned off" by the brain, and the stronger eye becomes dominant and retains good vision.

Six muscles are attached to the outside of each eye. If an object is to be perceived properly, these muscles must work in unison to focus the image on the center of the retina (macula) in the back of each eye. From the retina, the images then are relayed by the optic nerve to the vision reception area of the brain. Your brain "translates" these electrical messages from your two eyes into a single three-dimensional image which provides the depth perception of binocular vision.

No one knows why some children's eyes are misaligned, although it has been observed to run in families. Strabismus seems to affect boys and girls equally.

The eyes of some children are misaligned, a condition called strabismus. Two common forms of strabismus are esotropia (cross-eye) and exotropia (walleye).

Early Recognition

About 4 percent of children are affected by strabismus; if not treated before age 5 or 6, they risk permanent loss of visual acuity in the nondominant eye. Thus, the key to curing strabismus and amblyopia is early detection of the problem.

Strabismus is usually easy to recognize, but amblyopia may not be evident because the child usually does not realize that vision is poor in the eye. Tests of visual acuity may be needed to discover the amblyopia (see The Eye Examination, page 524).

The most common forms of strabismus in children are esotropia and exotropia. Esotropia (cross-eye) is characterized by the eye turning inward. Exotropia (walleye) occurs when the eye turns outward. Occasionally the eye will turn down or up. The deviation may be constant or occasional, such as when the child is tired and the muscles weakened.

Babies are born with the ability to see, but at first they are unable to focus. The nerve connections between the eyes and the brain have not yet become organized. During the first few weeks of life, your baby's eyes may

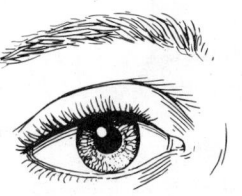
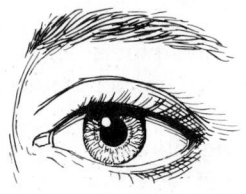

Normal pattern

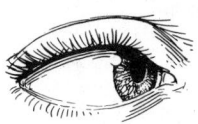
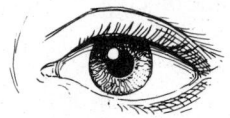

Cross-eye (esotropia)

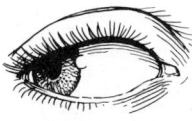
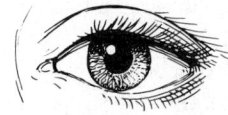

Walleye (exotropia)

appear to wander. At times they may appear to work independently, sometimes crossing and at other times roving outward. This is normal. By the end of the third or fourth month, however, your baby's eyes should appear to be working in parallel, and they should be able to focus on small objects.

Infants and toddlers often have a wide, flat nose and an extra fold of skin where the eyelids join the nose. These features may make your child appear cross-eyed. As the shape of your baby's features changes, however, the fold may disappear. Before you become alarmed that your child may have misaligned eyes—and before you dismiss the possibility—check carefully.

Begin by looking intently at your child's eyes. Is the point of light that you see in each eye symmetrically positioned with the other? If so, your child's eyes probably are aligned correctly.

The following is a list of other things to look for:

- Do your child's eyes work together? Test this ability by passing your hand across your child's field of vision. Look to see whether the eyes seem to move as one.
- Does each eye seem to follow objects, such as your face or a toy, if the opposite eye is covered?
- Is your toddler unable to gauge depth when handling or playing with objects?
- Does your child seem cross-eyed when playing with toys or other close objects but normal when looking into the distance?
- Does one eye squint when your child is in the sun?
- Does your child tend to tilt his or her head to one side?

A child with amblyopia usually closes the same eye or tilts his or her head to the same side in the latter two situations.

If you think that your child might have misaligned eyes, see your family physician or an ophthalmologist. It is never too early to have a child's vision tested for alignment—disorders can be diagnosed even in newborns.

The key to diagnosing amblyopia in a young child is to identify a difference in vision between the eyes. Your child's physician or ophthalmologist can test your baby by covering one eye and observing the baby's responses to the movement of various objects. If one eye is amblyopic, your child may try to remove the patch or otherwise object to its presence when it covers the favored eye.

By age 3, vision usually can be measured accurately. Poor vision in one eye does not necessarily mean that it is amblyopic. Reduced vision in one eye may be due to nearsightedness, farsightedness, or astigmatism, which your physician will test for. At the same time, your physician will examine the interior of the eye for signs of a cataract, tumor, inflammation, or other disorders.

Corrective Measures

Contrary to what many people believe, children do not outgrow strabismus and amblyopia, so prompt treatment is essential to prevent permanent vision impairment in the affected eye. Optical, medical, and surgical methods, alone or in combination, may be recommended.

Double Vision

Because of a nerve or muscle problem in the eyes, one eye may deviate from the other. The eyes will not focus in unison, and the images the brain receives from your eyes will be different from one another. This condition is called diplopia (double vision).

If the eye and brain connections have become well established (which usually happens by age 1 or 2), when a misalignment of the eyes occurs, the brain interprets the signals just as it receives them and produces two sets of images. Strabismus is the medical term used to describe eyes that deviate. The effect can be confusing and debilitating because objects appear twice in the field of vision.

Sometimes double vision is a sign of a more serious underlying problem such as diabetes mellitus (see The Eye and Diabetes, page 562), myasthenia gravis (see page 479), multiple sclerosis (see page 475), Graves' disease (see page 563), or brain injury.

In these cases, the underlying disease affects the nerves between the brain and eye muscles or the nerves of the eye muscles themselves. Double vision is usually only one of several symptoms of any of these disorders. If you develop double vision, contact your physician for a thorough examination.

In the meantime, you can alleviate the sensation temporarily by placing a patch over one eye. Treatment of an underlying disorder may resolve the double vision. If it does not, the condition sometimes may be corrected with prescribed eyeglasses. Occasionally, the condition is treated surgically to correct muscle misalignment.

Optical Approaches

If your child has strabismus associated with farsightedness (the eyes become crossed only when looking at close objects), eyeglasses may be enough to solve the problem. Sometimes the lenses are bifocal or have special prisms designed to compensate for the particular defect in the eye.

Medical Treatment

The nonsurgical form of treatment for amblyopia involves placing a patch over the normal eye in an effort to improve vision by forcing use of the weak eye. This stimulus seems to aid in the organization of the nerve connections between the eye and the parts of the brain that process visual perception. Normally, this organization and coordination take place for both eyes in the first year of life. If the stimulus of focusing an image is absent (such as in the nondominant eye of the child with strabismus), this organization fails to take place.

The same result sometimes can be achieved by treating the normal eye with medicated drops, called cycloplegics, which blur its vision temporarily and dilate the pupil. Some children with strabismus also may be treated with eyedrops called miotics which cause the pupil to constrict. These methods are most effective with young children.

Once vision in the weaker eye has improved, the treatment program will concentrate on bringing the eyes into parallel position.

Some practitioners advocate eye exercises for strabismus and amblyopia, but most ophthalmologists believe that they are of little value and thus do not recommend them.

In some cases, eyeglasses or surgery may be appropriate.

Surgical Treatment

Many children, particularly those with strabismus, require an operation to realign their eye muscles. The operation usually takes place on an outpatient basis in a hospital setting with the child under general anesthesia.

The surgeon will make a small incision in the tissue that covers the eye. One or more of the muscles of the eye are then repositioned to allow proper alignment. Depending on the complexity of the problem, more than one operation may be needed to bring the eye to normal position.

When treatment is completed before age 5 or 6, vision often is improved to near normal. The child not only will see better than before but also will appear normal. Looking like all the other kids can be of considerable importance during the impressionable years of personality development.

Eyelid Disorders

Our eyelids, although thin and delicate, are extremely important protectors of the eyes. Quick and powerful reflexes make the eyelids close when an object nears or when irritating particles are in the air. The eyelids also lubricate the eyes and wash foreign particles from them.

Lacrimal glands located above each eyeball produce tears, which are fed beneath the eyelids as a thin film. The tears drain away from the eyes through lacrimal ducts whose openings are located at the inner edge of each lid. The lacrimal ducts carry the tears to the nose, which is why whenever your eyes water or you cry, your nose waters too. The lids are lined with a transparent mucous membrane called the conjunctiva, which also covers the white surface (sclera) of the eye.

Occasionally the eyelids can be the site of problems. Most often such problems are infections, but they can be the result of muscle or nerve damage (see Eyelid Laceration, page 452).

Sties and Lumps

Signs and Symptoms

- Painful swelling on the eyelid margin
- Slightly blurred vision

A sty (hordeolum) is an infection near the root (follicle) of an eyelash. A sore similar to a boil or pimple develops as a result of bacterial infection. You may get more than one sty at a time or several in succession because

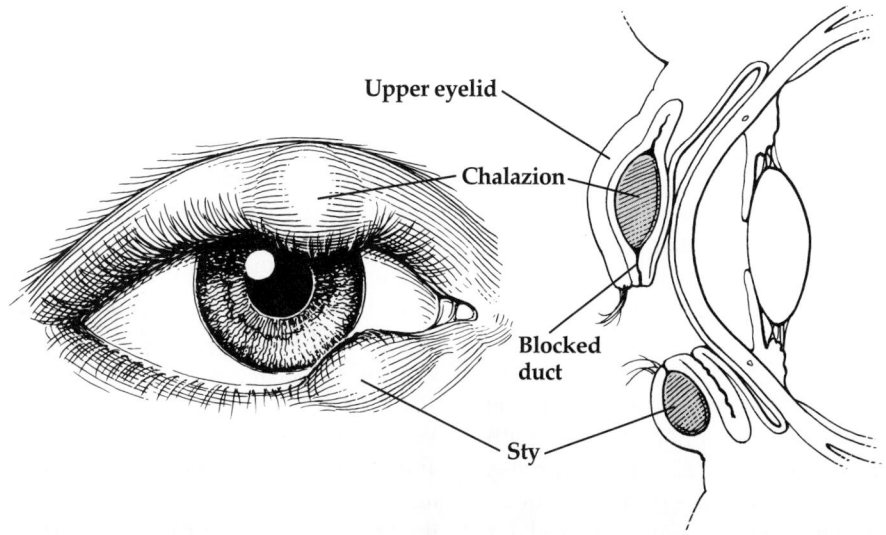

Upper eyelid

Chalazion

Blocked duct

Sty

A sty is an infection near the root of an eyelash. A blockage in one of the small glands in the eyelid can produce a similar swelling, called a chalazion.

the bacteria that initially infect one hair follicle spread and infect others.

Another form of swelling on the lid is a chalazion, which, unlike a sty, is relatively painless. A chalazion is the result of a blockage of one of the small glands (meibomian glands) that produce part of the tear layer. Bacterial growth may take place within the blocked gland. The chalazion is essentially an internal sty.

Diagnosis

A sty usually develops gradually, forming a painful red lump. Eventually the lump fills with pus and bursts. The release of pus relieves the pain, and after a few more days the sty usually disappears.

A chalazion develops a little farther up on and within the structure of the eyelid. In most instances it is only mildly uncomfortable, but it may be unsightly.

Sties and lumps are almost always harmless to the eye and general sight. However, if a sty interferes with your sight or does not disappear of its own accord or if you have successive infections, see your ophthalmologist. A chalazion probably will need to be treated by an ophthalmologist, although it might disappear without treatment. A presumed chalazion that persists despite treatment rarely is a tumor. A biopsy (in which a sample of the tissue is removed for laboratory analysis) may be required to make the diagnosis. (See page C-11 for color photographs of a sty and a chalazion.)

Treatment

You can treat a sty by applying a warm compress to the sore for about 10 minutes four times a day. To make a compress, soak a very clean cloth in warm water and wring it out before applying it to your eye. Using warm compresses will help relieve the pain.

Do not squeeze the sty in an effort to remove the pus. Let the sty burst on its own, then wash it thoroughly.

If the sty is stubborn, or you have successive infections, your physician may prescribe a topical antibiotic cream to apply to the eyelid. A particularly stubborn sty may be lanced and drained by your ophthalmologist.

A chalazion often will disappear without any treatment over time, perhaps a month or two. Applying warm compresses may help to speed the healing, as may application of an antibiotic corticosteroid ointment as prescribed by your physician.

If these methods prove unsuccessful or if the chalazion continues to enlarge, it can be removed in a simple surgical procedure. The operation can be performed in your physician's office with local anesthesia. After the procedure, the eye usually is covered with a patch for several hours.

Problems of Tearing

Tears often are thought of as a result of intense emotion. However, every time you blink—which you probably do every few seconds—tears lubricate your eyes. The fluid is essential for the proper functioning of your eyes.

When your eyes become irritated, extra tears form to help wash away foreign bodies. Occasionally, however, problems develop with the tear glands, and the results can be continuously watering eyes or dry eyes. Infection of the tear ducts also can cause tearing problems.

Dry Eyes

Dry eyes, caused by a lack of tears, can be a most uncomfortable sensation. The eyes may feel hot and gritty and may appear swollen and red. The condition is usually present in both eyes.

Dry eyes can be due to the presence of Sjögren's syndrome, a connective tissue disorder often found among people with rheumatoid arthritis (see Sjögren's Syndrome, page 920). Dry eyes may be a result of an allergy to eyedrops or ointment used for another condition; they also can occur for no apparent reason. They are most common among women after menopause. Although the condition is generally not a threat to sight, the sensation is so uncomfortable that medical treatment is usually necessary.

Treatment

If your eyes feel dry, if they swell, and if they feel hot and gritty, especially when you blink, consult your ophthalmologist. He or she will examine your eyes to determine the cause.

Your ophthalmologist probably will prescribe artificial tears that you can use to bathe your eyes whenever you want. If an allergic reaction to eyedrops is the cause, discontinue using them. However, the problem may not resolve and you may need to use artificial tears indefinitely.

Watering Eyes

Too much tearing can result from excessive tear production or inadequate drainage of the tear ducts. Other causes include irritations of the eye due to abrasion from foreign bodies, infection of the eyelid, inward-growing eyelashes, allergies, or nasal problems.

Improper drainage often is caused by blockage of a tear duct or drain, which occurs mostly among adults. However, about 5 per-

---

Eyedrops

Many brands of eyedrops can be purchased at your drugstore without a prescription. These fall into two general categories: those that act as artificial tears, and those whose active agent is a vasoconstrictor such as tetrahydrozoline.

Artificial Tears

These preparations contain substances, such as methylcellulose, that hold water and, indeed, resemble your own tears. One or two drops of these in each eye usually will provide lubrication and comfort for several hours. You may use artificial tears as often as you like.

Vasoconstrictors

In contrast, the products in this category contain a drug that causes the tiny blood vessels within the conjunctiva to constrict. If you have bloodshot eyes—redness and visible blood vessels—one or two drops in each eye will relieve the redness for several hours and often give comfort also. They may be useful for relieving the itchy eyes of people with hay fever, but they must not be used regularly.

Some of the eyedrops in this category also contain an antihistamine to provide added relief if you have hay fever. Use this type of eyedrop no more than two or three times a day, unless otherwise directed by your physician.

Reducing Complications

Each person has a different tolerance for drugs, and drugs affect different persons in different ways. Therefore, the risks of an unexpected response vary. Also, it is not possible to eliminate completely all of the effects from helpful and necessary eye medications. You can take a few steps to minimize the effects, however.

Use only the recommended dosage. Using some eyedrops more frequently than prescribed can lead to problems. After placing the medication in your eye, follow these simple steps.

Keep your eye closed for 30 to 60 seconds. This encourages absorption of the drug by your eye and minimizes drainage of the medication through your tear outflow canal into your nose.

Do not blink. Blinking tends to move the medication from your eye into your tear outflow canal.

Use your index finger to apply firm pressure for a minute or two over the junction of your lower eyelid and nose. This blocks the opening of your tear outflow canal and minimizes drainage.

Follow the Directions

Read the directions carefully for whatever eyedrops you use. Your pharmacist can help you understand the uses of these medications and also help you select the type that you need.

cent of babies are born with a tear duct that has failed to open. In most infants, the tear duct opens spontaneously within a few weeks. Usually only one eye is affected by continuous tearing.

If your eye or your child's eye tears constantly over a period of several days, see your ophthalmologist. The physician will examine the eye carefully for signs of blockage of a tear duct or of excessive tear production and ask you a series of questions to isolate other possible causes. Such causes include scarring of the tear duct caused by chronic sinusitis, chronic allergy, or injury to the nose.

Treatment

Your ophthalmologist may begin treatment by probing and irrigating the tear ducts. This method is most useful in infants and children. In some cases, an operation may be needed.

Infection of the Tear Duct

Occasionally the tear duct that leads to the nose can become blocked and infected. This condition is called dacryocystitis. When this occurs, the tissues between the inner angle of the eye (canthus) and the bridge of the nose become swollen, red, and tender. Tears then can no longer find their way into the nose and there will be excessive tearing. If you have these symptoms, see your ophthalmologist.

Treatment

Try applying a warm compress several times a day to the eye to relieve the discomfort. Soak a clean, lint-free cloth in warm water, wring it out, and place it over the affected eye for about 10 minutes.

Your physician may prescribe antibiotics. Once the acute infection has been treated, a new tear duct may need to be created surgically.

Blepharitis

Signs and Symptoms
- Sticky, crusty, and reddened eyelids
- Itchy, burning, swollen eyelids
- Conjunctivitis (see page 542)
- A granular feeling with blinking
- Loss of lashes

Blepharitis is an inflammation of the eyelid edges that often involves both seborrheic

dermatitis (see page 989) and a bacterial infection. When excess oil is produced in glands near the eyelashes, an environment favorable for the growth of bacteria develops. The result is a crusty inflammation that is uncomfortable and unsightly, but it is rarely threatening to sight.

People with blepharitis often have a history of recurrent sties and chalazions (see page 536). In severe cases, a corneal ulcer may develop as a result of the irritation (see page 547).

Diagnosis

If your eyelids become red and irritated and secrete an ooze that becomes crusty, you may have blepharitis. Do not be alarmed if you have to pry your eyes open in the morning, because the sticky secretions of the eyelids during the night often act to seal the eyes shut. In severe cases, small ulcers may develop on the edges of the lids, and the cornea can be scarred. Consult your ophthalmologist, who will examine your eyes and prescribe an appropriate course of action.

Treatment

Self-Help

Cleaning your eyelids carefully is important for treating blepharitis. In the morning, soak a clean lint-free cloth in warm water, wring it out, and place it over the eyes as a compress. This will loosen the scales. Then gently scrub your eyelashes and eyelid margins with a cotton-tipped swab that has been soaked in diluted baby shampoo. This will help remove the crusts and restore the normal lid environment.

Itchy Eyelid

Itching about the eyes often accompanies hay fever—but itchy eyelids may be a manifestation of contact dermatitis (see page 1036). If your fingers come in contact with some irritating or allergy-causing substance, it may be carried to your eyelids by your fingers. Cosmetics also may cause allergic reactions on the sensitive skin of the eyelids.

Do not rub or scratch your eyelids excessively because rubbing ultimately can result in lichen simplex chronicus (see page 988), with thickening patches of skin and persistent itching. If the skin of your eyelids is sensitive to certain cosmetics or other materials, avoid using them.

About That Twitchy Eyelid

From time to time you may experience the discomfort of a twitch in an eyelid. The involuntary quivering of the eyelid usually lasts only a few seconds but it can be irritating, and it can make you wonder whether something is wrong with your eyes.

Generally there is no need for concern because a twitch is almost always a minor ailment. The occasional twitch of a muscle in a hand, forearm, leg, or foot is a common experience, and eye twitches are closely related. These flutters, called fasciculations, last only a few seconds, although their occurrence can be frequent.

No one knows exactly what causes most twitches, although people often say that they seem to be related to fatigue and stress. Many people find them worrisome because they can be distracting, and some people fear that the condition may signal a more serious problem. Some people have eyelids that close involuntarily because of an unusual disorder called essential blepharospasm. Only very rarely are eye twitches a symptom of a serious disease. Serious facial tics, facial muscle spasms, and multiple sclerosis (see page 475) do involve the eyelids, but symptoms of those ailments are different enough that your physician will not confuse them with the ordinary twitchy eyelid.

Eye twitches are almost always harmless, but they can be irritating. Try gently massaging the affected eyelid. Many people find that this relieves the twitch significantly.

Medication

Your physician may prescribe an ointment or eyedrops containing both antibiotic and corticosteroid medications to clear the infection and reduce the swelling. If local treatment is unsuccessful, a course of antibiotics taken orally may be recommended.

Drooping Eyelid

Signs and Symptoms—Drooping of one or both upper eyelids

Drooping eyelid (ptosis) is a condition caused by a weakness of the muscle responsible for raising the lid. Some children are born with the condition, and for them surgical correction may be necessary to prevent amblyopia (see page 534). When present from birth, the condition usually affects only one eye. Drooping eyelid often runs in families.

In adults the condition usually is a normal effect of aging as the eyelid muscles lose tone; less often, it also can be the result of an injury or disease such as diabetes (see The Eye and Diabetes, page 562), myasthenia gravis, stroke, brain tumor, or cancer at the base of the neck or the apex of the lung, all of which can affect nerve and muscle responses.

Diagnosis

If you notice that your child's eyelids are noticeably uneven, especially to the degree that vision out of one or both eyes is obscured, see your ophthalmologist. Your physician will examine the eye and ask a series of questions regarding your child's general health. A complete physical examination may be recommended if a general health problem seems to be present.

If you suddenly notice that one or both of your own eyelids droop, see your physician. Again, a complete physical examination may be in order to determine whether a more general health problem could be the cause. If you notice the problem developing over several years, it may be due to the effects of aging.

Treatment

If your eyelid interferes with vision, see your physician. If the drooping is the result of a congenital abnormality, aging, or injury, an operation to strengthen the muscle may be performed. If a more general health problem such as myasthenia gravis, stroke, or diabetes is the cause, treatment of the underlying problem may help relieve the drooping eyelid.

A drooping of the upper eyelid is known as ptosis.

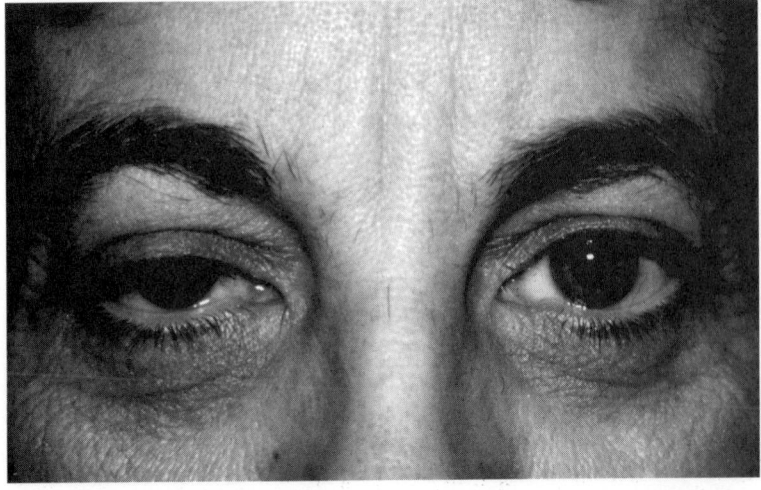

Cosmetic Surgery of the Eyelid

If your eyelids droop and the bags beneath your eyes sag, the problem may have developed as a result of heredity or as a natural part of aging. But whatever the cause, you may imagine that you always look tired. Perhaps the sagging skin even interferes with your peripheral sight. You decide to take action: you want the excess skin removed.

Blepharoplasty is a surgical procedure to remove excess skin and fat from the upper and lower eyelids. It is done routinely on an outpatient basis with a local anesthetic.

Procedure

Your surgeon makes an incision in the fold of the lid and just below the lower lash line. Excess skin, muscle, and fat are removed, and the incision is stitched.

Recovery

One of the most important elements in recovery is your follow-up care. This means you must follow directions from your surgeon in every detail.

Results

Blepharoplasty should not interfere with your vision, and you may wear your eyeglasses the day after the procedure. Wearing glasses can also help protect your eyelid from injury.

The recovery time is usually 2 to 4 weeks, by which time most swelling, tenderness, and pain should have subsided.

Complications

Blepharoplasty has fewer complications associated with it than most other forms of cosmetic surgery.

However, you may experience some temporary problems. Because many tiny blood vessels become disturbed during the operation, hematomas (blood under the skin) are always possible. These usually subside after a few days and leave no permanent sign.

During the operation the muscles of the eye may be disturbed slightly and cause temporary double vision, as can swelling of the conjunctiva. This usually subsides within the first few hours after operation. Many people report excessive tearing for a few days, but this usually disappears quickly.

Although rare, more serious complications can occur. One problem is ectropion, caused by removing too much skin from the lower eyelid. The eyelid turns out, causing tears to fall from the lid rather than passing over the conjunctiva and lubricating the eyeball. If severe, ectropion can be corrected surgically. Another rare but devastating potential complication is loss of vision from a severe hemorrhage.

Signs of Infection

If you experience any of the following symptoms after your eyelid operation, report them to your physician:

- Excessive swelling that does not disappear gradually
- Redness that becomes worse over several days
- Tenderness or pain in the eyelid that does not disappear gradually
- Problems with vision

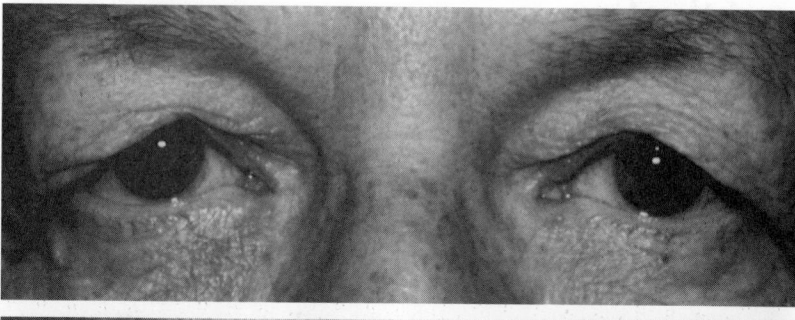
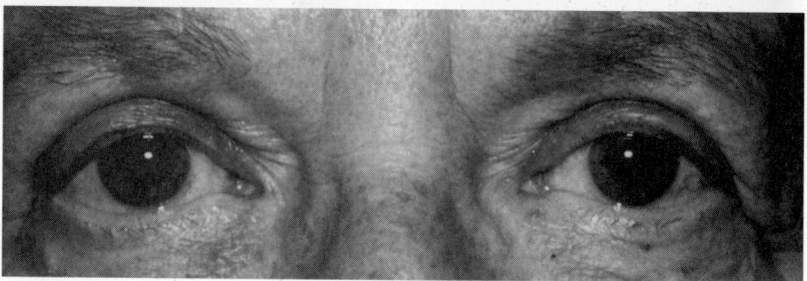

Blepharoplasty is a surgical procedure to remove excess eyelid tissue. Top, condition before surgery. Bottom, results of surgery on the upper eyelids.

Entropion and Ectropion

Signs and Symptoms
- Scratching of the eye by lashes
- Excessive tearing
- Eye irritation and matter in the eye on arising

Entropion and ectropion are problems often related to aging. In entropion, the upper or lower lid turns in, allowing the lashes to scratch the eye. In severe cases, an ulceration or scarring can occur on the cornea.

Ectropion is the reverse problem, and it is often the result of muscle weakness.

The lower lid turns out, sometimes causing the tears to flow out instead of lubricating the eye.

Although entropion and ectropion are usually the result of the aging process, ectropion can be due to an underlying condition such as atopic dermatitis (see page 1038) or lupus erythematosus (see page 918).

Diagnosis

One of the first signs of entropion is excess matter and irritation of the eyes in the morning. It usually clears later in the day. As the disorder advances, the irritation may become more frequent, if not constant. You may notice the lashes turning in toward the eyes.

With ectropion, you may notice the lower eyelid seeming to sag away from the eye, causing tears to run out of your eye rather than lubricating it and being absorbed by the eye.

In either case, see your ophthalmologist, who will examine the eye. In the early stages, entropion may not be obvious when you are sitting or standing, so one of the tests your physician may recommend may involve lying back and blinking forcibly.

Treatment

When ectropion causes tears to flow from the eyes, there are fewer tears to serve as lubrication, and the cornea may need to be kept moistened with artificial tears and lubricating ointments. A protective plastic shield often is worn at night to keep moisture in the eye.

Both entropion and ectropion can be treated surgically to reposition the muscles holding the lids in place. The procedures are fairly simple and are usually performed on an outpatient basis with a local anesthetic.

When an underlying condition is the cause of ectropion, treatment of the ailment is the first consideration.

Disorders of the Eye

Considering what a delicate and precise instrument the eye is, it is surprisingly tough. We tend to take our eyes for granted because most of the time they function flawlessly. However, the eye is susceptible to various disorders that, although not seriously affecting your ability to see, can be annoying or, over time, may present more serious risks.

These disorders include infections or inflammations of the conjunctiva (the mucous membrane that covers the inside of the eyelid and most of the outside of the eyeball itself), the iris, or the uveal tract within the eye. Other potential problems include eye hemorrhage and tumors (see Corneal Problems, page 546).

Conjunctivitis

Signs and Symptoms
- Redness in the eye
- Gritty feeling in the eye
- Itching of the eye
- Discharge in the eye that forms a crust during the night
- Blurred vision and sensitivity to light

Conjunctivitis is an inflammation of the transparent membrane (the conjunctiva) that lines the eyelids and the eyeball up to the margin of the cornea. Conjunctivitis can be caused by a bacterial or viral infection (commonly known as pinkeye), by an allergic reaction, or, in newborns, by an incompletely opened tear duct. Newborns are also susceptible to certain bacteria that can infect the birth canal. This form of conjunctivitis is known as ophthalmia neonatorum and must be treated without delay to preserve sight.

Both viral and bacterial conjunctivitis are common among children and are extremely infectious. Conjunctivitis can spread through a whole classroom of children in a matter of a few days.

Diagnosis

All forms of conjunctivitis share certain symptoms. The white of the eye becomes red or pink, and the eye feels gritty when you blink. The eye also produces a yellowish discharge that forms a crust during the night. This sticky crust can seal the eyes shut and you may have to pry the lids gently apart or to soak off the crusts.

Viral conjunctivitis usually produces a watery discharge, whereas bacterial conjunctivitis often produces a good deal of thicker matter. Some conjunctivitis also can be associated with a respiratory infection or with a sore throat.

Allergic conjunctivitis is a response to an allergen rather than an infection. When you come into contact with a substance to which you are sensitive, such as pollen, your body produces an immune response to ward off what it perceives as an invader. The result is usually intense itching, tearing, and inflammation of the conjunctiva. You will likely also experience some degree of itching and watery discharge from the nose.

If you have any of the symptoms of conjunctivitis, see your physician immediately. Your physician may take a sample from the conjunctiva for laboratory analysis to determine which form of infection you have.

(See page C-11 for color photograph of conjunctivitis.)

How Serious Is Conjunctivitis?
The inflammation of conjunctivitis makes it an irritating condition, but it is usually harmless to sight. However, because it can be highly contagious, it must be diagnosed and treated early. Occasionally conjunctivitis can cause corneal complications in adults (see Corneal Problems, page 546).

Treatment
You can soothe the discomfort of conjunctivitis by applying warm compresses to the affected eye or eyes. Soak a clean, lint-free cloth in warm water, squeeze it dry, and apply it to the eyes. Allergic conjunctivitis in particular is often effectively soothed with cool compresses. It also may be helped by specially formulated eyedrops that contain both an antihistamine and an agent that constricts blood vessels (see Eyedrops, page 538).

Medication
Your physician may prescribe antibiotic eyedrops if the infection is bacterial. Viral conjunctivitis disappears on its own.

Prevention
Because bacterial and viral conjunctivitis spread easily and quickly, good hygiene is the most useful method for controlling them. Once the infection has been diagnosed, the following steps may be useful:

1. Keep your hands away from your eyes.

2. Wash your hands frequently.

3. Change towel and washcloth daily.

4. Wear clothes once before washing.

5. Change your pillowcase each night.

6. Discard eye cosmetics, particularly mascara, after a few months.

7. Don't use other people's eye cosmetics.

8. Do not share towels or handkerchiefs with others.

Scleritis and Episcleritis

Signs and Symptoms
- Pain in one or both eyes
- Patchy redness on the eye
- Blurred vision

The outer part of the eyeball is composed of several parts. The sclera is a tough layer of tissue that covers most of the eyeball—the part commonly referred to as the white of the eye. The sclera, in turn, is covered by the episclera, a transparent tissue that stands between the sclera and the outer membrane (the conjunctiva). Occasionally, either the episclera or the sclera can become inflamed. (The conjunctiva is also subject to inflammation or infection; see Conjunctivitis, page 542.)

Inflammation of the episclera (episcleritis) is a mild and localized inflammation that most often occurs among young adults. Inflammation of the sclera (scleritis) is a more uncommon and serious disorder, one often associated with certain systemic autoimmune diseases such as rheumatoid arthritis (see page 909) or inflammatory bowel disease (see page 774). Scleritis occurs primarily among people between the ages of 30 and 60.

Diagnosis
Both scleritis and episcleritis are characterized by a red or violet patch or elevated nodule on the eye. In both disorders, tiny blood vessels of the tissue become inflamed. Scleritis may be accompanied by a dull pain. When scleritis occurs at the back of the eye, vision may be blurred. If you suspect you

Eye Hemorrhage

The conjunctiva is filled with tiny blood vessels. Occasionally one of them may break, appearing as a red spot or speck of blood on the white of the eye. This is called a subconjunctival hemorrhage, and it can be alarming when you first see it. It is nothing to worry about, unless your eye also hurts. If it does, see your ophthalmologist without delay.

Most simple eye hemorrhages disappear after 2 or 3 weeks. If hemorrhages recur, see your physician, who may recommend a more thorough physical examination to detect a possible underlying blood disorder or an excess of blood anticoagulant medication.

have either scleritis or episcleritis, consult your ophthalmologist for an eye examination. If you have scleritis, a more general examination also may be conducted because the ailment often is associated with another systemic disease.

Treatment

Episcleritis tends to disappear on its own after a week or two; it also tends to recur episodically. Your physician may prescribe steroids in drop or ointment form to help reduce the inflammation.

If you have scleritis, your physician likely will prescribe a course of corticosteroids in oral form or as eyedrops to help reduce the inflammation. A cycloplegic drug can be used to dilate the pupil by relaxing some of the muscles inside the eye, which lessens the chance for injury to the iris and reduces discomfort.

Uveitis and Iritis

Signs and Symptoms
- Redness of the eye
- Blurred vision
- Sensitivity to light

Uveitis is an inflammation of the uvea, the layer of the eye immediately beneath the sclera. The uvea consists of the iris (the colored portion of the eye), the ciliary body (which produces the fluid inside the eye and also helps control the movement of the lens), and the choroid (which lies just within the sclera and lines the eyeball from the iris all the way around the eye; see Choroiditis, page 560). Thus, inflammation of the uvea may include the area at the back of the eye in addition to the sides and the iris.

When the inflammation involves mainly the iris and the ciliary body, it may be called anterior uveitis. When it involves mainly the choroid, it may be called either choroiditis or posterior uveitis.

Uveitis may be a disordered immune reaction provoked by a systemic disease such as Crohn's disease (see page 774), ulcerative colitis (see page 777), sarcoidosis (see page 721), or another disorder. Uveitis also can occur in the presence of herpes simplex or herpes zoster (see Shingles, page 1011) infection.

Uveitis is potentially very serious. Early diagnosis and treatment are important to prevent permanent damage.

Iritis is any inflammation that primarily involves just the anterior portion of the eye.

An unusual but very serious form of uveitis is called sympathetic ophthalmia. If a seriously injured eye shows persisting inflammation for several weeks, there is a chance that an immune reaction may occur in the uninjured eye, with inflammation of the uvea and, ultimately, a substantial loss of vision in both eyes. This is the reason that an ophthalmologist may advise removal of an injured eye (enucleation) if the inflammation caused by the injury is not subsiding as expected.

Diagnosis

In uveitis, the eye is somewhat red, vision is blurred, and the eye is sensitive to light. Should you have any of these symptoms, see your ophthalmologist for an eye examination. A general examination also may be recommended to rule out the possibility of an underlying disorder.

Treatment

Uveitis and iritis can be treated medically with several drugs. Your physician likely will prescribe a cycloplegic drug to keep the pupil dilated. This relieves pain by preventing motion of the inflamed iris and lessens the chance of scars or adhesions between the lens and the posterior surface of the iris. Topical steroid ointment or drops may be prescribed to reduce swelling. Aspirin or an oral course of corticosteroids also may be prescribed to reduce swelling in more severe cases.

Proper treatment will lessen the chances of some of the potential complications such as glaucoma (see page 550), cataracts (see page 553), and fluid within the retina.

Orbital Cellulitis

Signs and Symptoms
- Pain in the eyes
- Decreased vision
- Displacement of the eyes
- Swelling of the eyelids
- General malaise

Orbital cellulitis is a rare, acute infection of the eye socket. It affects primarily children, and its onset is rapid and severe. Bacteria enter the orbit of the eye, often from an infection in the sinuses, a boil on the eye or eyelid, or a foreign object. The soft tissue lining becomes infected. In most cases, only one eye is affected.

The first signs of orbital cellulitis are usually swelling and redness of the eyelids, followed rapidly by pain and decreased vision. There may be noticeable displacement of the eye due to the swelling, resulting in an apparent protrusion of the eye from its socket. If your child exhibits these symptoms, call your physician and go to the nearest hospital emergency room.

Diagnosis
Your physician will conduct a series of tests to determine the nature of the infection. He or she will begin with an eye examination. Blood tests will be performed and specimens will be taken for laboratory analysis. A CT scan may be recommended to determine if the sinuses are involved or if a foreign object is present.

Treatment
Because orbital cellulitis is an acute and dangerous infection, your child most likely will be treated in a hospital. Your physician will determine a course of antibiotic treatment based on the particular infectious organism. Surgical drainage of any abscess may be necessary.

Retinoblastoma

Signs and Symptoms
- A white reflection visible in the pupil
- Crossed eyes
- Red, painful eye
- Poor vision
- Bleeding inside the eye
- Iris a different color in each eye
- White spots on the iris

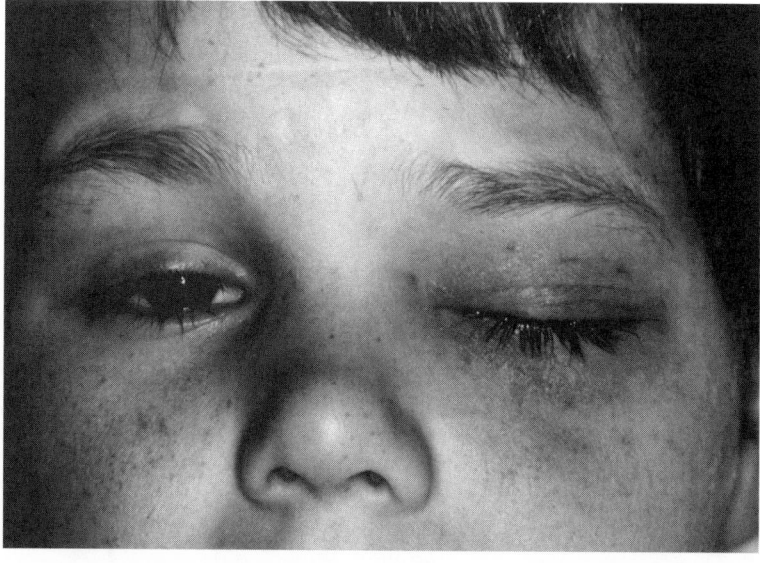

Orbital cellulitis is an infection that produces swelling and redness of the eyelid and eye socket. This requires immediate medical attention.

A tumor is an abnormal growth of tissue. Tumors can develop anywhere in the body and may be benign (self-limiting) or malignant (those that can spread and threaten life).

Retinoblastoma is a dangerous malignant cancer found in children, usually those younger than 5. One or both eyes can be affected. It is estimated that 30 to 40 percent of all retinoblastoma cases are hereditary. The prognosis for retinoblastoma is good, particularly when it is treated early. If someone in your family has had retinoblastoma, be sure to have your children tested early in life and then reexamined periodically.

Diagnosis
If you suspect that your child might have retinoblastoma, see your ophthalmologist immediately. The key to diagnosis is a thorough examination by a specialist experienced in diagnosing and treating retinoblastoma.

Examination is usually done with the person under general anesthesia in a hospital setting. The eyes are widely dilated to see whether growths are evident. Your ophthalmologist also may conduct an ultrasound examination and probably will recommend a CT scan of the head and eye orbits and globes.

Treatment
The treatment of retinoblastoma depends on the number and size of tumors, their location, and whether both eyes are involved. If the tumor is small, irradiation, laser therapy, or cryotherapy (freezing) may destroy it without damaging the eye. If the tumor has extended

outside the eye or has spread to other areas (metastasized), chemotherapy may be used. If the tumor is large and has impaired the vision or if it continues to grow despite other treatment, the eye may be removed.

Prevention
If you have a family history of retinoblastoma, seek genetic counseling before having children.

Melanoma of the Eye

Signs and Symptoms
- Brown or black spot on the iris or conjunctiva (membrane covering the white of the eye)
- Iris a different color in each eye
- Poor vision in one eye
- Red, painful eye

Melanoma usually is thought of as a cancer of the skin (see page 1005), but it can occur in the eye also, especially among elderly persons (see color photograph, page C-11).

Melanoma is often lethal. It is an espe-cially fast-growing and fast-spreading form of cancer, so early detection is essential. However, the signs are not always recogniz-able, and so early diagnosis is sometimes dif-ficult. The eye can be the primary site of the melanoma, or it may have spread (metasta-sized) from another location in the body.

Diagnosis
If you suspect you have a melanoma, see your ophthalmologist without delay. The key to diagnosis is a thorough examination by a specialist familiar with the clinical fea-tures and variations of eye tumors. In addi-tion to a thorough eye examination, your physician may recommend diagnostic tests to determine the extent of the tumor. These may include ultrasound examination, CT scanning (see page 1334), or MRI scanning (see page 1334).

Treatment
A small tumor often may be treated with radi-ation. Chemotherapy may be recommended if the tumor has spread. The eye may need to be removed surgically if the tumor continues to grow after other treatments.

Corneal Problems

The cornea is the curved, transparent cover-ing at the front of the eye. It works in concert with the lens to focus images on the retina, which in turn transmits "pictures" to the brain, where they are interpreted.

In some sense, the cornea is the window behind which the eye operates. Thus, being the most exposed part of the eye, the cornea is susceptible to a host of problems including various injuries, ulcers, and infections.

Corneal Injury

Signs and Symptoms
- Severe pain in the eye
- Red eye
- Swollen eyelids

Injuries to the cornea are fairly common. It takes little abuse to damage such a delicate tissue. A wind-borne speck of sand or saw-dust can scratch the cornea; wearing hard or soft contact lenses for too long also can abrade the cornea. The cornea can be burned from exposure to ultraviolet radiation after sitting in the sun or under a sunlamp for too long without proper eye protection.

Diagnosis
The moment injury to the cornea occurs, you may realize that something has happened to your eye. The tissue around the eye swells, and the eye itself reddens and begins to hurt intensely.

Alternatively, you may not feel the symptoms for several hours after injury, and then suddenly you find yourself in extreme discomfort for no apparent reason (see page 452).

If you experience the symptoms of corneal injury, see your ophthalmologist as soon as possible or go to the emergency room of the nearest hospital.

Your physician will examine the eye for signs of abrasion or burning and will determine the extent of damage. Using eyedrops containing a dye will help your physician identify damage to the cornea.

Treatment

Simple corneal injuries are treated by removing the foreign material (if any), covering the eye with a patch, and letting the eye heal itself. The cornea usually heals quickly, and within as little as a day or two your eye should be back to normal. Your physician may also apply an antibiotic ointment to prevent infection and prescribe a painkiller for the first day or two to relieve the discomfort.

A more serious corneal injury may require an operation to repair or replace it (see Corneal Transplantation, page 548).

Prevention

You can prevent future problems by wearing safety goggles when working with power tools and by wearing ultraviolet goggles when working with welding equipment, when sitting under a sunlamp, or when exposed to the sun's rays for long periods (see Protecting Your Eyes, page 532).

To ensure the health of your skin as well as your eyes, it is wise to take proper precautions and to limit the amount of time spent sunbathing either outdoors or under a lamp (see How to Avoid Sunburn, page 997).

Corneal Ulcers and Infections

Signs and Symptoms
- Impaired vision
- Pain in the eye
- Reddened eye
- Visible white patch on the cornea

A corneal ulcer is an open sore on the cornea. The ulcer can form as the result of an infection or, more commonly, from an abrasion or foreign body (see Corneal Injury, page 546) that may become infected. Eyelid problems, such as entropion (see page 541) and blepharitis (see page 539), also can cause a sore to form. Retraction of the lids, as in Graves' disease (see page 563), may permit exposure of the cornea so that it fails to be bathed in tears. This may result in ulceration of the cornea.

The infection itself can be viral, bacterial, fungal, or protozoan (another type of microscopic infectious organism). Viral infections are most frequently caused by the herpes simplex virus.

Diagnosis

The discomfort of a corneal ulcer probably will send you to an ophthalmologist. This physician will examine your eye and take a sample of the ulcer tissue for analysis to determine whether the cause is infectious.

The symptoms of a bacterial ulcer are generally more severe than those of a viral one. A bacterial ulcer also may be visible as a whitish patch over the cornea. A herpes simplex viral ulcer is usually invisible unless a test is performed in which a stain is placed on the cornea. The ulcer that appears will resemble the branches of a tree.

Treatment

Corneal ulcers are serious and should be treated as soon as possible by your ophthalmologist. Once your physician has determined the kind of ulcer you have, appropriate treatment will be prescribed.

Bacterial ulcers usually are treated with antibiotic eyedrops. If the ulcer is severe, an antibiotic may be injected near the eye for faster absorption. Topical application of corticosteroids sometimes is used to lessen the inflammation.

If your infection is viral, your physician may prescribe antiviral drops or ointment. These will help control the ulcer but, as with most other herpes infections, the ulcer may reappear.

If your corneal ulcer is caused by a fungus or protozoan organism, your ophthalmologist will prescribe specific drops for the eyes.

If left untreated, an ulcer may permanently damage the cornea. A deep ulcer can even erode through the cornea, thereby infecting the entire eyeball. If this happens, you will need surgery. A severely scarred cornea may require surgical replacement (see Corneal Transplantation, page 548).

Vitamin A Deficiency

Severe vitamin A deficiency in infancy and childhood may cause softening and deterioration of the cornea and permanent blindness. Lesser degrees of vitamin A deficiency will impair night vision (see Problems With Night Vision, page 239).

Vitamin A deficiency sufficient to cause eye problems is almost unheard of in the United States, but it is a major problem in some underdeveloped countries.

Corneal Transplantation

Surgical advances now offer a solution to severe corneal injury or scarring. If eyesight is greatly impaired by scarring or opacity of your cornea, transplantation may be possible. However, corneal grafting cannot be done if there is any infection in your eye.

Preparation

A normal transparent cornea is obtained, usually within a few hours of death, from a person who has made arrangements to be a donor. Often, tissue-typing is done to help ensure a good match between the recipient and the donor cornea.

Rejection is much less of a problem than with organ transplants such as kidney or pancreas because the cornea has few blood vessels. However, if evidence of rejection develops in the weeks (or even years) after the procedure, corticosteroid drops usually will control the problem.

Procedure

The donor cornea can be preserved in a special nutrient solution for several days, if necessary, before operation.

The operation is performed by removing the central part of the injured cornea with a trephine (a circular cutting instrument). Then, a graft of corresponding size is fashioned from the donor cornea. The graft is placed in the hole of the recipient eye and fastened into place with very fine sutures.

Your surgeon will give you detailed instructions in the care of your eye after the operation and will watch closely for signs of rejection in the transplanted cornea.

Warning Signs

If you note any of the following symptoms or signs, contact your physician:

- Increased discharge or redness in the eye
- Pain in the eye other than itching (which is normal)
- Worsening or any marked change in your vision
- Light flashes, multiple new floaters (dark or light spots, specks, or lines in the field of vision; see Spots and Floaters, page 561), or a gray film over your vision

Disorders of Vision

Disorders of vision can affect various parts of the eye. Some are refraction problems involving the shape of the cornea or muscle disorders (such as in strabismus and amblyopia; see Refraction Problems, page 522). Still others are the result of injury (due to burns, foreign objects, or abrasions; see Trauma to the Eye, page 531) or are caused by infection or inflammation (iritis, orbital cellulitis, uveitis, and others; see Disorders of the Eye, page 542).

Among the most serious disorders of vision are those related to the functioning of the eye itself. Some are the result of aging, a genetic tendency, or both. Such disorders include glaucoma (increased fluid pressure within the eye), cataract (clouding of the lens), and various retinal problems such as detachment, macular degeneration, retinal vessel occlusion, retinitis pigmentosa, and choroiditis.

New techniques and medications for detecting and treating glaucoma and cataract have made these two leading causes of blindness very treatable. In the case of glaucoma, early detection is the key to successful treatment. Today's modern surgical procedures make the treatment of cataracts among the most successful of all operations.

These diseases and disorders can be sight-threatening, particularly if not treated promptly.

Color Blindness

Signs and Symptoms
- Poor color vision, in which certain colors are muted and less discernible
- An inability to distinguish between certain shades of color
- In extremely rare cases, everything is seen in shades of gray

Although most people call it color blindness, life for a person with poor color vision is usually not black and white. In rare cases, everything is seen in shades of gray. However, most people with poor color vision are unable to distinguish between certain shades of color.

Your ability to view the world in hundreds of hues begins with three colors: red, blue, and green. As light rays pass through the lens and vitreous body (the transparent jelly-like substance of your eye), they interact with light-sensitive chemicals contained in specialized cells of your retina. These cells are called cones.

As long as the cones can accurately distinguish red, blue, and green, these colors can be further blended to produce a continuous band, or spectrum, of colors. However, if your cones lack one or more of these light-sensitive chemicals, you may see only two colors, such as either red and green, or blue and yellow.

The most common color deficiency is an inability to see red and green. Instead of a normal spectrum, a person with red-green color deficiency will have one or two neutral or gray areas where these two colors normally appear. Often, a person who is red-green deficient does not completely screen out both colors.

Defects can be mild, moderate, or severe, depending on the amount of light-sensitive substances missing from the cones. Also, a reduced sensitivity to red is seldom equal to a reduced sensitivity to green. Therefore, more people struggle to see green than red.

Interestingly, most persons with red-green deficiency are not aware of their problem. To them, leaves are green and roses are red, but they might not see the same colors as people with normal color vision. Their "green" may be what normal-sighted people call "yellow," but because they always have heard leaves called green, they interpret what they see as "green."

There are several causes of color vision deficiencies. The most frequent causes are described below:

Inherited. The genetic information that results in color vision deficiencies is passed along from a mother to her son. Because females usually possess genes that counteract the deficiency, the condition seldom afflicts women.

About 1 in 12 boys is born with some degree of color deficiency. This usually causes difficulty in accurately perceiving red and green. The gene that carries this defect also determines whether it will be mild, moderate, or severe. Whatever degree of color deficiency you might inherit, it remains the same throughout your lifetime. Usually, a person who has inherited a color deficiency will otherwise see normally.

Acquired. Color deficiencies can accompany various forms of eye disease. However, this occurs infrequently, accounting for less than 2 percent of the total defects in color vision. Acquired defects may affect your perception of blue and yellow as well as red and green. Whereas red-green deficiency is more commonly inherited, blue-yellow defects are more commonly acquired.

When the retina of the eye is affected by certain degenerative diseases, people often develop problems seeing blue and yellow. Disorders of the optic nerve (the nerve that transmits visual signals to your brain) also can affect your color vision. Optic nerve disorders, which can be caused by inflammation of the nerve or nutritional deficiencies such as a shortage of vitamin A, may make it difficult for you to recognize colors the way you once did. In the case of inflammation, one eye may perceive colors differently than the other. Cataracts can also impair your color perception.

Aging alone can bring on another type of acquired color deficiency. During childhood and adolescence, your ability to see and appreciate colors steadily improves and peaks in your 30s. Color vision then gradually deteriorates as a normal part of aging.

How Serious Is Color Blindness?

There is no cure for inherited color perception deficiency at this time, but the "hazards" of seeing color amiss are more inconvenient than dangerous. In instances of acquired color deficiencies, as the disease processes that cause them worsen, so does your color vision. However, treatments that slow or reverse the course of the disease often improve color vision.

Diagnosis

If you have trouble seeing certain colors, your physician can quickly and easily test to see if you have a color deficiency. Many ophthalmologists use a book entitled *Ishihara's Tests for Colour-Blindness*. This book, which contains several multicolored dot pattern tests, provides a simple and accurate assessment of color vision deficiencies of congenital origin.

Treatment

There is no cure for color vision deficiencies. In some cases, a colored filter over eyeglasses or a colored contact lens can be used to enhance perception of contrasts. However, these types of lenses do not enhance your ability to discern colors. And because they usually are worn over only one eye, they also can distort depth perception.

To help people who have been diagnosed with color vision deficiencies, many communities have recently added more blue color to green traffic lights to make them more easily discernible. Also, traffic lights have a universal top-to-bottom design (red-yellow-green), which makes familiarity helpful.

If you have problems discerning shades of color, your best approach is to find out the type of color deficiency you have and be certain there is no associated eye disease.

Glaucoma

In the United States, glaucoma is a leading cause of blindness. About 3 percent of Americans older than 65—about 2 million people—are affected. Of those, about 60,000 are legally blind. If detected and treated early, however, glaucoma need not cause blindness or even severe vision loss.

Glaucoma is not a single disease but rather is a group of diseases of the eye. However, the group has a single feature in common: progressive damage to the optic nerve due to increased pressure within the eyeball. As the optic nerve deteriorates, blind spots develop. If left untreated, the result may be total blindness.

The term "glaucoma" is derived from the Greek word *glauco*, which means "bright or sparkling." It may have been used to distinguish blind people with clear pupils from those whose eyes were clouded from cataracts. The term has evolved to mean vision loss associated with increased pressure within the eye.

The space between the lens and the cornea in the eye is filled with a fluid called the aqueous humor. This fluid circulates from behind the colored portion of the eye (the iris) through the opening at the center of the eye (pupil) and into the space between the iris and the cornea. The aqueous humor is produced constantly, so it must be drained constantly. The drain is at the point that the iris and the cornea meet, known as the drainage angle, which directs fluid into a channel (canal of Schlemm) that then leads the fluid to a system of small veins outside the eye.

When the drainage angle does not function properly, the fluid cannot drain and pressure builds up within the eye. Pressure also is exerted on another fluid in the eye, the vitreous humor behind the lens, which in turn presses on the retina. This pressure affects the fibers of the optic nerve, slowly damaging them. Over time, the result is a loss of vision.

The group of diseases known as glaucoma can be divided into two forms, acute and chronic. Of the two, the chronic form is far more common, affecting about 95 percent of people with glaucoma. Both types are discussed in detail below.

There also are several rare forms of glaucoma that do not fit into the two main categories.

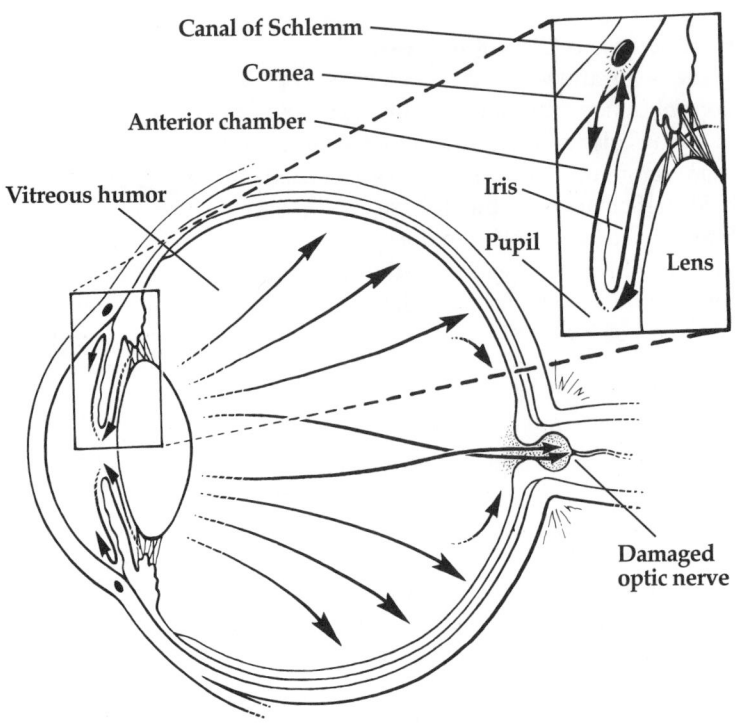

The vision loss of glaucoma results from the pressure of built-up fluid within the eye. Fluid normally passes through a narrow space between your iris and lens (see inset), then drains out of your eye through the canal of Schlemm. If this outward flow is blocked, pressure can damage your optic nerve and reduce vision.

Acute Glaucoma

Signs and Symptoms
- Blurred vision, usually in one eye
- Halos appearing around lights
- Pain in the eye
- Eye becomes red

Acute (closed-angle) glaucoma is less common than chronic glaucoma; it occurs primarily among elderly persons who are farsighted (see Farsightedness, page 525). Acute glaucoma often runs in families, as does farsightedness.

As we age, the lens in each of our eyes becomes gradually larger and tends to push the ciliary body and iris forward. This change gradually narrows the angle between the iris and the cornea; eventually, the narrowing is sufficient to close off the passage of aqueous humor to the extent that there is a sudden increase in pressure. Sometimes this closure is provoked by eyedrops that are used to dilate the pupil for examination of the interior of the eye. This is the reason ophthalmologists are cautious about dilating the pupil in older, farsighted persons.

Diagnosis
Attacks of acute glaucoma can develop suddenly or with warnings (preliminary attacks) weeks or months ahead. The attacks usually occur in the evening when the light is dim (and the pupil is dilated), and they last as long as the angle is closed. Your vision becomes blurred, you may see halos around lights, your eye becomes red, and you may have pain.

In a full-blown attack the symptoms are similar but are more severe and persistent. The pain may be extreme, causing vomiting. The cornea appears hazy, even gray and granular. The eyeball may be painful and hard.

How Serious Is Acute Glaucoma?
An attack of acute glaucoma is an emergency that should be treated immediately. If you suspect that you are having such an attack, contact your ophthalmologist without delay or go to your local hospital emergency room.

Treatment
Acute glaucoma often is treated with an emergency operation, known as an iridotomy, to create a drainage hole in the iris. New lasers allow eye specialists to form this opening in the iris without making an incision in the eye. The laser iridotomy technique is an office procedure that avoids many of the risks associated with conventional surgical treatment. With laser treatment, you often can resume normal activities the same day.

Chronic Glaucoma

Signs and Symptoms—Gradual loss of peripheral vision

Chronic glaucoma, unlike the acute form, often goes undetected for years. In chronic glaucoma the drainage angle is not blocked by the iris (as in acute glaucoma) and hence it also is called open-angle glaucoma. Still, fluid does not drain properly from the front chamber. As a result, the pressure within the eye increases gradually over months or years and slowly damages the optic nerve and retina.

The cause of the impaired outward flow seems to be some fault in the mechanism of absorption of the aqueous humor. Persons who are vulnerable to chronic glaucoma may have an increase in pressure within the eye after the use of eyedrops or systemic medications that contain corticosteroids. (For a more detailed discussion of glaucoma's effect on the eye, see Glaucoma, page 550.)

Diagnosis
Chronic glaucoma has no early warning signs. Your central vision will remain normal until the last stages of the disease. You gradually

---

Risk Factors for Chronic Glaucoma

Many people do not notice any symptoms of chronic glaucoma until significant, permanent damage has occurred. For this reason, it is particularly important to be aware of the risk factors for chronic glaucoma.

Age
After age 40, your chances of developing chronic glaucoma increase. The disorder is uncommon among children and young adults.

Family History
Glaucoma runs in families. About 20 percent of people with glaucoma have close relatives who have the problem.

Diabetes
If you have diabetes, your risk of developing glaucoma is 3 times greater than that for people who do not have diabetes.

Race
If you are black, your chance of developing glaucoma is significantly higher than that for other races.

The presence of several of these risk factors suggests that you and your physician should be especially alert for indications of glaucoma.

lose your peripheral vision, so that eventually only a narrow section of your visual field remains clear.

The only way to diagnose glaucoma early is to have regular eye checkups once you reach age 40. Certain tests can be performed by a general physician, although others must be performed by an eye specialist.

The earliest detectable abnormality of chronic glaucoma is increased pressure in the eye. A tonometry test is an inexpensive and painless test that allows your physician to determine the pressure within the eye (see Tonometry and Your Eyes, page 553). Your

The sequence of photographs suggests the progressive narrowing of the field of vision characteristic of chronic glaucoma.

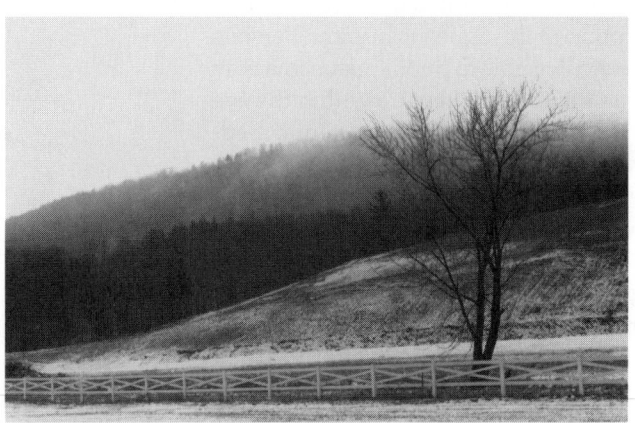

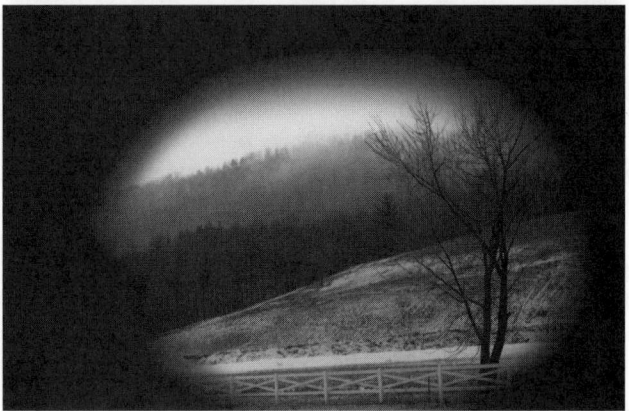

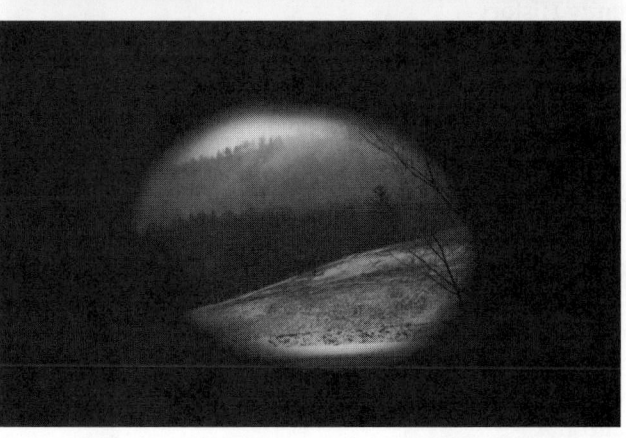

physician may include an ophthalmoscopic examination as part of a routine checkup. The ophthalmoscope, a small handheld device, allows a clear view of the eye's interior and can show damage to the optic nerve, a sign of glaucoma (see The Eye Examination, page 524).

Your peripheral vision also can be tested. Larger defects in peripheral vision can be detected by asking you to look into the eyes of the physician while he or she moves a hand off to one side and then up and down and asks whether you can see it. More detailed testing is done with computer-assisted devices. The tests can reveal optic nerve damage long before you become aware of any vision loss.

This test is not part of a routine eye examination. Rather, it is more likely to be used when your physician suspects glaucoma or another disease of the eye or brain.

How Serious Is Chronic Glaucoma?

Chronic glaucoma is a leading cause of blindness. Because the only symptom is a gradual narrowing of vision, it often goes undetected for years. Early detection through regular checkups can prevent blindness.

Treatment

It is not always necessary to treat slightly increased eye pressure. If no evidence of optic nerve damage is found, a modest increase in intraocular pressure does not necessarily require therapy. Instead, your physician may suggest careful monitoring of the condition by examination several times a year.

In most cases, chronic glaucoma is treated with eyedrops to help decrease the pressure in the eye. For years, the most popular eyedrops to treat glaucoma were those containing epinephrine or pilocarpine to increase the outflow of fluid. However, these drugs sometimes have troublesome local side effects. As a result, the most common topical medications prescribed today contain a beta-adrenergic blocker.

Beta-adrenergic blockers are remarkably effective and generally safe drugs. Three such drugs commonly used are timolol, betaxolol, and bunolol. However, if enough of the drug enters the general bloodstream, side effects may result. Rarely, they may aggravate the symptoms of heart failure, asthma, or emphysema. They can disturb heart rhythm and worsen bronchial asthma symptoms. In some circumstances, they can

Tonometry and Your Eyes

Glaucoma is one of the leading causes of blindness in the United States. Early detection of glaucoma cannot restore lost vision, but prompt treatment can arrest deterioration and slow subsequent loss. A simple testing procedure, called tonometry, can alert you and your physician to the possibility that you have glaucoma.

Tonometry is a method of measuring the pressure within the eyeball. Normal intraocular pressure is approximately 8 to 22 millimeters of mercury. If tonometry reveals higher pressure, further tests can be performed to determine whether you have glaucoma.

Applanation Tonometer

Your ophthalmologist may perform a sensitive test with an applanation tonometer. The applanation tonometer is a sophisticated device that usually is fitted to a slit lamp, a common instrument for eye examination. Your eyes are anesthetized with drops and the tonometer is placed directly on your eye. The readings from the device denoting eye pressure are very accurate. After the anesthesia wears off, your eyes may feel scratchy for a short time.

Air-Puff Tonometer

Optometrists, who are not physicians, often use the air-puff tonometer to test for glaucoma. This device, which uses air to measure eye pressure, is not as accurate as the applanation tonometer, but it is useful for glaucoma screening.

Tonometry should become a routine part of your general medical examination after age 40. If you have a family history of glaucoma, are nearsighted, or have diabetes, you should also be tested periodically before you reach 40.

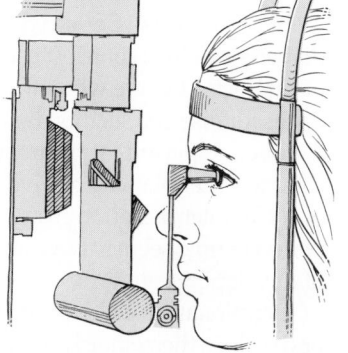

For a precise measurement of eye pressure, your physician may use an applanation tonometer.

---

leave you feeling fatigued, drowsy, depressed, or confused. They can cause temporary impotence. If you have diabetes and use insulin, a beta-adrenergic blocker may cause your blood sugar concentration to decrease unexpectedly (see Eyedrops, page 538).

Another form of treatment involves medications taken by mouth. Certain drugs, such as acetazolamide, can lower the pressure within your eye by decreasing the formation of normal eye fluid. This type of medicine also can cause general side effects. Long-term use of these drugs typically is avoided.

Your ophthalmologist understands the possible side effects and probably will tell you what you should look for. If you experience such problems, contact your ophthalmologist or your general physician. Your dosage may be adjusted or you may be given alternative treatment. When you see your physician, take the medication with you.

Surgery

If medical treatment is unsuccessful, your physician may recommend operation. Several options are available. In one, a laser beam is used to open blocked drainage channels in the front chamber of the eye. This fairly simple procedure can be done in your physician's office.

In more severe cases, an operation known as a filtration procedure may be recommended. In this operation, a drainage passage is surgically created between the interior of the eye and the conjunctiva to relieve the pressure within the eye.

Cataracts

Signs and Symptoms
- Blurred vision
- Impaired vision at night or in very bright light
- Halos around lights
- Second sight (the ability to read without glasses; often occurs with increasing age)

Cataracts are a major cause of vision loss worldwide: almost 20 million people are blind because of the condition. In the United States, more than 1 million cataract operations are performed each year.

Many people find the idea of cataracts alarming, assuming that if they develop them they will become blind. In truth, however, cataracts are one of the least serious eye disorders because surgery can restore lost sight in most instances.

A cataract is a clouding of the normally

clear lens of the eye. The lens, one of the two main focusing mechanisms of the eye, lies just behind the pupil. The clouding of the lens blocks the passage of light needed for sight. Although a cataract often starts in only one eye, usually both become involved. Cataracts are accompanied by changes in the chemical composition of the lens, but the cause of these alterations is unknown.

Everyone develops some clouding in the eye lenses with aging. In this sense, most people older than 60 have some degree of cataract formation.

Age is not the only factor in the development of cataracts. Certain diseases, such as diabetes mellitus, contribute to the formation of cataracts. People who take corticosteroid drugs for diseases such as rheumatoid arthritis over a period of years may develop cataracts. People who receive high amounts of ultraviolet radiation from the sun over a period of time seem to have an increased risk of developing cataracts.

Occasionally a child is born with cataracts or develops them shortly after birth. Certain eye disorders such as iritis (see page 544) or an injury to the eyeball also can contribute to the development of cataracts. Cataracts tend to run in families.

Diagnosis

Because everyone experiences changes in eyesight later in life, you may not even notice the gradual clouding of a lens. You may first discover a problem when you have trouble passing a vision test to obtain a driver's license.

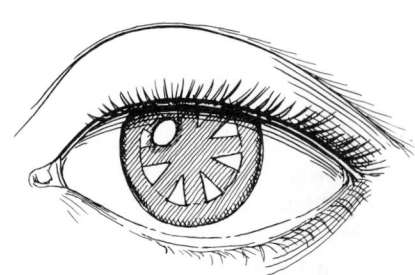

Cataracts (clouding of the eye's normally clear lens) are of several forms. Above: a nuclear cataract. Below: wheel-spoke-patterned peripheral cortical cataract. Almost all cataracts can be effectively treated by surgery.

You may notice a gradual change in your vision. This change often is described as a film-like covering over one or both eyes; the sensation may be rather like looking through fog. Your vision may be worse in dim or bright light (which results in narrowing of the pupil opening).

You may begin to have problems with night vision, particularly when driving. Glare and halos around oncoming lights make driving uncomfortable and dangerous. Some people notice a change in sight when reading. They find that they can read without their eyeglasses, a condition known as second sight. As the degree of clouding increases, the temporarily improved reading ability decreases.

Second sight is caused by a form of cataract known as nuclear sclerosis. Nuclear sclerosis is the most common form of cataract among older people. As the name implies, the cataract is located in the center (nucleus) of the lens. In early stages of development, the cataract serves to increase the focusing power of the lens.

People with nuclear sclerosis may find that they need a change in prescription glasses more frequently than in the past.

If you notice changes in your vision, see your ophthalmologist for a complete examination. Cataracts are often not visible to the observer until they are quite advanced. Your physician will conduct a complete eye examination, including a slit-lamp examination, and may use ultrasonography (see page 1335) to evaluate the posterior part of the eye to discover whether there are other abnormalities that cannot be seen through the ophthalmoscope because of the opacity of the cataract.

Treatment

The most effective treatment for a cataract is surgical removal. However, before such a major step is taken, a few simpler approaches can help temporarily.

Eyedrops to widen your pupil may help if you have small cataracts near the back of your lens. Repositioning a workroom light to avoid glare on the clouded lens also may help. Keeping your prescription for glasses up to date may make a difference too.

Surgery

At some point you probably will have to face the question of surgery (see When Is Cataract Surgery the Right Choice? page 555). An operation usually is appropriate when your failing vision seriously interferes with your normal activities. The decision to have the procedure varies with each person, depending on age, occupation, and lifestyle.

In some instances, surgery may be recommended early if there is risk that the cataract may lead to other eye complications. In earlier years, people with cataracts were often advised to postpone surgery until the cataract had "ripened" (totally clouded the eye). Allowing the cataract to become too advanced also can (rarely) cause complications. With recent advances in the procedure, physicians no longer recommend waiting that long.

Years ago cataract surgery was a major operation. You may have received general anesthesia, stayed in the hospital for several days, and spent part of that time on your back with your head immobilized in sandbags. Today, with improved techniques, cataract surgery is done in about an hour or less, under local anesthesia, with no hospital stay. The lens is removed from the eye and, in most cases, is replaced with an artificial lens. Alternatives to an artificial lens include contact lenses or thick-lensed eyeglasses (see Alternatives to Intraocular Lens Implant, page 556).

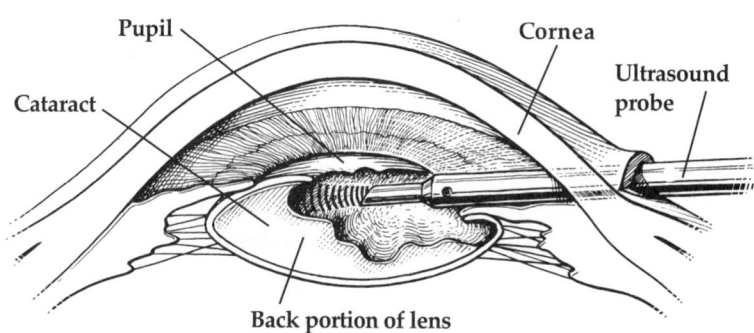

During phacoemulsification, sound waves emitted from an ultrasound probe break up the cataract, which is then suctioned out.

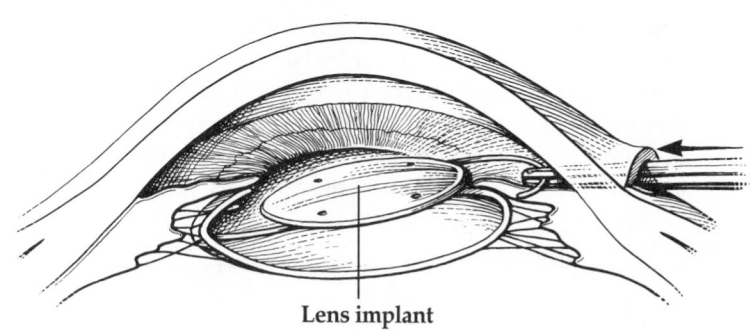

After removing the cataract, the surgeon inserts a plastic lens. The lens has two spring-like extensions that position it within the back portion of the lens capsule.

When Is Cataract Surgery the Right Choice?

Cataract surgery restores good vision to thousands of Americans every day—it is the most common surgery for Americans 65 or older. But some medical experts and government officials are concerned that a few ophthalmologists perform this surgery too often and too soon.

The U.S. Department of Health and Human Services published guidelines stressing that the decision to have surgery is yours and should be based on whether your cataracts interfere with your quality of life. In general, consider surgery when your vision problems hamper your lifestyle.

If you have cataracts and agree with one or more of the following statements, you may be a candidate for cataract surgery:

Because of my vision:

1. I don't feel confident when driving.

2. I can't do my best work.

3. I can't read comfortably.

4. I can't do things I like to do.

5. I'm afraid I'll bump into something or trip and fall.

6. I'm not as independent as I'd like to be.

7. I don't see well enough, even with my glasses.

With cataracts, time is on your side. A cataract can increasingly cloud your lens, but it rarely damages other structures of your eye. Waiting to have cataract surgery will not jeopardize the success of the operation.

Still, if you believe having a cataract lowers your quality of life, and you're willing to have surgery, discuss your surgical options with an ophthalmologist. Like all surgical techniques, cataract surgery is constantly being improved. Talk to an experienced eye surgeon who can help you choose the type of surgery best suited to your type of cataract.

Alternatives to Intraocular Lens Implant

Alternatives to the implantation of an intraocular lens include eyeglasses and contact lenses.

Eyeglasses

Until recently, thick-lensed eyeglasses were necessary. Although they are helpful, they do have significant drawbacks, including excess magnification, reduced side vision, and limited depth perception.

Contact Lenses

Contact lenses provide better vision than thick glasses. They are especially helpful if the lens of only one eye must be removed. Recent advances in the design and manufacture of contact lenses have made them more convenient and comfortable. Extended-wear contact lenses often are prescribed after cataract operation. However, contact lenses often are not recommended for older people, particularly those who have arthritis in their hands, because these lenses can be difficult to insert and to remove. (See What You Should Know About Contact Lenses, page 528, and Caring for Your Contacts, page 530.)

The most common type of cataract surgery is extracapsular cataract extraction. This surgery involves making about a half-inch incision on your eye's surface to remove the clouded lens. The membrane that forms the back portion of the lens capsule remains intact. (Rarely, surgeons use a procedure that removes the lens and the capsule.)

Increasingly, eye surgeons are removing cataracts by using a new form of extracapsular extraction called phacoemulsification. Phacoemulsification requires an incision less than half the size of traditional surgery, and recovery is quicker. But both procedures offer good long-term results and are about 95

Vision Problems After Cataract Surgery

After a cataract operation, your vision may gradually decrease because a thin membrane within your eye (the posterior lens capsule) may become clouded. The posterior lens capsule is left in the eye during most cataract operations because it is safer for the eye and it supports the implanted lens. If the capsule is causing your vision to cloud, this problem often can be solved with a laser. Usually the procedure is performed in the ophthalmologist's office or on an outpatient basis at a hospital.

It is important to remember that there can be many other reasons for decreased vision. Consult your ophthalmologist.

percent successful when done by experienced surgeons.

At times, cataracts can be removed successfully but vision does not improve. This may be the result of macular degeneration (below), which cannot always be diagnosed initially because of the presence of the cataracts—they preclude your physician from "looking in" in the same way that they affect your ability to "see out."

Macular Degeneration

Signs and Symptoms—Increasingly blurred central vision

Involutional macular degeneration is the most frequent cause of legal blindness in the United States and Great Britain. (The criteria for legal blindness may vary from state to state. A common standard is a vision of 20/200 or less in the better eye while using well-fitted glasses.) This disorder most often affects the elderly.

The macula, from the Latin meaning "spot," is located in the central portion of your retina. The macula is responsible for your central vision. In early stages of macular degeneration, small deposits form and blood vessels grow in the macular region between the retina and its supporting layer of choroid tissue. If these vessels leak plasma or blood, the retinal cells responsible for central vision are damaged. Eventually a scar may develop, producing considerable impairment of central vision.

Diagnosis

Early diagnosis of macular degeneration is vital to successful treatment. The disease usually develops gradually and painlessly. It typically affects both eyes, either simultaneously or one after the other.

A damaged or diseased macula causes difficulty in reading small print and seeing distant objects such as street signs. Fortunately, side vision is retained, so that if you have the ailment, you can walk about and even cross streets unaided. If you notice any decrease in your central vision, see your ophthalmologist as soon as possible. Better yet, have your eyes examined once a year once you reach age 50.

Your physician can test for macular degeneration during a routine examination.

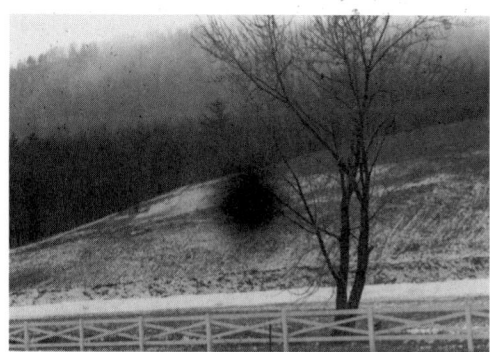

Progression of macular degeneration can cause this central blind spot.

He or she may perform a test known as fluorescein angiography to evaluate the blood vessel pattern in the eye and detect the presence of abnormal blood vessels. In this test a special dye is injected into a vein of the arm, and it then flows to the vessels of the eye. A series of photographs of the retina is then taken and the dye identifies any problems with the blood vessels.

Treatment
The only well-established treatment for macular degeneration is laser therapy to coagulate abnormal (leaking) blood vessels to prevent or slow further loss of vision. Such therapy is useful for a minority of persons during only the early stages of the disease.

Your ophthalmologist may ask you to use an Amsler grid to help prevent loss of vision from macular degeneration. By checking the pattern of the grid daily with each eye, subtle changes in your vision may be apparent. These changes may be due to fluid leaking from blood vessels. If changes occur, see your ophthalmologist without delay.

Retinal Detachment

Signs and Symptoms
- Sensation of flashing lights
- Many floaters in the eye
- Blurred vision
- Shadow over a portion of the field of vision

The retina is a thin, transparent membrane in the back portion of your eye. The retina contains the rods and cones that are sensitive to light. In addition, the retina contains the nerves that carry impulses from the rods and cones to the optic nerve, which, in turn, leads to the brain. The retina is essentially the film that processes the images projected by the cornea and lens.

Behind the retina is a layer of tiny blood vessels. This layer supplies oxygen and nutrients, which are essential for your eye to function properly. Retinal detachment results if the retina separates from this layer of blood vessels.

Most cases of retinal detachment are associated with a tear or hole in the retina. This defect, which may be caused by trauma to the eye or by changes in the vitreous fluid of the eye due to aging, allows fluid from the vitreous to leak under the retina and lift it from the underlying layer. Occasionally a tumor or an inflammatory disorder affecting the back portion of the eye is responsible for a detached retina.

Each year approximately 20,000 people in the United States suffer a retinal detachment. There are several risk factors. Nearsighted people are more prone to retinal detachment than others. The condition is more common among men than women, and it is more common among whites than among people of other races. The problem occasionally affects more than one member of the same family, so there may be a genetic factor.

Diagnosis
Retinal detachment is a medical emergency requiring immediate attention (see page 452). The condition is painless. However, symptoms almost always appear before the retina detaches. As the vitreous shrinks and sags, it may tug on the retina, producing the sensation of flashing lights. If the tugging is strong enough and causes a retinal tear, small blood

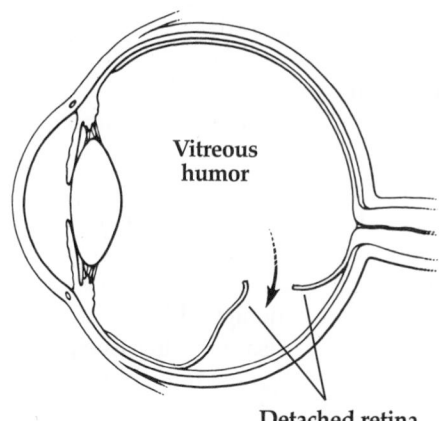

Vitreous humor

Detached retina

Your retina is a thin membrane attached to the back of your eye. If it develops a hole or tear, the jelly-like vitreous humor may flow behind your retina and detach it (detached retina).

vessels may be damaged, allowing blood to seep into the vitreous and causing hazy vision and the sudden appearance of new floaters (dark or light spots or specks or lines in the field of vision; see Spots and Floaters, page 561).

Not all tears or holes in the retina progress to a retinal detachment. If a detachment does occur, however, the portion of your visual field corresponding to the detached part of the retina becomes lost. You will perceive this vision loss as a shadow or curtain moving over your eye.

If you have any of these symptoms, see your ophthalmologist immediately or go to the emergency room of your local hospital. The physician will examine your eye and may use ultrasonography to get a precise picture of the condition of your eye.

Treatment
Surgery is the only effective therapy for retinal detachment. If a tear or hole is treated before detachment develops or if a retinal detachment is treated before the macula (the portion of the retina responsible for central

Lasers and Eye Disease

During the past 10 years, advances in laser technology have made possible effective treatment of various eye ailments. Sometimes lasers are used to seal a tear or to cauterize a blood vessel.

Diabetic Retinopathy
One of the more frequent applications of laser therapy is for diabetic retinopathy. This condition seems to be caused mainly by a reduction of the oxygen supplied to the tissues of the retina due to blood vessel deterioration consequent to diabetes.

By making numerous small burns in the periphery of the retina with the laser, the amount of retina that uses up oxygen is reduced and the remaining retina then has an adequate supply of oxygen. At each of the small burns there is, of course, no vision, but because they are mainly around the periphery, they cause only minimal impairment of vision.

For the most part, the results of laser therapy in persons with diabetes have been very good. The treatment should begin as soon as retinopathy threatens vision.

If you have diabetes, be sure to get regular examinations by an ophthalmologist.

Glaucoma
Physicians use a technique called laser iridotomy in treating acute glaucoma (a sudden increase of pressure within the eye). In this procedure, which can be done in a physician's office, a small opening is made in the iris to relieve built-up pressure between the iris and lens. Chronic glaucoma also can be treated with laser therapy to reduce intraocular pressure (see Glaucoma, page 550).

Retinal Detachment
Lasers are used to treat retinal detachment. Retinal detachment is a very serious disorder in which the retina located at the back of the eye becomes partially detached from the choroid tissue that nourishes it. If the retina is not reattached quickly, severe loss of vision may result. Lasers are now used to help seal the retinal tears that precede detachment (see Retinal Detachment, page 557).

Macular Degeneration
In its early stages, macular degeneration can be treated with laser therapy, although results are often disappointing (see page 556). In this disorder, blood vessels grow between the central portion of the retina (macula) and the choroid tissue. These vessels often leak blood, causing scarring and loss of vision. If the condition is diagnosed early, lasers can seal the blood vessels.

Secondary Cataract
After a cataract operation (see Cataract Surgery, page 556), vision may decrease gradually because a thin membrane within the eye (the posterior lens capsule) sometimes clouds up. The posterior lens capsule is left in the eye during most cataract operations because it is safer for the eye and it supports the intraocular lens implant.

If the posterior lens capsule causes blurred vision, the problem often can be solved with a laser beam. The procedure is usually performed in the ophthalmologist's office or on an outpatient basis at a hospital.

Orbital and Eyelid Tumors
New types of lasers are sometimes helpful for treating tumors around the eye. Your ophthalmologist will advise you as to whether this is indicated.

vision) has detached, your vision probably can be saved.

When a retinal tear or hole has not yet progressed to a detachment, your physician may use one of two techniques. A laser procedure is often used to prevent further detachment. In this process, known as photocoagulation, a laser beam is directed to the damaged area of the retina. The treated area then forms a scar, which usually holds the retina to the underlying tissue. The other method, known as cryopexy, uses intense cold. An ice probe is applied to the outer portion of the eye that covers the defect. This produces an inflammation that leads to formation of a scar (as in laser therapy), which holds the retina to the underlying tissue.

A major advantage of photocoagulation and cryopexy is that they can be performed on an outpatient basis. If your retina does become detached, however, you may be admitted to the hospital for further operation.

Surgical reattachment of the retina is usually performed by pushing the scleral layer of the eye back against the retina with a technique called scleral buckling. In this procedure the wall of the eye (sclera) is indented (buckled) over the defect. Silicone, either in the form of a soft sponge or a solid piece, is stitched to the outer surface of the sclera. When there are several tears or holes or an extensive detachment, scleral buckles sometimes are placed around the entire circumference of the eye.

Occasionally scar tissue forms in the vitreous, either before or after operation, and prevents reattachment of the retina. When this happens, the scar must be removed surgically and scleral buckling must be performed. In some complicated cases, injection of air or other gases or silicone oil into the vitreous cavity helps push the retina back against the wall of the eye. You may need to avoid strenuous activities for 3 to 4 weeks after the operation.

Retinal Vessel Occlusion

Signs and Symptoms—Sudden blurring or loss of vision in a portion or all of the visual field of one eye

The retina of the eye functions rather like the film in a camera, processing images from without and transmitting the information to the brain. Cells of the retina are nourished by tiny blood vessels. On rare occasions these retinal arteries and veins can become blocked by a blood clot or fatty deposit. If a retinal artery is blocked, the retina stops functioning, and blindness results in part or all of the eye.

Blocking of a retinal artery is an emergency because without a blood supply the rod and cone cells of the retina die. Blockage of a retinal vein is less threatening to sight than blockage of an artery. However, the blocked vein may rupture and spill blood and fluid into the vitreous humor, blurring and clouding vision.

These conditions, known collectively as retinal vessel occlusion, are more commonly found among elderly people. Often they are symptoms of another disorder such as hypertension or diabetes.

Diagnosis
An acute blurring of vision is the only symptom of retinal vessel occlusion. If the blockage is in an artery, the upper or lower field of vision may be affected. If a retinal vein becomes blocked, blood and fluid in the vitreous humor may cause blurring and clouding of vision over a period of several hours.

If you experience the symptoms of retinal vessel occlusion, contact your ophthalmologist immediately. This physician will examine the eye to determine an appropriate course of action. He or she probably will recommend a thorough general medical examination to identify any underlying systemic disorder such as hypertension or diabetes.

Regular eye and general examinations are most helpful for early detection of a possible problem.

Treatment
In many cases, little can be done to treat retinal vessel occlusion, although in some cases the spilled blood may be reabsorbed by the eye and sight will be restored. If the blood is not reabsorbed, the blurred vision will be permanent. Laser therapy may be used to treat glaucoma or swelling of the retina that may occur after retinal vein occlusion.

If an artery is involved, emergency treatment is the only chance of improving impaired vision. Administration of anticoagulant drugs to prevent further growth of a clot, or even an emergency operation to dislodge a blockage in the carotid artery (the major artery in your neck, supplying blood to your eyes and brain), may be helpful. Often, however, vision is only partially restored, if at all.

Optic Neuritis

Signs and Symptoms
• Acute loss of vision in one eye
• Pain on movement of the eye

Optic neuritis, an inflammation of the optic nerve, may be the result of a viral illness or of multiple sclerosis.

When the condition affects the portion of the optic nerve visible through the ophthalmoscope, it is known as papillitis. (An ophthalmoscope is a handheld instrument that illuminates the back of the eye.) When the inflammation occurs in the orbital portion of the optic nerve, it is known as retrobulbar neuritis.

Diagnosis
In optic neuritis, the optic nerve swells, blocking signals to the brain. The result is a gradual or sudden loss of vision. In the case of papillitis, the loss of vision is usually the only symptom. When retrobulbar neuritis is present, the loss of vision may be accompanied by pain on moving the eye. Nearly complete loss of vision in the eye can result within a day or two.

If you experience any of these symptoms, see your ophthalmologist, who will conduct a series of tests to determine the nature and extent of the problem. Your eyes will be examined with an ophthalmoscope, and you may have your visual field and color vision tested. Because optic neuritis often is associated with multiple sclerosis in young adults, your physician may recommend a complete medical examination.

Treatment
In many cases optic neuritis disappears on its own within 2 to 8 weeks, and sight is fully restored. Your physician may recommend corticosteroid medications in the form of tablets. This may hasten the resolution of the inflammation, but such treatment is controversial.

Optic neuritis can recur, especially when associated with multiple sclerosis, and each time more damage may be done to the eye.

Optic Neuropathy

Optic neuropathy is a painless swelling of the optic nerve due to loss of blood supply to the nerve. It may be associated with temporal arteritis or hypertension and usually resolves minimally. Both eyes can be involved.

The treatment is that of the underlying condition and may involve the use of corticosteroids.

Coloboma

A coloboma is a rare congenital defect in the development of the eye. This ailment occurs before birth. Often the iris, ciliary body, and other structures of the eye are absent. If the optic disc is involved, the optic nerve fibers are absent.

Depending on the extent of the defect, there may be partial or even complete loss of vision in the affected eye. Sometimes both eyes are affected. If either partial or complete vision is lost in an eye, it is imperative that protective glasses be obtained for your child as soon as possible to protect the unaffected eye from injury.

Choroiditis

Signs and Symptoms
• Blurred vision in one eye
• Pain or discomfort in the eye

The choroid is the layer made up mainly of blood vessels that lie between the retina and the sclera of the eye. Blood vessels in the choroid nourish the retina.

When this layer becomes inflamed (choroiditis), the retina may also become inflamed. This condition is then called chorioretinitis. When the inflammation subsides, the choroid and retina may be scarred and vision may be impaired.

Because the inflammation tends to occur in a spotty fashion, the loss of vision that corresponds to the scars therefore also is spotty. Each area of scarring will have a corresponding area of blindness, which can be discovered through testing of your visual fields. In many persons, the scarring left from choroiditis poses no handicap to vision because the spots of blindness (scotomas) are small.

The condition occurs among both children and adults. The cause is often unknown, although occasionally it may be associated with infections such as histoplasmosis or toxoplasmosis (see Histoplasmosis, page 711, and Toxoplasmosis, page 191).

Diagnosis

If you experience blurred vision with or without pain or discomfort in your eye, see your ophthalmologist. Your physician will examine the eye with an ophthalmoscope (an instrument that illuminates the back of the eye) and may recommend testing by fluorescein angiography to identify areas of inflammation. In this test, dye is injected into a vein of the arm, and it then flows to the blood vessels of the eye. A series of photographs of the retina are taken at close intervals.

Your physician also may recommend a general medical examination to rule out the possibility of a serious underlying disorder.

Treatment

Your physician may inject a corticosteroid drug near the eye to reduce the swelling. Treatment of any underlying disorder may help to reduce the inflammation of the choroid.

Retinitis Pigmentosa

Signs and Symptoms

- Difficulty seeing at night or in reduced light
- Poor central vision
- Loss of peripheral vision

Retinitis pigmentosa, most commonly known as night blindness, is sometimes an inherited disorder, but often it occurs for no apparent reason. The retina slowly degenerates in both eyes. The rods in the retina are affected most, causing defective night vision. As the disease progresses, peripheral vision also is lost, producing so-called tunnel vision.

The disease is uncommon. It leads to legal blindness in many cases. The criteria for legal blindness may vary from state to state, but generally a visual acuity of 20/200 or less in the better eye while wearing glasses is a standard.

Diagnosis

Retinitis pigmentosa often can be detected in childhood. Reduced night vision may become evident by age 10 years. If there is a history of the disorder in your family, have your child tested early.

Your ophthalmologist will conduct a series of tests and will ask for a thorough family history.

On examination, your physician may see dark pigmentation of the retina, hence the name pigmentosa. Tests to determine the presence and extent of the disease include electroretinography (which records the actions of the retina in response to light stimuli) and dark adaptation (to determine how the eyes adjust to reduced illumination).

Spots and Floaters

Just about everyone occasionally sees what appear to be specks, hairs, and transparent strings floating freely in the fluid of the eye. These vitreous floaters dart in and out of your field of vision. They are often leftovers from the prenatal growth of the eye.

Changes in the Vitreous

As you age, you may notice more and different floaters because the vitreous of your eye may partially liquefy. The vitreous is a jelly-like substance located behind the lens of your eye. It is composed almost entirely of water and accounts for three-fourths of the weight of your eye. At the back of the eye, the vitreous is attached to the retina, the light-sensitive part of the eye.

When some of the vitreous liquefies, it creates the appearance of spots, specks, hairs, or strings floating freely in the fluid. Common age-related floaters appear gradually over time and are rarely of medical importance. There is no effective treatment for the condition. The floaters may be annoying, but they tend to become less conspicuous with time.

Vitreous Collapse

If you are nearsighted or elderly, partial liquefaction of your vitreous may cause additional problems. The back portion of your vitreous may sag inward, causing a small portion of it to detach from the retina. This vitreous collapse is a common condition and also may cause the appearance of a floater or flashes of light when your eyes are closed or you are in a darkened room. These "lightning flashes" occur when your eyes move and the shrunken vitreous gently pulls on your retina, initiating a nerve impulse that you perceive as light.

Danger Signs

The sudden appearance of floaters or flashes of light may indicate a serious eye disorder. Possible causes include retinal tear, which can lead to a detachment, hemorrhage, and infection. If floaters or flashes of light appear suddenly, consult your ophthalmologist immediately.

As the disease progresses, night vision becomes increasingly poor and both peripheral vision and central vision are gradually lost, particularly during and after middle age.

Treatment

There is no effective treatment for retinitis pigmentosa, although there is some suggestion that vitamin A supplements may slow disease progression. The use of magnifying lens devices may be helpful.

Some researchers suggest using sunglasses to protect the retina from the effects of visible and ultraviolet light in an effort to preserve vision. Experimental glasses that widen the field of vision may prove helpful in the future.

Genetic counseling is the best hope for preventing retinitis pigmentosa.

The Eye in Systemic Diseases

The eyes provide a direct view of a portion of the circulatory system when the back of the retina is examined. Changes that take place in the blood vessels of the retina can help in diagnosis of certain systemic diseases such as diabetes and hypertension and even the possibility of stroke. However, these diseases and others also affect sight either in the long-term, as with diabetes and hypertension, or in the short-term, as with stroke, Graves' disease (a thyroid disorder), and cranial arteritis (a circulatory problem).

The Eye and Diabetes

Signs and Symptoms

- Blurred vision
- Fluctuating vision
- Sudden loss of vision
- Eye pain, in advanced cases

Both your vision and the movement of your eye may be affected in diabetes (for a detailed discussion of Diabetes Mellitus, see page 925).

Diabetic retinopathy, the medical term for a deterioration of the blood vessels of the retina, is a leading cause of blindness in the United States. It usually occurs in both eyes.

As the name implies, the disorder is a complication of diabetes, and it is commonly found among people who have had the disease (particularly the insulin-dependent variety) for at least 10 years. Almost all persons with diabetes show signs of retinal damage after about 30 years of living with the disease. The changes of diabetic retinopathy can be seen by your physician with an ophthalmoscope.

In diabetic retinopathy, there are poorly understood metabolic changes that lead to a relative lack of oxygen in the retina. The small blood vessels (capillaries) in the retina leak some of the protein and fats from the blood plasma to form deposits. The capillaries tend to close off, thus contributing to the lack of oxygen. The process of diabetes also weakens the walls of the vessels, which tend to become enlarged (microaneurysms). These microaneurysms appear as tiny red dots at the back of the eye. Sometimes these small blood vessels break, causing hemorrhages within the retina or extending into the vitreous, and these hemorrhages cloud vision. Often the blood is absorbed by the retina, but scars that decrease vision may remain.

New blood vessels also can grow over the retina and into the vitreous humor (the jelly-like material within the back portion of the eye). When this occurs, the disorder is known as proliferative retinopathy. These blood vessels also can swell and burst, causing loss of vision. The blood sometimes is reabsorbed but the retina can detach (see Retinal Detachment, page 557).

Diagnosis

Diabetic retinopathy is not a symptom of the onset of diabetes but is rather a long-term complication of the disease. It is separate and distinct from the changes in refraction that result from fluctuating blood sugar values (see Refraction Errors Due to Changing Blood Sugar Concentration, page 527). If you have diabetes, your eyes should be monitored and examined by an ophthalmologist annually.

Your physician will examine the retina with an ophthalmoscope (an instrument used to shine a bright light into the back of the eye), looking for signs of dilated blood vessels and microaneurysms. He or she also may use fluorescein angiography, in which a dye is injected into a vein of your arm and a series of retinal photographs are taken to detect signs of leaky blood vessels. This test allows your physician to pinpoint areas that threaten hemorrhage.

Treatment

Treatment begins with controlling the diabetes and the high blood pressure that may accompany diabetes. This may involve insulin or other diabetes medications, nutrition, and exercise programs.

Specific treatment for diabetic retinopathy may include laser therapy (see Lasers and Eye Disease, page 558). If a vein has leaked into the vitreous humor and scarring has occurred, a vitrectomy may be recommended. In this procedure, a part of the vitreous is removed along with the scar tissue. If the retina becomes detached from scarring, an operation may be required to reattach it.

Graves' Disease and Eye Problems

Signs and Symptoms

- Bulging or a feeling of pressure about the eyes
- Blurred or double vision
- Tearing
- Sensitivity to light
- Retraction of the eyelids
- An increased nervousness and heat intolerance
- Increased appetite, accompanied by weight loss

Graves' disease is a disorder of the thyroid gland in which too much of the hormone thyroxine is produced. An excess of thyroxine causes a wide range of symptoms, including jitters or nervousness, heat intolerance, weight loss despite a healthy appetite, rapid and irregular pulse, and a fine tremor of the hands (for a more detailed discussion of Graves' disease, see Hyperthyroidism, page 947).

The same abnormal immune mechanisms that stimulate the thyroid to excess activity also may cause eye problems. Changes in the muscles that control your eyes and eyelids can cause double vision and a wide-eyed

---

Third Nerve Palsy

Third nerve palsy is a common condition in diabetics. In this disorder there may be a rather sudden onset of pain around the eye and double vision. The affected eye turns downward and outward. The pupil usually continues to react normally, enlarging in darkness and contracting in light. The upper eyelid often tends to droop.

It is easy to think that such symptoms might imply a stroke, and in fact the disorder is the result of a temporary interruption of blood flow to the third cranial nerve, which governs the action of some of the muscles that control the position of the eyeball. Ordinarily, there are none of the other symptoms of stroke (see page 564). The pain lasts a few days and the eye recovers its normal function in 2 to 3 months.

(or pop-eyed) appearance. The eyes may actually protrude because of an increase in volume of the muscles, fat, and other tissues in the orbit behind the eye. This condition is called Graves' ophthalmopathy. In some cases, the optic nerve may be compressed by the enlarged tissues and may be seriously threatened. If retraction of the lids is extreme, the cornea may be exposed enough to cause severe drying or even a corneal ulcer (see Corneal Ulcers and Infections, page 547).

Once the disease is diagnosed, drugs or radioactive iodine can slow the gland's production of hormones, or surgeons can remove part of the gland to diminish its function. Sometimes, however, even after the excess production of thyroid hormone is corrected, eye problems persist or become more severe. Until recently, treatment was limited for people with Graves' ophthalmopathy. Today, however, it can be treated effectively.

Diagnosis

If you have protruding eyes and the distance between the upper and lower lids seems to be widening, your appearance is likely to be so distinctive that the diagnosis can be made quickly.

Sometimes, however, the eye changes can begin subtly and slowly so that the cause is not readily apparent. At times, only one eye will seem to be affected, giving the appearance of a tumor or infection from a sinus behind the eye. Sometimes irritation of the conjunctiva may be the most apparent symptom, and the problem may at first be regarded as a stubborn conjunctivitis or an allergic reaction.

Occasionally, the eye changes develop a year or more before or after the beginning of the abnormal thyroid action. Ordinarily, if the thyroid has just shown evidence of being abnormal, your physician will automatically look for the eye changes. However, if the thyroid is producing no symptoms, the physician may be less likely to think of Graves' disease as a cause of any eye symptoms. Double vision may be the first symptom, and a neurologic disorder, such as myasthenia gravis, may be considered initially.

The degree of protrusion of the eye can be measured by the ophthalmologist with an exophthalmometer. This is of more use for determining whether the protrusion is worsening (or, if it is being treated, whether it is improving) than for establishing the diagnosis.

A CT scan of the orbit (see CT Scanning, page 1334) usually shows enlarged muscles within the orbit and helps eliminate the diagnosis of a tumor or infection as a cause for the protruding eyes.

Treatment

In many cases, Graves' ophthalmopathy is a mild disorder that requires no treatment. Sleeping with the head elevated may lessen eyelid swelling.

If the symptoms are mild, topical ointments and artificial tears may be all that are needed to soothe the eyes. For some people, temporary oral treatment with cortisone drugs can help. Glasses with side guards also can be used to help protect the eyes from dust and drying wind.

In more severe cases, systemic corticosteroids, orbital radiotherapy, or surgery may be needed to correct the condition. To accommodate the swollen tissue behind the eyes, a surgeon may create extra space in the nearby sinus cavity. This allows the eye to settle back into a more natural position within the eye socket. This procedure often corrects the optic nerve changes, which can seriously threaten vision. The surgeon later may also reposition the enlarged muscles that control eye movement, thus correcting the double vision. Eyelid procedures can usually help the retraction of the eyelids.

Overactivity of the thyroid gland should be treated as soon as it is identified. Although there does not seem to be a clear connection between how the thyroid hyperactivity is treated and the condition of the eyes, it is desirable to eliminate the overactivity of the thyroid promptly and completely. If the treatment results in underactivity of the thyroid, replacement therapy with thyroxine tablets is initiated.

Hypertension and Vision

The ophthalmologist can make a remarkably accurate assessment of the seriousness of hypertension (high blood pressure) by examining the retina with an ophthalmoscope (for a full discussion of High Blood Pressure, see page 647).

The small blood vessels in the retina constitute a sample of all of the blood vessels in the body and have the advantage of being readily visible for your physician's inspection. Narrowing of the arteries, small hemorrhages, and exudates (accumulation of protein that has leaked from affected blood vessels) are evidence of hypertension. It is very unusual for hypertension to impair vision, but this can occur as a result of severe constriction of the retinal arteries and swelling (edema) of the retina, which occur in a hypertensive crisis. Treatment of the hypertension is the only way to reverse the loss of vision that may occur in a hypertensive crisis (for a more detailed discussion of treatments for hypertension, see page 651).

The Eye and Warning Signs of Stroke

Signs and Symptoms
- Sudden loss of vision in one or both eyes
- Double vision

The term stroke is used to describe several disorders related to a disturbance in the blood supply to the brain. The cause may be an insufficient supply of blood due to a blocked brain artery (known as an ischemic stroke) or a rupture of an artery and subsequent bleeding into the brain (known as a cerebral hemorrhage) (see Stroke and Vascular Disorders, page 461).

In most cases there are no warning signs for stroke. Only when you are experiencing one do you notice the symptoms of headache, paralysis, sudden weakness, and double vision or loss of vision.

However, certain ischemic strokes often

are foreshadowed by a series of small incidents known as transient ischemic attacks (TIAs). These attacks, which last for a few seconds or as long as a few minutes, are most often related to the disease atherosclerosis, which develops when fatty deposits form inside arteries (see Atherosclerosis, page 636).

Risk factors for stroke or TIAs include hypertension, some types of heart disease, diabetes, smoking, and advanced age. Most strokes occur in people 60 to 80 years old and are a major cause of death (see Transient Ischemic Attack, page 463).

Diagnosis

If you experience any sudden loss of vision or double vision or any other symptoms such as sudden weakness on one side of the body, speech difficulty, or incoordination in an attack that lasts up to a few minutes, see your physician immediately. You may experience these incidents over several days.

Your physician will examine you with an ophthalmoscope, an instrument used to examine the arteries of the retina. Tiny cholesterol-containing plaques in the retinal blood vessels can warn of an impending stroke. Two other tests, known as ophthalmodynamometry and oculoplethysmography, also may be performed to measure the amount of blood flowing through the arteries of the eyes. A general medical and a neurologic examination also may be recommended.

Treatment

Medicine

If atherosclerosis is found to be causing the attacks, you may be given anticoagulant medication to keep the blood from thickening and forming clots. This may include warfarin (Coumadin) or perhaps a combination of aspirin and dipyridamole. Treatment for hypertension may alleviate the symptoms and prevent a stroke as well (see High Blood Pressure, page 636).

Surgery

In some cases, surgery may be required if a carotid artery appears to be narrowed or blocked (see Carotid Endarterectomy, page 467). Some of the debris from atherosclerotic plaques in the lining of the affected artery is removed to restore blood flow.

Cranial Arteritis and Vision

Signs and Symptoms

- Acute loss of vision in one eye
- Jaw pain when chewing
- Pain in the temples
- Headache
- Sore scalp
- Poor appetite
- Muscle ache, particularly about the neck and shoulders
- Weight loss

Cranial arteritis, often known as giant cell arteritis or temporal arteritis, is an inflammation of an artery in the head, often near the temple (see Vasculitis, page 921).

The inflammation is probably a form of a disordered immune reaction. This reaction can thicken the lining of the affected artery, blocking blood flow to various parts of the body, most commonly the eyes. If left untreated, the disorder can cause partial or total blindness in one or both eyes.

Until recently, up to 30 percent of those suffering from cranial arteritis became blind in one eye. Today, medications offer effective relief, and blindness and other disabilities can be prevented.

Cranial arteritis is a condition of older people—usually between 60 and 75—and most frequently affects women. Blacks and Asians rarely develop the disease.

Diagnosis

Diagnosis is sometimes difficult because the symptoms of cranial arteritis can mimic the symptoms of other ailments. The symptoms may be vague—some people often feel just "run down." You may have fever and poor appetite or muscle and joint aches (particularly in the morning). You also may have the more usual symptoms of throbbing headache, loss of vision, pain over the temples, a painful jaw when chewing, and sore scalp. If you have any of these symptoms, see your physician for a thorough examination.

There is only one sure way to determine the diagnosis of cranial arteritis. A segment of artery, usually the temporal artery, must be removed for study. The procedure is often done as an outpatient procedure with a local anesthetic. Sometimes more than one segment is needed and so the procedure must be repeated.

Treatment

Cranial arteritis can be treated orally with a corticosteroid. At first your physician probably will prescribe a large dose to be taken daily. After several weeks the dosage may be reduced. The symptoms should decrease soon after treatment begins, and the risk of loss of vision is greatly reduced. Treatment often continues for a year or more.

The corticosteroid drug is used in the smallest dose that will control almost all of the symptoms of cranial arteritis. Occasionally, if symptoms are mild, aspirin can be used instead of the corticosteroid medication.

The disorder will run its course gradually in a year or more, and then use of the drug can be discontinued.

Chapter 21

Your Ears, Nose, and Throat

Contents

Understanding Your Ears, Nose, and Throat, 568
Your Ears, 568
Your Nose, 569
Your Throat, 569

Disorders of the Ear, 570
Swimmer's Ear, 570
Benign Cysts and Tumors, 571
Foreign Objects in Your Ear, 571
Ruptured or Perforated Eardrum, 572
Occupational Hearing Loss, 572
    Noise and Sound Levels, 573
    How to Protect Your Ears, 573
Barotrauma, 574
Acute Ear Infection, 574
Chronic Ear Infection, 575
    The Pros and Cons of Ear Tubes in
    Children, 576
Cholesteatoma, 577
Mastoiditis, 577
    Hereditary Deafness, 578
Otosclerosis, 578
Age-Related Hearing Loss, 579
    Communicating With a Hearing-
    Impaired Person, 579
    Hearing Loss and Hearing Aids, 580
Tinnitus, 582
Acoustic Trauma, 582
Meniere's Disease, 582
Labyrinthitis, 583

Acoustic Neuroma, 584
Benign Paroxysmal Positional Vertigo
    (BPPV), 584
Protruding Ears, 585
Wax Blockage, 585

Disorders of the Nose and Sinuses, 586
Nosebleed, 586
    Beware: Nose-Drop Addiction, 587
Nasal Obstruction, 588
Juvenile Angiofibroma, 589
Rhinophyma, 589
Loss of Sense of Smell, 589
    A Simple Remedy for a Runny
    Nose, 589
    Postnasal Drip, 590
Sinusitis, 590

Disorders of the Throat, 592
Pharyngitis, 592
    Lump in Your Throat, 593
    Tonsillectomy and Adenoidectomy, 593
Tonsillitis, 594
Epiglottitis, 594
Peritonsillar Abscess, 595
Laryngitis, 595
    Vocal Cord Problems, 596
    Proper Use of Your Voice, 597
    Speech After Laryngectomy, 598
Cancers of the Throat, 599

Understanding Your Ears, Nose, and Throat

Despite the small areas they occupy, your ears, nose, and throat are responsible for a remarkable number of functions. Your ear and its associated nerve mechanisms enable you to hear and to keep your balance. Your nose makes it possible for you to inhale air and filter it and also, simultaneously, to smell your surroundings. Your throat enables you to eat and drink, to speak, and even to sing.

Your ears, nose, and throat are interrelated in their functions and in the disorders that affect them. An infection of your throat or nose can spread to your ears. A cold or hay fever may affect your nose, throat, and ears. So it is not surprising that the same specialist, called an otorhinolaryngologist (from the Latin terms for ear, nose, and throat), treats your ears, nose, and throat. This medical discipline, known as ENT, is a subspecialty of surgery. Otologists are otorhinolaryngologists who are specifically interested in the ear.

Your Ears

The two main responsibilities of your ear are hearing and balance. Your ear has three parts: outer ear, middle ear, and inner ear. The pinna (or auricle, the folds of skin and cartilage usually referred to as the ear) and the outer ear canal, which delivers sound to your middle ear, make up your outer ear, the part we see. Within the outer ear canal are wax-producing glands and hairs that protect the middle ear.

The function of your middle ear is to deliver sound to your inner ear, where it is processed into a signal that your brain recognizes. Your middle ear is a small cavity, with the eardrum (tympanic membrane) on one side and the entrance to your inner ear on the other. Within your middle ear are three small bones (the ossicles) known as the hammer (malleus), anvil (incus), and stirrup (stapes) because of their shapes. These bones act like a system of angular levers to conduct sound vibrations into your inner ear. The hammer is attached to the lining of your eardrum, the anvil is attached to the hammer, and the stirrup links the anvil to the oval window, the opening to your inner ear.

Your middle ear is connected by a narrow channel, the eustachian tube, to your throat. Ordinarily, the eustachian tube is closed, but when you swallow or yawn, it opens briefly to allow an exchange of air, thus equalizing the air pressure within your middle ear and the air pressure outside.

Your inner ear contains the most important parts of the hearing mechanism—two chambers called the vestibular labyrinth and the cochlea. The vestibular labyrinth consists of elaborately formed canals (three semicircular tubes that connect to one another), which are largely responsible for your sense of balance. The cochlea, which begins at the oval window, curves into a shape that resembles a snail shell. Tiny hairs line the curves of the cochlea. Both the labyrinth and the cochlea are filled with fluid.

When sound waves from the world outside strike your eardrum, it vibrates. These vibrations from your eardrum pass through the bones of your middle ear and into your inner ear through the oval window. Then they disseminate into the cochlea, where they are converted into electrical impulses and are transmitted to your brain by your auditory nerve.

Structures of Your Ear

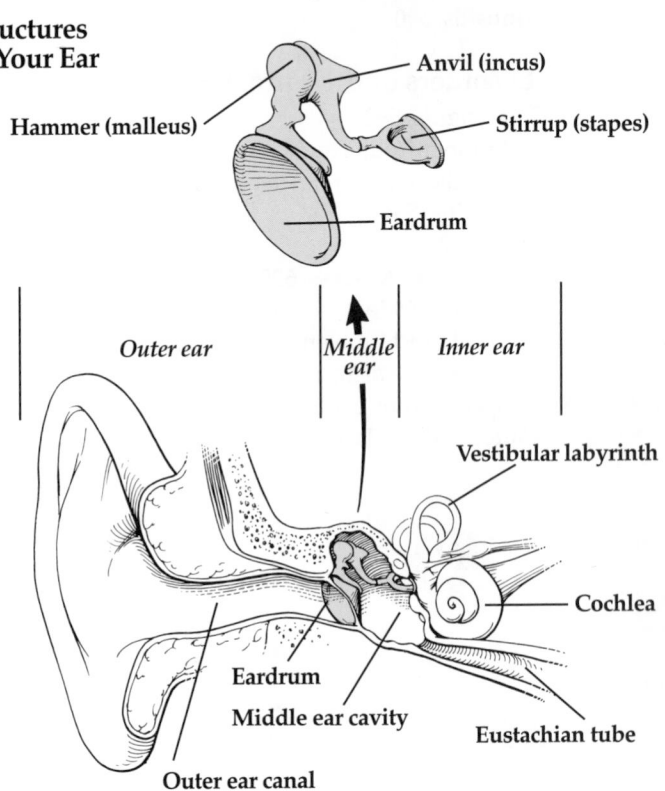

Hammer (malleus)
Anvil (incus)
Stirrup (stapes)
Eardrum

Outer ear   Middle ear   Inner ear

Vestibular labyrinth
Cochlea
Eardrum
Middle ear cavity
Eustachian tube
Outer ear canal

Your Nose

Your nose is the gateway to your respiratory system. Air that enters your nasal passage runs along the top of your palate (the structure that separates your nose from your mouth). As you inhale, air passes through to the intersection of your mouth and throat and continues its journey to the rest of your respiratory system (see page 700).

Your nose is divided into two identical chambers, your nostrils, which are separated by a partition composed of cartilage and bone and covered by a layer of mucous membrane. This wall is known as the septum. Thin pieces of bone, called turbinates, covered by mucous membrane curve in from the outer part of your nose toward your septum and act as baffles in your nasal passage. Your nasal passage also connects to your sinuses, air-filled cavities in your skull. Your adenoids are aggregations of tissue in the very back of your nasal passage.

Inside the front of your nose are protective hairs that filter the air you breathe. The main cavity of your nose is lined with a mucous membrane that warms and moistens the air.

In addition to warming and filtering air, your nose is responsible for your sense of smell and, to a large degree, your sense of taste. In fact, most of your ability to taste depends on your sense of smell. Smell begins with your olfactory nerve, which is found in the upper portion of your nose. This nerve contains very fine, sensitive fibers that transmit signals to your olfactory bulb, a structure located at the front of your brain, just behind your nose.

Your Throat

Your throat (pharynx) is part of the system that delivers air to your lungs, food and drink to your stomach, and sounds from the vocal cords to your mouth. Each time you inhale, air passes through your throat on its way to your windpipe (trachea) and lungs. When you swallow food, the muscles at the top of your throat help move the food from your mouth to your esophagus on its way to your stomach.

Several organs are located in your throat. Your voice box (larynx) in your trachea contains your vocal cords, which are responsible for most of the sounds of speech. (When you

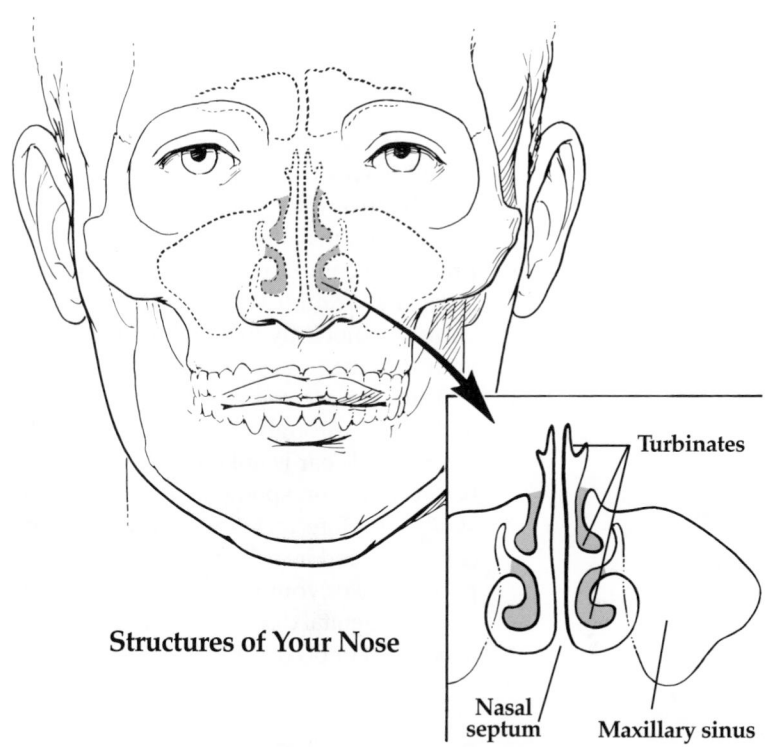

Structures of Your Nose

Turbinates

Nasal septum   Maxillary sinus

speak, your throat also helps you shape the sounds you make.) Your tonsils are on both sides of the back of your mouth along with your adenoids; these structures help protect children from infections. The epiglottis acts as a sort of lid for your trachea, closing when you swallow to keep water and food from entering your windpipe.

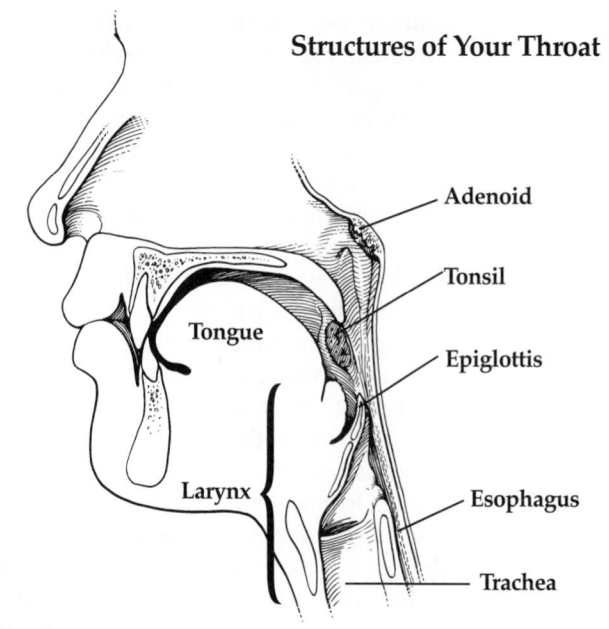

Structures of Your Throat

Adenoid

Tonsil

Tongue

Epiglottis

Esophagus

Larynx

Trachea

Disorders of the Ear

Your ear is a biologic marvel. It transfers sound waves from the air through elaborate channels into your inner ear and turns them into signals that your brain can interpret. The complex mechanisms, particularly in your middle and inner ear canals, allow you not only to hear but also to keep your balance.

Your ears are connected with your nose and throat through your eustachian tube. Your middle ear is linked to the mastoid, a honeycomb- or sponge-like part of your skull. Therefore, an infection in your middle ear can extend into the mastoid. This complexity makes your ear susceptible to infections, congenital disorders, and damage due to accident or occupational exposure.

Swimmer's Ear

Signs and Symptoms
- Itching of your outer ear canal
- Pain in your ear
- Oozing of yellowish or yellowish green, foul-smelling pus from your ear
- Pain in your ear produced by movement of your head
- Hearing loss

Swimmer's ear (external otitis) is a state of persistent irritation and inflammation of your outer ear canal. You also may have an infection. Eczema, the scaly shedding of skin layers (see page 989), develops in the canal. Your skin breaks, often as a result of scratching the itch of your eczema, and bacteria and fungi invade the tissues of the ear canal.

Swimming in polluted water is only one way to contract external otitis. It also may develop after you attempt to clear wax from the canal with a hairpin or similar "tool," causing irritation and itching or tears in your skin. This, in turn, may lead to more manipulation with your favorite "tool," although you risk perforating your eardrum with these instruments. Hair spray and hair dyes also can irritate your ear canal.

Occasionally a fungus, usually *Aspergillus niger*, causes external otitis. The symptoms are the same as for furunculosis, a condition of recurring boils (see page 1009). In furunculosis, a hair follicle in your ear canal becomes infected. People who have furunculosis tend to experience it repeatedly.

External otitis occurs most commonly in young adults.

Diagnosis
If you experience ear itching, flaking skin inside your ear, or pain in your ear canal, you may have external otitis. Yellowish or yellowish green pus often oozes from your ear, and sometimes this oozing seems to relieve the pain. It occasionally affects your hearing if the pus or swelling blocks your ear canal.

Your physician diagnoses the presence of external otitis by using an otoscope, a hand-held instrument that allows examination of your ear canal. If pus is present, a sample may be taken for laboratory analysis.

While most outer ear infections are bothersome, they are not usually dangerous to your general health if you treat them properly. Left untreated, particularly in diabetic persons, infections can spread and damage underlying bones and cartilage.

Treatment
If you suspect that you have swimmer's ear, there are some things you can do to relieve the pain before you see your physician. Placing a warm (not hot) electric heating pad over your ear may help, as will taking aspirin or another analgesic.

After the diagnosis is made, your physician probably will clean your ear canal with a suction device or a cotton-tipped probe. This will help relieve irritation and pain. Then your physician will prescribe treatment by one of various methods.

Frequently, physicians prescribe eardrops containing a corticosteroid preparation (to relieve itching and decrease inflammation) and an antibiotic (to control infection) (see page 1058). Occasionally, physicians prescribe drugs that you take orally. If you are in severe pain, your physician may prescribe a painkiller. Take care that no water gets into your ear while it is healing.

If the external otitis shows no marked improvement after 3 or 4 days, your physician may prescribe an oral antibiotic. Your physician can select a drug specifically for the organism causing your infection if a laboratory test has identified the organism.

Physicians often treat external otitis caused by a fungus with a dusting of sulfanilamide powder. Your physician will treat furunculosis with antibiotics, which you take either by mouth or as eardrops.

The condition may recur several times over a period of months, especially if it is caused by a fungus.

Prevention

External otitis often can be prevented. Avoid swimming in polluted water. Dry your ears after bathing and swimming because moisture in your ear canal can make it susceptible to infection. Place balls of lamb's wool, which repels water, in your ears while applying hair spray or hair dye.

Benign Cysts and Tumors

Signs and Symptoms
- A lump in your ear canal or in front of or behind your ear
- Accumulation of wax
- Discomfort in your ear
- Hearing loss

Sebaceous cysts are thick sacs filled with cheesy material produced by skin glands. They commonly develop behind your ear or in your scalp. Sebaceous cysts are benign and usually are not even noticeable.

Benign tumors of the ear canal (exostoses), which are caused by an overgrowth of bone, also may occur. Such tumors can grow large enough to block your ear canal and thus trap wax and interfere with hearing. Such exostoses grow very slowly, however, and often present no problem.

Diagnosis

Frequently you are not aware that you have a cyst. You may feel a semi-soft lump on your mastoid (the bony protrusion behind your ear) or in front of your ear. Such cysts outside your ear rarely cause any sort of discomfort, although they can become infected. If such a cyst becomes sore, you should visit your physician, who will probably prescribe antibiotic treatment.

In the case of a benign tumor, people are often unaware they have one, and the bony or wart-like growth usually poses no problem. Occasionally, however, such a growth may partially obstruct your ear canal. If your ear hurts or you experience hearing loss, con-

sult your physician. Your physician will examine your ear canal with an otoscope, which allows full viewing of your outer canal.

Treatment

When a benign tumor grows enough to block your outer ear canal, your physician will recommend that it be removed surgically. The procedure is a minor operation but is tricky because the skin covering the exostosis must be left intact; the skin is left because it is more resistant to infection than the skin that would grow in its place. Benign cysts and tumors pose no general health problem.

Foreign Objects in Your Ear

Signs and Symptoms
- Pain in your ear
- Hearing loss
- Sensation of something present in your ear

The assortment of objects that physicians remove from ears is astonishing—from marbles, tiny toys, and jewelry to insects, seeds, bits of paper and plastic, and even earplugs. Because of the complicated structure of your ear, any small object that you put into your ear can become lodged there.

Diagnosis

Usually, you know when something has gotten stuck in your ear. Your ear hurts or feels full, and it may affect your hearing. The problem can be a little harder to diagnose when a small child is affected. Ask the child if the ear hurts and if he or she was playing with any small objects. Look into the ear for a foreign body. If you do see the object, do not try to remove it. Your efforts can damage the delicate tissues of the ear or may force the object deeper. See your physician or go to a hospital emergency room for treatment.

How Serious Are Foreign Objects in Ears?

Most foreign objects do not cause a lasting problem. However, if an object is pushed into your eardrum, it may rupture, and your middle ear may be damaged, a potentially serious situation.

Treatment

After examining your ear, perhaps with an instrument that allows full viewing of your ear canal, your physician will remove the object by using a tiny tool called alligator forceps. Sometimes, physicians use gentle suction to withdraw the object or flood your ear with fluid to flush the object out. If the object is an insect that is still alive, you can try adding a few drops of mineral oil to your ear to immobilize the insect. This may decrease the discomfort until you get to a physician.

Ruptured or Perforated Eardrum

Signs and Symptoms
- Earache
- Partial hearing loss
- Slight bleeding or discharge from your ear

One reason for the advice that you should never put anything into your ear is the risk of breaking your eardrum. You may puncture your eardrum when you clean or scratch your ear with cotton-tipped swabs or with a small, sharp object. Other causes of a punctured eardrum are a slap on your ear and an explosion—both of these produce a sudden change in the air pressure in your ear.

An infection of your middle ear (otitis media, see page 574) may cause inflammation and even destruction of part of your eardrum. This is the most common cause of a hole in an eardrum. Small holes may heal, but larger ones stay open and permit infectious agents to enter your middle ear.

Pain in your ear, hearing loss, and a discharge from your ear may indicate a rupture (perforation) of your eardrum (tympanic membrane).

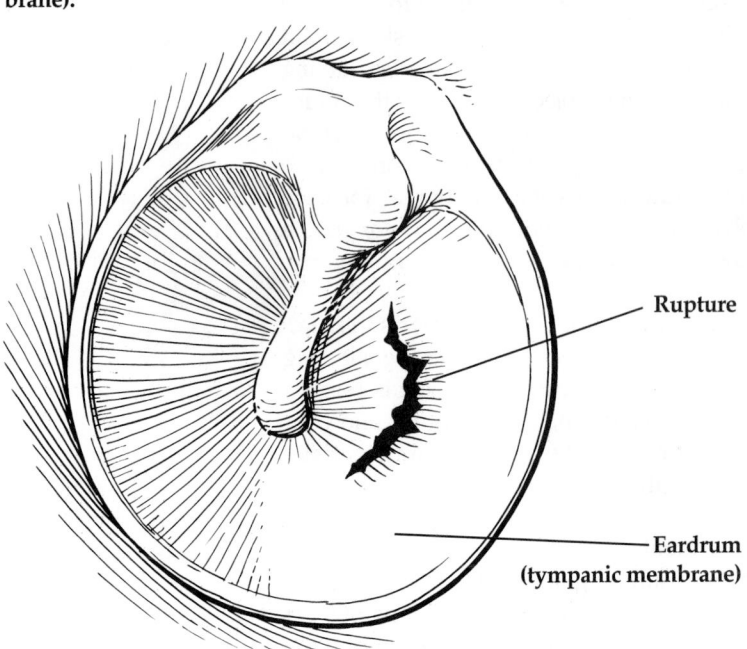

Rupture

Eardrum (tympanic membrane)

Diagnosis
If you experience increasing pain and hearing loss in your ear over a period of a day or so, followed by a discharge of blood or fluid (with subsequent relief of the pain), you may have a ruptured eardrum as a consequence of otitis media. See a physician promptly.

Your physician will examine your ear with an otoscope, an instrument that allows full viewing of your ear canal. If your eardrum is punctured, your physician will see the torn area or the bones of your middle ear behind it.

How Serious Is a Ruptured Eardrum?
A ruptured eardrum can be a painful condition, particularly at first. Sometimes the rupture heals by itself without complications and with little or no permanent hearing loss. Larger perforations may cause recurring otitis media.

Treatment
If you suspect that you have ruptured an eardrum, see your physician as soon as possible. In the meantime you can relieve the pain with aspirin or other analgesic drugs. Placing a warm (not hot) electric heating pad over your ear will help also.

Your physician may prescribe an antibiotic to make sure that no infection develops in your middle ear. Sometimes a plastic or paper patch is placed over your eardrum to seal the opening while it heals. Also, keep your ear dry until it heals.

Your eardrum will often heal within 2 months. If it has not healed in that time, your physician may recommend a minor surgical procedure to repair the tear.

Occupational Hearing Loss

Signs and Symptoms—Progressive hearing loss

Prolonged exposure to noise at 90 decibels (dB) or louder can damage your ear. The intense vibration caused by the loud sound waves damages the hair cells that line the cochlea of your inner ear. This kind of damage causes a condition known as sensorineural hearing loss because it affects the workings of your inner ear. Sensorineural hearing loss usually cannot be corrected.

The noise level of normal conversation typically is about 60 dB. The level is nearer

Noise and Sound Levels

Your ear interprets waves of varying air pressure as sound. These waves, composed of alternating peaks of high pressure and troughs of low pressure, can produce sounds that are loud or soft and of high or low pitch. When these sounds become unpleasant or interfere with other activities, they're referred to as noise.

The loudness of sound is measured in units called decibels (dB). Soft sounds are barely audible. Very loud ones can cause pain in your ear. Between these levels is the range of sounds to which you are exposed on a regular basis.

You may take for granted most of the everyday sounds you hear. Only when they interfere with what you are doing do you notice noise as a problem. Loud noise such as a heavy truck passing by is annoying, but after it is gone you may think no more about it. However, very loud noise, such as the continuous operation of a nearby jackhammer, chain saw, or other tool, can cause pain and ringing in your ears.

As a rule, if you have to shout to make yourself heard, the noise can damage your hearing. Under such conditions, decrease the noise, leave the area, or wear ear protectors. The charts show the average decibel levels for certain activities and the maximum job noise exposure per day allowed by law.

Maximum Job Noise Exposure Allowed by Law

Duration, Hours Daily	Sound Level, Decibels
8	90
6	92
4	95
3	97
2	100
1½	102
1	105
30 minutes	110
15 minutes	115

Sound Levels of Common Noises

Decibels	Noise
	Safe range
20	Watch ticking; leaves rustling
40	Quiet street noise
60	Normal conversation; bird song
80	Heavy traffic
	Risk range
85-90	Motorcycle; snowmobile
80-100	Rock concert
	Injury range
120	Jackhammer 3 feet away
130	Jet engine 100 feet away
140	Shotgun blast

How to Protect Your Ears

You cannot control the world around you, but you can take steps to protect your ears from unnecessary damage. If you work with or near heavy machinery or are bombarded by other loud or continuous noise, you are at risk of developing sensorineural hearing loss. Because this kind of loss generally is irreversible, it is very important to prevent it. Use the following strategies if you are at risk of hearing loss.

Wear Protective Plugs or Earmuffs in Your Workplace

Proven methods include protecting your ears with specially designed earmuffs that resemble earphones. These bring most loud sounds down to acceptable levels. They can close out the outside world, or they can be fitted with miniature speakers and a microphone so that you can communicate with others. Commercially available or custom-molded earplugs made of plastic or rubber effectively protect against excessive noise. Cotton balls are not adequate and can become lodged deep in your ear canal (see Foreign Objects in Your Ear, page 571).

Have Your Hearing Tested

Do this regularly if you work in a noisy environment. Early detection of hearing loss will allow you to take precautions to prevent further damage. Your employer may be responsible for providing ear protection. Ask about the kind of protection your company provides.

Beware of Recreational Risks

Sensorineural hearing loss related to recreation is becoming more common. Activities with the greatest risk are trapshooting, driving snowmobiles and some other recreational vehicles, and, in particular, listening to extremely loud music. Music noise can be a factor beyond attending too many rock concerts or cranking up the stereo so that it shakes the walls. Many people now use earphones to listen to music, often from small portable tape cassettes or radios, which, despite their small size, can produce extremely high sound levels.

Protect your ears from loud music by turning down the volume on the stereo or tape player. If you attend rock concerts, wear earplugs.

The roar of a subway train also can damage your ears. Again, wearing earplugs or even covering your ears with your hands can help protect you.

70 dB in a noisy restaurant and 90 dB for the sound of a large diesel truck about 5 yards away (see also the table on page 573).

Noisy work in heavy construction is a common cause of hearing loss. Airline ground crew members who refuse ear protection are at high risk, as are farm tractor operators. Rock musicians are at great risk, too, and so are the people who listen to rock music played very loudly.

Diagnosis

If you notice that your hearing has become less sensitive, see an ear, nose, and throat specialist and an audiologist. Your physician will examine your ears, and the audiologist will perform a series of tests to determine the nature of your hearing loss. After these examinations, specialists can recommend a proper course of action.

Treatment

If your hearing loss appears to be the result of an occupational hazard, wear proper protective equipment to prevent further deterioration of your hearing (see How to Protect Your Ears, page 573).

If your hearing loss causes communication problems, your physician or audiologist may have suggestions to help you overcome the difficulties. This may include use of a hearing aid (see page 580).

Barotrauma

Signs and Symptoms
- Moderate to severe pain in your ear
- Stuffy feeling in your ear
- Slight hearing loss
- Dizziness
- Tinnitus (noise in your ear)

The air pressure in your middle ear usually is the same as that in your outer ear, because of your eustachian tube. This tube is a narrow channel that connects your middle ear to the back of your nose. When you swallow or yawn, it opens and allows air to flow into or out of your middle ear.

If your eustachian tube is blocked, differences in pressure can occur between the two sides of your eardrum. This condition is known as barotrauma or barotitis media.

Diagnosis

If you fly or scuba dive while you have a congested nose (allergy, cold, or throat infection), you may experience the symptoms of barotrauma. Pain in one ear, slight hearing loss, or a stuffy feeling in your ears may be caused by your eardrum's pressing inward as a result of a change in air pressure.

A more serious problem can occur if the air pressure change is great or if your eustachian tube is entirely blocked. The small capillaries of your middle ear may rupture and bleed, filling your ear with blood and producing a hearing loss and a feeling similar to that of being underwater.

The symptoms of barotrauma usually disappear within a few hours after they begin. Barotrauma is not a serious condition and does not produce permanent hearing loss. However, if you think you have barotrauma, consult your physician, who will examine your ear and monitor your condition to help prevent an infection.

Treatment

If you must fly when you have a congested nose, try taking a decongestant or antihistamine an hour before takeoff and an hour before landing. This may prevent blockage of your eustachian tube. During your flight, suck candy or chew gum to encourage swallowing, which helps keep your eustachian tube open. Another way to open your eustachian tube is to inhale and then gently exhale while you hold your nostrils closed and keep your mouth shut.

If your symptoms do not disappear within a few hours, see your physician. Treatment may involve a surgical incision in your eardrum (myringotomy) and removal of the fluid that is there. Your physician also may prescribe a course of antibiotics to prevent infection within your middle ear.

Acute Ear Infection

Signs and Symptoms
- Feeling of fullness in your ear
- Severe earache
- Fever and chills
- Nausea and diarrhea
- Hearing loss

Acute ear infection (otitis media) occurs in four basic forms: serous otitis media, otitis media with effusion, acute purulent otitis media, and secretory otitis media. In the mildest form, serous otitis media, fluid gathers in your middle ear as a result of blockage of your eustachian tube or excessive production of fluid in your middle ear. There may be discomfort and temporary hearing loss, but usually no infection is present.

The second form, otitis media with effusion, includes both fluid accumulation and an infection. This often develops in conjunction with an upper respiratory infection, enlarged adenoids, or both. This form of otitis can lead to the third, and most serious, form, acute purulent otitis media.

In acute purulent otitis media, pus fills your middle ear. The pressure of the pus may burst your eardrum, causing a discharge of blood and thick pus. Acute purulent otitis most often affects children. The infection can be viral or bacterial.

Occasionally, recurrent or prolonged episodes of otitis media may cause a change in the lining of your middle ear. Then a thicker fluid in great quantities is produced. This results in secretory otitis media.

Diagnosis

When there is a sharp continuous pain in your ear with hearing loss and fever, chances are good that you have an infection of your middle ear. (In addition to crying, infants often tug at their ear if they have an ear infection.) See your physician without delay. If fluid or pus is visible in your ear canal, your physician may take a sample of it for culture in the laboratory to determine the kind of organism that is causing your infection.

How Serious Is Acute Otitis Media?

Serous and secretory otitis media are inconveniences, but usually do not cause permanent hearing loss. If not properly treated, the more serious forms of otitis media can produce infections that can spread to the mastoid process and, on rare occasions, to your inner ear. Permanent hearing loss can result from damage to your eardrum, middle ear bones, or inner ear structures.

Treatment

Until you see your physician, you can relieve some of the pain of acute otitis media by taking aspirin or some other analgesic and by placing a warm (not hot) heating pad over your ear.

Medication

In the case of serous otitis media, your physician may only prescribe decongestants to improve nasal breathing and increase the flow of air into and from your middle ear through your eustachian tube. Your physician may prescribe a course of antibiotics to fight the infection that is present in otitis media with effusion and acute purulent otitis media. Your physician may extend this antibiotic treatment if the infection fails to clear up.

Your physician may prescribe nasal decongestants or antihistamines if nasal congestion or nasal allergies are contributing to the development of your otitis media.

Surgery

If there is great pressure on your eardrum, you may need a surgical incision in your eardrum (myringotomy) to relieve the pressure. In children, surgeons generally perform a myringotomy in the hospital under general anesthesia. The eardrum heals within 1 to 2 weeks.

Chronic Ear Infection

Signs and Symptoms
- Earache
- Periodic seeping of pus from your ear
- Hearing loss

Any of the forms of acute otitis media—serous, otitis media with effusion, purulent, or secretory (see page 574)—can become chronic. A chronic ear infection (chronic otitis media) can be more dangerous than an acute one because its slow, long-lasting effect can result in permanent damage. An acute infection develops suddenly and usually is treated quickly. A chronic condition may not cause enough discomfort to warrant immediate action; thus, you may not notice it until it is well established.

Chronic serous otitis media occasionally can be due to a persistent swelling or inflammation of the adenoids in the very back of your nasal passage. The swelling blocks your eustachian tube. Problems with adenoids most often occur in children. When adults have the condition, it results from recurrent blockage of the eustachian tube or scarring of the eustachian tube from previous infections, nasal allergies, or masses in the back of the nose and throat.

Chronic otitis media with effusion and chronic purulent otitis are more serious. It appears that in some cases an initial acute infection never completely clears, and a low-level infection survives even after treatment. Such an infection can spread to the mastoid process, the honeycomb-like bone behind your ear. Infection in your mastoid is more difficult to eradicate.

The Pros and Cons of Ear Tubes in Children

One way of treating otitis media is to surgically insert a small plastic tube through your eardrum, which allows pus to drain out of your middle ear. However, discuss this procedure in detail with your ear, nose, and throat physician. Among the arguments for and against the procedure are the following points.

For the Procedure

1. The procedure usually results in a decrease in the frequency and severity of episodes of otitis media.

2. Hearing is restored.

3. The operation allows ventilation of your middle ear, thereby decreasing the risk of permanent changes in the lining of your middle ear—changes that might occur with prolonged infection.

Against the Procedure

1. The procedure requires brief general anesthesia, although on an outpatient basis.

2. You must avoid getting water in your ears while the tube is in place.

3. In rare cases, severe scarring or a permanent hole in the eardrum may result.

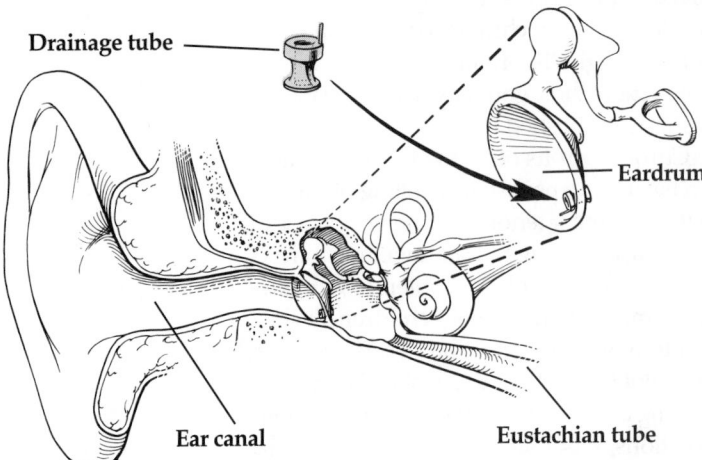

Drainage tube

Eardrum

Ear canal

Eustachian tube

In persistent cases of ear infection, your child's physician may insert a small tube into the eardrum to allow drainage of pus.

Sometimes an initial acute infection clears up but leaves the site more vulnerable to future infections. When a chronic infection then takes hold, the pus it produces can cause perforation of your eardrum or damage to the small bones in your middle ear.

Diagnosis

If pus is seeping from your ear canal and if your ear hurts or you notice a hearing loss, see your physician. He or she will examine your ear with an otoscope to identify the source of infection and also may arrange for X-rays or a CT scan (see page 1334) of your head to determine if the infection has spread to your mastoid process.

How Serious Is Chronic Otitis Media?

Chronic secretory otitis media is uncommon and, although uncomfortable and inconvenient, it rarely causes permanent harm. Left uncorrected, chronic purulent otitis media can cause permanent damage to hearing.

Treatment

Medication

Physicians usually treat chronic secretory and serous otitis media with antihistamines and decongestants if they are associated with nasal congestion or nasal allergies. Usually, chronic otitis media with effusion and purulent otitis media are treated with oral antibiotics. If your eardrum is intact, eardrops will not help because they cannot reach the site of infection.

Surgery

If the situation does not improve and adenoids are the cause of the problem, your physician may recommend surgically removing them.

Another method for treating the problem is to insert a small plastic tube through your eardrum to allow your middle ear to drain (see The Pros and Cons of Ear Tubes in Children, this page). Your ear must not become wet for the entire period of treatment, which may be several months to years. This can be difficult for anyone but particularly so for children.

If you have chronic serous or purulent otitis media and your mastoid process becomes infected, your physician may recommend a mastoidectomy, an operation in which the mastoid process is removed surgically to prevent recurrence and spread of the infection.

Cholesteatoma

Signs and Symptoms
- Hearing loss
- Pus seeping from your ear
- Headache or earache
- Dizziness
- Weakness of facial muscles

Cholesteatoma is a disorder of the mastoid process and your middle ear. It occurs as a result of a blocked eustachian tube. The air pressure in your middle ear lessens and your eardrum bends inward. It can also occur when ear canal skin grows into your middle ear through a hole in your eardrum. In your middle ear, the skin cells (epithelial tissue) that would normally be shed are caught and form a cyst or tumor known as a cholesteatoma. The cholesteatoma then erodes the bone that lines the cavity and damages the small bones of your middle ear.

In some cases this is a congenital problem in which skin cells have become trapped behind the eardrum during fetal development. When a cholesteatoma develops in the ear of a child, it may grow quickly. In adults the problem usually develops more slowly.

Diagnosis
Your physician will examine your ear with an otoscope, a small instrument that allows a full view of your ear canal, and will ask if you have a history of ear infections. If your physician suspects a cholesteatoma, he or she may refer you to an ear, nose, and throat specialist, who will perform a more complete examination and may give you a hearing test.

How Serious Is Cholesteatoma?
A cholesteatoma is benign and will not spread to other sites. But it can cause permanent hearing loss. It can also affect your facial nerve and, in rare cases, cause meningitis if left untreated.

Treatment

Surgery
The condition is chronic and can only be treated surgically. If the cholesteatoma is very small, your physician may remove it in a minor operation. A larger or more advanced cholesteatoma may require a more extensive operation or series of operations to correct damage to the bones of your middle ear. The procedure requires meticulous care

to remove every bit of the cyst. Repeat operations may be required because the cyst can grow back.

The operation also may include rebuilding of the bones of your middle ear to restore hearing. Transplanted ear bones from donors or artificial (prosthetic) devices may be used to reconstruct your middle ear.

In severe cases, your physician may perform a radical mastoidectomy. This leaves a cavity that can be cleaned out periodically. It does not restore damaged bones or lost hearing.

Mastoiditis

Signs and Symptoms
- Redness, swelling, and tenderness of the mastoid process behind your ear
- Earache
- Fever
- Discharge of pus from your ear

If acute otitis media is not treated (see page 574), the infection may spread to the mastoid process, the bone that is behind your outer ear and is connected to your middle ear. When mastoiditis occurs, the infection moves from your middle ear to the mucous membrane lining the mastoid process and the honeycomb-like bone within. If the infection is severe, it can destroy this bone and even spread further.

Diagnosis
If you notice any of the symptoms of otitis media or mastoiditis, consult your physician. Your physician will examine your ear, take a sample of any pus apparent in your ear canal, and may arrange for head X-rays or CT or MRI scan (see page 1334) to determine how far the infection has spread. Your physician may refer you to an ear, nose, and throat specialist.

Before the availability of antibiotics, acute mastoiditis was a leading cause of death in children. Now it is treated successfully with antibiotics, and the health risk is vastly reduced.

Treatment
Your physician will prescribe antibiotics to cure the infection of the mastoid. Lack of easy drainage of infected material from the mastoid cells makes it difficult to cure this infection. It may take several weeks of high-

Hereditary Deafness

Inherited abnormalities may cause deafness. It may accompany hereditary nephritis (Alport's syndrome, see page 833), a kidney disorder that runs in families. There are numerous other forms of deafness that run in families. These include deafness with goiter (Pendred's syndrome); deafness associated with malformation of the external ears, face, or neck; deafness associated with skin abnormalities; and deafness associated with mental retardation, retinitis pigmentosa (see page 561), and peripheral neuropathy.

There also are unusual forms of deafness that are not associated with other abnormalities. These forms of deafness are not common. If one has been identified in your family or in your child, seek genetic counseling (see page 42). You should initiate appropriate treatment and training if you have a deaf infant or child.

A mother who has rubella (see page 191) during pregnancy runs a high risk that it will also affect the developing infant. If rubella (German measles) occurs during the first 3 months of pregnancy, your child will probably be born deaf and have several other serious problems such as cataracts, heart defects, and brain or nervous system impairment. Rubella occurring later in your pregnancy also can cause hearing loss but is less likely to cause some of the other defects.

Prematurity, lack of oxygen during or shortly after birth, blood incompatibilities, and meningitis can cause hearing loss early in life.

dose antibiotic therapy to eradicate the infection. If antibiotic treatment does not solve the problem, your physician may recommend a mastoidectomy, in which part or all of the mastoid bone is surgically removed.

Otosclerosis

Signs and Symptoms
- Gradual hearing loss in one or both ears
- Tinnitus (noise in your ear)

In otosclerosis, the bony wall of your inner ear becomes disorganized and an abnormal growth of spongy bone occurs at the entrance to your inner ear. The stirrup, the tiny bone that vibrates to pass sound waves into your inner ear, may become immobile, causing conductive hearing loss. Conductive hearing loss is failure of the mechanism that passes vibrations through your middle ear via its connective bones. Unlike sensorineural hearing loss (see pages 572 and 579), conductive hearing loss often is reversible.

Otosclerosis is the most frequent cause of middle ear hearing loss in young adults, affecting about 10 percent of the American

population to some degree. Otosclerosis tends to run in families and is more common in women than in men. It appears more often in people who are white than in people who are black, Native American, or Asian.

Symptoms usually become apparent between the ages of 15 and 35. The condition tends to be slowly progressive and can affect one or both ears. The hearing loss may be slight or pronounced. In women with otosclerosis, the rate of hearing loss may increase during pregnancy.

Diagnosis
If you notice that your hearing seems to be gradually decreasing, see your physician. He or she will examine your ears, conduct hearing tests, and ask if any close relative experienced early hearing loss.

How Serious Is Otosclerosis?
Otosclerosis does not endanger your general health, and it often can be corrected. However, the isolation and emotional distress that deafness can cause may require difficult mental and lifestyle adjustments.

Treatment

Surgery
In most cases, otosclerosis can be treated successfully with an operation called stapedectomy. This is a surgical procedure in which your physician cuts the skin of your ear canal and lifts your eardrum out of the way to remove your stirrup (stapes) and replace it with a tiny wire or stainless steel prosthesis. Your eardrum is then replaced and usually heals in a week or two. In some instances, your physician may use a laser to create a small hole (stapedotomy) in the bottom of your stirrup (stapes) bone to allow for placement of the prosthesis.

You may experience temporary dizziness for some hours after your operation. Hearing usually improves quickly, and you will be back to normal activities within a few weeks. Occasionally, a blood clot that blocks sound conduction will form in your middle ear. Such clots usually disappear within a few weeks without treatment.

Stapedectomy can help most people with otosclerosis, but 1 to 2 percent of those who undergo the procedure lose all hearing in the ear. This is a matter for consideration before proceeding with the operation. If you have otosclerosis in both ears, you might consider having surgery on one ear and then waiting a year to gauge the results before having the other ear done. If your inner ear is damaged, a stapedectomy may not help the problem.

Medication

Treatment with tablets of sodium fluoride, calcium, and vitamin D is commonly used to prevent the progressive bony changes and further hearing loss by hardening the spongy bone, but there is continuing debate as to its value.

Hearing Aids

Hearing aids are another effective means of overcoming the hearing loss associated with otosclerosis. If you have otosclerosis in one or both ears, your physician may refer you to an audiologist for a hearing aid fitting (see page 580).

Age-Related Hearing Loss

Signs and Symptoms

- Gradual hearing loss
- Tinnitus (noise in your ear)

Hearing impairment is common among people older than 65 years. Almost a third of the people in this age group have a noticeable hearing loss. Some lose very little hearing, and others become quite hard of hearing.

When hearing loss is severe, we call it presbycusis (from the Latin *presby*, meaning "old," and *cusis*, meaning "hearing"). Typically, it begins between ages 40 and 50 and often worsens progressively. It affects the hearing in both ears, particularly for high-frequency sound. It affects men more often and more severely than women.

Presbycusis is a kind of hearing loss caused by changes in your cochlea or in nerves attached to it. Cells within your cochlea, the snail-shaped cavity in your inner ear, carry thousands of tiny hairs that convert sound vibrations into electrical signals. These signals go to the brain, where they are interpreted as sound. When some of these hairs become damaged or other changes take place in your cochlea, the signals are not transmitted as efficiently, and a loss of hearing results.

This form of hearing loss is known as sensorineural, referring to damage in the inner ear. Hearing loss as a result of aging is permanent and cannot be reversed surgically.

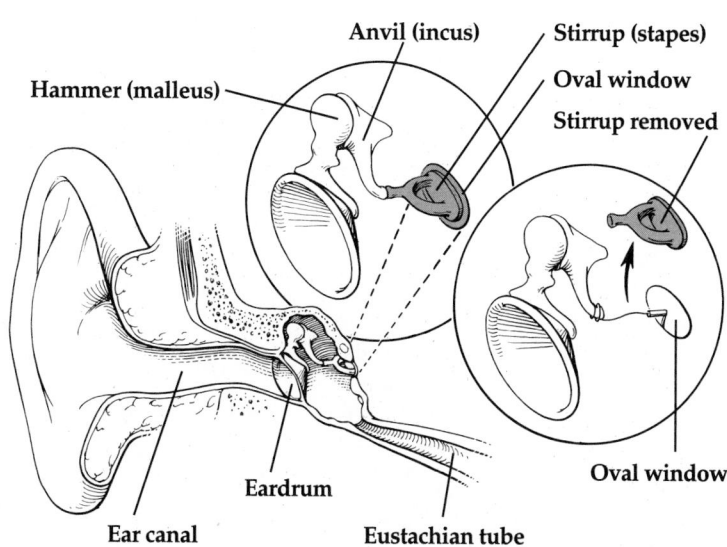

Hammer (malleus) · **Anvil (incus)** · **Stirrup (stapes)** · **Oval window** · **Stirrup removed** · **Eardrum** · **Ear canal** · **Eustachian tube** · **Oval window**

In a stapedectomy, the malfunctioning stirrup (stapes) of your middle ear is replaced with a tiny wire or a stainless steel prosthesis to transmit sound vibrations.

Diagnosis

If you or a family member notices that you are hearing less well, see your physician. He or she can arrange to have a series of tests done to determine whether the loss is sensorineural or conductive (see page 578). Often, you may deny that a problem exists. Occasionally, irritating tinnitus (noise in the ear) encourages people to consult a physician.

Communicating With a Hearing-Impaired Person

Here are a few suggestions for communicating effectively with a hearing-impaired person:

- Speak at a normal conversational level if the person is wearing a hearing aid. If the person is not, speak a little louder than normal but do not shout—it is irritating and unnecessary.
- Speak naturally but more slowly than you usually do. Add more pauses than normal in your speech pattern. Rapid speech is more difficult for a hearing-impaired person to understand.
- Before speaking, make sure you have your listener's attention. If he or she is watching your face, visual clues can help in understanding your words. Also, watch your listener's face for signs of incomprehension.
- Decrease competing background noise. Turn off the television set or stereo, and close the windows to traffic noises.
- Move within 2 to 3 feet of the person with whom you are conversing, so that your speech will be louder than most of the background noise.
- If you cannot reduce background noise, move to a quieter area to talk.

Hearing Loss and Hearing Aids

An estimated 25 million Americans could benefit from using hearing aids—yet only a fifth of that number wear them regularly. Some people do not realize, or refuse to believe, that their hearing is impaired. Others are skeptical that a hearing aid would help them or feel that the cost of a hearing aid is prohibitive. Still others are wary of hearing aids because of the experience of a friend for whom a hearing aid did not work out well or who may have been taken advantage of by an unscrupulous hearing aid dealer.

Set aside your fears. Current models are technologically advanced, simple to operate, and smaller than those of only a few years ago. You must shop carefully to find the hearing aid best suited to your needs, but for most kinds of hearing loss a hearing aid can be helpful.

Get an Examination

If you suspect that you have a hearing loss, see your physician. He or she may refer you to an otorhinolaryngologist (a physician specially trained in ear, nose, and throat problems) or an audiologist (a professional trained in hearing evaluation), who will conduct a complete examination and a series of hearing tests. Sometimes medical treatment or surgery can correct a hearing problem, particularly if the problem is in the outer or middle ear. However, if the problem is in your inner ear, it usually is not treatable medically. A hearing aid cannot make the problem disappear, but it can improve your hearing.

Use What's Best for You

Hearing aids now are compact and capable of providing a wide range of power. Most people wear in-the-ear aids, although behind-the-ear styles are still common. Even people with severe to profound hearing loss can use behind-the-ear models. Only rarely and in special circumstances are body-mounted hearing aids used. For those units, the earpiece is attached by a cord to a microphone and amplifier located in a small box that you carry in your pocket.

Cochlear Implant

Some children and adults who have very profound hearing losses, and who do not benefit from hearing aid use, may benefit from a cochlear implant. The surgeon implants an electrode into your inner ear for direct nerve stimulation. Implant recipients gain the ability to hear and recognize speech and many environmental noises. Almost all show improved ability to understand speech when they combine hearing through the implant with lipreading. More than half of the adults can understand speech without lipreading. Some have limited ability to use the telephone.

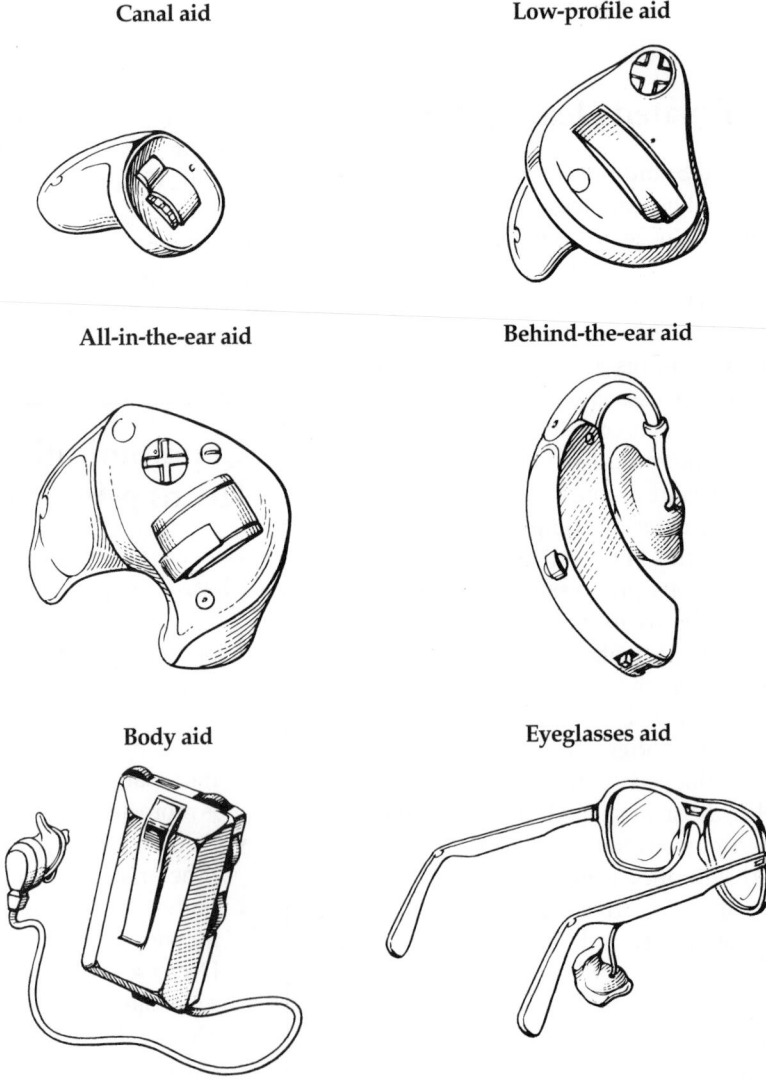

Canal aid

Low-profile aid

All-in-the-ear aid

Behind-the-ear aid

Body aid

Eyeglasses aid

From Hearing Aids for Hearing Problems (patient education brochure). By permission of Mayo Foundation.

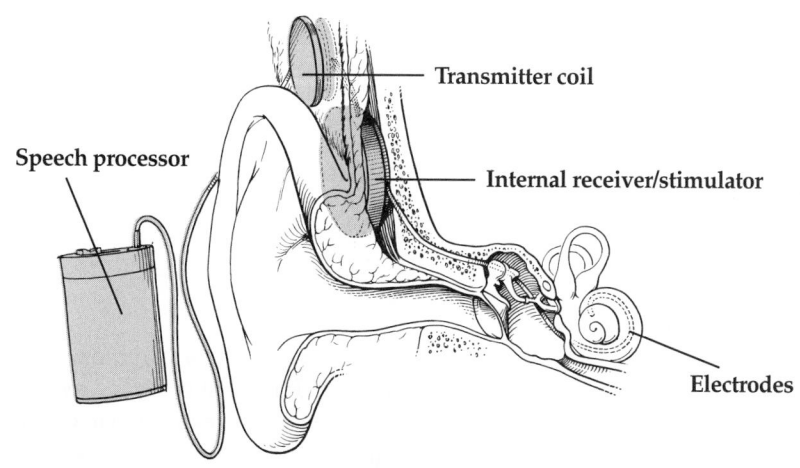

Speech processor

Transmitter coil

Internal receiver/stimulator

Electrodes

The cochlear implant includes external and internal parts. Sounds enter the ear-level microphone (not shown). The speech processor next codes the sounds and sends them by means of a transmitter coil to an internal receiver/stimulator and then on to electrodes in your inner ear (cochlea).

Get a Custom Fit

Hearing aids must be custom-fitted to ensure comfort and performance. First, a mold is made of your ear canal, so that the earpiece will fit exactly and be both comfortable to wear and capable of passing sound efficiently into your ear.

As you learn to wear the hearing aid, remember that your hearing will not return to normal. A hearing aid can only amplify sounds around you. For this reason, it may take a bit of adjustment on your part before you feel comfortable with your hearing aid.

Most likely you will need to practice tuning out background noise. Try wearing your hearing aid in quiet surroundings at first. This will allow you to become accustomed to the "new" sounds you are hearing. Wear your hearing aid daily. Make it a part of your routine.

Get Help With the Cost

The cost of hearing aids varies, but if cost is a problem, check with local civic and community groups. Some have programs to help people meet this cost.

When you select a hearing aid

(or two hearing aids, one for each ear), make sure there is a trial period before your purchase becomes final. Typical periods are 30 days, which should give you enough time to try the hearing aid. If the hearing aid is uncomfortable or does not seem to improve your ability to hear, ask the dispenser to adjust it.

If your hearing aid does not help you enough to warrant the purchase, return the unit for a refund. You may need to pay a rental fee for the time you used the hearing aid.

If you have any doubts about a hearing aid dispenser, check the credentials of the business with the Better Business Bureau. Beware of high-pressure sales techniques and "free" consultations. If you are not satisfied with your hearing aid or hearing aid dispenser, ask your otorhinolaryngologist or audiologist for additional recommendations.

Take Proper Care of Your Hearing Aid

Treat your hearing aid carefully. Avoid exposure to chemicals, such as hair spray, or to extremes of heat or cold. Wipe the ear mold portion daily with a dry tissue. Never immerse your hearing aid in water. (It is not waterproof.)

Sometimes people with presbycusis find that it is more difficult to hear high-frequency voices of women and children than lower voices of men. You also may find that it is more difficult to understand conversation in a group than conversation with a single individual. Severe hearing loss is not a health threat, but it can cause isolation and be socially debilitating.

Treatment

Presbycusis cannot be treated surgically or medically. A hearing aid is the only method

of treatment. Your physician will send you to an audiologist, who will conduct a thorough series of tests and may fit you for a hearing aid.

You may also learn certain useful techniques. These include lipreading, facing the speaker, decreasing background noise (for example, turning off the television set or dishwasher or shutting the windows to avoid street noise), and making maximum use of nonauditory clues such as gestures and facial expressions to help understand what people are saying.

Tinnitus

Signs and Symptoms
- Noise in your ear, such as ringing, buzzing, roaring, whistling, or hissing
- Hearing loss

Tinnitus, the annoying sensation of noise in your ear when no sound is present, is common. It can be a symptom of almost any ear disorder as well as other diseases, including cardiovascular disease and anemia. Scientists don't understand the mechanism that causes you to hear the sounds. Tinnitus usually is associated with hearing loss.

Diagnosis
If you hear ringing, buzzing, whistling, or other sounds when there is no apparent source of such noises, you probably have tinnitus. Such noises can be continuous or intermittent, and they can vary in loudness. They may be in synchrony with your heartbeat.

When testing for tinnitus, your physician will be looking for signs of ear disorders such as infectious diseases, ear obstructions, otosclerosis (see page 578), Meniere's disease (this page), acoustic trauma, hereditary deafness, or occupational hearing loss.

Your physician may examine your ears, test your hearing, and conduct a series of tests to determine the cause of noise in your ears. Your physician may also recommend a CT or MRI scan (see page 1334).

Treatment
Ear noise can be very annoying but is not in itself a threat to health. In some cases, the cause of tinnitus is easily treated, and the noise stops. Such is the case when ear wax, a foreign object, or mild middle ear infection is the cause. Hearing loss also may be reversed.

In many cases, however, treating the underlying cause of the symptom may or may not have an effect on the ear noise. One form of treatment is to cover up the unwanted sound with competing music (for example, a clock radio at night) or, in some cases, by using a tinnitus masker (a device worn like a hearing aid that produces noise more pleasant than that in your ear). Among those whose hearing is impaired, hearing aids also help decrease ear noise while amplifying outside sounds. If you have tinnitus, you should avoid loud noises, nicotine, aspirin, caffeine, and alcohol. Any of these may aggravate your condition. Often, you must learn to tolerate this annoying symptom.

Acoustic Trauma

Signs and Symptoms
- Hearing loss
- Tinnitus (ear noise)

Acoustic trauma is a common form of hearing loss. It is most often the result of a blow to your ear or an explosion in which air pressure changes drastically and suddenly, causing damage to the delicate bones and other mechanisms of your ear. Long exposure to loud machinery or excessively loud music can also cause it (see Occupational Hearing Loss, page 572).

Diagnosis
Hearing loss after a nearby explosion or a blow to your ear is fairly common. High-pitched tinnitus (ringing or other sounds in the ear) may be accompanied by partial deafness. Your physician will determine what kind of hearing loss you have sustained by using a series of tests.

Treatment
The only effective treatment for severe sensory hearing loss caused by trauma is a hearing aid (see page 580). However, other strategies can help you make the adjustment to partial deafness easier. These include the use of visual clues (like facial expressions) and lipreading.

Prevention
If you know you will be exposed to loud noise such as that from a jackhammer at a work site, protect yourself with specially designed earmuffs. These devices block out almost all external sound and can be fitted with microphones and receivers to let you communicate with others.

Meniere's Disease

Signs and Symptoms
- Severe attacks of vertigo accompanied by nausea and vomiting
- Tinnitus (ear noise)
- Muffled or distorted hearing
- Hearing loss

The symptoms of Meniere's disease were described more than a century ago by a Frenchman, Prosper Meniere. The typical symptoms he described included episodic vertigo with fluctuating hearing loss, a ringing in the ears (tinnitus), and a sensation of pressure in the affected ear.

Meniere's disease usually affects one ear first, and in about 25 to 50 percent of the cases, it eventually affects the other ear. Its cause is unknown. There seems to be an increase of fluid in the part of your inner ear called the labyrinth. This excess fluid causes pressure within the membranes of your labyrinth, distorting and occasionally rupturing them. This produces severe disruption in the sense of balance and often in the sense of hearing.

Diagnosis

Periodic attacks mark Meniere's disease. Between attacks—periods that may range from several hours to months or even years—there are no symptoms. The attacks themselves may last from a few hours to most of a day or longer.

The symptoms may range from mild to serious but, in varying degrees, usually involve vertigo (often so severe that it causes nausea and vomiting), tinnitus (ear noise such as buzzing or ringing), and muffled or distorted hearing or hearing loss, particularly in the low frequencies. The attacks can become increasingly severe.

If you experience any of these symptoms, consult your physician without delay. Your physician will conduct a test to measure how well you hear sounds of various frequencies. If this test is inconclusive, further tests may be needed to diagnose the problem.

One such test (called electronystagmography) involves flooding your ear with cold or warm water. Normally, this causes you to feel a whirling sensation that makes your eye movements flicker. This flicker is studied. The procedure is repeated with water of different temperatures. The responses to the flooding of each ear are recorded and compared with each other and with normal responses to determine if the balancing function of the inner ear is operating normally.

How Serious Is Meniere's Disease?

For most people, the disorder is primarily an inconvenience, and they have only rare attacks. For a few, however, Meniere's disease can cause complete deafness, and the vertigo and accompanying nausea can be frequent and debilitating.

Treatment

If you experience the vertigo of Meniere's disease, lie as still as possible to ease the symptoms. When the immediate symptoms have subsided, consult your physician.

Medication

Your physician probably will prescribe medication to combat the vertigo and its accompanying nausea and vomiting. Other treatments that seem to help some people include the use of diuretics and a low-salt diet to decrease the fluids in the body. Cutting down on your use of caffeine and nicotine may help. Also, avoid alcohol.

Your physician may prescribe sedatives to relieve the severe anxiety that a serious attack can cause. It is difficult to tell when drug therapy has been useful over long periods because Meniere's disease tends to go into remission and spontaneously disappear.

Surgery

When medical treatment fails to control the frequency and severity of attacks, your physician may recommend surgery. The operation may involve a procedure to relieve the pressure within your inner ear and its distended membranes. Sometimes the nerve that controls balance is cut.

When hearing loss is severe or complete in the affected ear and your vertigo is very serious, your physician may recommend a procedure in which your entire inner ear is destroyed. Then your other ear and muscle impulses and sight handle the balance function.

If you have Meniere's disease in both ears, treatment is more difficult. You may have surgery on the poorer of your two ears to stop the most debilitating attacks. You may receive streptomycin or gentamicin, antibiotics that are toxic to your ear, in carefully controlled amounts to disrupt the balance portion of your inner ear while preserving your hearing.

Labyrinthitis

Signs and Symptoms

- Extreme vertigo (loss of balance and a sensation that either you or the room is spinning)

- Nausea and vomiting
- Involuntary movements of your eyes

Labyrinthitis is an infection of the labyrinth, the fluid-filled chamber of your inner ear that controls balance and hearing. The infection may be either bacterial (the result of spreading from acute otitis media or purulent meningitis) or secondary to a viral meningitis (see pages 433, 481, and 574). With a bacterial infection, the hearing loss in the affected ear usually is total.

Diagnosis

If you experience sensations such as nausea and vertigo, your eyes move slowly to one side and then flick back to their original position, and you have lost all hearing in one ear, you may have labyrinthitis. Your physician will examine your ear and ask questions, including whether you recently had a middle ear infection.

The symptoms of labyrinthitis can be frightening, but the condition itself is not dangerous if you receive proper treatment.

Treatment

Your physician will prescribe antibiotics if you have bacterial labyrinthitis. For both bacterial and viral labyrinthitis, your physician may recommend an antinausea drug and a sedative to combat the effects of the vertigo. You may need to rest in bed for several days.

The severe symptoms of vertigo usually pass within a few days to a week. Feelings of imbalance may persist for several weeks or even months, particularly with quick movements. Recurrence of episodes of labyrinthitis is rare.

Acoustic Neuroma

Signs and Symptoms
- Mild dizziness
- Tinnitus (ear noise)
- Hearing loss

An acoustic neuroma is a very slow-growing benign (noncancerous) tumor of the eighth cranial nerve, usually near the point at which the nerve leaves the cranial cavity and enters the bone structures of your inner ear. Because this site is in an angle formed by some of your brain structures (cerebellum and pons) and a part of your skull, it is sometimes called an angle tumor.

Diagnosis

If you experience mild dizziness, loss of balance, ringing or other noises in one ear, and gradual hearing loss, you may have an acoustic neuroma. The dizziness does not occur in distinct episodes as it does in Meniere's disease.

Your physician will conduct an audiometry test and a neurologic examination and likely will order MRI or CT scans (see page 1334) of your skull to discover if a neuroma is present.

Treatment

Although benign in character and slow in growth, this tumor can be a serious threat, because it is located within your skull adjacent to a number of vital brain structures. As it grows, it creates pressure on these structures which can damage them. It must be surgically removed.

Benign Paroxysmal Positional Vertigo (BPPV)

Signs and Symptoms
- Abrupt onset of vertigo (sensation that either you or the room is spinning) lasting less than a minute when you move your head to certain positions
- Involuntary eye movements accompanying the vertigo

This disorder is characterized by sudden, extreme vertigo when you lie on one side or the other, or when you lean your head back to look at something above. Unlike other forms of vertigo, it is the position of your head, not the movement, that causes the vertigo. The problem lies in the vestibular labyrinth, the fluid-filled chamber of your inner ear that controls balance. The cause is unknown.

Diagnosis

If your surroundings seem to be spinning or you feel like you are floating while lying on one side or the other or with your head tipped back, and your eyes move from side to side involuntarily when this is happening, you may be experiencing positional vertigo. The symptoms usually decrease in less than a minute. See your physician, who may conduct a series of tests to determine what form of vertigo you have and whether your disorientation is a symptom of another disorder.

Treatment

Positional vertigo is an inconvenience but rarely a serious problem, unless you are in an occupation in which even short episodes of vertigo may be disruptive. The most common treatment is to avoid those positions or activities that cause the symptoms.

In recent years physicians have found a new, increasingly successful treatment for positional vertigo. Called the canalith repositioning procedure, it involves five simple maneuvers for positioning your head.

First, move from a sitting to a reclining position. Extend your head over the end of a table at a 45-degree angle. Turn your head to the side. Roll over onto your side, keeping your head slightly angled while you look down at the floor. Return carefully to a sitting position. Tilt your chin down.

Each position progressively moves debris from the posterior semicircular canal into a tiny bag-like structure called the utricle. Here debris likely attaches to sticky membrane walls where it no longer can cause dizziness.

One treatment often eliminates dizziness immediately. If not, a repeated attempt may loosen debris that remains trapped in your semicircular canals. Repeat the procedure if dizziness recurs.

After the procedure, you must keep your head upright for 48 hours, even as you sleep. This allows time for the particles to settle inside your utricle. You also may need to wear a neck collar to prevent tilting your head.

Protruding Ears

Signs and Symptoms—Ears that project an abnormally large distance from your head

Ears that protrude from the sides of your head are neither more efficient nor less efficient for hearing than are ears that lie flat against your head. Thus, the problem is largely cosmetic. It is fairly uncommon. The protrusion may vary from slight to extremely obvious. Sometimes, such ears may become the basis of an emotional problem, if you feel a sense of shame, ridicule, or unattractiveness.

Treatment

A popularly held misconception about protruding ears is that you can train them to grow closer to your head by taping or strapping them to the side of your head at night. This may make you think you are doing something about the problem, but it doesn't work. If you have mildly protruding ears, changing to a hairstyle that calls less attention to your ears is a more effective approach to the problem.

Surgery

A simple surgical procedure can correct protruding ears. The surgeon makes an incision near the fold of skin behind your ear. The surgeon then removes a strip of skin and, in some cases, cartilage, pulls your ear flat against your head, and closes the incision. The scars are hidden behind your ear. However, the procedure should not be done in children under age 4 because their ears are still developing. Usually, to avoid teasing, children have this procedure done just prior to beginning school.

Wax Blockage

Signs and Symptoms
- Partial hearing loss
- Ringing in one or both ears
- Earache
- Sensation that your ear or ears are plugged

Your outer ear canal is lined with hair follicles and glands that produce a wax called cerumen. These hairs and wax trap dust and other foreign particles to prevent them from entering your ear, thus protecting the delicate mechanisms of your ear.

Normally, the small amount of wax that forms makes its way over time to the opening of your ear, where it falls out or is removed as you wash. New wax is produced in the canal. Some people, however, produce or accumulate an excessive amount of wax. This extra wax hardens and blocks your ear canal. Wax blockage is one of the most common causes of hearing loss among people of all ages.

Diagnosis

If you experience progressive hearing loss over a period of a few weeks or months, your ears feel full, you have an earache, or you hear constant or occasional noises such as ringing in your ears, contact your physician. The first thing he or she will do is look for signs of earwax blockage.

Treatment

There is an old but wise saying: "Never put anything smaller than an elbow into your ear." Your ear canal and eardrum are very delicate and you can damage them easily by poking around with such common items as cotton-tipped swabs, bobby pins, paper clips, and twisted pieces of paper. These usually do not remove problem wax and, more importantly, can easily damage your ear canal or eardrum. Generally, you don't need to remove earwax. Do not attempt to irrigate your ears if you've had a perforated eardrum or mastoid surgery.

If your ear is healthy and excessive earwax persists, a few drops of baby oil, mineral oil, or glycerin placed in your ear with an eyedropper generally will loosen the wax. Use a few drops twice a day for several days. Although there are over-the-counter preparations, they are more expensive and often less effective.

Once you soften the wax well, you can attempt to remove it. Fill a 3-ounce rubber bulb syringe with body-temperature water. (If the water is much cooler or warmer, this procedure may cause severe, but brief, dizziness.) With your head tilted down, pull your outer ear up and back to straighten your ear canal. With the other hand, gently squirt water into the canal, exerting mild pressure but not causing pain. Then turn your head to allow the water to drain into a sink or bowl. You may need to flush your ear several times before the wax, usually in the form of a plug, falls out. Dry your outer ear with a towel. Dry your ear canal by inserting one full eyedropper of rubbing alcohol into the canal. This will absorb the water and destroy bacteria and fungi. Tip your head to the side to drain the alcohol.

Your physician uses a similar procedure to cure wax blockage or may scoop the wax out with an instrument called a curette or use a suction device.

Disorders of the Nose and Sinuses

Your nose is the main gateway to your respiratory system. Normally, your nose filters, humidifies, and warms the air as it moves from your nasal passage into your throat and lungs, 12 to 15 times a minute.

Occasionally, your nose is the site of conditions such as nosebleed, cold, hay fever, or a sinus infection. Luckily, most disorders of the nose and sinuses are temporary and easy to cure. Even loss of smell is rarely permanent. The following pages address the common disorders of the nose and its adjacent cavities, the sinuses.

Nosebleed

Signs and Symptoms—Sudden bleeding from one nostril

Most people experience a nosebleed at one time or another. Sometimes the cause is a hard impact on the nose, but often a nosebleed is simply the result of a cold, sinus infection, dry air, or a scab being knocked off. Sometimes there may be no apparent reason.

Among children and young adults, most nosebleeds begin on the septum, the cartilage that separates the two nasal chambers. This form of nosebleed is not serious and usually is easy to stop. The front of your septum, just inside your nostril, contains many fragile blood vessels. These vessels are easily damaged, either directly as from a blow or indirectly from crusting in your nose produced by breathing very dry air. A head cold or an allergy can also cause crusting.

In older people, nosebleeds may begin on the septum or deeper in the nose. These deeper nosebleeds, which are rare, often are harder to stop.

Diagnosis

In most cases, you can stop a nosebleed easily, and there is no need for further examination. However, when the bleeding is hard to stop or occurs frequently, you should visit your physician.

Your physician will examine your nose with a special instrument and light to see precisely where the problem lies. If the problem appears to be deep in your nose, your physician will look for other, more serious, problems such as a tumor in the back part of your nose.

Treatment

Use these easy steps to stop the common nosebleed:

1. Sit up or stand—don't lie down. An upright position decreases the blood pressure in the veins of your nose, which slows the flow of blood.

2. Pinch your nose with your thumb and index finger and breathe through your mouth. Do this for 5 to 10 minutes—the pressure on your bleeding septum should stop the flow of blood.

Some people apply an ice bag to their nose to constrict the blood vessels and stop the bleeding. This method is harmless, but it does not help to stop the bleeding—the cold reaches the vessels on the outside of the nose, not those on the septum.

If a nosebleed is difficult to stop or occurs frequently, you should see your physician. Treatment may involve several steps. First, a suction device removes excess blood. Then you will have a medicated cotton ball placed in your nose. The medication anesthetizes and shrinks your nasal linings.

Cautery

If the bleeding still continues, your physician may recommend chemical or electric cautery. For this procedure, the physician applies a topical anesthetic to the inside of your nose and then burns the affected blood vessels with a chemical or with a tiny electric instrument (cautery) to promote coagulation of the blood.

If the bleeding persists after cautery, your physician will gently pack your nostril with medicated gauze. The packing, which is left in place for several days, exerts pressure on the bleeding site to stop the blood flow. When the packing is removed, your vessels may be cauterized again to discourage recurrence of the bleeding.

Surgery

Nosebleeds caused by an underlying disease, such as hypertension or arteriosclerosis, or

that occur far back in your nose are often the most difficult to stop. Your physician will probably recommend the help of a specialist who can place a special pack in your nasal cavity. Its placement requires a special technique and sedation. This procedure is done in a hospital, where you will need to stay 2 or 3 days for observation. This procedure may be uncomfortable, but it usually is effective in stopping the bleeding.

In rare instances, the standard techniques do not work, and you may lose a large amount of blood. This can be dangerous and may require surgery to block the arteries that supply blood to the nosebleed site. The operation requires a hospital stay of several days.

Prevention

If you have frequent nosebleeds, you can take steps to prevent or decrease the frequency of their occurrence. Apply petroleum jelly to your nasal septum once or twice each day. Increase the humidity of the air you breathe by using a humidifier or vaporizer. Don't pick your nose, and avoid blowing your nose for several hours after a nosebleed. Blowing your nose increases pressure on the damaged vessels and can lead to another bloody nose.

Beware: Nose-Drop Addiction

Your local drugstore sells many products designed to relieve nasal congestion, including nasal sprays and nose drops. These products reach a large area of the mucous membrane directly, so they provide quick decongestion. But use them carefully and only for a limited period, if at all. They can be addicting.

Use nonprescription nasal sprays or nose drops no more than 3 or 4 times a day over a period of no more than 3 to 4 days. If you use them frequently over several weeks, they can have a rebound effect, causing your nose to become even more congested between applications of the medication. As a result, you will need greater and more frequent doses of the spray or drops.

Prolonged use of nasal sprays and drops can cause irritation of your mucous membrane, a stinging or burning in your nose, and a chronic inflammation of the mucous membrane known as rhinitis medicamentosa.

The only way to treat the problem of nose-drop addiction is to stop using nose drops. Your nose may become more congested than ever at first, but after a few weeks the congestion should gradually wear off as the inflammation subsides. If the initial problem of congestion remains, consult an allergist or an ear, nose, and throat specialist (see Allergic Rhinitis, page 1040).

Nasal Obstruction

Signs and Symptoms—Inability to breathe through your nose

Nasal obstruction is a physical blockage of the air passageways of your nose. Everyone experiences a certain amount of temporary blockage when suffering from a cold or an allergy. A real obstruction is more than a passing occurrence, however, and usually results from one of two causes: a deviated septum of your nose or chronic use of over-the-counter nasal sprays. Nasal polyps, nasal tumors, and enlarged adenoids are other potential causes.

Your septum is the cartilage and bony partition that separates your two nasal chambers. Although we usually think it divides the nose equally, few people have a septum that runs perfectly straight. Most variations are small, but in some people the septum veers significantly to one side or the other, creating the blockage. Such deviations are most often the result of an injury such as a blow to your nose. The deviation can also cause a disposition to nosebleeds (see page 586) or sinusitis (see page 590).

The other common cause of nasal obstruction, overuse of nasal decongestant sprays, often begins when you start using these as a way to unblock your congested nose. However, frequent use of decongestants results in a long-term tendency to more congestion. This begins a cycle in which you use more spray more frequently to keep your nasal passages clear. This is sometimes called nose-drop addiction or rhinitis medicamentosa.

Diagnosis

You may suspect that you have a nasal obstruction if you find that you have trouble breathing through your nose in the absence of a cold or an allergy. When you consult your physician, he or she will examine your nose for the cause of the obstruction and will ask questions regarding possible injury, allergies, and other symptoms as well as your use of nasal sprays.

Your physician may sometimes use a lighted flexible fiberoptic endoscope to assist in diagnosing nasal disorders or to better visualize the recesses of your nose during surgery.

Treatment

For many people, a deviated septum poses little or no inconvenience. However, if your condition causes a blockage that makes it difficult to breathe normally, a septoplasty may be the answer. Septoplasty is a surgical procedure that realigns your septum. It can be done either under local anesthesia on an outpatient basis or under general anesthesia during a brief hospital stay.

If overuse of nose drops or sprays causes the blockage, the treatment is simple: stop using these medications. Your condition may become worse for a while, but over a period of weeks your breathing should become more nearly normal as the ill effects of the nose drops wear off (see Beware: Nose-Drop Addiction, page 587).

If chronic nose congestion remains a problem, your physician can examine your nose and sinuses and recommend a program of therapy. Your physician may refer you to an allergist who will conduct a series of tests to determine if you are allergic to specific elements in your environment. If the physician finds an allergy, he or she may prescribe a course of therapy that may include antihistamines to help combat the problem (see page 1034).

Your nasal septum separates your nasal chambers. A deviated septum (see arrow) may be a cause of nasal obstruction.

Deviated septum

Juvenile Angiofibroma

Signs and Symptoms—Frequent nosebleeds

An angiofibroma is a benign tumor of your nose that occurs at puberty in boys and, in rare instances, in girls. It may shrink on its own after puberty, but it can grow rapidly, producing obstruction of nasal passages and sinuses and causing frequent and often severe nosebleeds. Rarely, it may put pressure on your brain.

Diagnosis

If your physician suspects juvenile angiofibroma, he or she will examine the inside of your nose for evidence of a tumor. A CT scan (see page 1334) can determine the size and location of the tumor. If the tumor does not shrink on its own, you may need to consider treatment.

Treatment

Usually, physicians surgically remove tumors that obstruct your airway or cause nosebleeds. Occasionally, your physician may use a procedure called embolization, either alone or just before the surgical removal. During embolization, your physician injects small pellets of a glue-like substance into blood vessels of the tumor. The pellets help block the blood supply to your tumor.

Rhinophyma

Signs and Symptoms—Large, bulbous, ruddy appearance of your nose

Rhinophyma involves the upper layer of skin—the epithelium—on your nose. This skin thickens greatly, causing your nose to appear large and bulbous. Why rhinophyma occurs is not clearly understood. Rhinophyma is not a threat to breathing or to your general health.

An exaggeratedly large and distended nose once was thought to result from heavy drinking. Now we know that alcohol consumption has nothing to do with it. People who drink moderately and those who abstain completely can have rhinophyma.

Diagnosis

If the skin of your nose gradually becomes excessively thick, causing your nose to take on a large, bulbous shape, rhinophyma is probably the cause.

Treatment

The only effective treatment for rhinophyma is surgery. In this procedure, the surgeon slices excess tissue off the outside of your nose, under general or local anesthesia in a hospital setting. As it heals, your nose usually resumes its normal shape.

Loss of Sense of Smell

Signs and Symptoms
- Decreased ability to detect odors
- Difficulty breathing through your nose

While suffering from a head cold, most people temporarily lose their sense of smell. When it is lost without any apparent cause, however, the condition is known technically as anosmia. The latter condition occurs when an obstruction in your nose prevents odors from reaching delicate nerve fibers in your nose that lead to the olfactory area (the area of your brain dealing with smell), when the nerves in your olfactory area are damaged, when your olfactory nerves and fibers

---

A Simple Remedy for a Runny Nose

While in the throes of a cold, who doesn't yearn for a foolproof method to cure a congested nose? Dozens of ads tout products that promise magical cures, but such products rarely match up to their billings. Even when they do relieve the congestion in your nose, they may produce unpleasant side effects such as drowsiness or dry mouth.

Sometimes your nose becomes too dry, making it hurt more than a runny nose. When the remedy contains an antihistamine, the mucus in your head may thicken, becoming a better trap for virus particles that can move along to your ear or throat. When you have a cold, you need to keep the mucus as liquid as possible. This is one reason it is important to drink lots of fluids.

One of the best temporary remedies for a stuffy nose does not cause complications or cost money. Breathing steam can loosen the mucus and clear your head. To set up a steam source, bring a kettle or pan of water to a boil and inhale the steam for several minutes, taking care not to get so close that it scalds you. Some people like to make a tent of a towel over their heads while inhaling the steam. This method is useful for loosening the mucus in your chest, too. Similarly, people often report feeling their heads clear when they take a steaming shower.

are destroyed, or when the area of your brain dealing with smell is damaged.

Nasal polyps, tumors, or swelling of the mucous membrane most often cause obstructions. Viral infections (a major cause of anosmia in older adults) and chronic nose infections or allergies commonly cause damage to the nerves of the olfactory area (see page 569). Damage to your olfactory nerves and fibers also can be due to a head injury, nasal surgery, or tumor.

Most people with anosmia can distinguish salty, sweet, sour, and bitter tastes (which are sensed on the tongue), but they cannot distinguish more subtle flavors (sensations provided by taste and smell).

Diagnosis

If you lose your sense of smell and you do not have a cold, consult your physician. Nasal polyps (see page 1041) and chronic nasal allergy are the most common causes of anosmia. Your physician will check for tumors of the nasal passages.

Most often, anosmia is an inconvenience. Occasionally, it can be a symptom of a more serious condition. Rarely, people experience brief episodes during which they smell odd or foul odors. In such cases, upon finding no relevant nasal condition, your physician may refer you to a neurologist for an examination and diagnostic tests to discover if the problem is in your brain.

You may need to have a CT or MRI scan (see page 1334) to check for a brain tumor or signs of a head injury. Trauma can damage your olfactory nerves—the nerves that carry smell sensations from your nose to your brain. If you lose your sense of smell after a concussion or other head injury, the blow may be the cause of your anosmia.

Treatment

If the cause is a nasal condition such as allergic rhinitis (hay fever) or nasal polyps, it can be treated easily, and your sense of smell is restored. Physicians usually treat allergic rhinitis with antihistamines. Your physician can remove nasal polyps and tumors surgically.

When the cause is not readily apparent, as is often the case when a virus is involved, your sense of smell may return when the tissues of your olfactory area regenerate on their own.

Sinusitis

Signs and Symptoms
- Pain about your eyes or cheeks
- Fever
- Difficulty breathing through your nose
- Toothache (uncommon)

Your sinuses are cavities in the bone around your nose. There are four pairs of sinuses: the frontal (in your forehead), ethmoid (between your eyes), sphenoid (deeper in your head, behind your eyes), and maxillary (in your cheekbones). They are connected to your nasal cavities by small openings. Normally, air passes in and out of your sinuses and mucus drains through these openings into your nose.

Sinusitis is an infection of the lining of one or more of these cavities. Usually, when your sinus is infected, the membranes of your nose itself also swell and cause a nasal obstruction. Swelling of the membranes of your nose may close off the opening of your sinus and thus prevent drainage of pus or mucus. Pain in your sinus may result from inflammation itself or from the pressure within your sinus that results from closure of the opening.

The infection can be bacterial, viral, or fungal. A common cold is the most frequent precipitating factor in sinusitis. Because the mucous membranes of your nose extend into and line your sinuses, a bacterial infection in your nose easily spreads into your sinuses.

Secondary infections from colds are the

Postnasal Drip

Mucus produced in your nose and sinuses travels in a thin film to the back of your throat. It serves to protect your lungs by trapping dust and other particles that you inhale. Generally, you are unaware of this process and swallow the mucus and the impurities it captures. Swallowing this mucus does no harm. It does not need to be spit out.

Normally, your nose and sinuses produce a cupful or more of mucus daily. However, when smoke or other irritants aggravate your nose, the amount of mucus will increase. This extra mucus, secreted to remove more irritants, is often the cause of the discomfort commonly referred to as postnasal drip.

In a sense, mucus is nature's ointment, because it helps soothe an irritated nose. You may become more conscious of it when the air is dry because then the mucus in your nose and throat may become thicker and more difficult to expel.

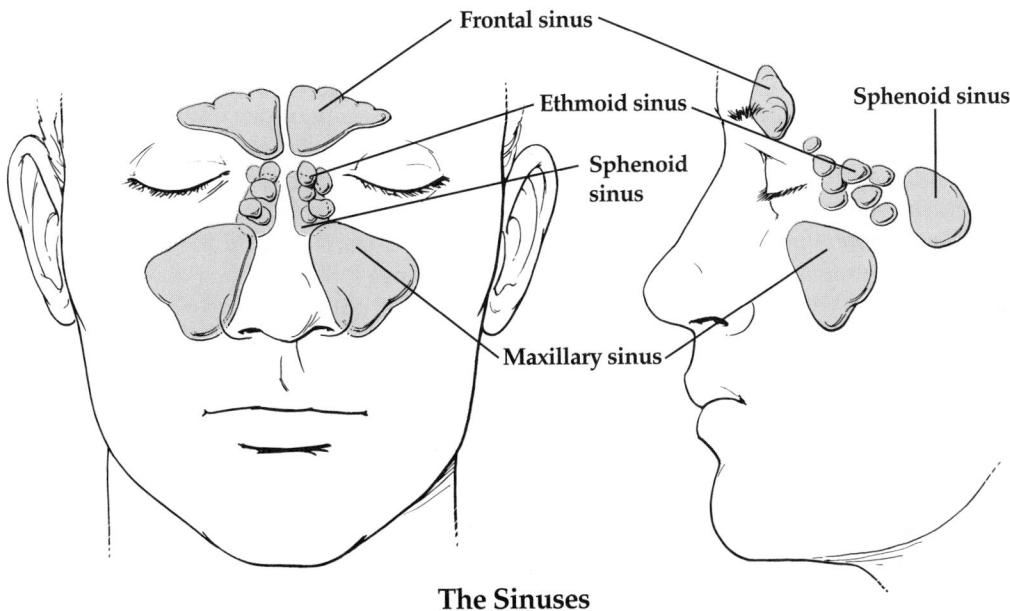

The Sinuses

most common causes but not the only ones. Chronic allergic rhinitis (hay fever) can cause sinusitis because infections can easily form in the mucus present in your nose and spread to your sinuses (see page 1040). A severely deviated septum can lead to sinusitis by obstructing your sinus openings. A dental abscess can extend from the root of an upper tooth to infect your sinuses (see page 607).

There are two forms of sinusitis, acute and chronic. Acute sinusitis is more common by far and usually is a bacterial infection. Examples include an infection after a cold, a dental abscess, and a deviated septum.

Chronic sinusitis is most often the result of repeated or untreated acute infections. The opening of your sinus becomes narrowed or closed due to scarring from previous infections, making it difficult for your sinus to drain.

Some people never get sinusitis. Others seem to get it every time they have a cold. In some, it develops as a result of jumping into water so that their noses and sinuses are suddenly flooded. The irritation and contamination result in sinusitis.

Diagnosis

If you experience symptoms of sinusitis, see your physician. If you have repeated or chronic sinusitis, your physician may recommend X-rays or a CT scan (see page 1334) to discover how serious your infection is. Your physician may take a sample of the mucus or pus, if present, for laboratory analysis.

How Serious Is Sinusitis?

Before the advent of antibiotics, sinus infections commonly spread into the bones of the face and occasionally into the brain. Today, sinusitis is unpleasant, but it rarely is a threat to general health. If left untreated, however, sinusitis can become chronic, making it more difficult to treat.

Treatment

There are a few things you can do yourself to lessen the symptoms. Stay indoors in an even temperature. Refrain from bending over with your head down—this movement usually increases the pain. Try applying warm facial packs or inhale steam from a kettle or basin of boiling water. (Be careful not to scald yourself.) Drink plenty of liquids to help dilute the secretions.

Medication

If your infection is bacterial, your physician will prescribe a course of oral antibiotic therapy lasting 10 to 14 days. You may take over-the-counter decongestants in the form of drops, sprays, or tablets to open the passages and encourage drainage of your sinuses. However, take care when using decongestants. They can do more harm than good by drying out your nose too much. Use them only on recommendation of your physician, and follow instructions carefully.

Surgery

Occasionally, sinusitis will persist despite

medical treatment. If this happens, an experienced surgeon may perform a new surgical procedure called endoscopic sinus surgery. It offers relief with no external incisions or scarring, the option of local anesthesia, and minimal pain and swelling. The procedure gets its name from the instruments that ear, nose, and throat specialists use for the operation. Endoscopes are pencil-thin instruments of various sizes. They are equipped with viewing devices and used with tiny cutting tools. This surgery clears a tiny, yet critical, nasal passage that, when blocked, causes recurrent sinus infections. Yet this procedure often requires no hospital stay, and you can sometimes return to work the next day.

Endoscopic surgery leaves your sinuses basically undisturbed and restores natural drainage. In a pre-surgery evaluation, your physician takes 5 to 10 minutes to view the interior of your nose with an endoscope, using a local anesthetic. Your physician may also request a CT scan (see page 1334) of your sinuses to refer to during surgery. After you're sedated and given a local anesthetic, your physician inserts an endoscope and delicate cutting tools into your nostrils and blocked sinuses. From the image projected on a monitor by the endoscope, your physician removes infected sinus membranes, polyps, and small bone fragments that block your sinuses, enlarges the sinus opening, and inserts a small vacuum to drain trapped fluids. The procedure takes 30 to 90 minutes. As a rule, you have no headaches, numbness, or swelling from the operation, although you may need antibiotics and pain medication. During the first 2 weeks, it's normal to have some discomfort and bleeding from your nose. You'll also have to make weekly visits to your physician for about 3 weeks to have dried blood and secretions removed. Occasionally, sinus blockage redevelops, and surgery must be repeated. Complications, although rare, can be serious, so choose an experienced surgeon.

If endoscopic surgery is not available or cannot be performed, conventional surgery using local anesthesia may be considered. The surgeon makes a small opening in the bone between the nose and infected sinus, and then the sinuses are flushed out with sterile water.

Disorders of the Throat

Your throat is in constant use, carrying food to your digestive tract and air to your lungs and making it possible for you to speak. With this heavy workload, it is subject to occasional problems.

Like other parts of your respiratory system, it is susceptible to infection, both bacterial and viral. Such infections occasionally are limited to your throat, as in the case of laryngitis. More commonly, they affect your entire system, as in pharyngitis or tonsillitis.

Your throat also is susceptible to abuse, ranging from heavy alcohol consumption or smoking to improper use of your voice while singing or speaking. These can cause a range of problems from chronic laryngitis to growths on your vocal cords.

Pharyngitis

Signs and Symptoms
- Sore throat
- Difficulty swallowing
- Fever

Your pharynx is the segment between your tonsils and your voice box—what you commonly think of as your throat. Thus, pharyngitis is another name for a sore throat, an inflammation that can be either acute or chronic.

A bacterium (often, beta-streptococcus) or a virus causes acute pharyngitis. If caused by the beta-streptococcus bacterium, the infection is commonly called strep throat.

The chronic form can be caused by a continuing infection of your sinuses, lungs, or mouth that spreads to your pharynx.

Constant irritation such as from smoking, breathing heavily polluted air, or consuming too much alcohol can also cause chronic pharyngitis.

Diagnosis

Your throat will be red and raw, making it difficult to swallow and sometimes even to breathe. Pus may be present. You may feel feverish.

If your sore throat lasts more than a few days, consult your physician. Your physician will examine your throat and will use a swab to take a specimen for laboratory analysis (culture) to determine if the infection is bacterial. Your physician will also look for signs of other illness such as nasal or respiratory infection.

Treatment

Most often, treatment is unnecessary. However, if you have a bacterial infection, your physician will prescribe a course of antibiotic therapy. If the infection is viral, antibiotics will not help.

Lump in Your Throat

Sometimes you have the sensation of a lump in your throat that feels like a little ball. It is present even if you aren't swallowing. Efforts such as clearing your throat and drinking water or swallowing hard won't get rid of it. The medical term for this common condition is globus sensation or globus syndrome.

Originally named globus hystericus, this condition shows the relationship between your emotional system and your throat. When you feel anxious, depressed, or stressed, the small muscular opening (pharynx) in the lower part of your throat begins to grow tense. That tension in your throat tells your brain that something is there, even when nothing is actually there.

If the condition persists, your physician may have you see an ear, nose, and throat specialist to examine your throat and larynx. The specialist will use a mirror to look for any other cause of this sensation.

This condition generally resolves on its own or occasionally with efforts directed at relieving stress or anxiety.

Get plenty of rest. You can relieve the pain of pharyngitis with aspirin or an aspirin substitute and by gargling with warm salt water (½ teaspoon of salt in a glass of warm water) several times a day. Throat lozenges can

---

Tonsillectomy and Adenoidectomy

Your tonsils and adenoids are lymph node tissues in your throat. (For a discussion of the lymph system, see page 968.) Your tonsils are located at the back of your mouth. Your adenoids are in the top of your throat.

Both the tonsils and adenoids act to filter infections from your body. Tonsils and adenoids are particularly useful in infants and children up to about 3 years old.

As you grow through childhood, the glands shrink. By puberty, your adenoids have almost disappeared and your tonsils have shrunk to the size of almonds.

Often, children older than 3 (and occasionally adults) come down with tonsillitis, a bacterial infection. Occasionally, the adenoids swell, too, giving the child's voice a nasal quality. When the glands become infected frequently (three or more times a year) and severely, your physician may recommend tonsillectomy and perhaps an adenoidectomy.

In the past, practically every child had his or her tonsils removed (often the adenoids as well) whether or not they became infected frequently. Now, the use of antibiotics makes the treatment of tonsillitis much easier. Most often, surgery is unnecessary.

However, in some cases the tonsils become so enlarged that they affect breathing and swallowing. In addition, the back of your nose and your eustachian tube may be blocked by enlarged and inflamed adenoids, thus causing middle ear infection (see page 574) as well as nasal obstruction.

Tonsillectomy and adenoidectomy are surgical procedures in which your tonsils and adenoids are removed. Tonsils do not grow back, but adenoids can, although they rarely cause a second problem.

After the procedure, your child usually is observed for several hours and then sent home. He or she will experience a very sore throat that will last for several days after the operation.

Tonsillectomy and adenoidectomy do not guarantee freedom from throat infections. The same organisms that cause tonsillitis, usually streptococci, can infect your throat. However, the frequency of throat infections usually is lessened after removal of these glands.

provide relief as well. You may want to switch to a soft or liquid diet to avoid irritating your throat.

Tonsillitis

Signs and Symptoms
- Sore throat
- Headache
- Fever and chills
- Sore glands of your jaw and throat

Tonsils are similar to lymph nodes. They are located at the back of your mouth, one on either side. Among other functions, they filter out harmful microorganisms that could infect your body.

Occasionally, when the tonsils become overwhelmed by a bacterial infection, they swell and become inflamed. This infection is known as tonsillitis. It is common, particularly among children.

Diagnosis
Symptoms of tonsillitis are similar to those of the flu. The primary symptom is a sore throat that makes it difficult to swallow. Others are headache, fever, and chills.

Your tonsils become visibly red and swollen. You may also notice specks of white discharge on your infected tonsils. The lymph nodes in the area, such as those under your jaw and in your neck, may be enlarged and tender.

If the symptoms last more than 48 hours or you or your child has a history of tonsillitis, see your physician. He or she will examine your throat and take a culture to determine if the infection is caused by the beta-streptococcus bacterium (strep throat).

These days, tonsillitis is primarily an uncomfortable nuisance. Do not leave it untreated, however, because it can lead to formation of an abscess in or around your tonsils.

Treatment
Get plenty of rest. Also drink soothing fluids. Gargling with warm salt water several times a day often helps lessen the pain. Aspirin, or an aspirin substitute such as acetaminophen for children, may be helpful.

Medication
If a bacterial infection is the cause of your sore throat, your physician will prescribe a course of oral antibiotic therapy (usually for 10 days). The symptoms should disappear within a few days after you take the first tablets.

Certain strains of streptococci that can cause tonsillitis and pharyngitis (see page 592) can also cause nephritis (see page 836) or rheumatic fever (see page 677). This is an important reason for completing your course of antibiotic medication as prescribed and not just stopping when your pain is relieved.

Epiglottitis

Signs and Symptoms
- Sore throat
- Fever
- Difficulty swallowing
- Hoarseness

Emergency Symptoms—Difficulty with breathing

Epiglottitis is an inflammation of the lid-like cartilage that covers your windpipe. The condition is most common among children between the ages of 2 and 5, although adults can get it too. It is more common among males than females and among whites than other races.

Epiglottitis usually is the result of a bacterial infection. Certain conditions, such as Hodgkin's disease, leukemia, and immunosuppressive diseases, can predispose adults to epiglottitis.

Diagnosis
The symptoms of epiglottitis can be similar to those of pharyngitis (see page 592) and tonsillitis (see this page) in that you or your child will have a sore throat and swallowing will be painful. Children often are feverish and hoarse.

If the sore throat lasts more than a few days, see your physician. Your physician will examine your throat and take a specimen for culture. If the result of the culture is positive for bacterial infection, your physician will prescribe an appropriate course of antibiotics. Also, your physician may want to take an X-ray of your throat.

This infection can begin swiftly, reaching an acute stage in hours. When your epiglottis swells, it can obstruct your windpipe, making it difficult to breathe.

It is common for the person who has epiglottitis to sit leaning forward, neck outstretched, to make breathing easier. If you or your child has difficulty breathing, call an ambulance or seek emergency treatment.

Treatment
Most cases of epiglottitis are treated with antibiotics to destroy the bacterial organism that causes the inflammation. Severe difficulty in breathing is treated as an emergency, requiring insertion of a tube into your trachea for breathing (tracheostomy).

Peritonsillar Abscess

Signs and Symptoms
- Sore throat and sore soft palate
- Severe pain on swallowing
- Fever
- Tendency to hold your head to one side, away from the pain

Peritonsillar abscess, also known as quinsy, is associated with tonsillitis. One of your tonsils becomes infected, and an abscess (a collection of pus) forms between this tonsil and the soft tissues around it.

The infection may spread over your soft palate (the soft area at the back of the roof of your mouth) before the abscess forms, making it possible for the abscess to cover a large area. The infection can spread to your neck and even down into your chest. Peritonsillar abscess is most common in young adults.

Diagnosis
If your throat becomes sore and the discomfort spreads to the soft tissues at the back of the roof of your mouth (soft palate), you may have a peritonsillar abscess. Your physician will examine your tonsil and palate, looking for an inflamed tonsil that has been displaced by swelling of the soft area of your palate.

How Serious Is a Peritonsillar Abscess?
If not treated properly, peritonsillar abscess can be serious: the infection can move to your neck and eventually into your chest, where it can infect the membrane covering your heart or the tissue between your lungs. Occasionally, the swelling can be so severe that the roof of your mouth is pushed against your tongue, blocking air flow and making swallowing very difficult.

Treatment
Your physician will treat the infection with antibiotics. If pus is present and does not drain quickly as a result of the antibiotics, your physician may drain the abscess surgically.

Because abscesses can recur, your physician may recommend a tonsillectomy. Your physician usually will perform the tonsillectomy soon after the antibiotic treatment is started or about 6 weeks after your acute infection has healed.

Laryngitis

Signs and Symptoms
- Hoarseness
- Tickling and rawness of your throat
- Constant need to clear your throat

Laryngitis is an infection or irritation of your larynx (voice box), which is located at the top of your trachea (windpipe). When the vocal cords of your larynx become inflamed or irritated, they swell, and this distorts sounds produced by the air passing over them. Your voice then sounds hoarse. In some cases, your voice can become so soft as to be undetectable.

There are two forms of laryngitis: acute and chronic. The symptoms and treatment are often the same for both forms.

Usually, a virus causes acute laryngitis, but it also can be the result of a bacterial infection. When caused by a virus, acute laryngitis usually disappears without treatment.

Structures of Your Larynx

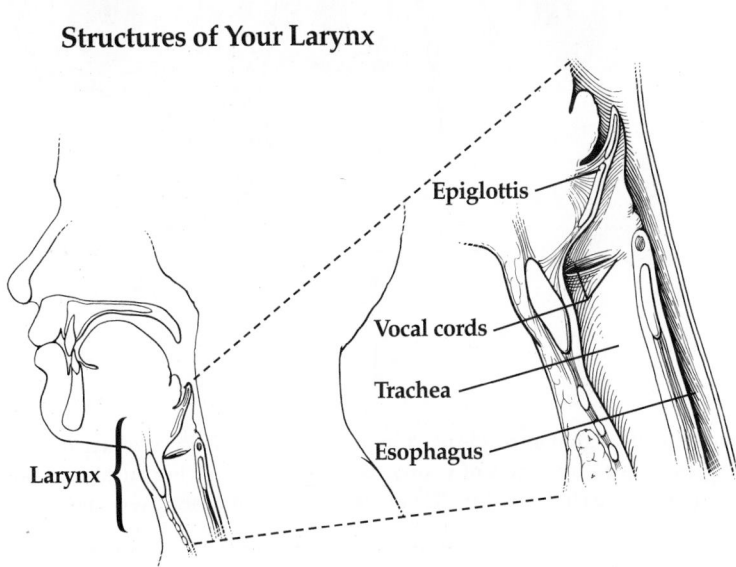

Epiglottis

Vocal cords

Trachea

Esophagus

Larynx

Vocal Cord Problems

The production of sounds by your larynx is called phonation. Within your larynx are two vocal cords that produce sound (phonate) by vibrating. The muscles of your larynx control the length and tension of the cords, which transmit their vibrations to the column of air that passes through your larynx. Your vocal cords also help to prevent food and water from entering your lungs during swallowing.

Your vocal cords are one vital element in the act of speaking or singing. They are susceptible to problems, including those caused by misuse or abuse. Such problems range from polyps to nodules to ulcers.

Polyps

Polyps are small swellings in the mucous membranes covering your vocal cords. As they grow, they take on a rounded shape. They may run the full length of your vocal cords or be localized.

A polyp can develop on your vocal cords as a result of abusing your voice through prolonged or repeated screaming, shouting, or speaking in a very low, unnatural tone. A polyp can also develop as a chronic allergic reaction or as a result of breathing irritants such as cigarette smoke or industrial fumes.

Polyps can make your voice become breathy-sounding and harsh. Sometimes your physician will remove them during the course of a special examination called laryngoscopy. Your physician may perform a biopsy of the polyp to be certain that there is no cancer. Frequently, your physician will recommend voice therapy after removal of a polyp to correct the underlying cause.

Singer's Nodule

People who use their voices a great deal, such as professional singers, teachers, auctioneers, and members of the clergy, are prone to have nodules on their vocal cords. Like polyps, nodules develop as a result of excessive use of your voice.

If you have such nodules, your voice will become breathy and hoarse. A nodule differs from a polyp in that it is a growth of the epithelium that covers the mucous membrane, not of the mucous membrane itself. Thus, it has a structural resemblance to a corn on a toe or a callus on your hand.

Resting your vocal cords by allowing little or no speaking for several weeks may permit the nodules to shrink. Sometimes biopsy and surgical removal are necessary. Voice therapy is essential in eliminating your vocal abuse and habits that are responsible for nodule formation. Children occasionally have screamer's voice nodules. These usually are treated with voice therapy alone.

Contact Ulcers

Your vocal cords also are subject to development of sores called contact ulcers. This ailment often results from improper use of your voice. Damage to your vocal cords (for example, due to the frequent regurgitation of gastric juices or after intubation for general anesthesia) is another common cause.

Contact ulcers appear where the two pieces of cartilage that hold your vocal cords in place touch each other. Symptoms include mild pain when swallowing or speaking and hoarseness.

Your physician will ask a series of questions to determine how you use your throat and what your eat-

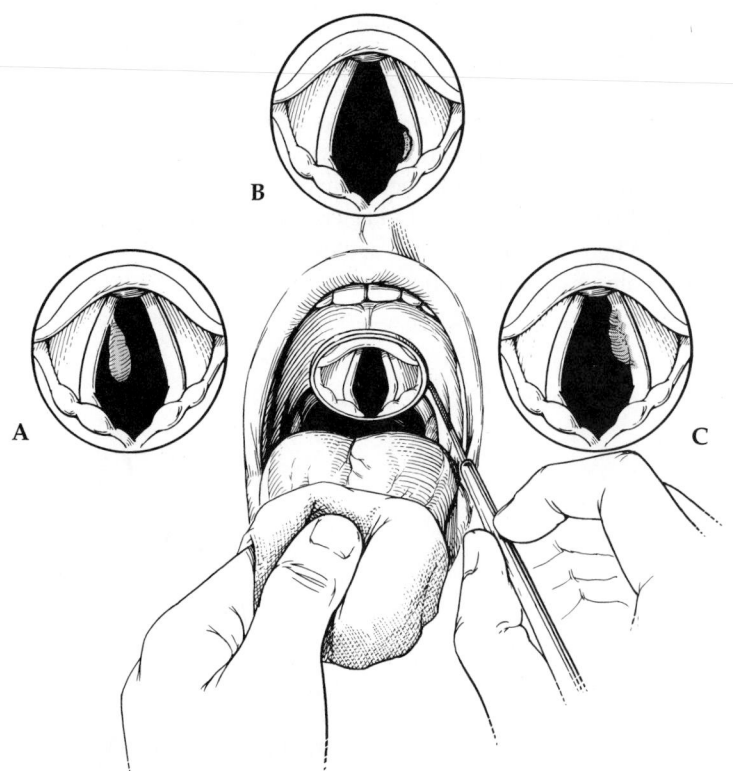

A small, angled mirror is used in performing indirect laryngoscopy, which provides a direct view of your vocal cords. (A) depicts a vocal cord polyp. (B) shows a contact ulcer. (C) reveals vocal cord cancer (see page 599).

ing patterns are. He or she may take a sample of the ulcerated tissue for laboratory testing to be certain there is no cancer present.

The primary treatment for contact ulcers is rest of your voice—often for 6 weeks or more—to allow the sores to heal. Retraining of your voice may be necessary to prevent the ulcers from recurring.

If gastric juices are the cause of your ulcers, there are several techniques for avoiding recurrence. Your physician may recommend an antacid, eating no more than 2 to 4 hours before retiring, and having the head of your bed raised on 4- to 6-inch blocks (see Esophageal Reflux, page 742).

Leukoplakia

Leukoplakia, literally white (*leuko*) patches (*plakia*) in Latin, can appear on one or both vocal cords. They can be associated with cancer. Your physician will remove them for laboratory study as soon as they are discovered. Leukoplakia (see page 618) is often the result of smoking.

Juvenile Papillomas

Many children have warts, benign growths believed to be caused by viruses. A few children, primarily boys, develop them on their vocal cords (juvenile papillomas).

They are not malignant, and they usually disappear at puberty.

In the meantime, however, these warts can be troublesome. They can grow in clusters, making them difficult to remove without damaging the larynx.

On rare occasions, juvenile papillomas can grow very fast and in large quantities, thus obstructing breathing. When this happens, they must be treated quickly to keep the air supply from being cut off entirely.

Laser treatment has become the preferred procedure. It is more effective and less harmful than excision with a blade.

Juvenile papillomas frequently recur, making repeat treatments necessary.

Laryngitis can occur in the course of another illness such as an ordinary cold, bronchitis, flu, or pneumonia. Irritations such as excessive talking or singing, allergic states, and breathing of irritating substances such as certain chemicals also can cause hoarseness and loss of your voice.

Constant irritation such as excessive drinking of alcohol or heavy smoking or reflux of stomach acid into the esophagus and laryngeal area most often causes chronic laryngitis (see Esophageal Reflux, page 742).

Diagnosis

The primary symptom of laryngitis is hoarseness. Changes in voice can vary with the degree of infection or irritation, ranging from mild hoarseness to almost total loss of voice, so that your vocalization becomes little more than the sound of a soft whisper. Your throat may tickle or feel raw, and you may have a frequent urge to clear your throat.

Simple viral laryngitis usually clears up within a few days. If your laryngitis persists for more than 2 to 3 days or you have other symptoms, see your physician.

How Serious Is Laryngitis?

For most people, laryngitis is a temporary problem that either resolves itself or can be

Proper Use of Your Voice

Here are a few practical recommendations that may help you avoid vocal cord problems:

- Excessively loud or raucous talking, yelling, screaming, or singing at a pitch that is too high for you can cause contact ulcers and vocal cord nodules. Lowering the pitch and speaking in a more normal range will lessen the strain on your voice.
- Also, a prolonged, hacking cough or persistent throat tickle that requires frequent vigorous throat clearing can damage your vocal cords. Treat these conditions promptly.
- Some men and boys try to lower the pitch of their voices to sound more masculine. When you speak for any length of time in this manner, your throat quickly becomes tired, causing pain and even contact ulcers.
- A less obvious recommendation regarding the use of your voice has to do with overall health and well-being. Everyone experiences the effects of physical fatigue and emotional stress at one time or another. When emotional stress or fatigue occurs, the muscles of your larynx and neck may become tense. Occasionally, such stress may cause vocal cord problems including hoarseness, breathiness, or even loss of voice. Thus, your voice can be a clue to your emotional health. Examine your life. If necessary, make changes to reduce unnecessary stress. It can contribute to the way you live—and sound.

Speech After Laryngectomy

Anyone who has had a laryngectomy must learn to speak again without a larynx. Not having a voice does not mean you must remain speechless, but your new speech will not sound the same as your voice did before.

Artificial Voice Aids

Using an artificial larynx is one method of vocal communication after laryngectomy. These devices produce sound that can be transmitted to the vocal tract. They are often used soon after surgery and in conjunction with learning esophageal speech or when using a voice prosthesis after tracheoesophageal puncture (TEP). Some people choose to use an artificial larynx as their only method of vocal communication.

The two main kinds of artificial larynxes are neck type and intraoral. Neck-type devices are handheld, battery-driven, electronic, vibrating machines. You hold the head of the device against your neck. The vibrations penetrate neck tissues and resonate in your throat and mouth, where you can convert them into speech by using your tongue, teeth, lips, and palate.

Intra-oral devices deliver sound directly into your mouth. A tone generator delivers sound into your mouth through a flexible tube. You can manipulate the sound with your tongue, lips, teeth, and palate to produce speech. Some intra-oral devices are battery operated and others are not. The latter use lung air to vibrate a reed or plastic disk that produces "voice" that is directed into your mouth and articulated into speech. Battery-operated neck-type devices can often be adapted for intra-oral use.

Esophageal Speech

Some people learn to speak again by a technique called esophageal speech. You swallow, or pump your tongue, to force air into your esophagus, then immediately expel the air. The walls of your esophagus vibrate, making a low-pitched sound similar to a belch. You can form this esophageal sound into words by using your tongue, teeth, lips, and palate. With training by a speech pathologist and much practice, some people become excellent speakers.

Tracheoesophageal Puncture (TEP) and Voice Prosthesis

Another method of vocal communication after laryngectomy is with a voice prosthesis. This essentially provides a bridge between the trachea and the esophagus. Your surgeon makes a small opening (stoma) in the rear wall of your trachea and the front wall of your esophagus and places a small silicone tube, called a voice prosthesis, in the opening.

You produce voice by exhaling and placing your thumb or finger over your tracheostoma. Air moves from your lungs, through the voice prosthesis, into your esophagus, which vibrates to produce voice. A valve sometimes can be placed over the stoma. This allows you to speak without using a thumb or finger. Not all people with laryngectomies are candidates for tracheoesophageal puncture and a voice prosthesis.

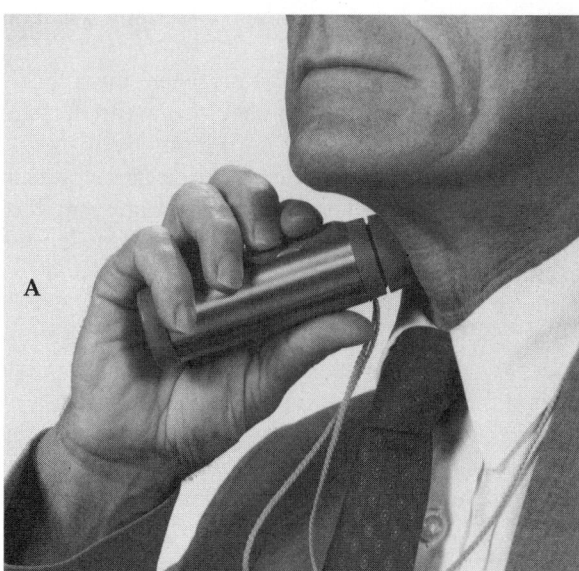 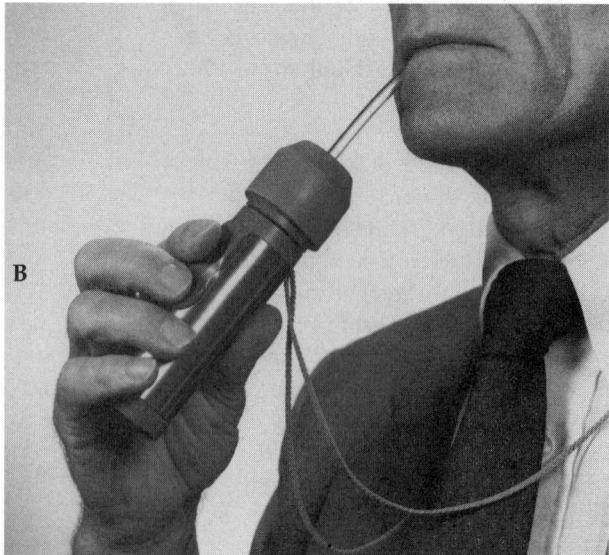

The two main types of artificial voice aids are the neck type (A) and the intra-oral device (B).

treated with antibiotics. When the hoarseness is due to alcoholism, chronic bronchitis, or workplace exposure, you need to correct the underlying problem.

Treatment

Medication

Your physician will determine whether your laryngitis is bacterial or viral by taking a throat specimen for laboratory analysis. If the cause is bacterial, your physician may prescribe a course of antibiotics. The symptoms should disappear shortly after you take the first tablets.

Laryngitis caused by a virus or inhaled irritant substance cannot be treated with antibiotics. The best treatment is to rest your voice as much as is practical, inhale steam (from a bowl of hot water or a teakettle), and drink warm, soothing liquids. This program of rest, steam, and liquids is useful for treating all forms of laryngitis.

For the problem to be solved, you must treat the underlying cause of chronic laryngitis. If you smoke, stop. If chronic bronchitis is the underlying cause (see page 714), antibiotic treatment should resolve the problem. If alcoholism is the cause, that must be treated. Treat allergy with antihistamines. For advice concerning treatment of esophageal reflux, see page 742.

Cancers of the Throat

Signs and Symptoms
- Hoarseness
- Pain or difficulty swallowing
- Swelling in your neck

Almost everyone experiences occasional hoarseness. It may be only one symptom of a cold or tonsillitis. If you have laryngitis, hoarseness may be your only symptom. Whether you have a cold or laryngitis, your voice usually returns to normal within a few days.

Hoarseness is also the key symptom of most other vocal problems and the only early symptom of vocal cord cancer. Most throat cancers occur as tumors on the vocal cords or in or around the larynx. Difficulty and pain on swallowing are signs of other forms of throat cancer, as is a large swelling in your neck.

If you smoke cigarettes, cigars, or a pipe, you are at greater risk of developing throat cancer than people who do not. If you drink large quantities of alcohol, you are at greater risk as well. The combination of drinking and smoking is particularly conducive to the development of cancer of your larynx. Throat cancers usually develop at around age 60, and men are 10 times more likely to develop them than women.

When hoarseness is your only symptom, and it has no obvious cause and lasts more than 2 weeks, consult your physician without further delay. If swallowing is difficult or painful for several weeks or if you notice a swelling in your neck, see your physician.

Diagnosis
Your physician will examine your throat and conduct an examination called a laryngoscopy. There are two kinds of laryngoscopies: indirect and direct.

Indirect laryngoscopy is a method of looking at your throat by using a mirror. This simple procedure usually can be done in your physician's office. You will be asked to open your mouth and breathe through it. Your tongue will be pulled forward gently to help open your airway. A local anesthetic may be sprayed on the back of your throat and soft palate, particularly if you have a strong gag reflex. Your physician will then place the mirror toward the back of your throat. As you say "ah" and "eee," your larynx will rise and your physician can view its interior in the mirror. The presence of tumors or other abnormalities will become visible in the mirror. Your physician may also use small, flexible fiberoptic instruments to view your voice box area.

Direct laryngoscopy is a more elaborate procedure that allows a more complete inspection of your larynx. A throat specialist usually performs the procedure in a hospital, because it requires local or general anesthesia. During a direct laryngoscopy, the physician inserts an instrument into your throat and often removes a tissue sample from a vocal cord for laboratory analysis.

How Serious Are Throat Cancers?
Most cancers of your throat are curable if detected early. Do not ignore them, because they can spread to other parts of your throat and, ultimately, to other parts of your body.

Treatment

Physicians treat tumors of your throat in one of several ways. Frequently, radiation therapy or a surgical procedure limited to only part of a vocal cord or the larynx can often cure cancers that are detected early. Usually, your physician can remove the tumor without removal of your larynx, but more advanced tumors may require complete removal of your larynx, a procedure known as a laryngectomy.

If you need a laryngectomy, surgical placement of a prosthesis can restore your voice (see Speech After Laryngectomy, page 598), or you can work with a speech therapist to learn a new method of speaking.

Chapter 22

Dental and Oral Disorders

Contents

Your Healthy Teeth, 602
Tooth Development, 602
The Parts of the Tooth, 602
Your Checkup, 603
Dentists and Their Specialties, 604

Tooth Decay, 605
How Tooth Decay Develops, 605
Treatments for Tooth Decay, 606
Tooth Abscess, 607
Prevention of Tooth Decay, 608

Periodontal Disease, 609
Gingivitis, 610
Periodontitis, 611
Trench Mouth, 612
Prevention of Periodontal Disease, 613

Developmental Disorders, 614
Impacted Teeth, 614
Misshapen or Discolored Teeth, 614
Treatment for Developmental
  Disorders, 615

**Infections and Diseases of the
Mouth, 617**
Canker Sores, 617

Gingivostomatitis, 618
Oral Thrush, 618
Leukoplakia, 618
Oral Lichen Planus, 619
Tongue Disorders, 619
  Bad Breath, 620
Oral Cancer, 621

Salivary Gland Problems, 622
Salivary Gland Infections, 622
Salivary Duct Stones, 623
Salivary Duct Tumors, 623

**Facial and Mandibular Trauma and
Fractures, 623**
Broken or Dislocated Jaw, 623
Loss of a Tooth (Avulsion), 624
Temporomandibular Joint Problems, 624

Prosthodontics, 626
Partial Dentures, 626
Dentures, 626
Denture Problems, 627
  Proper Care of Your Dentures, 627
  Osseointegration of Teeth, 628

Your Healthy Teeth

Few parts of your body play as many roles in everyday life as your mouth and teeth do. Many of the most important acts of self-expression—such as speaking, singing, and simply smiling—utilize the teeth to shape the sounds we make and help form our appearance. Crucial to health, the mouth and teeth are responsible for the first phase in the process of digesting food.

Our teeth may seem only minor health concerns, but tooth and oral disorders can disrupt almost every aspect of our lives.

Tooth Development

We are born toothless—or so it appears. In actuality, tooth development is well advanced by the third month of pregnancy, and by the fourth month there is evidence of enamel and dentin, the hard tissues of the primary or deciduous teeth (the baby teeth).

The first teeth appear in the mouth 6 to 7 months after the baby is born. The time these first teeth emerge varies greatly from child to child, but in most children the teeth have broken through the gums before the end of the first year.

In general, the first teeth to emerge are the incisors (the front teeth) in the lower jaw, followed by the front teeth in the upper jaw. Next come the canines, and last to appear are the molars. Most children have a full set of primary teeth by age 3.

There are only 20 primary teeth. Each primary tooth is normally replaced by one permanent tooth, incisor-for-incisor, canine-for-canine, and premolar-for-molar. The permanent first molars erupt behind the primary molars.

For many children, the emergence of permanent teeth begins at about age 5 to 6. The lower front incisors tend to come in first, followed by the upper front incisors and first molars. Permanent premolars and canines emerge later.

The process of shedding primary teeth to be replaced by permanent teeth usually lasts through the elementary school years. By age 14, 28 permanent teeth should be in place. The last four molars, the wisdom teeth, usually emerge in early adulthood, around age 20, to complete the permanent set of 32 teeth.

We have several kinds of teeth. From the center of the mouth toward the back on the top and bottom jaws, there are 8 incisors (4 in each jaw), 4 canines (cuspids), 8 premolars, and 12 molars.

The Adult Mouth

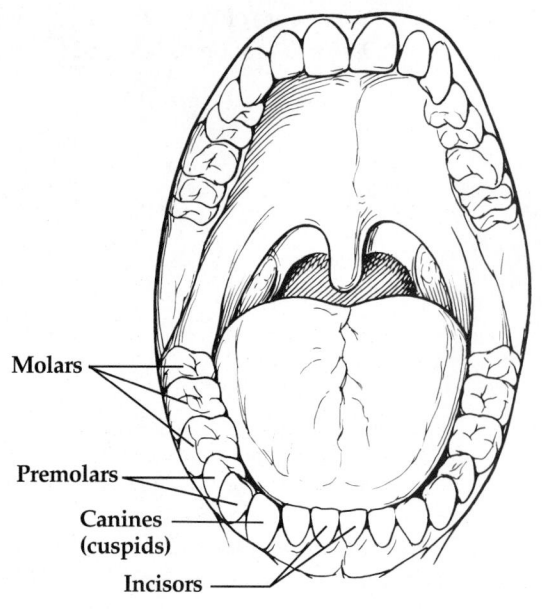

Molars

Premolars

Canines
(cuspids)

Incisors

The Parts of the Tooth

The basic structure of every tooth is essentially the same. The part of the tooth that is visible, the crown, is covered with enamel. The crown extends from just beneath the gum line to the top of the tooth. The hard enamel protects the structures of the tooth beneath. The enamel coating has no sensation and cannot heal after an injury.

Just beneath the crown lies the largest portion of the tooth, the dentin. The dentin is composed of millions of tiny cells arranged in tubules. It is a hard material (but not as hard as the enamel) and, unlike the outer layer, the dentin is sensitive to temperature and touch. Below the gum level, the dentin is covered by a layer called cementum. A connective tissue called the periodontal ligament connects the cementum to the bone that forms the socket.

Parts of the Tooth

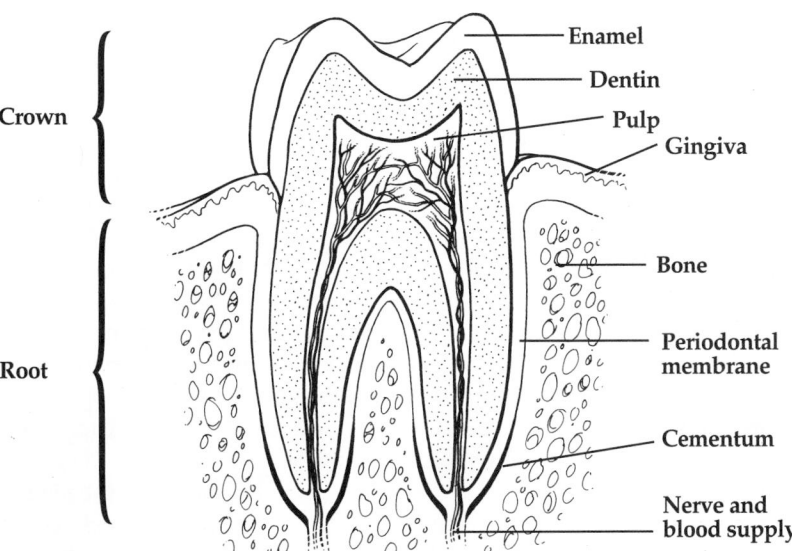

Crown

Root

Enamel
Dentin
Pulp
Gingiva
Bone
Periodontal membrane
Cementum
Nerve and blood supply

Inside the dentin, at the center of the tooth, lies the pulp chamber and the pulp. The pulp includes the blood vessels that feed the tooth and the nerves of the tooth. The nerves and blood vessels enter the teeth from the end of the roots.

This chapter describes disorders and diseases of the teeth and mouth. Many people experience some of these problems during the course of their lives; in fact, one of the most common human diseases is dental caries (tooth decay). Another very common disorder is periodontal disease, which contributes to the loss of teeth in adults.

Tooth decay and periodontal disease lead the list of oral disorders, but many others exist. These include other bacterial and fungal infections, oral cancers, salivary gland problems, problems of malformed and misaligned teeth, loss of teeth, and facial trauma.

Your Checkup

One of the important steps in preventing tooth decay (see Prevention of Tooth Decay, page 608) is to visit your dentist regularly for a thorough checkup.

How Often Should I See My Dentist?
You and your children (beginning at age 3, or earlier if symptoms appear) should visit the dentist usually twice a year. You may need to see your dentist more frequently if certain conditions or problems exist.

People who have several cavities per year and who pay little attention to oral hygiene at home may need to see their dentist more often, perhaps every 3 months, for treatment and cleaning. Adults older than 35 who are still getting cavities, take only moderate care of their teeth, and smoke and drink alcohol to excess also may need to visit the dentist frequently. Even people without natural teeth should see their dentist periodically.

Adults who have few cavities, take very good care of their teeth, and do not smoke or drink may need to visit their dentist only once a year. Your dentist will determine your examination schedule according to your specific needs.

Medical History
Before your dentist asks you to "Open wide, please," he or she probably will ask a few questions about your general health. The answers can have a direct bearing on your treatment.

For example, certain kinds of heart conditions make people susceptible to an infection of the heart valves when their gums are manipulated, such as in a thorough dental cleaning or when a tooth is filled or extracted. Therefore, these people usually take an antibiotic before dental treatment (see Infective

Endocarditis: Protection and Prevention, page 679). People who are allergic to penicillin can have a reaction when it is prescribed for tooth infections. Persons with diabetes whose disease is poorly controlled can become ill after the stress of dental treatment. People who have been ill with jaundice occasionally can carry the hepatitis virus without knowing it. Your dentist or dental assistant will probably also ask if you are on any medications, so that the dentist can avoid prescribing any that could cause harmful interactions.

Examination

Once the preliminary questions are over, your dentist will begin examining your mouth and teeth. Your gums and the soft tissues of your mouth will be examined first for signs of gingivitis (see page 610), periodontitis (see page 611), and less common disorders such as leukoplakia, oral lichen planus, or oral cancer (see pages 618, 619, and 621). If you have dentures, your gums will be examined for signs of pressure and uneven wear, indicated by patches of thickened skin, soreness, or reddened areas.

The next step is examination of each tooth by using a needle-shaped probe and a small mirror. Your dentist will be looking for signs of decay, including discolored areas and small fissures in the tooth enamel. Existing fillings will be checked for deterioration and for signs of new cavities around their edges. Your dentist will use a probe to check for periodontal disease around the base of your teeth.

Sometimes your dentist may suspect the presence of a cavity even when the enamel looks intact. He or she may then take X-rays of the area to check the teeth and surrounding tissue and bone. In addition, X-rays are often necessary if you have periodontal disease or have had the root canal of a dead tooth filled. X-rays can determine the status of wisdom teeth or, in younger people, of other unerupted permanent teeth. Your dentist will also check your soft tissues, tongue, and lips for lesions or other abnormalities.

Cleaning Process

Your dentist or dental hygienist also may clean your teeth (a process called dental prophylaxis). This is an essential step in maintaining the health of your teeth and gums. Plaque is a sticky substance that collects on teeth as a result of improper brushing or flossing. Calculus, often referred to as tartar, is plaque that has hardened and adheres tightly to the teeth.

Your dentist or dental hygienist can remove calculus in one of two ways. The traditional method involves scraping the deposits from your teeth with a sharp instrument known as a scaler. Some dentists also use an ultrasonic device that loosens the tartar through vibration. Whatever method is used, you may experience some bleeding of the gums. In some people, calculus develops quickly and must be removed every few months.

Once the calculus has been removed, the teeth are polished. Smooth teeth slow down the deposit of plaque. Polishing is done with a special toothpaste applied by a device with rotating rubber heads. With children, dentists often finish checkups with an application of fluoride to help prevent dental caries (see Tooth Care, page 363).

Dentists and Their Specialties

Just as there is no one type of physician who can handle all possible health problems, dentists also have specialties. General practitioner dentists may have special expertise in several areas, but for certain problems out of their training, you may elect to see or may be referred to a specialist. These include the following:

Periodontists, who diagnose and treat disease of the tissues supporting and surrounding the teeth (gums and bone)

Pediatric dentists, who specialize in treating children from birth through adolescence

Orthodontists, who diagnose and correct malpositions of the teeth and jaws

Endodontists, who diagnose and treat diseases and injuries of the tooth pulp and surrounding tissues

Oral and maxillofacial surgeons, who extract teeth and who diagnose and treat injuries, diseases, and defects of the jaw, face, and mouth

Prosthodontists, who create and fit artificial replacements for defective or missing teeth, including crowns, bridges (fixed partial dentures), and dentures

Tooth Decay

Tooth decay (caries) is a bacterial disease of the teeth. It is one of the most common of all human disorders. Dental caries affects children and young adults most frequently, although it remains a problem for many people throughout their lives.

Decay is the primary cause of tooth loss among people of all ages. Almost half of all American children have tooth decay by age 4, and many even earlier, despite great improvements in prevention through diet, the use of fluoride, and proper oral hygiene (see Tooth Care, page 363).

In the past, few people had their own teeth past middle age. Today, however, use of fluoride and better dental care, nutrition, and hygiene allow people to keep their teeth longer. This makes a relatively new problem, root caries, more common. Root caries is the decay of tooth roots and is an increasing problem among older people. A lifelong program of appropriate dental care, preventive nutrition, and good oral hygiene are keys to combating this form of dental caries.

How Tooth Decay Develops

Tooth decay is the result of three interacting factors: bacteria, dietary sugar, and vulnerable tooth surface.

Your mouth, like many other parts of your body, is host to bacteria. These bacteria convert some of the sugars and carbohydrates you eat into acid. The bacteria and the acids they form become part of the sticky deposit, called dental plaque, that clings to the surfaces of your teeth.

In addition to bacteria, plaque is composed of mucus and food particles. You can feel the plaque when you pass your tongue over the surface of your teeth several hours after brushing. The texture is slightly rough and is particularly noticeable on the surfaces of back teeth. Plaque adheres most strongly in pits and fissures of the molars and premolars, in the areas just above the gum line and between teeth, and at the margins of dental restorations (fillings).

The decay-producing acid that forms in plaque attacks the mineral in the tooth's outer enamel surface. The erosion caused by the plaque leads to the formation of tiny cavities (openings) in the enamel, which you probably will not notice at first. Indeed, the first sign of decay may be a sensation of pain when you eat something that is sweet, very cold, or very hot.

Once the enamel has been penetrated, the softer dentin beneath becomes vulnerable. The dentin contains tiny canals leading to the pulp at the core of the tooth. Inflammation results if bacteria reach the sensitive pulp. Blood vessels within the pulp swell and, because there is no room within the rigid tooth to expand, you experience pain. In addition, your body sends white blood cells to counteract bacterial invasion from the tooth into the surrounding tissues.

This kind of bacterial infection is known as a tooth abscess. Blood vessels around the tooth enlarge. The enlarged vessels press on nerves in the area, causing even more pain. Often, despite the body's efforts to fight it off, the infection overwhelms the pulp, and the nerve and blood vessels die. The toothache will cease, but the tooth will become vulnerable to the formation of an abscess later, sometimes years later.

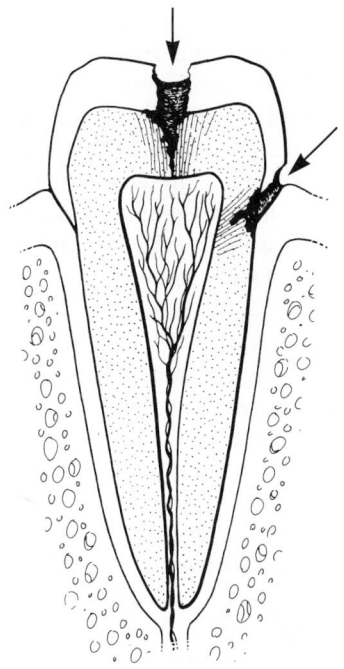

Dental cavities (caries) are common causes of tooth loss.

Tooth decay takes time to develop, often a year or two in permanent teeth but less in primary teeth. The initial formation of acid occurs within the first 20 minutes after you eat. Fortunately, you are not totally vulnerable to the effects of bacteria, acid, and the foods you eat. The chemistry and the mechanics of the mouth provide a certain amount of protection: your saliva and the actions of your tongue will wash away some of the destructive material. Today's dentistry also provides treatment and preventive measures to lessen the effects of dental caries (see Prevention of Tooth Decay, page 608).

Treatments for Tooth Decay

Most cavities are discovered during a dental examination because the early stages of decay usually are painless. Detecting and treating tooth decay early can save pain, expense, and, most importantly, your teeth.

The sooner a cavity is detected, the less painful the situation is likely to be because the outer parts of the tooth, the enamel and dentin, are far less sensitive to pain than is the pulp. One way of ascertaining whether you have a cavity is with dental X-rays. Your dentist will determine, on the basis of your dental history and the current condition of your teeth, whether and how many X-ray examinations are appropriate.

Even if you have a seriously decayed tooth, modern dentistry is equipped to deaden the discomfort of the treatment process and often can save the tooth through such procedures as dental fillings (restorations) or root canals (in which the diseased portion of a tooth is removed, leaving the unaffected portions of the root and tooth in place, covered with a crown).

Fillings

Most often, you have not noticed symptoms but when you visit your dentist for a regular checkup he or she finds a cavity. In some cases, however, you may notice mild pain in one tooth when you eat something that is sweet, very hot, or very cold. This is likely to be the earliest symptom of tooth decay that you will experience. If you feel a sharp pain when eating sweet, hot, or cold foods, this may signal a more seriously decayed tooth.

In each of these instances, the decay process usually can be halted by removing the decayed portion of the tooth (drilling) and replacing it with a restorative material (filling).

If the decay seems to be extensive or you are especially sensitive, you may be offered a local anesthetic (injected into the gums) to keep you from feeling pain. On occasion, some dentists will offer nitrous oxide gas to decrease discomfort and anxiety. If you are taking any medications, mention this to your dentist before accepting any anesthetic because certain medications and anesthetics taken together can produce adverse reactions.

Once the affected area has been cleared of decay, your dentist will prepare to restore the tooth. The kind of filling used depends on the location and function of the tooth. Molars, which do most of the work of chewing, experience the most stress and require more durable materials than do front (anterior) teeth. In addition, if possible, a filling in a front tooth should blend in color with the tooth itself.

Sometimes when decay is extensive, a temporary filling is inserted to provide your dentist an opportunity to observe the tooth's response and sensitivity to treatment. After several weeks, if there are no adverse signs or symptoms, your dentist removes the filling and replaces it with a permanent one.

The most common restorative material is silver amalgam, which is used in the back teeth. Such fillings are actually alloys of mercury, silver, and other metals. The recent addition of copper to the standard mixture makes today's "silver fillings" far more durable than those of even a few years ago.

Gold inlay, a more expensive restoration, is sometimes used in place of amalgam where more strength and support are necessary. Such a filling does not readily tarnish.

Fillings in front teeth need to be as invisible as possible. Silicate, a form of porcelain cement which resembles tooth enamel, was the standard choice until recently. Now, plastic resins are being used with increased frequency. Both forms can be tinted to match the color of the tooth that is filled. In the future, composite materials may be made strong enough to be used for the chewing surfaces of the molars and premolars.

Occasionally, gold foil is used as a restorative material for small cavities in front teeth. It is more expensive than porcelain or plastic composite materials but is more durable.

If your tooth is so decayed that it cannot support several fillings or a single large one without danger of breaking, your dentist may remove the decay, fill the site with cement or amalgam, and fit a porcelain crown, a metal crown, or a combination metal and porcelain crown over the tooth to restore it. A model is usually made from an impression of your tooth, and a crown is fabricated in the laboratory. This crown is then fitted, shaped, and finally cemented in place on what is left of the tooth.

Root Canal

If you have a tooth that is so severely decayed or infected that it is in danger of being lost, your dentist or an endodontist will perform a root canal. This procedure involves removal of the nerve and vascular tissue (pulp) from the root and pulp chamber as well as any associated decayed tooth structure. It allows for the root and base of the tooth itself to remain in place.

A root canal is performed as an office procedure and often requires local anesthesia. In this multistage procedure, the pulp is removed and the cavity that is created is then sterilized and filled with an inert material (gutta-percha) and cement. The remaining tooth structure will be more brittle than before and therefore will require permanent restoration, most often with a crown.

Tooth Abscess

Signs and Symptoms

- Persistent aching or throbbing pain in a tooth
- Sensitivity to hot or cold foods or liquids
- Pain on chewing
- Swollen lymph nodes in the neck
- Fever and general malaise

Some people do not view tooth decay as a potentially serious health problem, but if not dealt with promptly and properly, it can lead to a more troublesome ailment.

Decay can allow bacteria to infect the pulp of a tooth. The infection may spread to the root and into the surrounding bone. This is known as an abscess. If the infection reaches the bone, the tooth may loosen. The infected root and swollen tissue cause pain. If the tooth dies, the pain will go away, but the infection may remain, slowly destroying adjacent bone. The resulting breakdown material (pus) that forms as part of the infection can erode a channel through the jaw and form a swelling or boil on the gum.

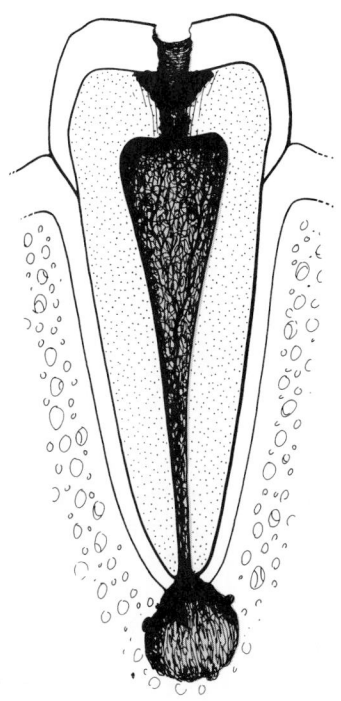

A tooth abscess occurs when bacteria enter through a decayed area and spread inward, infecting the pulp, root, and even bone surrounding the tooth.

Diagnosis

If you have persistent throbbing pain in a tooth, find chewing painful, or are sensitive to hot or cold foods or liquids, you may have an abscessed tooth. You may have a slight fever and swollen lymph nodes in the neck and feel generally unwell.

A swelling that forms on the gum near the sore tooth may at some point burst, releasing into your mouth a quantity of thick liquid material with a foul taste and smell; simultaneously, the pain probably will be relieved. If you experience any of these symptoms, see your dentist immediately. Your dentist will examine the tooth and decide on a proper course of action.

Treatment

Before you get to your dentist, you can help relieve the pain of an abscess by taking aspirin or another pain reliever. Do not apply aspirin directly to the tooth or surrounding tissue. Rinsing your mouth with warm, salted water every hour or so may be soothing but is not curative.

In the past, the only treatment for an abscessed tooth was extraction. Under certain conditions, extraction still is appropriate. However, dentists today often can save abscessed teeth.

As a first step, your dentist probably will prescribe an antibiotic to clear up the infection and keep it from spreading to other parts of your body. He or she can also prescribe pain relief medications to make you more comfortable.

To save the tooth, your dentist may anesthetize the area and then open a hole into the pulp chamber of the tooth. This will release the pressure. The pulp chamber can then be cleared out, disinfected, and filled with an inert material. If swelling persists after an abscessed tooth has been removed, your dentist may want to obtain special cultures to rule out a condition called actinomycosis.

Next, your dentist will place a temporary filling in your tooth. After the infection has cleared (usually within a few weeks), your tooth can receive a permanent filling.

Your dentist most likely will want to see you again in a few months, at which time X-rays will be taken of the tooth to determine whether bone and tissue are growing into the pocket left by the abscess. If the pocket appears to be healthy, the treatment is finished. If the infection persists, additional treatment is necessary and your dentist may refer you to a specialist who will perform a surgical procedure to remove the remaining diseased tissue, sometimes including a small portion of the root tip.

Prevention of Tooth Decay

A successful plan of decay prevention involves three steps: taking good care of your teeth; proper diet; and, in the case of children, application of sealants to the chewing surfaces of back teeth and application of fluoride to all teeth. Such a plan involves thorough brushing and flossing on a daily basis, seeing your dentist regularly for checkups, controlling the intake of sugar and carbohydrates in your diet, and using fluoride and sealants to help prevent caries.

In an ideal world, everyone would brush their teeth after each meal and all snacks. A more realistic goal is to brush at least twice each day—in the morning and before retiring—and to floss once. Much decay-causing activity occurs at night when your mouth is dry from lack of saliva and your tongue is inactive in cleaning your mouth. Brushing and flossing before retiring are important because they eliminate foods and bacteria that otherwise can cause decay.

Another strategy is to rinse your mouth with water after snacks (see page 366 for a discussion of proper methods for brushing and flossing teeth).

A key to developing lifelong good dental habits is to start early. Teach your children the ritual of brushing even before they have a full set of teeth. Similarly, your child's dentist will demonstrate the proper methods of flossing.

Control Sugar and Carbohydrate Intake

The concept that sugar contributes to tooth decay is not new. But the evidence points to all fermentable carbohydrates, not just sugar, as foods that cause tooth decay. Fermentable carbohydrates include all sugars and most cooked starches.

Because carbohydrates are an important part of a healthy diet, do not cut down on them. Instead, the following tips may be helpful in discouraging tooth decay. This does not mean that you may never allow yourself or your child to have ice cream, cake, pie, or candy. The amount of sugar you eat is less important than how and when it is eaten. Sweets eaten between meals do more harm than those eaten with a meal.

Try to incorporate the following strategies into your eating habits and your children's:

1. Avoid chewy, sticky foods, particularly as snacks. Such foods as candy, candy-coated nuts, sticky dry cereal, doughy bread, raisins, and dry fruit cling to your teeth. Do not eliminate raisins and dried fruit; just brush within 20 minutes after eating them (acid production by the bacteria that promote tooth decay is most active after this time), or rinse your mouth with water.

2. Choose snacks carefully. Snacking on foods that promote tooth decay is worse than eating the same foods during meals. Nibbling on snacks throughout the day allows bacteria to produce a constant supply of acid on your teeth. Do not constantly sip sugar drinks, suck on hard candies, sugar-sweetened breath mints, or cough drops, or chew gum.

Even babies are at risk of tooth decay. Babies put to sleep with a bottle of milk (or juice) are at risk of damaging teeth. Both contain sugars. If your baby needs a bottle to settle down, fill it with water.

The Value of Fluoride

Persons living in parts of the country where the public water supply naturally contains an optimal amount of fluoride have almost no dental caries. In a few communities, the natural fluoride content of drinking water is so high that brown stains appear on the teeth. Correct knowledge of the action of fluoride enables communities to avoid this cosmetic risk. There is no evidence that fluoride, whether added to water supplies or occurring naturally, is a health risk.

Fluoride is especially helpful when it is ingested by children whose teeth are developing. The fluoride is incorporated into the enamel structure and offers continuing protection.

Many communities in the United States add small amounts of fluoride to their water systems because the water supply is deficient in fluoride. This approach is both cost-effective and safe. If your municipal water supply is not treated, ask about fluoridation for drinking water in your children's schools. Supplemental fluoride drops or tablets are available by prescription from your dentist or physician.

Children, adolescents, and elderly people are most susceptible to tooth decay. For them, topical application of fluoride, including fluoride toothpastes, is desirable. Fluoride mouthwashes can also be useful. Many dentists also treat children's teeth with a fluoride solution as a part of regular checkups.

Fluoride is most effective in preventing caries on the smooth, nonchewing surfaces of your teeth. Consequently, most cavities occur on the chewing surfaces. The reason: these surfaces of your back teeth (premolars and molars) have depressions and grooves (pits and fissures) that are almost impossible to clean with a toothbrush.

Tooth Sealants

Besides good oral hygiene, the single best method to prevent decay of the chewing surfaces of back teeth is use of dental sealants. Sealants provide a thin plastic-like coating, usually clear or white.

The application is painless and easy. First, your dentist cleans the chewing surface of your premolars and molars. Then these surfaces are etched with a mild acid to improve adhesion. The teeth are thoroughly washed and dried. Then your dentist paints sealant onto each tooth in much the same way fingernail polish is applied. The sealant hardens into a shield that prevents accumulation of plaque in the pits and fissures.

Dental sealants can last up to 10 years, although various conditions may shorten their effectiveness. Regular visits to the dentist permit necessary touch-ups to extend the life of the sealant. If the sealant layer is lost, it can be replaced. If the sealant is damaged, the underlying tooth surface is at no greater risk for cavities than it would be if the sealant had never been applied.

Sealant protection is most appropriate for children. It should be applied when the first permanent molars erupt, at about age 6, and again when permanent second molars and premolars erupt, around ages 11 to 13. Older people, the disabled, those who live in institutions, and people with a high incidence of cavities also can benefit from sealants.

Periodontal Disease

Tooth decay (dental caries) is the primary cause of tooth loss. After age 35, periodontal disease also becomes an important cause of tooth loss. Many people experience periodontal disease in some form over the course of their lives, although they will not necessarily lose teeth.

The tissue in which the disease occurs is called the periodontium. This includes the gums (gingiva), the periodontal ligament, and the alveolar bone (tooth sockets). These structures support your teeth.

Periodontal disease is neither a disease that develops in 1 day nor an ailment that, with prompt attention, can be cured, never to appear again. Rather, periodontal disease results from a combination of factors involving bacterial plaque—the sticky substance found in everyone's mouth—and its long-term effects on the periodontium. It can take several forms, but the result is weakened tooth support.

The two most common forms of periodontal disease are gingivitis (inflammation of the gums) and periodontitis. Gingivitis is often a precursor of the more serious condition of periodontitis. Both of these diseases are discussed in the following pages, as is trench mouth and ways to prevent periodontal disease.

Gingivitis

Signs and Symptoms
- Swollen, soft, red gums
- Gums that bleed easily

The term gingivitis refers to inflammation of the gingiva or gums. It can be caused by deposits of plaque, the sticky film that forms on the exposed portion of teeth and irritates the gums.

Many people experience gingivitis first in puberty and then at various degrees of severity throughout life. Mild forms of the disease are very common among adults. People with uncontrolled diabetes and pregnant women are particularly prone to the development of gum inflammation.

Diagnosis
Healthy gums are firm and pale pink. If you notice that your gums are swollen, very tender, and bleed easily, you may have gingivitis. Often, people first detect a change in their gums when they notice that the bristles of their toothbrush are pink after brushing, a sign that their gums are bleeding even with the gentle pressure of brush bristles. Further examination usually reveals red, inflamed gums. Gingivitis often causes no direct pain or discomfort and thus is frequently overlooked.

If your gums seem swollen and red, consult your dentist. He or she will examine your gums carefully, looking for inflammation and excess deposits of plaque at the base of your teeth. As the gum margin swells, more plaque can be trapped, thus irritating the gum further.

How Serious Is Gingivitis?
Gingivitis often goes unnoticed because it usually is painless. If left unchecked, however, gingivitis can lead to periodontitis, a more serious disease that affects not only the gums but also the other supporting structures of the teeth, leading to tooth loss.

Treatment
Your dentist will treat your gingivitis by using several techniques. The first step is a thorough cleaning of the teeth to remove the plaque and calculus (a chalky material com-

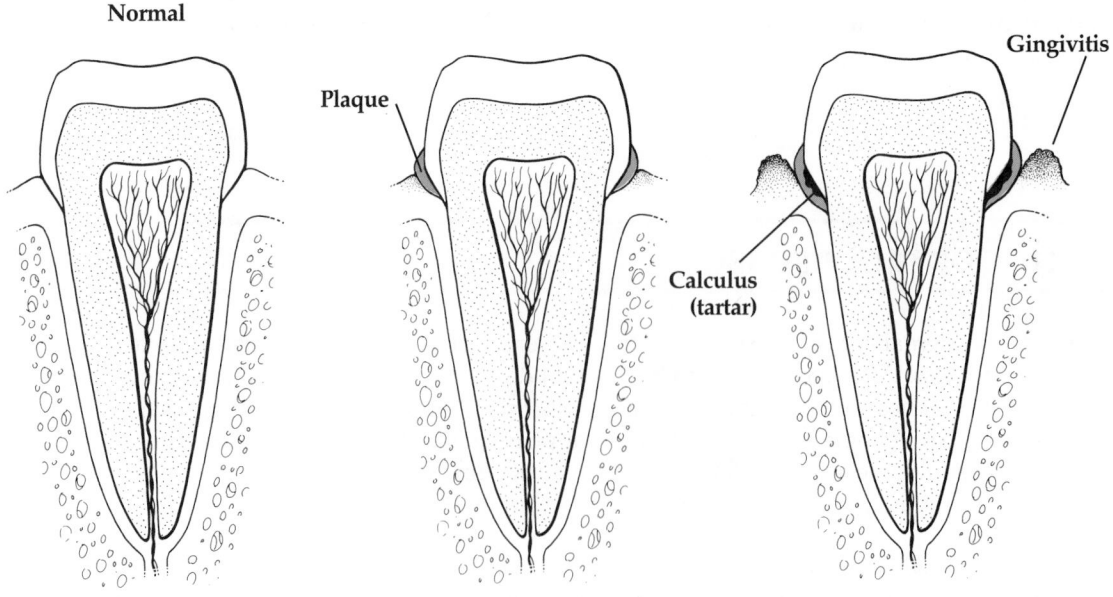

If plaque accumulates on a normal tooth and is not removed promptly, it can harden into a mineral deposit called calculus (tartar). Gradually, the nearby gums become inflamed and swollen, a disorder known as gingivitis.

posed of mineralized plaque, often called tartar). This cleaning can be uncomfortable, particularly if your gums are sensitive or if your teeth are encrusted with plaque and calculus. The removal procedure, known as scaling, is designed to remove the deposits of bacteria, plaque, and calculus.

Sometimes the inflammation is made worse by misaligned teeth, overhanging fillings, or poorly contoured restorations such as crowns and bridges that make plaque removal more difficult. Teeth can be straightened to minimize plaque accumulation, fillings can be replaced, and restorations can be recontoured.

Prevention

Gingivitis most often is the result of poor dental hygiene. If you take good care of your teeth, with thorough, daily brushing, regular flossing, and frequent professional cleaning, your chances of serious gingivitis developing are greatly decreased (see Prevention of Periodontal Disease, page 613).

Once you have gingivitis, a strict program of oral hygiene is necessary to keep the disease from becoming worse. This includes flossing as well as brushing. Your dentist or dental hygienist will show you how to brush and floss properly (see Proper Flossing and Brushing Techniques, page 366).

At first your gums may bleed after brushing. This should last only a couple of weeks. Soon your gums should be pink and firm, a sign of their improved health. The program must be followed indefinitely, however, for your gums to remain healthy.

Periodontitis

Signs and Symptoms
- Swollen or recessed gums
- Unpleasant taste in mouth
- Bad breath
- Pain in a tooth when eating hot, cold, or sweet foods
- Dull sound when a tooth is tapped
- Loose teeth
- Change in your bite

If gingivitis goes untreated or treatment is delayed, periodontitis may develop. Periodontitis gets its name from the Latin *peri* meaning "around," *odont* meaning "tooth," and *itis* for "inflammation."

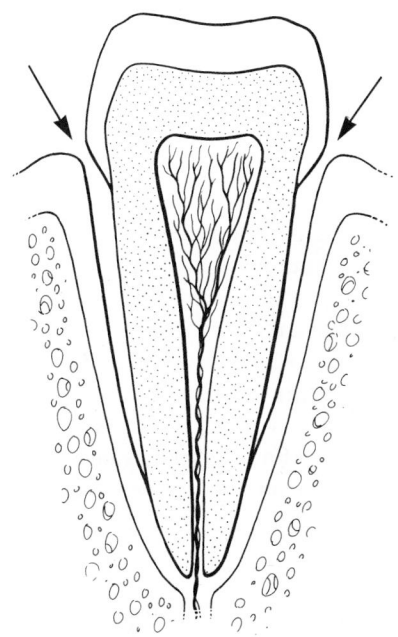

Untreated gingivitis can result in periodontitis, in which the inflamed gums gradually withdraw from the tooth (arrows); the tooth loosens and eventually may fall out.

In this disease, which was formerly known as pyorrhea (Greek for "flowing pus"), not only are the gums affected but also there is inflammation of the periodontal ligament and alveolar bone (tooth sockets), which help hold the teeth in place.

In periodontitis, plaque-filled pockets are formed between the teeth and gums. The gums become inflamed, enlarging the pockets and trapping increasing amounts of plaque. The prolonged and increasing inflammation also damages the periodontal ligament of each affected tooth. Over time, the gums gradually detach from the teeth. Pus forms in response to infection from invading bacteria and may, in severe instances, ooze from around the teeth.

The result of such long-term infection is an erosion of the bony socket housing the tooth. The tooth loosens and eventually may fall out.

Despite its long-term risks, periodontitis usually is painless. In some cases, however, an acute infection forms as an abscess in one or more of the pockets. This produces pain and eats away at bone even more quickly than the chronic condition does.

Generally speaking, the younger a person is when bone loss begins, the less the chances of saving the tooth. People who grind their teeth also may have more periodontal problems than those who do not.

Diagnosis

If your gums are swollen, if you have an unpleasant taste in your mouth and odor to your breath, if you experience pain on eating hot, cold, or sweet foods, or if you notice that a tooth is loose, see your dentist.

Your dentist will examine your teeth and gums for signs of periodontitis. Your gums will be examined for inflammation and deposits of plaque and calculus at and below the gum line and for erosion or withdrawal from the teeth. You may also be asked a series of questions to determine if a systemic disorder such as diabetes is present. If such indications are found, you may be referred to a physician for a thorough examination and treatment.

Treatment

Conservative (nonsurgical) therapy is the first step in treating periodontal disease. This includes meticulous cleaning of the root surfaces of your teeth by your dentist or hygienist. A strict program of oral hygiene also is required. This includes flossing as well as brushing. Initially, your gums may bleed after brushing, but this unpleasant condition should disappear within 2 weeks.

Your dentist will evaluate the condition of your teeth and gums after several weeks. Generally, gums respond to the flossing and brushing by becoming pink and more firm. If you are able to maintain your gums and teeth in this condition, you may be able to avoid surgical treatment.

Orthodontic Treatment

If your teeth are malaligned and crowded, plaque accumulation may be increased and removal of it may be more difficult, but the arrangement of the teeth does not cause periodontitis. Orthodontic treatment can correct the positions of the teeth. Uneven biting and chewing surfaces can be recontoured to decrease pressure. If you grind your teeth during sleep (bruxism), you can be fitted with a device to protect your teeth from excessive pressure; however, bruxism may have other causes that may have to be identified.

Surgery

In more advanced cases, your dentist may perform a surgical procedure. For example, a flap procedure is sometimes done to clean calculus from teeth, remove infected tissue, and recontour bone. The gum tissue surrounding your teeth is lifted, the area around the teeth and bone is cleaned and recontoured, and the tissue is replaced and sutured in place.

Another technique, known as gingivectomy, may be performed under local anesthesia. In this procedure, the gums are trimmed to decrease the depth of the pockets. After the procedure, the gum line is covered with a protective putty-like packing to allow your gums to heal. The dressing should not interfere with normal eating and drinking. If it does, call your dentist or the specialist who performed the surgery.

A similar procedure, a gingivoplasty, sometimes is performed to remove excessive gum tissue and to reshape the gums to enable them to stay self-cleaning.

Sometimes an operation on the underlying bone may be performed to correct anatomic deformities or damage caused by periodontal disease. Grafting with bone or a bone substitute is often used to replace lost bone. Guided tissue regeneration allows bone to regrow itself.

Prevention

In addition to techniques your dentist or periodontist can perform, you will be instructed in the proper care of your teeth. The goal is to prevent periodontitis from progressing or recurring. Good dental hygiene is paramount in the control of periodontal disease (see Prevention of Periodontal Disease, page 613).

Trench Mouth

Signs and Symptoms

- Profuse bleeding from and pain in the gums after slight pressure
- Grayish film on the gums

Trench mouth, also known as necrotizing ulcerative gingivitis or Vincent's infection, is a painful form of gingivitis. It affects young adults most often; it can be mild or severe. This condition received the name trench mouth because during World War I it occurred in soldiers who were living in trenches under conditions of poor hygiene and poor nutrition.

Trench mouth is characterized by profuse bleeding at the slightest pressure or irritation. The condition is the result of an infection with bacteria that normally inhabit the mouth. It is not passed from one person to another.

The onset of this disease is often sudden. The points of gum between teeth (the papillae) are usually damaged, leaving craters that collect plaque and food debris. The area is covered with a grayish layer of decomposing gum tissue. The inflammation and infection also may involve other parts of the mouth.

Diagnosis

If you have gum pain and profuse bleeding after slight irritation or pressure on the gums, see your dentist immediately.

Treatment

Your dentist will begin by gently and thoroughly cleaning your gums. Irrigation of the mouth with salt or peroxide solution often helps to relieve symptoms. Your dentist may recommend a nonprescription pain reliever to lessen discomfort. You will also be advised to get plenty of rest, eat a balanced diet, and avoid irritation from smoking or eating spicy foods. Antibiotics may be prescribed if you have a high fever.

Prevention of Periodontal Disease

Periodontal disease (including gingivitis and periodontitis) is due in large part to poor dental hygiene. Inadequate care of your teeth will allow plaque to form and to become anchored to your teeth.

Some plaque is removed by the action of your tongue and saliva when you chew. However, in certain areas of the teeth, particularly near the gum line and between teeth, sticky plaque and hard calculus (calcified plaque, also known as tartar) collect and tend to adhere to your teeth.

Thorough brushing and flossing of teeth are your best techniques for keeping plaque and calculus from forming. Brush at least twice daily. Floss once daily. Many dentists recommend brushing and flossing after every meal. Be sure to brush at bedtime because the action of plaque is most damaging at night when the amount of saliva in your mouth decreases (see Proper Flossing and Brushing Techniques, page 366).

In some people, plaque develops in unusual quantities or especially quickly. If you have this problem, your dentist may recommend special toothpicks, stimulators, or toothbrushes. Devices that irrigate with water under pressure can be used to flush the toxic products found in plaque out from between the teeth. Such devices do not remove the plaque but they can help neutralize some of its effects.

Although electric toothbrushes have not been found to be superior to regular toothbrushes in removing normal development of plaque, they can be useful to people with special needs, such as in those whose manual dexterity is impaired, people who develop large amounts of plaque quickly, and those who wear dental appliances. Electric toothbrushes are often preferred by caregivers.

Over-the-counter mouth rinses that are claimed to decrease plaque have yet to be proven more beneficial than brushing and flossing. The slick feel that some of these products impart to teeth is not due to the absence of tartar and plaque but rather to the glycerine included in the rinse.

For people with chronic periodontal problems, one plaque-fighting rinse, chlorhexidine, is effective. It is available by prescription only. It is superior to over-the-counter rinses but has not cured gingivitis, even in Europe where it has been available for several decades. Side effects include an unpleasant taste, irritation of the soft tissues of the inner mouth, and staining of the teeth. For this reason, chlorhexidine may be undesirable for routine dental hygiene over a prolonged period.

Recently there has been promotion of and subsequent demand for toothpastes that claim to control calcified plaque (tartar). The effectiveness of these products in the prevention of periodontal disease has yet to be proven. Antitartar toothpastes may prevent the formation of tartar on the surfaces of teeth and make your teeth more cosmetically appealing. However, they do not help remove tartar below the gum line and between teeth, where periodontal disease develops (see Controlling Tartar, page 368). One side effect of antitartar toothpastes is that they often cause teeth to become sensitive to cold.

No matter how careful you are, you are bound to have some plaque and calculus. The calculus must be removed by your dentist or dental hygienist with various instruments or an ultrasonic device that vibrates the deposits from your teeth. Visit your dentist every 6 to 12 months for such treatment; visit your dentist more often if you have periodontitis or if you develop large amounts of calculus quickly.

Developmental Disorders

In most people, the mouth and teeth develop in a fairly orderly and normal manner (see Tooth Development, page 602). However, problems may occur, often as a result of improper prenatal development or sometimes environmental or genetic factors.

Modern dentistry and oral surgery often can minimize the effects of the developmental disorders discussed in the following pages.

Impacted Teeth

Signs and Symptoms
- Pain in the gums
- Recurrent infection of partially buried tooth
- Bad breath
- Unpleasant taste

Teeth emerge through the gums primarily at three times during life. The first time is when the baby or primary teeth emerge after the first year or so; the second is when permanent teeth emerge during early school years; and the third is when the last teeth, the so-called wisdom teeth or third molars, appear during the late teens or early twenties.

The wisdom teeth frequently have trouble emerging properly as a result of an inappropriate size of the jaw. Wisdom teeth often are too large for the jaw and thus become rotated, displaced, or tilted as they attempt to emerge. This can cause pain and occasionally infection when the tooth traps food debris in the soft gum tissue surrounding it. If the tooth comes in at an angle, it can push on the adjacent tooth, sometimes damaging it and sometimes causing pain and possibly some shifting of the bite.

Diagnosis
Impacted teeth do not always cause discomfort. When they do, the experience is unpleasant. The tissues overlying the third molars may enlarge.

If you feel pain in your gums or have an unpleasant taste when you bite on or near where a wisdom or other unemerged adult tooth should be, you may have an impacted tooth. The tooth may be partly visible and the surrounding gums may be infected. The impacted tooth may press on other teeth, causing pain. Consult your dentist.

Treatment
Before you see your dentist, you can help relieve the pain by taking an analgesic such as aspirin or by rinsing your mouth with warm salt water.

Your dentist will examine your mouth for signs of unemerged teeth and infection. X-rays will be taken to determine the exact location and position of the tooth. If you have an infection around the tooth, called pericoronitis, your dentist may prescribe an antibiotic.

The usual treatment for an impacted wisdom tooth is removal. Wisdom teeth that emerge crooked can compromise your bite. Also, wisdom teeth are difficult to clean because they are so far back in the mouth and thus are prone to decay and periodontal disease.

Your dentist may remove the tooth or teeth in the office under local anesthesia. If your case is more complicated, your dentist may refer you to an oral and maxillofacial surgeon for the removal. If the tooth lies at a difficult angle or you have several teeth impacted, the procedure may require general anesthesia or may need to be done in a hospital.

Misshapen or Discolored Teeth

Signs and Symptoms
- Misshapen teeth
- Discolored enamel on primary or secondary teeth

If a tooth does not emerge through the gum, it is said to be impacted. This most often occurs with the wisdom teeth at the back of the mouth.

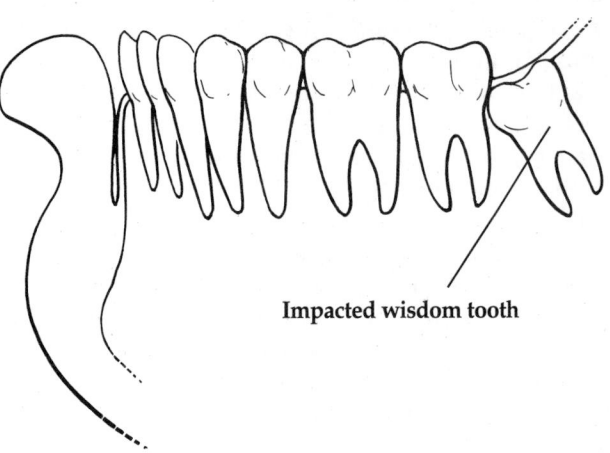

Impacted wisdom tooth

In rare cases, a child's teeth may not be normal in shape or color. Such abnormalities can be caused by many factors, including early illness or trauma, hereditary predisposition, or an environmental factor such as excessive fluoride in the drinking water or the mother's ingestion of tetracycline drugs during pregnancy and nursing. Enamel is completely formed on all but the wisdom teeth by about 8 years of age. Therefore, physicians do not prescribe a prolonged course of tetracycline treatment for pregnant women or children under age 8.

Most often, abnormalities affect both primary and secondary teeth. Misshapen teeth are caused most often by infection, high fever, or malnutrition during infancy or early childhood. The eight front teeth and the 6-year molars are the teeth most frequently affected because these develop first. The crowns of the teeth can be pitted or grooved and may be discolored. In rare cases, misshapen teeth are related to serious disorders such as syphilis (see page 1089) or Down syndrome (see page 44).

Occasionally, the enamel covering the teeth will be imperfect. Although this can be caused by several factors, most often it is the result of a genetic trait that recurs in families. The enamel may be discolored, thin, or even absent. Discoloration also can be caused by living in an area with fluoride content in drinking water of more than 2 parts per million. This amount of fluoridation is not a result of added fluoride but rather occurs naturally in some areas.

Treatment

Misshapen teeth can be treated by adding a restorative material or by covering them with crowns. Teeth without a complete covering of enamel and some very discolored teeth also may be treated in this manner. Sometimes this is done on primary teeth if the enamel is so malformed that serious cavities or wearing down of the teeth occurs. In these instances, the molar teeth often are fitted with stainless steel crowns.

Treatment for Developmental Disorders

Orthodontics

Few people have a perfect bite and pearly white, symmetrical teeth. For some of us, our teeth are slightly misaligned, perhaps where the uppers and lowers clamp together to form the bite or, in some cases, in the front, where the teeth are most visible.

Some misalignment or crowding may be minor, requiring little or no attention. However, a significant number of children and adults have problems that do require treatment. Most of us are familiar with the term orthodontics, the branch of dentistry that deals with the correction of misaligned (maloccluded) teeth.

In general, orthodontists are concerned with producing a normal (even) bite, with the teeth aligned and balanced within the jaws and face. Such manipulation of the teeth usually requires the use of appliances (braces) that gradually move the teeth into the desired positions in the jaw.

Identifying the Problem

In the ideal bite, the teeth of the upper jaw slightly overlap those of the lower jaw. The points of the molars fit into the grooves of the opposing molars. In the ideal jaw there is room for all teeth to fit neatly, neither crowded nor spaced. There are no rotations of teeth or any teeth that twist or lean forward or backward.

When teeth do not fit together properly, they can cause chewing problems (and therefore eating and digestion difficulties). Increased tooth decay also can result. The abnormal forces on the improperly fitting teeth may be a contributing factor in periodontal disease. Misaligned or protruding teeth can cause emotional distress if they affect appearance. Jaw surgery sometimes is needed to correct serious problems when both the teeth and the jaws are misaligned.

Your child's dentist will monitor the development of the secondary teeth and recommend consultation with an orthodontist if problems seem imminent. Most problems of alignment become apparent once the secondary teeth begin to erupt, often as early as age 6. In some instances the problems can be appropriately treated earlier.

Your orthodontist will thoroughly examine your child's mouth. He or she may take a series of X-rays. Some of the X-rays are used to determine the position of teeth, both erupted and yet to erupt. Special X-rays of the head may help to determine the size, position, and relationship of the jaw and teeth.

If the lower jaw is significantly smaller than the upper jaw, the upper teeth may protrude excessively over the lower (a condition called overbite). Similarly, if the lower jaw is larger than the upper, the upper front teeth can bite behind the lower ones (underbite). When significant discrepancies exist between the upper and lower jaws, an operation (orthognathic surgery) may be desirable. However, most often these problems can be corrected with various appliances. Similarly, teeth that are rotated, overlapped, or spaced are candidates for correction.

Today, more and more adults are seeking orthodontic correction of problems that were not treated when they were younger. Although in adults the treatment time often is longer because tooth movement is slower, the results usually are pleasing. More corrective jaw surgery is performed on adults than on children.

Other possible diagnostic studies include making impressions of your upper and lower teeth from which plaster models are constructed. Your dentist will ask you to bite down on a thin, wax-like material to make an impression that can be used to position plaster models accurately to represent the actual bite of your upper and lower teeth. Photographs of your teeth and face and other measurements and recordings also may be made.

Making Changes

If severe overcrowding is the main problem, certain permanent teeth, usually premolars, can be extracted to create room, and the remaining teeth are realigned by fitting appliances (braces) to them.

Fixed braces, usually made of an alloy, are either ring-like bands that encircle the molar teeth or bonds that are attached only to the outside surfaces of the premolar and anterior teeth. Clear or tooth-colored ceramic or inside braces are other options for fixed braces.

Wires, springs, and other force-producing devices place a tension on the teeth that gradually shifts them into new positions. The jaw responds to the pressure by dissolving bone in front of the moving tooth and laying down new bone behind it. Occasionally, tension will be drawn from the opposite jaw, usually achieved with elastic bands placed on upper and lower teeth and connected to an opposite tooth.

Sometimes extra anchorage or support is needed outside the mouth. In these instances, special head or neck gear is designed for attachment to the appliances within the mouth. Such appliances are often worn only at night or for specific periods during the day.

There may be times, particularly in the growing child, when certain removable appliances may be appropriate. These appliances may be designed to move certain individual teeth or groups of teeth.

Routine treatment time with braces ranges from approximately 6 months to 2 years or more. The correction is made during this time, but this is not the end of treatment. The teeth then must be stabilized for months, years, or sometimes indefinitely to keep the moved teeth in place.

To accomplish this stabilization, the teeth are usually fitted with one or more of various devices called retainers. Examples of retainers include positioners (rubber-like mouthpieces the person wears at night and bites into for a few hours during the day), removable retainers (with plastic material on the inside and wires on the outside of the teeth), removable, clear plastic retainers (completely cover the sides and biting surfaces of the

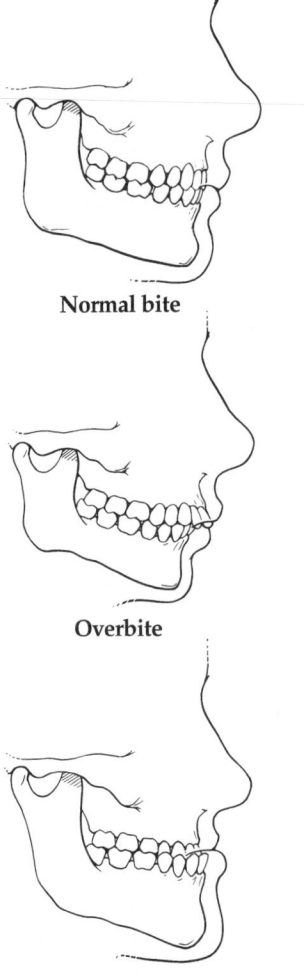

Normal bite

Overbite

Underbite

teeth), and semi-rigid wires (most often are adapted to and bonded on the inside of the front teeth).

Oral Hygiene

Take special care to clean your teeth regularly during the course of orthodontic treatment. Food and plaque accumulate around orthodontic appliances. If you do not remove these deposits, demineralization occurs and may leave permanent whitish marks (scars) on your teeth. Brush with a fluoride toothpaste and rinse with a fluoride mouthwash recommended by your dentist. Although somewhat more difficult, flossing is also recommended.

Corrective Surgery

In extreme cases when conventional orthodontic treatment is not enough to correct a problem, your dentist may recommend corrective surgery. This is more common in adults than in children.

Protrusion of the upper or lower jaw can be corrected by removing a section of bone and setting the remainder in its correct position. Conversely, short jaws can be lengthened; or the height of the lower face can be shortened or lengthened to provide better facial esthetics and function. Surgery can adjust other misaligned bites that may not respond fully to orthodontic treatment alone. Surgery may shorten the overall time of orthodontic treatment.

Corrective surgery usually requires hospitalization for a few days, usually is performed under general anesthesia, and has a relatively short recuperation period. The jaws may be wired together for a few days to a few weeks during the initial healing. During healing, chewing and other activities involving the jaws must be curtailed to some extent.

Infections and Diseases of the Mouth

Almost everyone occasionally experiences some sort of infection or disease of the mouth. Often we are not even aware of the problem, as in the case of gingivitis (see page 610), or it is so minor that it is merely a mild and passing irritation, as with the occasional canker sore or cold sore.

Other problems are more debilitating, as in the case of certain tongue, jaw, and salivary gland problems. Still others, such as oral cancer, can be life-threatening. We discuss each of these infections and diseases in the following pages.

Canker Sores

Signs and Symptoms—Small, painful, white ulcers in the mouth

Canker sores (aphthous ulcers) are common, annoying infections of the mouth. They occur singly or in clusters on the inside surface of the cheeks and lips, on the tongue, at the base of the gums, and on the soft palate (the movable flesh at the back of the roof of the mouth).

The cause of canker sores is unknown, although there seems to be an inherited disposition to them. Recurrent canker sores seem to occur in association with an injury to the mouth, such as that caused by a prick, puncture, or irritation, as from orthodontic appliances. Physical and emotional stress also seem to trigger attacks of canker sores, as do dietary deficiencies in some people. People lacking iron, folic acid, vitamin B_{12}, or a combination of these nutrients often are susceptible. In some women, canker sores develop just before the onset of menses.

Treatment

Canker sores develop quickly and disappear quickly, usually within 7 to 10 days. They can be treated with soothing over-the-counter ointments. If they become infected, see your physician or dentist, who may prescribe antibiotics to clear the infection. If a canker sore lasts more than 14 days, consult your dentist (see Cold Sores and Canker Sores, page 1010; color photograph, page C-10).

Gingivostomatitis

Signs and Symptoms
- Mouth and gum sores
- Bad breath
- Fever and a feeling of malaise

Gingivostomatitis is a common infection of the mouth among children. The condition is a viral infection and often accompanies an upper respiratory infection such as a cold or the flu.

Gingivostomatitis infections range from mild to severe. Generally they last about 2 weeks.

Diagnosis
If your child has sores on the gums or on the insides of the cheeks, has bad breath, runs a fever, and feels generally unwell, consult your dentist or physician. Your physician will examine your child's mouth and will check for any underlying infection, particularly of the chest or throat. A sample may be taken for culture.

Treatment
Treatment of any underlying infection or disorder will help clear the mouth infection. A medicated oral rinse may help relieve the pain and promote healing. Good oral hygiene and a nutritious diet of soft foods and plenty of fluids are important. Use of a mouthwash made of half a teaspoon of salt dissolved in 8 ounces of water, or an over-the-counter mouthwash, may be soothing.

Oral Thrush

Signs and Symptoms—Creamy-white sore patches in the mouth or throat

Your mouth houses many different kinds of microbes in very small numbers. One of them, the fungus *Candida albicans* (which is also found elsewhere in the body), on occasion can reproduce uncontrollably to produce an infection known as oral thrush. Thrush may extend downward into the esophagus (see Other Causes of Esophageal Inflammation, page 747).

This fungus is the same microbe responsible for the vaginal yeast infections that many women experience. Oral thrush tends to occur most often when your natural resistance to disease has been weakened by illness or when your mouth's natural balance of microbes has been upset by medication such as antibiotics, immunosuppressive drugs, or corticosteroid drugs.

Many people experience an outbreak of oral thrush at some point in their lives. The infection is most common among babies and young children and the elderly, although it can occur at any time of life.

Oral thrush can be painful, but ordinarily it is not a serious disorder. However, it can interfere with eating and thereby impair your nutrition. It can be treated by your physician or dentist, but it tends to recur.

Diagnosis
If slightly raised, creamy-white sore patches develop in your mouth or on your tongue, you may have oral thrush. The patches may be brushed off when you clean your teeth or eat. Brushing may make them sore and they may bleed slightly. The infection can spread to the roof of your mouth, to your gums or tonsils, and into your throat (see color photograph, page C-10).

If you have any of these symptoms, see your dentist or physician, who will examine your mouth and throat and will determine whether there may be an underlying cause for the condition.

Treatment
Your dentist or physician will prescribe a course of oral antifungal medication, often to be taken for 7 to 10 days. Any underlying disorder must be treated as well.

Prevention
After using inhaled corticosteroids for asthma, rinse your mouth thoroughly to reduce your risk of acquiring oral thrush.

Leukoplakia

Signs and Symptoms—Thickened, hardened, white patch on a cheek or tongue

The term leukoplakia comes from a Greek word meaning white plate, an apt description of the white patches that characterize this disorder. Ill-fitting dentures or a rough tooth rubbing against the cheek or gum is a common cause (see color photograph, page C-10).

When white patches develop in the mouths of smokers as the body's natural protection against the heat of tobacco smoke, the condition is called smoker's keratosis. Patches of leukoplakia also occur if a cud of chewing tobacco or snuff is held within the mouth for extended periods.

You can have leukoplakia at any time during your life, but it is most common among the elderly.

Diagnosis

You may notice a white or grayish patch that develops on the inside of one cheek or on your tongue over the course of several weeks. At first it may not be noticeable. After a while it may become rough and sensitive to hot or spicy foods.

If you observe such a patch, see your dentist or physician. If the patch persists after treatment, your physician or dentist may take a biopsy specimen of the area for examination under a microscope. About 3 percent of such patches are early signs of mouth cancer.

Treatment

Most treatment of leukoplakia involves removing the source of irritation. If a rough tooth or denture is the cause, the offending tooth will probably be filed down or replaced. If the patch is linked to smoking or chewing tobacco, you will be advised to quit the habit. Once the source of irritation has been removed, the patch may clear up, usually within weeks or months.

Oral Lichen Planus

Signs and Symptoms
- Small, pale pimples that form a lacy network on the tongue or cheeks
- Shiny, slightly raised patches on the tongue or cheeks
- Sore, dry mouth with a metallic taste

Oral lichen planus may be limited to a network of pale pimples or shiny, red, raised patches. Both are found on the sides of the tongue or inside the cheeks, or it may advance into a painful erosive lesion. Your mouth may be sore and dry and have a metallic taste. Some people experience no symptoms other than the raised pimples or bumps (see color photograph, page C-10).

The cause of oral lichen planus is uncertain. Emotional stress seems to trigger the response in some people. At other times, oral lichen planus is a side effect of certain medications. Any adult can have this rare disorder, but it affects middle-aged women more frequently than any other group.

There seems to be a relationship between the oral form and the skin form of lichen planus (see Lichen Planus, page 993) because almost half of those with the oral version also have it on the skin.

If you notice any of the signs described above, see your dentist.

Treatment

Sometimes treatment is unnecessary. If the cause is a certain medication, your dentist may advise you to discontinue its use. If you are experiencing discomfort, your dentist will prescribe appropriate medication.

Tongue Disorders

Signs and Symptoms
- Tongue becomes smooth, dark red, and sometimes sore
- Tongue becomes discolored black or dark brown
- Tongue appears hairy or furry

Glossitis is an inflammation of the tongue. Normally, the surface of your tongue is covered with small hair-like projections (papillae) of tissue. When glossitis occurs, the papillae are lost and a range of changes may occur, including discoloration. Specifically, the tongue loses its usual pink and velvety character. It may become sore.

Glossitis can be caused by various factors, including bacterial or fungal infection, iron-deficiency anemia (see page 957), and pernicious anemia (see page 958). Most tongue problems are minor, but if the symptoms persist for more than 10 days, visit your physician or dentist for an examination.

Acute Glossitis

This condition can occur as the result of a local infection, burn, or trauma. It may develop quickly and produce swelling and tenderness; it may cause difficulty in chewing, swallowing, and speaking.

If your tongue swells a great deal, it can obstruct your air passages. If this happens, call an emergency medical team (see Choking, Breathing Emergencies, and Resuscitation, page 406). Immediate corticosteroid treatment usually relieves the swelling.

Bad Breath

Just about everyone would like to have breath that always is "kissing sweet." Because fresh breath is important to us, manufacturers of mints and mouthwashes harvest substantial profits from this multi-million dollar industry.

Advertisements for many of these products maintain that your breath can be made wonderfully fresh; the accompanying implication often is of an increased attractiveness to the opposite sex. Sad to say, these products do not always succeed in curing your bad breath (halitosis)—or have any effect on your social life.

At best, these products are only temporarily helpful in controlling breath odors. They actually may be less effective than simply rinsing your mouth with water, brushing and flossing your teeth, or just eating a meal.

What Causes Bad Breath?

There are many causes of bad breath. First, your mouth itself may be the source. Bacterial decomposition of food particles and other debris in and around your teeth can produce a foul odor. Pockets of infection, as in periodontitis (see page 611), are obvious causes of odor. A dry mouth, such as occurs during sleep or as the result of some drugs or smoking, will enable dead cells to accumulate on your tongue (coated tongue), gums, and cheeks, and these will undergo bacterial decomposition.

Another cause of bad breath is eating foods containing volatile oils with a strong, distinctive odor. Onions and garlic are the best-known examples, but there are other vegetables and spices that also may cause bad breath. After this food is digested in your stomach and small intestine and the volatile substances are absorbed into your bloodstream, they are carried to your lungs and are given off in your breath. (Alcohol behaves in the same fashion, thus allowing measurement of blood alcohol levels by tests of the breath. Alcohol itself has almost no odor, however. The characteristic smell on the breath is mainly the odor of other components of the beverage.)

Lung disease can cause bad breath. Chronic infections in the lungs, such as bronchiectasis (see page 708) or lung abscess (see page 708), can produce very foul-smelling breath. Usually, much sputum is produced in these cases. If you have impaired motility of your stomach you may have bad breath from fermentation of the stomach contents. Belching may produce the odor. Esophageal reflux also can be a cause of bad breath (see page 742).

There are several general health problems that can cause a distinctive odor to the breath. Kidney failure (see page 852) can cause a urine-like odor; liver failure (see page 804) may cause an odor sometimes described as "fishy." Acetone in the breath causes a fruity odor and may occur in persons with diabetes who are developing ketoacidosis (see page 928) or commonly in children with childhood illnesses who have eaten poorly for several days.

Treating Your Halitosis

Odors coming from the mouth itself (these are the most common kinds) often can be eliminated by good oral hygiene: brush your teeth after every meal; floss to remove any food particles; have gum diseases treated and corrected; keep your mouth moist with frequent sips of water; and brush your tongue if it is coated (see Tooth Care, page 363).

Avoiding the foods that cause bad breath is another obvious precaution. However, no amount of toothbrushing or use of mouthwashes can do more than partially disguise any odors of garlic or onion that come from your lungs.

Causes such as lung disease, impaired emptying of the stomach, liver failure, and kidney failure must be corrected by treatment of the underlying conditions.

Geographic Tongue

This disorder is characterized by absence of papillae in patches, which makes the tongue appear smooth and bright red within those patches. In some cases, soreness or burning is an accompanying symptom. The cause is not completely understood.

Geographic tongue varies from day to day and may be persistent. There is no specific treatment. Avoiding hot or spicy foods, tobacco, and alcohol may help relieve the soreness of geographic tongue.

Hairy Tongue

Occasionally, hair-like papillae on the tongue grow profusely, producing a condition in which the tongue looks as though it is covered with hair. The tongue usually is not sore, but its appearance can be alarming.

Hairy tongue often is a result of antibiotic therapy, excessive use of certain mouthwashes, decreased saliva flow, or lack of adequate oral hygiene. The condition is not serious, and it usually clears after discontinuing use of the antibiotic or the offending mouthwash or when the fever breaks. You can remove the hair-like growths by brushing gently with a toothbrush (see color photograph, page C-10).

Discolored Tongue

Bacteria normally live in the mouth and are part of your body's natural balance. Occasionally, however, these bacteria can grow excessively and accumulate on the papillae or in the fissures of the tongue. The tongue then appears black or dark brown. Bismuth-containing medications (Pepto-Bismol) also can cause black tongue.

The discoloration can be caused by antibiotic therapy, a fungal infection, smoking, or chewing tobacco. You can help remove the discoloration by brushing your tongue with a toothbrush gently twice each day. You may wish to dip the brush in an antiseptic mouthwash. If the condition persists, see your dentist or physician.

Oral Cancer

Signs and Symptoms—Small, pale lump or discolored thickening along the side or on the bottom of the tongue, on the floor of the mouth, inside the cheeks, or on gums, roof of the mouth, or palate

Cancer of the mouth is common. As with most kinds of cancer, early detection is important to successful treatment.

The vast majority of oral cancers are of the squamous (scale-like) cell type. Sometimes the cause is unknown, but use of tobacco and excessive alcohol consumption are well-known risk factors (this includes chewing tobacco and snuff as well as smoking).

Oral cancer is less common in people who do not use either tobacco or alcohol. Chronic irritation from jagged tooth surfaces or poorly fitting dentures also may play a role.

Diagnosis

Most oral cancers occur along the side or on the bottom of the tongue or on the floor of the mouth. The tumors usually are painless at first and often are visible or can be felt with a finger.

Periodic examination of the soft tissues of the mouth is essential for early diagnosis. If you notice any persistent change from the usual appearance or feel of the soft tissues in your mouth, consult your dentist or physician. He or she will examine your mouth carefully. If an oral cancer is suspected, a local anesthetic will be applied to the area in question, and a small amount of tissue (biopsy) will be taken for laboratory study.

How Serious Is Oral Cancer?

If treated early, oral cancer often can be cured. Unfortunately, more than half of all mouth cancers are well advanced at the time of their detection. Often they spread into nearby lymph nodes of the neck. This requires treat-

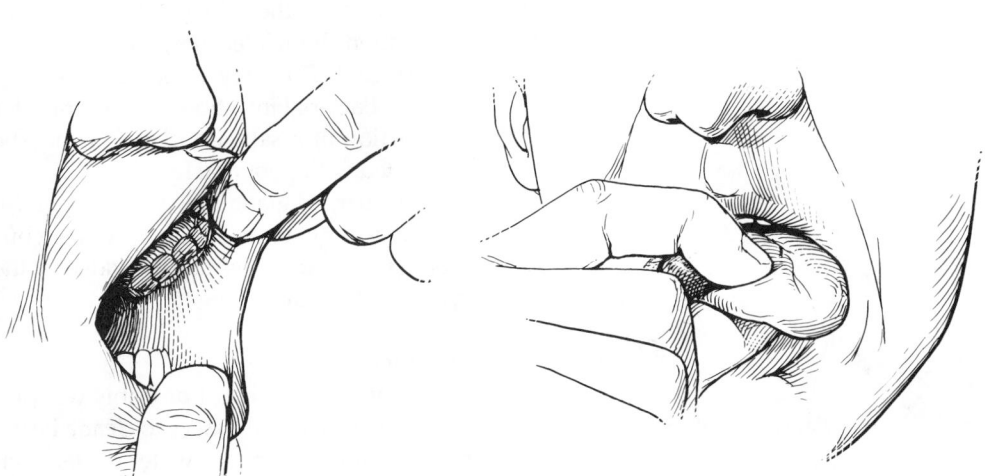

Routine self-examination of your mouth and tongue may enable you to see or feel an oral cancer when it is small and treatment may be most effective.

ment that is more extensive. The chance of a cure is diminished. Almost 25 percent of people with oral cancer die because of delayed discovery and treatment.

Treatment
Early surgical removal of the tumor gives the best chance of cure with the fewest side effects. Radiation therapy is an alternative to surgery and is particularly useful for tumors too large for surgical removal.

After the operation, rehabilitation programs can help restore comfort, speech, chewing ability, and a more normal appearance. Again, early detection and treatment offer the best chance of complete recovery.

Salivary Gland Problems

The saliva produced by your salivary glands serves several purposes. It aids in the mechanical cleaning of your mouth and teeth, it aids in swallowing, and it contains enzymes that aid in digestion and help control infection.

There are three major sets of salivary glands as well as numerous smaller glands located throughout your mouth. The parotid glands are located on each side of your mouth. The submandibular glands are under your jaw at the front of your mouth, and the sublingual glands also are in the floor of your mouth. Secretions from these glands drain into the mouth.

Possible malfunctions of the salivary glands include excessive secretion (sialorrhea) and decreased salivation (xerostomia, or dry mouth). An excess of saliva is characteristic in childhood, when certain oral infections are present, and often in mentally retarded persons. Too little saliva may result from use of certain drugs, radiation treatment, certain systemic diseases, and the aging process.

Salivary Gland Infections

Signs and Symptoms
- Swelling in the floor of the mouth, under the jaw, or in front of the ears
- Decrease in saliva flow
- Peculiar tastes in the mouth
- Pain in the mouth

Infections of the salivary glands are not uncommon. Viral infections, such as mumps (see page 1077), may affect the salivary glands. Bacterial infections may occur after obstruction of a salivary gland or may be associated with poor oral hygiene.

The enlarged gland may be quite painful and may limit your ability to open your mouth wide. Also, pus may be evident at the opening of the duct.

Treatment
Your physician or dentist probably will prescribe a course of antibiotics to clear a bacterial infection. Warm salt water rinses often will aid in removal of the pus.

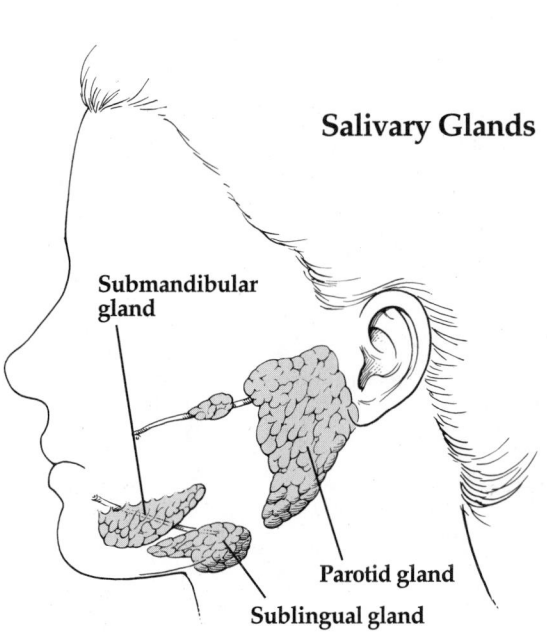

Salivary Glands

Submandibular gland

Parotid gland

Sublingual gland

Salivary Duct Stones

Signs and Symptoms
- Swelling under the chin or in front of the ear, particularly at mealtimes
- Lack of saliva, particularly when eating
- Pain in the mouth

The submandibular glands on the floor of the mouth can become blocked. Such blockages are caused by the formation of a small hard particle (a stone) composed of chemicals from the saliva that harden into a solid material. When this stone partially blocks the duct, pain may be produced, particularly during mealtimes when large quantities of saliva are needed. The engorged gland also may become swollen.

Diagnosis
If you notice a swelling under your chin or in front of your ear, especially at mealtimes, you may have a blocked salivary duct. You also may notice a lack of saliva and pain in the bottom of your mouth. See your dentist or physician, who will probably order an X-ray of your mouth to identify a duct blockage.

Treatment
A stone in a salivary duct can be removed by one of two methods: manipulation or excision. Your physician may be able to push the stone out of the salivary duct. If not, the stone can be removed by a surgical procedure.

In occasional instances, a gland that has had repeated infections and recurrent salivary duct stones may need to be surgically removed.

Salivary Duct Tumors

Signs and Symptoms—Swelling under the chin or in front of your ears

Rarely, the cells in one of the salivary glands, usually one of the parotid glands (in the cheeks) or submandibular glands (under the jaw), multiply to form a tumor. In most cases the growth is benign and self-contained. Such tumors develop over a period of years and cause the gland to swell gradually. Swelling usually is the only symptom.

Treatment
If one of your salivary glands seems swollen, see your dentist or physician, who will examine it and possibly refer you to a radiologist for a special X-ray called a ptylogram or sialogram. This test helps determine the nature of the problem.

Treatment usually involves surgical removal of the gland. If the tumor is malignant, and thus likely to spread (metastasize), radiation therapy or additional surgery may be recommended as well.

Facial and Mandibular Trauma and Fractures

When an accident happens, the most likely dental and oral injury is a dislocated or fractured jaw or having a tooth knocked out (tooth avulsion). Such traumas to the jaw are usually medical emergencies that should be attended to without delay.

Broken or Dislocated Jaw

Signs and Symptoms
- Teeth do not come together normally
- Jaw cannot be closed or when moved causes intense pain

Emergency Symptoms
- Obstructed airway
- Profuse bleeding

Most jaw trauma involves the mandible (lower jaw). If you sustain an injury to your mouth or face, seek help from your physician, an oral and maxillofacial surgeon, or the nearest hospital emergency room immediately for a diagnosis of the extent of the problem and appropriate treatment.

Diagnosis
Your physician will examine your jaw and

take a series of X-rays to determine if the bone is fractured. CT (see page 494) may be performed to be sure that no other bones of the face have been fractured. If the blow has been strong enough to break other bones of your face, there also may be damage to your neck and back.

Emergency symptoms include an obstructed air passage and profuse bleeding or both.

A fracture is suspected if you are unable to close your mouth, if your teeth are misaligned when your mouth is closed, or if you experience tenderness or numbness around your jaw. An upper jaw that can be moved is a definite sign of fracture. If you are unable to close your mouth, your jaw may be dislocated. Swelling and bruising are likely to accompany all jaw injuries.

Treatment

If you have any of the above symptoms after an accident involving your jaw, go to the nearest hospital without delay. If breathing is difficult or much blood is present, call for emergency medical service or 911. The emergency medical technicians may insert a tube to make breathing easier (see Choking, Breathing Emergencies, and Resuscitation, page 406). If your lower jaw is hanging free, cradle it very carefully in your hand until you reach the hospital.

Jaw Dislocation

If your jaw is dislocated, it may be treated by moving it back into place by manually manipulating it, sometimes after administration of an anesthetic.

Once the jaw is reseated, it may be stabilized with a bandage to keep your mouth from opening too wide and causing another dislocation. Avoid opening your mouth very wide for up to 6 weeks after the injury. When you feel a yawn coming on, place your fist under your chin to keep your mouth from opening wide.

If you have dislocated your jaw more than once, consult an oral and maxillofacial surgeon (a surgeon who specializes in problems of the jaw and the bones of the face) for possible treatment.

Jaw Fracture

The first step in treating a jaw fracture is to immobilize the jaw by using a bandage. Once you have been examined, a course of action will be chosen. In many cases this involves surgery to realign the bones and allow them to heal. Often the jaw will need to be immobilized for 6 to 8 weeks, perhaps by wiring it to the other jaw. During this time you will be able to eat only soft or liquid foods, and talking may be difficult.

Loss of a Tooth (Avulsion)

When a permanent tooth is accidentally knocked out (avulsion), appropriate emergency medical care is required, whether a child or an adult is involved (see Tooth Loss [Avulsion], page 453).

Temporomandibular Joint Problems

Signs and Symptoms
- Tenderness of your jaw muscles
- Dull aching pain in front of your ear
- A clicking sound or grating sensation on opening your mouth or chewing
- Locking of the joint, making it difficult to open or close your mouth

Your temporomandibular joints (TMJ) are the hinged joints that connect both sides of your lower jaw (mandible) to your skull. As with other joints, the bony surfaces are covered with cartilage and are separated by a small disc that prevents the bones from rubbing against one another. Muscles that enable you to open and close your mouth also serve to stabilize these joints, which are located about one-half inch in front of each ear canal.

As with other joints, the TMJ is susceptible to various disorders such as osteoarthritis, rheumatoid arthritis, and other forms of inflammation. In rare instances, tumors may arise in this area.

When you open your mouth, the mandible moves downward and forward. For normal jaw function, your left and right TMJs must work in synchrony. If the movement of both joints is not coordinated, the disc that separates the lower jaw from the skull can slip out of position, resulting in malfunction of the jaw. Should your mouth be forced open rapidly or too far, dislocation also can result.

Overuse of the joint by grinding your teeth (bruxism) or trauma to the side of your face also can cause TMJ pain. Extreme jaw clenching can lead to pain in your TMJ as well as over the temples. This occurs because the muscles that control jaw movement are also attached to a nearby bone of your skull.

In some people, headaches or pain in the side of the face or jaw is related to the abnormalities of the temporomandibular joint.

Diagnosis

Tenderness over the joint (with or without movement), a clicking or grating sensation when you open or close your mouth, and locking of the joints (making it difficult to open or close your mouth) when accompanied by pain may suggest a TMJ problem. See your dentist or physician.

He or she may order X-rays or an MRI scan (see page 494); in many cases they are normal. Your dentist or physician will also examine your bite to see if there are abnormalities in the alignment of your teeth and in the movement of your jaw. Such conditions as a high filling, a tipped tooth, teeth displaced due to earlier loss of other teeth, or certain inherited characteristics may produce such misalignments.

Bruxism can exist without your being aware of it. Often, the grinding occurs during sleep. Your dentist can determine the presence of a tooth-grinding habit by noting excessive wear on the biting surfaces of your teeth.

Another result of excessive grinding and jaw clenching is a dull discomfort in your jaw and head areas on awakening in the morning. This is called a musculoskeletal headache or tension headache (see page 501).

Treatment

For most people, pain in the area of the TMJ is not serious. Discomfort may be temporary or chronic in nature. It often goes away with little or no treatment.

Most cases of TMJ disorders are the result of inflammation within the joint. In these instances, physical therapy and medications (such as aspirin or other nonsteroidal anti-inflammatory drugs) used for treating similar symptoms in larger joints work effectively. Occasionally, a corticosteroid drug can be injected into the joint to reduce severe pain and inflammation.

If abnormalities in the alignment of your teeth are present, your dentist may correct this by balancing biting surfaces, replacing missing dentition, or replacing defective fillings or crowns.

If your TMJ is misaligned, your dentist may recommend a plastic bite plate (splint) to promote better alignment of jaw bones. This corrective device is worn over your teeth and helps to reestablish proper alignment. The device may need to be adjusted periodically by your dentist.

Splints typically provide relief from jaw locking, pain, and noise. In addition, your dentist may recommend modifications in your chewing habits. For example, he or she may discourage chewing of gum or of firm foods such as caramels, nontender meats, raw carrots, and celery as well as excessive mouth opening during yawning.

If symptoms continue and the use of a splint is unsuccessful, a specialist in oral and maxillofacial surgery may need to repair or to remove the disc that separates the adjacent bony surfaces of the TMJ, or portions of the bones themselves, or both.

Bruxism can be a difficult habit to break, especially if it occurs while you sleep. However, your dentist may provide either a soft or a firm appliance that you can insert over your teeth at bedtime to offset the effects of the clenching or grinding and to protect your teeth from excessive wear. In addition to these "nightguard appliances," biofeedback/relaxation therapy, physical therapy, and other behavior modification efforts can be of great help.

When symptoms of TMJ disorders occur without evidence of a physical abnormality, psychological factors could be responsible for the pain. For example, chronic tension and anxiety might cause you to maintain a clenched jaw, leading to TMJ disorder. In these situations, biofeedback/relaxation therapy may provide relief (see page 1121).

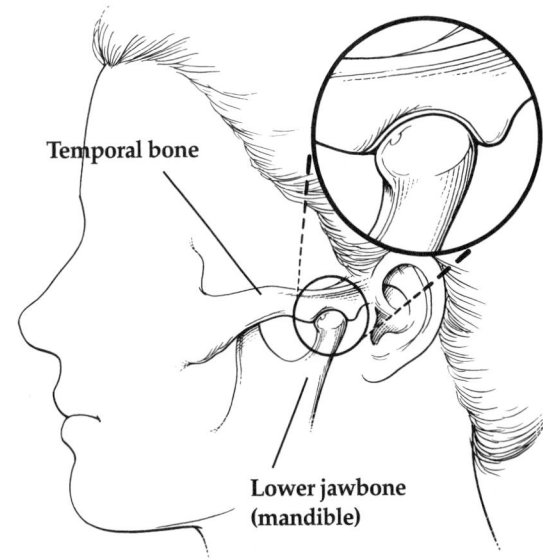

Temporal bone

Lower jawbone (mandible)

Your temporomandibular joint (TMJ) is a hinged joint situated on each side of your head where the lower jawbone (mandible) connects with the temporal bone of your skull. Inflammation, injury, or dislocation of this joint can cause pain.

Prosthodontics

We have all seen the picture of George Washington with a slightly pained look on his face. And most of us have been told that his expression was due to a pair of ill-fitting wooden dentures.

Before modern dentistry, losing one's teeth was an inevitable part of aging. Rare was the person who by old age had any teeth left. In the 18th century, the very fact that Washington had dentures at all shows that he was one of the lucky few who were able to take advantage of the then latest advances in dentistry.

Today, however, the story is different. Fewer and fewer people need to have their teeth removed and replaced with dentures. If you lose an adult tooth, a prosthodontist can make a replacement tooth.

Partial dentures (bridges) may be placed permanently (fixed) in your mouth or may be removable, depending on conditions in your mouth. Partial dentures may be made when one or more teeth need replacement. Replacement of all teeth is achieved with complete dentures, removable sets of artificial teeth. Dental implants may also be used to replace as few as one or as many as all the teeth in a jaw.

Partial Dentures

Once a permanent tooth has been lost, it should be replaced without delay. Your teeth are positioned such that every tooth holds its position and helps the adjacent teeth retain their proper positions, too. If you lose a tooth and do not replace it, the teeth on either side can gradually drift or tilt toward the open space. This can alter your bite, sometimes making it more difficult to chew.

Your dentist will determine what sort of partial denture, also called a bridge, is best suited to your needs. If you have healthy teeth on each side of the missing tooth or teeth, a fixed partial denture may be made. In this procedure, the healthy teeth on each side of the missing tooth or teeth are decreased in size to receive a retainer. The retainers and an artificial tooth are then joined together, and the retainers are cemented to the supporting teeth.

Another type of prosthetic device is known as a removable partial denture. This prosthesis has artificial teeth attached to a metal or plastic base. Clasps or other retainers are also incorporated into the partial denture, which secure it to some of the remaining natural teeth. Removable partial dentures are less costly than fixed partial dentures, and more teeth can be added to the denture if you lose neighboring teeth.

You must be very careful to keep all prosthetic appliances clean because they are all particularly prone to plaque buildup. If the partial denture is fixed, be sure to floss and brush it carefully. If it is removable, remove the prosthesis and brush it and surrounding teeth carefully after every meal. Also, remove partial dentures at bedtime.

Dentures

If, as a consequence of serious periodontal disease or decay, you need to have all of your teeth removed—a decision to be made in concert by you and your dentist—your dentist or prosthodontist will make a set of artificial teeth (dentures).

Dentures can never replace the function and feeling of natural teeth but certainly are a better alternative to no teeth at all. You will lose some sensation in eating because your hard palate (roof of your mouth) is covered by the upper denture. Also, you may be limited in regard to what foods you can eat. Foods such as corn on the cob, whole apples, and hard candies may be difficult to eat because pressures exerted by biting or chewing such foods can cause dentures to loosen in your mouth.

Accustom yourself to different methods of food preparation such as cutting corn kernels from the cob and slicing apples.

The chewing pressure you can exert with dentures is much less than you can exert with your natural teeth (which are anchored in your jaw). Well-fitted dentures usually do not require use of denture adhesives.

Fitting Dentures

There are two standard methods for fitting dentures. The teeth can be extracted and then the gums and jaw be allowed to heal before dentures are fitted. The other method is to prepare dentures in advance and insert them immediately after the extraction.

Not everyone is eligible for immediate dentures. Your dentist will be able to assess the conditions in your mouth and recommend the best approach for you.

Immediate dentures save you the inconvenience of being without teeth for a period of time. However, they often must be refitted once the jaw heals, and occasionally new ones must be made if the jaw changes shape significantly after extraction.

A full set of dentures usually consists of complete upper and lower bases that fit over the gums, but there is a variation known as an overdenture. When a few acceptable teeth remain in the jaw, the denture can be constructed to cover them. The covered teeth may need to have the nerve removed (root canal therapy) and be covered with a restoration prior to construction of the overdenture.

An overdenture may be somewhat more stable than a regular denture, and thus reduce potential soreness in your mouth. The remaining teeth under the denture must be carefully and regularly maintained to keep them healthy. Your dentist or prosthodontist will advise you on the possibility of using an overdenture.

Whatever kind of removable denture you have, it will need periodic fitting to keep it comfortable and to help prevent bone loss and mouth sores.

Denture Problems

Signs and Symptoms
- Persistently loose denture
- Pain in the mouth when dentures are in place
- Inflamed gums
- Sores in the mouth at denture pressure points

Because dentures are foreign to your mouth, the chances are good that you will experience a problem with them. Problems are more common with a lower denture than an upper denture. A denture may be loose-fitting, or sores may develop, or your gums may become inflamed. The lower denture usually does not remain in place by itself, and successful use may depend upon your ability to control a denture with the muscles surrounding it.

Many people in the United States suffer from ill-fitting dentures. Your natural teeth are supported by a specialized type of bone in your upper and lower jaws. When teeth are lost, the supporting bone begins to shrink. This bony shrinkage may be accelerated by the aging process and also by wearing ill-fitting dentures.

The result may be loose dentures. Loose dentures cause soreness during chewing and may become dislodged when you are talking or laughing. Changes in the bone make it difficult for your dentist to construct a properly fitting denture unless something can be done to improve the foundation on which it rests.

A loose denture is only one of the problems you may encounter as a result of the pressure that your dentures place on your gums. The denture rests on soft tissues in your mouth. In some areas, this tissue is more vulnerable to injury (less resilient) than in other areas. Your denture may cause

---

Proper Care of Your Dentures

A denture or removable partial denture (prosthesis) can last from 6 months to 5 years or more, depending on how well it fits, the condition of your jaw, its material, and how well you maintain it.

For a removable prosthesis to be comfortable and durable, you must care for it properly. Good maintenance is not difficult, particularly if you take these steps:

1. Make sure your prosthesis fits properly. If it seems uncomfortable after the initial adjustment period, see your dentist or prosthodontist.

2. Remove your prosthesis each night at bedtime. Your gums need a period of rest in order to remain healthy.

3. Store your removed prosthesis in water to which a denture-cleaning agent may be added when needed. Dentures not stored in water can warp, making them uncomfortable to wear. Removable partial dentures with metal bases should not be left to soak in cleaning agents longer than 15 minutes.

4. Clean your prosthesis each day, according to your dentist's instructions. Food particles and plaque must be removed regularly.

5. Brush and floss your remaining natural teeth each day. It is imperative to keep the remaining teeth and gums as healthy as possible, particularly because they often are the support to which a partial denture is secured.

6. Clean and massage your mouth and gums each day using a brush, cloth, or your finger. It is as important to keep the gums and soft tissues of your mouth clean and stimulated as it is to keep your teeth clean.

Osseointegration of Teeth

More than 40 percent of Americans age 65 or older and 4 percent of employed adults ages 18 to 64 have lost all of their natural teeth. Technology has come a long way since George Washington's legendary ill-fitting dentures, but dentures still can be troublesome.

The development of a dental implant technique called osseointegration (*osseo* means "bone"; *integration* means to "unite with something else") may help to diminish the problems of dentures in the future. The procedure was developed in Sweden in the 1960s and became available in this country in the early 1980s. In this procedure, titanium fittings are implanted in the bone of the jaw. Fixed or removable dentures, replacing some or all of the teeth or individual teeth, can be attached to the fittings. This procedure is often used for people who cannot tolerate standard dentures because of physical or emotional reasons.

In osseointegration, artificial teeth are attached to the bones of the lower or upper jaw. Conventional dentures rest upon a thin layer of gum tissue, which can become sore or infected. Osseointegration anchors the artificial teeth in the upper or lower jaw in much the same fashion as normal teeth are held in place. Chewing pressure, therefore, can be nearly normal, whereas with conventional dentures the chewing pressure generally is much less. In this way, osseointegration helps to prevent deterioration of the jaw.

The Procedure

The procedure involves several steps over a period of months. It is expensive. The surgical phase may require a general anesthetic and 1 or 2 days in the hospital in complex cases. For routine cases, the surgery may be performed in the dental office.

Holes are drilled in your upper or lower jaw (or both), and cylinders made of titanium are placed in the holes. The bony tissue of your jaw heals and grows around the implanted cylinders. Your old dentures can be adjusted for use during this healing period.

Several months after the operation, solid metal posts are screwed into the cylinders. After 2 to 4 weeks you return to have a cast made of your jaw with the posts in place. Then, artificial teeth are constructed and attached firmly to the posts with cement or tiny gold screws.

The success rate for some implant procedures is more than 90 percent. Such high success rates are derived from the skill and painstaking care with which osseointegration is performed and the discipline of patients in caring for their mouths.

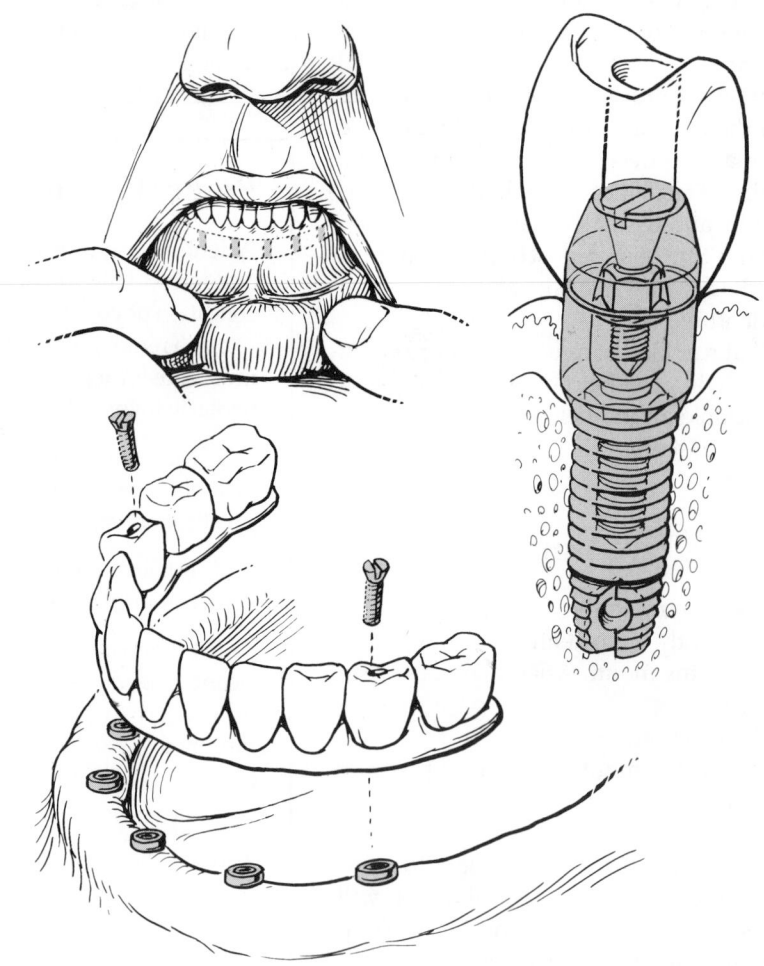

Osseointegration is a process whereby artificial teeth are permanently anchored into your mouth using titanium cylinders implanted in your jawbone.

pressure over this less-resilient tissue. This pressure is uncomfortable and can lead to the formation of sores and mouth ulcers.

Partial dentures place pressure not only on the ridges but also on the natural teeth surrounding the denture. Partial dentures can trap food, particularly when they do not fit properly. Good oral hygiene is important because retained food particles lead to plaque, calculus, periodontal disease, and decay of the natural teeth.

Diagnosis

If your dentures are uncomfortable for more than the initial few minutes after you put them in, if you experience pain when chewing, or if you notice that your gums are red and swollen or have sore white patches, see your dentist for an examination. Your dentist will study both the state of your jaw and the condition of your dentures and gums.

Treatment

Your dentist may be able to adjust your dentures to relieve the pressure on your gums or, if necessary, make a new set of dentures that conform to the current shape of your bones and gums. If your gums are red and swollen because of a fungal infection, your dentist can prescribe an antifungal medication.

If your jaw has shrunk and your dentist has trouble making dentures that will fit well, several surgical techniques are now available that may provide a better foundation upon which a new denture can be constructed. These techniques include operations to build up the soft tissue of your gum or hard tissue of your jaw. Sometimes a metallic support can be implanted in the bone.

Chapter 23

Your Heart and Blood Vessels

Contents

Your Healthy Heart and Blood Vessels, 633
Parts of Your Heart, 633
The Cardiac Cycle, 634
The Vascular System, 634
Listen to Your Heartbeat, 634
Disorders of the Heart and Blood Vessels, 635
Congenital Heart Disease, 635

Disease of the Heart and Blood Vessels: Living With the Risks, 635
Atherosclerosis: What Is It? 636
Chelation Therapy, 637
Controllable Risk Factors, 638
Cholesterol and Dietary Fats, 639
Limitations of Home Cholesterol Testing, 639
What Do Measurements of Blood Fats Mean? 640
Diet and Blood Fat Levels: What You Eat Can Make a Difference, 641
Drugs for Treatment of Abnormal Blood Fat Levels and Atherosclerosis, 642
Obesity, 643
Diabetes, 643
Lifestyle, 643
Uncontrollable Risks, 644

Cardiovascular Fitness, 644
Aerobic and Anaerobic Exercise, 645
How Challenging Should My Workouts Be? 645
How to Measure Your Pulse, 645
How Often Do I Need to Work Out? 646
What Is the Best Kind of Exercise? 646
Walking and Aerobic Exercise, 647
Just Starting Out? 647
Warm Up and Cool Down, 647

High Blood Pressure, 647
The Newest Classification and What It Means, 648
Normal Blood Pressure, 648
Causes of High Blood Pressure, 648
How to Take Your Own Blood Pressure, 649

Complications of High Blood Pressure, 650
Hypotension, 650
Isolated Systolic Hypertension, 651
Drug Treatments for High Blood Pressure, 651
Establishing Your Drug Therapy, 652
What You Can Do for Your Hypertension, 653

Coronary Artery Disease, 654
Common Diagnostic Tests, 654
The Exercise Tolerance Test, 655
Scans and Coronary Angiogram, 656
Angina Pectoris, 657
Congestive Heart Failure, 659
Pulmonary Edema, 660
Heart Attack, 661
The Coronary Care Unit, 662
Aspirin: Does It Prevent Heart Attacks? 663
Cardiopulmonary Resuscitation (CPR), 664
Coronary Artery Bypass Surgery, 665
Coronary Angioplasty, 666
Sexual Activity After a Heart Attack, 667
Cardiac Rehabilitation, 668

Disorders of Heart Rate and Rhythm, 669
Heart Arrhythmias, 669
Sick Sinus Syndrome, 670
Twenty-Four-Hour Cardiac Monitoring and Event Recording, 671
Internal Cardioverter-Defibrillator, 672
Heart Block, 672
Electrophysiologic Testing, 673
Sudden Cardiac Death, 674
Fainting Spells, 674
Artificial Cardiac Pacemakers, 675
Medications for Rhythm Control of Your Heart, 676

Disorders of the Heart Valves, 677
Rheumatic Fever, 677
Infective Endocarditis, 678
Infective Endocarditis: Protection and Prevention, 679

Mitral Valve Problems, 680
Heart Valve Valvuloplasty, 681
Mitral Valve Prolapse, 682
Aortic Valve Problems, 682
The Echocardiogram: Images Made With Sound, 683
Heart Valve Surgery, 684
Tricuspid and Pulmonary Valve Problems, 685

Diseases of the Heart Muscle and Pericardium, 686
Cardiomyopathy, 686
Myocarditis, 687
Pericarditis, 687
Heart Transplantation, 688

Circulatory Problems, 690
Arteriosclerosis of the Extremities, 690
Risk Factors for Arteriosclerosis of the Extremities (Intermittent Claudication), 691
Gangrene of the Extremities, 692
Arterial Embolism, 692
Aortic Aneurysm, 693
Thrombophlebitis, 694
Varicose Veins, 695
Lymphedema, 695
The Value of Support Stockings, 696
Raynaud's Disease, 697
Buerger's Disease, 698
Frostbite, 698

Your Healthy Heart and Blood Vessels

For generations, poets have endowed the human heart with a wide range of emotional abilities. Yet the plain truth is a good deal simpler: the heart is a pump—no more, no less.

But it is an extraordinary pump. Every minute of your life, your heart beats approximately once a second, and considerably more often when you are exercising. It weighs only about a pound but manages to pump 5 or more quarts per minute. In a single day, your heart will pump about 2,000 gallons of blood through your circulatory system.

When functioning normally, your heart pumps blood to the tissues to provide the cells with the oxygen and nutrients they need. This circulatory system consists of arteries and veins. The arteries take the blood to the tissues; the veins bring it back to the heart to be cycled through the lungs before it is returned to the tissues.

When the pumping of your heart, and the resultant circulation of the blood, is interrupted for more than a few minutes, life ends. In fact, all too often the first sign of heart disease is sudden death. It is for this reason that in recent years so much emphasis has been given to prevention (see Disease of the Heart and Blood Vessels: Living With the Risks, page 635).

Parts of Your Heart

The heart actually has two pumps. Each pump consists of a pair of chambers formed of muscles. It is the contraction of these muscles that causes the blood to be pumped. In each pump, the lower chamber is called a ventricle and the upper chamber is called an atrium. The four chambers of the heart are separated by valves.

The tissue of the heart consists of three layers. The exterior layer is the thin epicardium. In the middle is the myocardium, the heart muscle itself (from the Greek *myo* for "muscle" and *kardia* for "heart"). The inner lining of the heart is the endocardium, a thin, smooth structure. Protecting the whole package is the pericardium, a fibrous sac with a very smooth lining. In the space between the pericardium and the epicardium there is a small amount of fluid.

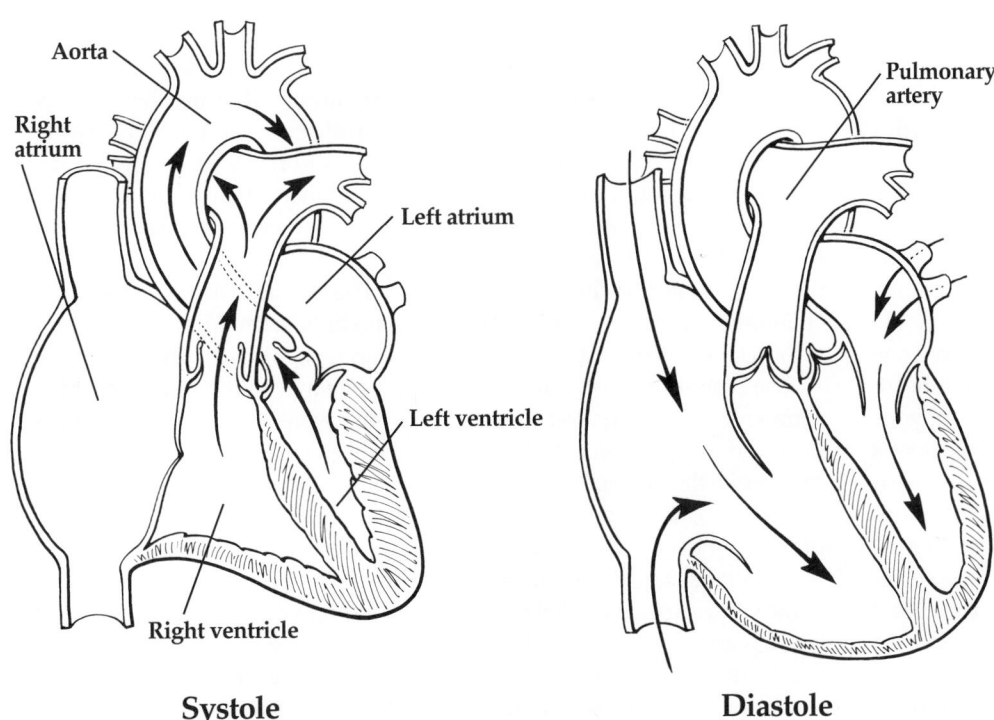

Systole

Diastole

The heart pumps in two stages. The ventricles contract during systole to pump blood out; they relax during diastole so that blood can reenter the heart.

The Cardiac Cycle

The blood entering the right side of the heart is returning from the tissues and has been delivered by the veins. The receiving chamber is the right atrium. This atrium also is a low-pressure pump, and it moves the blood into the right ventricle through the tricuspid valve.

The right ventricle has thicker, stronger walls than the right atrium. The right ventricle pumps the oxygen-poor blood through the pulmonic valve into the lungs, where the blood gives up the carbon dioxide it has carried from the tissues. At the same time, the blood is absorbing oxygen. The pumping action moves the blood from the lungs to the receiving chamber on the other side of the heart, the left atrium, which pumps the blood into the left ventricle through the mitral valve. The left ventricle exerts a powerful pumping action to send the oxygen-enriched blood into the aorta, the principal artery that subdivides and delivers the blood to the body's tissues, including the brain, organs, and extremities.

The contraction of the ventricles of the heart that forces blood out is called systole; the relaxation of the ventricles to allow blood to enter is diastole. The right and left chambers contract and relax simultaneously.

The rate at which the heart pumps varies, depending on the body's activities at the moment. When you are at rest, your heart pumps more slowly; when you run or climb stairs, the pace of your heart increases to provide your muscles and other tissues with the additional oxygen they need.

The typical heart rate is 72 beats per minute, and at each beat 2 to 3 ounces of blood is pumped into the arterial system. At this rate, the heart beats 104,000 times daily.

The Vascular System

The vascular system consists of the blood vessels in your body; its name comes from the Latin *vasculum* for "small blood vessel."

The vessels become smaller as they extend farther from the heart. The aorta delivers

Listen to Your Heartbeat

For most of us, the feel of the cold stethoscope on our chest is familiar. Less familiar is the bass-drum thumping your physician hears through the other end of that hearing device. The interpretation of that drumbeat can provide your physician with considerable knowledge about your heart and your health.

When listening to your heart, your physician will ask you to breathe in and out naturally or perhaps in a deliberately rhythmic fashion. He or she will move the stethoscope in small steps from one location to another over your heart.

During this examination, your physician can interpret the sounds he or she hears. The normal heartbeat has a consistent pattern represented by the syllables "lubb" and "dubb." These sounds correspond to closure of the heart valves. "Lubb" is followed by a short pause; "dubb" is followed by a longer pause. Differences in the

intensity of these heart sounds may provide clues to disease involving your heart or lungs. Obesity, emphysema, or fluid around the heart may seem to muffle the heart's pumping sounds.

Other sounds also may be detected. Murmurs are the result of turbulence in the blood during the heartbeat. Depending on the location, the character, and the relationship of the murmur to the lubb-dubb sounds, your physician often can identify the structural change in the heart valve that is responsible for the turbulence.

The presence of abnormal sounds (known as gallop sounds) during the relaxation phase (diastole) while the ventricles are filling suggests an alteration in the function of the heart muscle. Sounds heard during contraction (systole) of the ventricles, called clicks, combined with a murmur identify specific types of valve alterations.

A murmur may be a symptom

of anemia, a leaky valve, or a heart infection such as endocarditis (see Infective Endocarditis, page 678). In children, murmurs that are not the result of a structural abnormality often are heard. Called innocent murmurs, these typically are very faint, often are heard only intermittently, and usually are detected in only a small area of the chest. Innocent murmurs are harmless and often disappear by adulthood.

The echocardiogram (see The Echocardiogram: Images Made With Sound, page 683) has improved the physician's ability to interpret the significance of what he or she hears through the stethoscope by allowing comparison of what is heard to the actual flow of blood through the various compartments of the heart.

When your physician listens to your heartbeat, he or she is gathering clues to the health of your heart or to understanding what ails it.

blood to the large arteries; they, in turn, branch off several times and eventually blood flows into smaller vessels called arterioles. The arterioles supply the tiny capillaries that nourish tissues. Oxygen is given up from capillaries to the tissues, and carbon dioxide from the tissues is taken up into the capillaries. The arteries have to be strong as well as flexible because of the pressure of the blood being pumped through them.

From the capillaries, the blood begins its trip back to the heart by way of the venous system. The veins increase in size closer to the heart. As part of circulation, the blood travels through the liver and kidneys, which remove waste products. The veins, under less pressure, are less muscular and less elastic than the arteries.

Disorders of the Heart and Blood Vessels

Because of the constant activity of the heart and blood vessels, there is a wide range of potential problems and disorders. The two most common disorders are coronary artery disease (see Coronary Artery Disease, page 654), the principal cause of heart attack, and hypertension (see High Blood Pressure, page 647). Yet there are other kinds of problems that can affect the health of the valves (see Disorders of the Heart Valves, page 677), the heart muscle (see Diseases of the Heart Muscle and Pericardium, page 686), the rhythm of the heart (see Disorders of Heart Rate and Rhythm, page 669), or the ability of your blood vessels to circulate the blood to your tissues (see Circulatory Problems, page 690). Some problems, called congenital, are present at birth; others occur as the result of infection, hereditary factors, problems with the action of thyroid hormone on your heart, lung diseases that affect your heart, or trauma.

In the following pages, we will consider individually several dozen heart and blood vessel disorders, as well as some of the remarkable advances made in recent years in diagnosis and treatment for heart and circulatory problems. (Certain congenital heart ailments are discussed elsewhere in this book; see Congenital Heart Disorders, page 51.) But before considering the problems, it is important to understand something about the basic interaction between the lives we lead and our health.

What we eat, our exercise patterns, whether we smoke, and a number of other lifestyle considerations have an impact on the health of our hearts as well as on other organ systems. So we will begin with the risk factors for coronary artery disease and what we can do to use that knowledge for longer, healthier lives.

Your primary care physician may treat some heart and circulatory disorders. However, your physician may refer you to a cardiologist, a specialist who has had additional training in the diagnosis and management of heart and blood vessel disorders.

Congenital Heart Disease

There is a range of minor to serious heart ailments that are evident at or shortly after birth. Some involve malformations of the heart itself, and some involve malformations involving major vessels connecting the lungs and heart. (For a detailed discussion of Congenital Heart Disorders, see page 51.)

Disease of the Heart and Blood Vessels: Living With the Risks

Whether you are 80 years old and have survived a heart attack or are 18 years old and have no signs of heart disease, a sensible strategy of avoiding, minimizing, or living with the various risk factors for cardiovascular disease may be important to your future.

Our century has seen a rapid increase in the prevalence of cardiovascular disease. Today it is the leading cause of death in the United States, accounting for more than 950,000 deaths a year. Approximately 60 million Americans have some form of cardiovascular disease.

The positive side of the recognition that cardiovascular disease is our principal killer is that a tremendous amount of research has been and is being done on understanding, treating, and, perhaps most important, preventing heart disease in its various forms.

Since World War II, many scientists have been investigating the cause-and-effect relationships between our behavior, genes, and aging processes and the ways our hearts function (or malfunction). The Multiple Risk Factor Intervention Trial, the Framingham Heart Study, and many others have brought us to a new level of understanding.

The findings are persuasive. A remarkably high percentage of heart attack victims have a history of exposure to certain risk factors. A risk factor is a behavior or condition that places you at greater risk of having a disease than if you were not exposed. The fact is that people with high blood pressure, smokers, diabetics, and those who consume quantities of foods high in fats are more likely to have a heart attack than are those who avoid those risk factors.

Your sex, age, and heredity are other factors that also are in the equation. Rarely, acute, overwhelming stress can also result in a heart-related death (see Sudden Cardiac Death, page 674). In general, however, chronic stress probably does not cause coronary artery disease, although it can make you feel that life is not worth living. Contrary to earlier ideas, there does not appear to be any specific type of personality or behavior that predisposes you to coronary artery disease.

The good news is that both the prevalence of coronary artery disease and deaths from coronary artery disease have significantly decreased since the mid-1960s. Some of this decrease is associated with a decline in risk factors.

As you read the discussions of risk factors that follow, remember that they are to be considered together rather than separately. In fact, the different risks have a multiplier effect on one another. One finding of the Multiple Risk Factor Intervention Trial conducted by the National Heart, Lung, and Blood Institute makes the point effectively. According to this study, of about 13,000 white men between 30 and 60 years old, only 2 percent had a heart attack if they kept their cholesterol and blood pressure levels within reasonable limits and did not smoke. If one of these behavior controls was abandoned, the risk of heart attack increased to 5 percent; two risk factors produced an increase to 10 percent; and among those who smoked and failed to maintain healthy cholesterol and blood pressure levels, 20 percent had a heart attack.

There are few absolute answers, however. There are conflicting findings. Some studies suggest that there are causal relationships between certain dietary habits or laboratory findings and heart attacks; others conclude that the evidence is not so clear-cut. Yet, one message is paramount: how you live your life may have an important impact on your cardiovascular health.

In the following pages we will discuss the key risk factors. They are divided into two categories: those that you can do something about and those that you cannot change, such as having a parent who experienced a heart attack at an early age. However, recognizing the uncontrollable risk factors can be valuable. If you know your risks are high, you can take special measures in regard to the other risk factors that you can control.

Atherosclerosis: What Is It?

Healthy arteries are like healthy muscles. They are flexible, strong, and elastic. Their inside lining is smooth so that the flow of blood through them is unrestricted.

Atherosclerosis describes the condition in which fatty deposits accumulate in and under the lining of the artery walls. The name comes from the Greek word *ather*, meaning "porridge," because the fatty deposits are soft and resemble porridge.

Blood cells called platelets often clump at microscopic sites of injury to the inner wall of the artery. At these sites, fat deposits also collect. Initially, the deposits are only streaks of fat-containing cells but, as they enlarge, they invade some of the deeper layers of the arterial walls, causing scarring and calcium deposits. Larger accumulations are called atheromas or plaques and are the principal characteristic of atherosclerosis.

The greatest danger from these deposits is the narrowing of the channel through which the blood flows. When this occurs, the tissues (heart muscle, brain, muscles of the legs, or others) that the artery supplies will not receive their full quota of blood. Pieces of the fatty deposits also may be dislodged, travel with the blood flow, and finally obstruct an artery at some distant point (see Arterial Embolism, page 692).

The term arteriosclerosis means hardening of the arteries (from the Greek *sklerosis* for "hardening"). This often accompanies atherosclerosis and is not clearly separated from it. The walls of the artery become more rigid and often contain calcium deposits. Sometimes, the arteries in the forearms can be felt and may resemble small, hard pipes. In combination with atherosclerosis, arteriosclerosis also may lead to weakening and enlargement of an artery, a condition called an aneurysm (see page 693).

Atherosclerosis may be discovered in the course of a routine physical examination. During your physician's stethoscope examination of your neck, abdomen, or groin area, he or she may hear a blowing sound (a bruit) if a narrowing and roughening of the lining of the arteries at one or more of these points causes turbulence of the blood flow. He or she also will estimate the amount of blood flow by feeling for pulsations in the arteries at the wrists, legs, and feet. A decrease in pulsations is a reason to suspect partially obstructed blood flow.

More elaborate tests of circulation using sound waves often help in establishing the presence and degree of decreased blood flow (see Ultrasonography, page 1335). A CT scan or ultrasound scan of the abdomen (see CT Scanning, page 1334) often is used to identify a suspected aneurysm of the aorta in the abdomen.

Another test for locating the sites of plaques that narrow blood vessels is arteriography. In this test, a dye that shows on X-rays is injected into a catheter inserted through an artery in the groin, and several X-rays of the organ or limb are taken. In many cases, the diagnosis is not suspected until the artery is completely obstructed and you have experienced a stroke, heart attack, or arterial thrombosis in some other organ or extremity.

To some extent, the body can protect itself from narrowing of a particular artery by developing, with time, additional arterial connections that detour blood around the narrowed point. This is called collateral circulation.

If you have a significant amount of atherosclerosis in one part of your body, you are more likely to have some degree of impairment of arterial circulation in another part. For instance, the person who has poor arterial circulation in the legs may be vulnerable to angina or a heart attack because of some narrowing of the coronary arteries.

The details as to how atherosclerosis can

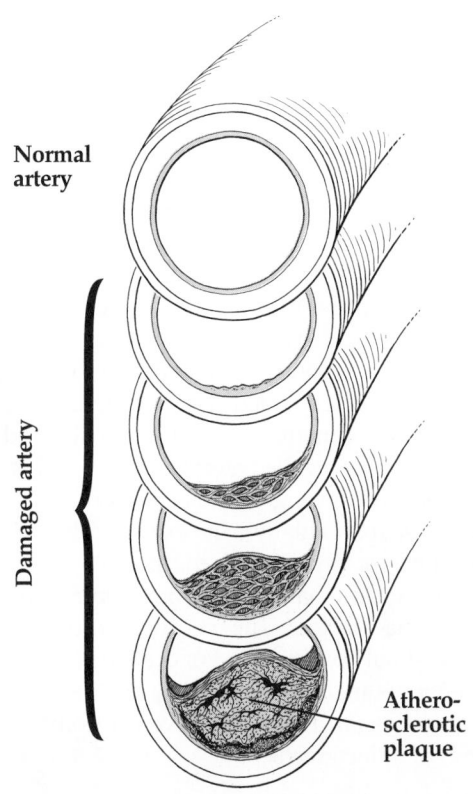

Normal artery

Damaged artery

Athero-sclerotic plaque

In atherosclerosis, plaque deposits gradually build up in the lining of the arteries. As plaque accumulates, blood circulation decreases. This increases the risk of heart attack, stroke, and other serious vascular problems.

cause difficulty will be described in the sections on stroke (see page 461), coronary artery disease (see page 654), and arteriosclerosis (see page 690).

Chelation Therapy

You may have heard the sales pitch: chelation therapy is a kind of chemical Roto-Rooter that can clear obstructing plaques from your arteries.

The truth is that although chelation therapy has its uses—for example, for ridding your body of toxic amounts of minerals or heavy metals—it has not been proved to be of value in treating arteriosclerosis, atherosclerosis, or other cardiovascular disorders.

Nevertheless, there are clinics across the country that make such claims. Chelating agents (the name comes from the Greek word meaning "claw") are able to attach themselves to some toxic substances. One agent, called edetate disodium (EDTA), proponents say, can bind to the calcium in the plaque in your arteries and then remove it. The treatment cycles typically involve 30 to 40 sessions over a number of weeks during which EDTA is administered intravenously. The cost usually runs to several thousand dollars.

We strongly advise against this "therapy." Neither your insurance company nor Medicare will pay for it. It is of no proven worth in preventing or treating cardiovascular disorders. In addition, it can be hazardous. Serious kidney complications and even death have resulted in some cases.

Controllable Risk Factors

Several factors may contribute to the development of atherosclerosis. These risk factors exert their effects over a period of years. High blood pressure has a multiplying effect on the harm of an increased cholesterol level. Keeping the blood pressure under control by limiting salt consumption and taking prescribed medications regularly lessens the chance of significant atherosclerosis developing. Smoking is a very strong promoter of atherosclerosis and is to be avoided. Diabetes accelerates the development of atherosclerosis and should be controlled as closely as possible. Obesity has an aggravating effect on atherosclerosis, particularly if the excess body fat is located mainly around the middle of the body. You can have at least some control over all of these factors. The precautions you take now should be continued over a long time or, better yet, indefinitely. Avoid all of these risk factors as far as possible, even if doing so might be inconvenient.

High Blood Pressure

Hypertension is the term physicians use for high blood pressure. This term does not describe a state of emotional tension, and the term should not be applied to brief increases in blood pressure such as those that occur with exercise or stress.

There are many causes of high blood pressure and many effective treatments; both are discussed at length later in this chapter (see High Blood Pressure, page 647).

High blood pressure is an important risk factor for heart disease (see pages 650 and 654). Over a period of years, high blood pressure can damage the arteries throughout the body so that the artery walls become thickened and stiff, a condition called arteriosclerosis. In persons with high concentrations of fats in their blood, fatty deposits will further narrow the arteries (see Atherosclerosis: What Is It? page 636).

The result of this arterial damage is a decrease in blood flow to vital organs such as the brain, heart, and kidneys. The body responds to this threat by increasing blood pressure to maintain an adequate flow of blood. This increase in blood pressure will lead to further blood vessel damage, and thus a vicious cycle is set in motion. This cycle exacts a toll on your heart, too, because it is forced to work harder. In some cases, the size of the heart muscle actually increases to accommodate its added load, a condition called cardiac hypertrophy. High blood pressure may eventually lead to congestive heart failure and even heart attack (see Congestive Heart Failure, page 659, and Heart Attack, page 661).

A typical blood pressure reading is 120/80 millimeters of mercury (mm Hg). This means that the heart is creating a maximum pressure of 120 mm Hg during its pumping effort (systole); when it is at rest between beats (diastole), the blood pressure is 80 mm Hg (see How to Take Your Own Blood Pressure, page 649).

There is considerable disagreement on what value represents the beginning of high blood pressure, but there is some agreement that if you consistently have a reading of 140/90 mm Hg or higher you have high blood pressure (see The Newest Classification and What It Means, page 648).

It is estimated that as many as 50 million Americans have high blood pressure, undiagnosed in many of them. The disorder has no evident symptoms. Having high blood pressure will not make you feel more nervous or tense; nor will it cause headache or nosebleeds (except in some very exceptional circumstances). In many cases, the problem is discovered during a physical examination when your health care provider routinely measures your blood pressure. Often there is no identifiable cause, although in some cases an association can be made with a family history of hypertension, kidney disease, or, in those sensitive to it, a high consumption of salt.

However, even if you have normal blood pressure, if you have close relatives who do have high blood pressure you would do well to limit your use of salt and to avoid weight gain. Have your blood pressure measured at least once a year.

Rarely, hypertension may be the result of a tumor of the adrenal gland (see page 937) or of an abnormality of the arteries that supply blood to a kidney (see Kidney Disease, page 650). However, in 95 percent of cases, high blood pressure has no identifiable cause. This form is termed "essential" hypertension.

There are many effective treatments for high blood pressure. In fact, the long-term complications that affect the kidneys, eyes, brain, and heart can be avoided with proper care, which may include drugs, cessation of smoking, reduction of salt, alcohol, and fat intake, and other strategies (see pages 651 and 653).

Smoking

About three decades ago, the Surgeon General of the United States announced that smoking cigarettes is a health hazard. Subsequently, a printed warning of the hazards of smoking was required on every package of cigarettes sold in the United States. In the years since, that warning has been made more emphatic—and an immense amount of clinical, statistical, and other research has reinforced the original point.

Smoking is bad for you—not only because of the association between smoking and lung cancer but also because smoking is near the top of the list of risk factors for heart disease. Smoking doubles the risk of sudden cardiac death (see page 674). It increases the risk of heart attack (see page 661). If a smoker stops smoking, the risk of heart attack returns to that of a nonsmoker within about 2 years.

Smoking a cigarette causes your adrenal glands to secrete a hormone that temporarily increases your blood pressure and makes your heart work harder. Smoking decreases the amount of oxygen available to your heart. As a result, every cigarette places a small but unnecessary load on your heart and blood vessels.

Smokers also have more atherosclerosis than nonsmokers do. This is probably because smoke increases the clumping of platelets and, through a series of steps, this clumping is a stimulus for the deposit of cholesterol in the arteries. Over time, smoking—especially in combination with other factors—can exact a significant toll.

Tobacco smoke contains carbon monoxide gas. When inhaled, the carbon monoxide binds to the hemoglobin in the blood, taking the place of valuable oxygen. The result is that the blood traveling to all parts of your body has less oxygen to deliver to your cells. Often, as much as 8 percent of a smoker's hemoglobin may be occupied by carbon monoxide and thus is unable to carry out its normal function of transporting oxygen.

Other research suggests that carbon monoxide also may have a direct, degenerative effect on the heart muscle itself, on the blood vessels, and perhaps even on the clotting of your blood. Low-tar, low-nicotine cigarettes also form carbon monoxide and thus cannot be considered to be safe (see Low-Tar, Low-Nicotine Cigarettes, page 318).

Because the process of atherosclerosis is accelerated with both high blood pressure and smoking, probably as a result of the harmful effects of nicotine and carbon monoxide on blood vessels, a smoker who has high blood pressure is at much greater risk of atherosclerosis.

Recent research suggests that there is a risk to nonsmokers from "passive" or "secondhand" smoking, the inhalation of tobacco smoke from nearby smokers. Even if you are not actually smoking, the presence of the smoke in the air around you can cause heart disease (see Secondhand Smoke, page 320).

The bottom line is simple: you will be doing your health a favor if you quit smoking and avoid places where there is tobacco smoke. The cumulative effect of smoking on your lungs, heart, and vascular system argues convincingly for quitting. (For specific advice on how to go about breaking the tobacco habit, see How to Stop Smoking, page 321.)

Cholesterol and Dietary Fats

We should all be aware of our blood cholesterol concentration because it may have a strong influence on whether we will, at some time, experience one of the complications of atherosclerosis. These include coronary artery disease with angina or a heart attack (myo-

---

Limitations of Home Cholesterol Testing

A home cholesterol test is convenient, inexpensive ($15 to $25), and may alert you to a high cholesterol problem, but a laboratory test ordered by your physician is more complete and accurate. Home tests have these limitations:

- They measure only total cholesterol. They don't measure high-density lipoprotein (HDL) cholesterol or low-density lipoprotein (LDL) cholesterol. Even if your level of total cholesterol is in the desired range, low HDL cholesterol increases your risk for cardiovascular disease.
- They are less sophisticated than laboratory tests. Results may be misleading if you have a disorder such as chronic liver disease or multiple myeloma that causes abnormalities of lipoproteins.

Frequent testing of your cholesterol usually isn't necessary, unless you have high cholesterol. The National Cholesterol Education Program recommends routine testing every 5 years.

cardial infarction) (see page 661), stroke (see page 461), and arteriosclerosis obliterans (see page 690).

If any of your blood relatives has or had a high cholesterol level, a heart attack, or stroke at an early age, you have a greater chance of having difficulties from atherosclerosis. Coronary artery disease tends to develop earlier in men than women. There is nothing you can do to change your heredity or gender, but you can take the precautions of having your blood cholesterol measured from time to time, of following a prudent, preventive diet, of controlling your weight, and of avoiding tobacco.

The problem of abnormal blood fat values is often discussed solely under the designation "cholesterol." Actually, several blood fats ordinarily are measured—namely, total cholesterol, high-density lipoprotein (HDL) cholesterol, low-density lipoprotein (LDL) cholesterol, and triglycerides. Knowing the levels of these blood fats will help your physician to identify abnormal states, to plan treatment, and to monitor the results of treatment. Still another test, called a lipoprotein profile, may be used to identify some of the uncommon blood fat abnormalities.

Serum total cholesterol and HDL cholesterol values may vary somewhat from day to day, or even from laboratory to laboratory. Tests done on blood obtained from the finger are more likely to give an erroneous result than are those done on blood obtained from a vein in the arm. Do not conclude that you have abnormal blood fats on the basis of a single measurement. Nor should you be completely reassured. Before coming to any conclusion, either that you do or do not have a problem, get at least two sets of measurements that are in essential agreement with each other.

Triglyceride (TG) values vary more widely than do total or HDL cholesterol values. Alcohol use and poorly controlled diabetes tend to increase the triglyceride levels.

If a direct blood measurement is unavailable, LDL cholesterol can be calculated from the three primary measurements by the formula

LDL cholesterol =
total cholesterol - (HDL cholesterol + TG/5)

However, direct blood measurement is more accurate (see Limitations of Home Cholesterol Testing, page 639).

What Do Measurements of Blood Fats Mean?

One test is not enough. Blood fats (total cholesterol, HDL cholesterol, LDL cholesterol, and triglycerides) should be measured on two or more occasions. Wide differences in results suggest a laboratory error.

Once you have two sets of values that are in agreement, how do you evaluate these numbers?

The National Cholesterol Program published the following guidelines in 1993 for the use of total cholesterol measurements. In individuals free of coronary artery disease, a desirable total cholesterol is designated as less than 200 mg/100 mL. If your value is in this range, you need to have measurements made only at 5-year intervals. Borderline-high cholesterol is in the range 200 to 239 mg/100 mL; dietary measures are advised for

those whose value is in this range. If, in addition, you have some of the other risk factors for coronary artery disease or are known to have coronary artery disease, you will need further studies and perhaps your physician will advise more stringent dietary restrictions (see page 641) and possibly drug therapy (see page 642).

High total cholesterol is 240 mg/100 mL or above. Drug therapy may be advised if this value remains above 240 mg/100 mL in spite of dietary efforts.

High-risk LDL cholesterol is greater than 160 mg/dL, borderline high-risk LDL cholesterol is from 130 to 159 mg/dL, and desirable LDL cholesterol is less than 130 mg/dL. It is generally recommended that persons with known

coronary artery disease have an LDL cholesterol of less than 100 mg/dL.

An HDL cholesterol level of less than 35 mg/dL, even if you have a normal total cholesterol level, may be an indication for further treatment, including exercise and weight loss initially. If there is no response, drug treatment may be recommended.

A family history of coronary artery disease, or the presence of it, and other risk factors are issues that physicians consider in evaluating older persons. Regardless of age, smoking cessation and control of diabetes and high blood pressure should be attempted before any medication for treatment of high blood fat levels, such as total cholesterol, is started.

The LDL cholesterol value roughly parallels the total cholesterol value. High values for these two categories are an indication that you may be vulnerable to atherosclerosis. In simple terms, the LDL cholesterol can be thought of as contributing to atherosclerosis in the same manner that hard water can cause a buildup of lime inside pipes—it is a simple matter of the cholesterol depositing into and onto the lining of the blood vessel.

Diet and Blood Fat Levels: What You Eat Can Make a Difference

To decrease a high blood fat level, start with dietary changes. If your triglyceride level is significantly high, avoid alcohol. If you are overweight, trim down. Try to achieve a distinctly lean weight. Avoid simple sugars such as syrups, table sugar, and sugar-sweetened soft drinks.

If your primary problem is an increase in total or LDL cholesterol, avoid foods that are high in cholesterol and saturated fats (they are often the same), decrease the total amount of fat in your diet, and increase the amount of complex carbohydrates (cereals, vegetables). How stringent your attempts are to do this and the details of how you can change your diet should be determined by your physician working together with a registered dietitian.

Know Your Fats
Some oils, such as palm and coconut oil, contain no cholesterol because they are of vegetable origin, but they tend to promote atherosclerosis because they are largely saturated. Hence, the statement "No Cholesterol" on a food label does not necessarily mean that the food is a good choice if your cholesterol value is high.

The process of hydrogenating an oil (such as making margarine from corn oil or safflower oil, or treating peanut butter so that the oil will not separate) will convert some of the polyunsaturated fats to monounsaturated fats and, to a lesser extent, saturated forms. The change to saturated forms increases somewhat their tendency to cause atherosclerosis. On the other hand, usually only a small proportion of the polyunsaturated fat is converted to a saturated form, and the margarine of safflower or corn oil origin, for instance, can be used by persons with a high blood cholesterol value despite the label "hydrogenated."

There is no advantage to deliberately increasing the amount of polyunsaturated fats in your diet but, if you want to use an oil or fat as part of a recipe or dish on a menu, polyunsaturated or monounsaturated forms are preferable to saturated forms. While convenient, such generalizations are not always accurate. For example, stearic acid is a saturated fat found in meats but probably does not cause atherosclerosis. Thus, the relationship between diet and atherosclerosis is not an entirely simple matter.

Myths and Maybes
Folklore has it that garlic and onions are useful in controlling blood pressure and preventing heart attacks, but there is no evidence to support this.

Much has been said and written about the potential benefits of increasing the amount of fiber in the diet. Fiber takes many forms, however, and it is mainly the fiber derived from oat bran and the soluble fibers in guar gum (a filler in ice cream and some other foods) and pectin (found in fruits and vegetables) that may promote lowering of blood cholesterol. However, as a practical matter, it takes substantial amounts to cause a decrease in your cholesterol level (see page 286). Also, large amounts of fiber in the diet may bind and lessen the availability of calcium and some essential trace minerals. Calcium, in particular, is bound by the phytate in oat bran and is made unavailable.

No Magic Answers
Consuming fish oils containing a high proportion of omega-3 unsaturated fatty acids has been proposed as an easy way to lower the risk of heart attacks. Fish that have a higher proportion of such fat are found in colder waters—the most common examples are tuna and salmon. These oils tend to lower the blood triglyceride level. However, they may increase the total cholesterol level. When consumed in large amounts, such fish oils interfere with the function of blood platelets in starting the process of blood clotting. Eskimos in Greenland who consume large amounts of these oils appear to have fewer heart attacks but have more strokes than do Europeans. They also bruise easily and have a tendency to bleed excessively.

Because fish oils can be considered a food supplement, they escape the ordinary supervision given to drugs by the Food and Drug Administration. Various forms have been widely promoted. Some of these have contained large amounts of vitamins D and A, toxins, or chemical residues. We suggest that you incorporate fish into your diet when convenient and feasible, but avoid the use of capsules or other medicinal forms of fish oil.

HDL cholesterol, the so-called good cholesterol, can be thought of as a scavenger or "cleanup" form that decreases the amount of the undesirable form, LDL cholesterol. Higher values of HDL cholesterol mean a lower risk with respect to development of atherosclerosis. The HDL cholesterol level tends to increase with exercise and weight loss, but considerable amounts of exercise may be needed before definite results are seen. A low HDL cholesterol level may be an indication for treatment if weight loss and exercise fail.

Higher levels of triglycerides are thought to favor development of atherosclerosis, but this relationship is not nearly as clear as that for LDL cholesterol and total cholesterol values. (Some physicians think that the triglyceride level is of little significance in the development of atherosclerosis.). Very high levels of triglycerides can lead to pancreatitis (see page 818).

Drugs for Treatment of Abnormal Blood Fat Levels and Atherosclerosis

The decisions about the degree of dietary modification and whether or not to use a drug for correction of abnormal blood fat levels must be made by your physician, who knows all the aspects of your health. After treatment begins, your physician will monitor your blood fat levels with periodic blood tests to judge effectiveness of the treatment and to determine whether additional measures are needed (such as increasing the dose of or changing the medication).

The following are the principal medications used in lowering abnormally high levels of blood fats.

Cholestyramine and Colestipol
These two drugs are resins that bind bile acids in the intestinal tract, thereby causing the liver to increase its manufacture of bile acids. Because some of the same mechanisms are used to make cholesterol, less cholesterol is made. Like all medicines intended for control of blood fats, these must be used daily, for months and years, to have a favorable effect on atherosclerosis. These resins are somewhat unpleasant to take, are expensive, and tend to cause constipation and bloating.

Nicotinic Acid
Nicotinic acid is one of the vitamin B complex. When taken in amounts many times larger than needed for its vitamin function, it becomes a drug. It has a favorable effect on triglyceride, HDL cholesterol, and LDL cholesterol. It is inexpensive but has the drawbacks of causing flushing, changes in liver function test results, and a tendency toward diabetes. Taking an aspirin tablet 20 to 30 minutes before taking the nicotinic acid may lessen the flushing.

Gemfibrozil
This medication is more convenient to take and, like nicotinic acid, has a favorable effect on HDL cholesterol, triglycerides, and LDL cholesterol. It may have some adverse intestinal effects.

Probucol
Probucol also is convenient to take and lowers total cholesterol. However, it also lowers your HDL cholesterol level, and this is an undesirable effect.

Statins
Lovastatin, pravastatin, simvastatin, and fluvastatin are statins that directly interfere with the manufacture of cholesterol. Thus, these drugs are particularly effective in reducing total cholesterol and LDL cholesterol. Statins may also promote the resorption of cholesterol deposits, which would make possible the reversal of atherosclerosis. Recent studies have shown that these drugs can significantly reduce deaths from coronary artery disease.

Blood Fat Level and Blood Pressure Drugs
Blood fat level may have a bearing on the selection of a medicine to control high blood pressure. Thiazide diuretics tend to increase total cholesterol and triglycerides. They may decrease HDL cholesterol.

Some beta-adrenergic blockers may increase LDL cholesterol and triglycerides and decrease HDL cholesterol, all adverse effects. If LDL cholesterol increases and HDL cholesterol decreases, there may be no change in total cholesterol. Calcium antagonists and alpha-adrenergic blocking agents may have favorable effects on both LDL and HDL cholesterol.

Aspirin
Through its effects on blood platelet function, aspirin lessens the likelihood of clots to form. Your physician may advise its use if you are at risk for stroke or heart attack (see Aspirin: Does It Prevent Heart Attacks? page 663).

Is Age a Factor?
There is some suggestion that abnormal blood fat levels are somewhat less harmful in older persons. However, high values should not be neglected. Discuss a high cholesterol or other blood fat finding with your physician.

Hereditary factors can produce abnormal blood fat values. One rare hereditary disorder causes such high levels of cholesterol that the affected person may die of a heart attack in childhood. Those who inherit a lesser form of this disorder have very high cholesterol levels and often have heart attacks in mid-adult life or sooner. The trend to high triglyceride levels may also be in one's genetic makeup.

Associated diseases such as hypothyroidism (see page 948), poorly controlled diabetes (see page 925), and kidney failure (see page 852) may influence blood fat levels. Some medications such as beta-adrenergic blockers or thiazide diuretics used for hypertension may have an adverse effect. As a first step in treating high blood fat concentrations, it is necessary to identify and correct, as far as possible, any associated disease.

An exercise program emphasizing aerobic exercise is reasonable if the HDL cholesterol level is low (see Cardiovascular Fitness, page 644). Alcohol intake should be significantly reduced or stopped if the triglyceride level is high. Although some studies suggest a somewhat lower frequency of coronary artery disease among people who take one or two drinks a day than among teetotalers, one should not regard this as a reason to take those one or two drinks per day.

The decision to lower an elevated cholesterol level depends on an assessment of your risk of developing coronary artery disease or atherosclerosis.

Obesity

If your weight exceeds your ideal weight (see chart of ideal weights, page 259) by 20 percent or more, you are obese by most definitions. If you are very muscular, you may be an exception because the norms of the height and weight table are not for heavily muscled people with relatively little body fat.

Obesity is not a specific risk factor unless it is associated with or contributes to a high cholesterol level in the blood. In addition, obesity may be associated with other risk factors such as high blood pressure and diabetes. Overweight people tend to have lower levels of the "good" HDL cholesterol, and weight loss tends to increase the HDL cholesterol level.

In short, if you are overweight, you may be increasing your risk of coronary artery disease

and heart attack. A sensible program of dietary adjustment and exercise to reduce your weight can help you reduce your risks (see Weight Control, page 277).

Diabetes

Diabetes is characterized by a lack of insulin, resulting in the body's inability to process the sugars in the diet. The use of insulin or other antidiabetic drugs has made the disorder manageable, but diabetes remains an important risk factor for heart disease.

Increased blood sugar level often is accompanied by increased fat level, which leads to atherosclerosis (see page 929) and other blood vessel problems. Male diabetics have about twice the normal risk of coronary artery disease and female diabetics have a five times greater risk.

If you have diabetes, careful management of your blood sugar level must be a key component of your strategy to minimize heart and blood vessel problems. A combination of dietary measures, weight control, exercise, and insulin or other antidiabetic drugs can help (see Diabetes Mellitus, page 925). The person with diabetes who smokes is at particular risk. If you are a person with diabetes who smokes, it is doubly important that you quit (see page 639).

Lifestyle

If your lifestyle is sedentary—that is, if you get no regular exercise—you may be allowing your heart to become deconditioned. Like any muscle, the heart requires exercise to maintain its tone, endurance, and ability to circulate blood efficiently through your body.

As yet, there is no proof that exercise can prevent coronary artery disease. However, exercise does affect other risk factors. Regular exercise can help decrease your normal heart rate, lower your blood pressure, decrease the level of fats in your blood, and help you keep your weight down.

Keep in mind, however, that not all physical activities are equally beneficial. Aerobic exercise—that is, exercise that involves continuous, rhythmic movements such as running or swimming and which increases the rate and depth of your breathing—enhances heart health. Isometric exercises (like weightlifting) that do not increase breathing are not as helpful to the health of your heart, despite the benefits of increasing muscle strength and bulk (see Cardiovascular Fitness, this page).

Remember, too, that if you are over age 40, have had a heart attack, are obese or have diabetes, or have another serious disease, discuss any exercise program with your physician before embarking on it.

Uncontrollable Risks

Your gender, age, and genetics cannot be changed: they are part of what you are. Nevertheless, be aware of what these factors mean to you and your risk of heart disease.

Age

The aging process itself does not cause coronary artery disease, yet as you age your risk of heart attack and related disorders increases.

Gender

Men tend to develop heart disease earlier than women. However, over time women and men are equally likely to die of a heart attack.

After menopause women become increasingly likely to have heart attacks and other related problems. It is thought that the hormone estrogen has a protective effect, so that after its disappearance at menopause the risks increase. Estrogen tends to increase the HDL cholesterol and lower the LDL cholesterol levels (see Cholesterol and Dietary Fats, page 639). Thus, estrogen replacement therapy for osteoporosis may have a beneficial effect on preventing coronary artery disease after menopause as well.

Until puberty, boys and girls have roughly the same levels of HDL cholesterol. However, during puberty, the levels in men decrease, which may explain the difference in rate of coronary artery disease.

Middle-aged men are the most likely candidates for heart attack; after age 60, the difference in risk between men and women narrows. But, as our society has changed in recent years and as women's roles and behavior have changed (specifically, there has been an increase in smoking in women), women have shown an increased frequency of heart attack, especially at earlier ages.

Heredity

The subject of genetic inheritance is complex. In simple terms, if your father or another close relative had a heart attack at a young age, then your risk of coronary artery disease is significantly greater than that in someone whose family has no history of cardiac problems. In short, the tendency to coronary artery disease runs in families, so you and your physician should be interested in the health of your parents and other immediate relatives. The risk includes not only the risk from genetic inheritance but also the risk from other influences such as smoking and a high-fat diet.

But, if your father died prematurely of a sudden heart attack, you are not necessarily destined to suffer the same fate. This is simply another piece of information to help you decide how you want to live your life. It argues strongly, however, for taking every preventive advantage offered, especially dietary and exercise regimens intended to minimize risks you can control.

If you do not have a family history of heart disease, you can still have heart disease. Therefore, pay attention to controllable risk factors.

Cardiovascular Fitness

Your overall health can be enhanced by regular physical exercise. Whether you have the resilience of youth or are feeling the toll the years take, whether you are male or female, tall or short, rail-thin or heavyset, whether you love or avoid competition, your heart—and virtually all your body systems, including your muscles and bones—will serve you better if you get regular exercise. A program of exercise can help you lose excess weight, decrease tension, become physically stronger, and even feel better about yourself. In addition, it may decrease your risk of cardiovascular disease (see Exercise and Fitness, page 289).

By definition, cardiovascular exercise involves the heart (from the Greek *kardia*) and blood vessels (from the Latin *vasculum* for "small vessels"). It is exercise that strengthens your heart by making it pump harder. Your muscles increase their ability to use oxygen as well. More oxygen is supplied to the heart muscle itself. More oxygen also is delivered to your muscles and other tissues, and this increases your overall capacity for work. Over time, cardiovascular exercise will make your heart more efficient. Paradoxically, working the heart harder during exercise means it will beat more slowly while you are at rest or exercising.

Another good effect of exercise is that it increases the amount of "good" cholesterol, high-density lipoprotein (HDL) cholesterol, in your blood, which seems to protect against heart attack.

Aerobic and Anaerobic Exercise

Not all types of exercise are equal. Aerobic exercise enhances cardiovascular health. It is essentially "exercise with oxygen." See your physician before you begin such an active exercise program.

An aerobic workout is one that causes your body to use extra oxygen and calories continuously. Jogging, bicycling, swimming, and walking are good examples. They increase your rate and depth of breathing (you begin to puff). Your body becomes warm. If the exercise is sufficiently long and vigorous, you will perspire.

Anaerobic exercise can be healthful, too, but it does little for the health of your heart. Anaerobic exercise is intense exercise of short duration. Weight-lifting is a classic example: strong muscles may be the end result of a weight-lifting program, but lifting heavy barbells a few times offers little challenge to your heart and lungs to deliver oxygen in a sustained fashion to your body's tissues. Workouts with light weights of sufficient duration may be aerobic, as evidenced by increased breathing and perspiration.

How Challenging Should My Workouts Be?

There is a direct relationship between your heart rate and the intensity and duration of your exercise. The harder you exercise, the higher your heart rate (pulse) goes, until you reach your maximal heart rate.

Your physician can calculate a target heart rate for you. Your target heart rate is the rate at which you must exercise regularly and continuously for 20 to 30 minutes if you wish to achieve an increase in cardiorespiratory fitness. It will be lower than your maximal heart rate. Several techniques are used to calculate target heart rate and are based on fitness level, age, and personal interest in an exercise program. For example, exercising at approximately 70 percent of your age-adjusted maximum heart rate for 20 to 30 minutes three to five times a week will improve your fitness remarkably. Your age-adjusted maximum heart rate is calculated by subtracting your age from 220. For exam-

---

How to Measure Your Pulse

Knowing your pulse rate can help you evaluate an exercise program. If you are taking heart medications, recording your pulse and reporting the results to your physician can help him or her determine whether the drugs prescribed are effective. If you have had a pacemaker implanted in your chest, pulse rate is a key indicator of how it is functioning.

These are the steps for determining your pulse in the radial artery in your wrist:

1. Stop your exercise.

2. Using the tips of your index and third fingers, locate the area between your wrist bone and tendon on the thumb side of either wrist. You will feel the pulsing of the artery when you have positioned your fingers properly.

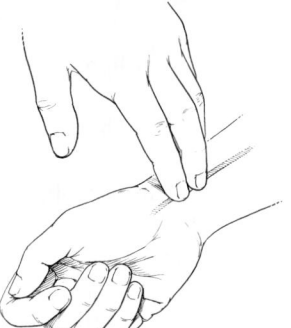

3. Make sure not to press so hard on the blood vessel that the flow of blood is obstructed.

4. Count your radial pulse for 10 seconds and then multiply by 6 for your pulse rate per minute.

ple, if you are age 50: 220 - 50 = 170; 70 percent of 170 = 119 beats a minute. (Note: Some persons with very irregular heart rates should not use the target heart rate method to regulate intensity of exercise.) (See How to Measure Your Pulse, page 645.)

The target heart rate calculation gives a heart rate that will fall somewhere within 50 to 80 percent of your exercise capacity. Some individuals with very irregular heart rates cannot use the heart rate method to regulate exercise intensity. In addition, certain medications such as beta-adrenergic blockers (see page 676) may interfere with this method.

Another way of judging how challenging your workout should be is through a rating of perceived exertion (see below). This refers to the total amount of physical effort experienced and takes into account sensations of exertion, physical stress, and fatigue. When using the rating scale, do not become preoccupied with any one factor, such as leg discomfort or labored breathing, but try to concentrate on your total inner feeling of exertion. A rating of 6 indicates a minimal level of exertion, such as sitting comfortably in a chair. A rating of 20 corresponds to a maximal effort—for example, jogging up a very steep hill.

Your physician will prescribe a specific perceived exertion range for you. A rating of 13 generally corresponds to 70 percent of maximal exercise capacity and would be considered near ideal for most people.

Another way of judging your workouts is the simple "talk test." During exercise you should be able to carry on a conversation with a companion. If you cannot do this, you are probably pushing too hard and should slow your exercise pace.

In general, if your exercise heart rate or perceived exertion rating is below the level recommended for you, you may increase your intensity. If your heart rate or perceived exertion level is above the recommended level, you should decrease your intensity. Additional fitness benefits gained from high-intensity exercise are small, and you increase the risk of muscle or joint soreness or injury.

A moderate exercise program should not cause discomfort. Stop exercising and consult your physician if you begin to have chest discomfort or pressure, severe shortness of breath, bursts of very rapid or slow heart rate, irregular heart rate, excessive fatigue, marked joint or muscle pain, dizziness, or fainting.

If you are just beginning, increase the duration and rate of your workout slowly over a period of 4 to 6 weeks. By monitoring your pulse rate, you can achieve this slow increase.

How Often Do I Need to Work Out?

The consensus among cardiologists is that at least three to five vigorous aerobic workouts per week are required to accomplish physical conditioning. Your heart rate should be in your target zone (70 to 80 percent of your age-adjusted maximum heart rate) for the duration of each workout. Each workout should last from 20 to 45 minutes. Include warm-up and cool-down activities (see Elements of Exercise, page 292).

It does not necessarily follow that this amount of exercise is enough to cause a readily measurable decrease in your total blood cholesterol level or an increase in HDL cholesterol. Nevertheless, an exercise program is likely to have some positive effects on your blood fat levels.

What Is the Best Kind of Exercise?

Ideally, you want an exercise program that involves continual activity but as little stress on your muscles and joints as possible. Walking, swimming, cycling, jogging, skating, and cross-country skiing are excellent. Tennis, basketball, and dancing can be aerobic, too, but each involves periods of inactiv-

Perceived Exertion Scale

Score	Perceived Exertion
6	
7	Very, very light
8	
9	Very light
10	
11	Fairly light
12	
13	Somewhat hard
14	
15	Hard
16	
17	Very hard
18	
19	Very, very hard
20	

ity, which decreases their aerobic value (see page 645).

Try to find a form of exercise that you enjoy; if you are bored at the end of the first week, you may not be able to keep at the exercise indefinitely. Establishing a consistent pattern of workouts is essential.

The intensity of exercise in any particular activity or sport can be judged by the increase in pulse rate and the general feeling of needing to breathe more heavily. The faster the pulse and breathing, the greater the intensity of the exercise. You can use walking at the rate of 3 to 4 miles per hour (a moderate degree of exercise) as your basis for comparison.

Walking and Aerobic Exercise

Walking appeals to many because it requires no special athletic skills. Best of all, it can be fun, convenient, and inexpensive and is a form of exercise that you can enjoy alone or with friends.

Walking briskly on a regular schedule improves your body's ability to consume oxygen during exertion. Thus, it can be an excellent form of aerobic exercise. It can help lower your resting heart rate and reduce your blood pressure. It helps burn calories.

To reap these benefits, you must walk briskly (raising your heart and breathing rates) for at least 20 to 30 minutes without interruption and regularly, at least three days each week (see Walking, page 297).

Just Starting Out?

If you are older than 40 years, sedentary, obese, diabetic, or a smoker, if you have hypertension, a kidney disorder, or other serious health problem, or if a close relative died of a heart attack before age 50, consult your physician before starting an exercise regimen. Your physician may have you undergo an exercise tolerance test (see page 655).

If at any time during a workout you experience chest pain, faintness, shortness of breath, or irregular heartbeat, stop your workout and consult your physician.

Warm Up and Cool Down

Each exercise session should open and close with some stretching exercises, perhaps easy jogging or walking. Your muscles, as well as your heart, need to be allowed to adjust to the change in pace (see Elements of Exercise, page 292).

High Blood Pressure

Throughout this book we identify medical disorders by giving their symptoms: this or that pain or shortness of breath suggests that you may have this or that ailment. With high blood pressure, however, that approach does not work.

Most affected persons have no symptoms. Even a physician cannot readily tell that you have high blood pressure until he or she actually measures the pressure by using an instrument called a sphygmomanometer (cuff and pressure gauge). Some think that headaches, dizziness, or nosebleeds are symptoms of high blood pressure, but this is not necessarily true.

"High blood pressure" and "hypertension" are interchangeable terms that refer to the fact that your blood is traveling through your arteries at a pressure that is too high for good health.

The incidence of high blood pressure increases with age. In addition, high blood pressure is more common in blacks than in whites. More men than women have high blood pressure in young adulthood and early middle age; thereafter the situation reverses.

Although high blood pressure generally is symptomless, this does not mean that it is not dangerous. High blood pressure has

The Newest Classification and What It Means

Don't be surprised if your physician no longer uses the terms "mild" or "moderate" to define hypertension. Here's the newest way to classify high blood pressure for healthy adults at least 18 years old:

Condition	Systolic (top number)	Diastolic (bottom number)	What to Do
Normal	Less than 130	Less than 85	Recheck in 2 years
High-normal	130-139	85-89	Recheck in 1 year
Hypertension			
Stage 1	140-159	90-99	Confirm within 2 months
Stage 2	160-179	100-109	See M.D. within a month
Stage 3	180-209	110-119	See M.D. within a week
Stage 4	210 or higher	120 or higher	See M.D. immediately

Note: Blood pressure conditions are based on the average of two or more readings taken at two different visits to your physician, in addition to the original screening visit.

been termed the "silent killer" because about 50 million Americans have it, but a third of them do not know they have it. The risk lies in the long-term damage the ailment can cause to your heart, brain, kidneys, and eyes, causing problems that can lead to major illnesses or even death.

There has been remarkable progress in detecting, treating, and controlling hypertension. During the past 20 years, there has been a substantial increase in the number of individuals who are aware of their hypertension and are taking medicine to control it. At the same time, the incidence of coronary artery disease and stroke has significantly decreased, partially as a result of progress in the detection, treatment, and control of high blood pressure.

Normal Blood Pressure

A typical normal blood pressure reading is 120/80 mm Hg. This means that the pressure in the arterial blood vessels is 120 mm Hg during the pumping phase of the heart (systolic pressure); when the heart is between beats, the blood pressure (diastolic pressure) is 80 mm Hg (for a discussion of blood pressure and how to take it, see How to Take Your Own Blood Pressure, page 649).

Blood pressure is determined by the amount of blood your heart pumps and the resistance to blood flow in the arteries (peripheral vascular resistance). Resistance to blood flow is affected by the diameter of the small arteries (arterioles). In general, the more blood the heart pumps and the smaller the arteries, the higher the blood pressure. A number of other things can influence these key factors and affect your blood pressure. In practice, a wide range of considerations enter into the equation. Blood pressure should be measured in a relaxed setting. A high reading should be confirmed with subsequent measurements during the next several weeks.

Your kidneys regulate the volume of water circulating in your body and the amount of salt your body contains. These two features have direct effects on your blood pressure. More salt in your body means that more water is being retained in your circulation and may cause an increase in blood pressure. More salt in your body also may increase the tendency for blood vessels to become narrow. Less salt means a trend to lower pressure. In someone who does not have high blood pressure, there is little effect on blood pressure over a wide range of salt intake. Other considerations are your nervous system, the blood vessels themselves (in particular, the smaller arteries called arterioles), and a number of hormones.

Causes of High Blood Pressure

The principal characteristic in most cases of high blood pressure is an increase in resistance to blood flow. This can occur if the diameter of your arterioles becomes smaller. Your heart has to work harder to pump the same amount of blood, and the pressure at which the blood is pumped increases.

How to Take Your Own Blood Pressure

If you have high blood pressure, monitoring your blood pressure can be a necessary part of your treatment. You can take your own blood pressure at home. Various devices, called sphygmomanometers, are available for measuring blood pressure. There are mechanical models with gauges and electronic ones with digital readouts. Discuss the purchase with your physician; he or she may recommend one model over another.

The most common model measures pressure without using mercury; this design measures the pressure in the cuff by its effect on a metal diaphragm. Another kind, a mercury gauge device, resembles a thermometer and consists of a vertical glass tube with a reservoir of mercury at the base. This is the kind used in many physicians' offices and hospitals. With either type, a rubber inflatable bladder encased in a cuff and a rubber squeeze bulb are the other constituent parts. A stethoscope may be attached or may be a separate element of the package.

The standard cuff fits most people. However, if you have a large

or a small arm, a special cuff may be necessary. If you purchase a blood pressure monitoring device, bring it to your physician and have it calibrated to make sure that it records blood pressure accurately. Recalibrate your blood pressure device every 6 to 9 months.

Do not take your blood pressure if you have a full bladder, have just consumed coffee, or have smoked a cigarette. These situations increase your blood pressure.

Sit quietly for 5 minutes before obtaining a blood pressure reading. Then follow these steps:

1. Position your arm at heart level, perhaps resting it on a tabletop or the arm of your chair. Right-handed people should measure the pressure in their left arm; left-handers do the reverse.

2. Apply the cuff of the sphygmomanometer to your bare upper arm. It should fit snugly, with its lower edge approximately 1 inch above the bend of your elbow.

3. Place the disc of the stethoscope face down under the cuff and immediately above the bend of your elbow (see illustration at right).

4. Squeeze the hand bulb rapidly. When the pressure gauge reading is 30 mm Hg above your anticipated systolic blood pressure, stop pumping. You should not hear any pulse sound.

5. Deflate the cuff slowly (the pressure should decrease approximately 2 to 3 mm Hg per second). As the pressure falls, listen for the pulse sound. Note the reading on the gauge when the beating first becomes audible: this is your systolic pressure (the highest pressure

produced by the contraction of your heart).

6. Continue deflating the cuff. Note the reading when the heartbeat can no longer be heard: this is your diastolic pressure (the lowest pressure reached during the relaxation of your heart).

7. Your blood pressure is written as systolic pressure/diastolic pressure.

8. Repeat the procedure at least one more time to confirm the accuracy of your reading.

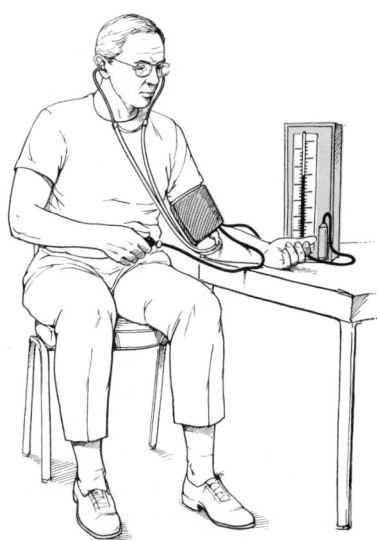

Proper position of the arm when obtaining a blood pressure reading using a mercury-gauge sphygmomanometer.

Electronic sphygmomanometers are becoming increasingly popular. They are more expensive but are easier to use because there is no stethoscope. A sensing device detects your pulse and transmits this information to an electronic chip. A digital readout provides your blood pressure reading.

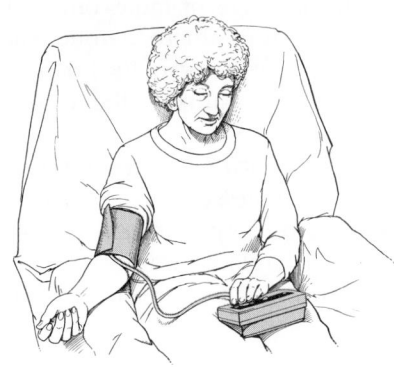

An electronic sphygmomanometer enables you to take your own blood pressure without the use of a stethoscope. Your blood pressure appears on a digital readout.

In general, the diagnosis of high blood pressure is made if your blood pressure is consistently 140/90 mm Hg or higher (see The Newest Classification and What It Means, page 648). Why it reaches or exceeds this level may not be identifiable. In fact, a specific disease or health problem is identified as the cause in fewer than 1 case in 20 of high blood pressure. When a cause cannot be determined, high blood pressure is categorized as essential hypertension.

When the cause can be clearly established, the term secondary hypertension is used because the increased pressure is the result of some other condition. These specific causes may include medications such as oral contraceptives, kidney disorders such as renal failure (see page 852), glomerulonephritis (see page 836), and certain adrenal gland problems (see page 937).

Complications of High Blood Pressure

Over a period of years, the excessive pressure of high blood pressure, left untreated, can lead to damage in various parts of your body.

Hypotension

Hypotension is low blood pressure. If blood pressure falls to dangerously low levels (shock), it can be life-threatening. Shock may result from significant loss of fluid or blood and rarely from serious infections. One of the goals of emergency treatment for hypotension will be to bring your blood pressure up to more normal levels.

Chronic low blood pressure (your blood pressure is below average but not hazardously so) is not uncommon. It can result from medications given for high blood pressure or from pregnancy, diabetes, or arteriosclerosis.

Postural Hypotension
One potentially dangerous manifestation of low blood pressure is called postural hypotension. Dizziness or faintness that occurs on standing up quickly from a seated position is the key symptom.

Typically, this is not a serious problem. Sensible precautions will often avoid future incidents. Stand up slowly from a seated position. If episodes seem to occur when you have been in the sun for prolonged periods or after a time of fasting, avoid such circumstances.

However, if you experience persistent fainting spells, consult your physician. Your physician will determine whether there is some underlying cause of the problem.

Heart attack, kidney damage, stroke, loss of vision, and other complications can result.

Hypertensive Heart Disease
The major cause of death in people with high blood pressure is one or more complications of coronary artery disease. High blood pressure accelerates the process of atherosclerosis (see page 636). This may affect the arteries that supply blood to the heart muscle. If these vessels become obstructed and the heart muscle is deprived of oxygen, a heart attack may occur.

When the blood pressure is elevated, the heart is forced to work harder to maintain blood flow to the tissues. Over time, the heart muscle may hypertrophy (enlarge) in order to keep pushing blood out of the heart into narrower vessels that have increased resistance. The left ventricle is the chamber of the heart that pumps blood to the rest of the body. Thus, this condition is termed "left ventricular hypertrophy." Left ventricular hypertrophy is associated with a higher risk of sudden death (see page 674) and heart attack (see page 661).

In addition, the heart's pumping muscles become less efficient over time, and congestive heart failure may result. The heart cannot pump out all of the fluid returning to it from the body. Thus, fluids accumulate in the lungs, legs, and other tissues as the blood "backs up" (see Congestive Heart Failure, page 659).

Stroke
When a blood vessel in the brain ruptures (cerebral hemorrhage) or, more commonly, a clot or fragment of atherosclerotic plaque blocks blood flow to part of the brain (cerebral thrombosis), a stroke is the result (see Stroke, page 461).

Strokes are much more likely in people with high blood pressure. In fact, hypertension is the most important risk factor for stroke. When the blood pressure is decreased by appropriate treatment, the risk for stroke is decreased as well.

Kidney Disease
About a fifth of the blood pumped by the heart goes to the kidneys. The kidneys filter out waste products and help to maintain proper blood chemistry values. They also control the balance of salts, acids, and water.

High blood pressure can injure the kidneys, thus impairing their ability to perform normal functions. Also, because some of the

Isolated Systolic Hypertension

Your blood pressure reading has two numbers. The top (systolic) number records the maximum pressure your heart uses to pump blood. The lower (diastolic) number refers to the minimum pressure in your arteries when your heart is at rest. If you have isolated systolic hypertension (ISH), your top number is high (160 or more) but your bottom number is normal. There are no symptoms or warning signs. ISH affects two-thirds of older people with high blood pressure. Four million people have the condition today, with an estimated eight million expected to develop it by the year 2025.

Physicians once thought ISH was a benign result of aging. They were reluctant to treat it because of lack of evidence of benefits, possi-ble side effects, and cost. However, a 5-year study of systolic hyper-tension in the elderly convinced researchers that treating this form of high blood pressure can help prevent 24,000 strokes and 50,000 incidents of severe cardiovascular problems each year—with savings of half a billion dollars.

Researchers at 16 clinical cen-ters studied 4,736 men and women 60 years of age or older with iso-lated systolic hypertension. On average, participants had systolic readings of 170 or more and dias-tolic levels less than 90. One group received drug treatment for ISH (chlorthalidone, a diuretic costing about 10 cents a day, and if systolic pressure didn't drop below 160, a small dose of a beta blocker, atenolol); the other group received an inactive medication (placebo). Participants tolerated the medica-tions well.

The treatment group had 36 percent fewer fatal and nonfatal strokes. In fact, the treatment group had fewer deaths from all causes, including cardiac and cardiovascu-lar problems. This was the first study to confirm the benefit of treating high blood pressure in people older than 80 years.

If you've been diagnosed with ISH, get accurate, regular readings of your blood pressure. Ask your physician about medications to control the problem, and follow the prescription carefully. Also, address the lifestyle factors that can add to your risk of ISH: smoking, obesity, a high-sodium diet, and use of alcohol.

---

kidneys' normal functions help control blood pressure, damage to the kidneys can worsen high blood pressure.

This can produce a destructive cycle that, ultimately, results in increasing blood pres-sure and a gradual failure of the kidneys to remove impurities from the blood (see Kidney Failure, page 852).

Drug Treatments for High Blood Pressure

Lifestyle changes regarding weight loss, exer-cise, and dietary adjustments (see What You Can Do for Your Hypertension, page 653) are preferred over long-term use of antihyper-tensive drugs. However, in many cases, a combination of lifestyle changes and anti-hypertensive medications is needed.

Your physician will determine which drug or combination of drugs may be best suited for you. Important considerations include how a drug works and the fact that some drugs work better than others at dif-ferent ages or in certain races. In addition, your physician may consider the cost, side effects, the interaction between multiple drugs, and how the drugs affect other ill-nesses. There may be several steps in the selection process because the first drug may not lower your blood pressure. A second, third, or even fourth drug may be tried either as a substitute or an additional drug.

The groups of drugs your physician may choose from in treating high blood pressure are described here.

Diuretics

Often, the first choice of drug, especially when your blood pressure is not very high, is a diuretic. Diuretics act on the kidneys to help the body eliminate salt and water. Diuretics may increase cholesterol, triglyc-erides, blood glucose levels, and uric acid (a cause of gout, see page 916).

Low doses are well tolerated and often are associated with minimal potassium loss. Your physician may suggest eating more foods such as orange juice or bananas, and he or she occasionally may prescribe a potas-sium supplement to correct any potassium deficiency. Careful restriction of dietary sodium both increases the effectiveness of the diuretic drug and decreases the tendency to eliminate potassium.

Establishing Your Drug Therapy

If your hypertension treatment involves medications, the chances are that you will be taking such medications continuously for the rest of your life.

Because each case of high blood pressure is different, your physician may have to adjust dosages or even change medications several times before finding the right drug combination.

Taking Your Blood Pressure

Because high blood pressure has no symptoms, the only way to be sure your medication is working is to measure your blood pressure.

At first, do it three or four times a day. Blood pressure tends to vary throughout the 24 hours. Sometimes it will increase gradually through the day, decrease while you sleep, and begin to increase shortly before you awaken. When you measure your blood pressure, be sure to record the time of day as well as the date and blood pressure reading. The goal is to keep your blood pressure in a good range around the clock.

Once your blood pressure returns to a satisfactory range, check it once or twice a week but try to do this at different hours (see How to Take Your Own Blood Pressure, page 649).

Do not stop taking your medication when your blood pressure reaches an acceptable level. The drug is needed to help keep your blood pressure at that level. However, if your blood pressure goes up again despite your drug therapy, consult your physician.

Side Effects

If you have side effects, consult your physician before you stop taking the drug. There may be alternatives available, and your physician probably can change the dose or choose another medication to meet your needs with fewer or no side effects.

Make It a Habit

As obvious as it sounds, you must take the drugs regularly and on schedule for them to work properly. At first, it may seem foreign to you, but establish a regimen so that swallowing your pills becomes a part of your daily routine.

It is sometimes helpful to use a plastic pillbox with one to three compartments for each day of the week. You can "load up" once a week for the 7 days to come, and if you are not sure whether you have taken your pill for a given scheduled time, you can see what pills remain in the box.

Beta-Adrenergic Blockers

These drugs are sometimes used as the initial drug treatment for hypertension. They work by blocking many of the effects of adrenaline (epinephrine) in your body, in particular the stimulating effect that it has on your heart. The result is that your heart will beat more slowly and less forcefully while the blocker is active in your body.

A common side effect is lethargy and a sense of fatigue, which limits the usefulness of these drugs. Certain of these classes of drugs also may decrease the blood level of HDL cholesterol, the "good" cholesterol (see page 642). Commonly used beta-adrenergic blockers include atenolol, metoprolol, propranolol, and timolol.

If use of a diuretic drug does not bring your blood pressure down, your physician may prescribe a beta-adrenergic blocker, perhaps in combination with a diuretic.

Calcium Channel Blockers

The calcium channel blockers function by blocking the entry of calcium into your cells. This effect decreases the tendency of your small arteries to become narrow. Examples of these drugs include diltiazem and verapamil.

Angiotensin-Converting Enzyme Inhibitors (ACE Inhibitors)

Like the calcium channel blockers, these inhibitors help prevent narrowing of arteries. The mechanism is different, however, in that these drugs block the formation of a natural body chemical, angiotensin II. This allows your blood vessels to dilate, and thus your blood pressure is decreased. Examples include captopril, enalapril, and lisinopril. These may be used alone or in combination with diuretics.

Other Drugs

Alpha-receptor blockers (such as prazosin and terazosin) and alpha-beta blockers (such as labetalol) occasionally are used as single agents or in combination with other hypertensive drugs.

Hydralazine and diazoxide are used for severe high blood pressure; nitroprusside may be used in emergency situations when an extremely high blood pressure threatens life.

What You Can Do for Your Hypertension

Often the precise cause of high blood pressure remains unknown. Still, the condition can be effectively treated. In fact, through proper treatment, the pressure can be brought down to manageable or normal levels, and most or all of the potentially dire consequences of hypertension can be avoided. If you have high blood pressure, follow the therapy your physician prescribes. This can decrease your blood pressure to normal—and keep it there. You will have a normal or nearly normal life expectancy.

Many physicians believe that the best strategy is to begin your treatment with changes in lifestyle: shed any extra weight, adjust your diet, restrict use of alcohol and caffeine, stop smoking, and increase physical exercise. If, after 3 to 6 months, your blood pressure has not dropped to healthier levels, a program of medication may be required (see Drug Treatments for High Blood Pressure, page 651). Even with drug treatment, however, lifestyle changes continue to be important.

Diet
The food you eat has an impact on your overall health, but especially on your heart and blood vessels. Reduce your intake of saturated fat and cholesterol to reduce your cardiovascular risk (see page 639). In particular, the moderation of one ingredient—salt—can decrease blood pressure almost immediately in sensitive people.

Salt Restriction
Excessive salt in the diet has been the focus of much study in recent years. The evidence is convincing: salt causes the body to retain fluids and thus, in many people, is a factor in causing high blood pressure. If you decrease your total salt intake (the salt contained in foods such as bread and butter as well as salt from a saltshaker) to an amount less than 1 teaspoon each day, you will probably decrease your blood pressure.

Salt (sodium chloride) is found in virtually all plants and animals. Some salt is necessary for the normal functions of your body. We need perhaps half a gram (500 mg) daily (roughly a quarter teaspoon of salt), but the average American consumes between 2 and 3 full teaspoons of salt every day.

Do not add salt to your food at the table; use only limited amounts (less than half a teaspoon a day) in preparing your food. Avoid highly salted foods such as chips and foods that are pickled. Remember that highly processed foods are often high in salt, including cheeses and cheese products, luncheon meats, bacon, and ham; condiments such as ketchup, mustard, and soy sauce; "fast foods"; and canned soups.

Get in the habit of reading food labels: monosodium glutamate (MSG), sodium chloride, and baking soda all represent salt. Recent studies suggest that even if you have normal blood pressure, reducing salt in your diet may prevent the development of hypertension. Maintaining an adequate intake of calcium, magnesium, and potassium also may lower your blood pressure. If you have questions, consult your physician or dietitian.

Weight Reduction
If you are more than 10 percent above your ideal body weight and have high blood pressure, shed those extra pounds. A loss of as few as 10 pounds may reduce your blood pressure significantly. In fact, in some people, weight loss alone is sufficient to avoid the need to take antihypertensive drugs (for specific guidance on weight control, see page 277).

Exercise
An appropriate regimen of exercise is good for your heart (see Cardiovascular Fitness, page 644). It also may help you to lose excess weight. Although the exact role aerobic exercise can play in treating high blood pressure has yet to be defined, hypertensive people who exercise regularly have had a decrease in their blood pressure. However, before embarking on an exercise program, consult your physician.

Other Factors
Smoking and drinking caffeinated beverages can have a short-term effect in increasing blood pressure. There is conflicting evidence that smoking and the use of caffeine contribute to sustained high blood pressure. However, the use of tobacco can accelerate the process of atherosclerosis in people with high blood pressure (see Atherosclerosis: What Is It? page 636). Quitting smoking is the healthiest strategy. If you need help in doing so, see Tobacco (page 315).

Heavy drinking also can lead to high blood pressure. A decrease in your alcohol intake can lower your blood pressure and may help prevent the development of hypertension. So limit your consumption of alcoholic beverages to no more than two drinks a day (see page 328).

Coronary Artery Disease

Coronary artery disease is our nation's leading cause of death, accounting for about 600,000 deaths each year. Although the condition may develop slowly over many years, its impact is instantaneous in nearly a third of the cases—death, without warning, is its only manifestation.

The blood vessels (coronary arteries) that provide oxygen and nutrients to the muscles of the heart are small. These arteries encircle the heart like a crown (hence the name "coronary") and send branches downward to the tip of the heart. In coronary artery disease, there is a buildup of material—cholesterol, scar tissue, calcium, and other substances—in the lining of these arteries. This accumulation, called atheromatous plaque, is the principal characteristic of atherosclerosis (see Atherosclerosis: What Is It? page 636). The effects can vary, from recurring chest pain called angina (see page 657) to congestive heart failure (see page 659) and heart attack (see page 661).

Atherosclerosis usually occurs in a somewhat irregular fashion, so there will be considerably more narrowing at some points than at others. The roughening of the lining of the arteries over the atheromatous plaques favors the development of a blood clot. Usually, in a heart attack, the final closure of the narrowed segment occurs as the result of a clot forming in this location.

The same factors (for example, smoking, high blood cholesterol levels, high blood pressure) that contribute to the development of atherosclerosis in other parts of the body also favor occurrence of atherosclerosis in the coronary arteries.

The walls of the coronary arteries include muscle fibers. At times, these may go into spasm—that is, contract and cause further narrowing of the channel. Such spasm may occur without apparent cause, but it also may result from strong emotional stress or exposure to cold.

Coronary artery disease is treated with a wide range of techniques, medications, and lifestyle adjustments. The diagnosis and treatment of coronary artery disease have seen a great deal of innovation in recent years. There are tests to determine if your symptoms are due to coronary artery disease (see The Exercise Tolerance Test, page 655). Other tests are available for those who have already experienced coronary artery problems (see Scans and Coronary Angiogram, page 656). In the operating room, bypass operations can direct blood around narrowed or blocked arteries (see page 665). In some situations, specialized procedures can open narrowed arteries (see Coronary Angioplasty, page 666).

The frequency of coronary artery disease appears to be decreasing slowly, because of a growing attention to the controllable risk factors (see page 638). The introduction of medications and new procedures and operations to improve the flow of blood to the heart muscle have proved helpful in minimizing symptoms and, to a lesser extent, have lengthened life in those who have had symptoms of coronary artery disease.

Common Diagnostic Tests

Narrowing or blockage of arteries in your heart can cause chest pain (angina pectoris),

An electrocardiogram (ECG) records electrical activity of your heart. Electrodes convey impulses to a device that produces a graphic representation of your heart's activity. This can be studied for patterns and abnormalities.

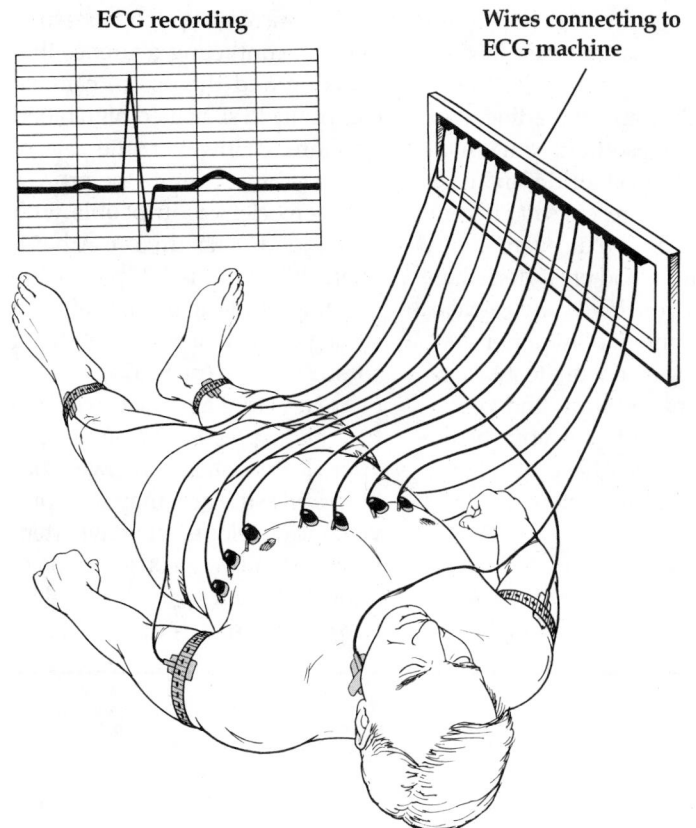

ECG recording

Wires connecting to ECG machine

heart attack, or even death. One of the challenges to your physician is to detect coronary artery disease before such consequences occur and to help you avoid or minimize the consequences.

Your physician cannot detect blocked coronary arteries simply by listening through the stethoscope, but there are clues to be heard (see Listen to Your Heartbeat, page 634). Your physician will also take your pulse and measure your blood pressure. But there are more specialized tests to be used as well.

Electrocardiography
Electrocardiography—also known as ECG or EKG (the "K" is for the Greek word *kardia* for

---

The Exercise Tolerance Test

The exercise may be on a treadmill or a stationary bike; the test may be called an exercise tolerance test or a stress test or a treadmill test. Whatever the exercise or the name, the principles are the same.

It is important to take an exercise tolerance test before you embark on a program of vigorous exercise, particularly if there is a history of heart disease in your family or if you are older than 40 and have other heart risks (see Disease of the Heart and Blood Vessels: Living With the Risks, page 635). The test is not done routinely, but your physician may advise it if you have symptoms that suggest coronary artery disease. If you already have had a heart attack, he or she may also order the test to determine the extent of your coronary artery disease.

The test accurately identifies the presence of coronary artery disease in nearly three-fourths of those with the disorder; it also identifies most of those without significant coronary artery disease.

Electrodes are placed on various parts of your chest and a blood pressure cuff is placed on your arm. Then you mount a treadmill or bicycle. The workout that follows will become progressively more demanding, and your heart rate will increase. The physician overseeing the test will be monitoring your heart rate, blood pressure, and electrocardiographic tracings and also will be watching for symptoms.

The test takes about half an hour, time well invested if you have one or more of the classic cardiac risk factors, which include smoking, diabetes, high blood pressure, high cholesterol level, or family history of stroke or heart disease. If you have already had a heart attack, your response on the test can help your physician to devise an exercise program for you that will enhance your recovery. Even if your heart reveals no signs of artery disease, the test can be useful in designing an effective workout program.

If the exercise tolerance test indicates that your heart's activity was constant and strong during the stress, the chances are excellent that your heart will function properly when you work out on your own. If there are signs of problems, the test results will be useful in establishing exercise limits and developing a special fitness program for you. If the exercise produces any abnormal patterns on the electrocardiographic tracings, your physician may advise additional evaluations, which may include angiography, radionuclide scanning with exercise (see Scans and Coronary Angiogram, page 656), or echocardiography (see page 683).

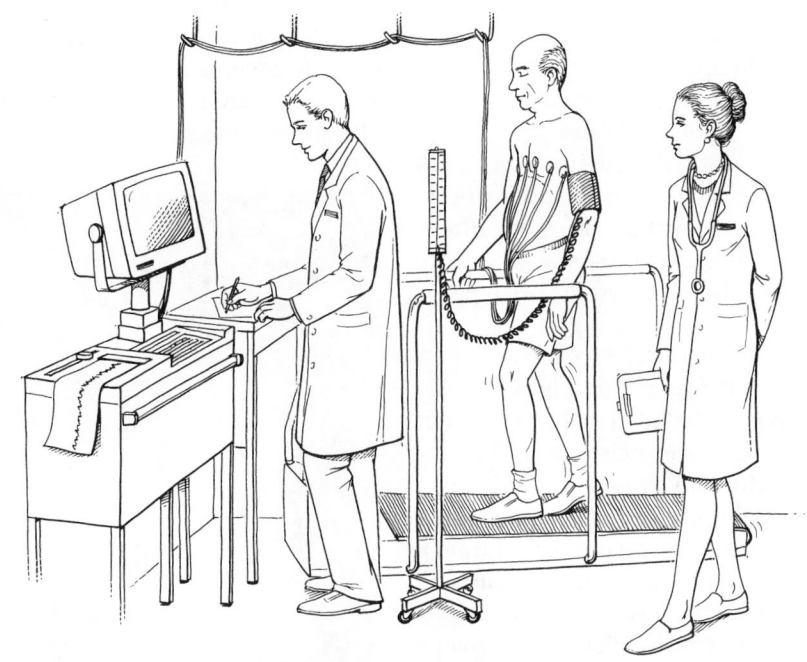

A treadmill test measures the activity of your heart while you exercise.

Scans and Coronary Angiogram

In diagnosing coronary artery disease, it often is invaluable to be able to "see" the coronary arteries and the shape and function of the heart chambers. Today, this can be done best by one of two basic approaches, either entirely from outside the body (noninvasive) or by inserting catheters or other instruments into the body (invasive). In general, images made by scanning devices are noninvasive methods to study heart function; coronary angiography, however, is an invasive procedure.

If your exercise ECG is abnormal, your physician may suggest a noninvasive radionuclide scan to help confirm the diagnosis of coronary artery disease. These tests are highly accurate, are easy to perform, and do not require a stay in the hospital. The radiation exposure is slight, and such a scan may eliminate the need for an angiogram.

A different approach uses sound waves to re-create the shape of the heart and large blood vessels. Heart ultrasound scans (echocardiograms) allow your physician to see the movement of your heart (see The Echocardiogram: Images Made With Sound, page 683).

Radionuclide Scans

Radionuclide scans can cost up to 4 times the amount of a treadmill exercise test, but they also provide more information. These studies are noninvasive, and there are two types:

Thallium Exercise Scan

One type of radionuclide examination of the heart is the thallium or sestamibi exercise scan. This procedure involves the injection of a small dose of radioactive isotope into a vein in your arm during a treadmill test. A special scanning device then records a series of pictures of the locations of this isotope in the region of your heart. Dark areas on the scans indicate portions of your heart to which blood flow

is impaired. However, this does not provide a picture of the actual blocked artery.

Radionuclide Angiogram

For this procedure, you receive an injection of a radioactive isotope that labels your blood cells. You are then placed on an exercise table (either supine or semi-upright) with your feet on the pedals of a bicycle. As you work the pedals, scans are made to locate the isotope in the region of your heart. A key finding would be impaired expansion or contraction of the heart wall, a signal that narrowed arteries are not carrying sufficient amounts of oxygen-rich blood (see page 1339).

Exercise Echocardiogram

Ultrasound or inaudible sound waves can be used to create two-dimensional images of the heart (see page 1335). When a portion of the heart muscle receives insufficient blood flow during exercise, it develops an abnormal contraction pattern that can be recognized by comparing the images of the contractions at rest (before exercise) and immediately following exercise. Either bicycle or standard treadmill testing can be used for this purpose. It is usu-

ally less expensive than radionuclide scanning.

Coronary Angiogram

Coronary angiography involves insertion of a catheter (a hollow, flexible tube) into an artery at your groin or elbow. This catheter is guided through your main artery, the aorta, into your heart. Then it is guided into a coronary artery. A dye that is opaque to X-rays is injected through the catheter to make the artery visible on an X-ray picture.

Angiography can be done on many blood vessels in the body, but when it is done on heart arteries (coronary arteries) the test is called coronary angiography. A variation of this procedure is used to treat narrowed coronary arteries (see Coronary Angioplasty, page 666).

In addition, the catheter can be placed in the left side of the heart, where the function of the mitral and aortic valves can be studied; the shape and function of the left ventricle of the heart also can be observed. To study the right atrium and ventricle and its valves (tricuspid and pulmonic), a catheter can be inserted into a large vein and advanced into the right side of the heart.

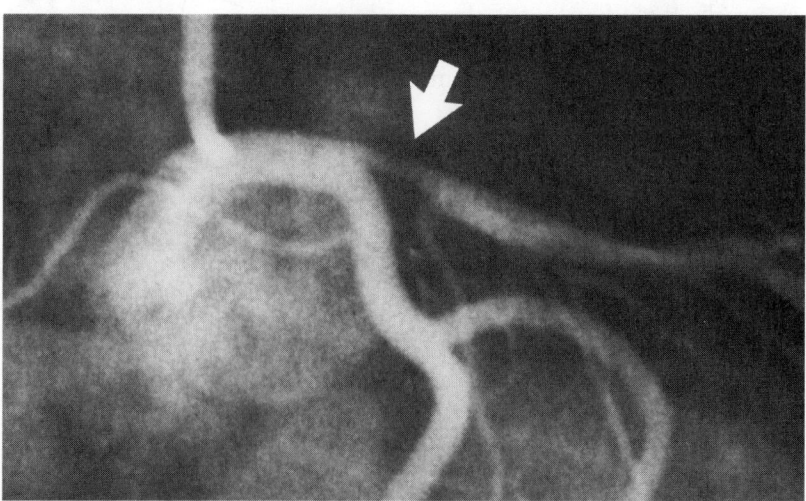

A coronary angiogram outlines major arteries of your heart. The arrow shows narrowing due to a buildup of atherosclerotic plaque.

"heart")—is an important tool in detecting heart disease and in pinpointing where difficulty lies when a problem is present.

An electrocardiogram is a graphic representation of the electrical forces at work in your heart. During the cardiac cycle, a pattern of changing electrical pulses reflects the action of your heart. These pulses can be recorded through electrodes attached to the surface of your body. The activity of the heart—represented by characteristic waves—can then be evaluated instantaneously on a television monitor or studied later on graph-paper printouts.

The ECG procedure is painless. While you are relaxing motionless on a bed or on an examining table, 12 to 15 electrodes are attached to the skin of your legs, arms, neck, and trunk. Then the recording process begins and is over in a few minutes.

The analysis involves looking for indications of heart rhythm abnormalities, of an old or a recent heart attack, or other trouble. Your physician may want to record an ECG of your heart when you are between 30 and 40 years old and in good health. This will provide a basis for comparison later if any heart problems develop.

Since its invention at the turn of the century, the ECG has proved to be an invaluable tool for the cardiologist. Most often, it is used on stationary, relaxed subjects. It also is a key part of the exercise tolerance test (see page 655). With a portable version, the Holter monitor, an ECG can be recorded from your heart during a 24-hour period while you go about your regular activities. This provides your physician with a day-long "diary" of your heart's functions, an especially useful tool in attempts to diagnose heart rhythm disturbances (see Disorders of Heart Rate and Rhythm, page 669).

Blood Tests

A sample of your blood may be taken for analysis. Among the measurements made will be your cholesterol level. Too much LDL cholesterol or too little HDL cholesterol puts you at greater risk of atherosclerosis, an accumulation of fats in your blood vessels (see Cholesterol and Dietary Fats, page 639). Other tests will include measurement of blood sugar level (for indications of diabetes) and of thyroid hormone (an overactive or underactive thyroid gland can produce heart abnormalities).

Chest X-Ray

A chest X-ray produces a picture that includes your heart and blood vessels and can be useful in identifying certain results of heart disease, including an enlarged heart. A wide range of new scanning methods allows further inspection of your heart (see Scans and Coronary Angiogram, page 656).

Angina Pectoris

Signs and Symptoms

- Pain (tight, band-like, crushing, suffocating sensation) that usually is centered beneath the breastbone (sternum) and may spread to the throat, jaw, or one arm
- Sensation of heaviness or tightness that is less than pain
- Attacks generally brought on by exercise or emotional stress

Angina pectoris gets its name from the nature of the pain: the Latin *angere* for "choke" describes the characteristic suffocating sensation, and *pectoralis* for "chest," where it is located.

The discomfort usually lasts for a minute or two, sometimes as long as 10 to 15 minutes. The pain may be severe and may be accompanied by a constricting feeling behind the breastbone (sternum) that may extend into the throat, jaw, or one arm. It may also be a mild heaviness, tightness, or burning discomfort.

Angina usually is brought on by exertion such as heavy lifting, sexual activity, or strenuous exercise. It is relieved by rest. Extreme cold or emotion such as intense fear, anger, grief, or frustration can cause it, as can ingestion of a heavy meal.

Angina is the direct result of insufficient blood reaching your heart muscle (ischemia). When you exert yourself, your heart requires more oxygen to do the extra work. When the coronary arteries that serve your heart are narrow and unable to accommodate the increase in flow of blood demanded by the exercise, nerves in your heart transmit pain messages to your brain.

Angina is a symptom, not a disorder. It can be the result of arteries narrowed by a passing spasm. More likely, a limitation of blood flow is the result of atherosclerosis (see page 636), in which the arteries are narrowed by an accumulation of deposits of fatty plaque.

Thus, angina often is one of the warning signs of coronary artery disease. When the attacks come frequently and are not linked to physical activity, they may be warning signs of an impending heart attack and require special treatment (see Heart Attack, page 661).

Angina is quite common. In men, it usually occurs after age 30; in women it tends to appear later. The cause in most cases is atherosclerosis.

Diagnosis

Most often, the discomfort occurs after strenuous physical activity or an emotional upset. However, it also can occur after mild exercise or even while you are asleep. The nature of the distress has been described as tight, band-like, crushing, burning, suffocating, and, occasionally, sharp. Sometimes it is mistaken for indigestion.

The duration of the pain is variable. If the chest pain is prolonged beyond 5 to 10 minutes, the risk of damage to the heart muscle increases. The pain may also be "referred," a term used to describe pain impulses confused by your brain. It may feel as if your jaw, neck, or arms are in great pain when in fact it may be the pain of angina that is being perceived as stemming from one or more of these locations.

There is no specific laboratory test for the diagnosis of angina. Your physician may want to obtain an electrocardiogram to see if damage has occurred. He or she also may order certain blood tests (heart enzymes) to rule out heart damage. In addition, your physician may want to obtain blood tests to make sure thyroid abnormalities (see page 945) or anemia (see page 956) are not present. Both of these disorders may force your heart to beat faster, use more oxygen, and, therefore, precipitate angina.

How Serious Is Angina?

The decrease in blood flow to your heart is partial and temporary, so damage does not occur. This is in contrast to the blockage of a heart artery that may result in permanent damage to a part of the heart muscle (see Heart Attack, page 661). When there is damage to the heart muscle, the term "heart attack" is often used. In some cases, angina may serve as a "warning sign" for a future or impending heart attack. Individuals with angina should be under a physician's care.

Treatment

If you experience angina, try to stop the activity that precipitated the attack. This should lessen the load on your heart and reduce its need for oxygen. The distress should improve within a few minutes. If the discomfort does not cease within a few minutes or if the frequency or severity of the attacks increases, seek immediate medical attention.

If you smoke, stop. Lose the extra pounds if you are overweight. Eliminating obesity or smoking may decrease or even eliminate your symptoms. Lowering cholesterol by diet, exercise, and, in some cases, cholesterol-reducing drugs may improve coronary artery plaques (regression), which may prevent or delay future problems.

Exercise

Having angina does not need to make you a sedentary person. In fact, exercise is a key part of dealing with your angina. The exercise must be compatible with the limitations imposed by your pain. Your own body and your physician will help you determine how much exercise is appropriate.

Medication

The classic treatment for acute attacks of angina is the drug nitroglycerin. Nitroglycerin opens (dilates) the coronary arteries, allowing more blood to flow to the heart muscle. Usually it is taken as a tablet that is allowed to dissolve under the tongue (sublingual). A form of nitroglycerin that is sprayed under the tongue is available. In a remarkably short time—within a few minutes—the discomfort will ease.

One side effect of nitroglycerin is that it causes headaches in some people. Usually the headaches are temporary and mild. If your physician prescribes nitroglycerin, keep your drug supply fresh because the tablet form of the drug loses potency in a matter of months. Also, keep the tablets out of direct sunlight, which causes loss of potency.

Long-acting nitrites (similar to nitroglycerin) also may be helpful in decreasing the frequency of angina attacks.

Calcium channel blockers are drugs that interrupt the normal flow of calcium through channels in your heart muscle. This produces dilation (a widening) of the coronary and other arteries in your vascular system, which results in increased blood flow to the heart muscle. The work required of the heart is also decreased and its demands for oxygen are lessened. The calcium channel blockers also decrease blood pressure.

The beta-adrenergic blockers decrease heart rate and blood pressure. Both (sometimes in combination) are useful in reducing the symptoms of angina.

Your physician will select an appropriate medication for your particular symptoms.

Surgery

If the angina continues in spite of the use of medications or occurs more often or with greater intensity, your physician may consider coronary angioplasty or coronary artery bypass surgery (see pages 665 and 666).

Congestive Heart Failure

Signs and Symptoms

- Swelling (edema) in the ankles; if bedridden, swelling in lower portions of back
- Breathlessness
- Weakness and fatigue

Congestive heart failure is a serious condition in which your heart loses its pumping efficiency. At times this can be life-threatening. In the most common forms, the heart fails to pump blood effectively. This decreases blood flow to tissues and organs throughout the body.

With failure of the left side of the heart, blood backs up into the lungs, which causes them to become congested with fluid (see Pulmonary Edema, page 660). This congestion is responsible for the sensation of breathlessness which is common in congestive heart failure.

If the right side of the heart fails, blood backs up into the legs and into the liver, which becomes congested. This produces a swelling (edema) that usually is most obvious in the lower legs and ankles. Often both left and right sides of the heart fail simultaneously.

Lack of adequate blood flow to the kidneys leads to accumulation of excess fluid and water in your body, an additional factor that increases the edema. Inadequate blood flow to the muscles reduces endurance. Therefore, people with congestive heart failure often experience early fatigue when they exert themselves physically.

The loss of pumping efficiency of the heart in congestive heart failure may be the result of weakened muscle tissue in the heart due to damage from a heart attack, of diseases directly affecting the heart muscle (see Cardiomyopathy, page 686), of a mechanical problem in the valves of the heart (see page 677), of prolonged high blood pressure, or of external constriction of the heart.

Diagnosis

At first, congestive heart failure produces a feeling of weakness, fatigue, and breathlessness. Routine physical activities may become more and more difficult to perform. At first, breathlessness appears only after exercise, but as the disease progresses the shortness of breath may occur while resting or after going to bed. Breathing may be more difficult when you are lying down. You might need to elevate your head on several pillows in order to be able to sleep.

The breathlessness is a sign of a failure of the left side of your heart. At its worst, the difficulty may awaken you at night. Such episodes usually are relieved by sitting up.

If your physician suspects heart failure, he or she will listen to your heart and lungs with a stethoscope to detect the sounds associated with heart failure. Your physician also will look for swollen or distended neck veins, an enlarged liver, and swelling (edema) of the feet, all of which may be signs of heart failure. Blood and urine tests will reveal whether your kidneys are properly removing waste products. An electrocardiogram (ECG; see Common Diagnostic Tests, page 654) will be recorded to investigate the rate and rhythm of your heartbeat and to look for evidence of a previous heart attack and a disturbance in the pathways that conduct electrical messages within your heart. A chest X-ray may reveal enlargement of the heart and congestion in the lungs. Echocardiography will allow your physician to detect weakened heart muscle or valve problems (see The Echocardiogram: Images Made With Sound, page 683).

How Serious Is Congestive Heart Failure?

If untreated, congestive heart failure can be fatal. However, lifestyle adjustments and proper drug treatment can improve heart function and relieve symptoms. Although medications do not cure the condition, they can be used long-term and in some cases will permit a nearly normal lifestyle.

Treatment

Once your physician has confirmed that you have heart failure, the first new rule of your life is to get plenty of rest to help you conserve energy. However, this does not mean you should retire to your bed. On the contrary, maintaining your mobility, or in some cases, even an exercise regimen, is a key component of the treatment program. Motion helps to keep your circulation moving. Given the effect of gravity, you may also find that a comfortable chair is better than your bed for resting.

Diet

Your physician may give you specific nutritional guidelines to follow but, in general, you should restrict the amount of salt you consume. Sometimes the need to restrict salt consumption is such that a dietitian may need to give you special dietary instructions that will include the use of salt-free bread and salt-free margarine or butter. Avoid alcoholic beverages. Reach and maintain a weight appropriate for your height and build (to determine your ideal body weight, consult the chart on page 259).

Medication

Most cases of congestive heart failure are treated with drugs in addition to appropriate dietary measures. The three most commonly used medications are angiotensin-converting enzyme inhibitors (ACE inhibitors), diuretics, and digitalis.

A recent form of drug therapy for heart failure involves use of drugs that dilate arteries (vasodilators). Examples include angiotensin-converting enzyme inhibitors (ACE inhibitors) (see page 652), hydralazine, and nitrates. In patients with heart failure, ACE inhibitors have been shown to reduce the need for subsequent hospitalization for heart failure and to prolong life. Not all patients can tolerate this drug, and sometimes drugs such as hydralazine and nitrates are used instead or in combination with ACE inhibitors. With heart failure, dilating the arteries reduces the work the heart has to do, which allows it to pump blood more effectively. These drugs also are used for high blood pressure.

Diuretics, which also are often used in treating mild cases of high blood pressure (see page 651), are sometimes called water pills. These drugs increase the rate at which your body eliminates urine and salt. This decreases the congestion in your lungs (thus relieving the breathlessness) and the swelling in your legs. Diuretics have few side effects, although you may urinate more frequently and more immediately after consuming fluids. In addition to salt loss, potassium is also eliminated. Your physician will monitor your blood potassium level and, if it is found to be depleted, may prescribe a potassium supplement.

Digitalis preparations affect the heart directly. They increase the strength of the heart's pumping action and are especially useful if your heart failure is the result of certain disturbances of heart rhythm (see page 669).

Whatever drug you are taking, it is extremely important to take the prescribed doses regularly. The dose of digitalis is often determined by blood tests, including measurement of the amount of the drug in your blood. The doses of the other drugs are determined by clinical response (that is, degree of improvement), effect on blood pressure and kidney function, and the presence of bothersome side effects. For example, ACE inhibitors may cause cough, and hydralazine and nitrates may cause headache or nausea.

Surgery

Occasionally, surgery is required. For example, if your cardiologist determines that you have a defective valve in your heart or a small area of damaged cardiac tissue, surgical repair may be appropriate. If you have a diseased heart valve, replacement of the valve may be necessary (see Heart Valve Surgery, page 684). For persons with myocarditis or cardiomyopathy, heart transplantation may be an option (see Heart Transplantation, page 688).

Pulmonary Edema

Emergency Signs and Symptoms
- Severe shortness of breath
- Restlessness and anxiety, feeling of suffocating
- Pink, frothy sputum
- Sweating
- Pallor

Pulmonary edema occurs when the back

pressure within the veins of your lungs becomes so high that large amounts of fluid are rapidly forced out of the veins and into the air sacs (alveoli) of your lungs. This produces fluid (edema) in the lungs.

Pulmonary edema is usually caused by an extensive heart attack, mitral or aortic valve disease, or, although rare, exposure to high altitude.

Diagnosis

Severe shortness of breath is the primary symptom of pulmonary edema; you feel as if you are starving for air or are drowning. This feeling of suffocation is accompanied by anxiety and restlessness. Other symptoms include sweating, pallor, and a cough that commonly brings up pink, frothy sputum. In some people the fluid causes wheezing. Thus, these people are said to have "cardiac asthma."

How Serious Is Pulmonary Edema?

Pulmonary edema is a life-threatening condition. Immediate hospitalization and treatment are required.

Treatment

Treatment consists of receiving oxygen through a mask. If you are having extreme difficulty breathing, it may be necessary to insert a breathing tube into your trachea and provide temporary mechanical ventilation.

Medication

A diuretic usually is given intravenously to remove fluid from your lungs. Morphine sulfate also is effective in relieving pulmonary congestion. If the pulmonary edema is due to a decrease in pumping function of your heart, medications that will strengthen the heart muscle (such as digoxin) may be given intravenously. If hypertension is present, your doctor may prescribe an intravenous vasodilator drug.

Heart Attack

Emergency Signs and Symptoms

- Intense, prolonged chest pain, often described as a feeling of heavy pressure
- Pain may extend beyond the chest to the left shoulder and arm, back, and even teeth and jaw
- Prolonged pain in upper abdomen

- Shortness of breath
- Fainting episode
- Nausea, vomiting, fainting, and intense sweating may occur
- Frequent angina attacks that are not the result of physical exertion (unstable angina)

The technical term for heart attack is myocardial infarction. *Myo* means "muscle"; *kardia* means "heart"; an *infarct* is an area of tissue that has died because of oxygen starvation.

Heart attack is the unscientific term that is applied to the event that occurs when a blood clot (thrombus) blocks the flow in one or more of your coronary arteries. When the clot blocks the blood supply to a heart muscle region, the oxygen supply to the cells in that area is cut off. Just as in angina pectoris (see page 657), this usually produces pain. The difference is that the interruption to the blood flow is temporary in angina, but in a heart attack the blood supply to a portion of the heart muscle is completely or nearly completely shut off. The result is that the heart muscle in the affected region dies.

Most often the clot that causes a heart attack forms in a coronary artery narrowed by the thickening of its walls by the fatty deposits of atherosclerosis (see page 636).

By definition, a heart attack is a medical emergency: if you think you are having a heart attack or are with someone who is, seek immediate medical attention. If your com-

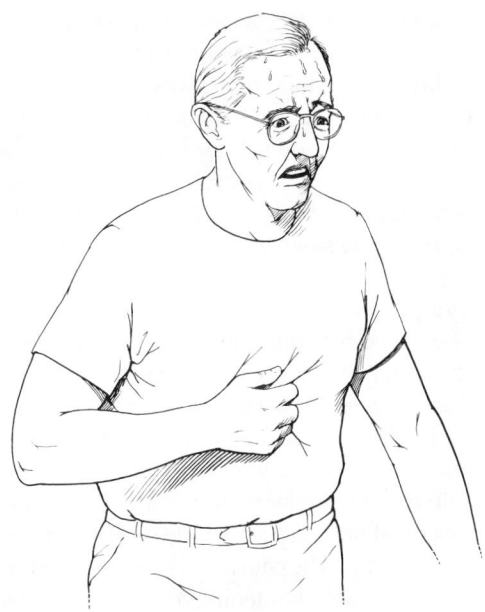

The pain of a heart attack varies from person to person, but typically there is a profound squeezing sensation in the chest, accompanied by profuse perspiration. Pain may radiate to the left shoulder and arm, to the back, and even to the jaw.

The Coronary Care Unit

If you have just had or are about to have a heart attack, the best place for you is in a hospital coronary or cardiac care unit (CCU).

The combination of constant cardiac monitoring and nursing observation in a CCU allows early detection of signs and symptoms and virtually instant attention when you need it. Such specialized care is required for people who have had a recent heart attack or who have severe angina (see page 657), disturbed heart rhythms (see page 669), or congestive heart failure (see page 659).

The Team
A cardiologist heads the CCU team; in some hospitals, a resident physician is available at all times as well. Highly trained nurses manage the monitoring and other care tasks and, often, the emergency procedures that must be done at a moment's notice.

The Equipment
Electrodes applied to your skin will connect you to a cardiac monitor (ECG, see Common Diagnostic Tests, page 654), which continuously monitors the rhythm and rate of your heartbeat. Your blood pressure will be monitored. Through a needle inserted into a vein in your arm, you may receive fluids and medications intravenously. Oxygen may also be provided.

More dramatic steps may be necessary if you actually experience a "coronary event" while in the CCU. Such events may be a problem with the rhythm of your heartbeat (see Disorders of Heart Rate and Rhythm, page 669), your heart actually stopping (cardiac arrest), or your heart beating rapidly but ineffectively (fibrillation). Electroshock equipment, cardiopulmonary resuscitation (CPR), and specialized drugs may be used in such emergency circumstances.

---

panion's heart attack has caused him or her to stop breathing, immediate cardiopulmonary resuscitation is necessary (see page 664).

Do not delay in seeking medical help. Delay is a mistake that takes thousands of lives every year. You may think the pain will disappear of its own accord; at other times, a heart attack can be confused with so-called heartburn (see page 742). Get immediate help. It may save your life.

Symptoms
The powerful squeezing sensation in your chest may be the chief symptom. Some describe it as the feeling of an enormous fist enclosing and squeezing their heart; others recall an accompanying sense of doom. The pain may be similar to that of angina, but it is sustained and responds little or not at all to nitroglycerin. The pain may be a discomfort or an inexplicable tightening, or it may feel as though an elephant has stepped on your chest.

A heart attack may be preceded by a series of angina attacks or it may occur suddenly with no advance warning. Unlike angina, however, the pain does not cease when the exercise or stress that caused it is discontinued. The pain may be constant or it may come and go.

Occasionally, the pain does not fit any particular pattern. This is especially true in the elderly and in persons with diabetes mellitus. Any prolonged pain in your chest or upper abdomen is cause for concern. Seek prompt medical attention. Do not attribute this pain to indigestion.

In some persons, a primary symptom of a heart attack is sudden onset of shortness of breath, which may or may not be associated with chest pain. In approximately 10 percent of cases, the only symptom of a heart attack is a sudden fainting spell (see Fainting Spells, page 674).

In elderly people and in diabetics, it is not unusual for a heart attack to occur with no accompanying pain or other symptoms. These "silent" heart attacks may be detected only when a routine electrocardiogram reveals a change in the pattern of transmission of electrical impulses through the heart.

Diagnosis
In the emergency vehicle or when you reach the hospital and professional medical care, your blood pressure will be taken and an electrocardiogram will be recorded (ECG; see Common Diagnostic Tests, page 654). In fact, you may be attached to this machine for much of your hospital stay so that your physicians and nurses can constantly monitor your heart's condition, perhaps within the confines of a special section of the hospital specifically for patients with heart conditions, called a coronary care unit (see this page).

At the hospital, other tests may be ordered including blood tests for enzymes that are released by damaged heart tissue, scans, and angiograms (see page 656). You will be observed carefully for several days. If there are no setbacks, you will be permitted to increase your activity gradually. The time in the hospital varies but ordinarily is 7 to 14 days.

How Serious Is a Heart Attack?
If the area of the damaged tissue (infarct) is small and the electrical system that controls your heart is not damaged, your chances of

surviving a heart attack are good. However, roughly a third of those who suffer heart attacks die before they receive medical care. Only a few years ago, the statistics were much worse—only about one in two survived. This improvement is due in part to the implementation of a wide variety of techniques, including cardiopulmonary resuscitation (CPR, see page 664), special tests (angiography and scanning, among others), and improved emergency care in ambulances or emergency vehicles or in cardiac care units designed to meet the immediate and continuing needs of persons having heart attacks.

The frequency of sudden death is a key reason why it is imperative that medical attention and, if necessary, CPR be provided as quickly as possible to the person who is having the heart attack. Most of those still alive 2 hours after a heart attack will survive; however, there is a range of possible complications.

Complications of a Heart Attack

Cardiac Arrhythmia
The system that controls your heartbeat is electrical. In some people, damage to the heart tissue from a heart attack can result in arrhythmia problems such as ventricular fibrillation. In this condition there are very rapid and uncoordinated contractions of the ventricles, resulting in insufficient blood flow to vital organs (see Heart Arrhythmias, page 669).

In some persons, the arrhythmia may be a heartbeat that is too slow. This may require temporary or, occasionally, permanent placement of a pacemaker (see Artificial Cardiac Pacemakers, page 675).

Congestive Heart Failure
In some cases the amount of damaged heart tissue (infarct) may be so extensive that the remaining heart muscle cannot do an adequate job of pumping the blood out of the heart. This can result in congestive heart failure (see page 659).

Death
In about one of every four people who die suddenly of a heart attack, there were no previous symptoms of heart disease. The immediate cause of death is thought to be underlying arrhythmia such as ventricular fibrillation (see Sudden Cardiac Death, page 674). The vast majority of persons who die

have severe disease of more than one coronary artery and the pumping action of their left ventricle is impaired, which, in turn, causes the arrhythmia. If no evidence of coronary artery disease is found, the cause of ventricular fibrillation often remains unknown.

Treatment
If you have symptoms that suggest a heart attack, call for emergency medical service or

---

Aspirin: Does It Prevent Heart Attacks?

In a recent study, male physicians took either one aspirin every other day or a placebo. Those who took the aspirin had fewer heart attacks.

Does this mean that taking an aspirin should be an every-other-day event for you, too? Not necessarily.

Aspirin and Platelets
Aspirin affects the way your blood clots. When you bleed because of an injury to a blood vessel, blood cells called platelets accumulate at the injury site. The platelets form a sticky plug that seals the opening in the blood vessel. Aspirin decreases the accumulation of platelets and impairs the formation of the clot when bleeding occurs.

Aspirin and Heart Attack
Because a heart attack is the result of blockage of a coronary artery by a blood clot, the effect of aspirin on clotting is beneficial during the first hours of a heart attack. Daily aspirin intake is beneficial for most persons with coronary artery disease, including those recovering from bypass surgery (see page 665).

Aspirin and Stroke
When you have had a bleeding event such as rupture of a small artery in your brain (hemorrhagic stroke, see Stroke, page 461), the aspirin-a-day regimen may be dangerous. The clotting ability of the blood is diminished by the aspirin, so the bleeding will be less likely to be stopped by the clotting of your blood.

Aspirin and Your Health
If you have coronary artery disease or if you have undergone coronary artery bypass surgery, aspirin may help decrease your risk of a subsequent heart attack. However, if you have high blood pressure, a history of stroke in your family, a bleeding disorder, ulcers, or impaired liver or kidney function or if you are taking the drug warfarin (Coumadin), avoid aspirin.

In any case, before taking aspirin regularly, discuss the matter with your physician.

(Note that aspirin—its chemical name is acetylsalicylic acid—is different from aspirin substitutes such as acetaminophen. Aspirin has an effect on clotting; acetaminophen does not.)

Cardiopulmonary Resuscitation (CPR)

As a bystander, you're a crucial link in responding to a heart attack emergency. Yet only about one-third of adults are trained in CPR, most in younger age groups. And only 25 percent of people who have a family member with heart disease have been trained.

To resuscitate someone, you must start cardiopulmonary resuscitation (CPR), or mouth-to-mouth breathing and chest compression, within 1 to 4 minutes. Could you?

First call 911. If the person is unconscious, a 911 dispatcher may advise you to begin CPR. Even if you're not trained, a dispatcher can instruct you in CPR until help arrives.

CPR training is critical if you're older or likely to respond to a heart attack emergency within your family. Ask your local Red Cross, county emergency services or public safety office, or state American Heart Association for the CPR training sites near you (see page 408).

911 for immediate help. If you think you are having a heart attack, do not try to drive to the hospital yourself.

Once you reach the hospital, the diagnostic tests discussed earlier will be initiated. You also may be given oxygen.

Medication

In some cases, a drug will be administered to dissolve the clot that is blocking the flow of blood. Clot-dissolving drugs (thrombolytic agents) such as streptokinase or tissue plasminogen activator may be delivered through a vein in the arm or directly to the clot by the use of a catheter. Your physician may also give you an anticoagulant drug orally to prevent further clotting.

There is a wide range of drugs your physician may prescribe depending on your condition and your rate of recovery. These are described here.

1. Pain Killers. If your condition is stable but your pain is great, you may be given an analgesic drug such as morphine to relieve the pain.

2. Nitrates. These drugs work by decreasing the oxygen requirement of your heart muscle. The best known of them, nitroglycerin, is placed under your tongue at the onset of angina pain (see Angina Pectoris, page 657); other forms are applied to the skin as an ointment or as a medicated patch or taken as long-acting tablets. Nitroglycerin often is given through a vein during or after a heart attack to produce a continuous decrease in oxygen requirements.

3. Beta-Adrenergic Blockers. These block the stimulating effect of the hormone epinephrine (adrenaline) on your heart. The result is that your heart will beat more slowly and less forcefully and thus will require less oxygen to continue its work.

4. Calcium Channel Blockers. These drugs interrupt the normal flow of calcium through channels in your heart muscle. Although they are not used routinely in treating heart attacks, occasionally physicians prescribe one of these medications to decrease the heart's demand for oxygen.

5. Aspirin. Because aspirin helps dissolve blood clots, it is frequently administered as soon as a heart attack is diagnosed. Aspirin often is used in combination with heparin (a drug that prevents clotting).

Recovery

When you are hospitalized, your activities will be limited and carefully monitored by the hospital staff. When you are released, follow your physician's instructions exactly.

Every day that passes means that you and your heart are recovering. The longer the time elapsed since your heart attack, the greater your chances of avoiding a second one and living a normal life.

Remember that you are not necessarily disabled. In fact, regular exercise—within the guidelines your physician suggests—can contribute to the return of your good health. Subject to your physician's guidance, you can return to work.

Do not be anxious about the possibility of another heart attack. Instead, try to channel anxiety into positive energy. Quit smoking (an absolute for anyone with heart disease). If you are unable to stop smoking (nicotine can be addictive), consider participating in a smoking cessation program. Medications that combat nicotine dependence may be used to help you through the early phases of nicotine withdrawal (see page 323). Establish a sensible exercise program and use it to keep your weight down. Decrease the fat content in your diet. Consider the other controllable risk factors in your life (see Disease of the Heart and Blood Vessels: Living With the Risks, page 635).

Coronary Artery Bypass Surgery

Heart attacks, angina, and other problems occur as the result of narrowed or blocked coronary arteries, the arteries that supply blood to the heart muscle. In certain situations, coronary artery bypass surgery or a coronary angioplasty is appropriate to relieve obstruction (see Coronary Angioplasty, page 666). These situations include cases in which the symptoms do not respond to optimal medical treatment or when blockage of the coronary arteries is severe.

Procedure

Bypass means an alternate route. A coronary bypass operation involves taking a short length of vein, usually from the thigh or lower leg (the saphenous vein), and using it to allow blood to bypass the blockage in a coronary artery. One or as many as eight or nine segments of these arteries may

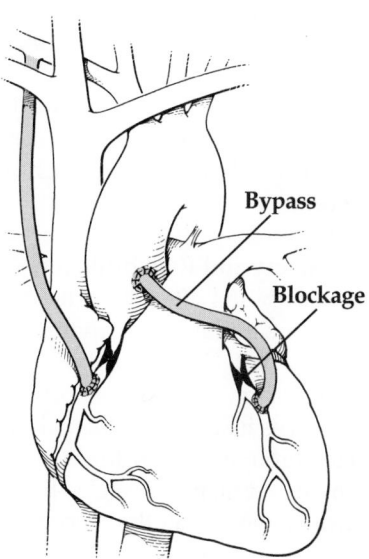

Bypasses around blockage sites can be surgically constructed out of veins taken from the leg (saphenous veins) or from arteries arising near the collarbone (internal mammary arteries).

receive bypasses, although four or five is average.

With time, these saphenous vein segments tend to develop blockages similar to those present initially in the coronary arteries. This may require medical treatment or another operation. More recently, the internal mammary artery has been used as the bypass. This artery lies inside the front of the chest. There is one on each side of the breastbone. The lower end of this artery is freed and sewn to the coronary artery beyond the blockage. The other end is left attached. Blood is thus rerouted into the coronary arteries.

The major advantage of this type of graft is its tendency to resist later buildup of atherosclerosis. Sometimes these arteries are unable to be used and sometimes both can be used.

For the operation, you will be given a general anesthetic. For a portion of the operation, the functions of your heart and lungs will be assumed by a heart-lung machine. The duration of the operation is 2 hours or more, depending on how much work is required.

Results

Adequate blood flow to the heart muscle is reestablished. This often relieves the angina or other coronary artery problem. Your physician may recommend preventive changes in lifestyle after you have bypass surgery. He or she may also recommend that you take one baby aspirin a day to help prevent obstructions from forming in your bypass vessels.

Recovery and Rehabilitation

A 6- to 7-day stay in the hospital is usual. After the operation, you may spend 24 to 36 hours in a spe-

cial cardiac care unit (CCU; see page 662). There the rate and rhythm of your heart and other vital signs will be closely monitored. Food and water will be provided intravenously; a tube will allow drainage from the site of the surgery. Oxygen or a respirator may be required.

Your physician and surgeon will advise you about your activities for the next several weeks of recovery and the gradual resumption of normal activity.

Bypass operations are done frequently and safely by an experienced surgical team. However, as with any operation, there are risks. In general, if you are under age 65 and have a normal left ventricle (the major muscle pump of the heart) and you are in relatively good health, your risk of dying during the operation and hospitalization is less than 1 percent.

Who Is a Candidate for Coronary Artery Bypass Surgery?

If you have mild exertional angina or have recovered from a heart attack with no continuing symptoms, you are probably best treated by medication or other means rather than by a bypass or other operation.

Although there have been controversial aspects of coronary artery bypass surgery, especially in the early days of its use, the consensus now favors this treatment in appropriate situations: for those with a blocked left main coronary artery, for those with disease in multiple vessels and poor function of the left ventricle (the main pump of the heart), and for those with debilitating angina. For these persons, a bypass procedure is of clear value in most cases and life is prolonged.

Coronary Angioplasty

Narrowed or blocked arteries may produce a heart attack, angina, or other problems. In some cases a special diet or medication or both may be the best treatment for such arterial problems; in other cases, bypass surgery (see page 665) or coronary angioplasty may be the best answer.

The full name for coronary angioplasty is percutaneous transluminal coronary angioplasty (PTCA). This means that, through the skin (percutaneous), a procedure is performed inside an artery (transluminal) of the heart (coronary) that reshapes (angioplasty) that artery.

The procedure is simpler than its name. PTCA is performed with local anesthesia while you are awake. This procedure is quite like the diagnostic procedure called coronary angiography (see Scans and Coronary Angiogram, page 656).

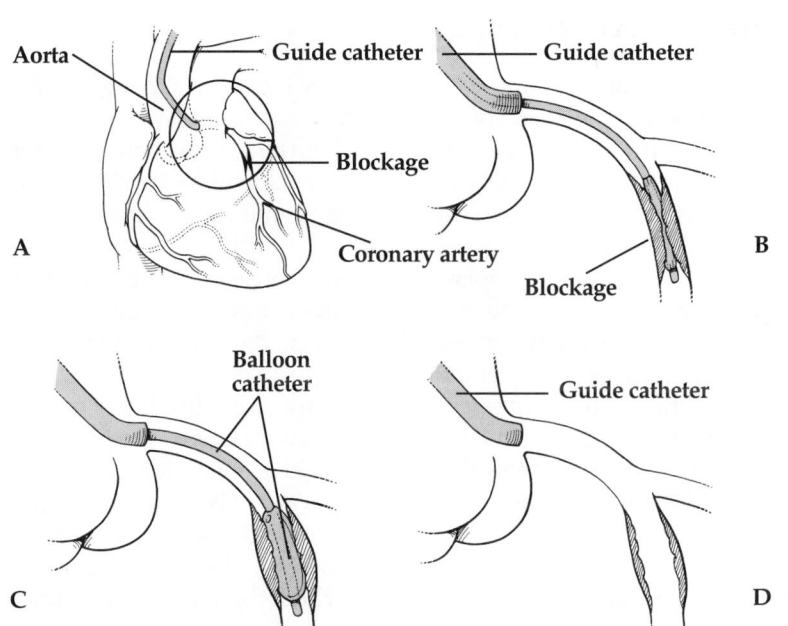

Percutaneous transluminal coronary angioplasty (PTCA) opens narrowed coronary arteries. A catheter inserted in an artery in the groin or shoulder is threaded to the affected artery (A). A second catheter is then inserted inside the first one (B). When it reaches the narrowed area, a balloon on its tip is inflated to reopen the artery (C). The catheters are then withdrawn (D).

Procedure

After a local anesthetic is injected into your groin or shoulder area, the physician inserts a hollow, flexible tube, called a guide catheter, into a leg or arm artery. While watching on a TV monitor that displays an X-ray image of the blood vessel and catheter, the physician guides the catheter into the narrowed coronary artery. A small amount of radiopaque dye may be delivered to the area through the catheter, in order to enhance the clarity of the angiogram and help the physician be sure of the exact location of the blockage.

A smaller catheter is then inserted inside the guide catheter. This one has a balloon at its tip. When the catheter tip reaches the area of obstruction in the coronary artery, the balloon is inflated for about half a minute to widen the obstructed part of the artery. While it is inflated, you may feel chest pain; when it deflates, the pain will fade. Several inflations and deflations usually are necessary. Then the balloon catheter is removed, and more X-rays (angiograms) are taken to see how blood flow has improved.

The entire process usually takes between 30 and 90 minutes. The procedure also may be used to treat blocked arteries elsewhere in the body, including the legs.

Results

Improved blood flow, increased blood pressure in the affected artery, compression or splitting apart of the blockage itself, and stretching or enlargement of a portion of the artery wall are the hoped-for results. In a small percentage of cases, the procedure is unsuccessful and bypass surgery is necessary; usually, a surgical team is available to proceed immediately. When the angioplasty alone is successful, the need for major surgery and the use of a heart-lung machine is avoided. The costs are considerably less and the hospital stay is days rather than weeks.

Recovery and Rehabilitation

For 24 hours after the procedure, your heart rate and rhythm and other vital signs will be closely monitored. Because the procedure involves insertion of a small catheter through the skin, the incision is small and many people go back to work a week after the procedure.

Who Is a Candidate for PTCA?

People whose angina has not been relieved by medications are candidates for this procedure. The ideal candidate has only one narrowed artery, although many persons with several areas of narrowing can undergo PTCA. The decision to recommend PTCA rather than bypass surgery is based on the location, number, and severity of blockages as well as on the overall function of the heart.

However, the procedure does not cure the underlying disease. In fact, the procedure may have to be repeated to reopen the same or another coronary artery that becomes blocked.

New Treatments Using PTCA

Several new treatments for opening blocked coronary arteries have been used with increased frequency. The procedural approach (a catheter) is very similar to that used in PTCA, but instead of using a balloon, the physicians use a laser, a tiny rotating blade, or a little metal "scaffold" to widen the obstructed artery.

Lasers use high-energy light to remove plaque from the vessel wall. Typically, a balloon is used after the use of the laser catheter to open the narrowing further.

Atherectomy devices mechanically remove plaque with tiny rotating blades. Some devices actually cut away the plaque so it can be removed from the body through the catheter. Other devices pulverize the plaque into microparticles that wash downstream in the circulation like flour being put down a drain. These microparticles are then cleared from the small blood vessels. As with laser treatment, a balloon inflation typically is used to complete the procedure.

Metallic coils or stents can act as a scaffold to mechanically hold the vessel open. They can be used to treat some complications of other procedures such as PTCA and also to decrease the chance of re-narrowing (re-stenosis). Stent use is increasing rapidly. Some patients with stents require blood thinners (anticoagulants) to prevent blood clots from forming on the metallic surface. The need for this is temporary (usually about 6 weeks). Other patients may not require anticoagulants.

One of these newer devices may be selected instead of PTCA, depending on your specific arterial blockage (stenosis), other factors relating to your condition, and the experience of your physician.

Sexual Activity After a Heart Attack

In short, no, it is not necessary to forgo the pleasures of sexual activity forever. However, a sensible lapse is in order, perhaps for 30 days after your heart attack.

The demands placed on your heart when you have sexual relations are roughly the same as taking a brisk walk or climbing a flight or two of stairs. Your heart rate, breathing rate, and blood pressure increase, so sexual activities should be approached as any other physical activities: sensibly, with caution but without fear.

At First, Take It Easy

Before the resumption of sexual intercourse, it makes sense to content yourself with lesser contacts, at first confining your intimacies to kissing or caresses. As your confidence grows in the health of your heart, gradually resume your usual sexual patterns.

In order to minimize the stress on your heart, it is sensible strategy to resume sexual relations with your usual partner under your usual circumstances: you will probably feel more relaxed and natural making love in a familiar setting. If you find certain positions less strenuous than others, take the less taxing route, at least at first.

The Importance of Communication

Talk to your partner, too, both before and after, to reassure yourself and that person. Shared fears and concerns may be alleviated if lines of communication are open.

Talk to your physician if you have fears or concerns. It is quite normal for your needs to have changed temporarily: you may experience an increased or reduced desire for sexual activity.

Recognize Warning Signs

If you experience chest pain, extreme shortness of breath, or irregular heartbeat during sexual activity, stop. Do not try to go too far too fast.

Again, it is time to go on with your life, but it is wise to do it sensibly and with the help and guidance of your physician and the loved ones around you.

Cardiac Rehabilitation

Recovery from a heart attack or "coronary event" may require a wide variety of rehabilitation strategies. To help you implement them, an equally varied group of professionals may be needed, including physicians trained in cardiology (cardiologist) and rehabilitation medicine (physiatrist), nurses, dietitians, occupational and physical therapists, an exercise physiologist, a psychologist, a smoking cessation counselor if appropriate, a pharmacist, and a rehabilitation coordinator.

The process of cardiac rehabilitation has three key stages. First are the immediate activities involved in saving your life and over which you have little control. Second is the ongoing medical attention, including medication and perhaps surgery; most of the decisions concerning this part of the process are made by you and your physician.

However, as a patient, you must take charge of the third stage, which includes the lifestyle adjustments you need to make as you recover. These begin with mental adjustments and carry through to changes in personal exercise, diet, smoking, and other habits. Below are listed some of the key matters you must address, often in conjunction with the appropriate professional help.

Stress

The psychological component of heart disease is still somewhat of a mystery, but there is a clear consensus that many people exert unnecessary pressures on themselves as they go about living their lives. After a heart attack, avoid such pressures.

Some individuals temporarily experience insecurity and even depression following a heart attack or coronary artery bypass surgery. Your cardiac rehabilitation team is experienced in these issues and will work with you to deal with these emotions.

Recovering from a heart attack does not necessarily mean you should change your job, avoid all of life's challenges, or make other radical changes. Decreasing the stress in your day-to-day activities, however, may involve rethinking workaholic habits, avoiding frustrating commuting or high-pressure deadlines, and working to minimize stressful events in your life.

Exercise

The prevailing wisdom used to be to advise the heart attack survivor to retire from an active life. This is not the approach today for most people.

As you recover, you may be given an exercise tolerance test (see page 655) to assess your heart's responses to physical activity. Your physician will advise you on what to do and not do, but in general your heart will grow stronger as you recover; exercise will enhance that strengthening process.

You will not go back to full-speed activities on day 1, but enrolling in a cardiac conditioning course may help you get started. If you were sedentary before your heart attack, a carefully planned exercise program is especially important.

While you are still in the hospital, a physical therapist may begin to help you get your body moving again and to regain your confidence in your heart and health. The therapist will instruct you in the initial phases of an exercise program and advance the program during your convalescence. An occupational therapist may provide you with instructions for a home program once you are dismissed from the hospital.

Ask your therapists for help in planning and establishing new exercise patterns appropriate to your lifestyle and condition. Also, outpatient supervised exercise rehabilitation programs are appropriate for many persons who have had a heart problem. Sometimes YMCAs or YWCAs offer them. Ask if one is available in your community.

Diet and Weight Control

If it was true before your heart attack, it is even truer now: keeping your weight down and avoiding saturated fats and cholesterol-rich foods are very important. Losing those extra pounds will decrease the stress on your heart. A change in eating habits to avoid fats will help limit the further accumulation of fatty plaque in your arteries.

Discuss your dietary habits with a registered dietitian at the hospital. This professional can help you draw up a plan to decrease intake of fats and to learn to think before you eat in restaurants and as you go about your day (see Nutrition and Health, page 251).

Stop Smoking

Every cigarette you smoke affects more than your blood pressure and heart rate. It accelerates the process of atherosclerosis (see page 636). Use the experience you have just had as an impetus to quit (see How to Stop Smoking, page 321).

Where to Get Help

Ask your physician or other professional helpers about where to turn for further cardiac conditioning programs or counseling after you leave the hospital. Check with the local YMCA or chapter of the American Heart Association in your area.

The message of cardiac rehabilitation is risk factor modification and instruction in exercise to resume a normal lifestyle (see Controllable Risk Factors, page 638). Listen! It may prolong your life.

Disorders of Heart Rate and Rhythm

The pumping of your heart must be constant and continuous; if the process becomes disordered or interrupted, your heart may fail to deliver the blood your tissues require for life.

Your heart itself is essentially two pumps, each of which consists of a pair of hollow chambers formed of involuntary muscle. The contraction of the muscle causes blood to be pumped.

The control mechanism for the heart rate involves electrical impulses. One of the four chambers of the heart, the right atrium, contains a group of cells called the sinus node. The sinus node acts as a pacemaker, producing electrical impulses that signal the muscle of the heart to contract in the pumping cycle.

Your heart rate varies depending on your activity at any given moment. When you are at rest, your heart pumps more slowly and at a regular rate, about 60 to 80 beats a minute. When you run, climb stairs, or otherwise exert yourself, the sinus node issues electrical "instructions" to increase the pace of your heart in order to provide your muscles and other tissues with the necessary additional blood and its supply of oxygen. Your heart rate may increase up to 200 beats a minute if you exert yourself strenuously.

If something goes wrong with the functioning of the sinus node and the normal pacing of your heart is disturbed, one of a number of rhythmic disorders of the heart may occur. Too rapid a heartbeat is termed tachycardia; too slow a heart rate is bradycardia.

Your heart rate may be affected by various factors including tobacco use, caffeine-containing foods, alcohol, and a number of drugs, both prescription and nonprescription. In addition, the cardiac disorders discussed in the following pages may produce heart rate problems.

Heart Arrhythmias

Signs and Symptoms
- None
- Palpitations or skipped heartbeats
- Spells of light-headedness or unconsciousness
- Chest discomfort
- Shortness of breath

If the rhythm of the beat of the heart is disturbed, the problem is termed arrhythmia. Depending on the nature of the arrhythmia, the symptoms vary. You may be entirely unaware of the problem or you may experience one or more of the symptoms listed above.

Almost everyone experiences an occasional skipped heartbeat or minor palpitation. In general, such an event is not an indication of a problem. However, if the discomfort is great or if the problem recurs, consult your physician. The problem may be quite minor or it may be serious; no treatment may be necessary, or a regimen of medication or other intervention may be required. Your physician's approach will depend on your age, physical condition, presence of underlying heart disease, and the precise nature of the disorder.

Ectopic Atrial Heartbeat
The least serious of the cardiac arrhythmias is an ectopic atrial heartbeat (from the Greek *ektopos* for "misplaced"). This problem involves a small variation in an otherwise normal pulse. In fact, the old cliché "my heart skipped a beat" may well have been coined to describe an ectopic heartbeat.

An ectopic atrial heartbeat is often termed extrasystole. The extrasystole may show up on a routine electrocardiogram. If there is

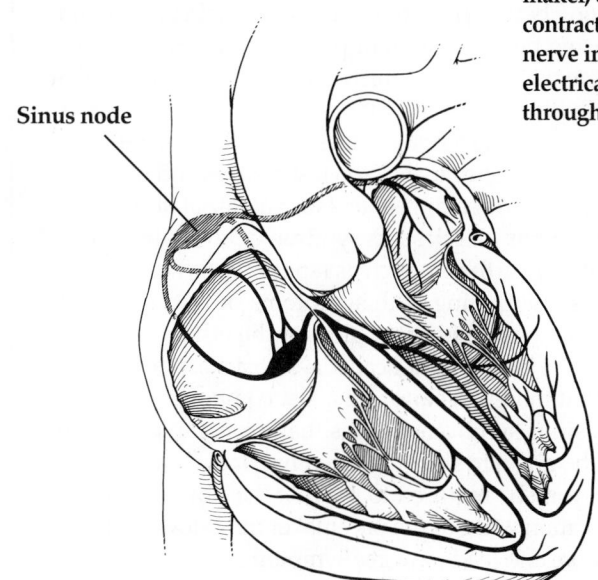

Sinus node

The sinus node, located in the right atrium, acts as your heart's pacemaker, controlling its contractions by issuing nerve impulses along electrical pathways throughout the heart.

concern that the ectopic beats are causing some of the symptoms listed above, an event recorder that you trigger at the first sign of symptoms or a 24-hour Holter monitor can be used.

In most cases, an ectopic heartbeat is harmless and requires no treatment. Often the problem is precipitated by excessive use of tobacco, alcohol, or caffeine-containing foods and beverages. Try decreasing or eliminating the use of these substances if you have an ectopic heartbeat.

In some cases your physician may prescribe a medication that will control the rhythm of your heart.

Atrial Fibrillation and Flutter

When functioning normally, the atria (see The Healthy Heart and Blood Vessels, page 633) contract at a rate coordinated with the rates of the other chambers of the heart, the ventricles. In some people, however, the atria may begin to contract much too often, a condition called atrial flutter. The ventricles tend to beat at every second atrial beat.

When the muscles making up the atrial walls are contracting in an ineffective and uncoordinated manner, the condition is called atrial fibrillation. In atrial fibrillation, the electrical impulses are transmitted to the ventricles in an irregular fashion, often more rapidly than normal. Both atrial flutter and atrial fibrillation tend to occur in episodes, with occasional attacks separated by long periods of normal heart rhythms. However, either may become persistent and chronic.

In atrial flutter or atrial fibrillation, the ventricles may fail to pump enough blood. The result is faintness and weakness. With atrial fibrillation, you may be aware of the irregularity of your pulse and heartbeat. The failure of the atria to contract normally (meaning that the chambers fail to empty completely) can allow a clot to form in an atrium. If the clot breaks loose and is carried in the bloodstream to the brain, it may cause an embolus (see Arterial Embolism, page 692), which can damage the brain (see Stroke, page 461) and other organs or extremities.

Atrial flutter is most often associated with a heart attack or a lung or heart operation. Atrial fibrillation may occur without heart disease or be produced by one of several disorders, including coronary artery disease, rheumatic heart disease (see page 677), malfunction of the mitral valve of the heart (see Mitral Valve Problems, page 680), heart infection (see Pericarditis, page 687), and various other lung and heart disorders. An excess of thyroid hormone also can result in the disorder (see Hyperthyroidism, page 947), but there may be no apparent cause for either arrhythmia, in particular among younger people.

Treatment

To establish the diagnosis, your primary physician or cardiologist will obtain an electrocardiogram (ECG). If the rhythm disturbance is intermittent, you may be provided with a portable electrocardiograph machine, called a Holter monitor or event recorder, that records your heart rate while you go about your normal activities (see Twenty-Four-Hour Cardiac Monitoring, page 671). Other tests also may be required, ranging from simply taking your blood pressure to performing an echocardiographic examination (see The Echocardiogram: Images Made With Sound, page 683) and, rarely, angiography (see Scans and Coronary Angiogram, page 656).

Once the diagnosis has been confirmed, the treatment depends on the cause. Most

---

Sick Sinus Syndrome

The function of the sinus node is to regulate your heartbeat. Sometimes the sinus node fails to perform adequately in this role as your heart's pacemaker. When this occurs, the condition is called sick sinus syndrome.

In this condition, the sinus node initiates beats too slowly, pauses too long between beats, or stops producing beats. If it stops producing beats, a different part of the heart must take over the pacemaker function, which it usually does at a rate that is substantially slower than normal.

To further complicate the situation, sinus nodes that are "sick" may also have a tendency to beat too fast at times and occasionally they beat in an irregular fashion (such as atrial fibrillation). Thus, the symptoms of sick sinus syndrome can be those associated with slow heartbeats (such as fatigue, light-headedness, and blackouts) alternating with symptoms of fast heartbeats (such as palpitations). Either the slow or the fast rhythms can cause shortness of breath, light-headedness, blackouts, or fatigue.

The fact that there is a slow and a fast component in many cases of sick sinus syndrome makes therapy complex. Medications may be given to slow the rapid heartbeat. In addition, a pacemaker may be required to prevent the slow heartbeats. Giving medication without the pacemaker may slow the heartbeats even more and lead to worse symptoms.

often, a medication will be prescribed that will control the rhythm of your heart (see Medications for Rhythm Control of Your Heart, page 676).

In some cases an electrical stimulus called electrical cardioversion may be given to help restore normal rhythm. First you may receive a drug treatment to limit the risk of an embolism. Then, after you have been anesthetized by a short-acting painkiller, an electric shock will be delivered from two "paddles." This mild shock will interrupt the pattern of arrhythmia and may allow your heart to reestablish a normal rate and rhythm.

Paroxysmal Atrial (Supraventricular) Tachycardia

If you feel your heart suddenly race, you may be experiencing an attack (paroxysm) of tachycardia (the word comes from the Greek words *tachys* for "rapid" or "swift" and *kardia* for "heart"). During such an attack, which may last for minutes or as long as a day or two, your heart rate may range between 140 and 240 beats a minute. Some people report an accompanying sensation of doom or anxiety.

Paroxysmal atrial tachycardia is not a life-threatening disorder, although some individuals will develop light-headedness. Repeated attacks may increase the risk of heart failure developing (see Congestive Heart Failure, page 659). Consult your physician when an attack occurs because he or she will be able to understand your condition better when able to examine you during an attack. An electrocardiogram examination may also be conducted (see Twenty-Four-Hour Cardiac Monitoring and Event Recording, below).

Treatment

Several self-help treatments are effective in returning the heartbeat to its normal rate. Holding your breath and straining (exerting pressure as if you were blowing up a balloon) while sitting with your upper body bent forward may help. Your physician can instruct you in other helpful techniques after he or she has examined you to make sure the techniques would be safe.

You also may be able to prevent future attacks by making some small changes in your lifestyle. Excessive use of tobacco and consumption of alcohol and caffeine-containing beverages (coffee, tea, and cola drinks) may increase your risk of such attacks. Try to limit their consumption.

Twenty-Four-Hour Cardiac Monitoring and Event Recording

The electrocardiogram (also known as ECG) is an important tool in detecting and diagnosing different types of heart rate and rhythm disorders.

An ECG is a graphic representation of the electrical forces of your heart. As the cardiac cycle repeats itself every second or so, there is a pattern of electrical pulses that reflect the action of the heart. These pulses can be recorded by electrodes attached to the surface of your body. The activity of the heart—represented by characteristic waves—can then be read instantaneously on a television monitor or studied later on graph-paper printouts.

The ECG has proven to be an invaluable tool for the cardiologist. A portable version, designed by J.J. Holter and called a Holter monitor, has been in use since 1961.

Electrodes attached to your chest are linked to a small box containing a recording device. As you go about your normal activities, the device records the activity of your heart. When you return to your physician a day or two later, he or she will have a day-long record of your heart's activities.

The Holter monitor is an especially useful tool for diagnosing heart rhythm disturbances that may occur at odd and unpredictable times. Together with a written diary you may be asked to keep regarding your activities and symptoms, the ECG from the Holter monitor may allow your physician to relate your symptoms to actual variations in your heart's rhythms.

Occasionally, a 6-hour recording is sufficient for diagnostic purposes. Unfortunately, sometimes the suspicious symptoms may not occur while the Holter monitor is attached. Under such circumstances, your physician may provide you with a transtelephonic monitor or event recorder. Transtelephonic event recorders can be worn for extended periods (weeks to months). You activate the device when you have a symptom, such as a palpitation. The device records the ECG, which is then transmitted by telephone to a reference laboratory. This increases the chances of making a correct diagnosis about your heart rhythm's relationship to the symptoms.

Your physician may use other means to slow down your heart rate during an attack. Certain medications may be used, but other methods may be appropriate. Among them may be the gentle application of pressure to the arteries in your neck. In some cases, an electrical stimulus, called electrical cardioversion, may be given to restore normal rhythms (see Atrial Fibrillation and Flutter, page 670).

Radiofrequency catheter ablation is now widely used to treat paroxysmal atrial tachycardia. Some types of paroxysmal atrial tachycardia, especially those associated with a rare condition called Wolff-Parkinson-White syndrome, may be permanently cured by placing a catheter in the vein and advancing it to the area of the heart where the abnormal heart rhythm originates. The abnormal tissue is then destroyed (ablated) with the catheter. This approach eliminates the need to take medications on a daily basis.

Ventricular Tachycardia and Fibrillation
Ventricular tachycardia is the term used to describe too-rapid contractions of the ventricles. It usually is associated with heart disease (see Coronary Artery Disease, page 654) or occurs in the several days immediately after a heart attack (see page 661).

Ventricular fibrillation describes a condition in which the muscle fibers of the ventricles contract in an uncoordinated and inefficient manner so that the pumping action virtually ceases. If a normal, organized pumping action is not restored in a matter of minutes, death results (see Sudden Cardiac Death, page 674).

Treatment
The first approach is to control the ventricular arrhythmia. Various medications will be administered and in some cases an electric shock may be delivered in a procedure called electrical cardioversion to restore normal heart rhythms. Occasionally, such arrhythmias can be treated surgically, with catheter ablation, or by the use of special autonomic defibrillators that can be implanted in the body somewhat like a pacemaker.

Other Arrhythmias
Among other (and usually minor) arrhythmias are ventricular premature complexes (VPCs). These resemble ectopic atrial beats. Ectopic ventricular beats are observed in the electrocardiograms of nearly two of every three adults monitored over a period of hours (see Twenty-Four-Hour Cardiac Monitoring, page 671). VPCs usually require no treatment unless they are associated with other symptoms or are occurring frequently.

However, there is an association between certain patterns of VPCs and sudden cardiac death (see page 674). Thus, if your physician notes VPCs in your electrocardiogram, he or she may recommend use of an anti-arrhythmia drug (see Medications for Rhythm Control of Your Heart, page 671).

Heart Block

Signs and Symptoms
- None
- Breathlessness and feeling of exhaustion

Internal Cardioverter-Defibrillator

Ventricular fibrillation is a life-threatening rhythm disturbance. Unfortunately, people who experience ventricular fibrillation are at risk of recurrence. In addition, individuals with ventricular tachycardia may have serious symptoms such as loss of consciousness, and the tachycardia may proceed to the more dangerous ventricular fibrillation. Because no medication is 100 percent effective for managing any recurrence, special measures are often warranted. Internal cardioverter-defibrillators are increasingly being used to fulfill this need.

Like pacemakers, internal cardioverter-defibrillators are battery-driven devices that are implanted in the body. Since they are slightly larger than pacemakers, they are implanted beneath the skin and muscle of the abdomen. The devices can also be used for pacing just like a regular pacemaker should the need arise.

Wire electrodes attach the pulse generator to the heart. Some of the wires are inserted through veins into the inside of the heart and can sense the heartbeat. Other wires may be attached to the outside of the heart. These are used for delivering the shock to the heart when it is required to correct the rhythm disturbance.

Internal cardioverter-defibrillators can sense the heart's rhythm and respond in a fashion that is designed to convert the heart to a normal rhythm. Some of these devices can detect when ventricular tachycardia occurs and then attempt to correct the rhythm with a small electrical pacing current. If several of these attempts are unsuccessful, or if ventricular fibrillation develops, then the internal cardioverter-defibrillator shocks the heart directly.

The shock may feel different for each person in each event. It may feel like a kick or a thump in the chest. Your physician will discuss indications for this procedure and its potential risks and complications.

Electrophysiologic Testing

In some situations, an electrocardiogram and other related tests used to check the electrical function of the heart are inconclusive, particularly in individuals who have experienced unexplained dizziness, fainting spells, or palpitations. In these cases, electrophysiology (EP) tests may be done in a controlled hospital setting to find out where the problem is and what can be done to fix or control it.

The procedure is done in a special laboratory that has equipment for recording the heart's electrical signals and for electrically stimulating the heart. The preparation is similar to that for a heart catheterization (see page 1340).

In EP tests, electrode catheters are inserted through blood vessels (usually veins) into the heart chambers, most commonly the right atrium and ventricle. These catheters sense electrical impulses in various regions of the heart and measure how the heart conducts impulses from one area to another. By determining where and when impulses occur, your physician can construct a "map" of the electrical system of your heart.

The electrodes can also pace the heart with a small electrical current just like a pacemaker electrode. Pacing the heart can help in the mapping procedure and can also be used to try to trigger the abnormal heart rhythms causing your symptoms. If this happens, you are in a controlled environment within the laboratory with special equipment and experienced personnel available to handle any problem. Observing the rhythm problem enables your physician to detect what may be causing the rhythm disturbance. During the test, various medications can be given to see whether the drugs prevent the problem. Pacemakers are also used to prevent some rhythm problems, and your response to pacing can be tested during EP tests.

During the EP test, your physician may stimulate your heart with tiny electrical impulses. These may trigger the rhythm disturbance that has been causing your symptoms.

The risk of a complication is less than 1 in 100. There may be bleeding, bruising, blockage, or infection at the site where the wires were inserted. There is also a small risk of perforation of the heart, tearing or separation of the lining of a blood vessel, or stroke. All of these are rare. In addition, risks stem from the fact that the test induces abnormal heart rhythms. In very rare situations, ventricular fibrillation may occur and require defibrillation. If this happens, you will be put to sleep briefly with a short-acting general anesthetic before the defibrillator is used.

Emergency Symptoms
- Extreme breathlessness and weakness
- Loss of consciousness, convulsions

Your heart rate is controlled by electrical impulses issued by the sinus node in the right atrium. These pacemaker cells produce electrical impulses that travel throughout both atria, causing the muscular walls of the atria to contract.

The electrical impulses travel from the atria through a small bed of specialized tissue called the atrioventricular node to specialized fibers (bundle of His) that conduct them to the muscle fibers of the ventricles. These muscles then contract.

In heart block, the electrical impulse passes through the atrioventricular node and bundle of His slowly, intermittently, or not at all. This condition can result from various causes including scarring in the path of the specialized conduction fibers, coronary artery disease (including a heart attack), congenital heart disease, the effects of certain drugs (including heart medications such as digitalis and the beta-adrenergic and calcium channel blockers), infections such as Lyme disease (see page 1067) and mononucleosis (see Infectious Mononucleosis, page 1064), and other disorders.

Diagnosis
In many people with heart block, there are no obvious symptoms. In severe cases, there may be a sudden loss of consciousness.

Heart block is classified by degrees. First-degree heart block is asymptomatic (without symptoms) and is evident only on the electrocardiogram as a delay in the transmission of the impulse from the atria to the ventricles.

In second-degree heart block, some of the impulses fail to reach the ventricles. The result is an irregular pulse. In many cases, second-degree heart block is a result of an excess of certain heart drugs, and the heartbeat returns to normal with the withdrawal of the medication. In others, the use of an artificial cardiac pacemaker is necessary (see Artificial Cardiac Pacemakers, page 675).

In third-degree heart block, no impulses reach the ventricles and the ventricles are forced to beat with their own intrinsic rhythm. The beating of the heart at this intrinsic rate is often so slow that the flow of blood to the brain and other parts of the body is insufficient. Loss of consciousness may result.

Treatment

First-degree heart block and many forms of second-degree heart block are not serious conditions. Only observation or withdrawing or reducing the medication that produced the heart block is necessary.

When the heart is no longer able to pace itself, a procedure to implant an artificial cardiac pacemaker is required (see page 675).

Sudden Cardiac Death

Signs and Symptoms
- Immediate loss of consciousness for no apparent cause
- No pulse

To many, having a heart attack is their most terrible fear. Yet a different ailment—called sudden cardiac death or cardiac arrest—is actually the leading cause of death in young and middle-aged men (it is more than 3 times as common in men as in women).

Modern medicine is only beginning to understand how the heart of an apparently healthy person suddenly stops beating or beats in an uncontrolled fashion. At times this has been associated with alcohol, the use of illicit drugs such as cocaine, and exercise.

The blood flow to the brain instantly

Fainting Spells

A fainting spell can be frightening, both for you and for those around you. Most often, however, there is no reason to panic.

A fainting spell—the medical term is syncope—is a symptom, not a disorder. When you pass out or faint, it means that your brain is not getting sufficient oxygen to function properly. The signs of impending syncope may include nausea, perspiration, or a "graying-out" of your vision. The key sign, however, is a loss of consciousness.

What Are the Causes?
Syncope usually is the result of a malfunction in either the cardiovascular or the nervous system.

Various heart problems can produce fainting spells. Among them are arrhythmias of the heart, especially an excessively rapid heart rate. In this case the heart pumps insufficient blood to the brain, resulting in syncope (see Heart Arrhythmias, page 669). A narrowing of the valve that feeds blood from your heart to your main artery (see Aortic Valve Problems, page 682), sudden decreases in blood pressure, and slowing of the heart also can produce syncope.

The involuntary (autonomic) nervous system controls the pumping of your heart and the pressure in your blood vessels. When it fails to function properly or if too little blood is being pumped, the autonomic nervous system may malfunction and fainting spells may occur.

What Are the Risks?
Once you are lying flat, blood flow is quickly restored, and you usually regain consciousness. Recovering consciousness quickly after a fainting spell means that little or no damage is sustained by your brain due to the shortage of oxygen. In fact, the most serious risk of syncope is usually from the fall itself: fractures or head injuries may result.

What Is to Be Done?
If you experience a fainting spell, consult your physician. He or she will first identify the cause of the syncope. Your physician then will treat the cause with appropriate means, which may mean heart medications or, rarely, a pacemaker. If the problem involves the autonomic nervous system, garments that constrict the circulation in your leg veins may help maintain an adequate supply of blood to your heart.

ceases, and loss of consciousness results. Ventricular fibrillation is most often the cause of sudden cardiac death. In turn, the fibrillation is usually caused by coronary artery disease (see Heart Arrhythmias, page 669).

However, in a significant number of cases, the cause of sudden cardiac death is unknown.

The ventricles are the lower two chambers of the heart and are largely responsible for pumping the blood to all parts of the body.

Artificial Cardiac Pacemakers

If your heart is unable to maintain a fast enough heartbeat or if it occasionally pauses, the solution may be an artificial cardiac pacemaker. This may be short-term treatment or a permanent solution.

Symptoms that may suggest a problem that will require a pacemaker include blackout spells, near faints, shortness of breath (especially during physical activity), and undue fatigue. Slow heartbeat or pauses can occur with various types of heart disease and even in an otherwise apparently normal heart.

An artificial pacemaker is an electrical device that causes the heart to beat by releasing a series of electrical discharges. It replaces the function of your heart's own control system, the sinus node and conduction system (see Disorders of Heart Rate and Rhythm, page 669). The implanted pacemaker mimics the electrical impulses of a healthy heart and restores a sufficiently fast heartbeat. At times, your heartbeat may be fast enough on its own; the pacemaker then automatically goes on standby.

Equipment
The pacemaker itself is small (weighing about 1½ ounces) and is powered by a lithium battery that lasts up to 10 years. Other models that are generally used only for short periods are not implanted but are carried outside the body (external pacemakers).

Procedure
The pacemaker usually is implanted beneath the skin on the front side of your chest just below your collarbone. The pacemaker is

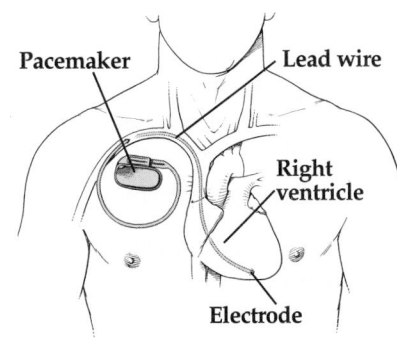

If your heart's internal pacing system fails to control your heartbeat, an artificial pacemaker may be surgically implanted. The battery-powered pacemaker is located beneath the skin of your chest. Flexible wire leads are threaded into the right side of the heart to deliver controlling electrical impulses.

connected to one or two insulated, flexible wire leads. These usually are passed, via a large vein beneath the collarbone, into the right side of the heart. There, an electrical contact (electrode) discharges impulses to the inner surface of the right side of the heart to stimulate its contractions when the heart rate slows.

Applications
The artificial cardiac pacemaker is not a solution to all heart problems, but it can be used to treat a number of heart disorders. Its primary application is to control or prevent slow arrhythmias of the ventricles. Many pacemakers prevent the heartbeat from ever going below a certain rate; this lower limit can be set by the physician even after the pacemaker is implanted. Other

pacemakers are designed to increase the heart rate automatically during activity or stress, just as in the normal heart.

Two-wire pacemakers (with one wire in the top chamber, or atrium, of the heart and one wire in the bottom chamber, or ventricle) are called dual-chamber devices. They ensure that the heart beats in a normal sequence—atrium first, followed quickly by the ventricle.

Some very specialized pacemaker devices can be used to treat specific types of fast arrhythmias when medicines are not effective.

Living With a Pacemaker
There have been major technologic advances in recent years, but modern pacemakers may still be affected by outside electrical interference. If you have a pacemaker, avoid arc-welding and mechanical work on a running car engine, because electromagnetic fields may interfere with your pacemaker's function. If you use a cellular phone, hold it to the ear farthest from your pacemaker, and don't carry your phone in a pocket over your pacemaker. In addition, avoid electromagnetic fields such as those found near a high-voltage transmission line or substation.

Pacemakers can also pose problems if you are undergoing an MRI scan (see page 1334) or if you have an operation in which electrocautery is used to control bleeding. Avoid hard contact to the pacemaker, such as might occur while playing football or firing a rifle from the shoulder near the pacemaker. Modern pacemakers are not affected by microwave ovens.

Medications for Rhythm Control of Your Heart

In treating your heart rhythm disturbance (arrhythmia), your physician may prescribe one or more of a group of drugs. Some work to slow down the pace of the heart; others increase it.

Digitalis

Digitalis preparations (for example, digoxin) may be prescribed to treat atrial arrhythmias. Digitalis slows the transmission of the heart's electrical impulses, thereby helping restore normal heart rate and rhythm. Digoxin also is used to increase the efficiency of the pumping action of the heart.

Calcium Channel Blockers

These drugs decrease the frequency and force of the heart's contractions, resulting in a decrease in its oxygen needs. They function by blocking the entry of calcium into your cells. Two of the calcium channel agents, verapamil and diltiazem, are used to treat arrhythmias.

Atropine

This drug is used to increase the heart rate. It may be used in treating the decreased heart rate (bradycardia) that results from heart attack or other disorders.

Beta-Adrenergic Blocking Drugs

These drugs block the stimulating effect the hormone epinephrine has on your heart. In treating disorders of arrhythmia, the beta-adrenergic blockers slow the speed at which the nerve impulses travel from the sinus node to the rest of the heart muscle.

Adenosine

This drug slows conduction in the atrioventricular node and is used to terminate paroxysmal atrial tachycardia.

Other Drugs

Quinidine, procainamide, disopyramide, mexiletine, flecainide, propafenone, sotalol, and amiodarone are new drugs that work to control abnormal heart rhythms, including atrial fibrillation, atrial flutter, paroxysmal atrial tachycardia, and ventricular tachycardia. Each of these drugs functions by stabilizing the heart rhythm to prevent episodes of tachycardia.

When the control system of the heart malfunctions and causes the ventricles to quiver very rapidly and ineffectively (fibrillate), the blood flow stops and sudden cardiac death can result.

When ventricular fibrillation occurs in someone in a hospital and prompt treatment is available, this rhythm disturbance sometimes can be corrected. However, in most cases of sudden cardiac death, the event occurs beyond the immediate reach of appropriate care and the victim dies before treatment can be given.

Treatment

If the heart ceases to function, cardiopulmonary resuscitation (see page 664) should be used to maintain some oxygenation of the blood and some flow of blood to the brain.

CPR may restore a heartbeat, but, in the event of ventricular fibrillation, an electrical shock delivered to the heart may be required. A device called a defibrillator is used to shock the heart, which stops the ventricular fibrillation and allows a normal heart rhythm to return. After resuscitation, drugs may be used to prevent episodes of ventricular fibrillation from recurring (see Medications for Rhythm Control of Your Heart, this page). Certain individuals who have survived an episode of cardiac arrest may receive an implantable cardioverter-defibrillator (see page 672), which monitors the heart rhythm. If it detects ventricular tachycardia or ventricular fibrillation, the device delivers a shock to terminate the arrhythmia.

Prevention

As we learn more of the causes of sudden cardiac death, it is becoming apparent that in some cases we can identify persons who are most at risk. Certain arrhythmias and other factors have been shown to produce ventricular fibrillation in some people. This is one reason why many cardiologists recommend having a so-called baseline electrocardiogram at about age 30.

People who have already had one heart stoppage are at increased risk for sudden cardiac death.

Disorders of the Heart Valves

The human heart consists of four chambers and four valves. Two of the valves (the mitral and tricuspid valves) regulate the flow of blood from the upper chambers (the atria) to the ventricles (the pumping chambers); the other two valves (aortic and pulmonary valves) regulate the flow of blood out of the ventricles for circulation to other parts of the body. The valves allow blood to flow in only one direction.

The mitral valve links the atrium to the ventricle on the heart's left side; also on the left the aortic valve opens to allow blood into the main artery for the body, the aorta. On the right side, it is the tricuspid valve that regulates flow from the atrium to the ventricle and the pulmonary valve that allows blood to exit from the heart to the lungs via the pulmonary artery.

Each valve consists of two or three thin folds of tissue. When closed, the valve prevents blood from flowing to the next chamber or from returning to the previous one.

When the valve opening becomes narrowed and flow through it is limited, the condition is termed stenosis. Each of the heart's valves may be subject to stenosis or obstruction. In some cases, a valve will lose its shape and begin to sag (prolapse) or will fail to close completely, causing a backflow of blood (regurgitation).

Valve problems may occur as a result of infection, congenital abnormality, or other causes. In the following pages, we will discuss a range of such disorders.

Rheumatic Fever

Signs and Symptoms

Major (two of the following must be present for the diagnosis to be made):
- Inflammation of the heart (carditis), sometimes manifested by weakness and shortness of breath
- Arthritis that tends to migrate from one joint to another
- Uncontrolled movement of limbs and face (chorea)
- Raised, red patches on the skin
- Lumps under the skin (subcutaneous nodules)

Minor (presence of one major and two minor criteria and evidence of a throat infection suggest the diagnosis of rheumatic fever):
- Joint aches without inflammation
- Fever
- Previous rheumatic fever or evidence of rheumatic heart disease
- Abnormal heartbeat on electrocardiogram (ECG)
- Blood test indicating presence of inflammation

Not long ago, many experts were making claims that rheumatic fever had virtually disappeared. Subsequent outbreaks of rheumatic fever among children in several cities in the United States indicate that the disease has made a comeback.

Rheumatic fever appears to be the result of an immune reaction of the body to specific strains of streptococcal bacteria. A week or two after a streptococcal throat infection, the initial symptoms of rheumatic fever may appear. Vigorous and complete antibiotic treatment of streptococcal sore throats will largely prevent the occurrence of rheumatic fever.

One of the problems in preventing rheumatic fever is that sore throats that result from harmless viral infections are often difficult to distinguish from those caused by streptococci. To be sure that streptococcal throat infections are treated properly, throat cultures are obtained to identify the organ-

Each heart valve consists of two or three folds of tissue. When closed, a valve prevents blood from flowing to the next chamber or from returning to the previous one. When open, blood flows freely.

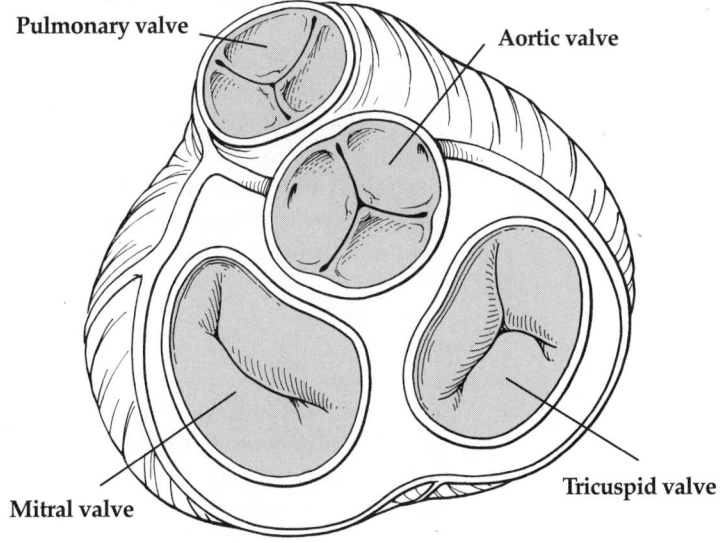

Pulmonary valve

Aortic valve

Mitral valve

Tricuspid valve

isms. If the throat culture result is positive, your physician will institute appropriate antibiotic treatment.

If the antibiotic is administered orally, all of the prescribed drug must be taken, even though the sore throat disappears within the first day or two.

Rheumatic fever occurs relatively rarely. The vast majority of streptococcal throat infections do not lead to rheumatic fever. When rheumatic fever does occur, it usually occurs in children.

Diagnosis

The signs and symptoms detailed above provide quite distinctive criteria for your physician's diagnosis of rheumatic fever.

How Serious Is Rheumatic Fever?

Rheumatic fever can result in inflammation in one or several organs. Most often, several joints are affected with an arthritic swelling, redness, and the sensation of heat.

The heart inflammation may resolve with no permanent effects. However, there may be permanent scarring of one or more valves, which may result in obstruction to blood flow (stenosis) or reversed (backward) flow of blood (regurgitation or insufficiency). Sometimes, over a period of months or years, valve function is seriously compromised and surgery ultimately may be required to repair or replace the damaged heart valve or valves. In rare instances, the heart muscle itself is overwhelmed by the inflammation and death from heart failure occurs (see page 659).

If acute rheumatic fever affects the brain, uncoordinated or uncontrolled movements of the limbs or facial muscles may occur. Such movements are described as chorea, a word derived from the Greek word meaning to dance. In the past, it was common for people to refer to this complication of rheumatic fever as Saint Vitus dance.

Rheumatic fever also can produce disc-like raised and red areas on the skin, called erythema marginatum. Lumps or nodules may form beneath normal-appearing skin.

Treatment

Prevention

Rheumatic fever is avoidable. Pay close attention whenever your child develops a sore throat, especially if it persists for more than 24 hours and is accompanied by a fever. Consult your physician (see page 86).

Throat Culture

If your physician suspects the presence of a streptococcal throat infection, he or she will collect a specimen by wiping the back of the throat with a cotton swab. This specimen then will be used in laboratory tests.

If certain types of streptococci are detected, your physician can prescribe an appropriate antibiotic drug. In many cases, this will be penicillin.

Medication

Antibiotics are given to eliminate any remaining streptococcal organisms. Usually, some kind of a suppressive schedule of antibiotics is continued for several years to prevent second attacks of rheumatic fever. Large doses of aspirin, and sometimes cortisone-like drugs, may be given to suppress the inflammatory process of acute rheumatic fever.

Remember, a sore throat is a common, and usually minor, problem. However, if a streptococcal infection is present and left untreated, serious lifelong heart complications may result from a bout of rheumatic fever.

Infective Endocarditis

Signs and Symptoms
- Fever
- Unusual fatigue or loss of appetite
- Heart murmur
- Night sweats, chills

The endocardium is the membrane that covers the interior of your heart's four chambers and valves. For infective endocarditis to occur, your heart must have a place where the infecting organism can lodge and reproduce; thus, if you have a normal, healthy heart, you are unlikely to contract infective endocarditis. However, you are at risk for this disease if you were born with a malformed heart or heart valves or if your heart valves have become scarred from rheumatic fever (see page 677). Such problems may mean that you have a roughened and abnormal surface within your heart where the infecting organisms can congregate, multiply, and potentially spread to other parts of your body.

Certain bacteria that commonly inhabit the mouth and upper respiratory tract may cause endocarditis. They may enter the bloodstream during a dental or surgical procedure such as a tooth extraction, tonsillectomy, or other operation that involves

Infective Endocarditis: Protection and Prevention

You are susceptible to infective endocarditis if you were born with a malformed heart or heart valve, your heart valves were scarred by rheumatic fever, or you have an artificial heart valve. Even if the cardiac problem is minor and has never caused any difficulty or if the cardiac defect has been repaired and you feel entirely healthy, you still are at risk for this potentially life-threatening infection.

Antibiotics offer protection from infective endocarditis by destroying or controlling bacteria. Use of such drugs may be advisable before and after certain procedures during which bacteria could enter your bloodstream, travel to your heart, and cause an infection there.

If you are at risk, follow these recommendations, which are adapted from the American Heart Association preventive regimens:

Dental Procedures and Oral or Respiratory Tract Surgery

If you are to undergo any procedure on your mouth or throat that may cause bleeding, your physician or dentist probably will prescribe amoxicillin for oral administration. Take the amoxicillin 1 hour before the procedure and again 6 hours afterward.

If you are allergic to amoxicillin (a type of penicillin), an alternative antibiotic such as erythromycin may be substituted. If you have already had heart valve surgery, an injectable antibiotic may be necessary.

Urologic or Gastrointestinal Surgery or Examination With Instruments

The intestinal bacteria (enterococci) often are resistant to penicillin. Appropriate preventive measures may include a combination of injectable antibiotics just prior to and again 8 hours after the procedure. Occasionally, oral antibiotics are sufficient.

Lung and Skin Infections

Antibiotic treatment may be appropriate as a prophylactic measure if a lung or skin infection develops.

Think Prevention

Daily oral hygiene is vital. So is regular, professional dental care. Get regular checkups, and routinely brush and floss your teeth and gums (see Tooth Care, page 363).

Be sure your dentist and each of your physicians know that you are at risk for endocarditis.

---

bleeding in the mouth or throat. Intestinal bacteria, called enterococci, may enter your bloodstream during an instrumental examination or surgery in areas such as the prostate, bladder, rectum, or female pelvic organs. Drug addicts who inject drugs into a vein with unsterilized needles also are vulnerable, even if they have normal valves.

Diagnosis

Endocarditis may develop rapidly, usually with fever and chills, but this is not always the case, especially in elderly people. You may experience any one of various other symptoms including night sweats, malaise, fatigue, loss of appetite and weight, and joint inflammation.

When the infection develops more slowly, your physician will look for such symptoms as an abnormally rapid heart rate (tachycardia), enlargement of the spleen, pallor or a yellow-brown color to the skin, tiny red spots on the skin and mucous membranes, and heart murmurs. Your physician will order a series of blood cultures to determine which microorganism is causing the infection.

How Serious Is Infective Endocarditis?

Infective endocarditis can be fatal without treatment and elimination of the infection. Because the illness usually occurs in people who already have heart disease, the outcome depends largely on whether complications occur. Even if you are cured of the bacterial infection, you may have continued heart symptoms for years after treatment due to additional valve damage from the endocarditis. Complications such as cardiac or renal failure may develop as well.

Treatment

Prevention

Even with the availability of powerful modern antibiotics, treatment can be difficult and the results uncertain. Thus, prevention is the best approach (see Infective Endocarditis: Protection and Prevention, this page).

Medication

Antibiotic therapy depends on the type of microorganism causing the disease. Cultures of the blood are used to determine which antibiotic is appropriate; often, a combination of antibiotics is used, with penicillin commonly being one of them. The medication is often injected directly into a vein and may be given continuously over a period of several weeks to eradicate the infection.

Surgery

If the infection causes major damage to the heart valves, valve replacement may be necessary (see Heart Valve Surgery, page 684).

Mitral Valve Problems

Signs and Symptoms

- None
- Breathlessness, especially after exercise
- Easy fatigability
- Frequent bouts of bronchitis
- Chest discomfort or palpitations

On the left side of your heart, the mitral valve links the upper chamber, the atrium, to the ventricle below. When the opening of the mitral valve becomes narrowed and the passage of blood through it is restricted, the condition is termed mitral valve stenosis (from the Greek *stenosis* for "narrowing"). When the mitral valve fails to close properly and blood flows back into the atrium from the ventricle, the disorder is called mitral valve regurgitation or incompetence.

Mitral valve stenosis is almost always due to rheumatic fever. In the United States, serious mitral valve regurgitation is most commonly due to a condition called myxomatous degeneration—which causes the mitral valve to become floppy. Worldwide, rheumatic fever remains the most common cause of mitral valve regurgitation.

Mitral Valve Stenosis

Obstruction of the mitral valve results in too much blood accumulating in the left atrium because of the narrowing of the exit valve. The atrium becomes enlarged as the pressure in it increases; blood also backs up into the lungs, leading to lung congestion (pulmonary edema). Mitral valve stenosis commonly leads to atrial fibrillation (see page 670).

Mitral Valve Regurgitation

A different problem occurs when the mitral valve does not shut tightly during the contraction of the left ventricle. Because blood flows back into the atrium, the flow to the rest of the body is decreased. The left ventricle (the main pumping chamber) then pumps harder in an attempt to compensate for this decreased flow of blood. Thus, the left ventricle may become enlarged. Eventually, the left ventricle may wear out and become flabby.

There are several possible causes of mitral valve regurgitation. It can be the result of damage sustained during a bout of rheumatic fever, but mitral valve regurgitation also may be present from birth. Mitral valve regurgitation can result from a ballooning out (prolapse) of the mitral valve (see Mitral Valve Prolapse, page 682).

Diagnosis

If you experience breathlessness, especially on mild exertion or at night, your physician may suspect mitral valve stenosis. In advanced cases, the backing up of blood may lead to accumulation of fluid (edema) in the ankles, causing them to swell. In cases of mitral valve regurgitation, many of the symptoms are similar to symptoms of mitral valve stenosis.

To confirm the diagnosis, your physician or a cardiologist will listen to your heartbeat to try to detect the sound of a characteristic heart murmur. A chest X-ray and electrocardiogram will be obtained (see Common Diagnostic Tests, page 654). An echocardiogram (see The Echocardiogram: Images Made With Sound, page 683) can define the configuration of the valve along with abnormalities of blood flow through it.

How Serious Are Mitral Valve Problems?

When the valve disease is mild, you may remain well or have only minimal symptoms for decades. However, the fatigue and breathlessness that eventually may occur can be disabling over time if the deformity of the valve is severe. There also is the risk of atrial fibrillation, in which the atrium beats in a rapid and uncoordinated fashion (see Heart Arrhythmias, page 669). This can lead to the dangerous formation of a blood clot (thrombus) that can travel (embolize) to other parts of the body (see Arterial Embolism, page 692).

Treatment

Prevention of Complications

Some mitral valve problems can be prevented by treating strep throat to prevent rheumatic fever (see page 677). Mitral valve problems put you at risk of infective endocarditis, so take proper precautions before undergoing oral or lower gastrointestinal examinations (see Infective Endocarditis: Protection and Prevention, page 679).

Medication

The excess accumulation of fluid (edema) in your lungs or lower extremities may be treated by use of a diuretic drug. Often called water pills, these drugs will increase the rate and volume of your urine formation, helping to decrease excess fluid in your body. Other medications may be used to help the heart to pump blood through the circulation more efficiently.

If you experience atrial fibrillation, a drug (digoxin) may be prescribed to slow the rapid heart rate. In addition, an anticoagulant may be prescribed to prevent blood clots.

Surgery

In cases of mitral stenosis, when other treatments are unsuccessful, your physician may recommend a procedure called balloon valvuloplasty. In this procedure, the constricted valve opening is enlarged using a catheter with a balloon on its tip (see Heart Valve Valvuloplasty, below). If the valve is too calcified, the balloon procedure may not be safe or feasible, and the valve will have to be replaced surgically. Some cases of mitral regurgitation, particularly from a myxomatous mitral valve, can be corrected by repair-

---

Heart Valve Valvuloplasty

If you have a narrowed heart valve (stenosis), it may limit blood flow and lead to such complications as an enlarged heart. The problem may be treated by open heart surgery (see Heart Valve Surgery, page 684), but another treatment option your physician may recommend is balloon valvuloplasty.

Heart valve valvuloplasty is used when the opening of a heart valve has narrowed. This may occur due to conditions that cause fusion of the valve leaflets, such as prior rheumatic fever (see page 677).

If you have symptoms of mitral valve stenosis (see Mitral Valve Problems, page 680), mitral balloon valvuloplasty is sometimes used as an alternative to surgery. The decision to proceed with mitral valvuloplasty is based on the risk of the procedure versus the risk of surgery. Less calcified and less severely deformed valves represent a very low risk.

If you have symptoms of aortic valve stenosis (see Aortic Valve Problems, page 682), aortic balloon valvuloplasty is sometimes used but generally only if aortic valve surgery is thought to be too risky for you or if you have some other serious medical problem that requires treatment prior to when the surgical replacement of an aortic valve could be performed.

Procedure

Balloon valvuloplasty of the mitral valve is a nonsurgical procedure in which a catheter is inserted through a vein, most often in the groin area. This catheter is advanced through your blood vessels to the right side of the heart.

The catheter is passed from the right atrium, through the common wall shared by the atria, to the left atrium, and then through the mitral valve, where the balloon is inflated to widen the valve opening.

The procedure for aortic valvuloplasty is similar except that a catheter is inserted into an artery in the groin area and advanced backward across the aortic valve. When the tip arrives in the opening of the diseased valve, the balloon is inflated. The narrowed valve is thus enlarged, improving blood flow. Sometimes inflation of two balloons is required to enlarge the opening.

Recovery

As with any heart procedure, there are risks. However, the result may be an immediate relief of such symptoms as breathlessness. The hospital stay and recovery are also substantially less—typically only a few days—than with open heart procedures.

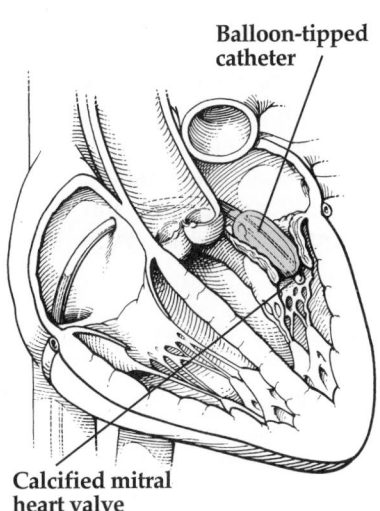

Balloon-tipped catheter

Calcified mitral heart valve

Mitral valve stenosis can often be effectively treated by threading a catheter with an inflatable balloon through a vein and across the atrial septum (which is carefully punctured). It is positioned through the tight mitral opening. Then the balloon is inflated, pressing the valve leaflets apart, producing a wider opening.

ing the valve surgically; other cases require replacement of the mitral valve.

Surgical replacement of the mitral valve can be accomplished with tissue prepared from certain animals or with a manufactured mechanical version (see Heart Valve Surgery, page 684). In selected situations, a heart valve valvuloplasty can be done for mitral stenosis (see Heart Valve Valvuloplasty, page 681).

Mitral Valve Prolapse

Signs and Symptoms
- None
- Brief episodes of rapid heartbeat (palpitations)
- Chest pain
- Breathlessness
- Easy fatigability

Located on the left side of your heart, the mitral valve links the upper chamber, the atrium, to the ventricle below. When functioning normally, the mitral valve, which consists of two leaflets, controls the movement of blood between the chambers. In some people, however, one or both of the valve leaflets balloon out (prolapse).

The prolapse of the valve may result in clicking sounds that your physician can detect when listening to your heart with a stethoscope. The condition may also result in failure of the valves to close properly, and blood may leak back (regurgitate) into the atrium during pumping by the ventricle. This flow of blood back into the atrium produces a sound called a murmur. The combination of these sounds has led to one of the names for mitral valve prolapse, the click-murmur syndrome.

This generally harmless condition may be found in as many as 1 in 10 Americans, more often in women than men. It also is more common in women who have scoliosis or certain other skeletal abnormalities (see page 906).

Diagnosis
Your physician probably will diagnose mitral valve prolapse with the aid of a stethoscope. Your physician or a cardiologist may do a confirming test called an echocardiogram (see page 683).

How Serious Is Mitral Valve Prolapse?
Often, mitral valve prolapse is discovered during a routine stethoscope examination of your heart. The condition is rarely a cause for concern.

In a small percentage of cases, however, this condition may cause episodes of rapid heartbeat (palpitations), chest pain, and significant valve leakage, which may require regular medical attention or even surgery.

Treatment
The vast majority of people with this condition live normal lives, have normal life expectancies, and are not required to make adjustments in their lifestyles. For most, the condition is best regarded as nothing more than a harmless variation from normal.

A rare complication of mitral valve prolapse, particularly in middle-aged or older individuals, is rupture of one or more of the supporting tendons (chordae). Portions of the valve (leaflets) may "flail" and allow leakage of blood, requiring urgent surgical repair.

Prevention
Mitral valve prolapse may put you at greater risk of infective endocarditis. As a precaution, prophylactic use of antibiotics before dental and certain surgical procedures is appropriate (see Infective Endocarditis: Protection and Prevention, page 679).

Medication
If you are among the few people who have mitral valve prolapse that produces frequent and troubling palpitations, your physician may prescribe a beta-adrenergic blocker. These drugs block the stimulating effect the hormone epinephrine has on your heart.

Aortic Valve Problems

Signs and Symptoms
- None
- Weakness on exertion
- Breathlessness
- Chest discomfort (angina)
- Fainting spells

The aortic valve permits the flow of blood from the main pumping chamber (the left ventricle) into the main artery of the body, the aorta, which, in turn, conducts the oxygen-carrying blood to progressively smaller arteries and to the tissues of the body. The valve itself consists of three cusps (cup-

The Echocardiogram: Images Made With Sound

Until the development of echocardiography (sometimes referred to as diagnostic cardiac ultrasound examination), your physician or cardiologist had to rely on physical examination, a graphic display of the heart's electrical activity (ECG), or an X-ray to evaluate the condition and function of your heart. Now it is possible to "look" directly at your heart without ever penetrating your skin.

This device uses reflected sound (echo) of the heart (cardio) to record (graph) an image. Special vibrating crystals generate harmless, high-frequency sound waves (they are inaudible to the human ear) that are aimed at and reflected from the tissues of your heart. The machine records the pattern of the reflection to compose an image of the heart on a monitor screen.

The heart can be seen in action. On a monitor screen, your physician can observe the heart's main pumping chamber, its movement (contractility), the shape and thickness of the chamber walls, the valves, the heart's external covering (pericardium), and large veins and arteries that lead into and out of the heart. The velocity and direction of blood flow through the heart valves and chambers can also be recorded by a device called a Doppler ultrasound to determine narrowing and leakage of the valves.

Procedure

Echocardiography is noninvasive and usually is painless. You will be asked to lie on your back and perhaps turn slightly to your left. Special jelly will be applied to your chest to increase the conductivity of the ultrasound waves.

The transducer (which contains the crystals that produce the waves and receive the echo) will be maneuvered to the best position on your chest. This transducer is linked by a cord to the monitor screen and other electronic components. If your physician needs a clearer picture, the transducer may be threaded down your throat into your esophagus and stomach to enhance the resolution of the images, because the heart and the major vessel in your chest (aorta) are located very close to the esophagus. This procedure is called transesophageal echocardiography.

Advantages

No X-ray exposure is necessary; the procedure is safe and noninvasive. The equipment is also portable, so the study can be done at your hospital bedside, in your physician's office, or even in the operating room.

Diagnosis

Echocardiography can be used to diagnose various heart ailments. Among them are coronary artery disease, heart attack, valve disorders, weakened heart muscles, fluid around the heart (pericardial effusion), abnormalities in the aorta, and congenital heart defects in infants as well as in children and adults. In addition, it has been particularly useful in evaluating function of the left ventricle, the main pumping chamber of the heart.

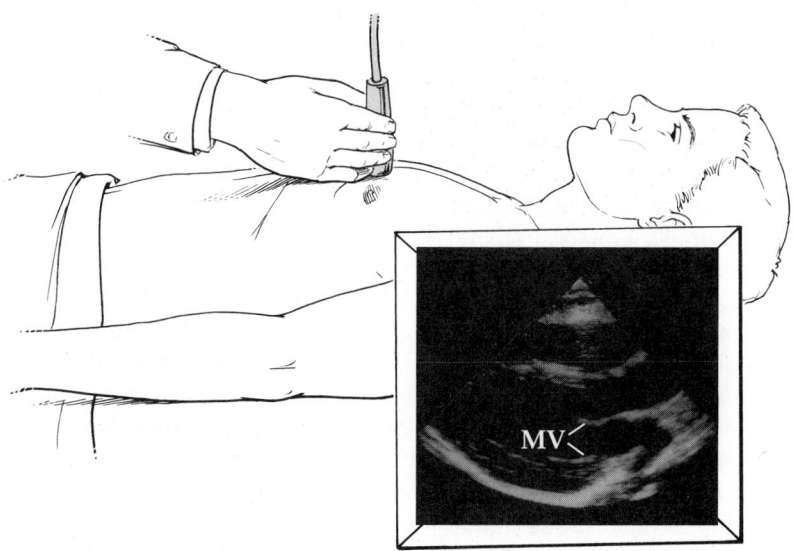

In echocardiography, a wand (transducer) that generates sound waves is positioned over the heart. Reflected sound waves are processed to produce continuous images of the heart tissues on a monitor screen. This echocardiogram shows a normal mitral valve (MV).

shaped folds of tissue) that come together to prevent blood from flowing back from the aorta to the ventricle between contractions.

Aortic Stenosis

When the opening of a valve becomes narrowed and passage through it is limited, the condition is termed stenosis. Such a narrowing in the aortic valve means the left ventricle (the main pumping chamber of the heart) has to pump harder to maintain a normal output of blood. This often results in the muscle of the left ventricle becoming thickened, a condition called left ventricular hypertrophy.

Heart Valve Surgery

In some cases, heart valve problems require no treatment. If treatment is necessary, it may include medications or a procedure called balloon valvuloplasty (see Heart Valve Valvuloplasty, page 681). Occasionally, however, open-heart surgery is the best option.

The term open-heart surgery implies opening the chest and using a heart-lung machine to support the patient while the abnormality of the heart is being repaired. Open-heart procedures include coronary artery bypass surgery (see page 665), correction of congenital abnormalities of the heart (see Congenital Heart Disorders, page 51), heart valve surgery, and removal of some heart tumors.

Valve Repair

If your natural valve can be repaired, the result is usually better and longer lasting, and you may not require additional medications such as anticoagulants that may be necessary with artificial valves. For example, if medications are no longer effective for mitral regurgitation, surgical repair may be indicated. Sometimes this is accomplished by repair of the valve itself and the tendons (chordae) that anchor it to the heart muscle. Sometimes repairing the valve includes "cinching" the surrounding ring of heart tissue tighter to ensure that the leaflets of the valve close adequately.

Mitral commissurotomy is a surgical revision during open-heart surgery in which the surgeon cuts between the valve leaflets that have become "stuck" together in some people with mitral stenosis. However, mitral balloon valvuloplasty (see page 681) is usually as effective as mitral commissurotomy, so operations are being used less frequently.

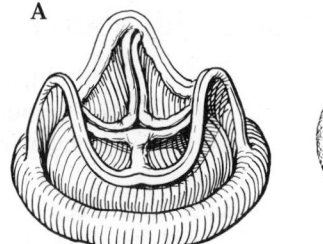 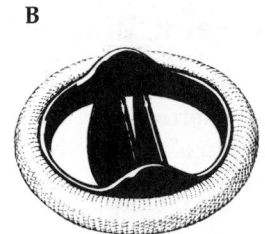 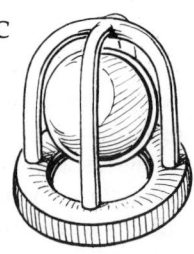

Three commonly used replacement heart valves are (A) valve made from animal tissue, (B) bileaflet valve (open), and (C) caged-ball valve.

Valve Replacement

Replacement of the mitral valve is necessary if either repair or balloon valvuloplasty is judged to be unlikely to provide a satisfactory result. Valve replacement is also the treatment of first choice for aortic valve disease that needs treatment beyond medications. To replace a damaged heart valve, the surgeon removes it and sutures an artificial (prosthetic) valve at the site.

Your surgeon and cardiologist will discuss with you what type of prosthetic valve would be best for you. Each type has particular advantages and disadvantages.

Mechanical prosthetic valves are constructed from metal and synthetic materials. Mechanical prostheses include ball valves, tilting disc valves, and double-tilting half-disc (bileaflet) valves. The advantage of all of these is that they are extremely durable. The disadvantage of mechanical valves is that you will need to take an anticoagulant such as warfarin (Coumadin) for the rest of your life, because blood has a natural tendency to clot on the valve. This clotting could either plug the valve or result in an embolism (a clot that moves to another part of the body such as the brain).

Bioprostheses are made from animal or human tissue. An animal tissue bioprosthesis is usually made from a pig's heart valve, or it is fashioned from the pericardium or outer lining of the heart of a cow. A human tissue bioprosthesis (homograft) consists of a heart valve donated from someone who has died. Unlike heart transplants, the valves can be preserved and are no longer living tissue. They also do not cause rejection. The advantage of bioprostheses is that they usually do not require anticoagulation. However, they are not as durable as mechanical valves.

All prosthetic valves are prone to infection, which is difficult to treat with antibiotics once it develops. Therefore, it is extremely important to take appropriate precautions (infective endocarditis precautions, see page 679) before any dental or surgical procedure if you have a prosthetic valve.

Procedure

You will be given a general anesthetic. Through an incision the length of your breastbone (sternum), your heart is exposed and connected to a heart-lung machine that will assume your breathing and blood circulation during the procedure. The damaged heart valve will be removed and replaced.

Recovery

After the operation (which lasts several hours) you will spend one or more days in a coronary or intensive care unit, where your heart function and general recovery will be closely monitored.

During recuperation, physical therapists, dietitians, and patient educators will assist you in your recovery and return to a productive life.

Over time the left ventricle muscle becomes less efficient, enlarged, and flabby.

Aortic Regurgitation

A different sort of problem occurs when the aortic valve fails to shut tightly between contractions. Called aortic regurgitation or aortic incompetence, this condition means that blood tends to leak back into the ventricle. Consequently, flow of blood to the rest of the body decreases and the heart must pump harder in an attempt to compensate for the decreased blood flow. As a result, the left ventricle often becomes enlarged. With time, the muscle of the ventricle may wear out and become flabby.

Both aortic stenosis and aortic regurgitation can result from damage sustained by the aortic valve from rheumatic fever or as the result of a congenital abnormality. In the United States, aortic stenosis most commonly occurs in elderly persons due to degeneration and calcification of the aortic valve. Aortic stenosis is much more common among men than among women.

Diagnosis

Your physician may discover either of these disorders while listening to your heart with a stethoscope. He or she then may order one of several other tests, including a chest X-ray (to determine if your heart has become enlarged), an electrocardiogram (ECG) to look for evidence of left ventricular hypertrophy, and an echocardiogram (see The Echocardiogram: Images Made With Sound, page 683).

How Serious Are Aortic Valve Problems?

The most serious risk with aortic valve problems is posed by the overwork of the left ventricle. This may result in angina (see page 657), congestive heart failure (see page 659), or fainting spells (see page 674).

Aortic valve problems are insidious and may develop without symptoms until they reach a hazardous phase. Prompt treatment (such as aortic valve surgery) may be necessary.

Treatment

In most cases, aortic stenosis or regurgitation does not mean you need to adopt a passive lifestyle. While strenuous activity is to be avoided, reasonable physical activity is usually encouraged.

Prevention

Aortic valve problems put you at greater risk of infective endocarditis. As a precaution, preventive use of antibiotics prior to dental and certain surgical procedures is appropriate (see Infective Endocarditis: Protection and Prevention, page 679).

Surgery

If your aortic valve is badly deteriorated, the only long-term solution may be surgical replacement or reconstruction of the valve (see Heart Valve Surgery, page 684).

Tricuspid and Pulmonary Valve Problems

The blood flows out of the four chambers of the heart through valves. Earlier we discussed the most common valve problems, those that concern the aortic and mitral valves in the left side of the heart. Rarely, the pulmonary and tricuspid valves also develop serious malfunctions.

Blood flows from the upper chamber, the right atrium, through the tricuspid valve to the right ventricle below. Then, through the pulmonary valve, it exits from the right ventricle to the pulmonary artery, which carries the blood to the lungs for oxygenation.

Both the tricuspid valve and the pulmonary valve (like the aortic and mitral valves) can have problems in which the valve opening narrows, restricting the flow of blood (conditions called tricuspid stenosis and pulmonary stenosis). In some cases, the valve fails to close properly, allowing blood to flow back through the valve when it is supposed to be closed (such disorders are termed incompetence or regurgitation).

Often, these ailments are discovered by physicians during routine examinations; treatment may not be required. However, if the function of the valve is badly deteriorated, valve repair or replacement may be necessary (see Heart Valve Surgery, page 684). In certain situations, the valve may be opened by stretching it with a balloon catheter inserted through a vein in the leg and advanced to the heart.

These valve problems also may put you at greater risk of infective endocarditis. As a precaution, preventive use of antibiotics prior to dental and certain surgical procedures is appropriate (see Infective Endocarditis: Protection and Prevention, page 679).

Diseases of the Heart Muscle and Pericardium

There are three layers of heart tissue: the epicardium, a thin, very smooth covering on the outside; the myocardium, the heart muscle itself (the name comes from the Greek *myo* for "muscle" and *kardia* for "heart") in the middle; and the endocardium, the inner lining, a very smooth layer in contact with the blood. Protecting the whole organ on the outside is the pericardium, a fibrous sac.

The heart muscle and its associated lining are subject to disease. Although relatively rare, diseases that damage the heart muscle (cardiomyopathy) do occur, both as an isolated problem and as a consequence of disorders that affect other organs as well. Inflammations of the myocardium (myocarditis) and the pericardium (pericarditis) also may occur.

Cardiomyopathy

Signs and Symptoms
- Brief episodes of rapid heartbeat (palpitations)
- Breathlessness
- Weakness
- Chest pain
- Fainting
- Fluid retention (edema)

When the muscle of the heart is damaged or defective, the disorder is termed cardiomyopathy, or heart muscle disease. The term "cardiomyopathy" comes from Greek roots for "heart" (*kardia*), "muscle" (*myo*), and "disease" (*pathos*). Cardiomyopathy may appear in one of several forms.

Forms of Cardiomyopathy

Dilated Cardiomyopathy
In dilated cardiomyopathy (also referred to as congestive cardiomyopathy), the heart muscle is weakened and is unable to pump efficiently. This may produce symptoms of congestive heart failure (see page 659) including breathlessness and retention of water, which results in a swelling (edema) that is most evident in the feet and ankles. Dilated cardiomyopathy also causes enlarged heart compartments and may lead to the formation of clots (thrombi) within the enlarged compartments. The clots may travel to other parts of the body (emboli). Dilated cardiomyopathy may occur at any age and run in families.

Alcoholic Heart Disease
Alcoholics may develop dilated cardiomyopathy after they have consumed large quantities of alcohol over many years. If the problem has not advanced to the point of heart failure, cessation of the drinking may halt the progression of the disease.

Hypertrophic Cardiomyopathy
If you have this form, the muscular walls of your left ventricle (the main pumping chamber of your heart) become thickened and stiff. This may impair the flow of blood into your heart as well as the ejection of blood out of it. This disorder often runs in families.

Restrictive Cardiomyopathy
This condition is characterized by stiffening of the heart muscle and a decreased ability to expand and fill with blood between contractions (the portion of the cardiac cycle termed diastole). Development of blood clots within the heart chambers, water retention (edema), and a tender liver are other common signs.

Diagnosis
In diagnosing cardiomyopathy (heart muscle disease), your physician will consider your symptoms, especially breathlessness and chest discomfort, and may perform X-ray and electrocardiographic examinations. Your physician also may obtain an echocardiogram to observe the motions of your heart at work (see The Echocardiogram: Images Made With Sound, page 683). The echocardiogram often can determine what form of cardiomyopathy is present. In some cases, a heart catheterization (see page 1340) may be performed by passing a flexible catheter through a large vein into your heart. Your physician may also obtain a biopsy specimen (tissue sample) from your heart for microscopic examination during this procedure.

How Serious Are Cardiomyopathies?
In most cases, there are no symptoms of car-

diomyopathy until the disease is quite advanced. Sometimes, sudden death is the only indication of the presence of the problem (see Sudden Cardiac Death, page 674).

Often, drug and other treatments can be used to ease the symptoms and improve life expectancy. There may be improvement over time. In some instances when the heart is badly damaged, heart transplantation is an option (see Heart Transplantation, page 688).

Treatment
Although it may be valuable to maintain a good level of overall fitness, strenuous exertion should be avoided. Treatment must be individualized to the type of cardiomyopathy.

Medication
The choice of drugs for treatment depends on which type of cardiomyopathy is present. The possible drugs include diuretics (water pills to decrease water retention), calcium channel blockers (see Calcium Channel Blockers, page 652), blood vessel dilators, drugs to control irregular heart rhythm (see Heart Arrhythmias, page 669), and digitalis and beta-adrenergic blockers.

In some cases, heart muscle disease is a secondary result of another ailment, and the symptoms may improve after effective treatment of the primary problem. Examples of this include hypertension, sarcoidosis, and hemochromatosis (see pages 647, 721, and 806).

Prevention
Certain of the cardiomyopathies may put you at greater risk of infective endocarditis. As a precaution, prophylactic use of antibiotics prior to dental and certain surgical procedures is appropriate (see Infective Endocarditis: Protection and Prevention, page 679).

In cases of alcoholic heart muscle disease, complete and permanent abstinence from alcohol is essential (see Alcohol Abuse and Alcoholism, page 325).

Myocarditis

Signs and Symptoms
- Fever
- Vague chest pain
- Joint pain
- Abnormally rapid heartbeat
- Breathlessness
- Fluid retention

The muscular layer of heart tissue is the myocardium. As its name suggests, the myocardium is the heart muscle itself (the word comes from the Greek *myo* for "muscle" and *kardia* for "heart").

Acute myocarditis is an inflammation of that muscle and usually occurs as a complication during or after one of various infectious diseases (such as coxsackie virus), rheumatic fever, or exposure to radiation, certain chemicals, or drugs. Accompanying pericarditis also may develop (see this page).

Diagnosis
In diagnosing the disease, your physician probably will use an electrocardiogram and an X-ray. Often, a heart muscle tissue examination (biopsy) is performed because this is the only way to confirm the diagnosis.

Myocarditis can be very serious, but the outcome depends on the type of infection. Severe cases can lead to cardiac failure and death, but most often the inflammation clears and good health follows.

Treatment
Therapy consists of avoiding vigorous exercise until the pattern of your heart's activity has returned to normal. A proper diet emphasizing salt restriction and treatment of the underlying cause, if it can be identified, are important.

If your physician observes abnormalities in your heart rhythm, he or she may recommend hospitalization, electrocardiographic monitoring of your heart with an ECG, and appropriate antiarrhythmia medications (see Medications for Rhythm Control of Your Heart, page 676) until your heartbeat returns to normal. In severe situations, your physician may consider heart transplantation (see page 688).

Pericarditis

Signs and Symptoms
- Chest pain radiating to the left side of the neck, shoulder, back, or upper and middle abdomen
- Breathlessness
- Swelling of the abdomen

Heart Transplantation

Heart transplantation has become a routine procedure in many medical centers during the past 25 years. Approximately 2,200 heart transplants are carried out each year in the United States. Results have improved so that the current 1- and 5-year survival rates at Mayo Clinic Rochester are 95 and 80 percent, respectively. Most transplant patients enjoy a full and active life, and many return to full-time employment.

Who Qualifies for a Heart Transplant?

Any patient from before birth to 70 years of age with end-stage heart disease not amenable to more conventional medical or surgical therapy can be considered for heart transplantation. Potential heart transplant candidates should be psychologically stable with good function of all other vital organs, including the liver, kidney, and lungs. Candidates should also be free of other noncardiac diseases, such as certain types of cancer, blood disorders, or severe diabetes, that would reduce life expectancy. Transplant recipients must be willing to accept a lifelong commitment to participate in their medical care, which involves many medications, regular participation in research studies, and scheduled physician and hospital visits. Most potential heart transplant candidates have a limited life expectancy, with symptoms of heart failure such as breathlessness, weakness, fluid accumulation, or cardiac rhythm irregularities.

Heart Donation

There is a shortage of donor hearts for transplantation. As many as 17,000 to 35,000 patients per year could benefit from cardiac replacement in the United States. Only 2,000 to 2,500 donor hearts are available each year. Up to 30 percent of people waiting for a heart transplant die before a donor heart becomes available. Many members of the general public are not yet aware of the vital need for organ donation. Therefore, educational efforts to inform more people of the need for healthy donor hearts is a high priority. Although no one would wish for another person to die so that a heart would be available for transplantation, when deaths occur the families often find comfort in helping another person or persons through organ donation. A single donor may provide lifesaving organs (heart, lungs, kidneys, liver, and pancreas) for six or more recipients.

Families should talk about this issue before the situation arises. The decision to donate a loved one's organs is much easier if families know beforehand what the person would want. Many states now have laws and regulations that promote the process of seeking permission for acquiring donor organs.

Procedure

Before the operation, a donor heart must be found. Most often, this heart comes from the body of a healthy person who died in an accident but did not sustain heart injuries.

The donated heart is transported in a special cold solution to the recipient hospital. The recipient's chest cavity is opened and the diseased heart is removed; then, the new organ is put in its place. During this portion of the procedure, the pumping of oxygenated blood to the body is taken over by a heart-lung machine, as is done routinely in many kinds of heart surgery.

What Is Rejection?

All transplanted organs are susceptible to rejection. The body's immune system recognizes the transplanted tissue as foreign and produces antibodies to attack the "intruder."

To minimize the risk of rejection of a transplanted heart, drugs that suppress the body's normal immune response are given. Some of these "immunosuppressive drugs" are used for a short time and discontinued shortly after the operation. Others are taken for the rest of a patient's life. Well-known medications in this class include cyclosporin, prednisone, and azathioprine. These drugs have side effects and can decrease the body's ability to recognize and resist infections. Medication dosages must be monitored carefully to minimize side effects. A biopsy of your heart tissue will aid your physician in assessing rejection. The biopsy specimen is obtained via a catheter that is placed in a vein and then advanced to the heart.

Recovery

Most successful recipients of heart transplants recover to carry on relatively normal lives. Approximately 90 percent of those who have received heart transplants are alive and active 1 year after the operation; many have lived for more than a decade and some have lived for more than 20 years following their heart transplantation.

Recent Developments

The major challenge in heart transplantation is solving the serious donor shortage. It does not appear that there will ever be enough donors to satisfy the need; thus alternative strategies are being explored clinically and experimentally.

One such effort involves the use of a left ventricular assist device to perform the work of the main pumping chamber of the heart (the left ventricle). Weakness of the left ventricle is the cause of heart failure symptoms in most patients. Assist devices are currently being used in a selected number of major centers to keep heart transplant candidates alive while they wait for a donor heart. The devices are proving very effective and ultimately offer hope for long-term treatment of patients with heart failure.

Another approach in the laboratory is the development of genetically engineered animals, particularly pigs, whose organs would not be rejected by a human (xenotransplantation). This work is in its early phases but may prove a long-term solution to the donor problem.

The pericardium can be described as the bag that encloses the heart. Essentially a sac, it has a very smooth inside surface; outside is the tough (fibrous) parietal pericardium.

Acute Pericarditis

Pericarditis is an inflammation of the pericardium; it may be caused by bacterial or viral infection. It occurs primarily in men between the ages of 20 and 50, often after a respiratory infection. As a result of the inflammation, pain is felt when the pericardium and the outer layer of the heart rub against each other. There may be an accumulation of excess fluid between the pericardium and the heart.

Cardiac Tamponade

When a great deal of fluid accumulates in the pericardium and presses on the heart, so that the heart cannot fill properly, the condition is termed cardiac tamponade. Injury to the pericardium at surgery or in an accident can cause an accumulation of blood and cardiac tamponade. Tuberculosis, tumors, or acute viral infections may result in fluid accumulation and also produce cardiac tamponade. The result can be a restriction of blood flow to the lungs and the rest of the body. Acute cardiac tamponade is a medical emergency.

Constrictive Pericarditis

In some cases, a permanent thickening, scarring, and contracture of the pericardium occur, often without apparent cause. Occasionally, a previous inflammation such as would be caused by tuberculosis may be responsible. The result again is a decrease in the ability of the heart muscle to expand between contractions and fill with blood (the portion of the cardiac cycle termed diastole).

Diagnosis

If you have acute pericarditis or tamponade, your physician may take an X-ray and record an electrocardiogram and an echocardiogram in order to differentiate pericarditis from a heart attack. Blood tests also may be obtained. Although recurrences are common, most patients recover completely from acute pericarditis in 2 weeks to 3 months. The diagnosis of constrictive pericarditis may require, in addition, CT scans of the chest (see CT Scanning, page 1334) or heart catheterization (see page 1340).

For both diagnosis and treatment of cardiac tamponade, a procedure called pericardiocentesis may be required. This involves draining the excess fluid from the pericardium by using a small tube (catheter).

Treatment

Medication

Treatment of pericarditis may include analgesics to relieve the pain. If water retention (edema) and swelling are present, diuretic drugs also may be given.

If an underlying cause such as tuberculosis or other bacterial infection is identified, antituberculosis or antibiotic drugs may be prescribed to treat that cause.

Surgery

In cases of chronic constrictive pericarditis, surgery may be required to cut out (resect) the portions of the pericardium that have grown stiff and are limiting the working of your heart. The procedure is called pericardiectomy. Although the pericardium is thought to serve various purposes, your heart will continue to function normally even if the entire pericardial sac is removed.

Circulatory Problems

The vascular system, the circuit through which your blood travels, consists of the blood vessels in your body. Its name is derived from the Latin *vasculum* for "small blood vessel."

The circulatory system consists of two loops. The shorter loop (pulmonary circulation) begins at the right side of your heart, delivers blood to your lungs, and then returns the oxygenated blood to your heart. The longer loop (systemic circulation) begins at the left side of the heart, where it receives the blood that was oxygenated in the lungs.

From the left side, the blood is pumped to the tissues of your body through a sequence of smaller and smaller blood vessels: arteries branch off into smaller arterioles, and the arterioles branch into tiny capillaries that deliver blood to the tissues. After the blood in the capillaries collects carbon dioxide and other waste products from the tissues, it begins its trip back to your heart via small venules and, eventually, veins. Blood circulates through your liver and kidneys, where waste products are removed or processed; then it returns to your heart.

The total amount of blood within your body is essentially constant (about 7 percent of your body weight); the distribution of blood within blood vessels varies considerably with exercise and exposure to heat and cold. During exercise, for example, the blood flow to active muscles is increased; after you eat, your stomach and intestines draw more blood to assist in the digestive process. Changes in the surrounding temperature also affect the flow of blood: warmer temperatures produce increased flow to the outer layers of your skin (which helps you to dissipate heat); alternatively, your body responds to cold by redistributing blood flow into the inner vessels (in order to conserve heat).

This flexible system is subject to a wide range of malfunctions. Some are the result of heart disorders; others occur because of disorders that directly affect the blood vessels, such as diabetes. The problems range from weakened blood vessel walls that balloon out (aneurysm) to blockages or narrowings that limit or stop the flow of blood (atherosclerotic blood vessel disease). These blood vessel problems can lead to life-threatening events such as stroke and heart attack.

Arteriosclerosis of the Extremities

Signs and Symptoms
- Leg pain, especially in the calves and feet, which develops during activity and resolves shortly after the activity is stopped (intermittent claudication)
- Numbness or pain in the foot or toes when at rest
- Ulcers or gangrene on the foot or toes

The effects of arteriosclerosis are most likely to appear first in your legs or feet (see Atherosclerosis: What Is It? page 636, and Disease of the Heart and Blood Vessels: Living With the Risks, page 635). In one of its forms, arteriosclerosis obliterans, the major arteries that deliver blood to your legs and feet become narrowed and blood flow decreases. Smaller blood vessels assume some of the load, but the physical activity of walking a block or two can produce cramps in your legs or feet; the cramps disappear within a few minutes after you discontinue the exercise. This sequence of walk-pain-rest is also termed intermittent claudication.

When some of the blood vessels actually become blocked (occluded), your foot may become pale, cold, and painful. Sometimes the final blockage develops gradually and

The circulatory system consists of two loops. In the shorter loop, called pulmonary circulation, blood is pumped from the right ventricle to the lungs. From there, oxygenated blood returns to the left atrium. In the longer loop, called systemic circulation, blood is pumped from the left ventricle through the arteries to tissues of the body. It returns through veins to the right atrium.

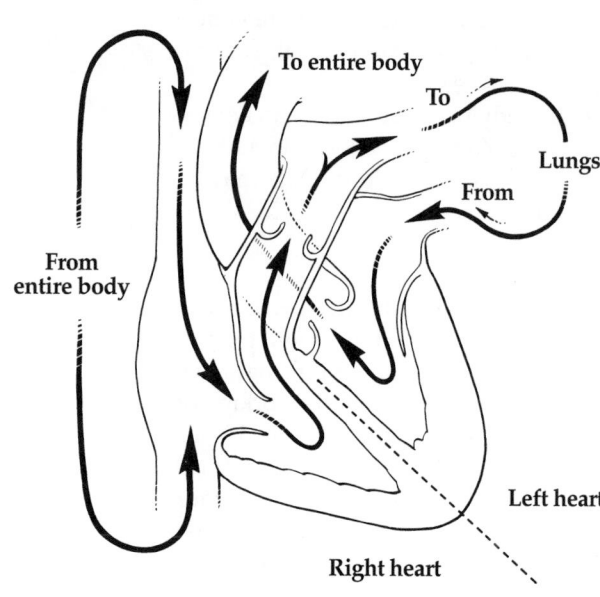

To entire body

To

From entire body

Lungs

From

Left heart

Right heart

your foot becomes vulnerable to even minor injury and infection.

Gangrene consists of the actual death of tissue and usually appears as a spot or area of black, shrunken skin near the tips of your toes or about your heel (see Gangrene of the Extremities, page 692). If the blockage occurs suddenly, as when a fragment of plaque or a clot lodges at a fork of your leg artery (commonly, at your knee), there is sudden and severe pain as well as paleness and coldness below the level of the blockage (see Arterial Embolism, page 692).

The limitation in blood supply often will cause inflammation and damage to the nerves (neuritis), which is manifested by burning, pain, and numbness.

These circulation problems are common in persons with diabetes; they also may have diabetic neuropathy. The decreased sensation that often accompanies diabetic neuropathy makes the person more likely to injure the affected foot (see Diabetes Mellitus, page 925).

Diagnosis

The key aspect to diagnosis is the nature and timing of your discomfort. Does the pain occur only with exercise? Is it relieved by rest? Does it recur when activity is resumed? If so, your physician may suspect arteriosclerosis of your extremity.

Your physician may take your blood pressure in the affected extremity. Other tests, including an ultrasound scan of the area, also may be ordered. Angiography (an X-ray examination during which a dye is injected into the artery that supplies the affected area) will tell your physician exactly where the blockage is and whether surgical repair can be attempted.

How Serious Is Arteriosclerosis of the Extremities?

For many people, arteriosclerosis of the leg is not a serious problem. For most, conservative care will prevent severe disability or loss of a limb; among diabetics, the problem occurs somewhat more often. Poor arterial circulation can blunt sensation to heat or cold, making you more susceptible to both burns and freezing. Take care in applying items such as a hot water bottle or heating pad to cold feet. In addition, do not expose your foot to freezing temperatures. If gangrene develops, surgical amputation may be necessary (see Gangrene of the Extremities, page 692).

Risk Factors for Arteriosclerosis of the Extremities (Intermittent Claudication)

Your risk for arteriosclerosis of the extremities (intermittent claudication) increases if you:

- Smoke
- Are a man
- Are a woman past menopause
- Are at least 60 years old
- Have high blood pressure
- Have high blood cholesterol
- Are overweight
- Are sedentary
- Have diabetes

Not smoking is the best way to prevent and reduce intermittent claudication. Exercise can improve blood flow in your leg's smaller arteries and condition your muscles so they require less oxygen.

Treatment

Self-Help

In most cases, physical activity is a useful element in treatment of limited arterial blood supply to the legs. Your physician will help you devise an appropriate regimen of daily walking or other exercise. Over time, the amount of activity required to cause pain will increase. The circulation can improve with time because collateral vessels that bypass the blocked segment will develop.

Smoking

Smokers are at particular risk for arteriosclerosis. Smoking contributes to the deposition of platelets on the inner layer of arteries. Cholesterol then accumulates. If you have limited arterial circulation, stop smoking.

Proper Foot Care

Foot care is essential. Wear shoes that fit properly. Even minor cuts or scrapes require immediate attention because the decreased circulation means that the tissues heal slowly. If left untreated, even a minor injury to the skin of your lower leg or foot can lead to infection, gangrene, and amputation (see Caring for Your Feet, page 931).

Medication

Your physician may prescribe aspirin or another analgesic if the pain continues even at rest. Your physician also may prescribe a

Gangrene of the Extremities

When the supply of blood to any tissue is severely impaired, the supply of oxygen and nutrients is also restricted. If the flow of blood is not restored in time, the tissue may die. Gangrene is the term used for dead (necrotic) tissue.

The blood flow to the legs may cease abruptly (see Arterial Embolism, this page) or slowly. In either situation, the foot becomes pale and cold. The pain is variable. Calf pain with walking (claudication) is almost always present, and minor injuries tend to cause an infection that may burrow deeply in the foot and involve the bones (see Osteomyelitis, page 899). As the circulation to the extremities ceases, the blood-starved tissues die and gangrene results.

Forms of Gangrene

There are two types of gangrene: wet and dry. Tissue with dry gangrene has died but has not become infected; areas affected with wet gangrene have died and become infected with bacteria.

Dry Gangrene

Tissue affected with dry gangrene is cold to the touch and gradually becomes black. At first, the tissue is painful but, as the affected tissue dies, the pain fades. Over time, the tissues will dry and drop off, but the gangrene will not spread. However, there is some risk of wet gangrene developing (see below).

Dry gangrene may occur in persons who have had diabetes (see page 930) for a long time or who have hardening of the arteries (see Arteriosclerosis of the Extremities, page 690) or Frostbite (see page 698).

Wet Gangrene

Also termed moist gangrene, this type involves bacterial infection. At first, the involved tissues may be red and hot as a result of inflammation. With time, the tissues become cold and blue; pus may ooze from the area. Eventually, the tissue with wet gangrene begins to fall off.

Because of the bacterial infection, wet gangrene tends to spread rapidly. The bacteria contribute to tissue breakdown. Some bacteria produce a gas that has a strong, disagreeable odor as it destroys the tissue (gas gangrene). If not promptly treated, the person with gas gangrene may die in a matter of days (see Gas Gangrene, page 1016).

Prevention

If you are a person with diabetes or have advanced arteriosclerosis, you must take special care of your feet (see Caring for Your Feet, page 931). Even minor injuries must be treated with special attention. Careful control of blood sugar level is important in diabetics. If you smoke, stop; every cigarette causes additional damage to blood vessels.

Whether you have diabetes or not, if you sustain a wound or injury, be sure it is properly treated. If virulent bacteria are present, wet gangrene may result from even a minor injury of a limb in which the blood supply is decreased. Proper care early can prevent wet gangrene later.

Treatment

If you think you may have gangrene, consult your physician. Treatment should be initiated immediately. Surgery to open or bypass blocked arteries may be necessary. Tissues affected by dry gangrene may shrivel up and not be a problem, but surgical removal of the dead tissue often is needed.

Antibiotic drugs usually will be prescribed to prevent or to treat wet gangrene. Tissue affected by wet gangrene may have to be removed surgically.

---

drug called pentoxifylline to improve the blood flow to your limbs, but its effectiveness is controversial.

Surgery

A surgical approach may be appropriate if one of the larger arteries in your leg becomes blocked. In some cases, a balloon device to expand the narrowed artery (balloon angioplasty) may be used (the procedure is similar to that used in heart surgery; see Coronary Angioplasty, page 666). Occasionally, lasers and other devices are used to open blocked arteries. Surgery to remove the damaged artery or to bypass it with an artificial vessel made of Dacron may be required.

Surgery is usually reserved for persons with severely impaired walking ability, pain, or breakdown of skin or for those who have the potential for loss of a limb.

Arterial Embolism

Signs and Symptoms

- Pain in the affected area
- Pale, cool skin
- Numbness

An embolus is a clot that has moved from its point of origin to a new location and is blocking the flow of blood. (The embolus is distinguished from a thrombus in that the latter is a clot that forms in the vessel and remains stationary and the former is a clot that travels to another location in the body; see Heart Attack, page 661.)

Emboli may be multiple and small, or they may be single and massive. Emboli can be life-threatening, such as when they lodge in the brain (see Stroke, page 461), or can lead to tissue death in an arm or leg if not treated within a few hours. Arterial emboli may originate in the left atrium if you are experiencing atrial fibrillation (see page 670) or in the left ventricle after a heart attack.

Diagnosis

When embolization occurs, the flow of blood to the legs and feet may stop abruptly or can slow gradually over weeks and months. If a clot or some debris from an atheromatous plaque in the aorta is carried with the flow of blood through the arteries in the thigh, it may plug the arteries at the level of the knee where the larger artery splits into several small ones. This obstruction causes sudden pain and pallor in the lower leg and foot.

If the clot or debris is not removed by surgery within a matter of hours, the tissue below that level may die and amputation might be necessary. When embolism occurs, it is important to protect the leg from any injury by wrapping it loosely with a soft blanket and gauze. Because the foot is very cold, it is tempting to apply heat, but this may damage the already compromised tissue. However, protecting the leg from loss of heat by using a blanket, gauze, or other wrap is important.

Your physician will measure the blood pressure in the affected limb and also may try to localize the embolus by an ultrasound examination or by injecting a dye into the affected blood vessels and taking an X-ray (arteriogram).

How Serious Is an Arterial Embolism?

If the flow of blood is not restored within a few hours, the affected limb could be permanently damaged and amputation may be necessary.

Treatment

Medication

When your physician concludes that the diagnosis is arterial embolism, he or she may immediately give you a drug to break up the embolus, perhaps delivering it directly to the affected artery through the use of a catheter. This is called thrombolysis. Long-term use of aspirin or a so-called blood thinner (anticoagulant drug) may be appropriate in order to prevent the development of more clots.

Surgery

If the health of a limb is in danger, immediate surgical removal of the clot may be required. This usually can be performed by using a balloon-tipped catheter inserted into the artery. As it is being withdrawn, the inflated balloon pulls the clot out. Occasionally, replacement or bypass of the blocked vessel is necessary.

Aortic Aneurysm

Signs and Symptoms

- Often, none
- Pulsating sensation in the abdomen

An aneurysm is an abnormal widening of an artery. A weakened wall of an artery is stretched as the blood is pumped through it, often creating an egg-shaped ballooning.

An aneurysm can occur in any blood vessel, including major ones in the brain (see Stroke, page 461) and minor ones anywhere in the body, but it is most likely to occur in the aorta, the main blood vessel that carries blood from the heart. A common site for an aortic aneurysm is immediately below the kidneys but above the junction of the abdominal aorta and arteries to the legs.

Abdominal aneurysms are thought to be largely the result of atherosclerosis. Complicating factors such as high blood pressure (hypertension) may contribute to the development of an aneurysm.

In addition to the expansion of the arterial wall, an aneurysm also characteristically has an accumulation of cholesterol, calcium, and even small blood clots. The weakened muscle fibers of the artery wall become fragmented and are replaced by scar tissue. Despite all these changes, the size of the artery's central channel may remain roughly normal.

Abdominal aortic aneurysms most often strike people over age 60, and men are more commonly affected than women.

Diagnosis

Often there are no symptoms. However, in

An aneurysm, an abnormal widening of an artery, can occur in any location, but commonly occurs in the abdominal aorta just below the kidneys. The weakened wall of the aorta balloons out over time, usually growing at a rate of ⅛ to ¼ inch a year.

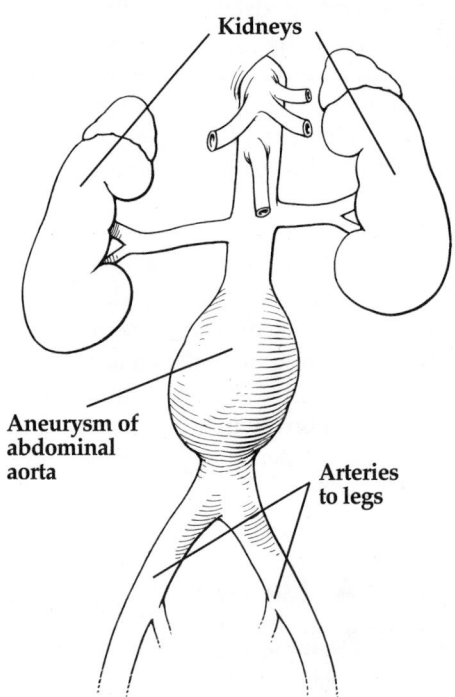

Kidneys

Aneurysm of abdominal aorta

Arteries to legs

advanced cases, pain may be present in the abdomen and lower back. Aneurysms tend to grow at a rate of about ⅛ to ¼ inch a year and often do not cause symptoms until blood begins to leak from the ballooning wall of the artery. If the aneurysm ruptures, shock, loss of consciousness, and death may be the catastrophic result.

Your physician may feel the pulsating vessel on routine examination of your abdomen. In some cases, an X-ray taken for another reason will reveal an aneurysm. Its presence is usually confirmed with an ultrasound examination or a CT scan (see page 1334).

How Serious Is an Aneurysm?

An abdominal aortic aneurysm can be life-threatening; all too often, the ailment is discovered during autopsy. Like heart disease, abdominal aortic aneurysm can be considered a silent killer. However, if discovered in time, there is a highly effective surgical procedure available to treat this disorder.

In some people, the layers of tissue that compose the wall of the aorta separate (dissect). Immediate treatment is required for this disorder; often surgical removal of the affected artery is necessary.

Treatment

Drugs are not of value in treating an abdominal aortic aneurysm. If the aneurysm is

small and no symptoms are apparent at the time it is discovered, your physician may recommend a watch-and-wait approach. No changes will be required in your physical activities, but periodic ultrasound examinations or CT scans will be done to determine if the aneurysm is expanding.

Surgery

In an emergency or as a preventive measure, your physician may recommend an operation to replace the diseased portion of aorta with an artificial artery made of synthetic material.

The risk of the aneurysm rupturing—a potentially life-threatening event—increases as the aneurysm grows. The operation is relatively safe when performed prior to rupture, but less than half of those operated on after rupture survive.

Thrombophlebitis

Signs and Symptoms
- Tenderness and pain in the affected area
- Redness and swelling

When a clot and associated inflammation occur in a vein, the disorder is termed thrombophlebitis. The name comes from Greek words for clot (*thrombos*), vein (*phleps*), and inflammation (*itis*). Often the name is conveniently shortened to phlebitis; if the inflammatory component is minor, it may be termed thrombosis.

Phlebitis usually occurs in an extremity and is most common in leg veins. It may affect either the deep or the superficial veins. The cause often is traceable to prolonged bed rest after an operation, paralysis, a malignancy, or the use of the female hormone estrogen. Sometimes prolonged sitting during a long car or airplane ride will cause thrombosis of a vein.

Diagnosis

Superficial Thrombophlebitis

When the clot and inflammation occur in a readily visible vein near the surface of the skin, the diagnosis is superficial thrombophlebitis. Your physician can make the preliminary diagnosis on the basis of the discomfort you have in the area and the hard, usually tender, clot that can readily be felt and seen.

Deep-Vein Thrombosis

When the phlebitis occurs in a vein deep within the leg (or, more rarely, in the arm), the condition is termed deep-vein thrombosis. To reach this diagnosis your physician may choose to perform one or more special tests including an ultrasound examination and making an X-ray after injection of dye into the veins of the leg (venogram).

How Serious Is Thrombophlebitis?

Superficial thrombophlebitis rarely leads to serious complications. However, with deep-vein thrombophlebitis, the principal danger is pulmonary embolism (see page 734). If you have several episodes of deep-vein thrombosis, a permanent obstruction could develop in the vein with persistent leg swelling.

Treatment

Treatment of superficial thrombophlebitis usually is limited to the application of heat to the affected area, elevation of the limb, and use of an anti-inflammatory drug. Deep-vein thrombophlebitis is treated by elevating the leg and using anticoagulant medications. Often, hospitalization is required.

Medication

An anticoagulant drug (most likely heparin) may be prescribed for treating the more serious deep-vein thrombophlebitis. It is likely to be administered intravenously. Later, warfarin (Coumadin) may be given orally, perhaps for several months. The purpose of the anticoagulant therapy is to prevent further growth of the clot. Rarely, drugs to dissolve the blood clots may be used.

Surgery

Your physician may recommend surgical treatment. The affected vein or the main vein in the abdomen (vena cava) may be tied off surgically to prevent the clot from coming free and lodging in the lung, causing a pulmonary embolism (see page 734). Sometimes, filters can be inserted into the veins to prevent movement of a blood clot to the lungs.

Varicose Veins

Signs and Symptoms

- Enlarged veins readily seen under the skin of the legs

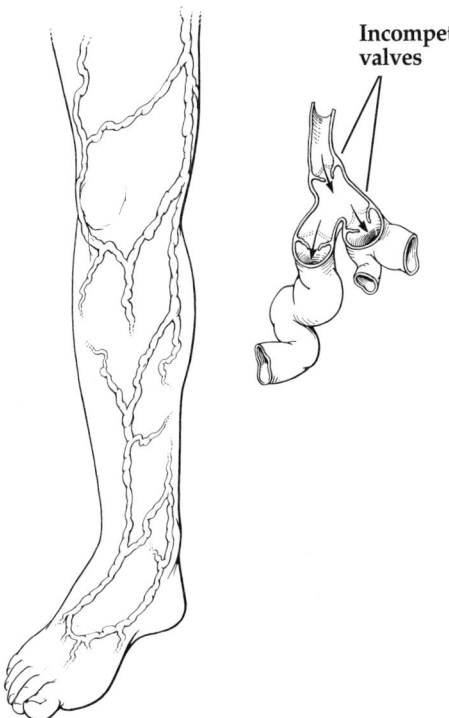

Incompetent valves

Varicose veins are enlarged veins that are easily seen beneath the surface of the skin of the legs and feet. These twisted veins may be caused by incompetent valves.

- Brownish gray skin discoloration on the ankle
- Skin ulcers near the ankles

Varicose veins are twisted and enlarged veins close to the surface of the skin. Any vein may become varicose (the name comes from the Latin root *varix* for "twisted"), but the areas most likely to be affected are the legs and feet.

About 1 in 10 Americans has varicose veins. Women are about twice as likely as men to have this disorder.

Lymphedema

Lymphedema is an abnormal accumulation of lymph fluid in the extremities. It causes painless swelling, which usually starts in the toes and foot and progresses toward the trunk. This form of edema may improve with bed rest and elevation of the leg initially, but as it progresses, the improvement may be marginal.

In some situations, the cause is obvious, for example after some type of traumatic injury, an operation, or radiation therapy. Occasionally lymphedema may be caused by an infection, particularly in tropical climates. A more serious cause of lymphedema is a cancer that obstructs the flow of lymph fluid back into the abdominal cavity. Thus, if you develop lymphedema for unexplained reasons in an extremity, your physician may perform tests to rule out a malignant cause.

The Value of Support Stockings

If you have varicose veins or deep-vein malfunction, an important component of your self-help program involves wearing the right clothing. You may find that appropriate support hose provide immediate and lasting relief. Use of support stockings also may be appropriate during pregnancy. Elastic bandages or support hose compress the varicosities and provide needed support.

Your physician may prescribe specially fitted stockings; they will provide the most pressure in the lower portions of your legs. Put them on first thing in the morning, even before you get out of bed. Make sure, however, that the stockings you wear are not tight around your groin or the calf of your leg.

A possible explanation for the disparity in the occurrence of varicose veins between men and women is the effect of pregnancy. Varicose veins occur as a result of a malfunction of the valves in the veins. Normally, the valves help prevent blood from flowing backward, but the valves can become stretched as a result of pregnancy, previous thrombophlebitis (see page 694), congenital weakness, obesity, or other causes. When the valves are weakened and are no longer able to close normally, blood pools in the veins. As a result, the veins enlarge and become varicose.

A condition that frequently occurs with varicose veins is the spider-burst leg vein. Although not usually medically significant,

Spider-burst veins are common and are only of cosmetic importance.

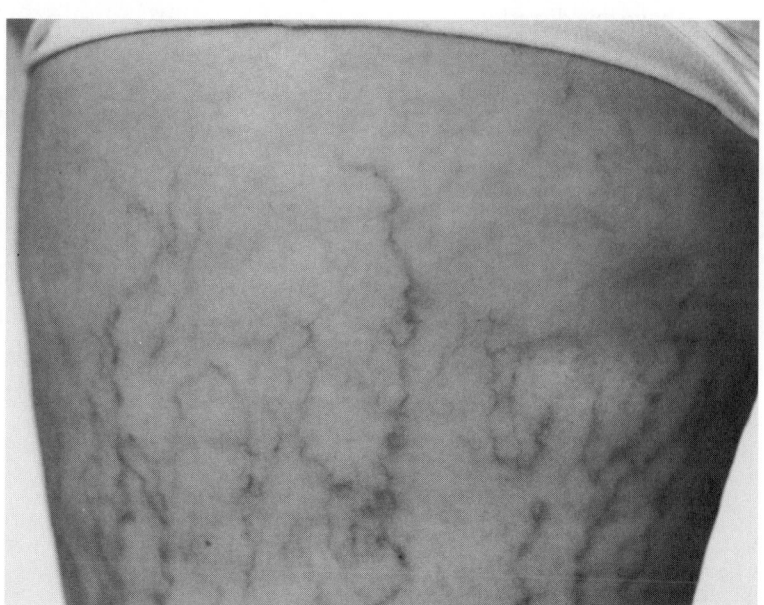

the vein patterns seen through the skin may be of cosmetic concern (see Spider Veins, page 1001).

Diagnosis
Superficial varicose veins are dilated, twisted, and usually dark blue. You may or may not have mild aching of your legs. Occasionally, the veins deep within the legs are involved. In such cases, your limbs may have significant swelling; occasionally skin ulcers will develop.

Your physician will examine your legs while you are upright and also will look for swelling, another indication of a malfunction of the vein valves.

Sometimes, ulcers form. Ulcers caused by varicose veins or malfunction of the valves within the vein ordinarily are located near the ankles and are the result of long-term "waterlogging" of these tissues as the result of increased pressure of blood within the affected veins. Brownish pigmentation usually precedes the development of an ulcer.

How Serious Are Varicose Veins?
Varicose veins tend to become increasingly prominent over time. However, self-help measures may limit their progression and discomfort. In some cases, surgery may be required to correct varicose vein ulcers.

Treatment

Self-Help
Avoid standing or sitting for long periods. If your lifestyle is essentially sedentary, be sure to flex your legs and ankles frequently—get up and walk around. At the end of the day, you will find that elevating your legs at least 12 inches above the level of your heart will help relieve any swelling.

A pattern of regular exercise also is valuable. Walking, biking, or swimming will help decrease the pressure in the veins and ease your discomfort. Another important strategy is wearing appropriate hose or stockings (see The Value of Support Stockings, this page). If a skin ulcer caused by an incompetent vein is present, your physician may place a specially treated piece of gauze over the site to aid in healing.

Medications
A paste-like medication can be made from a person's own blood platelets to heal skin

ulcers. When smeared on an open sore, growth factors in the platelets cause skin tissue to form over the ulcer. The medication reduces the risk of an ulcer recurring as well as the risk of gangrene.

Surgery

In severe cases, the skin near the varicose veins may become itchy or ulcerated or the pigmentation may change. If inflammation or bleeding occurs, consult your physician.

Some surgeons recommend stripping or injections to remove the veins, which may include removal of the varicose tributaries in addition to the main vein. The long-term benefit of varicose vein surgery in appropriate persons is high; in one study, 85 percent of patients were getting along very well at 10 or more years after the operation. Occasionally, if a skin ulcer fails to heal, your surgeon may elect to remove the ulcer and use a skin graft to assist healing.

Raynaud's Disease

Signs and Symptoms—Fingers or toes turn white on exposure to cold, with an accompanying stinging pain; the skin may turn blue or red before it recovers

Named after the French physician who described it more than a century ago, Raynaud's disease results from changes in the circulation in the hands or feet. It is a normal physiologic reflex mechanism for the blood vessels in your extremities to narrow when exposed to cold. However, for unknown reasons, in the person with Raynaud's disease this response is exaggerated.

Not only the fingers and toes but also the cheeks, nose, and ears may be affected. About 1 in 20 Americans has Raynaud's disease. Women are 4 to 5 times more likely to develop the problem as men. Typically, the first episode occurs before age 40.

(See page C-16 for color photograph of Raynaud's disease.)

Raynaud's Phenomenon

Raynaud's disease is an independent ailment and is not associated with any other problem or disease. In contrast, Raynaud's phenomenon may be a consequence of scleroderma (see page 919), exposure to certain chemicals (especially vinyl chloride, used in the rubber industry), or long-term use of vibrating tools such as pneumatic drills, jackhammers, or chain saws. The signs and symptoms of Raynaud's phenomenon resemble those for Raynaud's disease.

Acrocyanosis

Another related disorder, acrocyanosis, involves persistent coldness of the fingers, toes, or other affected tissues. Like Raynaud's disease, it is not a consequence of another disorder but, unlike Raynaud's disease, the affected areas are almost always cold. Excessive perspiration often accompanies the feeling of cold.

Treatment

For most people, Raynaud's disease is more a nuisance than a disability. Only rarely are there any long-term, serious consequences such as gangrene or ulcers of the fingertips.

Prevention

To avoid attacks of Raynaud's disease, adequate protection from the cold is essential. Dress warmly when exposed to cold, protecting the entire body, head, hands, and feet.

Other preventive measures include the following. Do not smoke. The nicotine in tobacco decreases blood flow in your skin. Use insulated glasses for cold drinks. Keep a pair of mittens or gloves adjacent to the freezer to use when handling cold containers. Run your car heater for a few minutes before driving in cold weather.

In cases of acrocyanosis, further treatment is rarely necessary.

Medication

Avoid over-the-counter cold remedies and diet pills containing the drug phenylpropanolamine. If you use birth control pills, switch to another method of contraception because these drugs affect your circulation and may make you more prone to attacks.

If these measures are not sufficient, your physician may prescribe a drug to prevent the blood vessel spasms that lead to Raynaud's disease.

In extreme cases, a surgical procedure to cut the nerves that control the blood vessels may be done, but the operation (known as sympathectomy) is not always successful and usually is a last resort. A similar procedure called sympathetic blockade can be performed by using an injection of various chemicals into the appropriate sympathetic nerves.

Buerger's Disease

Buerger's disease, named after the American physician Leo Buerger who identified its symptoms in 1908, is a rare disorder in which the blood vessels of the hands and feet become diseased. The skin of the hands and feet becomes tender and, over time, pain and ulcers develop and eventually amputation is needed. This occurs because of blockages that form in the blood vessels supplying the extremities.

The disease characteristically strikes men between 20 and 40; for unexplained reasons, there appears to be a direct link between smoking or chewing of tobacco and Buerger's disease.

The avoidance of tobacco usually results in a cure. However, many men with Buerger's disease seem to find it difficult to quit, and amputation of affected areas is the inevitable long-term result.

Frostbite

Signs and Symptoms
- Hard, pale, cold skin after prolonged exposure to cold
- White patches of skin
- Lack of sensitivity in the area
- Flesh is red and painful after thawing

When your skin and the underlying tissues freeze, the condition is called frostbite. The affected areas of the body most often are the hands, feet, nose, and ears.

Frostbite can occur to anyone exposed to very cold temperatures for a sustained period of time (several hours or more), but people with circulatory problems such as atherosclerosis are at greater risk (see page 636).

How Serious Is Frostbite?
In severe cases, the flow of blood to the affected area has stopped and the blood vessels have been damaged. In many cases, immediate treatment can reverse the damage, but in some instances amputation of the frostbitten areas is required.

Treatment

Prevention
The wearing of proper clothing in cold conditions can prevent most episodes of frostbite. Be sure to protect your hands, feet, nose, and ears. Avoid consuming large amounts of alcohol when you are exposed to prolonged cold.

If you are arriving in a cold climate and your body is used to a warmer one, your body requires some time to adjust to the change. Try gradual ventures into the colder temperatures, allowing your body, and your circulatory system in particular, time to decrease the blood flow to the surface of your skin and to maintain the heat within.

Warming Process
If your fingers or other areas are frostbitten, prompt treatment is essential. Seek professional care. Never immerse the affected part in hot water (see Frostbite, page 416, for treatment of less-serious frostbite).

Further Treatment
In severe cases in which infection is present, after the affected area has been warmed, antibiotics may be necessary. Bed rest and physical therapy may be appropriate. Do not smoke cigarettes during recovery.

Chapter 24

Your Lungs and Respiratory System

Contents

Normal Ventilation, 700

Respiratory Infections, 701
Bronchiolitis, 701
Acute Bronchitis, 702
  The Cough, 703
Pneumonia, 704
Tuberculosis, 705
Legionnaires' Disease, 707
Bronchiectasis, 708
Lung Abscess, 708
  Postural Drainage and Chest
  Percussion, 709
Empyema, 710
Pleurisy and Pleural Effusions, 711

Fungal Diseases of the Lungs, 711
Histoplasmosis, 711
Aspergillosis, 712
Cryptococcosis, 712
Coccidioidomycosis, 713

Chronic Lung Conditions, 714
Chronic Bronchitis, 714
Emphysema, 715
  Breathing Techniques, 717
  The Controlled Cough, 717
  Your Home Supply of Oxygen, 718
  Smoking and Chronic Obstructive
  Pulmonary Disease, 719

Asthma, 720
Cystic Fibrosis, 720
Sarcoidosis, 721
Interstitial Lung Disease, 721
Atelectasis, 723
Pneumothorax, 723
Lung Cancer, 724
  Smoking and Lung Cancer, 725
  Bronchoscopy, 726
  Lung Removal, 727

Occupation-Related Lung
Disease, 728
Asbestosis, 728
  Asbestos Removal From Buildings, 729
Pneumoconiosis and Silicosis, 730
Occupational Asthma, 731
Allergic Alveolitis, 731
Byssinosis, 731
  Fumes, Gases, Air Pollution, and
  Smoke, 732
Industrial Bronchitis, 733
Farmer's Lung, 733
Silo-Filler's Disease, 733

Your Lungs and Cardiovascular
System, 734
Pulmonary Embolism, 734
Cor Pulmonale, 735
  Lung and Heart Transplantation, 736

Normal Ventilation

The primary function of your lungs is to provide oxygen to your blood and to remove carbon dioxide from it. Your lungs are suspended within your chest (thoracic cavity), which is enclosed on all sides by your ribs, cartilage, and the muscle between them. Your diaphragm, which consists of sheets of muscle, separates your thoracic cavity from your abdominal cavity.

Your lungs are soft and spongy. If you are healthy, your lungs probably are a mottled pinkish gray color, although even healthy lungs can become blackened from carbon particles in polluted air. Your right lung is divided into three sections (lobes). Your left lung has two lobes. Your heart is between your lungs, nestled over one corner of your left lung.

To reach your lungs, air enters through your mouth and nose and then travels through the back of your throat (pharynx), through your voice box (larynx), and down your windpipe (trachea). The trachea branches into two main bronchial tubes, or air passageways. Each bronchial tube then branches into smaller passageways (bronchi), which divide several times more, finally forming much smaller tubes (bronchioles). The branching creates the appearance of an upside-down tree. The smallest bronchioles end in tiny closed elastic air sacs called alveoli. Your blood is carried to these air sacs by tiny blood vessels. The vessels, called pulmonary capillaries, release carbon dioxide from your blood into the air sacs and at the same time absorb oxygen from the air sacs into your blood. Your lungs contain approximately 300 million such alveoli. If they could be stretched out on a flat surface, they would cover an area approximately the size of a tennis court.

The pleura, a double-layer membrane with a very thin lubricating layer of fluid between the two layers, covers the outside of your lungs and the adjacent chest wall. This membrane allows your lungs to move easily within the chest cavity as you breathe.

When you inhale, the muscles of your ribs contract, causing your ribs to move upward and outward. At the same time, your diaphragm contracts, pushing down toward your abdomen. These two actions increase the size of your chest cavity and thus cause your lungs to expand and air to be sucked into them. The individual alveoli also expand with air. During normal breathing, a healthy adult can draw about a pint of air into the lungs with each breath. However, during heavy breathing, you can draw as much as 3 to 6 quarts of air into your lungs.

When you exhale, your diaphragm and rib muscles relax and return to their original positions. This decreases the size of your chest cavity, compressing your lungs slightly and forcing the stale air, now carrying carbon dioxide, out of your body. The whole process of breathing in and out occurs automatically without your thinking about it.

Your respiratory system has several defense mechanisms that prevent foreign material from entering your lungs. Hairs in the nose filter out the larger particles. Special cells in your trachea and bronchial tubes secrete mucus that helps keep the airways moist and lubricated and also catches bacteria, dust, and other foreign material. Tiny hair-like projections called cilia line your airways. These cilia continuously beat the mucus upward toward your throat to help keep the air passageway clean. Some substances may interfere with their function. For example, inhaling cigarette smoke causes the cilia to stop beating.

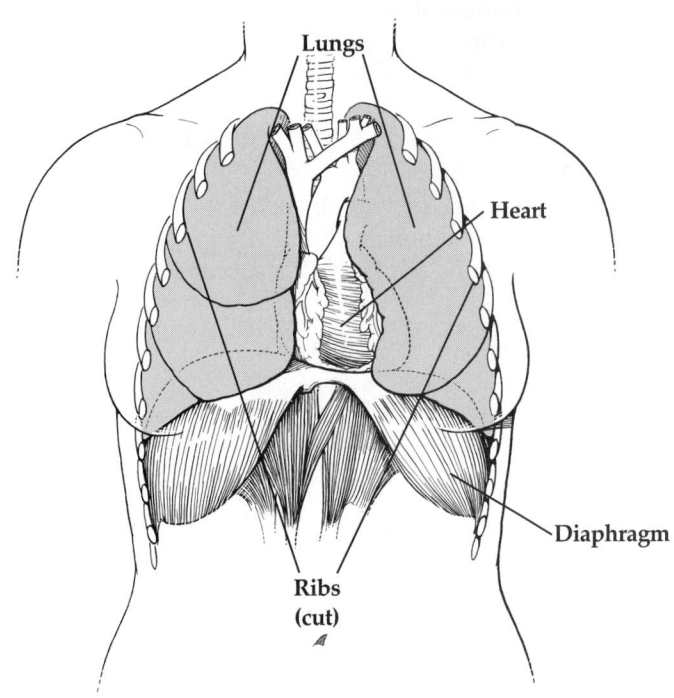

Lungs

Heart

Diaphragm

Ribs
(cut)

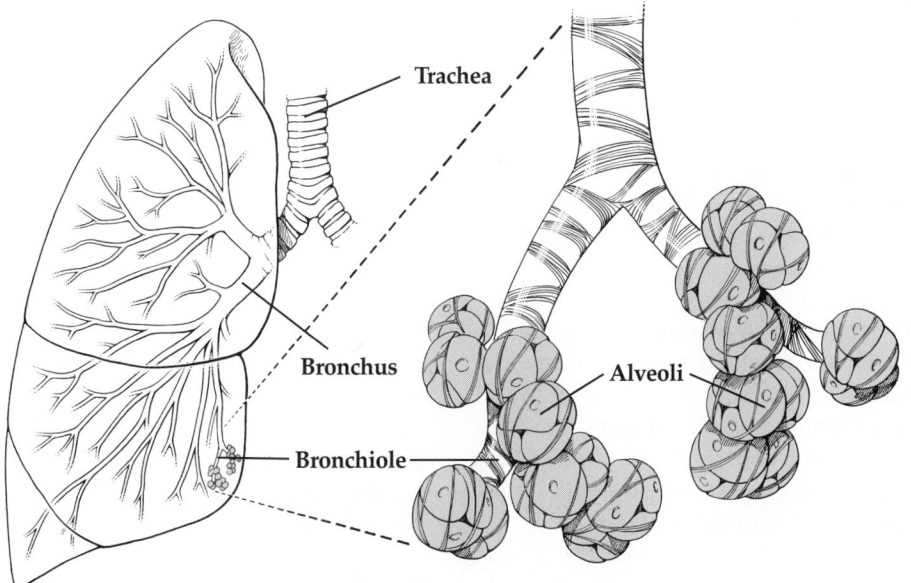

Trachea

Bronchus

Alveoli

Bronchiole

Enlargement of lung segment shows bronchioles and alveoli (air sacs). Within these air sacs, carbon dioxide is released from the blood as oxygen is absorbed by the blood.

Your lungs are connected to your heart by the pulmonary veins and arteries (the term "pulmonary" comes from the Latin word *pulmo* for "lung"). Your blood travels throughout your body, returns to your heart, and is pumped by the right ventricle (the bottom right chamber of the heart) through the pulmonary artery to your lungs. The blood then passes through the arteries of the lungs into smaller and smaller vessels, similar to the branching of the bronchi. Finally, it flows into the smallest blood vessels, called capillaries, which are located in the membranes lining the alveoli. Capillaries are so tiny that often the cells of your blood have to pass through them single file (see Your Healthy Heart and Blood Vessels, page 633).

After gases are exchanged in the alveoli, the blood, now carrying oxygen, passes into the smallest veins. These veins merge to form larger and larger vessels until the pulmonary veins are formed. The pulmonary veins carry oxygenated blood from the lungs back to the heart, from which it is pumped out again to deliver oxygen to the cells of your body and to remove carbon dioxide.

Respiratory Infections

If bacteria, viruses, or fungi enter the lungs and become established there, they can cause several diseases, ranging from common and usually benign illnesses such as colds (see Common Viral Colds, page 1071) and flu to more serious illnesses such as pneumonia, bronchitis, and tuberculosis.

Bronchiolitis

Signs and Symptoms
- Wheezing
- Exhaling heavily
- Rapid breathing and rapid heartbeat
- Sputum-producing cough
- Fever
- Bluish skin (cyanosis)

Cause
A respiratory infection such as that caused by the influenza virus or a bacterium may cause your bronchioles (the small airways in the lungs) to become inflamed and to secrete an excessive amount of mucus. Bronchiolitis is fairly common, especially during the winter, in children younger than 2 years, but it can occur in young adults under special circumstances. It usually is caused by a viral infection, often contracted from someone in the infant's household. In infants or families with a history of allergies or in infants with recurring bronchiolitis, an allergic reaction may be the cause.

Diagnosis
Usually, bronchiolitis is preceded by mild

nasal congestion for a day or two. Gradually, breathing becomes more and more difficult and may become more rapid with more vigorous exhalation. Wheezing, rapid heartbeat, and a cough may also occur. Fever may or may not be present.

In some cases, the infant may develop cyanosis (the lips and the beds of the fingernails become blue).

How Serious Is Bronchiolitis?

Bronchiolitis usually is not serious in older children and adults, but in an infant the air passages are much narrower than in an adult and may become partly or completely blocked. This makes it very difficult for the infant to inhale and exhale.

Treatment

Hospitalization might be needed, especially for an infant who is younger than 2 months, has cyanosis, has had repeated attacks, or is breathing very rapidly and shallowly. Treatment consists of providing warm, moist air, perhaps with extra oxygen. Medications will depend on the nature and severity of the symptoms.

Most infants recover within 2 days to a week, although in rare cases an infant will not survive. About half of the children who contract bronchiolitis will have later episodes of wheezing and may be more susceptible to respiratory infections.

Acute Bronchitis

Signs and Symptoms

- Soreness and feeling of constriction in the chest
- Breathlessness
- Wheezing
- Sputum-producing cough
- Chills
- Overall malaise and slight fever

Cause

When the mucous membranes that line the main air passageways of the lungs (trachea and large bronchi) become inflamed, the condition is called bronchitis or tracheobronchitis. An occasional occurrence of acute bronchitis is to be expected. Virtually everyone has bronchitis at some time, much as everyone has the common cold.

In most cases, this common ailment is the result of viral infections similar to those that cause the common cold (see Common Viral Colds, page 1071). The infection spreads to the bronchi, producing the deep cough that, in turn, tends to bring up a yellowish gray sputum from your lungs.

Diagnosis

If you have fever, your chest discomfort leaves you breathless, or you cough up blood or yellow or green sputum, call your physician. He or she will listen to your chest (using a stethoscope) and may obtain a chest X-ray, sputum culture, or other tests to rule out other causes. If you have chronic lung or heart problems (including asthma, emphysema, or congestive heart failure) and think you have bronchitis, you should also consult your physician.

How Serious Is Acute Bronchitis?

In virtually all cases, acute bronchitis disappears in a matter of days and there are no lasting effects. However, a pattern of recurring bronchitis can represent a more serious health concern (see Chronic Bronchitis, page 714).

Treatment

Because bronchitis most commonly is the result of a viral infection, your physician probably will be able to do relatively little to hasten your recovery. Rest, aspirin for fever, drinking extra liquids, and a nonprescription cough medicine are the cornerstones of treatment for acute bronchitis.

Avoid other irritants to the airways, such as tobacco smoke. Remember that the act of coughing also is irritating to the trachea and bronchi, so make attempts to suppress your cough (see The Cough, page 703). You do not have to confine yourself to bed while you have acute bronchitis, but it is wise to remain in a warm environment in which the air is somewhat humid, perhaps from use of a vaporizer.

Your physician may prescribe a bronchodilator drug to open narrowed passages in your lungs. If your sputum becomes yellow or green, your physician may prescribe an antibiotic.

Prevention

If you have repeated attacks of bronchitis, you may be able to trace their occurrence to the conditions in which you live. Cold, damp environments combined with excessive air pollution can make you more susceptible to acute bronchitis, so lifestyle changes may be advisable.

The Cough

A cough is a normal protective reflex, designed to defend your respiratory system against irritants. However, a forceful or nagging cough can be painful and bothersome. Some of these coughs need your physician's attention. Others respond to simple self-care and the right medicine.

What Causes a Cough?
Here are some typical irritations that cause coughing:

- Infections, such as colds and flu
- Postnasal drip—an overproduction of mucus that slowly trickles from the back of your nose down into your throat
- Environmental irritants, such as cigarette smoke, smog, dust, home aerosol sprays, and cold or dry air
- Asthma, which inflames and constricts the air passages
- Gastroesophageal reflux—the backup of stomach acid into your esophagus (or, in rare cases, your lungs) when you lie down
- Medications, such as inhaled corticosteroids or certain medications prescribed for high blood pressure and heart disease
- Coughing itself. Sometimes there is no medical explanation for a cough. Some people cough to release nervous tension, gain attention, or express anger. Whatever the reason, one cough can irritate your throat and lead to another, setting up a vicious cycle

Treatment

Dry, Hacking Coughs
These generally go away within 1 to 2 weeks. But if a persistent cough irritates your throat, suck on hard candy or cough drops, or drink tea sweetened with honey.

If a cough caused by gastroesophageal reflux disrupts your sleep, raise the head of your bed 6 to 8 inches. To temporarily reduce the frequency of your cough, take an over-the-counter cough suppressant. Although codeine is one of the most effective cough suppressants, it is a narcotic, so cough formulas containing codeine are available only by prescription in most states. Dextromethorphan is nearly as effective as codeine, with less risk of side effects.

Productive Coughs
A cough that brings up mucus helps remove irritants from your lungs and air passages. To thin mucus and make it easier to cough up, drink plenty of water. Using a humidifier or a vaporizer may also help loosen mucus.

It is best not to suppress a productive cough. However, if your cough continually disrupts your sleep, you can take just enough cough suppressant to decrease the frequency and severity of your cough, but not to get rid of it altogether.

Antihistamines may help dry up secretions associated with allergies, sinusitis, and postnasal drip, but they can make you sleepy. Do not take antihistamines in combination with alcohol or tranquilizers, or when you need to stay alert.

Serious Coughs
If your cough lasts longer than 2 or 3 weeks, see your physician. Managing a chronic cough requires careful evaluation and identification of a specific cause.

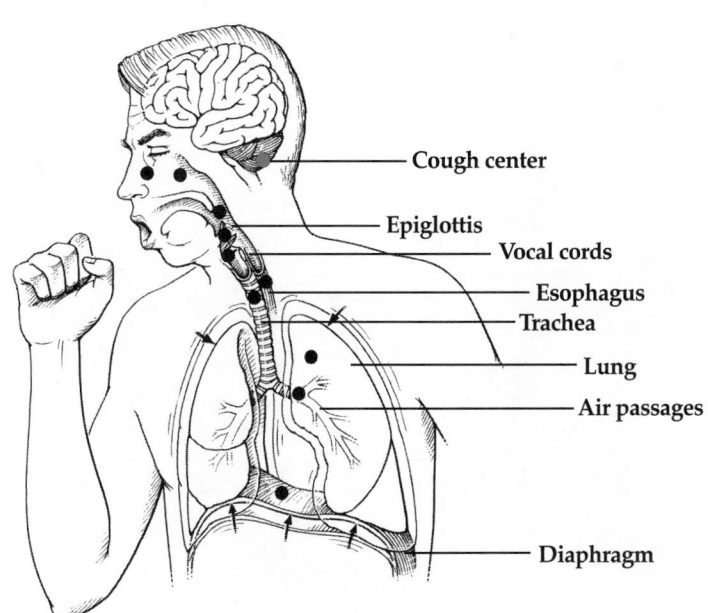

A cough begins when an irritant reaches one of the cough receptors in your nose, throat, or chest (see dots). The receptor sends a message to the cough center in your brain, signaling your body to cough. After you inhale, your epiglottis and vocal cords close tightly, trapping air within your lungs. Your abdominal and chest muscles contract forcefully, pushing against your diaphragm. Finally, your vocal cords and epiglottis open suddenly, allowing trapped air to explode outward.

Pneumonia

Signs and Symptoms
- Cough that produces bloody sputum
- Breathlessness
- Pain in the chest
- Chills
- Bluish skin (cyanosis)
- High fever
- Mental confusion

Pneumonia describes an inflammation of the tissues of your lungs. Rather than being an individual ailment, however, what your physician calls "pneumonia" actually can be any one of more than 50 different diseases. They range in seriousness from the mild discomfort that accompanies a cold to life-threatening conditions.

Causes
One key reason for this range of severity is that there are many causes of pneumonia. Among them are bacteria such as pneumococci, staphylococci, and streptococci; influenza and other viruses; and chemical irritants.

To make the subject of pneumonia more easily understood, the many varieties are classified into subtypes. For our purposes, three categories are useful: community-acquired, hospital-acquired, and aspiration pneumonia.

Community-Acquired Pneumonia
Community-acquired pneumonia gets its name from the way it is acquired—from the community at large rather than in the hospital. Common causes of community-acquired pneumonia are pneumococci, mycoplasma, and the influenza virus.

Hospital-Acquired Pneumonia
If you acquired your pneumonia while you were in the hospital, the types of possible infecting agents are much greater and possibly more severe than if you were infected in the course of normal, everyday life.

Aspiration Pneumonia
This type of pneumonia is the result of foreign matter being aspirated into the lungs. Most commonly this occurs when the contents of your stomach enter your lungs after you have vomited.

Diagnosis
The symptoms vary depending on the kind of pneumonia you have. Pneumonia may appear to be a cold at first or may develop as a complication of a cold. A cough typically accompanies most kinds, as does a fever.

Your physician will listen to your chest to detect distortions in your breathing that suggest the presence of the infection. Chest X-rays also may be obtained to identify the location and extent of the infection.

A sample of your sputum may be tested to identify the infecting agent. Usually, the sample that you produce by coughing will be sufficient for this test, but in some cases, other means, including the insertion of a bronchoscopy tube (see page 726) into the windpipe, may be necessary. Blood tests may also be conducted.

How Serious Is Pneumonia?
Pneumonia is a common ailment, occurring in more than 1 in every 100 people annually. In fact, it is likely that everyone inhales certain causative agents with some frequency. The seriousness of this disorder depends largely on your overall health. The healthy person has sufficient defense mechanisms to be able to neutralize the infections. In young people, pneumonia is often a passing discomfort that may remain undiagnosed and

Chest X-ray reveals pneumonia in upper lobe of lung (arrows).

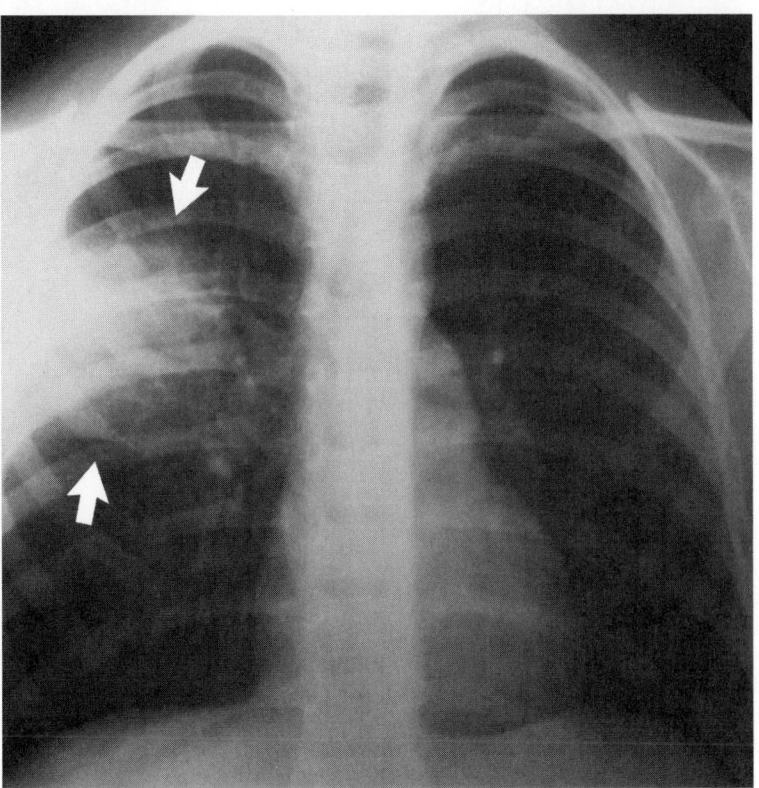

be regarded as simply a cold. If your defense mechanisms are impaired by alcoholism, aging, injury, use of immunosuppressant drugs, or other causes, you may be more susceptible to pneumonia. In people weakened by disease (especially heart failure or lung ailments such as chronic bronchitis, asthma, or emphysema) and in the elderly, death can result—sometimes in 24 hours. Proper medical care, bed rest, and careful monitoring are essential.

Treatment

Consult your physician because there is little you can do on your own, and serious pneumonia can be life-threatening. The treatment your physician will provide depends on the cause (whether bacterium, virus, or other agent) and the severity of your symptoms.

Medication

If the cause is bacterial, your physician will prescribe antibiotic drugs. Penicillin or erythromycin often is the drug of choice, but your physician may consider other antibiotics, too.

Other Therapies

Hospitalization may be necessary in severe cases; oxygen may also be administered.

Prevention

Pneumococcal pneumonia may be prevented by injection of a pneumococcal vaccine (see page 382). At present, it appears that this might give some degree of lifelong immunity to the disease, but the vaccine has not been in use for sufficient time to be certain.

Pneumonia is common in certain groups of people. We recommend vaccination against the *Pneumococcus* organism for healthy adults age 65 or older or for people with an immune deficiency disease or chronic illness such as heart disease, chronic lung disease, or alcoholism, or for people whose spleen has been removed. If you are in one of these groups, ask your physician about this vaccine. You probably should have it.

Tuberculosis

Signs and Symptoms

- Minor cough or cough that produces discolored or bloody sputum
- Slight fever
- Fatigue
- Loss of appetite and weight
- Night sweats
- Pain with breathing or coughing, and pain in the spine or large joints

Tuberculosis, often called "TB," has been present since antiquity. Although its incidence declined greatly during most of this century, there has been a significant increase since the early 1980s. This has been especially evident among the homeless living in inner city areas and those infected with the AIDS virus. TB continues to remain a health problem for infants and the very elderly. The disease has been occurring more frequently in certain areas of the country where it has been linked to the arrival of refugees from Asia and Central America.

Cause

This disease is a chronic bacterial infection that can develop after you inhale droplets sprayed into the air (as from a cough or sneeze) by someone infected with *Mycobacterium tuberculosis*. Your risk of contracting the disease varies directly with the frequency of your contacts with persons who have TB. The number of organisms released in a cough or sneeze is rather small, and the spread of infection to others is not as common as is the case with the common cold. Good ventilation and exposure to sunlight decrease the risk of exposure.

Diagnosis

If you are exposed to the TB bacterium, the organism may gain entry to your lungs. If you are infected, usually no symptoms are apparent initially, although there may be a mild cough and slight fever.

The spread of disease generally is limited or contained by your lymph nodes. The TB organism can spread through your lymph nodes and blood to almost any organ in your body. The areas commonly affected include the lining of the lungs, the bones of the spine or large joints, and your kidneys (you may experience symptoms suggestive of a bladder infection; see Cystitis, page 842).

The preliminary diagnosis of TB often is based on review of your chest X-ray. Usually within 2 to 3 months after the initial infection, a spot may be noticeable on an X-ray of your chest. This spot persists indefinitely and usually is no cause for concern. The tuberculin skin test converts from negative to positive at this time.

The tuberculin skin test is used to tell whether you previously have been infected with the TB organism. A common way of performing this test is to inject a small amount of tuberculin purified protein derivative (PPD) into your skin. If you have been infected by the TB organism, this injection will cause a reaction in your skin within 48 to 72 hours. The results of this test will be interpreted by your physician or a trained nurse 2 to 3 days after the injection. When a very active infection is going on in your body or if your immune system is suppressed, the tuberculin test reaction may be falsely negative.

In addition to the chest X-ray, your physician may obtain a sample of material from your sputum for staining and examination under the microscope. Your physician also may use a new molecular technique called polymerase chain reaction (PCR) to see if you have been infected with the TB organism.

The diagnosis is confirmed by growing the organism in culture in the laboratory. The easiest source of material to obtain for culture is sputum. Other common sources are urine and stomach secretions (obtained by placing a tube into the stomach). Your physician can obtain results from a staining test within 24 hours, but culture results may not be available for up to 6 weeks because the TB bacterium grows slowly.

The culture results also give information as to how well (or poorly) the bacterium will respond to treatment. Unusual forms of the TB-like organism are common and may require different or more intensive treatments.

How Serious Is TB?

In the United States, more than 95 percent of those acquiring an initial or primary TB infection have complete healing with no subsequent evidence of disease except the healed spots seen on a chest X-ray and a positive tuberculin skin test.

Sometimes tuberculosis develops within weeks after the initial exposure. More often, the TB organism may lie dormant for many years before disease becomes apparent.

The disease may be reactivated under conditions in which the immune system is weakened, including old age, malnutrition, alcoholism, immunosuppressive therapy, or certain illnesses such as AIDS or malignancies of the lymph or blood system.

Treatment

In the past, sanitariums often were used for persons who had active TB. This no longer is necessary unless you are unable to care for yourself. With modern therapies, hospitalization, enforced rest, or diet changes are seldom required to cure the disease.

Medication

If you have active TB, whether confined to your lungs or present in other areas of your body, your physician may prescribe at least two different medications to prevent the development of resistance to a single drug.

The drug regimens often include combined use of isoniazid and rifampin, although other combinations also can be used. Once these drug regimens are begun, symptoms often are relieved within 2 to 3 weeks, with improvement seen on the chest X-ray thereafter. In addition, generally after 2 to 3 weeks, you are no longer infectious. At times, the drug regimen needs to be changed or another drug added, depending on your response to therapy.

All medications used for TB have some toxicity, and your physician will discuss this with you. Both rifampin and isoniazid may cause a noninfectious form of hepatitis (the key symptom is jaundice; see page 803). This generally is reversible if you stop the medication. Rifampin may cause your urine, sweat, and tears to take on an orange or brownish color. If you are pregnant, your physician will discuss the potential effects of the medications on your pregnancy.

In recent years, an increasing number of tuberculosis organisms have been encountered which are resistant to the usual drugs used in treatment. This is a particularly frequent occurrence among inner city populations, AIDS patients, and certain immigrant groups. It therefore becomes important to determine the sensitivity to antituberculous drugs in every newly diagnosed case, so that appropriate drugs are prescribed.

Prevention

If you have a positive tuberculin skin test, especially if you recently have been in close contact with a person with TB, your physician may consider giving you medication to decrease the risk of activation of the organism. Isoniazid often is prescribed to be used for up to a year.

In addition, your physician may consider giving isoniazid or a similar medication to others who live in your household or to persons who are known to have been exposed in the past year.

Vaccines have been administered to millions of people worldwide and are known to be safe, although questions remain as to their value. Your physician may want to consider these vaccines if you are a high-risk individual, but they are of no value in a person whose tuberculin skin test is positive.

Legionnaires' Disease

Signs and Symptoms
- Malaise
- Slight headache
- Fever and shaking chills
- Cough that produces mucus or blood
- Shortness of breath
- Chest, muscular, and abdominal pain
- Nausea and vomiting
- Diarrhea

Legionnaires' disease was first identified when a sudden, virulent outbreak of pneumonia occurred at a convention hotel in Philadelphia in July 1976, primarily among delegates to an American Legion convention—hence its name. More than 200 people came down with a severe respiratory illness of unknown cause; 34 people died.

Cause
The cause eventually was identified as a previously unknown bacterium that subsequently was named *Legionella pneumophila*. The bacterium was then identified as being responsible for several earlier, smaller outbreaks of pneumonia, the earliest of which occurred in 1957. Children have come down with the disease, but most cases have occurred in middle-aged or older adults.

Legionella bacteria have been identified all over the world in all types of water-related environments. What is most important so far as disease is concerned is that the bacteria can thrive in warm, moist areas of the air-circulation systems of large buildings. They have been isolated from the evaporative coolers of large air-conditioning systems (the source of the outbreak in Philadelphia). In buildings, the bacteria can be spread through air ducts. Although these organisms have been found in a wide variety of places, the vast majority of similar sources are free of them, and thus legionnaires' disease is uncommon.

Diagnosis
Legionnaires' disease usually begins with a slight headache and a feeling of malaise, followed in less than a day by a rapidly increasing temperature. Within 24 to 48 hours, the fever reaches 104° Fahrenheit in about half of the affected persons, and many have shaking chills.

A mild, dry cough usually begins early and gets worse over several days. The cough usually produces mucus. About 20 percent of affected persons also cough up some blood in the mucus. About a quarter of those with the disease have gastrointestinal symptoms.

The disease usually gets progressively worse for the first 4 to 6 days. Another 4 or 5 days may pass before recovery begins, although in some persons the illness is milder. The lungs usually continue to be congested for some days after the fever disappears.

To diagnose legionnaires' disease, your physician will take chest X-rays and obtain samples of your blood and sputum to identify the presence of the bacterium.

How Serious Is Legionnaires' Disease?
Typically, legionnaires' disease is a very virulent disease, causing pneumonia severe enough to require hospitalization. Although most people recover, some hospitalized patients suffer from acute respiratory failure, which is fatal in about 15 percent of the cases.

Treatment
Hospitalization may be required. You also may need intravenous administration of fluids, because of the fluid loss due to the high fever. You also may need supplementary oxygen.

Medication
Various antibiotics appear to be effective against legionnaires' disease. Erythromycin seems to be the safest and most effective antibiotic.

Bronchiectasis

Signs and Symptoms
- Persistent mild or severe cough that produces large amounts of thick, foul-smelling sputum, usually gray-green, and may be streaked with blood
- Appetite and weight loss
- Anemia and general weakness
- Recurring attacks of pneumonia

Cause
Bronchiectasis is a chronic, abnormal expansion (dilation) of the walls of the bronchial tubes. The same condition occurs in persons who have chronic bronchitis, but in bronchiectasis the dilation of the bronchial tubes is more pronounced. Some people are born with the condition but, in most, bronchiectasis develops as a complication of cystic fibrosis (see page 720) or diseases such as whooping cough, pneumonia, and tuberculosis.

Diagnosis
If allowed to settle, the sputum produced by the chronic cough separates into three layers—a thick bottom layer containing pus, a middle layer of greenish fluid, and a top layer of froth.

Your physician may use X-rays or a CT scan (see page 1334) to confirm the diagnosis. (A CT scan is a useful, noninvasive way of diagnosing bronchiectasis.) Bronchography (an X-ray of the lungs obtained after injecting a material that appears opaque in the bronchial tubes on a chest X-ray) is not usually necessary unless surgical treatment is being considered and there is a need to define the extent of the disease precisely.

How Serious Is Bronchiectasis?
Bronchiectasis occurs primarily in children and young adults. The illness usually is diagnosed within the first 20 years of life. It is much less common since the introduction of antibiotic treatment for pneumonia.

Treatment
Your physician may suggest chest physiotherapy, which includes postural drainage and chest percussion (see Postural Drainage and Chest Percussion, page 709). A health care professional will teach you breathing exercises to help improve the functioning of your lungs.

Avoid dust, smoke, and other respiratory irritants. Get plenty of exercise because deep breathing helps raise secretions. Eat a nutritious diet. Drinking lots of fluids helps to dilute the sputum in your lungs.

Medication
Because bacterial infections are associated with production of pus in bronchiectasis, antibiotics are usually prescribed. Unless a specific antibiotic is indicated by tests of your sputum, ampicillin, tetracycline, or a similar drug is usually given. If you are allergic to penicillin-type drugs, your physician will prescribe a different medication. Your physician also may prescribe a bronchodilator to counteract the spasms in your bronchial tubes.

Antibiotics usually are prescribed for intermittent use. A common regimen requires taking the antibiotic for 7 to 10 consecutive days each month. Seldom should it be necessary to use an antibiotic continuously. At times it may be advisable to alternate among two or three kinds of antibiotics to prevent the development of a resistant bacterial strain.

Surgery
If you have no response to other treatments or if you are coughing up blood, surgical removal of the affected portion of the lung may be necessary. However, this is an option only if the disease is localized in one or two areas of the lungs.

Lung Abscess

Signs and Symptoms
- High and irregular fever
- Sweats and chills
- Shortness of breath
- Cough that produces sputum containing pus and sometimes blood
- Malaise
- Loss of appetite and weight
- Chest pain

Cause
A lung abscess is a cavity in your lungs that is filled with pus. It usually occurs when infectious material from your mouth or throat is inhaled and an infection becomes established in your lungs. Dental disease often is the source of the infection.

Postural Drainage and Chest Percussion

With bronchiectasis (see page 708), cystic fibrosis (see page 720), lung abscess (see page 708), and certain other lung problems, a large volume of secretions may accumulate in the lungs. Especially if you have cystic fibrosis, your physician may recommend one or both of the strategies called postural drainage and chest percussion to help empty your lungs of the unwanted secretions.

Postural Drainage

This process uses gravity to clear the lungs. You position yourself so that the secretions are moved to your windpipe (trachea) and you can cough them out. Because the branches of your lungs point in various directions, it may be necessary for you to assume different positions to drain different areas of the lungs.

Some physicians recommend a time-consuming series of positional changes to raise secretions in cystic fibrosis, a childhood disease (see page 720). Others have found that compliance with these instructions decreases as the child who has cystic fibrosis ages. Therefore, many physicians limit their recommendations to positions that drain areas of the lungs where secretions are most likely to lodge. (Usually these positions will be those that drain the lower portions of the lungs.)

Cystic Fibrosis
If you have cystic fibrosis, see your physician or a trained therapist at a cystic fibrosis center for specific instructions. Remember to cough during each position change to aid in raising the sputum.

Bronchiectasis
This condition is uncommon in upper lobes of the lungs because these lobes drain well when you are in an upright position. In these conditions, postural drainage may be simpler. You may drain lower portions of your lungs quite well by kneeling or lying on a bed, chair, or couch and putting your hands on the floor. Stay in that position for about 10 minutes, and cough periodically.

Collect the expectorated sputum and note its color and approximate amount. If no sputum is produced, stop postural drainage until it becomes worthwhile. If you are taking antibiotics, remember that these work better and will be effective for a longer period if you keep your airways as free of secretions as possible.

Chest Percussion

Chest clapping (percussion) is another means of loosening secretions in your lungs.

Lie on your back on a firm surface. Cup your hands and rapidly strike your chest wall with one hand and then with the other. You may want to protect your skin with a bath towel. Be careful not to strike the heart area, breasts, lowest ribs, shoulders, or kidneys.

Your physician may recommend a sequence that coordinates both chest percussion and postural drainage for maximum effect.

Parents and others concerned with a child's care should learn this technique, which also can be applied to the back. Adults also may need help when applying the procedure to the back, which may be the most important area.

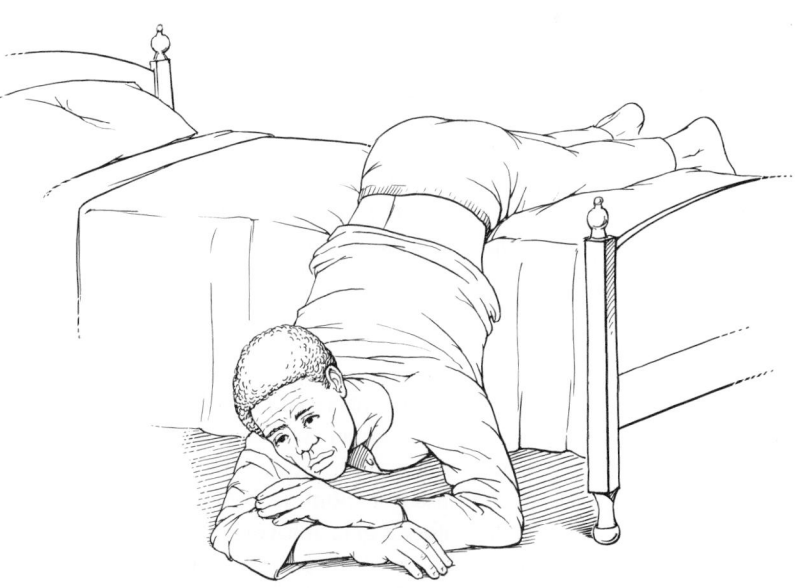

The postural drainage technique uses gravity to help clear lungs of unwanted secretions. The position shown here is designed to clear the lower lungs.

Infectious organisms in the mouth usually are inhaled when a person is unconscious as a result of excessive alcohol consumption, general anesthesia, excessive sedation, or a disease of the central nervous system. In middle-aged or older persons who smoke, lung cancer may cause a lung abscess by blocking a bronchial tube. Sometimes a lung abscess occurs as a complication of pneumonia. Other, rarer, causes of lung abscess are infections caused by tuberculosis or by fungal or parasitic organisms. In most cases, only a single abscess develops in the lung, although occasionally multiple abscesses appear.

Diagnosis

Symptoms of a lung abscess develop slowly over several days or weeks. Initially, they are similar to those of pneumonia. A cough is present after the abscess ruptures into a bronchial tube. Depending on the type of organism causing the infection, the sputum may be foul-smelling.

In addition to a physical examination, your physician will have a series of chest X-rays taken if a lung abscess is suspected and will take a sample of your sputum to check for bacteria or other organisms. Such information can lead to more effective treatment with specific antibiotics or other therapy.

How Serious Is a Lung Abscess?

Lung abscess is generally an acute disease, although if not treated adequately it can become chronic. With correct treatment, most people with an acute abscess recover completely without surgery.

Treatment

Medication

Antibiotics are necessary. The particular antibiotic prescribed will depend on what bacterium your physician finds to be the cause of the infection. If the abscess is the result of other organisms, your physician will advise other specific treatment (see Tuberculosis, page 705, and Fungal Diseases of the Lungs, page 711).

Other Therapies

Postural drainage and chest percussion may be used to drain the lung abscess (see page 709). If your lung abscess does not respond to antibiotics or drainage and percussion, bronchoscopy (see page 726) may be appropriate. Surgery may be advisable if the abscess has been present for several weeks, if it has a thick wall, or if it has spread into the pleural space (see Empyema, this page). Chest X-rays are often taken during the course of the disease to monitor progress.

Empyema

Signs and Symptoms

- Dry cough
- Fever and night sweats
- Weight loss
- Shortness of breath
- Chest pain on deep breathing
- Pleurisy (inflammation of the pleural membrane)

Normally, only a tiny amount of lubricating fluid is present in the pleural space, the space between the two layers of the pleural membrane that surrounds your lungs. Empyema (pus in the pleural space) occurs if infection is present.

Cause

Usually, empyema occurs as a complication of bacterial pneumonia, lung abscess, or certain other respiratory infections or after trauma to the chest or chest surgery.

Diagnosis

The buildup of infected fluid—up to a pint or more—puts pressure on your lungs. Pain due to pleurisy (see page 711) usually occurs early in the course of the disease but may disappear after more fluid is formed. If the accumulation of fluid is small, you may have no symptoms at all.

To confirm a diagnosis of empyema, your physician may perform thoracentesis. In this procedure, a needle is inserted through your chest wall to remove a sample of fluid from your pleural cavity.

Treatment

Treatment consists of antibiotic therapy and draining of the infected fluid from the chest. Your physician will prescribe the antibiotic that is most effective based on the results of culture of the infected matter.

Surgery

If the fluid in the pleural space flows easily, repeated thoracenteses may remove it. However, a thoracostomy—in which an incision is made in the chest wall under local anesthesia and a tube is inserted for drainage—is often necessary to ensure adequate removal of the fluid.

If this is unsuccessful, thoracotomy—opening the chest wall—may be performed under general anesthesia to permit thorough removal of the infection. If expansion of the lung is restricted because of thickening of the pleura (similar to a thick orange peel), surgery may be advisable to remove the thickening so that the lung can expand again.

Pleurisy and Pleural Effusions

Signs and Symptoms
- Shortness of breath
- Chest pain
- Dry cough
- Fever and chills

Pleurisy is inflammation of the pleura, the double membrane that surrounds each of your lungs. Pleural effusions are accumulations of fluid in the pleural space (between the lung and the chest wall).

Cause
Pleurisy and pleural effusions occur as complications of an underlying disease such as tuberculosis, pneumonia, pulmonary embolism, pancreatitis, cancer, or congestive heart failure or of trauma to the chest or other serious conditions.

In pleurisy, the two inflamed layers of the membrane rub against each other when you inhale and exhale. This produces a sharp, fleeting pain in your chest that is made worse by coughing, sneezing, movement, and deep breathing. The pain is relieved when you hold your breath or, sometimes, when you apply pressure over the painful area.

When pleural effusions develop, the pain usually disappears because the fluid serves as a lubricant. However, if enough fluid accumulates, it puts pressure on the lungs and interferes with their normal function, causing shortness of breath. A dry cough, fever, and chills sometimes occur as well, particularly if the fluid in the pleural space is infected (see Empyema, page 710).

Diagnosis
Your physician may suspect the diagnosis on the basis of your symptoms, findings on examination of your chest with a stethoscope, and the results of a chest X-ray. Sometimes physicians inject a local anesthetic and insert a needle through the chest wall (between the ribs) to remove fluid for analysis.

At the same time, a sample of tissue for microscopic study may be obtained, particularly if your physician is concerned that the fluid collection may be caused by a cancer (see Lung Cancer, page 724), a chronic condition such as tuberculosis (see page 705), or sarcoidosis (see page 721).

How Serious Is Pleurisy?
The outcome of pleurisy generally depends on the seriousness of the underlying disease.

Treatment
First, it is important to treat the underlying condition or illness that is causing the pleurisy or pleural effusion. However, in some cases the pleural effusion needs to be drained for several days by means of a chest tube.

Medication
Analgesics and anti-inflammatory drugs are generally prescribed. Sometimes codeine is prescribed to control the cough.

Fungal Diseases of the Lungs

Yeast and the spores of certain fungi, if inhaled, can become established in the lungs, causing disease. Most of these cause flu-like symptoms including fever, cough, and a general feeling of malaise.

Histoplasmosis

Signs and Symptoms
- Fever
- Cough

- General malaise
- Enlargement of liver, lymph nodes, or spleen
- Oral or gastrointestinal ulcers
- Difficulty breathing

Men are more likely than women to contract severe cases of this disease. In the United States, it is most common in the Mississippi and Ohio River valleys.

Cause

Histoplasmosis results from inhaling dust, particularly from chicken houses, bat-infested caves, and pigeon droppings, that contains the spores of the fungus *Histoplasma capsulatum*.

Diagnosis

There are four forms of histoplasmosis. One form, the mildest form, is almost indistinguishable from other diseases such as the common cold.

If the fungus spreads from the lungs through the blood, it causes the second form. This type is characterized by enlargement of the liver, lymph nodes, or spleen and, less often, by oral or gastrointestinal ulcers.

The third form, a chronic form, produces an illness similar to chronic tuberculosis.

The fourth form of histoplasmosis, the most serious form, is the disseminated (widespread) form, which can occur in persons with weakened immune systems.

To confirm histoplasmosis, your physician will obtain specimens of sputum, lymph nodes, bone marrow, liver, blood, urine, or oral ulcerations in order to check for the presence of the fungus.

It is common to see one or more spots on the lung on chest X-rays in persons who have had histoplasmosis in the past which went unrecognized or was symptomless.

How Serious Is Histoplasmosis?

In its mild form, histoplasmosis usually is benign and requires no treatment. The more serious forms of the disease can lead to death.

Treatment

Medication

If you have no symptoms, treatment usually is unnecessary. If symptomatic, oral antifungal agents such as ketoconazole or related drugs may be prescribed by your physician.

For severe infections, it may be necessary to administer amphotericin B, which must be given intravenously. If your lungs are affected, treatment will eliminate the fungus, but the lesions it produces in your lungs will remain.

Aspergillosis

Aspergillus is a genus of fungi that is found virtually everywhere. It may be present in nasal discharges and respiratory secretions of people who are exposed to it regularly (from the soil or farm dust), but it rarely causes problems in this group of people.

In persons with asthma (see Asthma, page 720), *Aspergillus* can produce a form of allergic response. In other susceptible persons, it can cause an unusual form of pneumonia. Both of these conditions, which are called aspergillosis, can be treated effectively with corticosteroids.

In persons whose lungs have been previously damaged, *Aspergillus* may collect within the lungs and cause coughing (which may include blood), weight loss, and mild fever. Often, surgery is needed to control bleeding.

If aspergillosis occurs in a person who has cancer of the blood (leukemia), the prognosis is poor, even with intravenous therapy with amphotericin B, an antifungal medication.

Cryptococcosis

Signs and Symptoms
- Low-grade fever
- Chest pain
- Cough that may produce sputum
- Lesions in the lungs
- Increasingly severe headaches
- Nausea
- Vertigo
- Loss of appetite
- Vision disorders
- Mental deterioration

Cause

Cryptococcosis is caused by the yeast *Cryptococcus neoformans*, which lives in soil and on pigeon droppings. Disease results when a person inhales the organism.

Diagnosis

In some cases, only mild symptoms occur. More serious cases resemble bronchitis, and lesions develop in the lungs. The yeast may remain in the lungs, or it may spread, especially to the central nervous system.

Your physician may take an X-ray to detect changes in the lungs and samples of sputum, pus, or spinal fluid to check for the presence of the yeast.

How Serious Is Cryptococcosis?

People who have weakened immune systems, such as those with leukemia, Hodgkin's disease, or AIDS, or people taking corticosteroids are most susceptible. Some mild cases clear without treatment, but in those people whose immune systems are already greatly weakened, cryptococcosis can lead to death, especially if it spreads from the lungs.

Treatment

Medication

Optimal treatment for those with immune system suppression consists of intravenous amphotericin B and oral flucytosine. Milder cases will respond to oral medications such as ketoconazole. Surgical removal of the nodules that form in the lungs may be advisable.

Coccidioidomycosis

Signs and Symptoms

- Fever and chills
- Backache and headache
- Chest pain
- Red, spotty rash
- Swelling of knees and ankles
- Cough
- Nasal congestion

Cause

Coccidioidomycosis is caused by breathing in spores from the fungus *Coccidioides immitis*, which exists in the soil in certain arid parts of the southwestern United States, Mexico, and Central and South America. In the United States, it was first discovered and is very prevalent in California's San Joaquin Valley, and hence its more popular names, San Joaquin or valley fever.

Diagnosis

Most commonly, coccidioidomycosis does not have any symptoms. Nine of every 10 people who have moved into the desert areas of the southwestern part of the United States test positive for this fungus within 4 to 5 years after their move. In approximately 10 percent of these people, chest pain develops. This pain, in addition to fever, chills, and other flu-like symptoms, usually begins 10 to 30 days after being exposed to the fungus. Nasal congestion and a mild cough may be followed by bronchitis. One to 2 days after the fever begins, a red, spotty rash, similar to the rash of measles, appears, and your knees and ankles may swell.

How Serious Is Coccidioidomycosis?

It may affect anyone, but if you are pregnant or if your immune system is weak, you are especially vulnerable. The disease tends to be more serious in dark-skinned people.

Usually the disease clears up without complications, although in some cases the lesions formed in the lungs may be difficult to cure and, in rare cases, the disease may recur after weeks or months. Occasionally the infection spreads throughout the body, causing lesions in the lungs, bones, and other organs.

Treatment

If you have no symptoms, treatment usually is unnecessary. If you have flu-like symptoms, treat these and rest in bed until the fever disappears.

Medication

Your physician may prescribe amphotericin B. Given intravenously, it helps in most cases. Ketoconazole, or another similar drug, taken orally is less effective but may be used between courses of amphotericin B in treating a recurrence of the disease.

Surgery

In severe cases, surgical drainage of lung abscesses or pleural fluids may help.

Chronic Lung Conditions

There are three chronic lung disorders in which obstruction to the flow of air out of the bronchial passages is a prominent symptom. In one, chronic bronchitis, there is a persistent inflammation of the lining of the bronchial passages, commonly, but not always, associated with obstruction to the outflow of air. Another, emphysema, is characterized by enlargement of the air sacs (alveoli) and destruction of the walls between them. There is almost always some degree of bronchitis associated with emphysema, and chronic obstruction to the outflow of air is prominent. Physicians often refer to emphysema and chronic bronchitis as chronic obstructive lung disease (COLD) or chronic obstructive pulmonary disease (COPD).

In the third disorder, asthma, the trachea and bronchial passages are prone to narrow too much and too easily in response to a wide variety of provoking stimuli. Obstruction to the outflow of air tends to be variable and episodic, often occurring in "attacks" (see Asthma, page 720).

Chronic Bronchitis

Signs and Symptoms
- Chronic cough that produces mucus
- Shortness of breath

This disorder consists of chronic inflammation and thickening of the lining of your bronchial tubes. There may be enough narrowing of these air passages to interfere with breathing and often to induce spells of coughing. In addition, the inflammation causes the glands of your bronchial tubes to produce excessive amounts of mucus, increasing the congestion in your lungs and further hampering your ability to breathe. It is a persistent disease, lasting for long periods and recurring often, and it may become permanent.

Most people with chronic obstructive pulmonary disease (COPD) have a combination of chronic bronchitis and emphysema, but one of these diseases is usually dominant. Those with chronic bronchitis tend to be over age 35 and often are overweight or obese.

Cause
Smoking is the major cause of chronic bronchitis. However, air pollution and dusts or toxic gases in the environment (smog, for example) or the workplace also can cause bronchial irritation and chronic inflammation. The disease is more prevalent in men than in women. About 20 percent of men have chronic bronchitis. However, because more women are smoking, the number of women with the disease is increasing.

Diagnosis
The primary symptom of chronic bronchitis (as distinct from emphysema) is a chronic cough that produces large amounts of mucus and has persisted for at least 3 months of the year for more than 2 consecutive years. Initially, the cough usually appears during the winter months. Then, over the years, it becomes almost continuous. As the disease worsens, relapses of the cough become more frequent and more severe, and you may experience shortness of breath.

In diagnosing chronic bronchitis, your physician will take your medical history,

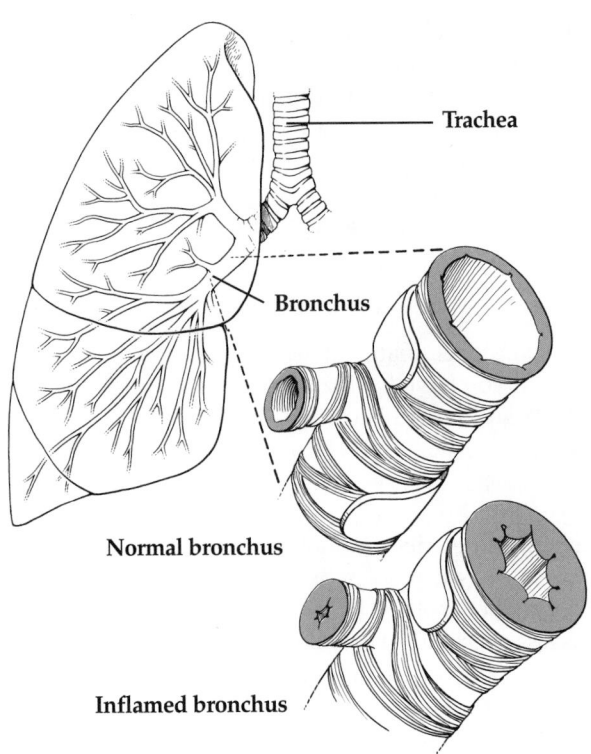

Trachea

Bronchus

Normal bronchus

Inflamed bronchus

In bronchitis, the main branches of the airway to the lungs (the bronchi) become inflamed and thickened. This restricts air flow.

perform a physical examination, and obtain lung function tests and a chest X-ray.

How Serious Is Chronic Bronchitis?

Chronic bronchitis is a serious disease. In people with severe disease, the likelihood of long survival is poor. However, if the disease is detected early and the affected person does not smoke, the outlook is more optimistic.

Treatment

If you smoke cigarettes, stop smoking. Other primary goals of therapy are relief of symptoms and avoidance of respiratory infections. Also, your physician will teach you how to deal with the disease.

One of the things you can do to prevent aggravation of your cough is to avoid fumes such as paint odors, exhaust fumes, and even certain cooking odors and perfumes. Avoid dust, extremely humid or dry air, and cold air. During the winter, use a humidifier in your home, particularly in the bedroom.

If at all possible, avoid exposure to anyone who has a cold because such an infection may severely aggravate your bronchitis. Make sure you dress appropriately for the temperature, and avoid large groups of people during the winter when colds and flu are common. If you do come down with a respiratory infection (typical symptoms include cough, a change in color or amount of sputum, and fever), call your physician promptly.

Unless your physician advises against it, get a flu shot (see Flu Shots, page 1066) yearly and be vaccinated against pneumococcal pneumonia (see Immunizations, page 1079). Note, however, that the pneumonia vaccine (Pneumovax) provides lifelong immunity against common strains of *Pneumococcus*. Seldom is a second vaccination necessary.

Drinking large quantities of fluid helps to dilute the thick mucus in your lungs and so may make removal by coughing easier. Keep in mind, however, that beverages containing caffeine and alcohol tend to remove fluid from your body, so limit the amounts you consume.

Medication

Your physician may prescribe a 7- to 10-day course of broad-spectrum antibiotics (antibiotics that are effective against many kinds of bacteria; examples are ampicillin, erythromycin, and tetracycline). These will be used if your sputum changes in color, volume, or thickness, changes that may indicate the onset of a respiratory infection. Your physician also may prescribe a bronchodilator if lung tests indicate the presence of spasm of your airways.

If your body's ability to get oxygen from your lungs into your blood is significantly impaired, your physician may prescribe oxygen therapy on either a continuous or supplemental basis. Devices are now available that permit oxygen delivery both in the home and in portable containers to allow maximum mobility.

Emphysema

Signs and Symptoms

- Shortness of breath
- Chronic, mild cough that may produce sputum
- Weight loss

The term emphysema is used as a synonym for chronic obstructive pulmonary disease (COPD).

Cause

Emphysema is quite common and in most cases is caused by smoking over a long period, although heredity and preexisting asthma may have some effect. Emphysema is most likely to develop in cigarette smokers, but cigar and pipe smokers also are at risk. Emphysema is more common in men than in women, but this difference is changing because more women are smoking.

Normally, your lungs contain 300 million elastic air sacs, called alveoli, in which oxygen is added to your blood and carbon dioxide is removed from it. Emphysema occurs when the alveoli lose their natural elasticity, become overstretched, and rupture. Several adjacent alveoli may rupture, forming one large space instead of many small ones. This process occurs slowly and does not affect all of the alveoli to the same extent, but it does prevent the lungs from functioning efficiently. Smoking may cause the elastic fibers that make up the walls of the alveoli to dissolve, damaging cells that produce a substance necessary for maintaining healthy elasticity.

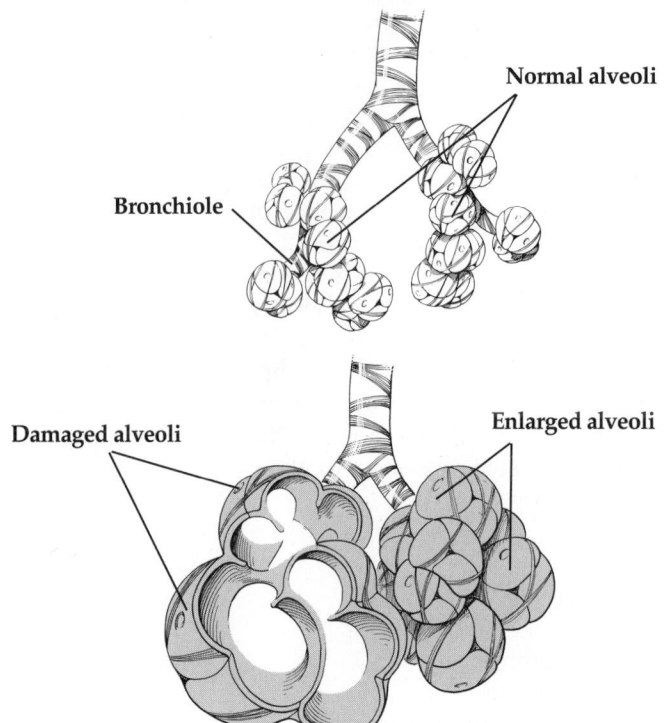

In emphysema, the air sacs of the lungs (alveoli) lose elasticity, enlarge, and may rupture. This decreases the exchange of oxygen and carbon dioxide in your blood.

Emphysema is characterized by damage to the smaller bronchial passages. This leads to a narrowing of these passages, especially when you breathe out or exhale. As a consequence, it takes longer for air to leave the lungs than is normally the case. This leads to slowing of the process of air exchange and to a sensation of shortness of breath.

Shortness of breath is the main symptom of emphysema, but it usually is not due to poor transfer of oxygen and carbon dioxide within the lungs. Rather, it results from decreased efficiency of breathing and the associated increased effort to breathe. This explains why supplemental oxygen is neither necessary nor particularly useful for treating shortness of breath in this disease, unless there is also a significantly reduced blood oxygen level.

In some persons, emphysema is caused by an inherited deficiency of an enzyme, called alpha$_1$-antitrypsin, which normally protects the integrity of the elastic fibers in the walls of the alveoli. On testing of their blood, such persons will be found to have low levels of this enzyme and likely will have severe emphysema in the third or fourth decade of their lives. Although unproven, smoking may block the action of this enzyme and thereby produce emphysema in persons without the inherited trait.

Diagnosis

As emphysema develops, you become less and less able to tolerate exercise or even mild exertion. Shortness of breath can slowly worsen over time, becoming severe, especially after respiratory infections. A change in the color, volume, or thickness of your sputum may signal the onset of a respiratory infection. Your physician will make a diagnosis of emphysema on the basis of your symptoms, medical history, lung function test results, and chest X-ray findings. He or she often will notice an increase in the size of your chest.

How Serious Is Emphysema?

Emphysema is a serious, chronic disease. The outcome can be poor if the involvement is extensive. There is no specific treatment for reversing the changes of emphysema.

However, if detected early, emphysema is largely a preventable disease—so stop smoking. If you stop before symptoms are present, you may prevent further progression of the disease.

People with emphysema are particularly prone to pneumonia, acute bronchitis, and other serious respiratory diseases.

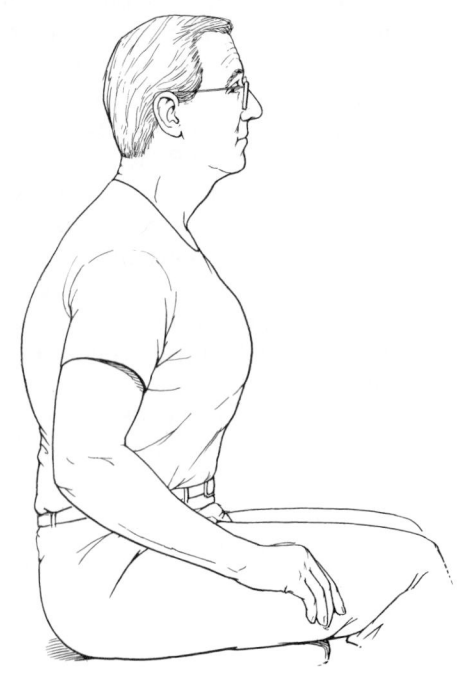

An enlarged chest can be one characteristic sign of emphysema.

Breathing Techniques

If you have emphysema or another chronic lung disorder, you may be helped by practicing some simple breathing exercises. You can develop a new breathing pattern in which you control emptying your lungs (expiration) by using your abdominal muscles. You can also increase the efficiency of your lungs and your inspiratory (inhaling) muscles. With your physician's guidance, develop a regimen of breathing exercises. Do them 2 to 4 times daily.

Diaphragmatic Breathing

Lie on your back with your head and knees supported by pillows. Begin the exercise by breathing in and out slowly and smoothly in a rhythmic pattern. Relax.

Now, place the fingertips of one hand on your abdomen, just below the base of your rib cage. As you inhale slowly, you should feel your diaphragm lifting your hand.

Practice pushing your abdomen against your hand as your chest becomes filled with air. Make sure your chest remains motionless while you do this. Try this while inhaling through your mouth and counting slowly to 3. Then purse your lips and exhale through your mouth while counting slowly to 6.

Practice diaphragmatic breathing on your back until you can take 10 to 15 consecutive breaths in one session without tiring. Then practice it on one side and then on the other. Progress to doing the exercise while sitting erect in a chair, while standing up, walking, and, finally, while climbing stairs.

Pursed-Lip Breathing

Try the diaphragmatic breathing exercises with your lips pursed as you exhale, that is, with your lips puckered (the flow of air should make a "ssssss" sound). Inhale deeply through your mouth and exhale. Repeat 10 times at each session.

Deep-Breathing Exercise

This exercise is simple but is a good discipline. While sitting or standing, pull your elbows firmly backward as you inhale deeply. Hold the breath in, with your chest arched, for a count to 5 and then force the air out by contracting your abdominal muscles. Repeat this deep breathing 10 times.

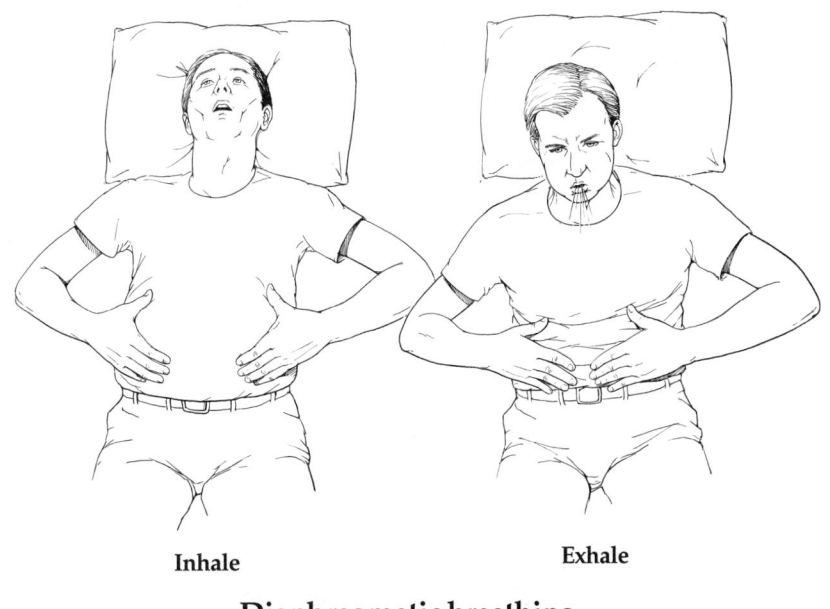

Inhale   Exhale

Diaphragmatic breathing

The Controlled Cough

If you have a chronic lung disorder that causes an accumulation of secretions in your lungs, you must clear them out to prevent infection. There are several simple ways to accomplish this, including postural drainage (see Postural Drainage and Chest Percussion, page 709) and the controlled cough.

Sit on the edge of a bed or chair. Lean slightly forward. Your feet should be on the floor, and you should be confident of your balance.

Inhale a deep breath through your nose, hold it for a moment, and then cough twice. Try two short and sharp coughs—do not try to do it all at once with explosive, uncontrolled coughs because they tend to collapse your airways, trapping mucus and air. This, in turn, may lead to shortness of breath.

Relax for a moment, then repeat this procedure. Keep a box of tissues close at hand in case your cough produces sputum.

By starting with gentle coughing and working up to harder coughs, you will develop a skill at clearing your lungs of secretions.

Treatment

Treatment cannot restore your lungs to normal, but therapy can keep your disease from getting worse and can teach you how to use your damaged lungs most efficiently.

The most important step is to stop smoking (for help, see Tobacco, page 315). If you do not stop, your disease almost certainly will get worse.

Also, avoid other respiratory irritants that may cause shortness of breath or tightness in your chest. These include fumes from paint and automobile exhaust, some cooking odors, certain perfumes, dust, cold air, and extremely humid air.

During cold weather, wear a soft scarf or a cold air mask (obtainable from any pharmacy) over your mouth and nose to warm the air that is entering your lungs. For the same reason, breathe through your nose because cold air can cause spasms of the bronchial passages. Using a humidifier in your home also may help. Finally, avoid exposure to persons with respiratory infections such as a cold or flu.

Your physician may prescribe a 7- to 10-day course of broad-spectrum antibiotics (antibiotics such as ampicillin, tetracycline, and erythromycin that are effective against many bacteria). Bronchodilators may be useful if you experience bronchial spasms as well.

To increase the efficiency of your lungs, first take the medications your physician prescribes. Second, exercise regularly. Less strenuous exercise such as walking or cycling can increase your exercise tolerance. Third, practice breathing techniques prescribed by your physician. Some people are able to improve their tolerance of exercise through this special training of the muscles that control inhalation and exhalation. The training can improve the strength and endurance of these muscles. Your physician will teach you how to do it correctly (see Breathing Techniques, page 717). Finally, see your physician promptly if your condition worsens or if a respiratory infection develops.

Sometimes physicians prescribe home

Your Home Supply of Oxygen

If you have a chronic lung disease, your physician may prescribe the use of supplemental oxygen at home. This has become common practice, provided appropriate testing reveals a significant lack of oxygen in your blood. The amount of inhaled oxygen (in liters of flow per minute) required to restore the blood oxygen to a satisfactory level should also be determined.

Even though supplemental oxygen may ease shortness of breath and improve your sense of well-being, it is prescribed primarily to support the heart. It is heart function that is most disturbed by an inadequate supply of oxygen. Therefore, whenever supplemental oxygen is prescribed, it should be used only as directed to achieve maximum benefits.

Taking Proper Precautions
Fire burns faster in an oxygen-rich environment, so take special care when using oxygen in your home. Keep objects that produce sparks, flames, or intense heat well away from the area where the oxygen is located. These include smoking materials, matches, lighters, electric radiant heaters, and electrical appliances such as heating pads, radios, and hair dryers. Keep flammable materials away from the area too. These include alcohol, aerosol sprays, combustible liquids, and any petroleum-based household substances including Vaseline and perfumes.

Never expose the oxygen tank and its attachments to temperatures above 125° Fahrenheit.

Handling the Equipment
Be sure that the oxygen cylinders are well secured to prevent them from tipping over. They are heavy and hazardous. When not in use, seal the tanks properly with protective caps.

When installing the regulator, follow the technician's instructions precisely. Before the regulator is attached, open the valve slightly and then close it immediately. This clears out dust or combustible material.

Using a Traveling Tank
If you require oxygen 24 hours a day, your physician may also recommend use of a portable oxygen device that allows you to travel beyond the reach of the large tank and its hose. The rules and regulations cited above apply equally to portable tanks. Portable containers carry only a limited amount of oxygen. Longer trips (more than several hours) require more preparation to ensure a continuous oxygen supply.

Smoking and Chronic Obstructive Pulmonary Disease

Smoking is the primary cause of chronic obstructive pulmonary disease (COPD) such as emphysema and chronic bronchitis. Deaths caused by chronic bronchitis and emphysema are significantly more frequent among people who smoke heavily than among nonsmokers.

By the time symptoms of COPD appear—typically, cough, shortness of breath, and difficulty tolerating exercise—damage has already occurred to your lungs. If you do not stop smoking, your disease will get worse. Stopping smoking tends to slow or halt progression of the disease but cannot reverse damage already done.

Tobacco Smoke
Tobacco smoke contains a mixture of chemicals, gases, and tiny droplets of tar. Thousands of substances have been identified in tobacco smoke. The toxic effects of many of them remain unknown. Some components are filtered off when you draw the smoke through the remaining unburned tobacco. However, as the cigarette burns, these chemicals are vaporized again and each puff of smoke thus contains more of the components. Most smokers inhale the cigarette smoke, which makes it even more dangerous.

Cigarette smoke contains 2 to 6 percent carbon monoxide. Carbon monoxide is a toxic gas that combines with hemoglobin (carboxyhemoglobin). When this occurs the hemoglobin molecule cannot transport oxygen to the tissues. Many smokers have carboxyhemoglobin levels of 8 to 10 percent in their blood whereas a nonsmoker commonly has only up to 1.5 percent. (A person dying from acute carbon monoxide poisoning has blood carboxyhemoglobin levels of 30 to 40 percent.) Thus, your tissues are deprived of needed oxygen.

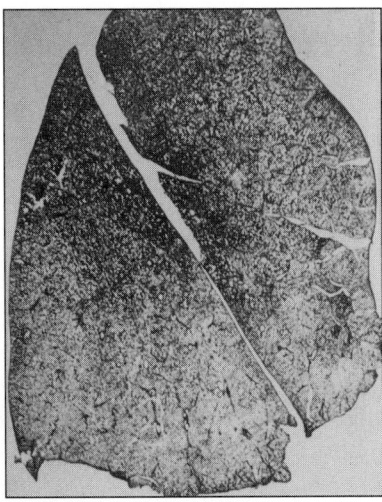

Normal lung

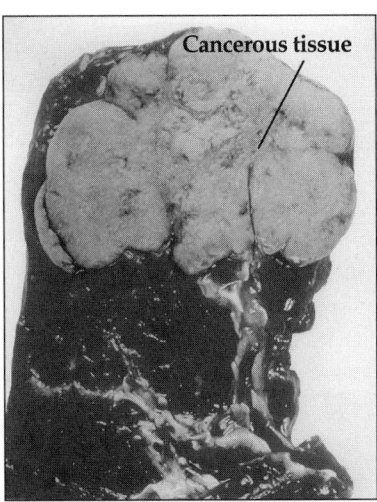

Cancerous tissue

Lung cancer

The tar found in cigarettes contains substances that cause cancer. Irritants in tobacco smoke cause your air passages to constrict and your bronchial tubes to produce excess mucus, and they cause you to cough. These irritants also may impair the function of the immune system cells in your lungs and upset the normal balance of pulmonary enzymes, which makes you more susceptible to respiratory disease. Finally, inhaled tobacco smoke stops the action of the cilia in your airway. Cilia are tiny hair-like projections in your windpipe and bronchial tubes. They help expel foreign material from your lungs.

Cigar and Pipe Smoke
Cigarette smoking is not the only cause of chronic respiratory disease. Although less dangerous than cigarette smoking, cigar smoking and pipe smoking are not innocuous. Because this smoke is more irritating, you are less likely to inhale.

Marijuana Smoke
Marijuana smoking also can lead to chronic respiratory disease. It contains many of the same irritants found in tobacco smoke. It also contains substances that are not present in tobacco smoke, such as delta-9-tetrahydrocannabinol. Some of them are respiratory irritants.

Marijuana usually is smoked in ways that make it more dangerous than cigarette smoking. Marijuana smokers usually inhale deeply and hold the smoke in their lungs, or they use a specially constructed pipe that concentrates the smoke and sends it into the lungs under pressure. Studies show that this inflames the airways and causes carcinogenic (cancer-prone) changes in the respiratory cells. In addition, it makes the lungs more susceptible to infection by any fungi or bacteria that might be present in the marijuana. Researchers have found significant decreases in the lung capacity of people who smoke marijuana daily. These smokers are at risk for COPD as well as laryngitis and chronic rhinitis.

Quit Smoking
If you are a smoker—stop (see Tobacco, page 315). Many people do not quit until they have symptoms of respiratory disease.

oxygen therapy on either a continuous or supplemental basis (see Your Home Supply of Oxygen, page 718).

Asthma

Signs and Symptoms
- Shortness of breath
- Cough
- Tightness of the chest
- Wheezing

Asthma is characterized by episodes of narrowing of the bronchial tubes of your lungs. Normally, these tubes narrow only as a protective reaction to prevent harmful substances from entering your lungs. With asthma, the bronchial tubes narrow too much, too often, and too easily in response to a variety of substances that ordinarily would not damage the lungs (see Asthma, page 1044).

Cystic Fibrosis

Signs and Symptoms
- Chronic cough
- Decreased energy and exercise intolerance
- Recurring pneumonia
- Shortness of breath
- Poor appetite
- Chronic diarrhea and malnutrition
- Salt depletion and heat exhaustion in hot weather

Cause
Cystic fibrosis is an inherited disease that affects both the respiratory and the digestive systems. It is the most common fatal hereditary disease in white children in the United States, affecting approximately 1 in every 2,000 infants. It also is one of the more common causes of chronic lung disease in children.

The disease seldom affects black, Asian, or Jewish children. It occurs in boys and girls equally. It is inherited on a recessive basis, which means that a child can have cystic fibrosis if both parents are carriers of the disease. (In this case the parents will have no symptoms themselves.)

Cystic fibrosis affects the mucus and sweat glands of the body. The first symptom in a newborn infant may be blockage of the intestine due to thick, clay-like meconium (the dark-green material present in an infant's intestine that makes up its first stool).

As the infant grows older, chronic respiratory disease may develop, including bronchitis, bronchiectasis (chronic, abnormal dilation of the bronchial tubes), collapsed lung due to blockage of the airways, pneumonia, or fibrosis of the lung.

These problems occur because the mucus in the child's lungs is very thick and sticky. Instead of serving as a lubricant, it clogs the respiratory system and allows bacteria and other microorganisms to grow within it, impairing the body's natural defenses. The pancreas may not provide the enzymes needed to digest fats and proteins completely, resulting in chronic diarrhea and malnutrition. The child's sweat glands also are affected, causing the sweat to be extremely salty.

Diagnosis
If your child has chronic respiratory or pancreatic disease, your physician may perform lung function or stool tests or may also order a sweat test to measure the amount of salt in your child's perspiration. This test is often performed on 2 consecutive days for an accurate diagnosis. If the test is positive and your child has siblings, test them also.

How Serious Is Cystic Fibrosis?
Cystic fibrosis is very serious and ultimately fatal. About half of the individuals with this disease live beyond age 26, although as techniques to treat cystic fibrosis have improved, some people have survived beyond their 30s. Mild forms of the disease may not produce symptoms until adulthood.

Treatment
Treatment is a long-term process, and frequent checkups are important.

If bowel symptoms are present, your child should receive a high-protein, low-fat diet. For instance, give skim milk instead of whole milk. Other than that, no special diet is required so long as the child is given a pancreatic enzyme preparation to supply the missing digestive enzymes. This comes as a capsule or powder to be taken with solid food. If your child is deficient in sodium or perspires heavily because of fever or hot weather, salt supplements may be given.

There are special exercises that parents can help their child perform to loosen and promote drainage of the mucus (see Postural

Drainage and Chest Percussion, page 709). Your child should do these exercises 1 or more times daily. A health practitioner can provide instruction on how to do them correctly.

Medication
Because the disease weakens the immune defenses against respiratory disease, it is important that vaccines be given against all respiratory diseases including whooping cough (pertussis), measles, and influenza. Respiratory infections also require prompt treatment with the antibiotic appropriate for the bacteria causing the illness.

Occasionally, oxygen supplementation is needed. Treatments with corticosteroids, aerosolized antibiotics, or amiloride, or with a substance that can dissolve mucus, are being tested.

Prevention
If you have a child with cystic fibrosis, each additional child will have a 25 percent chance of having the disease, a 50 percent chance of being a carrier, and a 25 percent chance of having normal genes. Since the recent description of the cystic fibrosis gene, our understanding of the cause, diagnosis, and treatment of this disease is rapidly changing. Specialists in cystic fibrosis can advise you on the latest developments.

Sarcoidosis

Signs and Symptoms
- Malaise
- Fever
- Shortness of breath, especially with exercise
- Weight loss

Cause
The cause of sarcoidosis is unknown. It can affect nearly any part of your body, including your skin, eyes, peripheral nerves, liver, lymph nodes, and heart, but in 90 percent of cases, it affects the lungs.

Sarcoidosis appears to involve the immune system. The T-helper lymphocytes, one of the types of white blood cells that protect your body from disease, seem to overrespond, causing a buildup of inflammatory cells in your tissue. In the lungs, this accumulation of cells distorts the walls of the alveoli (the small air sacs of your lungs), the bronchial tubes, and blood vessels, altering the normal diffusion of oxygen into blood in your lungs.

Sarcoidosis occurs in a higher percentage of blacks than whites in the United States, although all races are affected. Women are affected more often than men. It occurs primarily in individuals between the ages of 20 and 40, although in rare cases it can develop in children and elderly people.

Diagnosis
Usually, there are no symptoms with sarcoidosis, especially early in the disease. Many times, sarcoidosis is first suspected on a routine chest X-ray. To confirm the diagnosis, your physician may perform a lung biopsy using a fiberoptic bronchoscope to obtain tissue for examination (see Bronchoscopy, page 726). Sometimes, biopsy of skin, lymph nodes, or sclera of the eye is simpler if these structures are involved. Occasionally, the blood calcium level is higher than normal, and this may be a clue to the eventual diagnosis.

How Serious Is Sarcoidosis?
Sarcoidosis usually is a slow or chronic disease. Most of the affected persons recover completely or with only minor lasting effects, even without treatment. Some, however, have chronic disease that stays active or comes and goes intermittently for many years. Rarely, sarcoidosis leads to death, usually after many years.

Treatment

Medication
If you have pronounced symptoms or if the disease does not resolve spontaneously after 4 to 6 months, your physician may prescribe corticosteroids, which are then tapered off over several months or even years as the condition improves, as judged by chest X-rays or other tests. If the disease reappears, another course of corticosteroids may be required. However, this course of corticosteroids is likely to continue for a longer time than the initial treatment cycle because results generally are not as good with a second course of treatment.

Interstitial Lung Disease

Signs and Symptoms
- Shortness of breath, particularly with exercise
- General fatigue and malaise

- Loss of appetite and weight
- Cough with chest discomfort

Interstitial lung disease refers to a group of more than 180 diseases that are chronic, nonmalignant, and noninfectious. These diseases are characterized by infiltration of inflammatory cells into the walls of alveoli (the air sacs of your lungs), which causes abnormal formation of scar tissue in the connective tissue that supports the alveoli. If the disease progresses, scarring develops to the point such that the lungs may be destroyed. In most interstitial lung disorders, the causes are not known. These ailments generally affect people older than 50.

A major consequence of the formation of abnormal scar tissue is impairment of the transfer of oxygen to the blood.

Diagnosis

Your physician may suspect an interstitial lung disease based on your symptoms and the sounds he or she hears on examination of your chest with the stethoscope. He or she will probably order chest X-rays and lung function tests, both of which generally reveal significant abnormalities. Bronchoscopy with biopsy may be performed for confirmation of the diagnosis (see Bronchoscopy, page 726) or to rule out an infectious or malignant condition that may mimic the disease on chest X-ray.

If bronchoscopy is not diagnostic, thoracoscopy may be advised. This is a procedure in which a tube is inserted through the chest wall, usually under general anesthesia, to enable a biopsy specimen of the lung to be obtained under direct vision.

Alternatively, an "open" biopsy of the lung may be undertaken to establish a diagnosis. This is a surgical procedure, performed under general anesthesia, in which the chest wall is opened and a small sample of lung tissue is removed for examination under the microscope.

How Serious Is Interstitial Lung Disease?

These diseases have variable courses, depending on their cause. Some are progressive and ultimately fatal. Others become stable or have a fluctuating course.

A common type of interstitial lung disease is sarcoidosis (see page 721). Other types of interstitial lung diseases are idiopathic pulmonary fibrosis, pulmonary alveolar proteinosis, and Goodpasture's syndrome.

Idiopathic Pulmonary Fibrosis

This is a chronic noninfectious, nonmalignant disorder that causes progressive shortness of breath. Average duration of life after the onset of symptoms is 4 to 5 years, but many affected persons live much longer. Males and females are equally affected; the disorder commonly develops in the middle years of life, but it can occur at any age.

The diagnosis can be strongly suspected when certain typical sounds are heard through the stethoscope and certain characteristic patterns are seen on the chest X-ray and in results of lung function tests. However, lung biopsy, by bronchoscopy, thoracoscopy, or "open" surgery, also may be required. If there is a history of occupational exposure to asbestos (see Asbestosis, page 728), there could be a coexisting lung cancer.

Treatment may consist of corticosteroids, but only a small percentage of affected persons are helped. Lung transplantation has been used for this disorder.

Pulmonary Alveolar Proteinosis

This rare disorder occurs when material builds up within the alveoli (air sacs of the lungs). It occurs primarily in men, usually between the ages of 20 and 50. The cause is unknown.

In pulmonary alveolar proteinosis, the shortness of breath is minimal compared with the extent of involvement seen on the chest X-ray. (In contrast, in idiopathic pulmonary fibrosis the shortness of breath is greater than would appear likely from the relative lack of disease evident on the chest X-ray.) The problem may worsen over time or may disappear spontaneously.

Sometimes material from within the alveoli can be removed from the lung under general anesthesia. In this procedure (whole lung lavage), the material is literally rinsed from the lung—first from one lung and then from the other at a later date. Persons with this disease usually recover, although occasionally the disorder may recur.

Goodpasture's Syndrome

The precise cause of Goodpasture's syndrome is unknown, although it is more likely to occur in smokers. It occurs most often in young men. It causes hemorrhage of the lungs and glomerulonephritis (a type of inflammation of the kidneys; see page 836).

Although the hemorrhage itself can be

life-threatening, the lung symptoms can range from mild to severe. The diagnosis is made by biopsy of either lung or kidney. The course of the disease varies widely.

Your physician may prescribe corticosteroids or cyclophosphamide to control the disorder. In addition, your physician may elect to remove antibodies in your blood that may play a role in causing this disease.

Atelectasis

Signs and Symptoms
- Shortness of breath
- Fever
- Decreased blood pressure and rapid heartbeat
- Shock
- Pain on side of affected lung
- Severe, hacking cough

Atelectasis consists of a collapse of portions of a lung or sometimes of an entire lung.

Cause
It is caused by obstruction of bronchial passages in the lungs (commonly, by a plug of mucus), by accidental inhalation of a foreign object, or by outside pressure from a tumor, aneurysm, or enlarged lymph node. Sometimes it occurs as a complication after abdominal surgery when breathing may be shallow and portions of the lung are not expanded. It also may be associated with a bacterial infection. When obstruction occurs, the air beyond the obstruction is absorbed by the blood and that part of the lung collapses.

Diagnosis
Atelectasis can come on slowly (as with a growing tumor), or a massive, sudden collapse of the lung can occur. In making a diagnosis, your physician will look for an airless area on your chest X-ray.

Treatment
The first goal is to remove the cause of the obstruction. If coughing, suctioning, or other therapeutic measures do not work, bronchoscopy (see page 726) may be performed. Ampicillin or other medication may be prescribed to eliminate infection.

Prevention
Atelectasis is much less likely to occur after you have had an operation if, during post-operative recovery, you are encouraged to take deep breaths frequently and are up and walking as soon as possible. Commonly, an apparatus to teach you rapid, forceful inspiration is prescribed.

If you smoke or have chronic bronchitis or emphysema, you are less likely to have atelectasis after your operation if you discontinue smoking at least 3 to 4 days before your surgery. For several days before surgery you also can use bronchodilator medications (administered by an inhaler) and you can inhale an aerosol moisture periodically. Your physician may prescribe preventive use of an antibiotic that is effective against various organisms.

Pneumothorax

Signs and Symptoms—Breathlessness

Pneumothorax is the presence of air in the pleural space outside the lung but inside the chest wall. It also is referred to as collapsed lung.

Cause
When it occurs spontaneously, pneumothorax usually is thought to be due to rupture of a bleb (a blister containing air) on the surface of the lung. This spontaneous pneumothorax is most frequent in people younger than 35 or 40.

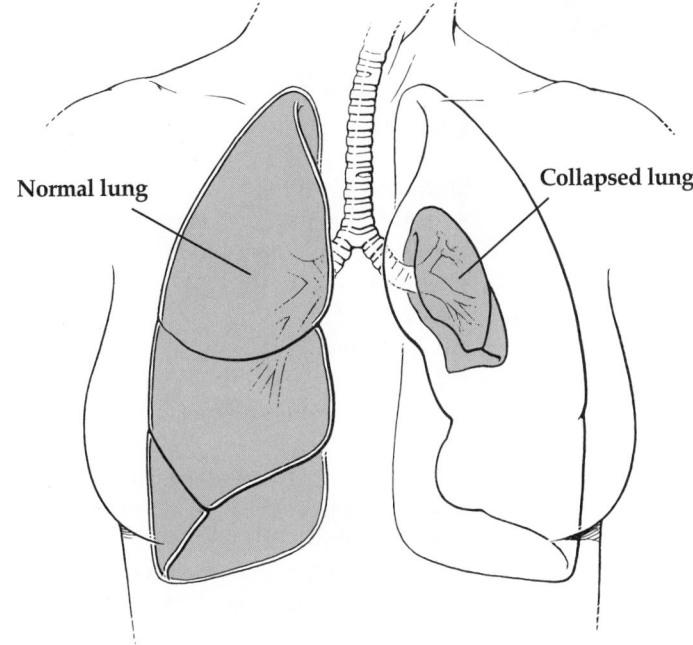

A collapsed lung (pneumothorax) results if air escapes from the lungs but is retained in the chest cavity.

Normal lung

Collapsed lung

Air also can enter the pleural space by other means. Air can enter the mediastinum (the space in the center of the chest between the lungs), especially during an asthmatic attack, and then rupture into the pleural space, causing a pneumothorax. When a lung biopsy specimen is taken at the time of bronchoscopy (see page 726) or during thoracentesis (removal of fluid from the pleural space), the pleura lining the lung may be penetrated, causing a leak of air which then may cause a pneumothorax.

Diagnosis

If the pneumothorax is small (a small amount of air in the pleural space), there may be no symptoms. If your physician suspects a pneumothorax, a chest X-ray may be taken to confirm the diagnosis and to determine the amount of air present.

Treatment

If your lung is less than 20 to 25 percent collapsed, your physician may choose to watch the progress by a series of chest X-rays until the air is completely absorbed or the lung is completely re-expanded.

If collapse of the lung exceeds 25 percent or if you are short of breath at rest, your physician may recommend removing the air through your chest wall. This can be done with a needle, but it is better performed by inserting a tube and applying constant suction for 24 hours or more. The latter procedure also helps to prevent recurrence of pneumothorax. Recurrent pneumothorax may require more aggressive surgical treatment.

Lung Cancer

Signs and Symptoms

- Cough that produces sputum containing pus and sometimes blood
- Shortness of breath
- Fever
- Chest pain
- Hoarseness
- Loss of appetite and weight

Lung cancer is the leading cause of cancer death in the United States in both men and women. About 100,000 men and 60,000 women die of lung cancer each year, and the number is increasing. The number of women dying of lung cancer is increasing because of increased smoking in this group over the past 30 years. Lung cancer occurs mainly in people between ages 45 and 70.

Cause

Cigarette smoking accounts for 85 percent of all lung cancers. Other risk factors for lung cancer include exposure to asbestos and other industrial carcinogens, secondhand smoke (see page 320), and high concentrations of radon (see The Radon Risk, page 378). Primary lung cancer is uncommon in nonsmokers, but cancer of the breast, colon, prostate, testicle, kidney, thyroid, bone, or other organs may spread (metastasize) to the lungs.

Benign (nonmalignant) tumors such as hamartomas are occasionally seen in the lungs. At times, these tumors have to be removed surgically if they are causing symptoms or if the diagnosis is uncertain.

More than 20 types of malignant and benign tumors have been identified as originating in the lungs. A benign tumor is a mass of abnormal tissue that does not spread and can be completely removed surgically. It is not life-threatening and is not likely to recur. A malignant tumor, however, is an abnormal growth of cells that can invade and destroy nearby tissue or organs and can spread (metastasize) to other parts of the body.

Almost all primary malignant cancers of the lung are one of four types: squamous cell carcinoma, adenocarcinoma, large cell carcinoma, and small cell carcinoma. About 60 percent of squamous cell carcinomas arise from the cells lining the central bronchi (the largest air passages of the lungs), making this one of the easier cancers to identify early through examination of your sputum. Squamous cell lung cancer accounts for 25 to 30 percent of primary lung cancers.

Adenocarcinoma usually arises in the lining of the smaller bronchi (air passages). It is now the most common type of primary lung cancer, causing about 35 percent of cases. It is named for the glandular structures that the tumor cells form (*adeno* means "gland"). It may spread to the lymph glands in that particular area of the lung and then, through the bloodstream, to other organs. Because it tends to arise in the periphery of the lung it is more difficult to identify early by sputum testing than is squamous cell carcinoma.

Smoking and Lung Cancer

Approximately 85 percent of the cases of lung cancer that occur each year can be traced to smoking. People who smoke more than 1 pack a day have a 20 times greater risk of lung cancer than do those who have never smoked. A person who has smoked 2 packs of cigarettes or more daily for 20 years has a 60- to 70-fold increased risk of cancer compared to a nonsmoker. Your risk of lung cancer decreases if you quit smoking.

Currently, lung cancer is more common in men than in women; however, because more women are smoking, their incidence of cancer is increasing rapidly. Lung cancer now surpasses breast cancer as the most common cause of cancer death in women. The American Cancer Society estimates that, by the year 2000, almost equal numbers of women and men will die from lung cancer.

Your risk of lung cancer increases with the number of cigarettes you smoke each day, the number of years you smoke, the amount of smoke you inhale, and the amount of tar and nicotine in the cigarettes you smoke.

Cigarette smoke contains a number of toxic gases plus tiny droplets of tar. Tar contains numerous carcinogens (substances that cause cancer) as well as co-carcinogens (substances that accelerate the production of cancer cells). Small (oat) cell carcinoma and squamous cell cancer are most strongly associated with cigarette smoking. Small cell cancer is a particularly aggressive cancer that spreads rapidly. It is most common in men who are heavy smokers. It seldom occurs in nonsmokers.

Cigarette smoke contains 2 to 6 percent carbon monoxide, a toxic gas that interferes with the ability of your body to transport and use oxygen. Irritants in cigarette smoke impair the function of the tiny microscopic hairs (cilia) that remove unwanted substances in your lungs and upset the normal balance of pulmonary enzymes, making you more susceptible to respiratory disease.

By 10 years after they quit smoking (see Tobacco, page 315), the death rate of those who smoked more than 20 cigarettes a day decreases by two-thirds, but still does not reach the level of those who have never smoked. Unfortunately, however, many people do not quit until they already have symptoms of respiratory disease or have developed cancer.

Bronchioloalveolar cell carcinoma, a subtype of adenocarcinoma, accounts for less than 5 percent of cases. It seldom spreads beyond the lungs; it affects the alveoli (air sacs) of your lungs.

Undifferentiated large cell carcinoma also appears in the periphery of the lung and spreads through the bloodstream. It accounts for 15 to 20 percent of lung cancers.

Finally, small (oat) cell carcinoma also develops in the central areas of the lung, making it easier to identify. Named for the small, round or oval shape of the cancer cells that resemble oats when viewed under the microscope, it is one of the more aggressive cancers. It tends to cause narrowing of the bronchi by compressing them. Small cell carcinoma accounts for 20 to 25 percent of lung cancers.

Diagnosis

A small proportion of asymptomatic lung cancers are detected on chest X-rays taken for

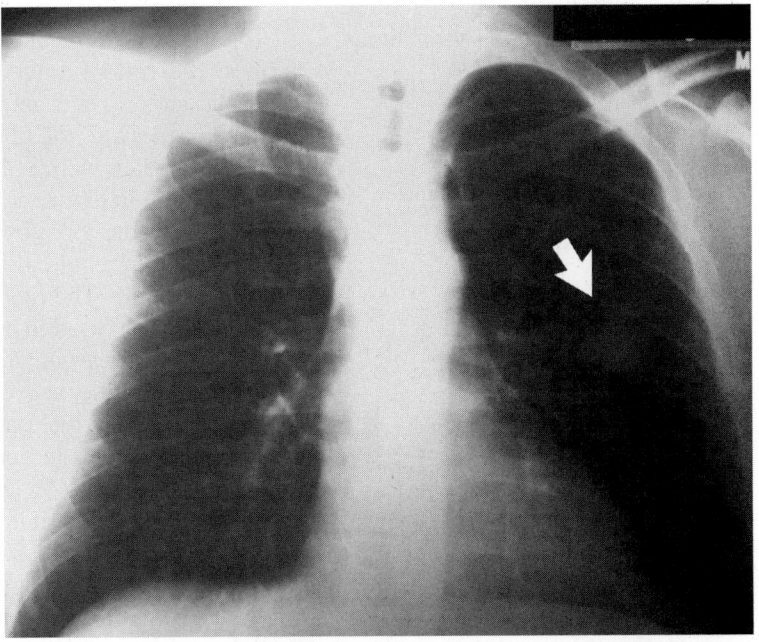

Chest X-ray reveals an abnormal mass in lung (arrow). Subsequent biopsy revealed this to be lung cancer.

various reasons other than detection of lung cancer. Many physicians recommend that middle-aged and older cigarette smokers have yearly chest X-rays because of their increased risk of lung cancer.

Examination of the sputum for cancer cells may sometimes detect a squamous cancer before symptoms appear. If symptoms are apparent, the location of the tumor may determine the nature of the symptoms you experience.

In many cases, a cough develops because an enlarging cancer is beginning to block an air passageway. Coughing up large amounts of blood is rare but, when it does happen, it indicates that the cancer has invaded a large blood vessel.

Persistent chest pain suggests that the tumor has invaded the chest wall. Infection in a lung because of blockage of an airway may cause fever, chest pain, and loss of weight. If the main bronchi are blocked by a tumor, that portion of the lung may lose volume (see Atelectasis, page 723). Various other symptoms may develop as the cancer spreads to such organs as the liver, brain, bone, heart, and adrenal glands.

Generally, lung cancer is first suspected either because of your physical symptoms or because an abnormal mass appears on a chest X-ray. Your physician may compare old and new chest X-rays to help determine if an abnormal finding on the new chest X-ray was present previously and if it has changed in size. In addition to a regular chest X-ray, tomograms (special chest X-rays that give a highly localized view of the lung) or other special studies such as a CT scan (see page 1334) may be obtained. A CT scan is useful for revealing very small lesions and determining if the cancer has spread to other sites.

Bronchoscopy (see below) may be per-

Bronchoscopy

Bronchoscopy is a procedure in which a specially designed tube is passed down your airway to allow your physician to see the inside of your air passages. Your physician can look for tumors, foreign objects, areas of internal bleeding, and abnormalities of your lungs

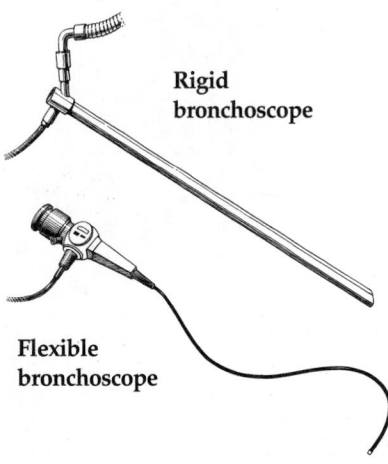

Rigid bronchoscope

Flexible bronchoscope

In bronchoscopy, your physician can see the inside of your air passages by passing a rigid or flexible tube (bronchoscope) into your airway.

and air passageways. The bronchoscope also has an open central channel through which your physician can remove excess secretions, obtain biopsy specimens, and introduce saline to rinse your lungs (lavage).

There are two types of bronchoscopes: the rigid bronchoscope, which is larger, rigid, and more difficult to use; and the fiberoptic bronchoscope, which is flexible and 3 to 7 mm in diameter.

Most bronchoscopic examinations in children require use of the rigid instrument. The rigid bronchoscope is often used in adults if a foreign body is present, dilation is required, or a laser is to be used in the tracheobronchial passages. Otherwise, the flexible fiberoptic instrument is used. It contains glass fibers that transmit light and return a magnified picture of the passageways of your lungs. Your physician can watch the progress of the bronchoscope on a small television-like screen.

You should not eat for at least 6 to 12 hours before bronchoscopy is performed. Fiberoptic bronchoscopy usually is performed under local anesthesia, but may be done under general anesthesia. The anesthetic agent, which depresses your cough and swallowing reflexes, usually is administered through your nostrils or mouth. Your physician also may give you a sedative to help you relax. The bronchoscope is then inserted through either your mouth or your nose. The procedure may be performed while you are sitting or lying down. Lidocaine jelly is used as an oral anesthetic and as a lubricant to protect your air passages.

When the flexible fiberoptic bronchoscope is used, the procedure is painless and there seldom are complications. After the procedure, you should not eat or drink anything for about an hour because your swallowing and cough reflexes still are depressed.

Lung Removal

Surgical removal (resection) of the tumor is the preferred treatment for people who have lung cancer that has not spread (metastasized) to other parts of the body. Depending on the extent of the cancer, people with squamous cell carcinoma, large cell carcinoma, or adenocarcinoma are candidates for surgical treatment. Surgery seldom is performed for small cell carcinoma because this type of cancer spreads too rapidly and too extensively to be totally removed surgically.

The Outlook

In those whose cancer is detected early enough so that surgical removal can be done, approximately 80 percent survive 1 year, and 50 percent are alive at 5 years after the operation. If the cancer recurs, however, the outlook generally is poor, although chemotherapy or radiation therapy may decrease the size of the tumor, prolong life, and relieve pain and other symptoms.

The Procedure

The tumor and the tissue immediately surrounding it, such as a lobe or even an entire lung, are removed. Usually, the lymph nodes draining the involved lung are removed as well. Radiation therapy sometimes is used in conjunction with removal. Normally you will be hospitalized for a week to 10 days after the operation, although it will take much longer before you recover completely. Many people are able to resume their normal activities in 4 to 6 weeks. However, the rate and degree of recovery depend on the general condition of your lungs and the amount of lung tissue removed as well as your overall health.

The Risk of Recurrence

After resection, be sure to have regular medical checkups to detect recurrence of the cancer, either within your lung or in other parts of your body.

---

formed to view the air passages and to obtain a biopsy specimen (sample of tissue for examination of the tumor). Your physician also may perform a complete blood cell count and liver function tests.

How Serious Is Lung Cancer?

Lung cancer is a very serious disease and has a very poor outlook. Overall, about 13 percent of people survive for 5 years. However, the outcome depends on the extent of the disease when it is discovered, your general health and age, the cell type of cancer, how rapidly it grows, and what type of therapy is given. Only 20 to 25 percent of all lung cancers can be removed surgically at the time of initial diagnosis. Once symptoms of lung cancer appear, the disease may be fairly well advanced and not treatable by operation.

Small cell cancer is very serious because of its tendency to spread early, often before symptoms are apparent. The 5-year survival after diagnosis is approximately 5 percent. Of those for whom surgery is an option, approximately one-third of people with squamous cell carcinoma and one-fourth of those with adenocarcinoma or large cell carcinoma survive 5 years after surgery.

Treatment

Basically, there are three treatment options for lung cancer: surgery (removal), chemotherapy, and radiation therapy. Laser surgery can be used to restore breathing when tumors obstruct central air passageways. Usually, this is done only when surgical removal of the cancer is not possible.

Surgery is the preferred treatment (see Lung Removal, above). Small cell cancer usually cannot be removed surgically, so other forms of treatment are used. Because lung cancer commonly occurs in people who have smoked heavily for many years, the lung not involved with cancer may be severely damaged by emphysema. Therefore, the surgeon cannot always remove the cancerous lung safely because the other lung may not be able to meet the person's oxygen needs. This situation can be clarified by breathing tests before the operation.

Radiation therapy, in which a beam of radiation is focused on the tumor at doses that destroy the cancer but do not harm surrounding tissue, is used in some patients. Chemotherapy, usually involving more than one drug, is the preferred treatment for people with small cell carcinoma. Radiation therapy may be added to the treatment program.

Occupation-Related Lung Disease

Hazardous materials in the workplace can cause lung disease if inhaled in quantity over time. Perhaps the best known of these diseases is asbestosis, which has numerous manifestations. Coal miner's disease and silicosis (caused by inhaling silica dust) also are well known. In addition, various industrial and agricultural dusts and some fungi cause diseases, usually named after an occupation or the type of dust inhaled.

Asbestosis

Signs and Symptoms
- Chest pain
- Shortness of breath
- Decreased exercise tolerance
- Cough

Asbestos was used extensively as an insulation in building construction for many years until 1975 when it was replaced by other materials such as fiberglass and slag wool. There are four types of asbestos fibers—chrysotile, amosite, anthophyllite, and crocidolite—and all can cause respiratory disease. Disease may result when large amounts of the fine asbestos fibers accumulate in your lungs.

More than 9 million workers are estimated to be at risk of this respiratory disease. People exposed to asbestos include workers in mining, milling, manufacturing, and installation of asbestos products. Trades that install asbestos products include pipe fitters, boiler makers, shipbuilders, and construction workers. Asbestos was sprayed on steel girders of buildings to prevent buckling in a fire. Asbestos also was used in fire-smothering blankets and safety clothing, as filler for plastic materials, in brakes and clutch linings, and in cement and floor tiles. Demolition workers and do-it-yourself home renovators working on older buildings are at risk.

You do not need to handle the material yourself to be exposed to the fibers. Electricians, painters, and others who worked next to the person installing asbestos insulation are at risk, as is the person who shook out and washed the clothes of someone who worked with it.

Occasionally, groups of cases have occurred in neighborhoods and communities near asbestos plants and mines. Avoid further exposure if possible.

Diagnosis
Asbestos exposure may cause asbestosis (a form of interstitial fibrosis or pneumoconiosis), mesothelioma (a cancer of the lining of the lung or abdomen), or lung cancer. Pulmonary asbestosis may result when the fibers accumulate around your bronchioles, the smallest air passageways. Your lungs react to the fibers by covering them, forming small masses of scar tissue. Symptoms appear when the scar tissue causes your lungs to lose their elasticity. The first symptom of asbestosis may be the gradual appearance of shortness of breath on exertion.

The severity of disease is directly related to the duration of your exposure and to the amount of fiber inhaled. Usually, at least 10 years of moderate to severe exposure must occur before symptoms of asbestosis appear. On your chest X-ray, the scar tissue will appear as small, scattered, opaque areas. They are first evident in the lower parts of your lung but gradually spread upward as the disease gets worse. Eventually, your entire lung may be affected, producing a honeycombed appearance.

Provide your physician with a detailed history of your work activities and any other sources of possible exposure to toxic dusts. Tell your physician about the availability and use of dust masks and other respiratory protection devices. An abnormal chest X-ray may suggest that you have been exposed to asbestos but does not necessarily mean you have asbestosis. The disease itself is diagnosed only if you have a history of exposure, suggestive chest X-ray and physical findings, and symptoms of debilitating pulmonary fibrosis (the abnormal development of scar tissue).

Another result of prolonged exposure to asbestos may be the development of pleural plaques around your lungs. These areas of thickening of the pleura, the double membrane that surrounds your lungs, usually occur along the lower part of the chest wall or near the diaphragm. The presence of pleural plaques is strong evidence that you have been exposed to asbestos but does not

Asbestos Removal From Buildings

Up to the early 1970s, asbestos commonly was installed in buildings as an all-purpose, low-cost insulation and fire-resistant fiber. It was sprayed onto beams, used as insulation for floors and ceilings, mixed into cement and floor tiles, and placed around pipes and boilers in schools, office buildings, and shopping malls. It is expensive to remove.

Asbestos in the Air

The problem is friable asbestos—asbestos that is flaking off. When disturbed during routine maintenance work, the tiny fibers can easily be released from the surface. These loose fibers may stay airborne for some time. The vast majority of the people who work in or go into buildings containing friable asbestos have a very small risk of contracting respiratory illness from the fibers, but what level of asbestos exposure is safe has not yet been determined.

Various federal, state, and local government regulations now require asbestos control or removal, particularly in schools. Many insurance companies will not finance buildings that contain asbestos.

The Removal Process

The first step in removing asbestos from a building is to determine the extent of the problem by obtaining counts of the asbestos fiber in air within the building. Owners of the building can hire an environmen-

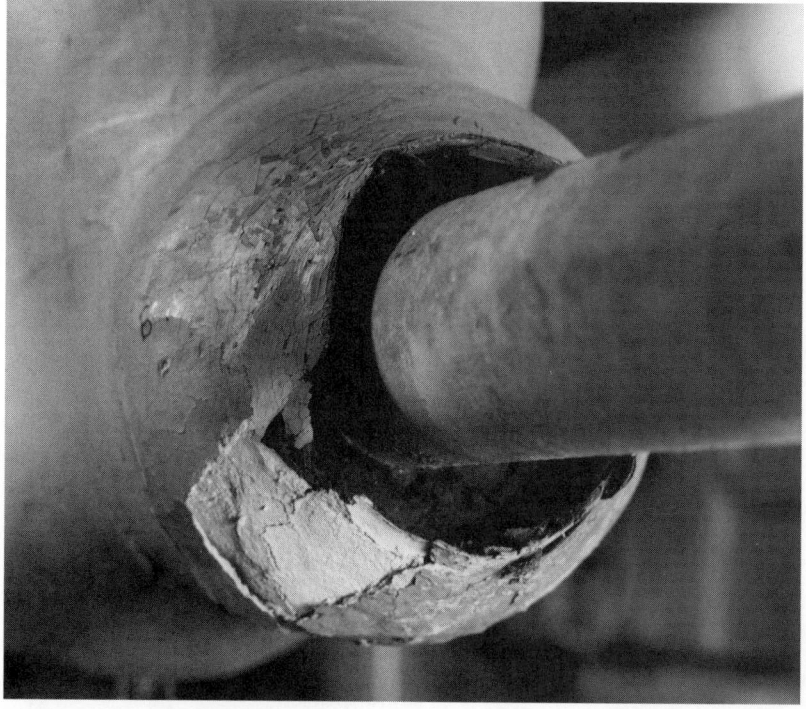

Asbestos used in this pipe covering can be hazardous to your health. Removal requires care and expertise.

tal consultant who specializes in asbestos to survey the building. The consultant should not be involved with anyone in the business of removing asbestos.

Asbestos removal is safest, easiest, and cheapest when the building is empty, although this is not always possible. In a building with tenants, the ideal removal plan consists of removing the material from those areas that are exposed because of maintenance work or renovations and then cleaning out the rest when the building is empty

before complete renovation or demolition. Until complete removal is possible, maintenance workers should be taught how to recognize and avoid the hazardous material. Also, the air should be monitored continuously if the asbestos is disturbed.

Removal of asbestos is a job for experts. Buildings should be demolished only after the portion to be torn down on a given day is dampened with water to prevent formation of dust clouds containing asbestos.

mean that your lungs are impaired unless you have other symptoms or signs.

Mesotheliomas, malignant tumors arising from the pleura, are a relatively rare type of cancer. Mesotheliomas may develop 20 to 40 years after the exposure to asbestos fibers and can occur even if the exposure was for only 1 or 2 years or even less. Many persons

with mesothelioma have no history of exposure to asbestos. The symptoms include chest pain, gradual appearance of shortness of breath, and weight loss. In about half of those with mesothelioma, the disease spreads, producing tumors in other parts of the body. In other cases, the tumors are limited to the chest. Pleural effusion, the buildup of fluid between the two layers of the pleural membrane, often contributes to shortness of breath and chest pain. The disease usually is fatal within 8 to 14 months; 75 percent of patients with mesothelioma die within a year after diagnosis.

Finally, if you smoke and have been exposed to asbestos, you have a much greater chance of developing lung cancer than does someone who smokes but has not been exposed. If you do not smoke, your chance of getting lung cancer from exposure to asbestos is much less. If you still smoke, quitting will help decrease your chance of getting cancer.

Treatment

There is no effective treatment for asbestosis.

Pneumoconiosis and Silicosis

Signs and Symptoms
- Shortness of breath
- Cough that produces sputum

Two types of pneumoconiosis, coal worker's pneumoconiosis and silicosis, are both caused by inhaled industrial particles that become permanently deposited in the lungs.

Coal worker's pneumoconiosis, also known as black lung disease or anthracosis, is caused by inhaling coal dust for prolonged periods, usually at least 10 years. Coal worker's pneumoconiosis is much more common in miners of anthracite coal (located primarily in the eastern United States) than in miners of bituminous coal (located primarily in the western United States).

Silicosis is caused by the inhalation of free silica (crystalline quartz). It is a severe disease caused by inhalation of industrial dust particles. Mining, stone cutting, quarrying (especially of granite), blasting, road and building construction, industries that manufacture abrasives, and farming are occupations that produce exposure to free silica. It usually takes 15 to 20 years of exposure before symptoms develop. However, unprotected workers in occupations with intense exposure to silica, such as sandblasting in confined spaces, tunneling through rock with a high quartz content, and manufacturing abrasive soaps, may develop silicosis in less than a year.

Diagnosis

In most cases, both coal worker's pneumoconiosis and silicosis cause no respiratory symptoms unless you are a cigarette smoker. These diseases are diagnosed when small, irregular, opaque areas are seen on your chest X-ray and you have a history of exposure to coal dust or silica. With long-term exposure, these irregular areas become larger and combine into more regular, small, rounded nodules.

However, both coal worker's pneumoconiosis and silicosis may develop into progressive massive fibrosis, also called complicated pneumoconiosis. Only a small percentage of those with coal worker's pneumoconiosis develop massive fibrosis. The mechanism that causes it is unknown. Those with silicosis, however, are likely to develop progressive massive fibrosis.

Fibrosis is diagnosed when an opaque area with a diameter larger than 1/2 inch is seen over the smaller opaque spots on your chest X-ray. The opaque areas combine so that they may cover the entire lobe of the lung. At this stage, the disease has progressed to cause shortness of breath and a cough that produces mucus. The symptoms are often more severe than the chest X-ray appearance suggests.

How Serious Are Coal Worker's Pneumoconiosis and Silicosis?

In their early stages, coal worker's pneumoconiosis and silicosis do not cause respiratory impairment. However, if massive fibrosis develops, which it ultimately does in silicosis, respiratory impairment occurs and, despite avoidance of further exposure, death results. Survival may be less than 2 years. In addition, persons with silicosis have a 3 times greater than average risk of tuberculosis.

Treatment

There is no specific treatment for either of these diseases. If you have either condition, avoid additional exposure to the causative dust. If you smoke, by all means stop. Limit your exposure to all respiratory irritants—cold air, dry air, extremely humid air, and irritating fumes.

If you have silicosis and your tuberculin skin test is positive, you will need treatment for tuberculosis, even if symptoms are not present.

Prevention

Prevention is the best course of action. Wear a dust mask and take other steps to prevent exposure to the dust if you are working in an occupation that puts you at risk of developing one of these diseases. In addition, do not smoke.

Occupational Asthma

Signs and Symptoms
- Shortness of breath
- Cough
- Tightness of the chest
- Wheezing

Cause

In 2 to 5 percent of people with asthma, the cause is related to occupation or environment. Some agents that are known to cause asthma are paints, wood dust, grain dust, pollens, synthetic dyes, gum arabic, and rosin (soldering flux). Inhalation of one of these agents does not mean you will develop asthma, however. A small percentage of the population seems to be genetically disposed to allergies that may be provoked by exposure to one of these agents.

Diagnosis

The symptoms are the same as those of non-occupational asthma. The diagnosis of occupational asthma depends primarily on your medical history and the results of pulmonary function tests, possibly including a bronchial provocation test in which you are exposed to the allergic substance in a laboratory and your reaction is measured.

Treatment

Treatment consists of bronchodilators, anti-inflammatory medications such as corticosteroids, and avoiding the substance that causes your asthma. Sometimes, you may have symptoms of asthma for years afterward even though you are no longer coming into contact with the offending agent (see Asthma, page 720).

Allergic Alveolitis

Signs and Symptoms
- Persistent cough that produces large amounts of sputum
- Wheezing
- Shortness of breath
- Decreased pulmonary function

Causes

This lung disease is caused by exposure to organic dusts. It goes by many names, usually relating to the occupation in which it is acquired. The best known are farmer's lung and byssinosis (see below). Grain dust can cause illness in farmers and in those who work in grain elevators.

Other illnesses include humidifier lung, which is caused by humidifiers, heating systems, and air conditioners that are contaminated by a fungus. Bagassosis results from fungi in moldy sugarcane fiber (called bagasse), and suberosis is caused by inhaling moldy cork dust. Sequoiosis is caused by moldy redwood sawdust. Maple bark stripper's disease is caused by rotting maple tree logs and bark. Finally, mushroom picker's disease is caused by moldy compost, and detergent worker's lung is caused by dust containing spores from enzyme additives.

Diagnosis

All of these dusts cause the same symptoms in those who are sensitive. Pulmonary function tests can help make the diagnosis.

How Serious Is Allergic Alveolitis?

In all cases, those who smoke are more susceptible and have more serious symptoms than nonsmokers.

Treatment

Generally, avoiding the irritating dust relieves the symptoms. Drink plenty of liquids and use a non-contaminated humidifier. If necessary, your physician may prescribe a bronchodilator.

Byssinosis

Signs and Symptoms—Chest tightness

Cause

This asthma-like disease sometimes is found in workers who produce cotton or, to a lesser extent, flax, jute, and hemp yarn and rope. Also known as brown lung and Monday fever (although it does not cause a fever), it is caused by inhaling dust from the raw

Fumes, Gases, Air Pollution, and Smoke

Exposure to high concentrations of toxic fumes and gases, air pollution, both outdoors and indoors, and smoke can cause various respiratory symptoms.

Industrial Fumes and Gases

Long-term low-level exposure or accidental exposure to high levels of industrial toxic chemicals can cause various temporary and sometimes chronic respiratory symptoms. Usually, the lower respiratory tract is affected, causing symptoms such as shortness of breath, cough, and chronic bronchitis (see page 714). A sampling of toxic chemicals includes ammonia, cyanides, formaldehyde, acid fumes, hydrogen sulfide, diazomethane, halides, nitrogen dioxide, isocyanates, ozone, phosgene, phthalic anhydride, and sulfur dioxide.

The industrial process of heating certain metals, such as cadmium, chromium, nickel, and beryllium, to high temperatures and then cooling them quickly releases fumes that can cause various respiratory diseases if inhaled. These include bronchitis, inflammation of the lungs, lung cancer, and metal fume fever. Metal fume fever is a flu-like illness that can result from exposure to fumes from copper, magnesium, zinc, and certain other metals. The symptoms usually appear several hours after work and then clear up within 24 hours. However, they return when the worker is exposed to the fumes again.

If you work in an industrial trade that uses high heat, such as welding, brazing, smelting, pottery making, and furnace work, you are most at risk. Using nonhazardous compounds, ensuring that ventilation is adequate, and using safe machinery and work practices can help prevent exposure to toxic fumes.

In all cases, workers who are exposed to these fumes and gases and who also smoke have a greatly increased risk of lung cancer.

Air Pollution

Outdoors

Given the right atmospheric conditions, air pollution caused by automobiles, power plants, and factories can result in increased levels of ozone and sulfur dioxide in the air. This often causes wheezing in people who have asthma and may cause shortness of breath in elderly people, young children, and persons with chronic cardiopulmonary disease. On days when the ozone level is high, usually after a long stretch of hot, humid weather, it is best that those at risk stay indoors.

Indoors

Indoor air pollution also can be a problem, especially because concerns about energy efficiency have resulted in construction of houses that are more tightly sealed. Therefore, fumes that once were of little concern tend to build up in the house instead of escaping to the outside. One example is cigarette smoke, which, besides having major health effects on the smoker, also affects nonsmokers who are exposed to it. For instance, passive cigarette smoking (the inhalation of tobacco smoke by nonsmokers) has been shown to cause increased respiratory infections and decreased lung function in children whose parents smoke. When ventilation is poor, wood smoke and fumes from kerosene floor heaters can aggravate asthma.

Another potentially hazardous agent is formaldehyde. It is present in urethane foam insulation and in some types of flooring used in construction of new houses, mobile homes, and furniture. When the products are new there may be a pungent odor due to formaldehyde fumes, which may irritate the eyes, nose, throat, and airways (trachea and bronchi). The formaldehyde gradually evaporates so that within a few months it should cause no problem. People with asthma may note worsening of the problem during these weeks or months.

Smoke

More fire fighters and fire victims die from smoke inhalation than from burns. Smoke inhalation has several effects on the lungs. It usually causes some degree of inflammation of the lower respiratory tract, which can develop into pulmonary edema if the exposure is severe enough.

Whenever anything burns, carbon monoxide is produced and, when inhaled, interferes with transportation of oxygen by the blood. All smoke contains this odorless gas. Be careful, therefore, when you have any fire indoors that produces smoke (such as indoor barbecuing).

The effects of inhaling carbon monoxide are so subtle as to be unnoticeable, and you can become unconscious without realizing anything is happening.

Smoke that contains a heavy concentration of floating particles also irritates the lungs.

Many plastics, polyurethanes, and other synthetic materials used in home furnishings give off various toxic gases when they burn. They are particularly dangerous to the lungs and may cause a severe, although temporary, illness. Long-term exposure, as in firefighters, may increase the risk of chronic illness, although this is difficult to measure.

plant bales. Those who work with cotton and other fibers during the cleaning processes that precede spinning—blowing, mixing, and carding (straightening)—are at greatest risk.

Diagnosis

The disease may develop soon after first exposure or after years of working in the industry. You may feel a tightness in your chest toward the end of the day on Monday, the first day after the weekend. At first, the symptoms do not appear during the rest of the week, but in 10 to 25 percent of affected persons the chest tightness gradually begins to persist for several days and eventually throughout the week and into weekend and vacation periods.

How Serious Is Byssinosis?

Byssinosis generally is not serious. If the disease persists or gets worse, however, it can lead to chronic illness such as emphysema and chronic bronchitis. Thus, you probably should stop working in the industry. When exposure to the fibers stops, the illness will clear up.

Treatment

Bronchodilators and antihistamines help clear up the symptoms.

Industrial Bronchitis

Signs and Symptoms

- Shortness of breath
- Chronic cough that produces sputum

Cause

Bronchitis in coal miners and workers exposed to cotton, flax, or hemp dust is called industrial bronchitis. Fumes from ammonia, strong acids, certain organic solvents, chlorine, hydrogen sulfide, sulfur dioxide, and bromine also may cause bronchitis. It remains unclear whether the bronchitis in these workers is caused by the dusts to which they are exposed or whether the exposure aggravates bronchitis from other causes, such as smoking.

Treatment

Industrial bronchitis is an acute disease. It clears up with rest, plenty of liquids, and elimination of exposure to the irritant. Sometimes use of a humidifier or vaporizer also helps.

Farmer's Lung

Signs and Symptoms

- Fever
- Chills
- Cough that produces sputum
- Worsening shortness of breath on exertion
- Fatigue
- Nausea and vomiting
- Loss of appetite and weight

Cause

Farmer's lung is a type of lung disease that results from repeated inhalation of dust from moldy hay containing the spores of a fungus. Only a small percentage of people exposed to the spores actually develop the disease, and then only after considerable exposure. Asthma does not predispose you to being susceptible. In fact, people with asthma or hay fever are unable to tolerate exposure to the quantity of dust required to cause farmer's lung.

Diagnosis

Your physician will review your medical history and may perform a physical examination, chest X-ray, and pulmonary function tests to confirm the diagnosis. Blood tests for antibodies associated with the disease are strongly suggestive but not diagnostic.

How Serious Is Farmer's Lung?

In acute cases, if you avoid exposure to moldy hay, your symptoms will usually decrease in severity within hours, although it may take weeks before you recover completely. The disease can be chronic, particularly if you are continuously exposed to low levels of the fungus over long periods.

Treatment

If you avoid exposure to the fungus, the acute disease does not develop. If you cannot avoid moldy hay, your physician can recommend a special type of protective dust mask. Also, it may be possible to prevent the growth of the fungus by using chemicals. In severe cases, corticosteroids may be prescribed.

Silo-Filler's Disease

Signs and Symptoms

- Runny nose
- Cough
- Breathlessness

Cause

Silo-filler's disease is an acute illness that results from inhalation of fumes given off by moist silage. The gas given off is nitrogen dioxide. When inhaled, it is irritating to the bronchi and lungs.

How Serious Is Silo-Filler's Disease?

The severity of the illness depends on the length of time the farmer is in the silo. Farmers sometimes die in silos filled with the yellowish gas and acrid odor of oxides and nitrogen. With less exposure, there may be only irritation of the respiratory tract. However, see your physician soon. Often, irritation of the lungs leads to pulmonary edema (a collection of fluid in the lungs), which can be serious and result in permanent damage to the lungs. There may be an associated bronchiolitis (inflammation of the tiny airways near the alveoli), which also may cause permanent damage to your lungs.

Treatment

Many physicians give corticosteroids to try to avoid permanent damage to the lungs.

Your Lungs and Cardiovascular System

The workings of your heart and lungs are interrelated. Blood travels through your lungs to be oxygenated each time it passes through your heart. Thus, if a blood clot forms in your veins and then travels through your bloodstream, the clot eventually may block an artery in your lungs, resulting in pulmonary embolism or death of tissue (infarction). Chronic lung disease can lead to heart failure (cor pulmonale).

Pulmonary Embolism

Signs and Symptoms

- Sudden shortness of breath
- Chest pain
- Anxiety
- Cough that produces blood-streaked sputum
- Excessive perspiration

Emergency Symptom—Sudden loss of consciousness

An embolus is a clot of foreign material—usually a blood clot but sometimes a globule of fat, an air bubble, tissue from a tumor, or a clump of bacteria—that is carried into and blocks an artery.

Cause

Most emboli come from blood clots (called thrombi) in the veins of the lower extremities or pelvis. They are carried by the bloodstream through the right side of the heart to the lungs. They also may arise from the walls of the heart. If a clot arises in the left side of the heart, the embolus will not go to the lungs but instead to the brain or some other part of the body. Tissue death (infarction) occurs when the blood supply to the tissue is blocked.

An embolism (sudden blockage caused by an embolus) can occur in any small artery, but the lungs are particularly vulnerable because all of the blood in your body passes through your lungs every time it circulates.

Diagnosis

The symptoms depend on the size of the embolus and how healthy your cardiopulmonary system is. Pulmonary thromboembolism may be difficult to diagnose, particularly if you have underlying cardiopulmonary disease. Your physician may order a chest X-ray, lung scan, or pulmonary angiogram (dye is injected into a vein of the arm or leg and then flows into the arteries of the lung so that they are highlighted on the X-ray).

Pulmonary angiography is the most accurate test for detecting emboli in the lung. However, it requires a high degree of experience to perform and interpret correctly. Your physician may recommend other tests as well.

How Serious Is Pulmonary Embolism?

Pulmonary embolism can be very serious; about 10 percent of affected persons die within the first hour. However, if you survive the initial attack and have appropriate diagnosis and treatment, the outlook is good. You should return to normal in a few weeks unless other serious disease is present.

Pulmonary embolism affects as many as 500,000 persons in the United States yearly and may cause as many as 50,000 deaths each year. In persons younger than 45, it occurs more often in women than in men. After that age it occurs equally in both sexes.

Surgery, prolonged bed rest, or inactivity (such as prolonged sitting when on an airplane trip), stroke, heart attack, obesity, and hip or leg fracture increase your risk of having a pulmonary embolism. Also, anything that increases the tendency of your blood to clot may make you more susceptible.

Treatment

Medication

Your physician may prescribe anticoagulant therapy to prevent further blood clots from forming or clots already present from enlarging. Heparin usually is the drug that is given, often in conjunction with warfarin (Coumadin). Other medications may be given to dissolve existing clots. All of these medications have side effects. Their use must be closely monitored.

Surgery

Surgery is rarely necessary, but it may be helpful in persons with recurring emboli for whom other treatments have not been effective or persons with a sudden, massive embolus.

Prevention

After an operation, you will be encouraged to get up and move around as soon as possible or to perform active and passive leg exercises. When on a trip, walk periodically or at least wiggle your toes and move your feet while sitting. If you are immobilized, keep your legs elevated and perhaps wear support stockings. All of these can help prevent pooling and clotting of blood in your legs, a frequent cause of emboli.

In some cases, if you are at risk for recurrent pulmonary embolism, you may be helped by taking low doses of heparin, warfarin, or antiplatelet drugs such as aspirin.

Cor Pulmonale

Signs and Symptoms
- Chronic cough that produces sputum
- Shortness of breath with exercise
- Wheezing
- Weakness and easy tiring
- Bulging of the veins in the neck
- Swelling of the lower extremities
- Enlargement of and tenderness in the liver

Cause

Cor pulmonale is enlargement and eventual failure of the right ventricle (the lower right chamber) of the heart due to pulmonary disease. Because the heart and lungs are closely associated in function and physical location, diseases of the lungs often affect the heart as well.

Blood goes from the right side of the heart into the lungs, where carbon dioxide is removed from and oxygen is added to the blood. Normally, it does not take a great deal of pressure to push the blood into the lungs, so the muscular walls of the right ventricle are not as strong as those on the left side, which pumps blood out to the rest of the body. However, when the lungs are impaired by emphysema, fibrosis, or other severe chronic lung disease, it takes more effort to pump blood into them. Although the heart is able to compensate for a while, eventually it fails, making this a very serious disease.

Diagnosis

To diagnose cor pulmonale, your physician will probably do a physical examination and take your medical history, perform a pulmonary function test, take a chest X-ray, and record an electrocardiogram.

How Serious Is Cor Pulmonale?

Life expectancy for people with cor pulmonale is generally the same as it is for people who have only the underlying pulmonary disease. Once symptoms appear, on average the survival is 2 to 5 years. If the underlying cause is uncomplicated emphysema, survival may be considerably longer.

Treatment

Your physician may arrange specific treatment for the underlying respiratory disease. In addition, he or she may advise the use of oxygen, restriction of salt and fluid intake, and diuretics.

Lung and Heart Transplantation

Lung transplantations were first performed in the early 1960s; however, after 10 years of poor results, lung transplantation was abandoned. Then, in the late 1970s, a new immunosuppressant drug called cyclosporine was introduced. This revived the possibility of successfully performing lung transplantation. Studies in animals, however, found that the supply of blood to the new lungs was insufficient and that the transplants did not heal adequately.

In the 1980s, a solution was found—transplant the lungs and heart together. In 1981, the first successful heart-lung transplantation was performed. Transplanting both organs together helps ensure that the new lungs and trachea receive enough blood to be able to heal.

The list of problems and limitations is long. Finding donor lungs and hearts can be very difficult because the lungs of brain-dead accident victims often are damaged. To be usable, lungs must match the recipient's body size, blood type, and tissue. Recently, by using new immunosuppressant drugs and new procedures, many double-lung and single-lung transplantations have been successfully performed, opening up the possibility that a donated heart and lungs can help save the lives of up to three people instead of only one. If a lung transplant recipient's heart is healthy, it often can be donated to someone in need, in a double transplantation.

Lung transplantation is a risky, expensive, and very complicated procedure that is performed only on patients whose only hope for survival is transplantation and who have a high probability of success.

Most recipients of successful lung transplants recover to carry on relatively normal lives in the short term. The long-term outcome is not yet known.

Chapter 25

Your Digestive System

Contents

Your Digestive System at Work, 739
Esophagus, 739
Stomach, 739
Small Intestine, 740
Large Intestine, 740
Liver, 741
Gallbladder, 741
Pancreas, 741

Esophageal Problems, 741
Heartburn (Esophageal Reflux), 742
Hiatal Hernia, 743
Other Causes of Esophageal Inflammation, 744
Hiccups, 745
Swallowing Problems, 745
Esophageal Motility Studies, 746
Gastrostomy, 747
Esophageal Stricture, 748
Foreign Bodies, 749
Esophageal Tumors, 750
Esophageal Varices, 750
Esophageal Rupture, 751

Stomach Problems, 751
Indigestion, 752
Peptic Ulcer, 753
Ulcers: Are Antibiotics an Answer? 754
Zollinger-Ellison Syndrome, 757
Gastritis, 758
Drug-Induced Stomach Problems, 758
Gastrointestinal Tract Bleeding, 759
Upper Gastrointestinal Endoscopy, 760
Stomach Tumors, 761
The Barium X-Ray, 762
Stomach Dilation, 764
Ménétrier's Disease, 764
Eosinophilic Gastroenteritis, 764

Disorders of the Small and Large Intestines, 765
Infections of the Gastrointestinal Tract, 766

Antibiotic-Associated Diarrhea, 769
Food Poisoning, 769
Malabsorption Problems, 770
Diabetic Intestinal Disorders, 772
Acute Appendicitis, 772
Meckel's Diverticulum, 773
Intussusception, 773
Protein-Losing Enteropathy, 774
Primary (Idiopathic) Intestinal Pseudo-Obstruction, 774
Carcinoid Syndrome, 774
Crohn's Disease, 774
Ulcerative Colitis, 777
Colostomy and Ileostomy, 777
Tumors of the Small Intestine, 779
Ileo-Anal Anastomosis, 780
Diverticulosis and Diverticulitis, 781
Irritable Bowel Syndrome, 782
Fiber in Your Diet, 783
Fiber Supplements, 784
Chronic Constipation, 784
Laxative Abuse, 785
Intestinal Gas, 785
Fecal Impaction, 786
Colon Polyps, 786
Colonoscopy, 788
Colon Cancer, 789
Screening for Colon Cancer, 790
Megacolon, 791
Peritonitis, 792
Familial Mediterranean Fever, 793
Intestinal Obstruction, 793
Vascular Problems of the Bowel, 794

Anorectal Disorders, 795
Hemorrhoids, 795
Anal Itch, 796
Anal Fissures and Fistulas, 796
Rectal Bleeding, 797
Anorectal Abscess, 798
Anal Pain, 798
Proctitis, 798

Fecal Incontinence, 799
  Sexually Transmitted Infections of the
  Rectum, 799

Liver Disease, 800
Acute Viral Hepatitis, 801
  Hepatitis Vaccine, 802
Alcoholic, Toxic, and Drug-Related Hepatitis, 803
Chronic Hepatitis, 804
Cirrhosis, 804
  Liver Biopsy, 807
Liver Tumors, 808
Enlarged Liver, 809
Liver Abscess, 810
  Liver Transplantation, 811
Genetic Liver Problems, 811

Gallbladder and Bile Duct Disorders, 812
Gallstones, 812

Bile Duct Obstruction, 814
  Percutaneous Transhepatic Cholangiography
  (PTHC), 815
  Endoscopic Retrograde
  Cholangiopancreatography (ERCP), 816
  Laparoscopic Surgery, 817
Choledochal Cysts, 817

Pancreatic Diseases, 818
Acute Pancreatitis, 818
Chronic Pancreatitis, 819
Malignant Pancreatic Tumors, 820
Congenital Pancreatic Abnormalities, 822

Hernias, 822
Inguinal Hernia, 822
Other Abdominal Hernias, 823
  Hernia Surgery, 823

Your Digestive System at Work

Your digestive system consists of many parts. Among them are the esophagus, stomach, and the small and large intestines, tubular structures through which food and waste products pass and in which digestion takes place. Two large glands, the liver and the pancreas, furnish some of the enzymes and other substances needed for digestion. Your gallbladder, a hollow organ located just under your liver, stores bile manufactured by your liver.

The food you eat is propelled through your digestive tract by muscular contractions that for the most part are automatic (involuntary). The process of digestion changes the components of food into a form that eventually can be absorbed into your bloodstream. After the nutrients are absorbed, your digestive tract eliminates unwanted material.

Digestion begins when you chew your food. The food is broken into smaller pieces by your teeth and, at the same time, is mixed with saliva secreted by your salivary glands. Your saliva contains an enzyme, called ptyalin, that begins to change starches (carbohydrates) into sugars. Chewing reduces the food to a mushy consistency. When you swallow, the food is propelled into the back part of your throat, past the opening of the voice box (larynx), and into the upper part of your esophagus. Food is prevented from entering your larynx by a flap of soft tissue (epiglottis) that closes as food passes into the esophagus. When the epiglottis fails to close completely, a minor coughing fit may result. Such an episode is said to be the result of the food "having gone down the wrong way."

Esophagus

Once you swallow food, it moves down into the esophagus, a tube approximately 10 inches long that leads directly into the stomach. The food is moved into your esophagus by muscles in the back of your throat (pharynx). When it enters the main part of the esophagus, muscles there undergo a series of wave-like contractions, called peristalsis, to move the food into your stomach. Peristalsis is the mechanism by which the food is moved throughout the remainder of its trip

through your digestive tract until the waste products reach the muscles of the anus.

A muscle that encircles the bottom portion of the esophagus (lower esophageal sphincter) is critical in the passage of food into your stomach. When this valve-like sphincter relaxes, it opens and permits food to enter your stomach. It then closes, which prevents any food from flowing back (regurgitating) into your esophagus. When this sphincter muscle fails to work properly, stomach contents regurgitate into the esophagus. Called esophageal reflux, this partial regurgitation may be damaging to the sensitive lining of your esophagus by allowing stomach acid to come into contact with it. If this occurs, you may experience the symptoms of heartburn and have a condition called esophagitis (see Heartburn, page 742, and Other Causes of Esophageal Inflammation, page 744).

Stomach

The walls of your stomach consist of various layers of powerful muscles. These muscles serve an important mechanical function as they cause the stomach to churn, breaking the food into smaller and smaller pieces. In addition, gastric juices manufactured by the glands that line your stomach mix with the food particles. These juices contain pepsin, a digestive enzyme that begins to break down proteins in the mixture, and hydrochloric acid, which creates the proper environment for pepsin to work.

Although it serves a useful function, your stomach is not vital to the breakdown of food and its subsequent absorption. Only small amounts of such food as alcohol, simple sugars, and some medications are actually absorbed in the stomach.

There is a delicate balance in your stomach between the acid produced by its glands and the resistance of your stomach lining to that acid. If this balance is upset, the result may be damage to the stomach lining, such as a peptic ulcer (see page 753) or gastritis (see page 758).

Food leaves your stomach in two phases. The upper portion of your stomach contracts first, pushing the more liquid material into your small intestine. The more solid food

Gastrointestinal Tract

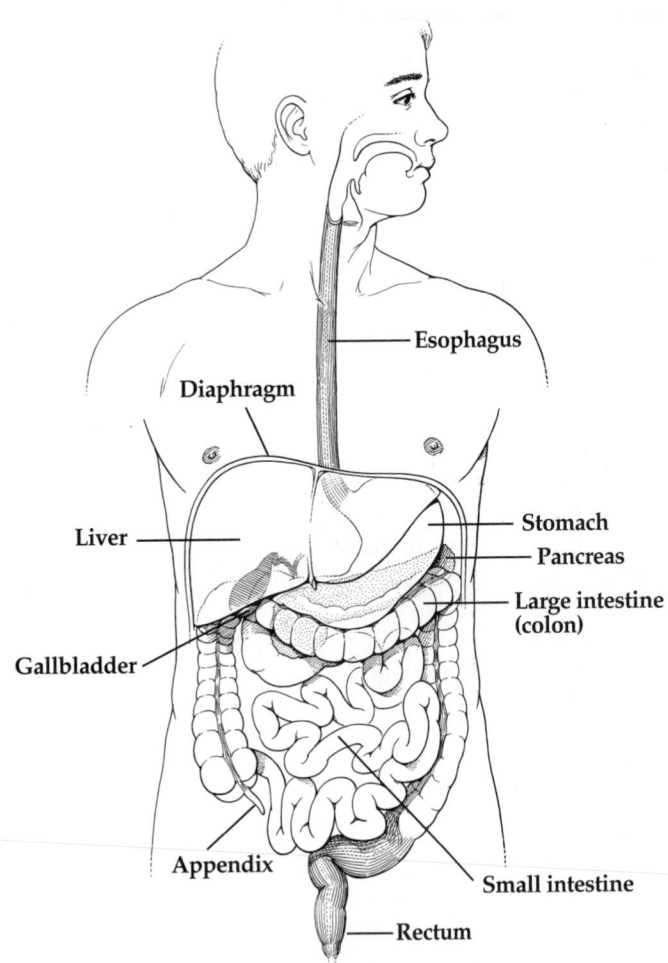

Esophagus

Diaphragm

Liver

Gallbladder

Stomach

Pancreas

Large intestine
(colon)

Appendix

Small intestine

Rectum

of absorption takes place. The final section of the small bowel, the ileum, has some absorptive function (for vitamin B$_{12}$, for example) in addition to being responsible for the passage of food into the large intestine.

The duodenum contributes to the mixing of food material and also neutralizes acid coming from your stomach. Bile ducts from the liver and gallbladder and the pancreatic duct from the pancreas empty their digestive juices into the duodenum to aid in preparing the chyme for maximum absorption.

As the semisolid food continues its movement downward through your small intestine, it undergoes further digestion by various enzymes. In this process, the food is broken into smaller particles that then can be readily absorbed through the lining of the small intestine into your bloodstream. The starches (carbohydrates) are broken down into simpler sugars, and proteins are broken down into amino acids. Fats are broken down by enzymes from the pancreas. Because of their detergent-like properties, bile acids from the liver render the fat molecules soluble in water so that they can then be absorbed into your bloodstream. In addition, minerals, vitamins, water, and electrolytes (such as sodium and calcium) are absorbed through the wall of the small intestine into your bloodstream.

By the time the food is ready to pass into your large intestine, almost all its nutrients have been absorbed.

Large Intestine

At this point, the role of your digestive system changes. Now its job is to remove the waste, consisting mainly of undigested and nonabsorbed food, fiber, and water.

The liquid (primarily water) from the small intestine is carried into the large intestine (colon) where most of it is reabsorbed. Your colon is extremely efficient in this process—of the 10 quarts of fluid that enter it every day, approximately 9.9 quarts are reabsorbed before reaching the anus.

The rest of the waste material moves through the three major segments of your colon—right, transverse, and left descending colon—then into the S-shaped sigmoid colon in the left lower abdomen, and finally into the rectum, the last 4 to 6 inches of the colon. It is here that the material collects until defecation.

leaves later, primarily by the action of the muscles in the lower part of your stomach. The partially processed food (called chyme) then travels through the pyloric canal into the first portion of your small intestine, the duodenum.

Small Intestine

The small intestine (or small bowel) is an elongated tube whose length in adults varies from 12 to 22 feet, depending both on the tone of its muscular wall and on the way it is measured.

The small intestine is divided into three parts. The duodenum is the smallest part, and it is here that the absorption process truly begins. The jejunum, the largest portion of the small bowel, is where the majority

Liver

Your liver produces bile, a fluid containing cholesterol and bile acids. Bile flows from the liver through the cystic duct to your gallbladder, where it is stored. It is eventually emptied into the duodenum, where it performs its major function of assisting in the absorption of fats through the lining of the small bowel into the bloodstream. The bile acids are then reabsorbed in the small intestine and cycled into the liver to be used again.

The liver has other functions also. One is the storage of glycogen, a complex carbohydrate that is converted to sugar for release into your bloodstream when your blood sugar level falls. Glycogen is deposited in the liver when the level of sugar in the blood increases. Many proteins also are synthesized in the liver.

The liver helps determine the amount of nutrients that are sent to the rest of your body. It also serves as a clearinghouse to eliminate some foods and substances that have served their purpose but are no longer useful. In addition, your liver breaks down some medications to enable them to be eliminated in the stool. Alcohol also is metabolized in the liver to supply energy or to be deposited as fat.

Gallbladder

The gallbladder is a pear-shaped organ that sits beneath the liver. It is a storage site for much of the bile that is produced in the liver. The bile passes into the gallbladder through a duct (cystic duct) and is stored until it is needed for the digestion of fats that have passed into the small intestine. It is discharged through the cystic duct into the lower portion of the bile duct and then into the duodenum.

Usually, the amounts of bile acids and cholesterol are balanced, but sometimes the concentration of cholesterol becomes too high. The result may be the formation of gallstones.

The gallbladder serves a useful function but is not vital to maintaining your normal body functions because bile can be delivered directly from the liver into the duodenum.

Pancreas

Shaped somewhat like a banana, the pancreas stretches from your duodenum, to which its head is attached, to the spleen. This vital organ produces two kinds of secretions. One is pancreatic juice, which passes through the ducts of the pancreas into the duodenum, where it aids in the digestion of fats and proteins. The other kind includes the hormones insulin and glucagon, which pass directly into your bloodstream and help regulate the metabolism of glucose and protein in the liver and other tissues.

Given the numerous parts and the complexity of the gastrointestinal tract, it is hardly surprising that many types of disorders and diseases can occur. In discussing the normal functions and dysfunctions of the stomach, intestines, and the rest of the system, this chapter will follow the same path as the food you eat. First, we will explore problems associated with the esophagus and stomach. We will then proceed to problems of the intestines and then to anorectal diseases. Finally, we will discuss diseases of the liver, gallbladder, and pancreas.

Esophageal Problems

When you swallow food, muscles at the back of your mouth (soft palate) form the food into a soft mass called a bolus. The epiglottis, a leaf-shaped structure at the root of your tongue, folds over the top of the windpipe to protect your trachea and airway. The food is propelled from the back of your mouth into your esophagus.

Your esophagus is a muscular tube, approximately 10 inches long, that leads directly into your stomach. The food automatically travels through the esophagus as a result of wave-like muscular contractions called peristalsis.

At the lower end of the esophagus is an area of specialized muscle called the lower esophageal sphincter. This opens to allow the food to pass into the stomach. The lower esophageal sphincter then closes to prevent return (reflux) of food and stomach juices (including acids) from the stomach back into the esophagus.

This section will discuss problems of the esophagus. The most common problem is heartburn, which, incidentally, has nothing to do with the heart but is the result of stomach acid returning (refluxing) back to the esophagus.

Other problems covered in this section include inflammation of the esophagus, swallowing problems, constriction of the esophagus, tumors, and rupture.

Heartburn (Esophageal Reflux)

Signs and Symptoms
- A burning sensation in the chest that may start in the upper abdomen and radiate into the neck
- Regurgitation of sour or bitter-tasting material into the throat and mouth, especially when lying down or sleeping

Heartburn (esophageal reflux) is a frequent discomfort. About 1 in 10 adults has heartburn at least once a week; 1 in 3 has the problem at least once a month. Moreover, because of hormonal changes and increased pressure within the abdomen, one in four pregnant women experiences heartburn daily.

Most infants are born with an incompetent lower esophageal sphincter. This allows stomach contents to back up (reflux) into the esophagus. By age 12 months, the lower esophageal sphincter has matured in most infants and reflux becomes a less common occurrence.

Heartburn occurs when acid-containing stomach contents are allowed to regurgitate back into the esophagus. Under normal circumstances, food passes into the stomach from the esophagus and is prevented from traveling back up the esophagus by the lower esophageal sphincter, which remains tightly closed except when you swallow food. Sometimes, however, the sphincter muscle becomes lazy and relaxes (opens), allowing acidic stomach contents to move back up the esophagus, producing the symptoms of heartburn.

Diagnosis
Usually a description of your symptoms will be all your physician needs to establish the diagnosis of heartburn.

However, if your symptoms are particularly severe or do not respond to treatment, tests such as a barium X-ray of the esophagus and stomach (see The Barium X-Ray, page 762) or an endoscopic examination (see Upper Gastrointestinal Endoscopy, page 760) may be necessary. In an infant with severe reflux, a barium X-ray of the esophagus may be done.

A hiatal hernia (a protrusion of part of the stomach through the diaphragm) often is found on barium X-ray in people with heartburn, but many hiatal hernias cause no symptoms and require no treatment (see Hiatal Hernia, page 743).

How Serious Is Heartburn?
Occasional heartburn can be uncomfortable but is not a serious problem. However, if your heartburn occurs frequently, there is a chance of esophagitis, an irritation (inflammation) of the esophageal lining caused by stomach acid. If the esophagitis becomes severe, the result can be bleeding and difficulty in swallowing because of a constriction (stricture) of the esophagus. Some people with severe esophagitis develop Barrett's esophagus (see Other Causes of Esophageal Inflammation, page 744).

In infants with heartburn, complications are rare. These complications include pneumonia (due to the aspiration of stomach contents into the lungs), delayed growth and weight gain, and iron-deficiency anemia (see page 957).

Treatment
There are several lifestyle changes that can help prevent or relieve heartburn.

If you are a smoker, stop smoking. Cigarettes relax the lower esophageal sphincter and predispose you to heartburn.

Eat three balanced meals a day but cut down on the size of the portions. Do not eat anything in the 2 to 3 hours before you go to bed. Retiring on an empty stomach decreases the amount of acid your stomach produces and lessens the chance for nocturnal reflux.

If you are overweight, lose weight. A leaner abdomen decreases the pressure on your stomach, which in turn may lessen reflux.

Hiatal Hernia

Your chest is separated from your abdomen by a domed sheet of muscle called the diaphragm. To reach your stomach, your esophagus has to pass through an opening (the hiatus) in the diaphragm.

When the tissue around the hiatus weakens, part of the stomach may protrude through the opening into the chest cavity. This is termed hiatal hernia. Hiatal hernia is believed to be caused by a weakening of the anchoring tissues of the gastroesophageal junction to the diaphragm, perhaps due to increased pressure within the abdomen such as sometimes results from obesity or, rarely, trauma.

Hiatal hernias are common. About 25 percent of all persons older than 50 have a hiatal hernia. Because the majority of such hernias produce no symptoms, they usually go undetected. They are frequently found in patients with heartburn who undergo barium X-ray studies, and are then an incidental finding. It is unlikely that a small hiatal hernia will cause you any problems and, by itself, is not a dangerous ailment.

However, hiatal hernias are found more commonly in persons with heartburn than individuals who do not have this symptom. Malfunction of the lower esophageal sphincter is the most important factor in allowing heartburn to occur, but the presence of a hiatal hernia is a contributing factor also.

Large hernias (a substantial part of the stomach is above the diaphragm) can cause slow bleeding and iron-deficiency anemia (see page 957).

One potential danger of a very large hernia, when almost all of the stomach protrudes through the diaphragm into the chest cavity, is strangulation. The herniated stomach can become so tightly constricted that its blood supply is severely compromised. If this occurs, you will feel persistent chest pain and have difficulty swallowing. This is a medical emergency and may require prompt surgery. Strangulation of the stomach in large hernias is uncommon, but surgical repair may be advisable to avoid emergency operations in more risky circumstances.

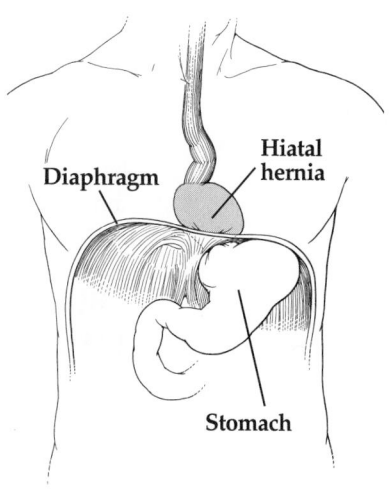

In hiatal hernia, a portion of the stomach protrudes through the diaphragm into the chest cavity.

Elevate the head of your bed at least 6 inches by using blocks or a foam wedge. This assists gravity in keeping your stomach acid where it belongs.

Avoid tight clothing and tight belts.

Decrease the amount of alcohol, chocolate, fats, and peppermints you consume. These substances relax the lower esophageal sphincter.

Be aware that medications such as birth control pills, antihistamines, antispasmodics, some heart medications, and asthma medicines may aggravate heartburn because they decrease the strength of the lower esophageal sphincter.

For many who experience heartburn occasionally, the use of liquid antacids whenever heartburn occurs, especially after meals and at bedtime, gives significant relief.

If your infant has a mild case of heartburn, the condition may improve by keeping the child on his or her stomach with the head and shoulders elevated. It also helps to reduce the volume in each feeding. Try feeding your baby more often and thicken the feedings with cereal. In more severe cases, the baby's head should be kept elevated at all times.

For more significant heartburn in adults, drugs such as cimetidine, ranitidine, famotidine, or nizatidine, which block acid production in the stomach, may be necessary. Another strategy your physician may try is to increase the strength of the esophageal sphincter with a drug such as cisapride. However, no prescription drug should be used until the other methods have been given a chance.

Omeprazole is a newer medication with a different mechanism of action from the other drugs. It is a more powerful inhibitor of acid production and relieves heartburn more effectively. However, its long-term safety is not proved, and it is only approved for short-term use in the United States (many European countries, however, have approved it for longer-term use). Also, when use of any of these medications is stopped, heartburn usually returns.

Surgery

Few adults who have heartburn require surgery. Only about 5 percent continue to have severe symptoms or have complications despite medication and lifestyle changes. In these cases, surgery is a viable alternative. The procedure, called fundoplication, involves creating a high-pressure zone in the lower esophagus which prevents reflux. This is sometimes done by laparoscopy, a minimally invasive procedure (see page 817).

When an infant fails to respond after 6 weeks of intensive medical treatment and has complications of reflux, surgery may be indicated. Consult your infant's physician.

Other Causes of Esophageal Inflammation

In addition to heartburn from a weakened lower esophageal sphincter, many other disorders can result in inflammation of your esophagus.

Barrett's Esophagus

Persistent reflux of acid from the stomach may damage the normal skin-like lining of the esophagus, which is then replaced by a lining that resembles the lining of the stomach. This new lining usually can resist the gastric reflux, but inflammation at the upper end of the new lining may narrow (stricture) the interior passageway of the esophagus.

Ulcers may occur in the stomach-like lining, and these can bleed and perforate the esophageal wall. In addition, there is a slightly increased risk of cancer occurring in Barrett's esophagus. Your physician may want to evaluate the lining of your esophagus periodically by upper gastrointestinal endoscopy (see page 760) and biopsy to increase the chance of detecting and treating abnormal cells at an early stage.

Scleroderma of the Esophagus

Scleroderma is a disease characterized by an overgrowth of scar-like tissue; the result is a stiffening and hardening of tissues. The esophagus is commonly affected. (Besides the gastrointestinal tract, scleroderma can affect organs such as the lungs, heart, and kidneys, as well as the skin; see Scleroderma, page 919.)

Scleroderma can weaken the lower esophageal sphincter, allowing acid to reflux into the esophagus and cause the symptoms and complications associated with reflux (see Heartburn, page 742). At times, a stricture (narrowing) develops in the esophagus, making swallowing more difficult.

Your physician may prescribe an acid-reducing medication such as cimetidine, ranitidine, famotidine, or omeprazole, which may lessen the amount of reflux. He or she will also instruct you in measures to prevent reflux (see page 742). If the narrowness of the esophagus prevents or retards the passage of food, an esophageal dilation may be performed (see page 748).

Herpes Simplex Esophagitis

Infection by herpes simplex virus can cause inflammation and ulcers in the esophagus. People who have such a viral esophagitis are usually debilitated from another disease or, for other reasons, their immune system is exceptionally depressed. Herpes blisters coupled with other symptoms of an esophageal infection strongly suggest a viral esophagitis.

Antibiotics are not effective in treating viral esophagitis, but the antiviral drug acyclovir may be helpful in herpes simplex esophagitis.

Candida Esophagitis

A fungus, *Candida* or *Monilia*, growing in the esophagus can produce an inflammation of the esophagus with associated pain on swallowing. This is called *Candida* esophagitis. This type of infection often occurs in people whose immune systems are depressed, for example as a result of drugs used to fight cancer. There are several antifungal medications that can be used in treatment.

Radiation Esophagitis

This inflammation of the esophagus occurs commonly as a result of radiation treatment for lung (see page 727) or esophageal cancer (see Esophageal Tumors, page 750). The symptoms are heartburn and pain on swallowing. The likelihood of this disorder increases in direct relation to the amount of radiation you receive. With the help of medication, the inflammation usually resolves once the radiation treatment is stopped.

Hiccups

Holding your breath . . . swallowing water from the "wrong" side of the glass . . . breathing in and out of a paper bag . . . inhaling pepper or ammonia . . . eating a spoonful of sugar . . . having someone startle you.

These all are common—and not consistently successful—methods of getting rid of the hiccups, a generally minor complaint that has afflicted almost everyone at one time or another.

For the most part, hiccups are a harmless, minor annoyance. Sometimes, however, hiccups persist for days or even weeks. When this occurs, they can interfere with eating and sleeping. After major surgery,

a prolonged case of the hiccups can impede the healing of an abdominal wound. In rare instances, persistent attacks can be a symptom of a serious disorder.

Although almost everyone has had hiccups, few people know exactly what they are. Very simply, hiccups are repeated, involuntary contractions of your diaphragm. The abrupt closure of your voice box checks the inflow of air: the result is a hiccup.

The phrenic nerves control the smooth, coordinated, normal contraction of the two leaves of the diaphragm, the membrane that separates the chest from the abdomen. The phrenic nerves extend

from the neck to the chest. Hiccups may result from irritation anywhere along the path of a phrenic nerve. Reflex contraction of the diaphragm similarly can be the result of irritation to nerves.

Hiccups are more likely to occur when your stomach is distended, typically after eating a big meal or drinking an overabundance of alcohol.

As for a cure, try this: massage the back portion of the roof of your mouth with a cotton-tipped swab, moving the swab gently back and forth for a minute or so. We cannot guarantee this method, but it does work much of the time.

Pill-Induced Esophagitis

Acute pain in the front of the chest made worse by swallowing is occasionally caused by pills or capsules that stick and dissolve or break open before reaching the stomach. Most likely, the causes of these symptoms are tetracycline antibiotics, potassium and iron medications, and some arthritis drugs. This is preventable by washing down medications with a glass of water and not lying down just after taking medication. If a pill-induced esophageal ulcer does occur, it usually gets better within a few days.

Swallowing Problems

Signs and Symptoms
- Liquids and solid foods stick in the throat or chest
- Regurgitation of food
- Gurgling sound in the throat
- Chest discomfort on swallowing

Emergency Symptoms—Complete blockage—unable to swallow liquids or solids (drooling saliva)

Swallowing problems produce different symptoms for different reasons. Food may get stuck in your throat, or it may take longer than normal to swallow your food. You may

experience what seems to be heartburn, or you may have a severe chest pain.

The causes of persistent swallowing problems vary. Damage or malfunction of the muscles in the wall of the throat or esophagus will cause swallowing difficulties. Ulcers or scar tissue (stricture) in the esophagus as the result of stomach acid reflux (see Heartburn, page 742) may make it difficult and sometimes painful for you to swallow. Pouches, called diverticula, may form in the esophageal lining and interfere with the movement of food down the esophagus.

Swallowing problems are also associated with certain diseases such as myasthenia gravis (see page 479) or esophageal cancer (see Esophageal Tumors, page 750).

Swallowing problems may be transient and unimportant, but it is always possible that such problems could be an indication of a serious medical problem. Therefore, see your physician if you continue to have pain or any difficulty swallowing. Early diagnosis is important.

Some types of swallowing problems are described below.

Achalasia

This is a rare disorder of the esophagus. It is caused by the lack of coordinated movement (peristalsis) of the muscles of the esophagus and by the failure of the sphincter muscle at the lower end of the esophagus to relax. This makes it very difficult for food to pass into the stomach. The underlying reason for the condition is not fully known.

The primary symptom of achalasia is failure of liquids and solid foods to pass through the esophagus. Food is often regurgitated. Sometimes, particularly in the early stages, drinking a large amount of liquid helps to "push" the food into the stomach. Eventually, however, this fails to provide relief (in fact, in some people certain liquids, especially if very hot or very cold, also may seem to stall in the esophagus from the start). Some chest discomfort or pain may also occur.

If you have the symptoms of achalasia, your physician will order a series of tests including a barium X-ray (see page 762) or an esophageal motility study (this page) to determine whether the esophageal muscles are functioning properly. Often, upper gastrointestinal endoscopy (see page 760) is done to be sure there is no cancer present that may be causing the symptoms of achalasia.

If achalasia is left untreated over the course of several decades, esophageal cancer may develop. Malnutrition, weight loss, and aspiration of food into the lungs, which can lead to pneumonia, are other problems associated with achalasia.

Medication may be somewhat helpful in some cases of achalasia, but it often has little effect.

Esophageal Motility Studies

If your swallowing problem is thought to be caused by abnormal contraction of the muscles of your esophagus, your physician will arrange for an examination called an esophageal motility study. This diagnostic test records movement and pressures in your esophagus. After the recording tube is passed through your mouth or nose into your esophagus, continuous recordings of the pressures are made over a period of 10 to 15 minutes. These recordings demonstrate the strength and coordination of the peristaltic waves along your esophagus when you swallow.

These studies can show whether there is excessive pressure in the esophageal sphincter, if it is functioning properly, and if there are poorly coordinated peristaltic waves that can cause high-pressure readings in several areas of the esophagus at the same time. These studies can confirm the presence of achalasia, esophageal spasm, or pharyngeal paralysis (see Swallowing Problems, page 745).

Another treatment for achalasia is mechanical stretching of the muscles. A slender tube with a balloon attached is passed down the esophagus to the narrowed area. Then the balloon is filled with air or water under pressure to expand the balloon and open (dilate) the passageway. To lessen the discomfort when the tube is inserted, you will be sedated with a medication injected into a vein; also, a spray will be applied to your throat and pharynx to anesthetize them. The balloon dilation weakens the lower esophageal sphincter so that food can pass down the esophagus by gravity. After this treatment, coordinated contractions in the esophagus do not return to normal but most people can swallow adequately.

Also, the surgical procedure called esophagomyotomy can be used. In this procedure, the surgeon opens the chest to reach the esophagus. The muscles at the lower end of the esophagus are then partially cut to allow the food easier passage. The risks of this operation are low and long-term results generally are excellent.

Diffuse Spasm

Multiple high-pressure, poorly coordinated contractions of the esophagus are referred to as diffuse spasm. They usually occur after a swallow. This is another rare disorder of the esophagus that affects the smooth (involuntary) muscles in the walls of the lower esophagus. The cause for diffuse spasm is not known.

Initially, the diagnosis may be difficult. The symptoms can be mild and may even disappear without treatment. It is possible that you might mistake its symptoms for simple heartburn. But if the cause of the apparent heartburn is diffuse spasm, the symptoms often continue intermittently over a period of years. They may become more severe with time. The symptoms almost invariably are associated with food and liquids being delayed in the esophagus.

Esophageal dilation (see page 748) may produce relief initially. Surgery occasionally may be necessary.

Pharyngeal Diverticula

When muscles in the wall of the throat (pharynx) weaken, especially with aging, pouches called diverticula are formed. They can become large enough to trap food.

If pouches form, you may regurgitate food particles shortly after eating. Your throat will become irritated, and you may notice a gurgling sound. As the pouches grow larger, the food that is retained for days may give you bad breath.

There is the risk that fluid and undigested food will be regurgitated and passed into the lungs during the night (aspiration), increasing the risk of a lung infection.

Surgery is the treatment for diverticula that are producing uncomfortable symptoms. Pouches (diverticula) can also occur in the esophagus, but they rarely cause any problems in this location.

Pharyngeal Paralysis

The principal symptoms of pharyngeal paralysis are weakness and incoordination of the muscles of the pharynx which cause difficulty in swallowing. Persons with this problem have difficulty in getting food from their mouth into their throat and esophagus. In addition to swallowing difficulty and throat discomfort, this disorder also may result in inhalation of food (aspiration) into your windpipe or regurgitation of food into your nose.

As with so many swallowing disorders, it is believed that the symptoms are the result of a faulty transmission of nerve impulses to the muscles in the pharynx. This occurs in various neuromuscular disorders such as

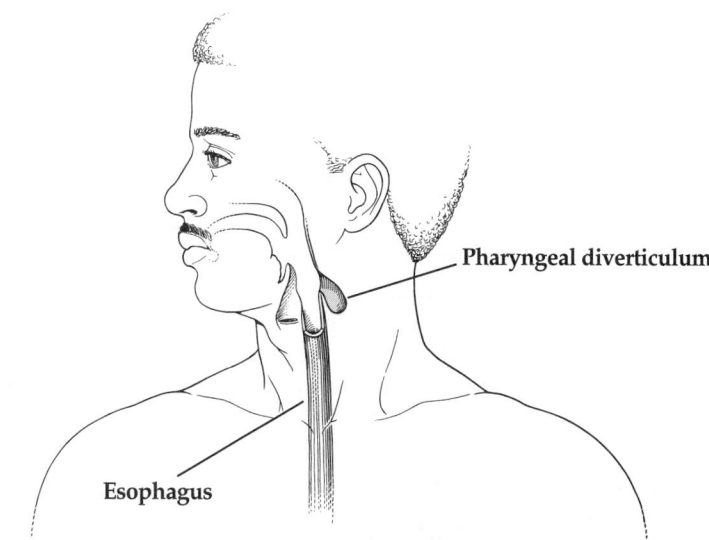

Pharyngeal diverticulum

Esophagus

myasthenia gravis (see page 479) and amyotrophic lateral sclerosis (see page 477) and neurologic conditions such as some types of brain tumor or stroke (see Brain Tumor, page 492, and Stroke, page 461). Food poisoning in the form of botulism may cause the rather abrupt onset of pharyngeal paralysis (see Botulism, page 488).

Tests to establish the diagnosis of pharyngeal paralysis may include a barium X-ray (see page 768) and an esophageal motility study (see page 746). Upper gastrointestinal endoscopy (see page 760) also may be done to eliminate other possible causes.

If the muscular wall of your throat (pharynx) weakens, a small pouch, called a pharyngeal diverticulum, may form and trap food or liquids.

Gastrostomy

Sometimes you are unable to swallow foods properly, such as when the swallowing mechanism of your throat or upper esophagus is disabled. The result is an inability to consume sufficient food for adequate nutrition. If the cause is the result of a neurologic problem (such as stroke) or of surgical removal of the swallowing apparatus because of a cancer of the pharynx or larynx, you will need another way to deliver food into your small bowel.

This can be done by the surgical placement of a tube into the stomach. The tube bypasses the swallowing mechanism of the pharynx and esophagus. Nutrients can be infused directly through this tube into the stomach, from where they pass into the small bowel for diges-

tion and absorption. Sometimes an extension of this tube is placed into the small bowel. With this type of feeding mechanism, adequate calories can be instilled to maintain growth and nutrition.

In recent years, gastrostomy feeding tubes have been placed by using upper gastrointestinal endoscopy (see Upper Gastrointestinal Endoscopy, page 760), eliminating the need for general anesthesia and surgery. At times, these feeding gastrostomy tubes can be placed while you are an outpatient. Your physician or dietitian will instruct you in proper feeding techniques, including the amount of calories to be infused in specially prepared formulas to ensure adequate nutrition.

In some people, the ability to swallow returns and these feeding gastrostomy tubes can be easily removed.

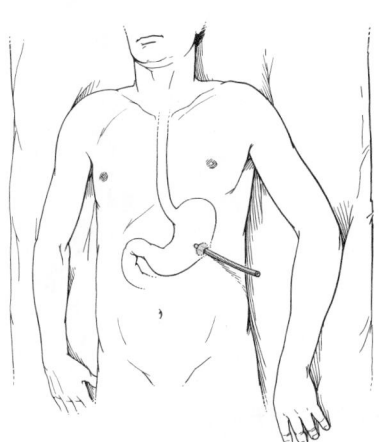

A gastrostomy tube allows you to receive food directly into your stomach.

If the paralysis is due to a disease such as myasthenia gravis, it usually will respond to treatment for the disease. People recovering from a stroke often experience improvement over time.

Many people with pharyngeal paralysis require temporary feeding and therapy through a nasogastric tube (a tube running through the nose to the stomach). Surgery is rarely effective. Sometimes, a tube is placed directly through the abdominal wall into the stomach for feeding (see Gastrostomy, page 747). This bypasses the affected area in the pharynx or esophagus and allows use of the remaining intestine for proper digestion.

Other Disorders

Swallowing difficulties may result from other conditions such as tumor, scar tissue, or congenital disorders. Some people experience the sensation of a lump in their throat without having any actual problem in swallowing their food. This disorder is called globus. At times, this particular swallowing problem may be the result of stress.

If your physician suspects that the problem is globus, as part of the examination he or she may ask you to identify any possible source of stress that could be responsible. In most cases, relief of your emotional distress will eliminate the problem.

Esophageal Stricture

Signs and Symptoms—Difficulty swallowing

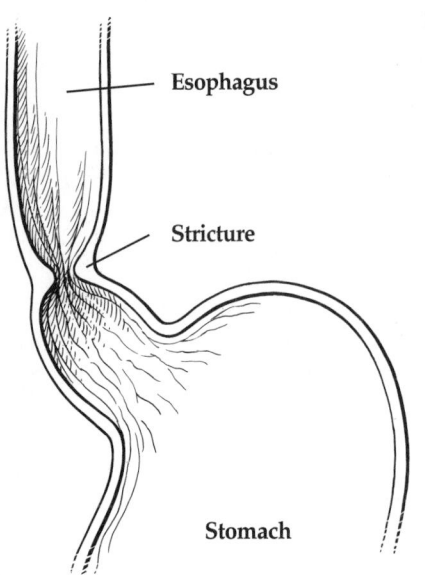

Esophagus

Stricture

Stomach

Narrowing of the passageway of the esophagus is called an esophageal stricture. This can cause difficulty in swallowing.

Esophageal stricture is a narrowing of the passageway of the esophagus so that solid food or even liquids cannot pass through without difficulty. In most adults the principal cause of a stricture is excessive exposure of the esophagus to gastric acid as a result of reflux of stomach contents into the esophagus (see Heartburn [Esophageal Reflux], page 742). Reflux causes scar tissue to form, and this tissue narrows the passageway. Scar tissue also can result from previous esophageal surgery or ingestion of caustic chemicals. The swallowing of caustic chemicals is preventable. Proper identification and storage of caustic materials in the household will help prevent such accidents (see Preventing Poisonings, page 351).

An esophageal web also can narrow the upper end of the esophagus. For unknown reasons, these webs are more likely to appear in middle-aged women and may be associated with iron deficiency. The difficulty in swallowing usually is restricted to solids.

Another esophageal constriction is a mucosal ring. This may occur near the lower esophageal sphincter. Again, this disorder causes occasional difficulty in swallowing solids.

Diagnosis

Your physician may perform a barium X-ray (see page 762) and an endoscopic examination (see Upper Gastrointestinal Endoscopy, page 760) to be sure that an esophageal or stomach cancer is not the cause of your swallowing difficulty.

Treatment

If the stricture is a result of chronic esophagitis or previous ingestion of caustic material, of esophageal webs, or of mucosal rings, the restricted passageway may be opened up with an esophageal dilator. The dilator stretches open the stricture, web, or ring. This is sometimes called esophageal bougienage.

Before this procedure, you will be required to fast for at least 6 to 8 hours. A topical anesthetic will be applied to the lining of your throat. You may also receive a sedative. A thin, flexible instrument called a fiberoptic endoscope is inserted into your esophagus (see Upper Gastrointestinal Endoscopy, page 760).

In one commonly used method, a guidewire is inserted through the endoscope and then the endoscope is withdrawn. Progressively larger dilators are threaded along the length of the wire and through the stricture, to force open the passageway. At times, balloons are attached to the guidewire and are moved to the point of the narrowing. There they are inflated, which may help open the passageway.

An esophageal dilator usually is quite safe, but you may feel a little tightness or discomfort in your chest or some pain when you swallow for a few hours after the procedure. The benefit of dilation is that it permits blocked food and fluids to move freely through the esophagus and into the stomach.

Rarely, a surgical procedure is needed for these disorders.

Foreign Bodies

Signs and Symptoms
- Difficulty in swallowing
- Complete inability to swallow liquids or solids, often accompanied by drooling of saliva

Emergency Symptoms
- Inability to breathe or to utter a sound
- Pale and clammy skin

If you swallow something and it becomes lodged in your throat, your esophagus may be partially or totally obstructed. The likelihood of an obstruction occurring is increased among those who have problems with esophageal strictures (see page 748), tumors (see page 750), or abnormal muscle contraction (peristalsis) of the esophagus.

When the esophagus is narrowed by any of these conditions, the risk of food, especially a large piece of meat or bone, becoming lodged is increased. Others who have problems with foreign body obstructions are elderly denture wearers and those who have difficulty in chewing their food properly. Children are prone to swallowing pins, coins, pieces of their toys, or other objects that can obstruct their esophagus.

Blockage of the throat by a large piece of meat lodged in it may cut off the airway and is a medical emergency. This situation may result in inability to breathe or to utter a sound. You may turn blue and lose consciousness in a minute or two. The Heimlich maneuver may dislodge the offending piece of food (see The Heimlich Maneuver, page 407). This event sometimes is called a café coronary in that it occurs in a restaurant after a person has eaten a large piece of meat (and, often, has consumed alcoholic beverages).

The more common situation occurs when food is stuck farther down your esophagus, at a point where it can block the passage of food into your stomach. If the obstruction is total, you will keep on spitting out saliva. Go to your local emergency room to have the foreign body removed (see Upper Gastrointestinal Endoscopy, page 760).

Whatever its size or shape, a lodged foreign body always is a serious matter. If stuck in the lower pharynx, it can inhibit your ability to breathe. Farther down your esophagus, the object can block the passage of food into your stomach. It also may create swelling at the spot in which it is lodged, which aggravates the obstruction. If an object manages to reach your small intestine before becoming stuck, it can cause an infection, ulceration, or hemorrhage.

Many foreign objects actually may pass into the stomach and through the gastrointestinal tract without delay. However, if the object is sharp-edged, it may scratch or perforate the esophagus, stomach, or intestine on the way through.

Depending on the location and degree of obstruction caused by the lodged object, you may have virtually no symptoms or you may find it almost impossible to swallow. In addition, other symptoms may occur, including sweating, nausea, rapid pulse, and cold, pale, or clammy skin. These symptoms suggest the possibility of perforation or hemorrhage.

Diagnosis
Your physician may perform a barium swallow examination (see The Barium X-Ray, page 762) or an endoscopic examination (see Upper Gastrointestinal Endoscopy, page 760).

Treatment
A foreign object in the esophagus usually is removed with a fiberoptic endoscope. Before the instrument is inserted, you may receive a sedative, and your pharynx will be anesthetized. Through the endoscope your physician can retrieve most objects in the esophagus.

Your physician may elect to push the object into the stomach if he or she thinks that it will pass all the way through the digestive tract. Once the object has been removed from the esophagus and the swelling subsides, your physician will want to inspect your esophagus and to treat any identifiable abnormality that may have contributed to the obstruction.

Esophageal Tumors

Signs and Symptoms

- Progressive difficulty in swallowing
- Weight loss
- Regurgitation
- Vomiting of blood

Most esophageal tumors form in the middle or lower part of the esophagus; nearly 90 percent of esophageal tumors are malignant.

The principal symptom of an esophageal tumor, whether benign or malignant, is progressive difficulty in swallowing. The difficulty will begin with solid foods, but eventually it will be difficult to swallow even liquids. As the condition worsens, you will probably lose weight, your breath may become foul-smelling, and you may begin to regurgitate food.

Malignant tumors are twice as likely to occur in men as in women; heavy smokers and drinkers between the ages of 50 and 60 are at the highest risk.

Because swallowing becomes progressively worse over a period of time, many people delay seeing a physician. Consequently, in many cases by the time help is sought, the cancer has spread beyond the

Barium X-ray reveals narrowing of the esophagus (see arrows) caused by a malignant tumor.

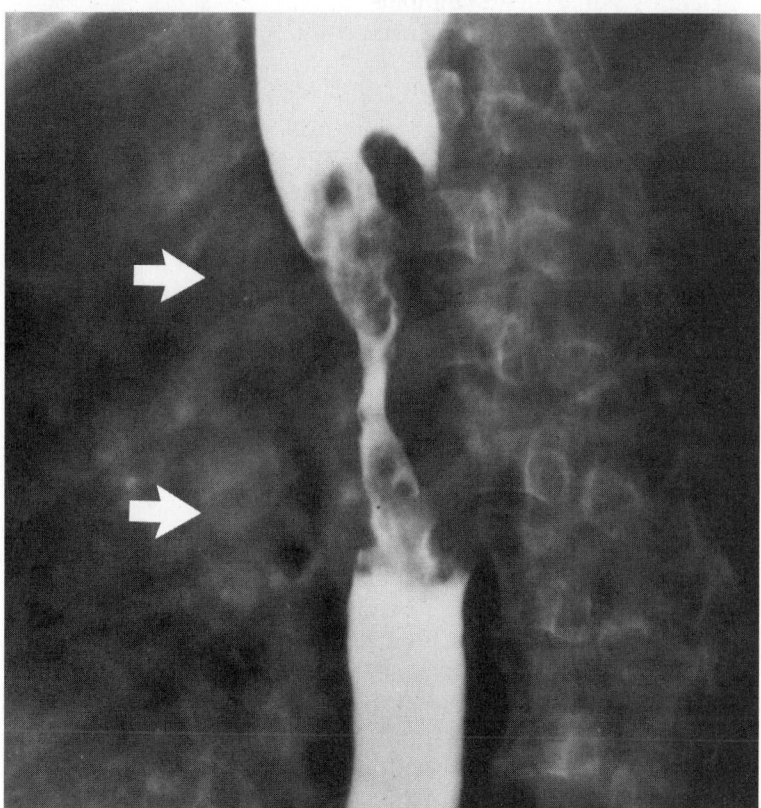

esophagus. Successful treatment depends on early detection.

Diagnosis

Any difficulty swallowing requires immediate attention from your physician. The diagnostic tests may include a barium X-ray (see page 762) and an endoscopic examination (see Upper Gastrointestinal Endoscopy, page 760). In some cases, your physician may take a sample from the esophagus for laboratory analysis (see Biopsies, page 1332). Your physician also may order a CT scan (see page 1334) to determine the extent of the tumor beyond the esophagus.

How Serious Is an Esophageal Tumor?

Most tumors in the esophagus are malignant. Because the disease usually is far along in its development before the diagnosis is made, the survival rate is poor.

Treatment

Surgery

If you have a malignant tumor of your esophagus that has not spread beyond that organ, surgery (at times combined with radiation therapy) or radiation therapy alone may be the initial treatment. However, if surgery is ruled out, there are treatments that can relieve the obstruction caused by the tumor. These include removing part of the obstructing tumor with a laser directed through an endoscope (see Upper Gastrointestinal Endoscopy, page 760), or inserting a prosthesis, a hollow plastic tube, into the esophagus past the cancer. Although these procedures do not cure the tumor, they often temporarily relieve the inability to swallow by increasing the opening through the obstructing cancer. This allows you to eat.

Esophageal Varices

Emergency Signs and Symptoms

- Vomiting of blood
- Faintness, sweating, and pallor (shock)

Esophageal varices are rare. In this condition, blood vessels (veins) become abnormally dilated or enlarged in the wall and lining of the esophagus. The pressure within the expanded blood vessels may cause them to rupture. If they hemorrhage and the bleeding is heavy, you can go into shock.

Varices frequently occur in people who have liver disease (see Cirrhosis, page 804).

How Serious Are Esophageal Varices?
Bleeding from a varix is a life-threatening situation.

Treatment
After an endoscopic examination (see Upper Gastrointestinal Endoscopy, page 760), your treatment will depend in large part on the location of the bleeding and how severe it is. Often, drugs are used initially to control variceal bleeding.

Your physician may choose to place a special tube into the stomach. This tube (often called a Sengstaken-Blakemore or Minnesota tube) has balloons attached at the levels of the esophagus and the stomach. When the tube is in place, one or both balloons may be inflated to compress the varices. This may temporarily stop the bleeding, and then the tube with the attached balloons can be removed.

Through the endoscope, your physician may place small rubber bands over the enlarged veins to stop bleeding. Another procedure is to inject a solution into the vein, which initially obliterates and then inflames and scars the varix. This procedure is called variceal sclerotherapy. These methods often stop the bleeding but may need to be repeated.

Yet another procedure is called transcutaneous intrahepatic porto-systemic shunt (TIPS). A guidewire is passed through the skin into the liver under local anesthesia. A tube passed over the wire is left within the liver to shunt blood away from and thereby decompress the esophageal varices.

If these methods fail, your physician may refer you to a surgeon who may advise an operation to shunt blood away from the ruptured varices (see Cirrhosis, page 804).

Esophageal Rupture

Emergency Signs and Symptoms
- Chest pain
- Rapid and shallow breathing
- Sweating
- Blood in vomitus

The lower esophagus can be torn by an episode of forceful vomiting. This is called esophageal rupture and is a medical emergency.

It is also possible that the lining of the esophagus can be injured during a diagnostic procedure in which an instrument is inserted into the esophagus (see page 748). You might sustain the same sort of injury swallowing a foreign object (see Foreign Bodies, page 749).

An esophageal rupture may produce some blood in your vomitus, and you may think you are having a heart attack because of the pain in your chest. Your physician can diagnose the problem with a chest X-ray, possibly after you swallow contrast material to show the point of the rupture radiographically (see The Barium X-Ray, page 762).

Treatment
An esophageal rupture generally requires surgical treatment. Often, the rupture leaks food into the tissue around the esophagus or into the chest cavity. This area needs to be examined and cleaned out during the operation.

In some situations, the tear is not extensive and the wound will heal without surgery. Antibiotics are given in these situations to prevent bacterial infection. A tube is inserted through your nose into your esophagus or stomach to assist in draining secretions. You will receive nourishment through a vein (intravenous feedings), or a feeding tube placed in your small bowel, until the tear has healed.

Stomach Problems

Shaped like a gourd, the stomach rests in the left central section of your upper abdomen, just below your rib cage. The stomach receives food from the esophagus, and its churning, mixing action reduces the food to a semi-liquid mixture. In addition, the stomach secretes acid, which in turn activates some enzymes that aid in the digestive process.

Most of the stomach's contents trickle into the small intestine for further digestion and absorption.

The stomach does not always function

smoothly. We all experience occasional indigestion and painful heartburn. These discomforts usually pass without requiring special medical attention. However, if such commonplace problems persist, they can indicate a more serious underlying problem.

Such problems often involve the lining of the stomach, which generally is remarkably resistant to injury. However, at times its resistance may break down and a small hole (ulcer) may develop in the lining. Ulcers, gastritis, and other stomach problems are discussed in the following pages.

Indigestion

Signs and Symptoms
- Discomfort or feeling of fullness in the upper abdomen
- Heartburn
- Nausea
- A sensation of bloating, often relieved by belching

Indigestion (dyspepsia) is a nonspecific term used to describe many symptoms associated with abdominal distress, particularly after eating.

Indigestion itself is not a disease. Rather, it is a common symptom that most people have at one time or another. Some have indigestion only when they eat certain foods or drink excessive amounts of alcohol. Others have episodes daily. Often, despite diagnostic tests, no specific cause of the indigestion is ever found.

However, this does not mean that you should ignore your indigestion, particularly if it occurs often. Indigestion can be a symptom of a serious disease such as peptic ulcer, gastritis, gastric cancer, or gallbladder disease.

Diagnosis
Indigestion is a vague description—that is why it is so important for you to be specific about your symptoms. Your physician will ask you to describe the discomfort. Where does it typically occur? Does it occur before, during, shortly after, or several hours after a meal? Because indigestion can be caused by problems anywhere in the digestive system, these questions are your physician's initial attempt to pinpoint the affected area.

For example, if the discomfort is below your umbilicus (navel), it is unlikely to be a problem in your esophagus, stomach, duodenum, or gallbladder. However, if the discomfort is above the umbilicus, these sites may need to be considered further to eliminate disorders that may be mimicking the symptoms of indigestion.

The timing of the symptoms also may offer a clue. If the discomfort occurs when you are eating, this suggests esophagitis or gastritis (see pages 742 and 758). A discomfort that occurs several hours later may suggest an ulcer in your duodenum (see page 753).

Once your physician has determined the pattern of your symptoms, he or she may want to check for blood in your stool (see Screening for Colon Cancer, page 790). Whether or not other tests are done depends on your age, the duration of your symptoms, and their severity. Because of the risk of cancer, older people with symptoms are more likely to have further diagnostic tests. If you are younger than 30, your physician may want to try antacids or other medications for a short time to see if your symptoms are relieved. If they are not, your physician may order additional studies.

Abdominal symptoms can be evaluated with barium X-ray studies of the esophagus, stomach, small intestine, and colon (see The Barium X-Ray, page 762). Your physician also may consider an ultrasound or CT scan of your pancreas, liver, and gallbladder (see Ultrasonography, page 1335, and CT Scan, page 1334). Another test that may be helpful is an endoscopic examination (see Upper Gastrointestinal Endoscopy, page 760). The particular tests your physician orders depend on your specific symptoms.

How Serious Is Indigestion?
In itself, indigestion is more a discomfort than a serious problem. However, because it can be a symptom of a major underlying disease, indigestion should be taken seriously, particularly if it is of new onset or is not responsive to medication.

Treatment

Medication
At times, no cause for your indigestion may be found in spite of extensive testing. Your physician may elect to try a few weeks of treatment with antacids or an acid-reducing medication such as cimetidine, ranitidine, nizatidine, or famotidine, or he or she may try to use a medication such as sucralfate that

probably works by coating and thereby protecting the lining of the stomach. Another possible medication is metoclopramide, which enhances the emptying of the stomach. These medications have various degrees of success.

Lifestyle Adjustments

Your physician also might advise elimination of certain foods, such as alcohol, that may be causing your indigestion. He or she also might discourage the use of cigarettes, which may be contributing to indigestion. In addition, your physician may inquire as to whether tension or stress in your life may be contributing to your symptoms. If so, efforts should be directed at changing those factors, which, in turn, may relieve your symptoms.

If a specific cause such as a peptic ulcer, gastritis, or duodenitis is found, your physician will recommend specific therapy.

Peptic Ulcer

Signs and Symptoms
- Burning, aching, gnawing, or hunger discomfort in the upper abdomen or lower chest that is relieved by milk, food, or antacids
- Black, tarry, foul-smelling stools
- Bloated feeling after meals
- Nausea and vomiting

Emergency Symptoms
- Shock: cold, clammy skin and fainting, suggesting excessive blood loss
- Vomiting of fresh blood (bright red)

Peptic ulcers are holes or breaks in the inner lining of the esophagus, stomach, or duodenum. Peptic ulcer generally occurs in the lower part of the stomach, in the initial portion of the duodenum, and occasionally in the lower esophagus.

The cause of ulcers is not fully known. Normally, the linings of the esophagus, stomach, and duodenum are kept intact by a balance between the acid and stomach juices and the resistance of these linings to injury. When the balance breaks down, the result may be a peptic ulcer.

If your stomach produces a great deal of acid, you may not necessarily develop an ulcer; likewise, if you have low acid production, it is no assurance that you will never have an ulcer. What appears to be decisive is the balance between the amount of acid and the quality and quantity of the protective lining.

The most common peptic ulcer, a duodenal ulcer, is one that appears in the duodenum, the initial portion of the small intestine. A gastric ulcer (stomach ulcer) is usually found on the lower portion of the stomach, and an esophageal ulcer is usually located in the lower section of the esophagus.

Peptic ulcers are not uncommon in our society. Statistics suggest that 1 of every 10 people will have a peptic ulcer during his or her lifetime. Typically, the age at diagnosis peaks between 40 and 50 for duodenal ulcers and between 60 and 70 for gastric ulcers. Frequently, ulcers recur within 1 year after healing, sometimes without symptoms.

There is some evidence that some people may have an inherited disposition to ulcers. Peptic ulcers are 3 times more likely to occur in families of patients with duodenal ulcer than in the general population. And relatives of people with gastric ulcers are likely to have the very same kind of ulcer.

Contrary to popular belief, there is no clear evidence that people who are under a lot of stress or eat hurried, irregular meals are more likely to have ulcers. Furthermore, ulcers do not affect primarily high-level business executives any more than those in other occupations. Ulcers affect people of all socioeconomic levels.

Duodenal Ulcer

There is no one symptom that will tell you that you have a duodenal ulcer. A relatively

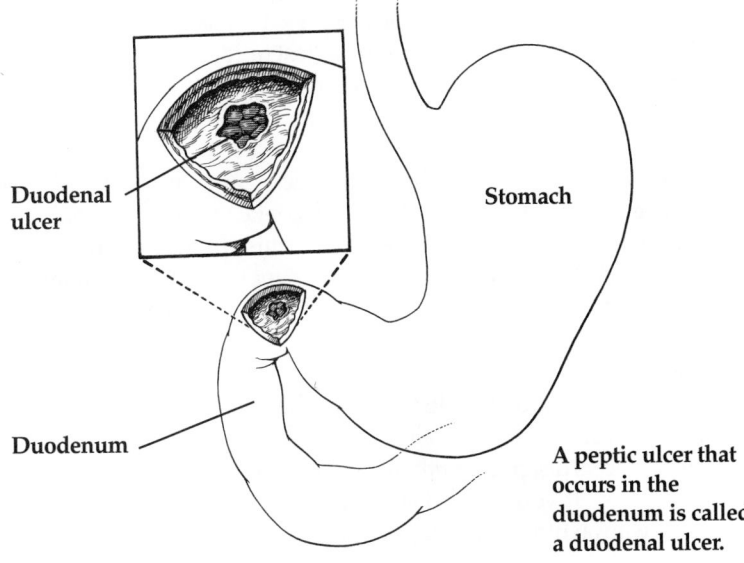

Duodenal ulcer

Stomach

Duodenum

A peptic ulcer that occurs in the duodenum is called a duodenal ulcer.

reliable indication, however, is a burning, aching, gnawing, or hungry sensation in the upper middle section of your upper abdomen or a pain under your breastbone that comes and goes. If the ulcer is located on the back wall of your duodenum, it is possible that you will feel pain in your mid-back. At times, you may feel bloated and nauseated after meals. If the scarring that results from a long-standing ulcer obstructs the pylorus (the opening from the stomach to the small intestine), you may feel distended after meals and even vomit or regurgitate.

In some cases, you may not experience any pain with your ulcer. Bleeding may be the initial sign. The stools may be black, tarry, and foul-smelling. Less common is vomiting of red or coffee-ground material or passing maroon stools.

A condition in which tumors form in the pancreas or duodenum, Zollinger-Ellison syndrome, will cause excessive production of a hormone (gastrin) that stimulates gastric acid secretion in the stomach. Peptic ulcer may develop in the stomach and duodenum or other areas of the small intestine. These tumors are sometimes malignant (see Zollinger-Ellison Syndrome, page 757).

Cigarette smoking may be associated with duodenal ulcers. These ulcers not only are more likely to develop in heavy smokers but also are less likely to heal as quickly as in nonsmokers. The relationship between smoking and ulcer formation is not fully understood, but it is thought that the nicotine somehow inhibits the alkaline secretions of the pancreas that are partially responsible for neutralizing stomach acid.

Recent research has shown that many ulcers may be secondary to bacteria called *Helicobacter pylori (H. pylori)* (see Ulcers: Are Antibiotics an Answer? this page).

Gastric Ulcer

Excessive gastric acid may contribute to the formation of a gastric ulcer. However, in most cases it is believed that a gastric ulcer develops because the mucus and protective lining of the stomach are defective and unable to resist the usual amount of stomach acid. Because excess acid secretion is not the primary cause of a gastric ulcer, smaller doses of either liquid antacids or acid-reducing medications than are required for duodenal ulcers may be effective. Certain medications, including analgesics such as aspirin, can cause gastric ulcer or gastric erosions. The reason why they do this is unclear but may involve a weakening in the protective lining of the stomach.

It is not easy to distinguish between a duodenal and a gastric ulcer on the basis of pain symptoms. The pain from a gastric ulcer may be less likely to be relieved by eating; in some cases, eating actually may make the pain of a gastric ulcer worse.

There are several potentially dangerous complications associated with peptic ulcers. Sometimes an ulcer will hemorrhage, necessitating hospitalization. One danger of severe hemorrhage is shock (see Recognizing and Treating Shock, page 442). Another is that, if the bleeding is only slight but continues over a period of time, an iron-deficiency anemia may develop (see page 957).

Perforation, another serious complication, occurs when the ulcer erodes through the wall of the stomach or duodenum into the abdominal cavity. This produces the sudden onset of an intense and persistent pain. If this occurs, see your physician at once. Most often, emergency surgery is required.

Obstruction at the outlet of the stomach is a complication in individuals with long-standing duodenal or pyloric channel ulcers.

Ulcers: Are Antibiotics an Answer?

Many people with ulcers harbor *H. pylori* bacteria, which can be effectively treated with antibiotics. Twelve months after treatment, most people show no ulcer recurrence, while recurrence is more common after using standard ulcer medications. Although not yet considered standard treatment, antibiotics are gaining acceptance among physicians, many of whom still reserve them for recurrent ulcers or ulcers that don't respond to typical approaches.

Your physician may order a special test or identify the organism from a biopsy at the site of the ulcer, using an endoscopic procedure (see page 760). Antibiotics may need to be combined with standard medications.

There are drawbacks to using antibiotics. Large doses of medication are required. You may be asked to take up to 12 to 15 pills daily for 10 to 12 days. For some people, this approach is inconvenient and difficult to maintain. Also, over time, *H. pylori* may become resistant to antibiotics; using a combination of antibiotics, however, makes this less likely.

Side effects are another disadvantage of using antibiotics. About 20 percent of people who take them experience nausea and diarrhea.

Some ulcers disappear without treatment. Others go away with H_2 blockers. If you've tried standard treatments and still have trouble with an ulcer, ask your physician about antibiotic treatment.

This results in dilatation or enlargement of the stomach. Vomiting of easily recognized food ingested hours earlier may occur.

Diagnosis

If your physician suspects that you have an ulcer, he or she may conduct several diagnostic tests. The two major tests are a barium X-ray (see page 762) and an endoscopic examination (see Upper Gastrointestinal Endoscopy, page 760). If the barium test is negative yet your symptoms continue, an endoscopic examination may be performed. If the ulcer is in your stomach, your physician may take a sample of tissue for laboratory analysis (biopsy) to rule out a malignancy. Duodenal ulcers are rarely malignant.

How Serious Are Peptic Ulcers?

With early detection and proper treatment, most people recover from their ulcers within a few weeks. However, early treatment does not guarantee a cure because more than half of all persons treated for ulcers have a recurrence within 2 years.

Treatment

The goals of treatment are to relieve symptoms, heal the ulcer, prevent relapse, and avoid complications.

Medication

The vast majority of persons with peptic ulcer disease respond well to medication. The key to treatment is either decreasing the amount of acid present or strengthening the protective lining of the stomach or duodenum. The mainstay of treatment is a class of drugs that decrease the amount of acid produced in the stomach. These drugs are called H_2 blockers. These medications include cimetidine, ranitidine, nizatidine, and famotidine. Your physician also may consider omeprazole, which is a more potent inhibitor of stomach acid than H_2 blockers. The usual course of therapy lasts approximately 6 weeks.

Once your ulcer has healed, your physician may advise you to take a smaller dose of one of these medications on a daily basis, particularly if you have had recurrences in the past. Other useful medications include sucralfate, which may coat the lining of your stomach and duodenum. Another recently released drug is misoprostol, which is believed to have similar properties. Antacids sometimes are used to supplement these medications.

Surgery

In recent years, the number of operations performed for peptic ulcer disease has steadily decreased, primarily because the availability of more effective medications has alleviated the need for surgical treatment in many cases.

However, if you have an ulcer that does not respond to medical treatment or you have serious complications such as hemorrhage, obstruction, or perforation, you may be a candidate for surgery. Understand, however, that surgery is not a panacea. There are many side effects associated with this operation.

The Procedure

Various procedures are used in the surgical treatment of ulcers. If you have an acute perforation, most likely you will need an immediate operation. Depending on his or her evaluation at the time of the operation, your surgeon may only close the hole (perforation) in the stomach or duodenal wall where the ulcer eroded through into the abdominal cavity.

For uncontrollable acute bleeding, the small artery that is the source of the bleeding is identified and tied off. Generally, this is at the base of an ulcer. The entire ulcer also may be cut out.

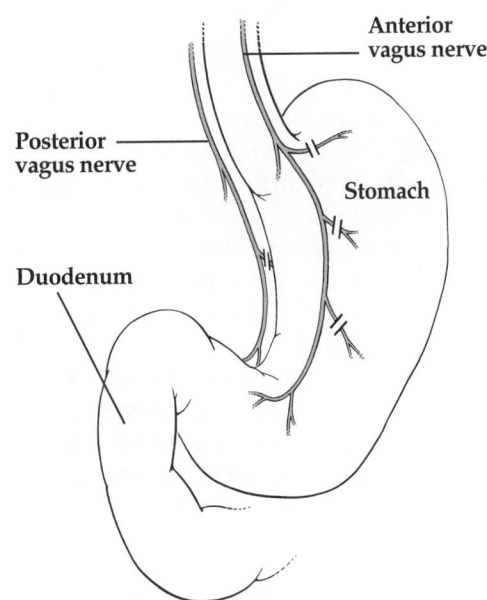

If treatment of your ulcer requires surgery, the surgeon may sever nerves that control acid secretion in your stomach. There are several surgical options; one is called proximal gastric vagotomy (shown above), in which branches of the vagus nerve are severed.

In addition to these emergency steps, if your surgeon thinks your condition is safe enough to warrant a more extended operation, he or she will perform a surgical procedure to decrease acid production in your stomach. This is similar to what he or she would perform if operating in a non-emergency situation.

Potential Complications
Several complications are associated with peptic ulcer surgery.

Ulcer Recurrence. Ulcers recur in about 5 percent of patients who have undergone surgery. The vast majority of these recurrences are seen with duodenal ulcers. The most common symptom of a recurrent ulcer is abdominal pain. Sometimes, a recurring ulcer does not respond well to medication, and a second surgical procedure may be necessary.

Alkaline Reflux Gastritis. A small number of people experience abdominal discomfort, loss of appetite, and vomiting of bile-colored (yellowish or greenish) material that is thought to be due to the reflux of duodenal contents back into the stomach. Often, a severe iron-deficiency anemia is present (see page 957). Medical treatment of this problem generally is not successful. Sometimes, additional surgery is recommended.

Dumping Syndrome. After peptic ulcer surgery, some persons experience one or more of the following symptoms: light-headedness, sweating, abdominal discomfort, vomiting, and diarrhea after meals. This is called the dumping syndrome. The dumping syndrome occurs within 60 minutes after a meal and is thought to be the result of the too-rapid emptying of stomach contents into the small intestine.

Treatment of the dumping syndrome includes the elimination of liquids at mealtime (consume liquids between meals), limiting sweets, and eating frequent small meals rather than three large meals.

Diarrhea. Some people who have undergone peptic ulcer surgery have diarrhea unrelated to dumping, usually within 2 hours after a meal. The cause is not clear.

Hypoglycemia. Palpitations, light-headedness, and sweating may occur more than 1 hour after eating and are thought to be due to a decrease in blood sugar concentration caused by the insulin produced in response to rapid absorption of sugar.

To avoid these symptoms, reduce your intake of sweets at meals. The symptoms of hypoglycemia respond to sugar taken by mouth, best in the form of a fruit juice.

Hematologic Complications. People who have all or part of their stomachs removed invariably have malabsorption of certain food elements. Iron deficiency is the most common deficiency after peptic ulcer surgery and may be the result of blood loss or iron malabsorption (see page 957). The anemia that results from iron deficiency usually takes several years to develop, except when it is caused by acute blood loss. Chronic iron deficiencies can be treated with medications taken orally.

In addition, the stomach produces a substance (called intrinsic factor) that is necessary for the absorption of vitamin B_{12}. If this factor is missing or significantly decreased in amount because of the removal of a portion of your stomach, you may acquire pernicious anemia (see Pernicious Anemia, page 958). Treatment is a monthly injection of vitamin B_{12} underneath your skin. Oral preparations of vitamin B_{12} are not helpful because they will not be absorbed.

General Malabsorption. Mild malabsorption is common after ulcer surgery. Weight loss is more likely to occur in persons who have part of their stomach removed.

Nutrition
One traditional treatment approach, the bland diet with plenty of milk, is no longer considered important or effective in the treatment of ulcers. Drinking large quantities of milk is discouraged, in fact, because foods rich in protein and calcium tend to stimulate acid production.

Another change from past dietary rules is that your physician may recommend that you avoid foods that make you feel worse. At the same time, your physician will probably caution you about eating peppers, garlic, cloves, chili powder, caffeine, and alcohol. Avoid even decaffeinated coffee because it promotes acid production.

Prevention
The delicate balance between the acid and the protective lining in your gastrointestinal

tract can be disrupted by alcohol, aspirin, and some other medications. Aspirin and certain other anti-inflammatory drugs have this disruptive effect, but acetaminophen does not (see Drug-Induced Stomach Problems, page 758).

If you smoke, stop. Smoking probably contributes to the development of an ulcer and retards or prevents healing.

If you have a history of ulcer, mention this problem whenever a physician prescribes a medication for you. If aspirin or a potentially ulcer-provoking drug is absolutely necessary, the danger of an ulcer developing can be greatly lessened by the simultaneous use of either an acid-reducing medication such as cimetidine, ranitidine, nizatidine, or famotidine or a protective agent such as sucralfate or misoprostil.

Zollinger-Ellison Syndrome

Signs and Symptoms
- Ulcer-like symptoms in the upper abdomen (see Signs and Symptoms of Peptic Ulcer, page 753)
- Symptoms may be severe, persistent, and not relieved by antacids
- Diarrhea

Zollinger-Ellison syndrome is a condition in which tumors, called gastrinomas, form in the pancreas or duodenum. The tumors secrete a substance called gastrin that causes excessive acid secretion in the stomach.

As a result, between 90 and 95 percent of persons with Zollinger-Ellison syndrome have peptic ulcers at some point during their disease. Ulcers associated with this syndrome are typically more persistent and respond less well to treatment than do typical peptic ulcers (see Peptic Ulcer, page 753). It is estimated that this syndrome is responsible for up to 1 percent of all peptic ulcers.

Zollinger-Ellison syndrome may occur at any age, but the symptoms are more likely to appear between ages 30 and 60.

Diagnosis
If you have the symptoms of Zollinger-Ellison syndrome, your physician will perform blood tests to see whether the gastrin level in your blood is increased. Generally, a person with Zollinger-Ellison syndrome has an abnormally high serum gastrin level in addition to producing excessive amounts of acid. Your physician may also order a barium X-ray of your stomach, duodenum, and, sometimes, jejunum (the middle section of the small intestine) or upper gastrointestinal endoscopy to detect the presence of ulcers (see The Barium X-Ray, page 762, and Upper Gastrointestinal Endoscopy, page 760).

Because these gastrinomas are often very small and difficult to locate, treatment previously was directed at solving the ulcer disease rather than dealing directly with the tumor. However, recent advances in high-quality ultrasound (see page 1335) that can be used in the operating room and nuclear medicine scans that use a tiny dose of radioactive material that attaches to the tumor and shows as a "hot spot" on the scan have increased the successful identification of these tumors.

How Serious Is Zollinger-Ellison Syndrome?
Zollinger-Ellison syndrome may be a serious disease. In half to two-thirds of the patients, the gastrinomas are malignant and slowly spread, most commonly to the lymph nodes and liver. Moreover, the ulcer disease associated with this syndrome usually is severe and not easily treated with conventional ulcer medication or surgery. As with most serious diseases, the earlier the condition is diagnosed, the better the chances of a favorable outcome.

Treatment
Typically, the ulcer disease in Zollinger-Ellison syndrome is resistant to standard doses of ulcer medication and conventional surgery (see Peptic Ulcer Surgery, page 755). Especially if you are young, your physician may elect to perform an operation to identify and remove the tumor responsible for the excess production of acid. Sometimes these tumors are small or multiple in nature and therefore cannot be located or removed.

If your surgeon is unable to remove the gastrinoma, you will need to take an acid-reducing medication. The most effective drug is omeprazole, which has the advantage of virtually eliminating acid production for a period of time with small doses. Other beneficial medications include famotidine, ranitidine, nizatidine, and cimetidine. You may need to take doses of these medications which are larger than the usual doses and to take them more often than you would need to for an ordinary peptic ulcer. These medications generally need to be taken indefinitely to prevent recurrence of symptoms.

If the gastrinoma is malignant, your physician will need to watch carefully for growth of this tumor in addition to treating its effects on acid production.

Gastritis

Signs and Symptoms
- Upper abdominal discomfort
- Nausea and, occasionally, vomiting
- Diarrhea

Emergency Symptoms—Bleeding

"Gastritis" is a general term that means inflammation of the lining of the stomach. It can result from a number of causes, each of which may produce somewhat different symptoms.

Gastritis can occur as a result of acid-induced damage to the lining of the stomach when no ulcer is present. Excessive smoking or alcohol consumption both are known to produce mild gastritis or to aggravate existing gastritis symptoms.

Gastritis also can be a side effect of a number of prescription drugs (see Drug-Induced Stomach Problems, this page). One form of the ailment, erosive gastritis, is often associated with the ingestion of aspirin or similar medications. Severe stress due to burns, trauma, surgery, or shock may produce gastritis.

In most cases, the symptoms of gastritis are relatively mild and short-lived, pose no real danger, and have no lasting effect. Occasionally, gastritis may cause bleeding, but it is rarely severe.

Paradoxically, gastritis is also seen in some persons whose stomachs do not produce acid. In these cases, the lining of the stomach is atrophied (hence the name atrophic gastritis). This condition may be associated with vitamin B_{12} deficiency (see Pernicious Anemia, page 958) and occurs in many older people.

Gastritis affects virtually everyone at some time in their lives. Even very healthy people may experience gastritis with some regularity. The incidence of gastritis increases with age, and more women than men are affected.

Diagnosis
Your physician may be able to make the diagnosis on the basis of your description of your symptoms. He or she may obtain a barium X-ray of your stomach (see The Barium X-Ray, page 762). Often, the results of this study are normal. The diagnosis normally can be confirmed by gastroscopy (see page 760), which reveals the typical lesions.

How Serious Is Gastritis?
Gastritis generally is not serious except for the discomfort it produces. Rarely, it results in gastrointestinal bleeding.

If you appear to have gastritis, your physician will inquire about your eating habits. Your physician also will want to know if you are a heavy drinker or smoke regularly. If the gastritis appears to be a side effect of drug use, your physician may recommend that the medication be taken at very specific times of the day or be replaced with other drugs.

Treatment

Medication
Antacids in liquid or tablet form are a suitable and common treatment for mild gastritis. If you are troubled by excessive acid and antacids fail to provide relief, your physician may give you a prescription drug such as cimetidine, ranitidine, nizatidine, or famotidine, which decreases the amount of acid produced by your stomach.

Medication to protect the lining of the stomach, such as sucralfate or misoprostil, also may be used. If you are deficient in vitamin B_{12}, you will need to take vitamin B_{12} injections on a monthly basis indefinitely.

Drug-Induced Stomach Problems

Signs and Symptoms
- Heartburn
- Indigestion
- Constipation
- Diarrhea
- Change in the color of your stool (see Gastrointestinal Tract Bleeding, page 759)
- Iron-deficiency anemia (see page 957)

Drugs have been, and continue to be, an indispensable part of the medical treatment of many ailments. The federal government and the pharmaceutical industry try to ensure that the drugs marketed in this country are effective and relatively safe. Part of this task involves identifying what, if any, are the potential hazards of the use of prescription and over-the-counter medications.

The obvious goal of drug therapy is to obtain the greatest possible relief with a minimum of side effects. Yet, virtually all drugs produce some unwanted effects. Terms such as "side effects" and "adverse reactions" are used to describe these harmful effects. Therefore, when taking a medication it may be necessary to accept the minor annoyance of some unwanted side effects in order to gain the more important therapeutic effect.

Side effects range from very mild to extremely severe. Some are very common and can be tolerated if the benefits outweigh the discomfort or harm. Others are rare and may be severe enough to be life-threatening. Your physician may want you either to decrease the dosage of the drug or to stop taking it altogether in the event of such unwanted effects.

Perhaps the principal offenders are anti-inflammatory drugs, of which many are used to treat the inflammation characteristic of arthritis. These include aspirin and a class of medications known as nonsteroidal anti-inflammatory drugs (NSAIDs) that include indomethacin, ibuprofen, naproxen, tolmetin, sulindac, piroxicam, diflunisal, and fenoprofen.

Aspirin (acetylsalicylic acid) is one of the most effective and safest drugs available when it is used prudently. However, persons who take more than two or three tablets a day may experience microscopic gastrointestinal bleeding.

If you are susceptible, aspirin and the other anti-inflammatory drugs may cause an erosion, gastritis, or gastric ulcer in your stomach—despite the fact that you may have no history of stomach ulcer. However, generally these medications do not cause duodenal ulcer.

It is not clear how aspirin and similar drugs produce gastric ulcers. These medications appear to decrease the protective properties in the lining and mucus of the stomach.

In addition to causing gastrointestinal problems, aspirin can inhibit the function of platelets, which serve as plugs to stop bleeding every time you cut yourself or sustain any type of laceration. Because of this interference, you should discontinue the use of aspirin prior to any operation. Moreover, pregnant women should not take aspirin because it increases the likelihood of significant bleeding during pregnancy, particularly during delivery.

Gastrointestinal Tract Bleeding

Signs and Symptoms
- Blood in the stool
- Vomiting of blood

The Cause
The most common causes of gastrointestinal bleeding are peptic ulcer, gastritis (often associated with alcohol abuse or the overuse of drugs such as aspirin or other anti-inflammatory drugs, see page 758), variceal bleeding in the esophagus, small tears in the lower esophagus and upper stomach (Mallory-Weiss tears), tumors, polyps and diverticula in the colon, and hemorrhoids.

Red or maroon stool can indicate several problems, such as colonic polyps (see page 786), cancer of the colon (see page 789), Crohn's disease (see page 774), and ulcerative colitis (see page 777). It may also mean blood from the stomach or duodenum, particularly if the bleeding is considerable. If you see blood in your stool or in the toilet, consult your physician. The source of the blood simply may be hemorrhoids (see page 795), but other potential sources should be evaluated.

Vomited blood clearly suggests that the bleeding is from the esophagus, stomach, or duodenum. Any blood that enters the intestines below the duodenum usually does not reflux back into the stomach but passes in the stool. One of the more common explanations for heavy bleeding in the stool in people older than 60 is a painless hemorrhage from a diverticulum in the colon (see page 781).

Vomiting of bright red blood indicates that the bleeding began shortly before you vomited. If the blood is dark red or appears brown and has the texture of old coffee grounds, the blood has been in your stomach for a longer time. Bleeding that occurs in the stomach or duodenum and exits through the rectum often results in black, sticky, and foul-smelling stools that resemble tar. Licorice or ingestion of iron or bismuth subsalicylate (such as Pepto-Bismol) may also turn your stool black.

The Diagnosis
Often, blood in the stool can be detected only by diagnostic tests because the amount is too little to see (occult blood) (see Screening for Colon Cancer, page 790). Over time, the un-

Upper Gastrointestinal Endoscopy

Upper gastrointestinal endoscopy (esophagogastroduodenoscopy), sometimes shortened to gastroscopy, gives your physician a direct view of the upper part of your digestive tract. A device called a fiber-optic endoscope is inserted through your mouth into your esophagus, stomach, and duodenum. This thin, flexible tube equipped with a lighting and lens system enables the specially trained physician to examine the interior of your digestive tract. A channel within the gastroscope permits the passage of instruments that allow the physician to take samples of tissue (biopsy) and fluid and to perform certain treatments.

The Procedure

As with the barium X-ray examination (see The Barium X-Ray, page 762), you must fast or restrict yourself to liquids for several hours prior to the examination. This procedure usually is done on an outpatient basis. If a sedative is used, do not drive that day.

Before the physician inserts the tube, a local anesthetic may be sprayed into your mouth and throat to dull the gag reflex that may be produced by the pressure of the tube on the back of your tongue and throat. You also may be given an intravenous injection of medication to sedate you partially. You may feel some mild discomfort or fullness as the tube is inserted or when air is introduced.

Your physician will pass the instrument through the esophagus, into the stomach, and then into the upper portion of the small bowel (duodenum) in order to examine the upper gastrointestinal tract. Some air will be passed through the instrument to open these regions for an adequate examination.

The Uses

In recent years, endoscopy has proved its usefulness in the diagnosis of many gastrointestinal diseases by permitting both direct observation and biopsy. The channels in the endoscope also allow the passage of devices that can remove small growths, polyps, or swallowed foreign bodies. Special catheters can be inserted to scar (sclerose) or clip bleeding varices (see page 750). Also, devices can be passed through the channels of the gastroscope that allow electrical current or laser light to be used to stop bleeding lesions or destroy tumor tissue. Narrowed areas (strictures), especially in the esophagus, may be stretched (dilated) to improve swallowing (esophageal dilation, see page 748).

Gastroscopy is very safe. However, it should be done only by physicians experienced in the use of the endoscope. Very rarely, bleeding or perforation injuries may occur.

When Is It Done?

Endoscopy is often used for the following conditions:

Esophagitis. This is one of the most common benign diseases of the upper gastrointestinal tract (see page 742). It occasionally cannot be diagnosed with an X-ray but can be seen clearly with an endoscope. Obviously, not everyone who complains of heartburn needs to undergo endoscopy. However, when symptoms persist despite treatment, when swallowing is a problem, or when an X-ray reveals a narrowing, mass, or ulcer in the esophagus, endoscopy is advised. The abnormal area can be assessed better through the gastroscope, and biopsy specimens can be obtained.

Swallowing Difficulties. Besides scarring of the esophagus, other problems of the esophagus also can affect swallowing. These include motility problems caused by inability of the esophagus to propel food normally into the stomach. Your physician may perform an endoscopic examination in order to obtain a better understanding of the nature of your problem.

Peptic Ulcer. Endoscopy is more accurate than a barium X-ray in detecting most peptic ulcers and may be used as the first test when ulcers are suspected. However, because it is less expensive and not as uncomfortable, many physicians still

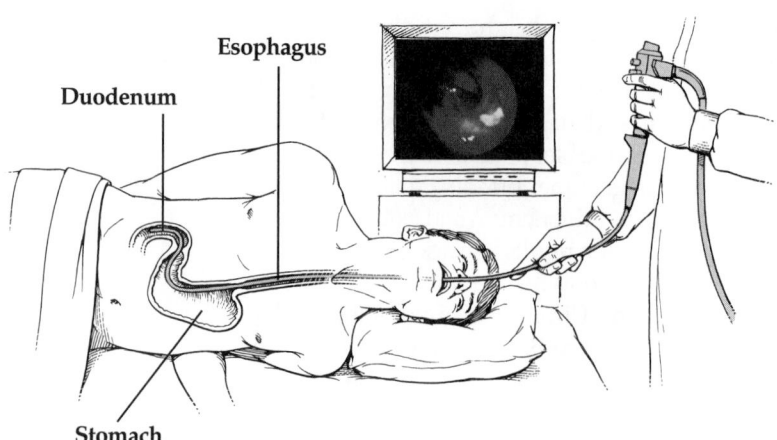

Esophagus

Duodenum

Stomach

A fiberoptic endoscope can give your physician a direct view of your upper gastrointestinal tract (esophagus, stomach, and a portion of your duodenum). The image on the screen shows a peptic ulcer.

use a barium X-ray for persons whose symptoms suggest an ulcer. Endoscopy usually is then performed when the barium X-ray is either inconclusive or shows a definite abnormality, especially in the esophagus or stomach. When bleeding from an ulcer or cancer is suspected or ulcer surgery is going to be performed and there is need to see if there are other lesions, endoscopy may be recommended.

Cancer. When cancer is suspected, the endoscope may be used both to examine suspicious-looking masses seen on the barium X-ray and to take a biopsy sample of that tissue. Persons who have gastric ulcers should have follow-up endoscopic examinations to ensure that the ulcer has healed. Gastric ulcers are more likely to be cancerous than other types of ulcers, and an X-ray cannot always correctly identify whether an ulcer is indeed cancerous.

Upper Gastrointestinal Bleeding. Endoscopy is the most accurate method of determining the actual site of upper gastrointestinal bleeding. Many physicians believe that endoscopy should be done on anyone who has continued gastrointestinal bleeding (see page 759) that may require surgery. Although in the majority of cases the upper gastrointestinal bleeding stops spontaneously, there is no way of predicting the cases in which hemorrhage will continue.

Thus, endoscopy is usually recommended.

In addition, in persons who continue to bleed or who are suspected to be at risk of bleeding again soon, the use of devices inserted through an endoscope to permit electrocautery, laser treatment, or injection of a sclerosing (scarring) agent may slow or stop the bleeding and eliminate the need for surgery.

Surveillance Examination. Certain chronic conditions of the upper gastrointestinal tract, such as Barrett's esophagus (see page 744), may predispose to the development of cancer. In such cases, regular endoscopic examinations may be helpful to look for the earlier signs of malignancy.

---

detected microscopic bleeding can produce an iron-deficiency anemia that may leave you tired and weak from the loss of hemoglobin and iron in the stool (see Iron-Deficiency Anemia, page 957).

If your physician suspects that the bleeding is from the upper part of the gastrointestinal tract, he or she may pass a nasogastric tube into your stomach to see if there is blood in it. Endoscopy (see Upper Gastrointestinal Endoscopy, page 760) may be done to find the source of bleeding. If your physician believes that the bleeding is from the colon, he or she may obtain an angiogram of the colon (see page 656) or perform colonoscopy (see page 788), depending on the amount of blood found at the site.

Treatment

Often, the bleeding stops spontaneously; sometimes blood transfusions are necessary. Treatment depends on the cause and severity of the hemorrhage.

If the bleeding is due to an esophageal varix, the continuous intravenous infusion of a drug such as vasopressin is often successful, at least in stopping the loss of blood temporarily. Sometimes delivery of a scarring (sclerosing) agent, or clipping the vein via an upper gastrointestinal endoscope, may stop the bleeding.

If the bleeding is from a diverticulum in the colon, a drug injected directly into the artery that supplies that portion of the colon may stop the bleeding. At times, the use of an electrical current or laser light delivered through an endoscope may stop bleeding in the stomach, duodenum, or colon. If the bleeding resists these treatment methods, surgery may be required.

Stomach Tumors

Signs and Symptoms
- Discomfort in the upper or middle region of the abdomen not relieved by milk or antacids
- Black, tarry stools
- Vomiting of blood
- Vomiting after meals
- Weight loss
- Anemia
- Bloated feeling after meals

Emergency Symptoms—Shock: cold, clammy skin and fainting suggest excessive blood loss

Most gastric tumors are malignant. They affect twice as many men as women, usually between the ages of 50 and 70. It is rare to

The Barium X-Ray

The barium X-ray enables your physician to examine your upper gastrointestinal tract and small bowel for the presence of ulcers, tumors, strictures, and other abnormalities. It also allows visualization of motor or motion abnormalities of the esophagus, stomach, and small bowel and assessment of gastroesophageal reflux.

A barium enema permits visualization of the lining of your rectum, colon, and often the terminal portion of the small bowel (ileum) on the X-ray, aiding in the diagnosis of diseases such as colon cancer (see page 789), Crohn's disease (see page 774), ulcerative colitis (see page 777), and polyps (see page 786).

The Preparation

Before the examination, you will fast overnight. For the ingestion of barium, you will be asked to drink a chalky liquid that may be flavored to make it more pleasant tasting.

If you are having a barium enema, you will probably be given a laxative the night before to help empty your colon. You also will be in-

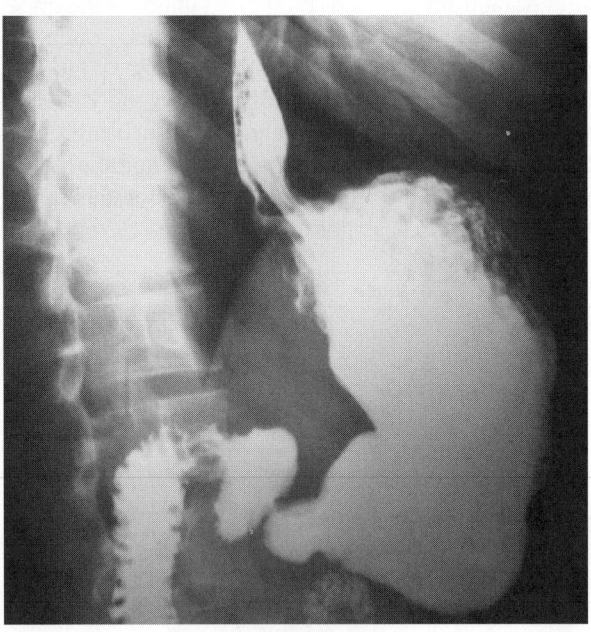

Normal stomach

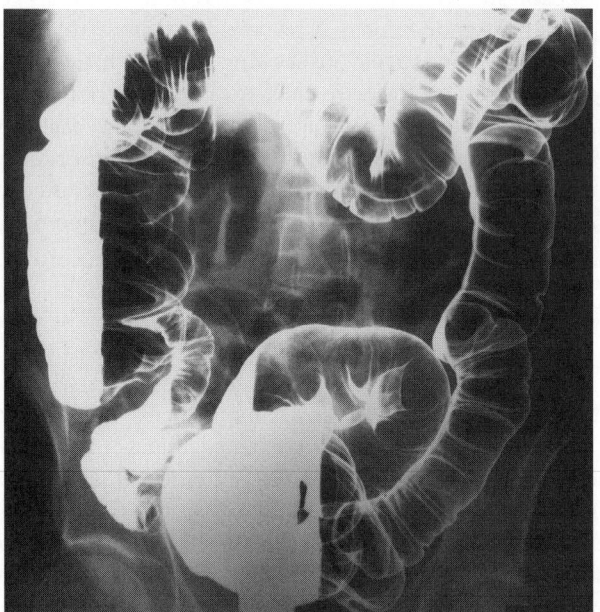

Normal colon

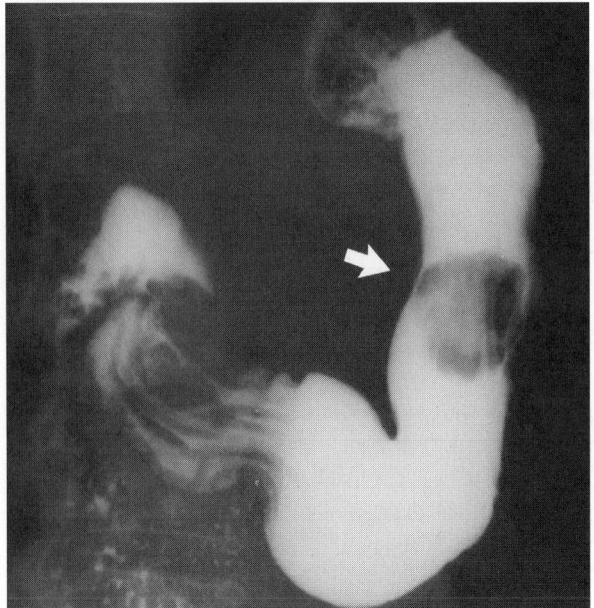

Stomach cancer (arrow)

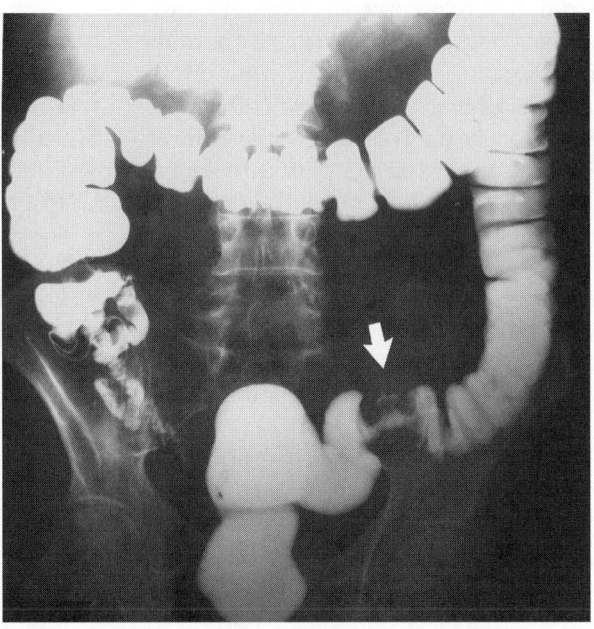

Colon cancer (arrow)

structed to take a cleansing enema an hour or two before the procedure.

For the barium enema, the material is infused into your rectum. Although you will feel the urge to run to the bathroom, it is important that you hold the barium in so that X-rays can be taken.

The Procedure

X-rays do not pass through the barium mixture. Once the mixture coats and fills in the hollows of your digestive tract, an X-ray picture reveals a clear silhouette of the shape and condition of these organs.

A fluoroscope is used to visualize this image. This device contains a fluorescent screen that converts the X-ray image into visible light. The fluoroscope is also capable of providing a conventional X-ray picture at any point during the procedure.

After the barium is ingested, it moves down the esophagus into your stomach and small bowel. The fluoroscope permits the examining physician to watch this process. A narrowing of the column of barium in the esophagus usually means that the passageway has been narrowed because of stricture, tumor, or varices (see Esophageal Problems, page 741). If the column appears to be abnormal in its contour, it suggests a muscular dysfunction in the esophageal walls. If the barium leaks out, it means that the esophagus has been perforated, which is a very serious matter.

For an even clearer picture of the stomach, occasionally you might be asked to take a powder or pill that releases gas into your stomach. The gas will expand your stomach to provide a more detailed picture of the digestive tract.

The examination may last several hours if your small intestine is to be examined as well (an upper gastrointestinal examination, involving only your esophagus, stomach, and duodenum, takes about 15 minutes). The extra time is required because the additional X-rays of the small intestine will be taken at 15- to 30-minute intervals.

For the barium examination of the colon, the radiologist delivers the barium through the rectum. He or she will place you in various positions and palpate your abdomen as the barium flows through your colon. He or she will attempt to force the barium into the small bowel at the time of this examination. At times, the radiologist may instill some air into your colon to obtain better delineation of fine features of its lining. This is particularly effective in detecting changes of ulcerative colitis or Crohn's disease or in finding very small polyps. The radiologist also may take an X-ray of your colon after you have expelled the barium.

Side Effects

The barium suspension is excreted in the stool and normally should cause no ill effects. Taking a laxative is commonly advised after a barium study of the small bowel to ensure prompt passage of the barium. However, a barium enema has been known to aggravate ulcerative colitis or even precipitate a perforation in the colon, so the test should never be taken lightly.

For several days after the test, your stool will be light pink or white. You should be able to eat a normal diet immediately after the examination, but drink plenty of liquids during the remainder of the examination day.

find this type of cancer in people younger than 40.

As few as 1 of 10 stomach tumors is benign. Like the malignant tumors, the most common early symptom of a benign tumor may be microscopic bleeding that can be detected only by laboratory examination of your stool.

The cause of malignant gastric tumors is unknown. Genetic factors may have some influence. They are 2 to 4 times more common in members of the immediate family of people with the disease. Stomach cancer is much more common in some countries, such as Japan. However, the children of Japanese who migrate to the United States have a much lower incidence of stomach cancer, suggesting that environmental influences such as diet may be potential causes.

Diagnosis

There is no one symptom that will suggest that you have a malignant gastric tumor. One of every four persons with a malignant tumor has the same symptoms as someone with a peptic ulcer (see page 753). Approximately 5 percent of stomach cancers are lymphomas. The symptoms of lymphoma are very similar to those of stomach cancer (see Lymphomas, page 968).

If persistent indigestion develops for the first time in your life along with unexplained weight loss and nausea, your physician may want to obtain a barium X-ray (see The Barium X-Ray, page 762) or an endoscopic examination (see Upper Gastrointestinal Endoscopy, page 760).

In most cases, these procedures will determine whether your symptoms are due to a malignant tumor or to some other abnormality such as a peptic ulcer (see page 753). If your physician believes it is warranted, he or she may remove a small piece of tissue from your stomach with the endoscope for laboratory analysis (biopsy). If a malignancy is found, your physician may also want to obtain a CT scan (see page 1334) to determine whether the disease has spread to other organs.

How Serious Are Malignant Tumors?

This form of cancer is difficult to treat. If the cancer is confined to the stomach, the chance of cure is good. However, the disease often has spread, and the chance of cure is then significantly decreased.

Treatment

Surgery

If the tumor is malignant, surgical removal offers the only chance for a cure. The likelihood of success depends almost exclusively on whether the cancer has spread (metastasized) to other areas of the body. If the cancer is caught early and it is determined that surgery can remove all of the affected areas, full recovery is possible. Even when surgery may not be able to effect a cure, it still may be recommended to help alleviate pain, bleeding, or obstruction.

Medication

In addition to surgery for malignant tumors, your physician may choose chemotherapy as an additional treatment, using a number of anticancer medications. Radiation is sometimes used, but both radiation and chemotherapy can only relieve the symptoms; they do not cure the cancer. If the cancer is too far advanced for chemotherapy or surgery to be effective, analgesic drugs may be used to reduce pain.

Stomach Dilation

Signs and Symptoms—Distended abdomen with constant feeling of fullness

This is an uncommon condition in which the stomach becomes extremely bloated (dilated). Dilation occurs most often after a person has had gastric surgery or from an obstruction at the pylorus (see Pyloric Stenosis, page 55). It also can be a complication of some diseases such as pneumonia (see page 704) and diabetes (see page 925), or it may occur for no discernible reason. In any case, the most effective treatment for stomach dilation is nasogastric suction, a procedure in which a tube is inserted through the nose into the stomach. The underlying cause needs to be treated.

Ménétrier's Disease

Signs and Symptoms

- Stomach pain
- Vomiting, nausea
- Weight loss
- Possible intestinal bleeding
- Swelling of the hands, feet, or legs

This is a disease of unknown origin in which the lining of the stomach grows to the point that it creates large folds and these folds may contain tiny breaks (erosions). The erosions can develop into ulcers, and some people experience intestinal bleeding. Protein may be lost from these folds. As a consequence, swelling in your extremities may occur.

If you have Ménétrier's disease, X-rays will reveal the enlarged stomach folds. To rule out any possibility of cancer, your physician may perform upper gastrointestinal endoscopy and biopsy (see page 760). Under certain conditions, your physician may opt to perform a laparotomy (a surgical opening of the abdomen) to confirm the diagnosis.

There is no single treatment for this disease, although in all likelihood your physician will urge you to eat only small meals. If you suffer from associated problems such as ulcers or protein deficiency due to the disease, they will be treated separately. The use of acid-suppressing medications may be helpful, particularly if erosions or ulcers are present (see Peptic Ulcer, page 753). These drugs also may decrease the protein loss in the stomach. In some cases, surgery may be necessary to remove all or nearly all of your stomach.

Eosinophilic Gastroenteritis

This is a rare gastric disease in which the lining of the stomach and the intestinal tract becomes infiltrated with eosinophils (a type of white blood cell). The diagnosis can be made by biopsy, and treatment with corticosteroids usually is effective.

Disorders of the Small and Large Intestines

The small intestine consists of three parts: the duodenum, the jejunum, and the ileum. It is within this 12 to 22 feet of thin tubing coiled in the abdomen that most of the nutrients are absorbed from the food you eat.

Before food can be absorbed, it must be digested. The food that was broken down into smaller particles in the stomach and thoroughly mixed into a semiliquid material slowly flows into the small intestine in small portions. There the digestion process goes into full swing and the nutrients are absorbed.

The breakdown products of digestion are absorbed into the bloodstream mainly through the lining of the small intestine. This lining has numerous small projections called villi, and these projections significantly increase the surface area available for food to be absorbed. Bile (from the liver) and pancreatic juices assist in the process of digestion.

In the large intestine, the waste from the digestive process is solidified and prepared for evacuation. Also referred to as the colon, the large intestine is about 4 to 6 feet long.

The large intestine is connected to the small intestine at the ileocecal valve. Through this valve, the semi-liquid waste material passes into a chamber of the large intestine called the cecum. Attached to the cecum is the appendix; its function is unknown but it causes problems when it becomes inflamed (see Acute Appendicitis, page 772).

The shape of the large intestine resembles a bridge in that it runs up, across, and down in the abdomen. The ascending colon section of the large intestine starts on the right side of the abdomen in the cecum and moves up toward the liver. The portion of the colon that crosses the abdomen from right to left is referred to as the transverse colon. The descending colon is the section that moves downward into the sigmoid colon. Shaped like the letter "S," the sigmoid colon curves toward the pelvis, where it joins the rectum. The rectum is a relatively straight 4- to 6-inch tube that leads to the anus.

The nutrients of the food you eat are almost all absorbed in the small intestine, so what passes through the ileum into the large intestine is a mixture of the unabsorbed nutrients, fiber, water, and electrolytes such as sodium. As this mixture continues through the large intestine, much of the water and salt is reabsorbed through the lining of the large intestine. Once the water is removed, the waste becomes a semi-solid mass that is more easily passed through the anal canal and out the anus. By the time the waste products reach the anus, more than 90 percent of the liquid that originally entered the colon has been reabsorbed.

This reabsorption of water and sodium is critical to good health because both the water and the sodium are required in the functions of the body. If the body's need for water increases or the body's stores become depleted,

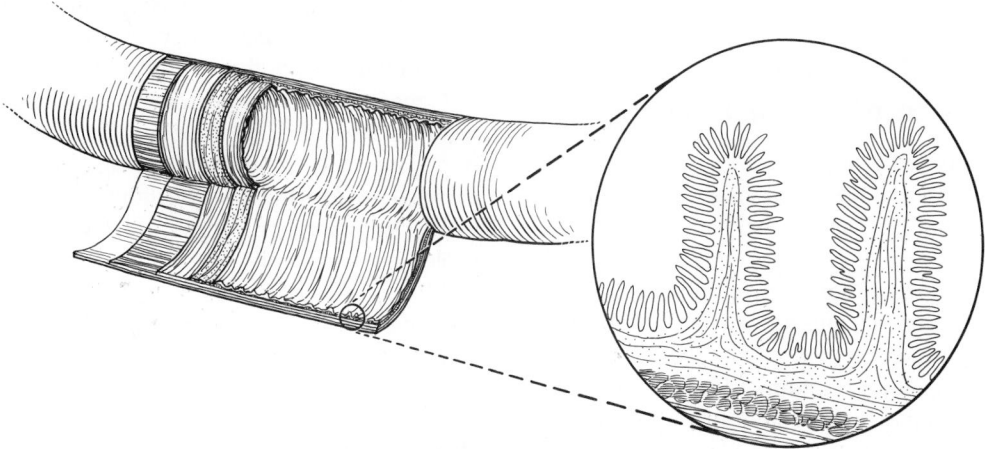

The wall of your small intestine is lined with many small projections called villi (see inset). Villi serve to increase the surface area available for food to be absorbed by the small intestine.

The Large Intestine

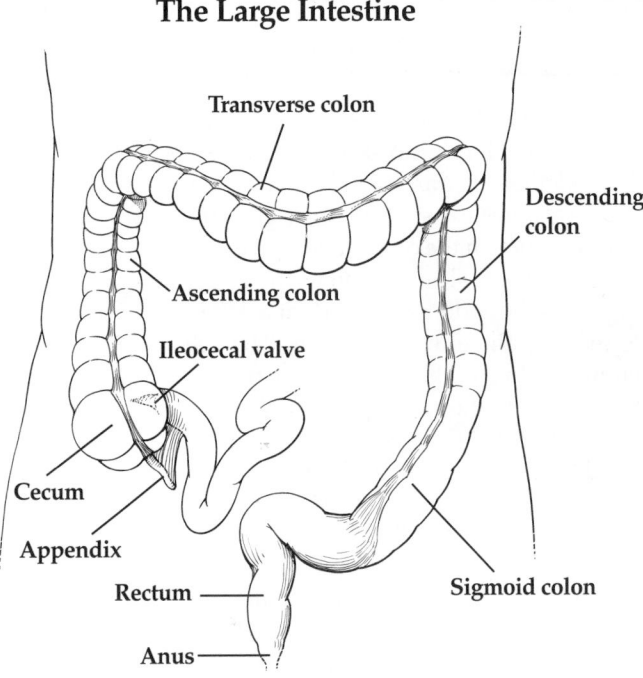

more water may be reabsorbed, leaving the stool uncomfortably hard. The value of dietary fiber is especially important because it not only increases the bulk of the feces but also keeps the feces relatively moist because the fiber absorbs fluid.

Microorganisms in the colon break down some of the dietary fiber and other waste products in the stool that are not digested by the stomach and small intestine. A part of the waste product of this digestive action is rectal gas.

The large intestine on occasion may become inflamed or infected. For various reasons, this part of the digestive tract is also subject to more tumors and polyps than any other.

Infections of the Gastrointestinal Tract

Signs and Symptoms

- Watery diarrhea, at times bloody
- Cramping abdominal pain
- Low-grade fever
- Nausea or vomiting or both
- Occasional muscle aches and headaches

Emergency Symptoms—Profuse diarrhea to the point of causing light-headedness

Infections of the gastrointestinal tract are extremely common throughout the world.

In developing countries, diarrhea caused by infection is the leading cause of death in children.

Improvements in sanitation and hygiene have had a significant impact on preventing many of these infections, particularly those transmitted by contaminated food and water. Even so, the Centers for Disease Control estimates that more than 25 million infections of the gastrointestinal tract occur each year in the United States and cause more than 10,000 deaths.

Viruses account for well over half of the infections of the gastrointestinal tract. In addition, there are infections by bacteria and infestations by parasites. In this section, we describe the common causes of infections of the gastrointestinal tract.

Viral Infections

Acute viral gastroenteritis is the second most common disease in the United States, upper respiratory tract infections being the most common. Normally, the symptoms consist of diarrhea, nausea, vomiting, low-grade fever, abdominal cramps, and muscle pains.

Acute viral gastroenteritis may be severe and may cause death in infants, in elderly or debilitated persons, or in persons whose immune systems are suppressed by disease or certain medications. Viral gastroenteritis also may occur in older children and adults and may be the cause of considerable discomfort and of time lost from school or work.

Many of these viruses are passed by fecal to oral transmission. Hand washing is a key to preventing transmission of the virus to others.

For practical purposes there are no specific tests, including "stool tests," to diagnose these illnesses. Your physician will often make the diagnosis based on your symptoms and similar cases in the community.

Generally, in these persons the infection resolves over time. Antibiotics are not effective. The use of antidiarrheal drugs is to be avoided because these medications may prevent elimination of the virus and, thus, may prolong the infection.

Many types of viruses can cause acute viral gastroenteritis. However, the most common are those caused by the rotavirus and the Norwalk virus.

Rotavirus

Rotavirus is the most common cause of infectious diarrhea in developed countries such as the United States. It is a frequently identified cause of diarrhea in children younger than 2. It also is the most common source of diarrhea in children attending child-care centers. Rotavirus occasionally causes epidemics of infection among the elderly in nursing homes. The peak frequency of rotavirus infections in the United States is during the winter. The virus is transmitted from one person to another.

The incubation period is 1 to 3 days. Typical symptoms include watery (nonbloody) diarrhea, vomiting, and low-grade fever lasting 5 to 8 days.

There is no specific treatment for rotavirus gastroenteritis. Current research centers on the development of a vaccine.

Norwalk Virus

The Norwalk virus is an important cause of outbreaks of gastroenteritis in families and communities, particularly in older children and adults. This disorder also is called winter vomiting disease, a reflection of the most common accompanying symptoms (vomiting) and the time of the year when most cases occur. In addition to diarrhea, nausea, and vomiting, many persons with this disorder experience muscle aches.

This virus usually is found in contaminated food or drinking water. The incubation period from the time of ingestion of the contaminated food or water to the onset of symptoms ranges from 4 to 72 hours.

Other Causes of Viral Gastroenteritis

Cytomegalovirus is a common cause of diarrhea in immunosuppressed persons. This virus is not uncommon in those with AIDS (see AIDS, page 1060). Gancyclovir is sometimes effective in treating cytomegalovirus-induced diarrhea.

Gastrointestinal infections with herpes simplex virus are frequent in homosexual men, heterosexual women who engage in anal intercourse, and immunosuppressed individuals. Generally, persons infected with the herpes simplex virus experience anal pain, constipation, and bloody diarrhea. These persons also may have neurologic symptoms, particularly posterior thigh pain or numbness or tingling of the buttock or anal area. Treatment generally is supportive, consisting of analgesics, warm sitz baths, and stool softeners. The antiviral drug acyclovir can decrease the severity of the initial attack and the chance of later relapses.

Bacterial Infections

Bacterial causes of infectious diarrhea often are easier to identify than viral causes. Most outbreaks of infectious gastroenteritis caused by bacteria are self-limiting and do not need specific treatment. In some cases, antibiotics are useful.

Many kinds of bacteria can cause diarrheal disease. In this section we will discuss some of the more common varieties.

Campylobacter

Campylobacter infections occur in all age groups, but the largest percentage occurs in children younger than 1 and in young adults. Campylobacter may be the most common bacterial cause of infectious diarrhea in young adults. Infections with this organism generally occur in the summer and fall.

The most common source of Campylobacter appears to be contaminated food, particularly raw milk and poultry.

The incubation period from exposure to onset of symptoms is 2 to 4 days. The illness may have an abrupt onset, with the appearance of abdominal pain, nausea, low-grade fever, headaches, and muscle pains. If you become infected, you may experience many bowel movements per day. In severe cases, the stools may be bloody.

This illness rarely lasts longer than 1 week. Occasionally, you may experience a relapse or a prolongation of your illness. Because the illness is self-limited, antibiotic treatment often is not necessary. Antidiarrheal agents should not be used because they may delay clearing of this organism from your system and thus prolong the symptoms. If the symptoms are severe, an antibiotic such as erythromycin or tetracycline can be given.

Salmonella

Salmonella has been implicated as responsible for about a third of the cases of diarrhea from contaminated food. Salmonella generally originates within the food itself (as opposed to from the hands of infected food handlers). The population thought to be at greatest risk are those at the extremes of age—the very young and the very old. Salmonella infections generally occur in the summer and fall.

Recently, some evidence has been found to suggest that Salmonella occurs in animals treated with antibiotics. The use of tetracycline for growth promotion in animals may increase the risk of a Salmonella infection in individuals who consume meats from these animals. The potential risk to consumers is now an area of intense investigation.

The *Salmonella* bacteria commonly are found in meats, poultry, eggs, unpasteurized cheese and milk, chocolate made from contaminated cocoa beans, and contaminated marijuana. Pet turtles also are a common source of infection. The disease can be passed by the fecal-oral route. For example, if you change your infected baby's diaper, fail to wash your hands properly, and then sit down to dinner, you could become infected. When *Salmonella*-infected food is not cooked adequately or thawed properly, you may acquire the infection. The symptoms of *Salmonella* include abdominal cramps, diarrhea, nausea, vomiting, and fever.

If you have the symptoms of *Salmonella* infection, your physician may test your stool for the organism. In most cases, the infection clears on its own and only supportive treatment (hydration) is needed. In some people, *Salmonella* can cause a severe and prolonged illness, and antibiotic treatment is necessary. In these cases, the stool is tested to make sure that an effective antibiotic is chosen for the particular type of *Salmonella*.

Shigella

Shigella is an important cause of bacterial gastroenteritis in the developing world and in travelers to these areas. It also occasionally occurs in outbreaks in the United States. This disorder is most common in children ages 1 through 5.

Shigella is transmitted primarily from person to person by the fecal-oral route. Outbreaks can occur in child-care centers. Occasionally, outbreaks can be caused by contamination of food by infected food handlers.

The usual symptoms are watery diarrhea associated with cramping, abdominal pain, and fever. Occasionally, you may pass blood and mucus.

Generally, the disease is self-limited. Antibiotics may be effective in shortening the duration of the diarrhea and in eliminating *Shigella* from the gastrointestinal tract. The usual drug of choice is ampicillin, and it can be given orally after appropriate stool cultures have been obtained. Alternative medications include trimethoprim-sulfamethoxazole and tetracycline.

Escherichia coli

There are various subgroups of the organism called *Escherichia coli* (*E. coli*). The source for this infection usually is contaminated food and water. Incompletely cooked hamburgers at fast food restaurants have been the source of disease caused by a relatively newly described *E. coli*.

If the diarrhea is mild, generally no treatment is necessary other than rehydration. For more severe or prolonged symptoms, an antibiotic such as trimethoprim-sulfamethoxazole, sulfamethoxazole, or ciprofloxacin often is prescribed. Antidiarrheal medications should not be used because they delay elimination of the organism.

Parasitic Infestation

Parasitic infestations are the least common of the three major causes of diarrheal diseases.

Giardia lamblia

This parasitic organism causes giardiasis, which is probably the most common parasitic cause of diarrhea in the United States. Outbreaks of giardiasis can occur in communities where the water supply is contaminated by raw sewage. Giardiasis also may be contracted by drinking water from lakes or mountain streams far from human habitation, in which case beavers are often thought to be the source of infection.

As many as two-thirds of the persons with giardiasis have no symptoms. However, they may pass the infestation to others. Those who do develop symptoms typically have watery diarrhea, abdominal cramps, and weight loss. Generally, these symptoms occur 1 to 3 weeks after exposure. The stools may be foul-smelling, greasy-looking, and floating. Bloating and distention also may occur. Low-grade fever may be present. These symptoms usually last for 5 to 7 days, although some people have problems for months.

This infestation can be diagnosed by examining the stool under the microscope to look for the characteristic organism. Giardiasis is treated with metronidazole or quinacrine hydrochloride. Follow-up stool examinations are important because the medications frequently do not eliminate the parasite entirely.

Entamoeba histolytica

Entamoeba histolytica is a common cause of diarrheal disease throughout the world, although it is relatively uncommon in the United States. Infection generally occurs from person to person through the fecal-oral route. This organism is a common cause of diarrhea in homosexual men.

If this organism is identified as the cause of diarrhea, your physician may recommend treatment with metronidazole. Other drugs sometimes are used.

Cryptosporidium

Cryptosporidium is a common cause of diarrhea in patients with acquired immunodeficiency syndrome (AIDS) (see page 1060). It can also cause illness in otherwise healthy persons. Epidemics have occurred as a result of contaminated public water supplies. If you are infected with this parasite you can experience prolonged watery diarrhea with up to 25 bowel movements per day. The diagnosis is based on examination of the stool. In otherwise healthy individuals, the infection resolves without treatment in 1 to 2 weeks. In persons with AIDS, the infection usually is chronic. There is no effective treatment, although several promising drugs currently are undergoing study.

Treatment

As noted in the descriptions above, most of these infestations of the gastrointestinal tract are self-limited. The primary danger is dehydration following the loss of fluids and electrolytes in the stool. Therefore, the primary goal of treatment is replacement of fluids and these essential electrolytes.

Recently, it has been learned that replacement of fluids orally may be more effective than replacement of fluids through a vein. Thus, your physician may recommend fluid replacement by mouth if this can be tolerated. At other times, particularly if there is severe dehydration or vomiting, he or she may recommend intravenous therapy.

For most infections, the use of antidiarrheal agents is not appropriate. These agents may retard the elimination of the causative organism and thus prolong the disease. However, there are some situations, particularly in mild diseases, in which your physician may recommend their use (see Traveler's Diarrhea, page 383).

Antibiotic-Associated Diarrhea

Signs and Symptoms

- Diarrhea occurring during or shortly after antibiotic therapy
- Abdominal cramps
- Fever

Antibiotics, most commonly clindamycin, ampicillin, cephalosporins, and the aminoglycosides, can cause diarrhea. Usually, the diarrhea is a result of the antibiotic altering the environment of the bowel, which permits certain bacteria to flourish. This may cause inflammation of the colon.

Antibiotic-associated diarrhea is fairly common, affecting up to 25 percent of clindamycin users and up to 10 percent of those who take ampicillin. The most serious form of antibiotic-associated diarrhea is pseudomembranous colitis.

Typically, the symptoms of diarrhea begin 4 to 10 days after the antibiotic treatment is begun. However, in as many as 25 percent the symptoms do not develop until the antibiotic has been discontinued. The symptoms usually abate after the drug is discontinued.

Diagnosis

If your physician suspects that your diarrhea is related to the use of antibiotics, he or she

---

Food Poisoning

Food poisoning is caused by the ingestion of contaminated food. Its symptoms usually include diarrhea and nausea. Vomiting, loss of appetite, and stomachache also may occur.

The most common cause of food poisoning is due to the toxin produced by the bacterium *Staphylococcus aureus*. When this organism contaminates certain foods (often via the hands of a food handler), it multiplies rapidly. This explains why staphylococcal food poisoning often occurs in outbreaks, especially when cream pastries, mayonnaise-containing foods, or potato salad is the vehicle for the bacterium.

Other potential causes of food poisoning include *Bacillus cereus*, *Clostridium botulinum* (see Botulism, page 488), *Salmonella*, *Escherichia coli*, *Campylobacter jejuni*, and Norwalk virus (see Infections of the Gastrointestinal Tract, page 766).

What to Do

In most cases, the discomforts of food poisoning pass in a few hours. After the vomiting or diarrhea ends, consume clear liquids for the first 12 hours; then, limit food intake to bland foods for the following 24 hours. For very young children, the elderly, or persons who are ill with other ailments, consult your physician.

Prevention

The best strategy is to avoid food poisoning. Keep all meats and leftovers refrigerated. Beware of any food contaminated by uncooked meat juices; wash it thoroughly before eating it. Do not eat foods contaminated with molds.

will perform tests on a sample of stool. If you have pseudomembranous colitis, a toxin from a common causative organism, *Clostridium difficile*, may be found.

How Serious Is Antibiotic-Associated Diarrhea?

Many people do well after discontinuing the antibiotic; others become extremely ill and have persistent diarrhea and dehydration. On occasion, pseudomembranous colitis may develop into a life-threatening situation.

Treatment

Your physician will stop treatment with any antibiotic that may be causing your diarrhea.

If your symptoms are mild, your physician may prescribe cholestyramine, which binds to and therefore eliminates the offending toxin of the *Clostridium difficile* organism. For more severe cases, either vancomycin or metronidazole can be used.

Relapses are not unusual and usually require one or more additional courses of treatment.

Malabsorption Problems

Signs and Symptoms
- Weight loss
- Diarrhea
- Abdominal cramps, gas, and bloating
- General weakness
- Foul-smelling or grayish stools that may be fatty or oily

If the process of digestion is to go smoothly, the nutrients contained in the food you eat must be broken down (digested) into molecules that can be absorbed into your bloodstream. Sometimes, for various reasons, these nutrients are not completely digested or their absorption is impaired. When this occurs, vital nutrients that should be used by your body instead are eliminated in the stool. The result of this malabsorption can be malnutrition.

Malabsorption can be caused by many different problems. If there is disease of the pancreas, enzymes necessary to digestion may be absent, and malabsorption may be the result. This is often called maldigestion. Because most of the absorption takes place in the small intestine, a disease here may lead to the loss of vital nutrients in the stool.

A principal sign of malabsorption is steatorrheal stools. This results from an excessive loss of fat in the stool. The stool may be gray or pale and somewhat larger than normal. The excessive fat content may cause the stool to be more malodorous than normal. In addition to fat, protein is also lost in the stool, resulting in wasting of the body's tissues.

Malabsorption may cause a deficiency of vitamins A, B_{12}, D, E, and K and folic acid because these valuable nutrients are lost in the stool. Low blood levels of vitamin B_{12} and folic acid strongly suggest malabsorption. With continued loss of fat in the stool, calcium may be lost in excessive amounts and two rather unexpected consequences may occur: urinary stones of calcium oxalate form (see page 844), and a demineralizing state of the bones called osteomalacia develops (see page 896).

Some of the most likely causes of small bowel malabsorption are discussed below. For another common cause of malabsorption, see Chronic Pancreatitis, page 819.

Celiac (Nontropical) Sprue

Celiac (nontropical) sprue is a common cause of malabsorption. This disease is caused by a sensitivity to gluten, a protein found in wheat, rye, oats, and barley. The intolerance to gluten causes the lining of the intestine to lose its tiny folds (villi) through which nutrients are absorbed. In addition, digestive enzymes are no longer produced in the intestinal lining in adequate amounts. The common symptoms are foul-smelling diarrheal stools, bloated abdomen, and anemia.

Celiac sprue often occurs in children. In these children, the most dramatic symptoms are weight loss and failure to grow. The bony changes of rickets may be seen in children; in adults, osteomalacia may occur with bone pain and tenderness (see Osteomalacia and Rickets, page 896).

In addition to examining your stool to see if it contains excessive amounts of fat, if your physician suspects celiac disease, he or she may order a barium X-ray of your small bowel (see The Barium X-Ray, page 762). Biopsy of the lining of the small intestine is also usually done by using a device inserted through the mouth. The specimen is examined under the microscope for the characteristic changes of nontropical sprue.

Celiac disease usually is treated by eliminating from the diet those foods containing gluten. To correct certain nutrient deficiencies, initially you may be given vitamin and mineral supplements. Your physician or dietitian will instruct you in a proper gluten-free diet. They may also give you the names of gluten-free diet cookbooks and of support groups in your area.

If a gluten-free diet is carefully followed, the villi of the small intestine will resume their normal shape and absorption ability over a period of several months. Your stools will return to normal, and you will stop losing weight. The gluten-free diet must be followed indefinitely or the symptoms will return (see page 285).

Tropical Sprue

This is another disease that causes malabsorption. It affects visitors to tropical regions of the world. The symptoms can appear many months or even years after the affected person returns from the tropics. The cause of this disease is uncertain but it may be an infectious microorganism.

People with tropical sprue may suffer from diarrhea, weight loss, anemia, and inability to gain weight.

The diagnostic tests are basically the same as those for celiac sprue.

Treatment for tropical sprue generally consists of a folic acid and vitamin supplement and an antibiotic such as tetracycline. Usually, no special diet is required. Depending on the severity of the disease, you may be on antibiotics for as long as 6 months.

Bacterial Overgrowth

Normally, overgrowth of bacteria in the small intestine is not a problem because the constant muscular movement of the intestine (peristalsis) removes the bacteria. However, under certain conditions, intestinal bacteria may grow to a point such that they cause malabsorption. This condition may be a factor contributing to the diarrhea in diabetics with bowel involvement.

The cause of bacterial overgrowth most often is an impairment of peristalsis which allows bacteria to accumulate. Bacterial overgrowth also is seen after bowel surgery in which segments of the small bowel are bypassed. The diagnosis is made by cultures of samples taken from the small bowel or sometimes by indirect tests that involve collections of blood, breath, or urine. The treatment is antibiotics, often given in a cyclical fashion, such as 1 week out of each month.

Scleroderma

When scleroderma affects the intestine, it causes atrophy of its muscular walls, which can impair both absorption of nutrients and movement of the intestine. Scleroderma also may affect the muscular lining of the esophagus and cause heartburn (see Scleroderma of the Esophagus, page 744).

Because the disease is progressive and can spread to other organs, clinically it is known as progressive systemic sclerosis (PSS) (see page 919). The cause of this chronic disease is unknown. It may be associated with severe diarrhea caused by bacterial overgrowth. Antibiotics given in cyclical fashion (such as for 1 week of each month) may be helpful.

AIDS

Another disease that produces problems of malabsorption is AIDS, acquired immunodeficiency syndrome (see page 1060). The primary symptoms, diarrhea and weight loss, in patients with AIDS are thought to be the result of infections in the small intestine and colon.

Whipple's Disease

This malabsorption disorder primarily affects men older than 45. The disease is caused by an infectious organism that was only recently identified. Symptoms such as diarrhea, abdominal pain, progressive weight loss, and a darkening of the skin may occur as well as arthritis that may date back several years. The bacterial infection also may produce a low-grade fever. The diagnosis is made by a biopsy of the small bowel.

The long-term (12 to 18 months) use of antibiotics typically is effective in correcting malabsorption due to Whipple's disease.

Amyloidosis

This is a disease produced by the presence of a protein, called amyloid, that has starch-like qualities. Depending on where the unwanted deposits of this protein appear in the body, the consequences can be either insignificant or severe. For example, a buildup of amyloid in the small intestine will make the lining rubbery, firm, and waxy and result in serious malabsorption. The diagnosis of this condition is made by small bowel biopsy.

There is no known method of preventing the formation of amyloid deposits. Treatment is geared toward relieving symptoms or treating an underlying disorder that may be responsible for the amyloidosis (see page 974). Such disorders are tuberculosis, Hodgkin's disease, and rheumatoid arthritis.

Lactose Intolerance

Lactose, the principal sugar in cow's milk and found only in milk and dairy products, requires the enzyme lactase for its digestion. Lactose intolerance occurs when the lining of the walls of the small intestine produces reduced amounts of this enzyme.

Lactose intolerance causes abdominal cramps, bloating, diarrhea, and excessive gas when more than a certain amount of milk is ingested. Small amounts of milk usually do not produce symptoms. A low level of lactase in the lining of the small intestine actually may be the normal state in that 70 percent or so of the world's population is affected. Lactose intolerance is uncommon in Northern and Western European whites and their descendants in the United States. Lower levels of lactase occur more commonly in the United States among people of Mediterranean, African, or Asian origin. It is believed that more than 30 million Americans have some degree of lactose intolerance.

Low lactase levels may occur in association with other malabsorptive diseases such as nontropical or tropical sprue, viral or bacterial infection of the small intestine (see pages 770 and 771), and cystic fibrosis (see page 720).

If you have lactose intolerance, you need not eliminate dairy products totally from your diet. Rather, decrease your consumption of milk products, drink milk only during meals, and try to get your calcium from cheese and yogurt, dairy products that are lower in lactose than milk is. Another alternative is to buy a commercial lactase preparation, such as Lactaid or Dairy Ease, that can be mixed into your milk. These preparations convert lactose into simple sugars that can be easily absorbed.

Short-Bowel Syndrome

After surgical removal of a significant portion of the intestine, some persons have malabsorption problems. This condition is referred to as short-bowel syndrome. Because different nutrients are absorbed in different areas of the small intestine, the effect surgery has on nutrient absorption depends on how much and what part of the intestine was removed. Unless some critical part of the bowel was removed, the remaining portion usually is capable of adapting to accommodate more absorption and thus prevent the malabsorption of nutrients. The exception is the lower part of the small intestine just before it joins the colon. Removal (or significant disease) of a small segment of this area may result in diarrhea.

Acute Appendicitis

Signs and Symptoms

- Pain starting in the upper abdomen or around the navel and settling in the lower right side of the abdomen
- Nausea and vomiting
- Urge to pass stool or gas
- Lack of appetite

The appendix, a worm-shaped structure that projects out from the first section of the large intestine, is about 3½ inches long and

---

Diabetic Intestinal Disorders

Long-standing diabetes may result in decreased function of the nerves that control the muscular activity of the stomach and the remainder of the intestinal tract.

A condition called diabetic gastroparesis results, and there is diminished mixing in and propulsive activity by the stomach. Over time, the stomach begins to resemble a limp bag and gradually enlarges. If affected, periodically you may vomit rather large amounts of fluid and partially digested food that has been consumed as much as a day or two before. The unpredictability of the movement of food from the stomach into the intestine makes regulation of the diabetes very difficult. Drugs such as metoclopramide or cisapride sometimes are effective in treating this disorder.

When the intestines are the primary site of deterioration of nerves, the propulsive action of the intestine is impaired. The diarrhea tends to occur at night and, because of impaired sensation and function of the anal sphincter, there may be fecal incontinence during sleep. Some degree of malabsorption may be seen, but this may be the result of the simultaneous occurrence of bacterial overgrowth (see page 771), nontropical sprue (see page 770), or pancreatic insufficiency (see Chronic Pancreatitis, page 819).

In some instances, administration of antibiotics in a cyclical fashion (such as 1 week of each month) will control the diarrhea. This suggests that bacterial overgrowth in the poorly moving small intestine is responsible.

At other times, the diarrhea may be the result of impaired function of the nerves to the gut. Occasionally, a medicine called clonidine is effective in this situation.

has a cavity running down its center. It has no known function or importance in humans. It is not clear as to why on occasion the appendix will become inflamed, swollen, and filled with pus, producing appendicitis.

Those most likely to have an acute appendicitis attack are between the ages of 10 and 30, although it can strike at almost any age. Death due to acute appendicitis is rare. Appendicitis often is more difficult to diagnose in infants and the very old.

Diagnosis

Your physician will ask you questions about your symptoms, including whether you have lost your appetite, have discomfort on urination, or have an unusual urge to pass gas or move your bowels. Your abdomen will be examined carefully, and a rectal examination will be performed. Abdominal tenderness is an important sign.

If you have acute appendicitis, you will be admitted to a hospital immediately. Depending on your symptoms, a blood test and a urine analysis may be done.

How Serious Is Appendicitis?

Peritonitis, a serious infection of the lining of the abdominal cavity (peritoneum), may develop if the appendix bursts.

Treatment

Surgery

The standard procedure is to remove the infected appendix surgically. Removal of the appendix does not affect digestion.

Meckel's Diverticulum

A diverticulum is a sac or pouch that forms in a weakened section of the wall of the bowel. Meckel's diverticulum is an example of a congenital type of diverticulum. This pouch generally forms in the lower part of the small intestine (ileum). Typically, such diverticula are about 2 inches long.

Although this common disorder frequently presents no symptoms, the diverticulum can become inflamed and bleed. In some cases, especially among young children, bleeding may occur as the result of an ulcer that has formed at the same site. If inflammation of a Meckel diverticulum becomes severe, it can obstruct the intestine or perforate the intestinal wall. The treatment

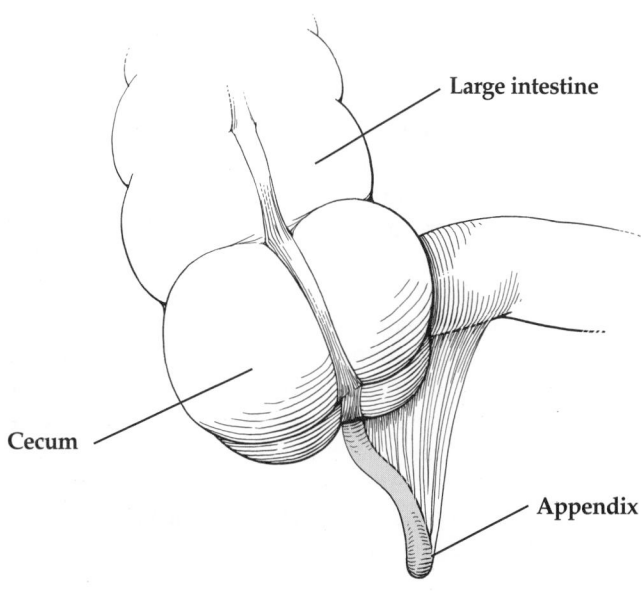

Large intestine

Cecum

Appendix

The worm-shaped appendix is attached to the cecum; it has no known function in humans. The appendix can become inflamed and lead to a medical emergency.

of any of these complications is surgical removal of the diverticulum.

Intussusception

Signs and Symptoms

- Sudden severe abdominal pain
- Weakness and lethargy
- Vomiting, often with bile
- Bloody stools that may resemble currant jelly
- Shallow breathing
- Shock

Intussusception is a rare disorder in which a portion of the intestine, usually of the small intestine, telescopes into another segment of the intestine. This is the most common cause of intestinal obstruction in children between the ages of 3 months and 6 years.

The cause is unknown, but in some cases there has been a correlation between intussusception and certain viral infections.

Typically, intussusception strikes abruptly in a previously well child. The child suddenly has a severe pain that occurs at frequent intervals. At first, the child may play normally between the pains but soon becomes weaker and lethargic.

Diagnosis

If your child has these symptoms, do not delay in calling your physician. The symptoms and physical findings may be sufficient to establish the diagnosis. Often, however, further tests such as an abdominal X-ray or a barium X-ray may be done (see The Barium X-Ray, page 762).

How Serious Is Intussusception?

If left untreated, intussusception may be very serious. Most children recover, however, if treatment is begun within 24 hours after the initial symptoms.

Treatment

The barium enema used for diagnosis may be sufficient to push the telescoped intestine back into its proper place. The recurrence rate after this "treatment," however, may be as high as 10 percent. In many cases, surgery is necessary; generally there is no recurrence after surgery.

Protein-Losing Enteropathy

Signs and Symptoms

- Blood in the stool
- Generalized swelling of tissues

Some gastrointestinal disorders cause protein in the blood (plasma protein) to be discharged into the gastrointestinal tract and excreted in the stool. Plasma protein may pass into the gastrointestinal tract through an inflamed or ulcerated intestinal lining such as in cases of regional enteritis and ulcerative colitis (see page 777).

The result of loss of protein in the stool is low blood protein, which in turn can cause a generalized swelling (edema) of tissues.

Intestinal lymphangiectasia is a type of protein-losing enteropathy in which swelling of the lymph channels of the small intestine leads to loss of protein and fat from the lymph channels into the gut. Children and young adults are most commonly affected by this disorder.

The principal treatment is a low-fat diet.

Primary (Idiopathic) Intestinal Pseudo-Obstruction

Signs and Symptoms

- Sudden attacks of abdominal pain
- Nausea and vomiting
- Weight loss

Although not truly an intestinal obstruction, the intestines function improperly, as if

they were obstructed. They become distended and you may experience acute attacks of abdominal pain, nausea, and vomiting. Malabsorption (see page 770) may accompany this disorder, with subsequent weight loss. Because the cause is unknown, physicians sometimes call this condition idiopathic intestinal pseudo-obstruction. If an underlying disease such as scleroderma (see page 771) or diabetes (see page 725) is the cause, the term "secondary intestinal pseudo-obstruction" is used.

Treatment of intestinal pseudo-obstruction is difficult. Special diets are ineffective. If the disorder is severe, liquid nutrients can sometimes be administered into a vein, thus bypassing your stomach. This can be done on a temporary basis in the hospital or on a permanent basis in your home (home parenteral nutrition).

Carcinoid Syndrome

Signs and Symptoms

- Flushing of the skin
- Diarrhea

Carcinoid tumors are slowly growing malignancies, usually in the ileum, the lower section of the small intestine. These tumors may spread to the liver and also may metastasize to the lungs and other organs.

Occasionally, carcinoid tumors can cause flushing of the skin and diarrhea (carcinoid syndrome). With this complication, detection of excessive levels of a normal body chemical in the urine is an important biochemical indicator of this type of tumor.

The objective of treatment is to decrease the mass of the tumor by either chemotherapy or surgery. Depending on how soon the cancer is detected and where it is located, some people fully recover after surgical treatment. Many live 5 to 10 years after the cancer has spread (metastasized) because the tumor grows slowly. Death usually results from heart or liver failure when the cancer reaches these organs.

Crohn's Disease

Signs and Symptoms

- Chronic diarrhea
- Low-grade fever
- Fatigue

- Weight loss
- Abdominal cramps and pain around the navel or on the right side of the abdomen
- Joint pain
- Skin lesions

Inflammatory bowel disease is a term generally used to describe two disorders that involve the gastrointestinal tract and for which no cause has been found. These disorders are Crohn's disease and ulcerative colitis (see page 777).

Crohn's disease, sometimes referred to as ileitis, regional enteritis, or granulomatous colitis, is a chronic inflammation of the intestine. It mainly involves the ileum (the lower part of the small intestine). However, it also can affect your colon or any other part of your digestive tract. The inflammation often involves the entire thickness of the bowel wall.

Crohn's disease is uncommon, occurring in about 1 to 5 per 10,000 people. Children and adults may be affected.

Heredity or environmental influences may play a role in the development of Crohn's disease. About 1 out of 4 patients with Crohn's disease has a relative with Crohn's or ulcerative colitis.

With proper nutrition and medical management, people with Crohn's disease usually can lead normal lives.

Diagnosis

The symptoms of Crohn's disease may include persistent diarrhea, abdominal pain, fever, and general fatigue. Occasionally, there may be blood in the stool. Often, a significant weight loss occurs.

Barium X-rays of the small intestine and of the colon usually reveal abnormal areas. Segments of intestine appear irregular and less flexible than normal (see The Barium X-Ray, page 762). Sometimes your physician may use a colonoscope (see page 788) to visualize the lining of your colon and the last several inches of your ileum.

How Serious Is Crohn's Disease?

The course of Crohn's disease varies greatly from one person to another. Many people with Crohn's disease remain completely without symptoms (asymptomatic) after the initial one or two episodes of disease. However, many others have recurrent episodes of abdominal pain, diarrhea, and low-grade fever.

The diarrhea itself can be debilitating to the point of significant malnourishment. Episodes of abdominal pain, reflecting gradually increasing bowel obstruction, may reach the point such that you avoid eating because of discomfort.

The complications of Crohn's disease are many and varied. Progressive obstruction, particularly of the small bowel, is the most common reason for surgical treatment in Crohn's disease. Obstructive symptoms generally develop gradually over a long period.

Fistulas and fissures in and around the anal and rectal areas also are common. A fistula is an abnormal passage between two segments of the intestine or from the intestine to the skin. Fistulas can develop from the intestine to the vagina or bladder. An anal fissure is a crack or cleft in the anus or skin around the anus (see Anal Fissures and Fistulas, page 796). When internal fistulas develop, food bypasses areas of the bowel necessary for absorption. In external fistulas, there can be continuous drainage of bowel contents to the skin. Sometimes infections occur in these areas. Bleeding also may occur with Crohn's disease, although it generally is not massive in nature.

Often, the progressive obstruction, the inflamed mass of tissue, or the fistula does not respond to medical therapy and may require surgery. Perforation of the bowel or massive bleeding is rare.

If you have Crohn's disease, it is not uncommon to have symptoms and signs apart from the digestive tract but related to the

Barium X-ray shows Crohn's disease. Arrow indicates narrowing of the lower portion of the small intestine (ileum).

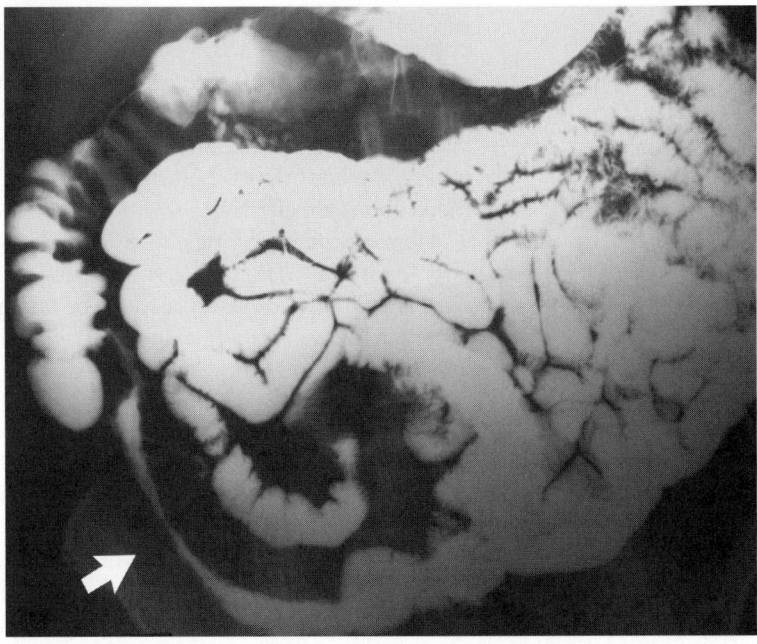

bowel disease. These may involve arthritis, particularly of large joints, or inflammation involving the eye or skin. Occasionally, inflammation of the bile ducts may be associated with Crohn's disease (see Primary Sclerosing Cholangitis, page 814). In addition, the development of kidney stones is common with Crohn's disease. Crohn's disease is chronic, but there may be periods of remission.

Treatment

Medication

There is no cure for Crohn's disease. If your Crohn's disease is asymptomatic or in remission, treatment may be unnecessary. If your symptoms are mild, perhaps involving several loose stools per day, your physician may prescribe an antidiarrheal pill or a bulk former that contains vegetable fibers.

If your disease is more active, your physician may consider anti-inflammatory medications such as sulfasalazine and corticosteroids. Sulfasalazine is particularly effective if your colon is involved.

If sulfasalazine is not tolerated or is ineffective, mesalamine tablets can be used. Mesalamine contains the agent 5-ASA, which is also the active ingredient in sulfasalazine, but in a higher dose. Mesalamine is also available as a suppository and as an enema for use when the Crohn's disease is limited to the lower part of the colon.

Corticosteroid enemas are also useful in Crohn's disease of the lower colon. Oral corticosteroids are reserved for more significant flare-ups of the disease. They are effective for both colonic and small bowel involvement. Some physicians may recommend a course of immunosuppressive therapy with drugs such as azathioprine or 6-mercaptopurine. It takes a few months of therapy before these medications are effective.

Metronidazole may be effective, particularly for fistulas or fissures in the anal region. Generally, this medication needs to be taken indefinitely not only to heal the fistula or fissure but also to prevent recurrence. At times, metronidazole is used for Crohn's disease of the colon. Metronidazole may cause numbness or tingling in the fingers and toes if used for many months at a time. If this occurs, discuss it with your physician.

None of these medications cure Crohn's disease. They are used as anti-inflammatory agents to provide relief from symptoms.

Currently, investigators are studying new preparations of corticosteroids and other medications that have fewer side effects and more potent anti-inflammatory activity.

Nutrition

The ability to absorb adequate nutrients often is limited in people with Crohn's disease, particularly if the disease affects significant portions of the small bowel or if portions of the small bowel have been removed surgically.

Your physician may advise specific replacement of certain vitamins or minerals if there is evidence of deficiency. It is not uncommon that persons with Crohn's disease have a deficiency of vitamin B_{12}, which is absorbed in the lower segment (ileum) of the small bowel. If this occurs, vitamin B_{12} can be easily replaced with monthly injections through the skin.

Bile acids also are absorbed in the lower portion of the small bowel. If the bile acids are not absorbed in the small bowel, they may cause diarrhea by interfering with the absorption of water in the colon. At times, the use of a bile acid binder, such as cholestyramine, is effective in decreasing the amount of stool.

Some physicians advocate the use of elemental diets consisting of liquid preparations that contain simple sugars, amino acids, and minerals, particularly for active Crohn's disease if you are malnourished. Some affected persons need to receive their nutrition intravenously for weeks, or even months, during severe bouts of Crohn's disease. Avoiding oral intake of food allows the bowel to rest.

Surgery

Approximately 70 percent of those with Crohn's disease require at least one operation at some point. These operations usually are performed for complications such as obstruction, abscesses, or perforation. Although surgical treatment may alleviate the symptoms for several years, it is not a cure. Most often the disease recurs.

In people with Crohn's disease limited to the colon, removal of the large intestine may be recommended, particularly if medical treatment fails. In this operation, the entire colon, rectum, and anus are removed, and the end of the ileum (the last section of the small intestine) is brought out through the abdominal wall for the passage of stool. This is called an ileostomy. A plastic pouch into which the stool is evacuated is attached to the skin around the opening (stoma) (see Colostomy and Ileostomy, this page).

When the disease is limited to the small intestine, surgery typically involves removing the diseased segment of bowel and rejoining the two ends of healthy intestine.

Ulcerative Colitis

Signs and Symptoms
- Bloody diarrhea that may contain mucus
- Abdominal pain
- Painful, urgent bowel movements
- Fever
- Weight loss
- Joint pains
- Skin lesions

Ulcerative colitis is one of two disorders that are termed inflammatory bowel disease (see Crohn's disease, page 774). The causes of inflammatory bowel disease are unknown. Unlike Crohn's disease, which can involve any portion of the intestinal tract, ulcerative colitis is confined to the colon.

Ulcerative colitis is a chronic condition in which an inflammatory reaction characterized by tiny ulcers and small abscesses is limited to the inner lining (mucosa) of the colon. The inflammatory reactions almost always involve the rectum and extend into the rest of the colon. The amount of colon affected by the inflammatory process varies from person to person. If the inflammation is limited to the rectum, the term ulcerative proctitis sometimes is used.

Although this disease can strike at any

Colostomy and Ileostomy

Colostomy and ileostomy are surgical treatment options for diseases such as cancer or Crohn's disease. This alters the normal route for the elimination of waste. An opening (stoma) is created in the abdominal wall. A portion of intestine is brought out through the opening, and the stool is eliminated into a pouch (appliance) worn securely over the opening.

The main distinction between the two procedures is that during a colostomy a portion of the colon or large intestine is pulled through the abdominal wall, whereas an ileostomy involves bringing the end segment of the small intestine (ileum) through the opening.

Colostomy
During a colostomy, the surgeon makes an incision that permits examination of the colon and possibly removal of diseased areas. Sometimes the anus and rectum are also removed and the anal area is closed. A separate incision is then made in the abdomen, and a section of colon is pulled through this opening. A pouch is then securely fastened over the opening.

The feces then flow into the pouch, which is emptied periodically.

There are different types of colostomies, depending on what section of the colon is used. The consistency of the stool also de-

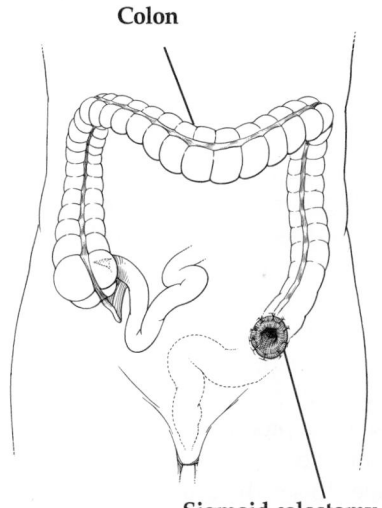

Colon

Sigmoid colostomy

In performing a sigmoid colostomy, the surgeon alters the normal route for waste excretion. The remaining intestine is brought through an opening (stoma) in the abdominal wall. Stool can be eliminated into a pouch worn securely over the opening.

pends on where the digestive process has been interrupted. For example, if the initial portion of the colon empties into the pouch, the stool will be loose; if the lower end of the colon is brought through the stoma, the stool will be formed because more of the liquid has been absorbed in the colon.

Although many stomas are permanent, sometimes a temporary stoma is done to allow a part of the bowel to heal after injury or disease. After the area is healed, the stoma is closed and the bowel is reconnected so that the normal elimination process can continue.

Ileostomy
This procedure is done when the entire colon and rectum are removed, often because of Crohn's disease.

During the conventional ileostomy, a portion of the small intestine is brought out through the opening created in the abdominal wall. As in the colostomy, the ileostomy requires that a pouch be worn over the stoma to collect the waste, which in this case has a liquid consistency because the digestive process has been halted before the colon, where much of the liquid normally is absorbed.

A variation of the ileostomy is being done in some medical centers. Called a continent ileostomy, or Kock pouch, this operation involves the creation of an internal pouch and valve for waste, the pouch and valve being constructed of a portion of the small intestine. This pouch can store your waste internally for several hours at a time, eliminating the need for an outside pouch. At your convenience, you insert a catheter (a thin tube) into the opening that has been created in your abdomen and drain the liquid feces from the internal pouch. The valve prevents the pouch from leaking at any other time.

Although most patients are squeamish at first about using the catheter, they soon get used to it, and it is painless. Initially, the pouch is emptied every few hours but after a while two to four times a day usually is adequate. The time required for the emptying usually is no more than if you were having a bowel movement.

The ileal pouch or Kock pouch

procedure is done in some situations if you have ulcerative colitis (see page 777) or hereditary polyposis (see Colon Polyps, page 786) and an ileo-anal anastomosis (see page 780) cannot be done. This procedure is not done if you are known to have Crohn's colitis.

Adjusting to the Change
No matter what type of colostomy or ileostomy you require, there will be a period of adjustment. A stomal therapist can be helpful in this period. In most situations, you can continue to lead a full and active life.

Physical Activity
In the 6 to 8 weeks immediately after the operation, avoid lifting, pushing, or pulling more than 5 to 10 pounds. As you begin to resume normal activities, the best single guide for what to do and not to do is what you were comfortable with prior to your operation. In general, walking, swimming, and simple exercise are good activities that will help firm your muscles and keep your digestive tract working properly.

Bathing
You may bathe or shower with or without the appliance over the stoma. However, long, hot baths or showers are to be avoided with the appliance attached. You may find that keeping the appliance above the water level in the bath or covering the area with a border of tape in a picture-frame shape will be helpful.

Sexuality
Most physicians advise abstention from sexual activity for a while after this operation. Sexual relations can be resumed thereafter: do not assume that your partner no longer cares for you sexually. Be patient and talk about the feelings each of you has.

You may find that certain positions are more comfortable than others. Sexual dysfunction is not uncommon immediately after the operation. If pain in the vagina or inability to achieve erection occurs, it may be temporary. If the problem continues after several months, discuss it with your physician.

Guidelines for driving a vehicle and other activities will be discussed with you by your physician.

---

time of life, its peak incidence is between the ages of 15 and 35. It is more common among whites. Like Crohn's disease, ulcerative colitis tends to run in some families.

Diagnosis
If you have the symptoms of ulcerative colitis, your physician will perform a flexible proctosigmoidoscopy, a procedure in which an instrument is inserted into the rectum to allow the examiner to see the lining of the lower portion of the colon and rectum (see Screening for Colon Cancer, page 790). A biopsy specimen can then be taken from the area. A barium X-ray (see page 762) or colonoscopy (see page 788) may also be done.

How Serious Is Ulcerative Colitis?
At times, ulcerative colitis may be without symptoms. At other times, inflammation of the colon may occur, causing bloody diar-

rhea. Such flare-ups may alternate with periods of remission.

For approximately 15 percent of persons with ulcerative colitis, the disease process may be quite serious, with inflammatory changes involving the entire colon. The symptoms are severe bloody diarrhea, fever, and abdominal pain. These symptoms may even constitute a medical emergency because there is a risk of dilation of the colon (toxic megacolon) or perforation of the markedly inflamed colon.

Ulcerative colitis also may be associated with various symptoms in other areas of your body. These may include pain or inflammation of large joints, most often the knees, ankles, and wrists. In some cases, ankylosing spondylitis (see page 914) may be associated with ulcerative colitis. Skin abnormalities that occur with ulcerative colitis include erythema nodosum (tender bumps that turn into dark areas that look like bruises) and pyoderma gangrenosum (chronic ulcers of the skin). Acute inflammation of the eye may also develop. Although uncommon (occurring in about 1 in 20 people with the disease), flow of the bile from the liver can be partially obstructed (see Primary Sclerosing Cholangitis, page 814).

In addition, for people whose colons are completely or almost completely involved by ulcerative colitis, there is an increased risk of cancer of the colon after the disease has been present for at least 8 to 10 years. In those persons who have lesser degrees of involvement (such as colitis involving only the left side of the colon) the risk is less and not apparent until 15 to 20 years after the onset of colitis. The risk of cancer increases with time. However, this risk is not dependent on the degree of inflammation. That is, cancer can develop despite the symptoms of ulcerative colitis being minimal.

Treatment

The goal of treatment is to control the inflammatory process, relieve the symptoms, and prevent complications.

Medication

The principal drugs used in the treatment of ulcerative colitis are the anti-inflammatory agents sulfasalazine, mesalamine, olsalazine, and corticosteroids.

Sulfasalazine is generally used for minor flare-ups of the disease and also in maintaining remissions. Mesalamine and olsalazine, are derivatives of sulfasalazine and contain the active ingredient 5-ASA. These drugs can be used if you can't tolerate sulfasalazine or if it is ineffective. Mesalamine is also available as a suppository or enema. Corticosteroids (see page 919) are used for more severe episodes of bloody diarrhea. If the inflammatory process is confined to the rectum, a corticosteroid enema may be useful in suppressing the inflammation and alleviating symptoms.

When the diarrhea is massive, hospitalization may be required to begin medical therapy, to provide hydration through a vein, and to place the bowel at rest by not using oral feedings. Recently, cyclosporine, a potent immunosuppressive agent, has shown promise in the treatment of severe ulcerative colitis.

Immunosuppressive therapy, with medications such as azathioprine or 6-mercaptopurine, is used occasionally with careful supervision by your physician.

Nutrition

No food has been shown to make ulcerative colitis better or worse. It's best to simply avoid foods that promptly cause discomfort.

Surgery

Approximately 20 to 25 percent of those with ulcerative colitis require surgery at some time. These are the people who do not respond to medication or who have severe complications. The present trend is to perform surgery earlier in the disease process, when it appears that the inflammation of the colon is unresponsive to medication, instead of waiting until the patient becomes debilitated. The operation most commonly done is total removal of the colon and rectum with ileo-anal anastomosis (see page 780). Unlike prior techniques, this is not disfiguring, preserves the passage of stool through the anus, and usually is well tolerated by most of those selected for the operation.

If you have had extensive ulcerative colitis for more than 8 to 10 years, your physician may recommend the elective removal of your entire colon for prevention of cancer (see Ileo-Anal Anastomosis, page 780). As an alternative, he or she may suggest periodic examination of your colon by colonoscopy (see page 788) to look for changes suggesting a transformation to malignant cells in your colon and to biopsy random areas.

Tumors of the Small Intestine

Signs and Symptoms
- Abdominal cramps and pain
- Bloody stools
- Nausea and vomiting
- Weight loss

Tumors of the small intestine are relatively uncommon—they represent only 3 to 6 percent of all abnormal growths in the gastrointestinal tract. Intestinal tumors can be benign or malignant.

Most tumors of the small bowel are benign and usually are discovered between ages 40 and 60. The most frequent symptoms are pain, nausea and vomiting, and bleeding. There are several types of benign tumors, including lipomas, leiomyomas, angiomas, and adenomas. These tumors do not spread.

Ileo-Anal Anastomosis

Not long ago, persons who underwent operation for ulcerative colitis had no choice but to have an ileostomy, a procedure in which the entire colon and rectum are removed and an opening in the abdominal wall is created for the passage of stool. After an ileostomy, these people need to wear a pouch over the opening at all times.

Now, the most common surgical procedure for ulcerative colitis is the ileo-anal anastomosis. During this procedure the entire colon and rectum are removed but the anal sphincter muscles are preserved. A pouch is made in the ileum (the last segment of the small intestine) and is brought down and sutured to the anus.

A temporary ileostomy (see Colostomy and Ileostomy, page 777) usually is created to allow the ileal pouch and its attachment to the anus to heal. After a period of time, this temporary ileostomy is closed and the feces are then expelled through the anus. This eliminates the need for wearing an external bag to collect the feces.

It should be noted that ileostomy is still done for some people with ulcerative colitis, particularly for elderly persons or those with weak anal sphincters.

How Is It Done?

During an ileo-anal anastomosis, the colon and rectum are removed through an incision in the abdomen. Then your surgeon removes the inner lining from the anus but carefully preserves the sphincter muscles.

A small pouch is then made at the end of the ileum to collect the fecal material to decrease the number of bowel movements you have. This creation of a pouch may not be necessary in children and young adults because the ileum can often adapt itself.

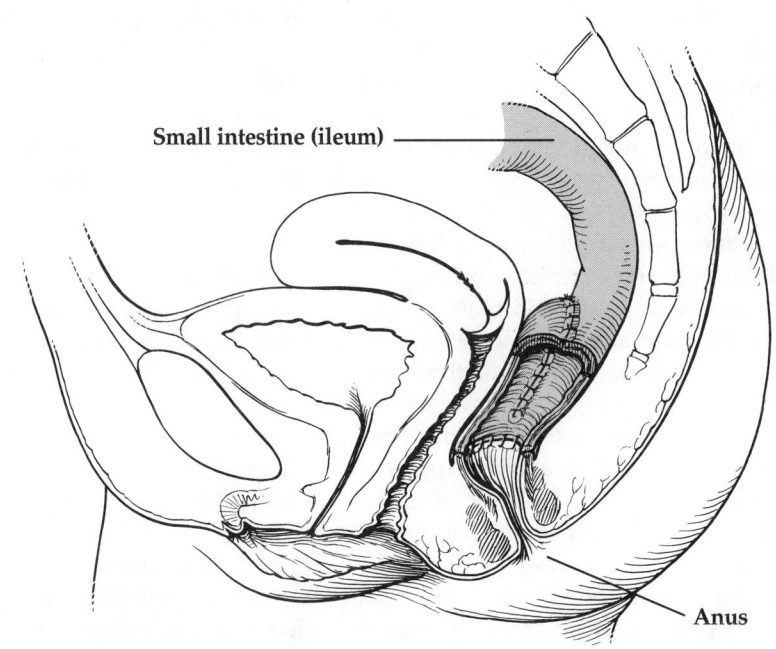

In the surgical procedure known as ileo-anal anastomosis, the diseased colon and rectum are removed but the anal sphincter muscles are left intact. The small intestine (ileum) is then stitched directly to the anus. This procedure allows for near normal passage of stool rather than the permanent use of an ileostomy bag.

A temporary ileostomy is necessary to allow time for your intestines to heal. In this procedure, an opening (stoma) is made through the abdominal wall and a loop of the ileum is brought out. Fecal material will then be expelled through this opening and into a pouch that you will wear around it. Unlike a permanent ileostomy, the temporary one is closed in 2 to 3 months. Then, you will no longer need to wear a pouch on your side.

Recovery

After some initial pain, you should start feeling better soon. Many patients who have been debilitated from their disease are surprised to gain weight and strength so quickly following their operation. By the time they return to the hospital to have the ileostomy closed, they often feel better than they have in years.

Once the ileostomy is closed, expect to have frequent bowel movements for several months. Usually, the first bowel movement occurs about 3 days after the stoma is closed. The pouch made at the end of the ileum slowly increases in size. As this pouch becomes larger, it can store more stool and the number of bowel movements per day will decrease.

Initially, you may get discouraged. During the first few weeks, it may seem like you are spending all your time in the bathroom, and your anus may become sore from frequent bowel movements. You may even have episodes of incontinence. Your physician may prescribe a medication to slow down your bowel and thicken the consistency of the stool if that is a problem.

Usually, determination and patience will pay off. The number of stools will often decrease to about 5 or 6 a day and the urgency and incontinence will go away.

They often are an incidental finding on an X-ray made because of another problem, although some benign tumors can cause bleeding.

A small percentage of tumors of the small intestine are malignant. The most common malignant types are adenocarcinoma, leiomyosarcoma, carcinoid tumor, and lymphoma.

If you have a malignant tumor in your small intestine, your symptoms may include weight loss, abdominal pain, nausea and vomiting, and bleeding. Your physician may feel an abdominal mass.

Bleeding, perforation, and obstruction are common manifestations of a leiomyosarcoma, whereas a carcinoid tumor may cause no symptoms before it spreads (see page 774).

Diagnosis
The diagnosis of a tumor in the small intestine is often made with a barium X-ray (see page 762).

How Serious Are Tumors of the Small Intestine?
Benign tumors are not life-threatening, but they can cause dangerous symptoms such as bleeding and obstruction. Like any malignancy, cancer of the small intestine is a dangerous and life-threatening illness and requires prompt treatment.

Treatment
Surgery is usually recommended for all benign tumors that cause symptoms and for

malignancies that have not become too widespread for surgical treatment. At times, the X-ray examination of the intestine cannot distinguish a benign from a malignant tumor, and surgical exploration of the abdomen and removal of the tumor are necessary before the diagnosis can be made. When a tumor has metastasized to such an extent that surgery will not be effective, steroid medications, chemotherapy, and radiation—either individually or in combination—may be used.

Diverticulosis and Diverticulitis

The development of multiple pouches that project outward from the wall of the colon is termed diverticulosis. When inflammation occurs in or around these small pouches, or if they rupture, the condition is called diverticulitis.

Symptoms
Most people with diverticulosis have no symptoms. Typically, diverticulosis goes undiscovered or is an incidental finding during a barium enema performed for other reasons (see The Barium X-Ray, page 762).

Diverticulitis is more likely to occur in the lower (sigmoid) portion of your colon. A diverticulum becomes inflamed or infected, probably as a result of undigested food and bacteria lodging in it. This compromises the blood supply to the diverticulum, making it susceptible to an invasion by bacteria. The

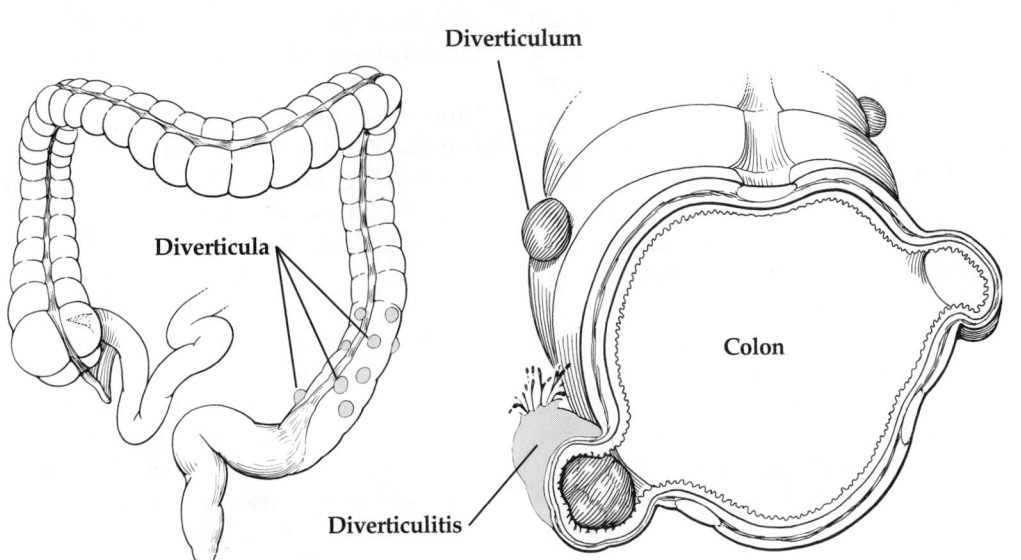

Diverticulum

Diverticula

Colon

Diverticulitis

Diverticula are small pouches of the large intestine (left drawing). When these pouches produce no discomfort, the condition is termed diverticulosis. If the diverticula become inflamed, or if they rupture, the problem is called diverticulitis (right).

result can range from a small abscess to a massive infection or perforation. The process resembles that of appendicitis (see Acute Appendicitis, page 772), except that it occurs in the lower left side of your colon.

If you have diverticulitis, you may have severe cramping pains, usually more severe on your left side. The pain may be severe or it may be mild for several days before getting worse. Fever and nausea commonly are present.

Sometimes the inflamed diverticulum ruptures, spilling intestinal material into the abdominal cavity. This causes peritonitis, a medical emergency. Hemorrhage is a less frequent complication (see Peritonitis, page 792).

What Is the Cause?

The cause is unknown, but diverticular problems are much more common in industrialized nations such as the United States, leading some physicians to speculate that the relatively low intake of fiber in the Western diet may be a major factor. The risk of diverticular disease increases with age, with the frequency in Western countries ranging from 20 to 50 percent in persons older than 50.

Treatment

Treatment for diverticulitis may involve simple bed rest, stool softeners, a liquid diet, and antibiotics when the inflammation is mild and the diverticulum has not ruptured. When rupture or widespread infection has occurred, intravenous antibiotic therapy may be necessary. Hospitalization usually is required, and surgery may be necessary.

If you experience a series of attacks, surgical removal of the involved segment of the bowel at a time when no symptoms are present may be advised. Surgery also may be required if you do not respond to intravenous antibiotic treatment during an acute attack. Often, in these more acute situations a temporary colostomy (see Colostomy and Ileostomy, page 777) is performed. At a later date the bowel may be reattached during a second operation.

With diverticulosis, many physicians believe treatment is unnecessary when there are no symptoms. Others prescribe a high-fiber diet and, if there are some minimal symptoms, an antispasmodic medication. Often, symptoms of an irritable bowel (see Irritable Bowel Syndrome, this page) are incorrectly blamed on diverticulosis.

Irritable Bowel Syndrome

Many Americans periodically have symptoms of irritable bowel syndrome. Because people with irritable bowel syndrome often suffer in silence without taking their complaint to a physician, the number with this disorder is unknown.

Symptoms

Abdominal pain and a change in bowel habits are the main symptoms. The pain can occur anywhere in your abdomen, and it can be severe. Indigestion, heartburn, and nausea also may occur.

Typically, the symptoms occur after a meal and are temporarily relieved by a bowel movement. Persons with irritable bowel syndrome frequently complain of feeling bloated and passing an excessive amount of gas, which also relieves the discomfort.

Constipation also is a frequent complaint. The bowel movement may be pellet-like or in small balls or ribbons. Often, those with irritable bowel syndrome abuse laxatives because of chronic constipation. Diarrhea also may occur but is a less frequent symptom.

What Is the Cause?

Irritable bowel syndrome often is called "spastic colon." It probably is the result of abnormal muscular activity of the intestinal wall. The causes of this abnormal activity vary. At times it may be aggravated by a specific food, but in many persons who have irritable bowel syndrome, chronic stress and depression may be the primary cause or at least contribute to flare-ups of symptoms.

Irritable bowel syndrome often begins in adolescence or in young adulthood. It occurs more frequently in women than in men.

Minimizing Your Symptoms

Irritable bowel syndrome is a chronic condition that may occur on and off throughout your life, but there are things you can do to minimize the symptoms:

1. See your physician. The symptoms of irritable bowel syndrome may mimic the symptoms of a serious disease. It is important that you undergo a complete examination, particularly if the symptoms have appeared only recently, to be sure your problem is not being caused by something more serious. An examination of your rectum (see Screening for Colon Cancer, page 790) and a

barium enema (see The Barium X-Ray, page 762) may be done. Knowing that your symptoms are not due to a dangerous disease may ease your mind—and possibly decrease the stress that may make your irritable bowel syndrome worse.

2. Select foods carefully. If a specific food appears to bring on your symptoms, eliminate it from your diet. Sometimes a high-fiber diet including consumption of fresh fruits, vegetables, and fiber supplements is helpful; in some people, however, it can increase bloating and gas.

3. Do not eliminate a food just because it appears to cause symptoms on a single occasion. Be sure that the food produces symp-

---

Fiber in Your Diet

In recent years, Americans have become increasingly aware of the need for more fiber in their diets. A high-fiber diet decreases your chance of constipation and also may decrease your risk of colon cancer.

But before you buy one of the high-fiber supplements on the market, look in your refrigerator and cupboards. The chances are that you have everything you need right in your kitchen to increase the fiber content in your diet.

What Are High-Fiber Foods?
High-fiber foods—often referred to as bulk or roughage—include whole-grain products, fruits, vegetables, and legumes. These are generally better sources of fiber than anything you can buy at the drugstore.

Fiber and Digestion
Unlike foods that are broken down and absorbed during digestion, fiber is not affected by the digestive enzymes. Thus, it passes virtually unchanged through the stomach and small intestine and into the colon. In the colon, some forms of fiber are fermented by bacteria and others resist fermentation and are expelled in the stool unchanged.

Fiber increases the weight and size of the stool, in addition to softening it. The bulky stool is easier to pass, lessening the chance of constipation.

Advantages and Disadvantages
Fiber may decrease your risk of colon cancer. Some physicians believe fiber may help to clear the colon of substances that may be changed by bacteria into cancer-promoting chemicals. They base this belief on the low incidence of colon cancer in countries where a high-fiber diet is the norm. Others argue that fiber itself does not protect against colon cancer but that people who eat high-fiber diets tend not to consume as much fat; and, they believe, animal fat may promote colon cancer.

Many forms of dietary fiber promote bowel regularity. Fiber may decrease the chances of complications in the event of diverticular disease. In addition, fiber may decrease the size of hemorrhoids and prevent hemorrhoidal bleeding. If you have loose, watery stools, fiber may help to solidify the stool, because it absorbs water.

Other benefits of eating fiber include a possible lowering of cholesterol level and, in diabetics, a slowing of the absorption of sugar, which may decrease the need for insulin in some people with diabetes.

Fiber does have a few disadvantages too. It can produce excess gas. Also, some sources of fiber—oat bran and wheat fiber, for example—can remove minerals such as calcium, iron, and zinc from your body. If you eat a balanced diet and take a reasonable amount of milk with your oat bran and high-fiber cereals, this is usually not a problem.

Strategies to Consider
To help ensure adequate dietary fiber, follow these suggestions:

1. Get your fiber from food. Sometimes people assume that if they take a fiber supplement, they need not pay attention to their diet. A supplement is not a good substitute for fiber from your food.

2. Eat a varied diet, including high-fiber foods such as grains, vegetables, fresh fruits, and legumes. High-fiber snack foods include nuts, seeds, popcorn, fresh and dried fruits, and whole-grain crackers.

3. Limit your consumption of processed foods, which often have little fiber. The refining process removes the outer coat (bran) from grain; thus, this highly desirable form of fiber is lost. This is why whole-grain products are higher in fiber content than those made of refined flour. In a similar fashion, removing the skin from fruits and vegetables decreases their fiber content. An orange contains considerably more fiber than the juice squeezed from it. So think twice before peeling fruits and vegetables or even squeezing the juice from them if you want to increase the fiber content of your diet.

4. Increase your fiber intake gradually.

toms consistently before giving it up. Many persons with irritable bowel syndrome restrict their diet to just a few selections and feel the worse for it. They often feel better when they return to a more varied diet. Some foods will seem to cause distress when consumed in larger amounts but do not when taken in small helpings or as part of a meal.

4. Bulk formers, which contain the natural vegetable fiber psyllium, are available without a prescription and may help relieve your constipation and diarrhea. Your physician also may want to try an anti-spasm medication occasionally. This medication may improve your problem temporarily but should not be used for a long period.

Biofeedback techniques also may be helpful in relieving stress.

Remember, irritable bowel syndrome does not predispose you to more serious disorders.

Fiber Supplements

Fiber supplements can be convenient and sometimes even necessary. For example, some people have trouble eating foods rich in fiber. They develop abdominal pain, cramping, and gas. Although these side effects tend to disappear after a few weeks, fiber supplements may be an alternative if you can't tolerate high-fiber foods. Here are tips on selecting and taking a fiber supplement:

- A psyllium-based supplement can satisfy your appetite like any high-fiber food. Take it before meals if you're overweight; after meals if you're underweight.
- Drink at least 8 ounces of water or juice with each dose.
- If you're on a calorie-controlled diet or you have diabetes mellitus, select a supplement that has no added sugar. Examples include sugar-free Metamucil, Fiberall powder, and Konsyl (but not Konsyl-D).
- If your diet restricts sodium, shop for a sodium-free supplement. Most supplements are low in sodium anyway, containing less than 10 milligrams. It's always a good idea to check the nutrition label.
- Drink a liquid supplement soon after you mix it. Most fiber supplements contain psyllium as their main active ingredient. When mixed in liquids, psyllium gels. If you wait too long, taste and texture may be unappealing. Also, although rare, psyllium allergies have been reported in people who have eaten psyllium-containing cereal or inhaled psyllium powder from medications.

Chronic Constipation

Signs and Symptoms
- Passage of hard stools less than three times a week
- Occasionally, abdominal bloating and discomfort

Many people believe that constipation is the inability to have a bowel movement daily. In fact, it is not necessary to have a bowel movement every day. For some, regularity means having a bowel movement three times a week; for others, it is part of their daily routine.

What Is the Cause?
As your colon removes water from the waste products, a stool is formed and moved through the intestine by muscular contractions. Alterations in the speed at which the waste passes through the colon or in the amount of water removed can affect normal bowel function.

The Diagnosis
If the constipation is a recent development or your stool habits differ from what you consider normal, see your physician. He or she first will rule out such causes of constipation as obstruction (see Intestinal Obstruction, page 793) and hypothyroidism (see page 948). In addition, consideration will be given to your medications. Some medications may cause constipation, including those used to treat Parkinson's disease, depression, hypertension, or some heart disorders.

Your physician may want to perform a flexible proctosigmoidoscopic examination (see Screening for Colon Cancer, page 790) and a barium study of your colon (see The Barium X-Ray, page 762) to rule out other causes of disease within the colon.

Are Laxatives the Answer?
Many people with constipation rely heavily on laxatives to relieve their problem. Paradoxically, laxatives can lead to constipation when not used properly. They also can damage your bowel and disrupt your body's normal balance of minerals.

If constipation is a problem, take these steps before trying a laxative:

1. Drink at least six to eight glasses of water or other liquids every day.

2. Increase the fiber content of your diet by eating more fresh fruits and vegetables.

3. Incorporate regular physical exercise into your daily regimen.

4. Add to your diet a bulk former that contains the vegetable fiber psyllium.

5. Set aside a specific time every day for trying to have a bowel movement.

6. Do not resist the urge to move your bowels.

7. Consider adding a fiber or bran supplement to your diet.

8. If constipation continues, it may be reasonable to use milk of magnesia or mineral oil occasionally at bedtime, but avoid regular use of it.

9. Avoid irritating enemas such as those containing soapsuds. Such enemas are advised in preparation for certain X-ray or endoscopic examinations of the colon but have no place in daily life.

10. Avoid enemas in general. A thorough "cleansing" of the colon, by either an enema or a laxative, actually contributes to the problem of constipation.

11. If your constipation does not improve, see your physician.

Intestinal Gas

Most intestinal gas (flatus) is produced in the colon. Usually the gas is expelled during a bowel movement. All people pass gas, but some people produce an excessive amount of gas that bothers them throughout the day.

What Is Gas Made of?

Intestinal gas is composed primarily of five substances: oxygen, nitrogen, hydrogen, carbon dioxide, and methane. The foul odor usually is the result of small traces of other gases such as hydrogen sulfide and ammonia and other substances.

Nitrogen and oxygen are in the air we breathe and may be in intestinal gas when swallowed air travels through the digestive system. Some carbon dioxide is produced by

---

Laxative Abuse

It is rare for anyone to need a laxative on a daily basis, yet many people find reasons to overuse laxatives.

Some have an irrational fear that they will be ill if their bowels do not move each day and so they take laxatives daily to ensure a daily bowel movement. Others take large amounts of laxatives regularly as a preventive measure, even though they have no evidence of constipation. Still others take laxatives in an attempt to purge their systems in order to lose weight.

Kinds of Laxatives
One of the oldest laxatives is castor oil; it undergoes chemical transformation within the colon to become an acid that prevents the intestinal wall from absorbing water. Prolonged use of castor oil can damage the cells that line your intestinal tract. Phenolphthalein is a laxative that acts by irritating the bowel wall; it is the active ingredient in many of the small chocolate or candy-like tablets that are laxatives. Other laxatives work by increasing the water content within your colon and are less irritating to your bowel; these include milk of magnesia and stool softeners.

Bulk-forming laxatives or so-called natural laxatives expand when they come into contact with water in the colon. These laxatives prevent the formation of hard stools.

What Are the Risks of Overuse?
Excessive use of laxatives is harmful. When taken in excess, laxatives will flush out necessary vitamins and other nutrients before they can be properly absorbed. Laxatives also contribute to an excessive excretion of water, sodium, and potassium. Furthermore, habitual use of laxatives tends to weaken the muscles in the intestine and make them flabby and less able to function properly. As a result, once you stop taking a laxative on a regular basis, your constipation not only will return but also may be worse.

Excessive use of laxatives can bring about diarrhea or real constipation by inducing lazy bowel syndrome. This is a condition in which the bowels fail to function properly because they have begun to rely on the laxative to do the work of elimination. Laxatives also can interfere with the effectiveness of other medications your physician might prescribe.

Fecal Impaction

A fecal impaction is a mass of hardened stool that cannot be eliminated by a normal bowel movement. It can occur after an extended period of constipation and most often poses a problem for elderly people, especially those who are bedridden, and for young children.

The main symptoms are an intense desire to have a bowel movement and pain in the anal region, rectum, and center of the abdomen. Nausea and vomiting may occur, and you may lose your appetite.

Causes

Inadequate consumption of dietary fiber, complex carbohydrates, and liquids can lead to a fecal impaction. Other possible causes include:

- Prescription and over-the-counter drugs (such as codeine-containing pain relievers, antidepressants, and aluminum-containing antacids), and inappropriate (excessive) use of laxatives
- Immobility, especially bed rest
- Health problems such as hemorrhoids, kidney failure or transplantation, cancer, cardiovascular disease, spinal cord injuries and neurologic conditions such as Parkinson's disease and amyotrophic lateral sclerosis (Lou Gehrig's disease)
- Failing to heed the call when your body tells you it's time for a trip to the bathroom. This is common among young children, who may prefer play to a bathroom visit

Prevention

To reduce your risks of a fecal impaction:

- Drink two or more glasses of water with each meal and one between meals
- Eat a high-fiber diet
- Heed the first urge to defecate
- Don't use laxatives on a regular basis
- If possible, avoid prolonged bed rest and medications that increase your risks of fecal impaction

A fecal impaction can generally be removed manually, by a nurse or physician.

---

a chemical reaction in the small intestine. Hydrogen, carbon dioxide, and, in many persons, methane are produced in the large intestine by bacterial fermentation of carbohydrate that has not been digested and absorbed in the small intestine.

Swallowed air makes up a small fraction of intestinal gas. Carbonated drinks may release carbon dioxide in the stomach and may be a source of gas.

How Can You Prevent It?

Although potentially embarrassing and certainly annoying, excess intestinal gas is not a serious condition. Here are a few self-help measures you can try:

- Avoid or limit gassy foods. Worst gas-formers are beans and other legumes, wheat and wheat bran, cabbage, onions, Brussels sprouts, sauerkraut, apricots, bananas, and prunes. Milk and other dairy products can also cause gas if you have reduced amounts of lactase, the enzyme needed to digest lactose, the main sugar in milk.
- Eat fewer fatty foods. Fatty meats, fried foods, cream sauces, and gravies tend to increase gas and bloating.
- Limit sugar substitutes. Up to half of healthy people poorly absorb the sorbitol and mannitol contained in some sugar-free foods, candies, and gum. The amount of sorbitol contained in five sticks of sugar-free gum can cause gas and diarrhea.
- Don't rely on antacids. They neutralize stomach acid to relieve heartburn, but they don't reduce gas.
- Do try some anti-gas products. Adding Beano (a food enzyme) to high-fiber foods reduces the amount of gas they make. Lactaid and Dairy Ease reduce excess gas caused by lactase deficiency. Products with simethicone are rarely effective.

Sometimes excessive gas is attributable to a disease of the digestive tract, and treatment for that disease often decreases the amount of gas produced in the intestines. In most cases, however, excessive gas is not the result of disease.

Colon Polyps

Signs and Symptoms

- Often none are apparent
- Recent change in bowel movements
- Blood in the stool
- Mucus discharged from the anus
- Microscopic amounts of blood in the stool

Benign (nonmalignant) tumors of the large intestine are not uncommon. It is believed that two of every three Americans older than 60 has some type of growth (or lesion) in their colon.

Most of these tumors are polyps that arise from the lining of the colon. They usually are harmless and are discovered accidentally, often during a screening test for colon cancer (see Screening for Colon Cancer, page 790) or during a test to diagnose another disorder.

Types of Polyps

Several different varieties of polyps are found in the colon. The most common is a hyperplastic polyp that generally is less than ¼ inch in diameter. These tiny polyps are not a health risk although, if such polyps grow to be larger than ½ inch in diameter, they should be removed for an accurate diagnosis under the microscope.

Juvenile polyps occur during childhood. Your child may experience rectal bleeding or the polyp may even be seen to drop down through the anal canal during defecation. These polyps can be easily removed with a colonoscope (see Colonoscopy, page 788). These polyps also do not degenerate into a malignancy.

Inflammatory polyps are thought to result from injury to or inflammation of the lining of the colon such as after a bout of ulcerative colitis (see page 777). These also are not a significant health risk.

The other major category of polyps are adenomas. These are classified into three varieties based on features seen under the microscope: tubular, tubulovillous, and villous. The most common are tubular adenomas, which generally are less than ½ inch in diameter. Villous adenomas are less common. More than half of them are at least 1 inch in diameter. Often, with these tumors you may experience significant mucus discharge in the stool along with blood. Tubulovillous adenomas contain characteristics of the two other types.

The adenomatous polyps have the potential for malignancy, and this potential usually increases as the size of the polyp increases and when more villous characteristics are present. Thus, these polyps should be removed, most often via colonoscopy (see Colonoscopy, page 788), to prevent the development of cancer. At times, even if the polyp shows microscopic cancer in a few cells, the removal via colonoscopy is curative.

At other times, if there is concern about the spread of cancer from the polyp itself, your physician may recommend an operation to remove a section of the colon that includes the polyp and surrounding tissue and lymph nodes.

Most colon polyps are not considered hereditary, but there seems to be a tendency for them to appear in several members of a family. Also, if a colon polyp develops in a person, he or she may have others later in life.

One type of disorder in which colon polyps are present is believed to be strongly hereditary. Called familial adenomatous polyposis, this rare disorder is characterized by the appearance of numerous (often 1,000 or more) polyps throughout the entire colon. These polyps can be asymptomatic (without symptoms) or may cause rectal bleeding. Typically, this condition appears during childhood or adolescence.

Gardner's syndrome refers to the existence of multiple colon and other intestinal polyps along with other nonmalignant tumors such as lipomas, fibromas, and osteomas in other regions of the body.

Cancer of the colon inevitably occurs in these hereditary forms of colonic polyposis. Therefore, removal of the colon (total colec-

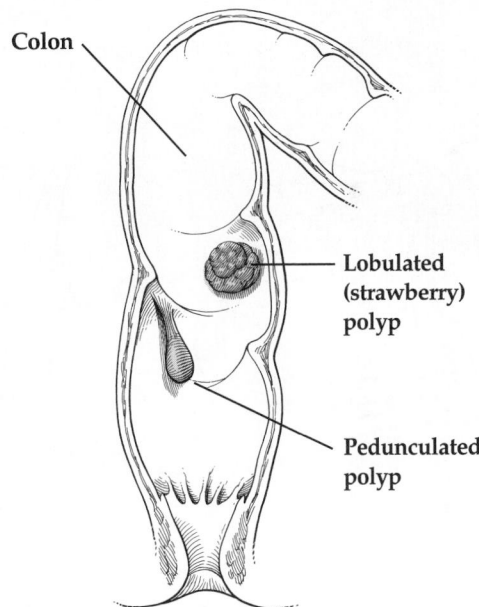

Colon

Lobulated (strawberry) polyp

Pedunculated polyp

Polyps are small growths that may appear in the large intestine. In most cases, they are benign (nonmalignant). They may assume various shapes. Pedunculated and lobulated (strawberry) are two common forms.

Colonoscopy

Colonoscopy is the examination of the entire colon by using a fiberoptic endoscope. This flexible instrument transmits light, allowing the specially trained physician to examine the lining of the colon from the anus to the cecum, the junction of the small and large intestines. Sometimes, the last several inches of the small intestine can be examined as well.

Applications

Colonoscopy is the most accurate method of examining your colon for polyps or other small lesions. In persons known to be at risk for these abnormalities, periodic colonoscopy may be very useful.

Other common uses include biopsy and removal of polyps (polypectomy) that have been de-tected during a barium enema or proctoscopy; searching for a cause of chronic or acute bleeding when a cause cannot be established by other tests; screening for cancer when there is a history of other diseases or a family history that increases a person's risk of colon cancer; differentiating colitis caused by Crohn's disease from ulcerative colitis; assessing the extent of involvement due to colitis prior to surgery; and identifying the cause of diarrhea when other tests or examinations offer no clear diagnosis.

A laser beam can be directed through a channel of the colonoscope and applied to a bleeding lesion or one that has the potential to bleed. Electrocoagulation through the colonoscope can be used for similar purposes.

The Procedure

If you are scheduled to have colonoscopy, you will need to adhere to special dietary instructions, usually beginning the day prior to the test. You will be given a laxative or liquid solution the night before the procedure and often an enema that morning. You also may be given a sedative just prior to the examination.

Risks

The main complications of the test are hemorrhage and perforation, but the risk is very low. Colonoscopy is not recommended if you are having an episode of acute di-verticulitis (see page 781), have vascular disease in the bowel, or are in the midst of an acute phase of colitis.

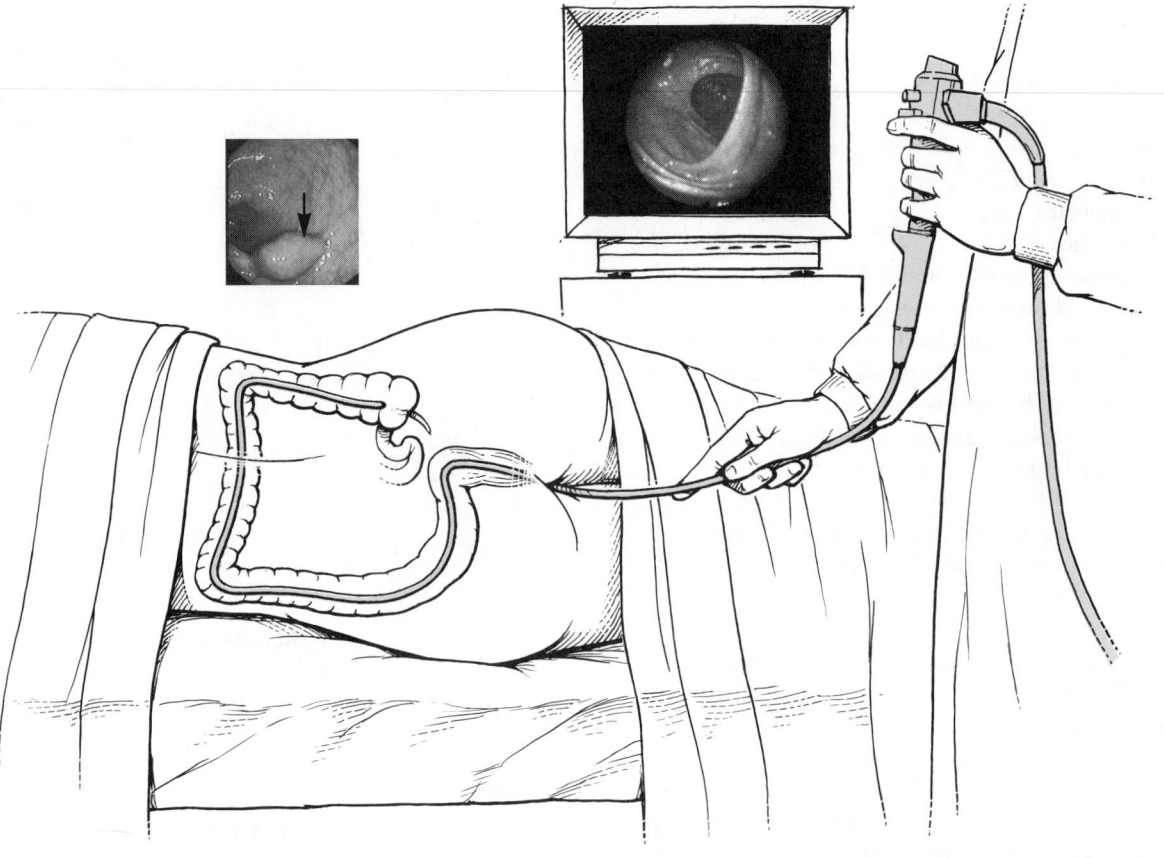

A colonoscopy examination involves gently inserting a fiberoptic colonoscope into your rectum and large intestine to view your lower gastrointestinal tract. Screen on monitor shows a normal colon. Inset: colon polyp.

tomy) is advised as soon as the diagnosis is established. It is also important for blood relatives to be examined at a relatively young age (approximately 10 to 12 years) so that appropriate treatment can be carried out if they also have colonic polyposis.

Diagnosis

Most frequently, colon polyps are discovered during an examination for another colon problem or during evaluation of microscopic blood in the stool (see Screening for Colon Cancer, page 790). Then, you may have a barium enema (see The Barium X-Ray, page 762) and a proctosigmoidoscopic examination (see Screening for Colon Cancer, page 790). Alternatively, colonoscopy may be performed to examine your colon and to treat any detected lesions. In the future, new, noninvasive techniques such as computed tomography colography and virtual colonoscopy may be available.

How Serious Are Polyps?

An adenomatous polyp has the potential to become cancerous. Most, if not all, colon cancers seem to develop from polyps. Moreover, sometimes they may cause problems such as bleeding and obstruction. The removal of polyps plays a significant role in the prevention of colon cancer.

Treatment

The removal of most of these benign polyps is a relatively simple procedure. They usually are removed when detected because this eliminates the chance that they will ever become malignant. Commonly, the polyp is removed during colonoscopy. If the tumor cannot be removed by this means, a laparotomy (a surgical opening of the abdomen) and opening of the colon will be required to remove the polyp.

If an adenomatous polyp is found at the time of colonoscopy, your physician may recommend periodic examination of the colon because of the likelihood of further adenomatous polyps developing.

If you have familial adenomatous polyposis, the likelihood of colon cancer is virtually 100 percent by age 40. Thus, physicians usually recommend that the entire colon be removed to prevent cancer. The procedure normally done is a colectomy with ileostomy (see Colostomy and Ileostomy, page 777) or an ileo-anal anastomosis (see Ileo-Anal Anastomosis, page 780).

Colon Cancer

Signs and Symptoms

- Rectal bleeding
- Altered bowel habits
- Abdominal cramps or pain
- Microscopic amounts of blood in the stool
- Unexplained anemia
- Unexplained weight loss
- Sometimes, none

Cancer of the colon and cancer of the rectum are two of the more common forms of cancer among adult men and women. These two cancers are jointly referred to as colorectal cancer.

Factors that increase your risk of colorectal cancer include a family history or prior history of adenomatous colon polyps, familial adenomatous polyposis (see Colon Polyps, page 786), colon cancer, or ulcerative colitis (see page 777).

Although the precise cause of colon cancer is unknown, some studies suggest that diet plays an important role. It has been suggested that the higher proportion of animal fat in our diet may account for the large amount of colorectal cancer in the United States compared with countries such as Japan where the dietary emphasis is on vegetables, poultry, and fish.

Diagnosis

If you have rectal bleeding, do not assume that you just have hemorrhoids. Your physician will want to perform a rectal examination using a gloved finger. You may have additional studies, such as a barium enema (see The Barium X-Ray, page 762), proctosigmoidoscopy (see Screening for Colon Cancer, page 790), or colonoscopy (see Colonoscopy, page 788), depending on the results of the other tests and your symptoms. The diagnosis of colon cancer sometimes is made after investigation of the cause for anemia or for the finding of microscopic blood in the stool (see Screening for Colon Cancer, page 790) or a change in bowel habits.

Recent discoveries have included identifying the gene responsible for some types of familial colon cancer. Tests may soon be available to assist in screening these individuals to assess their risk of developing colon cancer.

How Serious Is Colon Cancer?

Colon cancer accounts for about 20 percent

Screening for Colon Cancer

Cancer of the rectum and colon is the second leading cause of cancer deaths in the United States. More than 150,000 Americans each year are found to have this disease; roughly 60,000 die.

Often, colorectal cancer is discovered too late for cure. However, this does not always have to be the case. When discovered in its early stages, colorectal cancer usually is curable by surgery. Thus, it is important that you be aware of symptoms of this disease and the diagnostic tests that can detect colorectal cancer in its early, and most curable, stage.

Family History
If a parent or sibling has had colon cancer or an adenomatous polyp (see Colon Polyps, page 786), you also may be at an increased risk for colon polyp or cancer. In this situation, your physician may want to perform regular examinations of your colon, such as by colonoscopy (see page 788) or by barium X-ray (see page 762).

Symptoms of Colon Cancer
Early detection starts with being aware of the symptoms of colon cancer. This includes any change in your normal bowel movement, especially the frequency of your stools, rectal bleeding, lower abdominal pain, and unexplained, persistent urges to defecate. The latter symptom may be caused by a mass in the rectum.

Screening Tests Important
In addition to seeking medical attention for symptoms, consider having periodic screening tests such as stool blood testing and proctosigmoidoscopy. These simple tests can be used to discover early cancer or polyps before they cause symptoms.

Stool Blood Tests
These tests measure hidden (occult) blood in stools. Numerous stool blood tests are available. They vary in cost and accuracy. The most widely used type involves smearing a sample of stool onto a chemically treated paper card. The card is then mailed to a laboratory or given to your physician for interpretation of results. The accuracy of home kits has not been established.

Annual stool blood testing may lower (by about one-third) but not eliminate the risk of dying from colorectal cancer. The problem is that many cancers do not bleed and will not be detected by this method. Also, most positive test results are due to bleeding from trivial sources, like hemorrhoids, or to interfering substances in stool. A positive test result would require a colonoscopy (see page 788) or barium X-ray (see page 762) to determine its significance.

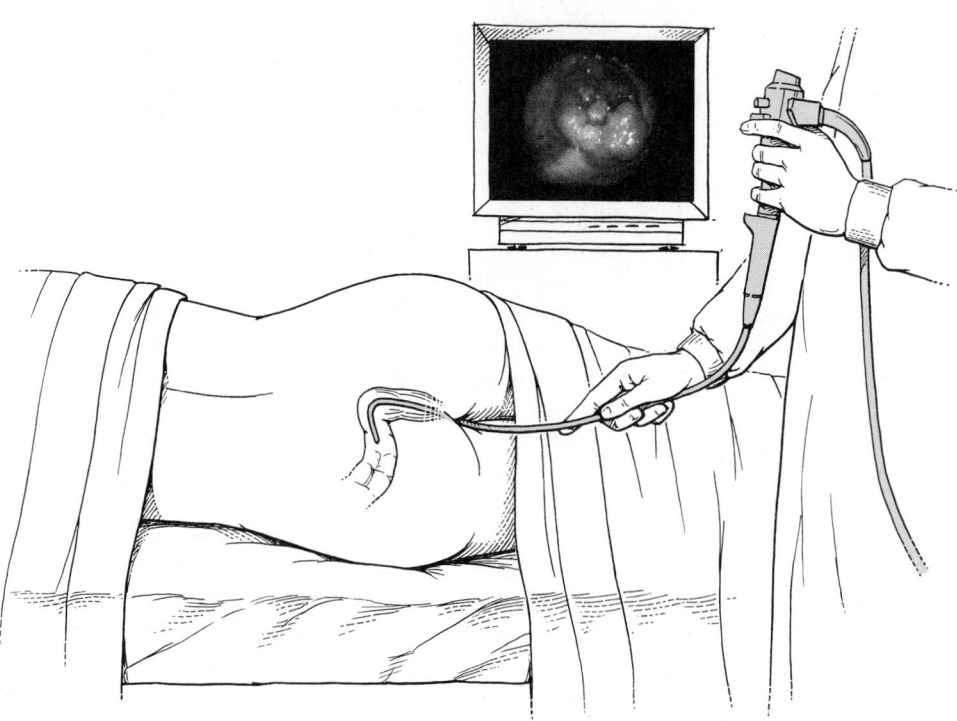

Your physician uses a flexible fiberoptic proctosigmoidoscope to examine your rectum and sigmoid colon. The image on the screen shows colon cancer. This common screening examination can also help identify other colon problems.

Proctosigmoidoscopy

Another test that often is recommended is a flexible proctosigmoidoscopic examination. The test requires one or two enemas for preparation, no sedation, and about 5 minutes to perform. This test examines the lower portion of the colon (sigmoid) and rectum by using a flexible, lighted tube called a flexible proctosigmoidoscope. Approximately 50 percent of all colorectal cancers or polyps can be seen during such an examination. In addition, diagnosis of other diseases such as Crohn's or ulcerative colitis can be made with this instrument. Samples of tissue can be taken through the instrument for later examination under a microscope (biopsy).

The frequency with which this test should be performed has been a subject of debate. Our recommendation is that, in the absence of any family history of colon cancer, this examination should be done initially at age 45 and every 3 to 5 years thereafter. For those who have had a previous polyp or have a family history of polyps, more frequent examinations by colonoscopy (see page 788) may be appropriate.

In some situations, an inflexible hollow instrument is used to inspect the rectum and the lower portion of the sigmoid colon. Often, this is done in conjunction with a barium examination of the colon or to diagnose specifically, and at times treat, anal disorders. This procedure commonly is called rigid proctoscopy.

Future Screening

Several innovations on the horizon could improve the effectiveness and lower the cost of colorectal cancer screening. Stool tests designed to identify specific substances shed from cancers or polyps, rather than to detect blood, may increase the accuracy of early detection.

There is growing evidence that some individuals are predisposed to developing colorectal cancer. In the future, it may be possible to identify the abnormal gene responsible for this predisposition and intensify screening efforts in persons with such genes.

Finally, improved techniques may allow more complete and comfortable visualization of the colon and rectum. These include special ultrasound techniques and a promising, non-invasive X-ray method based on a computer-generated three-dimensional image of the colon called "virtual colonoscopy."

---

of the deaths due to malignant disease in this country. When detected and treated at an early stage, these cancers are considered to be curable. Unfortunately, many people do not seek medical attention when such warning signs as rectal bleeding or a change in bowel habits become evident.

Treatment

Surgery

The present approach to the treatment of colon cancer is surgery. In about half of the cases, surgery can cure this form of cancer.

Before the operation, you may have a blood test and a CT scan (see page 1334) to help determine whether the cancer has spread (metastasized) beyond the location of the tumor. If the cancer has spread, surgery may be ruled out except to relieve bowel obstruction or bleeding.

Other Treatments

After surgery, your physician may recommend additional treatment, especially if you are at high risk for a recurrence. For example, your physician may recommend chemotherapy with drugs such as 5-fluorouracil (5-FU), levamisole, or 5-FU and leucovorin. These drugs decrease the chance of tumor recurrence and improve survival in persons with colon cancer that has spread only to nearby lymph nodes. However, to be effective, this treatment must begin within 4 weeks after surgery. (When used in combination with radiation therapy, these drugs also can be effective as the sole treatment for rectal cancer.) If a bowel obstruction is present or if there is bleeding, laser therapy through a colonoscope may help relieve symptoms. Your physician will advise you as to whether this additional treatment may be useful.

Megacolon

Signs and Symptoms
- Severe constipation
- Malnutrition

From either congenital or acquired causes, the colon can become so enlarged that it becomes unable to move feces. This condition is referred to as megacolon or giant colon. Nerve damage in the colon or rectum frequently is the cause of megacolon.

Hirschsprung's disease is a congenital disorder in which babies are born without ganglion nerve cells in a segment of their rectum. These infants are unable to have a bowel movement because the segment of the colon nearest the anus is unable to relax to permit the passage of feces. Symptoms are massive abdominal distention, absence of bowel movements, and impaired nutrition. Hirschsprung's disease occurs more often in males and often runs in families. The diagnosis is made by biopsy of the rectum under general anesthesia.

A type of acquired megacolon is psychogenic megacolon, which develops usually at the time of toilet training. It creates severe and chronic constipation.

In Central and South America, an infection called Chagas disease causes megacolon. The infection destroys the ganglion cells of the colon to create a condition similar to Hirschsprung's disease (see page 57) except that it occurs in adults rather than in children.

Some other conditions that can cause megacolon are severe neurologic disorders such as spinal cord injury and Parkinson's disease (see page 472) and use of some medications including narcotics.

Diagnosis
Your physician will examine your rectum with a proctoscope (see page 791) and probably with a barium enema (see The Barium X-Ray, page 762). For the diagnosis of Hirschsprung's disease, the physician will obtain a biopsy specimen of your infant's rectum under general anesthesia. For most cases of acquired megacolon, no biopsy is needed.

Treatment
The best treatment for Hirschsprung's disease is surgery because it usually will restore normal bowel movements. In the case of acquired megacolon, the key is education on proper bowel habits (see Chronic Constipation, page 784).

Your physician also may suggest the use of enemas or laxatives (such as mineral oil) to help retrain your bowel. Treatment of any underlying problem or decreasing the use of narcotic-containing medication may be appropriate.

Peritonitis

Signs and Symptoms
- Increasing abdominal pain
- Distended abdomen
- Nausea and vomiting
- Inability to pass feces or gas
- Fever
- Low blood pressure
- Thirst

Peritonitis is an inflammation, either confined to one area or widespread, of the peritoneum, the membrane that covers the abdominal organs.

Peritonitis most often is due to bacteria in the peritoneal cavity. Typically the bacteria enter from a perforation in the gastrointestinal tract or from trauma of the abdomen, as with a penetrating wound. Peritonitis also can be the result of a severe reaction from the release of enzymes from the pancreas, digestive enzymes, or bile due to injury or perforation.

Persons with systemic lupus erythematosus (see page 918) also may have bouts of peritonitis due to inflammation without perforation.

The most frequent causes of peritonitis are perforations due to appendicitis (see page 772), diverticulitis (see page 781), or peptic ulcer (see page 753). Obstruction of the small bowel with subsequent gangrene and bowel perforation (see Intestinal Obstruction, page 793) may cause peritonitis.

Diagnosis
If your physician suspects peritonitis, you will be hospitalized; peritonitis is a medical emergency that must be treated immediately. Blood tests and X-rays may be done to help establish the diagnosis.

Treatment
Surgery usually is necessary, either for the removal of the tissue that has caused the problem (such as appendicitis) or to repair an injury such as a perforation in the stomach or intestine.

To fight the infection, antibiotics are given through a vein. Because the intestines temporarily do not function during an episode of peritonitis, a tube will be placed through your nose into your stomach to drain secretions or air that accumulates and is not spontaneously passed. This tube is called a nasogastric tube. It can be removed when the bowel resumes its normal function.

Familial Mediterranean Fever

Signs and Symptoms
- Fever
- Abdominal pain
- Chest pain
- Pain in the joints
- Skin lesions on the lower part of the legs

Familial Mediterranean fever is an inherited intestinal disorder that is characterized by recurrent fever and inflammation. Because of the inflammation that occurs in the abdominal cavity with this disorder, familial Mediterranean fever is also called periodic peritonitis.

In most people who have familial Mediterranean fever, symptoms begin between the ages of 5 and 15. Fever is present during most attacks. In addition, there may be inflammation of the lining of the abdominal cavity, chest cavity, or joints, producing symptoms that resemble those of peritonitis (see page 792), pleurisy (see page 711), or arthritis (see page 913), respectively. Approximately one-quarter of people with familial Mediterranean fever have a painful red area of swelling in their lower legs. Persons affected by this disorder generally have recurrent attacks that may vary in severity and site from one episode to another.

The cause of familial Mediterranean fever is unknown. Most affected persons are symptom-free between attacks.

Diagnosis
Your physician will need to know whether any member of your family has ever had this disorder. He or she also will want to know how long your attacks last and how often they occur, because familial Mediterranean fever episodes usually last between 24 and 48 hours and occur at intervals of 2 to 4 weeks.

There is no one laboratory test that will be decisive in the diagnosis, although your physician probably will have your blood analyzed. In fact, diagnosis is a process of elimination in that your symptoms may initially suggest a number of other possible diseases, such as appendicitis (see page 772), acute pancreatitis (see page 818), or intestinal obstruction (see page 793).

Treatment
Many different treatment programs, including the use of antibiotics or corticosteroids, have been tried, but none has proved effective. The use of colchicine has resulted in a dramatic decrease in the number of attacks in many persons. Your physician will discuss with you the potential side effects of the chronic use of colchicine.

Intestinal Obstruction

Signs and Symptoms
- Abdominal distention
- Spasmodic pain or cramping in the mid-abdomen
- Vomiting
- Inability to pass feces or intestinal gas

Intestinal obstruction is partial or complete blockage in either the small intestine or the colon. This obstruction prevents the products of digestion from completing the journey through the intestines.

If you have a blockage in your small intestine, you may feel cramp-like pain in the middle of your abdomen and have bouts of vomiting. Failure to pass feces can occur no matter where the obstruction is located. If your lower colon is totally blocked, you will not even be able to pass gas. A partial intestinal obstruction may stimulate your intestine to secrete fluid, which may result in diarrhea.

A dramatic feature of intestinal obstruction is abdominal distention. The abdomen will protrude more and more as the condition worsens. The swelling is produced by intestinal gas and fluid trapped within the obstructed segment of the intestine.

Several things can cause an obstruction. The most common cause of obstruction in the small intestine is adhesion (scar tissue) from a prior operation. Hernias (see page 822) and volvulus (a knotted or twisted intestine) are also common causes of obstruction in the small bowel. In the colon, a cancer and other disorders can cause obstruction.

Sometimes the obstruction is nonmechanical and results from failure of the intestines to move material along. This is called adynamic ileus and sometimes occurs after injury to or operation on the abdomen.

Diagnosis
No one symptom is a sure sign of intestinal obstruction, nor will any one symptom reveal the precise cause of the obstruction. However, a significant sign of complete blockage would be your inability to pass gas or have a bowel movement.

If your physician believes that your symptoms point to an intestinal obstruction, he or she will arrange for an X-ray that may detect the obstruction. He or she may also conduct a sigmoidoscopic examination (see Screening for Colon Cancer, page 790), colonoscopy (see page 788), or a special X-ray study of the colon (see The Barium X-Ray, page 762) to see where the obstruction is located. Sometimes just these test procedures will relieve the obstruction.

How Serious Is Acute Intestinal Obstruction?

If the obstruction blocks the blood supply to the intestine, the tissue may begin to die. This will increase the possibility of gangrene or a perforation of the intestine. These are both life-threatening situations.

Treatment

If your physician suspects an intestinal obstruction, he or she may place a tube through your nose into your stomach or initial portion of your small bowel. Suction will be applied to remove intestinal secretions and air through the tube. Called nasogastric suction, this technique often will relieve the distention of the abdomen. Lost fluids must be replaced with intravenous feedings.

At times, the cause of an obstruction will resolve spontaneously after the distention has been relieved. If the obstruction does not resolve after nasogastric suction, an operation may be necessary. In most cases of adynamic ileus, correction of the underlying disorder will correct the obstruction.

Vascular Problems of the Bowel

The abdomen is fed by a vast network of blood vessels. Unfortunately, sometimes this necessary blood supply is inadequate. When this happens, the affected area becomes deficient in nutrients and oxygen, and the result can be tissue death.

The vascular disorders of the bowel are described below.

Mesenteric Ischemia

In this disorder, there is partial or complete lack of blood flow to the gut. This commonly occurs over a period of time as a result of the accumulation of cholesterol on the lining of the arteries leading to the intestines (see Atherosclerosis: What Is It? page 636). This deposition of cholesterol is similar to what

happens in the coronary arteries of persons who have angina; thus, it is hardly surprising that coronary artery disease may be found in persons who have impaired arterial blood supply to their intestines.

The main symptom of partial blockage is severe, cramping abdominal pain, most often around the navel, which is aggravated by eating and relieved by fasting. The pain can mimic the discomfort of angina pectoris (see page 657) and is sometimes called abdominal angina.

A clot (embolus) that passes from the heart to the arteries supplying the intestine can cause sudden, complete blockage of the supply of blood to a portion of the gut. If you have a complete blockage of the arteries in the intestine, severe pain will begin immediately. You may pass bloody stools.

Examination of the blood vessels, called angiography (see page 656), determines the site of obstruction. This generally is followed by an emergency operation to remove the segment of intestine that has lost its blood supply. If there has not been permanent damage to the intestine, the clot can be removed or the affected artery can be reconstructed.

Ischemic Colitis

In ischemic colitis, the blood supply to the colon is decreased, although usually the affected vessels are not major arteries. This condition most often affects the elderly. The symptoms include lower abdominal pain and rectal bleeding.

Surgery may be required in severe cases, but most often the problem resolves spontaneously. Later, a narrowing of the colon (stricture) may occur at the site of the episode of ischemia.

Angiodysplasia of the Colon

This is dilation, distortion, or thinning of blood vessels in the colon. It is more common in the elderly. Rectal bleeding is a common symptom. The diagnosis of angiodysplasia of the colon requires an angiogram of the colon (see page 656) or direct visualization of the lesions at colonoscopy (see page 788). The hemorrhage can be halted by blocking the affected vessel during a diagnostic procedure called arteriography (see page 656) or by cautery or laser treatment of the lesion through the colonoscope (see page 788). When there is massive bleeding or bleeding is from multiple sites, surgical removal of the affected part of the colon may be necessary.

Anorectal Disorders

The anus is the 1½-inch-long canal that is the outlet for the rectum. A ring of muscles, the anal sphincter, controls the movement of the solid waste products of the digestive process through the anus and thus out of the body.

The anus is a relatively simple structure in contrast to the other parts of the digestive system. Generally, the anorectal disorders are hemorrhoids, crack-like sores (fissures), abscesses, and inflammations.

Hemorrhoids

Signs and Symptoms
- Bright red blood on the toilet paper, in the water of the toilet bowl, or on the stool itself
- Protrusion of soft tissue at the anus
- Tenderness, especially during a bowel movement

Hemorrhoids (often referred to as "piles") are clusters of veins located in the anus, just under the membrane that lines the lowest part of the rectum and anus. Sometimes, often as a result of straining during a bowel movement, these veins become swollen. This forms the hemorrhoid. Because these veins are thin and easily ruptured, bleeding may occur during a bowel movement. Hemorrhoids are also common during pregnancy because increased pressure in the veins causes them to swell.

Hemorrhoids can occur internally (near the beginning of the anal canal) or externally, outside the orifice itself. Both types are common, and both may bleed.

Hemorrhoids can become especially painful if a blood clot forms. These hemorrhoids are referred to as thrombosed (from thrombosis, for clot). These generally occur in external hemorrhoids and cause a painful lump at the anal opening.

Itching and anal pain generally are not symptoms of hemorrhoids unless associated with a complication such as thrombosis or erosion of the overlying surface.

Diagnosis
Visual examination of your anus by your physician usually reveals whether you have external hemorrhoids. The anus can be examined with a rubber-gloved finger but, because a hemorrhoid is very soft, a definite diagnosis may not be made. Your physician may also examine the area with a proctoscope or anoscope (see Screening for Colon Cancer, page 790). Your examination may also include a barium enema (see The Barium X-Ray, page 762) or colonoscopy (see page 788).

All episodes of rectal bleeding should be investigated. Do not assume that rectal bleeding is from hemorrhoids until other potential sources of bleeding, such as a colon polyp or colon cancer, have been ruled out.

Treatment
Most people with hemorrhoids are so little bothered by the problem that they ignore it. For others, however, the symptoms are too bothersome to be easily dismissed.

If your hemorrhoids are producing only mild discomfort, your physician may suggest over-the-counter creams, ointments, or pads containing witch hazel, or a topical anesthetic agent. This, in combination with daily warm baths or showers, may relieve your symptoms. More liquids and fiber in your diet can help soften your stool and make constipation less likely, which may decrease the chances of further hemorrhoids developing.

If possible, avoid prolonged standing or sitting. If you must sit for long periods, don't use an inflatable "donut" cushion to pad your chair.

If you have a persistent or recurrent protruding or bleeding internal (inside the anal canal) hemorrhoid, your physician can perform a corrective procedure right in his or her office. This involves tying off the internal hemorrhoid with a rubber band. In a few days, the hemorrhoid painlessly falls off. This method is effective in about 75 percent of cases.

When a blood clot has formed within an external hemorrhoid, your physician can remove the clot, which should provide prompt relief.

Other techniques include injecting a shrinking agent into an internal hemorrhoid or destroying the hemorrhoid by infrared photocoagulation, a technique in which the affected tissue is destroyed.

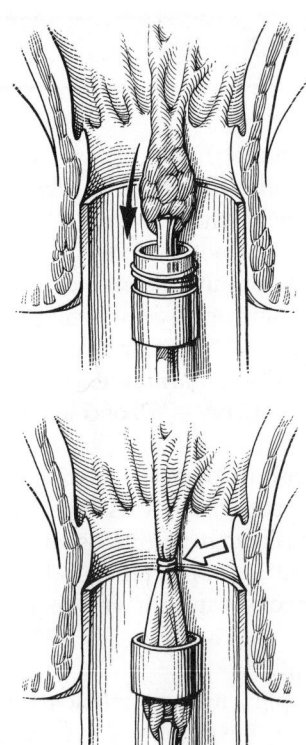

To remove an internal hemorrhoid with a rubber band, the physician first attaches a special instrument to the hemorrhoid and stretches it downward (top). Then a rubber band is placed around the hemorrhoid (arrow) to cut off its blood supply. Both the hemorrhoid and the rubber band are eliminated later with body waste.

Large hemorrhoids are removed surgically in a procedure called hemorrhoidectomy. The more extensive the removal of hemorrhoidal tissue, the less chance of recurrence but the greater the discomfort in the several days after the operation. Laser surgery shows promise, but the value and cost-effectiveness of this approach are unproved.

Anal Itch

Anal itching, also called pruritus ani, is a distracting, potentially embarrassing, and common problem; almost everyone is afflicted at one time or another.

A persistent anal itch is a more common problem for children and the elderly. In children, it may be due to the presence of a common parasite called pinworms (see page 1082). Among the elderly, the cause usually is aging dry skin.

For most of the rest of the population, the cause of the problem is not always easily established. In evaluating your anal itch, your physician will look for signs of a skin ailment such as psoriasis, skin cancer, or a yeast infection. He or she will also examine you for hemorrhoids, anal fissure, or anal fistula, each of which may cause itching and irritation. These disorders rarely are a cause of anal itching. In fact, often the precise cause remains a mystery.

Here are some additional factors that may predispose you to anal itching: some people, in an effort to be squeaky clean, scrub their rectal area with a harsh soap and rough washcloth, which causes itching, burning, and irritation. Some people use over-the-counter medication to relieve the itching. These drugs, in fact, may sensitize the skin and cause irritation, with itching and burning. Some physicians believe that stress may be a factor, although this has not been proved. The muscles that normally keep the anal canal closed tightly can become lax, allowing stool-containing mucus to seep out and irritate the surrounding skin. If the anal area is not cleansed adequately after a bowel movement, bits of stool will cling to the skin and cause irritation and itching.

Treatment

If anal itching is a problem for you, try the following self-help measures:

1. Stop scratching. As hard as this may be, summon your will power and try it. Continued scratching leads to persistent inflammation and damage to the delicate tissue. The more you scratch, the more you itch. Try a cold pack and a 0.5 percent hydrocortisone cream or ointment (available without a prescription) to relieve the discomfort.

2. Keep the area clean. Cleanse the area gently in the morning, in the evening, and after a bowel movement. Use moistened, unscented, white toilet paper or cotton balls.

3. To prevent skin irritation from the leakage of mucus, place a cotton pad between your buttocks, up against the anus. Replace the pad as necessary.

4. Taking an antihistamine tablet at bedtime may lessen the itch. Drugs such as diphenhydramine or chlorpheniramine are available without a prescription.

If these measures do not relieve your problem, see your physician for a thorough evaluation.

Anal Fissures and Fistulas

Signs and Symptoms
- Pain during and after bowel movements
- Bright red blood on the stool or toilet paper

An anal fissure is a relatively minor cut or crack in the lining of the anal canal in an area adjacent to the tailbone, scrotum, or vagina. It starts at the anal opening and extends up into the canal.

An acute anal fissure may heal with the addition of fiber to the diet; a medication that softens the stool also may help. If the cut is deep, the pain may be more intense, both during and after defecation, because the tissue may cause the anal sphincter muscle to go into spasm. Again, the addition of fiber, a stool softener, or a bulk former containing psyllium will help relieve the pain (see Chronic Constipation, page 784). A warm bath will relax the muscle and reduce the spasm that causes the pain.

If the pain continues, your physician may decide to operate. This is usually a minor surgical procedure that does not require an overnight stay in the hospital.

An anal fistula is an abnormal tube-like passageway from the anal canal to a hole in the skin around the opening to the anus. The fistula is usually the result of an anorectal abscess that has drained (see Anorectal Abscess, page 798). Sometimes a fistula may result from inflammation or previous surgery of the lower colon.

If the opening in the skin becomes obstructed, pus and debris can collect in the fistula tract, causing pain and swelling. This will often drain spontaneously and symptoms resolve until the opening again becomes clogged.

At times, an anal fistula or anorectal abscess indicates the presence of Crohn's disease (see page 774) or is the result of previous operation in this area. A rectal examination, colonoscopy, and small bowel X-ray (see Colonoscopy, page 788, and The Barium X-Ray, page 762) may be done.

Treatment of fistulas usually consists of cutting the skin, fat and muscle overlying the fistula tract. The wound is left open and usually heals in 4 to 6 weeks. Abscesses are drained by cutting the skin overlying the collection of pus.

Rectal Bleeding

Rectal bleeding can be a sign of cancer, but it does not always signal disease. More often it indicates a problem in the digestive system that isn't life-threatening and responds well to treatment. Causes of bleeding in the lower gastrointestinal tract are listed here:

- Proctitis—an inflammation of the inner lining of the rectum. It can be caused by infection or radiation treatment, or the cause may be unknown. If a bacterial infection is the cause, your physician may prescribe an antibiotic (see page 798)
- Colon or rectal polyps—rectal bleeding may be the initial sign of a rectal or colon polyp, or even cancer (see page 786)
- Hemorrhoids—enlarged veins in the lining of the anus (see page 795)
- Anal fissure—a tear in the lining of your anus (see page 796)

- Anal fistula—an abnormal channel that develops between the anal canal and the skin around the opening to the anus (see page 796)
- Rectal prolapse—a portion of the rectum protrudes through the anus. This can be caused by continued straining to defecate. As you age, your rectal muscles weaken, so prolapse can become chronic in later years. Surgery often can correct the problem
- Diverticular disease—small sacs or pouches (diverticula) commonly form on the large intestine. They uncommonly cause bleeding, sometimes without other symptoms. Your physician may perform tests to establish the site of bleeding, or you may need surgery if the bleeding persists (see page 781)

Although eating beets can produce a reddish stool that sometimes is mistaken for blood in the stool, don't attempt self-diagnosis. Rectal bleeding requires prompt evaluation by your physician to establish its cause and, more importantly, to rule out cancer.

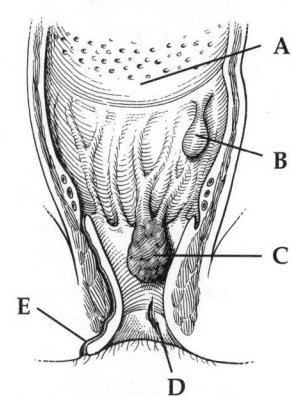

Cross-section view of anus and rectum shows causes of rectal bleeding: **(A)** proctitis, **(B)** polyp, **(C)** hemorrhoids, **(D)** anal fissure, and **(E)** anal fistula. (Not shown: Rectal prolapse and diverticular disease.)

Anorectal Abscess

Signs and Symptoms
- Discharge of pus
- Fever
- Discomfort in or around the anal opening
- Swelling and redness near the anus

Anorectal abscesses affect the area immediately around the anus. Most anal abscesses are the result of infected anal glands.

An abscess that is easily accessible near the anus can be lanced and drained, either in your physician's office or at a hospital outpatient service. However, if you have a fever and sharp pains accompanied by a sense of pressure between your anus and coccyx (the coccyx is the tailbone, at the base of your spine), your physician may suspect an abscess higher up into your rectum. These deep abscesses are less accessible, their diagnosis is more difficult, and their potential complications are more serious.

Deep rectal abscesses warrant careful attention because they could be caused by an intestinal disorder such as Crohn's disease (see page 774), ulcerative colitis (see page 777), or diverticulitis (see Diverticulosis and Diverticulitis, page 781).

Diagnosis
If there is a possibility of a deep anorectal abscess, your physician will perform a thorough examination of your rectum, which may include proctosigmoidoscopy (see Screening for Colon Cancer, page 790) and a barium enema (see The Barium X-Ray, page 762), and possibly a CT scan or ultrasound (see pages 1334 and 1335). If you are too tender to examine adequately, your physician may do these examinations while you are under anesthesia.

Treatment

Surgery
Once the abscess has been identified, you will be hospitalized and the abscess will be lanced and drained. In addition, you may be given an analgesic for your pain. Antibiotics are given if the infection is severe.

Proctitis

Signs and Symptoms
- Blood, mucus, or pus in the stool
- Constipation
- Diarrhea
- Severe rectal pain
- Fever

Proctitis is an inflammation of the rectum that may result from an infection (bacterial or viral). It also may be a feature of ulcerative colitis (see page 777) or Crohn's disease (see page 774). In some instances, proctitis is due to anal intercourse. A person with proctitis due to a sexually transmitted infection can spread the disease to other sexual partners (see Sexually Transmitted Diseases, page 1087). Radiation treatment such as for prostate cancer can also cause proctitis.

Some of the symptoms associated with proctitis are a clue to the possible cause of the infection. Mucus, blood, or pus in your stool may suggest an inflammation caused by gonorrhea. If herpes simplex virus has caused the proctitis, there is extreme anal pain along with ulcers or blister-like elevations around your anus. In both cases, the skin around your anus may burn and itch.

Anal Pain

Have you ever had a sharp, severe pain in your rectum awaken you from a sound sleep?

This painful condition is called proctalgia fugax. The cause is not well understood, but it is believed to be due to an intense spasm of the muscles in the lower pelvis and rectum. The pain resembles the discomfort you experience from a cramp in your calf.

Typically, the pain occurs at night while you are asleep. You awaken to this intense and unrelenting pain. Within a few minutes to half an hour the pain subsides. It can recur at irregular intervals, with the frequency varying from twice a week to a few times a year. Sometimes the spells disappear entirely.

Although this can be very frightening, rest assured that the pain is not serious. It is not caused by cancer, hemorrhoids, or other diseases of the rectum.

What should you do? First, see your physician. He or she can perform the diagnostic tests that will rule out any serious disease. This will help ease your mind; intense pain is not necessarily equated with serious illness.

Here are some tips to try the next time you have the pain.

1. Sit in a bathtub full of warm water.

2. Try to have a bowel movement; this sometimes eliminates the pain.

3. Drink warm water or eat crackers; this may stimulate normal contractions in the intestine that will relieve the spasm.

A repeated urge to defecate or an inability to move your bowels may develop. If the source of the infection is not just in the rectum but deeper in your bowel (proctocolitis), the symptoms are likely to be more severe anorectal pain and fever.

Diagnosis

Your physician will examine the skin around your anus, analyze the stool for infection, and conduct a proctosigmoidoscopic examination (see Screening for Colon Cancer, page 790).

How Serious Is Proctitis?

Depending on the cause, the inflammation may or may not be easily treated. Bacterial infections respond to antibiotics but viral infections do not.

Treatment

Medication

The initial treatment for bacterial proctitis is an antibiotic such as ciprofloxacin. There is no medication available that will cure proctitis caused by herpes simplex virus, although your physician will prescribe agents that can control the spread of the infection and ease the symptoms. Proctitis can be treated with 5-ASA or corticosteroid enemas (see Crohn's Disease, page 774, and Ulcerative Colitis, page 777). These agents can also be used in radiation-induced proctitis. If they are ineffective, laser treatment may be considered.

Fecal Incontinence

Fecal incontinence refers to the inability to control bowel movements. When this disorder occurs in any healthy adult, the problem is usually due to some type of underlying condition (see Encopresis, page 1098, for a discussion of a similar condition in children).

Diagnosis

Your physician will question you carefully to determine if there is a precipitating cause of your incontinence, such as sneezing or coughing, if it occurs only at night, and if there are any associated symptoms. He or she also will examine your anal sphincter to determine whether the muscles in this area are intact. Your physician may also order special studies including electromyography (EMG, see page 1344) or the use of special devices to determine various pressures in your rectal and anal regions.

Causes

Fecal incontinence may be caused by an abscess or inflammation in the rectum, anus, or perianal area. It can be the result of a previous operation in this area or of trauma or complications occurring at the time of delivery of an infant. Particularly if the anal sphincter is intact, fecal incontinence can be due to an injury or a disorder of the nervous system, particularly one affecting the spinal cord.

Fecal incontinence occurs often in the elderly. As you age, the muscles and ligaments that control urination and defecation become less efficient and thus are more readily disturbed by a physical ailment. However, incontinence is not an inevitable part of getting older.

Fecal impaction, particularly in the elderly, can be a cause of incontinence. This generally occurs in people who experience constipation. The impaction does not totally obstruct the bowel so that the more liquid portions of the stool seep past the area of impaction, causing incontinence.

Treatment

In some adults with fecal incontinence, a bowel retraining program can be begun, particularly if the anal sphincter is intact. At times, this may include the use of a bulk former (see Chronic Constipation, page 784).

Sexually Transmitted Infections of the Rectum

Several infectious diseases are transmitted sexually through anal intercourse (see Sexually Transmitted Diseases, page 1087). Specifically, proctitis caused by gonorrhea (see page 1087), herpes simplex virus (see page 1090), and anal warts (see page 1092) usually is communicated through rectal intercourse (see Proctitis, page 798).

Sexually transmitted rectal infections can be serious because of the risk of complications, particularly bleeding, the later development of a narrowing or stricture of the rectum, or, rarely, cancer.

Many such bacterial infections are clinically considered to be mild and pose no threat to other systems of the body. However, if you experience the symptoms of any sexually transmitted infection, see your physician for proper treatment. Your physician may want to screen for the AIDS virus if a sexually transmitted infection of the rectum is present.

Your physician may advise you to sit for a certain period of time each day for defecation; this often results in continence during the remainder of the day. He or she also will advise you to increase your hydration and emphasize eating fresh fruits and vegetables. This sometimes helps to produce a more normal stool and decreases the number of times you have to defecate.

At times, your physician may recommend a surgical procedure on the anal sphincter, particularly if the sphincter has been damaged by trauma.

In most people, particularly in the elderly, there is no surgical procedure that will result in consistent improvement. However, if the sphincter has been damaged by surgery, trauma, or childbirth, a surgical repair of the sphincter may result in significant improvement.

Liver Disease

Apart from the digestive tract itself, the organs of the digestive system include the liver, the gallbladder, and the pancreas (see Gallbladder and Bile Duct Disorders, page 812, and Pancreatic Diseases, page 818).

The liver not only is the largest single internal organ in the body but also is the most complex. Weighing as much as 4 pounds, the liver performs many complicated tasks that are essential to the proper functioning of the entire body. These functions may be grouped into three categories: regulation, metabolism, and detoxification.

The liver regulates the composition of your blood, in particular the amounts of glucose (sugar), protein, and fat that enter the bloodstream. The liver also removes from the blood a substance called bilirubin, which is a residue from the breakdown of red blood cells. Once the bilirubin enters the liver it is chemically changed so that it becomes soluble in water. Then it is added to the bile, enters the intestinal tract, and is eliminated.

If, for any reason, the liver is unable to remove the bilirubin from the blood, the bilirubin level will build up and the bilirubin eventually will be deposited in the skin, causing a yellow appearance known as jaundice.

The liver processes most of the nutrients that are absorbed from the intestine. Besides converting many of these nutrients into forms that can be used by the body, the liver also serves as a storage center for some nutrients such as vitamin A, iron, and other minerals. It manufactures cholesterol, vitamin A, blood clotting substances, and specific proteins.

The liver also detoxifies the blood. This means it removes drugs, alcohol, and potentially harmful chemicals from the bloodstream and treats them chemically so they can be excreted in the feces and urine.

Daily, the liver manufactures about a quart of bile, a yellow fluid. The bile travels through the liver ducts and then through the cystic duct to the gallbladder where it is stored temporarily. After you eat a meal, the gallbladder expels the bile so that it travels through the common bile duct and empties into the duodenum. The bile acids in the bile facilitate the digestion of fats. Spicier fatty meals tend to cause more vigorous contraction of the gallbladder and common bile duct.

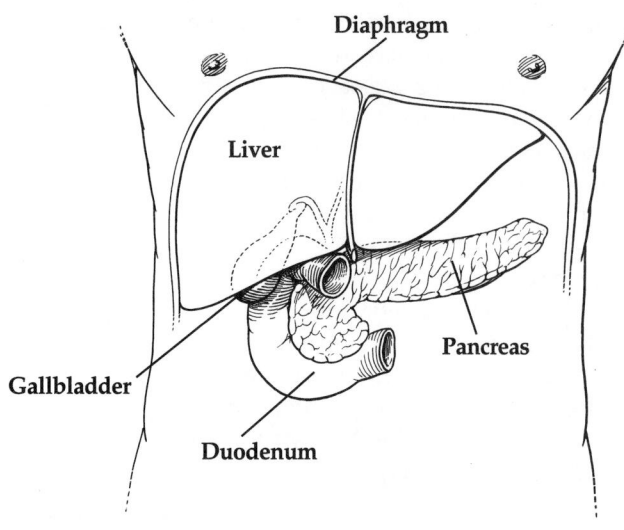

Diaphragm

Liver

Gallbladder

Pancreas

Duodenum

Because of the complexity of the liver and its exposure to so many potentially harmful substances, it would be reasonable to believe that it is especially vulnerable to disease. However, nature protects the organ in several ways. First, the liver is capable of regeneration—it can heal itself by repairing or replacing injured tissue. It also is constructed so that many units are responsible for the same task. Thus, if tissue in one section of the organ is injured, by trauma or disease, other cells will perform the functions of the injured section indefinitely or until the damage has been repaired.

Despite this built-in protection, the liver does suffer from many diseases, especially inflammatory conditions that can threaten its health and the health of its host.

Acute Viral Hepatitis

Signs and Symptoms
- Jaundice (yellowing of the skin and eyes)
- Fatigue
- Lack of appetite
- Nausea and vomiting
- Alterations in senses of taste and smell
- Low-grade fever

Hepatitis is an inflammation of the liver caused by a virus or, less commonly, by certain medications or toxins (see Alcoholic, Toxic, and Drug-Related Hepatitis, page 803).

Three main types of viral hepatitis have been identified: hepatitis A, hepatitis B, and hepatitis C. The symptoms are similar.

An acute viral hepatitis can range from being without any symptoms whatsoever to being fatal; the latter is rare. If you have hepatitis, you may feel better within a few days after your initial symptoms disappear, but it may take months for your liver to recover completely.

Acute Hepatitis A
This is a highly infectious form of hepatitis and is the most common form. The disease is transmitted mainly by contaminated food or water. If you have hepatitis A, the virus will be in your stools, blood, and bile for 2 to 3 weeks before any symptoms develop. The virus disappears once jaundice develops or within 2 to 3 weeks afterward. Thus, anyone who comes into contact with your blood or feces, even before you have symptoms, may become infected with the virus.

The symptoms of hepatitis A often are similar to those of intestinal flu. But because the infected liver is unable to filter bilirubin from your blood, your skin and eyes may become yellow, and the bile excreted in your urine may turn it tea-colored.

The vast majority of persons with hepatitis A recover completely. Within 1 to 2 months, your liver is completely healed. Hepatitis A does not develop into chronic hepatitis (see page 804) or cirrhosis (see page 804), nor does the hepatitis A virus remain in your body even if no symptoms are present (carrier state).

Acute Hepatitis B
Hepatitis B is potentially a more serious form of viral liver infection. Its symptoms are much the same as those of hepatitis A but can be more severe and last longer. As a result, there is a greater possibility of liver damage. A complication in up to 10 percent of hepatitis B cases is the development of chronic hepatitis.

The hepatitis B virus commonly is acquired through exposure to contaminated blood. Those most likely to contract the virus are intravenous drug users who share contaminated needles. Sexual contact with a person who has hepatitis B also can spread the disease. Other persons who may acquire hepatitis B virus include health-care workers exposed to blood and persons who need repeated transfusions of blood products (for example, hemophiliacs; see Hemophilia, page 975). However, testing of donor blood before transfusion has virtually eliminated the risk of acquiring hepatitis B from a blood transfusion.

A pregnant woman may pass the virus to her developing fetus. There are some infected people (carriers) who never have symptoms but are capable of passing the virus to others. And some persons who have had hepatitis B remain carriers. Ninety percent of those with uncomplicated hepatitis B recover within 3 to 4 months.

Hepatitis C
Hepatitis C may produce symptoms that resemble hepatitis A and B, except that they are often less severe and jaundice may not be present. In fact, the majority of persons with hepatitis C are either asymptomatic or have only mild fatigue. Often an abnormal result on a routine liver test will alert a physician to the possibility of hepatitis C.

Hepatitis C virus can now be identified with a blood test. Before blood tests to screen for hepatitis C were available, blood transfusions were a major cause of hepatitis C. Now this is rare. You can also acquire hepatitis C from sharing contaminated needles, as with intravenous drug use or, although uncommon, tattoos. Often, the source cannot be identified. Hepatitis C frequently leads to chronic liver disease. Although infrequent, it can also cause liver scarring (cirrhosis).

Occasionally, hepatitis may be caused by other viruses, notably cytomegalovirus or Epstein-Barr virus. Sometimes, no virus can be identified in an individual whose illness suggests viral hepatitis. It is likely that some viral causes of hepatitis have not yet been identified.

Diagnosis

If you notice that your skin is becoming jaundiced or that you have any other symptoms of hepatitis, your physician may conduct a blood test. In addition to a careful medical history, your physician will ask you a number of questions about your sex life, the medications you have taken in the past few months, and whether you have had any blood transfusions (or contact with fresh blood) during the same period.

How Serious Is Hepatitis?

Virtually all persons who are healthy prior to contracting hepatitis A recover from the acute illness; 90 percent of individuals with hepatitis B also recover. Hepatitis C often gives rise to chronic hepatitis (see Chronic Hepatitis, page 804).

If you are elderly or have medical problems such as diabetes, congestive heart failure, or severe anemia, recovery is apt to take longer, and the risk of complications is greater. Your physician may advise treatment in a medical center specializing in liver disorders.

Treatment

There is no specific treatment for acute hepatitis. Bed rest is not essential, although you may feel better if you restrict physical activity. It is important to maintain an adequate intake of calories. You may find you feel better if most of your day's calories are consumed in the morning.

You will be asked to abstain from any alcohol, at least during your recovery, because both alcohol and drugs make excessive demands on the already damaged liver.

In severe cases, hospitalization may be required, particularly if you are unable to eat solids or drink fluids needed for adequate

Hepatitis Vaccine

If a member of your family has hepatitis B or you work in a profession that exposes you to the hepatitis B virus, your physician may suggest that you be immunized. Americans considered to be at high risk for hepatitis B virus infection include people who inject illicit drugs with needles, people with multiple sex partners, sexually active homosexual and bisexual men, sexual partners of those with hepatitis B, people with hemophilia, people who undergo hemodialysis for kidney failure, dental and medical health professionals, and male prison inmates.

All infants should receive hepatitis B vaccine as part of their routine childhood immunization series. Preadolescents (starting at age 10), all adolescents, college students, and young adults also should receive the vaccine.

The Occupational Safety and Health Administration now requires some employers to offer hepatitis B vaccine at no cost to employees. Included are health care workers, public safety personnel, and other workers who might be exposed to blood.

Because hepatitis B is widespread in certain regions of the world, ask your physician about the vaccine if you plan to travel outside the United States and Canada (see Immunizations, page 380).

A hepatitis A vaccine is now available which offers protection against the most common type of the disease, hepatitis A. If you have been exposed to hepatitis A, you may be given an injection of an immune globulin that contains protective antibodies against hepatitis A virus. It is usually given immediately after (within 2 weeks) known exposure to contaminated food or contact with an infected person or before possible exposure to hepatitis A (for example, immediately before a trip to an area where the disease is common). Sometimes it does not actually prevent the infection but does make the disease state mild enough that you have no serious symptoms. The protection given by the immune globulin injection lasts for only a few weeks.

nutrition and hydration. Generally this is only for several days.

After hepatitis B or C, your physician may draw blood periodically for a few months to check for continuing inflammation of the liver or a return to normal. Interferon, an antiviral agent, has been approved for the treatment of persistent hepatitis B and C, but it produces lasting benefit in only a minority of individuals treated.

Although it is not necessary to isolate a person with hepatitis from the rest of the family, the entire household should be aware of how the virus spreads. Thus, stringent hand washing after going to the bathroom is important, as is thorough cleansing if there is any contact with the affected person's feces, blood, or any body fluid.

Prevention
See Hepatitis Vaccine, page 802.

Alcoholic, Toxic, and Drug-Related Hepatitis

Signs and Symptoms
- Jaundice (yellowing of the skin and eyes)
- Fatigue
- Lack of appetite
- Nausea and vomiting
- Alterations in senses of taste and smell
- Low-grade fever

Hepatitis can occur after excessive and chronic use of alcohol; it also can occur immediately after the inhalation or ingestion of a toxin or the use of certain medications.

In general, the symptoms and signs of alcoholic, toxic, and drug-related hepatitis are indistinguishable from those of acute viral hepatitis. The key difference is that the offending agent that caused the hepatitis must be identified and eliminated.

Treatment generally is supportive rather than specific and is designed to give the liver time to heal. This may involve just observation of your health and symptoms; at other times, you may be required to avoid eating protein (which cannot be broken down and eliminated by the liver during the acute phase of injury), and nutrients will be delivered through a vein to maintain calorie support and prevent dehydration.

Alcoholic Hepatitis
This form of hepatitis may produce virtually no symptoms or it can begin with mild flu-like symptoms. Sometimes it can lead to liver failure.

Someone with a severe case of alcoholic hepatitis may run a high fever and develop an enlarged liver (see page 809). Recovery often is slow. Even after complete abstinence from alcohol, recovery may take weeks, and abnormalities in the liver tissue can persist for 6 months or more (see Cirrhosis, page 804).

The development of fluid retention, particularly in the abdomen (characterized by an enlarging abdomen), and difficulty in maintaining your mental concentration are worrisome features and may indicate liver failure. It is imperative that, if you are to recover, you must abstain from alcohol permanently, and from some medications temporarily. Check with your physician before taking any medications.

Toxic and Drug-Induced Hepatitis
The liver can be damaged by chemical agents and industrial toxins such as carbon tetrachloride. But drug-induced hepatitis is a more common problem. Both prescribed medications and those purchased over-the-counter can produce hepatitis in susceptible persons.

Several widely used drugs can produce an adverse liver reaction. Isoniazid (used for the treatment of tuberculosis), methyldopa (a treatment for high blood pressure), and the pain reliever acetaminophen have been clearly associated with hepatitis. The anesthetic halothane is another.

Certain other drugs have been found to interfere with the flow of bile in some instances. Among them are the antibiotic erythromycin, the tranquilizer chlorpromazine, oral contraceptives, and anabolic steroids. Such liver complications usually subside within a few days or weeks after use of the drug is stopped. Do not use oral contraceptives if you have a history of jaundice during pregnancy. Both oral contraceptives and anabolic steroids have been associated with liver cancer in a small percentage of cases.

Because of these risks, inform your physician if you have any history of liver disease or liver problems before taking any medication. Furthermore, if you have any symptoms or laboratory findings that suggest hepatitis, your physician will want to know if you have been taking any medication in the previous 2 months.

Chronic Hepatitis

Signs and Symptoms
- Often, none
- Fatigue
- Lack of appetite
- Nausea and vomiting
- Persistent or recurring jaundice
- Low-grade fever

Chronic hepatitis comes in two major forms: chronic persistent hepatitis and chronic active hepatitis.

Chronic persistent hepatitis (which is simply a mild form of chronic active hepatitis) sometimes is the result of hepatitis B or C. Often, the cause is not apparent. Generally, this form of chronic hepatitis is nonprogressive. Liver failure does not occur, and cirrhosis of the liver rarely results.

Most people with chronic persistent hepatitis have no symptoms. However, some complain of fatigue, lack of appetite, and, occasionally, vomiting and nausea.

Chronic active hepatitis, however, is a progressive disease that may lead to liver failure, cirrhosis, or death. Chronic active hepatitis has various causes, the most common of which seems to be hepatitis B or C. A reaction to certain medications may cause this condition as well. In some cases, no specific cause is found. With chronic active hepatitis, fatigue is a common symptom, although there may be virtually no symptoms or there may be all of those associated with acute infectious hepatitis (see page 801).

Diagnosis
At first, you may appear to have acute viral hepatitis, but if your symptoms do not respond to rest and your blood test results continue to be abnormal, your physician may suspect chronic hepatitis. Besides blood tests, he or she may obtain a liver biopsy specimen (a small sample of liver tissue is removed for microscopic analysis; see page 807). Chronic active hepatitis is a serious disease and can be fatal. Chronic persistent hepatitis generally is well tolerated and may resolve spontaneously, although many months may be required for recovery.

Treatment
No specific treatment is required for chronic persistent hepatitis.

The treatment for some cases of chronic active hepatitis is corticosteroids. Your physician may consider the use of corticosteroids if your chronic active hepatitis was not the result of a virus and you have evidence of severe inflammation in your liver. As many as 60 to 80 percent of those treated with these drugs have a complete remission. You should begin to feel stronger and your appetite should return to normal within a few days to weeks after the treatment is begun. You may have no symptoms after a month or so of treatment, but it may be as long as 6 months to 2 years before your blood is free of all signs of the hepatitis. Even so, relapses are common after the corticosteroid regimen is discontinued.

At times, azathioprine is used in association with corticosteroids. These drugs are most effective when the chronic hepatitis is not caused by hepatitis B or C virus.

Although suppressing inflammation, the corticosteroids may not prevent progression to cirrhosis (see Cirrhosis, this page). Occasionally, if the disease is severe and fails to respond to treatment, your physician may consider liver transplantation (see Liver Transplantation, page 811).

Cirrhosis

Signs and Symptoms
- There may be none
- Loss of appetite
- Weight loss
- Nausea and vomiting
- General fatigue and weakness
- Jaundice (yellowing of the skin and eyes)
- Abdominal pain
- Intestinal bleeding
- Small, red, spider-like blood vessels under the skin or easy bruising
- Loss of interest in sex. Men may become impotent. Women cease to menstruate
- Itching
- Swelling of the abdomen and legs

Emergency Symptoms
- Vomiting or passing blood through the rectum
- Mental confusion

Cirrhosis is a condition in which liver tissue has been irreversibly and progressively destroyed as a result of infection, poison, or some other disease. The normal liver tissue is replaced by scarring and areas of regenerating liver cells.

As liver cells die, thick scar tissue may grow in their place. With the death of these cells, more and more of the complicated functions of the organ are handled by fewer and fewer cells. The liver initially may increase in size to compensate for cells no longer able to carry out their normal function. In time, with more scarring, the liver becomes smaller.

A healthy liver performs its various functions on the nutrients that have been absorbed in the gut and sent to it by the bloodstream. If the liver cells die and the liver itself contracts, it becomes increasingly more difficult for blood to flow to the liver. The blood flow may then reverse (portal hypertension) and actually bypass the liver, robbing it of important nutrients. Reversal of blood flow may cause the spleen to enlarge, and varices may develop in your esophagus, which are prone to bleed (see Esophageal Varices, page 750).

If the scarred or cirrhotic liver is unable to process the blood and remove breakdown products properly, these breakdown products may have an adverse effect on your brain. Often these products are excessive amounts of protein that normally are broken down and removed by the liver. Blood levels of these substances increase and may cause a tremor of the hands, mental confusion, and, finally, coma (encephalopathy).

Another cause of portal hypertension is development of a blood clot in the vein that brings blood into the liver (portal vein thrombosis). In some situations, there may be no discernible cause for the obstruction of this vein.

A blood clot that blocks blood flow out of the liver, a disorder called hepatic vein thrombosis or Budd-Chiari syndrome, is a far less likely cause of portal hypertension. This obstruction also causes the liver to become enlarged and extremely tender. It usually produces a serious form of water retention in the abdomen (ascites).

There are various causes and forms of cirrhosis.

Alcohol-Induced Cirrhosis

In the United States, alcoholic cirrhosis is the most common type. It usually occurs after many years of heavy drinking and develops in as many as 15 percent of alcoholics. Typically, people who develop cirrhosis from alcohol abuse have consumed a pint or more of whiskey or several quarts of wine daily for

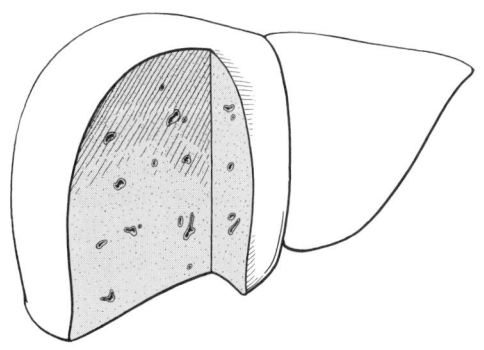

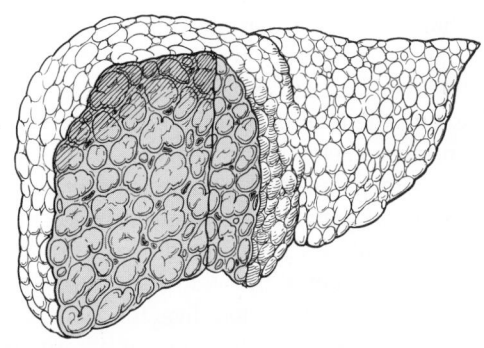

Shown in cross-section, the normal liver (top) shows no sign of scarring. The cirrhotic liver (bottom) has extensive scarring.

at least 10 years. As little as 3 ounces of 100-proof whiskey (45 grams of alcohol) every day for several years may be sufficient to cause liver damage.

Symptoms of cirrhosis are often silent in the alcoholic. For others, the symptoms begin slowly. These include lack of appetite, weight loss, easy bruising, weakness, and fatigue. Jaundice and esophageal bleeding may follow.

Treatment is directed toward the complications of the disease, such as bleeding or the accumulation of excess fluid in the abdomen (ascites). It is imperative that the alcoholic give up alcohol. This will not reverse the damage already done to the liver, but it will lessen further liver damage. The person who has cirrhosis and has stopped drinking will feel better and may live longer.

Cryptogenic Cirrhosis

Also known as post-hepatitic cirrhosis, this is the final stage of chronic liver disease that occurs as a result of hepatitis B virus, hepatitis C virus, or unknown causes. Most of the unknown causes are probably viral.

The symptoms are similar to those of other forms of cirrhosis. At times, people with cryptogenic cirrhosis have no symptoms, and the diagnosis of the disease is made at the time of an operation for another disorder or from a liver biopsy performed for unexplained liver enlargement (see Liver Biopsy, page 807).

Biopsy of the liver is used to confirm the diagnosis. There is no specific treatment for the cirrhosis itself. Rather, attention is directed to controlling fluid accumulation and to avoiding medications or excess protein that may contribute to mental confusion.

Primary Biliary Cirrhosis

The biliary tract consists of the ducts, within and leading from the liver, that deliver bile to the intestine. Primary biliary cirrhosis is characterized by chronic inflammation and scarring of the microscopic bile ducts within the liver. The cause is unknown. The result is that the liver is progressively destroyed and scarring (cirrhosis) develops.

Many people with primary biliary cirrhosis initially have no symptoms. Their condition usually is discovered during a routine physical examination that includes blood tests that relate to various liver functions. For unknown reasons, this form of biliary cirrhosis affects mostly women between the ages of 35 and 60.

The symptoms of primary biliary cirrhosis include severe itching (pruritus) on the hands and feet and eventually the entire body. Jaundice, dark urine, and darkening of skin exposed to the sun occur as the liver disease progresses. This slow progression results eventually in portal hypertension (see page 807), the accumulation of fluids, and eventually liver failure and death. Small collections of fat are often seen in the area around the eyes, a reflection of the high cholesterol values in these persons (see Xanthelasma and Xanthoma, page 1001).

The diagnosis usually is suspected on the basis of your clinical history and appearance and abnormal blood test results. A liver biopsy should be performed to confirm the diagnosis (see page 807). In addition, your physician may want to examine the bile ducts themselves by using X-rays, to exclude any obstruction in this area (see PTHC, page 815, and ERCP, page 816).

There is no specific therapy for primary biliary cirrhosis; however, several investigational agents appear promising. The goal generally is to relieve the symptoms. The drug cholestyramine may be effective in decreasing the itching. In addition, your physician may prescribe vitamin supplements because vitamins are inadequately absorbed in this particular disorder.

Increasingly, liver transplantation is being used for persons with severe liver failure from primary biliary cirrhosis.

Secondary Biliary Cirrhosis

Secondary biliary cirrhosis results from prolonged obstruction of the common bile duct or one of its branches. This may result from a previous operation that produces narrowing (stricture) in the bile duct area. In other cases, a chronic inflammation of the bile ducts (Primary Sclerosing Cholangitis, see page 814) may be the cause of chronic obstruction and the ultimate development of cirrhosis.

The signs and symptoms are similar to those of primary biliary cirrhosis. At times, fever and pain in the right upper portion of your abdomen may be present, reflecting an infection originating from the impaired flow in the bile ducts.

Your physician's diagnosis will be based on identifying the obstruction of the bile ducts. This is done either by using a combined endoscopic and X-ray approach or by inserting a long, thin needle into the liver and then into the bile ducts to introduce a contrast medium that will be visible on the X-ray and so show the obstructed duct (see PTHC, page 815, and ERCP, page 816).

The goal of treatment is to relieve the obstruction. This sometimes can be done with surgical reconstruction, although the recurrence rate is high. If the obstruction is in the portion of the bile duct within the liver, surgery may be quite difficult. A small hollow tube (stent) may be inserted to keep the strictured area open, perhaps at the time of percutaneous transhepatic cholangiography (see PTHC, page 815). If episodic bouts of infection persist, your physician may consider the use of antibiotics.

Hemochromatosis

This is an inherited disease that causes the body to store excessively high amounts of iron. The liver is most directly affected because it is the primary storage site for iron, and the accumulation of iron in the liver may cause cirrhosis. The excess iron also may affect the pancreas, endocrine glands, and heart.

Hemochromatosis primarily affects men between the ages of 40 and 60. The loss of iron in the menstrual flow tends to protect women from hemochromatosis. The disease may be accompanied by diabetes mellitus (see page 925) and increased skin pigmentation—thus the nickname "bronze diabetes."

The symptoms are weakness, fatigue, weight loss, and impaired sexual performance. Often, the disease is detected by blood tests in a person who is symptom-free.

If your physician suspects hemochromatosis, he or she will examine your blood for excessive iron content. Biopsy of your liver (see this page) may be done.

Generally, the best treatment is to remove the excess iron by withdrawing blood (phlebotomy) once or twice a week. Sometimes this treatment may be required for 1 to 2 years until the iron in the blood reaches a normal level.

When the disease is detected early, the outcome usually is good. However, if the disease is left untreated, cirrhosis will develop. If you have hemochromatosis, your blood relatives should be screened for the disorder.

Wilson's Disease

This is an inherited disorder in which copper accumulates in various organs of the body, especially the brain, eyes, kidney, and liver. This rare disease is characterized by tremors, liver disease, pigmentation of the cornea of the eye, and symptoms of chronic hepatitis (see page 804). If untreated, the liver disease leads to cirrhosis.

The treatment involves removing the deposits of copper by use of a medication called penicillamine. This treatment usually is continued for life. With proper treatment, the prognosis is good. If you have Wilson's disease, your blood relatives should be screened.

Alpha$_1$-Antitrypsin Deficiency

People with a deficiency of the enzyme inhibitor alpha$_1$-antitrypsin tend to have emphysema and liver disease in adult life. When liver disease develops during infancy, it is often related to this deficiency.

People with this disease often have cirrhosis with no apparent symptoms.

Diagnosis

The more visible signs of cirrhosis—jaundice, water retention (edema), and spider-like vessels on the skin—are not always present. (See page C-15 for color photograph of spider-like veins.) Even without these more recognizable symptoms, your physician may find an enlarged liver or spleen during a routine medical examination.

On the basis of these findings, your physician probably will order blood tests. The results may be normal or may reveal minor changes that are not necessarily definitive signs of cirrhosis of the liver. But a long history of heavy drinking would make such a diagnosis more likely. A definitive diagnosis would require a liver biopsy (a sample of liver tissue is examined microscopically; see this page). This will reveal the extent and nature, and possibly the cause, of the liver damage.

How Serious Is Cirrhosis?

Cirrhosis is very serious because the damage is irreversible. There is no cure for cirrhosis. Annually, at least 30,000 people die from alcohol-related liver disorders alone.

The serious complications that may occur are described below.

Portal Hypertension

This occurs in more than two-thirds of people with cirrhosis. It causes impairment of flow in the portal vein that supplies the liver. The pressure within the portal system increases, causing enlargement of the spleen and the development of dilated veins in the esophagus and stomach (see Esophageal Varices, page 750).

Liver Biopsy

In the course of diagnosing liver disease, your physician may perform a liver biopsy. This is a simple diagnostic procedure that is used in various liver disorders, including cirrhosis, hepatitis, and tumors.

The Procedure

You will be given a local anesthetic to prevent discomfort and will be positioned flat on your back. Your physician will insert a thin needle between or below your ribs into your liver and then will remove a small sample of tissue for laboratory analysis.

The Risks

Liver biopsy is safe and unlikely to have any complications. Occasionally, there is some pain or bleeding after the procedure.

The Results

The laboratory tests conducted on the tissues may reveal the presence (or absence) of certain disorders. If you are already known to have a liver disorder, the biopsy can be helpful in evaluating the progress of the disease.

Esophageal Bleeding

This may result from rupture of esophageal or gastric varices. This is a life-threatening emergency. Initial treatment may involve infusion of a drug (vasopressin) that may reduce the pressure within the varices and stop the bleeding, at least temporarily. In addition, a tube often is inserted through the nose into the stomach. Attached to this tube are both a stomach balloon and an esophageal balloon. These can be inflated to compress the varices in an attempt to stop the bleeding. If bleeding stops or slows, an irritating or sclerosing agent can be injected, by using a catheter placed through an endoscope (see Upper Gastrointestinal Endoscopy, page 760), directly into the vein. This is called esophageal variceal sclerotherapy. Other options include rubber band ligation and transcutaneous intrahepatic porto-systemic shunt (see page 751). In other cases, surgery is necessary to stop the bleeding, although the risk of death during surgery for acute esophageal or gastric variceal bleeding is very high.

Ascites

Ascites is an accumulation of excess fluid within the abdominal cavity. Treatment often includes a salt-restricted diet and the use of diuretics to eliminate water and salt through the urine.

Spontaneous Bacterial Peritonitis

This occurs when ascites fluid becomes infected. Abdominal pain along with a low-grade fever may be present. The diagnosis is made by inserting a catheter into the abdomen and removing fluid for laboratory examination to identify the infecting organism. The treatment is with antibiotics.

Hepatic Encephalopathy

This is a complication in which the brain is poisoned by the toxic elements from the liver, which is no longer capable of properly filtering the blood to remove toxins. Blood tests will be conducted to determine ammonia levels, which are an index of the degree of accumulation of such toxins. The persons who develop this may experience a change in their personality and may become mentally confused, drowsy, and tremulous (see Liver Disease, page 800).

Treatment

There is no specific treatment for cirrhosis. Treatment is largely confined to the complications of cirrhosis (see page 804).

If you have fluid retention, your physician will advise a salt-restricted diet. This needs to be followed carefully because even small increases in the amount of salt in your diet may produce a considerable amount of swelling. In addition, the amount of water in your diet may be somewhat restricted. Diuretics may be prescribed to hasten the removal of fluid from your system.

If there are signs of encephalopathy, your physician also may advise a low-protein diet. Your dietary instructions will provide adequate calorie intake.

Your physician also may prescribe vitamin supplements, particularly vitamins K, A, and D.

If itching becomes particularly troublesome, the drug cholestyramine may be prescribed. This medication may interfere with the absorption of other drugs and therefore should be taken separately.

Abstain from the use of alcohol and any other medication that is broken down by and eliminated through the liver. If some of these medications are absolutely needed, your physician may adjust your dosage.

In some situations, your physician may refer you to a medical center that specializes in liver diseases for consideration for liver transplantation (see page 811).

Liver Tumors

Signs and Symptoms

- There may be none
- Loss of appetite and weight
- Abdominal pain
- Nausea and vomiting
- General fatigue and weakness
- Enlarged liver
- Ascites (swelling in the peritoneal cavity)
- Jaundice (yellowing of the skin and eyes)

Most tumors that form in the liver are malignant. Usually they are cancers that have spread (metastasized) to the liver from another part of the body; they are referred to as secondary liver cancer. The liver is especially vulnerable to invasion by tumor cells and, with the exception of lymph nodes, it is the most common site of metastasis.

The malignant liver tumor that originates in the liver or bile ducts is called primary liver cancer (hepatocellular or cholangiocarcinoma). In the United States, primary liver cancers account for only 1 to 2 percent of the malignant tumors found during autopsy. Liver cancer occurs 2 to 4 times more frequently in men.

Certain factors tend to predispose a person to primary liver cancer. These include chronic liver disease such as cirrhosis, hepatitis B infection, and exposure to certain toxins.

Benign, or nonmalignant, liver tumors also occur. The most common is the hemangioma. Hemangiomas are often discovered incidentally during study of the liver for another reason. Normally, treatment is not needed. Hepatic adenoma (another benign tumor) occasionally occurs in women who take oral contraceptives over a long period. Adenomas may regress or become smaller when use of the birth control pill is discontinued. Hepatic adenomas may cause pain and may even rupture and require surgical removal. Another condition, focal nodular hyperplasia, sometimes occurs with the long-term use of oral contraceptives. This disorder generally has no symptoms.

Liver cysts are very common and usually are found incidentally when the liver is examined by CT or ultrasonography (see page 1334). Liver cysts carry no risk of malignancy, and symptoms are rare. Treatment is unnecessary except in the rare instances when they cause significant abdominal discomfort.

Diagnosis

Many benign tumors of the liver are asymptomatic and thus are never discovered. If they grow large enough, however, they may cause pain, liver tenderness, or internal hemorrhage.

If the tumor is cancerous, the symptoms are more evident because a person with liver cancer may become debilitated over time. If you have a history of liver dysfunction or liver disease and your health is failing, your physician may consider the possibility of liver cancer.

If a liver cancer is suspected, a thorough physical examination and blood tests may be the first step. In addition, you will probably have a CT scan (see page 1334) or an ultrasound examination (see page 1335); either can reliably detect a mass in the liver. Liver biopsy, in which a sample of liver tissue is removed for laboratory analysis, provides more information (see page 807). An ex-

ploratory abdominal operation may be required if the liver biopsy does not provide a definitive diagnosis.

How Serious Is Liver Cancer?

Liver cancer usually is fatal. Most patients do not live beyond 6 months to a year after diagnosis.

Treatment

In some cases, chemotherapy is used to relieve the symptoms, but this treatment only infrequently improves the outcome.

In the case of multiple, spreading (metastatic) tumors, surgery is of little or no value. However, it may be recommended if a benign tumor is very large and causes discomfort or when a primary liver cancer is small and localized.

If a solitary metastatic tumor nodule from a distant site (such as the colon) is found and there is no evidence of spread of the cancer to other locations, surgical removal may be attempted in hope of a cure.

Enlarged Liver

Signs and Symptoms

- Often none, other than mild tenderness over the liver
- Pain in upper right portion of the abdomen
- Varying degrees of jaundice

Diagnosis

An enlarged liver, called hepatomegaly, is usually discovered during an examination of

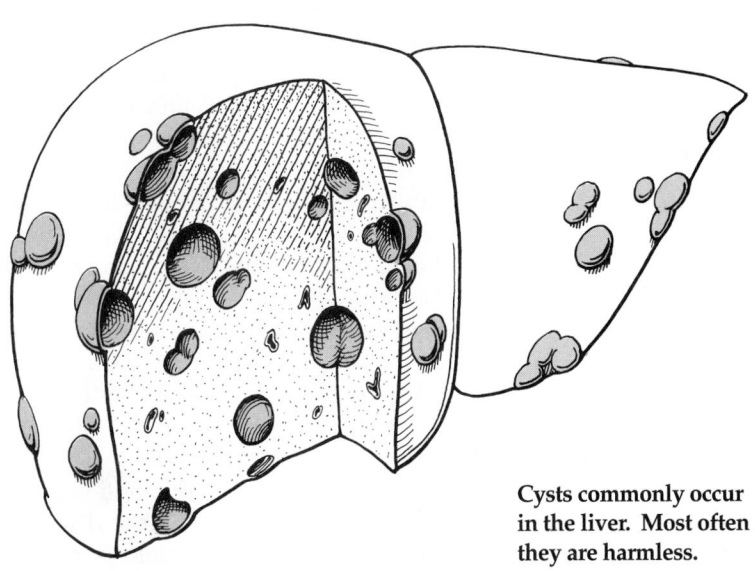

Cysts commonly occur in the liver. Most often they are harmless.

the abdomen by your physician. The normal liver is rather soft and is located beneath the ribs on the right side of your body. Your physician sometimes can feel your liver by placing his or her hand just below your rib margin and asking you to take a deep breath (the deep breath causes your liver to descend so that your physician can feel its edge).

An enlarged liver or one that is firmer than normal often can be felt readily during this maneuver. This is the same technique used to detect enlargement of the spleen (splenomegaly), which is located beneath the left rib margin. Enlargement of the liver or the spleen is more difficult to detect in an obese person.

A CT scan (see page 1334), ultrasound examination (see page 1335), or MRI scan (see page 1334) of the liver will reveal the size, configuration, and texture of the liver and also will determine whether a tumor is present within the organ.

Causes

Perhaps the most common cause of an enlarged liver is the accumulation of fat. In the United States, a fatty liver commonly is part of chronic alcoholism or sometimes of ordinary obesity. This condition also can occur as a complication of prolonged corticosteroid use. Reye's syndrome (see page 484), an acute illness almost exclusively of children, has as one of its features the presence of fatty deposits within liver cells.

The liver may increase in size because of too much glycogen, as a result of a glycogen storage disease. Glycogen is a starch that is stored in and transformed by the liver into glucose, a form of sugar that the body is able to use for energy. Accumulation of glycogen results from many of the disorders that cause fatty infiltration of the liver. In addition, excessive glycogen accumulation may occur in children and teenagers with poorly controlled diabetes (see page 925).

Amyloidosis is a disorder that deposits an excess of a protein called amyloid in the liver and other parts of the body. The amyloid makes the liver enlarged, pale, and rubbery in consistency; swelling due to water retention (edema) is also a frequent problem with this disorder. The principal means of diagnosis of amyloidosis is a blood test and biopsy of the liver (see page 807).

The liver is vulnerable to infiltration by tumors or lesions caused by other diseases. One example is miliary tuberculosis (miliary refers to the seed-like tumors it generates). Another such disease is sarcoidosis, a disease of unknown origin that causes lesions in many organs of the body, including the liver.

Treatment

Treatment for enlarged liver generally is determined by the underlying cause. Elimination of alcohol intake and loss of weight, if necessary, are advised.

Liver Abscess

Signs and Symptoms
- Persistent fever
- Chills
- Nausea and vomiting
- Weakness
- Weight loss
- Tender liver
- Jaundice

Abscesses sometimes form within the liver as a result of infection by bacteria or ameba. Those of bacterial origin generally have a more rapid course with fever and chills; those from amebiasis progress more slowly.

Diagnosis

If your physician believes that you may have a liver abscess, he or she may arrange for a CT scan (see page 1334) or an ultrasound examination of your liver (see page 1335). From the image that is produced, he or she may be able to determine the size, location, and number of the abscesses. Blood tests also may be helpful, particularly if your physician suspects that the cause of the abscess is a parasite.

Insertion of a needle into the abscess, using the CT scan or ultrasonogram for guidance, will allow withdrawal of some of the fluid for laboratory analysis. However, if your physician suspects that the cyst is caused by a parasite (Echinococcus), he or she may refrain from inserting a needle.

How Serious Are Liver Abscesses?

A liver abscess, particularly from a bacterial cause, is a potentially fatal problem. Even when the liver abscess is correctly diagnosed and properly treated, many affected persons do not survive.

Treatment

If the liver abscess is caused by a bacterium, your physician may advise catheterization for drainage and the use of antibiotics given through a vein for several weeks. At times, surgical exploration and drainage of the abscess or even removal of the portion of the liver containing the abscess is required.

If the cause is ameba or Echinococcus, your physician may advise specific medications.

Genetic Liver Problems

Some inherited liver abnormalities cause high concentrations of bilirubin in the blood, a condition called hyperbilirubinemia. This produces jaundice (yellowing of the eyes and skin).

Gilbert's Syndrome

Gilbert's syndrome is an inherited disorder in which bilirubin is not properly processed in the liver for excretion in the feces. Bilirubin has to combine (conjugate) with another substance in the liver in order to make the bilirubin water-soluble and capable of being excreted through the bile. Bilirubin is usually unconjugated or unprocessed in Gilbert's syndrome because of a deficiency of the enzyme necessary to accomplish this conjugation.

Gilbert's syndrome may be the most common cause of hyperbilirubinemia. The jaundice it causes is rather mild but may be aggravated by fasting. In some cases, the dis-

Liver Transplantation

During the past decade, liver transplantation has become an increasingly acceptable therapy for severe liver disease. Transplantation is limited only by the number of donor organs available. In 1994, approximately 3,500 liver transplantations were performed in the United States. Since 1981, the survival rate for people who receive a liver has steadily improved. Today, almost 90 percent are alive 1 year after transplantation, and 80 percent are alive 3 years after the procedure.

Advances in the preservation of donor organs have improved survival rates, as have refinements in surgical technique and postoperative care. However, the most important advances have come in the use of drugs that discourage rejection of the donor organ.

Medications

Cyclosporine decreases your body's natural tendency to reject a donated organ. In effect, it alters the action of your immune system, reducing (suppressing) its effectiveness, and is therefore called an immunosuppressant. Specifically, cyclosporine prevents white blood cells (lymphocytes) from damaging the transplanted liver.

More recently, FK506 (tacrolimus) was added to the expanding list of immunosuppressive medications. This drug enables physicians to more rapidly reduce doses of corticosteroids, which are also used to prevent rejection.

Newer antibiotic and antiviral drugs are playing important roles in preventing and treating infection of the transplanted liver. Ganciclovir, for example, can be used for prevention or treatment of a cytomegalovirus infection.

Who Is a Candidate?

People who have severe (potentially fatal) liver disease are candidates for transplantation, as are those who have an unacceptable quality of life. Children and adults under age 65 are the best candidates. Those selected generally have liver disease that is progressive and incurable by other medical or surgical treatments. There should be no evidence of cancer. Children selected often are young and have congenital abnormalities of the liver.

The Procedure

Liver transplantation is a lengthy, complex operation. It can take 6 to 10 hours and is mainly done at large medical centers where experienced personnel and extensive facilities generally yield the best results.

Surgeons can split livers, transplanting a single organ into two recipients. A child can receive a lobe of a liver donated by a parent; the results are similar to a whole-organ transplant from an unrelated donor.

There is increasing evidence that timing of liver transplantation may affect the success of the surgery. Earlier transplantation may improve survival while lowering costs by reducing blood loss and the need for hospital care following the operation.

Recovery

Family support is important to rehabilitation, which may require up to 4 months. Lifelong therapy with immunosuppressive drugs can help prevent rejection of the new organ. However, use of these drugs requires lifelong monitoring for complications.

order is detected only during a routine blood test. Gilbert's syndrome does not lead to liver damage; treatment is unnecessary.

Crigler-Najjar Syndrome

This rare, inherited disorder causes two types of hyperbilirubinemia: type I and type II. Type I, the most severe form, is due to an absence of the enzyme needed to conjugate the bilirubin. Type II is less severe because there is only a partial enzyme deficiency.

There is no treatment that will cure type I Crigler-Najjar syndrome. The infant born with it usually dies within the first year.

Type II hyperbilirubinemia, however, can be treated successfully with medication, usually phenobarbital.

Dubin-Johnson Hyperbilirubinemia

Some disorders cause both conjugated and unconjugated hyperbilirubinemia. One such inherited disorder is Dubin-Johnson syndrome, otherwise known as chronic idiopathic jaundice. People with this disorder often will have no symptoms or only vague gastrointestinal symptoms. In some cases, their liver is enlarged. This disorder can be successfully treated with medication.

Gallbladder and Bile Duct Disorders

The gallbladder is a pear-shaped sac 3 to 4 inches long and roughly 1 inch in diameter that generally lies underneath the liver on your right side. The gallbladder stores the bile that is produced in your liver and then discharged through the bile duct into the duodenum, usually after a meal. Bile facilitates the digestion of fats.

Gallstones

Signs and Symptoms
- Intense and sudden pain in upper abdomen
- Pain may last 30 minutes to several hours
- Pain may move around to the right shoulder blade
- Often nausea and, sometimes, vomiting

Gallstones are a common problem; an estimated 1 million new cases are diagnosed yearly in the United States.

Gallstones are crystalline structures that can be as small as a grain of sand or larger than a golf ball. They can be smooth and round or irregular with many edges. Some people have only one gallstone; others may have several or even hundreds.

The stones that collect in the gallbladder may produce no symptoms. But a gallstone that obstructs the cystic duct (leading from the gallbladder to the bile duct) or the bile duct itself (the conduit into the duodenum from both the liver and gallbladder) may produce a painful spasm and inflammation at the site of the obstruction.

The pain of a gallbladder attack (biliary colic) normally begins quite suddenly and may persist for several hours. The pain is severe and constant, often accompanied by nausea and vomiting. After the pain subsides, there may be a mild aching sensation or soreness in the right upper abdomen, which may last for up to a day.

True pain from a gallbladder attack is infrequent, generally occurring no more than one to three times per year. Belching, bloating, intolerance of fatty foods, or frequent abdominal pain should not be attributed to gallstone disease.

If you become jaundiced, especially if the yellowing of your skin is accompanied by pain, this suggests migration of a stone into the common bile duct (see Bile Duct Obstruction, page 814). The presence of a high fever or shaking chills usually implies an underlying complication such as inflammation of the gallbladder (cholecystitis), acute pancreatitis (see page 818), or infection in the bile duct due to obstruction (cholangitis). Sometimes the symptoms of gallbladder disease (biliary colic) may be precipitated by eating a fatty meal, but they occur during the night.

Not all gallstones are made of the same material. Eighty percent of the stones in persons residing in the United States are composed primarily of cholesterol; the remaining 20 percent contain mostly calcium salts of bile pigment. Normally, the bile acids in bile keep cholesterol from becoming too concentrated and thus forming gallstones. However, if the amount of cholesterol in the bile increases beyond the ability of bile acids to maintain this balance, the cholesterol crystallizes and, in some people, stones eventually will form. Although rare, extreme, rapid weight loss can lead to gallstone formation.

About 1 in 10 Americans has or will have gallstones. Autopsies show that gallstones develop in 20 to 30 percent of women by the age of 70, which is more than twice the number found in men. The likelihood of gallstones increases with age and obesity. Although gallstones develop in many people, they usually do not cause symptoms. The chance of symptoms or complications developing from stones is probably less than 20 percent over a long period.

Diagnosis

If a severe and lasting pain develops in your upper abdomen, your physician may suspect gallbladder difficulties. Your physician will conduct a physical examination to look for jaundice and will palpate your abdomen to see if your gallbladder is tender or has become distended because of an obstruction.

If your physician believes the cause may be gallstones, you may have a blood test and an ultrasound examination (see page 1335).

Treatment

If you have gallstones and no symptoms that can be attributed to the stones, your physician may elect only to observe and not recommend any specific treatment.

Surgery

If you are having gallbladder pain (biliary colic or acute cholecystitis), your physician may recommend surgical removal of the gallbladder (cholecystectomy). This is a very safe operation with a very small risk of complications and is the preferred approach for treating most persons with gallbladder disease. In most circumstances, this can be performed using a laparoscope (laparoscopic cholecystectomy) (see page 817).

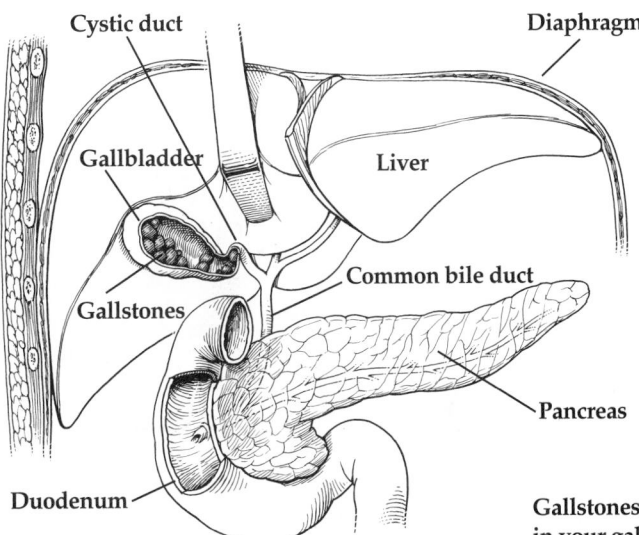

Gallstones may form in your gallbladder. If a stone obstructs your cystic duct, you may experience a painful gallbladder attack.

Stone Dissolution

An option that has been developed in the last couple of decades is stone dissolution. This applies only to cholesterol stones. A bile acid (chenodeoxycholic or ursodeoxycholic acid) is given in tablet form. The medication works by decreasing the cholesterol concentration within the gallbladder, which enables the bile acid to bring the solid cholesterol stone back into solution. This drug works best if the cholesterol stones are small (less than half an inch in diameter) and are the floating type.

If you have a pigment or calcified stone, you are not a candidate for this type of medication, nor is this drug recommended for pregnant women with gallstones because of possible damage to the fetus.

The dosage is based on body weight. If you are obese, you may require a larger dose. It generally takes many months or even years for the bile acid treatment to dissolve the stone. Thus, this is not a practical approach if you are having frequent bouts of gallbladder pain. In addition, after the drug therapy ends, there is a 50 percent chance of more gallstones developing because the underlying problem of excess secretion of cholesterol into the gallbladder is still present.

Other Treatment Options

Additional treatment methods have been developed in the past several years, especially for persons who have other serious medical problems and for whom surgery might be dangerous. One involves the delivery of methyl tert-butyl ether (MTBE) via a catheter

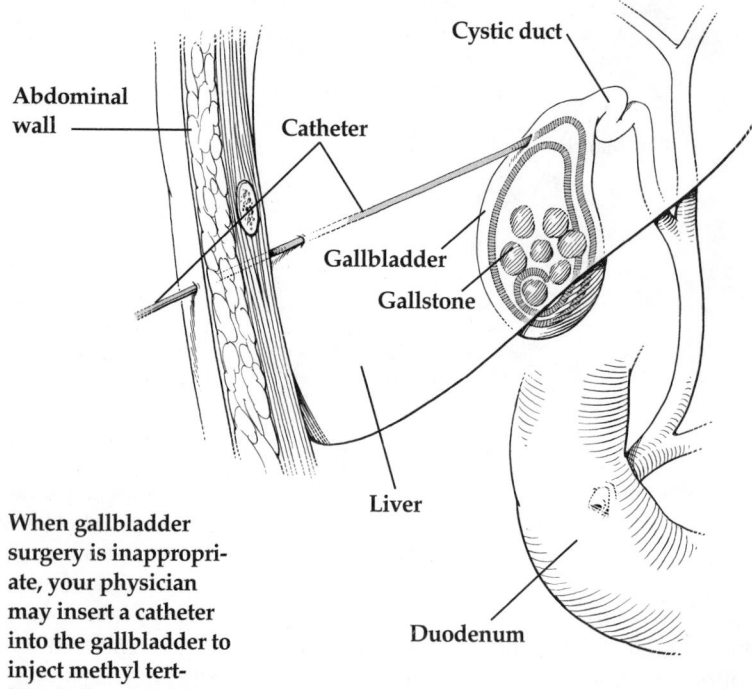

Abdominal wall ——

Catheter

Cystic duct

Gallbladder

Gallstone

Liver

Duodenum

When gallbladder surgery is inappropriate, your physician may insert a catheter into the gallbladder to inject methyl tert-butyl ether (MTBE), a solvent that dissolves the stones.

directly into the gallbladder. For this to be effective, the stones have to be cholesterol in nature. Often, this may dissolve the stones after 1 to 2 days of constant treatment. The gallbladder remains in place, and your physician may prescribe chenodeoxycholic or ursodeoxycholic acid tablets indefinitely to prevent formation of new stones within the gallbladder.

A method under investigation for several years is stone fragmentation with high-frequency sound waves (biliary lithotripsy). However, this has been found to be of limited use for gallbladder stones.

Bile Duct Obstruction

Signs and Symptoms
- Jaundice (yellowing of the skin and eyes)
- High fever with chills
- Clay-colored stools
- Tea- or coffee-colored urine
- Abdominal pain in the upper abdomen

Emergency Signs
- Shock: cold, clammy, pale skin with weak or rapid pulse
- Mental confusion

The presence of gallstones in the common bile duct (the conduit into the duodenum for bile from both the liver and the gallbladder)

is the most common cause of bile duct obstruction (see Gallstones, page 812). After surgical removal of the gallbladder (cholecystectomy), in a small percentage of cases a stone remains in the common bile duct. These stones may obstruct the narrow common bile duct and cause episodic pain in the upper abdomen. Often, spiking fevers with shaking chills (cholangitis) and jaundice also are symptoms of acute bile duct obstruction.

Because the common bile duct and pancreatic duct are joined in most persons, an obstruction in the common bile duct may lead to an obstruction in the pancreatic duct and subsequent pancreatitis (see Acute Pancreatitis, page 818). Obstruction of the common bile duct is an emergency situation requiring immediate relief of the obstruction.

Other Causes
Obstruction of the bile duct also can be caused by a stricture or narrowing of the duct, inflammation of the duct, or cancer.

Trauma
Narrowing (stricture) of the common duct is a potential complication of gallbladder surgery. The stricture may develop immediately after gallbladder surgery or may be delayed for several years. In either event, an additional operation often can correct the problem.

Hemobilia
Blood in the bile duct (hemobilia) can lead to a clot that can obstruct the duct. Hemobilia is a rare condition that may occur as a result of trauma to the liver or bile duct during surgery. People with hemobilia often have abdominal pain, jaundice, and occult blood in their stool. Often, the clot dissolves spontaneously. At other times, surgical removal is needed.

Primary Sclerosing Cholangitis
In some people a chronic disorder called primary sclerosing cholangitis (PSC) develops. Sclerosis is hardening and thickening of tissue, in this case of the bile duct wall. PSC can produce a partial blockage of the duct. This obstruction can produce much the same symptoms as gallstones in the bile duct, including jaundice, pain in the right side of the abdomen, episodes of fever and chills, itching, and fatigue. In addition, sclerosing cholangitis may cause cirrhosis, liver failure, or hemorrhage from esophageal

varices (see Cirrhosis, page 804). Frequently, sclerosing cholangitis is associated with an underlying disease such as ulcerative colitis (see Ulcerative Colitis, page 777).

Bile Duct Cancer

A malignant tumor in the bile duct can cause obstruction. If you have the symptoms of bile duct cancer (which include jaundice, itching, weight loss, and clay-colored stools), your physician may order an ultrasound examination or a CT or MRI scan (see page 1334), which then may be followed by cholangiography (see ERCP, page 816, and PTHC, below).

Other Disorders

Sometimes the bile duct can become partially or completely obstructed if it is subjected to pressure on its outside wall. This often can be caused by a complication of either acute or chronic pancreatitis (see pages 818 and 819, respectively), cancer of the pancreas (see Malignant Pancreatic Tumors, page 820), lymphoma (see Lymphomas, page 968), or cancer that has metastasized (spread) from another part of the body. The principal symptom is jaundice. Treatment is directed at the underlying disorder. At times, it may be necessary to cut the bile duct and place it in another location on the small bowel to bypass an obstructed segment of intestine.

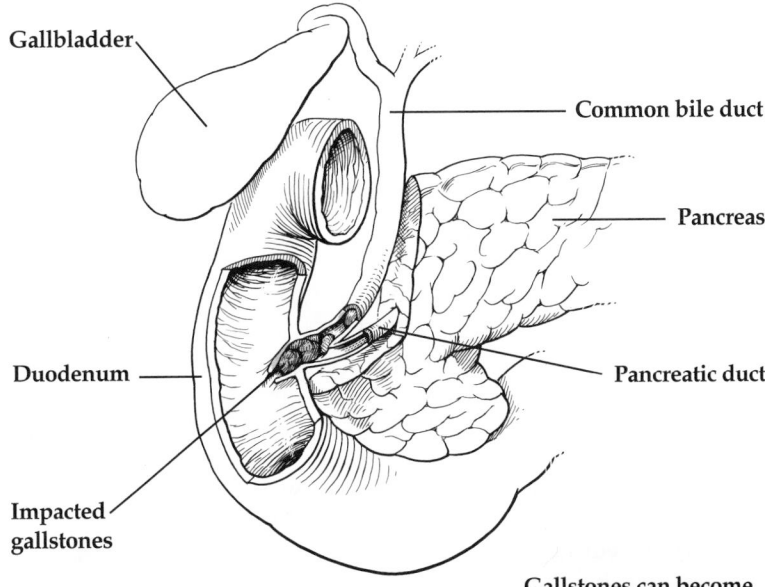

Gallbladder — **Common bile duct** — **Pancreas** — **Duodenum** — **Pancreatic duct** — **Impacted gallstones**

Gallstones can become impacted in the common bile duct at the entrance to the duodenum. This obstruction is a potentially life-threatening condition requiring immediate treatment.

Diagnosis

Because the initial symptoms of a bile duct obstruction are similar regardless of the cause, your physician will conduct many of the same diagnostic tests that would be used for gallstones. He or she also may inject a contrast material into the bile duct for either endoscopic retrograde cholangiopancreatography (see ERCP, page 816) or percutaneous

---

Percutaneous Transhepatic Cholangiography (PTHC)

PTHC is a contrast X-ray procedure that provides pictures of the bile duct. It is used to diagnose the cause of upper abdominal pain after gallbladder surgery or unexplained jaundice when a bile duct obstruction (such as from a gallstone) is suspected.

The Procedure

You will be asked not to eat for 8 hours prior to the test. You will lie down on a tilting X-ray table that can be rotated into vertical and horizontal positions. A tube will be inserted into a vein in your arm for administration of medication for

sedation and of an antibiotic. Then, the skin over your liver will be cleansed with an antiseptic and a local anesthetic will be injected into the skin. The rest of the procedure begins when you feel numb where the anesthetic was injected.

A long, flexible needle is inserted into your liver. In most instances you will not feel the needle pass into the liver. However, if you should, the feeling of fullness or pain will be only temporary. When the X-ray image indicates that the needle has reached the bile duct, contrast medium is injected through it.

At this point, a series of X-rays

are taken as you and the table are rotated to different positions to provide different views of your liver. When the procedure is completed, the needle is removed and a dressing is applied. Your physician probably will ask that you lie in bed on your right side for at least 6 hours after the test. In addition, you may be given pain medication.

The procedure takes between 45 minutes and 1 hour and is usually done in a hospital. Many physicians prefer that you stay in the hospital overnight for monitoring in case bleeding or infection should develop.

Endoscopic Retrograde Cholangiopancreatography (ERCP)

One of the principal methods of evaluating your bile and pancreatic ducts involves viewing the ducts through their opening into the intestinal tract by using an endoscope. The purpose of ERCP is to identify bile duct stones (gallstones), long-standing inflammatory disease of the pancreas, or obstruction of either of these two ducts. The obstruction may be from scar or inflammatory tissue or from tumors, usually cancers.

The Procedure

You will be asked not to eat or drink for 8 to 12 hours before the test. Just before the procedure begins, an intravenous tube will be placed into a vein in your hand; a sedative and a medication that relaxes your stomach and intestines will be given through this tube. An anesthetic drug will be sprayed into the back of your throat to eliminate gagging when the endoscope is passed into your throat. You will be lying on your left side. At this point, the flexible endoscope is passed into your mouth, down your throat, through the length of your stomach, and into your duodenum. Throughout this entire process the physician views the passage of the endoscope.

Air is used to inflate the intestinal tract in order to identify the tiny opening through which the bile and pancreatic ducts drain their fluids into the duodenum. Once this opening is found, you will be placed on your stomach. A fine hollow tube (or catheter) is passed through the endoscope and into the bile and pancreatic ducts. A dye or contrast solution is injected through this catheter into the ducts to fill them. X-ray pictures are then taken.

Other types of catheters can be placed through the endoscope to treat specific abnormalities identified on the X-rays. A catheter fitted with an electrical cautery wire can be used to enlarge the opening of the bile duct to permit the extraction of a stone. The extraction can be performed with a specialized balloon or basket catheter. If there is concern over a possible tumor, another type of catheter can be placed into the bile duct to obtain samples of tissue for testing. Finally, strictures (narrowings) from scarring or tumors can be stretched or opened with a dilating balloon catheter, and a hollow tube (stent) then can be inserted through the endoscope into the narrowing to maintain free passage of bile into the duodenum.

There are possible side effects. The medications given to you during the procedure may make you feel tired, dizzy, dry-mouthed, and sometimes slightly nauseated. The air placed into your intestines may leave you feeling gassy and bloated for several hours.

Do not eat or drink anything until your gag reflex returns. Your throat may feel sore for a day or so; for this you may use lozenges or salt-water gargles.

The entire ERCP procedure takes 30 minutes to 1 hour. It can be done on an outpatient basis.

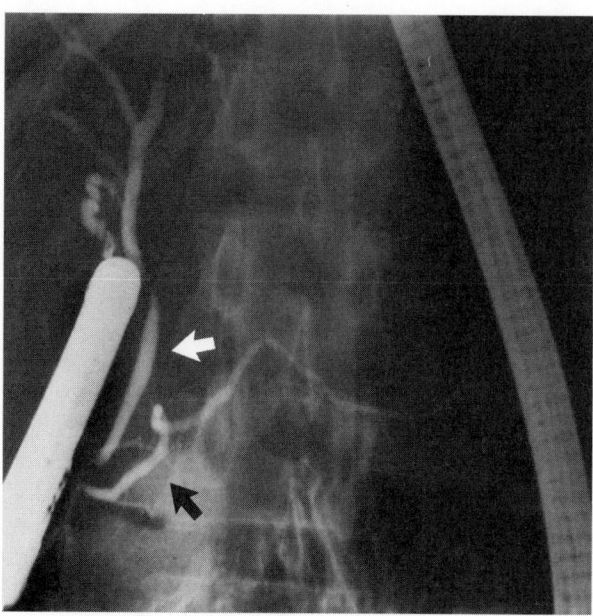 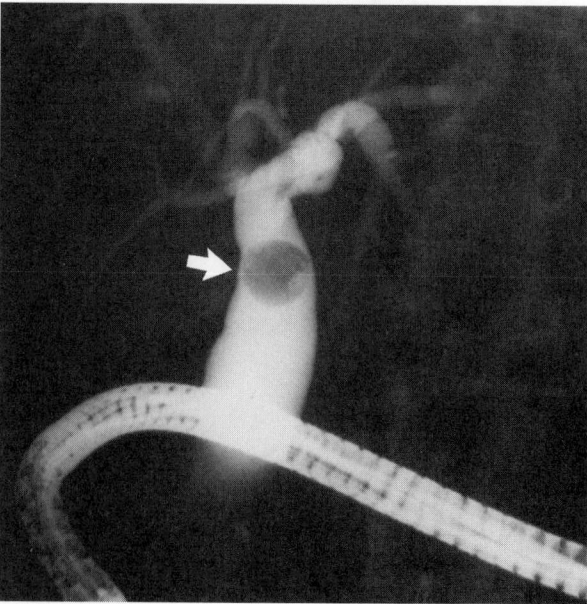

ERCP studies. At left is a normal common bile duct (white arrow) and pancreatic duct (black arrow). At right is a dilated common bile duct with a stone (white arrow).

transhepatic cholangiography (see PTHC, page 815).

How Serious Is Bile Duct Obstruction?

Bile duct blockage is a serious and often life-threatening problem and requires prompt treatment. Cultures of your blood during episodes of fever may reveal the presence of bacteria that have leaked into the bloodstream from the obstructed bile duct. Blood infection (sepsis) can lead to shock.

Treatment

The principle of the treatment is to relieve the blockage of your bile duct.

Surgery and Endoscopic Treatment

If the cause of the obstruction is stones within the bile duct and, in addition, you have stones in the gallbladder, your physician may recommend surgical removal of both the stones and the gallbladder. At other times, particularly if the risk of operation is great or if you have had your gallbladder removed previously, your physician may recommend a special procedure called an ERCP (see page 816). At the time of the ERCP, a cutting device can be inserted through the entrance of the bile duct at the level of the small intestine. This entrance can then be enlarged to permit the passage of the obstructing stone.

If the obstruction is the result of a stricture or narrowing of the bile duct, a surgeon skilled in biliary tract repair can reconstruct the bile duct. At other times, particularly if previous unsuccessful attempts at bile duct repair have been made or if there are multiple strictures, an alternative approach may be recommended. A hollow tube (stent) can be inserted into the bile duct across the narrowed area to permit the free passage of bile.

If the cause of the obstruction is bleeding in the bile duct, surgery is often required to tie off the bleeding vessel.

There generally are multiple areas of narrowing of the bile ducts (strictures) in primary sclerosing cholangitis. Thus, attempts at operation or placement of a stent often are unsuccessful. There is currently no specific treatment for primary sclerosing cholangitis that will reverse or remove the multiple strictures. If this disorder results in severe liver failure, liver transplantation may be considered (see Liver Transplantation, page 811).

If the cause of the bile duct obstruction is external pressure such as from a malignant tumor, treatment initially will be directed at

---

Laparoscopic Surgery

Increasingly, surgeons perform operations through tiny incisions, using remote-controlled instruments. If the gallbladder is to be removed, the operation is called laparoscopic surgery or, more precisely, laparoscopic cholecystectomy.

Laparoscopic cholecystectomy is done through four small (keyhole-size) incisions. The incisions are made below the breastbone, near the navel and beneath the rib cage on the right side.

Tubes are placed in the incisions and instruments are slipped through them. One instrument contains a tiny video camera that shows internal anatomy and guides progress. Another instrument enables the surgeon to remove the sac-like gallbladder with a laser or electric cutting device while viewing the anatomy on a television screen.

The operation takes about an hour and requires a general anesthetic. Unlike conventional gallbladder surgery, which requires a hospital stay of a week, the procedure is often done as same-day (outpatient) surgery. Occasionally an overnight stay in the hospital is required.

Laparoscopic surgery may not be an option if you have large stones in your bile duct, a bleeding disorder, stones that obstruct your bowel, adhesions on your gallbladder, or conditions that substantially increase your risk for general anesthesia.

---

the primary disorder. At times, the placement of a stent (see page 816) also is effective in relieving this obstruction.

Medication

Itching is often a predominant symptom with chronic obstruction of the bile ducts. It can be managed by use of the drug cholestyramine. Your physician also may prescribe vitamins, such as vitamins K, A, and D, that are poorly absorbed in persons with bile duct obstruction.

If fever and chills are present, your physician may want to treat these symptoms with antibiotics, often given through a vein.

Choledochal Cysts

Cysts sometimes form in the bile duct, leading to an abnormal expansion of the duct (choledochal cyst). As a result, the secretions from the pancreas may return (reflux) into the common bile duct, causing inflammation and, at times, narrowing (stricture) of the duct.

Because the process is gradual, many people have occasional symptoms of abdominal pain and irritation for years before an obstruction develops. The cyst and the associated complications can be diagnosed with such tests as ultrasonography, CT scanning, or cholangiography (see ERCP, page 816, and PTHC, page 815).

Treatment
Once it has been identified, the cyst is removed surgically. People who have had a choledochal cyst have an increased risk of biliary duct cancer developing later.

Pancreatic Diseases

The pancreas lies horizontally behind the lower part of the stomach. Its head rests against the wall of the duodenum; its tail reaches toward the spleen.

The pancreas is a gland, meaning it has the ability to manufacture a secretion that is used in another part of the body. In fact, it actually is two glands.

As an exocrine gland, it produces and secretes digestive enzymes and alkaline material (sodium bicarbonate) directly into the pancreatic duct. Then these materials flow into the duodenum. The alkaline secretion makes it possible for the enzymes from the pancreas and small intestine to break down nutrients in the gut to smaller units, enabling the nutrients to be absorbed through the small bowel into the bloodstream.

As an endocrine gland, it primarily produces and secretes the hormones insulin and glucagon into the bloodstream. These hormones are important in the metabolism of carbohydrates and fats.

Infections, injury, and tumors can cause enough damage to the pancreas to affect its functions. If the secretion of the hormone insulin is diminished, diabetes mellitus occurs (see page 925). Another disorder that may affect the pancreas, cystic fibrosis, is discussed at length on page 720.

Acute Pancreatitis

Signs and Symptoms
- Abdominal pain that is intense and lasting and may radiate to the back and chest; it often begins 12 to 24 hours after a large meal or bout of heavy drinking
- Low-grade fever
- Nausea or vomiting
- Clammy skin
- Abdominal distention and tenderness

Pancreatitis is an inflammation of the pancreas. The inflammation may be acute or chronic (see Chronic Pancreatitis, page 819).

Many factors are associated with or may be a cause of acute pancreatitis, such as alcohol use, gallstones, increased triglyceride or calcium level in the blood (found in blood tests), viral and bacterial infections, and drugs. The mechanisms by which any of these conditions triggers pancreatic inflammation are not well known. Nevertheless, there are several theories as to what happens and why.

The principal theory is that the enzymes of the pancreas eat away at the gland itself. This process is called autodigestion. These powerful digestive enzymes normally are secreted by the pancreas in inactive forms but somehow may be activated inside the gland rather than in the intestine. As a result, the enzymes begin to digest the tissue of the pancreas.

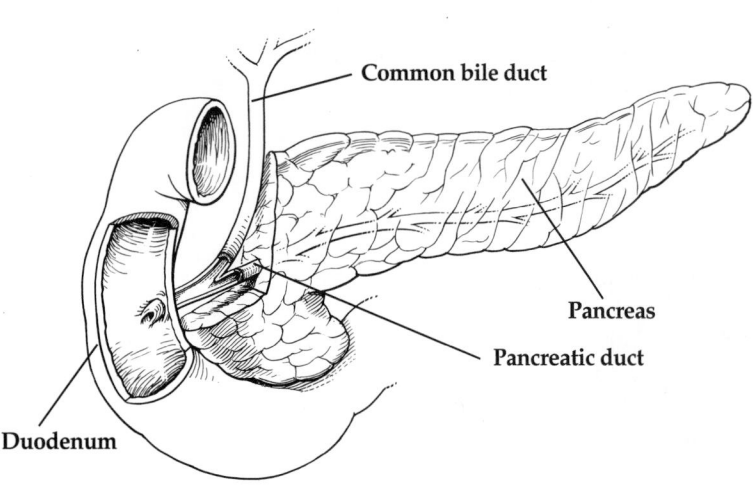

Common bile duct

Pancreas

Pancreatic duct

Duodenum

In addition to digesting pancreatic tissue, it is believed that certain enzymes, especially trypsin, set off a chain reaction by activating other enzymes. These reactions then increase the number of enzymes that are digesting the gland.

Autodigestion causes swelling (edema), hemorrhage, and damage to the blood vessels. The process also releases certain substances (histamines) that cause the blood vessels to enlarge. If unchecked, this series of reactions can produce a very serious case of acute pancreatitis.

Diagnosis

If you have an intense, constant pain in your upper abdomen that may radiate through to your back, chest, or flank, your physician may suspect acute pancreatitis. The pain is often worse when you lie flat and relieved when you sit up or bend forward. You may notice that you do not pass gas and that your abdomen is tender and is distended.

During your physical examination, your physician may elicit pain by palpating the abdominal area. He or she also will look for low-grade fever, low blood pressure, and accelerated heartbeat.

A sample of your blood may be taken for analysis for specific abnormalities such as excessive levels of certain enzymes from the pancreas, a high white blood cell count (leukocytosis), high blood sugar (hyperglycemia), and low calcium level (hypocalcemia). You may also have an X-ray taken of your abdomen and chest. An ultrasound or CT scan (see page 1334) of the abdomen may be obtained to examine the pancreas and to look for a bile duct problem, stone, or destruction of the gland.

How Serious Is Acute Pancreatitis?

In most cases, the symptoms of acute pancreatitis subside within a week. However, severe acute pancreatitis can be life-threatening. The major complications of acute pancreatitis include destruction of the gland, development of an abscess in the pancreas, a cyst in the pancreas (pseudocyst), and leakage of pancreatic fluid into the abdomen.

Treatment

Medication

Treatment of mild acute pancreatitis centers on quieting your pancreas and decreasing the flow of pancreatic enzymes. To ease the pain, an analgesic usually is prescribed. If an abscess develops, you will be given antibiotics through a vein.

Part of the overall strategy is to prevent or reduce the release of pancreatic enzymes and thus protect the pancreas from further damage. Because eating may increase gastric secretion, you may be given nourishment intravenously while the pain is present. In some cases, it may be necessary to drain your stomach through nasogastric suction (by inserting a tube through your nose). Consumption of alcohol is to be stopped.

Surgery

If the underlying cause of the pancreatitis is gallbladder disease or an obstructed pancreatic duct, surgery may be necessary, but only after the pancreatitis has been brought under control. At times, an operation may be needed if complications of acute pancreatitis develop.

If a stone is present at the common entrance to the small intestine from the common bile duct and pancreatic duct, your physician may consider a procedure in which the duct is enlarged (sphincterotomy). An endoscope is inserted into the opening of the duct (see ERCP, page 816, and PTHC, page 815) and the duct can then be enlarged so that the obstructing stone can be removed.

Chronic Pancreatitis

Signs and Symptoms

- Abdominal pain that is intense and lasting and may radiate to the back and chest
- Fever
- Excessively foul, bulky stools
- Nausea or vomiting
- Weight loss
- Clammy skin
- Abdominal distention
- Onset of diabetes mellitus
- Symptoms appearing periodically over years in a pattern of acute attacks

This type of pancreatic inflammation differs from acute pancreatitis (see page 818) in that it develops over a period of years. A person with chronic pancreatitis may have recurrent attacks of acute pain along with chronic persistent pain. Chronic pancreatitis may also be present before the onset of painful attacks. Many people with chronic pancreatitis often have a history of alcohol abuse. In some, the cause is unknown.

If you have chronic pancreatitis, over time your pancreas becomes less able to secrete the enzymes needed for proper digestion and absorption of dietary fats. This inability to perform properly is called exocrine insufficiency and is a principal characteristic of chronic pancreatitis. Among adults, chronic pancreatitis due to alcoholism is the most common cause of pancreatic exocrine insufficiency; in children, cystic fibrosis is the most common cause (see page 720).

The pain of acute pancreatitis is steady and persistent for many hours or even several days. The pain of chronic pancreatitis may be constant and daily, indefinite or occasional, intermittent or absent altogether.

Pancreatic insufficiency (the failure to produce enzymes necessary for digestion and absorption of nutrients) results in weight loss, pale-colored stools (these are fat-containing stools, a condition called steatorrhea), and other signs of malabsorption. Also, with severe scarring of the pancreas, diabetes mellitus (see page 925) may develop.

Apart from steatorrhea, the key sign of chronic pancreatitis is small, hard deposits that form in the pancreatic duct or tissue. This condition is called pancreatic calcification and can be seen on an X-ray. Alcohol-induced pancreatitis is a common cause of this kind of calcification. Obviously, excessive drinking should be avoided, but even moderate but consistent social drinking over the years may produce significant pancreatic calcification.

Diagnosis

To confirm the diagnosis of chronic pancreatitis, your physician will take a sample of your blood and your stool. Patients with chronic pancreatitis often have a high fat content in their feces because fat is not being absorbed by the intestine. The analysis of your blood may not show the same high levels of certain enzymes characteristic of acute pancreatitis, but your physician will look for other blood abnormalities associated with chronic pancreatitis.

Your physician may obtain a CT scan (see page 1334) and have you undergo endoscopic retrograde cholangiopancreatography (see ERCP, page 816) to look for evidence of an obstruction of the pancreatic or common bile duct. Your physician also may inject a solution to stimulate the pancreas and then measure the gland's ability to discharge secretions into the duodenum. Called a stimu-

lation test, this is important in determining whether your pancreas is the cause of your malabsorption of nutrients and weight loss.

Treatment

The therapy for chronic pancreatitis usually centers on two problems: pain and malabsorption.

Medication

If you have intermittent pain, you may be given a nonnarcotic pain reliever (analgesic) to avoid becoming addicted to medication.

In addition, your problem of malabsorption may be treated with pancreatic replacement therapy. This therapy requires that you take an enzyme preparation with every meal. This preparation replaces the enzymes that are not being secreted into the duodenum by your pancreas. Generally, eight tablets with meals are prescribed (two after eating a few bites, four during the meal, and two at completion of the meal). Three such tablets may be taken with snacks.

Diet

You may be told to avoid fatty foods and alcohol.

Surgery

If the pain cannot be relieved by drugs, surgery may be necessary to drain the pancreatic duct, remove the damaged pancreatic tissue, or deaden nerves that are transmitting the pain.

Malignant Pancreatic Tumors

Signs and Symptoms
- Abdominal pain that may radiate to the back
- Lack of appetite and weight loss
- Jaundice (yellowing of the skin and eyes)
- Itching (pruritus)
- Nausea and vomiting
- Intestinal bleeding

Cancer of the pancreas ranks just behind lung cancer, colon cancer, and breast cancer as the most common cause of death by cancer. It is more common among men, and men between the ages of 60 and 70 are most at risk. The cause of pancreatic cancer is unknown.

The most common symptoms are weight loss, abdominal pain, and jaundice. Weight loss, the causes of which are not fully understood, usually is significant. The average loss is about 25 pounds. Jaundice occurs if the cancer blocks the common bile duct.

Diagnosis

If you have an unexplained loss of more than 10 percent of your normal body weight and upper abdominal pain with unexplained back pain, see your physician. Among other things, your physician will be looking for signs of an enlarged liver and abdominal tenderness.

If pancreatic cancer is suspected, he or she may order an ultrasound (see page 1335) or CT scan (see page 1334). Your physician also may arrange for endoscopic retrograde cholangiopancreatography (see ERCP, page 816). A biopsy of the pancreas may be done by using the ultrasound or CT scan for guidance to obtain tissue for examination under a microscope. At times, surgical exploration may be required to make the diagnosis.

How Serious Is Pancreatic Cancer?

The survival rate with pancreatic cancer is poor. By the time the malignant tumor is identified, it often has spread (metastasized) to other parts of the body. The median survival is little more than 3 to 6 months from the time of the diagnosis.

Treatment

Surgery

Surgical removal of the tumor often is required. However, at the time of operation, your surgeon may not be able to remove the tumor, either because it has invaded vital structures that cannot be removed or because it has spread to distant sites.

Your surgeon may elect to bypass a portion of the intestine if he or she is concerned that the tumor may be causing an obstruction in this area. In addition, if you have jaundice, he or she may also bypass the area of obstruction in the common bile duct.

Other Therapies

If it is judged impossible to remove the tumor, your physician may advise an ERCP (see page 816) to insert a thin, hollow tube (stent) to relieve the obstruction and allow the resumption of bile flow into the small bowel.

Chemotherapy with or without radiation therapy may be considered. Pain can be relieved with strong analgesics or by destruction of nerves that lead to the pancreas (celiac ganglionic block). Pancreatic enzymes can reduce malabsorption and weight loss.

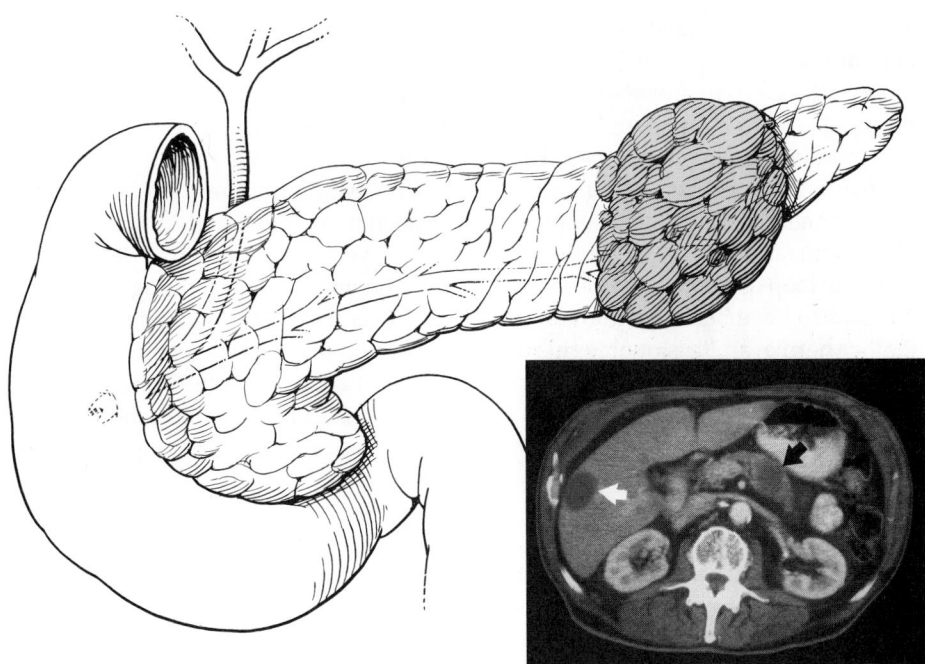

Illustration shows cancer of the pancreas. Computed tomography scan (inset) is cross-section image, revealing large, malignant tumor in pancreas (black arrow) that has spread (metastasized) to the liver (white arrow).

Congenital Pancreatic Abnormalities

Annular Pancreas

An annular pancreas is a ring-shaped formation of pancreatic tissue that grows around the duodenum and may cause intestinal obstruction. Annular pancreas occurs in both children and adults.

This pancreatic abnormality will make you feel exceptionally full after meals, and later you may have pain in the pit of your stomach that might bring on nausea and vomiting. Because the symptoms are mild and tolerable, many people go for years before this condition is properly diagnosed.

Your physician will consider other possible disorders in evaluating your condition, because people with an annular pancreas often have complications such as pancreatitis (see page 819) and peptic ulcer (see page 753). The potential for these complications makes it necessary that the problem be corrected surgically (bypass the obstruction) once it has been diagnosed.

Pancreas Divisum

This is a congenital defect in which parts of the pancreas fail to grow together. In this event, the pancreas must drain its secretions through a smaller secondary duct. Some physicians believe that this causes partial obstruction, pain, and a possible inflammation of the pancreas (see Acute Pancreatitis, page 818), but this is controversial.

Hernias

A hernia is often thought to be the result of heavy lifting and the person with the hernia a man who has lifted too much. In fact, hernias often have no apparent cause, and anyone—even a newborn baby—can have one.

If any part of an abdominal organ protrudes through a weak point or tear in the abdominal wall, it is considered to be a hernia.

There are several types of hernias that commonly affect the general area of the abdomen: inguinal, femoral, paraumbilical, and incisional hernia. Another hernia, called a hiatal hernia, is a protrusion of part of the stomach through the esophageal opening of the diaphragm (see page 743). If the blood supply to the loop of trapped intestine is cut off, it is said to have become strangulated. Yet another hernia, an incisional hernia, occurs when a surgical incision in the abdominal wall does not heal properly.

Inguinal Hernia

In men, a hernia commonly develops in the region where the spermatic cord and blood vessels to the testicles pass out of the abdominal cavity and into the scrotum. The area where these structures pass through the abdominal muscles is called the inguinal canal. Inside the abdominal cavity, the opening into the inguinal canal is called the internal ring. The opening of the canal on the outside of the abdominal muscles is called the external ring.

A weakness in the tissues can allow a loop of bowel to pass out of the abdomen by following the course of the spermatic cord. This is an indirect inguinal hernia. Sometimes the weakness occurs between the internal ring and the pubic bone. A bulge originating in this area is called a direct inguinal hernia. Both indirect and direct inguinal hernias probably account for four of every five hernias in men. Less often, an inguinal hernia can develop in a woman at the point where the connective tissue binding the uterus exits from the abdomen to join with the tissue surrounding the vaginal opening.

Signs and symptoms of an inguinal hernia include discomfort while bending over during lifting and a tender lump in the groin.

How Serious Is an Inguinal Hernia?

A hernia that cannot be forced back into the abdomen by application of pressure is possibly trapped (incarcerated). Without treatment, the hernia can strangulate because the blood supply has been compromised. The result can be gangrene, a life-threatening condition requiring immediate surgical attention.

Diagnosis

Your physician can diagnose a hernia by feeling the area of the internal ring with an examining finger. If there is a bulge in this area, it is usually due to a hernia.

Many hernias cause a noticeable bulge near (to the left or right of) the pubic bone. If the bulge persists and is accompanied by nausea and vomiting, the hernia may have become obstructed or strangulated. Many minor hernias are uncovered during routine physical examinations.

Treatment

Surgery

If surgery is needed, the best treatment for an inguinal hernia is an operation in which the intestine is pushed back into the abdomen and the weakened muscles in the abdominal wall are sewn together. After surgery, it will be about a month before you will be able to return to any strenuous activities.

Other Therapies

Wearing a corset or truss is not an acceptable form of treatment for a hernia. Your physician may have you wear one prior to operation as a precaution against the problem growing worse. But this is not a permanent solution.

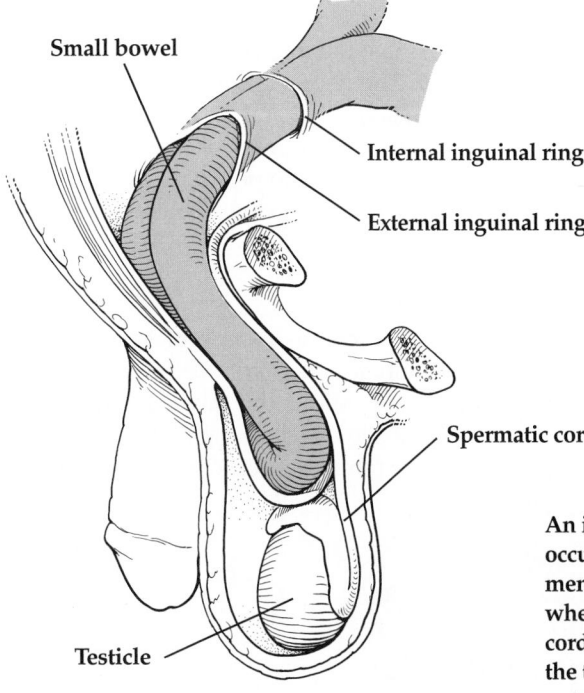

Small bowel

Internal inguinal ring

External inguinal ring

Spermatic cord

Testicle

An inguinal hernia occurs commonly in men at the point where the spermatic cord that suspends the testicles passes out of the abdomen into the scrotum.

Other Abdominal Hernias

Although less common, other types of abdominal hernias may need surgical correction, particularly if they cause discomfort.

Femoral Hernia

A femoral hernia forms along the canal that

Hernia Surgery

Surgery is the preferred treatment for most abdominal hernias, with the exception of an umbilical hernia in an infant (a condition that occurs as a result of incomplete development of the abdominal wall), which usually corrects itself in a year or two.

The Procedure

Hernia surgery is relatively simple. It consists of pushing the protruding intestine back into the abdomen and then surgically repairing the weakened or torn muscle or tissue to prevent the intestine from breaking through again.

Surgery may be postponed if you have a cold and cough because the spasmodic pressure in the ab-

domen may weaken the incision before it can heal properly.

Before the operation you will be given an anesthetic—local, spinal, or general, depending on the type and severity of the hernia. A small incision is then made in the groin and the herniated tissue is returned to the abdominal cavity. If the herniated intestine is strangulated and gangrenous, that section of the intestine will be removed (resected) and the nongangrenous ends will be sutured together. The operation is concluded by closing the defect in the tissue or muscle of the abdominal wall. The operation usually takes less than an hour.

Your surgeon may elect to strengthen a weakened abdominal

wall with a prosthetic or synthetic material (such as Dacron or Gore-Tex). At times this operation can be done as outpatient surgery. Your surgeon may elect to repair your hernia using a laparoscopic technique (see Laparoscopic Surgery, page 817).

The Recovery

After the operation you will be urged to move about as soon as you are able, usually within the first day. You will be permitted to eat whatever foods and liquids agree with you. However, if you notice any redness or discomfort around the site of the incision, report it to your physician. It may be a sign of infection.

carries the principal blood vessels (femoral artery) into the thigh (the femur is the thigh bone). This hernia usually produces a bulge that is slightly lower than where an inguinal hernia usually appears. A femoral hernia is more likely to become strangulated than is any other type of hernia. Femoral hernias are more common in females.

Paraumbilical Hernia

A far less common type of hernia is the paraumbilical hernia. In this instance, a bulge appears at the navel because of a weakness in the abdominal wall surrounding the umbilicus. Some newborn children are found to have a similar problem, called umbilical hernia, because part of their bowel has remained within the umbilical cord rather than returning to the abdominal cavity (see page 17). These hernias often are without symptoms (asymptomatic).

Incisional Hernia

A surgical incision in the abdominal wall that did not heal properly can produce a hernia. Such hernias usually pose a relatively small risk of causing any problems, although, at times, portions of your intestine may exit (prolapse) through the hernia and cause discomfort.

Chapter 26

Your Kidneys and Urinary Tract

Contents

Your Kidneys and Urinary Tract, 826

Congenital Kidney Disorders, 827
Anatomic Abnormalities, 827
    The Kidney X-Ray, 829
Medullary Sponge Kidney, 830
Vesicoureteral Reflux, 830

Inherited Kidney Disorders, 831
Polycystic Kidney Disease, 831
Cystinuria, 832
    Blood in the Urine, 832
Renal Tubule Defects, 833
Alport's Syndrome, 833
Congenital Nephrotic Syndrome, 833
Sickle Cell Disease, 833

Injury and Inflammation of the
Kidneys and Urinary Tract, 834
Injury of the Kidney and Ureters, 834
Traumatic Injury of the Bladder and
    Urethra, 835
    Toxic Injury of the Kidney, 835
Acute Interstitial Nephritis, 836
Acute Glomerulonephritis, 836
Chronic Glomerulonephritis, 838
Nephrotic Syndrome, 840

Urinary Tract Infections (UTI), 841
Acute Pyelonephritis (Kidney Infection),
    841
Cystitis (Bladder Infection), 842
    Interstitial Cystitis, 842
Urethritis, 842

Stones, Cysts, and Tumors, 843
Kidney Stones, 843
Bladder Stones, 845
    Kidney Stone Lithotripsy, 846
Kidney Cysts, 847
Cancer of the Kidney or Ureter, 847
Bladder Cancer, 848
    Cystoscopy, 849

Blood Vessel Problems, 850
Acute Arterial Occlusion, 850
Renal Artery Stenosis, 851
Malignant Hypertension, 852
Renal Vein Thrombosis, 852

Kidney Failure, 852
Acute Kidney (Renal) Failure, 853
Chronic Kidney (Renal) Failure, 854
End-Stage Kidney (Renal) Disease, 855
    Kidney Dialysis Treatments, 856
    Kidney Transplantation, 857

Your Kidneys and Urinary Tract

The kidneys and urinary tract form a complex system whose primary function is removal of excess fluid and waste material from the blood. In addition, the kidneys function as glands by producing hormones that are important in the production of red blood cells, in the regulation of blood pressure, and in the formation of bone.

The system has the following structures: kidneys, ureters, bladder, and urethra. Your kidneys, a pair of bean-shaped organs, are located against the back of the abdominal wall on either side of the spine at the level of the lowest ribs. Each kidney is generally about the size of your fist. Your ureters are muscular tubes, one from each kidney, that propel the urine to the bladder, a muscular bag that stores the urine. Your urethra is the narrow tube through which the urine leaves the bladder during urination.

Most of us were born with two functioning kidneys. However, some are born with a single kidney that is entirely capable of sustaining normal life.

The kidneys are able to vary their activities from day to day to adjust to the daily changes in kinds and amounts of food and fluids that are consumed. For example, suppose that one day you happen to drink large amounts of water or other beverages and on the next you drink almost none. Your kidneys are able to adapt accordingly, neither allowing your tissues to be flooded on the one day nor depleted on the next. They do this by carefully controlling the amounts of fluid and salts that are excreted in your urine. Although other organs such as skin, lungs, and intestine also remove fluids, the kidneys are by far the most important organ for fluid excretion.

This is how the process works. Blood enters each kidney from its renal artery, a major branch of the aorta, the body's main artery. Although together the kidneys account for less than 1 percent of the body's weight, 20 percent of the blood pumped from the heart at any given time passes through them.

Once inside the kidney, the blood passes through a set of filtering systems called nephrons. These are the main functioning units of the kidney. Each kidney contains more than 1 million such units, each consisting of a tuft of small blood vessels, called a glomerulus, and some tubules.

First, the blood passes through the glomeru-

The Kidneys and Urinary Tract

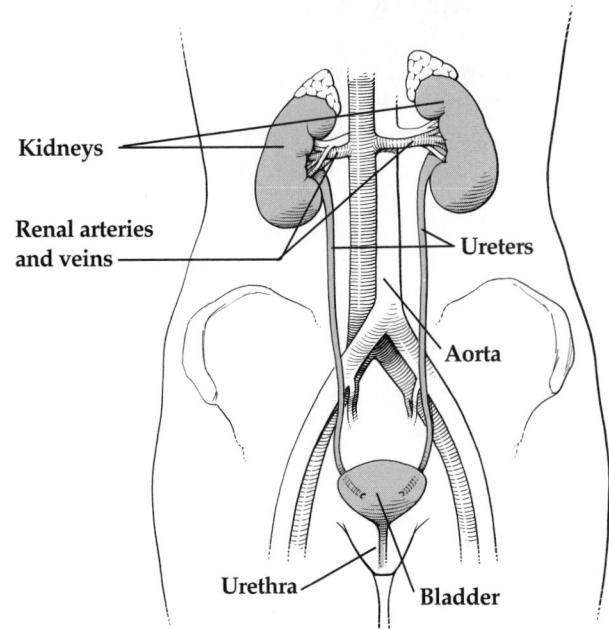

Kidneys

Renal arteries and veins

Ureters

Aorta

Urethra   Bladder

Kidney (Cross-Section)

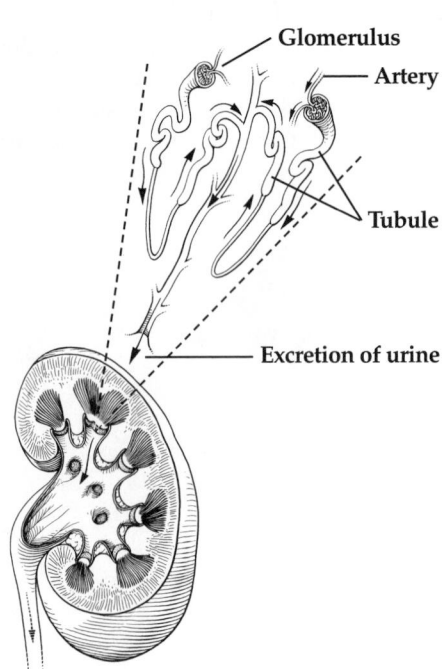

Glomerulus

Artery

Tubule

Excretion of urine

lus. The blood cells, proteins, large particles, and some of the water remain in the bloodstream. Everything else, including a large volume of water, filters out and passes into the tubule.

In the tubule, an important process occurs to control what will be excreted in the urine and what will be reabsorbed into the blood. Waste products (such as urea, creatinine, and uric acid) and excess salts, water, and calcium remain within the tubule. The other substances are absorbed, in precisely the amounts needed by the body, by the cells that make up the walls of the tubules. These absorbed substances are then returned to the bloodstream. Thus, the composition of the urine is determined by both the need to get rid of unwanted substances and the need to retain other substances.

The urine that has remained in the tubule emerges from its lower end, enters the ureter, and goes to the bladder, where it is stored. When the nerves of the bladder signal a feeling of fullness, the urine is voided through the urethra. On average, about 1.5 quarts of urine is excreted every day. But this is only a small fraction of the amount of fluid initially filtered through the glomerular capillaries into the tubules.

The blood that leaves the kidney contains salts, protein, sugar, calcium, and other substances vital to maintaining normal body function. This blood travels through the renal vein and recirculates throughout the body.

Most of the time this cleaning process is performed flawlessly. Sometimes, however, problems occur in the kidney's ability to filter. For example, if the tubules are defective, valuable substances that ordinarily are returned to the bloodstream instead may be excreted in the urine. Or the glomeruli may leak protein into the urine, a condition called nephrotic syndrome (see page 840). Injury, hypertension, exposure to toxins, kidney stones, tumors, and even infections in other parts of the body can cause kidney damage. Unfortunately, many kidney diseases often have no noticeable symptoms until they have done substantial and irreparable damage.

A good indication of whether the kidneys are functioning properly is obtained by a urinalysis, a simple test that is often performed during routine physical examinations. The urinalysis is the first step in determining the presence of kidney or related disease and in separating major problems from minor ones. Infection can be detected, and the bacteria causing it can be identified, by growing a culture from the urine, so that the correct antibiotic can be prescribed (see page 1347).

Your primary physician is often the first to detect a kidney or urinary problem. He or she then may refer you to a nephrologist if the problem is in the function of your kidneys or to a urologist if the problem is with the urinary tract.

The remainder of this chapter will examine the diseases and disorders of the kidneys and urinary tract. Conditions specific for either females or males will be covered in the chapters Women's Health (see page 1139) and Men's Health (see page 1195).

Congenital Kidney Disorders

Because human beings need only one functioning kidney, many infants born with an abnormal or even a single kidney can lead normal lives.

Many of the following anatomic abnormalities cause no symptoms and may often go undetected, at least initially, or are detected when tests are done for other purposes.

Anatomic Abnormalities

Solitary Kidney
This term is used for the situation in which one kidney is missing. The other kidney performs the work of two, usually with no problems.

Horseshoe Kidney

In this condition, the bottom ends of the two kidneys are connected, forming a horseshoe appearance. Horseshoe kidney often goes undetected unless an ultrasound scan (see page 1335) or a kidney X-ray (intravenous pyelogram, or IVP, see page 829) is taken. Blood in the urine, kidney stones, urinary obstruction, and increased susceptibility to infection are complications of horseshoe kidney. These can be treated if and when they occur. The condition itself rarely leads to kidney failure.

Duplication of Kidney

The pelvis (the urine-collection portion) of the kidney is divided into separate compartments, each with its own ureter. This may occur in one or in both kidneys. There may not be any symptoms, but this disorder carries with it an increased risk of infection or urinary obstruction.

Floating or Dropped Kidney

In this unusual condition, the kidney moves up or down in the flank, depending on body position. In the past, various symptoms have been blamed on this condition, but it now is thought that a floating or dropped kidney usually is not a matter of concern and does not require any further testing or treatment.

Congenital Ureteral Pelvic Junction (UPJ) Obstruction

This disorder involves an obstruction in the area where the ureter enters the kidney. Typically, this occurs on only one side. Obstruction is often detected in children after the passage of bloody urine (often after a blow to the area of the kidney). At other times, abdominal pain or infection will lead to the diagnosis. Sometimes this disorder is detected at the time of an ultrasound during the prenatal period. Pressure due to the obstructed kidney drainage leads to scarring of the kidney and may progress to loss of function on the affected side. Surgery is usually required to eliminate the obstruction and prevent further kidney damage.

X-ray of kidneys reveals duplication of the ureter on one side (white arrow).

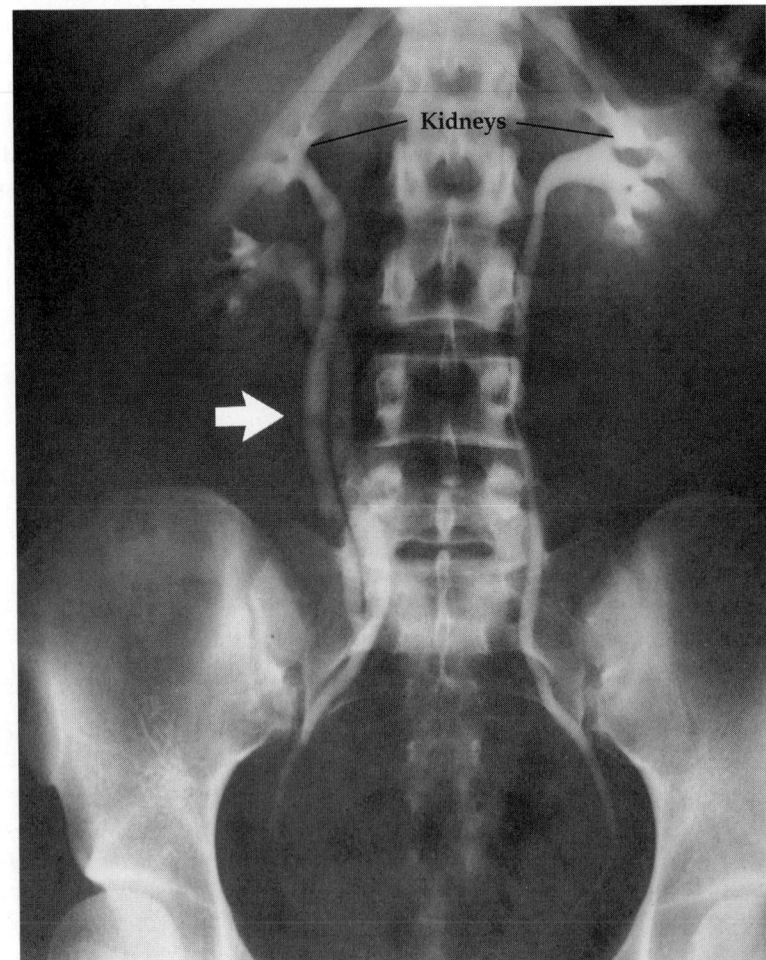

Multicystic Dyplasia

This disorder is usually detected on prenatal ultrasound. The affected kidney commonly functions poorly, if at all. The disorder may spontaneously regress with time. The other kidney typically functions satisfactorily, so the child grows and develops normally.

Congenital Hydronephrosis

While the fetus is still in the uterus, its kidneys may become distended with urine as a result of an obstruction to urine outflow that may persist after birth. There are many causes of such urinary obstruction. One of the most common in males is an obstruction in the urethra, just below the bladder. Ultrasonography (examination with ultrasound) can detect this condition in the fetus. After birth, the cause of the condition can be determined by various special X-ray methods including intravenous pyelography (see this page). Infection may be the first indication of obstruction. An operation may be necessary to relieve the obstruction and thus prevent

---

The Kidney X-Ray

Intravenous pyelography, also known as IVP or as excretory urography, is an X-ray examination used to provide a detailed picture of the kidney and lower urinary tract. The IVP does not give the physician detailed information about kidney function.

If you are to undergo IVP, you will be instructed not to eat or drink for 6 hours before the test. You may be given a laxative to clean out your colon. (This makes it easier to see your kidney.)

The examination begins with the injection of a contrast agent (a substance opaque to X-rays) into a vein in your arm. Your bloodstream will rapidly deliver it to your kidneys, where it is filtered through each glomerulus into the renal tubules. Later, it flows throughout the kidneys, down the ureters, and finally into the bladder. Throughout this approximately hour-long procedure, a series of X-rays is taken.

There is a related procedure called voiding cystourethrography. During this procedure, a catheter is inserted through the urethra into the bladder and X-rays are taken while the bladder is filled with fluid and subsequently emptied. This gives clear evidence of whether the fluid stays in the bladder or flows back up (refluxes) to the kidney.

If your physician suspects that you have an abnormality of your kidney or urinary tract, IVP is often one of the first radiologic tests done. It also is useful for determining the presence of congenital abnormalities, tumors, scarring of the kidneys, and stones in the urinary tract. An ultrasound or CT scan often is used to further define any abnormal IVP findings.

IVP depends on the ability of each kidney to move the material throughout the urinary system. Thus, it is difficult to obtain a good IVP study when the kidneys do not filter properly.

Except for emergencies, pregnant women should not have an IVP because the radiation may harm the fetus.

Most of the time there are no side effects after IVP, although some people report nausea, vomiting, or pain in the arm where the injection was made. Allergic reactions to substances injected into the body occasionally do occur, so you should advise your physician of any allergies you may have. Of special concern are allergies to iodine, seafood, or radiologic contrast agents.

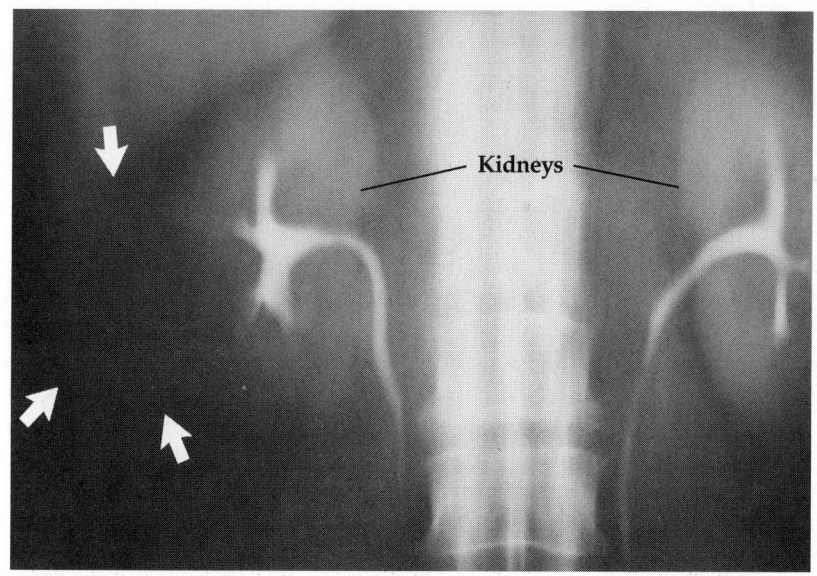

Intravenous pyelography (IVP) provides a detailed view of the kidneys. White arrows show tumor.

kidney damage. In many infants with congenital hydronephrosis, the condition may resolve spontaneously with time.

Medullary Sponge Kidney

Signs and Symptoms
- Flank pain
- Burning pain on urination or blood in the urine
- Kidney infection or stones

Medullary sponge kidney is the result of an abnormality in the way the collecting ducts of the kidney drain the urine into the kidney's pelvis (the urine-collection portion of the kidney). If there are symptoms, they typically occur in adolescence or in the 20 years thereafter. Often there are no symptoms. Medullary sponge kidney is only rarely associated with serious kidney problems such as blood in the urine, kidney infection, or kidney stones. The diagnosis can be made with a kidney X-ray (see page 829).

Treatment
The specific symptoms are treated. When there are no symptoms, physicians recommend drinking adequate quantities of water.

Vesicoureteral Reflux

Signs and Symptoms
- Recurrent urinary tract infections
- Scarring or stunted kidney growth revealed in kidney X-ray
- Protein in the urine
- High blood pressure

Vesicoureteral reflux is the single most common urinary tract problem in children. It often occurs when there are anatomic abnormalities of the urinary tract. During voiding, urine passes from the bladder back through the ureter to the kidney (refluxes) because the valve in the ureter does not function properly.

Reflux can be harmful to the kidney because it creates abnormal pressure and, most importantly, because it introduces bacteria from the bladder into the kidney. The kidney can become infected and, ultimately, damaged. Reflux is one of the most common causes of severe hypertension and end-stage kidney failure in children and young adults.

Diagnosis
If your child is having recurrent urinary tract infections, your physician may suspect vesicoureteral reflux. Reflux can sometimes be detected during a kidney X-ray, or IVP (see page 829). However, the definitive test for this problem is voiding cystourethrography.

During this procedure, the child is catheterized (a thin flexible tube is passed through the urethra to the bladder; see page 829) and X-rays are taken while the bladder is filled with fluid and then emptied. This shows whether the fluid stays in the bladder or flows back up (refluxes) to the kidney. It also allows an estimate of the severity of the problem, which is important in recommending treatment. A similar test, called radionuclide cystography, sometimes is used instead of the voiding cystourethrogram.

If your child does have reflux, renal radionuclide scanning or IVP may be done to determine whether the kidneys have sustained any scarring or other damage.

How Serious Is Vesicoureteral Reflux?
The reflux may be mild, moderate, or severe. If the reflux in your child is mild, there is a good chance that the problem will disappear as the child grows. Moderate or severe reflux is less likely to disappear with time.

Reflux should never be ignored. Damage to the kidneys is a real danger with this problem, particularly in infants and children younger than 5. Kidney damage due to reflux is responsible for about 6 percent of the cases of end-stage renal failure in children and young adults.

Treatment
Treatment for vesicoureteral reflux depends on its severity.

Medication
Initially, particularly when the reflux is mild to moderate, the child may be given low doses of antibiotics to keep the urine free of bacteria, thus preventing the refluxed urine from infecting the kidneys. Typically, this involves a daily dose of an appropriate antibiotic. Urine samples should be cultured at regular intervals to ensure that no bacteria are present.

Surgery
An operation may be considered for children who have severe reflux, moderate reflux that shows no sign of resolving as they grow older, urinary infections despite continuous antibi-

otic treatment, or other urinary abnormalities that make the resolution of reflux unlikely.

The operation for reflux involves reimplanting the ureter into the bladder. In 95 percent of cases, the reflux is abolished by this operation. However, urinary tract infections continue to occur in a small number of cases despite an apparently successful operation.

Children who undergo this operation should receive antibiotics for the first 3 months after the operation. At that time, another voiding cystourethrogram or radionuclide cystogram can be obtained to determine whether the problem has been corrected.

Inherited Kidney Disorders

There are some kidney disorders that seem to run in families. If your physician finds one of these diseases in a member of your family, he or she may also do tests on other family members, even if they have no symptoms, to see if they also have the disease.

Polycystic Kidney Disease

Signs and Symptoms
- Flank pain
- Blood in the urine
- Excessive urination at night
- Kidney stones
- Anemia (in children)
- Hypertension

In polycystic kidney disease, the kidneys contain clusters of cysts that interfere with function and enlarge the kidneys. It occurs in both children and adults. The disease is much more common in adults and usually does not cause symptoms or problems until the second or third decade of life or later. It is estimated that 500,000 adult Americans have this disease. The number may be even greater because some persons with polycystic kidneys may never have symptoms.

The childhood form is often diagnosed shortly after birth. Problems associated with this disease include high blood pressure, anemia, kidney failure, and liver disease in early to middle childhood.

Diagnosis
If the presence of polycystic kidneys is suspected, the examining physician probably will order an ultrasound examination (see page 1335) and perhaps a CT scan (see page 1334) or MRI scan (see page 1334). In certain situations, your physician will rely on analysis of chromosomes to determine whether you have the gene for polycystic kidney disease.

How Serious Is Polycystic Kidney Disease? With the adult form of the disease, hypertension and progressive loss of renal function often develop during adulthood. At times, bleeding into a cyst occurs and may be associated with flank pain. Renal stones occur more often in people who have polycystic kidney disease than in the general population. Most people with this disease reach end-stage renal disease by the time they are in their 40s or 50s, but some have end-stage renal disease earlier. Others may have only

Polycystic kidneys are enlarged from development of fluid-filled sacs. This condition can result in kidney failure.

Polycystic Kidneys

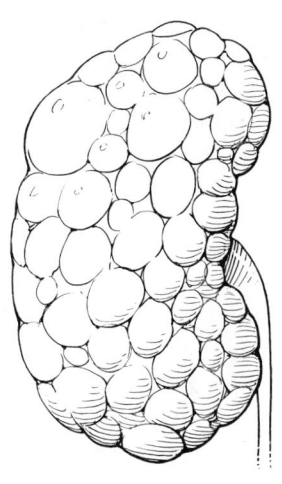
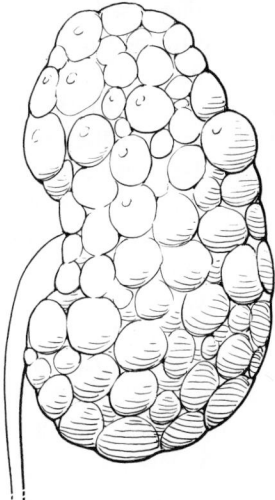

a mild to moderate loss of renal function throughout life. Once end-stage renal disease is reached, kidney dialysis or kidney transplantation is necessary to sustain life. Many of the adults with this disease also have liver problems, including liver cysts. The liver cysts can become infected, and this causes fevers and other symptoms.

The childhood form of the disease is very serious and may result in death in infancy or childhood. If there is a family history of brain aneurysms or if there are any neurologic symptoms, your physician may also investigate for the presence of a possible aneurysm.

Treatment

Currently, no treatment is available to prevent the cysts from forming and enlarging, but treatment is available for the symptoms and complications of polycystic kidney disease. Control of hypertension will help preserve what kidney function is remaining. Urinary tract infection must be treated promptly to prevent kidney damage. Puncture of cysts is sometimes necessary because of pain, bleeding, infection, or obstruction. In some cases, it is necessary for a surgeon to drain many cysts because massive enlargement of the kidneys may be affecting abdominal organs (for example, liver, pancreas, and intestines). Occasionally, cyst puncture and drainage may be performed to try to improve or stabilize kidney function. When end-stage renal disease ensues, kidney dialysis or transplantation has been successful.

The childhood form of the disease requires careful and consistent medical attention for the many complications. High blood pressure is common and usually requires medication. Most affected children will reach end-stage renal disease during childhood. Thus, dialysis or transplantation is used much earlier for this form of polycystic kidney disease. The associated liver disease is often severe.

Cystinuria

Signs and Symptoms
- Blood in the urine
- Pain
- Kidney stones

If you have cystinuria, your kidneys' tubules are not reabsorbing certain amino acids adequately. Excessive amounts of lysine, arginine, ornithine, and cystine are excreted in the urine. This inheritable disorder occurs in 1 of every 10,000 persons and is characterized by stones in the kidney, ureter, and bladder.

Blood in the Urine

Blood in the urine (hematuria) may be visible to the eye or, more commonly, apparent only when the urine is examined under a microscope. In the latter situation, hematuria is often diagnosed when a urinalysis is performed for some other reason, such as a screening test at the time of a routine or sports physical examination.

Hematuria may result from a wide variety of kidney or urinary tract problems such as infection, stones, glomerulonephritis, cysts, and tumors, as well as others. However, many people with hematuria have no evidence of any of these problems, despite careful evaluation; they have what is called benign hematuria.

Benign hematuria is not associated with any kidney damage or with any serious long-term effects. There are two forms of benign hematuria: a nonfamilial form and a familial or inherited form.

Nonfamilial benign hematuria (also called sporadic) typically is detected in childhood but may not become apparent until later. Aside from the presence of blood in the urine, all other findings related to the urine, blood, and kidneys are normal. Treatment is unnecessary. In many cases, the hematuria disappears gradually with time.

The familial form of benign hematuria is transmitted as an autosomal dominant trait. Therefore, several members of a family usually are affected, and screening of family members is helpful in establishing the diagnosis. In many cases, a kidney biopsy is necessary to confirm the diagnosis of benign familial hematuria and distinguish it from other conditions. Benign familial hematuria commonly is recognized in childhood. Typically, it persists throughout life but causes no kidney damage or other problems. No treatment is necessary.

In some children with isolated hematuria, a high concentration of calcium is found in the urine (hypercalciuria) and is believed to be the cause of the hematuria. These children may have an increased risk for having kidney stones.

Diagnosis

A special chemical analysis of the urine will reveal the presence of the substances found in cystinuria. If you pass a kidney stone, your physician will order a test to determine the exact composition of the stone. If the stone contains cystine, it is likely that you have cystinuria.

How Serious Is Cystinuria?

Cystinuria is a serious disease. Many who have it require daily medication for the rest of their lives and may need numerous operations because of the stones. People with cystinuria are likely to form cystine stones that may damage the kidneys by causing ureteral obstruction or infection. Most will make many such stones. Fortunately, cystinuria rarely leads to kidney failure and does not affect other organs.

Treatment

If you have cystinuria, a large fluid intake is recommended. Your best medicine is water. Because cystine is more soluble in alkaline solution, your physician may advise you to drink sodium bicarbonate or sodium citrate solutions in amounts needed to keep the urine alkaline. Those who do not respond to treatment with water and alkaline salts can be given other drugs that decrease cystine excretion. However, because of possible adverse effects, these should be used only if adequate fluid intake and alkalinizing solutions fail.

Renal Tubule Defects

Renal Tubular Acidosis

There are several inherited disorders in which the kidneys cannot properly remove acid from the bloodstream, or excessive bicarbonate (base) is lost in the urine. Under these circumstances, the kidneys also often lose an abnormal amount of potassium, calcium, and sodium in the urine. The blood becomes acidic, and chloride levels increase in the blood. In children, such tubular defects are often manifested by impaired growth. In adults, kidney stones may form and frequently lead to the diagnosis. Treatment generally consists of giving enough sodium biocarbonate or potassium bicarbonate to keep the blood in its normal range of alkalinity.

Vitamin D-Resistant Hypophosphatemic Rickets

This is an inherited disorder in which the kidneys are unable to retain phosphate normally. The result is impaired growth, rickets, and shortened adult stature (see Osteomalacia and Rickets, page 896).

Alport's Syndrome

Alport's syndrome is an inherited disease due to a defect in the collagen that helps to form the basement membranes of many organs of the body, including the kidneys, and the hearing apparatus of the inner ear. The syndrome affects men more severely than it affects women.

The usual course of this syndrome in males is progression to loss of kidney function. Eventually dialysis or kidney transplantation is necessary, usually between adolescence and age 40.

Females may have minimal or no symptoms but can pass on the gene for the disease to their children. Often, very similar inherited kidney disorders are not associated with hearing loss. These are referred to simply as hereditary nephritis.

Congenital Nephrotic Syndrome

Congenital nephrotic syndrome is evident shortly after birth and is most commonly found in families of Finnish origin. Its symptoms are low birth weight, a large placenta, large amounts of protein in the urine, and massive fluid retention. Infection, malnutrition, or renal failure may result in death during the first year of life. Early treatment, including transplantation, has been successful in some children.

Sickle Cell Disease

Sickle cell disease occurs most frequently in blacks. People with this disorder may have an abnormal hemoglobin molecule, delay in growth, and, in infants, failure to thrive. Kidney problems include susceptibility to urinary tract infection, blood in the urine, and loss of the kidney's ability to concentrate the urine, which results in dehydration or loss of salt in the urine.

A progressive loss of kidney function can occur, more often in older people. Both dialysis and transplantation can be complicated by sickle cell disease but may be performed successfully. Those with only the sickle cell trait may notice blood in their urine but typically do not have serious kidney disease (see page 960).

Injury and Inflammation of the Kidneys and Urinary Tract

There are many forms of injury of the kidneys and urinary tract. Because of their protected location within the body, traumatic injury is not common. However, the kidneys are quite susceptible to injury by toxic substances. Infection of the urinary tract is more common in women than in men. Inflammation of the kidney can be drug-induced, the result of an infection in the urinary tract or elsewhere in the body, or associated with disorders that also affect other organs.

This section is about problems common to both sexes. Problems affecting only males or only females are covered in the chapters Men's Health (page 1195) and Women's Health (page 1139).

Injury of the Kidney and Ureters

Signs and Symptoms
- History or evidence of physical injury
- Blood in the urine
- Severe pain in the flank
- Nausea, vomiting, and swelling of the abdomen
- Fever
- Internal bleeding
- Shock

Traumatic injury to the kidney and ureters is not common. It occurs mainly as a result of athletic activities or industrial or traffic accidents. Serious injury to the kidneys is relatively rare because they are protected by the rib cage and the heavy muscles of the back.

Diagnosis
If you have been in an accident and have symptoms or signs that could indicate kidney damage, your blood and urine will be examined. A kidney X-ray (see page 829) or a CT scan or MRI scan may be obtained. Another test that may be used is renal scanning to determine whether the blood flow to your kidneys has been jeopardized. If damage to or blockage of the renal arteries is suspected, a special X-ray study of the artery called arteriography or angiography probably will be done (see page 656).

How Serious Is Trauma to the Kidney and Ureters?
Most often, injured kidneys are merely bruised, and the bleeding stops spontaneously. Sometimes, however, complications such as severe hemorrhage, infection, and shock may develop. After an injury to its blood vessels, the kidney's ability to function may be destroyed within a few hours. Generally, kidney injuries require hospitalization.

Treatment

Emergency
As many as 20 percent of traumatic injuries to the kidneys require emergency operation because of massive hemorrhage.

Surgery
An injured kidney sometimes must be removed. Drainage of the space surrounding the kidney and repair of large kidney lacerations or a torn ureter may be necessary. Operation also is performed to remove clots or other obstructions.

Conservative Therapy
Often, treatment for kidney trauma consists of bed rest for 7 to 10 days and narcotics given for relief of pain. Within 6 months after

the injury, an examination with IVP is generally done to make sure that the kidney has healed properly.

Traumatic Injury of the Bladder and Urethra

Signs and Symptoms
- History of injury
- Inability to urinate
- Blood in the urine
- Pain in the lower abdomen
- Shock

Traumatic injury to the bladder is not common because of the organ's location within the abdomen. When the bladder is injured, most often it happens during an operation such as hernia repair. The bladder also can be ruptured by bone fragments produced by a sharp blow to the pelvis such as in an auto accident.

Rupture of the urethra, the narrow tube that carries urine from the bladder, is more common but less dangerous. Most such injuries are limited to cuts and bruises. In women, urethral damage is rare.

Diagnosis
If your history and symptoms indicate a possible bladder or urethral injury, your physician will do a thorough examination of your abdomen and rectum. An X-ray will be obtained to determine if your pelvis is fractured. The physician also may do a cystoscopic examination, which involves passing a special tube up the urethra into the bladder to permit visual inspection of this part of the lower urinary tract (see page 829).

Toxic Injury of the Kidney

The kidneys are particularly vulnerable to toxic injury because of the vast quantity of blood circulating through them at any given time. Thus, if you have been exposed to a toxin, the effect may be greater on your kidneys than on other organs.

The four most common types of toxic injury to the kidney are described here.

Analgesic Nephropathy
This condition occurs 3 to 5 times more often in women than in men and results from the long-term abuse of nonsteroidal anti-inflammatory drugs (such as phenylbutazone, indomethacin, and ibuprofen), and analgesic drugs that contain phenacetin. Some physicians believe that excessive amounts of acetaminophen may occasionally be harmful to the kidneys, but this has not been definitely proven.

Analgesic nephropathy is one of the most common causes of chronic kidney failure. Its signs and symptoms include pus in the urine, anemia, and hypertension.

Lead Nephropathy
In children, this usually results from ingestion of lead-based paint. Adults generally are poisoned from inhaling vapors produced when metal covered with lead-based paint is welded. Alcohol illegally distilled in an apparatus made from car radiators is another source of lead poisoning. If you have lead nephropathy, your symptoms may include gouty arthritis, hypertension, abdominal pain, and anemia (see Lead Poisoning, page 71).

Acute Uric Acid Nephropathy
Because it does not result from exposure to a toxin from outside of the body, this injury is unlike the previously mentioned toxic injuries. The cause is the body's overproduction of uric acid. It most often occurs in persons with bone marrow and lymph node disorders who have been treated with certain drugs. Its symptoms are diminished urine output and the presence of blood and uric acid crystals in the urine.

Nephropathy From Solvents and Fuels
Carbon tetrachloride and other solvents and fuels have the potential for causing damage to the kidneys. This is the reason for the warning on many commercial cleaners and sprays that they be used only in well-ventilated circumstances.

If your physician suspects that you have any of these toxic injuries, he or she will take a thorough medical history, paying particular attention to medications that you have taken and contacts that you have had with toxic substances. Blood and urine tests will be done. Toxic injury to the kidney may lead to chronic kidney failure if exposure to the toxic substance continues. Fortunately, most toxic injuries can be treated, and kidney function is restored simply by stopping exposure to the toxic substance at an early stage. Others, such as lead and urate nephropathy, require special treatment.

How Serious Is Trauma to the Bladder or Urethra?

These types of injuries usually require hospitalization. The most serious situation is a ruptured bladder that leaks urine into the abdominal cavity. This is a life-threatening situation because of the risk of infection, and it requires emergency surgery to repair the rupture and to remove the urine from the abdominal cavity.

The worst long-term complication of urethral injury is stricture, a severe narrowing of the urethra produced by stiffening of the scar that remains after the injured part of the urethra has healed.

Treatment

Emergency

The treatment of shock and hemorrhage takes priority (see page 441). These are treated by blood transfusions and fluid replacement given through a vein. Pulse rate and blood pressure are monitored constantly.

Medication

Antibiotics are given to prevent infection.

Surgery

An operation is necessary for a ruptured bladder. In the event of an injury to the urethra, a catheter (tube) may be passed through the urethra into the bladder to provide a route for the urine and left in place for several days. If a stricture or narrowing of the urethra persists, causing difficulty in urination, see your urologist.

Acute Interstitial Nephritis

Signs and Symptoms
- Blood in the urine
- Protein in the urine
- Hypertension
- Fever
- Rash
- Weight gain
- Swelling

Acute interstitial nephritis, an inflammation of the kidney, may affect the glomeruli, the tubules, or the spaces between. It is usually temporary and can be caused by several kidney diseases or by allergic reactions to drugs.

If you have acute interstitial nephritis, the inflammation is mainly confined to the spaces between the glomeruli and the tubules. This type of nephritis almost always is a result of an allergic reaction to a drug or to a disturbance in the immune system.

Occasionally, some commonly prescribed drugs may cause acute interstitial nephritis. For this reason, your physician will question you about the medications you are taking. The most common such drugs are penicillin, ampicillin, and nonsteroidal anti-inflammatory drugs (for example, indomethacin, ibuprofen, and naproxen).

Diagnosis

With acute interstitial nephritis or any other form of kidney inflammation, the kidneys are damaged and allow red blood cells and proteins to escape into the urine. Thus, a urinalysis is the first step toward making the diagnosis. Blood tests to assess kidney function also are needed. A kidney biopsy may be required to confirm the diagnosis and to evaluate the degree of damage.

How Serious Is Acute Interstitial Nephritis?

Fortunately, kidney damage that results from acute interstitial nephritis usually is reversible. If the cause is related to the use of a drug, once use of that drug is stopped the kidney begins to heal. Sometimes short-term dialysis is necessary (see page 856). Complete recovery is generally the rule, although progression to chronic renal failure may occur in rare cases.

Treatment

Avoidance of drugs known to cause acute interstitial nephritis is essential. Fluid retention and swelling may be treated by restrictions on salt and fluid intakes. A drug is prescribed to treat the hypertension. Restriction of dietary protein intake may be appropriate.

Dialysis may be necessary for a short time if the kidneys are not functioning adequately. In some cases of acute interstitial nephritis, corticosteroid drugs such as prednisone are prescribed.

Acute Glomerulonephritis

Signs and Symptoms
- Recent streptococcal or viral illness
- Cola- or tea-colored urine
- Hypertension

- Fluid retention
- Protein and red blood cells in the urine
- Mild anemia
- Headaches
- Blurred vision
- Generalized aches and pains

Acute glomerulonephritis, an inflammation of the glomeruli, most often occurs after an infectious disease but sometimes it can be caused by other diseases or it can be a primary kidney disorder. If acute glomerulonephritis occurs after an infectious disease, it may be called acute post-infectious glomerulonephritis. The most common infection leading to acute glomerulonephritis is that caused by streptococci. Other infections that cause it are endocarditis (an inflammation of the lining of the heart), typhoid fever, syphilis, dialysis shunt infections, and malaria. In addition, the kidney inflammation can be brought on by viruses such as those that cause mononucleosis, mumps, measles, or hepatitis or by echovirus or coxsackievirus. Acute glomerulonephritis is not actually a response to the infection or to the virus but is a result of the body's immune response elicited by the infection. Other causes are IgA (Berger) nephropathy, lupus erythematosus, vasculitis, Henoch-Schönlein purpura, and diseases of the glomeruli. These will be discussed in the following sections.

Acute glomerulonephritis rarely occurs after a streptococcal infection (strep throat or strep skin infection, called impetigo), but when it does it usually happens in children ages 6 to 10. Typically, the glomerulonephritis develops some time after the person seems to be well again. In cases of strep throat, it takes anywhere from 6 to 10 days after the cessation of throat symptoms for acute glomerulonephritis to emerge. For strep skin infection, the average latency period is 2 weeks. In contrast, IgA (Berger) nephropathy may cause glomerulonephritis and blood in the urine immediately after an upper respiratory infection.

However, most strep infections do not cause glomerulonephritis. Only a few strains (types) of strep have this potential. Also, not everyone who gets acute glomerulonephritis has symptoms. In families who have experienced an outbreak of strep infection by a strain that can cause glomerulonephritis, there typically are three or four nonsymptomatic cases of acute glomerulonephritis for every one that produces symptoms.

Diagnosis

If your recent health history and symptoms lead your physician to suspect acute glomerulonephritis, your throat or skin lesion will be cultured to determine if streptococcal organisms are still present. Blood studies will be done to identify your immune response, and a urinalysis will be obtained. If these tests suggest glomerulonephritis, a kidney biopsy may be used to determine the underlying cause.

How Serious Is Acute Glomerulonephritis?

In most cases of acute glomerulonephritis, particularly those related to infection, the fluid retention and hypertension resolve within a week. The abnormal urinary values may take several months to return to normal.

The prognosis appears to be better for children than for adults. Most children have a complete recovery and show no evidence of chronic renal disease later in life, although in a very small percentage of them a chronic form of glomerulonephritis may develop and slowly lead to renal failure. Adults do not do as well after acute glomerulonephritis, but no one understands the reasons for this. Adults who have had a particularly severe initial attack that leads to high blood pressure or large amounts of protein in the urine tend to be more prone to chronic kidney failure.

Those who have one attack of the disease generally do fine once the kidneys heal. Although recurrent attacks are unusual, a third to a half of those who have sporadic attacks have progressive renal deterioration.

Treatment

Your physician may advise you to stay in bed. Your salt and water intake may be restricted to minimize fluid retention and swelling. You will be given medication for your hypertension, and you may be placed on a special diet to restrict protein intake (if your serum creatinine or blood urea nitrogen value increases). If you have an active strep infection, your physician will prescribe medication such as penicillin. If the glomerulonephritis is caused by an organism other than strep, it will be treated with an appropriate antibiotic.

Henoch-Schönlein Purpura

This is an important cause of acute glomerulonephritis in children. The symptoms include a characteristic rash that is more prominent on the legs and buttocks, pain in joints with or without swelling or tenderness (especially in the ankles and knees), and abdominal pain. Some children have blood in their stools. Not all children with Henoch-Schönlein purpura have abnormalities involving the kidney. When such involvement is present, there is blood and sometimes protein in the urine along with fluid retention and high blood pressure. Most persons with Henoch-Schönlein purpura recover without kidney damage. However, progressive renal damage does sometimes occur. Most children recover completely without specific treatment, but many adults are left with permanent kidney damage. In some cases, drugs such as corticosteroids may be prescribed.

Hemolytic-Uremic Syndrome

This disease occurs mainly in infants and young children. It occurs much less often in older children and only rarely in adults. In its typical form, an illness with diarrhea (often due to a certain type of *Escherichia coli* bacteria) is followed abruptly by hemolytic anemia, a decrease in the blood platelet count, and rapid loss of kidney function. Other systems such as the central nervous system may be affected as well. Dialysis and blood transfusions often are required during the acute phase of the illness.

Most affected children have a complete recovery, but some are left with chronic kidney damage or damage to some other organs.

Chronic Glomerulonephritis

Signs and Symptoms
- Protein in the urine
- Blood in the urine
- Hypertension
- Gradual kidney failure

Chronic glomerulonephritis is frequently associated with a slow, progressive loss of renal function. There are several diseases of the glomeruli that impair the kidney's ability to retain protein and red blood cells, and these diseases can and often do lead to chronic glomerulonephritis.

Membranous Glomerulonephritis
Irregular deposits of immune-related protein occur along the wall of the glomerulus. More than 80 percent of persons with this disease have nephrotic syndrome (abnormal loss of protein—symptoms include swelling and weight gain from fluid and sodium retention, see page 840). Older men with large amounts of protein and high blood pressure are more likely to progress to kidney failure.

IgA Nephropathy
Also known as Berger's disease, this disease is characterized by recurrent episodes of blood in the urine. Young men are most often affected, but it can occur at any age, even in children. In the majority of cases, renal function remains well preserved even after years of disease. Long-term treatment with fish oils may help some individuals.

Focal and Segmental Glomerulosclerosis
This disease is characterized by scarring of some of the glomeruli. Persons with this disease may have nephrotic syndrome (see page 840). Males are slightly more likely to have this ailment. Both children and adults are affected. Many physicians are trying short courses of high-dose corticosteroids (pulse therapy) to reverse this disease. The condition can be associated with vesicoureteral reflux (see page 830).

Mesangial Proliferative Glomerulonephritis
In this rare chronic disease, portions of the glomeruli are enlarged. Blood and protein are found in the urine. It occurs slightly more often in males than in females. Older children and young adults are most commonly affected.

Diabetic Nephropathy
This may be the most common cause of end-stage renal disease in the United States. Approximately 50 percent of patients with insulin-dependent diabetes mellitus will have significant kidney disease within 12 to 20 years after the onset of their diabetes. This involvement of the kidney often is detected by routine urinalysis, which shows protein in the urine. It also is detected if nephrotic syndrome (see page 840) or hypertension develops or the blood creatinine level (a measure of kidney function) increases. Controlling blood pressure with medicine known as angiotensin-converting enzyme inhibitors (ACE inhibitors) may prolong the time before end-stage kidney failure develops. Once there is a significant amount of protein in the urine, end-stage renal disease usually follows within 5 to 10 years. Also, end-stage renal disease will usually result within 2 to

6 years after the creatinine value increases above normal or hypertension develops (see page 855).

Glomerulonephritis Due to Other Diseases

Several diseases that affect other organ systems can also damage the glomeruli. These include systemic lupus erythematosus (an immune disorder more common in women of childbearing age; see page 918), amyloidosis, myelomas, hepatitis C, and AIDS.

Diagnosis

If you have chronic glomerulonephritis, it may be detected when your physician finds urine abnormalities, impaired renal function, or hypertension during a routine examination or an examination for an unrelated illness. Blood and urine tests and diagnostic studies to visualize the kidney (IVP, ultrasound examination, CT scan) may be done. Renal biopsy may be necessary to determine which disease is causing the chronic glomerulonephritis.

How Serious Is Chronic Glomerulonephritis?

The outcome for chronic glomerulonephritis varies depending on its cause and the severity of the complications, particularly the high blood pressure and the protein loss in the urine.

Mesangial proliferative glomerulonephritis may or may not result in end-stage renal failure. If it does, this usually happens within 10 years after the diagnosis. If the leakage of protein into the urine can be controlled, there is a good chance of avoiding chronic renal damage. However, if there is no response to medication and the nephrotic syndrome persists, often the condition will progress to end-stage renal failure.

Children with focal and segmental glomerulosclerosis occasionally have spontaneous remission of their disease. In adults, however, spontaneous remission is not likely. Although the time for it to happen varies widely, most adults and children with this disease have a progressive decline in renal function. Those with large amounts of protein in their urine may progress to end-stage renal failure within months after the diagnosis. In at least 50 percent of those with focal and segmental glomerulosclerosis, end-stage renal failure develops.

Spontaneous remission of membranous glomerulonephritis is common among children but occurs in only 20 to 25 percent of adults with the disease. Those who have even a partial remission generally do not go on to end-stage renal disease. When it occurs, renal failure is most likely during the first few years after diagnosis. About 30 to 40 percent of those with membranous glomerulonephritis require dialysis or transplantation within 10 years after their diagnosis.

IgA nephropathy usually progresses slowly, if at all. Those with hypertension, large amounts of protein in their urine, and excess urea in their blood tend to have a worse outcome than do those with more moderate disease. In about a quarter of the persons who have this disease, end-stage renal failure develops within 25 years after diagnosis.

There are several glomerular lesions associated with lupus erythematosus. Some, such as minimal lupus glomerular lesion and mesangial lupus glomerulonephritis, generally do not cause substantial kidney damage. Others, such as diffuse proliferative lupus glomerulonephritis and membranous lupus glomerulonephritis, may produce end-stage renal failure, although this is becoming uncommon because of new treatment programs. About 85 percent of those with mild forms of the disease survive for at least 10 years.

Children with Henoch-Schönlein purpura usually do not have progressive kidney disease. However, when urinary abnormalities persist, kidney function may continue to deteriorate.

Treatment

If you have chronic glomerulonephritis, your treatment will be directed by the course of your illness. You will be given medication for your hypertension and a diet low in protein and phosphate, adjusted to what your impaired kidneys can handle. In some people, glomerular lesions are treated with corticosteroids. Others do not respond to this treatment. Many physicians believe that a reduction in your daily amount of protein may be of benefit in slowing the progression of kidney disease. In addition, your physician may consider using an angiotensin-converting enzyme inhibitor (ACE inhibitor), particularly if there is an excess of protein in the urine such as from focal sclerosis and membranous glomerulonephritis. Good control of your blood sugar may also be beneficial. In addition, if the cause of the glomerulonephritis is hepatitis C, your physician may consider treatment with interferon (see page 801).

When renal function deteriorates to the extent that maintenance of health or even life is not possible, dialysis or kidney transplantation must be considered (see page 855).

Nephrotic Syndrome

Signs and Symptoms

- Large amounts of protein in the urine
- Swelling of the eyelids, feet, and abdomen
- Increased weight from fluid retention
- Poor appetite

Nephrotic syndrome is the common feature of many diseases that affect the function of the glomerulus so that excess protein is excreted in the urine. The most common causes of the nephrotic syndrome include diabetes mellitus, drugs (for example, nonsteroidal anti-inflammatory drugs, gold), multiple myeloma, glomerulonephritis, and systemic lupus erythematosus (see pages 925, 973, 836, and 918). Diseases of the glomeruli often result in this syndrome—for example, mesangial proliferative glomerulonephritis, focal and segmental glomerulosclerosis, and membranous glomerulonephritis (see page 838).

In children, the average age at detection is 3 to 4 years. The majority of these children have a form of nephrotic syndrome called minimal change disease (also known as lipoid nephrosis, nil lesion, or foot process disease). About 15 to 20 percent of the adults who have nephrotic syndrome that cannot be traced to infection, drug exposure, malignancy, a disease that affects multiple systems in the body, or hereditary disorders also have this form of the syndrome. The most common lesion that can result in nephrotic syndrome in adults is membranous glomerulonephritis. It accounts for up to 40 percent of adult idiopathic (no known cause) nephrotic syndrome.

Diagnosis

If you have the symptoms of nephrotic syndrome, your physician will do blood and urine studies. If these show large amounts of protein in the urine, he or she may recommend a renal biopsy for establishing a more precise diagnosis and for formulating the best treatment plan. Children seldom require a renal biopsy for an accurate diagnosis.

How Serious Is Nephrotic Syndrome?

The seriousness of this syndrome depends on its cause and whether or not there are complications. As a rule, if you have minimal change disease (a glomerular disease that often results in nephrotic syndrome), you can expect both remissions and relapses of the proteinuria (excessive protein in the urine). Prior to the development of antibiotics, infection was a leading cause of death. Now, however, the mortality rate is extremely low. The vast majority of children and adults with minimal change disease do not go on to develop progressive kidney failure.

When the syndrome is caused by infection or drugs, it often resolves after the infection is cured or the drug use is discontinued.

Some of the other lesions that can cause nephrotic syndrome do not have such a favorable outcome. Many people with focal and segmental glomerulosclerosis or membranous glomerulonephritis progress to end-stage renal disease. The more persistent the nephrotic syndrome, the worse the long-term outcome.

Treatment

Regardless of the underlying cause, treatment of nephrotic syndrome is aimed at alleviating symptoms and preventing complications. The most important predictor of outcome appears to be whether the proteinuria can be reduced or eliminated.

If you have one of the types of nephrotic syndrome that responds to corticosteroids, your physician will probably prescribe prednisone to decrease the urine's protein content. In minimal change disease, corticosteroid therapy enhances the body's tendency toward natural remission. The treatment usually consists of daily oral doses of prednisone for 2 months. Those who are going to respond generally do so within the first month.

Relapse after the medication is discontinued is not uncommon and usually occurs within the first year. If you have a relapse, your physician will most likely prescribe prednisone again, but the dosage will be reduced gradually over 3 to 6 months instead of use of the drug being stopped abruptly.

Prednisone is a powerful drug and has significant side effects, the most common being increased appetite, weight gain, and facial puffiness (see Corticosteroid Drugs, page 919). Some children require so much of the drug that their growth is slowed temporarily. Cyclophosphamide is another drug that can be given if there is no response to prednisone. However, this medication can cause bone marrow problems, bladder irritation, or, occasionally, problems with reproduction, so it is not the preferred drug.

Nephrotic syndrome caused by focal and segmental glomerulosclerosis or membranous glomerulonephritis does not always respond to standard courses of corticosteroids (prednisone), and pulse therapy with higher doses of steroids may be necessary. In a few cases, encouraging results have

been obtained with the anti-inflammatory drug meclofenamate.

Other treatment measures used in nephrotic syndrome include a salt-restricted diet, medication for hypertension (if it is present), and diuretic drugs to control fluid retention. Some persons with nephrotic syndrome are especially susceptible to certain kinds of infections, and administration of pneumococcal vaccine is frequently recommended.

Recent experience with a class of drugs called ACE inhibitors (a type of blood pressure drug) indicates that these drugs may be useful in some persons with nephrotic syndrome.

Urinary Tract Infections (UTI)

Urinary tract infections are common, especially among females, and account for 6 million office visits annually in the United States. One to 3 percent of school-age girls have urinary tract infection; with the beginning of sexual activity, women have a marked increase in the frequency of infection.

The majority of urinary tract infections affect the lower tract—the bladder and the urethra. Most bacteria gain access to the urinary tract via the urethra. Under normal circumstances, these bacteria are flushed out of the body during urination. (Urine also has antibacterial properties that inhibit the growth of bacteria.) However, certain factors increase the chances that these bacteria will take hold and multiply into a full-blown infection. Sexual intercourse, pregnancy, urinary obstruction, and the virulent nature of some bacteria all contribute to the likelihood of such an infection.

Health care providers often use the term urinary tract infection (UTI) to describe infections that begin in the kidney, bladder, or urethra. These infections are called acute pyelonephritis, cystitis, and urethritis.

Acute Pyelonephritis (Kidney Infection)

Signs and Symptoms
- Flank pain
- High fever

- Shaking chills
- Vomiting
- Burning sensation during urination
- Increased frequency of urination

Sometimes bacteria travel up the ureters to the upper tract or kidneys, causing acute pyelonephritis (kidney infection).

Diagnosis
If your symptoms suggest a urinary tract infection, your physician will ask for a midstream sample of urine to determine the presence of bacteria. The combination of urinalysis followed by a urine culture if an abnormal bacterial count is found should reveal whether you have an infection. The presence of fever and flank pain suggests that infection has extended into the kidney itself, although there is no simple test to differentiate kidney infection from lower urinary tract infection.

How Serious Is Acute Pyelonephritis?
When properly treated, acute pyelonephritis rarely progresses to chronic renal disease, although it can be an immediate threat to life in an elderly or weakened person. It can also recur if the infection is not totally eradicated.

Treatment
Antibiotics are the first line of treatment. When recurrences are frequent or the kidney infection is chronic, there may be an underlying problem such as vesicoureteral reflux

(a condition in which the urine flows backward from the bladder to the ureter; see page 830). A kidney X-ray called an IVP (see page 829), renal ultrasound examination (see page 1335), or other diagnostic tests may be warranted.

Cystitis (Bladder Infection)

Signs and Symptoms
- Frequent and urgent urination
- Burning during urination
- Pressure in lower abdomen
- Blood in urine
- Malodorous urine

Often referred to as honeymoon cystitis, this bladder infection commonly occurs in women as a result of sexual intercourse. During sexual activity, bacteria are introduced into the bladder through the urethra. Once inside the bladder, the bacteria begin to multiply. Usually, the body can rid itself of such bacteria by the process of urination, but when it cannot, cystitis or bladder infection may occur.

Although sexually active women between 20 and 50 years of age are the most likely to have cystitis, even young girls are susceptible to lower urinary tract infections because the anus, a constant source of bacteria, is so close to the female urethra. More than 90 percent of cystitis episodes are due to *Escherichia coli*, a species of bacteria commonly found in the rectal area. Males who are under age 50 and have normal urinary tracts rarely contract urinary tract infection.

Diagnosis
If you have the symptoms of cystitis, your health care provider may want a urinalysis on a urine sample collected in a special way. To do this, you wash the vaginal area or the tip of the penis with a disinfectant, pass a small amount of urine into the toilet to cleanse the urethra, and then collect the next portion of voided urine in a sterile cup for examination. (This is a midstream collection.) If urinalysis reveals an abnormal bacterial count, a culture to determine the kind of bacteria may be done so that appropriate treatment can be initiated.

(Note: Blood in the urine without pain or discomfort may not be the result of an infection, and the possibility of a kidney stone or a bladder or kidney tumor should be considered. See pages 843, 847, and 848, and consult your physician.)

How Serious Is Cystitis?
Although very uncomfortable and annoying, cystitis is not a serious disease. Some minor cases resolve without treatment. However, because of its proximity to the kidneys, your physician probably will treat your bladder if it is infected and will obtain a urine culture for testing (1 to 2 weeks after treatment) to make sure that the infection is gone.

Treatment
Cystitis is often treated with a 3- to 5-day course of antibiotics, which are taken orally. More severe cases may require treatment for 7 to 10 days. The symptoms usually disappear within 24 to 48 hours after the first dose. Persons who have more than two infections within 6 months may need low-dose antibiotic therapy as a preventive measure indefinitely. Some women who are prone to bladder infection may benefit by taking a low dose of an antibiotic after sexual intercourse.

Urethritis

Signs and Symptoms
- Frequent urination
- Pain during urination
- Pus in the urine
- Penile discharge

Urethritis is an infection of the urethra, the

Interstitial Cystitis

Painful and frequent urination are the main symptoms of interstitial cystitis, an inflammation of the bladder wall that almost always affects only women in their childbearing years. The exact cause of this uncommon condition is not known, but it is not the result of an infection or cancer.

A urologist can diagnose interstitial cystitis using a cystoscope to visually examine the lining of the bladder (see page 849). The condition is not a sign of a more serious underlying disease.

There is no specific treatment for interstitial cystitis, but pain medications are helpful in some people. If your symptoms are more severe, a urologist may administer medication directly to the bladder wall through a cystoscope. However, these approaches only make symptoms more tolerable. Fortunately, the initial symptoms rarely worsen, and in some people, symptoms abate in time.

tube that transports urine from the bladder during urination. The same organisms that infect the kidney and bladder can infect the urethra. In addition, because of the female urethra's proximity to the vagina, sexually transmitted infections such as herpes simplex virus and *Chlamydia* also are possible (see page 1088).

In men, urethritis often is the result of bacteria acquired through sexual contact. The vast majority of such infections are caused by gonococci and *Chlamydia*. Reiter's syndrome is a combination of urethritis, arthritis, and an eye inflammation called conjunctivitis and is usually acquired through sexual contact (see page 913).

Diagnosis

It is difficult to differentiate urethritis from cystitis in women because their symptoms are similar. One clue is provided by urinalysis. Approximately 30 percent of women who have painful and frequent urination do not have a significant amount of bacteria in their urine. This indicates that the inflammation is in the urethra and that it may not be the result of an infection.

Your physician will question you about your symptoms. If the illness began gradually more than 7 days before the examination and there is no blood in your urine, the symptoms are likely to be from infection with *Chlamydia*, particularly if there has been a recent change in sex partners. Bloody urine, a sudden onset of illness of short duration, and a history of previous infection suggest that a bacterial infection is the cause.

In men, the physician will attempt to squeeze a sample of the discharge from the urethra when the bladder has not been emptied for several hours. If no discharge can be obtained, a small swab can be inserted into the urethra to procure a sample for examination.

How Serious Is Urethritis?

Never ignore urethritis. It is particularly dangerous because the symptoms may disappear without treatment. Because many cases are caused by sexual transmission, notify partners. When left untreated, conditions such as gonorrhea and *Chlamydia* infection can ultimately cause problems such as pelvic inflammatory disease, stricture of the urethra, sterility, arthritis, meningitis, and inflammation of the heart.

Treatment

Treatment depends on the cause. For *Chlamydia* infection, an antibiotic such as tetracycline is taken orally for 7 days. In most cases in which urethritis is caused by gonorrhea, penicillin is used. However, gonorrhea occasionally is resistant to penicillin, and a different medication may be chosen after appropriate laboratory tests. Antibiotics also are prescribed for other bacterial infections. In some situations, your physician will advise that your sexual partner also be treated.

Stones, Cysts, and Tumors

Kidney Stones

Signs and Symptoms

- Gradual development of pain that usually begins in the flank and moves downward to the groin, vulva, or testicle as the stone moves down the ureter
- Persistent urge to urinate
- Blood in the urine
- Family or personal history of stones

Few who have passed a kidney stone can forget the experience. Most people who have had this experience agree that it was one of the most excruciatingly painful episodes in their life. Occasionally, stones are passed with minimal or no symptoms.

Kidney stones (renal lithiasis) is a relatively common disorder. About 3 to 5 percent of women and 6 to 9 percent of men will have had at least one stone by the time they reach

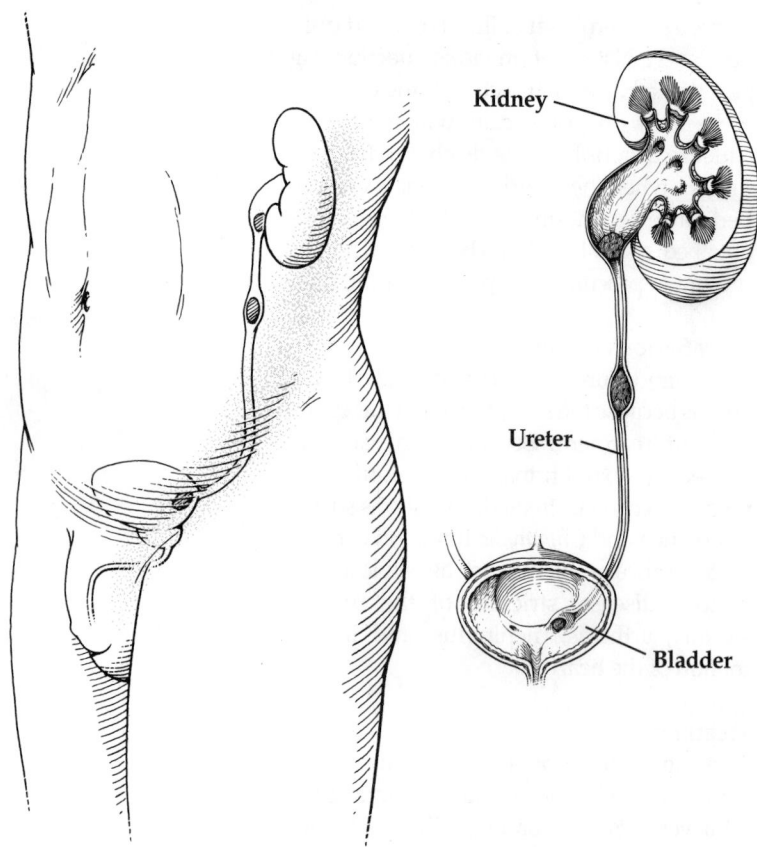

Kidney

Ureter

Bladder

Blue-tinted zone on torso is where the pain of kidney stones most often occurs. Stones originate in your kidneys and can move into the ureter and bladder.

age 70. There is some tendency for kidney stones to recur. The annual recurrence rate is 3 percent after the first stone and 6 percent after the second stone. The tendency to have certain types of stones runs in families. Some types are associated with other conditions such as overactive parathyroid glands, renal tubule defects (for example, renal tubular acidosis), bowel disease, or ileal bypass for obesity. However, the most common cause of kidney stone formation remains unknown—so-called idiopathic stone disease.

A kidney stone is the result of a chemical reaction that occurs when the urine becomes too concentrated. Calcium salts, uric acid, cystine, and other substances in the urine crystallize to form a hard mineral deposit, often the size of a small pebble.

The most common types of kidney stones in the Western Hemisphere are described here.

Calcium Stones

These account for 75 to 85 percent of all stones and are 2 to 3 times more common in men than in women. The first stone usually appears at age 20 to 30. Once you have had one calcium stone, you are likely to have another unless specific treatment is started.

These stones usually are formed by calcium combining with oxalate, phosphate, or carbonate. The most common type is the calcium oxalate stone. The oxalate may be present as a result of the consumption of certain foods. In addition, some people with diseases of the small bowel may have an increased tendency to form oxalate stones.

Uric Acid Stones

Also formed mainly in men, uric acid stones account for up to 10 percent of all stones. Half of those with uric acid stones also have gout.

Cystine Stones

Persons who form cystine stones have the hereditary disorder cystinuria (see page 832). Men and women are equally likely to have cystine stones. These account for only 1 percent of stones.

Struvite Stones

Formed mainly in women, struvite stones are the result of urinary tract infection with bacteria that produce a specific enzyme. These stones can grow very large, producing the appearance of a stag's horn. They can obstruct the urinary tract and cause kidney damage.

Not all stones produce symptoms. It is not uncommon for stones to be discovered during X-ray studies made for an unrelated problem. Generally, the pain occurs when the stone breaks loose and begins to work its way down the ureter.

Diagnosis

If your physician suspects that you have a kidney stone, he or she will request a chemical analysis of your blood and of a 24-hour collection of urine.

If you are having severe pain, you may be in the process of passing the stone, and your physician may prescribe a strong pain medication to help you through the episode. Often, a special kidney X-ray, an IVP, is obtained (see page 829). Hospitalization may be required.

Your physician will probably ask you to urinate through a strainer so that the stone can be recovered for analysis. Every effort should be made to determine the composition of your stone because this information suggests the cause and so allows the treatment to be planned accordingly.

How Serious Are Kidney Stones?
Although the process is painful, most kidney stones pass through the ureter and into the bladder without causing any permanent damage. However, the underlying cause must be determined and treated to avoid further stone formation.

It is important to avoid complications such as urinary tract infection and obstruction, both of which can lead to extensive kidney damage.

Treatment
The selection of treatment depends on the type of stone and whether there are complications. However, there is one rule that applies to all persons with kidney stones: drink at least six to eight glasses of water every day and also drink at least one glass of water at bedtime and another at some time during the night. Adequate fluid intake dilutes the urine, thus making it less likely that crystals will form. Your physician will often consult with a urologic surgeon who is skilled in the treatment of stone disease to decide on the proper treatment for kidney stones when they are detected.

Medication
Whether you will need to take a medication that inhibits the growth of stones depends on the severity of your disease. With certain types of calcium stones (usually associated with excessive calcium excretion), a thiazide diuretic usually is successful in preventing the formation of new stones. A phosphate-containing preparation also may be prescribed to inhibit stone formation in the urine.

The calcium stone formation resulting from distal renal tubular acidosis, a defect in the ability of the renal tubules to filter acids, may be prevented by keeping the urine alkaline (see page 833).

If you have a uric acid stone, your physician may prescribe allopurinol and a medicine to keep the urine alkaline.

When a struvite stone is found, the first task is to suppress the infection that caused it. Several types of antibiotics may be prescribed.

Surgery
Obstruction, infection, or serious bleeding indicates that an operation may be needed to remove a stone. In the past, stones were removed through an incision in the kidney, renal pelvis, or ureter or by passing an instrument up the ureter from the bladder. Now, a less invasive treatment that uses shock waves (generated by sound) to fragment the stone is often successful (see Kidney Stone Lithotripsy, page 846).

Some calcium stones are caused by abnormally active parathyroid glands. The treatment for this condition is removal of parathyroid tissue to avoid future renal damage (see page 950).

Nutrition
Dietary excesses or deficiencies may contribute to stone formation. Because specific factors vary, your physician may review your case and suggest appropriate dietary modifications.

Bladder Stones

Signs and Symptoms
- Infection
- Interruption of urine stream
- Pain in penis
- Inability to urinate except in certain positions
- Blood in the urine

Most bladder stones in Americans are the result of another urologic problem. Urinary infection and enlarged prostate are the most common causes. Ninety-five percent of all bladder stones occur in men.

Diagnosis
If you have the symptoms that suggest a bladder stone is present, your physician will perform a thorough examination including a rectal examination. Urinalysis usually will reveal infection and blood in the urine (hematuria). Generally, bladder stones can be seen on an X-ray of the bladder.

How Serious Are Bladder Stones?
Bladder stones usually pass without intervention. However, if they do not, they should be removed and the underlying cause should be identified and treated.

Treatment
Small stones can be removed with a cystoscope, a tube that is inserted into the bladder

Kidney Stone Lithotripsy

The majority of kidney stones pass without any intervention.

In the past, anyone with a kidney stone that could not be passed and needed removal had to undergo a major operation and a 2-week hospital stay and was left with a large scar. Today, thousands of kidney stone operations are avoided every year because of a technique called kidney stone lithotripsy. No incision or hospitalization is required.

This procedure was developed in West Germany and was approved for use in the United States in late 1984. The lithotriptor produces shock waves that pulverize the stones to small fragments, which then are easily passed in the urine.

If you are to undergo lithotripsy, you will be given a general anesthetic agent. (With newer machines, only a local anesthetic is needed.) Then you will be lowered into a large tub of water so that your body is submerged up to your shoulders. Two X-ray devices within the lithotriptor are used to locate your stone and to position you properly. Newer lithotripsy machines do not have tubs and may use ultrasound rather than X-rays to image the stone. However, these newer lithotriptors are less powerful and often require multiple treatments to fragment the stone.

Because your body has the same acoustical properties as water, your body is not hurt by the hundreds of shock waves that bombard you during the hour-long treatment. However, the kidney stone is so brittle that it crumbles. Although you will not feel the shock waves, there is a loud noise that resounds throughout the treatment room every time a shock wave is generated by the machine. You will be wearing earphones to protect your ears.

During the treatment, X-rays are made to determine the status of the stone. Typically, the stone begins to crumble after 200 to 400 shock waves. As many as 1,500 shock waves may be given during a treatment.

After the anesthetic wears off, you will be encouraged to walk about and to drink lots of water to wash out the small stone fragments.

This lithotripsy treatment is used for stones within the kidney itself or in the upper portion of the ureter. It cannot be used in the lower part of the ureter.

Stones that cannot be fragmented in the lithotriptor often can be treated by lithotripsy in other ways. In one such procedure, percutaneous ultrasonic lithotripsy, a small incision is made in the skin, and through it a cystoscope-like instrument is passed into the kidney. Then, a small ultrasound-producing unit is inserted to shoot sound waves at the stone. The physician removes the resulting fragments through the instrument.

In another variation of lithotripsy, a small instrument with an ultrasound-producing unit is passed up through the bladder and into the ureter (endoscopic lithotripsy). Other techniques to break stones in the ureter include laser lithotripsy and electrohydraulic lithotripsy. These work particularly well on ureteral stones that are inaccessible by the other methods.

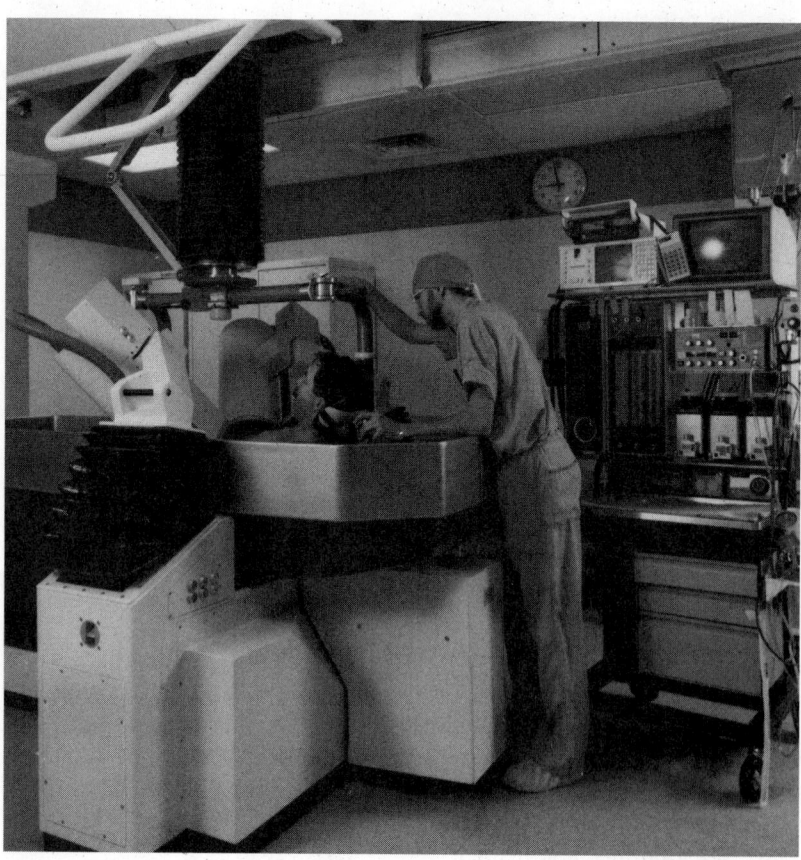

Kidney stone lithotripsy with bath.

through the urethra. Larger stones may require a procedure called electrohydraulic lithotripsy. In this procedure, an instrument that dispenses an electric charge is placed in the bladder through the urethra. The electricity breaks up the stone.

Sometimes a medication is used to dissolve bladder stones.

Kidney Cysts

Signs and Symptoms
- Flank pain
- Blood in the urine

Kidney cysts are noncancerous lesions of the kidney. They usually are round and hollow and contain water-like fluid. They vary from very small to some that contain quarts of fluid. Unlike cancer, a cyst generally grows slowly and ceases to grow after it has attained a certain size.

Cysts in the kidney are very common. At least half of the population over age 50 probably has at least one kidney cyst. Some researchers have found a higher incidence of cysts in women than in men. The fact that infants and children rarely have these cysts suggests that the cysts are not inherited.

Diagnosis
Usually, the cyst is found when an abdominal or kidney ultrasound examination (see page 1335) or CT or MRI scan (see page 1334) is done for some other reason. These methods usually can distinguish between benign cysts and cancer of the kidney.

How Serious Are Kidney Cysts?
Most kidney cysts do not cause symptoms. Only when a cyst is extremely large will it impair renal function. However, cysts do sometimes rupture and collapse. Hemorrhage within the cyst can occur. Sometimes an infection or, rarely, a cancer will begin in a cyst.

Treatment
Generally, no treatment is required. In rare instances, however, operation or aspiration by a needle through the skin is required to collapse or decompress a cyst to relieve the pressure or pain and to prevent damage to the kidney.

Cancer of the Kidney or Ureter

Signs and Symptoms
- Blood in the urine
- Flank pain
- Abdominal mass felt during examination
- Weight loss
- Fatigue
- Intermittent fever

There are several varieties of cancer of the kidney and ureter, some of which are described here.

Renal Cell Carcinoma
This is the most common cancer of the kidneys. It also is called renal adenocarcinoma or hypernephroma. It begins in one of the cells that form the lining of a renal tubule. More than 25,000 new cases are diagnosed each year in the United States, and approximately 11,000 deaths annually are related to this malignancy.

Renal cell carcinoma occurs twice as often in men as in women. The most common age at diagnosis is between 55 and 60.

Smokers, particularly those who smoke pipes or cigars, are at greater risk of renal cell carcinoma than are nonsmokers. In some instances, the disease appears to be hereditary. A large number of persons with von Hippel-Lindau disease, an inherited condition affecting the capillaries of a part of the brain, also have renal cell carcinoma. People on dialysis for end-stage renal disease also have a slightly higher incidence of this type of cancer.

Transitional Cell Cancer
These tumors can occur in the kidney or ureter and account for 10 percent of all kidney cancers. They may be associated with the abuse of analgesic drugs such as phenacetin. The painless passage of blood in the urine may be the only sign of this disorder. Transitional cell cancer typically affects middle-aged women.

Wilms' Tumor
Children with cancer of the kidney usually have Wilms' tumor. It accounts for 95 percent of the renal cancers in children under age 14 and occurs in approximately 8 of every 1 million children under that age. The majority of the children with it are less than

7 years old at the time of diagnosis. The tumor usually is asymptomatic and is found when palpation of a child's abdomen detects a mass.

Diagnosis

Any time blood is seen in the urine, see your physician. When one of these cancers is suspected, a special kidney X-ray, an IVP (see page 829), a CT or MRI scan (see page 1334), or an ultrasound examination (see page 1335) will be performed. Occasionally, additional tests are done, including a biopsy of the suspected mass (see page 1332).

Once the growth has been identified as a cancer, CT scanning often is used to determine its extent (see page 1334). Studies such as chest X-ray, bone scan, and liver tests also are done to ascertain whether the cancer has spread to other organs.

The presence of transitional cell cancer can usually be confirmed with an IVP (see page 829) followed by cystoscopy to determine the precise location of the tumor. A special examination of urine collected over a 24-hour period (cytology) may also identify cancer cells.

How Serious Is Cancer of the Kidney?

The outcome with renal cell carcinoma depends on the extent to which the tumor has spread. If the tumor is in its earliest stage, 60 to 75 percent of affected people will survive for at least 5 years. If the lymph nodes around the kidney have been infiltrated, the 5-year survival rate drops to 5 to 15 percent. When the cancer has spread to other organs, fewer than 5 percent survive for 5 years.

If a transitional cell cancer has not spread, the 5-year survival rates are very high. If the cancer has spread, the chance of surviving 5 years is 10 to 50 percent.

Children with Wilms' tumor generally have a good outlook if the disease has not spread. Overall, 85 to 90 percent survive for at least 5 years.

Treatment

When it appears that a renal cell carcinoma has not spread beyond the kidney, the best treatment is removal of the entire kidney. Some surgeons advocate also removing the surrounding lymph nodes. Sometimes, radiation therapy may be used to prevent spread of the cancer.

If the disease has spread, there is no universally agreed on method of treatment. Chemotherapy or immunotherapy for kidney cancer is still in its infancy but has been effective in some cases.

In an early stage, a transitional cell cancer and the surrounding area are removed and an attempt is made to save the kidney itself. If the tumor is larger, the kidney and ureter are removed along with the portion of the bladder that is connected to the ureter (to decrease the risk of bladder cancer).

A combination of treatments is used for Wilms' tumor. The mass is removed, and the child is given chemotherapy. Sometimes, radiation therapy also is used.

Bladder Cancer

Signs and Symptoms

- Blood in the urine
- Pelvic pain
- Difficulty in voiding urine

Men are 4 times more likely than women to get bladder cancer. Approximately 50,000 new cases of bladder cancer are diagnosed annually in the United States. The disease is responsible for more than 10,000 deaths each year.

Bladder cancer rarely occurs in persons younger than 40. It appears to be related at least partially to environmental factors. The disease is more prevalent among smokers and workers in the dye, chemical, leather, and rubber industries.

Diagnosis

The presence of blood in the urine without pain or discomfort is the most frequent early symptom. A common diagnostic error is to presume that blood in the urine means a bladder infection (see Cystitis, page 842). If you have symptoms that suggest a possible bladder cancer, your physician may have a sample of urine examined for malignant cells. A special kidney X-ray called an IVP (see page 829) may be obtained and a cystoscopic examination (see page 849) that will enable the physician to see into the bladder will be performed. During the cystoscopic examination, a small sample of the bladder lining will be removed to be examined under a microscope for malignant cells.

Cystoscopy

Cystoscopy is an important technique for direct examination of the urethra, the inside of the bladder, and, in men, the prostate gland.

If you are to have a cystoscopic examination, you usually will be given a local anesthetic and will remain awake during the brief procedure. (Children generally are given a general anesthetic.) The cystoscope, a narrow tube, will be inserted through your urethra into your bladder. This tube carries a special lens and a fiberoptic lighting system, so that the examining physician can actually see the structures through which the cystoscope passes.

It may be necessary to remove a sample of bladder tissue for examination for cancer or other diseases or even to remove a small stone. All of this can be done through the cystoscope.

Cystoscopy is useful for evaluating various bladder problems—including recurring infection and pain during urination—for which no cause can be found. One of its most important uses is in the detection of bladder cancer. In women, cystoscopy is useful for detecting chronic inflammation of the urethra or bladder (see page 1192). In men, it sometimes is used to evaluate the degree of obstruction that an enlarged prostate may cause (see page 1209).

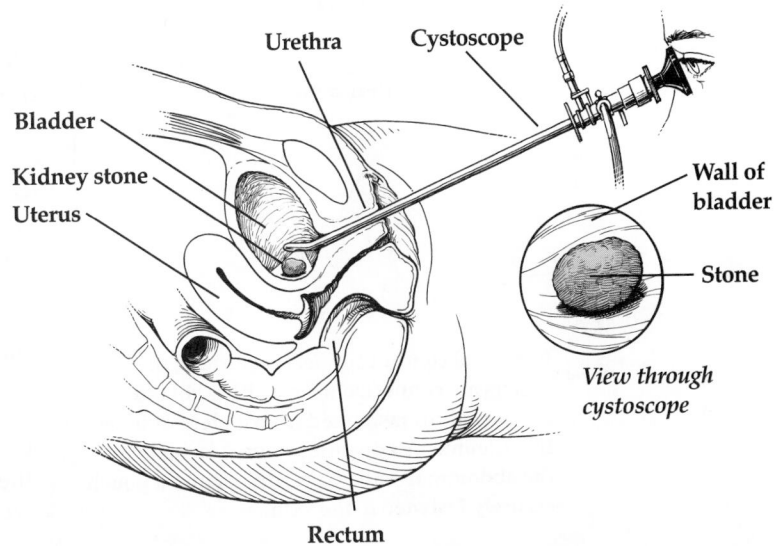

Cystoscopic examination reveals a kidney stone in the bladder. This simple procedure usually is done under local anesthetic on an outpatient basis.

If cancer is found, your physician may order a CT or MRI scan of the abdomen or pelvis to determine the stage of the cancer's growth (see page 1334). Tests to determine whether the cancer has spread beyond the bladder include a chest X-ray and blood studies.

How Serious Is Bladder Cancer?

If the tumor is small and has not invaded deeply within the bladder (that is, it is superficial), the chances of recovery are good. About 50 to 70 percent of people with this type of bladder cancer will have a recurrence within 3 years, but again the cancer will be superficial. About 12 percent of those whose initial disease is superficial eventually will have a more invasive cancer.

Approximately 45 percent of those whose cancer has invaded muscle or fat live at least 5 years, provided they have radiation therapy.

The vast majority of people whose bladder cancer has spread to other organs do not survive beyond 2 years despite treatment.

Treatment

For a superficial bladder cancer, treatment usually consists of removing the tumor itself. A major operation is not required because the surgeon is able to remove the tumor through a cystoscope.

After removal of a superficial tumor, cystoscopic evaluation with biopsy is repeated every 3 to 6 months for many years to detect recurrence of the cancer. If superficial disease recurs, the tumor again will be removed cystoscopically. This time, the bladder may be infused with cancer-fighting drugs to decrease the chance of future bladder cancer.

If the disease has progressed to invade the bladder muscle and fat, the bladder probably will be removed. In men, the prostate gland also is removed, which frequently causes impotence. Women with advanced bladder cancer usually must also undergo removal of the ovaries, uterus, and a portion of the vagina.

Removal of the bladder makes it necessary to create an opening through which urine can pass. There are various ways to do

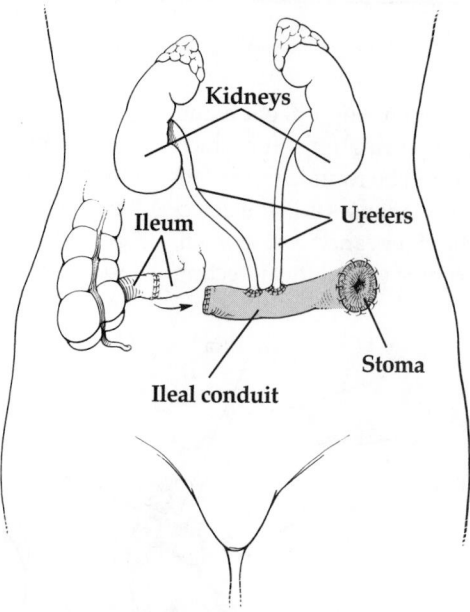

In an ileal conduit surgical procedure, the ureters are connected to an artificial bladder (ileal conduit) fashioned from a piece of intestine (ileum). An opening (stoma) is made in the abdominal wall. Urine drains into a pouch securely fastened to the skin.

this. In one of the more successful techniques, the ureters are connected to an artificial bladder fashioned from a piece of intestine. The new bladder is attached inside the body near the navel. Then, an opening is created through the abdominal wall to drain the urine into a pouch worn against the body under the clothes. This is called the ileal conduit procedure.

Some physicians recommend radiation therapy and chemotherapy after this operation for invasive bladder cancer. When lymph nodes, bone, or other organs have been infiltrated by the tumor, chemotherapy can be administered. In 30 to 70 percent of people with metastatic disease (cancer that has spread to other organs), chemotherapy is helpful in arresting the spread of cancer and in alleviating pain. However, the benefit usually does not last more than 6 months, and then the cancer continues to progress.

A combination of chemotherapy followed by radiation therapy or surgical removal of the bladder prolongs life for some persons with invasive disease.

Blood Vessel Problems

Blood enters the kidneys from the renal artery, a major branch of the aorta (the main artery from the heart). Twenty percent of the volume of blood pumped from the heart at any given time passes through the kidneys. After the kidneys perform their filtering function, the blood returns by way of the renal vein to the inferior vena cava, the major vessel that carries blood from all parts of the body back to the heart.

Disorders of either the renal artery or the renal vein not only can affect the way the kidneys function but also can be a major cause of hypertension. In addition to the disorders described below, preeclampsia and eclampsia (rare but serious conditions that occur in pregnant women shortly before they give birth, see page 204) and vasculitis (an inflammation of small arteries, see page 921) can result in blood vessel problems in the kidneys.

Acute Arterial Occlusion

Signs and Symptoms
- Abrupt onset of flank or abdominal pain
- Blood in the urine

Acute blockage of the renal artery may occur after injury to the abdomen or side. It also occasionally occurs in people known to have heart disease (primarily mitral or aortic valve disease, see page 677, or atrial fibrillation, see page 670). In such individuals, blood clots may travel out of the heart and through the aorta to lodge in the renal artery.

Diagnosis
The diagnosis often is made by arteriography (a form of angiography, see page 656). In this test, a catheter is inserted through the groin into the aorta and manipulated to reach the renal artery. Then a contrast agent is injected

and X-rays are made. Occasionally, a renal scan is used to make the diagnosis.

Treatment

There is no specific therapy. The danger is that the affected kidney may cease to function. But, if this happens, the other kidney can take over the process of eliminating wastes. If arterial occlusion occurs in a person who has only one kidney (see Solitary Kidney, page 827), renal failure may occur (see page 852).

Renal Artery Stenosis

Signs and Symptoms—Hypertension

Renal artery stenosis is a blockage of the renal artery before it enters the kidney. The result of this is development of chronic kidney failure or hypertension, which may be difficult to treat. Renal artery stenosis causes 1 to 2 percent of all cases of hypertension, but these are the most easily cured cases.

In the elderly, this condition most often results from atherosclerotic disease (see Atherosclerosis: What Is It? page 636). This disorder also occurs in women 20 to 40 years of age as a result of thickening of the artery wall (fibromuscular dysplasia).

Diagnosis

This condition is suspected when your physician hears a bruit (loud noise) with a stethoscope over the kidneys. Particularly for young persons with this bruit, a special kidney X-ray called an IVP (see page 829) is obtained. This may reveal decreased size of the affected kidney. A kidney ultrasound examination, which also measures arterial flow, may be helpful in identifying narrowing of the arteries. Then, an arteriogram is obtained to determine exactly where the blockage is located.

Treatment

Treatment is often indicated either to improve the control of hypertension or to arrest the progression of chronic kidney failure due to renal artery stenosis. Sometimes this condition can be treated surgically. This surgery is done to prevent progressive renal failure in addition to improving hypertension control. In the past several years, a new treatment has been successful, particularly in women with fibromuscular dysplasia. This consists of passing a special catheter into the renal artery and then inflating the balloon at the tip of the catheter to open the artery.

For some people, medication to control hypertension may be prescribed.

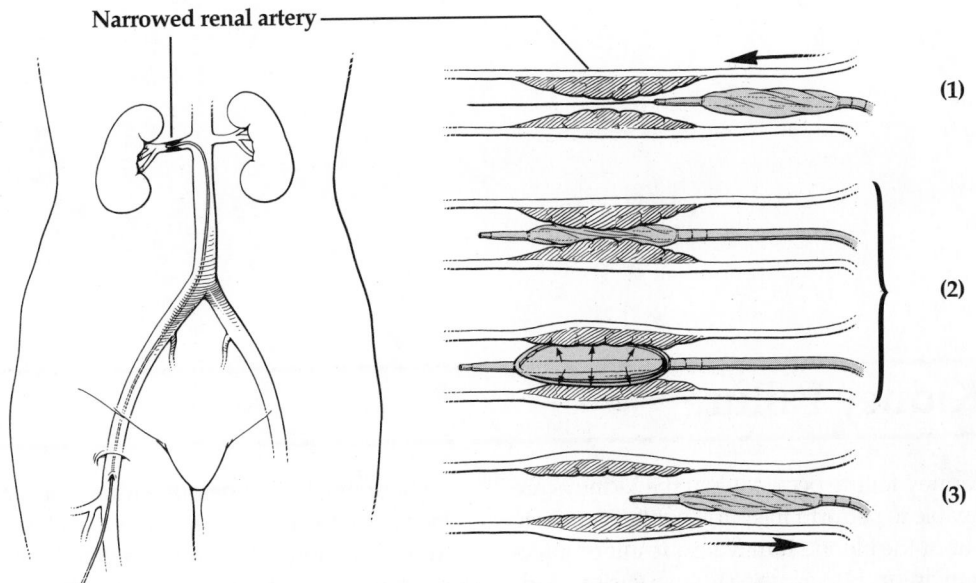

Narrowed renal artery

(1)

(2)

(3)

Percutaneous transluminal angioplasty can be used to open a narrowed renal artery. During the procedure, a catheter is threaded through an artery in the thigh up into the narrowed renal artery (1). The artery is then dilated with a balloon situated at the tip of the catheter (2), and the catheter is then removed (3).

Malignant Hypertension

Emergency Symptoms
- Rapid increase in blood pressure
- Blurred vision
- Severe headache
- Shortness of breath
- Chest pain
- Seizures

This is a potential medical emergency that generally occurs in individuals being treated for hypertension. For reasons that are not clearly understood, the blood pressure increases dramatically, and this causes the other symptoms.

Diagnosis
Your physician will find a very high blood pressure and also may see worrisome changes on ophthalmoscopic examination of your eyes (see page 564). In addition, standard urinalysis may show an excessive amount of protein in your urine.

Treatment
If this condition is treated promptly, the outcome is quite good. If it is not treated promptly, serious damage to the brain, eyes, heart, and kidneys may occur. The treatment may include hospitalization and intravenous administration of drugs to bring down the blood pressure. Then, the intravenous treatment is replaced by antihypertension drugs taken by mouth.

Renal Vein Thrombosis

Signs and Symptoms
- Severe pain in the lower back and flank
- Large quantities of protein in the urine

In this condition, a blood clot (thrombus) has developed in the vein leaving the kidney. It may occur shortly after significant trauma to the abdomen or back. It may be the result of a tumor blocking the blood flow in the renal vein, or it may be associated with the nephrotic syndrome (see page 840). In rare cases, this occurs after severe dehydration, particularly in infants.

Diagnosis
Your physician may inject a dye through the groin into your vena cava (the blood vessel that returns blood from all parts of the body to your heart) and then into the renal vein. This dye will outline the blood clot in the renal vein. The diagnosis can also sometimes be made with the use of an ultrasound technique called Doppler imaging, which can detect a blood clot in the vein.

Treatment
Most often the treatment is anticoagulant medications (blood thinners). Over time, the renal vein often reopens unless the obstruction is due to tumor growth into the vein from a kidney cancer.

Kidney Failure

Kidney failure occurs when the kidneys are unable to perform their task of filtering waste out of the blood. It may be a result of infection, injury, exposure to toxins, various kidney diseases, diseases such as diabetes, systemic lupus erythematosus, or sickle cell anemia, or obstruction to the flow of urine from the kidney by a stricture, cancer, or chronic obstruction of the prostate.

There are two types of kidney failure. One is acute kidney failure, a sudden loss of kidney function. This often is related to the severe decrease in blood pressure that may occur with severe trauma or complicated surgery (see Shock, page 441), with severe infection (see Septic Shock, page 444), or with a severe, complicated illness. Although acute kidney failure is a potentially serious condition that may require hospitalization and round-the-clock care, the kidneys themselves generally are able to resume normal function over a period of several weeks to a few months after the crisis.

The other type, chronic kidney failure, is a slow, progressive destruction of kidney function, usually as a result of disease. End-stage renal disease is said to occur when the kidneys are functioning at only 5 to 10 percent of their capacity. At this point, kidney dialysis or transplantation is necessary to preserve life.

Acute Kidney (Renal) Failure

Signs and Symptoms
- Fluid retention
- Gastrointestinal tract bleeding
- Seizures
- Coma

Acute kidney failure is the term used to describe a rapid deterioration in the kidneys' ability to remove waste products from the blood. Thus, the wastes accumulate within the body. If something is not done to rid the body of these wastes, the person will die.

Forty to 50 percent of all cases of acute kidney failure are related to surgery or trauma, with severe bleeding, severe dehydration, or shock. Exposure to certain drugs or toxins also may precipitate acute kidney failure. In some patients, acute kidney failure occurs as part of the symptom complex of multiple organ failure in which the heart, lungs, liver, brain, and kidneys may fail (totally or only partially). Another cause is obstruction to the flow of urine out of the kidney by a stricture, tumor, or chronic enlargement of the prostate (see page 1209).

There are many theories to explain how this kidney shutdown occurs. Some believe that cell debris obstructs the cavity of the tubule, thus interfering with its ability to filter out waste products. Others theorize that several factors combine to diminish blood flow through the glomeruli. We do know that many conditions can bring about acute kidney failure, including those described below.

Renal Ischemia
This is the most common actual cause of acute kidney failure. It is a deficiency of blood flow to the kidney as a result of obstruction or constriction of a blood vessel.

Nephrotoxic Agents
Many common and uncommon substances can be toxic to the kidneys (nephrotoxic).

Exposure to radiographic contrast agents such as those used during arteriography (see page 656) can precipitate acute failure. This is unlikely in a healthy person. But in 10 to 40 percent of those with an underlying kidney disease, especially diabetic kidney disease, this type of exposure can result in acute kidney failure.

Occasionally, a person with a life-threatening infection who is receiving an antibiotic such as streptomycin or gentamicin may go into acute kidney failure. The chance of kidney failure developing due to an antibiotic is greatly enhanced with age, underlying kidney disease, potassium depletion, liver disease, and the use of a diuretic or other nephrotoxic drug. In addition, the nonsteroidal anti-inflammatory drugs, even if used for a relatively short time, occasionally can cause acute kidney failure.

Extensive traumatic injuries can cause the release of the protein myoglobin, found in muscle, which frequently causes acute kidney failure. Heat stroke, severe exercise, drug overdose, infection, or excessive alcohol intake also can activate the release of myoglobin and result in acute kidney failure. Contact with heavy metals or various solvents can induce acute kidney failure.

Kidney Diseases
Diseases such as interstitial nephritis (see page 836) and glomerulonephritis (see page 838) may result in acute kidney failure.

Diagnosis
If you appear to have acute kidney failure and are not already in the hospital, you will be hospitalized. There, your physician will attempt to determine whether you have acute kidney failure or have some other kidney disease that affects kidney function.

How Serious Is Acute Kidney Failure?
Acute renal failure can be very dangerous. Only about half of the people who develop acute renal failure will survive to be dismissed from the hospital. The mortality rates are highest among people who enter the hospital with severe chronic medical problems such as lung disease, heart disease, or liver disease, or people who are using potent immunosuppressive medications. Mortality rates are 50 to 70 percent for people whose acute renal fail-

ure developed after an operation or a traumatic accident. The mortality rate is especially high (about 90 percent) in individuals who require mechanical ventilation for lung failure or medications to treat a very low blood pressure. Individuals who have had a recent stroke also do not do well.

Other factors that can affect the outcome of acute renal failure are old age, infection, and gastrointestinal bleeding.

Treatment

If you have acute renal failure, your physical condition will be monitored closely for evidence of complications such as infection, heart or neurologic problems, hypertension, or gastrointestinal bleeding. Your laboratory tests will be closely monitored for the development of uremic poisoning or other chemical imbalances. Should problems occur, they will be treated with the appropriate medication. Your physician also will alter your intake of fluid so that the intake is equal to the output.

Unlike chronic renal failure, acute renal failure can be reversible, and many people fully recover in 1 to 2 months. It may take as long as a year for full function to be regained, however. Your physician will monitor your diet and, in particular, protein consumption, plus any need for medications to protect you from the consequences of acute renal failure. Occasionally, people progress to chronic renal failure.

Nutrition

You will probably be put on a high-carbohydrate low-protein diet. Essential amino acids and glucose may be given intravenously if your nutritional status is doubtful. This treatment sometimes provides a quicker recovery. Salt and potassium intake may be restricted.

Chronic Kidney (Renal) Failure

Signs and Symptoms

- Abnormal urinalysis
- Hypertension
- Loss of weight
- Nausea
- Vomiting
- Malaise
- Headache
- Decreased urine output
- Fatigue
- Decreased mental acuity

- Muscle twitches and cramps
- Gastrointestinal bleeding
- Yellowish brown cast to the skin
- Itching

Unlike acute renal failure, chronic renal failure generally occurs over a number of years as the kidneys' nephrons are destroyed slowly and often imperceptibly.

Chronic renal failure is a particularly insidious disease because often there are no symptoms in its early stages. In many cases, no symptoms are apparent until kidney function has decreased to less than 25 percent of what is considered normal.

Several diseases initiate the chronic kidney failure process, the most common being glomerulonephritis in any of its several forms (see page 838). Other causes include polycystic kidney disease, hypertension, pyelonephritis, vesicoureteral reflux, and use of analgesics (see pages 831, 647, 841, 830, and 341, respectively).

The single most common cause of end-stage renal disease in the United States is diabetes mellitus: kidney damage (nephropathy) develops in approximately 50 to 60 percent of those with insulin-dependent diabetes (type I). Eventually, these people need dialysis or kidney transplantation.

If you have diabetes, you should have annual measurement of microalbuminuria (a protein filtered by the kidneys) as a screening test for the development of very early diabetes-related kidney failure (diabetic nephropathy). Your physician may recommend the use of angiotensin-converting enzyme (ACE) inhibitor medications (specifically captopril) to slow the progression of this disease.

If you are a young diabetic in otherwise normal health, and you have chronic renal failure, you may be a good candidate for combined pancreas and kidney transplantation. The pancreas transplant will cure the diabetes, and the kidney transplant will cure the kidney failure.

No matter what its cause, chronic kidney failure results in the buildup of wastes and fluid in the blood, which a properly functioning kidney would excrete into the urine. A person with chronic kidney failure is said to have uremia, a term used to describe not only the wastes in the blood but also a host of metabolic and endocrine functions that also are impaired.

There are very few systems in the body

that are not affected when chronic kidney failure occurs. The fluid retention that is common can cause congestive heart failure (see page 659) and swelling of body tissues. Other problems that could occur include weakening of the bones so that they become susceptible to fracture, anemia, ulcers in the stomach, miscarriage in pregnant women, and changes in skin color. Even the central nervous system can be damaged—the affected person finds it difficult to concentrate or to remember and may have difficulty with the nerves and muscles in the arms and legs.

Diagnosis

If your symptoms suggest chronic renal failure, your physician will want to establish that the condition is indeed chronic. X-ray studies can be used to determine if both kidneys are smaller than normal, a sign of chronic damage. Occasionally, X-ray dye can worsen renal failure. Your physician may use diagnostic studies that do not involve exposure to such dyes.

How Serious Is Chronic Renal Failure?

This condition eventually may progress to end-stage renal disease (see this page). When this occurs, the kidneys simply are not capable of sustaining life. If the person is to live, either dialysis or kidney transplantation is needed.

Treatment

Treatment is begun immediately after chronic renal failure is diagnosed. Although there is no cure, there are things that can be done to control the symptoms, to minimize the complications, and to slow the disease progression.

An important component of treatment is control of the underlying disease and its complications. Hypertension, congestive heart failure, urinary tract infections, kidney stones, abnormalities of the urinary tract, or the forms of glomerulonephritis that respond to therapy will be treated as appropriate. Severe anemia may require the administration of a medication called erythropoietin. In addition, a form of vitamin D, called calcitriol, may be administered to prevent the development of bone disease (see Osteomalacia, page 896), which can accompany kidney failure. A component of treatment not to be overlooked is education in preparation for when dialysis or kidney transplantation may be necessary.

Nutrition
A proper diet is extremely important so that you receive the appropriate amount of calories to avoid malnutrition. Recent studies have shown that moderate restrictions in dietary protein may be important in slowing the progression of chronic kidney failure. The problems of nausea, vomiting, and lack of appetite may be reduced with use of a low-protein diet. Adequate calorie intake can be provided by carbohydrates and fat. Restricting salt intake may decrease an abnormally high blood pressure. Water intake may need to be regulated carefully. As the disease progresses, restriction of phosphate and potassium may become necessary.

End-Stage Kidney (Renal) Disease

Signs and Symptoms

- Kidneys permanently ceasing to function
- Uremia and many resulting complications, which may include hypertension, congestive heart failure, anemia, bone disease, gastrointestinal problems, urinary infection, and dementia

When kidney function has deteriorated to between 5 and 10 percent of normal capacity, the condition is called end-stage kidney disease. This means that the kidneys are incapable of sustaining life and that their function must be provided by either dialysis or a transplanted kidney.

There are more than 185,000 persons in the United States on chronic dialysis and about 60,000 persons who are living with a functioning kidney transplant.

The largest group of persons with end-stage kidney disease are those with diabetes mellitus.

Diagnosis

End-stage kidney disease is the end of what generally is a long process of chronic kidney failure. Although chronic kidney failure may be silent initially, by the time the kidneys are functioning at only 20 to 25 percent of normal capacity, the symptoms usually have become overt. The person usually has been under the care of a physician for 10, 15, or even 20 years when end-stage kidney disease is diagnosed.

Kidney Dialysis Treatments

It has only been within the past 40 years that dialysis and kidney transplantation have given large numbers of people with chronic and irreversible kidney failure the opportunity to live long after their kidneys have ceased to function. Dialysis is an artificial means of removing the waste products and extra fluid from the blood when the kidneys are unable to do so on their own.

Dialysis can be used as a temporary measure during acute kidney failure. This prevents the debilitating and ultimately fatal buildup of wastes in the blood and allows the kidneys time to heal so they can resume their work. It also can replace part of the function of the kidneys when it is clear that chronic disease has rendered them useless.

When does a person with advanced kidney failure need dialysis? Every case is different. As a rule, however, most physicians try to manage chronic kidney failure for as long as possible with conservative measures (see Chronic Kidney [Renal] Failure, page 854).

Inevitably, however, there comes a time when the benefits of dialysis outweigh the risks.

For young and otherwise healthy people, transplantation is usually preferred over dialysis because it affords a better quality of life. Most of these individuals undergo dialysis until a suitable transplant donor is found. This will be discussed in detail in a later section (see page 857). However, transplantation is not an option for many people with kidney disorders because of their poor physical health and associated medical conditions.

In the United States, more than 185,000 persons are on dialysis. For acute situations, dialysis can be done in a hospital dialysis unit or in an intensive care unit. Most persons with stable kidney problems have their dialysis in outpatient centers or at home.

Many patients who are on dialysis have other chronic medical problems, which may lead to heart attacks, stroke, other circulation problems, and infections. Complications associated with various forms of dialysis include malfunction of the access to the bloodstream, infection of this access, and nutritional difficulties—particularly malnutrition, obesity, peritonitis, and hernias.

Dialysis is not a panacea, but it can be credited with prolonging life in thousands of persons and saving the lives of many others.

The several different types of dialysis are described here.

Hemodialysis

This form of dialysis removes extra fluid, chemicals, and wastes from your blood by filtering your blood through an artificial kidney (dialyzer). Before you can undergo hemodialysis, the most common form of dialysis, an access to the bloodstream must be created surgically, usually in your arm or leg. One form of access is a fistula, a connection between an artery and a vein. Another type of access is a tube of synthetic material inserted between an artery and a vein.

As a rule, most persons on dialysis require 6 to 12 hours of dialysis per week, usually divided into 3 dialysis sessions. However, an individual dialysis prescription ensures that each person receives an adequate amount of dialysis and proper nutrition.

When you are connected to the dialysis machine, your blood is pumped from the vascular access into the artificial kidney, which removes the waste products from the blood. The artificial kidney acts like the glomeruli because it makes the blood flow across membranes that let the waste compounds filter through. A solution in the machine helps to regulate the substances that are left in the blood and to remove excess fluid. Less than 1 cup of blood is outside your body at a time.

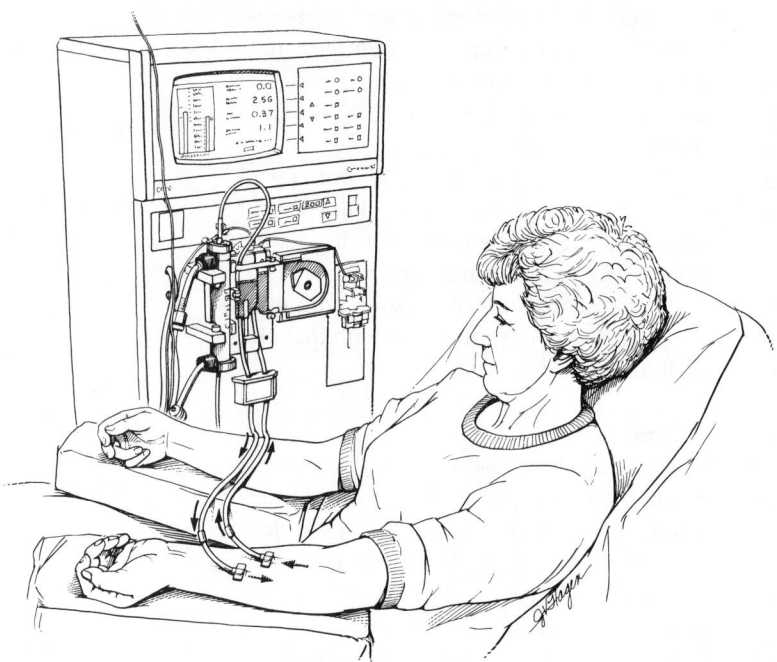

Dialysis machine artificially cleanses the blood of waste products in people whose kidneys no longer are able to do so on their own.

Peritoneal Dialysis

This form of dialysis uses your own peritoneal cavity (in the abdomen) to filter the blood. This cavity has a vast network of capillaries.

The first step is implantation of a catheter leading into the abdomen. Then, through this catheter, dialysis solution is repeatedly infused into and drained out of the abdominal cavity. The small blood vessels in the membrane that forms the inside surrounding lining of the abdomen filter waste products and water into the dialysis solution. This process is continued for as long as necessary.

Continuous Ambulatory Peritoneal Dialysis (CAPD)

Continuous ambulatory peritoneal dialysis is peritoneal dialysis in which the dialysis solution is exchanged 4 times a day, 7 days a week. The exchanges are spaced throughout the day (morning, noon, later afternoon, and before bedtime).

Dialysis occurs between exchanges while the dialysis solution is in the peritoneal cavity. This method can be performed by the person at home.

Continuous Cyclic Peritoneal Dialysis (CCPD)

Continuous cyclic peritoneal dialysis is peritoneal dialysis in which a cycler machine does the exchanges every night for 10 to 12 hours while you sleep. Dialysis occurs between exchanges while the dialysis solution is in your peritoneal cavity. In this variation, a machine automatically infuses dialysis solution into and out of your peritoneal cavity and drains several times over the course of the night while you sleep.

How Serious Is End-Stage Kidney Disease?

End-stage kidney disease is fatal unless dialysis is initiated or kidney transplantation is performed. Both of these methods have risks that can be life-threatening. Each individual is unique and should receive counseling from a physician who specializes in treating kidney disease (nephrologist) regarding the limitations of and expectations from these repeated treatments.

Treatment

Once a person has progressed to end-stage kidney disease, the conservative measures used to manage chronic kidney failure—dietary restrictions, medications, and treating complications and underlying cause—are not enough. In some cases, kidney transplantation is not in the best interest of the individual because of poor general health. Dialysis then becomes the only option.

Kidney Transplantation

Transplantation and dialysis (see page 856) are the only two treatment options for persons with end-stage kidney disease. In the past 15 years, nearly 100,000 kidney transplantations have been performed in the United States.

Not everyone with end-stage kidney disease is a suitable candidate for kidney transplantation. Those with infection, acute glomerulonephritis, unstable coronary artery disease, or other severe medical problems generally are considered not to be in good enough condition to undergo a major operation. They are more likely to have adverse reactions, including death, after transplantation than are healthier individuals.

However, when successful, transplantation provides a healthier and better-quality life.

The actual operation itself is not a complicated procedure. What can be complicated is finding the right donor, which is important to lessen the chance of rejection of the new kidney. Compatibility is determined by blood tests that provide information about both the donor and the recipient, such as blood type and the nature of the antibodies present in each. A brother or sister of the recipient generally is the most likely to have compatible tissue. Unfortunately, a sibling donor is not always available, especially for a very young recipient, because donors have to

be at least 18 years old to give their consent. Because of the shortage of kidneys, many transplant centers consider using less closely related donors, such as a grandparent, aunt, uncle, or cousin.

When a living donor is not available, tissue-typing centers throughout the country are called on to help locate acceptable donors from among accident victims and others who have offered to donate their kidneys after their death (cadaver kidney). A kidney from a cadaver must be transplanted within 48 hours after the death of the donor. Thus, some people have to undergo long periods on dialysis until a compatible cadaver donor is available.

After the transplantation operation, the person receives immunosuppressant drugs to keep his or her body from rejecting the foreign kidney. Recently, drugs such as cyclosporine, FK-506, and anti-lymphocyte preparations have greatly increased the chances of acceptance. If the donor is a blood relative of the recipient, the chances are 85 to 95 percent that by 1 year after the transplantation, the kidney will still be functioning. With a cadaver donor, the chances are about 80 percent that the kidney will still be working quite well by 1 year after the transplant operation.

In cases in which the transplanted kidney is rejected, a second or even third transplantation can be done. The rate of acceptance in these cases is significantly less than it is at the initial transplantation.

Improvements in preparing patients for transplantation and in monitoring their recovery have decreased mortality to as low as 5 percent in some medical centers.

Transplant recipients usually are hospitalized for 5 days to 6 weeks, depending on how well their body accepts the new kidney. The major hurdles are rejection and infection. Immunosuppressant drugs have greatly decreased rejection, but they make it harder for the body's immune system to fight infection. For this reason, your physician will often give antibiotics to prevent viral and fungal infection for the first few months after transplantation. This is the most likely period in which a serious infection may develop. Because transplant recipients must take an immunosuppressant medication for the rest of their lives, they are prone to have infections.

Kidney transplant recipients need careful medical follow-up to enhance the success of the operation and to ensure good general health.

Chapter 27

Your Bones, Joints, and Muscles

Contents

Your Musculoskeletal System at Work, 861
Your Bones, 862
Your Joints, 862
Your Muscles, 862

Common Problems, 863
Bone Fracture, 863
Dislocation, 866
   Sports Injuries, 867
Severed Tendon, 867
Pulled Muscle (Muscle Strain), 868
Sprain, 869
   Heat vs. Cold Treatment, 869
   P.R.I.C.E., 870
Shin Splint, 870
Muscle Cramp, 871
   Neck Pain, 871
Thigh Bruise, 872
Tennis Elbow, 872
Runner's Knee, 873
Achilles Tendinitis, 874
Baseball Finger, 874
Heel Pain, 874
   Principles of Sports Rehabilitation, 875
Knee Injuries, 876
   Other Causes of Knee Pain, 876
   Knee Swelling, 877
   Arthroscopy, 878
   Support Braces, 879

Absence or Loss of a Limb, 879
   Artificial Limbs, 879

Muscle, Tendon, and Soft Tissue Disorders, 880
Tenosynovitis, 881
Tendinitis, 882
Fibromyalgia, 883
Costochondritis, 883
Carpal Tunnel Syndrome, 884
Arthritis at the Base of the Thumb, 885

Ganglion, 886
Dupuytren's Contracture, 886
Reflex Sympathetic Dystrophy Syndrome, 887
Muscle Tumors, 888
Muscular Dystrophy, 888

Problems of the Feet, 889
Metatarsalgia, 889
Burning Feet, 890
   Shopping for Shoes, 890
Morton's Neuroma, 890
Corns and Calluses, 890
Bunions, 891
   Treating Calluses, 891
   Tired Feet, 892
Flatfeet, 892
Hammer Toe and Mallet Toe, 892
Ingrown Toenail, 893
Foot Ulcers, 893

Bone Diseases, 894
Osteoporosis, 894
Osteomalacia and Rickets, 896
Paget's Disease of the Bone, 897
   Endocrine Disorders and the Bones, 898
Fibrous Dysplasia, 898
Osteogenesis Imperfecta, 898
Osteomyelitis, 899
Bone Tumors, 899

Back Pain, 899
Strains and Spasms, 900
   Corsets: Comfort and Cautions, 904
Prolapsed Disc, 904
   Sciatica, 905
Spondylosis, 906
Lumbar Stenosis, 906
Scoliosis, 906

Joint Disorders, 907
Osteoarthritis, 907
   Baker's Cyst, 909

Rheumatoid Arthritis, 909
Juvenile Rheumatoid Arthritis, 911
   Joint Replacement, 911
   Joint Disorders of Childhood, 912
Inflammatory Arthritis, 913
Infectious Arthritis, 914
   Rheumatic Fever Arthritis, 915
Gout, 916
Acute Painful Shoulder, 917
Bursitis, 917

Immunologic Rheumatic Diseases, 918
Lupus (Systemic Lupus Erythematosus), 918
   Corticosteroid Drugs, 919
Scleroderma, 919
Sjögren's Syndrome, 920
Polymyositis and Dermatomyositis, 920
   Vasculitis, 921
Polymyalgia Rheumatica, 922

Your Musculoskeletal System at Work

As its name suggests, your musculoskeletal system consists of muscles (from the Latin word *musculus*) and bones (from the Greek word *skeletos*, which means "dried-up body"). The bones in your body are interconnected at junctions called joints. Most joints are essentially hinges that allow the bones to move within certain prescribed limits. Others move in a different way, such as the hip and shoulder, which are ball-and-socket joints, and the backbone (vertebral column), which has limited movement.

Besides providing mobility, your musculoskeletal system also protects your internal organs. Your ribs surround your lungs and heart. Your skull protects your brain. Until the system breaks down, whether due to accident, disease, or simply wear and tear over time, most of us take this miracle of mechanics for granted.

Breakdowns can occur at any time and for various reasons. This chapter discusses a range of potential problems, from ankle sprains and ailments of the foot and back to amputations, arthritis, and osteoporosis. We also discuss less common ailments such as lupus and gout. First, we briefly review your bones, joints, and muscles.

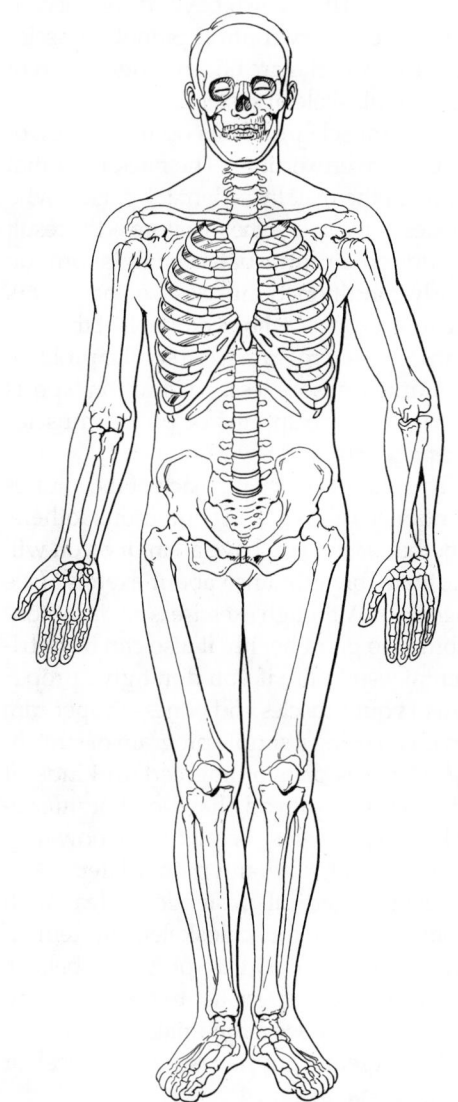

Your bones are living tissue and are always changing. They provide support for your body and function as your body's depository for important minerals.

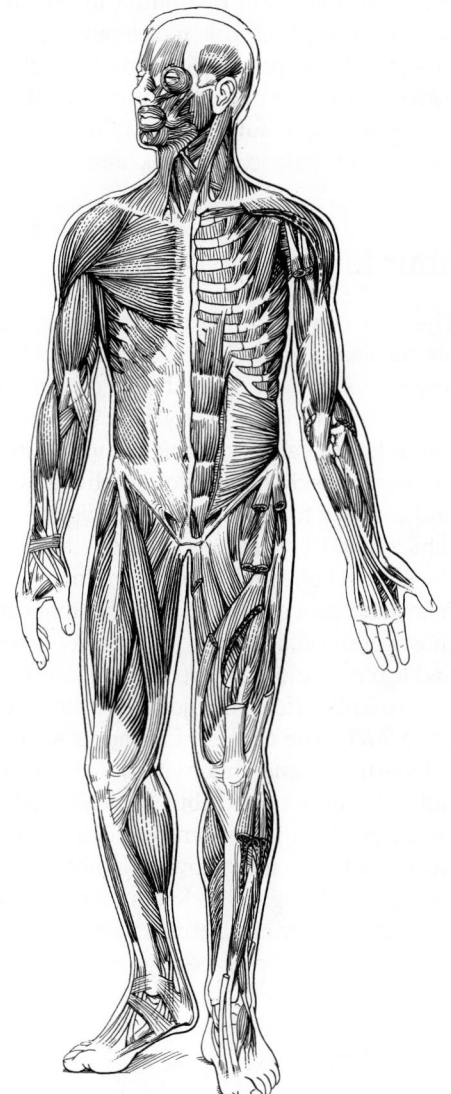

Many of your skeletal muscles are paired, enabling your body to move. Tendons connect these muscles to your bones.

Your Bones

There are 206 bones in your body. Your bones are composed of osseous tissue. Osseous tissue consists of various substances, among them proteins, minerals, and bone cells.

The proteins form a framework into which the minerals, especially calcium and phosphate, become incorporated. Bone cells monitor the ongoing process whereby the calcium phosphate mineral is deposited or withdrawn. Your bones are alive and always changing, providing support for your body and also functioning as your body's storehouse for these important minerals. Inside certain bones is the marrow, a soft core that manufactures blood cells (see page 955).

Problems with your bones may vary. Some are the result of trauma in which a bone is bruised or broken (see page 863) or dislocated (see page 866). Others, such as osteoporosis (see page 894) or osteomalacia (see page 896), result from a malfunction of the complex balance of bone chemistry.

Your Joints

The ends of your bones that meet in a joint are cushioned with a layer of cartilage, which absorbs some of the shock or weight involved in movement. Your joints also contain a liquid called synovial fluid, a membrane, a protective casing called the capsule, and bands of fibrous tissue called ligaments, which bind the parts of a joint together.

As with bone problems, joint ailments are many and varied. Osteoarthritis, perhaps the most common, is mainly the result of wear and tear on the joints (especially the cartilage) and usually affects one joint at a time (see page 907). The causes of ailments such as osteoarthritis and rheumatoid arthritis are not fully understood, but these disorders produce pain and discomfort in joints, with inflammation in the synovial membrane and cartilage (see page 909). Joints may also sustain injuries from trauma (certain knee injuries, for example; see page 876).

Your Muscles

There are some 650 muscles in your body. The muscles are fibers with an elasticity that sets them apart from other body parts. This key characteristic allows the muscles to shorten and lengthen and thus produce movement at the joints.

Virtually all muscles are paired. In your arm, for example, the contraction of your biceps muscle will cause your arm to flex, whereas a contraction of the opposing triceps muscle causes your arm to extend. Tendons connect muscles to your bones.

Not all muscles produce movement of your skeleton. In addition to the skeletal (striated) muscles, there are smooth (nonstriated) muscles. You can find these muscles in such internal organs as the stomach, uterus, and bladder and in the walls of blood vessels. They usually are arranged in sheets. Physicians call them involuntary muscles, because they are not under conscious control. Heart (myocardium) muscle is another type of muscle. This is also beyond the mechanism of voluntary control. Smooth muscles and heart muscles are not considered part of the musculoskeletal system.

Most muscle problems occur because of strain or overexertion. The back pain that occurs in the usually sedentary person who decides to rearrange the furniture is the result of sudden or unusual demands put on poorly conditioned muscles (see page 899). The rookie jogger who overdoes it at the start of an exercise program has a similar problem with muscle soreness. Common sports injuries include sprains or pulled muscles (see pages 868 and 869).

This chapter discusses each of the injuries mentioned above and numerous others. Whether or not you have an injury, you will find valuable guidance about exercise (see page 867). Although exercise is a critical contributor to good health, it also can be detrimental, especially if you don't give proper care to your muscles and bones. Proper care can mean using a simple program of stretching exercises or avoiding certain kinds of activities if you already have joint or musculoskeletal problems. Being careful now may save you pain, time, and money later.

Several medical professions deal with problems of the musculoskeletal system. If you or your primary care physician believe that you need a specialist to treat your ailment, you may see a rheumatologist, orthopedic surgeon, physiatrist, or physical or occupational therapist.

A rheumatologist is a physician who has special training in diseases of the musculoskeletal system (such as arthritis and other joint diseases). If you have rheumatoid arthritis, lupus, or a less common joint ailment, or if your arthritis is not responding to treatment, you may seek the care of a rheumatologist.

Orthopedics is the discipline concerned with preventing or correcting disorders of the body's moving parts, including the skeleton, joints, muscles, ligaments, and cartilage. An orthopedic surgeon is a physician with additional training in this specialty. An orthopedist may recommend physical, medical, or surgical treatment.

A physiatrist is a specialist in physical medicine and rehabilitation. The physiatrist is a physician who is specially trained to help restore the useful function of injured or damaged joints or limbs. The rehabilitation program the physiatrist recommends may include special clothing or equipment, exercise, pain control treatments, or other approaches.

A physical therapist is a licensed professional who helps you recover by using such measures as heat, water, light, massage, and exercise. An occupational therapist is also a licensed professional. Often, occupational therapists work in collaboration with physical therapists. These specialists in occupational rehabilitation can help you to accomplish tasks that your ailment or injury prevents you from doing.

Common Problems

Although the body's mechanical system is extremely durable, muscle and bone injuries are commonplace. Excessive stress can break the rigid bones and strain or damage the flexible muscles or joints when extended beyond their usual range. Whether we fall from an apple tree at 8 or tumble while playing tennis at 65, most of us experience a wide variety of musculoskeletal injuries in our lifetimes. A discussion of the most common of these injuries follows.

Bone Fracture

Signs and Symptoms
- A swelling or bruising over a bone
- Deformity of a limb
- Localized pain that is intensified when the affected area is moved or pressure is put on it
- Loss of function in the area of the injury
- In an open or compound fracture, the broken bone breaks through adjacent tissues and protrudes from the skin

A fracture occurs when a bone cannot withstand the physical force exerted on it. Simply put, a fracture is a broken bone. Fractures are common injuries. In fact, most people sustain one or more fractures during their lives.

Broken bones can be classified into several categories. A simple fracture is one in which the bone breaks but does not come through the nearby soft tissues. A comminuted fracture is one in which the bone fragments into several pieces. When the bone protrudes through the skin, it is termed an open (compound) fracture.

We also classify fractures according to the way the bone breaks. If the bone actually snaps into two or more parts, it is called a simple or complete fracture. When the break is limited to a crack and the bone is not separated into two parts, the fracture is termed incomplete. An impacted fracture occurs when one fragment of bone is embedded into another fragment of bone.

Another kind of fracture occurs in people with bones weakened by disease. Bone cancer (see page 899) or a bone disorder such as osteoporosis (see page 894) can result in weakened bones that fracture spontaneously or with only minor stresses exerted on them. Such breaks are termed pathologic fractures, because the principal cause is an underlying disease.

The risk of fracture varies with age. The skeleton is flexible in children, so their bones are more likely to bend than to break. As a result, when a child fractures a bone it is often a type of incomplete fracture called a greenstick fracture. The bone doesn't snap neatly like a dried twig but cracks more like a green stick.

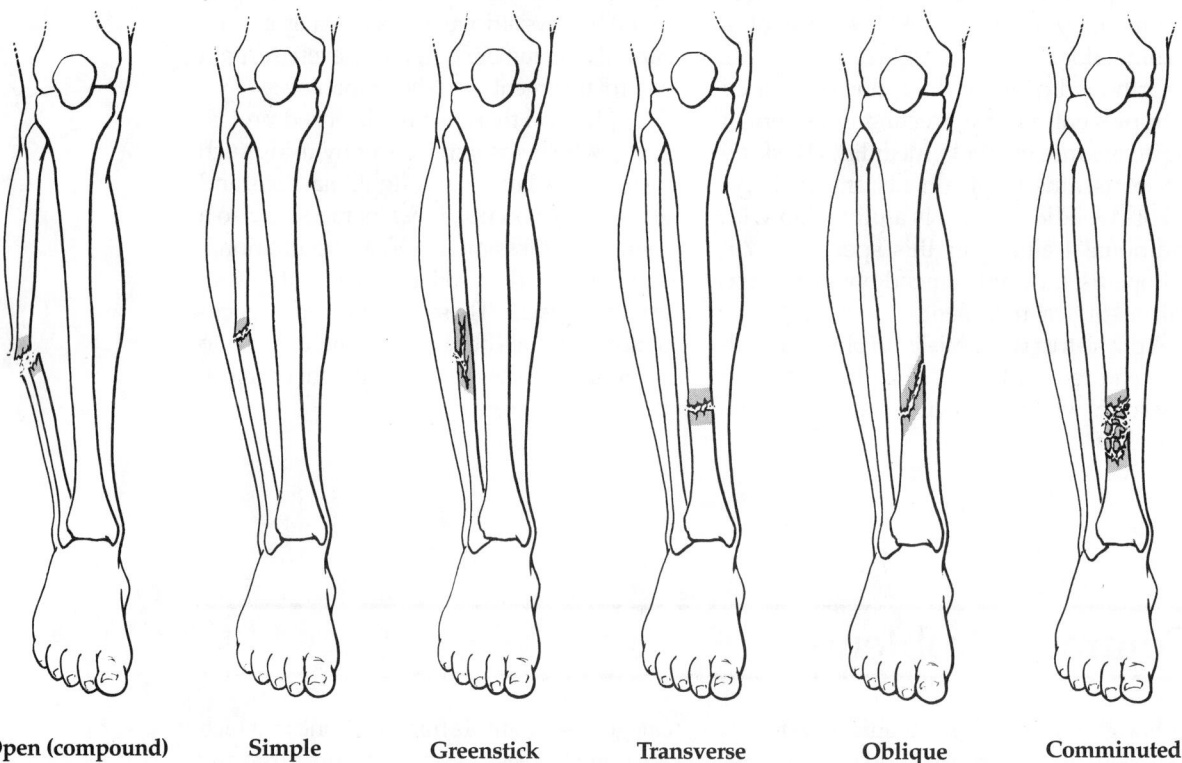

| Open (compound) | Simple | Greenstick | Transverse | Oblique | Comminuted |

Open fractures break through the skin. Simple fractures do not. Simple fractures are classified according to the way the bone breaks. Several varieties of simple fractures are included in the illustrations above.

Elderly people are more likely to have brittle bones, and falls or other events that would have no effect on younger bones can cause fractures.

Still another variety is the stress fracture. The stress fracture is really a hairline crack and often is invisible on an X-ray for up to 6 weeks after injury. The recommended treatment for stress fracture is likely to be rest, but may also include an operation or the therapies discussed below.

Diagnosis

Your physician will begin by taking a history, followed by a physical examination. In the event of an open fracture, the bone protruding from the flesh makes the diagnosis obvious. In some instances of simple and incomplete fractures, however, identifying the fracture isn't always easy. Severe sprains and incomplete fractures sometimes closely resemble one another.

An X-ray helps confirm the diagnosis, and X-rays will be taken from two or more different angles. In the case of suspected skull or vertebral fractures, the physician may also order a computed tomography (CT) or magnetic resonance imaging (MRI) scan (see page 494).

How Serious Is a Fracture?

The seriousness of a bone fracture depends on the location of the break and the damage sustained by the bone and adjacent tissues.

If you break certain minor bones of your hands or feet, your physician will recommend only that you avoid using the affected area. For more serious fractures, dangerous complications can occur if you don't receive treatment. In any fracture, your physician should examine the adjacent area carefully to establish whether blood vessel or nerve damage occurred. Injuries to the skull or spine bring the risk of brain injury (see page 451) or spinal cord damage (see page 506). Open fractures need treatment to ensure that the bone and adjacent tissues don't become infected (see Osteomyelitis, page 899).

The time required for recuperation from a broken bone varies with the age and health of the patient and the nature of the fracture. In children, a minor break may heal entirely within a few weeks. In elderly people, a serious fracture may require months to repair. Sometimes a fracture that is healing particularly slowly may require a procedure in which bone tissue taken from another bone is grafted onto the fracture. The source of bone for a graft is often the pelvic bone.

With prompt and proper treatment and a sound rehabilitation program, you can usually expect a complete recovery.

Treatment
All suspected fractures should be treated with proper first aid (see page 445) and examined by a physician, and an X-ray should be taken. (See also Sprain, page 869.) If it is to heal properly, a bone that has been displaced must be set in its proper position. Setting of the bone is called reduction. When it can be done without an operative procedure, it is termed closed reduction. You will receive an anesthetic, and your physician will reposition the bone using X-rays as a guide.

Surgery
If surgery is necessary, the procedure is termed open reduction. Appropriate anesthesia is used, and an incision is made to gain access to the broken bone so it can be set in its proper position.

A fracture that is unstable or is immediately adjacent to or extends into a joint may require a device such as a pin, plate, or screw—or even a special kind of glue—to hold it in place. During a surgical procedure, the physician fastens the device to the bone to properly position and stabilize the broken parts. Advantages of this approach include early mobility of the joint and use of the injured limb within a matter of weeks rather than months, because the device can carry some of the weight or stress on the bone.

In some instances it may be desirable to insert an artifical joint, especially in elderly persons with osteoporosis or another disorder that has led to a deterioration of the bone or joint (see Joint Replacement, page 911).

Immobilization
After the bone has been set, it is usually necessary to immobilize it and, in some cases, also the adjacent joints. Preventing motion between the two ends of the bone lessens pain and facilitates healing. Casts, splints, and occasionally traction can help accomplish this. In some cases, however, no such artificial means are necessary. The mass of chest muscles that surround a broken rib, for example, will hold it in place. Your physician may simply tape a broken finger to an adjacent digit.

Casts and Splints
Your physician may put a cast on your broken arm to immobilize it. First, a layer of soft material covers your arm to protect the skin from irritation. Then, bandages saturated with plaster are wrapped around the limb. When the plaster dries over a period of a day or two, the cast will be rigid. However, you should be careful to avoid changing the cast's shape during the drying process. Do not handle the cast with your fingertips, but use the palm of your hand to maneuver the cast. Since flattening the cast can put pressure on your skin beneath the plaster, do not rest the cast on a flat surface, but on pillows. Casts made of fiberglass or plastic dry more quickly (usually within 30 minutes) and are lighter and stronger than those made of plaster of Paris.

Occasionally, your physician may apply a splint. This device immobilizes, supports, and corrects injured, displaced, or deformed structures. Often splints are used instead of a full cast to prevent motion of a dislocated joint or of the ends of a fractured joint.

Traction
Sometimes it is difficult to immobilize a broken bone by other means, as with the thighbone, which a dense layer of muscles protects. Then a mechanical system of weights may hold broken parts of the bones in the proper position. Traction, the force created by this system, is especially useful for fractures in which surrounding muscles tend to pull ends of the broken bone over one another.

Rehabilitation
After the bone has been set in its proper position and immobilized, the next important part of any treatment program is rehabilitation. This process begins as soon as possible, even if the broken bone is still in a cast. Movement of adjacent tissues is important to blood flow, enhances the healing process, and prevents the formation of blood clots. Movement also helps maintain muscle tone. It also may limit wasting (atrophy) of the muscles and withering of the bones due to prolonged immobilization. In addition, it helps prevent the stiffness (loss of range of motion) that occurs in unused joints.

Medication
In most cases, your physician will limit medication to analgesics (to reduce pain) and sometimes antibiotics (to reduce the risk of infection).

Dislocation

Signs and Symptoms
- An injured joint that becomes misshapen and immovable, usually after it has been subjected to a blow, fall, or other trauma
- Swelling and intense pain

A dislocation is, simply, a joint that is out of place. This situation occurs when the joint ends of bones are forced from their normal positions. The joint will no longer function properly. In addition, the unnatural movement of the bones may cause damage to the structure of the joint and perhaps to the muscles, ligaments, nerves, and blood vessels.

In some cases, the cause of the dislocation is an underlying disease (such as rheumatoid arthritis; see page 909) or a congenital weakness. People who sustain repeated dislocations may have deficient ligaments and their joint may dislocate spontaneously.

Diagnosis
After you sustain a dislocation, it will become difficult or impossible to move your joint. The pain will likely be intense and become more severe if you attempt to move the joint. There usually is a visible change in the configuration of the joint, sometimes with swelling.

If your physician suspects that you have a dislocation, an X-ray will confirm the diagnosis and help determine whether you also have an accompanying fracture (see page 863).

Nursemaid's Dislocation
This common and often misdiagnosed dislocation of the elbow occurs in children younger than 5. It usually occurs when an adult suddenly pulls or jerks a child's arm. The immature elbow cannot withstand this stress, and a dislocation occurs.

The child typically experiences pain and limited mobility in the elbow. Generally, X-rays rule out any other problems. When the bones are returned to their proper position, the pain decreases or resolves.

How Serious Is a Dislocation?
If a vertebra is dislocated, there is a risk of spinal cord damage and, potentially, paralysis. Similarly, nerve damage is a risk when a shoulder or hip is dislocated.

In most cases, however, a physician can correct a simple dislocation without substantial nerve or tissue damage. The joint then will be immobilized for a short time (typically, 2 weeks). After a period of recuperation, the joint is likely to be nearly or fully normal.

When the joint has been weakened and spontaneous dislocations occur, a surgical procedure may be needed to tighten the ligaments of the joint and prevent recurrences.

Treatment
Any suspected dislocation should be treated with proper first aid (see page 449) and examined by a physician, and an X-ray should be taken. If you suspect a dislocated vertebra, however, don't move the injured person: wait for professional care (see Spinal Injuries, page 448). The displaced bones in the joint must be returned to their proper position. This setting of the bones is called reduction.

A dislocation needs treatment as soon as possible. If it remains untreated for more than half an hour, the swelling and pain are usually so severe that it is not feasible to treat the dislocation without an anesthetic. It is also crucial that only a person with proper training provide any treatment. Improper attempts at reduction can further damage the joint and surrounding structures.

Immobilization
After the joint is returned to its normal position, it is usually necessary to immobilize the joint, most often with a splint.

Rehabilitation
After the joint is back in its proper position and immobilized, rehabilitation begins. This may start even if the joint is in a cast. Movement stimulates blood flow in adjacent tissue, which enhances the healing process. Movement also maintains muscle tone and limits the wasting of the muscles and withering of the bones due to prolonged immobilization. It also helps prevent the stiffness in joints that results from extended disuse.

Be sure to follow your physician's advice about limiting the physical activity of the affected joint. Too rapid a return to normal activity puts you at risk of reinjuring the joint.

Medication
In most cases, the only medication used to treat a dislocation is analgesics to reduce the pain and an anesthetic if manipulation or an operation is needed. Antibiotics are used only rarely.

Sports Injuries

Most injuries that occur during athletic activity result from unusual demands put on bones, muscles, or other tissues. The novice runner who struggles to complete 5 miles the first day on the track will have undreamed-of aches and pains. The over-40 ex-jock who comes out of retirement for the company softball game is an excellent candidate for sprains and pains.

An injury-free life is an unrealistic goal. However, a few sensible rules will help you avoid inconvenient, painful, expensive, and, at times, disabling injuries.

Consult Your Physician

If you are older than 40, obese, or a heavy smoker; if you have had unexplained chest pains, heart problems such as a previous heart attack, irregular heart rhythms, or other serious health problem; or if you lead a sedentary life, consult your physician before you start a vigorous exercise regimen. Your physician may suggest a stress test (see page 655) to evaluate the condition of your heart and lungs and offer valuable do's and don'ts specific to your physical condition.

Warm Up Before Exercising

To avoid injury, stretch and loosen your muscles for at least 5 to 10 minutes. The increased blood flow of such a warm-up will reduce tension in your muscles, improve their range of motion, and may even increase your level of performance. Simultaneously, you reduce significantly the chance of muscle strains and other injuries.

Cool Down After Exercising

After your workout, it is just as important to allow your muscles to cool down. The muscles you use contract during a workout, and most repetitive activities also can cause them to become permanently shortened. To restore balance to your muscles, a session of stretching after the workout is critical. Muscles that aren't returned to normal in this manner are more likely to sustain strains and spasms (see page 868).

Pace Yourself

Sudden and unfamiliar exertion is most likely to cause injuries. If you are bent on improving your performance, do so—but at a sensible pace. Don't double your distance or duration overnight. Develop a program that allows your body to become conditioned to the activity, so that it can adjust to the challenges you offer it over time.

Select the Sport That Is Right for You

If you have a painful back or perpetually sore knees, the pounding of jogging is not for you; perhaps a daily swim or a ride on a stationary bicycle more nearly suits your needs. See page 294 for guidance in selecting the exercise most suitable for you.

Make It a Habit

Working out only once a week, no matter how vigorous the activity, puts you at risk of injury (and fails to provide you with maximal aerobic and conditioning benefits; see page 290). Try to establish a schedule of at least three 20-minute workouts a week.

Take Care of That Injury

When you sprain an ankle or twist a knee, make sure you get medical advice, and then follow it. A key element will likely be what physicians commonly refer to as the tincture of time. Allow the injury to heal before you test it too vigorously (see page 869).

Severed Tendon

Signs and Symptoms—A deep cut accompanied by an inability to move a finger, toe, or other joint

A severe cut of the tissues of the hand, foot, forearm, or calf may damage the tendons, the fibrous tissues that connect muscle to bone. Severing a tendon results in the inability to move the affected joint.

A severed tendon requires attention of two kinds. First, the wound must be closed immediately to aid healing and prevent infection. Second, the tendon must be repaired surgically. Sometimes both can be done in one procedure when the wound is initially treated. However, in some cases the cut must heal before the operation can be performed. Generally, however, reattachment is done within a week of the injury.

Diagnosis

The key symptom, the inability to move a finger, toe, or other joint, suggests that the tendon is severed. The muscle is no longer linked to the bone it usually maneuvers. This injury is different from a severed nerve, which may prevent muscle contraction.

Your physician may want an X-ray of the affected area if it appears that a fracture may accompany the injury.

How Serious Is a Severed Tendon?

In most cases, prompt repair of a severed tendon allows the affected area to return to nearly normal. However, you may experience some stiffness and a decrease in the range of movement.

Treatment

Surgery

If you suspect a severed tendon, seek immediate medical help. Tendons are stretched taut like elastic. When severed, the two pieces may snap back from the tear and be difficult to retrieve. As a result, an incision may be required to enlarge the cut. In some instances, physicians use tissue from another tendon to repair the damaged tendon.

Rehabilitation

After an operation, the area of injury usually is immobilized. Your physician may recommend an exercise program when it is time for you to resume physical activity. Physicians now often recommend passive exercise (principally flexing movements involving no stress on the injured area) to help decrease the long-term stiffness.

Pulled Muscle (Muscle Strain)

Signs and Symptoms
- Localized pain when an injury occurs, followed by tenderness and, in some cases, swelling
- Stiffness or tenderness that occurs during the 24 hours immediately after you sustain a pulled muscle (or muscle strain)
- If the muscle seems to have no function whatsoever, the muscle may have ruptured

If you place too great a demand on a muscle, you may experience a so-called pulled muscle (or muscle strain). A minor muscle pull results from overstretching or overworking the area. Your muscle will not lose its strength, but it will become sore.

A more serious muscle pull occurs when some of the fibers of a muscle actually tear, causing your muscle to contract and to bleed internally. Occasionally, the entire muscle may be torn apart, either partially or, in rare instances, entirely. When this occurs, your muscle is ruptured.

One of the most common muscle strains occurs to the hamstrings. A group of muscles at the back of the thigh, the hamstrings enable you to flex your knee and extend your thigh, motions that occur when you run. A muscle pain or weakness at the back of your thigh may indicate an injury to your hamstring muscles.

A second common muscle injury is the so-called groin pull (or strain). When you sustain a groin pull, the tendons and muscles of your groin (including abdominal, leg, and pelvic areas) may be stretched or torn. Repetitive overuse or a single traumatic event can cause pain or muscle spasms in the groin area.

Diagnosis

The discomfort in the area (which may include tenderness, muscle spasms, and swelling) is the key to diagnosis. An X-ray may be taken to rule out a bone injury as a cause of the problem.

How Serious Is a Muscle Pull?

If you treat muscle pulls with the simple measures described below and rest properly during recuperation, you can usually expect a complete and rapid recovery.

However, if you suspect that a muscle has ruptured or that a bone is fractured (see page 863), or if the pain persists for more than a few days, seek professional medical help. You may need an operation to repair the damage.

Treatment

Apply ice or cold packs to the injured area for the first 24 hours after injury. After that, use a heating pad or hot baths. At times, particularly if swelling is extensive, you can use cold packs throughout the entire recovery of a muscle injury. You may prevent or reduce swelling if you elevate the injured muscle and use a compression wrap such as an elastic (Ace) bandage, although you should not bind it tightly. Try not to use the injured muscle while it is painful, usually a period of no more than several days.

Medication

For minor muscle pulls, aspirin or another over-the-counter drug may help reduce the pain. For moderate or more severe muscle strains, consult your physician before taking medication. He or she may prescribe an anti-inflammatory drug to reduce the swelling, a muscle relaxant, or an analgesic for pain, depending on the injury.

Surgery

If the muscle is ruptured, an operation may be your best option.

Prevention

You can avoid many muscle pulls with appropriate conditioning and a routine of muscle stretching and loosening exercises before exercising (see page 292). If you experience recurrent muscle pulls, you may need a program of muscle development for chronically weak muscles.

Sprain

Signs and Symptoms

- Rapid swelling, sometimes accompanied by discoloration of the skin
- Impaired joint function
- Pain and tenderness in the affected area

Emergency Symptoms—If an audible popping sound and immediate difficulty in using the joint accompany the injury, apply ice and seek emergency medical care

Although we may use the term "sprain" to identify a wide range of injuries, a true sprain involves damage to the ligaments, the tough bands of elastic-like tissue that connect bone to bone in a joint. A sprain occurs when a traumatic event, such as a violent twist or stretch, causes your joint to move outside its normal range of movement and your ligaments stretch or tear.

Sprains most commonly occur in joints of the ankles, knees, and arches of the foot. In all three cases, a fall or stumble can cause the weight of your body to be placed on the joint in an unnatural position, resulting in a sprain.

Diagnosis

Any joint can be sprained. If the joint cannot function, the injury is more likely to be a fracture (see page 863) or a dislocation (see page 866) than a sprain. If you suspect bone or serious ligament damage in the joint, or if the pain and difficulty in moving the joint do not go away within 2 or 3 days, seek professional medical care. Your physician may order an X-ray to rule out a fracture.

How Serious Is a Sprain?

In general, the greater the pain, the more serious the injury, but sprains vary in severity from minor to those requiring surgery.

Heat vs. Cold Treatment

After you sprain a ligament or strain a muscle, it's best to use cold treatment for 1 to 3 days after the injury. This reduces swelling and inflammation. Swelling damages cells by decreasing the oxygen supply to surrounding tissues. Cold applications slow the metabolism within your cells and allow the tissue to survive a temporary lack of oxygen. This promotes the renewal or repair of cells and speeds healing. Cold also constricts blood vessels to control bleeding and relieves pain directly by acting as a local anesthetic.

Most bleeding associated with acute inflammation resolves within 1 to 3 days. To relieve muscle spasms, minor sprains, and strains, apply cold treatment intermittently for 24 to 48 hours. You may relieve pain by applying heat to your injury, rather than cold. However, this may complicate your recovery by causing more swelling and bleeding. Use heat only after swelling and bleeding have stopped. Heat is usually the best treatment for chronic pain, and it also helps prepare your muscles for strengthening exercises during rehabilitation.

Repeated minor sprains can also lead to a weakening of your joint. In most cases, a sprained joint will be able to bear weight within 24 hours and be fully healed within 2 weeks.

Degrees of Sprain

Your sprain may be mild, moderate, or severe.

Mild Sprain

A mild sprain occurs when fibers within ligaments become overstretched or torn slightly. You may feel minor to considerable pain and tenderness when you touch or move the joint. There is little or no swelling. You can usually put weight on the joint, and X-rays are normal.

Moderate Sprain

When ligament fibers tear but are not completely ruptured, you have a moderate sprain. Pain and tenderness are moderate, and you may experience some swelling and black-and-blue discoloration. It's difficult and painful to move your joint.

Severe Sprain

If one or more ligaments tear completely, you have a severe sprain. The area is painful, swollen, and black-and-blue. You can't move your joint normally or put weight on it.

Treatment

For a simple sprain, apply ice to reduce swell-

An ankle sprain occurs when ligaments that support your ankle are stretched or torn. The anterior talofibular ligament (highlighted in circle) is the one most often injured.

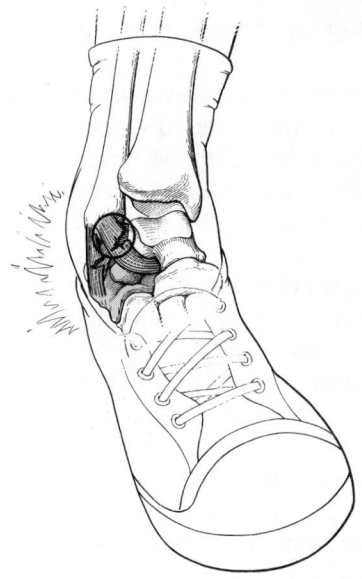

ing during the first 24 hours after your injury. Support the joint with a supportive wrap such as an elastic (Ace) bandage, and rest it in an elevated position. Resume normal activity slowly, testing the injured joint gradually after a day or more has passed.

P.R.I.C.E.

If you sustain a minor soft tissue injury, *p*rotection, *r*est, *i*ce, compression, and *e*levation are the words to remember—P.R.I.C.E. This self-help treatment can help speed your recovery.

Protection
Immobilize the affected area to encourage healing and to protect it from further injury. You may need to use elastic wraps, slings, splints, crutches, or canes.

Rest
Avoid activities that cause pain or swelling; rest is essential to tissue healing.

Ice
To decrease pain, muscle spasm, and swelling, apply ice to the injured area. Ice packs, ice massage, or slush baths all can help.

Compression
Since swelling can result in loss of motion in an injured joint, compress the joint until the swelling has ceased. Wraps or compressive (Ace) bandages are best.

Elevation
To reduce swelling, raise the swollen arm or leg above the level of your heart. It is especially important to use this positioning at night.

Medication

If you seek medical help, your physician may prescribe an anti-inflammatory drug. You may want to take aspirin or some other analgesic for pain.

Surgery

If your sprain is serious enough that the joint is unstable, an operation may be required to repair ligaments that are torn or detached from the bone. Your physician also may elect to immobilize the area of the sprained joint in a cast or splint. If these measures are necessary, carefully follow your physician's advice on rehabilitation. This may involve a supervised physical therapy program and an exercise program to strengthen the muscle surrounding the sprained joint.

Prevention

Taping, bracing, or wrapping knees, ankles, wrists, or elbows can be a convenient and efficient means of preventing recurrent sprains. Ankle devices that are laced and have supports on the inner and outer sides of the ankle seem to be as effective as taping for a chronically sprained ankle. Exercises can also be valuable for strengthening muscles weakened by recurrent injury.

Shin Splint

Signs and Symptoms—Pain on the shin (the front part of the leg above the ankle and beneath the knee)

When pain occurs on the front, inside portion of the large bone of your lower leg, the tibia, it may be the result of a shin splint. Shin splints occur when fibers of the membrane that ties muscles to the front and side of your tibia are irritated and inflamed, producing pain and occasional swelling.

Most often, shin splints are the result of the repeated pounding on hard surfaces that is characteristic of certain athletic activities (typically running or playing sports such as basketball or tennis) or long marches (by army recruits, for example).

Diagnosis
In addition to examining your leg, your physician may order an X-ray of the area to rule out a hairline crack or stress fracture of the tibia (see Bone Fracture, page 863).

Treatment

As with other minor musculoskeletal injuries, rest, ice, and protection (wrapping with elastic bandages or tape) are effective treatments for a shin splint. Sometimes you can reduce the discomfort with hot soaks or a warm whirlpool bath.

Medication

Your physician may prescribe aspirin or another over-the-counter anti-inflammatory medication.

Other Therapies

In some cases, a soft insert in your shoe also can reduce some of the shock you sustain in vigorous physical activity. Your physician may prescribe a similar but specially fabricated device (orthotic) if your foot has a structural abnormality.

You may eliminate the problem by avoiding exercise that involves a persistent pounding of the legs (such as running or basketball) for 2 weeks to 2 months in favor of bicycling or swimming.

Muscle Cramp

Signs and Symptoms
- Sudden and sharp muscle pain, often in the legs
- A distorted lump of muscle tissue visible beneath the skin

A cramp, sometimes called a charley horse, is actually a muscle spasm in which your tissue contracts, producing sudden and intense pain. A common variety of muscle cramp occurs in the calf muscles of your leg during sleep. But overuse, injury, muscle strain, or simply remaining in the same position may result in a muscle cramp.

Cramps commonly occur in an athlete who is overfatigued and dehydrated during sports that are played in warm weather.

Certain activities characteristically result in so-called professional cramps. Writer's cramp is the classic example—the thumb and first two fingers of the writing hand become cramped as a result of long periods spent gripping a pen or pencil. In the past, watchmaker's and seamstress's cramps were common afflictions.

How Serious Is a Muscle Cramp?

Almost everyone experiences a muscle cramp at some time. For most people, cramps are only an occasional inconvenience. For some, however, muscle cramps, especially at night, are a nagging problem. If you begin to experience frequent and severe cramps that interfere with sleep, consult your physician.

Intermittent claudication, a distinct form of cramps in the legs that is associated with exercise, is caused by an inadequate blood supply to the calves (see Atherosclerosis of the Extremities, page 690). Another form of exercise-related cramps in the legs is caused by nerve compression in the spine (see Lumbar Stenosis, page 906).

See your physician if you repeatedly have cramping in your legs when you exercise. Potassium loss in the urine from the use of diuretics (medication used for hypertension

Neck Pain

Your neck supports a weight equivalent to that of a bowling ball year after year. No wonder it's occasionally stiff and sore. When your neck is stiff or in pain, you automatically tense your muscles to prevent further movement. But tense neck muscles can cause painful spasms, restricted neck movements, strained ligaments, and radiating pain.

To combat a flare-up of neck pain, try the approaches described below.

Medication

Acetaminophen or a nonsteroidal anti-inflammatory drug such as aspirin, ibuprofen, or naproxen may provide temporary relief.

Rest

Lie down during the day to ease strain on your neck. But avoid prolonged inactivity, which may cause stiffness.

Cold, Then Warmth

A cold pack often dulls the sensation of pain in the first day or two. Apply cold several times a day, for 20 minutes or less each time. Don't use cold or hot packs if you have heart or circulation problems or a reduced sensitivity to temperature.

Collars

Although it's rarely necessary, you may find that a soft cervical collar soothes pain and reminds you to limit movement that causes pain. You can find the collars at a medical equipment store or pharmacy, or fashion one at home from layers of warm toweling. Wear it in the evening for 2 to 3 weeks during periods of acute pain.

If you have a pins-and-needles tingling or numbness radiating to your arms or legs, or if your neck pain does not improve after 3 to 5 days of self-care, call your physician.

to accelerate fluid loss) or from excessive sweating is often blamed for muscle cramps, but it is an uncommon cause.

Treatment

When a cramp occurs, gently straighten the limb, because stretching the contracted muscle usually will provide immediate relief. Try compressing and massaging the affected muscle. Immersion in a hot bath or the use of a heating pad also may provide relief. Cold packs also may reduce muscle spasm or relax a tense muscle. At times, you may reduce the intensity of pain by voluntarily contracting the muscles that are opposite to those that are cramped. For example, if you have a cramp in your calf, flex the front of your foot upward toward your knee and hold it there until the cramp lessens.

Prevention

Avoid dehydration, do stretching exercises before and after your workouts, and don't overfatigue your muscles.

Medication

If recurrent cramps disturb your sleep, your physician may prescribe diazepam or diphenhydramine.

Thigh Bruise

Signs and Symptoms—Pain and tenderness in the muscles at the front of the thigh which occur suddenly and are aggravated by movement

The set of four muscles on the front of your thigh which allow you to extend your leg at the knee is called the quadriceps femoris. When these muscles tear or are strained, especially from physical contact, the resulting injury is termed a thigh bruise or contusion.

Diagnosis

Pain and swelling of the front part of the thigh, along with an inability to bend (flex) the knee as much as your other knee without pain, usually indicate a thigh bruise or contusion. Often there is discoloration under the skin, beginning with a redness and progressing to the characteristic black-and-blue bruise. This injury can take anywhere from a week to months to heal. X-rays can exclude a fracture.

Treatment

You may obtain relief from the discomfort of the injury with some combination of rest and the use of ice immediately after the injury occurs. A supportive wrap (Ace bandage) and leg elevation help reduce swelling. Short-term use of crutches may help keep weight off the injured leg. Supportive wraps (or tape) will provide some protection when you resume activity, as will properly fitted pads if contact sports are involved.

Tennis Elbow

Signs and Symptoms
- Recurrent pain on the outside of the upper forearm below the crease of the elbow
- In some cases, pain extending down the forearm toward the wrist

The name tennis elbow is a misnomer, since many persons who experience it have never played tennis. Both tennis elbow and a related ailment called Little League elbow are elbow pains that probably result from repeated, tiny tears in the tendons that attach the muscles of your lower arm at the elbow.

The tears can result from a wide variety of activities that involve a repeated rotary motion of the forearm. Hitting a backhand in tennis, painting a house, or wielding a screwdriver all have been known to precipitate tennis elbow. Little League elbow usually occurs in youngsters, and often the cause is the strain of pitching a baseball.

Diagnosis

A physical examination will probably be sufficient for your physician to reach a diagnosis, but to rule out other complications, an X-ray of the painful area may be needed. If you have tennis elbow, the X-ray will be normal.

How Serious Is Tennis Elbow?

In most cases, the discomfort will fade over time, perhaps 6 to 12 weeks. Youngsters with Little League elbow should not use the arm if it is painful, since this can lead to growth plate injury.

Treatment

The application of ice to the elbow, massage, use of a splint at night, and rest are suitable treatment approaches.

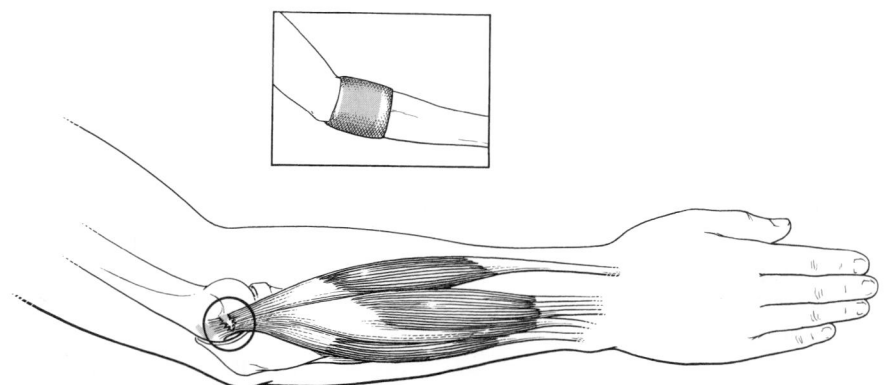

Tennis elbow produces pain on the outside of your forearm near your elbow when you exercise the joint. Tiny tears in tendon tissue cause the discomfort (see circle). In some cases, you can get relief from a forearm support band (see inset) worn just below your elbow.

Prevention
To avoid recurring episodes of tennis elbow, you may want to use a forearm support band. Worn just below the elbow, it can relieve stress placed on the inflamed tendons. You can do strengthening exercises with a hand weight (with your elbow cocked and the palm down, repeatedly bending your wrist).

Medication
Aspirin or another over-the-counter anti-inflammatory medication is effective for reducing the pain of tennis elbow. Your physician may inject a steroidal medication in certain instances. However, because these are powerful drugs, they should not be used in mild cases (see Corticosteroid Drugs, page 919).

Runner's Knee

Signs and Symptoms—Pain at the front of the knee, often accompanied by swelling

With the continuing popularity of jogging, many people have experienced runner's knee. The pain in one or both knees is caused by inflammation of the tendons (tendinitis). The inflammation is usually the result of overuse or misuse rather than a single traumatic event (see also Knee Injuries, page 876). The pain usually isn't constant, but you notice it when you move your knee.

Diagnosis
As a rule, your physician will make a diagnosis on the basis of the degree of discomfort and a physical examination. An X-ray will be normal and a surgical procedure is rarely necessary.

How Serious Is Runner's Knee?
Given proper rest and treatment, the pain of runner's knee will disappear over time, usually within a matter of weeks. However, if you do not address the cause of the problem, it may recur.

Treatment
Apply ice to the sore knee, and avoid the activity that caused the discomfort. Also avoid deep knee bends because they will stress the sore tissues.

Prevention
The most common cause of runner's knee is an improper training program. You may prevent recurrences by reviewing your training program and receiving instruction by a person knowledgeable in sports medicine. It may be necessary, however, to change your exercise program.

Some people switch from jogging to swimming or bicycling, activities that put much less stress on the knees. In some cases, orthotic devices may help correct flatfeet or other alignment problems in your legs.

If alignment problems seem to be causing your symptoms, your physician may refer you to a physiatrist, podiatrist, or physical therapist.

Support for your kneecap in the form of a light brace can also help. Another important strategy is a stretching and exercise program that helps maintain the balance and flexibility of your muscles (see Exercise and Fitness, page 289).

Medication
Aspirin and other anti-inflammatory drugs can effectively reduce pain and discomfort associated with runner's knee. Your physician may recommend an injection of an anti-inflammatory steroidal medication. However, steroids are used only in extreme cases (see Corticosteroid Drugs, page 919).

Achilles Tendinitis

Signs and Symptoms
- A dull ache or pain in the Achilles tendon, especially when running or jumping
- A mild swelling or tenderness may accompany the discomfort

Emergency Symptoms—Pain and inability to move the foot may require emergency treatment, usually a surgical procedure

Achilles tendinitis is an inflammation of the tendon that links your leg muscles to the bone at the back of your heel, commonly called the heel cord. The pain is the result of tiny tears in the tissue. Most often, they occur during strenuous exercise.

Diagnosis
An X-ray of the area will be normal if you have Achilles tendinitis.

How Serious Is Achilles Tendinitis?
Unless the Achilles tendon is severed, conservative treatments such as rest, ice, and perhaps a change in exercise program should be sufficient to allow the tendon to repair itself over a period of weeks.

Treatment
Resting the affected area is often the best treatment. You may want to switch to another form of exercise, at least temporarily. Applying ice to the Achilles tendon can also provide relief. An orthotic device that elevates the heel within the shoe may relieve the strain on the stretched tendon.

Surgery usually is required only when the tendon is torn completely (ruptured).

Medication
Aspirin and other anti-inflammatory drugs will reduce the pain and discomfort associated with Achilles tendinitis.

Baseball Finger

Signs and Symptoms
- Swelling and pain in the last joint of your finger
- Inability to straighten your finger

Also known as mallet finger or jammed finger, this injury occurs when the tendon that connects the muscles at the end of your finger is forcibly separated from the bone. This often results when the tip of your finger is struck by a thrown or batted ball.

Diagnosis
Because the injury is usually the result of a traumatic event, an X-ray will be taken of the injured joint. If your finger appears normal on the X-ray, your physician can rule out a fracture.

How Serious Is Baseball Finger?
With proper treatment, your injured finger can be used normally within approximately 8 weeks. However, you may have a permanent deformity of your finger.

Treatment

Immobilization
Baseball finger usually is treated by immobilizing the end of the affected finger with a splint. The last joint will be splinted in an extended position for approximately 6 weeks to allow the tendon to repair. After the splint has been removed, you should return your finger to normal use gradually. Your physician will recommend gentle range-of-motion exercises.

A surgical procedure is usually necessary only when a fracture accompanies the injury.

Medication
Use aspirin or another anti-inflammatory drug to relieve the discomfort of the injury.

Heel Pain

Signs and Symptoms—Pain in the heel of the foot when weight is placed on it

The heel pad consists of fibrous tissue that cushions the underlying structure of your foot when you put weight on it. Pain in the heel probably results from tears or inflammation of your heel pad where it attaches to your heel bone. Also called painful heel syndrome, this common ailment may cause mild to intense pain.

Diagnosis
Your physician will determine whether the pain is constant or whether it occurs only when you step down on your heel. An X-ray may rule out a stress fracture. However, stress fractures are often not apparent on an

Principles of Sports Rehabilitation

At its simplest, sports rehabilitation aims to return the injured athlete to normal physical activity, good health, and full function. The approach to, speed of, and eventual result after any rehabilitation are influenced by various factors, including your age, level of normal physical activity, body structure, and conditioning at the time of injury.

The four principal stages of the rehabilitation process are described below.

Stage 1
Stage 1 involves controlling the inflammation and pain of the injury. A P.R.I.C.E. treatment approach is usual (protection, rest, ice, compression, and elevation; see page 870).

Stage 2
The second step endeavors to restore the full range of motion to your injured joint. Your physical therapist may recommend exercises you can do alone or with an assistant moving the muscles surrounding a joint. Muscle strengthening exercises will follow, usually with isometrics (in which the extremity is not moved but the muscles are flexed). Then you may begin light weight training, perhaps with a rubber or elastic tube. When you have regained substantial strength and normal range of motion, additional exercises, perhaps using a stationary bicycle (for lower extremity injuries) or swimming (for upper body injuries) can be very helpful.

Stage 3
Only in stage 3 of rehabilitation do you return to biomechanical skill patterns related to specific sports. For example, a baseball pitcher recovering from an operation on the arm would resume throwing a baseball at this stage. Accompanying the gradual resumption of specific skill activities is a general cardiovascular endurance program, perhaps involving long-distance biking, swimming, or running.

Stage 4
With your return to normal activity and condition, your physician may prescribe a maintenance program, stage 4 of rehabilitation, to enable you to maintain flexibility, strength, and endurance. Skipping any of the steps in this process may put you at risk of reinjury or a prolonged recovery.

X-ray for up to 6 weeks after an injury.

Sometimes the X-ray shows a spur of bone projecting forward from the heel bone (the calcaneus). Although in the past these bone spurs have been blamed for heel pain (and then surgically removed), they are not ordinarily a cause of pain. Therefore, surgery is rarely appropriate.

Another type of image, called a bone scan (see page 1336), can often help confirm the diagnosis.

How Serious Is Heel Pain?
In most cases, the pain will fade or disappear in a matter of weeks. It can recur, however, especially if you wear improper footwear (poorly fitted athletic shoes or those that lack cushioning of the heel) when performing weight-bearing exercise. Wearing a different pair of well-fitted shoes each day may be helpful. Some people find that the only way to avoid a recurring problem is to modify their activity, switching from jogging or tennis to swimming or bicycling. In most patients, however, the prognosis is complete recovery.

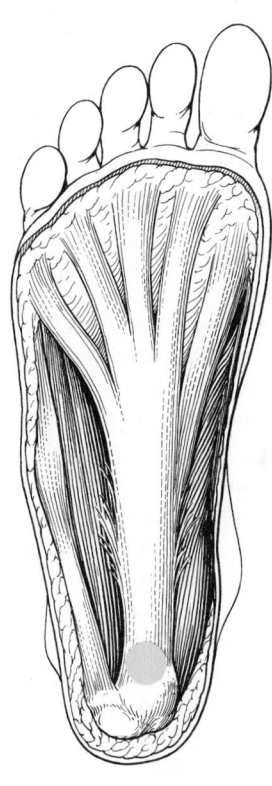

Heel pain may result from tears or inflammation of your heel pad where the tissue attaches to your heel bone (see circle). This pain rarely is caused by bone spurs.

Treatment

Apply ice to your sore heel. Massage and gentle stretching also may provide some relief. Soft-soled running shoes may help, as can inserting a rubber sponge pad into the shoe with the portion of the pad under the painful area removed. If the heel pain proves especially persistent, your health care provider may prescribe an orthotic device—a heel cup that is custom-made of molded polyethylene foam.

Medication

Try aspirin and other over-the-counter anti-inflammatory drugs first. If they do not help, consult your physician. Your physician may inject your heel with an anti-inflammatory steroid drug such as cortisone. However, these drugs should be used only when conservative measures are ineffective (see Corticosteroid Drugs, page 919).

Knee Injuries

Signs and Symptoms

- Pain and swelling in your knee
- Instability of the knee
- A popping sound, a snapping sensation, or a physical locking of the joint

Emergency Symptoms—If your knee locks rigidly in one position or a traumatic event produces intense pain and your knee ceases to function properly, seek emergency medical help

---

Other Causes of Knee Pain

Because your knee is a complex, vulnerable joint, many factors can cause knee pain. The most common sources of knee pain are injuries, genetic predisposition to knee problems, the constant stress of bearing excess weight, and general wear and tear. Osteoarthritis also commonly affects knees as the cartilage in your knee joint gradually deteriorates. You begin to feel an aching pain when you move your knee or put weight on it.

But other sources can cause knee pain as well. Chondromalacia, a softening and loss of smooth cartilage that covers the backside of your kneecap, is usually an early sign of deterioration, and it leads to pain when you move your knee, especially when you kneel or go down stairs. Popliteal cysts occur when the membrane containing fluid that lubricates your knee joint becomes inflamed, and a tender, bulging cyst forms behind your knee. Bending your knee may increase the pain.

Knee injuries result from a wide variety of causes. Acute knee injuries can occur during contact sports such as football, and the wear and tear of time can produce chronic knee problems.

Two key factors make your knee joint susceptible to injury. First, its location leaves it exposed, both to unexpected trauma and to practically nonstop use. Second, your knee is complex. It is more than a hinge. Its range of motion is unique among your body's joints: it must slide, glide, and swivel—as well as bend.

Diagnosis

If you sustain a knee injury, your physician may administer an anesthetic before the examination because the knee may be painful to touch, and it will need to be examined in a variety of positions.

One or more tests that often follow the external examination assess the joint's internal structure and the damage it has sustained. Traditional X-rays are one method of evaluating your knee. Others include arthrography, in which your knee is X-rayed after a dye is injected into the joint space (see page 1341), and magnetic resonance imaging (MRI), in which a computerized image of the structure of your knee is based on the tissue's response to a magnetic field. Arthroscopy also may be done. Here the physician examines the interior of your knee by inserting a tube and fiberoptic equipment through a small incision (see Arthroscopy, page 878).

How Serious Is a Knee Injury?

The severity of knee injuries varies, depending on the type of damage the joint sustains. There are several major categories into which most knee injuries are classified. All can produce pain and swelling of the joint.

Meniscal Tears

The meniscus is the crescent-shaped cartilage in your knee between the ends of the bones of your thigh and lower leg. Certain impact and twisting injuries can produce tears in the meniscus, causing pain in the joint. A popping sound sometimes occurs at the moment of injury.

Often the injury will cause you to collapse. In some cases, you will be able to get up and even resume activity, but more likely a cartilage tear in your knee will produce immediate swelling and continuing pain. Even if it heals over a period of weeks, it may recur.

Knee Swelling

Occasional isolated knee swelling may occur for no readily apparent reason. Sometimes this is associated with pain on movement of the knee joint. In addition, your knee may be tender and exhibit redness or inflammation. At other times, your knee may be swollen without pain, tenderness, or inflammation.

If your knee is inflamed, your temperature elevated, and it hurts to move your knee, consult your physician immediately. These symptoms may indicate an infection in the joint space of your knee. Occasionally they may be initial manifestations of gout (see page 916). If there is pain most of the time or on certain movements, this may represent an injury to the cartilage or ligaments that support your knee, a condition your physician should evaluate.

Sometimes the isolated knee swelling may be an initial symptom of a systemic disease such as rheumatoid arthritis (see page 909) or inflammatory bowel disease (see page 913). Your physician should direct treatment at the underlying disease. In young persons, knee swelling not associated with pain or inflammation may indicate a spontaneous event that resolves over several days. If resolution does not occur, see your physician again.

Ligament Tear

Ligaments are dense bands of tissue which surround a joint and provide stability. Occasionally these stretch and tear, causing immediate pain, tenderness over the site of injury, and swelling of the knee (see above).

Loose Bodies

Some knee injuries involve pieces shredded from the inner surface of the kneecap (the patella) or cartilage (meniscus) which are torn from their proper positions and float about in the joint cavity. The effect is similar to a pencil being caught in a door hinge.

Even a small piece of loose cartilage can become pinched in the knee joint and "lock" the joint or cause pain.

Treatment

The treatment required for a knee injury varies with each injury. For relatively minor knee injuries, the proper treatment approach is summarized by the acronym P.R.I.C.E.: protection, rest, ice, compression, and elevation (see page 870). Stop using your knee when you injure it. Use ice and compression to limit swelling. Keep your leg elevated to help reduce pain and swelling.

If your joint has sustained major damage, a reconstructive surgical procedure will be necessary. Dislocated or fractured bones may need to be reset, or torn or ruptured ligaments reattached. Often, minor damage can be repaired by arthroscopy; this surgery involves a small incision rather than a large opening and much greater tissue repair (see Arthroscopy, page 878).

Rehabilitation

After surgery, your physician may apply a splint, brace, or cast for your initial recuperation period. After you are allowed to move your knee, you will receive a program of exercises to follow to restore range of motion and strength to your joint. A physical therapist or rehabilitation specialist may oversee your recuperation.

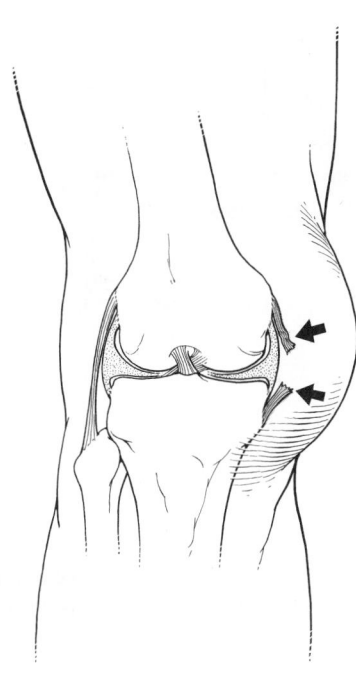

Arrows point to a torn ligament, a common form of knee injury. Swelling occurs and the joint becomes unstable.

Arthroscopy

Until the development of a device called the arthroscope in 1972, injuries of the knee and other joints often required an operation, an extended hospital stay, and a long and painful recuperation. Although some joint problems still require large incisions to open the knee or shoulder for reconstructive surgical procedures, physicians can now correct many less serious injuries with a device called an arthroscope.

The Instrument

The arthroscope (*arthro* for "joint," and *scope*, meaning "to view") consists of a tube, an optical system of magnifying lenses, and a fiberoptic light source.

The Procedure

After an anesthetic is administered (either local or general), the physician makes a small incision on one side of the kneecap (or shoulder or other joint to be examined). The incision is often so small that stitches are not required to close it after the procedure is complete.

The tube of the arthroscope is then inserted. Through the eyepiece or on a screen, the physician can look at the inside of your joint. A sterile fluid may be injected into the joint space to enlarge it and enhance visibility.

Options

Once inside the joint, the arthroscope offers an opportunity not only to examine the tissues but also, through the use of attachments, to take a biopsy specimen or even to perform minor surgery. Floating bits of cartilage can be removed, and minor tears and other disorders can be treated in this way. The arthroscope is also valuable in diagnosing various joint diseases.

Recuperation

Unlike traditional procedures in which the joint itself is opened, little time is needed for the joint to heal after arthroscopy. The procedure rarely takes more than an hour, and usually you can return home shortly thereafter.

Although you should not subject the joint to vigorous physical activity for several days, you can resume most normal activities immediately.

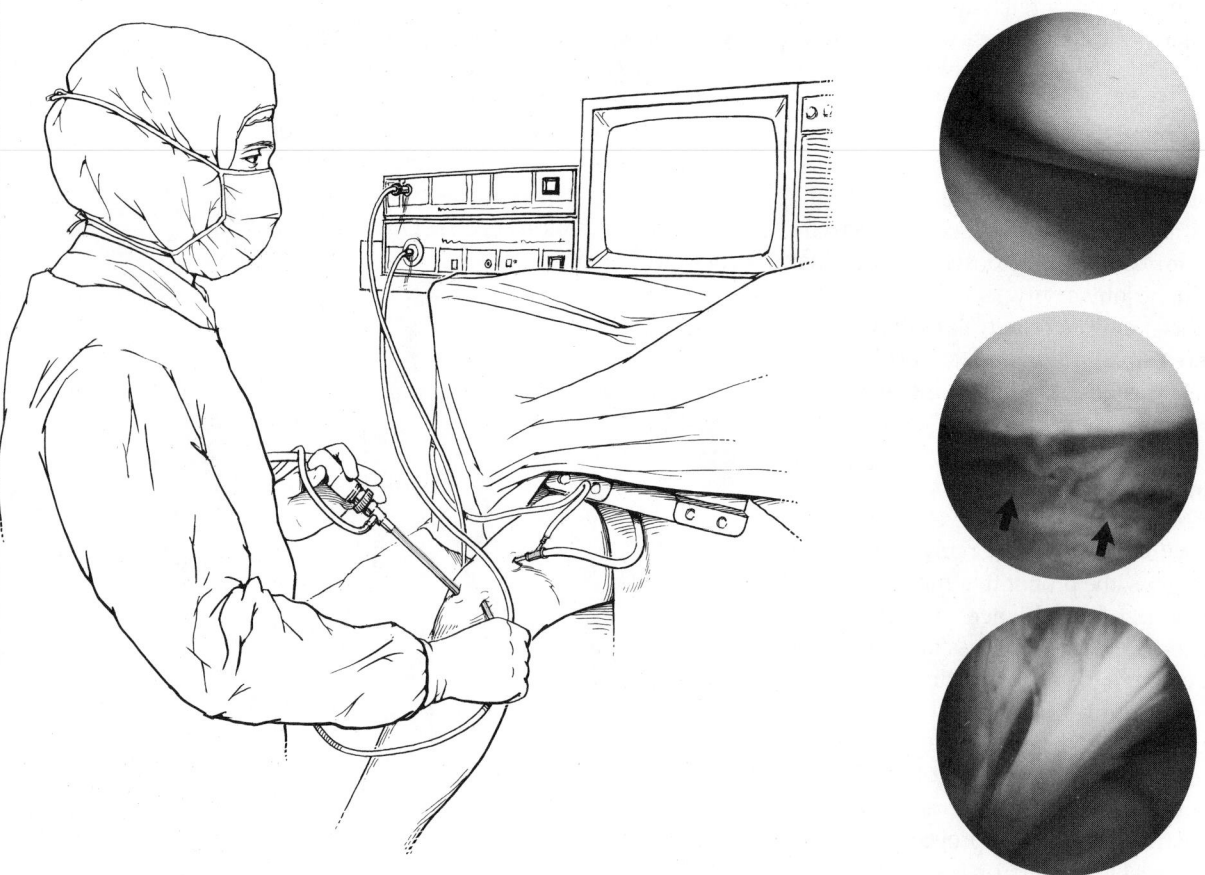

Using an arthroscope, your physician can see inside your knee or other joints and perform tests and repairs without major surgery. Right: arthroscopic views of normal meniscus (top), torn meniscus (middle, see arrows), and normal anterior cruciate ligament.

Support Braces

If your knee is unstable, you may wish to try one of several types of knee braces or support bandages available. You may find two types in an orthopedic supply store. One is a rubbery, neoprene sleeve that slips over your knee and has a hole to expose your kneecap. Relatively inexpensive prophylactic knee braces that don't require a prescription commonly have a hinge on the outer side—or both sides—of your knee. Both of these devices may seem to offer more support than they actually do. They do not protect against the most common knee injury, but the warmth and compression they provide can make your knee feel better.

If you tear your anterior cruciate ligament (the most common knee injury), your physician can prescribe a custom-made brace to help stabilize your knee. The decision of whether or not to do this is based on your age and lifestyle. If your injury prevents you from resuming your usual physical activity, a custom knee brace may stabilize your knee without the need for surgery. If surgery is necessary, a custom brace can protect your knee during recovery and aid in preventing reinjury.

Absence or Loss of a Limb

Some people are born without one of their limbs. Such congenital absences occur as the result of a developmental defect. The cause also may be a drug or other substance used during the pregnancy, but more often the cause is unknown.

The loss of a limb can be a catastrophic event. Such an amputation usually involves a major operation, whether it is precipitated by a traumatic event such as an automobile accident or by a considered medical decision to remove the limb because of a disease such as cancer or loss of blood supply.

In addition to drawing on the body's healing capacity, an amputation also requires a significant psychological adjustment. The adjustment involves not only learning to live with altered physical capacities but also accepting the change in your body image.

Your physician and other health care professionals can help you make the necessary adjustment. An artificial limb may be fitted to help you live as normally as possible (see this page). If you become depressed or have difficulty adjusting to an amputation, psychiatric help may be indicated.

Physicians perform surgical amputations for a wide variety of reasons. Some people with advanced diabetes (see page 930) develop poor circulation in the extremities, because of narrowing of the channels in the arteries. The ulcers and gangrene that can result lead to the need to amputate a foot or

Artificial Limbs

When cancer surgery, gangrene, an accident, or another illness or event results in the loss of a limb, a replacement part (prosthesis) may be substituted.

An artificial limb can never replicate the movement, flexibility, strength, and sensitivity of your original arm or leg. Yet, once you adjust to it, the prosthesis allows you to live a more complete life.

A physiatrist, orthotist, or physical therapist can help you recover. Exercises keep your remaining muscles in condition, and you receive a temporary prosthesis. At first, wear it for short periods. Gradually, you will be able to wear it all day long. After the tissues have healed fully and you have adjusted to the temporary prosthesis, a specially designed artificial arm or leg can be fabricated.

The permanent limb must be tailored to meet your specific needs. It will strike a balance between physical demands for mobility and strength and concern with appearance of the limb.

leg. Other circulatory problems also can produce gangrene (see page 692). The best treatment for certain bone cancers (see page 899) involves removing the tumor, which may require amputation of an arm or leg.

Sometimes an amputation is the result of an accident. When a finger or toe or larger body part is severed, it is an emergency requiring immediate medical attention.

How Serious Is an Amputation?
Amputation that results from an accident has various attendant risks, including blood loss and shock. As with any invasive procedure, there is also the risk of infection. The risk is greater if the amputation is accidental as opposed to surgical. In either case, your physician or surgeon will take all possible precautions to avoid infection.

In most cases, the amputation procedure itself isn't life-threatening. The problem, therefore, is dealing with the consequences of the amputation. These range from coping with the immediate pain of the amputation to adjusting your lifestyle. The loss of a leg, for example, will have a significant impact on your mobility and balance, to which you must adjust.

The surgical removal of a body part also can be an emotionally demanding event. There may be pain in the stump or the sensation, sometimes painful, that the limb or part of the limb is still present (so-called phantom limb sensation). In addition, your self-image, self-confidence, and self-worth may be affected. If you need an artificial limb, it will be tailored to your needs in both its function and its appearance.

When a physician surgically reattaches a severed body part, the usefulness of the part varies from case to case. In some instances, the reattached part regains most or all of its usefulness, whereas in others, sensitivity, flexibility, and strength remain impaired.

Treatment
In the event of a medical emergency involving a severed body part, you must take proper precautions to ensure that both the affected person and the part are properly cared for in advance of reattachment (see page 450).

Surgery
Physicians have made remarkable advances in recent years in reattaching severed fingers, hands, and even limbs. With the help of a microscope, fine surgical repairs and reattachments of tiny structures are possible. The results depend on many factors, but if the severed body part has had proper care and a trained surgeon is available, the chances for a successful reattachment are good.

Rehabilitation
A physician or a physical therapist will propose a program of rehabilitation. Frequently, a team approach involves physical and occupational therapists and orthotists under the guidance of a physiatrist (a physician who specializes in physical medicine).

Basically, the program consists of a plan for achieving as normal a life as possible, and it includes exercises to help maintain the strength of the remaining muscles. If you need an artificial limb or other equipment, the program may include other exercises, instruction on the use of crutches, counseling, and other aspects that allow you to return to normal activity. You usually are fitted for the artificial limb after the pain and swelling that follow the operation have abated. Then a training process helps you master the different movements involved in using the prosthesis or artificial limb (see Artificial Limbs, page 879).

Medication
Treatment may involve analgesics to reduce pain and antibiotics to fight infection.

Muscle, Tendon, and Soft Tissue Disorders

The tissues of your muscles are elongated and elastic, which allows them to extend and contract. When you move a limb, one muscle contracts to produce the movement; when you return the limb to its original position, the opposite muscle must contract.

Equally important to movement are the tendons, the tissues that connect the muscles to the bones. In most parts of your body, the tendons are interwoven with the muscles or are simply short connectors between the ends of the muscles and the bones. In your hands and feet the tendons are long and cord-like, but throughout your body the fibrous tendons convey the movement of the muscles to the bones. Thus, a muscular contraction causes the attached tendons and bones to move.

As with the rest of the musculoskeletal system, we tend to take our muscles and tendons for granted—until pain, stiffness, or immobility alerts us to their malfunctions. In the following pages, we consider a number of common muscle, tendon, and soft tissue disorders, from the discomfort of tendinitis to the paralyzing disorder muscular dystrophy.

Tenosynovitis

Signs and Symptoms
- Difficulty in straightening a finger or thumb: the finger seems to hesitate when you try to point it and straightens in a sudden, jerking motion
- Tenderness and pain in a finger
- Movements are accompanied by a crackling sound
- Pain when you move your wrist or shoulder

Emergency Symptoms—A joint that becomes heated and inflamed may be infected, and you should seek immediate medical help (see also Infectious Arthritis, page 914).

Long, cable-like tendons run through your hand and into each finger. Each tendon is protected by an individual membrane called the synovium, the same tissue that shields the joint cavity in your knee and other large joints (see page 862). In tenosynovitis, the membranous sheath becomes inflamed or infected.

The cause can be overuse and is common for factory workers or typists whose work involves countless repetitions of the same hand movements (see Carpal Tunnel Syndrome, page 884).

An infection from a puncture wound can cause tenosynovitis. Tenosynovitis also can occur in the wrist or, even more commonly, in the bicipital tendon in the shoulder.

One type of tenosynovitis is called trigger finger. The characteristic symptom of trigger finger is a clicking sensation in the finger as it is bent or straightened. If untreated, this can progress to an inability to straighten your finger. In a typical case, you decide to

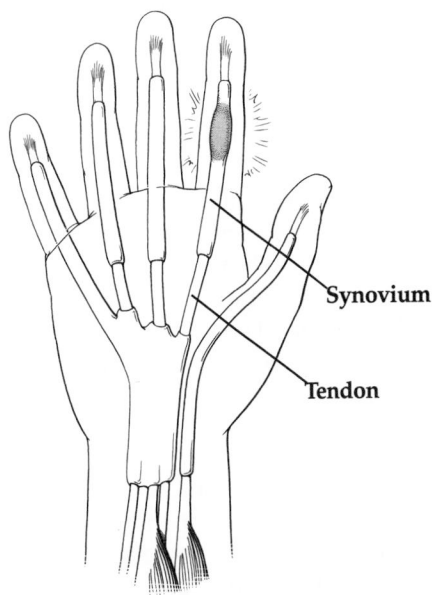

Synovium

Tendon

Each of the cable-like tendons in your hand is sheathed in a protective membrane called the synovium. When the synovium is inflamed or infected (see highlight), tenosynovitis can result. Treatment varies from rest to medication or even surgery.

straighten your finger, but it doesn't respond; then you glance down and suddenly it jerks into position.

This problem is most common in women at or beyond middle age. An X-ray can rule out any bone involvement.

How Serious Is Tenosynovitis?
If a bacterial infection causes tenosynovitis, you must receive treatment immediately because the infection may cause permanent functional damage to the affected tissues.

When tenosynovitis is the result of overuse, time and rest may produce a full recovery. If you resume the activity that led to the tenosynovitis, your symptoms will likely recur; thus, you may need to change your work habits.

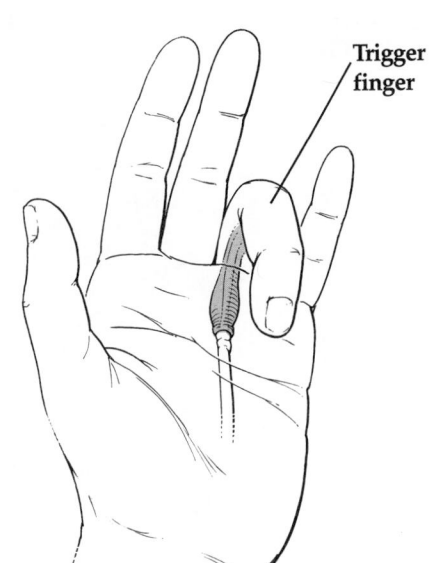

Trigger finger

One form of tenosynovitis is called trigger finger. The sheath that protects the tendon is inflamed and narrowed, making it difficult to straighten your finger. Opening the synovium surgically may restore full movement.

Treatment

Medication
If an infection is causing the discomfort, your physician will prescribe an antibiotic.

An analgesic or anti-inflammatory drug such as aspirin may reduce the pain of non-infectious tenosynovitis. In some cases, injection of a steroid drug such as cortisone may relieve the symptoms. However, steroid drugs are used only when more conservative measures fail (see Corticosteroid Drugs, page 919).

Surgery
If the diagnosis is infectious tenosynovitis, you may need an operation immediately. The operation will release the buildup of pus and limit the spread of the infection. When the cause is mechanical rather than an infection, a surgical incision in the membrane may relieve persistent tenosynovitis; this procedure may restore full movement.

Tendinitis

Signs and Symptoms—Pain and tenderness just outside a joint, especially your elbow or shoulder

A minor injury or excessive use can produce soreness in the shoulder or elbow. The cause is usually a small tear or inflammation of the tendon that links your muscles to your bone.

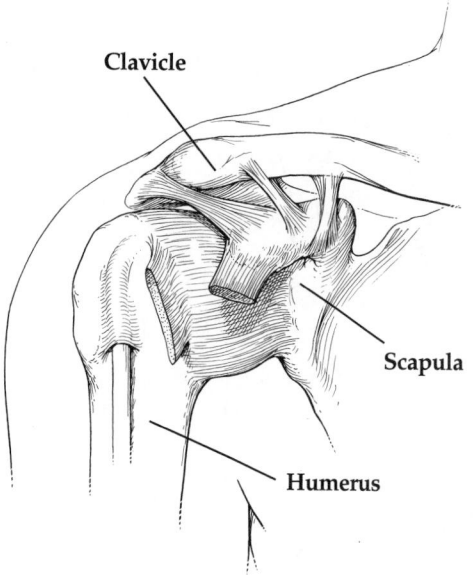

The shoulder joint is a complex structure. Strong tendons attach muscle to bone. Ligaments help hold the joint together.

Clavicle

Scapula

Humerus

Tendinitis is most common in the elbow (see Tennis Elbow, page 872) and the shoulder. An X-ray of the area of soreness can rule out any bone involvement.

How Serious Is Tendinitis?
Tendinitis can cause permanent damage to your tendons. The natural tendency to favor the painful area also can lead to stiffness. A vague discomfort at age 30 can, if the overuse is continued for years, lead to a loss of flexibility due to scarring of the tissues.

Sometimes the discomfort of tendinitis disappears within a matter of weeks, especially if you rest your elbow or shoulder. In elderly people and those who continue to use the affected area, tendinitis often heals more slowly and usually progresses to a chronic condition. The ligaments and tendons around your shoulder may gradually stiffen, a condition leading to a loss of movement; this is termed frozen shoulder (see Acute Painful Shoulder, page 917).

Treatment
Rest is essential. Do not use the affected area for several days. A sling is sometimes helpful, as is an Ace or other bandage that compresses the affected area. Also, elevate and apply ice to the area. This may help reduce discomfort and swelling.

Medication
An analgesic such as aspirin will help reduce the discomfort.

If tendinitis persists, your physician may inject the area with a steroid drug such as cortisone (see Corticosteroid Drugs, page 919).

Surgery
When a tendon is torn, a reconstructive operation may be necessary.

Exercise
Although rest is a key part of treating tendinitis, prolonged inactivity can cause stiffness in your joints. You should maintain flexibility of your joint by doing gentle range-of-motion exercises after a few days of resting the area. This can help prevent frozen shoulder.

Prevention
You can avoid a recurrence of tendinitis by warming up before exercising and cooling down after exercise (see page 292). Strengthen-

ing exercises also may help avoid further episodes of tendinitis.

Fibromyalgia

Signs and Symptoms
- Generalized aches and pains accompanied by stiffness
- Fatigue, associated with disordered sleep

Fibromyalgia is an ailment characterized by aches, pain, and stiffness in the joints and muscles. Other terms for this condition are fibrositis and tension myalgias.

The character of the pain may vary considerably. Aside from tenderness with pressure on various parts of the body, there is no related physical abnormality.

Fibromyalgia may be the result of emotional tension or stress. Other causes are far less common. Symptoms are likely to persist for many years.

You will feel the pain in your muscles and at the points where your muscles attach to your bones by the ligaments. Common tender points are at the front of your elbow and hip joint, the back of your knee or shoulder, the base of your neck, and along your vertebrae. Pain and soreness may result from muscle fatigue or prolonged tension, and it may be aggravated by motion.

Diagnosis
The diagnosis of fibromyalgia is based on the characteristic symptoms and the absence of evidence of any underlying disease that could account for the symptoms. No laboratory tests confirm or exclude a diagnosis of fibromyalgia, but your physician may order laboratory tests to rule out other conditions. The pain of fibromyalgia is very real.

How Serious Is Fibromyalgia?
This disorder is chronic but not crippling, and should not lead to disability. Many unfortunate patients spend large amounts of money investigating these symptoms to no avail.

Treatment
It's important to attend to disordered sleep and undertake efforts to produce more normal sleep. A program of physical therapy progressing to a program of recreational physical therapy is central to the treatment of this condition.

It is important to reduce stress as much as possible. Sometimes it is necessary to consult a psychiatrist and use psychoactive drugs.

Other Therapies
Environmental toxins do not cause fibromyalgia. Administering anti-rheumatic drugs or vitamins or altering the diet does not seem to help.

Medication
In most cases, fibromyalgia is treated with acetaminophen, although the use of this and other medications is far less important than the measures described above.

Costochondritis

Signs and Symptoms—Pain and swelling in the front of the chest where your ribs join your breastbone (sternum)

The name comes from the Latin word *costa* for "rib" and the Greek word *chondros* for "cartilage." Logically, then, this is an "inflammation" (*itis*) of the cartilage of the rib cage.

The pain and soreness result from an inflammation of the cartilage. The inflammation may be caused by a blow or trauma sustained by the rib cage, but often the cause is unknown. Movement of the ribs and pressure exerted directly on the affected area exaggerate the pain (see Chest Wall Pain, page 434).

When it first strikes, the pain of costochondritis often causes anxiety because it is confused with that of a heart attack. Costochondritis itself is not a medical emergency, but the sudden onset of especially severe and intense chest pains should prompt you to seek immediate medical help because of the dangers of a heart attack.

Costochondritis is also known as Tietze's syndrome, after the German surgeon who identified it.

Diagnosis
Tenderness at the junction of the ribs and breastbone suggests the diagnosis, but without actual swelling that you or your physician can feel, it is difficult to confirm the diagnosis. Your physician may want to use chest X-rays, electrocardiograms, and blood tests to exclude other unrelated disorders that could produce the same sort of pain.

Treatment

Given time and proper rest, the symptoms may disappear. Exercise may aggravate the symptoms, so avoid activities that worsen your discomfort.

Medication

Aspirin and other anti-inflammatory drugs may reduce your discomfort. Your physician may inject a steroid drug such as cortisone into the affected area (see Corticosteroid Drugs, page 919).

Carpal Tunnel Syndrome

Signs and Symptoms

- A numbness or tingling sensation in your fingers and hand
- Wrist pain that seems to shoot up into your forearm or down into the palm of your hand or surface of your fingers
- The numbness or pain may be worse at night, and it may awaken you. Often the discomfort will occur after a day in which you have used your hand or wrist forcefully. You may find relief by shaking your hand or getting up and walking about

The carpal tunnel is a passageway through your wrist (carpal is from the Greek word *karpalis*, which means "wrist"). Bounded by bones and ligaments, the carpal tunnel protects the nerves and tendons that extend into your hand.

Swelling or inflammation of the tissues that constitute the tunnel compresses the median nerve. Because this nerve provides sensation to your thumb, index, middle, and ring fingers, pressure on it produces the numbness and pain that characterize carpal tunnel syndrome. Often this ailment affects both wrists.

This syndrome is common to certain professions in which the wrist is subject to repetitive stresses and strains, especially those involving pinching or gripping with the wrist held flexed. Thus, blacksmiths have traditionally had a high incidence of carpal tunnel syndrome. The discomfort of carpal tunnel syndrome may also affect typists, carpenters, grocery clerks, factory workers, meat cutters, violinists, mechanics, and, occasionally, hobbyists such as golfers or canoers.

The problem isn't always an independent medical problem, however; it often accompanies other diseases or events. Some pregnant women find that their tendency to retain water and gain weight leads to carpal tunnel syndrome, but the symptoms usually disappear after childbirth. Carpal tunnel syndrome may also accompany some endocrine disorders such as diabetes and, rarely, hypothyroidism (see page 948) and acromegaly (see page 942) as well as rheumatoid arthritis (see page 909). In general, women approaching middle age are most likely to have carpal tunnel syndrome.

Diagnosis

A diagnostic key is that the numbness in your fingers does not include the little finger. Your physician may want an electromyogram or nerve conduction study (see page 1344) to indicate whether the electrical impulses traveling along the median nerve are slowed in the carpal tunnel, indicating that the nerve is being compressed. A test for Tinel's sign also may be done: the physician taps on the front of your wrist, and tingling or a shooting pain into your hand or forearm is usually a reliable indication that the syndrome is present. Atrophy or loss of bulk in the muscles of your thumb may be present as well.

How Serious Is Carpal Tunnel Syndrome?

With proper treatment, the pain and numbness can be relieved and no permanent damage is sustained by the hand or wrist.

Treatment

Conservative treatments include simply resting the joint and wearing a splint, which immobilizes your wrist but allows your hand to function almost normally so that you can carry on your usual activities. A splint often helps, especially in relieving the nighttime symptoms.

Medication

Your physician may inject the affected area with a steroid drug such as cortisone. But this treatment usually is used only when more conservative strategies have failed (see Corticosteroid Drugs, page 919). If the problem recurs after two injections of cortisone, your physician may recommend an operation.

Surgery

When the pain or numbness of carpal tunnel syndrome is persistent, an operation may be the best option. This involves dividing the ligament that is pressing on your nerve. At

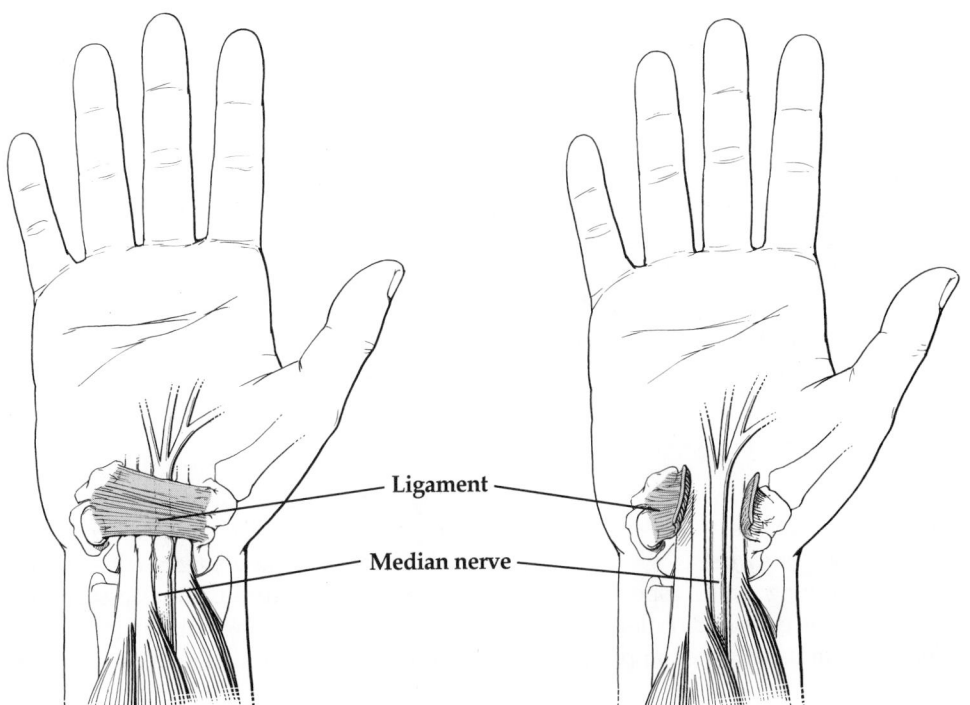

Ligament

Median nerve

A narrow tunnel through your wrist—the carpal tunnel—protects your median nerve, which provides sensation to your thumb, index and middle fingers, and the thumb side of your ring finger. When swelling or inflammation occurs in the tunnel, the median nerve can become compressed, producing pain and numbness. If conservative treatment is not effective, the carpal tunnel ligament may be severed (right) to relieve the compression.

times, this surgery can be done through an arthroscopic approach (see page 878). After recuperation, normal use of the wrist and hand usually returns within a few weeks to months.

Arthritis at the Base of the Thumb

Signs and Symptoms
• Pain and, possibly, swelling at the base of your thumb, especially when performing simple activities such as writing, opening a jar, or turning a key in a door
• Clumsiness or pain in the area when holding a small object

This common problem may affect anyone, and it is often the first sign of osteoarthritis in your thumb. Arthritis at the base of the thumb is caused by degeneration of cartilage and bone in the joints, and it is most common in women after age 55. Although wear and tear may be a factor, other contributors may be heredity, previous injury (such as dislocation of your thumb), rheumatoid arthritis (see page 909), gout (see page 916), and, frequently, repetitive activity (knitting, crocheting, or screwing a bolt, for example). These repetitive

movements can cause cartilage damage and weakening of the ligaments that support the joint. A physical examination and X-rays will reveal the extent of the problem.

Treatment
Simply limiting the use of your thumb usually allows swelling, inflammation, and pain to subside. You may need to take aspirin or other over-the-counter analgesics for discomfort. Medical supply stores carry splints that wrap and stabilize your thumb joint to reduce pain and stress on the joint; for a custom-designed fit, see an occupational therapist. You may devise other ways to perform the tasks that irritate the joint, or break them into shorter blocks of time with frequent rest periods. Ask your physician or occupational therapist about tools and utensils specially designed for people with arthritis (such as special scissors that close automatically after opening and padding on tool and utensil handles to make them thicker).

You can help keep your joint mobile with regular exercise. Every day, move your thumb around in a circle and bend the joint by touching it to your opposing fingers. Don't continue if it hurts. It's frequently best to do the exercise after washing dishes or taking a hot shower, when your joint is warm.

If your pain continues to be persistent and severe, your physician may recommend surgery. Ligament reconstruction may help in early-stage arthritis. If the joint surfaces are severely damaged, a surgeon may either implant an artificial device to replace the joint or remove the joint and replace it with a piece of tendon. A new procedure for replacing the thumb joint with an implanted metallic and plastic prosthesis to stabilize the joint and give greater mobility is currently under evaluation.

Ganglion

Signs and Symptoms

- A lump on your wrist
- Accompanying pain, especially when your wrist is extended or flexed, may be present, but usually the lump is painless

A ganglion is a swelling that appears beneath your skin, usually on the back of your wrist but in some instances on the top of your foot, on the front of your wrist, or in your fingers. It results from an accumulation of a jelly-like substance that has leaked from a joint or tendon sheath. Usually rubbery to the touch, a ganglion may vary in size.

Diagnosis

A physical examination will be done and, in some cases, other tests or an X-ray will be needed to exclude other problems. An ultrasound examination (see page 1335) is sometimes useful to confirm the diagnosis.

A ganglion is a swelling beneath the skin, usually on the back of the wrist. This is a harmless condition, but consult your physician to rule out more serious causes.

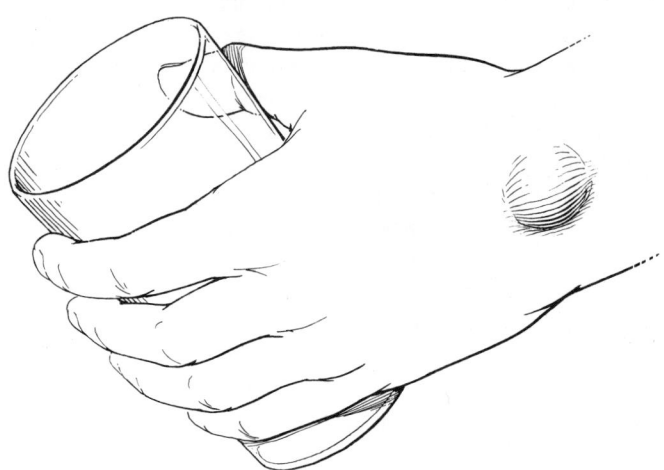

How Serious Is a Ganglion?

A ganglion is essentially harmless. However, if you observe a lump on your wrist or foot, seek your physician's counsel in order to rule out other more serious causes. If the ganglion is painful, your physician may be able to relieve the discomfort through surgical or other means, but in most cases the harmless, small lump requires no treatment and has no effect on your activities.

Treatment

Surgery
Your physician may burst the ganglion simply by putting pressure on it after puncturing it in several places with a needle or may drain the jelly-like contents with a needle. A surgical procedure is unnecessary in most cases, but if the ganglion is painful and does not respond to drainage, it can be removed surgically.

Dupuytren's Contracture

Signs and Symptoms

- An inability to straighten one or several fingers
- A small lump, cord, or area of tightness in the palm of your hand

This disorder is named after the early 19th-century French surgeon, Baron Dupuytren, who described it. It is characterized by a hardening of the lining of tissue beneath the skin of the palm of the hand (the palmar fascia).

Dupuytren's contracture usually isn't painful, but it may cause a progressive deformity of your hand. A similar hardening and shrinkage of tissue also may occur on the soles of your feet. Dupuytren's contracture is most common in the ring and little fingers, but it can affect any finger, the thumb, or the feet.

The cause of Dupuytren's contracture is unknown, but there appears to be a strong genetic component. Another common trait is that many persons with Dupuytren's contracture are middle-aged men, and some are alcoholic or have epilepsy. The reason for such linkage is unknown. The condition probably is not related to a single traumatic event.

Diagnosis

A physical examination is usually reliable for

diagnosing Dupuytren's contracture. Dimpling of the skin over the affected area is fairly characteristic. A cord of immobile tissue may also lie beneath the skin. A change in the position of the wrist does not affect a contracture.

After your physician diagnoses the condition, it is important to monitor its progression. To do so, your physician may ask you to place your hand palm down on a tabletop or other flat surface. If you are unable to hold your fingers and hand flat, treatment may be necessary. Even if you can perform this task, you should repeat it periodically. If the result indicates that your condition has worsened, surgical treatment may be in order.

How Serious Is Dupuytren's Contracture?
Although this common disorder is rarely painful, the decreasing flexibility of your fingers can be debilitating over time. In many cases, however, treatment is not required.

When an operation is necessary, most or all normal movement often can be restored, although in some people the problem may recur.

Treatment

Surgery
Surgical treatment involves removing the shrunken tissue and, in extreme cases, skin grafting or other surgical intervention. Your hand will be bandaged with the fingers in a straightened position for a few days or weeks, after which you will begin a course of physical therapy involving finger and hand exercises.

Reflex Sympathetic Dystrophy Syndrome

Signs and Symptoms
- Pain and tenderness in a hand or foot that develop in the weeks or months after an injury, heart attack, or stroke
- Tender, thin or shiny skin in the affected area, accompanied by increased sweating and hair growth

Reflex sympathetic dystrophy syndrome usually affects a hand or foot. The pain is usually of a burning quality, and accompanying symptoms will likely include swelling due to water retention and tenderness in your joints. Often the skin itself will be ten-

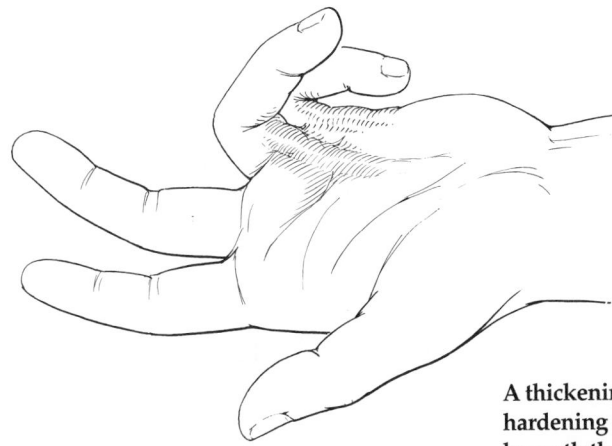

A thickening and hardening of tissue beneath the skin on the palm of your hand can lead to an involuntary, fixed contraction of one or more fingers. Called Dupuytren's contracture, surgery can correct this progressive deformity.

der. Sometimes the pain is so severe that any skin contact, even by a gentle breeze, can be painful. The syndrome usually advances over a period of months to a second phase in which the skin becomes cool and shiny. In some cases, contracture may follow.

In two-thirds of the cases, an accident, heart attack, stroke, or injury precipitates reflex sympathetic dystrophy syndrome. Most often, it occurs in people older than 50 years, and men and women are equally likely to be affected.

Diagnosis
Tests that measure skin sweating, temperature, or circulation can confirm the diagnosis. A commonly used test is the bone scan. This may show an increased circulation to the joints in the affected area. Skin temperature, circulation, and sweating tests may show abnormal patterns in response to cold or other stimulation. X-rays may also be useful. In later stages, they will reveal a loss of minerals from the bones. The syndrome can lead to irreversible damage to the affected area.

Treatment

Medication
You may use an analgesic to reduce the pain. A program of heat and cold and exercise also may help relieve the pain and tenderness. In some cases, your physician may prescribe a corticosteroid (see page 919). In other cases, injections of an anesthetic may be used to block pain fibers in affected nerves. Surgery is rarely helpful.

Muscle Tumors

Signs and Symptoms
- A lump in a muscle, perceptible on the surface of the skin
- Pain in the affected area
- A rapid increase in the size of the lump

Muscle tumors are rare, and when they do occur they are usually benign. However, a malignant muscle tumor (rhabdomyosarcoma) can be life-threatening and requires immediate treatment.

Diagnosis
If you observe any sort of lump under your skin, see your physician. Most lumps under the skin are lipomas. They consist of fat and are located between the skin and the muscle layer. Often they are identified easily with slight finger pressure and move readily. They are rubbery to touch and are not tender. It is not unusual to have several such collections. These lumps are rarely a cause for worry.

Your physician will examine the lump and, if concerned, may order a traditional X-ray, a magnetic resonance imaging scan, or a computed tomography scan of the area (see pages 494 and 1334). A biopsy of the tissue also may be necessary, in which a sample of tissue is removed for laboratory analysis.

Treatment
If the tumor is benign, it may require no treatment or will simply be excised. If it is malignant, however, surgical removal, radiation treatments, or chemotherapy may be necessary.

Muscular Dystrophy

Signs and Symptoms
- Muscle weakness, characterized by an apparent lack of coordination, clumsy gait, and an inability to elevate your arms over your head
- Progressive crippling, resulting in loss of mobility

Muscular dystrophy is a progressive disease in which muscles decrease in size and grow weaker. (The word dystrophy comes from the Greek prefix dys, which means "bad" or "painful," and the word trephein, which means "nourishment.") Literally, dystrophy means insufficient nourishment. The most common type of this rare ailment is called Duchenne's muscular dystrophy, or pseudohypertrophic muscular dystrophy.

We don't know why the muscles in persons with Duchenne's muscular dystrophy lack a key protein essential to muscle function. In the absence of this protein, the muscles grow progressively weaker, yet they may appear larger than normal, because fat tissue replaces the lost muscle.

The tendency to have this rare disease is inherited. Duchenne's muscular dystrophy usually strikes at an early age (often before the age of 5 years), and it affects only males.

Diagnosis
In the toddler, a decrease in mobility skills—walking or climbing stairs—or difficulty in lifting the arms over the head may indicate Duchenne's muscular dystrophy. The physician is likely to order a biopsy of the muscle tissue (a small sample of tissue is removed for laboratory examination).

How Serious Is Muscular Dystrophy?
Muscular dystrophy is a crippling disease. In most cases the arms, legs, and spine become progressively deformed; by the teenage years, most patients need a wheelchair. Because of their susceptibility to chest infection, most patients with muscular dystrophy die before adulthood, usually of pneumonia or other chest infection.

Treatment
There is no cure for muscular dystrophy. The best treatment regimen involves trying to minimize the deformities through physical therapy.

Prevention
Although we know little about treating Duchenne's muscular dystrophy, it is clear that the disorder is inherited in more than half the cases.

Because the affected genes are carried by females, any woman with a family history of muscular dystrophy should seek genetic counseling before considering pregnancy. The odds are 1 in 2 that a male child of a carrier will have this devastating disorder.

Problems of the Feet

Your feet take you where you want to go. They are affected by excesses of heat or cold, and they alert you when they are injured or mistreated. But, if you're lucky—and you wear properly fitted footwear—you'll spend almost no time worrying about them.

When your feet are sore, walking can be painful. If foot problems occur, you may want to seek guidance from your physician, an orthopedic surgeon, or a podiatrist. A podiatrist, although not a medical doctor, is a licensed professional whose area of expertise is the examination of the human foot and the diagnosis, prevention, and treatment of foot disorders.

In the following pages, we discuss common foot problems.

Metatarsalgia

Signs and Symptoms
- Pain in the front (ball) of the foot
- Frequently causes the sensation of "walking on pebbles"

The term metatarsalgia actually includes a group of foot disorders. Although it affects males and females, from adolescents to older adults, it is most common among middle-aged women. There are multiple causes, and simple treatments usually bring relief.

Diagnosis
Tough, cord-like ligaments hold together the 26 bones in each of your feet. As you walk, your muscles work the bones like levers, making movement possible.

"Meta" means between. You have five metatarsal bones in each foot. Each has a narrow shaft and a knobby tip. They link your ankle and heel bones (tarsals) with the bones of your toes (phalanges). Hinge joints between the metatarsals and phalanges let your toes move up and down and, to a lesser extent, sideways.

Narrow, high-arched feet can focus stress on the balls of your feet. If your legs are unequal in length, the metatarsal-phalangeal joints of the shorter leg receive additional stress. Bunions or tender calluses under your metatarsal-phalangeal joints often cause pain-

ful skin irritation. Other contributing factors can include rheumatoid arthritis, stress fractures, fluid accumulation, muscle fatigue, flat feet, excess weight from pregnancy or obesity, and excessive standing or walking.

Treatment
Simple measures usually reduce pain at the front of your foot. Avoid wearing tight, thin-soled, and high-heeled shoes. Consult your podiatrist or physician for a foot pad that relieves pressure on the metatarsal area. Physicians commonly prescribe nonsteroidal anti-inflammatory medications, such as ibuprofen or sulindac. Bunions or calluses can be treated with over-the-counter or prescription astringents, emollients, or ointments. Rarely, your physician may inject a corticosteroid into the tender area. Surgery is seldom necessary.

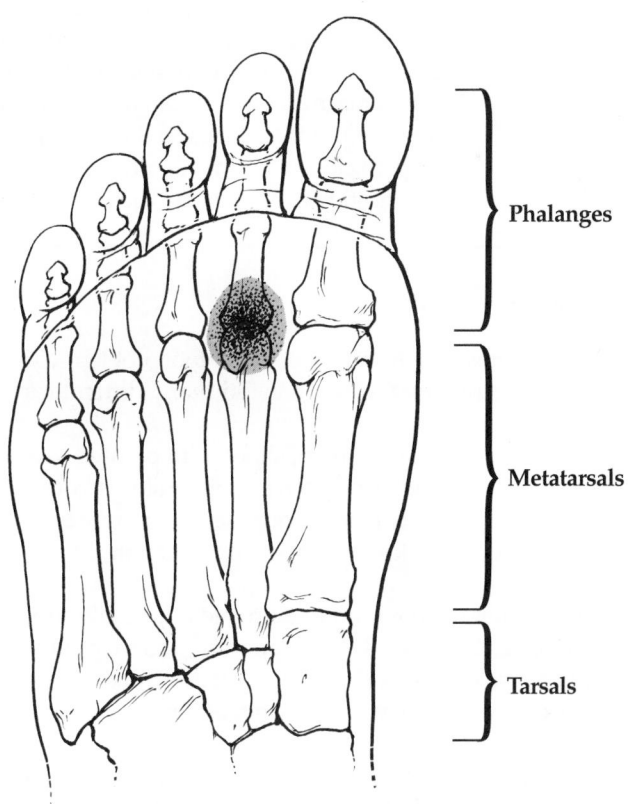

The pain of metatarsalgia can occur at any of the joints that separate the phalangeal and metatarsal bones in your foot. Highlighted area shows the joint most commonly affected.

Burning Feet

Signs and Symptoms—Nearly constant burning and stinging feet

Common among people older than 65 years, burning feet can cause discomfort ranging from mild irritation to severe pain. The disorder may be temporary. Possible culprits include irritating fabrics, poorly fitted shoes, a fungal infection such as athlete's foot, or an encounter with a toxic substance like poison ivy.

Diagnosis
Often, the cause of burning feet is difficult to pinpoint. Although generally not serious, it can signal a significant problem. If a nerve or blood disorder causes the symptoms, you may also have prickling, weakness, or change of sensation in your legs; nausea, diarrhea, loss of urine or bowel control, or impotence; or persistent symptoms. Other family members may also have burning feet.

Peripheral neuropathy, damaged or diseased nerves connecting your brain and spinal cord (central nervous system) to your sense organs, skin, muscles, glands, and internal organs, may cause a persistent condition. Nerve damage may result from more than 100 causes, including diabetes mellitus (see page 925), pernicious anemia, inherited disorders, poor nutrition caused by fad dieting or alcoholism, use of certain medications, exposure to poisons (arsenic or lead, for example), chronic kidney failure, or liver disease.

Your physician will first rule out superficial irritants, diabetes, or a blood disorder. Then he or she will consider a nerve disease, often with the help of a neurologist.

Treatment
Regardless of the cause, self-help measures may provide relief. Wear non-irritating socks made from synthetic fibers such as acrylic or polypropylene. Select well-fitting shoes made of natural materials that breathe. A specially fitted insole (if it's in good condition) may help. Reduce or eliminate activities that aggravate your condition (standing in one place for long periods, for example). Cool your feet in cold, but not icy, tap water for 15 minutes twice a day. Get enough sleep. Reduce your level of stress. Prescription and over-the-counter analgesics (such as aspirin or acetaminophen) may provide relief.

If nerve damage is the cause, it can take months for the symptoms to subside, because nerves heal slowly. Sometimes simply restoring an adequate diet may allow your nerves to heal.

Morton's Neuroma

Signs and Symptoms
- A burning sensation that radiates into the involved toes
- Soreness in your feet, even when you rest them

Morton's neuroma is a benign growth that develops on a nerve at the base of the toes.

Treatment
If you have symptoms of Morton's neuroma, remove your shoes periodically and gently massage the painful area. In severe cases, surgeons remove the growth responsible for the painful symptoms.

Corns and Calluses

Signs and Symptoms—A thickened layer of skin, often between the toes

Corns and calluses are the result of constant pressure or repeated friction on your skin, producing a thickening and hardening

---

Shopping for Shoes

Improperly fitted shoes are the source of many foot problems. If you shop carefully for shoes, you can avoid many difficulties later.

Buy shoes with adequate toe room; shoes with pointed toes can cramp your feet and lead to ingrown toenails, calluses, corns, and bunions. Select low heels, because high heels can cause back problems by forcing you to lean back to compensate for the forward tilt of your heel.

Laced shoes generally offer more room and adjustable support. Athletic shoes, strapped sandals, and soft, roomy pumps with cushioned insoles are good choices. Soft calfskin or suede allows your skin to breathe, whereas vinyl and plastic impair evaporation of perspiration.

Shop for shoes in the early afternoon to get a fit that will accommodate your foot as it swells throughout the day, yet is not too roomy. Measure the size of both feet. As you age or put on weight, your shoe size may change. Because your arches also tend to relax with age, you may need wider, larger shoes. Ask your shoe shop to stretch your shoes at any point that rubs.

of the skin. Corns are smaller (less than a quarter-inch long) than calluses.

Shoes that fit poorly are often the cause of corns or calluses on your feet (see also Bunions, this page). Calluses on your hands usually result from the pressure or friction of repetitive labor: if you use a shovel or other hand tool daily, you will find your hands lined with calluses over time. Friction and pressure can do the same to your feet.

How Serious Are Corns and Calluses?
Corns and calluses are common and rarely cause more than minor discomfort. However, if you have diabetes, infection and other complications can occur, so you need to take special care (see Caring for Your Feet, page 931). If a corn or callus becomes painful or ulcerated, consult your physician.

Treatment
In most people, curing a corn or callus is a matter of eliminating the cause. If improperly fitted footwear is the cause, wear shoes of soft leather and the proper shape. A little stretching of your shoe in the right places can do wonders. In a few weeks, the corn or callus should disappear. If the problem persists, your physician may refer you to a foot specialist (an orthopedic surgeon or podiatrist) who may remove the tissue.

Bunions

Signs and Symptoms
- A bony protrusion occurring at the base of your big toe
- Accompanying pain and limitation of motion

A bunion occurs when the big toe bends toward the next toe, sometimes overlapping it. The condition is called hallux valgus, from the Latin *hallux*, which means "big toe," and *valgus*, which refers to the angular deformity. It results in a minor deformity of the foot.

The base of the big toe is thrust out beyond the normal profile of the foot, producing the bump known as the bunion. The bunion often is subjected to constant rubbing that, in turn, results in a thickening of the skin (see Corns and Calluses, page 890).

This common but minor problem is several times as likely to occur in women as men. Although some people are genetically predisposed to develop the condition, more

---

> ## Treating Calluses
>
> You can gradually thin some of the thickened skin of corns and calluses by rubbing the skin with a towel whenever it has been softened by a shower or bath. The alkalinity of the soap, along with the soaking in water, softens your skin so you can rub off the upper layers.
>
> Use a pumice stone as a mild abrasive during or after bathing to reduce the thickness of callus tissue. This is not recommended, however, if you have diabetes or poor circulation.

often the ailment results from forcing the foot into a tight shoe with a pointed toe and a high heel.

Diagnosis
Your physician may request X-rays from several angles to confirm the visual diagnosis.

How Serious Is a Bunion?
A bunion usually causes minor discomfort. However, accompanying bursitis or osteoarthritis can develop, causing pain and stiffness (see pages 917 and 907, respectively). A bunion can make finding suitable shoes difficult, and often the shoes are unsatisfactory in appearance. If your bunion becomes very painful and annoying, consult your physician.

Treatment
Shoes that fit properly are often the best remedy and preventive for the discomfort of a bunion. The shoes should provide ample room for your toes. If bursitis develops, you may find that a hole cut in the upper surface of an old shoe in the area of the bunion will

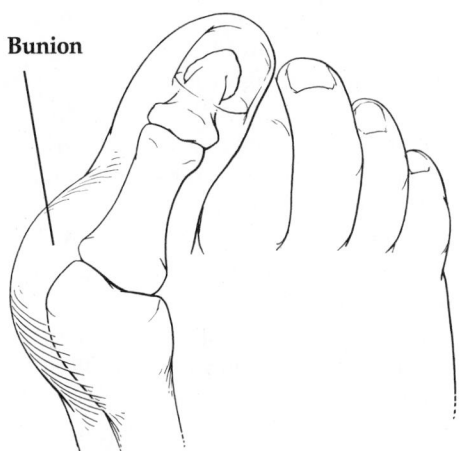

Bunion

When the base of your big toe extends beyond the normal profile of your foot, the bump that results is called a bunion. To prevent a bunion, avoid shoes with narrow toes or high heels.

Tired Feet

Each year, millions of Americans experience problems with their feet. The five most common foot problems are flatfeet, cavus feet (high arches that cause your heel to bend inward and your toes to claw), calluses or corns, hallux valgus (a deformity of the big toe that frequently leads to bunions), and hammer or claw deformities of the small toes.

Foot problems increase with age. As you age, the pad of fat under your heel becomes smaller and less spongy. This places more stress on the muscles and bones in your foot when you're standing or walking. Degenerative joint diseases make your feet less flexible, which can interfere with the normal bone movements within your feet and adversely affect your posture. Atherosclerosis can cause foot problems by reducing the circulation to your feet. Obesity, friction or pressure from ill-fitting shoes, or years of wearing high-heeled, narrow-toed shoes can compound the problems aging brings.

You can help your tired, aching feet by wearing properly fitted shoes. Sometimes, specially designed corrective shoes can help correct foot problems.

provide relief. Commercially available felt pads may be helpful. Surgery is generally not necessary for bunions, particularly if they do not hurt. In rare and extreme cases, an operation may be performed to realign the bones and remove excess bone tissue.

Flatfeet

Signs and Symptoms—No visible arches in your feet when you place your weight on them

Your feet are highly specialized structures. Each is made up of 26 bones held together with ligaments, muscles, and tendons. The intricate alignment of these structures results in the formation of metatarsal (side-to-side) and longitudinal (lengthwise) arches. As you walk, these springy, elastic arches help distribute your body weight evenly across each of your feet and lower limbs. Your arches also play an integral role in how you walk. They must act as rigid levels for proper mobility, but they must also be resilient and flexible to adapt to various surfaces.

Everyone has flatfeet at birth. Your arches are usually fully developed by age 12 or 13. Some people's arches never form properly. Left untreated, flatfeet can lead to muscular

imbalances and joint problems involving your ankles, knees, hips, and low back.

Most people develop arch problems as a result of ongoing stresses. Excessive weight, postural abnormalities, weakened supportive tissue, or overuse may weaken the ligaments and muscles supporting the arch that runs lengthwise in your foot, causing it to "fall." Activity on hard surfaces or prolonged stresses on the balls of your feet may cause a weak or fallen metatarsal arch, which normally runs side-to-side across the forefront of your foot. This places additional pressure on the nerves and blood vessels in the area, and commonly results in pain and irritation. Fallen arches may lead to other foot problems, including inflammation and pain in the ligaments in the bottoms of your feet, Achilles tendinitis, shin splints, stress fractures, bunions, and calluses.

Diagnosis

Your physician or podiatrist can readily diagnose fallen arches by a simple examination of your feet.

Treatment

If you experience chronic pain as a result of flatfeet, you may get effective relief by wearing a custom-designed arch support called an orthotic. Orthotics adapt to the contours of your feet and slip into your footwear. Corrective orthotics readjust your foot into a more ideal weight-bearing position. They also help control excessive inward or outward rotation of your longitudinal arch when you are walking, provide support, and absorb shock. Accommodative models provide foot and arch support for people who cannot tolerate the more rigid corrective orthotics. Orthotics may not fit in all of your shoes. Custom-made orthotics require a visit to your physician or podiatrist. Many major medical insurance plans cover a portion of the cost.

Hammer Toe and Mallet Toe

Signs and Symptoms

- A claw-like or mallet-like clenched appearance to a toe
- Accompanying pain and difficulty in movement

Unlike a bunion, which affects the big toe (see page 891), hammer toe may affect any toe (although most commonly the second toe is affected). The toe becomes bent and painful. Generally, both joints in a toe are affected, giving it a claw-like appearance. Hammer toe can result from wearing shoes that are too short, but the deformity also occurs in persons with long-term diabetes who have muscle and nerve damage as a result of the disease (see Caring for Your Feet, page 931).

A mallet toe has a deformity of the end of the toe that gives it a mallet-like appearance.

How Serious Are Hammer Toe and Mallet Toe?

Both hammer toe and mallet toe can be painful and make walking and other movements uncomfortable and more difficult.

Treatment

Your physician or a podiatrist may prescribe an orthotic appliance to position your toe properly and relieve the pressure and pain in your toe. Make sure you wear shoes that fit properly. A corrective surgical procedure is another possibility in some cases.

Ingrown Toenail

Signs and Symptoms—Pain, swelling, and redness around a toenail

An ingrown toenail is a condition in which the toenail grows into the flesh of the toe, often the big toe. It can result from unusually curved toenails, poorly fitted shoes, or toenails that are cut improperly. The tissue around the nail may become infected.

Treatment

If the tissue around the nail is infected, your physician will prescribe an antibiotic and may also trim the portion of the nail that has grown into the toe (a minor procedure that is done in the office). Your physician may also recommend warm soaks, a topical antibiotic, and rest.

Prevention

To avoid chronic recurrence of ingrown toenails, don't clip your nails too short; also, cut them straight across rather than curving them to match the shape of your toes. Wear socks and shoes that fit properly, and avoid excessive pressure on your feet and toes.

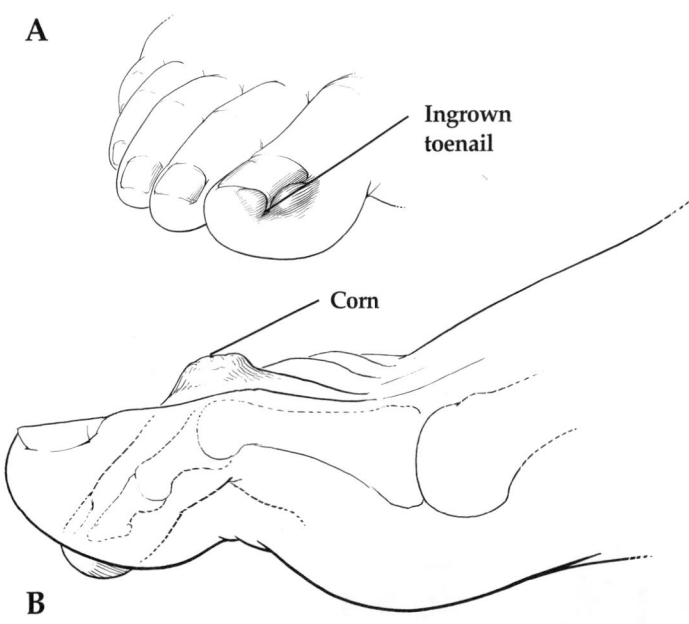

A

Ingrown toenail

Corn

B

To avoid an ingrown toenail (A), don't clip your toenails too short. Clip them straight across. When a toe takes on a claw-like, clenched appearance, it is termed hammer toe (B). This most often affects the second toe, which frequently develops a corn due to pressure on the shoe. An orthotic appliance inserted into the shoe may be sufficient to relieve discomfort. To help avoid hammer toe, wear shoes that fit properly.

Foot Ulcers

Signs and Symptoms
- An open sore on the skin surrounded by inflamed tissue
- If the tissue is infected, pus is discharged from the ulcer

People with diabetes, in particular, are at risk for foot ulcers. A foot ulcer can be the result of long-term blood vessel or nerve deterioration or even of bedsores from prolonged immobilization.

Diagnosis

If the ulcer is likely the result of arterial problems, your physician will check for the presence or absence of pulsation in the arteries of your foot. If necessary, you will have a special ultrasound test to check for blockage of the arteries to your leg. Particularly if there appears to be a need for an operation, arteriography also may be done to examine the blood vessels themselves and identify abnormalities (see page 656).

Ulcers from an inadequate arterial blood supply ordinarily occur at or near the toes, whereas ulcers produced from poor veins tend to be located near the ankle. Ulcers resulting from a nerve deficit are often on the soles, frequently at the site of a callus.

See your physician if you develop a foot ulcer.

Treatment

Surgery

Many foot ulcers will heal without an operation. However, sometimes an operation on the arteries or even an amputation is necessary.

Prevention

Your physician may recommend that you use special stockings or support hose to help circulation and prevent future ulceration. In the case of an ulcer from poor veins, your physician may recommend elevating your feet. This means that, as much as possible, your feet should be elevated above your heart to assist in drainage and to lessen the associated swelling.

If you have diabetes, inspect your feet daily. Look for sores or cuts. Use a mirror for surfaces you can't see, or get help.

Bone Diseases

The 206 bones in the human body consist of hard, rigid tissue. The bones are the skeletal framework to which your muscles are attached and within which your organs are located.

Our bones are made up of proteins, sugars, minerals, and other materials. They are living, changing tissues that produce blood cells and act as a storehouse for the minerals calcium and phosphate. Given the range of activities that take place within our bones, a range of problems and malfunctions can occur.

Some of the diseases that may affect bone, such as osteoporosis, are common, whereas others, such as fibrous dysplasia or Paget's disease, are uncommon or rare. However, they all result in failure of the function of the remarkable structural system we know as the skeleton.

Osteoporosis

Signs and Symptoms
- Back pain
- Loss of height over time, with an accompanying stooped posture
- A fracture of the vertebrae, wrists, or hips

Most cases of osteoporosis are the result of an acceleration of the normal changes our bodies undergo as we age. Unfortunately, 1 of every 4 women older than 45 years and 9 of 10 women older than 75 years have varying degrees of osteoporosis. These women have primary osteoporosis, which gradually depletes the store of calcium in the bones; this form usually becomes more evident after the onset of menopause. Men start with a larger reserve of bone minerals, and so their loss of bone density due to osteoporosis becomes evident later in life and to a lesser degree. A calcium-poor diet, smoking, a sedentary lifestyle, early menopause, and being underweight all heighten the risk of osteoporosis.

The term osteoporosis is from the Greek *osteon* for "bone" and *porus* for "pore" or "passage." Osteoporosis literally makes your bones more porous. The percentage of calcium stored in your bones decreases over time, causing your skeleton to weaken and leading, in some cases, to fractures. This demineralization has various causes.

Osteoporosis also can accompany endocrine disorders such as acromegaly and Cushing's syndrome (see pages 942 and 937) or can result from excessive use of drugs such

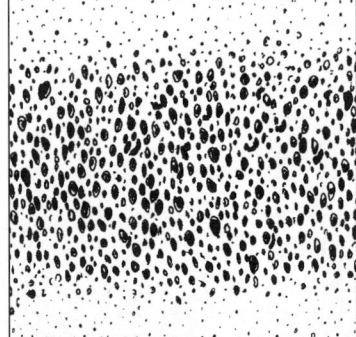 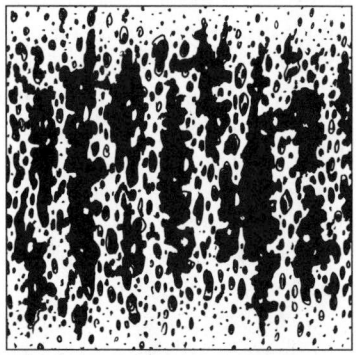

Left: Normal bone. Right: Osteoporotic bone, which is more porous and thus weaker and subject to fracture.

as corticosteroids. In such cases, the problem is termed secondary osteoporosis. The treatment must be directed at curing the principal ailment or not using the offending drug.

Diagnosis

Your physician may observe osteoporotic bone in a routine X-ray of your spine before you even know you have the disease. In many cases, however, the first symptom of osteoporosis is a fracture. A hip or wrist may break with a minor fall or accident (although in some cases spontaneous hip fractures precipitate the fall). In an X-ray of an osteoporotic bone, the bone's shape is the same as that of a normal bone (unless the bone is fractured) but it is less dense. The image is less distinct, which suggests a weaker bone.

If your physician suspects you have osteoporosis, appropriate blood or urine tests will exclude other causes for a loss of bone density. One or several X-ray-like tests, including CT (see page 1334) or photon absorptiometry, will define the degree of bone density loss.

How Serious Is Osteoporosis?

Fractures are the key consequence of osteoporosis. Although the fractures tend to heal normally, they often occur with very little or no unusual stress, and further fractures may occur once healing has taken place.

Osteoporosis also affects your lifestyle. For many people, living with osteoporosis means adopting more sensible dietary and exercise programs to minimize future bone loss. It also means taking a commonsense approach to daily activities to avoid putting your bones at risk.

The vertebral fractures characteristic of osteoporosis rarely require surgical treatment. Called compression fractures, they may cause minimal discomfort if they are minor; if they are more extensive, you may have a painful episode of backache. Commonly, the pain begins abruptly, centers in your back (but may radiate around the trunk), is aggravated by movement and relieved by heat, and gradually subsides over the next 1 to 2 months. Over a period of years, however, a sequence of spinal compression fractures can lead to dowager's hump (also called widow's hump) and an increasingly bent-over posture.

Osteoporosis can be crippling when your bones are weakened severely. The disorder also is associated with perhaps 40,000 deaths annually, largely from complications of surgery or immobilization after hip fractures.

Treatment

Exercise

A regular, reasonable exercise program is a crucial part of the battle against osteoporosis. Weight-bearing exercise (that is, exercise such as walking rather than swimming) may help the bones to regain calcium. In addition, exercise can improve your musculature, which may help avoid future falls and fractures.

Select your exercise carefully. Start out slowly and increase gradually. Appropriate exercises include walking, riding a stationary bicycle, and working out on a rowing machine. Paradoxically, the serious female competitive runner is often vulnerable to osteoporosis because of a decrease in estrogen production and scanty or absent menstrual periods that may accompany extreme leanness.

Prevention

Although there is little agreement among researchers as to whether you can fully prevent osteoporosis, there is an emerging consensus that the more calcium a woman has stored in her skeleton before menopause, the less her risk of developing significant osteoporosis. To that end, a young woman should adopt dietary and exercise programs that foster deposition of calcium in her bones.

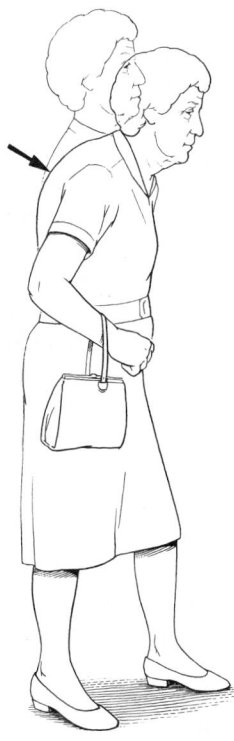

One of the long-term effects of osteoporosis can be a series of vertebral compression fractures that, over time, can produce the stooped posture commonly called dowager's hump.

Eat foods high in calcium, including dairy products, leafy green vegetables, beans, nuts, and whole-grain cereals. Many physicians advise you to take a calcium supplement if your dietary calcium intake is deficient. The value of this advice has yet to be proved adequately, but a calcium intake of approximately 1,000 milligrams per day from diet or supplements may help you maintain maximal calcium status. For an elderly woman with osteoporosis, the same strategies apply.

Weight-bearing exercise is important to women younger than 40 who are concerned about the risk of developing osteoporosis. Effective preventive exercises include jogging, walking, tennis, bicycling, dancing, rope-jumping, cross-country skiing, and almost any activity that combines movement with stress on your limbs, including weight training.

In general, adopting an exercise program that serves the basic goals for cardiovascular fitness (see page 644) will help you avoid bone loss.

Even though exercise, adequate consumption of calcium, and appropriate supplementation with estrogen and vitamin D are the most important elements in preventing osteoporosis, additional precautions may be beneficial. Limit caffeine consumption to no more than three cups of coffee per day. Avoid very large amounts of fiber in your diet because dietary fiber binds the calcium in your intestine and may interfere with absorption. Avoid consuming very large amounts of protein. Avoid excess alcohol, and stop smoking (see How to Stop Smoking, page 321).

Medication

When you begin menopause, your physician may recommend estrogen replacement therapy. This course of medication will replace the supply of estrogen as your ovaries cease to supply it, enabling your skeleton to slow its rate of absorption and retain calcium stores. Estrogen is the best treatment for prevention and improvement of osteoporosis. If your uterus is present, your physician also may prescribe progesterone to prevent the lining of your uterus (endometrium) from being overstimulated. You do not need progesterone if you have had a hysterectomy. Estrogen is available now in many forms, including oral tablets and an estrogen patch for the skin. Ask your physician which is best for you. In addition, your physician may recommend supplementary calcium.

Surgery

If a fracture occurs, you may need an emergency operation to set a broken wrist, hip, or other bone. Physical therapy is a key part of the recovery from any fracture.

Osteomalacia and Rickets

Signs and Symptoms
- Pain in the bones of your arms, legs, spine, and pelvis, with actual tenderness of the bones
- Progressive weakness

In Children
- In addition to the above symptoms, a child with rickets may have bowlegs and develop a pigeon breast (projection of the chest) and a protruding stomach
- A slight fever and restlessness at night

Osteomalacia means "softening" (*malakia*) of the bones. This softening occurs from a loss of the mineral calcium from the skeleton. The bones become flexible and gradually are molded by forces, such as bearing weight, that are exerted on them. Deformities can then result. When osteomalacia occurs in children, it is termed rickets.

One of the two most common causes of osteomalacia is malabsorption of fat, called steatorrhea. In this condition, your body does not absorb fats, and they are passed directly out of your body in your stool. The result of this problem is that vitamin D, which is usually absorbed with fat, and calcium are poorly absorbed. This poor absorption can be a result of digestive disorders such as nontropical sprue and short-bowel syndrome (see pages 770 and 772).

The other common cause of osteomalacia is an increased amount of acid in the body fluids as a result of faulty kidney function. Called renal tubular acidosis, this problem occurs in persons with congenital or acquired kidney disorders (see page 833). In simple terms, this increased acid gradually dissolves the skeleton (just as vinegar will soften an eggshell).

A less common cause of osteomalacia is a dietary shortage of vitamin D, a key component in the body's process of calcium absorption. Because milk is supplemented with vitamin D, and because even small exposures to sunlight result in the manufacture of vitamin D in your skin, in our society osteomalacia and rickets rarely result from a lack of vitamin D. However, if you or your child has trouble digesting milk products, your physician may advise taking vitamin D supplements to be sure that no deficiency occurs (see Lactose Intolerance, page 772). A long-term deficiency of calcium in your diet also can result in osteomalacia, but it usually causes osteoporosis. There is also a hereditary form of rickets with shortened adult stature, often called vitamin D-resistant rickets (see page 833).

Diagnosis

If your physician suspects osteomalacia or rickets, a blood test can measure the amounts of the minerals calcium and phosphorus. Your physician will X-ray the affected bones. Infrequently, a bone biopsy, in which a small sample of bone tissue is removed for analysis, also may be needed to confirm the diagnosis.

Once osteomalacia is diagnosed, the next and most essential step is to find out whether the cause is an intestinal problem (malabsorption) or a kidney defect.

How Serious Is Osteomalacia?

In most cases, when the mineral deficiency is eliminated, so are the symptoms. In children and adults, appropriate treatment can correct most of the mineral depletion in the bones, and the skeletal deformities disappear in time.

Treatment

Medication

Treatment is usually directed toward correcting the underlying problem. Calcium and vitamin D supplements may be necessary.

Surgery

In extreme cases, particularly in vitamin D-resistant rickets, skeletal deformities may require surgical correction.

Paget's Disease of the Bone

Signs and Symptoms

- Pain and a sensation of warmth over the involved bones
- Headache
- Bowing of a lower limb
- Hearing loss

The disorder called Paget's disease (also known as osteitis deformans) is named after a mid-19th century English surgeon. Paget's disease of the bone initially occurs when too much bone tissue is broken down. In response, the body increases the rate at which new bone forms. However, the new bone is laid down in a disordered pattern and may be softer and weaker than normal bone. The result of Paget's disease is somewhat like that of osteoporosis in that the bones grow weak and may become deformed and even fracture.

Most cases of Paget's disease of bone are diagnosed in persons between the ages of 50 and 70 years, although in rare instances it has been found in young adults. Occasionally, it runs in families.

Diagnosis

If your physician suspects that you have Paget's disease of the bone, blood and urine tests can determine whether the amounts of by-products from the bone breakdown process are higher than normal. Your physician may also order traditional X-rays and bone scans (see page 1336). Occasionally, a physician may do a bone biopsy to obtain a sample of affected bone tissue to aid in determining appropriate treatment.

How Serious Is Paget's Disease of Bone?

Many people with the disease have no symptoms. In fact, it may be discovered by accident with a routine X-ray or blood test.

In persons with symptoms, usually only one area of the body is affected, most likely the spine, skull, pelvis, thighs, or lower legs. However, multiple sites can be involved. The affected bones can become deformed and subject to fracture. In most cases, the disease tends to progress very slowly.

In rare cases, serious, long-term complications range from deafness to congestive heart failure. Rarely, a malignancy of the bone may develop.

Treatment

If you don't have symptoms, you probably won't need treatment. If you have symptoms, your physician may recommend a medication.

Medication

In its early stages, treatment to reduce pain and inflammation is all that is required. Aspirin and other mild analgesic and anti-inflammatory drugs are sufficient. If the dis-

Endocrine Disorders and the Bones

Your endocrine system controls various functions of your body. Consisting of glands that secrete hormones, the endocrine system affects virtually all body functions and parts. Your bones are no exception. Each of the following disorders affects the bone.

Acromegaly
This condition is the result of the pituitary gland secreting too much growth hormone. It occurs in adulthood. Persons with acromegaly have characteristically large hands, feet, jawbone, and skull (see page 942).

Gigantism
Gigantism is a rare ailment that also is caused by too much growth hormone. It occurs in children and results in accelerated growth and excessive adult height (see page 942).

Hypopituitarism
Children whose pituitary glands produce too little growth hormone suffer from hypopituitarism. This disorder results in dwarfism (see page 943).

Hyperparathyroidism
In this condition, the body produces too much parathyroid hormone. One result is that the bones release too much calcium, which may cause a weakening of the skeleton with cystic changes (see page 951).

however, the bone tissue is fibrous rather than bony. Typically, it first appears in childhood. The cause of fibrous dysplasia is unknown. This disorder may affect one bone or several bones. One form of fibrous dysplasia is associated with premature sexual maturation in girls (Albright's syndrome; see Sexual Precocity, page 135).

Diagnosis
Your physician will confirm the presence of fibrous dysplasia with X-rays of your bone or with a bone biopsy, in which samples of bone tissue are removed for laboratory examination (see page 1332).

Treatment
Although fibrous dysplasia is not curable, excess fibrous growths may be removed surgically from affected bones. Bone grafts also may be necessary.

Osteogenesis Imperfecta

Signs and Symptoms
- Fragile bones resulting in fractures
- The white part of the eyes (sclera) is deep blue or black
- Limb deformities, particularly bowing
- Flatfeet
- Short stature

Osteogenesis imperfecta is a rare inherited disease in which bones are abnormally brittle and fragile. Fractures may occur at birth or later when the child begins to walk. Hearing impairment is common during adolescence and later in life.

There are various forms of the disease. In the less severe forms there is often a marked reduction in the number of fractures once a child reaches adolescence.

Diagnosis
The diagnosis is made with X-ray studies of the bones.

How Serious Is Osteogenesis Imperfecta?
The most severe forms of osteogenesis imperfecta are often fatal. Many children with severe disease die of cardiorespiratory complications during infancy or childhood.

Treatment
The treatment for less severe forms of this disease involves reducing the risk of frac-

ease progresses, etidronate is an effective medication for mild pain or deformity. It is usually given in 6-month courses. In the near future newer and more effective drugs will be available. Calcitonin hormone is another effective medication but requires injection and is expensive.

Surgery
When deformities occur, an operation may be required. This, however, is uncommon.

Fibrous Dysplasia

Signs and Symptoms
- Bone pain, especially in the lower part of your leg
- Difficulty in walking
- Rarely, fractures and multiple bone deformities
- Often, fibrous dysplasia will cause no symptoms

This disorder bears some resemblance to Paget's disease (see page 897), because it is characterized by abnormal cystic growth of bone tissue. In the case of fibrous dysplasia,

tures. It is important to set all fractures promptly and to correct skeletal deformities. Genetic counseling should be considered before another pregnancy.

Osteomyelitis

Signs and Symptoms
- Intense pain and a sensation of heat at the site of the affected bone
- Tenderness and swelling
- Fever
- Fatigue

Osteomyelitis is an infection of bone caused by bacteria (or rarely fungi); it can lead to destruction of bone and surrounding tissue. The infection may be introduced as you sustain a wound, fracture, or other injury. It also may be carried to the bone via the blood.

Osteomyelitis is more common in children than adults, but it is now rare in the United States. It usually can be treated successfully with antibiotic drugs, but it can recur.

Diagnosis
If your physician suspects osteomyelitis, a blood test, traditional X-ray, a bone scan (see page 1336), or needle biopsy (see page 1332) may help with the diagnosis. Your physician also may need a surgical biopsy of the bone, in which a sample of the bone, pus, or other tissue from the deep abscess is removed for laboratory examination.

Treatment
An extended course (3 weeks or more) of antibiotics is the usual treatment. Bed rest and immobilization of the affected bones are also recommended. In some instances, it may be necessary to surgically remove the infected tissues.

Bone Tumors

Signs and Symptoms
- A hard lump on the surface of a bone
- Accompanying pain
- Fractures of the bone

Tumors that begin in bones are rare. If cancerous, the malignant cells often have traveled (metastasized) from a cancer elsewhere in the body. The exceptions are a blood cancer called multiple myeloma that begins in the bone marrow (see Multiple Myeloma, page 973) and osteosarcoma, which is the most common primary bone malignancy.

Both of these diseases are much less common than metastatic bone cancers. More often, bone tumors prove to be benign.

Diagnosis
X-rays are helpful, but they may not yield a firm diagnosis. In order to rule out a malignancy, your physician may do a biopsy, in which a small sample of the tissue is removed for laboratory examination.

How Serious Is a Bone Tumor?
A benign growth rarely presents any health risk. If the tumor is the result of a cancer that has metastasized from another site or is a bone malignancy, the survival rate varies.

Treatment
Benign tumors occasionally require surgical removal.

The cancerous bone tissue of osteosarcoma is removed surgically and anticancer drugs are prescribed. Sometimes the limb can be preserved by removing the diseased portion of the bone and reconstructing the arm or leg. This is followed by a program of rehabilitation.

Back Pain

More than 33 separate bones form your backbone, the flexible column that runs from the base of your skull to your tailbone. These bones, the vertebrae, are stacked on top of one another. In the spaces between your vertebrae are spongy cushions called discs, which have a strong, fibrous outer covering that protects a gel on the inside. The entire assembly of vertebrae and discs is held together by a network of ligaments and muscles.

The intricate structure of your back is a remarkable piece of engineering: it bends and twists and bears the weight of your body and the loads you carry. Your backbone also

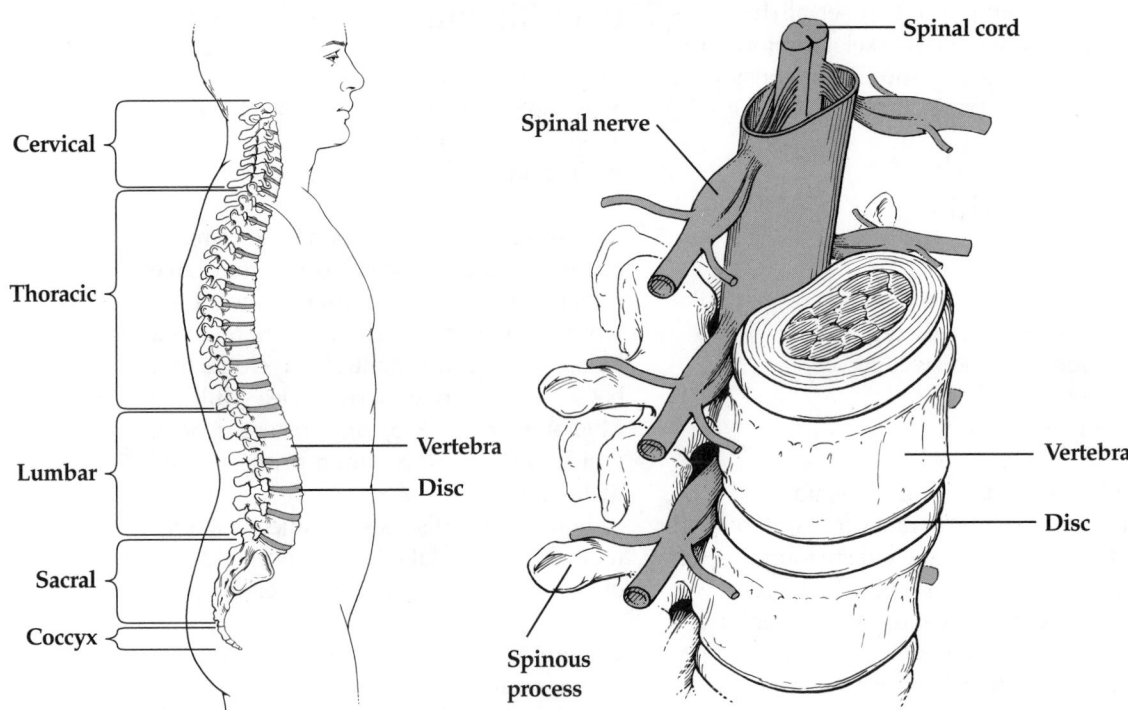

Cervical

Thoracic

Lumbar

Sacral

Coccyx

Vertebra

Disc

Spinal cord

Spinal nerve

Spinous process

Vertebra

Disc

protects your spinal cord, the main pathway for your central nervous system.

The complexity of the structure of your back contributes to the potential for problems. Seemingly minor changes in the alignment or balance of any part—whether a disc, a vertebra, or muscles—can make movements painful. When the nerves or spinal cord that travel through your backbone (spinal canal) are affected, there is a risk of pain or numbness in any part of your body, because virtually your entire skeleton is served by these nerves. If you injure your back seriously, you risk permanent damage to your spinal cord and resulting paralysis (see Spinal Injuries, page 448).

The following pages consider back problems from the simple backache nearly everyone experiences occasionally to rarer ailments such as spondylosis. We provide strategies to help you avoid back pain and injuries—and to deal with them if they occur.

Strains and Spasms

Signs and Symptoms—Back pain and stiffness

Most often back pain is caused by a simple muscle or ligament pull or strain. Lifting a barbell improperly can lead to back pain. So can a sneeze. Stress can be a factor. Sometimes there's no apparent cause.

Back pain can occur at any point on your spine, but the most common point is in the lower back. Back problems are among the most common ailments of humankind. Young or old, male or female, short or tall, most Americans experience some back discomfort in their lifetimes.

Diagnosis

Your physician will first review your medical history and perform a physical examination. If there's reason to suspect a spinal problem, your physician may recommend diagnostic studies to eliminate problems such as a prolapsed disc (see page 904) or spondylosis (see page 906).

Sometimes you may feel pain at the very moment you strain the muscle or ligament. At other times a gradual soreness may develop. You may even awaken to a discomfort. Regardless of how the pain develops, it is often difficult for your physician to determine the cause. Your physician will want to know whether you have a history of back problems.

How Serious Are Strains and Spasms?

There's no denying the discomfort that accompanies a sore back. Simply going about daily life can seem like agony, or you may be immobilized.

Usually, the problem will subside given time and rest, although recurring episodes of back discomfort are the rule rather than the exception. Every person is different, but a combination of simple preventive measures, including good posture, may help you to avoid, or minimize, future back problems.

Prevention

Certain everyday activities put your back at risk for injury. Lifting is one obvious example, but how you sleep and sit can also be critical to the health of your back. Here are some simple strategies to consider.

Exercise

Regular exercise is your most potent weapon against back problems. Activity can increase your aerobic capacity, improve your overall fitness, and help you shed excess pounds that stress your back.

Stretching and toning your back and other supporting muscles can help reduce wear and tear on your back. Stretching reduces your risk of injury by warming up your muscles. It also increases your long-term flexibility.

Strength training can make your arms, legs, and lower body stronger. In turn, your risk for falls and other injuries decreases.

Strong arms, legs, and especially abdominal muscles also help relieve back strain. If you have osteoporosis, back strengthening exercises may help prevent additional compression fractures (see Osteoporosis, page 894).

Ask your physician or a physical therapist for advice before beginning an exercise program, especially if you've hurt your back before or if you have other health problems, such as significant osteoporosis.

Start slowly. If you're out of condition from lack of activity, your back muscles may be weak and susceptible to injury. Pace yourself and don't overdo. As you become stronger, work up to 15 minutes of exercise daily.

Make smart moves. Generally, swimming and other water exercises are safest for your back. Because they're non-weight-bearing, these activities place minimal strain on your lower back. Workouts on a stationary bike, treadmill, or cross-country ski machine are less jarring to your back than running on hard surfaces. Bicycling is a good option, too. However, be sure to adjust the height of the seat and handlebars, so that you assume good posture while pedaling. If you golf, protect your back by shortening your backswing.

Avoid high-risk moves. You may need to avoid or modify activities, especially if you've had back problems. Avoid movements that cause you to exaggerate the stretch of your muscles. For example, don't try to touch your toes with your legs straight. Activities that involve a lot of twisting, quick stops and starts, and contact sports pose the greatest risks to your back.

Lifting

Bend your knees, not your back. Whether the object you want to pick up weighs a frac-

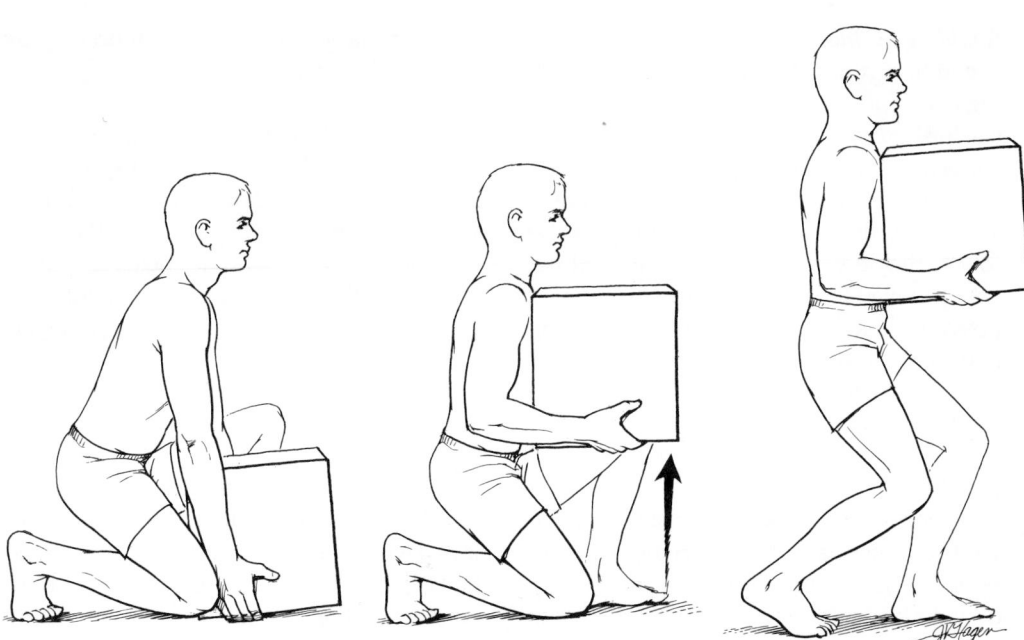

When lifting any object, let your legs do the work. Bend your knees rather than your back. Hold the object close to your body and lift gently. Avoid jerking or lunging upward.

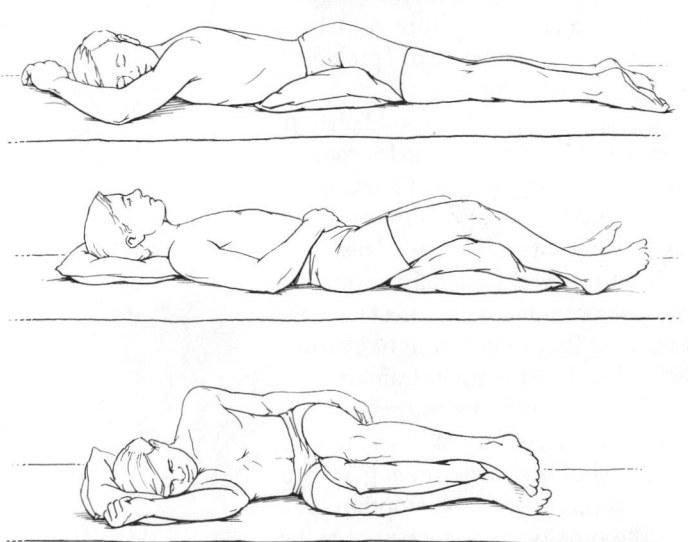

To avoid aggravating your backache when you sleep or lie down, sleep on your stomach only if your abdomen is cushioned by a pillow (top). If you sleep on your back, support your knees and neck with pillows (middle). Best option: sleep on your side with your legs drawn up slightly toward your chest (bottom), with a pillow between your knees.

tion of an ounce or a hundred pounds, squat with your back straight and let your legs do the lifting. Bring tension on your muscles gradually: don't jerk or lunge to lift the load.

Sleeping

Lying down provides relief for backache—and also an opportunity for backache prevention. Don't sleep on your stomach unless your abdomen is cushioned by a pillow; sleep on your side with your legs bent and drawn up slightly toward your chest. Make sure your mattress provides your back with proper support (use a bed board of ½-inch plywood under the mattress if the mattress is too soft or sags).

Avoiding Stiffness

If you find yourself seated at a desk, standing in one position, or behind the wheel of a car for hours every day, you are at risk for stiffness and muscle fatigue. Make it a point to break the routine at frequent intervals. When standing, shift your weight from one foot to the other periodically; when sitting, get up—even for a few seconds—as often as possible. Take frequent breaks when driving and get out and stretch. A small pillow placed at the base of your back can also help support your spine.

Weight Loss

One important cause of backache in the United States is being overweight: extra pounds at the midriff put strains and stresses on your back. If you are overweight, try to

reduce and to establish an appropriate exercise program (see page 289).

Posture

Parents, teachers, and drill sergeants alike are famous for ordering their wards to stand up or to sit up straight. Like it or not, it's excellent advice. People who both stand up and sit up straight all day, every day, are at less risk for backache because poor posture is one of the more common causes of backache.

What Is Poor Posture?

One extreme is the slouch, in which the shoulders are rolled forward (called kyphosis). In people who perpetually slouch, the muscles of the chest are shortened and flexibility is reduced. In the opposite postural extreme, the swayback (also known as lordosis), the stomach sticks out too far in front and the buttocks too far in the rear—and the backbone takes on an exaggerated curve between the pelvis and ribs (the lumbar region). Such a swaybacked posture puts much pressure on the lower back and contributes to back problems.

What Is Good Posture?

Imagine that strings connect your ears to the bones that protrude from your ankles. Now, starting with your knees bent and shoulders hunched, pull those theoretical strings taut by standing up. When you stand as straight as possible, the string should extend up your leg just behind the kneecap and across the meat of your thigh and pass by the tip of your shoulder.

Ways that you can achieve good posture are described below.

Attention! The military stance may seem a bit exaggerated, but you should apply some of its rules to your upright posture. Keeping your backbone straight is an obvious one; holding your shoulders back helps too. Don't forget to pull in your stomach and buttocks, trimming your profile, and pull in your chin.

Sit Up Straight! A slouched posture when seated can only aggravate back discomfort. In general, sitting puts more stress on your back than standing does.

Sit in chairs with either straight backs or low-back (lumbar) support. The seat should be high enough that your thighs rest horizontally on the seat. That way, your weight

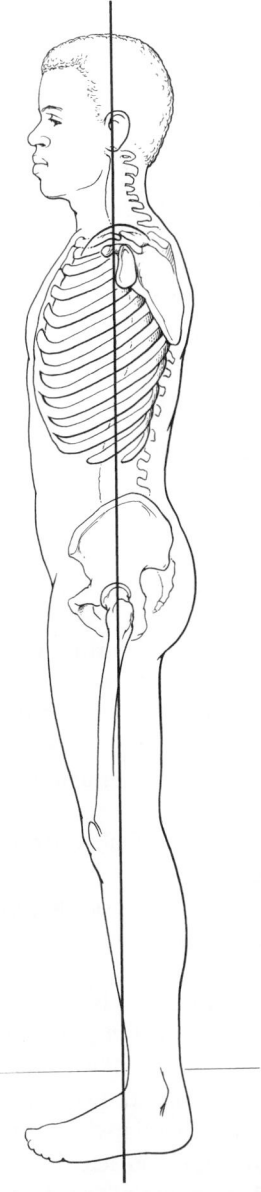

For proper posture, stand straight and imagine that a string extends from your earlobe to your instep.

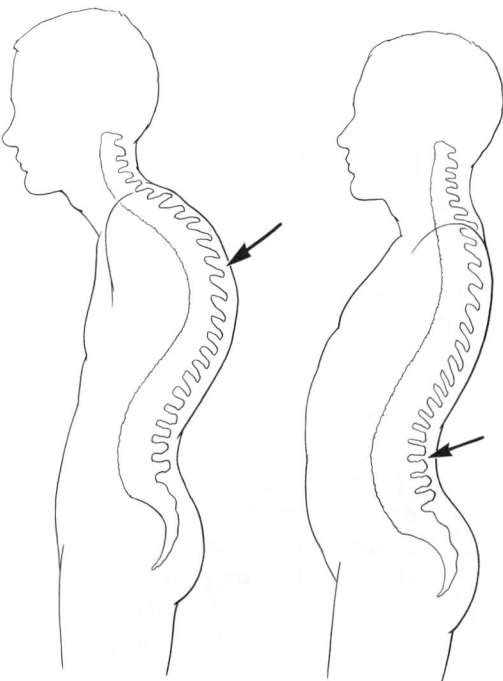

Common forms of improper posture are kyphosis, left, in which shoulders roll forward, and lordosis, right, sway-backed posture.

is more evenly distributed and your back isn't forced to assume a disproportionate amount of your weight.

Wear Proper Footwear. Wear shoes that provide good support. High heels, in particular, put stress on your back. So, to help avoid backache, wear shoes with low or flat heels.

Practice Good Posture. It isn't enough to know what good posture is. You have to practice it. Of course, it isn't easy to change years of bad habits, but you must concentrate on maintaining a proper upright posture at all times.

Treatment

The causes of back pain are numerous, ranging from minor strains and sprains to a slipped disc (see Prolapsed Disc, page 904) and various chronic problems of the spine. Although diagnosing the precise cause isn't easy, it is important to rule out certain potential underlying causes. Therefore, be sure to see your physician when you have back pain.

Most back spasms or simple strains require rest, and in a few days you will be able to return to normal activities. In the meantime, there are various possible treatments. Surgery is rarely the preferred treatment for backache, but if more conservative treatments such as rest or heat or ice and therapeutic exercise fail (see Self-Help, below), your physician may refer you to a neurologist, neurosurgeon, physiatrist, or orthopedic surgeon for a more comprehensive evaluation of your condition.

Self-Help

Because most back problems aren't life-threatening, physicians frequently recommend home treatment first. Episodes of back pain usually resolve within 2 weeks with simple measures such as rest and over-the-counter pain relievers. Regardless of the type of treatment, 80 to 90 percent of back pain resolves within 6 weeks. Strained ligaments or severe muscle strain may require up to 12 weeks to heal. But with time and proper care, even a herniated disc can repair itself.

Sources of heat and cold (hot baths, hot and cold compresses) can soothe sore and inflamed muscles. Use cold treatments first, several times a day, for no longer than 20 minutes each time. Use ice, wrapped first in a plastic bag, then in a cloth or towel (to protect your skin). After the acute pain subsides (usually 1 or 2 days), apply heat with a heating pad or heat lamp. Limit heat applications to 20 minutes, using care to avoid a burn.

Medication

Pain relievers such as acetaminophen, ibuprofen, or aspirin can help ease your pain. Depending on your diagnosis, your physician also may prescribe stronger pain killers or muscle relaxants. If the pain is localized in one definable area, your physician may inject a corticosteroid drug (see Corticosteroid Drugs, page 919).

Physical Therapy

Your physician or physical therapist can design specific treatment and exercise programs for you. An exercise that might help one person could harm another. So be sure to follow instructions.

Basic therapy includes application of alternating heat and cold and gentle massage to your back. For some disorders, braces, corsets, or mechanical traction can help. These measures may take some of the pressure off the affected area. In addition, exercises to stretch and strengthen the muscles of your back reduce the risk of future back

problems. Again, because needs vary, see your physician or physical therapist for specific instructions.

Surgery

If none of the other approaches provide relief, your physician may refer you to a neurologist, neurosurgeon, or orthopedic surgeon. Do not take spinal surgery lightly. Try the more conservative approaches first because an operation is required in less than 1 percent of all cases of back pain.

Prolapsed Disc

Signs and Symptoms
- Mild to severe pain in your back or neck
- If the prolapsed disc is in your neck, numbness or weakness of an arm or hand may occur; often, serious neck, shoulder, and upper extremity pain is present
- If the damaged disc is in the middle or lower part of your back, numbness or weakness may occur in the buttocks, legs, or feet
- A shooting pain that occurs if you cough, sneeze, or strain
- Usually one arm or one leg is affected significantly more than the other arm or leg

The discs are the pads located between the bones (vertebrae) of your spine. When one of the discs ruptures, the resulting condition is called a prolapsed disc. This disorder is also known as herniated disc or slipped disc (although there is no actual slippage).

The discs contain a soft, jelly-like substance. Age or strain may cause the disc to develop a bulge (herniate). This places pressure on nearby nerves, which causes pain, numbness, or weakness.

A prolapsed disc is most likely to occur in the lower back, although any disc can be affected. The condition rarely occurs in children.

Diagnosis
Your physician may order a series of X-rays, a CT scan (see page 1334), or an MRI scan (see page 1334) following a careful physical examination. These tests help to determine the extent of the injury and also to rule out other conditions that cause similar symptoms, such as a spinal tumor or a circulatory problem (see pages 508 and 690, respectively). The material protruding from the

---

Corsets: Comfort and Cautions

You can obtain back support braces and corsets either by prescription or over the counter at most full-service pharmacies and medical supply stores. Worn properly, they relieve strain by restricting motion in your lower back when you sit or stand. They also can provide warmth, comfort, and support to your back.

Unfortunately, to give enough support, many back braces and corsets have stiff stays and uncomfortable shoulder straps. They can be unattractive and expensive. Also, because the support comes from the corset rather than from your own muscles, a corset may actually weaken your back muscles, especially if you wear it for long periods. Most experts recommend using braces and corsets for short periods or only during back-straining activities.

disc is not visible on routine X-rays, but sometimes it can be seen on an MRI or CT scan. Another X-ray test called myelography (see page 510), which requires injection of a dye into your spinal column, may better define an abnormality suspected but not clearly seen on the CT or MRI scan.

An electrodiagnostic study of your nerve conduction pathways can confirm nerve compression caused by a herniated disc or spinal stenosis. This test is called electromyography (EMG) (see page 1344).

To rule out a bone tumor or a compression fracture caused by osteoporosis, your physician may recommend a bone scan.

To perform a bone scan, the physician injects a radioactive substance called a tracer into a vein, and a special camera is used to identify or rule out a tumor or fracture.

How Serious Is a Prolapsed Disc?
In many people, a prolapsed disc will repair itself if given time (usually 2 to 6 weeks) and proper rest (sometimes complete bed rest). In some instances, you may need an operation.

Treatment
The most common prescription for a prolapsed disc is decreased activity and, in some cases, bed rest. Physicians often recommend two weeks of such a regimen (see Strains and Spasms, page 900). After 1 or 2 weeks of markedly decreased activity, you can usually resume activity slowly and progressively. Conservative physical therapy measures such as the use of heat or ice, massage, gentle exercises, and sometimes traction may be helpful.

Surgery
Sometimes nerve compression from disc protrusion does not resolve with rest. In such cases, a surgical procedure called a laminectomy may be necessary to remove the disc or the part of the disc that is compressing the nerve.

In the lower back, this procedure usually is done by making an incision in the back, removing a small amount of bone covering the disc, and then removing part of the disc material. All of the disc cannot be removed when approached from the back.

Although a similar procedure is sometimes done in the neck or upper back, occasionally it is desirable to remove the disc by approaching it from the front of the torso. In

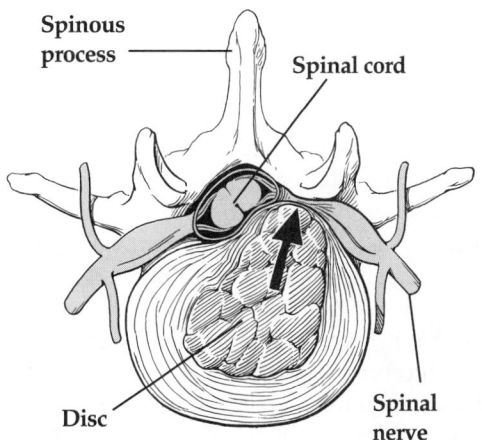

If one of the discs in your back ruptures, a portion of the disc's jelly-like interior can be displaced, putting pressure on a spinal nerve (as shown in cross-section at left) or on the spinal cord. This condition is variously known as a prolapsed, ruptured, herniated, or, more commonly, a slipped disc.

this case, it is not necessary to remove any bone, and a larger amount of disc can be removed. When this approach is used, physicians often consider fusing together the vertebrae on either side of the damaged disc.

These two operative procedures require an incision, leave a surgical scar, and, of course, require a period of wound healing. Nevertheless, they allow the surgeon to see directly the nerve that is being compressed and to remove the disc, ligament, bone, or other material that is compressing it.

Other Therapies
In an effort to avoid the surgical incision and decrease recovery time, physicians may try two other options for a carefully selected group of patients with nerve compression from disc protrusion.

Chymopapain, an enzyme derived from the tropical papaya tree, can be injected into the disc. It causes the disc to shrink, reduc-

---

Sciatica

Of 100 people with back pain, only 1 or 2 people may experience sciatica, named after the sciatic nerve that extends down each leg from your hip to your heel. Nerve inflammation or compression of a nerve root in your lower back can cause sciatica. You may feel the pain radiating from your back down through your buttock to your lower leg.

Tingling, numbness, or muscle weakness may also accompany nerve compression. Coughing, sneezing, and other activities that exert pressure on your spine can aggravate sciatica. Usually, the pain resolves on its own. However, severe nerve compression can cause progressive muscle weakness.

ing the pressure on the nearby nerve and, in many cases, eliminating the pain. The use of this procedure has decreased significantly during the past decade.

Another procedure, called percutaneous discectomy, allows the disc to be removed from between the vertebrae with a mechanical device that fits into a large needle. The physician inserts this large needle through the skin into the disc, much like the needle used to inject chymopapain into the disc.

Unfortunately, sometimes the nerve compression cannot be relieved with chymopapain or the percutaneous technique. In other patients, the nerve compression is not necessarily due to disc material. In these cases, the more conventional surgical procedure may be the only solution.

Spondylosis

Signs and Symptoms
- Back pain
- Tenderness and difficulty in moving your back
- Pain in the back of your thighs
- Mild cases of spondylosis are usually symptomless

Spondylosis is a disorder in which the spine, over time, becomes stiff and loses flexibility. The name is derived from the Greek words for "vertebra," *spondylos*, and "condition," *osis*.

The cause can be excessive use, injury, or simply the aging process. Whatever the cause, the discs between the vertebrae become worn, and the spaces between the vertebrae narrow. Bony spurs also can develop. The result is the pain and stiffness of spondylosis.

Spondylosis is sometimes referred to as degenerative joint disease or osteoarthritis of the spine. However, you should not confuse it with ankylosing spondylitis (see page 913).

Diagnosis
An X-ray of your spine will determine the condition of the discs and vertebrae. If you have had problems with prolapsed discs, you may be more susceptible to spondylosis.

How Serious Is Spondylosis?
For most people, living with spondylosis is a matter of developing strategies for dealing with the discomfort, although in rare cases,

spondylosis in the lower back can lead to difficulty in urinating, defecating, and walking (see Lumbar Stenosis, this page).

Treatment
Your physician is unlikely to be able to offer a simple solution. Likely recommendations include a combination of an analgesic drug such as aspirin, physical therapy, and other self-help approaches.

Lumbar Stenosis

Signs and Symptoms
- Pain in the buttock, thigh, and calf associated with walking and standing
- Pain stops with sitting or bending forward

Lumbar stenosis can result from either arthritic changes or a congenital narrowing of your spine that produces a compression of the lower end of the spinal canal. Symptoms can be similar to those caused by blockage of the arteries to the lower extremities (see Arteriosclerosis of the Extremities, page 690).

Diagnosis
Your physician will examine the arteries of your lower legs and may order special tests to make sure the arteries are functioning properly. If these vascular studies are normal, your physician may order a CT scan, an MRI scan, or a myelogram of the spine to determine whether your spinal canal is narrowed.

Treatment
If symptoms persist, you may need to consult a specialist to consider whether you need an operation (called a laminectomy) to relieve pressure on the spinal nerves.

Scoliosis

Signs and Symptoms
- A sideways curvature of the spine
- Asymmetric rib cage with one shoulder blade protruding

Scoliosis is a painless, abnormal curvature of the spine (from the Greek word *skoliosis*, meaning "curvature"). Usually a curve to one side develops, followed by a compensating bend in the opposite direction.

Congenital defects of the spine cause scoliosis in only a small percentage of cases. Most cases are of unknown origin, probably traceable to genetic factors. The deformity may begin during infancy (more often in boys) or in the preschool years and immediately after. Often, however, the signs go undetected until adolescence. Adolescent girls are more likely to have scoliosis than boys. Because the onset is gradual and not associated with pain, significant curvature can develop without the child or parent knowing it.

Diagnosis

A visual examination is usually sufficient to recognize the condition, although your physician may want to X-ray your spine to determine the extent of the curvature. Many schools have screening programs to detect this disorder.

How Serious Is Scoliosis?

Scoliosis may be a chronic and progressive disorder. Mild cases need close follow-up, generally cause few problems, and do not need treatment.

In more significant scoliosis, the vertebrae at the scoliotic curve may rotate, resulting in widely separated ribs on one side of the body and narrowed spaces on the other. In severe cases, lung problems may develop over a period of many years.

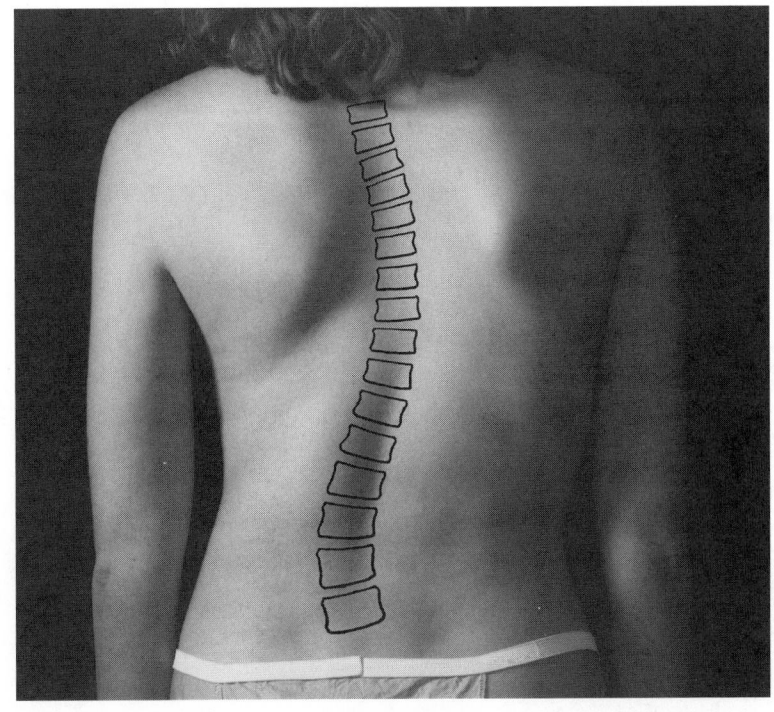

Treatment

Once scoliosis is diagnosed, close observation is required. In general, exercises have no effect on scoliosis. Small curves do not require special treatment. If curves become more pronounced, treatment with a brace will be required, especially in growing young people. More severe curvature may require surgery by a specialist in this disorder.

A sideways curvature of the spine is called scoliosis.

Joint Disorders

A layer of resilient tissue called cartilage cushions the ends of your bones that meet in a joint. The cartilage has a very smooth surface. Surrounding the joint space is a membrane called the synovial membrane. This membrane produces synovial fluid to lubricate the joint. Surrounding this membrane is a fibrous, protective casing called the capsule. Bands of fibrous tissue called ligaments bind all the parts of a joint together.

Problems that occur in the joints may be the result of mechanical failure of the parts (as with osteoarthritis, the so-called wear-and-tear arthritis). Often, however, the cause of joint disorders is an inflammation pro-

duced by infection, disease, or some unknown cause. Most joint ailments caused by inflammation are termed arthritis, from the Greek words *arthron*, for "joint," and *itis*, for "inflammation." The following pages outline the common and some of the more unusual varieties of arthritis.

Osteoarthritis

Signs and Symptoms

- Pain in a joint during or after use
- Discomfort in a joint before or during a change in the weather

Heberden's nodes are bony lumps at the ends of fingers. They occur most often in women and may be a sign of osteoarthritis. Although initially painful, Heberden's nodes are of little more than cosmetic concern.

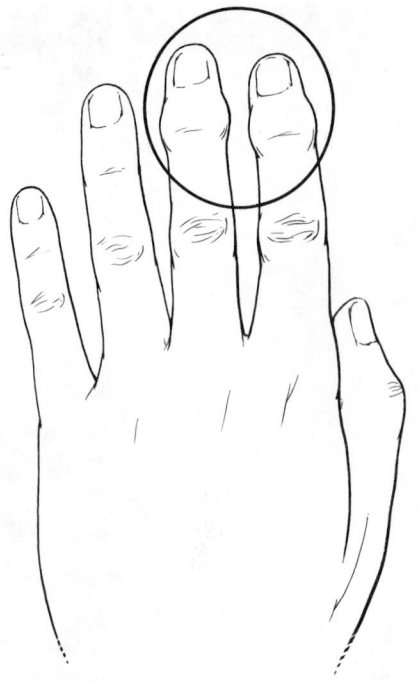

- Swelling and a loss of flexibility in a joint
- Bony lumps on the end joint of the finger (called Heberden's nodes) may develop. Similar lumps on the middle joint of the finger (called Bouchard's nodes) also may develop

Osteoarthritis is one of the most common disorders known to humankind. People have recognized it for centuries, and it affects tens of millions of Americans. Many elderly people have osteoarthritis but don't realize it until their physician recognizes it on a routine X-ray. Many affected persons have a family history of osteoarthritis.

If the knee or hip is involved, osteoarthritis initially strikes only one joint; if the fingers are affected, multiple joints often become arthritic.

Although we don't know the precise mechanisms, it is clear that wear and tear is a principal cause of osteoarthritis. This explains the alternative names for osteoarthritis: degenerative joint disease and wear-and-tear arthritis (osteoarthrosis, another term, is used interchangeably with osteoarthritis). Thus, the athlete who sustains joint injuries and the laborer whose joints are challenged every day by demanding physical activity are both at heightened risk of developing arthritic joints later in life.

Here's what occurs in the joint of a person with osteoarthritis. The cartilage that cushions the impact on the joint gradually deteriorates. Its smooth surface roughens, and it loses its cushioning effect. Over time, the ends of the bones also are affected, as bone grows along the sides of the bone to produce lumps. Each of the steps in this process produces pain.

Osteoarthritis commonly occurs in your neck or back. The usual progression involves the development of bone spurs on the sides of a damaged vertebra, as seen on X-rays of the bone. Osteoarthritis also commonly affects the knee and hip. In young people, osteoarthritis is relatively rare, although osteoarthritis of the knee is not uncommon in young adults.

Diagnosis

The presence of pain in either one or a few joints is a key to the diagnosis of osteoarthritis; the sheer prevalence of the disorder is another. Bone spurs (called osteophytes) may be evident in an X-ray of the affected joint, indicating the presence of osteoarthritis. Blood tests can exclude rheumatoid or other forms of arthritis.

Another clue may be the presence of Heberden's or Bouchard's nodes, bony lumps that appear over a period of years in the end and middle joints of your fingers. Your physician may inquire whether your parents also had them because there is apparently a genetic tendency for Heberden's nodes. Women have them about 10 times as often as men.

How Serious Is Osteoarthritis?

Osteoarthritis doesn't go away, although the pain tends to fade within a year of its appearance. Over time, the ends of the bones that rub together (after the breakdown of the cartilage) become polished in a process called eburnation. Still, the effects of osteoarthritis are crippling in only rare cases.

Age is a significant factor in the disorder: it is more likely in elderly people than in young people, and some joints tend to be more affected over time.

Treatment

Exercise

Although osteoarthritis is a wear-and-tear disease, appropriate exercise can be a valuable treatment approach. A physician or a physical therapist (if your physician refers you to one) should advise you on an exercise program, but range-of-motion and muscle strengthening exercises can help you prevent future problems and avoid stiffness.

Other Therapies

Consult your physician about the use of heating pads, hot water bottles, and hot baths. If your neck is affected by osteoarthritis, your physician may prescribe a cervical collar for acute episodes.

Weight control can be an invaluable adjunct to other treatments: excessive weight puts unnecessary pressure on the joints and can exacerbate the condition. Good posture also can be an aid, especially for osteoarthritis of the spine (see What Is Good Posture? page 902).

Medication

Aspirin is one of the most effective drugs for treating arthritis. If you don't tolerate aspirin well, many other anti-inflammatory drugs or acetaminophen can reduce the pain and discomfort.

If inflammation is severe, your physician may recommend an injection of a corticosteroid drug. This is most likely for cases in which a weight-bearing joint, such as a knee or ankle, is affected (see Corticosteroid Drugs, page 919).

Surgery

When long-term deterioration has occurred, a hip or knee replacement operation may create a useful joint (see Joint Replacement, page 911). If the joints in your hands have deteriorated significantly, an operation also may be appropriate.

Rheumatoid Arthritis

Signs and Symptoms

- Pain and swelling in the smaller joints of your hands and feet
- Overall aching or stiffness, especially after sleeping or periods of motionlessness
- Affected joints are swollen, painful, and warm to the touch during the initial attack and ensuing flare-ups

Rheumatoid arthritis, unlike the more common osteoarthritis (see page 907), is not the natural result of time and the wear and tear of normal use. Rather, it is probably an autoimmune disease in which your body's immune system attacks itself. We don't understand this well yet. Researchers suspect that an unidentified virus stimulates the immune system, but the disease-fighting cells inflame the joints.

Baker's Cyst

Rheumatoid arthritis can lead to the development of a painless cyst that appears on the back of your knee. If this occurs, the lining (synovium) of your knee joint is producing too much fluid. This synovial fluid can build up and break through the lining and move to the back of your knee, or push the lining out, creating the characteristic bulge of a cyst.

Baker's cyst was named after William Morrant Baker, a British surgeon. Other names include popliteal bursitis and synovial cyst of the popliteal space.

Your physician may draw the fluid out with a needle and syringe or remove it surgically after giving you a local anesthetic. Sometimes a drug to reduce inflammation (hydrocortisone) is injected to help prevent a recurrence.

Unlike osteoarthritis, which affects only the musculoskeletal system, rheumatoid arthritis is a systemic disease that, in some patients, affects such organs as the heart, lungs, and eyes. It also tends to affect more than one joint at a time, resulting in an overall stiffness and aching. It is generally symmetric in its assaults, affecting both feet or both hands. It also may produce small lumps, called rheumatoid nodules, under the skin near the elbow, the ears or nose, the back of the scalp, over the knee, or under the toes. They range in size from that of a pea to perhaps that of a walnut. Usually the lumps are not painful and present no physical problem.

The disease can strike at any time, but most often it develops between ages 20 and 50 years. (A variant of rheumatoid arthritis called juvenile rheumatoid arthritis is dis-

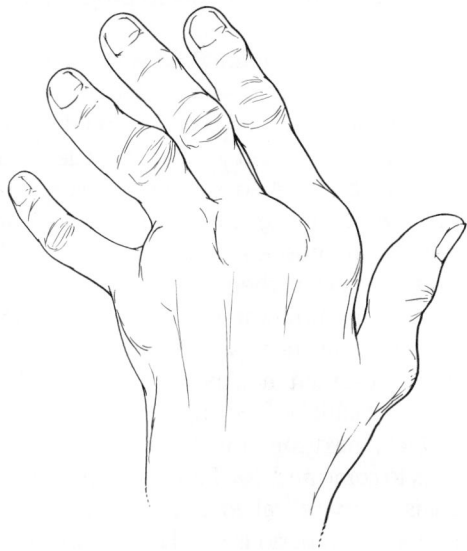

Rheumatoid arthritis can lead to a deformity in the fingers. The hand may lose strength and be painful during flare-ups of the disease.

cussed on page 911.) Roughly 3 times as many women as men have rheumatoid arthritis. An estimated 7 million Americans have the ailment.

Diagnosis

The principal area of attack of rheumatoid arthritis is the synovium, the membrane that lines your joints (for discussion of the configuration of a joint and its parts, see page 862). Rheumatoid arthritis causes this smooth membrane to become inflamed. Researchers have discovered that the disease-fighting cells of the immune system are especially active in the synovial tissues of patients with rheumatoid arthritis.

Accompanying the inflammation of the synovium are other changes in your joints. Tissue in the cartilage tends to proliferate, which also produces an erosion of surrounding tissues, including ligaments, muscles, and bones. In addition to contributing to the discomforts of rheumatoid arthritis, these changes also produce a looseness in your joints.

If your physician suspects you have rheumatoid arthritis, he or she will conduct a thorough physical examination. Your physician will try to establish whether you have discomfort on both sides of your body. If so, a diagnosis of rheumatoid arthritis is likely. Laboratory tests can confirm the diagnosis.

A special blood test that determines the erythrocyte sedimentation rate (see page 1331) helps confirm the presence of rheumatoid arthritis, as does another blood test for an antibody called rheumatoid factor. Four of five persons with rheumatoid arthritis have this abnormal antibody. As the disease advances, X-rays can follow its progression.

How Serious Is Rheumatoid Arthritis?

Rheumatoid arthritis is the most debilitating form of arthritis. People with this disease often have deformed joints, which lead to loss of mobility. Also, some people experience sweats and fevers along with loss of strength in muscles attached to affected joints. Yet, even when stricken with severe forms, the individual with rheumatoid arthritis usually retains flexibility in the joints and has less pain than the appearance of the deformed joints would suggest.

Often, the disorder is chronic, although it tends to come and go. Periods of increased disease activity, called flare-ups or flares, alternate with periods of relative remission, during which the swelling, pain, difficulty in sleeping, and weakness fade or disappear. It is difficult to predict how severe the disease will be in any one person. Persons who have more or less continuous symptoms for 4 or 5 years are more likely to have a lifetime of problems with the disease. Some of them will have "burned-out" rheumatoid arthritis after 10 to 20 years. Results of the sedimentation rate test will be more normal, but joint deformities will remain, as will some pain and impaired joint function.

The cyclic nature of rheumatoid arthritis presents researchers with one of the most confusing aspects of the puzzle. There is no cure, but with proper treatment, a strategy of joint protection, and changes in lifestyle, most people are able to live long, productive, and nearly normal lives after the disease develops. However, proper medical care is essential for dealing effectively with this chronic disorder.

Treatment

Rest and Exercise

The key strategy is to establish a proper balance of rest and exercise. The preservation and restoration of function to affected joints involve muscle-building, range-of-motion, and other exercises; yet, you must maintain a suitable balance of exertion and rest. At times, the use of a splint at night is helpful.

Because of the ebb and flow of the disease, strategies used during flares and periods of remission differ. The intense disease activity of a flare-up puts you at risk of joint damage, so a combination of rest, pain reduction strategies, and even immobilization of the involved joint is usual. During flares, keep exercise of the affected joints to a minimum to avoid damaging your joints. During periods of remission, you should exercise and carry on your normal activities. Still, it is equally important to recognize your limits and avoid undue fatigue. Follow the advice of your physician or physical therapist carefully. No specific diet is useful, but observe general principles of good nutrition and avoid obesity.

Medication

Anti-inflammatory drugs, in particular aspirin, are basic to treating the pain and inflammation of rheumatoid arthritis. Corticosteroid drugs such as prednisone may be very effective for relieving pain and inflammation, but they provide no lasting benefit and they should be used with great caution because of their numerous side effects. In fact, they relieve the pain so effectively that patients may overuse their joints and suffer lasting joint deformities. Prednisone is also an ingredient in some nonapproved arthritis cures. Although such cures may give momentary relief, they also may lead to long-term harm. (See also Corticosteroid Drugs, page 919.)

Sometimes physicians use a wide variety of other drugs in an attempt to suppress inflammation and the overactive immune system. These drugs may include non-steroidal anti-inflammatory agents, antimalarial drugs, methotrexate, gold salts, and experimental medications.

Surgery

When a joint has become badly damaged or deformed, an operation may restore usefulness. Occasionally, joint replacement (see this page) may be necessary for severely eroded joints.

Juvenile Rheumatoid Arthritis

Signs and Symptoms
- Swelling and stiffness in the joints
- Fever and rash
- Fatigue and irritability
- Associated inflammation of the eye

Juvenile rheumatoid arthritis resembles rheumatoid arthritis (see page 909) but also differs in significant ways. Differences include the age of the typical patients (juvenile rheumatoid arthritis affects children, and rheumatoid arthritis affects adults) and the long-term nature of the ailment. In most cases, juvenile rheumatoid arthritis is not a lifelong disorder and its symptoms fade after several months or years.

There are several subcategories of the disorder, each with its own distinguishing characteristics. When four or fewer joints are affected, it is termed pauciarticular juvenile rheumatoid arthritis; children with this type tend to have little or no disability after several years of disease. The form called polyarticular juvenile rheumatoid arthritis is more virulent and frequently causes chronic joint problems. About one-half of children with acute juvenile rheumatoid arthritis recover completely, and one-half have chronic

Joint Replacement

When a joint disorder such as osteoarthritis or rheumatoid arthritis cripples a hip or knee joint, a surgical procedure called arthroplasty may be the best treatment.

Arthroplasty is a re-forming of the joint. The operation may simply smooth the damaged lining of a joint, but a replacement arthroplasty involves an actual replacement of certain parts of the joint itself with a plastic or metal device.

The hip is the most commonly replaced joint. In a hip arthroplasty, a ball on a stem replaces the top of the thigh bone (femur). The cup of the pelvis is also replaced with a polyethylene cup. A special glue may fasten both implants. Recent developments include artificial joints covered with a material that allows bone tissue to grow into it and a short-stem hip replacement.

Prostheses can replace knees, finger joints, and other joints. The results are generally remarkable: people who were unable to walk before their hip arthroplasty frequently leave the hospital about a week later. Although the durability of these prostheses is not yet clear, evidence to date suggests that replacement parts are durable with moderate use.

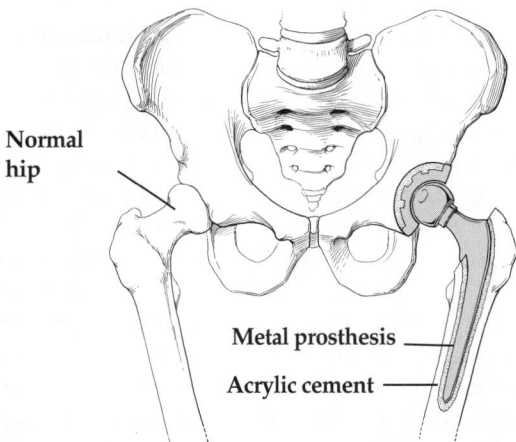

Normal hip

Metal prosthesis

Acrylic cement

At left is a normal hip. A prosthesis like the one highlighted at right can replace your joint when your hip is broken or deteriorates from arthritis or osteoporosis.

disease. The causes of juvenile rheumatoid arthritis are unknown.

Diagnosis
The disorder is diagnosed on the basis of observed symptoms, because there is no one test that confirms it. However, various blood tests may be conducted.

How Serious Is Juvenile Rheumatoid Arthritis?
As with rheumatoid arthritis, there is a risk of permanent joint damage from juvenile rheumatoid arthritis. In addition, however,

Joint Disorders of Childhood

There are numerous rare skeletal problems peculiar to children. Some of these are described below.

Legg-Calvé-Perthes Disease

This disorder (also called Perthes' disease) occurs more often in boys than in girls. It usually becomes evident between the ages of 5 and 9 years.

The result of Perthes' disease is a deterioration of the top portion of the thighbone (femoral head) due to defective circulation to that part. This is called avascular necrosis. The cause is unknown.

The child generally complains of pain in the hip and may walk with a limp. At other times, pain may be evident in the knee. An X-ray helps establish the diagnosis. In the early stages of the disease, however, conventional X-rays may appear normal. At times, an MRI scan (see page 1334) or a radionuclide study (see page 1336) is helpful.

Healing usually requires a period of 2 to 3 years. In years past, physicians recommended bed rest or a sling to keep weight off the leg and hips. More recently, because the outcome seems unrelated to these rather extreme restrictions, physicians recommend crutches or, at times, no treatment. Your physician may instruct you in physical therapy measures to keep the head of the thighbone (femur) in the hip socket. Tension, bracing, and surgery are occasionally necessary.

Most children with this disorder heal without significant deformity. Others, however, are left with a deformed hip joint that, in later adult life, may cause hip pain and

dysfunction (osteoarthritis, see page 907). In these individuals, surgery may be needed.

Slipped Capital Femoral Epiphysis

During the growth spurt just before puberty, the growth plate of the ball of the hip may slip. The thighbone rotates outward and slides upward relative to the ball of the hip. This unusual condition is called a slipped capital femoral epiphysis.

The major symptoms are pain in the knee, thigh, or hip and a limp that involves lurching to the side and outward turning of the foot. Symptoms usually evolve gradually over weeks or months, but they can also appear suddenly in association with an injury.

The capital epiphysis slips most commonly in boys between the ages of 11 and 14 years, particularly those who are overweight. In one-fourth of cases, it affects both hips.

A slipped capital epiphysis requires emergency hospitalization. If X-rays confirm the diagnosis, the child is put in traction in a hospital bed and prepared for surgery. If a slip is detected early, while it is still mild, it can be fixed with an operation in which metal pins are inserted to prevent further displacement. However, if the slip progresses until it is severe, it can deform the hip and interfere with normal walking. Even after extensive bone-cutting surgery to correct an advanced case, the child risks developing arthritis prematurely.

Osgood-Schlatter Disease

Children between 11 and 15 years,

especially boys, may have pain and swelling at the bony protuberance just below the kneecap, on the shinbone (tibia). This is the point at which tendons from the kneecap attach to the tibia. (It is also the point at which irritation from kneeling on hard surfaces can cause bursitis, known as housemaid's knee.)

Rest is usually the best treatment for Osgood-Schlatter disease and it usually resolves over time as the skeleton matures.

Congenital Dislocation of the Hip

In this condition, sometimes called developmental dysplasia of the hip, the hip socket (into which the head of the femur fits) is too shallow at birth, making the joint especially susceptible to dislocation. The problem can lead to an altered shape of the bones of the joint, which may require extensive surgery later in life.

Even if a baby appears to be entirely healthy, your physician should be on the alert for this condition during the first year of the child's life. Early diagnosis can permit simple treatment with splinting, which is usually successful. Congenital dislocation of the hip tends to recur in families, so alert your physician if you or your spouse had the condition.

Clubfoot

Technically known as talipes equinovarus, this deformity of the foot, which may be hereditary, is present at birth. It can be treated with casts or splints during the first few weeks of life, often with good results (see page 46).

the growing child also experiences abnormal bone growth. For example, the disease may accelerate growth in one leg bone but not in the other, producing one leg that is longer than the other.

Another risk is that a child will often instinctively keep an affected joint motionless to avoid pain. This can result in weakened and contracted muscles and even a deformity over time.

Treatment

In general, treatment for juvenile rheumatoid arthritis resembles that for the adult form (see page 909).

Medication

Your physician may prescribe ibuprofen, naproxen, or aspirin and other anti-inflammatory drugs.

Other Therapies

Range-of-motion exercises and splints to prevent loss of motion and deformity are used on affected joints.

There will be a delicate balance between maintaining some semblance of normal activity while providing sufficient rest to avoid fatigue and excessive stress on affected joints. During periods of severe disease activity, bed rest or tutoring at home may be necessary, but it is important, for psychological and physical reasons, to avoid isolating a child from his or her normal routine.

Surgery

If a child sustains severe joint damage, reconstructive procedures or joint replacement (see page 911) may be required, but in general it is advisable to wait until the affected joints have reached maturity.

Inflammatory Arthritis

Signs and Symptoms

Inflammatory arthritis may take one of several forms, each with somewhat different manifestations (discussed below):

Psoriatic Arthritis

- In the person with psoriasis (see page 992), an accompanying form of arthritis may occur, especially in the finger and foot joints

Reiter's Syndrome

- A form of arthritis often transmitted by sexual contact, which is characterized not only by pain in the joints but also by a penile discharge (urethritis), a painful inflammation of the eye (conjunctivitis), and a rash
- Some people inherit susceptibility, which is induced by infection transmitted by sexual contact or by ingestion of contaminated food or water

Ankylosing Spondylitis

- A form of arthritis that affects the joints of the body's trunk, including the hips, shoulders, and ribs, but especially the back and neck. Pain and stiffness are early signs, but in advanced cases a poker spine—a very stiff, inflexible backbone— is common

Arthritis of Inflammatory Bowel Disease

- In patients with inflammatory bowel disease, a characteristic form of arthritis also may occur. Most often, the disease affects peripheral joints—those of the knee, ankle, and elbow, in particular. As with almost all forms of arthritis, you will notice the pain and stiffness more frequently in the morning

All four of these forms of arthritis have a genetic factor. Each of them has characteristic gene markers that indicate a genetic predisposition to the disease.

A tissue-typing test can establish the presence of the marker, although the presence of a certain gene does not mean you will get these ailments. Rather, the gene confirms a tendency to the ailment and reinforces the observation that these disorders tend to recur within families. Why one of these disorders develops in one person and not another remains a mystery.

Psoriatic Arthritis

Psoriasis is a common skin disease in which areas of the skin assume an inflamed, reddish color (see page 992). The surface of the skin of the elbows and knees may become scaly. The fingernails may become pitted and discolored. Psoriatic arthritis accompanies psoriasis in about 1 in 10 people with the skin problem. More women than men have these ailments, and typically they strike persons in their 20s and 30s.

For most people, the effects of psoriatic arthritis are minor. It produces some pain and discomfort in affected joints but has little effect on overall health.

Treatment

In most cases, anti-inflammatory drugs such as ibuprofen, naproxen, and aspirin along with range-of-motion exercises are the basic treatments. Your physician may prescribe stronger drugs for more difficult cases.

Reiter's Syndrome

We don't understand this disease very well. Reiter's syndrome usually appears in stages.

First, the penile discharge occurs. Some time later (a few days or weeks), joint pain occurs, often in the knee, heel, or fingers. Skin lesions similar to those of psoriasis may also appear, as may an eye inflammation called conjunctivitis (see page 542).

Reiter's syndrome may appear once or episodically. Attacks tend to last a few weeks or months. It occurs mainly in persons with a genetic predisposition to it and primarily in whites (blacks rarely get it). Reiter's syndrome occasionally leads to permanent damage to the joints, although the inflammation of an acute attack can produce tenderness and pain. Reiter's syndrome is the most common cause of arthritis of the lower extremities in young men.

Treatment

Your physician will probably recommend anti-inflammatory drugs such as aspirin to treat Reiter's syndrome; but he or she may also prescribe stronger drugs.

Ankylosing Spondylitis

Persons with this disorder have the same gene marker that is found in persons with Reiter's syndrome. It tends to be an inherited disorder—some people who have ankylosing spondylitis have relatives who also have it.

Males are affected more often than females, generally during the third decade of life. Occasionally, the person already has inflammatory bowel disease (see Crohn's Disease,

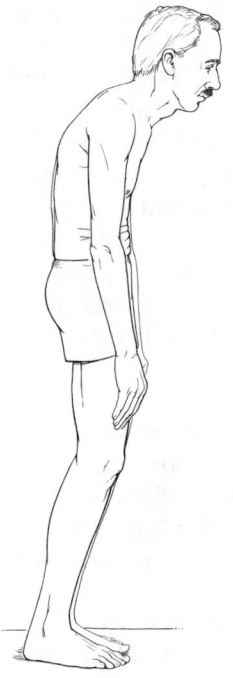

Ankylosing spondylitis can lead to this characteristically stooped-over posture.

page 774, and Ulcerative Colitis, page 777).

The name is derived from Greek words that identify the characteristic symptoms: "rigid" (*ankylosing*) "spine" (*spondyl*) with accompanying "inflammation" (*itis*). The usual disease course involves a soreness in the spine and other joints of the trunk. As the disease progresses, the affected bones begin to grow together, rendering the joints immovable. In addition, some people develop a peripheral arthritis resembling rheumatoid arthritis.

In most cases, ankylosing spondylitis is a mild condition, often going undiagnosed for decades; in rare cases, it can be crippling. In serious cases, eye, heart, and other complications may result.

Treatment

Anti-inflammatory drugs may relieve the chronic pain and stiffness. However, a program of physical exercise is essential to treatment. You should proceed with regular activity as much as possible. But you also need to perform range-of-motion and stretching exercises habitually to combat the tendency of ankylosing spondylitis to reduce flexibility.

Good posture is important (see page 902), and physicians particularly discourage smoking because of the long-term potential for the disorder to limit air exchange due to its effects on the rib cage. A surgical procedure may be an option in advanced cases.

Arthritis of Inflammatory Bowel Disease

In about 1 of 10 patients with ulcerative colitis (see page 777) and 1 of 5 with Crohn's disease (see page 774), one or more sore joints accompany the digestive disorder.

Treatment

In the short term, physicians usually treat the joint pain, often in the hands or feet, with aspirin or other anti-inflammatory drugs. Control or cure of the inflammatory bowel disorder is the long-term solution.

Infectious Arthritis

Signs and Symptoms
- Pain and stiffness in one joint, typically a knee, shoulder, hip, ankle, elbow, finger, or wrist
- The surrounding tissues are warm and red
- Chills, fever, and weakness

Emergency Symptoms—If you have all three of the above-described signs and symptoms, seek immediate medical attention

Bacteria, virus, or fungus can cause a joint infection. Typically, the infecting agent enters the body and spreads to the joint via the bloodstream. In some instances, an open wound or puncture provides the infection direct access to the joint.

Infectious arthritis, unlike other joint disorders, can occur in anyone at any time: the infecting agents are not limited by a person's age, sex, or race.

What Are the Types of Infectious Arthritis?

Lyme Disease
Lyme disease is named for the town on the Connecticut coast where it was first observed. It is contracted from a tick bite. Usually, a disc-shaped rash will develop around the bite, and other symptoms may follow, including fever, chills, sore throat, fatigue, and nausea. Some weeks later, stiffness and pain may occur in the joints.

Gonococcal
Roughly a third of those who contract gonorrhea, a sexually transmitted bacterial disease (see page 1087), experience pain in several joints. A rash also may result. This type of infectious arthritis is reported 10 times more frequently in women than in men.

Staphylococcal
When a boil or other infection releases the staphylococcal bacterium into your bloodstream, it can spread to a knee or other joint. The pain is usually intense and sudden.

Tuberculous
A small number of people with tuberculosis have accompanying arthritis. The symptoms are usually few, so it may go undiagnosed. If you have tuberculosis and experience slight joint pain, consult your physician.

Viral
Arthritis symptoms may occur in persons who have hepatitis B, rubella (German measles), mumps, and other diseases caused by viruses. In general, however, the arthritis requires no specific treatment but resolves

Rheumatic Fever Arthritis

The management of rheumatic fever is one of modern medicine's success stories. Once it caused serious heart problems in many children. The advent of prompt treatment of streptococcal infections with antibiotic drugs, however, markedly reduced its incidence.

However, a form of arthritis is a common manifestation of the illness. This form of arthritis characteristically occurs several weeks after a streptococcal infection, usually of the throat. Your joints become swollen, reddened, and painful to move. Typically, your joints are affected in a manner often described as migratory: first, one joint is painful for a time, and then the pain seems to migrate to another joint.

The arthritis of rheumatic fever is not strictly an infectious arthritis, but rather is a hypersensitivity reaction in the joints. In general, the treatment is the same as that for the rheumatic fever, although your physician may remove fluid from swollen joints with a needle in order to reduce the discomfort (see Rheumatic Fever, page 677).

with the treatment of and recovery from the underlying disease.

Diagnosis
If your physician suspects a form of infectious arthritis, he or she may remove fluid from the joint with a needle in order to conduct laboratory tests. You may also have blood tests.

How Serious Is Infectious Arthritis?
In most cases, prompt diagnosis and treatment of a joint infection result in a rapid and complete recovery.

Treatment
Because of the risk of permanent damage to the bone or cartilage, a joint infection needs to be treated immediately. Unless the cause of the infection is viral, your physician will prescribe an antibiotic drug. Hospitalization may be necessary. Your physician may use a needle to drain the infected joint, or the joint may be opened surgically and damaged tissues removed. If your joint is seriously damaged, it may be necessary to surgically reconstruct the joint.

During recuperation from an infection, the joint may be immobilized with a splint. After the infection is eliminated, physical therapy may be necessary to regain strength and mobility in the affected joint.

Gout

Signs and Symptoms

- Severe pain that strikes suddenly in a single joint, often at the base of your big toe
- Accompanying swelling and redness

Also called crystal-induced arthritis, gout occurs when uric acid crystals accumulate in the affected joint. Some uric acid is derived from a food substance in the diet known as purines, but the greater part is produced by our bodies daily. If you have gout, you lose the normal balance: your body produces too much uric acid or too little is excreted. When the amount of uric acid in your blood and body fluids increases, uric acid in the fluid around the joints (synovial fluid) forms crystals and gout results, typically in the joint at the base of your big toe.

Ninety percent of persons with gout are men older than 40; 1 in 4 has a family history of the ailment. Gout has long had a reputation as an illness that results from the excessive consumption of food and drink, which may be true, but gout also can strike at any time and for no apparent reason. People who are obese or who suffer from hypertension may be at greater risk for crystal-induced arthritis. The stress of an injury such as a fracture or a surgical procedure may provoke an attack. Thiazide diuretics, a common treatment of high blood pressure that reduces the water content of the body, may raise uric acid levels in the blood and provoke gout in the susceptible person.

Diagnosis

An episode of gout begins within a matter of hours. A joint that seemed entirely normal will become intensely painful, red, and swollen. The joint will remain very painful for several days. The discomfort will subside gradually over the next 1 to 2 weeks, leaving the joint apparently normal and pain-free. Even though the joint at the base of the great toe is involved most frequently, gout can affect other joints in the feet, ankles, knees, hands, and wrists.

To confirm the diagnosis, your physician may withdraw some fluid from the affected joint to look for crystals of uric acid within the white blood cells. Your physician also may do blood tests for levels of uric acid; but the tests can be misleading, because the levels may be nearly normal during an acute attack of gout. In addition, many people with high levels of uric acid never experience an attack of crystal-induced arthritis.

Sometimes, a long-term accumulation of uric acid may produce lumps, called tophi, just beneath the skin. The most common site is the cartilage of the ear. Infrequently, kidney stones may result from the build-up of uric acid.

What Is Pseudogout?

Pseudogout is a related ailment that involves the deposit of crystals of a calcium salt rather than uric acid in the joints. The affected joints are more likely to be knees, wrists, and ankles than those of the foot. Pseudogout strikes women and men with roughly equal frequency, but the age at onset is late, typically 70 years. The ailment is also known as calcium pyrophosphate dihydrate crystal deposition disease.

How Serious Is Gout?

Your physician can treat an acute attack effectively and prevent future attacks by giving you maintenance medication. After an attack has run its course (generally a matter of days and no more than a few weeks), the affected joint usually returns to normal. If you do not receive proper treatment, however, joint damage can be permanent and uric acid deposits may cause kidney problems or even stones.

Treatment

Medication

Colchicine, in use for centuries, is still valuable for acute attacks of gout. Indomethacin is also used for acute attacks. Between attacks your physician may use other drugs, including probenecid and allopurinol, to control the levels of uric acid in your body.

Physicians usually treat pseudogout with anti-inflammatory drugs, although colchicine is effective in some cases.

Nutrition

Although physicians no longer consider food and drink the main cause of gout, avoid excessive consumption of alcohol, maintain your weight within reasonable limits, and avoid foods that contain purines if you have gout. Purine-rich foods include sardines, anchovies, sweetbreads, liver, and kidney. Remember, attempts at rapid weight reduction may provoke an acute attack.

Acute Painful Shoulder

Signs and Symptoms
- Pain in your shoulder
- Limited range of motion
- Pain in your upper arm or neck

Also known as bicipital tendinitis and periarthritis of the shoulder, acute painful shoulder occurs at the point where the tendon of the biceps muscle passes, like a rope through a pulley, over the head of the humerus (upper arm bone). Inflammation can develop easily in this area, often for no particular reason, although excessive use of the shoulder may be the cause.

An acute attack may occur suddenly and remain painful for several weeks or more than a month. Pain may extend well into the biceps area.

Motion, particularly extending your arm to the side or putting on a coat, may produce pain. Sometimes people hold the affected arm close to their body and avoid moving it. However, if your joint is not extended through its range of motion with some frequency, even during the acute phase when it is painful to do so, ligaments and other tissues about the joint will stiffen and your shoulder will "freeze." Movement of the joint will then be very limited, even after the inflammation subsides.

Episodes of acute painful shoulder tend to recur. In some instances, the biceps will actually tear, requiring surgical repair. In such cases, there will be a visible distortion or bulge near the shoulder and accompanying pain.

In other cases, the ligaments that surround the shoulder joint (the rotator cuff) also may tear. The symptoms may resemble those of acute painful shoulder, but you can distinguish a shoulder cuff tear if your shoulder can be moved readily to the side and overhead by someone else, whereas you are unable to accomplish these motions. Again, your physician may need to surgically repair the tear.

Treatment

Medication
During the acute phase of frozen shoulder, your physician probably will prescribe anti-inflammatory drugs in generous amounts. In very severe instances, your physician may prescribe prednisone by mouth for limited periods. If pain and inflammation persist, a prednisone injection into the joint may be helpful (see Corticosteroid Drugs, page 919).

Other Therapies
Your physician will determine the amount of motion you should do each day. If, despite exercise, your shoulder remains too limited in its range of motion, the joint may be forcibly put through its normal range of motion while you are under a general anesthetic.

Bursitis

Signs and Symptoms—Pain and swelling in the area of your elbow, hip, knee, shoulder, big toe, or other joint

A bursa is a sac-like membrane found in many joints (there are actually 78 on each side of the body). The bursa acts as a cushion between the bone and the fibrous tissues of the muscles and tendons, facilitating movement by limiting friction. When a bursa becomes inflamed, the resultant disorder is termed bursitis.

Repeated physical activity often leads to bursitis: throwing a baseball and swinging a tennis racket are common causes. Job-related tasks also can lead to bursitis; for example, with housemaid's knee the front of the knee becomes inflamed. Although you usually can trace bursitis to events of overuse or pressure, there may be no such obvious cause.

Diagnosis
Your physician will conduct a physical examination and inquire about recent activities. By palpation, he or she may also identify tenderness in a localized area. If it appears that

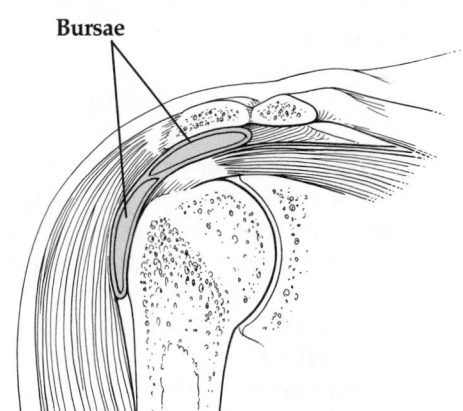

Bursae

Overuse of a joint can lead to bursitis, an inflammation of the bursa, which serves as a cushion between bone and fibrous tissue.

something else may be causing the discomfort, your physician may want an X-ray of the affected area; if bursitis is the cause, the X-ray images will be normal.

Treatment
Bursitis usually disappears within 2 weeks, given reasonable care of the painful joint.

Anti-inflammatory drugs such as aspirin may help relieve the discomfort. Your physician may give you a local injection of a corticosteroid drug (see Corticosteroid Drugs, page 919).

When bursitis occurs repeatedly in the same joint, the affected bursa may be removed surgically.

Immunologic Rheumatic Diseases

Physicians sometimes also call these diseases connective tissue diseases or collagen diseases. The terms are based on the knowledge of 50 years ago, and today some people still use them. Disorders within this group include lupus (systemic lupus erythematosus), scleroderma, and polymyositis—all caused by alterations in the immune system (see page A-16).

Common to all of these disorders is an inflammation of unknown cause that can affect almost all tissues in your body.

Lupus (Systemic Lupus Erythematosus)

Signs and Symptoms
- Joint pain, swelling, and redness that come and go from day to day, most often in your fingers and wrists
- Rashes, especially across your nose and cheeks
- Localized chest pain accompanied by coughing
- Sunlight sensitivity that produces rash and fever reactions
- Inexplicable fatigue
- Raynaud's phenomenon (see page 697)

Lupus (systemic lupus erythematosus) is a chronic disease of unknown origin. It typically affects the synovial membrane in your joints, producing pain and inflammation. Both the joint discomforts and the rash tend to be episodic, with alternating periods of remission and flares.

The typical person with lupus is a female between the ages of 15 and 35 years. Ten times as many women as men have lupus. Lupus sometimes appears for the first time during pregnancy, usually with little or no effect on the unborn child.

Diagnosis
Your physician will take your medical history and perform an examination to diagnose the condition. Physicians often order laboratory studies, such as an antinuclear antibody (ANA) test that may be positive. Normal, healthy people can also have a positive ANA, so your physician will not base the diagnosis on laboratory tests alone. Your physician may do a blood test for rheumatoid factor. You may also have a creatinine test because lupus can affect kidney function.

How Serious Is Lupus?
For many people with lupus, the disease is not a major illness. For some, however, it is a serious disease that must be managed carefully to avoid serious complications, especially kidney disease, joint damage, and complications of treatment. Typically, lupus is a lifelong ailment that comes and goes. It may affect virtually every organ system in your body.

Treatment

Medication
The treatment of lupus depends on its severity. In some cases, treatment is not necessary. At times, however, physicians use corticosteroids (see page 919) and other drugs.

Other Therapies
Your physician may recommend that you avoid excessive exposure to the ultraviolet rays in sunlight. Physical therapy and treatment of depression may be necessary. Because of long-term risks associated with

Corticosteroid Drugs

Corticosteroid drugs are modified forms of the hormones cortisone and hydrocortisone, which are made in the adrenal gland. This family of drugs has an important place in the treatment options of today's physician.

Uses

The corticosteroid drugs have a strong anti-inflammatory effect that reduces swelling, pain, redness, and heat of sore joints. In addition to their obvious value in treating disorders of the adrenal glands, corticosteroids can be invaluable remedies for a wide range of other ailments, including skin diseases, allergies, certain tumors, and numerous types of arthritis and other musculoskeletal problems.

You can take these drugs in tablet form for a sustained period (sometimes for years), apply them topically to your skin, place them into your eye with drops, or inject them directly into a localized area. They also are used for long periods to prevent rejection of the transplanted organ in persons who have had an organ transplant.

Risks

With sustained, long-term use of corticosteroid drugs, the risk of side effects is great. The adrenal glands tend to shrink (atrophy). Weight gain, a loss of bone mineral akin to that in osteoporosis (see page 894), muscle weakness, water retention, hypertension, a rounding of the facial features (commonly called moonface), thinning of the skin, and other problems also can result. No one has all of these side effects, of course, and with short-term use you have a good chance of having none. The risks with topically applied corticosteroid medications are regarded as so small that you can now obtain some preparations without a prescription.

For persons who take prednisone daily for 3 to 6 months or longer, particularly if side effects such as rounding of the face and thinning of the skin have occurred, the adrenal glands may have atrophied and the related function of the pituitary gland may have decreased. In such cases, the adrenal glands no longer can produce the needed amounts of hydrocortisone when your body is faced with the stress of surgery, severe infection, or injury, when lack of the hormone may even cause your death. When people whose bodies no longer produce enough hydrocortisone have a surgical procedure or sustain injury, physicians prescribe generous amounts of prednisone or other corticosteroid drugs intravenously or by muscle injection to provide for the temporary increase in hormonal needs.

If you take prednisone daily, keep this information readily available in case of an emergency.

Cortisone by Injection

Cortisone injections have remarkable effects for the treatment of such acute conditions as bursitis and tendinitis. Also, they are invaluable for relieving pain and swelling in individual joints affected by chronic osteoarthritis or rheumatoid arthritis. Often, a single injection will relieve an acute condition permanently, but more injections can be given if necessary. However, as few as six injections within a 12-month period can damage bone and joint structure, so your physician is unlikely to administer more than three or four within a calendar year.

Corticosteroid drugs differ from anabolic steroid preparations (male sex hormones), which sometimes are inappropriately used by athletes to increase muscle bulk (see page 345).

---

lupus, your physician will carefully monitor the status of the disease and the medications you use to treat it.

Scleroderma

Signs and Symptoms

- A thickening and tightening of the skin, especially on your arms, face, or hands, resulting in a loss of flexibility
- Puffy hands and feet, particularly in the morning
- Joint pain and stiffness
- Raynaud's phenomenon (see page 697)

Scleroderma, also known as progressive systemic sclerosis, means "hard" (sclero) "skin" (derma). This disorder leads not only to a hardening of the skin but also to a permanent shine and tightness of the affected tissues. It is not related to multiple sclerosis (see page 475).

As with other immunologically mediated disorders, and especially in scleroderma, in which tiny blood vessels are often involved, malfunction of almost every organ in the body can occur.

Most people with scleroderma contract it between the ages of 20 and 40 years, although it is not unheard of in children and elderly people. Women are about 4 times as likely to get scleroderma as men.

Diagnosis

The diagnosis is based on a careful medical history along with a physical examination (see color photograph, page C-16). Raynaud's phenomenon, a condition in which the skin color changes to a dead white pallor, then blue, and finally to a reddish color, occurs more commonly in scleroderma than in any of the other connective tissue diseases. Raynaud's phenomenon may occur with emotional stress or exposure to cold.

Your physician may do a biopsy, in which a tissue sample of the affected skin is removed for laboratory study.

How Serious Is Scleroderma?

The usual course of the disease involves an initial phase of approximately 2 years during which affected tissues harden and stiffen. After that time, the skin effects of the disorder are unlikely to progress and may even lessen somewhat, although in rare instances the hands may become permanently crippled.

In a minority of people, organ involvement can occur, producing hypertension, lung problems, kidney failure, and intestinal tract problems that can lead to malnutrition. In rare cases, these long-term effects can be life-threatening.

Treatment

Medication
The approach depends on the severity of the case, but there is no known treatment for this condition. Your physician may prescribe a blood vessel dilator if Raynaud's phenomenon is present; hypertensive drugs to treat high blood pressure; analgesics, such as aspirin, for joint pain; and antibiotics for intestinal problems.

Other Therapies
If your skin is affected, exercise is essential. Movement can limit the stiffening effects and help maintain blood flow.

Because nicotine causes the blood vessels to contract, physicians recommend cessation of smoking (see How to Stop Smoking, page 321).

Be sure to wear warm gloves for protection when your hands will be subjected to cold temperatures (such as when reaching into a freezer).

If heartburn occurs, you can use antireflux measures (see page 742) and you should avoid eating in the 3 to 4 hours before bedtime. Your physician may recommend an antacid medication to protect your esophagus (see page 744).

Sjögren's Syndrome

Signs and Symptoms
- Dryness in your eyes, characterized by a feeling of sandiness or grittiness
- Dry mouth

This disorder often accompanies rheumatoid arthritis (see page 909) or other ailments such as lupus (see page 918), scleroderma (see page 919) or polymyositis (this page). Most people who suffer from Sjögren's syndrome are middle-aged women.

The eyes become red, dry, and painful. They may feel as if a foreign body has become lodged in the eye but, on examination, none is found.

Treatment

Medication
Eyedrops may be useful for treating the discomfort in your eyes. You can relieve your dry mouth by stimulating the production of saliva. Your physician may prescribe corticosteroids or other drugs if your case is severe.

Polymyositis and Dermatomyositis

Signs and Symptoms
- Muscle weakness
- Pain, swelling, heat, and redness in the small joints
- Reddish patches of skin on the face, knuckles, elbows, knees, or ankles

Polymyositis is a disorder in which the "muscles" (*myo*) become "inflamed" (*itis*); when a particular skin inflammation accompanies the muscle weakness, the disorder is termed "dermatomyositis" (from the Greek word *derma* for "skin").

Adults between 30 and 60 years of age and children between 5 and 15 years old are most likely to have these disorders, but they can strike at any age. Women are about twice as likely to have polymyositis or dermatomyositis.

Vasculitis

Vasculitis is a term used to describe conditions caused by inflammation and damage to the blood vessels, especially the arteries. Inflamed arteries may cause various general symptoms such as fever, weakness, and malaise or, if a particular organ is involved, may cause more specific symptoms such as abdominal pain if the arteries to the gut are involved.

In general, no specific blood tests can diagnose the various forms of vasculitis, including polyarteritis, allergic angiitis and granulomatosis, hypersensitivity vasculitis, and cranial arteritis. With these ailments, the erythrocyte sedimentation rate is often elevated (see page 1331).

Your physician may confirm the diagnosis by removing a segment of an artery for laboratory examination (see Biopsies, page 1332).

Treatment usually involves corticosteroids, at the lowest dose that prevents symptoms. Occasionally, aspirin is also effective for treating the the conditions described below.

Polyarteritis

This serious disorder involves an "inflammation" *(itis)* of "many" *(poly)* arteries. Inflammation can result in obstruction of the vessels, reducing the supply of blood reaching the affected area.

The skin, intestines, kidney, and heart are at greatest risk. Typical symptoms include weight loss, fever, weakness, and fatigue. Occasionally, if the lung is affected, asthma symptoms may occur, or if the gut is involved, abdominal pain and bloody diarrhea may occur.

Middle-aged men are most likely to suffer from polyarteritis, although there is a juvenile form of the illness.

In the past, this disease was often fatal; but with proper treatment many people with polyarteritis can lead normal lives.

Allergic Angiitis and Granulomatosis

Also called Churg-Strauss disease, this ailment closely resembles a type of polyarteritis (nodosa), but the lungs usually are involved in allergic angiitis. Asthmatic attacks are common. Blood and erythrocyte sedimentation rate tests (see page 1331) may confirm the diagnosis.

Hypersensitivity Vasculitis

This form of vasculitis is the result of exposure to a drug or foreign agent. Occasionally, the skin is involved.

Cranial Arteritis

This disorder, described by Mayo Clinic physicians more than 50 years ago, occurs almost exclusively in people older than 50 and affects women more often than men. Also termed temporal or giant cell arteritis, this condition is characterized by headache and a tender, thickened artery that can be felt at the side of the head. Malaise, fatigue, loss of appetite, weight loss, and sweating are common accompanying symptoms. Occasionally, it causes pain on chewing and vision problems. Left untreated, it can lead to partial or total blindness.

The diagnosis is suspected from the medical history, and it may be confirmed by biopsy of the affected artery. Recovery is the general rule, although in some cases it requires 1 to 2 years of treatment with corticosteroid drugs or aspirin.

Diagnosis

Your physician will perform a careful medical history and physical examination, particularly of your skin and muscle strength.

Your physician may also order a series of blood tests to determine the presence of certain muscle enzymes. A test called electromyography can measure the electrical patterns of your muscles (see page 1344). In addition, a biopsy, in which a tissue sample is removed for laboratory study, may be conducted on affected muscles.

How Serious Are Dermatomyositis and Polymyositis?

The signs and symptoms of dermatomyositis and polymyositis most often persist for many months or even years. A particular danger is the potential effect on the muscles of the throat, which can make swallowing difficult. Lung problems also may occur.

Treatment

Medication

The primary treatment of polymyositis or dermatomyositis is medication. Your physician will probably use prednisone (see Corticosteroid Drugs, page 919) or aspirin. Occasionally, methotrexate, azathioprine, and intravenous immunoglobulin are other options.

Other Therapies

Once the medication begins to take effect, your physician will recommend an exercise program.

Polymyalgia Rheumatica

Signs and Symptoms
- Pain and stiffness in the muscles of your lower back, thighs, and hips, or neck, shoulders, and upper arms
- Slight fever, fatigue, and weight loss

The name of this ailment is from the Greek words that mean "many" *(poly)* "muscles" *(myo)* in "pain" *(algia)*. Rheumatica (or its equivalent, rheumatism) is an ancient word for muscle and joint soreness.

Polymyalgia rheumatica is likely due to an immunologically mediated inflammation of unknown cause. Most of the inflammation occurs in the hip and shoulder joints, which accounts for the pain and stiffness. But inflammation may occur elsewhere in the body as well.

It affects elderly people, usually those older than 50 years, and is more common in whites than in other races. It affects women more often than men.

Diagnosis
Information about the onset of pain is important for diagnosis. In polymyalgia rheumatica, the pain usually strikes suddenly and may involve most muscles, although the neck and shoulders are often the most painful. The discomfort is likely to be worse in the morning, but it may occur at night also. There are no specific tests to confirm the diagnosis, but certain X-ray or laboratory tests may eliminate other possible causes for the discomfort.

How Serious Is It?
Left untreated, polymyalgia rheumatica may lead to eye problems and weight loss. However, the typical disease course is about 5 years, after which it usually disappears. It may be associated with inflammation and tenderness in arteries just under the scalp (see Cranial Arteritis, page 921) or other major arteries in the body. A biopsy of an artery may be appropriate.

Treatment
Corticosteroids (see page 919) usually will produce improvement within a few days. Physicians use these drugs in the smallest dose that will control the symptoms until the disease runs its course. Your physician may prescribe aspirin and other anti-inflammatory drugs.

Chapter 28

Your Endocrine System

Contents

Your Endocrine System at Work, 924

Pancreatic Disorders, 925
Diabetes Mellitus, 925
  "Reactive Hypoglycemia," 929
  Caring for Your Feet, 931
  New Nutrition Guidelines, 932
  Updated Treatment Guidelines, 933
  Glucose Self-Monitoring, 933
  Insulin Injection, 934
Islet Cell Tumors of the Pancreas, 936

Adrenal Gland Disorders, 937
Cushing's Syndrome, 937
Addison's Disease, 938
Pheochromocytoma, 939
Aldosteronoma, 940
  Hirsutism, 940
Congenital Adrenal Hyperplasia, 941

Pituitary Gland Disorders, 941
Acromegaly/Gigantism, 942
Prolactinoma, 942
Nonfunctioning Pituitary Tumors, 943
Hypopituitarism, 943
Diabetes Insipidus, 944

Thyroid Disorders, 945
  Goiter, 946
Hyperthyroidism, 947
Hypothyroidism, 948

Parathyroid Gland Disorders, 950
Hyperparathyroidism, 950
Hypoparathyroidism, 951

Your Endocrine System at Work

The endocrine glands function as a control system for the human body. Unlike other organs and body parts that enable us to move, breathe, eat, or sense the world around us, the endocrine system influences the body's processes. Along with the nervous system, it coordinates the body's activities and responses to usual and unusual events.

The key mechanism of the system is the hormone. Different types of endocrine hormones are secreted by different glands. Most of these hormones are released into the bloodstream so that they can deliver instructions to various organs and tissues. The pancreas, for example, secretes the hormone insulin, which enables the body to regulate the amount of sugar in the bloodstream. In response to stress or other stimuli, the adrenal glands secrete adrenaline (also called epinephrine), which produces a sudden and remarkable burst of energy. Similarly, the pituitary, thyroid, parathyroid, and gonadal glands each influence certain body functions.

A hormone is a chemical messenger (the name itself comes from the Greek verb that means "urge"). Although hormones circulate throughout the body via the bloodstream, each influences only certain organs (target organs) or tissues.

As a rule, the greater the amount of a particular hormone in the bloodstream, the greater the activity of the target organ or organs of that hormone. Some hormones (such as several of those produced by the pituitary gland) control other glandular activity, but virtually every system in the body is subject to the influence of the hor-

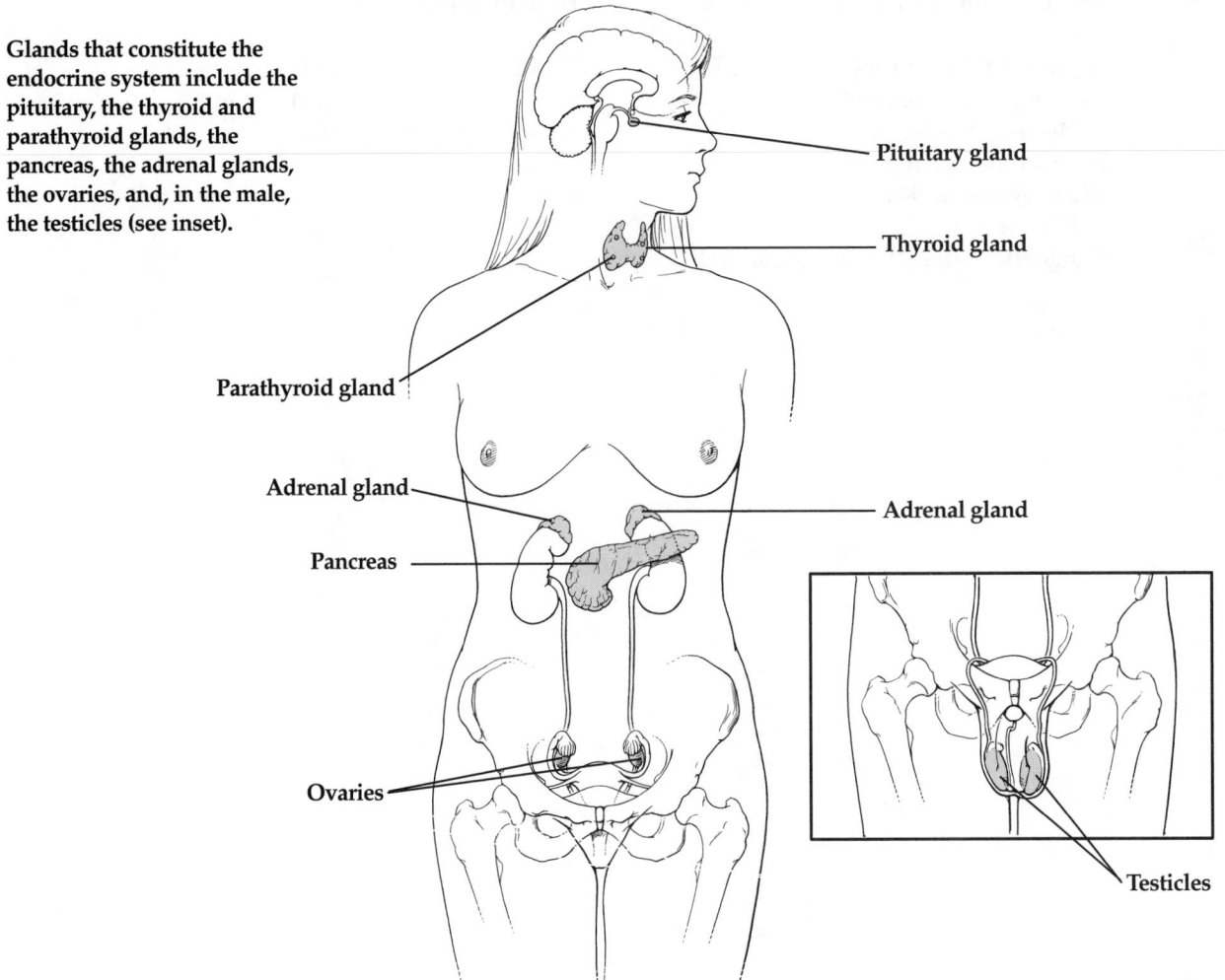

Glands that constitute the endocrine system include the pituitary, the thyroid and parathyroid glands, the pancreas, the adrenal glands, the ovaries, and, in the male, the testicles (see inset).

Pituitary gland

Thyroid gland

Parathyroid gland

Adrenal gland

Adrenal gland

Pancreas

Ovaries

Testicles

mones, either directly or indirectly. Reproduction and growth patterns are established by hormonal activity, as are the body's fluid and salt balances.

The endocrine system consists of several separate but interrelated glands or tissues that produce hormones. In most people, the pancreas, the adrenal, pituitary, thyroid, and parathyroid glands, and the ovaries or testicles work in tandem, controlling the ebb and flow of hormones so efficiently that the body's glandular activity goes virtually unnoticed. Occasionally, however, the endocrine system malfunctions.

Because of the complexity of the endocrine system, many problems, great and small, can result from a malfunction. For example, in diabetes, the most common endocrine disorder, there is an excess of a sugar, called glucose, in the blood. This can produce a variety of symptoms, including constant thirst and excessive urination. When a child's pituitary gland malfunctions, he or she may be at risk of gigantism or dwarfism if the disorder is not properly diagnosed and treated.

The physician whose principal concern is the function of the endocrine system is the endocrinologist. In the following pages, we will consider the hormonal problems that endocrinologists commonly encounter. These ailments involve the pancreas and the adrenal, pituitary, thyroid, and parathyroid glands. (The testicles are discussed in Men's Health, page 1195. The ovaries and breast disorders are discussed in Women's Health, page 1139.)

Pancreatic Disorders

Located behind your stomach, the pancreas is a long, thin organ roughly the length of your hand. It plays a key part in the digestive process, producing enzymes essential to the digestion of food (see Your Digestive System at Work, page 739). The other role of the pancreas, which might best be described as "fuel control," is the one that affects persons with diabetes.

The hormones produced by the pancreas enable your body to break down (metabolize) the food you eat. They regulate your body's use of glucose, a simple form of sugar that is an energy source for much of the daily activities of all of your cells.

When your pancreas is functioning normally, the glucose concentration in your blood changes in response to a wide variety of events, including meals, exercise, stressful situations, and infections, but it remains within set limits.

Three hormones are produced by the pancreas. The first is insulin, which is produced when the concentration of glucose in the blood increases. This normally occurs shortly after you eat a meal. Muscle and fat cells, among others, are stimulated by insulin to absorb the glucose they need as fuel for their activities. Surplus glucose is stored by the liver in the form of a starch called glycogen.

The second pancreatic hormone is glucagon. When needed, it breaks down the glycogen stored in the liver, causing it to be released as fuel into the bloodstream. In effect, this raises the concentration of sugar in the blood.

The third hormone produced by the pancreas, somatostatin, is thought to be a factor in regulating the production and release of both insulin and glucagon.

Diabetes Mellitus

Signs and Symptoms
- Increased thirst
- Increased urination, both in volume and frequency
- Weight loss despite increased appetite
- Fatigue, nausea, vomiting
- Vaginitis, skin infections, blurred vision, frequent bladder infections

Emergency Symptoms

- Diabetic ketoacidosis: symptoms develop over a period of hours. Increased thirst and urination, nausea, deepened and more rapid breathing, abdominal pain, and a slightly sweet-smelling breath are the symptoms that precede a gradual loss of consciousness from diabetic ketoacidosis. This condition is most likely to occur if you are insulin-dependent, often after you miss a dose of insulin or when you have an infection
- Hypoglycemic coma (insulin reaction): symptoms develop over a period of minutes. Trembling, weakness, or drowsiness followed by headache, confusion, dizziness, double vision, or lack of coordination are hallmarks of an insulin reaction. An intoxication-like state, and eventually convulsions or unconsciousness, may follow. Emergency care is essential
- Hyperosmolar coma: symptoms develop over a period of days. This is a gradual loss of consciousness, most often in an older person whose diabetes usually does not require insulin injections. Hyperosmolar coma often occurs in conjunction with some other illness, such as stroke

Sometimes the pancreas' balanced system of control fails. The amount of glucose in the bloodstream increases at times when the cells are unable to draw on it. The result is hyperglycemia (from the Greek *hyper* for "above," *glyk* for "sugar," and *emia* for "blood"). This condition is easily diagnosed by measuring the concentration of glucose in the blood. If it is high enough, some glucose will spill into the urine, where it can be detected easily.

When your body's cells are unable to use the glucose in the bloodstream because of a lack of insulin activity (absence of enough hormone or resistance to the hormone), diabetes mellitus results. The origins of the name are Greek, referring to sweetness or honey *(mellitus)* that passes through *(diabetes)*.

More than 10 million Americans have been diagnosed as having diabetes mellitus. It is estimated that at least another 5 million are unaware that they have the ailment. Often, mild diabetes causes no outward symptoms for years.

About 1 in 10 people with diabetes have insulin-dependent diabetes mellitus (IDDM), and the rest have non-insulin-dependent diabetes mellitus (NIDDM). Insulin-dependent diabetes mellitus is also known as type I, juvenile, ketosis-prone, or juvenile-onset diabetes. We will refer to it as IDDM, the name that most accurately describes the disorder.

IDDM can develop in anyone at any age. Persons typically affected are children and young adults (young males are at somewhat greater risk than young females). Most people whose diabetes is diagnosed before age 19 have the insulin-dependent variety of diabetes. Apparently heredity is a factor in the development of diabetes—about two of every three people with diabetes are from families with some history of the disease. Although genetics is an important factor, inherited characteristics alone are not sufficient to produce the disease without the influence of other factors that are not yet completely understood.

As the names suggest, IDDM is distinguished from NIDDM by the fact that insulin is needed for treatment. In the person with IDDM, the pancreas usually produces little or no insulin. The symptoms of IDDM usually develop rapidly, in a matter of months or even weeks. During the first year after diagnosis, there may be a time of improvement called the "honeymoon period," during which insulin is not needed or its dosage may be greatly decreased. In the fully developed state of IDDM, insulin injections are needed to prevent ketoacidosis and ultimately death.

Other terms used for NIDDM include adult-onset, stable, and type II diabetes. Typically, persons with NIDDM are more than 40 years old.

The problem they face is not an absence of insulin. Although they may have a modest shortfall of the hormone, they are equally likely to have normal or even elevated concentrations of insulin in their blood. Their bodies, however, are resistant to it. Greater amounts of insulin are needed to maintain normal amounts of glucose in the blood.

Most persons with NIDDM are overweight or obese. Excess weight worsens the state of the diabetes, and weight reduction has a favorable effect. In some instances, insulin injections will be required to keep blood glucose concentrations within satisfactory limits but, unlike the situation in IDDM, omission of these injections will not result in ketoacidosis. Medicines taken by mouth, called oral hypoglycemic agents, often are helpful in NIDDM. A weight-loss program often decreases or eliminates the need for insulin or an oral hypoglycemic medication.

A mild form of diabetes—gestational diabetes—develops in 2 to 3 percent of women who are pregnant. It usually can be treated with diet, and blood sugars return to normal after the baby is born. However, many pregnant women who develop gestational diabetes develop NIDDM later in life.

Because most pregnant women are young adults, nongestational diabetes that begins during pregnancy usually will be of the IDDM variety. Therefore, if you are pregnant and you develop diabetes, see a specialist.

A third, but much less common, type of diabetes is called secondary diabetes. This may behave like either IDDM or NIDDM, but it is distinguishable from them because its cause is another disorder such as acromegaly (see page 942), Cushing's syndrome (see page 937), hyperthyroidism (see page 947), or surgical removal of the pancreas.

Diagnosis

If you experience frequent urination and thirst, consult your physician, who will determine the concentrations of sugar in your blood and urine. Glucose in the urine is called "glycosuria"; a high glucose concentration in the blood is termed "hyperglycemia." These findings are evidence of both forms of diabetes, IDDM and NIDDM.

Testing the urine for substances called ketones may help distinguish between IDDM and NIDDM. Unless insulin is given in appropriate amounts, the person with IDDM frequently has substantial amounts of ketones in the urine, whereas in NIDDM only small amounts of ketones, if any, are found from time to time.

If the person with IDDM fails to receive insulin for a few days, ketoacidosis (see page 928) will almost certainly develop. This condition involves an accumulation of ketones in the blood and urine, deeper and more rapid breathing, and gradual loss of consciousness. Without prompt and vigorous treatment, death is likely.

NIDDM may develop gradually over a period of years. Often it is discovered unexpectedly during a routine urine or blood test conducted at the time of a physical examination. A substantial amount of glucose in the urine is required to produce the classic triad of symptoms: increased thirst, increased volume of urine, and weight loss.

How Serious Is Diabetes?

Until the discovery of insulin in 1921, the almost inevitable result of IDDM was death. However, modern medications administered in a carefully monitored program have made possible the effective management of both IDDM and its less severe variant, NIDDM.

Some people with IDDM experience extremes of high and low concentrations of sugar in the blood, a condition variously termed "brittle," "unstable," or "labile" diabetes. These individuals ultimately may require hospitalization to become stabilized. "Intensive insulin therapy" consists of three to four insulin injections a day, and is often used for unstable diabetes. However, a carefully controlled lifestyle, including proper dietary controls and a less-demanding schedule of insulin or oral medications, in most cases will enable a person with diabetes to live a normal, productive life despite the diabetes.

Both IDDM and NIDDM have potential short- and long-term risks. Short-term dangers are posed by insulin reactions (very low concentrations of glucose) and by very high concentrations of glucose in the blood, but these complications usually are resolved when a satisfactory program of diet, exercise, and, if necessary, adjustment in medication dosage is developed. Ketoacidosis is another short-term danger that a person with diabetes must avoid.

Diabetes has two types of long-term effects. These develop slowly and have few early symptoms. One type is associated with blood vessel involvement. Damage to the large vessels puts the person with diabetes at greater risk of stroke, heart attack, and gangrene of the feet. The other type occurs when small blood vessels sustain long-term damage, causing problems with the eyes, kidneys, or nerves. Recent research has shown that tight blood glucose control substantially reduces your risk of diabetes-related complications (see pages 461, 661, 691, 562, and 854).

Insulin Reaction (Hypoglycemia)

Insulin reaction occurs when the concentration of glucose in your blood falls below normal. Too little glucose circulates to the nervous system and other cells, which become energy-starved. Hypoglycemia can occur if the dose of insulin or oral hypoglycemic agent is too large, if you miss a meal, or as a result of extended or vigorous physical activity. In someone without diabetes, hypoglycemia can result from certain kinds of tumors or from drinking alcohol with minimal food intake.

Insulin reactions occur most often in people with diabetes who take insulin by injection, although such reactions also can occur in those who take antidiabetic tablets by mouth (oral hypoglycemic agents).

Symptoms

Hypoglycemia symptoms vary from one person to another, but commonly include weakness, trembling, and dizziness. You will often experience rapid heart rate and cold perspiration. Your skin appears pale or ashen. Nervousness, hunger, blurred vision, and a tingling sensation in your hands and feet may accompany the other symptoms.

If hypoglycemia is not corrected, headache and difficulty in walking may follow. You may exhibit unusual behavior patterns, appearing confused and sometimes stubborn or uncooperative. As the condition worsens, the lack of coordination may become more exaggerated, and you may seem intoxicated. In extreme cases, unconsciousness occurs (see hypoglycemic coma, page 926). Convulsions can result, particularly in children. In elderly people, strokes may occur but are extremely uncommon.

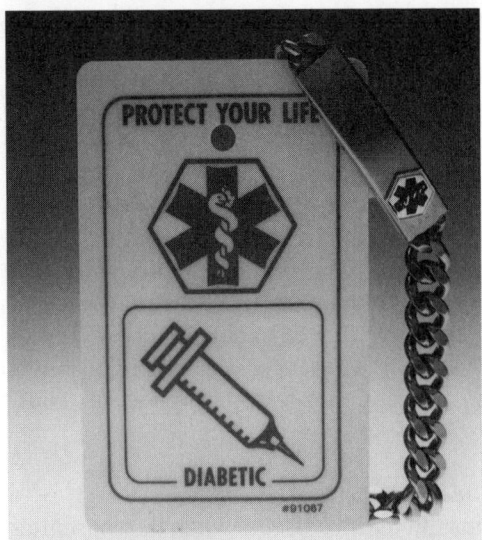

An alert-bracelet or identification card can be a lifesaver in an emergency. This identification will make medical personnel aware of your condition, helping them to reach a correct diagnosis and to provide you with appropriate treatment.

Recognizing the Symptoms

Part of the education process for people who take insulin or oral agents is learning how to recognize a hypoglycemic reaction and how to deal with it.

When symptoms begin to appear, stop all activity—bring the car to a halt, turn off the lawn mower, cease jogging—and treat the reaction. Carry a concentrated source of sugar with you at all times in case a candy or soda machine isn't within easy reach. Alert family and friends to the symptoms and the usual course of your hypoglycemia reactions. They should never attempt to feed you anything if you have lost consciousness, but they can assist you in the earlier stages or summon medical help if necessary.

Treatment

In most cases, a simple carbohydrate such as sugar will raise blood glucose levels within 10 or 15 minutes. Drink a small glass of orange juice or a soft drink (not sugar-free), or eat two or three sugar cubes or a piece of candy. If the symptoms do not disappear, have a second helping. Because panic attacks can closely resemble insulin reactions, test your blood for sugar to determine whether anxiety or an insulin reaction is causing the symptoms. If it is an insulin reaction, eat a snack to prevent recurrence.

Emergency Assistance

Insulin reactions are serious, but if recognized early and treated promptly they usually can be dealt with easily. However, if unconsciousness occurs, someone must inject either glucagon under your skin (as if it were insulin) or glucose into a vein. Because insulin reactions can occur any time or place, wear a medical-alert necklace or bracelet or carry a card that identifies you as a person with diabetes (see the illustration on this page).

Ketoacidosis

This acute complication of IDDM most often occurs when you fail to receive scheduled insulin injections or are under stress from illness or injury. (Psychological factors or emotional stress usually has little or no effect on blood glucose concentration.) Amounts of glucose and ketones increase in the blood, causing it to become more acidic.

Symptoms

Increased urination and an unquenchable

"Reactive Hypoglycemia"

During the past 25 years, thousands of people have diagnosed their poor appetite control, headaches, chronic fatigue, or anxiety as hypoglycemia. They say these symptoms appear after meals, and they often self-impose a sugar-free diet to relieve their distress. But this kind of hypoglycemia, called "reactive hypoglycemia" because of its relation to meals, is rare—if it exists at all. What many people call hypoglycemia usually involves psychological problems.

Between meals, the level of glucose (sugar) in your blood falls. But as long as you are healthy, that level remains within a normal range. In true reactive hypoglycemia, blood sugar levels fall below normal, triggering your body to release four hormones: epinephrine, glucagon, cortisol, and growth hormone. These release stored glucose (glycogen) from your liver and step up production of glucose. Epinephrine probably is responsible for the symptoms of hypoglycemia because it causes sweating, tremor, rapid heartbeats, anxiety, and hunger.

The only way to find out whether you have reactive hypoglycemia is to get a blood test 2 to 4 hours after you eat, while you're feeling hypoglycemic. Your blood glucose must measure below normal.

If true reactive hypoglycemia is so uncommon, then what is causing your symptoms? And why does giving up sugar make them go away?

Stress and anxiety probably are to blame. Anxiety triggers release of epinephrine, just as low blood sugar does. Your body responds by producing symptoms that resemble hypoglycemia.

Emotional stress can manifest itself in erratic eating behavior with a compulsion for sweets. Eliminating sugar from your diet has no physical effect, yet you may think it does. If you feel you are controlling your condition, your anxiety lessens and you feel better.

---

thirst will develop over the course of several hours (it may happen more quickly in a child). Weakness and drowsiness may follow, along with a flushed complexion, vomiting, diarrhea, or abdominal pain. Sometimes your breath assumes a sweet, fruity smell that may be confused with the odor of alcohol (it's actually another waste product, acetone, being expelled via the lungs). At an advanced stage, breathing becomes deeper and more rapid. If you lose consciousness, the condition is described as diabetic coma.

Treatment

These symptoms demand immediate treatment because death can result (government statistics suggest that ketoacidosis is the cause of about 1 in 10 deaths in persons with diabetes). Ketoacidosis is most likely to occur if your diabetes is undiagnosed or not well controlled. However, anyone with diabetes is subject to ketoacidosis under such circumstances as accidental injury, infection, or loss of large quantities of fluid through vomiting or diarrhea. In these situations, it is important to monitor closely the glucose concentration in your blood and the ketone concentration in your urine.

Ketoacidosis requires emergency medical treatment. This involves the administration of insulin and intravenous infusion of salt solutions to replace lost body fluids. Close monitoring of your blood glucose concentration and fluid status is needed until stability is established. Recovery from ketoacidosis is usually rapid and complete if prompt treatment is received.

Hyperosmolar Coma

Older persons with NIDDM who also have another illness (such as stroke) and who fail to consume enough water may develop a very high level of glucose in the blood. Ketones are found only in small amounts, if at all.

The result may be a loss of consciousness requiring hospital care. It is extremely important for persons who have even mild diabetes to drink a generous amount of water during illnesses. Elderly people, who may become confused and fail to ask for water, are particularly vulnerable to hyperosmolar coma.

Atherosclerosis, Hypertension, and Coronary Artery Disease

Changes in your body's small and large blood vessels are at the root of most complications of diabetes. Because your body doesn't process fats efficiently, fatty substances build up on the walls of your arteries, narrowing the channels through which blood passes. This is called atherosclerosis. By restricting blood circulation, it can lead to high blood pressure (hypertension), heart attack, stroke, or foot ulcers.

High blood pressure damages blood vessels, tissues, and organs through which the blood passes. Coronary artery disease involves atherosclerosis of the blood vessels that supply oxygen and nutrients to the heart.

All three of these complex, long-term disorders are substantially more likely to occur in persons with diabetes. You can reduce your risk of atherosclerosis by controlling your diabetes, limiting fat and calories in your diet, exercising regularly, maintaining reasonable weight, not smoking, and controlling high blood pressure. Your physician may prescribe medications to help control abnormal levels of blood fats. Refer to the detailed discussions of atherosclerosis (see page 636), hypertension (see page 647), and coronary artery disease (see page 654) for approaches to treatment and prevention.

Occasionally people with diabetes get cramps in their calves (claudication) while walking or climbing stairs. The cramps cease when the activity is stopped. Claudication, any unusual discoloration of the feet, skin ulcers, or wounds that do not heal should prompt an immediate consultation with your physician (see page 691).

Vision Problems

Diabetic eye disease is called diabetic retinopathy (see page 562). Tiny blood vessels at the back of your eye (retina) become more numerous, bulging, and weak. The subsequent bleeding, scarring, and retinal detachment can lead to blindness. Because diabetic retinopathy often is symptomless until well advanced, it is important to schedule annual eye examinations. Your physician will know when to begin laser treatments to seal damaged vessels and prevent further bleeding (see page 558). Approximately half of all people with diabetes develop diabetic retinopathy after 10 years, and such problems are almost universal in those who have had diabetes for 30 or more years. Cataracts (see page 553) and glaucoma (see page 550) occur frequently as well.

High blood glucose concentrations can cause a refractive error in the eye, which blurs vision. This may become much worse when diabetes treatment rapidly lowers blood sugar concentration. Glasses should not be fitted until the blood sugar value has been stabilized for 6 to 8 weeks.

Kidney Disease

Kidney disease eventually affects 30 to 40 percent of people with IDDM and 5 to 10 percent of those who have had NIDDM for at least 20 years. Either type can impair your kidneys' ability to filter wastes from your body (see Chronic Kidney [Renal] Failure, page 854).

To prevent or lessen the effects of kidney disease, keep your blood pressure under control. Get prompt treatment for urinary tract infections. Your physician will periodically examine your urine for loss of albumin or protein. Also, avoid regular use of pain medications containing phenacetin, because they can damage your kidneys. Your physician can recommend alternatives, and will limit your exposure to intravenous dyes in X-ray examinations.

Diabetic Neuropathy

High blood sugar levels can damage the nerves, affecting their ability to send messages. Your feet, and sometimes your hands, might tingle, burn, or feel numb (peripheral neuropathy). Over time, the affected areas become less sensitive and more subject to injury and infection. When complicated by impaired circulation to the extremities, ulcer formation and gangrene can result. To help avoid infection, practice good foot care (see Caring for Your Feet, page 931).

Diabetic neuropathy also can affect bladder control, the intestinal tract, and the blood vessels, and it can cause impotence.

Foot Problems

If you have diabetes, you are at risk for foot problems. Cuts, blisters, corns, calluses, and other conditions that are rarely more than minor irritations to someone without diabetes can rapidly become serious medical problems. Gangrene or infection can result and, in severe cases, amputation of the foot or leg may be required (see Diabetes Mellitus, page 925).

If you have insulin-dependent diabetes, the risk of foot problems is low in the first 10 years or so that you have the disease. However, be alert for symptoms of the potential complications outlined below and seek proper care if you observe them.

Caring for Your Feet

If you have diabetes or poor circulation to your lower extremities, you should spend a few minutes of each day caring for your feet. By doing so, you may minimize future foot complications. A few commonsense guidelines follow.

Keep Your Feet Clean

Wash your feet carefully every day, using warm water and mild hand soap or a cleanser recommended by your physician. Dry them thoroughly with a soft, clean towel. To prevent dry skin, apply a moisturizing lotion (not between the toes). Wear only soft, absorbent, clean socks or hose, and avoid shoes and socks that are tight enough to restrict circulation or cause your feet to perspire excessively. Avoid socks made from synthetic material because they do not allow evaporation of moisture.

Examine Your Feet Daily

Examine your feet carefully, including tops, bottoms, areas between the toes, and the toenails. You can use a small mirror if you have difficulty seeing the bottoms of your feet. Look for cuts and scrapes, cracks, calluses, bruises, corns, or signs of infection such as swelling or redness. Consult your physician if you notice any areas of soreness or infection. In any case, your physician should inspect your feet routinely at your regularly scheduled visits.

Trim Your Toenails Properly

Do not use scissors or rounded clippers because they can cause injury. With an emery board, file the nails straight across, rather than curving them to match the shape of the toes, and not too short. This will help avoid ingrown nails, a common ailment that, for someone with diabetes, is potentially serious.

Avoid Injury

Exercise increases circulation and helps maintain the health of your feet. However, in selecting your physical activities, consider the risk of injury. Also avoid extremes of hot and cold. When your feet or legs become tired, sit down and elevate them for a few minutes.

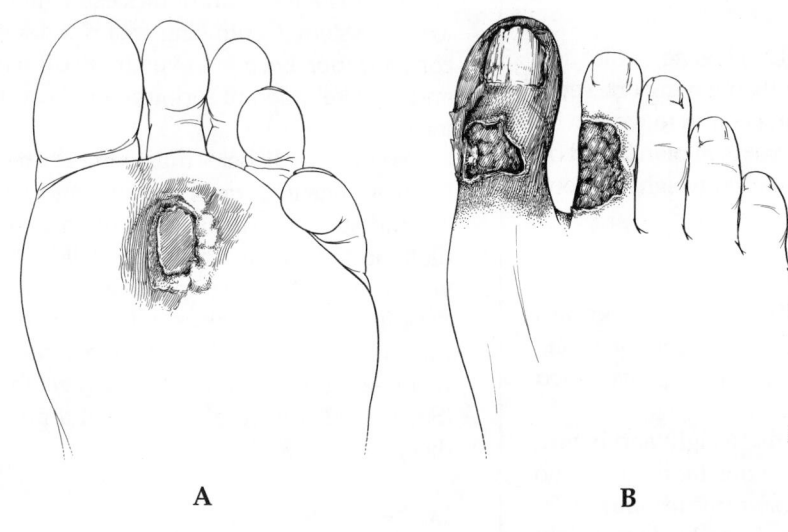

A   **B**

Over a period of years, diabetes can result in deterioration of nerves and blood vessels in your extremities. In such cases, minor wounds sometimes lead to development of neurotropic ulcers (A). In some instances, the deterioration of blood vessels can severely limit flow of blood, leading to gangrene (B).

Charcot's Joint

Another serious long-term complication of diabetic neuropathy is Charcot's joint. This uncommon problem occurs with long-standing nerve deterioration. The small bones of the arch of your foot gradually disintegrate, and your feet rather quickly become swollen and very flat. Charcot's joint can have crippling results, although there is little pain.

Treatment

Although medications are essential for people with IDDM and for many with NIDDM, the treatment of either disorder involves all-important lifestyle changes. Unlike certain other diseases that have no demonstrable link to patterns of physical activity and diet, the management and progress of diabetes are inextricably linked to behavior. Persons with diabetes must be prepared to adapt to the disorder in three ways: an appropriate diet and weight control plan, a sensible approach to physical activity, and medication (if necessary).

Various health care professionals may be involved in the care of the person with diabetes. The family physician, general pediatrician, general internist, or an endocrinologist or diabetologist probably will supervise the medical care, but consultations with podiatrists, ophthalmologists, and other professionals may also be needed if complications develop.

Yet, if you have diabetes, your role is as vital as that of any of the caregivers. Only you can assume responsibility for the day-to-day management of your illness. This means closely adhering to the medication, dietary, and exercise regimens recommended by your physician.

New Nutrition Guidelines

The American Diabetes Association (ADA) has new nutrition advice for people with diabetes. Rather than having one set of guidelines for everyone, the ADA encourages you to work with a registered dietitian to develop a personal meal plan based on your food preferences, health concerns (such as weight or blood cholesterol level), and insulin therapy.

Other changes are the following:

- Reasonable weight goals. Instead of striving endlessly toward your "ideal" weight, aim for a "reasonable" weight. Dropping as few as 10 to 20 pounds may be enough to improve blood sugar control.
- Flexible fat levels. If you're at a healthy weight and have a normal blood cholesterol level, keep your fat intake to no more than 30 percent of your total calories (the recommendation for all Americans). However, if you need to lose weight or if you have high cholesterol, 20 to 25 percent of calories from fat may be healthier.
- Calculated use of sugar. Sugar is no longer forbidden. New information shows that table sugar affects blood sugar about the same as complex carbohydrates like bread, rice, or potatoes. What's important is your overall amount of carbohydrate intake, not its source.

Meal planning for diabetes continues to be a nutritionally balanced, flexible style of eating. Greater flexibility, however, takes responsibility. More than ever, it's critical that you work with a registered dietitian and the rest of your diabetes team to learn how to enjoy more variety within the limits of your diet.

Nutrition

A proper diet is essential. In fact, for many with NIDDM, a program of weight control alone is sufficient to treat the disorder. A specific diet is tailored for each person, but the basic approach of dietary therapy involves weight reduction for the overweight individual and the establishment of regular eating patterns for the lean person. (For guidance regarding the ideal weight for your height and frame size, consult the chart on page 259. If your weight is 20 percent or more in excess of the number given and you are not unusually muscular, you are overweight.)

Alcoholic beverages tend to aggravate diabetes; therefore, limit your alcohol consumption. Furthermore, alcohol is a concentrated source of calories that can complicate your weight-control program.

The goal of a proper diet is twofold. First, it will help control your blood glucose levels. Second, and equally important, it will help you control or reduce your weight. Obesity increases your body's need for insulin because extra food contributes extra glucose to your system. Controlling your blood sugar concentration becomes even more difficult, and the likelihood of serious complications increases.

People with diabetes must carefully regulate their consumption of carbohydrates (sugars and starches), fats, and proteins. Your dietitian will create a program tailored for your needs. Avoid simple sugars, such as those in candy and cookies and sugary drinks. Include in your diet fiber-rich foods such as whole-grain breads, fruits, and vegetables. (See page 284 for a discussion of a proper diet.)

Exercise

Exercise is another part of the treatment program for diabetes. Regular exercise helps maintain overall health, but more important, it benefits the heart and blood vessels and may improve circulation. It is valuable in a weight-reduction program.

Because the muscles use more glucose during vigorous exercise, exercise helps decrease blood glucose concentration. In addition, exercise makes the cells throughout the body more sensitive to insulin, enabling them to use the available supplies of it more efficiently.

Your physician will help you establish guidelines for how frequently and how vigorously you should exercise. Chapter 10 discusses exercise programs in general (see page 289), but people with diabetes have several special concerns. Because exercise functions much like insulin in decreasing the blood glucose level, you have to be alert to the possibility of developing an excessively low concentration of blood glucose (see Insulin Reaction, page 927). Eating a light carbohydrate snack and drinking milk about 30 minutes before exercising may be a good practice. Carrying a fast-acting carbohydrate or glucose tablets is also recommended in the event you feel the nervousness, weakness, hunger, or other characteristic symptoms of hypoglycemia. If you have IDDM, try to time your physical activity so that it doesn't coincide with the times when your injected insulin has its maximal effect—this practice will lessen the risk of hypoglycemia.

Medication

Insulin is the drug used for IDDM. Oral hypoglycemic medications may or may not be used by people who develop NIDDM. However, a key factor in the use and dosage of insulin or another drug is the individual's willingness to follow the dietary and exercise guidelines discussed above.

The decision to use insulin or an oral hypoglycemic medication is based on the type and severity of the diabetes. For an obese person with NIDDM, careful regulation of food intake, accompanied by an exercise regimen, may be the solution. If such measures cannot control the disease, your physician may prescribe either oral medication or insulin injections. If you have IDDM, insulin shots are necessary. Dosage will depend, in part, on how carefully you follow your guidelines for diet and exercise.

Insulin

Insulin is available in various types and strengths. Some is obtained from the pancreas of cattle or hogs. Recombinant DNA technology has made possible the production of synthetic human insulin.

Some varieties of insulin act quickly, whereas others act for longer periods. The type of insulin, its amount, and the timing of administration are tailored to the person's individual needs and readiness to undertake a disciplined program. A mixture of regular insulin with intermediate insulin and additional injections at other times of the day may be needed. Persons with IDDM usually

Updated Treatment Guidelines

Can tight control of blood sugar delay complications from diabetes? For decades the answer was maybe. Now the National Institutes of Health says yes. Diabetes ultimately can result in blindness, kidney failure, and nerve degeneration. An NIH-sponsored study shows that tight blood-glucose control reduces, by about 60 percent, the risk for development and progression of these complications. If you have insulin-dependent diabetes mellitus (IDDM), tight control means:

- Checking your blood sugar more often, using finger pricks
- Adjusting insulin more frequently
- Keeping good records

If you don't take insulin, carefully control your blood sugar with diet, regular exercise, and, if prescribed, oral medication. The closer to normal you keep your blood sugar, the lower your risk of complications.

require multiple injections of insulin each day. Your physician will help determine which approach best suits your needs.

Many people with IDDM and even some with NIDDM can undertake a regimen called

Glucose Self-Monitoring

The key to treating diabetes is controlling the blood glucose concentration, and in order to manage it, you must monitor it. Glucose self-monitoring offers a way to determine whether adjustments in diet, medication, or exercise are necessary. It is especially important to the person who requires medication, whether it is insulin or an oral agent. Pregnant women with diabetes and whose glucose level is unstable would do well to check their concentrations several times daily. The same holds true for anyone with diabetes whose glucose is unstable.

In years past, urine testing was a common way to assess blood sugar. Today, blood tests are more accurate. Your physician will help you determine the timing, frequency, and methods to use. In general, blood tests should be conducted before meals and at bedtime, times when glucose levels should be relatively normal. In addition, your physician may order a special blood test (called a "glycosylated hemoglobin test") to determine how your sugar has been controlled during the previous 6 to 8 weeks.

Keep careful records of the results of each test. Taken individually and together, they will help you and your physician determine the effectiveness of your treatment program and whether changes in medication, diet, or exercise are necessary.

intensive insulin therapy. This consists of an injection of rapidly acting insulin before each meal, along with an injection of a long-acting insulin (the doses depend on the blood glucose concentration at the time). An insulin pump is another possibility. This battery-operated device holds a supply of insulin that is delivered continuously and automatically through a needle under the skin of the abdomen. Mayo Clinic physicians generally recommend the multiple-injection approach (intensive insulin therapy) rather than use of a pump.

Oral Hypoglycemic Agents

If you have trouble controlling your blood sugar with diet and exercise alone, your physician may recommend an oral hypoglycemic

Insulin Injection

All insulin is administered by injection (when taken orally, the digestive system destroys the hormone before the body can put it to use). It is important that this simple procedure be conducted properly:

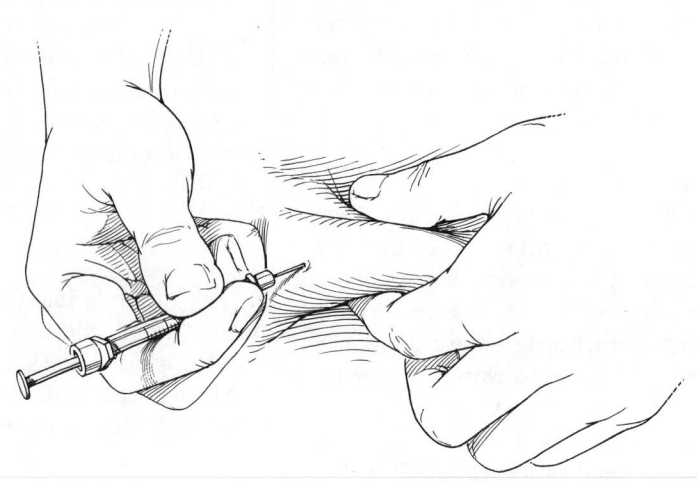

1. Remove the protective covering from the needle. Draw the plunger back to the mark on the syringe corresponding to the exact dosage of insulin you require.

2. Hold the bottle of insulin upright in one hand, and push the needle through the rubber stopper. Push the plunger down to empty the air from it.

3. Turn over the bottle and syringe together. Check that the tip of the needle is covered by the solution, then slowly pull the plunger back, drawing in slightly more than your prescribed dose.

4. To remove any air bubbles, tap the syringe until the bubbles rise to the needle end, then push the plunger until they return to the bottle. Adjust the solution in the syringe to your exact dose, and remove the needle from the bottle.

5. Using an alcohol swab or a cotton ball soaked with alcohol or soap and water, clean the area of the injection.

6. Hold the syringe as you would a writing utensil. With your other hand, pinch a 1- to 2-inch fold of skin.

7. Quickly insert the entire length of the needle into the fold of the skin.

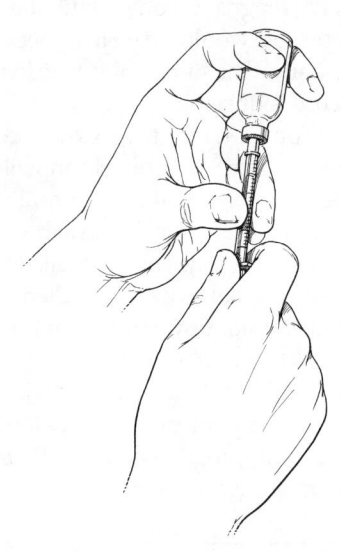

8. Release the pinched skin and inject the insulin by gently pushing the plunger all the way down at a steady, moderate rate. Note: If the plunger jams as you are injecting the insulin, remove the needle from the skin and note the number of units remaining in the syringe. Contact your health care provider for further instructions.

9. After injecting the insulin, cover the area of the injection with an alcohol swab or a cotton ball dampened with alcohol. Apply pressure to the area for a few seconds, but do not rub it because rubbing could cause the insulin to be absorbed into the bloodstream too quickly.

10. Dispose of the needle properly in a covered, puncture-proof container.

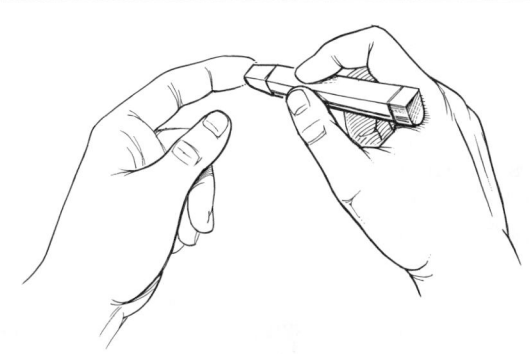

(1) The proper insulin dosage is essential to control diabetes. Blood sugar measurements are more accurate than analysis of urine. Spring-loaded devices with a needle activated by a button or other mechanism are quick and easy to use and reduce the discomfort of the pinprick.

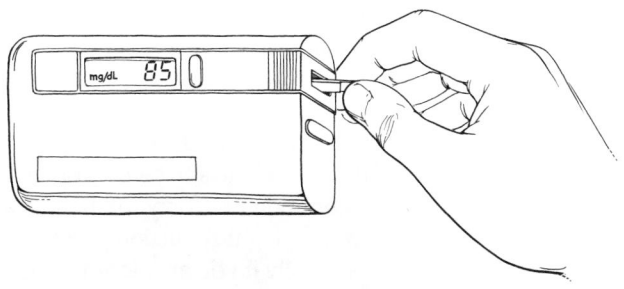

(3) Although direct-reading strips are available, blood glucose meters automatically analyze the sample and provide a single numerical reading rather than an estimated range.

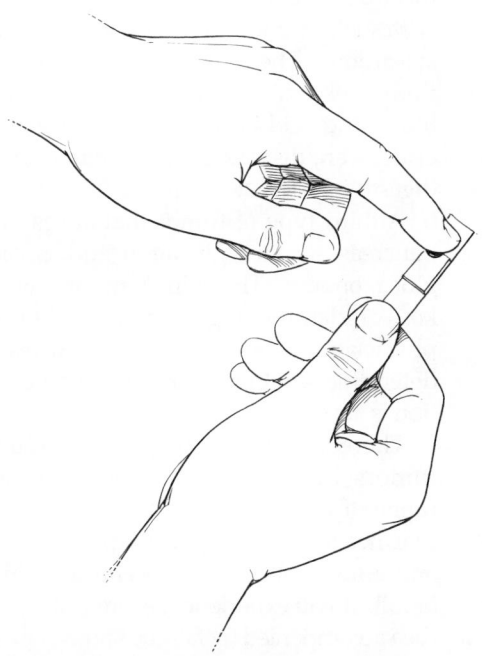

(2) In the glucose monitoring test, a drop of blood is applied to the chemically treated portion of a test strip.

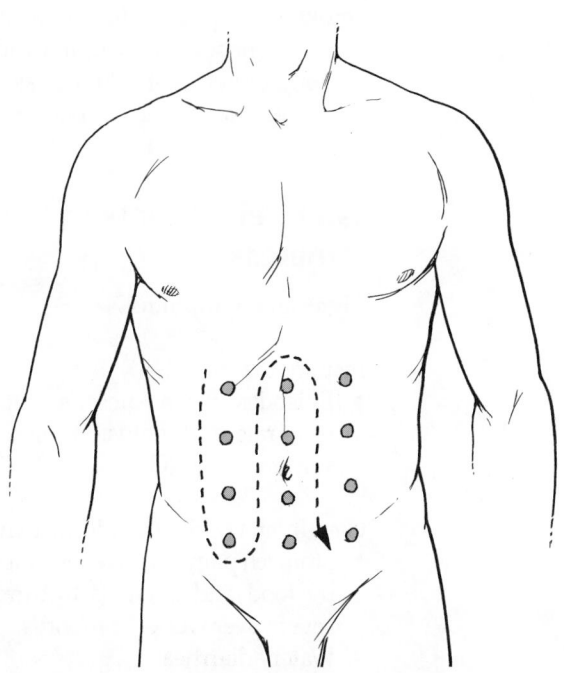

(4) Because insulin injected into the abdomen is absorbed more consistently, inject insulin into the abdomen rather than the thighs, arms, or buttocks, especially during physical activity. Change injection sites systematically. If too many injections are given in a small area, fatty tissue under the skin may become scarred. This can make absorption into the bloodstream erratic.

agent to stimulate your pancreas to make more insulin. These drugs also may help your cells use insulin and glucose more effectively.

An oral diabetes medication works well only if your pancreas still produces some insulin. You take the medicine once or twice daily, usually before meals.

Surgery

In some situations your physician may want to refer you to a medical center where a pancreas transplantation can be considered. This sometimes is performed at the same time as a kidney transplantation if diabetes has severely damaged your kidneys.

Prevention

There is no known prevention for IDDM, but obesity is closely associated with the development of NIDDM in persons older than 40 years. As a result, weight reduction may help forestall its development in some cases. If your weight is 10 percent or more over that recommended for your height and frame size, a weight-reduction program is in order, especially if you are older than 40 years and have a family history of diabetes (see page 1099 for a discussion of obesity).

Once you have been diagnosed as having diabetes, good control of your blood sugar can limit the development and progression of possible complications. A good exercise program is crucial. If you are a smoker, quit; smoking is especially hazardous to the person with diabetes and significantly adds to the long-term risk of heart disease and other side effects (see Smoking, page 639).

Islet Cell Tumors of the Pancreas

Signs and Symptoms

Insulinoma
- Episodes of weakness, sweating, rapid heart rate, and confusion; relieved by consumption of food

Gastrinoma (Zollinger-Ellison syndrome)
- Stomach pain that is relieved temporarily by food and antacids but grows more severe over weeks or months
- Watery diarrhea

Glucagonoma
- Rash that occurs on various areas of the body
- Sore tongue
- Weight loss

Most pancreatic tumors do not manufacture hormones, and many of them are malignant (see page 820). Some uncommon or rare tumors arise out of the islets of Langerhans, the clusters of cells in the pancreas that normally secrete the hormones insulin and glucagon. These tumors often secrete these hormones in excessive amounts, which, in turn, may produce serious effects.

The tumor may be named after the hormone it produces. The islet cell tumor that produces insulin is called an insulinoma and causes periods of hypoglycemia (low concentration of sugar in the blood). The symptoms are the same as those of insulin reactions that occur after insulin injections (see page 934). These symptoms tend to develop gradually over several months to a year and often occur with exercise, on an empty stomach, or before breakfast. Dietary therapy is of no permanent value, although frequent consumption of food may alleviate symptoms temporarily. Treatment is surgical removal of the tumor.

A second type of hormone-producing islet cell tumor is gastrinoma. Gastrin is a hormone that stimulates secretion of acid and digestive juices in the stomach. A tumor that overproduces gastrin will cause severe ulcer symptoms that respond poorly to standard ulcer treatments. The condition associated with such a tumor is called Zollinger-Ellison syndrome. The diagnosis is confirmed by finding excessive amounts of gastrin in the blood and acid in the stomach. Treatment options are discussed in the chapter on the digestive system (see page 757).

A third type of tumor that arises in the pancreas secretes glucagon and is called glucagonoma. The skin symptoms are the key for identifying glucagonoma, but your physician also will conduct blood tests to determine whether your glucose concentration is abnormally high.

There are other hormone-producing tumors, but these are rare and have a wide range of manifestations, including watery diarrhea (even during fasting), weight loss, and a low potassium concentration in the blood. If you experience severe watery diarrhea accompanied by fatigue and weight loss over a period of several weeks, your physician probably will want to do special stool, blood, and radiologic tests to rule out those rare conditions.

How Serious Are Pancreatic Tumors?

Like all tumors, pancreatic tumors demand immediate treatment. When diagnosed promptly, however, they often can be removed.

Treatment

Surgical removal of the affected tissues is usually the key component of treatment. Some of these tumors may be malignant. Medical therapy may be helpful in reducing symptoms due to excess hormone production, particularly if the tumor has spread.

Adrenal Gland Disorders

There are two adrenal glands, each located on top of a kidney and each about the size of the end section of your thumb. An adrenal gland consists of two portions: the inner core, called the medulla, and the outer layer, called the cortex.

The medulla produces two hormones—epinephrine (adrenaline) and norepinephrine (noradrenaline). The brain controls the production of these hormones. When secreted into the bloodstream, they increase your heart rate and blood pressure and affect other body functions. Physical and emotional stresses usually trigger the release of these hormones.

The cortex produces a group of hormones called corticosteroids, of which there are three kinds. One kind is the sex hormones. They include male hormones (androgens) and female hormones (estrogens), which affect sexual development and reproduction. (Note that sex hormones also are produced elsewhere in the body, by the testicles and ovaries, and that both male and female hormones are found in men and in women.) Another kind includes the hydrocortisone family of hormones (glucocorticoids). These influence the conversion of starchy foods into glycogen, a storage form of sugar, in the liver. The third kind is the mineralocorticosteroids. They control the body's use of the minerals sodium and potassium; aldosterone is the principal member of this group. All of the corticosteroids are under the control of a hormone from the pituitary gland, except that aldosterone mainly is controlled by a different hormone, renin, produced by the kidney.

The hormones of the adrenal glands affect virtually every system in the body to some degree. Their effects are complex, and some of their actions overlap. Disturbances and failures can occur in this intricate system, leading to the disorders described below.

Cushing's Syndrome

Signs and Symptoms
- The face becomes rounder and more red over a period of several months to years
- Hump-like collection of fat between and above the shoulder blades
- Striations on skin of lower trunk
- Fatigue and muscle weakness
- Water retention (edema)
- Hypertension
- Excess growth of hair
- Mood swings
- Impotence or cessation of menstruation
- Osteoporosis, especially in the spinal and pelvic bones
- Diabetes
- Easy bruising
- Obesity

This disorder occurs when excess glucocorticoid hormones circulate in the bloodstream. The excess may be the result of an overproduction by the adrenal glands or of extended use of steroid drugs for treating another ailment. The syndrome is named for Harvey Cushing, an early 20th-century American surgeon.

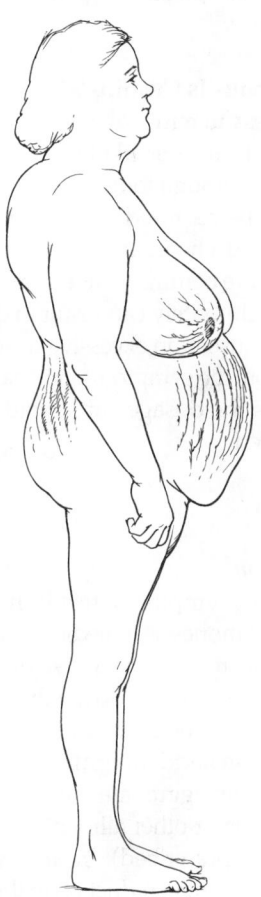

Cushing's syndrome occurs when excess glucocorticoid hormone circulates in the bloodstream. If Cushing's syndrome is untreated, the face can assume an exaggerated roundness, the back has a characteristic hump, and skin on the lower trunk shows striations.

Diagnosis

During the physical examination, the physician looks for characteristic changes in the head and shoulders. Roundness and redness of the face and an excess of fatty tissue above the collarbones and between the shoulder blades are clues to diagnosis. Frequent, or even spontaneous, bruising on the arms and legs is another symptom.

If you are taking a corticosteroid drug to treat another ailment (such as rheumatoid arthritis, asthma, or a skin disorder), the cause should be obvious to your physician. However, if the cause is overproduction of the hormones by the adrenal glands, further testing will be required. This overproduction may be due to a tumor of one adrenal gland, to enlargement of both glands, or to overproduction of the adrenal-stimulating hormone from a tumor in the pituitary gland, lung, or other organ. The exact cause is determined by measuring the hormones in blood and urine before and after taking a synthetic hormone (dexamethasone) in conjunction with scans (MRI or CT, see page 494 and page 1334) of the pituitary, adrenals, or lungs. Direct blood sampling from the veins draining the pituitary gland also may be necessary.

How Serious Is Cushing's Syndrome?

The successful removal of a benign pituitary or adrenal tumor is likely to result in a full recovery, although long-term hormone therapy may be required. Accelerated atherosclerosis with heart attacks and fractures of the spine are common. If left untreated, this disorder ultimately can result in death.

If the cause is an excessive dose of steroid medication, the symptoms gradually will disappear as the dosages of steroid hormones are reduced.

Treatment

Medication

When the symptoms result from taking steroid hormones as a medication, treatment consists of stopping their use or decreasing the dosage. However, do not discontinue this medication without consulting your physician because sudden termination of steroid treatment can aggravate the underlying disease (asthma or other ailments for which the steroid was prescribed). Your physician will prescribe a gradual reduction in the dosage of steroids. In some cases, another drug may be used in place of the steroid originally prescribed. For as long as a year after steroid medication is stopped, a physical stress such as injury, infection, or surgery may produce a dangerous insufficiency in production of adrenal hormone, requiring emergency treatment (see Addison's disease, this page).

Surgery

When Cushing's syndrome is the result of a tumor in the adrenal gland, pituitary gland, or lung, removal of the tumor or even of the entire gland is usually the best treatment. If surgery is not possible or not successful, treatment options include radiation and drugs to block adrenal hormone production. In childhood, radiation may be the primary treatment for a tumor in the pituitary gland. If the treatment renders the adrenal glands incapable of providing the hormones your body needs, your physician will prescribe oral drugs to replace the missing hormones.

Addison's Disease

Signs and Symptoms

- Weakness, lethargy, and anemia
- Weight loss and decreased appetite
- Darkening of the skin
- Low blood pressure
- Hypoglycemia
- Abdominal pains accompanied by diarrhea, indigestion, vomiting, or constipation
- Decreased sexual interest
- Joint and muscle aches

Emergency Symptoms—Acute adrenal failure (addisonian crisis): dehydration (precipitated by severe diarrhea and vomiting), shock, and loss of consciousness

In contrast to Cushing's syndrome (see page 937), Addison's disease occurs when the cortex of the adrenal gland fails to produce enough steroid hormones. The disorder is named for the 19th-century English physician who identified it, Thomas Addison. Sometimes it is called adrenocortical hypofunction.

This failure of the adrenal glands may be the result of the body attacking itself (as in an autoimmune disease) or a consequence of some other disease such as tuberculosis. The disorder can occur at any age, including infancy, and is equally likely in males and females.

Diagnosis

Usually, the symptoms of Addison's disease develop slowly, perhaps over a period of months, but they may appear suddenly. If your physician thinks you have this disorder, samples of your blood and urine will be analyzed to measure the amounts of corticosteroid hormones present. Measuring the body's response to synthetic adrenal stimulating hormone may be necessary.

How Serious Is Addison's Disease?

Immediate hospitalization is essential for acute adrenal failure, which may be provoked by physical stress, infection, injury, vomiting, diarrhea, or the use of diuretic drugs. Adrenal failure is a life-threatening condition that requires immediate medical care, including infusions of salt solutions and steroid hormones. However, when Addison's disease is diagnosed early, treatment requires only daily doses of steroid tablets and salt supplements, taken orally, for a normal, healthy life. The symptoms will disappear. Often, the skin will lose its dark color.

Treatment

Medication

If you have Addison's disease, your physician will prescribe one or more steroid drugs for use on a regular basis. Take this medication faithfully, according to your physician's instructions. It is your body's only source of these essential steroid hormones. Without them, acute adrenal failure can result.

A typical routine for taking the replacement hormones, usually one of the prednisone or hydrocortisone drugs, involves a dose in the morning and one in the late afternoon (to mimic your body's normal rhythm of steroid production). A second drug, called fludrocortisone, controls your body's sodium and potassium needs and maintains a normal blood pressure. Too large a dose of this drug may result in excessive salt retention, which causes high blood pressure and swelling in the feet. The amounts of drugs used to replace lacking adrenal hormones should not cause stomach ulcer problems, and so these drugs do not need to be taken with antacid medication.

The body's reliance on oral steroids means that it is not able to respond to stressful circumstances that require additional amounts of hormone. These stresses include events such as an operation, an infection, or even a minor illness. In the event of an unusually stressful situation, consult your physician about a possible change in dosage of the steroids. It is imperative that any person taking this type of steroid medication regularly wear a necklace or bracelet that states the need for the hormones in case of emergency with loss of consciousness.

Nutrition

Moderate amounts of salt should be consumed in the diet daily. A low-salt diet could provoke symptoms of acute adrenal failure.

Pheochromocytoma

Signs and Symptoms

- High blood pressure
- Excessive sweating
- Increased heart rate or sensation of pounding heart
- Headache
- Pale complexion
- Weight loss
- Constipation

Diagnosis

This tumor arises from cells in the medulla or core of the adrenal gland and overproduces the hormone epinephrine or norepinephrine. The increased blood pressure may be constant or come in episodes associated with sweating, headache, pale skin, and awareness of the heartbeat. Finding elevated levels of these hormones in the blood or urine, especially after an episode, strongly suggests the diagnosis of pheochromocytoma and the need for further testing.

How Serious is Pheochromocytoma?

Pheochromocytoma can be life-threatening if untreated, because trauma or surgery may provoke the tumor to release dangerously high levels of epinephrine. These tumors may be associated with other tumors of the endocrine glands, such as a medullary thyroid cancer. Most tumors are benign and do not spread, but some may be malignant.

Treatment

Surgical removal of the tumor usually is advised, and in most cases the symptoms disappear. Prior to surgery, medications are given to block the effect of the hormones and normalize blood pressure.

Aldosteronoma

Signs and Symptoms
- High blood pressure
- Muscle weakness or cramps
- Occasionally, excess urination and thirst

Diagnosis
Also known as Conn's syndrome, this tumor arises from the outer portion of the adrenal gland (cortex) and produces the hormone aldosterone in excess. This causes the body to maintain too much sodium and water and lose potassium, resulting in high blood pressure and low blood potassium levels. When this combination is found, further tests are done to confirm the diagnosis. Elevated aldosterone levels also may occur as the result of non-tumorous production from the adrenal glands.

How Serious Is Aldosteronoma?
Because these tumors are rarely malignant, the main concerns are the problems that arise from increased blood pressure (see page 647). Very low potassium levels may cause muscle and heart problems.

Treatment
If a tumor in one adrenal gland is found, surgery to remove that gland will improve blood pressure and normalize hormone and potassium levels in most people, but some may continue to need medication for high blood pressure. Medications that specifically block the effects of aldosterone can also be used and are effective.

Other Adrenal Tumors
Tumors in the adrenal gland can produce cortisol in excess and cause Cushing's syndrome (see page 937).

Very rarely, adrenal tumors can produce sex hormones of the opposite sex, which could result in impotence or enlargement of the breasts in men or abnormal hair growth,

Hirsutism

In some women, hair may begin to grow on the face, chest, ears, and other locations where typically only men have hair. Such hairiness, called hirsutism, can be caused by the use of drugs such as phenytoin (better known by its brand name Dilantin), which is used to treat some seizure disorders, and by some agents used to control hypertension. Certain tumors and other disorders of the adrenal glands and ovaries also can cause hirsutism.

In many cases, after tests and examinations, the physician finds no apparent explanation. These patients have what is known as idiopathic hirsutism—that is, hairiness of unknown cause.

Physicians believe that in most cases there is a slight increase in sensitivity to, or production of, androgen (a male hormone), which occurs for no known reason. Women with idiopathic hirsutism experience normal menstrual cycles, have normal ovaries, and have no evidence of tumors or abnormal adrenal gland function. With such factors ruled out, the condition poses no health risk but is a matter of cosmetic concern.

Potential drug treatments are available. No one drug has been approved specifically for the purpose of treating excess hairiness, but several—including cortisone-like hormones, a diuretic called aldactone, and oral contraceptives that contain the hormones estrogen and progestin—may prove effective for suppressing androgen levels and controlling hirsutism.

However, keep in mind that these are powerful drugs. They have possible side effects. Also, they are not uniformly effective in treating hirsutism, and even when successful may take several months to produce an effect. Cosmetic methods of control may be preferable (see page 1019).

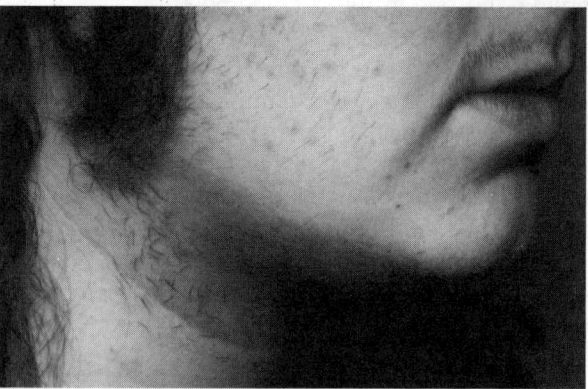

Excess hair on the face and other locations is termed hirsutism. It can occur as a side effect of certain prescription drugs, but often occurs for no known reason.

menstrual irregularities, and deepening of the voice in women.

Often an adrenal tumor is found when a scan of the abdomen is obtained for another purpose. Hormone studies will ensure that this tumor is not producing excess hormones. Scans have to be repeated over time to check for tumor growth. These benign tumors are termed non-functioning adrenal adenomas. Although cancer of the adrenal gland is rare, the chance that an adrenal tumor is cancerous increases with its size. Because of this, surgery may be recommended for larger or growing tumors.

Congenital Adrenal Hyperplasia

Signs and Symptoms
- Enlargement of the penis in male infants and of the clitoris in female infants
- Sometimes, acute adrenal failure (see page 938)
- High blood pressure (rarely)
- Growth is accelerated in early childhood but ceases early, resulting in short adult stature

This condition is the most common adrenal gland disorder in infants and children. It is the result of a genetic abnormality that causes an enzyme deficiency, which in turn causes the adrenal glands to produce a distorted pattern of steroid hormones. Some women have a partial or mild deficiency of the enzyme. They develop normally in childhood but as young adults can have problems with hirsutism, menstrual irregularities, or infertility.

Diagnosis
When the presence of congenital adrenal hyperplasia is suspected, the physician will examine the genitals carefully and conduct blood and urine tests to measure the hormones produced by the adrenal gland.

How Serious Is Congenital Adrenal Hyperplasia?
The first step is to rule out other causes for the symptoms. Once this disorder has been diagnosed, it usually can be treated with medication. The principal long-term risk is the side effects of the medication, so the physician will closely monitor skeletal and other growth patterns in young patients.

Treatment
In most cases the therapy consists of corticosteroid drugs taken orally on a daily basis.

Pituitary Gland Disorders

Located at the base of the brain behind the nasal passages, the pituitary gland is roughly the size and shape of a hazelnut. Despite its diminutive size, it is the most important of the endocrine glands. It serves as a control center for the body's long-term growth, day-to-day functioning, and reproductive capabilities.

The pituitary consists of two parts, the front (anterior) lobe and the rear (posterior) lobe.

The anterior lobe produces six distinct hormones, including prolactin to stimulate the production of breast milk and growth hormone to regulate the body's physical growth. The other four influence other parts of the endocrine system, stimulating activities in the thyroid gland, ovaries, testicles, and adrenal glands.

The posterior lobe produces two hormones: oxytocin and antidiuretic hormone. Oxytocin prompts contractions during childbirth and stimulates the breasts to release milk during breastfeeding. Antidiuretic hormone acts on the kidneys to control urine output.

Most abnormalities of the pituitary gland are caused by pituitary tumors. These can be classified as either functioning or nonfunctioning. The functioning tumors release excess amounts of one of the normal pituitary hormones, which in turn cause specific physical signs and symptoms such as Cushing's syndrome (see page 937).

Both types of tumors also can cause problems simply by pressing on neighboring vital tissues. Although the vast majority of pituitary tumors are not malignant and do not spread, they can lead to significant and even life-threatening problems.

Acromegaly/Gigantism

Signs and Symptoms
- Accelerated growth to excessive adult height (in gigantism only, with onset during childhood)
- Gradual enlargement of hands, feet, jaw, forehead
- Widely spaced teeth
- Large tongue
- Excessive perspiration
- Sleep apnea
- Carpal tunnel syndrome
- Pituitary mass effects (see Nonfunctioning Pituitary Tumors, page 943)
- Hypopituitarism (see page 943)

These symptoms usually result from the overproduction of growth hormone from a pituitary tumor. The changes occur slowly, usually over several years, and often are not apparent to the patient or family.

Diagnosis
The presence of certain physical features may suggest acromegaly. Your physician will ask specific questions regarding an increase in glove, shoe, or hat size, and the inability to fit into older rings. Old pictures may be examined to determine if there has been a change in appearance over time. Blood tests showing excessive amounts of growth hormone and other hormones under its control confirm the diagnosis. Measuring growth hormone after ingesting glucose also may be necessary. A specific test of peripheral vision may be done. A CT or MRI scan of the head may be obtained to pinpoint a tumor in the pituitary gland. Very rarely, a tumor outside the pituitary can cause this syndrome.

How Serious Is Acromegaly/Gigantism?
Excess growth hormone causes growth of not only the bones but also the internal organs. Other possible effects are high blood pressure, diabetes mellitus, arthritis, colon polyps, and loss of vision. If the condition is left untreated, the heart may become enlarged, leading to heart failure.

Treatment
Surgical removal of the tumor is the most common treatment. Radiation therapy may be used, especially if the entire tumor cannot safely be removed. Two medications may also be used to decrease growth hormone secretion: bromocriptine, taken as a pill, and octreotide, given as an injection under the skin. The normal pituitary gland may be damaged by the tumor or in the course of treatment, and if this occurs, hormone therapy will be necessary.

Prolactinoma

Signs and Symptoms

In Women
- Irregularity or cessation of menstrual cycles
- Milky discharge from the breasts
- Infertility

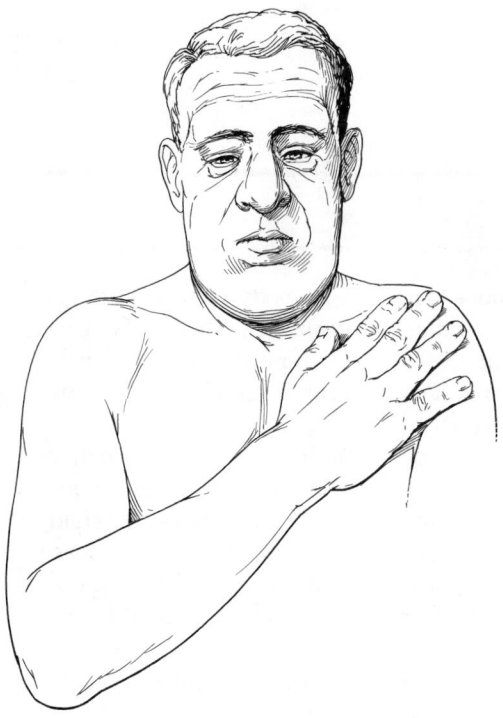

Acromegaly is caused by an excess of growth hormone in adulthood. The condition may result in an overgrowth of the hands, jaw, skull, and other bones, producing exaggerated body parts and coarsened features.

In Men
- Impotence, decreased sexual interest, decreased body hair
- Infertility

In Both Sexes
- Pituitary mass effects (see Nonfunctioning Pituitary Tumors, this page)
- Hypopituitarism (this page)

This pituitary tumor overproduces the hormone prolactin. Tumors can range in size from microscopic to several centimeters in diameter. In larger tumors, peripheral vision loss and other symptoms of a pituitary mass (see below) can occur. High prolactin levels can occur from causes other than prolactinomas, including several medications.

Diagnosis
Your physician will take a careful medical history and physical examination to exclude other causes of high prolactin. Your breasts will be examined for discharge. Blood tests will measure your level of prolactin and other hormones. A CT or MRI scan of the pituitary will determine if a tumor is visible.

How Serious Is Prolactinoma?
The major effect of increased prolactin levels is to decrease the normal levels of the sex hormones. Although such deficiencies are not life-threatening, you may require treatment to achieve pregnancy and to prevent long-term complications such as osteoporosis (see page 894).

Treatment
Both medication (bromocriptine) and surgery are acceptable treatment options for prolactinoma. Your physician will determine which is best for you.

Nonfunctioning Pituitary Tumors

Signs and Symptoms
- Loss of peripheral vision
- Double vision
- Drooping of an eyelid
- Headache
- Excessive thirst and urination
- Fatigue, light-headedness
- Intolerance to cold
- Constipation
- In women, irregular menstrual periods
- In men, decreased sexual interest, impotence, decreased body hair
- In children, slowed growth and development

Nonfunctioning tumors—tumors of the pituitary that do not produce a hormone in excess—cause symptoms by pressing on the tissues surrounding the pituitary. For example, the nerves that control vision and eye movement lie close to the pituitary and can be affected by a pituitary tumor. The normal function of the pituitary also can be affected, ultimately causing deficiencies of the thyroid, adrenal, growth, water balance, or sex hormones. Usually the symptoms progress gradually, but in rare cases they occur suddenly (pituitary apoplexy). Many times a tumor is found on a scan for an unrelated symptom.

Diagnosis
CT or MRI scanning confirms the presence of a pituitary tumor. Vision testing also will be performed. Your blood and urine will be tested to determine if you have any associated hormone excess or deficiency.

How Serious Is a Nonfunctioning Pituitary Tumor?
Several types of nonfunctioning tumors can develop in the pituitary gland. Two of the most common types are pituitary adenoma and craniopharyngioma. In some instances these tumors cause few, if any, of the problems listed above; in others, they cause serious and life-threatening hormone deficiencies or pressure on the brain.

Treatment
If you require treatment, the tumor usually is removed surgically. You may also have radiation therapy. Hormone deficiencies are treated with the appropriate hormone replacement.

Hypopituitarism

Signs and Symptoms

In Children
- Slowed growth and sexual development
- Hypoglycemia (see page 927)

In Adults

- In women, cessation of the menses, infertility, or inability to lactate after childbirth
- In men, decreased sexual interest and loss of beard or body hair
- Fine wrinkling of the skin adjacent to the eyes and mouth
- Fatigue
- Decreased appetite and sometimes weight loss

Emergency Symptoms—Fever and a decrease in blood pressure in response to stressful situations or infection

Hypopituitarism is a disorder in which your pituitary gland produces insufficient quantities of one or more of the pituitary hormones. The name is derived in part from the Greek prefix *hypo*, which means "under." Some people inherit a tendency toward hypopituitarism. Others acquire the ailment for unknown reasons. In many instances, however, the cause is identifiable.

The condition can be caused by a tumor or inflammation of the pituitary gland, or it can develop after a serious head injury. Some women experience hypopituitarism after childbirth because the gland, which normally increases in size during pregnancy, grows so large that the body is unable to provide it with the oxygen and other blood-delivered products it needs; some or all of the pituitary tissue then dies.

Because the pituitary gland also produces hormones that activate other glands, underproduction of those hormones can result in the symptoms of other disorders, including hypothyroidism (see page 948) and Addison's disease (see page 938).

Diagnosis

Hypopituitarism in a child will result in dwarfism. The key indication is abnormally slow growth. Your child's physician monitors the growth of infants, and this exaggeratedly slow growth pattern will be observed at your baby's regular checkups. This ailment is rare; very few children who are shorter than average have the hormone insufficiency.

If your physician suspects hypopituitarism in you or your child, he or she will conduct tests to measure hormone concentrations in the blood and urine. Subsequent testing may involve injecting insulin to induce low blood sugar concentrations (hypoglycemia; see page 927). This condition stimulates the pituitary gland to produce its hormones, and they can then be measured.

If test results indicate a shortage of pituitary hormones, further tests are done to determine the underlying cause. A tumor is one possibility (see pages 941 through 943).

How Serious Is Hypopituitarism?

If the hormone that controls adrenal function is impaired, your body will be unable to respond normally to physical stresses such as injury or infections. This can be life-threatening. Growth hormone deficiency results in short stature, which may be associated with subsequent psychosocial problems. Appropriate hormone replacement prevents these problems and other symptoms of hypopituitarism.

Treatment

If a cause for hypopituitarism is identified, specific therapy for this may improve the hormone deficiencies. If not, various hormone replacement therapies will be necessary, depending on the degree of dysfunction of the pituitary gland. In children, injections of a synthetic growth hormone can stimulate body growth. Estrogen for girls or testosterone for boys may be required for sexual development. Adults also may need sex hormone replacement for specific fertility treatments. In both you and your child, pills for thyroid hormone replacement and adrenal hormone replacement may be required. Adrenal hormones such as prednisone or hydrocortisone need to be taken daily, with higher doses during times of illness. You should then wear a bracelet or necklace indicating that you require hormone replacement.

Diabetes Insipidus

Signs and Symptoms
- Excessive thirst
- Increased urination

Emergency Symptoms—Dehydration, physical collapse, and low blood pressure may precipitate a comatose state

Despite the similarities in symptoms and in name, this disorder should not be confused with diabetes mellitus. Diabetes mellitus is the result of a deficiency of insulin, the hormone that enables your body to use and maintain glucose to provide its cells with energy. Diabetes insipidus results from a deficiency of antidiuretic hormone (ADH), which is secreted by the posterior lobe of the pituitary.

If there is a shortage of antidiuretic hormone, your body loses control of its water balance. Rather than reabsorbing the water required to maintain proper fluid levels, your kidneys simply pass the water out.

In almost half of the cases of diabetes insipidus, the cause of the disorder is unknown, although a pituitary tumor may become evident several years after the onset of symptoms. Identifiable causes include damage to the pituitary from a head injury or from surgery for pituitary tumors and other inflammatory conditions.

Diagnosis

The key symptom is the large volume of urine that is excreted; urine output of between 5 and 20 quarts within 24 hours is not uncommon. Urination throughout the day and night will be the rule, as frequently as every 30 minutes. The dehydration that results from such increased urination can dry your skin and almost certainly will result in an insatiable thirst.

If diabetes insipidus is suspected, your physician probably will conduct a water-deprivation test in which you consume no fluid for several hours. Urine produced during that time is analyzed. If you have normal amounts of antidiuretic hormone, the volume of urine will decrease; if you have diabetes insipidus, you will eliminate substantial volumes of water. Your physician may also conduct blood tests to determine water and salt balance.

How Serious Is Diabetes Insipidus?

Except for cases in which the underlying cause—a tumor or disease—presents difficulties, a person with diabetes insipidus can, with treatment, expect to lead a normal life.

Treatment

Your physician will have three goals: to determine the cause, to eliminate it (if possible), and to control the symptoms.

Medication

Antidiuretic hormone will be administered either in a nasal spray or by injection. This hormone therapy usually is lifelong. However, for cases in which the known cause is an injury to the head or the result of surgery, the gland may regain its normal function over a few months to a year; if so, the medication can be discontinued.

A diuretic drug in the thiazide family may also be prescribed. Despite the fact that diuretics ordinarily are used to increase urination, thiazides have been effective for treating diabetes insipidus.

Surgery

If a tumor in your pituitary gland is the cause, surgery or radiation therapy may be appropriate (see pages 941 through 943).

Nutrition

Because sodium restriction helps in some cases, your physician may advise limiting your dietary salt intake.

Thyroid Disorders

Shaped like a bow tie, your thyroid gland is located at the base of your neck. The gland wraps around your windpipe (trachea); a crossbar (isthmus) connects its pair of lobes.

The thyroid helps set the rate at which your body functions. It responds to instructions from your pituitary gland by secreting the hormone thyroxine, whose actions control the pace of chemical activity in your body. Such activities vary directly with the quantity of thyroxine present: the more hormone circulating in the bloodstream, the greater the speed at which chemical reactions occur. The thyroid also produces calcitonin,

Goiter

The term goiter, which is derived from the Latin *guttur* for "throat," is used to describe a wide variety of conditions. In fact, goiter means simply an enlargement of the thyroid gland. This enlargement can be a small, localized lump or it can be a more general swelling of both lobes.

The enlarged thyroid gland can produce normal, subnormal, or excessive amounts of its hormone. The enlargement can interfere with swallowing. In rare instances the enlargement will grow around the trachea (windpipe), causing it to narrow. Surprisingly, goiters generally produce little discomfort.

In the past, the most common cause of goiter was a shortage of iodine in the diet in areas where the soil was deficient in iodine. Goiter became more rare after iodized salt was introduced; also, our food supply now contains adequate iodine. Supplements are therefore unnecessary, although in other parts of the world iodine deficiencies are not uncommon.

Simple Goiter

Simple goiter is characterized by a soft, widespread enlargement of the gland. It is most common during pregnancy or adolescence, although it is relatively uncommon today. If the simple goiter enlarges to the degree that it becomes a cosmetic problem, thyroid hormone can be given to decrease its size.

Graves' Disease

Graves' disease usually produces a slight but generalized swelling of the thyroid, although the gland can become large (see Hyperthyroidism, page 947).

Adenomatous Goiter

Adenomas are aggregations of more or less normal thyroid tissue that wall themselves off from the rest of the gland. Infrequently, one or more adenomas produce excessive

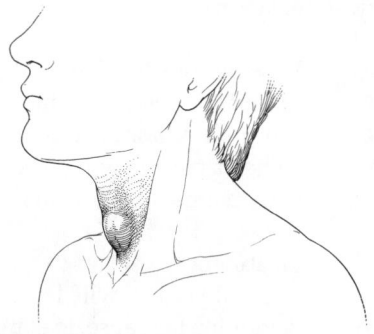

Goiter is an enlargement of the thyroid gland, most often due to a shortage of iodine in the diet. After iodized table salt was introduced, goiter became an uncommon ailment in the United States.

amounts of thyroid hormone, and hyperthyroidism results. Rarely, an adenoma partially blocks your windpipe (trachea) and produces breathing difficulty that superficially may resemble asthma (see Hyperfunctioning Thyroid Nodules, page 947).

Thyroid Cancer

Most thyroid cancers grow slowly. They tend to occur somewhat more frequently in persons who have had radiation therapy to the neck. The common types are papillary and follicular. The papillary type tends to spread to the lymph glands in the neck. The follicular type may go to your lungs and other more distant parts of your body.

Thyroid cancer begins as a small lump that cannot be distinguished readily from an adenoma. Tissue from a lump can be obtained through a needle for microscopic examination. Although this test does not always produce a clear answer as to whether the lump is cancerous, the information often is a good guide to your need for surgical removal of the lump.

If the lump proves to be malignant at operation (the pathologist can tell your surgeon within a matter of minutes whether the removed lump is malignant), your surgeon

will remove most of the thyroid gland. Under certain circumstances, radioactive iodine can be given after the operation to supplement surgical treatment. Thyroid hormone medication also is thought to retard growth of the remaining cancer cells.

Medullary Cancer of the Thyroid

In this unusual form of thyroid malignancy, the cancer cells secrete a hormone called calcitonin. The progress of the cancer can be followed by measuring calcitonin concentrations in the blood. Medullary carcinoma frequently occurs in members of the same family, and a person who has it also may have pheochromocytoma (see page 939).

Lymphocytic Thyroiditis

This type of goiter, sometimes called Hashimoto's disease after the Japanese pathologist who first described it, is one of the most common of all thyroid disorders. An abnormal antibody causes your thyroid gland to lose function, resulting in hypothyroidism (see page 948).

The gland usually becomes moderately enlarged and rather rubbery in texture. Blood tests for the antibody are helpful for diagnosis, and a thyroid needle biopsy confirms it. Thyroid hormone treatment usually causes the gland to shrink so that surgical removal is not needed.

Subacute Thyroiditis

This uncommon condition causes thyroid pain that is aggravated by swallowing. The gland is slightly enlarged and very tender. A sedimentation rate test may be conducted to help diagnose it (see page 1331). In cases of subacute thyroiditis, the sedimentation rate may be very high, and thyroid hormone values may be either high or low.

The thyroid generally returns to normal in a few months. Often, aspirin will control the symptoms, although your physician may prescribe corticosteroid medications if the symptoms are more pronounced.

a hormone that affects the amount of calcium in your blood.

Hyperthyroidism

Signs and Symptoms
- Weight loss despite increased appetite
- Increased heart rate and blood pressure
- Nervousness and sweating
- Swelling at the base of the neck (goiter)
- Increases in the frequency of bowel movements, sometimes diarrhea
- Muscle weakness
- Irritability

Emergency Symptoms—Thyrotoxic crisis: fever, very rapid pulse, agitation, and even delirium. Immediate care is required

Hyperthyroidism (also known as overactive thyroid disease) occurs when the thyroid gland produces excessive amounts of thyroid hormone. Its name is derived from the Greek *hyper*, which means "over," and *thyreos*, for "shield-shaped," describing the appearance of the thyroid gland. (Hypothyroidism, or underactive thyroid disorder, is discussed on page 948.)

The two forms of hyperthyroidism are Graves' disease (also known as toxic diffuse goiter) and hyperfunctioning nodular goiter (sometimes called Plummer's disease, named for an early physician at the Mayo Clinic). Both forms involve the excessive manufacture and release of the thyroid hormone thyroxine.

Graves' Disease
The functions of your thyroid gland ordinarily are controlled by a hormone secreted by your pituitary gland. In Graves' disease, your thyroid gland is stimulated excessively by an abnormal antibody, and the normal thyroid-stimulating hormone (TSH) from your pituitary cannot be detected in the blood. The production of thyroid hormones is abnormally high. The amount of thyroxine in your blood also is high.

Hyperthyroidism involves an increase in your body's normal energy expenditure (basal metabolic rate). One manifestation of this change is an increase in your appetite because your body demands more fuel for its added activity. This generates excessive heat, so you feel warm while others may be cool or comfortable. Your hands may tremble and you may have warm, sweaty palms. Your heart pounds forcibly at a rapid rate and occasionally develops a rapid irregularity (atrial fibrillation, see page 670). Sleep difficulties are common. The thyroid gland will be enlarged, but often so slightly that it isn't noticeable. Abnormalities in your immune system, which in Graves' disease may stimulate the thyroid, can affect your eyes. This causes widening of your lids, excessive tearing, and sometimes double vision.

Hyperfunctioning Thyroid Nodules
This form of hyperthyroidism results from excessive production of thyroxine by one or more adenomas of the thyroid. An adenoma is a portion of the gland that has walled itself off from the rest of the gland. It forms a lump, often half an inch or more in size, that you can feel and sometimes see.

Most adenomas of the thyroid produce little or no thyroid hormone, but occasionally an adenoma begins to manufacture an excessive amount of the hormone. This results in all of the symptoms of hyperthyroidism found in Graves' disease except that your eyes are not affected.

Diagnosis
Your physician will try to detect a slight tremor when you stick out your tongue and extend your fingers, and may inquire whether you have experienced diarrhea or other changes in your toilet habits. You may be asked whether you find yourself sensitive to increases in temperature and whether your symptoms are lessened in cooler temperatures. While you swallow, your physician will examine your thyroid gland.

The most evident physical signs of Graves' disease are protruding eyes, hand tremors, and a rapid heartbeat. Symptoms include sleeping difficulties.

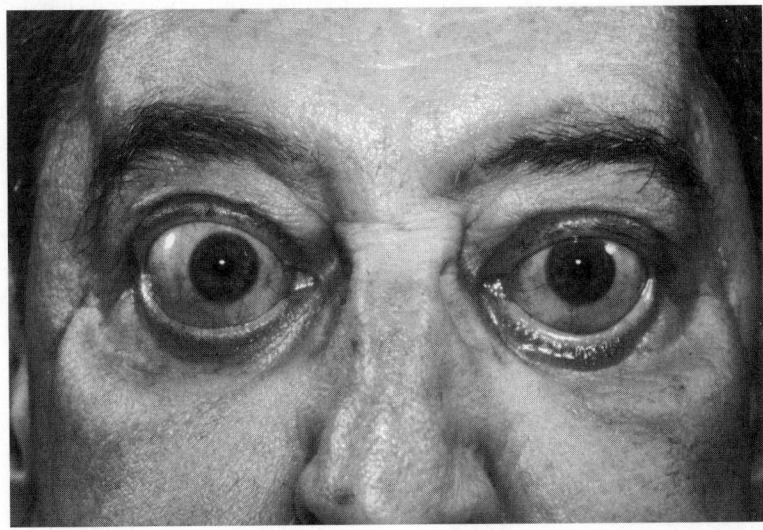

Because anxiety can cause symptoms like those of hyperthyroidism, psychological causes for the symptoms must be ruled out. Blood tests can detect an increase in the thyroxine concentration and low to absent amounts of TSH. A radioactive iodine tracer test usually is done to help establish the diagnosis and to aid in planning treatment.

In Graves' disease the thyroid gland usually has an abnormal "hunger" for iodine; a greater-than-normal amount of the radioactive iodine given with this test will collect in the thyroid within 24 hours. In the case of hyperfunctioning thyroid nodules, blood test results are similar to those in Graves' disease. Radioactive iodine tracer tests show that the iodine goes almost entirely to the overactive adenoma.

How Serious Is Hyperthyroidism?

Hyperthyroidism varies in severity. In some people, a brief cycle of treatment produces a complete and permanent cure. In others, relapses occur and a second or even third round of treatment is necessary.

If left untreated, the disorder is potentially fatal. In most cases of hyperthyroidism, however, normal health can be restored.

Treatment

Three types of treatment are available: a liquid form of radioactive iodine, an antithyroid medication in tablet form, and surgery. The proper course of treatment for you will be determined by your physical condition and age and by the nature and severity of your hyperthyroidism.

Medication

The most common treatment of hyperthyroidism involves drinking a liquid form of radioactive iodine. Your body will deliver the iodine (a key component of thyroid hormone) to the thyroid gland, and the concentrated radioactive iodine will cause the tissue in the gland to slow its production of hormones. The dose of radioactive iodine depends on the size of the thyroid gland and the findings on the tracer test.

The status of your thyroid will need to be reassessed in 2 to 3 months. At that time, a second dose of radioactive iodine may be required or thyroid replacement therapy initiated (see Hypothyroidism, this page). If thyroid function is normal, reassessments at 6- to 12-week intervals will be needed to monitor the gland's function.

Another treatment involves taking antithyroid drugs in tablet form. Within 6 to 8 weeks after this therapy is started, the symptoms of hyperthyroidism ordinarily disappear. However, the usual course of treatment requires that the tablets be continued for at least 9 to 12 months. When the year-long course of treatment is completed and the drug is discontinued, there is a substantial chance that the hyperthyroidism will return and another course of treatment will be needed.

Surgery

Treatment of hyperfunctioning thyroid nodules consists of surgical removal in most instances, but radioactive iodine and antithyroid drugs also are used in the same manner as for Graves' disease. During surgery, most or a portion of the thyroid gland may be removed, especially if symptoms recur after two or three courses of radioactive iodine therapy or of an antithyroid drug. In rare cases, the abnormality of the eyes is so severe that vision is threatened and an operation may be needed to relieve the pressure behind the eyes.

Nutrition

If you experience severe weight loss and muscle wasting, a diet providing supplemental calories and protein may be necessary.

Hypothyroidism

Signs and Symptoms

- Lethargy characterized by slowed physical and mental functions
- Slowed heart rate
- Intolerance to cold temperatures
- Constipation
- Dry skin and hair
- Goiter (in some patients)
- Heavy and prolonged menstrual periods
- Decreased sexual interest

Emergency Symptoms—Myxedema coma: intense cold intolerance and drowsiness followed by profound lethargy and unconsciousness. A myxedema coma may be precipitated by sedatives, infections, or other stress on your body, and requires emergency medical treatment

An underactive thyroid gland causes hypothyroidism (the opposite of hyperthyroidism, page 947). Its name comes from the Greek *hypo* for "under" and *thyreos* for "shield-shaped." The group of symptoms and findings that develop after several years of untreated hypothyroidism is termed myxedema.

The thyroid hormone has such significant effects on your growth and development that deficiencies can lead to a wide variety of health problems. Your body's normal function rate (basal metabolic rate) slows, leaving you feeling mentally and physically sluggish. In extreme cases, deficiency states can lead to developmental disabilities in infants and young children (see Cretinism, this page). Adults can exhibit a slowing of mental processes, an inability to maintain normal body temperatures, and even heart failure.

Hypothyroidism has various causes. The thyroid gland can gradually be destroyed by an abnormal antibody. The pituitary gland can fail to produce a hormone called thyroid-stimulating hormone (TSH). Hashimoto's disease (see Lymphocytic Thyroiditis, page 946) may be a cause of hypothyroidism. Occasionally, treatment for hyperthyroidism works too well, creating hypothyroidism. In rare instances, infants are born without thyroid glands.

Although not a common ailment, hypothyroidism is not unusual. It can occur in either sex and at any age. However, middle-aged women are most commonly affected, while those most likely to remain undiagnosed are the elderly.

Diagnosis

Hypothyroidism usually develops slowly over months or even years. If you have hypothyroidism, you may not notice the changes, but a friend or relative who has not seen you for some months may find the deterioration remarkable.

At first, your only symptoms may be constant fatigue with muscle aches and an inability to stay warm in cool or cold temperatures. You may become constipated. Your face becomes puffy, and your skin dries, thickens, and loses its luster. Your voice may grow hoarse, and you may experience hearing loss. Although weight gain often is considered to be a common symptom of hypothyroidism, your increase in weight is only slight, if present at all.

The most effective way to diagnose hypothyroidism is with laboratory tests. Blood samples are analyzed for different forms of the thyroid hormone and for thyroid-stimu-lating hormone (TSH) and antibodies. Low thyroid hormone and high TSH values suggest hypothyroidism, and a high antibody value suggests that Hashimoto's disease is the cause of the hypothyroidism.

How Serious Is Hypothyroidism?

In most people, hypothyroidism is neither chronic nor progressive, and its treatment results in a normal life. However, treatment is especially important in infants and in people with severe hormone deficiencies.

Myxedema Coma

Hypothyroidism is unlikely to be life-threatening, except when myxedema coma occurs. This rare condition is usually the result of long-term, undiagnosed hypothyroidism, and it may be provoked by sedatives, narcotics, illness, exposure to cold, accident or injury, or surgery. Myxedema coma requires immediate treatment, usually with hormone injections.

Cretinism

In infants, untreated hypothyroidism can result in dwarfism and mental retardation (cretinism). If the condition is diagnosed within the first several months of life (as it often is because of routine blood tests conducted immediately after birth), the chances of normal development are excellent. In a child with the arrested development characteristic of cretinism, typical signs include constant drooling, a swayback and potbelly, short stature, and irregularly placed, poorly formed teeth.

Treatment

Medication

The key treatment is daily consumption of thyroid hormone. Physicians generally prescribe a synthetic thyroxine and prefer brand names to generic preparations. In most cases, the condition improves noticeably within 2-3 weeks after the hormone therapy is begun. All symptoms disappear within a few months. However, the individual must continue this treatment for the rest of his or her life.

Nutrition

In some people, the lack of thyroid hormone results from a long-term shortage of iodine in the diet. The thyroid gland increases in size in an attempt to compensate, and goiter, a swelling at the front and base of the neck, results.

This condition is now rare in the United States because our table salt is supplemented with iodine and our food supply is generally rich in iodine. In other parts of the world where the soil lacks iodine, iodine deficiency remains a common cause of goiter. In such areas, the use of iodized salt is an effective public health measure (see page 946).

Parathyroid Gland Disorders

The thyroid gland is at the front and base of your neck; the parathyroid glands are located on its four corners. The parathyroid glands are small—each is about the size of a grain of rice. They produce parathyroid hormone. When too much of this hormone is produced, the resulting disorder is called hyperparathyroidism (the Greek prefix *hyper* means "above"). An underproduction is hypoparathyroidism (the Greek prefix *hypo* means "below").

Increased hormone secretion by one or more of the parathyroid glands increases the amount of calcium in your blood, mainly by releasing it from the bones and by increasing its absorption from the small intestine. The parathyroid glands maintain the level of calcium in your blood within very narrow limits by turning their secretion off or on (just as a thermostat controls a heating system to maintain a constant air temperature). Vitamin D is also necessary for regulating the amount of calcium in your blood. Another hormone called calcitonin, which is manufactured in the thyroid gland, plays an uncertain role.

Hyperparathyroidism

Signs and Symptoms
Hyperparathyroidism may be symptomless at first, unless pain from kidney stones develops. However, over several years, symptoms may appear:

- Kidney stones
- Fatigue
- Increased urination and thirst
- Indigestion or ulcer symptoms

When one or more of the parathyroid glands produce an excess of their hormone, the resulting disorder is termed hyperparathyroidism (the reverse disorder is hypoparathyroidism, in which too little of the hormone is produced; see page 951). When there is too much parathyroid hormone circulating in your body, the calcium concentration becomes exaggeratedly high and the phosphorus concentration is low.

In more than 80 percent of cases, the cause is a small growth in one of the parathyroid glands. In other instances, all four of the glands become enlarged and overproduce the hormone. The growths are usually localized and are unlikely to spread to other organs.

Once thought to be rather rare, this ailment is not uncommon among middle-aged people. Women are about twice as likely to have hyperparathyroidism as men.

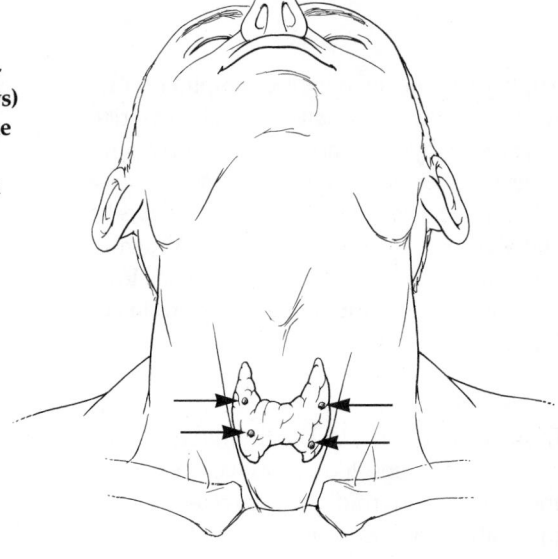

Located on your thyroid gland, the rice-sized parathyroid glands (arrows) produce a hormone that controls the level of calcium in your blood.

Diagnosis

About half of those with hyperparathyroidism have no symptoms. Frequently, the diagnosis is made accidentally when abnormally high calcium values are discovered during routine blood tests for some other disorder. Low amounts of phosphorus in the blood also are suggestive of the disorder. Direct measurement of the amount of parathyroid hormone in the blood helps confirm the diagnosis.

In hyperparathyroidism, excessive consumption of vitamin D can raise the blood calcium level (hypercalcemia). The use of certain diuretic drugs, called thiazides, is another possible cause of an increased blood calcium value. In rare situations your physician may conduct an ultrasound examination of the thyroid region in an attempt to locate tumors in the parathyroid glands. A condition called sarcoidosis (see page 721) also can increase the amount of calcium in the circulation and must be excluded. Some cancers of the lung, breast, and other organs sometimes secrete a substance that closely resembles parathyroid hormone, increasing blood calcium concentrations.

How Serious Is Hyperparathyroidism?

In some cases, treatment is unnecessary and your physician will simply monitor your condition. The condition of your kidneys will be followed closely to determine whether kidney stones are appearing and whether the kidney is disposing of waste substances normally.

There is a long-term danger to your bones: too much calcium in the blood means that much of the mineral is being released from the bones, which are the storage area for calcium in the body. Thus your physician may perform further tests, such as a bone mineral density, to assess the status of your skeleton.

You may require surgery on your parathyroid gland to remove the tumor if there is evidence that its effects are adversely affecting your skeleton. Occasionally, you may have peptic ulcers with hyperparathyroidism.

Treatment

A surgeon experienced in parathyroid surgery will be able to find and remove the tumor in most cases. If the tumor is not found in the usual location of the parathyroid glands, more elaborate techniques, such as surgical exploration of the region behind your breastbone (sternum), may be needed.

Hypoparathyroidism

Signs and Symptoms

- Muscle spasms or numbness, especially in your hands, feet, and throat
- Breathing difficulty
- Dry skin
- Yeast infections
- In children: vomiting, convulsions, and headaches

When the parathyroid glands produce too little of their hormone, the disorder that results is termed hypoparathyroidism. (The opposite disorder is called hyperparathyroidism, in which too much hormone is produced; see page 950.) Hypoparathyroidism is rare and is far less likely to occur than hyperparathyroidism.

Parathyroid hormone is crucial to your body's use of calcium. Without sufficient quantities of it, the amount of calcium in the blood falls below normal and the amount of phosphorus rises. A low blood calcium concentration can produce various problems, particularly muscle spasms and cramps. Over several years, cataracts and, rarely, convulsions may develop.

There are two types of hypoparathyroidism. Spontaneous hypoparathyroidism of unknown cause may be associated with a susceptibility to yeast infections and a failure of the ovaries or adrenal glands. Children are affected more often than adults.

The second type results from inadvertent removal of the normal parathyroid glands during surgery for goiter or as a surgical complication after removal of multiple overactive parathyroid glands.

Diagnosis

The key finding in the diagnosis of hypoparathyroidism is an abnormally low concentration of calcium in the blood (a condition known as hypocalcemia) and an abnormally high concentration of phosphorus.

How Serious Is Hypoparathyroidism?

The muscle spasms associated with hypoparathyroidism can be uncomfortable, and breathing difficulty can result from spasms of the muscles controlling your vocal cords. If the amount of calcium in your blood has been low for many years, cataracts and convulsions can occur.

Treatment

Your physician will prescribe vitamin D and calcium supplements. If certain symptoms are especially severe (in particular, the muscle spasms), you may be given an intravenous injection of calcium to provide immediate but temporary relief.

You must take calcium and vitamin D supplements for life in amounts consider-ably larger than those required for ordinary nutrition. Also, because your blood calcium concentration must be monitored, your physician will establish a schedule of blood tests for you. The supplements should re-store satisfactory health, but the regularly scheduled tests are important for maintain-ing normal levels of the essential calcium in your blood.

Chapter 29

Your Blood

Contents

Understanding Your Blood, 954
Enlarged Spleen, 954

Anemias, 956
Iron-Deficiency Anemia, 957
The Dangers of Too Much Iron, 958
Pernicious Anemia, 958
Folic Acid Deficiency Anemia, 959
Sickle Cell Disease, 960
Porphyrias, 961
Rare Hemoglobin Diseases, 961
Hemolytic Anemias, 962
Other Anemias, 962

Leukemias, 964
Chronic Myelogenous Leukemia, 964
Acute Nonlymphocytic Leukemia, 965
Chronic Lymphocytic Leukemia, 966
Acute Lymphocytic Leukemia, 966
Bone Marrow Transplantation, 967

Lymphomas, 968
Hodgkin's Disease, 969
Non-Hodgkin's Lymphoma, 970

Growth Disorders of the Bone Marrow, 971
Polycythemia Vera, 971

Agnogenic Myeloid Metaplasia, 972
Multiple Myeloma, 973
Monoclonal Gammopathy of Undetermined
Significance, 973
Amyloidosis, 974
Granulocytopenia and
Agranulocytosis, 974

Bleeding Disorders, 975
Hemophilia, 975
von Willebrand's Disease, 977
**Disseminated Intravascular
Coagulation, 977**
Thrombocytopenia, 978

Blood Transfusions, 979
The Donation Procedure, 979
Transfusion Types, 980
Blood Groups, 980
Adverse Reactions to Transfusions, 981
Safety of Blood Transfusions, 981
Transfusion With Your Own Blood, 982
Using Your Own Blood During
Surgery, 982
The Future: Synthetic Substitutes, 982

Understanding Your Blood

The blood that circulates throughout your body performs a number of crucial functions. In the tissues of your lungs, inhaled oxygen is picked up by your blood and delivered, by your arteries, to tissues throughout your body. At the same time, the blood removes carbon dioxide from these tissues and, through the veins, returns it to your lungs, where it passes into the exhaled air.

The blood also carries life-sustaining nutrients from your intestines to cells throughout your body. When waste products from these cells need to be removed, the blood transports them to the kidneys where they are excreted (see Your Kidneys and Urinary Tract, page 825).

By serving as the vehicle for long-distance messengers such as hormones, the blood helps the various parts of your body to com-municate with each other and to coordinate their functions. The blood acts as a medium for your immune system by carrying anti-bodies (proteins that help protect your body against foreign substances) and cells that fight infections (see page 1056). And it even helps to regulate your body temperature by dissipating the heat produced in the muscles.

These different functions are performed by blood cells and the liquid part of the blood, called plasma. Most of the cells are red blood cells (erythrocytes). These are the cells that contain hemoglobin, a red, iron-rich, complex substance. Hemoglobin binds to oxygen in the lungs in order to carry it through the bloodstream to tiny blood ves-sels (capillaries) where the hemoglobin releases the oxygen so that it can move out of the bloodstream to the cells that need it.

Enlarged Spleen

The spleen is located in the left up-per quadrant of the abdomen, pro-tected by the overlying rib cage.

The spleen has at least four ma-jor functions. First, it is part of the immune system, serving as a major site for clearing foreign organisms and antigens from the blood-stream; it also generates part of the antibody response to foreign anti-gens. Second, the spleen plays an important role in removing normal and abnormal blood cells from the bloodstream.

Third, the spleen also plays a role in regulating the blood flow to the liver. Fourth, under some con-ditions, the spleen may become a major site for the production of blood cells.

Normally, the spleen cannot be felt because of its position under the rib cage. However, in some situa-tions, the spleen enlarges (spleno-megaly) and often becomes palpable. Sometimes this enlargement occurs without any other symptoms. At other times it is accompanied by pain, particularly in the left upper outer aspect of the abdomen and occasionally in the left shoulder.

Acute enlargement of the spleen due to bleeding within the organ may occur after trauma to the left rib cage or upper abdomen, and often it is associated with pain. An enlarged spleen accompanied by fever may appear with diseases such as infectious mononucleosis, tuberculosis, histoplasmosis, bac-terial endocarditis, and malaria (see page 1055).

An enlarged spleen can also occur in certain diseases associated with disordered function of the im-mune system, such as rheumatoid arthritis, lupus (systemic lupus ery-thematosus) (see page 918), and im-mune hemolytic anemia (see page 962).

Because the spleen plays an im-portant role in flow of blood toward the liver, any disease that obstructs this process—such as cir-rhosis, obstruction of the major vein to the liver (portal vein), or conges-tive heart failure with backup of blood into the liver—can cause enlargement of the spleen. A num-ber of diseases in which abnormal red blood cells are present (such as thalassemia and sickle cell disease) may also cause an enlarged spleen.

Finally, either benign or malig-nant disease may cause infiltration of abnormal cells into the spleen, with subsequent enlargement. An example of a benign process is amyloidosis (see page 974). Malig-nancies such as leukemias, lym-phomas, Hodgkin's lymphoma, and metastatic tumors are other examples of conditions that infil-trate the spleen, causing enlarge-ment.

To evaluate an enlarged spleen further, your physician may order tests such as ultrasound or com-puted tomography, and treatment will be directed at the underlying cause.

White blood cells (leukocytes) defend your body against foreign matter, including infection-causing bacteria, viruses, and fungi. There are three main types of white blood cells. One type, the granulocytes (grainy cells), includes neutrophils, eosinophils, and basophils. These and the second type, the monocytes, respond to many different types of infection and also defend by engulfing foreign substances. The third type of white blood cells, known as lymphocytes, react to specific infecting agents. The lymphocytes include B cells and T cells. B cells produce antibodies, and T cells attack foreign and virus-infected cells. (For more on the immune system, see The Workings of Your Immune System, page 1056.)

Platelets (thrombocytes) are colorless blood cells that repair injured blood vessels. They stop loss of blood from the bloodstream by forming plugs in vessel holes. When any of your blood vessels is damaged, platelets gather to plug the site of injury. This is the first step in clot formation (coagulation), a process that is completed by proteins, called clotting factors, that travel in the plasma.

The plasma, a yellowish liquid, carries other proteins as well as the clotting factors. Plasma can be defined as what is left after the cells are removed from your blood. Serum is plasma from which the clotting factors also have been removed.

There is another circulatory system in your body, the lymph system, which carries a fluid called lymph. The lymph helps to return water and proteins from the tissues to the blood.

Most of the blood cells are produced in the bone marrow, a material in cavities inside many of your bones. Most of these cells continue to mature and develop further into specific types of blood cells within the bone marrow. However, for some blood cells this maturation process occurs in the spleen or lymph nodes.

When your physician suspects that you might have a blood disorder, he or she will have blood tests performed. Samples for these tests can be collected by drawing blood from a vein in an arm or from capillaries in a fingertip. Blood tests generally are part of the routine physical examination.

The most common blood cell test is the complete blood cell count (abbreviated as CBC). This involves counting the number of each type of blood cell in a given volume of your blood and examining the cells under a microscope to check for any abnormalities in

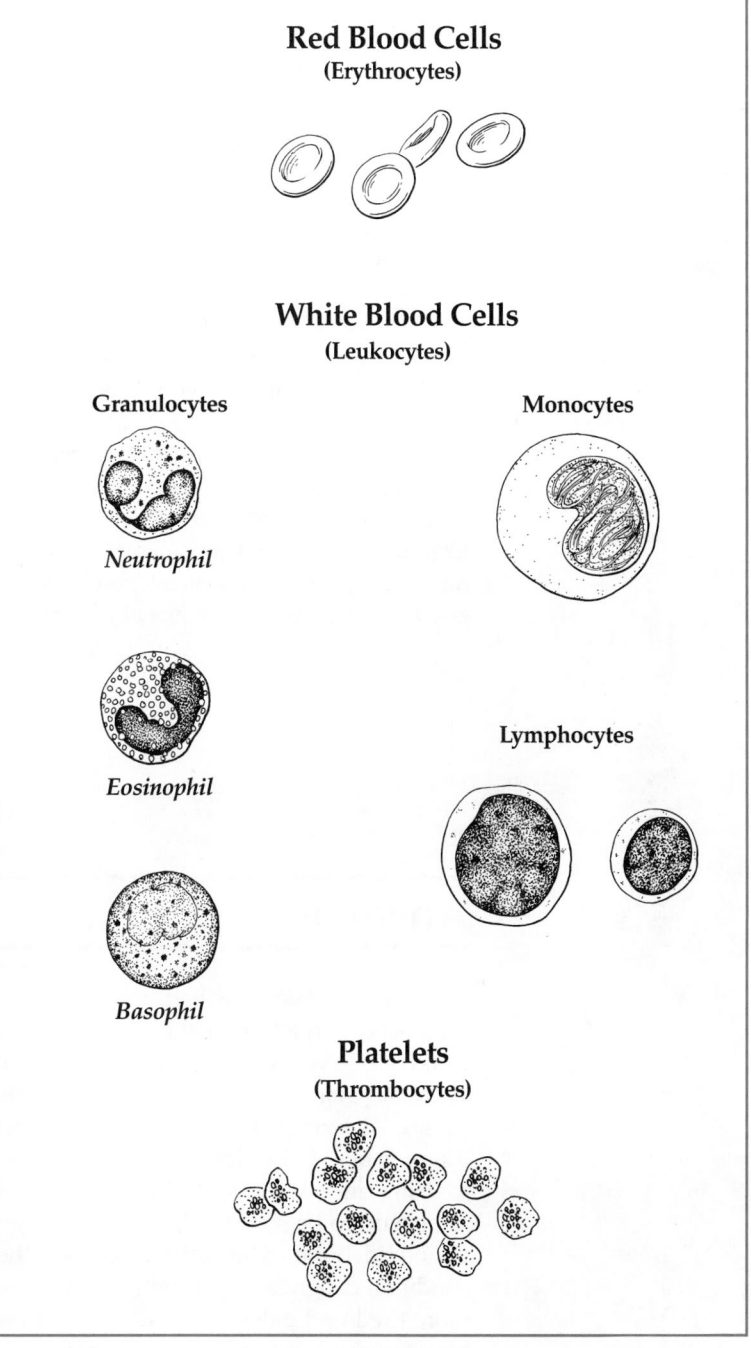

Red Blood Cells
(Erythrocytes)

White Blood Cells
(Leukocytes)

Granulocytes

Neutrophil

Eosinophil

Basophil

Monocytes

Lymphocytes

Platelets
(Thrombocytes)

Red blood cells (erythrocytes) are cells containing hemoglobin. White blood cells are called leukocytes, and there are three types: granulocytes, monocytes, and lymphocytes. They defend your body against foreign matter. Platelets (thrombocytes) repair injured blood vessels.

their size or shape. Part of the complete blood count is determining the hematocrit value, the percentage of your total blood volume that the red blood cells occupy. The hematocrit value normally is about 42 percent in women and 47 percent in men. Another part of the complete blood count is assessing the hemoglobin status (hemoglobin is the iron-rich molecule in the red blood cell that binds oxygen and delivers it to the cells of your body).

If your physician thinks you may have a disorder that involves a specific type of white blood cell, he or she will do a differential count. This determines the relative amounts of each kind of white blood cell. Other blood tests measure the number of platelets and the bleeding time (a useful indication of how well your platelets are functioning).

To study how well your body is making new blood cells, your physician may examine a sample of your bone marrow under a microscope. This marrow usually is taken from the back of the large pelvic bone or breastbone (sternum) (see page 1332).

Many problems with your blood can be treated by your family physician. Occasionally, you may be referred to a specialist in disorders of the blood, a hematologist.

Some blood disorders are a type of cancer. Examples include leukemia, lymphoma, and multiple myeloma. Hematologists or oncologists (cancer specialists) traditionally treat these types of cancer with drugs called chemotherapeutic agents. They cooperate closely with radiation specialists, who treat cancers with X-rays. Sometimes a physician will specialize in both oncology and hematology.

In the following pages, we will discuss various blood disorders. These are divided according to the part of the circulatory system in which they arise. The anemias are problems caused by too few red blood cells. Symptoms of anemia may include paleness as well as breathlessness and lack of endurance. Decreased numbers of white blood cells impair your body's resistance to infection. The leukemias are usually accompanied by too many white blood cells. The lymphomas involve the lymph nodes, spleen, and bone marrow. The clotting disorders result from defects in platelets or in clotting factors.

Anemias

Anemia is a state in which hemoglobin is diminished. In addition, the number of red blood cells (erythrocytes) usually is decreased. There are many anemias that have various causes. As a group, the anemias are the most common blood disorders.

When anemia starts, the signs and symptoms tend to be so mild that they often go unnoticed, but their severity increases as the condition progresses. At first, you may be more tired and paler than usual. The best places to check for pallor are your nail beds, the undersides of your eyelids and lips, and your palms. Anemia may cause the creases in your palm to be as pale as the surrounding skin. This occurs when the hemoglobin value is less than 7 g/dL. When you exercise, you may feel more out of breath than is usual. You also may be aware that your heartbeat is faster than normal.

Iron deficiency is the most common cause of anemia. Without enough iron, your body cannot produce adequate amounts of hemoglobin. When you have a shortage of vitamin B_{12} (as in pernicious anemia) or of folic acid (folic acid deficiency), you cannot make sufficient numbers of red blood cells. If you inherit a disorder such as sickle cell disease, thalassemia, or a rare hemoglobin disease, your body produces a defective form of hemoglobin.

In the hemolytic anemias, the red blood cells are broken down (hemolyzed) faster than the bone marrow can produce new red blood cells to replace them. The most common cause of hemolytic anemia is an immune response against your own red blood cells (autoimmunity). The second most common cause is drugs that you may be taking for other conditions such as infections or high blood pressure.

Inherited defects of enzymes such as glucose-6-phosphate dehydrogenase (G6PD) can cause hemolytic anemia. Many infections and chronic diseases, including some cancers, can interfere with the production of red blood cells and thus result in anemia (called anemia of chronic disease).

Despite the many similarities among the signs and symptoms of the following anemias, each of these disorders has a different cause.

Iron-Deficiency Anemia

Signs and Symptoms
- None are apparent early in this disorder
- Pallor
- Fatigue

Iron-deficiency anemia occurs when the amount of iron in the body is insufficient to permit manufacture of the amount of hemoglobin needed. There are several main causes of the deficiency, including insufficient consumption of iron-containing foods, poor absorption of iron by the body, and loss of blood.

Worldwide, iron deficiency is the most common cause of anemia. It occurs particularly frequently among women of childbearing age.

In nonpregnant women, the cause is the monthly menstrual loss of blood. Without iron supplementation, iron-deficiency anemia occurs in virtually all pregnant women because their iron stores have to serve the increased blood volume of the mother as well as be a source of hemoglobin for the growing fetus.

The condition may occur in infants, children, and adolescents. All three age groups go through spurts of rapid growth that require a great deal of iron for the manufacture of new muscle and hemoglobin. In addition, lead poisoning can contribute to iron-deficiency anemia in children (see Lead Poisoning, page 71).

In adults, the most common cause of the condition is blood loss from the digestive tract, which can occur with drugs such as aspirin and nonsteroidal anti-inflammatory drugs (NSAIDs), malignancy, and diaphragmatic hernia (see page 743).

Diagnosis
The symptoms of iron-deficiency anemia tend to appear so gradually that they are often hard to notice. As with other anemias, you may feel tired and less tolerant of exercise. Your skin, gums, nail beds, and eyelid linings may be pale. Eventually, the anemia may become severe enough that your heartbeat seems more rapid and noticeable.

Rarely, people with this condition develop a craving for substances that are not foods. This craving is called pica. They may eat ice, clay, or soil. Some of these substances will interfere with absorption of iron in the intestinal tract and thus may worsen the iron deficiency.

Your physician can use various blood tests to diagnose iron-deficiency anemia. The size of the individual red blood cells is diminished but the number of them may be nearly normal. The amount of hemoglobin in the cells is low and, under a microscope, individual red blood cells will appear pale.

When there is a question of blood loss from the digestive tract, special tests (see page 790) can precisely measure the amount of blood in the stool.

How Serious Is Iron-Deficiency Anemia?
This is a chronic condition. When iron-deficiency anemia is severe enough, it may interfere with work performance. However, this and other effects usually can be reversed quickly by iron replacement therapy. When iron-deficiency anemia is found, the cause of the deficiency must be uncovered. It may be the first symptom of a serious disorder such as cancer of the colon, colon polyps, peptic ulcer, or gastritis (see pages 789, 786, 753, and 758). It may be the result of other serious disorders. Do not be satisfied until the definite cause is found and treated.

Treatment
The key to prevention of iron-deficiency anemia not due to disease is adequate nutrition.

Nutrition
Foods rich in iron that your body can readily absorb include meats (especially liver), fish, poultry, eggs, legumes (peas and beans), potatoes, and rice. Many wheat products receive added iron when they are processed, but this iron is not in a form that your body can easily use. The iron in many vegetables is poorly absorbed. You can enhance your body's absorption of iron by drinking citrus juice when you take a supplement or eat an iron-containing food. In contrast, milk and tea decrease iron absorption.

Eating plenty of iron-containing foods is particularly important for people who have high iron requirements, such as children and pregnant or menstruating women. It is also crucial for those whose diets are low in iron, including strict vegetarians, people on weight-reduction diets, and infants.

Breast milk contains iron in a form that is particularly easy for the body to use. However, it does not contain enough iron to allow the maximal growth of an infant who is older than 4 months. So breastfed infants should start receiving supplemental iron drops or iron-fortified cereal at that age. Iron-fortified formula is available for formula-fed infants.

Iron supplements can be helpful during times of great need, such as growth spurts in children and pregnancy. However, be careful not to overdo it (see The Dangers of Too Much Iron, below).

Medication

To treat iron deficiency, your physician will recommend supplemental iron salts (ferrous sulfate or ferrous gluconate). These are usually taken orally, three times a day. Only rarely is it necessary to give iron by intramuscular injection.

Surgery

If the underlying reason for the iron deficiency is loss of blood from the digestive tract, such as in colon cancer, an operation will be required.

Other Therapies

Your physician may consider giving you a transfusion of packed red blood cells (see page 980), but only if you have extremely severe anemia is immediate correction needed.

Pernicious Anemia

Signs and Symptoms

- Usually, none are apparent early in the disease
- Reduced exercise endurance and rapid, noticeable heartbeat
- Sore tongue
- Poor appetite and loss of weight
- Disturbed walking gait and balance
- Mental changes, including memory loss, depression, and dementia
- Numbness in hands and feet

Pernicious anemia is caused by a deficiency of vitamin B_{12}, which is needed for normal production of red blood cells. It is often hereditary. The term pernicious was adopted when no effective treatment was known and the condition was inevitably fatal.

The foods that contain vitamin B_{12} are meat and dairy products. However, except in strict vegetarians, this disorder is not a result of not eating enough of these foods. Rather, pernicious anemia results from the failure of the digestive tract to absorb vitamin B_{12}. This impaired absorption is thought to be a complex process.

The cells that line a part of the stomach produce a substance called intrinsic factor (IF), which is necessary for absorption of vitamin B_{12} in the small intestine. Intrinsic factor attaches itself to vitamin B_{12}, and it is this combination that is absorbed in the lowest portion of the small bowel (ileum), just before the small bowel enters the colon. A vitamin B_{12} deficiency also can result when the ileum is diseased or removed in the course of surgery because then the intrinsic factor-vitamin B_{12} combination is not absorbed.

The condition is unusual. It occurs most often in older people. Men and women are affected in similar numbers. It is most common among people of northern European descent. Those with the disorder tend to be fair-haired.

Diagnosis

To check for pernicious anemia, your physician can perform various blood tests. One test measures the amount of vitamin B_{12} in your blood. Also, your blood is examined under a microscope to assess the size and

---

The Dangers of Too Much Iron

Too much of a good thing may be dangerous—so don't take too much supplemental iron.

Iron supplements are appropriate only when you need more iron than a balanced diet can provide. If you think you need an iron supplement, check with your physician before taking any because overloading your body with iron can be even more serious than iron-deficiency anemia.

You are especially likely to collect too much iron in your body if you have inherited one or two genes for a relatively common condition called hemochromatosis (see page 806). This disorder is caused by excessive absorption of iron by the digestive tract, and the consumption of iron supplements could greatly accelerate the course of the disease.

Excess iron accumulation can damage your liver and cause cirrhosis. You can get a type of diabetes called bronze diabetes in which your skin may turn a bronze-like color. Your heart may fail, or its rhythm may be disturbed if overloaded with iron. Iron deposits in your joints can cause arthritis. Injury to the testicles by iron accumulation can cause impotence and sterility. Hemochromatosis is treated by phlebotomy, the removal of 1 unit of blood (approximately a pint) once or twice a week.

If you are losing blood because of some serious condition such as colon cancer, taking an iron supplement may delay the diagnosis. Iron-deficiency anemia is an important diagnostic clue that should be pursued by your physician.

shape of red blood cells. If you have pernicious anemia, your red blood cells will be enlarged and there will be fewer of them.

Occasionally, it may be necessary to study a sample of your bone marrow, where the red blood cells are produced (see page 1332). Your physician may order a test to determine whether antibodies to intrinsic factor are present, an indirect way of telling whether intrinsic factor itself is present or absent. He or she also may order a Schilling test to determine whether you have a vitamin B_{12} deficiency due to a lack of intrinsic factor (and therefore pernicious anemia) or if there is a failure to absorb the vitamin for some other reason.

How Serious Is Pernicious Anemia?

This chronic disease progresses slowly but steadily if not treated. In the past, before proper treatment was developed, it eventually caused death after many years. Now, replacement therapy with adequate amounts of vitamin B_{12} corrects the deficiency and allows a normal life. However, if the condition progresses for a long time before detection, it may cause some damage to certain parts of the body, primarily the nervous and digestive systems.

Treatment

Recognition of the disorder's hereditary nature makes it possible to prevent the development of symptoms. If you have a relative who has pernicious anemia, inform your physician so that he or she can test your blood every few years, before any symptoms appear. If your physician decides that you do have pernicious anemia, he or she can treat you for it.

Medication

To treat pernicious anemia, vitamin B_{12} is injected. At first the injections may be done once daily, but after several days the injection can be given once a month.

These injections must be given indefinitely. Neither oral supplements nor dietary changes are useful treatments because the underlying problem is the inability of the digestive tract to absorb the vitamin.

Folic Acid Deficiency Anemia

Signs and Symptoms

- Usually none are apparent early in the disease
- Low exercise endurance and rapid, noticeable heartbeat
- Weight loss
- Diarrhea

As in pernicious anemia (see page 958), folic acid deficiency interferes with the production of red blood cells. Folic acid, which is also known as folate, is a member of the vitamin B group. Lack of it causes an anemia characterized by red blood cells that are large but few in number. Deficiency can result if you do not get enough folic acid in your diet to meet your body's demands or if your intestines cannot absorb it.

The disorder is not uncommon. Alcoholics often develop it if they become malnourished when drinking becomes their principal source of calories and their digestive tract does not absorb as well as it used to. The ailment sometimes develops in pregnant or lactating women and during the growth spurts of infancy and adolescence. At these times, the body's demand for folic acid may outrun its supply. Folic acid deficiency anemia is often present in malabsorption problems (see page 770). Certain anticonvulsant drugs and some other medications may induce folic acid deficiency.

Your physician may also consider other causes of folic acid deficiency, such as problems with the bone marrow, the effect of certain agents used to treat cancer, liver disease, thyroid disease, smoking, and hemolysis (see page 962).

Diagnosis

The symptoms of folic acid deficiency are similar to those of pernicious anemia, so your physician will perform various blood tests to distinguish between the two disorders. These include counting the cells in your blood, examining the cells under a microscope, and measuring the amount of folic acid in the blood. If folic acid deficiency anemia is present, your physician may perform more tests to look for an underlying cause.

Treatment

Depending on its underlying cause, folic acid deficiency may be chronic or acute. Proper treatment will let you lead a normal life.

Prevention

Most people can prevent folic acid deficiency by eating a balanced diet, limiting their consumption of alcohol, and taking prescribed supplements during pregnancy. If you have folic acid deficiency, it is important to eliminate the condition that was its underlying cause. For instance, if alcoholism was the reason folic acid deficiency developed, you must stop drinking.

Nutrition
In some cases, adequate nutrition is the remedy. The main food sources of this vitamin are raw fruits and vegetables, liver, and kidney. Folic acid is found in a wide variety of foods, but it can be destroyed by extensive cooking.

Medication
In almost all cases, supplemental folic acid is given orally every day. It is injected only if the underlying problem is a disorder of the intestinal tract that severely interferes with absorption.

Sickle Cell Disease

Signs and Symptoms
- Fatigue, breathlessness, and rapid heartbeat (as in other anemias)
- Delayed growth and development
- Susceptibility to infections
- Skin ulcers on the lower legs
- Vision problems when the retina is affected

Emergency Symptoms
- Attacks of pain caused by blocked blood vessels and damaged organs

Normal and sickled red blood cells. The sickled cells assume a crescent shape.

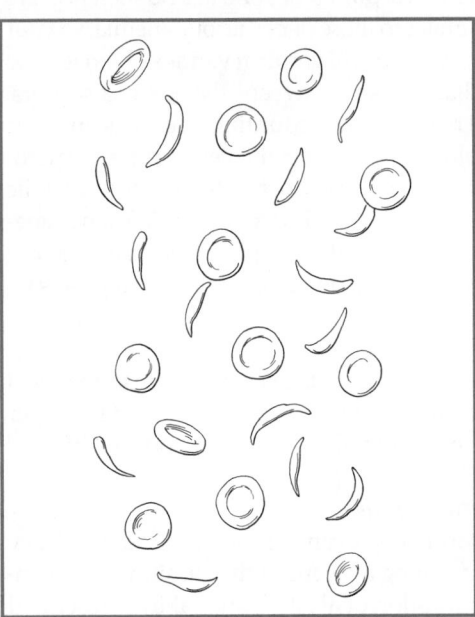

- Aplastic crises, in which the number of red blood cells decreases drastically
- Symptoms of anemia—severe shortness of breath, fatigue, light-headedness, particularly on standing

Sickle cell disease is the most common inherited disorder. In sickle cell disease, the red blood cells become rigid and shaped like crescents or sickles rather than being flexible and round. These changes in the red blood cells may precipitate attacks of pain. The disorder gets its name from this change of shape (sickling), which results from the presence of an abnormal type of hemoglobin known as hemoglobin S. These cells are fragile and tend to undergo hemolysis—that is, the red blood cell breaks up and its hemoglobin is released into the plasma, resulting in anemia. The disease is also called sickle cell anemia.

This is an inherited disorder and is relatively common in black people. If you have sickle cell disease, you received one gene for hemoglobin S from each of your parents. This gene is recessive, so if you have only one copy of it, you are a carrier of the sickle cell gene.

If you are a carrier, your red blood cells may be deformed but no symptoms occur unless you are at high altitude. Some carriers of sickle cell disease will experience symptoms during an unpressurized plane flight or while traveling in a car at high altitudes. The decreased level of oxygen renders the red blood cells more fragile and deformed, thus increasing their tendency to sickle and break up (hemolysis).

Diagnosis
To detect sickle cell disease, your physician will perform various blood tests. The test that confirms the diagnosis is hemoglobin electrophoresis, a laboratory procedure that isolates and identifies the telltale hemoglobin S.

How Serious Is Sickle Cell Disease?
It is a chronic disease that makes your body vulnerable to infection. You can limit its progression by avoiding infections or by getting them treated early.

Two types of acute, severe episodes can occur, spontaneously or when triggered by infection or other stress. These are the crises produced by acute sickling and may be associated with obstruction of small blood vessels, pain, and the breakdown of red blood

Porphyrias

The group of diseases called the porphyrias encompasses several rare blood disorders. They result from the body's inability to properly manufacture heme, the oxygen-carrying component of hemoglobin in the red blood cells. Heme is made in both the liver and bone marrow through an assembly line of chemical reactions. In each type of porphyria, one step in the production of heme is defective.

Sometimes concentrations of chemicals build up under the surface of the skin. Exposure to sunlight sometimes produces a toxic reaction that causes painful skin lesions. These can lead to permanent scarring and disfigurement such as loss of an ear or nose.

Some people with porphyria also develop excessive hair growth on the face, arms, hands, and legs. In some porphyrias, the chemical defect can cause teeth to develop a reddish hue. Fingernails and toenails may become deformed into a claw-like shape.

The skin damage can begin in childhood. If the toxins accumulate to high levels in other organs, such as the brain, the individual may survive only a few years. Occasionally porphyrias begin in adulthood. People with these forms usually are able to lead long, relatively normal lives.

No treatment exists to correct the chemical defect responsible for porphyria. Some relief from the progressive symptoms of the disease is provided by certain medications, frequent removal of blood (phlebotomy), and, in some cases, surgical removal of the spleen.

If porphyria exists in your family or your partner's, seek genetic counseling before having children, so you know the potential risk to your offspring.

---

cells. The crises can include bone and joint pain, central nervous system problems (such as strokes), acute chest pain, and infections. At times, there also may be a temporary failure of red blood cell development in the bone marrow that can result in exceptionally severe, life-threatening anemia. Repeated crises can produce increasing damage to the kidneys, lungs, liver, and central nervous system, at times resulting in death. During pregnancy, there may be an increase in both maternal and fetal mortality.

In contrast, the sickle cell trait is usually harmless except in situations of low oxygen level, and it is of concern primarily when you are considering marriage and children.

If you know that sickle cell disease runs in your family, genetic counseling may help you prevent passing it on to your children. If both you and your spouse carry the trait, the risk is 1 out of 4 that your child will have sickle cell disease. The disease can be detected before birth, and some couples choose to abort an affected fetus.

Treatment

Medication
Your physician may prescribe a daily oral supplement of folic acid, because the disease increases your body's need for this vitamin. Your physician will also be on the lookout for infections. Antibiotics are given to treat infections and sometimes to prevent them. Immunizations for pneumococcus, influenza, and *Haemophilus* should also be completed.

During crises, you will receive medications to relieve the pain and fluid to prevent dehydration. Oxygen is given if there is not enough oxygen in your bloodstream.

Antisickling drugs are being tested. Hydroxyurea, a chemotherapy agent, has been shown to decrease the number of sickling crises. In addition, hydroxyurea may lessen the need for blood transfusions.

Rare Hemoglobin Diseases

Rare hemoglobin diseases, also called hemoglobinopathies, are caused by the presence of variant forms of hemoglobin. Over 400 variants have been identified. These abnormal hemoglobins tend to be less efficient than the normal form at carrying oxygen to the cells of the body.

One example is hemoglobin S-C. In this case, the affected person inherits the sickle cell trait (hemoglobin S) from one parent and another variant (hemoglobin C) from the other parent. With this condition, life span is slightly decreased and mild to moderate anemia is persistent. However, affected persons occasionally can have attacks of pain as in sickle cell disease (see page 960).

Hemoglobin E disease tends to occur in people of Southeast Asian origin. It also causes mild to moderate anemia.

Other Therapies

Blood transfusions are the most effective means of replacement available. They may reduce the level of abnormal hemoglobin.

Hemolytic Anemias

Signs and Symptoms

- Fatigue
- Paleness
- Breathlessness
- Heartbeat faster and more noticeable, particularly on exertion
- Yellow-tinged skin
- Dark urine
- Enlarged spleen

Emergency Symptoms—Sudden onset of pain in the upper abdomen

The hemolytic anemias are conditions in which red blood cells are destroyed and the hemoglobin is liberated from these cells. In these disorders, old red blood cells are broken down faster than the bone marrow can produce new red blood cells. The word "hemolytic" comes from Greek roots meaning "destruction of blood."

There are inherited and acquired forms of hemolytic anemias. Hereditary hemolytic anemias may be caused by abnormalities in the red blood cell membrane or by red blood cell enzyme deficiencies. In one hereditary type, called spherocytosis, the red blood cells are small, round, and fragile. Other inherited hemolytic anemia disorders include deficiencies of enzymes (such as glucose-6-phosphate dehydrogenase and pyruvate kinase).

Hemolytic anemias can be caused by certain medications and infections. Sometimes they result from an immune response against your own red blood cells (autoimmunity). Some types of hemolytic anemia are hard to treat, but they seldom are fatal.

Diagnosis

If your physician thinks you may have a hemolytic anemia, he or she will have a sample of your blood examined to count the number of young red blood cells (called reticulocytes) and to see if the red blood cells are deformed. The number of young red cells is increased in hemolytic anemia. Your physician also will examine your upper abdomen to see if your spleen or liver is enlarged.

Treatment

Medication

If your hemolytic anemia was caused by a drug, your physician will have you stop taking that drug. If your condition resulted from autoimmunity, your physician can prescribe medications to treat this problem. Corticosteroid medications such as prednisone are often helpful in preventing the destruction (hemolysis) of red blood cells.

Surgery

Some cases, especially those involving hereditary spherocytosis and those caused by autoimmunity that are not responsive to corticosteroids, are treated by surgical removal of the spleen (splenectomy).

Other Anemias

In addition to the usual types of anemias discussed above, rarer forms may occur as the result of genetic factors or as a consequence of certain diseases or the use of certain drugs. Among these types of anemias are those described below.

Glucose-6-Phosphate Dehydrogenase Deficiency

This is the result of an inherited defect in an enzyme, glucose-6-phosphate dehydrogenase, in the red blood cell. Like hemolytic anemia (see this page), this disorder causes the untimely breakdown of red blood cells. It occurs commonly in people of Mediterranean ancestry and in black people.

The symptoms range from mild to severe, depending on which type of defective gene for the enzyme is present. In blacks the symptoms tend to be milder; in people of Mediterranean ancestry the symptoms tend to be more severe.

The gene for the enzyme is sex-linked (carried on the X chromosome). Therefore, like hemophilia (see page 957), this disease almost always affects boys and men (who have only one X chromosome) rather than girls and women (who have two such chromosomes).

Thalassemia

There are two types of this unusual disease. Both are based on inherited defects in hemoglobin. In alpha-thalassemia, not enough of the part of hemoglobin called alpha-globin is produced. In beta-thalassemia, beta-globin is lacking.

Alpha-thalassemia occurs most often in people of southeast Asian descent. Beta-thalassemia is also known as Cooley's anemia, after the American physician who described it, and as Mediterranean anemia, because it is common in that region. The name "thalassemia" comes from Greek roots for "sea" and "blood."

The genes for both thalassemias are recessive, so you have to inherit them from both parents to get the disease. If you have only one gene, you are said to carry the trait but you will have no symptoms. When inherited from both parents, thalessemia frequently causes severe chronic anemia with poor growth, enlarged spleen, and, sometimes, heart failure.

Without treatment, death occurs in early childhood. There is no cure, but therapy can prolong life into the 20s or 30s. The treatment is repeated transfusions of packed red blood cells. These cells carry a great deal of iron, which can overload the body's vital organs. To lessen this effect, a medication may be given to cause the iron to be excreted in the urine. A treatment that still is experimental is bone marrow transplantation (see page 967). Genetic counseling may help you to avoid passing the disorder on to your children.

A milder form of thalassemia, thalassemia minor (or thalassemia trait), is common. This disorder produces blood cells that look like those present in iron-deficient blood, but there are no symptoms. Iron therapy may be harmful because it causes iron overload. This disorder by itself does not cause problems.

Anemia of Chronic Disease
Occasionally, an anemia can develop as the result of a chronic disease. The important groups of chronic diseases most often associated with anemia include chronic inflammation, such as rheumatoid arthritis (see page 909); uremia, as in kidney failure (see page 852); chronic liver disease (see page 800); acute and chronic infections; and decubitus ulcers.

Anemia of chronic disease is curable only if the underlying disorder can be cured or made less severe.

Aplastic Anemia
Aplastic means a failure in development, and aplastic anemia is an anemia caused by a drastic decrease in the bone marrow's production of all types of blood cells. This unusual and serious disease can occur spontaneously or it can be triggered by certain medications or toxic substances.

The disorder may be acute or chronic. It always is progressive. The symptoms of the anemia, if severe enough, resemble the response of a normal person to high altitude. Because the platelet count also is low, easy bruising and bleeding may occur. The low number of white blood cells leaves you vulnerable to bacterial infection. Infection and hemorrhage are emergency symptoms.

To diagnose aplastic anemia, your physician will use the complete count of the cells in your blood and an examination of a sample of your bone marrow. Treatment starts with elimination of the cause, if it is known. Your physician will try to protect you from infections and will treat any that do occur aggressively with antibiotics. Transfusions of red blood cells and platelets may be considered. You may be a candidate for bone marrow transplantation (see page 967) if your case is severe and a suitable donor is available.

Prevention may be aided by avoiding exposure to organic solvents, volatile chemicals, cleaners, and paint removers, particularly in a confined space. Occasionally medications and some diseases can also be responsible.

Sideroblastic Anemia
Sideroblasts are young red blood cells that contain excess iron. The name is derived from the Greek roots for "iron" and "germ." Sideroblastic anemias are rare disorders in which the red blood cells are overloaded with iron, the blood contains a high concentration of iron, and hemoglobin production is defective.

The treatment depends on the cause. You can acquire this anemia as a result of exposure to drugs or toxins such as alcohol and lead. When the offending agent is removed, the anemia may disappear entirely. It is also associated with certain cancers such as leukemia (see page 964), lymphoma (see page 968), and myeloma (see page 973) and with inflammatory diseases such as rheumatoid arthritis (see page 909). In such cases, the underlying condition should be treated. There is also an inherited form of sideroblastic anemia.

In some cases, no cause can be identified. In these cases, blood transfusions may be needed, along with a drug to remove the iron (via the urine) that accumulates from the transfused red blood cells.

Leukemias

Leukemias are cancers of the body's blood-forming tissues, including the bone marrow and lymph system. These cancers cause the formation of large amounts of abnormal white blood cells. These abnormal white blood cells reach high concentrations in the bone marrow, lymph system, and bloodstream, and their accumulation can interfere with the functions of the vital organs. Eventually, they overwhelm the production of healthy blood cells, including white and red blood cells and platelets.

In addition to the overabundance of abnormal white blood cells, there is an insufficient number of healthy ones. Therefore, the body's ability to fight infections is decreased. The abnormal white blood cells interfere with the production of red blood cells and platelets in the bone marrow. The deficiency in red blood cells means that the body's organs do not receive enough oxygen; the shortage of platelets makes the blood clotting process less effective, leaving the body more vulnerable to bleeding and bruising. Because of all these effects, leukemia is fatal without successful treatment.

The causes of leukemia are not known. Researchers have proposed that certain chemicals and viruses might play a role. Susceptibility to leukemia may be inherited. The ailment runs in some families, and people with certain congenital disorders, including Down syndrome (see page 44), are at higher risk of developing it.

Leukemias are classified depending on which type of white blood cell is affected. Myelogenous leukemia is a cancer of the granulocytes, a type of white blood cell that is formed in the bone marrow. Lymphocytic leukemia involves the lymphocytes, a type of white blood cell produced in the lymph system and marrow.

Types of leukemia are further divided according to how quickly they progress and the maturity of the cells affected. Acute leukemia progresses quickly with proliferation of immature cells. These cells, called blasts, are early stages of more mature white blood cells. Chronic leukemia progresses more slowly and is characterized by overproduction of mature white blood cells as well as blasts. Both acute and chronic forms occur somewhat more frequently in men than in women.

Chronic Myelogenous Leukemia

Signs and Symptoms
- Symptoms of anemia (see page 956)
- Bone pain
- Fever and infections
- Weight loss
- Swollen lymph nodes
- Pressure under the left ribs from an enlarged spleen
- Bleeding and bruising
- In some cases, none

Emergency Symptoms
- Severe bleeding
- Sudden appearance of small red marks on the skin

Chronic myelogenous leukemia is characterized by an overproduction of cancerous versions of granulocytes, a type of white blood cell formed in the bone marrow. This type of leukemia also may be called myeloid, myelocytic, or granulocytic. The disorder tends to occur in middle-aged persons.

Diagnosis
The disease can develop insidiously. In about a third of the cases, there are no symptoms at the time of diagnosis. These cases are detected when routine blood tests give abnormal results.

To determine whether you have chronic myelogenous leukemia, your physician will perform certain blood tests. These include a complete blood cell count (see page 955), a differential count of the various types of white blood cells, and measurement of an enzyme called leukocyte alkaline phosphatase. A small sample of the bone marrow may be examined (see page 1332). Your physician will also determine whether you have an abnormal chromosome known as the Philadelphia chromosome; this abnormality is found in 96 percent of those with chronic myelogenous leukemia. Molecular genetic techniques identify the other 4 percent.

How Serious Is Chronic Myelogenous Leukemia?
Chronic myelogenous leukemia is a progressive disease that cannot be cured except by bone marrow transplantation (see page 967).

In most people with this disorder, an acute phase, called a blast crisis, develops within 3 to 5 years. The blast crisis is characterized by a high concentration of blasts (immature white blood cells) in the blood and by red pinpoints (petechiae) on the skin that result from bleeding as a consequence of a lack of platelets. Death ensues because the blast crisis is a form of acute leukemia that is particularly resistant to treatment. So far, the only treatments that have been found to alter the course of this disease are high-dose chemotherapy with total-body irradiation followed by bone marrow transplantation and the use of interferon.

Treatment

Medication

Treatment of the chronic phase generally is simple chemotherapy such as hydroxyurea given by mouth, or busulfan or interferon injected daily under the skin. High-dose chemotherapy, along with bone marrow transplantation (see page 967), sometimes is used in persons younger than 55.

Surgery

If your spleen is extremely enlarged, it may be removed surgically (splenectomy). This has not been found to increase the duration of survival and usually is done only to relieve pain and bleeding if the spleen ruptures.

Acute Nonlymphocytic Leukemia

Signs and Symptoms
- Fatigue and lack of feeling of well-being, due mainly to anemia
- Fevers
- Bruising, small red marks on the skin, or a rash
- Weight loss
- Overgrowth of the gums
- Blurred vision or loss of vision
- Headaches or seizures
- Swollen lymph nodes
- In some cases, none

Emergency Symptoms
- Bleeding from the digestive tract; altered state of consciousness or inability to talk or move an extremity
- Fever, with bacterial infection in the blood

Acute nonlymphocytic leukemia is a cancer that causes overproduction of immature white blood cells known as blasts; ordinarily, these cells would have gone on to become granulocytes. The word nonlymphocytic distinguishes it from leukemias that affect the lymphocytes or their precursors. This form of acute leukemia is also called myelogenous, monocytic, myelogenic, or myelocytic, in reference to the bone marrow, the site of origin of the affected cells. It is the most common type of leukemia in adults.

Diagnosis
Diagnosis of acute nonlymphocytic leukemia is based on a complete blood cell count (see page 1330), a differential count of the various types of white blood cells, and examination of a sample of bone marrow. Your physician also will look for certain chromosome abnormalities that can help establish the diagnosis or predict how your body will respond to the disease. In some cases, your physician also may have a sample of your spinal fluid analyzed.

How Serious Is Acute Nonlymphocytic Leukemia?
The onset of acute nonlymphocytic leukemia can be extremely rapid. Without treatment, death can occur within weeks. Treatment with combinations of certain drugs (chemotherapy) frequently produces remission, a condition in which the body is rid of all evidence of the disease. However, without further treatment, recurrences develop in more than 80 percent of the patients who enter remission. Thirty-five to 40 percent of individuals have prolonged remission when they are given further therapies and an initial remission is achieved.

Treatment

Medication

Combinations of different chemotherapeutic drugs are given under the direction of your physician. Therapy with antibiotics can help to prevent or can treat the bacterial infections that are frequent complications. Your physician will choose an appropriate antibiotic based on the results of cultures of the blood, sputum, or urine specimens.

Other Therapies

Bone marrow transplantation may be performed in remission, in relapse, or in second remission, if an appropriate donor can be found.

Chronic Lymphocytic Leukemia

Signs and Symptoms
- Swollen lymph nodes
- Fatigue and lack of feeling of well-being, mainly due to anemia
- Infection
- Weight loss
- Bleeding
- Night sweats
- Pressure under the left ribs from enlargement of the spleen
- In many cases, none

Chronic lymphocytic leukemia is a cancerous proliferation of the white blood cells known as lymphocytes. It is the most common leukemia in the Western world. Ninety percent of the cases are in people older than 50. The disease occurs 2 to 3 times more often among men than among women. This difference in frequency between the sexes is more marked in this leukemia than in the other leukemias.

Diagnosis
The onset of chronic lymphocytic leukemia tends to be insidious, with symptoms developing gradually. Most cases are detected by routine blood tests performed in people who have no symptoms. These tests include complete blood cell count (see page 1330) with a differential count showing a high proportion of lymphocytes.

If your physician finds that you have the disease, he or she may conduct further tests to establish what subtypes of lymphocytes have been affected. The results of these tests will help predict how rapidly or slowly the disorder will advance and how you should be treated.

How Serious Is Chronic Lymphocytic Leukemia?
The course of chronic lymphocytic leukemia varies widely. Because it is an overproduction of mature, functional lymphocytes, persons with this disorder may survive for many years, even without treatment.

In contrast, in some the disorder progresses more rapidly, and earlier treatment may be required and usually is very helpful.

Treatment
If your disease is not advanced, your physician may choose not to start any form of treatment but instead may just keep track of your condition with periodic complete blood cell counts.

Medication
Treatment for advanced disease includes appropriate chemotherapy. Corticosteroid drugs such as prednisone also may be used with chemotherapy.

Surgery
Rarely, removal of the spleen (splenectomy) may be performed if it has become massive or if immune complications have arisen and are resistant to treatment with drugs.

Acute Lymphocytic Leukemia

Signs and Symptoms
- Abnormal bruising, including small hemorrhages into the skin
- Bleeding from mucous membranes
- Fatigue and lack of feeling of well-being
- Fever
- Paleness
- Enlarged liver, spleen, or lymph nodes
- Bone pain

Emergency Symptoms
- Fever
- Bleeding

Acute lymphocytic leukemia is a cancer that produces overproduction of immature blood cells known as blasts (these cells would otherwise have become lymphocytes). This particular type of blast is also called a lymphoblast, so the disorder is also known as acute lymphoblastic leukemia. It has been called childhood leukemia because it most frequently affects children.

Diagnosis
The symptoms of acute lymphocytic leukemia may appear suddenly or may be present weeks or months before the diagnosis is made. If the disease is suspected, your physician will perform blood tests, including a complete blood cell count (see page 1330) with a differential count of the various types of white blood cells. If the results of these tests suggest acute lymphocytic leukemia, a sample of your bone marrow will be exam-

ined to see whether it contains a high concentration of blasts (see page 1332).

In most medical centers, further tests are performed to determine what subtypes of lymphoblasts are present. These and other tests on the leukemic cells can help your physician characterize the disease and choose the most appropriate treatment.

How Serious Is Acute Lymphocytic Leukemia?

Without treatment, bleeding and infection lead to death within months. Before current treatments were developed, this was the inevitable course of the disease. Today, however, one of the great success stories of cancer treatment is the treatment of this leukemia in children between the ages of 2 and 10.

The younger you are and the lower your white blood cell count at the time of diagnosis, the higher your chances are of being cured. With proper combination chemotherapy, up to 70 percent of children are in complete remission at 5 years after detection of the disease, and most are probably cured. However, the prognosis is not as good for older children and adults; only about 20 percent achieve long-term survival. The outcome also depends on the particular type of lymphoblast that is present.

Treatment

Medication

Treatment of acute lymphocytic leukemia has three or four phases.

First, an attempt is made to achieve remission, usually by administering anticancer drugs in combination. Using combinations of drugs maximizes the effect on the leukemic cells. Your physician also may inject an anticancer (chemotherapeutic) drug such as methotrexate into your spinal fluid. Unfortunately, however, adverse effects still can create problems because some of these drugs can interfere with the normal functions of the bone marrow, the immune system, and other organs. In addition, some chemotherapeutic drugs temporarily slow the growth of children, but these children usually catch up after treatment is finished.

Second, once remission has been achieved, your anticancer drugs may be continued and radiation therapy to your central nervous system also may be recommended. These treatments are designed to kill the cancer cells that may linger in your central nervous system beyond the reach of medications given orally or intravenously. If not destroyed, such cells could cause a relapse later on.

For some persons, additional courses of chemotherapy, at times with different drugs, are given during remission in the hopes of eliminating the last surviving leukemic cells.

Last, maintenance treatment may be used to ensure that the remission continues. This involves relatively low-dose chemotherapy over the course of several years.

Other Therapies

Bone marrow transplantation may be performed after a relapse or in persons deemed to be at high risk of relapse.

Bone Marrow Transplantation

Bone marrow transplantation offers hope to seriously ill people. Bone marrow transplantation permits use of higher doses of chemotherapeutic agents and thus an enhanced anticancer action.

Types of Transplants

Syngeneic
The donor of a syngeneic transplant is the identical twin of the recipient. Identical twins have the same genetic makeup so the recipient is not at risk for a severe reaction to the transplant, called graft-versus-host disease, or rejection of the transplant. However, few persons have identical twins.

Allogeneic
The donor is a brother, sister, or parent of the recipient. In order to establish the compatibility of the potential donor's bone marrow, a test for human lymphocyte antigens (HLA test) is done to determine whether there is an HLA match.

This test examines six proteins, the HLAs, found on the surface of the white blood cells and most other cells of the body. The odds of an HLA donor/recipient match are about 25 percent if two siblings in a family are tested, but they increase to about 75 percent if there are six.

Autologous
In autologous bone marrow transplantation, bone marrow is taken from the person with the cancer.

Then this person is subjected to high doses of chemotherapy and perhaps irradiation. After this treatment has been completed, the bone marrow is returned to the person. There is no risk of graft-versus-host disease in autologous bone marrow transplantation.

Unrelated Donors
This type of bone marrow transplantation uses unrelated donors for allogeneic bone marrow transplantation. These donors are selected on the basis of their HLA system being identical or nearly identical to that of the recipient. A National Bone Marrow Registry has been set up to help locate HLA-matched bone marrow donors who are not related.

Transplantation Process
Bone marrow donation is more complicated than blood donation. Bone marrow is removed from the donor's pelvic bone (ilium), under general anesthesia in the hospital, and injected into one of the recipient's veins. From there the bone marrow cells travel in the bloodstream to the bone marrow space, where they produce new cells.

Throughout the transplantation process, the recipient stays in a special hospital room that is ventilated with filtered air to minimize the risk of infection; intravenous treatment with antibiotics also is used.

In allogeneic and syngeneic bone marrow transplantation, the bone marrow generally is removed from the donor and injected into the recipient the same day. In autolo-gous transplantation, the bone marrow is stored frozen (these cells can remain frozen for months to years) until the person has completed the high-dose chemotherapy, with or without radiation therapy.

Bone marrow transplantation is a unique process of donation because the marrow that has been donated replaces itself, and the loss of bone marrow is not significant. Therefore, there is no long-term concern about having only one organ, such as there is in kidney transplantation.

When to Do Transplantation
The best results after allogeneic and syngeneic bone marrow transplantation have been obtained in cases of severe aplastic anemia (see page 963), chronic granulocytic leukemia (see page 964), and acute nonlymphocytic leukemia (see page 965). There have been clinical trials to evaluate bone marrow transplantation for treating acute nonlymphocytic leukemia in remission (see page 965), acute lymphocytic leukemia in remission (see page 966), lymphoma in remission (see this page), and neuroblastoma in remission (see page 493). People with these diseases have a very high risk of dying in a relatively short time unless they receive some form of treatment such as transplantation.

In autologous transplantation, the best results have been obtained in treating Hodgkin's lymphoma (see page 969) and non-Hodgkin's lymphoma (see page 970). Cur-rently, it appears that persons whose disease is responsive to chemotherapy or who again achieve complete remission after relapsing after chemotherapy are the best candidates for this procedure. Some programs are evaluating the use of bone marrow transplantation for tumors such as breast cancer and other cancers.

What Are the Risks?
The major cause of disease and death in bone marrow transplantation is graft-versus-host disease, not graft rejection. This complication can affect the skin, liver, gastrointestinal tract, and lungs. This is the major complication in allogeneic transplantation but is not a problem in syngeneic or autologous transplantation.

The mortality rate is 25 percent in the first 100 days after an allogeneic bone marrow transplantation, from infection or graft-versus-host disease. The second major problem is a type of pneumonia that can be caused by infection or other complications.

The Future
Additional techniques are being developed for treating leukemia and lymphoma. One is the use of specific antibodies (monoclonal antibodies) that are directed against the disease cells. After the marrow is removed, it is treated with the monoclonal antibodies, and possibly other chemotherapeutic agents, prior to being given to the patient. This has been utilized in autologous transplantation.

Lymphomas

Lymphomas are cancers of the lymph system. The lymph system includes the lymph nodes, or lymph glands, which are located throughout the body and are connected by small vessels called lymphatics. The spleen is also part of the lymph system. Often, the first symptom of lymphoma is enlargement of lymph nodes with no other obvious symptoms. Lymphomas may also occur outside the lymph nodes in virtually any part of the body.

Swelling of the lymph nodes, which are

normally the size of a bean, is not necessarily a sign of lymphoma; many other conditions can cause nodes to enlarge. However, if your glands stay swollen for more than 4 weeks, consult your physician.

Lymphomas are a diverse group of diseases. They include Hodgkin's disease and non-Hodgkin's disease, which are described below.

Hodgkin's Disease

Signs and Symptoms
- Painless swelling of lymph nodes in the neck, armpits, or groin
- Persistent fatigue
- Fever and chills
- Night sweats
- Weight loss and loss of appetite
- Severe itching

Emergency Symptoms
- Sudden onset of high fever from any cause
- Loss of bladder or bowel control
- Numbness or loss of strength in the arms and legs

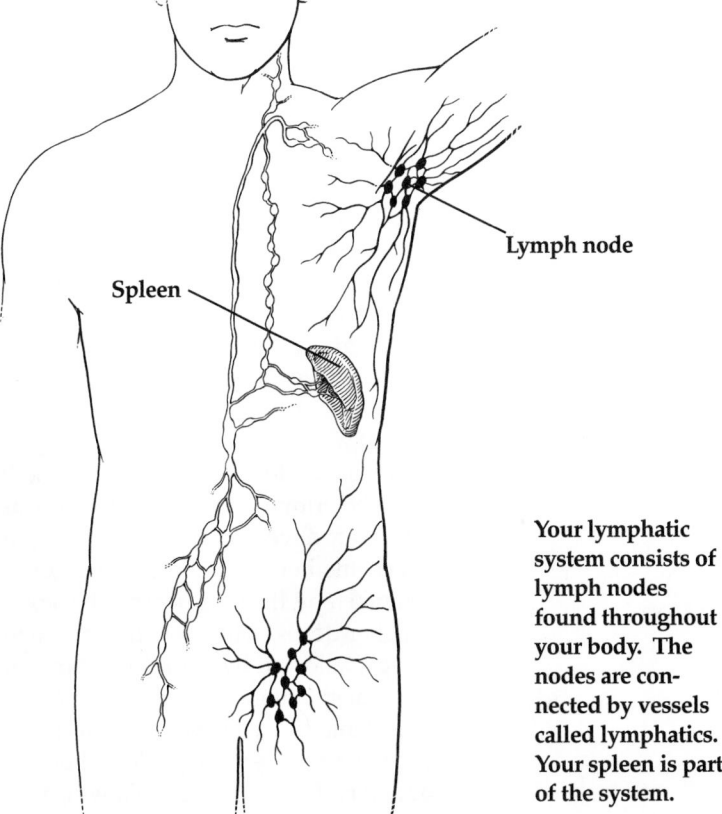

Spleen

Lymph node

Your lymphatic system consists of lymph nodes found throughout your body. The nodes are connected by vessels called lymphatics. Your spleen is part of the system.

Hodgkin's disease is named after Thomas Hodgkin, a 19th-century English physician. Four major types can be identified on the basis of the appearance of the tissue under the microscope (histologic subtypes).

The cause of Hodgkin's disease is not known. Fifty to 90 percent of individuals with this disease have Epstein-Barr virus in malignant cells (see page 1064). Whether this is the cause is not known. Individuals with AIDS are at high risk for the development of Hodgkin's disease.

Hodgkin's disease usually affects people between 15 and 35 years old, but it can occur in those older than 50. The presence of Hodgkin's disease often is suspected when an enlarged lymph node is detected.

Diagnosis
To determine whether you have Hodgkin's disease, your physician will ask about previous medical problems, conduct a thorough physical examination, take a chest X-ray, and obtain tests of your blood and urine.

Most important will be a lymph node biopsy, in which lymph node tissue is removed and studied for the presence of the

patterns typical of Hodgkin's disease. Occasionally, only a portion of the node is removed for examination under a microscope. The remainder of the node, still in place, is then used as a marker to evaluate your response to treatment.

If your physician finds that you have Hodgkin's disease, he or she will conduct more tests to find out how advanced the tumor is and to decide how best to treat it. This testing process is called staging the tumor and may involve a bilateral bone marrow biopsy (see page 1332), a computed tomographic scan of your abdomen and chest (see page 1334), a gallium scan (see page 1338), or an operation to explore the abdomen (a laparotomy).

How Serious Is Hodgkin's Disease?
When Hodgkin's disease is detected early and treated properly, as many as 90 percent of the cases can be completely cured. Years ago the disease was almost always fatal. Of patients with the most advanced stages of the disease, 50 to 80 percent have no disease 10 years after chemotherapy and are considered cured.

Treatment

Radiation Therapy
Radiation therapy is the main treatment when the spread of the disease is limited. Radiation therapy is sometimes used in combination with chemotherapy. When one lymph node region is involved, 90 percent of affected persons are disease-free after 10 years. For those who have two lymph node regions involved, either above or below the diaphragm, 70 percent are alive and disease-free after 10 years.

Medication
For advanced Hodgkin's disease, chemotherapy is the primary treatment. Two-thirds of persons are alive and disease-free long-term after chemotherapy. If there is a relapse after chemotherapy, the treatment can be repeated at higher doses, with or without radiation therapy, followed by autologous bone marrow transplantation (see Bone Marrow Transplantation, page 967). In this process, bone marrow is removed before chemotherapy and replaced afterward, allowing the use of larger doses of anticancer drugs.

Surgery
Occasionally, an operation will be performed to explore the abdomen (laparotomy) in order to determine the extent of the disease.

Non-Hodgkin's Lymphoma

Signs and Symptoms
- Painless enlargement of lymph nodes, with or without swelling of the abdomen
- Persistent fatigue
- Fever or chills
- Night sweats
- Loss of appetite

Emergency Symptoms
- Sudden onset of high fever, from any cause
- Severe constipation or profuse urination
- Mental confusion, drowsiness
- Involuntary loss of urine or stool
- Numbness or loss of strength in the arms and legs

Non-Hodgkin's lymphomas are a group of tumors that arise from the lymphocytes (white blood cells). These tumors are classified according to their cell size as seen under the microscope. They are also grouped into three broad categories by level of activity of the malignant cells: low grade, intermediate grade, and high grade.

These tumors are more common than Hodgkin's disease. They occur more frequently among people who have received organ transplants because their immune mechanisms are inhibited by immunosuppressive therapy. Individuals with AIDS (see page 1060) are at higher risk for developing this disorder. The disease typically is detected in persons from ages 45 to 70 and, unlike Hodgkin's disease, it often occurs in older persons.

Diagnosis
If your physician suspects that you have non-Hodgkin's lymphoma, he or she will do a physical examination and obtain laboratory tests on your blood and urine, a computed tomography scan of your abdomen (see page 1334), and a bone marrow study by aspiration and biopsy (see page 1332). Your physician will also perform a lymph node biopsy for classifying the disease.

How Serious Is Non-Hodgkin's Lymphoma?
Low-grade non-Hodgkin's lymphoma is not curable but the survival rate is good and it is very responsive to initial therapy. The 5-year survival rate is about 75 percent. If you have this disease but have no symptoms, your physician may recommend observation only.

In contrast, some of the intermediate- and high-grade non-Hodgkin's lymphomas are curable with aggressive treatments, but survival is usually less than 1½ years if treatment does not produce a complete remission. Sixty to 80 percent of affected individuals enter a complete remission with chemotherapy. The risk of relapse and death relates to your age and other factors.

Treatment

Medication
Chemotherapy with a combination of anticancer drugs is usually used.

Surgery
An operation to decrease the size of the tumor (debulking) has been used when the lymphoma involves the stomach or in cases of other unusual appearances of the disease, but it is not used in treating most people.

Other Therapies

Radiation therapy is used in some instances of low-grade and intermediate-grade non-Hodgkin's lymphoma.

Nutrition

To maintain your quality of life, it is important that you follow guidelines for proper nutrition. However, this has not been proved to increase the chances of survival.

Growth Disorders of the Bone Marrow

The marrow lies in spaces within your bones and normally produces all of your red blood cells and platelets and most of your white blood cells. When something goes wrong with your bone marrow, the consequences are serious. Production of cells is no longer orderly and deficiencies may occur, leading to anemia, bleeding disorders, and vulnerability to infections.

In a young child, all of the bones contain active marrow that forms blood cells. As the body matures, active blood-forming marrow is found only in the bones of the spine, skull, ribs, and pelvis. However, if for some reason the body requires extra blood cells, the bone marrow in the arms and legs may be stimulated to revert to active production.

If your physician thinks that you may have a bone marrow disorder, a sample of your bone marrow will be removed for study under a microscope. In a process called aspiration, a special needle is inserted into your hipbone or breastbone and a small amount of the marrow is withdrawn through it.

Often a biopsy of the bone marrow is obtained at the same time. The site of the biopsy is infiltrated with an anesthetic, a needle is inserted into the bone, and a small piece of bone marrow is removed for examination under the microscope (see page 1332).

Polycythemia Vera

Signs and Symptoms
- Weakness
- Itching, especially in a warm bath
- Dizziness
- Sense of fullness in the head and redness of the face and hands
- Fullness in the left upper abdomen

Emergency Symptoms
- Blood in the vomit or stool
- Stroke
- Blood clot in the legs

Polycythemia vera occurs when the bone marrow produces too many blood cells. The word "polycythemia" refers to "many cells in the blood"; "vera" means "true."

In this disorder there is a high concentration of red blood cells in the circulating blood, but white blood cell and platelet counts may also be increased. The condition is unusual, and its cause is not known.

Polycythemia vera generally appears in late middle age; it is extremely rare in children. It is slightly more common among men than women.

Diagnosis
The symptoms of polycythemia vera appear gradually. If your physician thinks that you may have it, he or she will order various blood tests including a complete blood cell

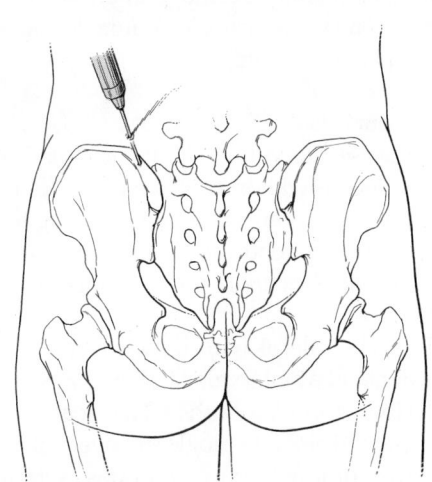

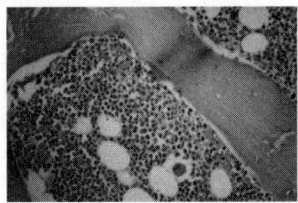

In a bone marrow biopsy, a needle is used to remove a sample of bone marrow for examination under a microscope (above).

count (see page 955) and possibly measurement of the vitamin B_{12} and certain other substances, such as leukocyte alkaline phosphatase, in your blood. The values often are unusually high in this disorder. Uric acid levels are also increased, which may cause attacks of gouty arthritis (see Gout, page 916).

Another sign is an increase in the volume of blood without much of an increase in its plasma component. Your physician can measure the increase with special blood tests.

Additional tests are used to differentiate polycythemia vera from secondary polycythemia, which has other causes such as heavy cigarette smoking, severe lung disease, abnormal hemoglobins, living at high altitudes, and certain tumors. It is especially important to exclude diseases such as kidney cancer which may have an associated elevated red blood cell count.

In secondary polycythemia, the blood's high content of red blood cells is a response to the low oxygen concentration in the air and therefore in the blood. Because there is less oxygen in the blood, the body attempts to overcome the deficiency by making more red blood cells until there are too many.

How Serious Is Polycythemia Vera?

Without treatment, the symptoms of polycythemia vera worsen and the risk of death from stroke (see page 461) or heart attack (see page 661) increases. The reason for this is that the high concentration of blood cells makes the blood thicker (more viscous) and so it has greater difficulty flowing through the blood vessels.

With proper treatment, you generally feel normal and the risk of stroke or heart attack lessens. Although there is no cure, most people live for more than 10 years with the disease. In a small percentage of those with polycythemia vera, acute leukemia develops after a period of years.

Treatment

To decrease the volume of the circulating blood, blood is withdrawn from a vein (phlebotomy). This is effective in decreasing the viscosity of the blood and lessening the danger of stroke. Generally this is the first treatment used.

The schedule of withdrawal is about a pint of blood at intervals of a few days initially to weeks or months. The goal is to maintain the blood hemoglobin level within the range of low to normal values. Often, blood withdrawal can be stopped for months at a time if the hemoglobin level remains in the required range.

Medication

If your blood has high white blood cell and platelet counts, in addition to a high content of red blood cells, your physician may prescribe a drug that cuts down blood cell production by the bone marrow, such as radioactive phosphorus. A disadvantage of radioactive phosphorus therapy is that it has been associated with transformation of normal white cells to leukemia cells, in some cases over a period of years. One advantage of it is that one treatment a year may be enough to control the disease.

Other medicines may be used on a daily basis to lower both the white blood cell count and the platelet count. Some other specific therapies are directed at the platelets.

Surgery

If your spleen becomes extremely enlarged, which happens in rare cases, your physician may consider surgical removal of it (splenectomy).

Agnogenic Myeloid Metaplasia

Signs and Symptoms
- Breathlessness on exertion
- Rapid heartbeat
- Paleness
- Enlarged spleen
- Night sweats
- Weight loss
- Stuffed feeling after eating

In agnogenic myeloid metaplasia, the bone marrow gradually becomes scarred and less able to manufacture blood cells. Then, blood cells are also produced outside of the marrow, in the spleen and liver, and both of these organs can become enlarged. The name of the disorder means "bone marrow transformation of unknown origin." It is also called idiopathic myelofibrosis.

Treatment

Medications are available, but there is no cure. Most affected persons become dependent on blood transfusions.

Enlargement of the spleen may cause pain or reduce the number of platelets in the blood (by trapping them in the spleen), and your physician may consider surgical removal of the spleen (splenectomy).

Multiple Myeloma

Signs and Symptoms
- Fatigue and weakness
- Back pain that progresses insidiously
- Unexplained bone fractures, especially in the vertebrae or ribs
- Vulnerability to infection
- Bleeding problems, such as nosebleeds and bleeding gums
- Bone fracture

Emergency Symptoms
- Severe constipation and profuse urination
- Excessive sleepiness or fluctuating level of consciousness
- Significant decrease in urine flow
- Incontinence of stool or urine
- Numbness or loss of strength in extremities

Multiple myeloma is a cancer that produces uncontrolled multiplication of a type of white blood cell in the marrow called a plasma cell. As these cells grow and take up more space in the marrow, the bones may weaken, causing pain, particularly in the back and ribs. As the bones become more fragile, they break more easily.

Eventually, the growth of plasma cells interferes with the production of normal red blood cells, white blood cells, and platelets by the bone marrow. Anemia, susceptibility to infection, and bleeding problems can result.

The name of this unusual disorder means a bone marrow tumor that occurs in many sites. The disease primarily affects persons older than 50, with the average age being 63 at the time of diagnosis. It occurs slightly more often in men than women, and it is almost twice as common among blacks as whites. This disease is not inherited.

Diagnosis
A common symptom of multiple myeloma is back or rib pain that is slowly progressive. The pain eases with rest and increases with movement. It eventually may also be felt in the neck and hips.

If your physician suspects that you have multiple myeloma, he or she will have a sample of your bone marrow examined for myeloma cells. X-rays of your skeleton will show whether your bones have any of the thinned-out areas that characterize the disease. Your physician also will have various blood tests performed, including a complete blood cell count (see page 1330) and measurements of calcium, uric acid, creatinine, and blood proteins.

Ordinarily, the plasma cells produce antibody proteins to fight infections. In this disorder, mutation of one such cell gives rise to a new line of abnormal cells. When this happens, another small molecule, called Bence Jones protein after the 19th century English physician who discovered the substance, may be produced. Therefore, your physician will check samples of your blood and urine for the presence of these proteins.

Increased amounts of protein from these abnormal cells are common in the blood of older people, and the discovery of one increased protein does not necessarily signify multiple myeloma. Such a state may be referred to as monoclonal gammopathy of undetermined significance (see this page). When such an abnormal protein is found, your physician will carry out examinations to exclude multiple myeloma. Occasional checkups thereafter may be advised.

How Serious Is Multiple Myeloma?
There is no cure. However, treatment can prolong your life for years and can relieve the

---

Monoclonal Gammopathy of Undetermined Significance

The finding of a monoclonal protein in the blood in older people is not uncommon. This protein is an abnormal antibody-like protein that comes from a single line (or clone) of plasma cells. Plasma cells are a type of white blood cell in the bone marrow. They produce the antibodies needed for normal immunity.

Monoclonal gammopathies are usually detected in the course of routine physical examinations. They occur in 1 percent of healthy persons older than 50 and in 3 percent older than 70.

In 75 percent of cases, the monoclonal gammopathies never cause a problem. However, in the remaining 25 percent, the amount of the abnormal protein in the blood eventually increases, indicating the presence of a disorder that will probably require treatment. Such conditions include lymphoma (see page 968), multiple myeloma (see this page), and amyloidosis (see page 974). Therefore, if you have a monoclonal gammopathy, your physician will want to check your blood to identify the protein and recheck you at intervals ranging from every 3 months to yearly or longer.

symptoms. Your physician will watch your progress to judge your response to treatment and to avoid complications.

Treatment

If you have multiple myeloma, remain active, drink plenty of fluids, and eat a balanced diet. Staying active helps to retain the calcium in your bones (not the blood), which keeps your bones strong. Some restrictions, such as avoiding heavy lifting, may be necessary. If pain is disabling, a back brace, cane, or other orthopedic support device may help you remain active. Drinking fluids prevents dehydration. The amount of protein you eat does not need to be restricted.

Medication

If your multiple myeloma is detected in its early stages, you may not need treatment. If treatment is required, however, your physician will prescribe appropriate anticancer medication, either by pills or by intravenous delivery. Analgesics can alleviate bone pain.

Surgery

If your bones become unstable, surgical repairs may be necessary to strengthen them.

Other Therapies

Radiation directed at specific sites, usually on the back and neck, can control severe pain and disease in that area.

Amyloidosis

Signs and Symptoms

- Fatigue or weakness
- Numbness of hands or feet
- Weight loss
- Shortness of breath
- Swelling of the legs
- Diarrhea

In amyloidosis, a protein called amyloid is deposited in sites throughout the body. The term "amyloidosis" is something of a misnomer because it suggests a condition involving a starch-like substance, but the material in question is a protein, not a starch. The disorder is rare.

Diagnosis

The diagnosis of amyloidosis hinges on the detection, by biopsy, of amyloid deposits in tissues in your body. The biopsy sites fre-

Granulocytopenia and Agranulocytosis

When your physician conducts tests of your blood, a wide variety of findings may emerge. Among the more unusual disorders may be granulocytopenia or agranulocytosis.

These uncommon problems are usually caused by other disorders, possibly leukemia (see page 964) or aplastic anemia (see page 963). They also may be side effects of certain medications.

Granulocytopenia

When the blood contains less than the normal number of a grainy type of white blood cell called "granulocytes," the condition is called granulocytopenia. Either the bone marrow does not produce enough of these cells or they are being destroyed at a rate that is higher than usual.

The condition is also known as neutropenia because the granulocytes that most often are affected are the neutrophils. The name neutrophil (neutral-loving) comes from the fact that it is stained about equally by acidic and basic dyes. This subtype of cell is considered to be the body's first line of defense against bacterial or fungal (but not viral) infection. Therefore, granulocytopenia increases the body's susceptibility to infections. Antibiotic treatment can help ward these off.

Granulocytopenia can be the first sign of leukemia (see page 964) or aplastic anemia (see page 963). Granulocytopenia that is due to another problem or to medication, such as chemotherapy, is more common than spontaneous occurrence of the ailment.

Agranulocytosis

This rare condition is a drastic decrease in the blood's content of granulocytes. Almost all of the neutrophils are destroyed, leaving the body particularly prone to infection. Therefore, people with this ailment must be watched carefully for the development of infections and must be treated with antibiotics.

Most often, the disorder occurs as a rare, acute response to exposure to certain chemicals, solvents, or hydrocarbons or to certain medications including penicillins, phenothiazines, and anti-inflammatory agents.

The usual treatment is to remove the affected person from additional exposure and to protect him or her from serious infection until the bone marrow can recover.

quently used include the gums, rectum, abdominal fat, and kidney. Biopsy of the heart, nerves, and bone marrow occasionally is performed to establish the diagnosis.

As in multiple myeloma (see page 973), the plasma cells may produce abnormal proteins. Your physician may check your urine for the presence of these proteins.

How Serious Is Amyloidosis?

No curative treatment has been found. The condition is chronic, progressing slowly and usually leading to death after a number of years.

The severity of the disorder depends on which organs are affected by the amyloid deposits. Potentially life-threatening situations, including kidney failure (see page 852) and congestive heart failure (see page 659), may occur. If the accumulations of amyloid are limited to less crucial sites, there may be no symptoms. Most cases are somewhere between these two extremes.

Treatment

Medication

Your physician may prescribe certain medications to see if they are effective. In addition, your physician may prescribe diuretics and other medicines if your heart is affected, and analgesics, if necessary, for pain. It is wise to avoid direct exposure to people with known infections.

Nutrition

Changing the amount of protein you eat will not affect the disease, but other special diets may be necessary, depending on which organs are affected. Your physician will discuss with you any dietary restrictions or nutritional supplements that may be necessary.

Bleeding Disorders

Bleeding disorders result from disruption of the body's elaborate process by which blood clots form. This coagulation process, which involves platelets as well as plasma proteins called clotting factors, begins when platelets stick to the site of injury to a blood vessel. An intricate cascade of enzyme reactions occurs to produce a web-like protein network that encircles the platelets and holds them in place (platelet phase) to form the clot (coagulation phase). In this cascade, each clotting factor is transformed, in turn, from an inactive to an active form.

Specialized laboratories can study the coagulation mechanism in an affected person's blood to pinpoint the place in the cascade at which the fault lies.

Problems with clotting factors cause bleeding disorders such as hemophilia, von Willebrand's disease, and disseminated intravascular coagulation. Bleeding disorders based on clotting factor problems generally tend to cause bleeding deep in the tissues and joints, although excessive bruising, severe nosebleeds, and other types of bleeding can occur as well.

When platelets are too few (thrombocytopenia) or fail to function, one result is red pinpoint hemorrhages known as petechiae, seen in the skin.

Hemophilia

Signs and Symptoms

- Many large or deep bruises
- Pain and swelling of joints, caused by internal bleeding
- Blood in the urine or stool
- Prolonged bleeding from cuts or injuries or after surgery or tooth extraction

Emergency Symptoms

- Bleeding into the head, neck, or digestive tract
- Sudden pain, swelling, and warmth of large joints such as the knees, elbows, hips, and shoulders and of the muscles of the arms and legs
- Bleeding from any injury (especially if you have a severe form of hemophilia)

Hemophilia, named from Greek roots meaning "fond of blood," includes several inherited disorders of specific clotting factors (the proteins in the plasma that cause the blood to clot). The most common is hemophilia A, also called classic hemophilia, in which there is not enough of clotting factor VIII. Hemophilia B (or Christmas disease), in which factor IX is lacking, makes up most of the remaining cases.

Both the A and B forms of the disorder have also been called the royal disease, because hemophilia was inherited by descendants of England's Queen Victoria and introduced into the royal houses of Spain, Germany, and Russia. Although hemophilia is one of the most commonly inherited bleeding disorders, it is still a rather unusual ailment.

Hemophilia A and hemophilia B are caused by genes that are recessive and sex-linked (carried on the X chromosome), so the disorder almost always occurs in boys, not girls (see page 42). Girls who inherit a hemophilia gene usually are symptomless carriers (they are said to have hemophilia trait) because they are protected by the normal gene on their other X chromosome. Most often, hemophilia occurs in families who have a history of the disease, which passes from grandfather to grandson through a mother who is a carrier. However, new cases sometimes occur in families in which the disease has not previously been apparent.

Diagnosis

The major problem for people with hemophilia is not superficial external cuts, which can be easily treated with pressure and a bandage, but is uncontrolled internal bleeding. The severity of bleeding varies from person to person. The more severe forms become apparent early in life. Newborns often show no signs of hemophilia unless they are circumcised, but marked bruising may develop beneath the skin as the child starts to crawl or walk. In more severe forms of hemophilia, excessive bleeding happens often and even spontaneously without any apparent cause. However, in its mild forms, hemophilia may not become apparent until later in life, and troublesome bleeding episodes may happen only after surgery, tooth extraction, or major injury.

Your physician can establish the diagnosis by using specialized laboratory tests that measure the clotting activity of factors VIII and IX (or other factors) and determine the presence or absence of an inhibitor of these factors.

How Serious Is Hemophilia?

With current medical treatment, people with hemophilia can have close to an average life expectancy. Although the disease is lifelong, it can be controlled with medication or by the administration of clotting factors, allowing a relatively normal life. Depending on the severity of the hemophilia, it may be necessary to take extra care to minimize bleeding as a result of physical activity or surgical or dental procedures. Sometimes the disorder becomes more difficult to control because antibodies develop to the clotting factor that has been used in the treatment.

Without treatment, recurrent bleeding into the joints can cause chronic pain and weakness and even can destroy the joint (through osteoarthritis, see page 907). Bleeding into muscles and soft tissue may put pressure on nerves, producing pain, stiffness, and numbness. Without adequate control, permanent nerve damage and muscle wasting eventually may occur. When blood collects in the head, neck, or digestive system, the condition is considered to be extremely serious. So it is important to stop these episodes promptly. To prevent joint destruction, all bleeding episodes should be treated promptly by infusion of a clotting factor replacement or, for mild hemophilia A, a medicine called desmopressin (see below). If you have hemophilia or think you may carry the trait, prenatal testing and genetic counseling can help you learn whether you could pass the disorder on to your children (see page 42).

Treatment

Despite having hemophilia, you may lead a relatively normal life.

Exercise

Physical therapy can help damaged joints to function better. Swimming, bicycle riding, and walking can build up your muscles, thus helping to protect your joints. Do not engage in contact sports.

Medication

If you have mild hemophilia A, your bleeding episodes may be treated with infusion (slow injection into a vein) of desmopressin (also known as DDAVP). This drug helps stop bleeding by stimulating the release of factor VIII and making blood vessels contract.

If you have hemophilia B or more severe hemophilia A, bleeding episodes may stop only after the missing clotting factor is replaced by infusion. These clotting factors are derived from donated human blood and are supplied as purified concentrates, as fresh frozen plasma, or as cryoprecipitate (a clotting factor concentrate derived from donated human blood). The clotting factor concentrates are now treated to prevent transmission of the AIDS virus (see AIDS, page 1060). In addition, recombinant factors have also been developed. With special training (available through your physician or a regional hemophilia center), you can learn to infuse DDAVP or some of these blood products yourself as soon as you show signs of bleeding. Do not use medications that might worsen bleeding, such as aspirin.

Surgery

If recurrent internal bleeding has destroyed any of your joints, you may choose to have that joint replaced surgically with an artificial joint (see Joint Replacement, page 911).

von Willebrand's Disease

Signs and Symptoms
- Nosebleeds or excessive menstrual bleeding
- Easy bruising
- Blood in the stool, characterized by a black or tarry appearance

This chronic bleeding disorder is caused by a defect in a clotting factor called von Willebrand factor. In many cases, there also is a deficiency of factor VIII. Ordinarily, these two factors combine to form the active complex that is needed to cause platelets to gather at the site of blood vessel injury. In von Willebrand's disease, the platelet aggregation and clot formation are impaired.

The disease is named after the early 20th-century Finnish physician who described it. It has also been called pseudohemophilia or vascular hemophilia. It is the most common hereditary bleeding disorder.

The severity of symptoms varies from person to person. The most severe form of the disease is rare, but milder forms are now recognized as being much more common. It affects both sexes in equal numbers. Before adolescence, a key symptom is nosebleeds that may be severe enough to require a visit to your physician or the emergency room. In women, the menstrual flow is heavy. Other symptoms are marked bruising, blood in the urine or stool, and bleeding during and after surgery or tooth extraction.

Diagnosis
To diagnose the disease, your physician will arrange for specialized blood tests. He or she will look for prolonged bleeding time, impaired platelet function, and a shortage of active von Willebrand factor and, in some cases, of factor VIII as well.

Treatment
If you have von Willebrand's disease, the treatment to prevent or to stop the bleeding may be infusion of the drug desmopressin, which stimulates release of von Willebrand factor and factor VIII from blood vessel walls. Transfusion of plasma or cryoprecipitate also may be used (cryoprecipitate is a clotting factor concentrate derived from donated human blood). Avoid medications that might worsen bleeding, such as aspirin. There is no prevention for this inherited disorder aside from genetic counseling of prospective parents who have it. If you are found to have von Willebrand's disease, it is possible that your brothers, sisters, or children also might have it. Therefore, they may want to seek appropriate testing and counseling (see page 42).

Disseminated Intravascular Coagulation

Signs and Symptoms
- Severe bleeding from many sites in the body
- None may be apparent

Emergency Symptoms—Severe bleeding, especially with trauma or at surgical incision sites

This is a nonhereditary bleeding disorder that actually results from excessive coagulation. It occurs when activated clotting factors are present throughout the bloodstream instead of being limited to sites of injury. These factors cause circulating platelets to clot (coagulate) in small blood vessels all over the body—hence the name disseminated intravascular coagulation.

So much of the body's supply of clotting

factors and platelets is used up by this inappropriate coagulation that not enough is available for the formation of clots at injury sites. The body also reacts by stepping up the system that dissolves clots, and this promotes generalized bleeding.

The disorder is also known by the acronym DIC, as intravascular coagulation and fibrinolysis, and as defibrination syndrome. It occurs only occasionally, almost always as a complication of one of a large variety of serious underlying diseases including infection and malignancy, or following trauma or surgery.

Diagnosis

If your physician suspects that you have disseminated intravascular coagulation, he or she will perform various blood tests. These include platelet count, prothrombin time, measuring the fibrinogen concentration in your blood, and other tests to confirm the diagnosis.

How Serious Is Disseminated Intravascular Coagulation?

The conditions that cause the disorder tend to be life-threatening, but if they are treated successfully the disseminated intravascular coagulation will stop. These include various obstetric emergencies, widespread cancer, massive trauma, shock, and bacterial sepsis (blood infection).

The severity of the disorder itself varies. When disseminated intravascular coagulation occurs with cancer or some other disorder, it can be chronic, being detected only in blood tests but not causing any spontaneous bleeding. More often, it is acute, causing severe bleeding from multiple sites such as surgical incisions. Clots may form in the legs or a stroke may occur. Rarely, it is serious enough to cause gangrene in the fingers, genitals, or nose.

Treatment

The only really effective approach is to treat the underlying condition that caused the disseminated intravascular coagulation. However, transfusion of various blood products also may be necessary to replace the clotting factors depleted by the widespread coagulation. Treatment with heparin (a drug that is given through a vein and prevents clotting) may be needed when there is evidence of clotting or when there is no response to blood product transfusions and bleeding continues.

Thrombocytopenia

Signs and Symptoms

- Easy or excessive bruising
- Measles-like rash, usually on the lower legs
- Nosebleeds
- Blood in vomit or stools
- Heavy menstrual flow
- Bleeding during surgery

Emergency Symptoms—Serious or widespread bleeding, including bleeding in the brain and digestive system

Thrombocytopenia, a common bleeding disorder, results from a shortage of platelets in the blood, hence its name, which is derived from Greek roots meaning "a poverty of clotting cells." The disorder is divided into two types: idiopathic and secondary. Most often it is an acquired condition rather than a hereditary one.

Idiopathic thrombocytopenia is also known as idiopathic thrombocytopenic purpura (ITP). Purpura (derived from the Greek word for purple) is a rash made up of small red marks (petechiae) caused by bleeding into the lower layers of the skin. Although idiopathic means "of unknown cause," most cases of idiopathic thrombocytopenia are a result of production by spleen and lymph tissue of antibodies against the body's own healthy platelets. These antibodies destroy the platelets prematurely. Because of this process of immunity against oneself (autoimmunity), the disorder is also called autoimmune thrombocytopenic purpura (AITP or ATP). It occurs most often in children and young adults but can occur at any age. It affects more women than men, but this condition is equally likely to occur in boys as in girls.

In isolated secondary thrombocytopenia, there is some other cause of the ailment. The underlying disorders include viral infections, systemic lupus erythematosus (see page 918), lymphoma (see page 968), chronic lymphocytic leukemia (see page 966), sarcoidosis (see page 721), cancer of the ovary (see page 1190), and overwhelming infection following transfusion and drugs. Drugs that sometimes cause thrombocytopenia include heparin, quinidine, sulfonamides, procainamide, rifampin, and chemotherapy drugs.

Diagnosis

To detect thrombocytopenia, your physician will obtain a platelet count and an examination of a stained smear of your blood under a microscope. If it appears that you have thrombocytopenia, your physician may proceed to special blood tests and a bone marrow examination to determine what is causing the concentration of platelets in your blood to be low (see page 1332).

How Serious Is Thrombocytopenia?
Particularly in children, idiopathic thrombocytopenia can sometimes go away without any treatment. In these cases, the bone marrow may make up for the shortening of the life span of the platelets by producing large numbers of new ones while the initiating cause appears to subside. The young platelets are especially active in clotting, so even though the total concentration of platelets is low, bleeding problems may not occur. Thus, your physician may decide that no special treatment is necessary.

In adults, acute thrombocytopenia often becomes a chronic ailment. It may vary in severity over time, and it can even recur after an apparently complete remission. The most serious complications, bleeding into the brain and digestive tract, occur only rarely.

Treatment
If you have secondary thrombocytopenia, your physician will treat the underlying condition or will stop the medications that may have caused it. In some situations, your physician may use thrombopoietin, a hormone that stimulates bone marrow cells to produce platelets.

Medication
Various medications that suppress or otherwise alter the immune system, including prednisone (a corticosteroid drug), are used to treat idiopathic thrombocytopenia. Do not use medications that impair the function of platelets, such as aspirin.

Surgery
Surgical removal of the spleen (splenectomy) is sometimes undertaken to relieve symptoms or to help cure chronic idiopathic thrombocytopenia that does not respond to corticosteroids.

Other Therapies
With severe bleeding, lost blood is replaced with transfusions of packed red blood cells. Occasionally, platelet concentrates (see page 981) are given after intravenous immunoglobulin administration.

Sometimes treatment is not needed. In such cases, despite the low concentration of platelets, no bleeding complications result and the condition simply may go away.

Blood Transfusions

Blood transfusions often are necessary to save the life of a person who has a blood disorder, some other disease, an accident, or surgery. Blood donations are always needed, so consider giving blood if you possibly can. Only a small percentage of people in the United States who are eligible to donate blood actually do so.

The Donation Procedure

If you are older than 17 and weigh at least 110 pounds, you may be a suitable blood donor. However, you must not donate if you have had certain diseases, such as hepatitis, or if you are a member of a risk group for AIDS (acquired immunodeficiency syndrome). (For more on these diseases, see pages 801 and 1060.)

To give blood, go to a blood donation center or a hospital. There, trained staff members will take a small sample of your blood to check whether you have enough hemoglobin; they also will ask some questions about your health. If your health is good and your hemoglobin concentration is normal, they will draw a pint of blood from a vein in your arm.

Giving blood is quick and painless. It also is completely safe, because a new, sterile, disposable syringe is used for each donor. Therefore, there is no risk of getting any disease by donating blood.

The average volume of blood in the body is 10 to 12 pints in men and 8 to 9 pints in women. The usual amount of blood taken during donation is 1 pint. If you are a healthy adult, you can spare this amount without affecting your own well-being. Within a few hours, your body will have replaced the fluid you have lost. Your red blood cells will have returned to their usual numbers well before you are eligible to give blood again (in 8 weeks).

Transfusion Types

When donated blood that has been stored as collected is infused, this is known as whole blood transfusion. More often, however, donated blood is separated into its various components—packed red blood cells, fresh-frozen plasma, cryoprecipitate, coagulation factor concentrate, granulocytes (a type of white blood cell), and platelets—and these components are given as needed.

Red Blood Cells

If you are deficient in red blood cells but not in the other components of blood, a transfusion of red blood cells, rather than whole blood, is best. This provides only the red blood cells you need, without any extra volume from the other blood cells and plasma.

Thus, the risk of increasing the circulating blood volume too high above normal is minimized.

Transfusions of red blood cells are often used to treat various types of anemia such as disorders that involve depression of the bone marrow's production of these cells. Red blood cells are also transfused during the acute crisis of such inherited anemias as sickle cell disease (see page 960), thalassemia (see page 962), or glucose-6-phosphate dehydrogenase deficiency (see page 962).

Red blood cells can be kept in storage in a liquid form for a maximum of 6 weeks. Frozen red blood cells may be stored for up to 10 years.

Fresh-Frozen Plasma

Fresh-frozen plasma can be used to treat clotting disorders, including mild forms of hemophilia and von Willebrand's disease, as well as serious burns. This blood product can be stored frozen for 1 year.

Cryoprecipitate

Cryoprecipitate is prepared from fresh plasma and stored frozen. It is enriched for three clotting factors: factors I and VIII and von Willebrand factor. Cryoprecipitate is used to treat clotting disorders includ-

Blood Groups

The blood groups were discovered around 1900, when it was observed that blood collected for transfusions was compatible in some recipients but not in others. It was found that each person spontaneously forms antibodies against antigens that his or her own red blood cells lack.

If you receive blood that contains blood group antigens different from your own, then your antibodies attack the cells in the transfused blood that carry these antigens—that is, foreign cells. The blood groups are based on which antigens (proteins) are carried on your red blood cells. Like other physical characteristics, which antigens you have is controlled through pairs of genes inherited from your parents.

There are four major blood

groups: A, B, AB, and O. Each of these groups is divided into two Rh types, positive and negative. The most common blood group in the United States is O positive, followed by A positive, B positive, O negative, A negative, AB positive, B negative, and AB negative. The four major blood groups are inherited in a consistent manner. They can be used to exclude paternity.

Today, the blood groups of donors and recipients are matched to make transfusions safe. If your blood group is A, your red blood cells are coated with A antigens, and your plasma carries antibodies against B. If your blood group is B, you have B antigens and antibodies against A.

If your blood is Rh-negative,

your red blood cells do not carry an antigen called the "rhesus factor" (Rh factor). You do not spontaneously produce antibodies against this factor. However, Rh typing is particularly important if you are a woman because you may start developing anti-Rh antibodies after exposure to Rh-positive blood at the time of your first pregnancy. Then, if you are exposed again to Rh-positive blood, serious complications and even death could result. (For information on pregnancy in Rh-negative women, see Women's Health, page 1139.)

Many other minor blood subgroups also occur that become important only in special circumstances such as organ transplantation.

ing hemophilia (see page 975) and von Willebrand's disease (see page 977).

Coagulation Factor Concentrate

Coagulation factor concentrates are freeze-dried preparations of specific clotting factors from plasma. Before being transfused, the concentrate must be reconstituted. It is used to treat clotting disorders such as hemophilia.

Granulocytes

Transfusions of granulocytes may be used to treat severe neonatal sepsis. These cells can be stored for only a few hours. These transfusions are rarely needed today because of the availability of modern antibiotics.

Platelets

Platelet transfusions can control bleeding in people who have lost blood by a process called massive blood replacement or from prolonged surgery or other reasons.

The production of platelets can be suppressed in leukemia (see page 964), lymphoma (see page 968), or thrombocytopenia (see page 978) that has been caused by treatment with chemotherapy or radiation. Therefore, affected persons often receive transfusions of platelets. However, platelet transfusions tend not to be useful for those with idiopathic thrombocytopenia because they induce destructive antibodies against these cells (see below).

Platelets can be stored for only about 5 days before they become nonfunctional.

Adverse Reactions to Transfusions

When you receive a blood transfusion, you are given donor blood that has been matched with your own blood group (see Blood Groups, page 980). Before the actual transfusion starts, the blood bank mixes a sample of your blood with some of the donor's blood to double-check that they are compatible.

Antibody Reactions

Despite the precautions, sometimes a transfusion recipient will be carrying antibodies against the donor's red blood cells, white blood cells, or platelets. An immune reaction results. If you receive incompatible blood, you may experience fever, shaking, chills, chest pain, low back pain, pain along the vein that received the transfusion, shortness of breath, pink urine, hives, and nausea. Shock,

---

Safety of Blood Transfusions

Because the AIDS epidemic has prompted changes in the way blood is donated, tested, and transfused, our nation's blood supply is safer than at any time in the past. Current approaches to selecting and testing potential donors minimize the risk of a transfusion-related disease. Developments that have enhanced the safety of the blood supply include:

- Confidential methods that allow donors who may be at risk for AIDS to disqualify themselves
- A highly sensitive test for HIV that is used for routine screening of all blood donations
- Newer methods for destroying HIV and other viruses in some blood products
- Routine screening of all blood donations for other viruses that can be transmitted through blood
- Expanded use of autologous (your own blood) donations

---

kidney failure, or intravascular coagulation can ensue and, rarely, even death may occur.

Your risk of having this kind of immune reaction is increased if you have received multiple blood transfusions in the past. As you are exposed to blood antigens from more and more different donors, you may develop antibodies against obscure blood groups.

Communicable Diseases

Blood transfusions can spread diseases such as hepatitis, cytomegalovirus infection, syphilis, malaria, toxoplasmosis, and AIDS. Various tests are performed on donated blood to minimize the risk of infection.

For AIDS, testing starts with the enzyme-linked immunosorbent assay (ELISA). If this test is positive, a more specific assay, a Western blot or immunoblot assay, is performed to confirm the result. If a blood bank determines that you have this virus, it will discard your blood and notify you. However, never donate blood if you think you may have the virus. Instead, see your physician.

Symptoms of hepatitis include fatigue, jaundice, dark urine, nausea, and vomiting (see page 801). Symptoms of AIDS include unexplained weight loss, diarrhea, swollen lymph nodes, and unusual skin cancers (see page 1060).

Other Reactions

There are other possible adverse reactions to transfusions. For instance, if you have heart trouble, you may have difficulty handling an increase in blood volume. In addition, if you

Using Your Own Blood During Surgery

It is possible to recover the blood a patient loses during an operation for return to that patient. In this procedure, known as intraoperative autologous transfusion, surgeons salvage blood cells from the wound while they are operating. The cells are washed free of debris from the wound and then returned to the patient.

receive repeated transfusions of red blood cells (200 transfusions or more), you may experience iron overload.

It is important to realize that the vast majority of persons who receive a transfusion have no adverse reactions or infections as a result. If you truly need a transfusion, you should not let unfounded or exaggerated fears prevent you from accepting it.

Transfusion With Your Own Blood

The safest blood for you to receive is your own. Your immune system will not react to your blood as foreign, and you cannot give yourself any infections that you do not already have. Giving one's own blood, also known as autologous transfusion, is becoming more popular.

In an emergency, you may have to rely on transfusions from random donors unless you are at a medical center that can salvage your own blood during surgery (see this page). However, if your physician is planning elective surgery for you, ask him or her if you can donate your own blood ahead of time. Usually, you give it over a period of a few weeks in advance of when your operation is scheduled. Your blood will be stored and used, if necessary, to replace blood that you lose during the operation.

It costs more to receive your own blood than to get a random donor transfusion. The reason is the extra work involved in specially labeling your own blood, storing it separately, and delivering it to you at the right time. However, many people consider the added expense to be well worth it.

You might assume that if, for some reason, you cannot donate your own blood, the next-best thing is to receive blood from a designated donor. This person is a friend or relative who has the same blood group that you do. However, a blood bank is much better than you are at selecting donors whose blood will not cause an adverse reaction. Blood from designated donors chosen by you may not be compatible with your blood type or as safe as you think.

Because there will always be situations in which using your own blood is impossible, the growth of the increase in autologous transfusion will not abolish the need for blood donors.

The Future: Synthetic Substitutes

Researchers at many centers are working on the development of synthetic substitutes for blood. There are several reasons for this effort. Having such materials could help to prevent transfusion complications such as infection and immunologic reaction as well as to overcome shortages of donated blood. However, these synthetic blood substances are still experimental. In addition, although they are designed to carry oxygen, they cannot perform any of the myriad other functions of the blood. Therefore, the best way to prevent adverse reactions to transfusions is to donate your own blood beforehand for your own use.

Chapter 30

Your Skin

Contents

Healthy Skin, Hair, and Nails, 984
Proper Skin Care, 986
What Is Your Skin Type? 986

Skin Disorders, 987
Contact Dermatitis, 987
Prickly Heat Rash, 988
Neurodermatitis, 988
Atopic Dermatitis, 989
Stasis Dermatitis, 989
Seborrheic Dermatitis, 989
Dandruff, 990
Overtreatment Dermatitis, 990
Acne, 990
Does Diet Affect Acne? 991
Rosacea, 991
Psoriasis, 992
Skin Care for People With Psoriasis, 992
Lichen Planus, 993
Pityriasis Rosea, 993
Dry Skin, 994
Anti-Drying Bathing Basics, 994
Ichthyosis, 994
Hives, 994
Pigmentary Changes, 994
Itching, 995
Drug Rashes, 996
Sunburn, 996
Photosensitivity, 998
Solar Elastosis, 998
Treatment for Aging or Damaged Skin, 999
Senile Skin, 1000
Wrinkled Skin, 1000
Spider Veins, 1001
Xanthelasma and Xanthoma, 1001

Benign Skin Tumors, 1001
Skin Tags, 1002
Seborrheic Keratosis, 1002
Actinic Keratosis, 1002
Birthmarks, 1002
Cherry Angioma, 1002
Liver Spots, 1003

Moles, 1003
Monitor That Mole, 1003
Keloids, 1003
Warts, 1003
Lasers, 1004

Skin Cancers, 1004
Basal Cell Cancer, 1005
Squamous Cell Cancer, 1005
Melanoma, 1005
Kaposi's Sarcoma, 1006

Skin Infections, 1007
Impetigo, 1007
Folliculitis, 1007
Boils and Carbuncles, 1009
Erysipelas and Cellulitis, 1009
Lymphadenitis and Lymphangitis, 1010
Cold Sores and Canker Sores, 1010
Blisters, 1010
Shingles, 1011
Molluscum Contagiosum, 1012
Fungal Infections, 1012
Insect Bites, 1014
Human Bites, 1015
Portuguese Man-of-War Stings, 1015
Wound Infections, 1016

Hair, 1017
Female-Pattern Baldness, 1017
Male-Pattern Baldness, 1017
Temporary Hair Loss, 1018
Can Lost Hair Grow Again? 1019
Hirsutism, 1019
Taking Proper Care of Your Hair, 1020

Fingernails and Toenails, 1021
Paronychia, 1021
Care of Ingrown Toenails, 1022
Fungal Infections of the Nails, 1022
Discoloration or Deformity of the Nails, 1023
Taking Proper Care of Your Nails, 1023

Healthy Skin, Hair, and Nails

Your skin is a unique and remarkable organ. The 2 square yards of skin that cover the average adult constitute approximately 15 percent of the body's total weight.

One square inch of your skin contains millions of cells and many specialized nerve endings for sensing heat, cold, and pain. In addition, each square inch contains numerous oil glands, hair follicles, and sweat glands. An intricate network of blood vessels nourishes this complex structure.

Your skin protects your vital organs. It also serves as your heat regulator. Capillaries and blood vessels in your skin dilate or constrict according to your body's temperature. When you are hot, you sweat, and the evaporation of the sweat on your skin lowers your body's temperature. When your body is chilled, these blood vessels become narrowed, and your skin becomes pale and cold. This constriction decreases the flow of blood through your skin, reducing the heat loss and conserving heat for the main part of your body. Your sweat glands also excrete waste products, such as urea. However, this is a minor pathway of waste disposal compared to your kidneys' production of urine.

By its texture, temperature, color, and clarity, your skin gives information about your general health. Sensory nerves send signals to your brain about hazards. A group of spe-cialized nerve endings in your skin can arouse your nerve and endocrine systems to sexual excitement.

The average thickness of your skin is 1/10th of an inch. However, it ranges from very thin on your eyelids and inner folds of your elbows to very thick on the palms of your hands and soles of your feet. Your skin is composed of three layers—the epidermis, the dermis, and the subcutaneous tissue.

The epidermis is the top layer, the skin you see. The outermost surface of the epidermis is made up of dead skin cells. Squamous cells lie just below the outer surface; basal cells are at the bottom of the epidermis.

It takes approximately 1 month for new skin cells, manufactured in the living epidermis, to move upward to the outer surface. As the cells move away from their source of nourishment, they become smaller and flatter, changing into a lifeless protein called keratin. Once on the surface, they remain briefly as a protective cover and then flake off as a result of washing and friction. Thus, the skin is a dynamic organ, constantly being replenished.

Cells that manufacture skin constitute about 95 percent of your epidermis. The remaining cells produce a black pigment, melanin. Melanin provides the coloring of your skin and helps protect it from ultraviolet light.

People of all races are born with the same number of pigment cells (melanocytes). However, the rate at which melanin granules are formed in these cells and their degree of concentration in the epidermis are inherited characteristics and major factors in skin color differences.

The dermis, found beneath the epidermis, makes up 90 percent of the bulk of your skin. It is a dense bed of strong, white fibers (collagen) and yellow, elastic fibers (elastin) through which blood vessels, muscle cells, nerve fibers, lymph channels, hair follicles, and glands are interspersed. The dermis gives strength and elasticity to your skin. As you age, the dermis becomes thinner, and the skin becomes more transparent. This accounts for the prominence of blood vessels in the skin of elderly people.

Beneath the dermis lies the subcutaneous tissue, which is composed largely of fat and through which blood vessels and nerves run.

Your Skin

Epidermis

Dermis

Subcutaneous tissue

This layer, which specializes in manufacturing fat, is unevenly distributed over your body. The roots of your oil and sweat glands are located here. Subcutaneous tissue thins and disappears with aging.

Oil glands (sebaceous glands) are distributed throughout your skin but are most concentrated in your scalp, face, mid-chest, and genitals. They are attached to hair follicles and secrete an oily substance (sebum) that rises through the follicle to the surface of the skin. The oily sebum—made up of fatty acids, cholesterol, various hydrocarbons, unsaturated alcohols, and waxes—lubricates and protects your skin.

You have two types of sweat glands. The eccrine glands are distributed throughout your body. However, your palms, soles, forehead, and underarms have the richest supply. The apocrine glands are specialized sweat glands that secrete sweat in times of stress or emotion. In the ear they form a portion of the earwax; elsewhere they produce body odor. They are most abundant under your arms and around your nipples and genitals.

The human being is a hairy animal; only the lips, palms, and soles are truly hairless. Your scalp hair, like your skin, protects your scalp from excessive sun exposure and your head from trauma. It is a visible indicator of your age and, to some extent, of your general health.

Each hair grows from a single live follicle that has its roots in the subcutaneous tissue of your skin. Oil from an oil gland next to the hair follicle provides gloss and, to some degree, waterproofing for the hair. Your hair follicles are nourished by minerals, proteins, vitamins, fats, and carbohydrates brought to them by tiny capillaries. Your hair, like the surface of your epidermis, is made up of the dead protein keratin. Hair also contains melanin. Just as the pigment cells determine your skin color, the number of melanin granules in your hair determines its color.

Your fingernails and toenails also are products of your epidermis and are composed of the protein keratin. Each nail grows outward from a nail root that extends back into a fold of skin.

Your fingernails normally grow at the rate of an eighth of an inch a month, approximately 2 to 3 times faster than your toenails. Growth slows in old age. Sudden or significant changes in the appearance of your nails can be a first signal of illness.

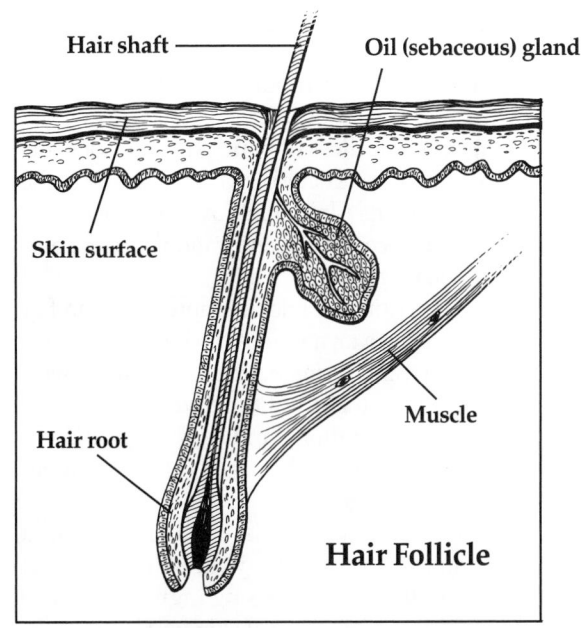

Hair Follicle

Severe malnutrition, injury, or some kinds of chemotherapy impair hair and nail formation. During a period of such impaired formation, the shaft of growing hair thins and even may break off. Similarly, an area of thinning of the nails may be evident. The width of this thin nail zone or length of the thin portion of the hair shaft varies with the duration of the injury or the use of chemotherapy. Contrary to common belief, the structure of your nails is not related to the structure of your bone. You cannot strengthen brittle nails by taking extra calcium or gelatin.

Problems such as acne, dermatitis, hair loss, fungal infections of your nails, and many other skin, hair, and nail conditions are usually best treated by a physician called a dermatologist. Good self-care habits can help prevent many skin problems.

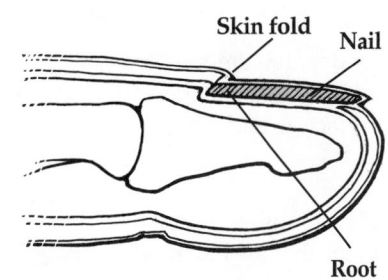

Your Fingernail

Proper Skin Care

The single most important goal in caring for your skin is to protect it against ultraviolet light. Regardless of your skin color or type, or your age, monitoring your exposure to the sun—and its ultraviolet rays—can help prevent unnecessary deterioration and, eventually, skin cancer.

Dark skin can tolerate more sun than fair skin. However, any skin can become blotchy, leathery, and wrinkled from continued overexposure to the sun. Protective clothing, sunscreen preparations, and daily lubrication or moisturizing can help (see How to Avoid Sunburn, page 997).

Proper cleansing is another important strategy in protecting your skin. The best procedures and cleansing ingredients vary according to the type of skin you have—oily, dry, balanced, or a combination of these.

What Is Your Skin Type?

The skin of your face is generally the best guide in classifying skin type. Examine your skin closely, especially the pores.

Oily Skin
Oily skin is caused by overactivity of the sebaceous glands. Oily skin is thick and has large pores. Oily skin has a greater tendency to develop acne but not wrinkles. Most people with oily skin also have oily hair.

Dry Skin
Dry skin can be caused by underactivity of the sebaceous glands, environmental conditions, or normal aging. Dry skin is usually thinner and more easily irritated. It often is associated with dry hair and small pores. There is a greater tendency to develop wrinkles but not acne. Your skin tends to become drier as you age.

Balanced Skin
Balanced skin is neither oily nor dry. It is smooth and has a fine texture and few problems. However, it has a tendency to become dry as a result of environmental factors and aging.

Combination Skin
Combination skin consists of oily regions—often on the forehead and around the nose—and regions that are balanced or dry.

If you use cosmetics, be sure to match them to your skin type: an oil base is suitable for dry skin and a water base is suitable for oily skin.

For women, the first step in facial cleansing is the removal of eye makeup products. Use cotton balls to avoid damaging the delicate tissue around your eyes.

When washing your face, use tepid (never hot) water and a facecloth or sponge to remove dead cells. Use a mild soap for your face and skin; a superfatted variety of soap may be better if your facial skin is dry. You may need to clean oily skin two or three times each day.

In general, avoid washing your body with very hot water or strong soaps. Bathing dries out your skin. If you have dry skin, use soap only on your face, underarms, genital areas, hands, and feet. After bathing, remove excess water from your skin by brushing it rapidly with the palms of your hands. Then, apply a bath oil and rub the oil-water mixture into your skin until it is dry. This is especially important in winter, when your legs, arms, and the sides of your body become particularly dry. The oil not only lubricates your skin, but it also prevents evaporation of water that your bath adds to your skin.

Shaving can be hard on a man's facial skin. You may have unusually sensitive skin. Or, you may injure yourself by the way you shave. If you shave with a blade razor, always use a sharp blade. Soften your beard by applying a warm facecloth for a few seconds; then use plenty of shaving cream. Pass the blade over your beard only once, in the direction of hair growth. If you reverse the stroke to obtain a close shave, you can cause a skin irritation called razor burn. If you use an electric razor too vigorously, you may also irritate your skin. You can buy various preparations to treat skin irritation caused by an electric razor.

Women who shave their skin for cosmetic purposes also need to avoid skin irritation. When you use a hair remover (depilatory) for the first time, determine whether the product is irritating to your skin by applying the preparation to a small area.

If a skin problem develops, do not neglect it. See your physician. The benefits of good skin care will become increasingly apparent to you and to others as you grow older.

Skin Disorders

Because it is a complex organ constantly exposed to the elements, your skin is susceptible to various problems. If you take care of your skin, you can prevent many skin disorders.

Your skin protects your body from the environment. It is surprisingly resistant to a wide variety of insults. However, it may become irritated and inflamed, a condition called dermatitis. Its capillaries may become enlarged as a result of sunburn, hives, or rosacea.

Any of the production activities within your skin can go awry—for example, too much oil (acne), too many new skin cells (psoriasis), or too much or too little melanin (pigmentary changes).

The skin disorders described below are not life-threatening or contagious. However, they can cause acute discomfort or make you upset about your appearance. Your symptoms may disappear in a week, may require surgery, or may call for a long-term treatment program.

The term dermatitis, which is used interchangeably with eczema, simply means an inflammation of the skin. It has many causes. It may appear as contact dermatitis, prickly heat rash, lichen simplex chronicus (neurodermatitis), atopic dermatitis, stasis dermatitis, and seborrheic dermatitis.

Contact Dermatitis

Signs and Symptoms
- Redness and itching
- Blisters and weeping from the sores in severe cases
- Skin changes limited to the area of contact with the causative agent

Direct contact with one of a number of substances can cause a skin inflammation called contact dermatitis (see color photograph, page C-3). The rash caused by exposure to poison ivy is a good example of this problem, although individual sensitivity varies considerably (see page 1036). If you are sensitive to material in a watchband or

ring, your skin beneath the object can become inflamed. Another example of contact dermatitis is red, sore eyelids that can result from your use of certain cosmetic products or from touching your eyelids with other materials on your fingers.

Diagnosis
Your dermatologist may suspect that your skin problem is the result of a contact sensitivity. Then, he or she may test your skin by applying small amounts of different substances to your skin under an adhesive covering and examining the site 48 hours later. This is called patch testing.

If your skin responds to one or more of these substances, the problem is known as allergic contact dermatitis. Relatively few persons have such a response. When virtually everyone who contacts a specific substance reacts with dermatitis, the ailment is known as irritant contact dermatitis. In contact dermatitis, only the areas of skin contacted by the offending substance react. The area with the greatest exposure reacts most severely.

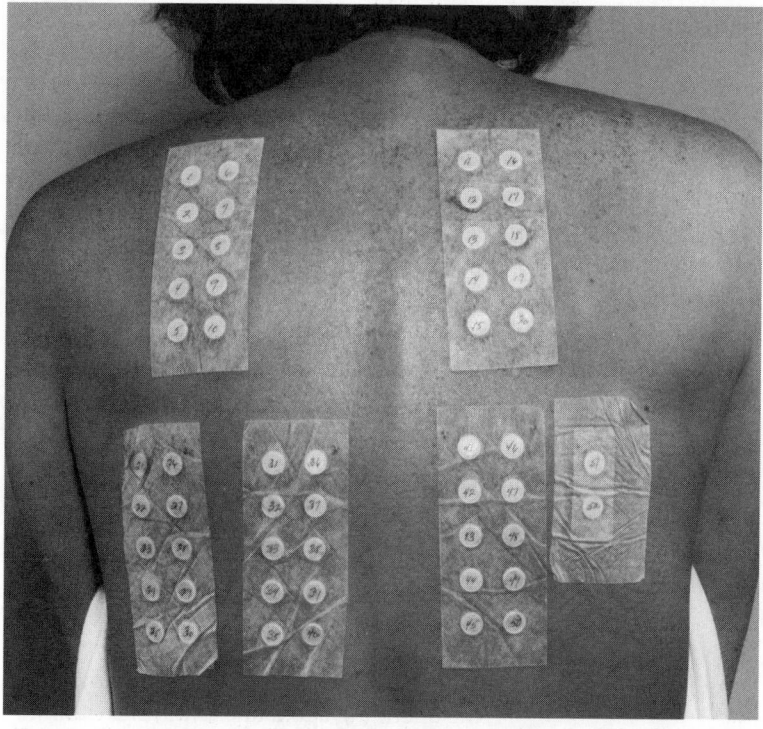

Patch testing can be helpful in determining whether you are allergic to a specific substance.

Prickly Heat Rash

To some of us, hot weather means the arrival of prickly heat rash. This condition is characterized by a rash of pinhead-sized bumps surrounded by a zone of red skin (see color photograph, page C-3).

Prickly heat itches intensely; often, there is an accompanying prickling, stinging sensation. Typically, it occurs on the neck, upper chest, groin, and armpits. The medical name for the most common variety of prickly heat is miliaria rubra.

Excessive perspiration produces prickly heat, because the moisture damages cells on the surface of your skin. These damaged cells form a barrier that blocks the free flow of sweat out to the surface of your skin. Instead, the sweat accumulates beneath your skin.

The best treatment for prickly heat is prevention. Avoid situations that lead to excessive perspiration. If you already have a prickly heat rash, keep the affected area cool and dry, and the problem probably will clear up spontaneously within a few days.

An air-conditioned environment can be most helpful. Also, avoid antiperspirants, lotions, insect repellents, or powders if you are still perspiring. After your skin is cool and dry, use a calamine-type lotion to help relieve the symptoms.

In allergic contact dermatitis, the allergen may be something that you have used for years with no problem. Mild chemicals such as hexachlorophene in soap and acetone in nail-polish remover can produce contact dermatitis if you use them repeatedly over a long period of time.

Other hard-to-identify causes include ingredients in medicinal lotions (antihistamines, antibiotics, or antiseptics), plants (ranging from trumpet creeper to mangoes), rubber, metals (such as nickel), dyes, cosmetics, and chemicals used in manufacturing (such as those used in making shoes or clothing).

Some substances cause dermatitis only when they contact your skin in the sunlight (see Photosensitivity, page 998). Typical examples include shaving lotions, sunscreens, ointments containing sulfa drugs, some perfumes, and coal-tar products. Other causes of contact dermatitis may be airborne, such as ragweed pollen or insecticide spray.

Treatment
Treatment consists primarily of identifying the offending agent and avoiding it. Sometimes, hydrocortisone-containing creams or slightly astringent wet dressings may help.

Neurodermatitis

Signs and Symptoms
- Itching, aggravated by nervous tension
- Small patches of thickened, leathery skin
- Scratch marks (excoriations)

Although they are not precisely the same condition, the names neurodermatitis and lichen simplex chronicus often are used interchangeably (see color photograph, page C-3). Simply put, these common skin disorders consist of small flat growths (plaques) of various sizes (1 to 10 inches in diameter) with definite margins that have become thickened and leatherlike (lichenified).

Lichen simplex chronicus is usually the result of something—often a tight garment—that rubs or scratches, or causes you to rub or scratch, an area of your skin. This leads to thickening of the skin, which, in turn, produces itching and thus encourages more rubbing or scratching. This problem also may occur in a plaque of psoriasis or in the skin around the anus.

Generalized neurodermatitis is closely related to localized neurodermatitis, but it tends to involve more of the body. The affected skin tends to be less leathery. Long-standing neurodermatitis may lead to brownish pigmentation. This condition often is associated with nervous tension and anxiety.

Treatment
The primary treatment for these skin problems is to stop the scratching. You may be able to avoid scratching the area when you understand that your scratching aggravates the condition. If you have trouble ignoring the area, a dressing that is difficult to remove, and that is left on for a week or more, may help.

Your physician may recommend hydrocortisone-containing lotions to decrease the itching and inflammation. These often can be purchased as over-the-counter preparations. If the inflammation is more severe, your physician may prescribe a stronger cortisone preparation. Also, the thickened plaques may be thinned by applying salicylic acid-containing ointments that have a peeling effect.

Sedatives and tranquilizers may help, but your physician will want to monitor your use of these substances because they can be addictive.

Atopic Dermatitis

Signs and Symptoms—Itchy, thickened, fissured skin, most often in the folds of the elbows or backs of the knees

Atopic dermatitis (infantile eczema, see color photograph, page C-2) is often associated with allergies such as asthma (see page 1044), nasal congestion (see page 1040), and hives (see page 1038). Frequently, it runs in families. It usually begins in infancy as areas of scaling and redness concentrated in the folds of the elbows or knees. This ailment causes severe itching.

Atopic dermatitis may wax and wane in severity during childhood and adolescence. It tends to become less of a problem in adult life (see page 1038).

Treatment

Treatment consists of applying hydrocortisone-containing lotions. If your skin cracks open, physicians sometimes prescribe wet dressings with mildly astringent properties. If itching is severe, antihistamines may help. Diphenhydramine has a substantial sedative action—in addition to being an effective antihistamine—and may be helpful at night.

Stasis Dermatitis

Signs and Symptoms—Thickening and itching of the skin at your ankles

Varicose veins, and other chronic conditions in the legs involving vessels other than arteries, can lead to buildup of fluid (edema) in tissues beneath the skin (see Varicose Veins, page 695). As a result, these areas are poorly nourished by blood and become fragile. Because your ankles have less supportive tissues, they are often the site of involvement. Your skin may become inflamed, or open ulcers may develop around your ankles and heal very slowly. This condition is called stasis dermatitis (see color photograph, page C-3). Although initially the skin may become thin, it later becomes irregularly thickened, perhaps in response to itching and continued scratching.

Treatment

Treatment consists of correcting the condition that causes water to accumulate in your ankles for extended periods. This may involve varicose vein surgery.

Another treatment option is to elevate your legs well above the level of your heart for a week or more. This is usually done in a hospital, under the direction of a physician specializing in the care of varicose veins. When you begin walking again, you may need elastic support stockings for your lower legs.

You also may use wet astringent dressings to soften the thickened, yet fragile, skin and to control infection.

Seborrheic Dermatitis

Signs and Symptoms
- Greasy-appearing, scaling, itching areas over your scalp, at the sides of your nose, between your eyebrows, behind your ears, or over your breastbone
- Stubborn, itchy dandruff

Seborrheic dermatitis (see color photograph, page C-3) is characterized by greasy scaling and a somewhat reddened appearance of the skin, predominantly over the scalp and in the folds at the sides of the lower portions of the nose, above the bridge of the nose, and over the breastbone. It also occurs beneath the breasts, in the folds of skin in the genital regions, and around the navel (umbilicus) in obese persons.

Some people are born with a tendency to have seborrheic dermatitis and will never completely get rid of it, although treatment can help keep it under control.

In folds of skin kept moist by contact with other skin (beneath your breasts or around your genitals, for example), secondary infections with yeast may complicate the condition. You may be more susceptible to these infections if you are taking antibiotics.

Treatment

Treatment consists of frequent shampooing of your scalp, followed by careful rinsing. Application of hydrocortisone-containing creams or solutions may soothe your skin. Your physician may recommend a specific shampoo. You also may need treatment for a secondary infection.

Dandruff

Everyone has some degree of scaling of the skin on their scalp because of the normal process of shedding the outer layer of cells. If the flaking becomes obvious on your hair and clothing, it is commonly called dandruff (see color photograph, page C-3).

The cause of dandruff is unknown. It is a mild form of seborrheic dermatitis (see page 989) and is considered to be caused by overactive oil glands or, perhaps, a yeast infection.

You probably can recognize ordinary dandruff. If your dandruff persists or you have very large flakes together with symptoms around your nose, ears, or chest, you may have a more severe form of dandruff or perhaps even psoriasis of the scalp (see page 992). If you have questions about its seriousness, consult your dermatologist.

Treating Your Dandruff

Over-the-counter dandruff shampoos usually contain sulfur, salicylic acid, selenium, or tar as their active ingredient.

Shampoo daily, leaving the lather on for a few minutes before rinsing. Sometimes flaking can be caused by a residue of shampoo in your hair, so you need to rinse very thoroughly. Finish up with a conditioner to help smooth out any tangles. A conditioner is an after-shampoo rinse that coats the hair to make it softer and more manageable. Neither your dandruff nor a daily shampoo will cause hair loss.

When your dandruff clears up, shampoo as needed. Occasional use of a dandruff shampoo can help keep a mild condition in check.

If your flaking persists despite home remedies, your dermatologist may prescribe a rub-on steroid lotion to suppress the flaking or a stronger salicylic acid or tar medication to loosen the scales so that you can wash them away more easily.

Overtreatment Dermatitis

Signs and Symptoms—Redness and sensitivity of the skin in areas aggressively treated for another skin disorder

A common skin problem actually is the result of overtreatment. Dermatologists often see people who have inflammation of the skin (dermatitis) that has persisted for several weeks or months and worsened, despite frequent application of several ointments or other treatments.

Typically, there is no way that the underlying disorder can be identified. The inflammation resulting from the excessive treatment obscures the underlying disease that may or may not still be present.

Treatment

In this situation, you must discontinue all treatment other than the most soothing measures for a week or two. This idea is often hard to accept. However, assessing the problem is possible only after all medications are withdrawn. Meanwhile, the problem may lessen considerably—or even disappear.

Acne

Signs and Symptoms
- Blackheads or whiteheads on face, neck, shoulders, or back
- Pimples ("zits")
- Cysts

Acne occurs when the hair follicles of your skin become plugged. Each follicle contains sebaceous glands that secrete a fatty oil (sebum) to lubricate your hair and skin.

When your body produces sebum and dead cells faster than they can exit from the pore, the two solidify as a white, cheesy plug. This plug may close the pore, causing the follicle wall to bulge, thus creating a whitehead. If the pore stays open, the top surface of the plug may darken, causing a blackhead. Blackheads are neither caused nor colored by dirt.

Pimples are infections that develop when whiteheads rupture the follicle wall. After the rupture, solidified sebum, dead cells, and bacteria invade your skin. Ruptures deep within your skin form boil-like infections called cystic acne (see color photograph, page C-9).

In some situations, the sebaceous gland continues to secrete material that does not rupture through the skin. Instead, a flattened, pliable lump forms under the skin. This is called a sebaceous cyst or wen. Sometimes the lumps can be an inch or more in diameter. Generally, there is no discoloration or pain unless the cyst becomes infected.

Three out of four teenagers have some acne. It is most prevalent in adolescence, because hormonal changes stimulate the sebaceous glands during these years, increasing sebum production and the chances of acne. Menstrual periods, the use of birth control pills or cortisone medications, and stress may aggravate acne in later life. Sudden onset of severe acne in a mature woman may be caused by a tumor that affects hormone production. This requires prompt medical attention.

Application of oil or grease to your skin can aggravate acne. This includes use of oil-based makeup, suntan oil, or hairdressing solutions, as well as oils from machinery or cooking.

Diagnosis

Acne usually is easy to diagnose. Pimple-like pustules alone, with no blackheads or whiteheads, may be another skin disease (see Rosacea, this page) or a reaction to medications such as corticosteroids.

How Serious Is Acne?

For many people, acne is a chronic problem from puberty through early adulthood. It eventually clears up in most cases, but permanent scars may remain. Medical treatment usually provides visible improvement within a few months, but the condition can affect self-esteem, confidence, personality, and social life.

Treatment

Your acne may require a lengthy, consistent treatment involving four basic steps. First, identify everything that aggravates your acne and avoid these things. Second, follow your physician's advice about removing blackheads and mature pimples, or have this done by a professional. Third, use a cleansing agent or soap that dries out your skin enough to cause minor shedding of skin so that the follicular plugs flake. Finally, promote skin peeling within your follicles, either by using one of the medications described below or by using a sunlamp (with proper caution).

Medication

Two types of medication can help acne. The first is topical, that is, you apply it directly to your skin. This lotion dries up the oil and promotes the skin's peeling. Over-the-counter lotions are mild and contain benzoyl peroxide, sulfur, resorcinol, or salicylic acid as the active ingredient. Stronger lotions containing these ingredients or a vitamin A acid (tretinoin or retinoic acid) require a prescription and supervision by your dermatologist.

The second type of medication is taken orally. For severe acne, your dermatologist may prescribe either an antibiotic (tetracycline) or—if your acne is severe—a new form of vitamin A acid (isotretinoin). Both can

---

Does Diet Affect Acne?

You may hear that some foods, such as chocolate or spices, add to acne problems. Actually, there is little or no scientific evidence to suggest this. However, if certain foods seem to make your acne worse, it may be best to avoid them. Discuss this with your physician.

---

cause side effects, and neither should be used during pregnancy. The vitamin A preparation, in particular, may cause birth defects. Because such harmful effects are likely to occur during the very early stages of pregnancy, even before you are certain you are pregnant, do not use this drug if you are not using birth control measures.

Surgery

Cystic acne and sebaceous cysts may require minor surgery (under local anesthesia) for drainage and removal.

Physicians may use cosmetic surgery to diminish scars left by acne. The main procedures are dermabrasion or peeling by freezing or chemicals. However, if your skin tends to form scar tissue (see Keloids, page 1003), these procedures can make your complexion much worse.

Peeling procedures eliminate superficial scars. Dermabrasion, usually reserved for more severe scarring, consists of abrading the skin with a rapidly rotating wire brush. Your physician will use a local anesthetic or topical freezing of your skin during the procedure. General anesthesia ordinarily is not required. Generally, dermabrasion is done as an outpatient procedure.

Rosacea

Signs and Symptoms

- Red areas on face
- Inflammation of cheeks, nose, forehead, and chin
- Red, bulbous nose

Rosacea (see color photograph, page C-9) is a chronic inflammation of the cheeks, nose, chin, forehead, or eyelids. The cause is unknown. The symptoms are due to enlargement of blood vessels just under the skin. This occurs most frequently in fair-skinned people who blush easily.

Rosacea usually begins between ages 30 and 50 years. Although it is more common in women, men are more likely to have the severe form, with a bright red, bulbous nose.

Because it may cause pimple-like pustules in the reddened areas, the condition used to be called acne rosacea. However, this name is misleading because the blackheads and whiteheads of acne are not associated with rosacea.

Treatment

Rosacea is not life-threatening, but it seriously affects your appearance. Sometimes you can minimize the redness by avoiding hot or spicy foods, hot beverages, and alcohol. Consult your physician if these avoidance measures do not decrease the redness to your satisfaction.

Long-term treatment with an antibiotic (such as tetracycline) almost always is effective in controlling rosacea. After decreasing the dose of the antibiotic gradually to maintain control, you may eventually discontinue the drug without recurrence of the rosacea. Later, laser treatment can eliminate persistent blood vessels and improve your complexion.

Psoriasis

Signs and Symptoms
- Dry, red patches of skin covered with silvery scales
- Small scaling dots (most commonly seen in children)

Emergency Symptoms—Reddening and scales affecting your entire skin

---

Skin Care for People With Psoriasis

You can help manage psoriasis with good skin care. Find a time that is best for you to care for your skin each day, following these guidelines.

Check your skin daily for dry, red, patchy skin with silver scales. Although some sunlight may be helpful, do not increase your risk of skin cancer by spending a lot of time in the sun. Do not become sunburned. Follow your physician's advice about sun exposure. Protect your skin from injury, scrapes, cuts, and constant friction, which may cause your psoriasis to flare.

Psoriasis, a common skin disease, apparently develops from a genetic predisposition that affects the life cycle of skin cells. Normally, it takes about a month for new cells to move from the lowest skin layer, where they are produced, to the outermost layer, where they die and scale off in tiny flakes. With psoriasis, however, the entire cycle takes only 3 or 4 days. As a result, dead cells accumulate rapidly, forming thick scales.

Psoriasis (see color photograph, page C-16) is characterized by flare-ups and partial remissions. The attacks can range from a few spots of dandruff-like scaling to large areas with major eruptions. Psoriasis most commonly affects your elbows, knees, trunk, and scalp; pits or ridges may develop in your nails.

The eruptions take various forms, including pustules, cracking skin, itching, minor bleeding, or aching joints. Psoriasis is not contagious.

Skin injuries such as a cut, burn, rash, or insect bite most frequently trigger psoriasis flare-ups. Other precipitating factors may include medications, viral or bacterial infections, excessive alcohol consumption, being overweight, lack of sunlight, a bad sunburn, stress, or constant friction on the skin.

Approximately 3 million Americans have psoriasis and 100,000 of these people have severe symptoms. It can strike suddenly at any age, but the onset usually is gradual and begins between ages 15 and 35. It is most common among white-skinned people.

Diagnosis

The diagnosis usually is by physical inspection. Your physician may need to obtain a skin sample (biopsy) for microscopic analysis to rule out other disorders or a fungal infection.

How Serious Is Psoriasis?

Psoriasis ranges from mild to severe and chronic. It cannot be cured. However, treatment for different levels of severity is generally effective when psoriasis flares up.

If almost all of your skin is affected, this is an acute attack, and you require prompt treatment. Acute secondary infections also can start during any flare-up. A secondary chronic condition of arthritis develops in nearly 1 out of 10 cases, more frequently in women (see Psoriatic Arthritis, page 913).

Treatment

Self-Help

If you have psoriasis, you can best help your-self by maintaining good general health. If you maintain a normal weight, psoriasis will be less aggravating when it occurs in creases or folds of your skin. You may be able to resolve some patches by exposing the psori-atic areas to sunlight.

Avoid scratching, rubbing, or picking at the patches of psoriasis. These habits cause thickening of the patches.

Medication

In mild cases, over-the-counter coal-tar soaps, shampoos, cleansers, or ointments used together with bath oils will suffice. Your dermatologist can help devise a treat-ment suited to your needs and, if necessary, may prescribe stronger coal-tar or cortico-steroid preparations.

If you have patches of psoriasis on your scalp, they will be more resistant to therapy and may require a phenol and sodium chlo-ride (salt) lotion or a stronger tar preparation in addition to a daily tar shampoo.

In disabling cases, physicians prescribe an oral anticancer drug, called methotrexate, to slow down the rapid production of skin cells. This drug is used only when no other ther-apy has worked, because it may cause liver damage after long-term use.

Phototherapy

Severe cases of psoriasis often require pho-totherapy at a hospital or psoriasis-care facil-ity for about 3 weeks. First, an application of coal-tar ointment (Goeckerman therapy) sen-sitizes your skin. Then, your skin is exposed to ultraviolet light. A new class of oral med-ications (psoralens), used with ultraviolet A light irradiation, controls the psoriasis in some people. This is called PUVA therapy.

Continuing Research

The Food and Drug Administration (FDA) recently has approved calcipotriene, a med-icated ointment containing a derivative of vit-amin D, for treating psoriasis. You apply a thin layer of this prescription ointment twice daily to psoriatic patches of skin (but not on your face or eyes). Its adverse side effects, while fewer than those of corticosteroids commonly used to treat psoriasis, include burning, itching, or other skin irritation.

Lichen Planus

Signs and Symptoms—Itchy spots on wrists, legs, torso, genitals, mouth, and lips

Lichen planus is a rare, recurrent, itchy rash characterized by shiny reddish purple spots on the skin and gray-white ones in the mouth (see color photograph, page C-10). Most commonly it appears in mid-life. The initial attack may persist for weeks or months, and recurrences can continue over many years. Oral symptoms, consisting of a dryness and metallic taste or burning in the mouth, may appear first and be the only evi-dence of the disease.

The cause of lichen planus is unknown. Flare-ups may be related to stress. The rash may produce ridges in your nails and leaves behind dark spots on your skin.

The diagnosis is by inspection or biopsy.

Treatment

Corticosteroid ointment may relieve itching. Corticosteroid tablets (prednisone) are pre-scribed for severe cases.

Pityriasis Rosea

Signs and Symptoms—Mildly itchy red spots on torso, upper arms, neck, and thighs

Pityriasis (scaling) rosea (rose-colored) is a common benign rash (see color photo-graph, page C-15). It most frequently affects young people.

A single scaly red patch on the torso may be the first sign. After several days, more spots appear. A virus probably causes pity-riasis rosea. The rash usually disappears in 3 to 12 weeks.

Your physician may perform blood tests to rule out other diseases.

Treatment

Treat the area gently, because irritating your skin may cause the eruption to spread to other areas of your body. Mild lubricants and anti-itching (antipruritic) lotions may control the itching. Hydrocortisone cream also may help.

Moderate sunbathing helps, but avoid sunburn. Your physician also may recom-mend antihistamine tablets.

Dry Skin

Signs and Symptoms—Itchy, scaly skin

Dry skin, also known as asteatosis or winter itch, is a common problem that occurs especially in older people (see color photograph, page C-15). It is particularly annoying in the winter, when the cold air outside and the heated air inside are low in humidity. Asteatosis is a common winter complaint in the Midwest.

The symptoms result from the loss of natural moisture and oil from the skin. Your skin may become cracked. Round patches of irritated skin may develop, resembling ringworm (see page 1013). The most common sites are the lower legs, upper arms, sides (flanks), and thighs.

Treatment
To help decrease the dryness that causes asteatosis, adjust your bathing habits in winter (see Anti-Drying Bathing Basics, this page). Moisturize your skin daily. Bathing does not contribute to dryness of your skin so long as you limit use of soap and lubricate your skin immediately afterward with a bath oil or other lubricant. Also, use a humidifier during the winter.

If your symptoms persist, apply an over-the-counter hydrocortisone (corticosteroid) cream to your skin. For a severe rash with itching, your physician may prescribe a stronger corticosteroid preparation to lubricate your skin and lessen the itching. If you have a general, persistent itching, consult your physician. This may be a symptom of other disorders.

Ichthyosis

Signs and Symptoms—Dry, scaly skin starting in early childhood

Ichthyosis is also called fish-scale disease, because of the appearance of its characteristic rash. Ichthyosis is the most common form of inherited skin disease (see color photograph, page C-15).

This disorder usually first occurs in childhood, between ages 1 and 4. Sometimes it disappears entirely for most of the adult years, only to return in later years.

You will notice the rash most frequently on your elbows, knees, and hands. It usually worsens in the winter. Ichthyosis may be associated with atopic dermatitis (see page 989).

Treatment
Rub white petroleum jelly (Vaseline) on your affected areas and wrap them in plastic overnight. Twice daily applications of lactic acid lotion or cold cream also help.

Hives

Signs and Symptoms
- Red or pink, itchy bumps on the skin
- Swelling of the skin

Hives, also called urticaria, is one of the more common skin diseases (see color photograph, page C-9). Typically, the condition appears as a reaction to internal or external allergens. A rare form of hives, called angioedema, can be life-threatening.

For a detailed discussion of Hives and Angioedema, see page 1038.

Pigmentary Changes

Signs and Symptoms
- Slowly growing white patches of skin
- Dark brown patches of skin

Anti-Drying Bathing Basics

Follow these tips to minimize the drying effects of bathing on your skin:

1. Bathe less frequently. Two or three times a week is often enough for most people. Limit yourself to 15 minutes, and use warm, rather than hot, water.

2. Choose superfatted, nonsudsing soaps that clean without removing natural oils. Soap substitutes in bar, gel, and liquid forms are less drying than deodorant and antibacterial soaps. Use soap only on your face, underarms, genital areas, hands, and feet—and use clear water elsewhere.

3. Brush your skin rapidly with the palms of your hands, or gently pat your skin with a towel after bathing. Seal in moisture, while your skin is still damp, with an oil or cream. Pay special attention to your legs, arms, back, and sides of your body. If your skin is already dry, a heavy, water-in-oil-formula moisturizer will last longer than a light cream with more water than oil.

Itching

The medical term for itching is "pruritus"—but no matter what you call it, it can be a miserable, distressing condition.

Causes

Itching can indicate a systemic condition such as liver disease with obstruction of the bile ducts, some blood disorders (see Polycythemia, page 971; Leukemia, page 964; and Hodgkin's Disease, page 969), and, rarely, cancer. Kidney failure (see page 852) may cause severe itching when there are high levels of urea and other waste products in the blood. Itching may also be caused when larvae of the hookworm family of parasites (see page 1084) penetrate your skin. This includes swimmer's itch, creeping eruption caused by the larvae of cat and dog hookworm, and ground itch caused by the true hookworm.

Many external skin disorders can have itching as a major problem, including insect bites, atopic dermatitis, hives (urticaria), lichen planus, and skin parasites (scabies) (see pages 1014, 989, 994, 993, and 1085, respectively). Aging skin often is more likely to itch. Some drugs—aspirin and codeine-related pain relievers, for example—can cause itching without causing a rash.

Neurodermatitis (see page 988) (lichen simplex chronicus) is characterized by itching and is perpetuated by the scratching of the itch. This rubbing produces an area of thickening (lichenification) of the skin. The thickened skin causes you to rub or scratch some more.

Emotional stress can contribute to or aggravate the sensation of itching, no matter what the underlying cause may be. If emotional factors are the primary cause, the condition is known as psychogenic itching. People may believe that a parasite is causing their itching. This may be associated with other symptoms, such as burning sensations in the tongue, and may constitute a major psychiatric problem.

Treatment

Although many medicines can moderate or relieve pain, no medicine will specifically lessen itching.

Antihistamines will relieve the itching of hives but not other forms of itching. Most antihistamines do have a mild sedative effect, however, and may help you get to sleep. Tranquilizers also may be helpful in this indirect manner.

Your physician may refer you to a psychiatrist for help if your itching is the result of stress or psychogenic causes.

Creams or ointments containing hydrocortisone may help control the itch of insect bites, atopic eczema, or neurodermatitis.

Perhaps the most common cause of itching is the dry skin associated with aging. Here are some self-help measures you can try: keep your bathwater lukewarm and limit the time of immersion; use minimal amounts of soap; lubricate your skin after bathing; avoid alcohol-containing lotions; apply bath oil daily and immediately after bathing to affected areas; keep room temperatures cool; keep humidity up by using a humidifier—just short of the point at which water condenses on your windows.

You can use Aveeno (a form of oatmeal soap available at your drugstore) in your bathwater for severe itching arising from dry skin. You can get much the same effect from an oatmeal bath or a starch-and-soda bath.

For the oatmeal bath, tie a handful of oatmeal into a piece of cotton cloth. Boil it just as you would cook the oatmeal. Then use this "oatmeal sponge" while you bathe in a tub half full of lukewarm water.

To prepare a starch-and-soda bath, add half a 16-ounce box of baking soda and one 16-ounce box of laundry starch to a tub half full of lukewarm water. Mix well, and then bathe, but do not use soap.

An Aveeno, oatmeal, or starch-and-soda bath sometimes will help you get through a difficult day or night when no other remedy seems to help.

Skin color is the result of the melanin pigment created by cells (melanocytes) in the skin. Occasionally, something happens to this mechanism. An area of skin may produce too much melanin and so becomes darker (chloasma) (see color photograph, page C-7). Or, when no melanin is produced, the patch of skin becomes white. When a white patch grows periodically, you may have a skin disorder called vitiligo (see color photograph, page C-7).

Chloasma patches are most common on the face and seldom spread very far. They often are associated with pregnancy or use of birth control pills in women. However, both men and women may get them for no apparent reason.

Although vitiligo patches can start at any age, they often first appear between ages 20 and 30. They may begin on your face above the eyes or on your neck, armpits, groin, hands, or knees. They are often symmetric and can spread over your entire body. Heredity is often a factor.

Sometimes the destruction of melanin-producing cells by the immune system causes vitiligo. In other cases, there are associated disorders, such as thyroid problems (see page 945) or pernicious anemia (see page 958).

Neither vitiligo nor chloasma is life-threatening. Cosmetics or skin dyes often are used to hide the patches. Because vitiligo patches sunburn easily, use of a sunscreen lotion is necessary.

Treatment

Repigmentation and depigmentation treatments are used to restore uniform skin color. Repigmentation of vitiligo patches is done by exposure to sun or ultraviolet light after sensitizing the area with topical or oral medications (psoralens). This type of treatment is referred to as PUVA therapy and is administered under the direction of your dermatologist.

Retin-A cream applied nightly and removed by washing may help to lighten the chloasma (see page 999).

Drug Rashes

Signs and Symptoms
- Skin changes, including redness, hives, blisters, and bleeding into the skin
- Itching

You may have an allergic reaction to any over-the-counter drug or to one prescribed by your physician (see color photograph, page C-15).

When a rash develops while you are taking any kind of medicine, you should suspect that medicine as the cause of the rash. Your family physician or a dermatologist can help sort out possible causes.

Drug reactions can involve more than an itch or rash. The signs and symptoms of a drug reaction may be extremely varied. You may experience fever, seizures, nausea, vomiting or diarrhea, heartbeat irregularities, difficulty breathing or asthma, or decreased urine flow. In addition, laboratory tests may demonstrate an effect on your hemoglobin value or white blood cell count.

Rashes take various forms. This makes it more difficult to determine the cause of the rash. Rashes from drugs usually occur during the first few days of taking the medication. This time relationship may alert you to further problems.

Fever is the earliest sign of many drug reactions. Fortunately, rashes usually appear early during the course of a drug reaction and will warn you that you may be experiencing a drug reaction. If you take multiple medications, a persistent rash is a warning to seek medical help (see Adverse Drug Reactions, page 1275).

Treatment

If your rash is caused by a medication, the signs and symptoms will usually cease when you stop taking the drug. However, if the drug was prescribed, consult your physician before discontinuing its use.

If your rash is itchy, oatmeal baths or wet dressings may soothe it (see Itching, page 995). Topical hydrocortisone cream also may help. Antihistamines sometimes relieve certain types of drug rashes.

Sunburn

Signs and Symptoms
- Red, tender, swollen skin
- Water blisters

Emergency Symptoms—Fever, chills, nausea, or delirium

Sunburn is the result of the skin's overexposure to the sun's ultraviolet radiation. It is a major cause of the dramatic recent increase in malignant melanoma, the most lethal form of skin cancer. A history of painful, blistering sunburns, especially in childhood, increases your risk of developing melanoma (see page 1005). But intense, brief exposure from "sun worship" on weekends is also a hazard, and a risk factor you can control. Whatever your age, there's no such thing as a "healthy tan."

Only short-wavelength ultraviolet light causes sunburn unless you become photosensitive (see page 998). The ultraviolet content of sunlight varies. It is greater at higher elevations because it is not filtered out by clouds or haze. Cold air does not reduce ultraviolet radiation from the sun. Reflected ultraviolet light from snow, sand, water, and other surfaces can burn as severely as direct sunlight.

Congestion in the capillaries that supply blood to your skin causes the swollen, red skin of a sunburn. Although any ultraviolet radiation can penetrate your skin, only short wavelengths affect the capillaries, under normal conditions. The darker your skin, the less these rays penetrate, because they are absorbed by the melanin pigment.

Mild sunburn or exposure to sun may stimulate your skin to produce extra melanin as protection against further ultraviolet penetration. More melanin means a deeper tan, if the additional pigment is distributed evenly. Otherwise, it forms freckles, liver spots, or discolored splotches. Your melanin production and dispersal are genetic. There is nothing you can do to change your tanning capacity.

Your skin type greatly influences how much sun you can tolerate before you suffer a sunburn. Consider what happens to your skin in 45 to 60 minutes of unprotected exposure to the sun. If you always burn easily and seldom or never tan, your skin is very sensitive. If you burn minimally or moderately and tan gradually, your skin is moderately sensitive. If you rarely or never burn and tan profusely or have deeply pigmented skin, your skin is minimally sensitive.

Although your skin type is an important factor in your susceptibility to sunburn, other factors also contribute. You are most likely to sunburn without tanning if you have light-colored skin, blue or green eyes, and blond or red hair. Resistance to sunburn and easy tanning are most likely if you have dark brown eyes, brown or black hair, and brown or black skin.

Diagnosis

Symptoms of sunburn do not appear until a few hours after exposure, but the pain, redness, and occasional blistering of sunburned skin are unmistakable.

How Serious Is Sunburn?

The effect of sunburn is like that of any burn, although its development is relatively slow rather than rapid (as from a heat burn). There is damage to your skin. If the sunburn is severe, skin cells die and blisters form. The skin then heals in a period of a week or two.

Damage to your skin cells from recurrent sunburn is cumulative, and continued overexposure to ultraviolet radiation produces long-term effects. These can include skin discolorations, actinic keratosis (see page 1002), and skin cancer (see page 1004). Ninety percent of all skin cancer is due to this irreversible damage.

Treatment

Medication

Treat your sunburn with cool tap water compresses and, if severe, hydrocortisone cream (available over-the-counter) several times daily. Leave the water blisters intact to speed healing. If they break open on their own, remove the skin fragments and apply an antibacterial ointment on the open areas to help prevent infections. Keep the wounds clean. And take aspirin several times daily.

If your sunburn is severe, contact your physician even before the symptoms and signs are fully developed. Your physician may elect to prescribe oral corticosteroid treatment to decrease the reaction and prevent some of the symptoms.

How to Avoid Sunburn

Years ago, a deep tan was considered fashionable, even glamorous. Physicians encouraged people to sunbathe. It was considered healthful. Today, we know that chronic overexposure to the ultraviolet radiation in sunlight causes your skin to age prematurely. Wrinkles form. But most importantly, skin cancer may develop in later years.

If you expect to be exposed to sunlight for lengthy periods, protect yourself. Wear a hat. Select shirts with long sleeves and avoid shorts. When possible, plan out-of-doors recreational activities for early-morning or late-afternoon hours to decrease ultraviolet radiation, which is most intense from 10 a.m. to 2 p.m.

Use a premium-quality sunscreen lotion whenever you are outdoors for sustained periods. A sunscreen can protect you from burning and allow some tanning. Coconut oil, cocoa butter, or baby oil do not make you tan faster, and they provide very little protection from ultraviolet radiation. Good sunscreens contain either para-aminobenzoic acid (PABA) or benzophenone. Some contain both. (PABA can cause a rash.) Alcohol-based sunscreens seem to penetrate deeper and afford the best protection.

Sunscreens are rated by their sun protection factor (SPF) in a range from 2 to 45. Follow your physician's instructions as to the correct rating for your type of skin. It's probably best to use a sunscreen with an SPF rating of at least 15. Your sunscreen will work best if you apply it at least half an hour before exposure. Reapply your sunscreen frequently during exposure. Protection diminishes as the sunscreen evaporates. Bathing and perspiration can wash it away. Sand, water, and other surfaces reflect light that can burn as severely as direct sunlight.

Also be sure to use a sunscreen for winter exposure. The greatest hazard in winter months is on cloudy days after a fresh snow. Skiers should always use a sunscreen. Radiation is greater at higher altitudes.

The delicate skin around your eyes, nose, and lips needs extra protection. Some people prefer a sun blocker, such as zinc oxide or titanium dioxide, which stops all radiation from reaching the skin. Others use a special lip sunscreen with an SPF rating of 15 or higher.

Avoid perfumes or after-shave lotion before sun exposure. Such preparations may produce discolored patches on your skin. If you have had sun-sensitive reactions in the past, read about photosensitivity (see below; for a list of sensitizing substances, see below). After your sun exposure, bathe or shower away perspiration, salt, pool chemicals, and sunscreen products. Then apply a lubricant to your skin.

Photosensitivity

Signs and Symptoms
- Redness
- Rash
- Blistering or swelling

Photosensitivity is a heightened reaction of skin to light from the sun or artificial sources, usually following consumption of medications or foods.

Certain medications cause photosensitive reactions in some people. These include anticancer drugs, water pills, tranquilizers, antibiotics of the tetracycline family, antidepressants, antihistamines, birth control pills, anticonvulsants, antidiabetic or high blood pressure (antihypertension) medications, sulfonamides (usually prescribed for urinary tract infections), and topical antiseptic creams.

Some skin products also can cause a reaction. This is called photocontact dermatitis.

Common photocontact sensitizers include plants (such as limes, parsley, celery, carrots, mustard, or figs), artificial sweeteners (cyclamates), antibacterial deodorant soaps, perfumes containing bergamot, sandalwood, lavender, or citron oils, skin-bleaching creams, shampoos or soaps with coal-tar ingredients,

sunscreens with para-aminobenzoic acid, medicated cosmetics, detergents, and after-shave lotions.

There are two categories of photosensitive reactions, photoallergic and phototoxic. A photoallergic reaction is a result of changes in your immune system. When this occurs, your skin will have a bad reaction each time it is exposed to sunlight.

Your skin becomes red (although not necessarily sunburned) and develops a bumpy rash similar to poison ivy. Discolored patches, blisters, or swelling also can occur. Symptoms can extend to areas not exposed to the light. Photoallergy can strike again, with suddenness, later in life. Once you are sensitized to a substance, you can react again and again. You also can react to substances that are chemically similar.

A phototoxic reaction, however, will look and feel like an exaggerated sunburn with inflammation, redness, blisters, and the characteristic discomfort. You may have this reaction any time a sufficient amount of the sensitizing chemical is present in your body and you are exposed to the activating wavelength of light.

Treatment
Your photosensitive reaction usually will disappear within a week after you begin protecting your skin from light exposure and avoiding the sensitizing substance, although in some cases the symptoms linger.

If you have had a photoallergic reaction, it is especially important to wear protective clothing and sunscreens when outdoors. For a severe reaction, your physician may prescribe a corticosteroid ointment or cream or hydroxychloroquine tablets to help suppress photoallergic reactions.

Solar Elastosis

Signs and Symptoms
- Loose, sagging, or wrinkled skin
- Dry, tough, leathery skin

Elastosis is a degenerative disease of the connective tissues of your skin. This degeneration happens slowly as a result of normal aging. Repeated exposure to ultraviolet radiation, however, can accelerate the rate dramatically by a process called photo-aging. The resulting condition is solar elastosis.

Your skin is comprised of two types of connective tissue. One type is a strong, white fiber (collagen); the other is an elastic, yellow fiber (elastin). Ultraviolet radiation penetrates skin and damages these tissues. The amount of collagen is decreased; the amount of elastin is increased but it loses its elasticity. The orderly structural arrangement deteriorates, and abnormal cell growth begins.

Each exposure to ultraviolet light causes slight but irreversible changes, so the damage within your skin accumulates over the years. The signs and symptoms of solar elastosis appear gradually as the skin loses its resilience, flexibility, and water-holding capacity. If you have had excessive sun exposure, by the time you are 30 years old the overexposed areas of your skin can look 15 to 20 years older.

If you sunburn easily and tan poorly, you are most susceptible to solar elastosis. This condition usually occurs in fair-skinned, blue- or green-eyed people with blond or red hair who are frequently exposed to intense

---

Treatment for Aging or Damaged Skin

The effects of time and aging can be markedly diminished in most people with procedures whose results last from months to many years (after that, a procedure may have to be repeated). Unless you have extra risk factors, all of these are done primarily on an outpatient basis. They are not covered by most health insurance policies.

If any of these procedures are performed by someone who isn't adequately trained, the results can be disfiguring. Make sure you go to a qualified physician.

Collagen Injections
Collagen is a type of fibrous molecule that makes up 90 percent of your skin. If you have only a few wrinkles, collagen from the skin of cows can be injected into them to fill them in. Because your body slowly absorbs the collagen, the procedure must be repeated every few months.

Risks
Some people are allergic to the collagen, so prior testing is recommended.

Retin-A
Retinoic acid is a form of vitamin A that can eliminate fine wrinkles on sun-damaged skin. You apply Retin-A cream nightly to your face, neck, upper chest, or hands. This causes peeling of the surface skin and stimulates new skin growth. It may even reverse some deterioration within the dermal layer. Most people also report better skin texture and a healthier glow.

Risks
Increased sensitivity, dryness, redness, and excessive peeling can result. Less-frequent applications (perhaps three times per week) would then be appropriate.

Avoid sun exposure while using this medication, or discontinue its use prior to exposure. Skin treated with Retin-A should not come into contact with dyes, hair-removal wax, or perfume.

Dermabrasion
This technique smooths fine wrinkles. It can be done on the entire face or just on problem areas, such as around the mouth. The top skin layer is "sanded" off, causing new skin to form. Redness lasts a week or two, pinkness for several weeks after that.

Risks
If you tend to get cold sores (fever blisters), they can flare up after the procedure. Any exposure to the sun will cause a bad burn that can permanently discolor the skin. Dermabrasion is not recommended for Oriental people and those with dark skin, because their pigmentation can end up blotchy.

Chemical Peel
A caustic chemical is used to burn the outer skin layer, which then peels, causing new, smoother skin to regenerate. You can have your entire face treated, or just spot areas, such as around your mouth or eyes. A brown, crusty scab lasts for 10 days, redness about 6 weeks, and pinkness for several months.

Risks
You can be left with small scars, or with severe scarring if the procedure is not done by a physician. Your skin will be permanently lighter, without sun-protecting pigmentation; this makes you more susceptible to sunburn and to developing skin cancer. This procedure is not suitable for Orientals, blacks, or other dark-skinned people, who can end up with blotchy pigmentation.

sunlight without protection. The risk is highest for sunbathers, farmers, sailors, and others who are often outdoors. Those who live in regions with intense sunlight are more at risk; such areas include higher elevations and the Western plains.

Diagnosis

You can see the effects of solar elastosis by comparing your protected skin to overexposed skin. Your dermatologist can confirm the diagnosis by examination, which may reveal other symptoms of sun-damaged skin (see this page), including solar keratosis (see page 998).

How Serious Is Solar Elastosis?

The photo-aging process causes cumulative effects. There is no medical treatment to reverse the damage or to rejuvenate your skin.

If your skin has been damaged enough to cause solar elastosis, your risk of acquiring skin cancer is increased. See your physician whenever you have a new growth or a change in an existing growth such as a mole.

Treatment

Your dermatologist may recommend lubricating creams to reduce dryness and soften your skin. Facial massages and masks can make your face feel better for a while by toning muscles and stimulating blood circulation. Collagen injections may smooth out minor wrinkles in the short term, perhaps for a month or so.

Wrinkled Skin

Wrinkling is a natural part of aging. As you grow older, your skin gets thinner, drier, less elastic, and more wrinkled, and it tends to lose its youthful color and glow.

Dryness is a result of decreased oil production within your skin. Deterioration in the connective tissue (elastin and collagen) in your dermal layer causes sagging, wrinkling, and thinning. Finally, as your blood supply slows, your rosy glow begins to fade.

Although aging of your skin is inevitable, it can be slowed by maintaining good general health and consistently using sunscreens whenever you are outdoors.

There is no cure for wrinkled skin. Overexposure to sun and excessive cigarette smoking accelerate wrinkling dramatically. Avoid them. Your physician may prescribe Retin-A (see Treatment for Aging or Damaged Skin, page 999).

Your physician also may recommend chemical peeling, dermabrasion, or a face-lift as a longer-lasting treatment. Retin-A, a derivative of vitamin A, is an effective peeling medication (see page 999). Dermabrasion is a surgical procedure that removes the outer layer of your skin with sandpaper or, more commonly, a wire brush. Face-lifting is the surgical removal of some facial skin so that the remaining skin is stretched more tightly.

To prevent further damage, avoid sunlight if you can. If you cannot, protect your skin (see page 997).

Senile Skin

Signs and Symptoms

- Skin discolorations including liver spots, freckles, and red, yellow, gray, or brown blotches
- Skin texture changes including coarse wrinkles, sagging folds, sallowness, roughness, excessive dryness, or leathery toughness
- Skin growths including scaly patches

The effects of aging on skin are gradual under normal conditions. However, the signs of age may appear faster if you are susceptible to sun damage and expose your unprotected skin to ultraviolet radiation frequently (see color photograph, page C-4).

Senile or sun-damaged skin is irreversible. The separate symptoms and treatments are described in sections on liver spots (see page 1003), solar elastosis (see page 998), and actinic keratosis (see page 1002), the three principal problems associated with senile skin.

Sun damage also increases your chances of skin cancer (see page 1004) significantly, so, as you age, watch for early signs of these malignant growths.

Your susceptibility to sun damage is greatest if you are green- or blue-eyed, are fair-skinned, have blond or red hair, and sunburn easily. Sun protection (see page 997) is critical if you spend time outdoors.

Treatment

For treatment of specific symptoms, see the sections referred to on page 414. In general, however, it is wise to apply adequate lubrication and sunscreen lotions. Also, consult your physician about new growths or changes in existing ones.

Spider Veins

These really have nothing to do with spiders. However, the pattern of bluish veins seen through the skin of the leg does look a bit like a spider. (See color photograph, page C-15.)

Both the cause and the prevention are unknown. Unlike more serious varicose veins (see page 695), spider veins generally are painful only to your vanity. For some people, wearing a skirt or shorts is no longer an option because of worries about the appearance of the purple-blue veins on the legs.

The easiest course is to ignore the veins. They are a common, mild, and medically insignificant variety of varicose veins. However, if the unsightly blood vessels do concern you or, more importantly, if they prevent you from taking part in activities you otherwise would enjoy, sclerotherapy is a treatment option.

What Is Sclerotherapy?
It is a procedure that scars the veins, preventing blood from flowing into them and eliminating the discoloration. The treatment has no significant effect on circulation in the leg.

The physician slowly injects a solution (most commonly saltwater or saline solution) into one or several of the visible veins. Treating each vein requires only a few minutes, and generally many veins can be injected in a single session. If you have many spider veins in different areas, you may need multiple treatments. Although sclerotherapy does not prevent new spider veins, one or more treatments generally eliminate 50 to 80 percent of the spider veins.

Are There Side Effects?
In most people, the color of the spider veins fades within a week or so and is gone within 2 months. In about one in three cases, a yellow-brown discoloration appears in the area and takes weeks or even months to fade. In rare instances, this discoloration persists longer.

Xanthelasma and Xanthoma

Signs and Symptoms—Soft, fatty bumps beneath the surface of your skin

Both xanthelasma and xanthoma are yellowish bumps that appear beneath the skin. These bumps have sharply defined margins.

Xanthelasmas (see color photograph, page C-11) are flat and appear in the skin of your eyelids near your nose. They do not hurt, and they may be harmless, but you should have your blood tested for increased concentrations of cholesterol and triglycerides.

Xanthomas are a symptom of an underlying metabolic disorder that increases the fat (lipid) concentration in the blood. Xanthomas can appear anywhere on your body but most commonly occur over joints or tendons. With certain disorders they often appear where your skin receives persistent pressure, such as on your knees, elbows, hands, feet, or buttocks. Xanthomas are flat and can vary from less than 1 inch to more than 3 inches across. They are associated with diabetes mellitus (see page 925), primary biliary cirrhosis (see Cirrhosis, page 806), some malignancies, and several inherited metabolic disorders such as familial hypercholesterolemia (elevated cholesterol).

Consult your physician if you want to have a xanthelasma or xanthoma removed. But be aware that they may reappear.

Benign Skin Tumors

Benign skin tumors are very common and usually are harmless. As you grow older you are likely to have a number of them. With the exception of actinic keratoses (see page 1002) and certain moles (see page 1003), benign tumors do not require removal unless they are irritating or cosmetically displeasing. As a precaution, however, consult your physician about any new growth or changes in old areas. Several kinds of benign patches, lumps, and bumps that can occur on your skin are described in the pages that follow.

Skin Tags

Signs and Symptoms—Small protrusions of skin on your neck, armpits, upper trunk, and body folds

Skin tags, also called acrochordons, are tiny benign tumors of unknown origin that protrude from your skin on a narrow stalk (see color photograph, page C-4). They are soft and normally skin-colored, but may appear darker.

Skin tags are common, especially after middle life. They usually are painless, but they can become irritated by friction from clothing.

Treatment
Treatment is unnecessary, unless the tag is bothersome. Your physician can remove it, without scarring, by freezing it with liquid nitrogen (cryotherapy), cutting it off, or burning it off with electricity.

Seborrheic Keratosis

Signs and Symptoms—Yellow, brown, or black growths on the face, chest, shoulders, and back

Seborrheic keratoses are benign skin tumors of unknown origin that commonly appear on light-skinned people after age 40 (see color photograph, page C-4). The oval growths have a waxy, wart-like, scaly, slightly elevated surface and range from ⅛ to 1 inch or more across. Their color varies from yellow to dark brown or black. They have a pasted-on appearance. Occasionally, they appear singly but most often are seen in large numbers. They are not caused by exposure to sunlight or by viruses.

Treatment
Seborrheic keratoses are normally painless and require no treatment unless they itch, irritate, or detract from your appearance. The growths are never deeply rooted, so removal is simple and nonscarring. Your physician can freeze them off with liquid nitrogen (cryotherapy) or can use a surgical procedure.

Actinic Keratosis

Signs and Symptoms—Gritty, scaly, gray-to-dark-pink patches on the face, scalp, and back of hands

Actinic or solar keratosis occurs mostly in fair-skinned persons with sun-damaged skin (see color photograph, page C-4). Initially, the keratoses are flat and scaling; later, they have hard, wart-like surfaces. Their sandpaper-like surface is more easily felt than seen. Actinic keratoses are considered to be benign tumors, but they may be signs of precancerous changes in your skin.

Treatment
Prompt medical attention is needed, because 20 percent of untreated keratoses develop into squamous cell skin cancer (see page 1005). Your physician can remove them by freezing with liquid nitrogen (cryotherapy) or by using topical medication, electrical burning, or surgery. A sample of the tissue is studied for signs of cancer.

Birthmarks

Signs and Symptoms—Skin marking that develops before or shortly after birth

Several kinds of common birthmarks are termed hemangiomas. They are benign, usually painless, markings of unknown origin caused by a proliferation of blood vessels at the site.

For a detailed discussion of birthmarks, see page 15.

Cherry Angioma

Signs and Symptoms—Small, smooth, cherry-red bump on skin

Cherry angioma is a benign skin tumor of unknown origin that appears most frequently after age 40 (see color photograph, page C-4). It can occur almost anywhere on your skin but most commonly is found on the torso. These tumors range from pinhead size to ¼ inch across. Large angiomas can bleed profusely when they are injured.

Treatment
A cherry angioma is painless and harmless, but you may want it removed for cosmetic reasons. It is superficial, so your physician can remove it easily by freezing it with liquid nitrogen (cryotherapy), applying laser treatment (see page 1004), or destroying it by a minor electrosurgical procedure.

Liver Spots

Signs and Symptoms—Flat, light-brown to black spots on your face or backs of hands

Liver spots, also known as senile lentigines, are harmless flat patches of increased pigmentation that range from freckle-size to a few inches across (see color photograph, page C-4). They are extremely common after age 55 and occur most commonly on the backs of the hands or the forehead. Although frequently associated with overexposure to sun, they also can occur from unknown causes.

Treatment

Most people seek no treatment. For cosmetic reasons, liver spots can be lightened with skin-bleaching products or can be removed by freezing with liquid nitrogen (cryotherapy). Recurrence or appearance of new spots can be minimized by using high-protection sunscreen lotion.

Moles

Signs and Symptoms—Flesh-colored, brown, blue, or black spots on the skin

Nearly everyone has moles (see color photograph, page C-5). These benign tumors are nests of pigment cells. They may contain hairs, stay smooth, become raised or wrinkled, and even fall off in old age.

Moles are usually harmless, but they can become cancerous. Consult your physician about changes in color or size, or if itching, pain, bleeding, or inflammation develops. Certain moles (in particular, those that are irregularly shaped, have a mixed brown and black color, are congenital, or are located around the nails or genitals) should be monitored by a physician (see Melanoma, page 1005).

Treatment

Treatment usually is unnecessary. For cosmetic reasons, a mole can be removed surgically. If changes develop in a mole, your physician may remove it for microscopic examination.

Keloids

Signs and Symptoms—Flesh- or lighter-colored nodular or ridged growths on the skin

A keloid is an overproduction of scar tissue, sometimes called hypertrophic scarring (see color photograph, page C-5). It occurs at the site of a skin injury (operation, vaccination, severe acne, burn, or even a minor scratch). It is fairly common on black skin and much less common on white skin.

Your keloid is harmless, but it may be tender, itchy, or displeasing. Some keloids stop growing or even disappear by themselves.

Treatment

Surgical removal often causes further scarring unless it is followed by X-ray treatment or injection of steroids at the site. Small keloids may be removed by freezing with liquid nitrogen (cryotherapy).

Warts

Signs and Symptoms—Small, hard, flesh-colored, white, or pink granulated lumps on the skin

The common wart, verruca vulgaris, is a benign tumor caused by a virus that stimulates rapid multiplication of skin cells (see color photograph, page C-5). Warts are con-

---

Monitor That Mole

Moles have no known purpose, and scientists don't know why they develop. Most moles are harmless, and you only need to remove them if they're irritated or unattractive. However, you do need to monitor them.

Examine your skin carefully on a regular basis to detect early skin changes that signal melanoma. Check for any of these signs that may indicate melanoma:

Size. Melanomas tend to be the diameter of a pencil or larger.

Color. Individual benign moles usually have one color. Multiple colors require evaluation.

Shape. Harmless moles typically have smooth edges. Look for irregular borders.

Height. Benign moles tend to be flat or dome-shaped. Be wary of moles that are partially flat and partially elevated.

Texture. Scales, shedding of skin, oozing, or mild bleeding can signal melanoma. So can hardening or softening of the colored area.

Sensation. Is there itching, tenderness, or pain?

Nearby Skin. Pay attention to swelling, redness, or other coloring that spreads into skin near the pigmented area.

Lasers

What Are Lasers?

Laser stands for *l*ight *a*mplification by *s*timulated *e*mission of *r*adiation. Each laser derives its name from the substance—solid, liquid, or gas—within the laser tube, which is stimulated to emit light. As the light reflects between mirrors to create a laser beam, it becomes stronger.

The wavelength of the beam is the key to the laser's effect on tissue. A major advance using pulsed laser light of various wavelengths provides safer treatment and better results.

Some lasers used to treat skin conditions can destroy all skin tissue. Others have wavelengths that target tissue of a particular color or pigment, such as the red hemoglobin that colors the port-wine stain. Lasers are accepted treatment for recurring warts around your nails and on the soles of your feet, some skin cancers, tattoos, bulbous nose (rhinophyma), pre-cancer of the lip, spider veins on the face, pigmented birthmarks, and hemangiomas (abnormal collections of blood vessels in the skin).

Lasers cause minimal bleeding and pain and reduce the risk of infection. Laser surgery for skin problems almost never requires a hospital stay, and you may have local anesthesia. But lasers are not magical, and treatments are expensive. Sometimes, when a medical facility makes the considerable financial investment lasers require, there's pressure to use the tools to recover the investment. Yet a laser isn't always the best choice.

Whenever a health care provider suggests laser treatment, investigate alternatives. They may be less costly, more readily covered by insurance, and offer the same (or possibly a better) result. Also ask how many times your physician has done the procedure you're investigating.

---

tagious by contact. They most commonly occur on the hands or feet (plantar warts).

Warts are harmless and many disappear by themselves within 2 years. Plantar warts, which occur on the bottom of your feet, however, are often painful from the pressure of standing on them.

Treatment

Treatment might be unnecessary. Over-the-counter medications may remove a wart. If this fails, your physician can prescribe stronger preparations or remove it by freezing (cryotherapy), electrical burning, minor surgery, or laser surgery.

Skin Cancers

If you observe any changes in an existing growth on your skin or a new growth that ulcerates without healing, seek medical attention. This could be skin cancer. The cure rate for skin cancer is high with early treatment, but neglect can lead to disability or even death.

More than 90 percent of skin cancers occur on areas regularly exposed to ultraviolet radiation, and this exposure is considered to be the chief cause. Other contributing factors include genetic predisposition (evidenced by light-colored skin, blue eyes, blond or red hair), chemical pollution, and X-ray radiation. Inorganic arsenics, which were used in medical treatments before 1970 and are still used in herbicides, may contribute.

Identification of skin cancer in its earliest stage allows for early treatment and a high cure rate. This section will help you become familiar with the various forms of skin cancer and show you how to check your skin periodically for such lesions and how to use sunburn protection routinely to guard against the development of skin cancer (see How to Avoid Sunburn, page 997).

Basal Cell Cancer

Signs and Symptoms
- Pearly or waxy bump on the skin of your face, ear, or neck
- Flat, flesh-colored or brown scar-like lesion on chest or back

Basal cell cancer is the most common form of malignant skin tumor, accounting for 75 percent of all skin cancers (see color photograph, page C-6). When the basal cells in your epidermis become cancerous, they form a painless bump or flat lesion that may ulcerate after a few months, enlarge slowly, and never heal completely.

These cancers usually occur on unprotected areas of skin. A primary cause is probably the repeated overexposure to ultraviolet radiation. Genetic predisposition also may be a contributing factor. Fair-skinned, blue-eyed, red-haired persons are the most vulnerable. Onset most commonly occurs after age 40.

Basal cell cancer remains a local growth and only very rarely spreads to other parts of the body. However, lack of medical attention can allow the growth to invade nearby tissues and underlying structures—including your nerves, bones, or brain.

Treatment
Diagnosis requires a skin biopsy of your bump or lesion. Treatment depends on the cancer's size, depth, and location and may include scraping and cauterization, surgical excision, cryosurgery, X-ray radiation, or a series of microscopically controlled shaved excisions (Mohs' surgery).

With early treatment, the cure rate exceeds 95 percent. However, you will need to use high-protection sunscreens diligently to avoid further growths. You also should have regular medical examinations.

Squamous Cell Cancer

Signs and Symptoms—Firm, red nodule or flat lesion with scaly or crusted surface on face, ears, neck, hands, or arms

Squamous cell cancer is a malignant tumor that arises from the midportion of the epidermal layer of the skin (see color photograph, page C-6). It is more aggressive than basal cell cancer. It can spread (metastasize) to other locations, including lymph nodes or internal organs.

The tumor initially is painless, although pain may develop if it ulcerates and never completely heals. It begins in normal skin, in a burn or scar, or at a site of chronic inflammation. It may originate from a precancerous skin tumor that occurs in sun-damaged skin (see Actinic Keratosis, page 1002).

This cancer appears most frequently on skin regularly exposed to sunlight, and ultraviolet radiation is likely the main cause. Genetic predisposition may be a contributing factor. Fair-skinned, blue-eyed, blond or red-haired persons are most vulnerable. The onset most commonly is after age 50.

Treatment
Diagnosis requires biopsy of your nodule or lesion. Treatment will depend on the cancer's size, depth, location, and signs of metastasis. Surgical removal of the tumor and the skin around it, together with X-ray treatment, may be necessary. You may need a skin graft to replace excised skin. For cancers that recur after surgical removal, Mohs' surgery (a series of microscopically controlled, shaved excisions) may be necessary.

With early treatment, the cure rate is approximately 95 percent. Persistent use of high-protection sunscreens will minimize further development of such lesions. Be sure to follow up with regular medical examinations for possible recurrence.

Melanoma

Signs and Symptoms
- Superficial spreading melanoma: small lesion with irregular border and red, white, blue, or blue-black spots on trunk or limbs
- Nodular melanoma: shiny, firm, dome-shaped bumps anywhere on skin
- Acral lentiginous melanoma: dark lesions on palms, soles, tips of fingers and toes, or mucous membranes
- Lentigo maligna melanoma: large brownish spot with darker speckles on skin overexposed to sun

Melanoma is the most deadly but least common skin cancer. It typically arises painlessly from cells that produce the skin's pigment (melanin). Approximately 70 percent of these cancers appear on normal skin; 30 percent arise from an existing mole that has undergone sudden changes (color, size, pain, itching, bleeding, swelling).

The cancer first spreads in the surrounding skin and is highly curable at this phase. If not treated, the tumor then spreads downward into other areas of the skin or to lymph nodes or internal organs.

Superficial spreading melanoma accounts for 70 percent of cases and strikes at any age. Nodular melanoma may ulcerate and fail to heal completely. It can develop anywhere on the skin, usually between ages 20 and 60.

Acral lentiginous melanoma accounts for 10 percent of the cases and is more common in old age. Lentigo maligna melanoma occurs in 5 percent of cases. It frequently afflicts elderly persons and is associated with senile skin (see page 1000). A benign brownish spot may appear several years before turning cancerous (see color photographs, page C-6).

Sunlight is the chief cause of melanoma. Fair-skinned, blue-eyed, blond- or red-haired persons are most vulnerable, and dark skin is the most resistant. Certain moles that may transform into melanoma can run in families. Other contributing factors are listed in the introduction to this section (see Skin Cancers, page 1004).

The incidence of melanoma has doubled among Americans during the past 20 years. In various forms, it can strike at any age. Men have a higher mortality rate.

Diagnosis

Your physician may suspect a melanoma from visual inspection. A skin biopsy is needed to confirm the diagnosis. If there is a possibility of the melanoma spreading to other locations, your physician may order further testing, including a complete physical examination with chest X-ray and CT scan (see page 1334).

How Serious Is Melanoma?

Prompt treatment in the early stages provides a cure in 85 percent of the cases. When the tumor has grown downward or spread to the lymph nodes or other organs, the 5-year survival rate is 30 percent.

Treatment

The usual treatment is surgical removal of the tumor with a wide margin of normal skin. In some cases it will be necessary to excise nearby lymph nodes. This may be followed by a skin graft to the site of operation. In the case of disseminated or widespread disease, other treatment may include anticancer drugs and immunotherapy. Immunotherapy involves injecting a vaccine that stimulates your immune system to destroy cancerous tissue.

A necessary part of the follow-up process for long-term management of this cancer is periodic medical examinations for evidence of recurring melanoma.

Kaposi's Sarcoma

Signs and Symptoms

- Aggressive form: red-purple nodules anywhere on the skin
- Indolent form: dark blue or purple-brown nodules on the toe or leg

Kaposi's sarcoma is a malignant condition sometimes associated with other cancers, including leukemia or lymphoma (see color photograph, page C-6). The early lesions are red to purple and resemble a birthmark (hemangioma). Older lesions become brown to black, are flatter, and occur with scarring of the skin.

The disease appears in two forms: aggressive and indolent. The aggressive form occurs both internally and externally. It is now occurring with greater frequency because of its association with acquired immunodeficiency syndrome (AIDS). If linked with the multiple disorders of AIDS (see page 1060), this is a dangerous cancer.

The dark tumors of the indolent form, which are caused by blood vessel involvement, can spread to your hands and arms or can produce fungus-like growths—or both. This cancer may penetrate your underlying tissue and invade bone, lymph nodes, and internal organs.

Treatment

After an examination and skin biopsy reveal Kaposi's sarcoma, your treatment may include X-ray therapy or chemotherapy. Elastic support hose may provide some relief by reducing swelling.

Skin Infections

Because your skin is your first line of defense, it often must deal with attacks from bacteria, viruses, fungi, and insect venom. If bacteria become established in a wound, they can cause a number of illnesses; bacteria or other foreign invaders may infect hair follicles or develop in skin, as in erysipelas (see page 1009) or shingles (see page 1011).

Skin infections range from localized, superficial infections (like impetigo) to widespread, life-threatening infections. The symptoms depend on where the infection develops and the organism that is causing it.

Impetigo

Signs and Symptoms—Itchy, red sores with yellow or gray crusts on the face, legs, or arms

Impetigo is a fairly common superficial skin infection caused by bacteria—staphylococci, streptococci, or both (see color photograph, page C-12). It may occur on normal skin, but the bacteria usually invade at the site of a skin abrasion, scratch, or insect bite—or as a secondary complication of other skin diseases, such as dermatitis (see page 987).

The infection starts as a red sore that blisters briefly and then oozes during the next few days to form a sticky crust. The sore tends to grow and is contagious through bacteria in the blister's fluid. Physical contact—including scratching—can spread the infection to other parts of the body or even to other people.

An ulcerating form of impetigo, ecthyma, appears as itchy, thick, brown-black crusts ringed by red skin. In rare instances, the bacteria may infect the bloodstream and, in children, lead to kidney disease (see Acute Glomerulonephritis, page 836).

The incidence of impetigo is highest among children who live in poor hygienic conditions. In adults it appears mostly as a complication of another skin problem.

Your physician will diagnose impetigo by examination and culture of tissue from your infection.

Treatment
Topical medications are effective in limited and minor infections. For more extensive infections, your physician may prescribe antibiotics (such as penicillin or erythromycin) to be taken orally. Wash the area several times each day with antibacterial soap or cleanser to soften the crusts, so that you can gently remove them. To avoid spreading the infection, do not share towels, clothing, and razors. Avoid skin contact until the condition clears. The sores heal slowly, but the cure rate is very high.

Folliculitis

Signs and Symptoms—Small, white-headed pimples around the hair follicles

Folliculitis is a superficial infection of the hair follicles (see color photograph, page C-12). These infections are common and usually are caused by staphylococci or fungi. They can occur anywhere on your skin as a result of clothing friction, hair follicle blockage, or injury. For example, shaving your neck or underarms can produce a rash of them that becomes chronic unless treated.

Barber's itch is a staphylococcal infection of the hair follicles of the bearded area, especially the upper lip near the nose. Itching may occur a day or two before the pinhead-sized pustules erupt. Shaving is a major aggravating factor.

A similar eruption due to a fungal infection is called tinea barbae. This requires antifungal treatment.

Pseudofolliculitis barbae occurs primarily in black males when the hair of the beard grows into an adjacent hair follicle and forms a small, curled-up mass within the follicle. Chronic infection is present.

Treatment
You can treat mild folliculitis with a topical antibiotic alone. For more extensive folliculitis, such as that involving the beard, you will need hot tap-water compresses and oral antibiotics. Use a new razor blade each day for shaving if you have folliculitis of the beard. Take care to avoid reinfections from contaminated clothing or reused razor blades.

Pseudofolliculitis barbae may respond only if the infected person does not shave.

Chapter 30 continued on page 1009.

Photographic Guide to Common Skin Disorders

The color and texture of your skin can reveal a great deal about the health of your skin and your health in general. Often, the first clue to illness is revealed in the form of a rash or a welt, a growth or a blemish. At other times, the skin disorder is in itself the only abnormality. The photographs that follow provide an overview of various skin disorders. Because skin ailments can vary widely in their manifestations, it is important to consult your physician if you are uncertain about the cause of any skin blemish.

Contents

Childhood Diseases. **C-1**

Skin Disorders at Birth and Infancy. **C-2**

Birthmarks (Hemangiomas). **C-2**

Dermatitis (Eczema) in Adults. **C-3**

Noncancerous (Benign) Skin Disorders. **C-4**

Skin Cancers **C-6**

Skin Color (Pigmentary) Changes, Hair, and Nails . . . **C-7**

Fungal Infections. **C-8**

Acne and Hives. **C-9**

Mouth (Oral) Disorders **C-10**

Eye Disorders. **C-11**

Skin Infections. **C-12**

Infestations and Bites. **C-14**

Other Skin Diseases. **C-15**

Childhood Diseases
All Highly Contagious

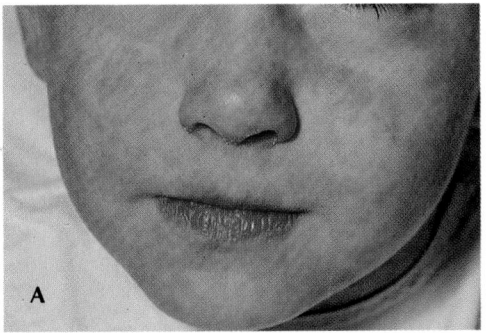
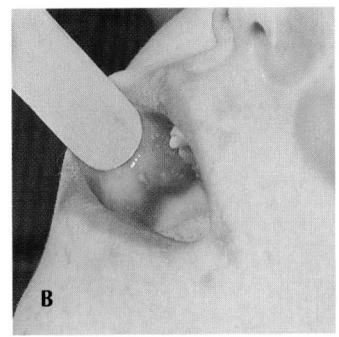

Measles (rubeola)—Red, blotchy rash first appearing on the face (A) or behind the ears, then spreading to the chest, back, and finally to the arms and legs. In addition, small white spots appear on the inside lining of the cheek (B) (see page 1073).

German measles (rubella)—Fine, pink rash that appears on the face, trunk (shown above), and then the arms and legs. It generally lasts 2 or 3 days (see page 1074).

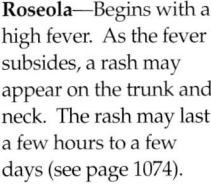
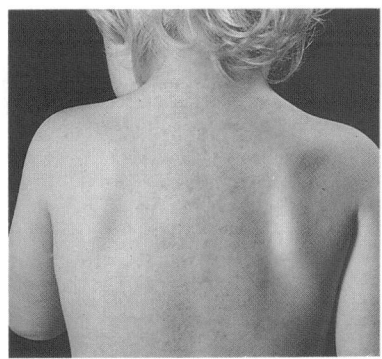

Roseola—Begins with a high fever. As the fever subsides, a rash may appear on the trunk and neck. The rash may last a few hours to a few days (see page 1074).

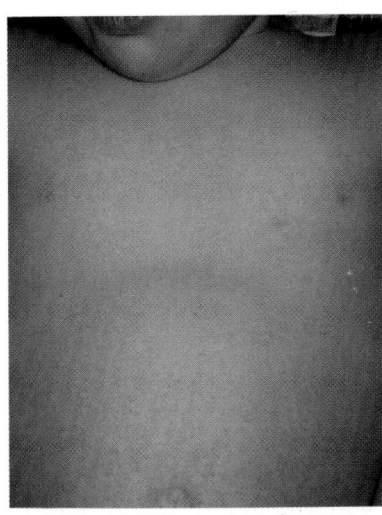

Scarlet fever—Rash appearing on the neck and chest (but not the face), then spreading to the entire body. The rash has a sandpaper consistency. Often, the rash is most severe on the armpits and groin (see page 1080).

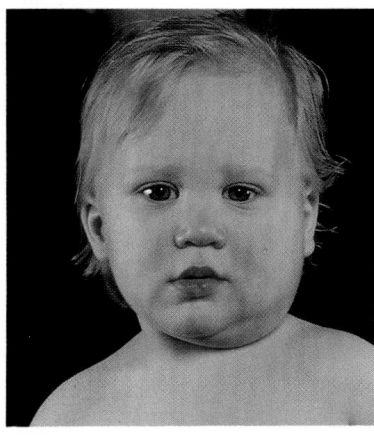
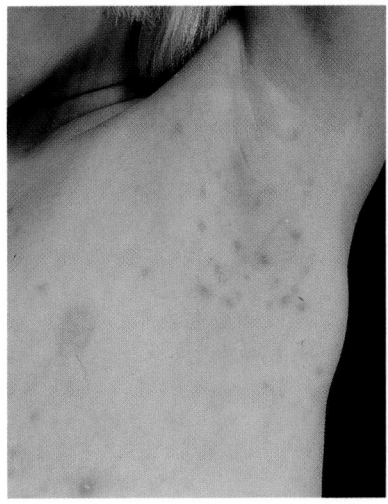

Mumps—Characterized by swollen, painful glands just beneath the angle of the jaw, causing the cheeks to puff out (see page 1077).

Chickenpox (varicella)—Itchy, red rash that breaks out on the face, scalp, chest, back, and, to a lesser extent, arms and legs. The spots quickly fill with a clear fluid, rupture, and then turn crusty. Spots at various stages of development may occur at the same time (see page 1076).

Skin Disorders at Birth and Infancy

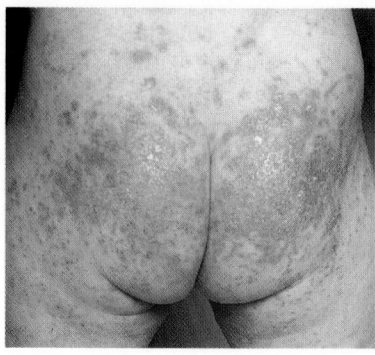

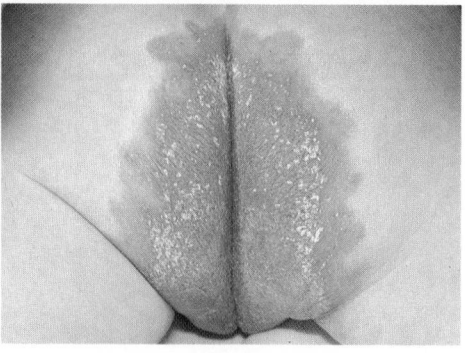

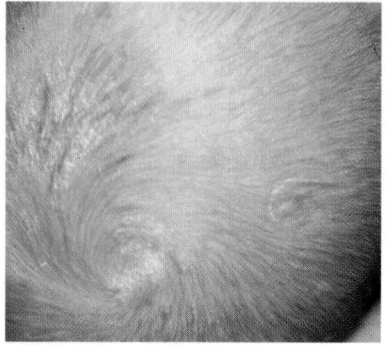

Diaper rash (diaper dermatitis)—Most often results from reaction of sensitive skin to contact with urine or stool. It often disappears without treatment (see pages 14 and 68).

Candidiasis—Fungal infection may appear on the buttocks and genitals as bright red spots that come together to form a solid red area with a scalloped border (see page 1013).

Cradle cap (seborrheic eczema)—Common problem that generally occurs in infancy. Dry, scaly patches give scalp a dirty appearance. A yellow crust may form over the scales. In addition, scaly patches may occur around the hairline, eyebrows, eyelids, nose, and ears (see pages 14 and 68).

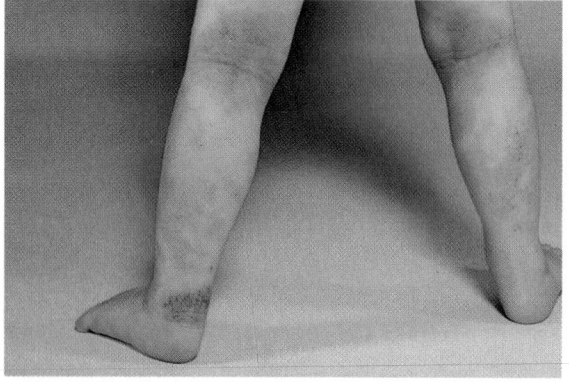

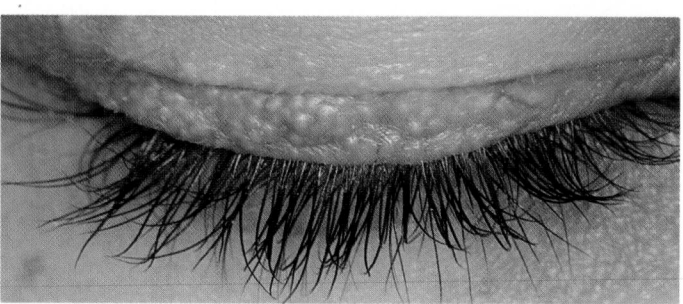

Infantile eczema (atopic dermatitis)—Rough, red, patchy rash usually associated with extremely dry skin. It may be a reaction to food or to an irritant such as clothing, baby powder, or urine. Itching is associated with the rash (see pages 14, 989, and 1038).

Milia—Small white bumps or cysts on a newborn's face or, less often, the trunk. They resemble whiteheads and usually disappear without treatment within a few weeks (see pages 15 and 69).

Birthmarks (Hemangiomas)

There are many forms of birthmarks. Hemangiomas are one common type. These are benign tumors made of newly formed blood vessels. They characteristically are bright red or sharply protruding lesions that may appear anywhere on the body.

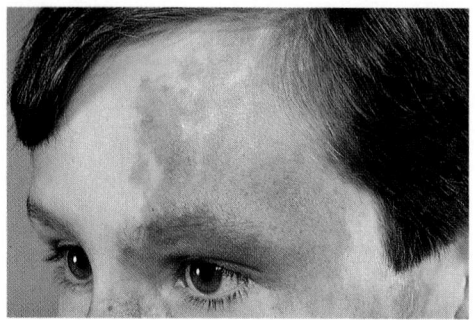

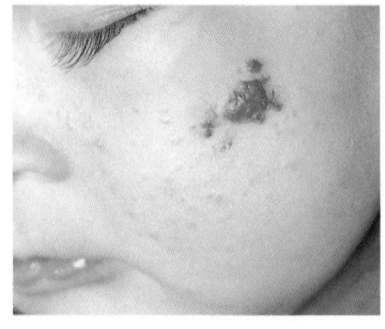

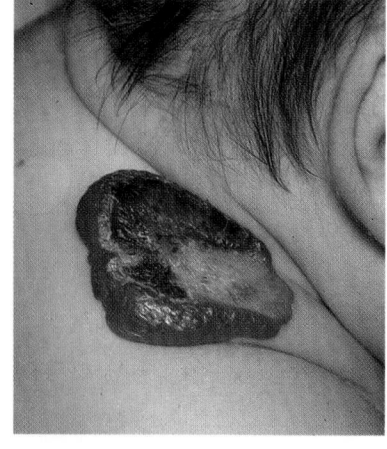

Port-wine stain—Maroon or red skin discoloration. The most common site is the face (see page 16).

Strawberry hemangioma—Often appears on the face, scalp, back, or chest, but may occur anywhere on the body (see page 15).

Cavernous hemangioma—Typically a red-blue spongy mass made up of tissue filled with blood (see page 16).

Dermatitis (Eczema) in Adults

The term dermatitis, which describes irritated, inflamed skin, may be used interchangeably with the term eczema. There are many forms, including those shown below.

Contact Dermatitis

Direct contact with any one of various substances can cause contact dermatitis. (See pages 987 and 1036.)

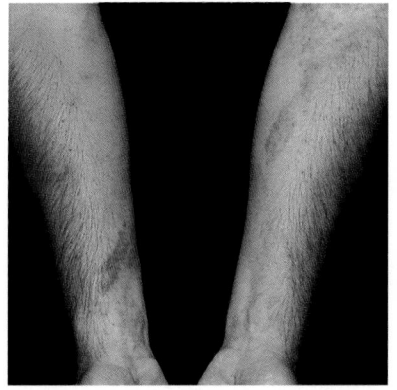

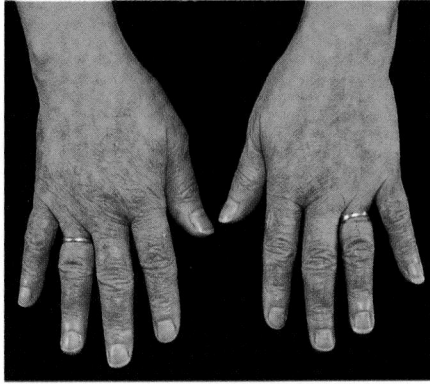

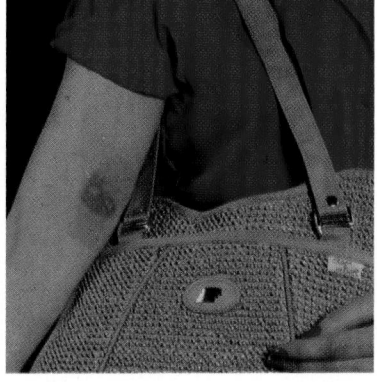

Poison ivy—Characterized by an itchy rash consisting of small bumps, blisters, and general swelling (see page 1036).

Dishpan hands—Common reaction to many household chemicals (see page 987).

Nickel dermatitis—Contact with chemicals such as the nickel contained in this purse-strap buckle causes this rash (see page 1037).

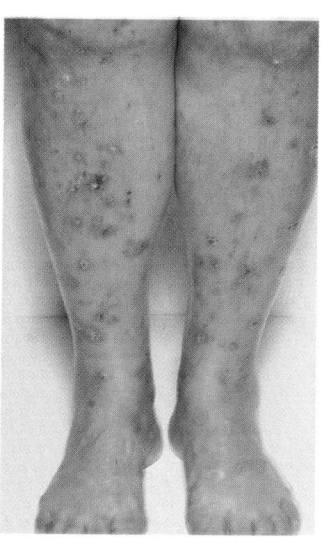

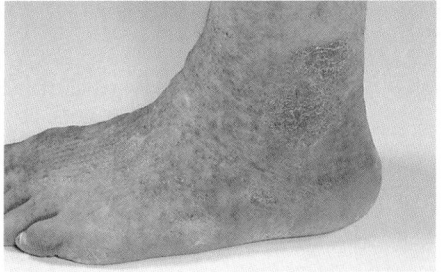

Stasis dermatitis—Thickening and itching of the skin at the ankles, often associated with varicose veins. At times the skin becomes inflamed, or open ulcers slowly develop around the ankles and heels. The skin often becomes irregularly thickened from continued scratching (see page 989).

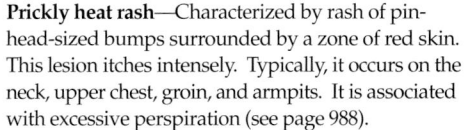

Seborrheic dermatitis—Greasy-appearing, scaly, itchy areas at the sides of the nose, between the eyebrows, behind the ears, or over the breastbone. Dandruff is mild seborrheic dermatitis of the scalp (see page 989).

Neurodermatitis—Characterized by scratch marks (excoriations) and small, flat growths (plaques) of various sizes, with definite margins. The growths become thickened and leather-like (lichenified). The condition is often called lichen simplex chronicus (see page 988).

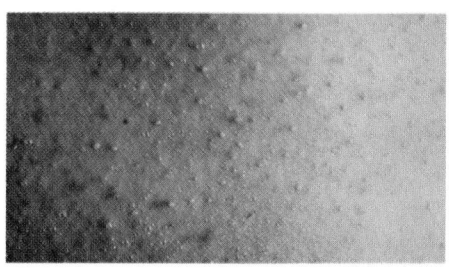

Prickly heat rash—Characterized by rash of pinhead-sized bumps surrounded by a zone of red skin. This lesion itches intensely. Typically, it occurs on the neck, upper chest, groin, and armpits. It is associated with excessive perspiration (see page 988).

Noncancerous (Benign) Skin Disorders

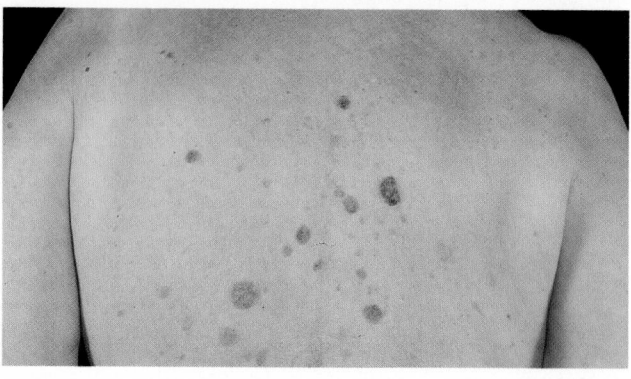

Seborrheic keratoses—Benign skin tumors that commonly appear after age 40. These oval growths have a waxy, wart-like, scaly, slightly elevated surface. Their color varies from yellow to dark brown or black. They have a pasted-on appearance. Occasionally, they appear singly but most often are seen in large numbers (see page 1002).

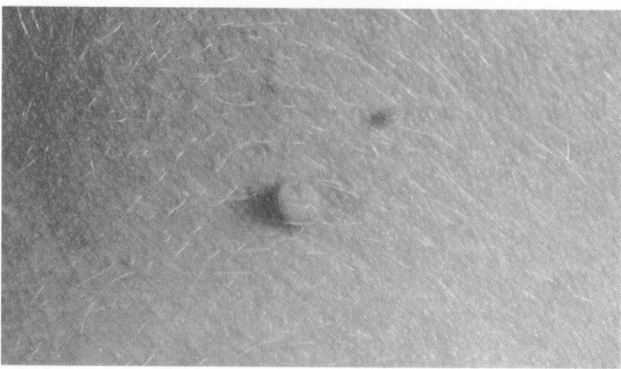

Skin tag (acrochordon)—Tiny, harmless, painless tumor that protrudes on a narrow stalk. It is soft and normally skin-colored but may appear darker (see page 1002).

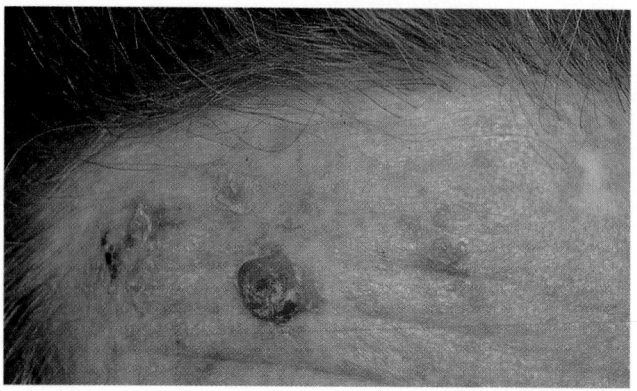

Actinic keratoses (solar keratoses)—Gritty, scaly, gray to dark-pink patches on the face, scalp, and back of hands. They have a sandpaper-like surface that is more felt than seen. The probable cause is long-term, excessive exposure to ultraviolet radiation in sunlight (see page 1002).

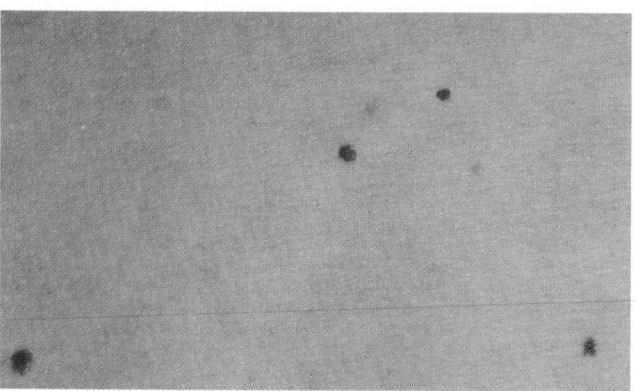

Cherry angioma—Benign skin tumor of unknown origin that appears most frequently after age 40. It is characterized by a small, smooth, cherry-red bump on the skin. It is most commonly found on the torso. It ranges in size from that of a pinhead to ¼-inch across (see page 1002).

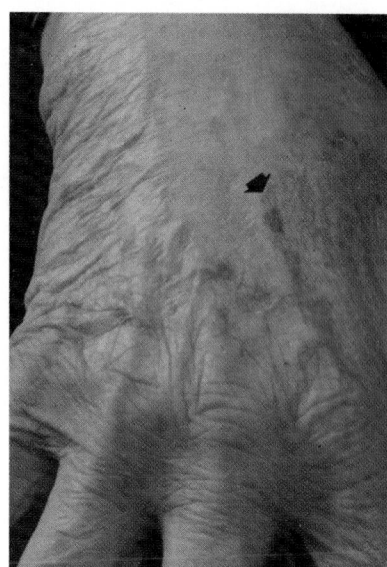

Liver spots (senile lentigines)—Harmless, flat patches of increased pigmentation that range from freckle-size (see arrowhead) to a few inches across. They are light brown to black and may occur on your face or the backs of your hands (see page 1003).

Sun-damaged skin—Characterized by coarse wrinkles, sagging folds, sallowness, roughness, excessive dryness, or leather-toughness. The cause is long-term, excessive exposure of unprotected skin to ultraviolet radiation (see page 1003).

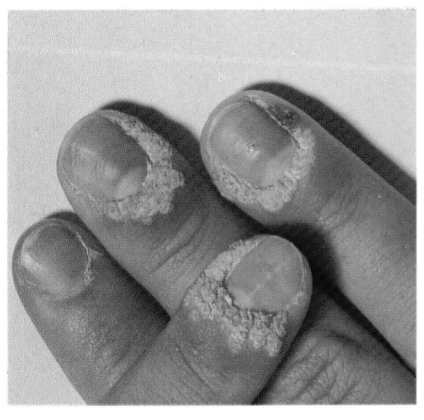
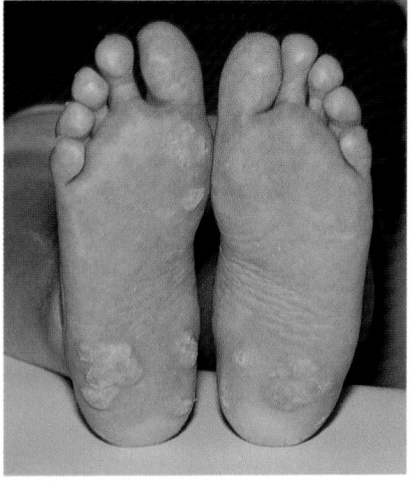
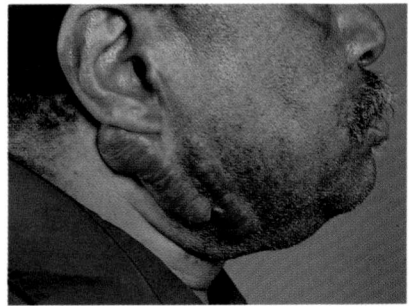

Wart (verruca vulgaris)—Benign tumor caused by a virus that stimulates rapid multiplication of skin cells. Warts are contagious by contact and most commonly occur on the hands or feet (see page 1003).

Keloid—Overproduction of scar tissue. Consists of flesh- or lighter-colored, nodular or rigid growths on the skin. A keloid is harmless but may be tender, itchy, or unsightly in appearance (see page 1003).

Moles (Pigmented Nevi)

Moles are benign accumulations of pigment cells. They may contain hairs, stay smooth, or become raised or wrinkled. It is important to consult your physician about any change in the color or size of a mole, or if itching, pain, bleeding, or inflammation develops. (See page 1003.)

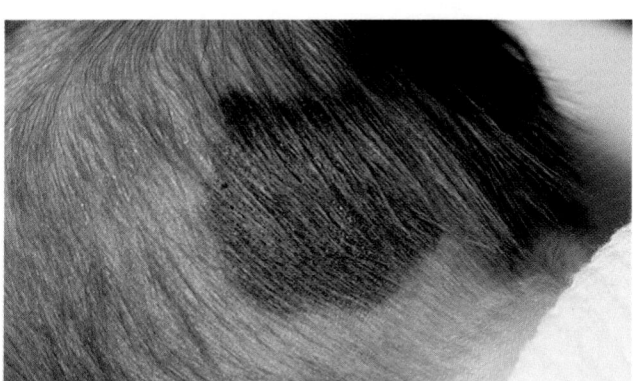
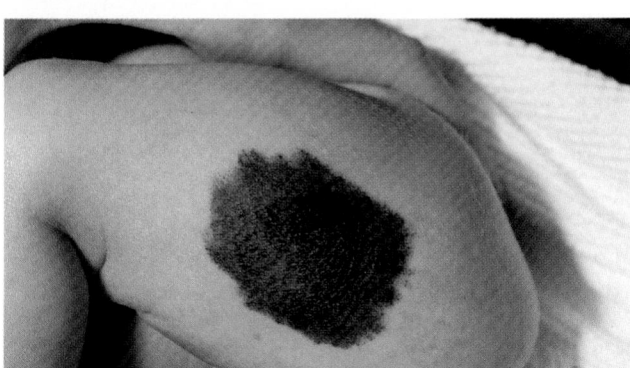
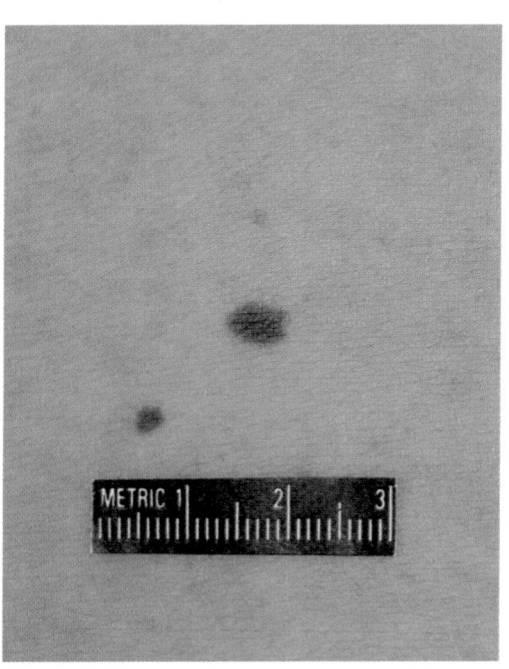

Skin Cancers

Melanomas
Melanomas are the most lethal forms of skin cancer. These skin growths require prompt diagnosis and treatment.

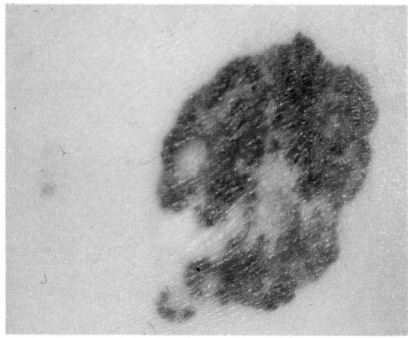

Superficial spreading melanoma— Characterized by variations in color and an irregular border. The most frequent sites for this common type of melanoma are the torso and limbs (see page 1005).

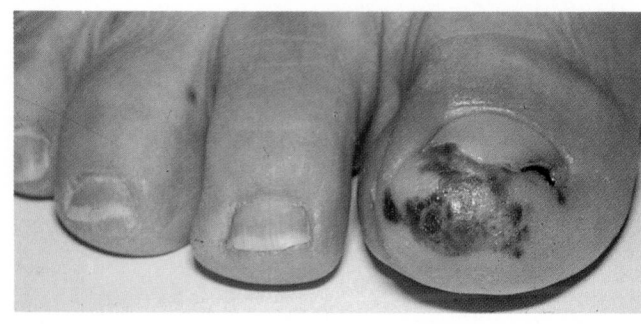

Acral lentiginous melanoma—Freckle-like melanoma of the extremity. The skin around or under a fingernail or toenail is commonly affected (see page 1005).

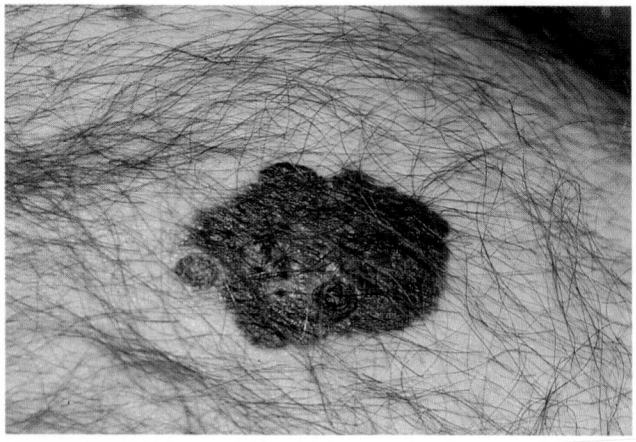

Nodular melanoma—From its inception, this growth is raised above the skin surface. There is no most-frequent site. Because invasion into the lower skin occurs early, prompt treatment is especially crucial (see page 1005).

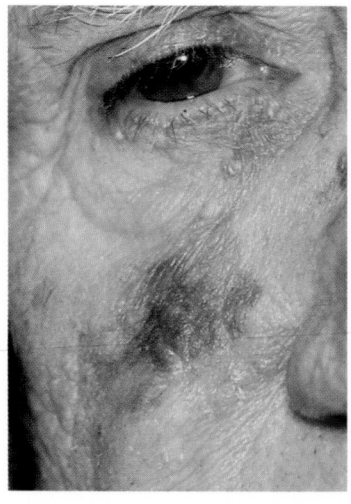

Lentigo maligna melanoma—Most often afflicts elderly people. It occurs primarily on sunlight-damaged skin of the face or backs of the hands. It is always preceded by lentigo maligna, a flat, tan to brown area that may exist for many years or decades before the cancerous cells begin to penetrate deep into the skin (see page 1005).

Other Skin Cancers

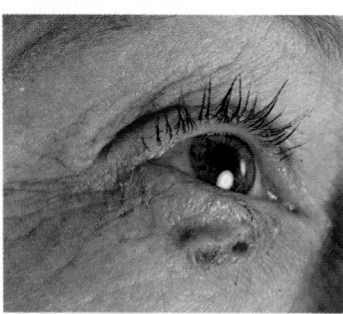

Basal cell cancer—The most common malignant skin tumor. It is characterized by a pearly or waxy bump on the skin of the face, ears, or neck, or it may be a flat, flesh-colored or brown, scar-like lesion on the chest or back (see page 1005).

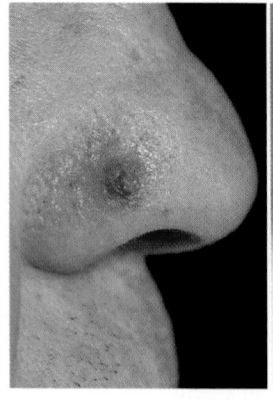

Kaposi's sarcoma—Red-purple nodules anywhere on the skin (above left), or dark-blue or purple-brown nodules on the toe or leg (above right). It is now occurring with greater frequency because of its association with acquired immuno-deficiency syndrome (AIDS) (see page 1006).

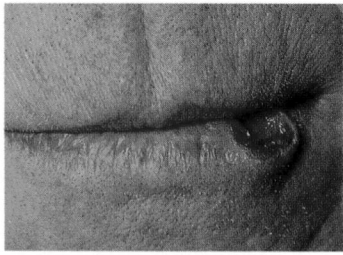

Squamous cell cancer—Normally painless unless it ulcerates. Generally, it occurs in areas regularly exposed to sunlight. The lesion is generally firm, red, nodular, or flat, with a scaly or crusted surface. It occurs most commonly on the face, ears, neck, hands, or arms (see page 1005).

Skin Color (Pigmentary) Changes, Hair, and Nails

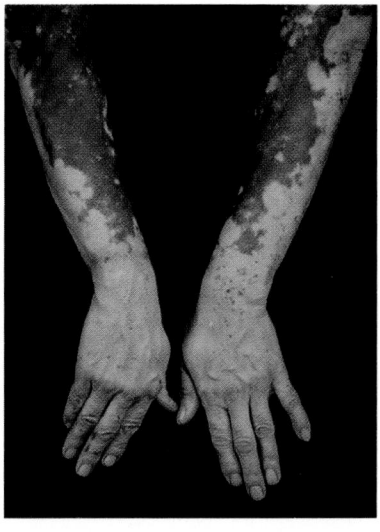

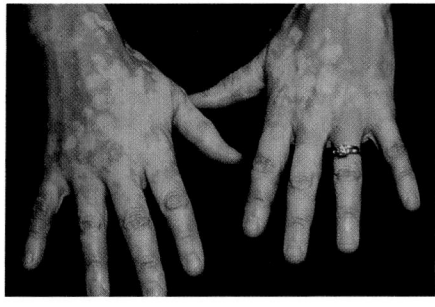

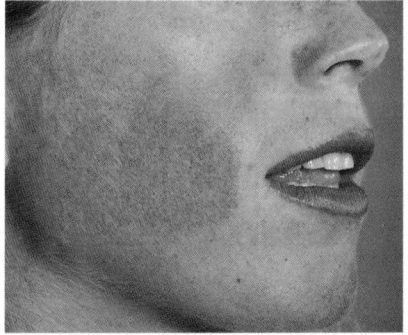

Vitiligo—If you have black skin, vitiligo can turn your skin patchy white (left). If you have white skin (above), you may first become aware of vitiligo during the summer, when depigmented areas of your skin become more noticeable as the rest of your skin tans (see page 994).

Chloasma—Patches of darker skin, most commonly found on the face. It may be associated with pregnancy or use of birth control pills. Chloasma results from excessive melanin in the skin (see page 994).

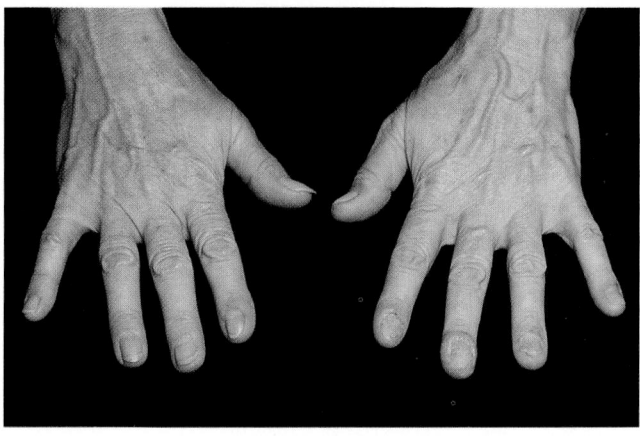

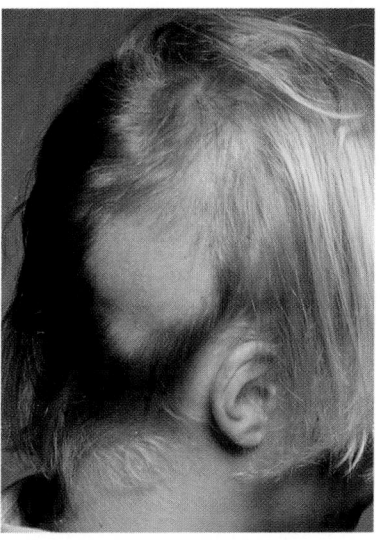

Paronychia—Superficial infection of the skin around the nails, most commonly caused by staphylococci or a fungus (*Candida*). The skin next to the nails becomes red and swollen (see page 1021).

Alopecia areata—Sudden hair loss. It usually starts abruptly with one or more circular bald patches that may overlap. The bald areas are smooth and painless. The cause is unknown (see page 1018).

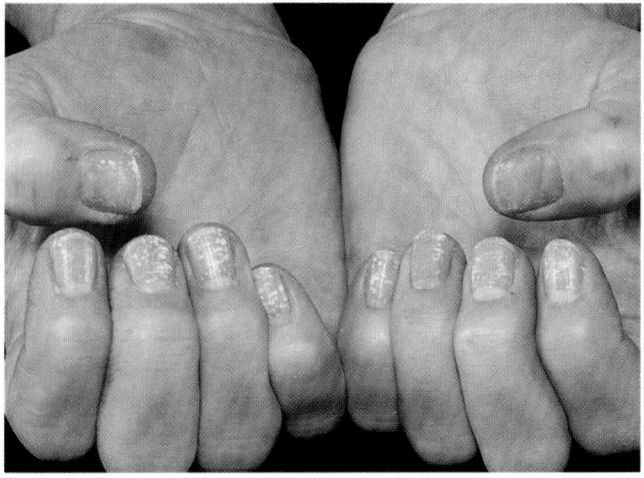

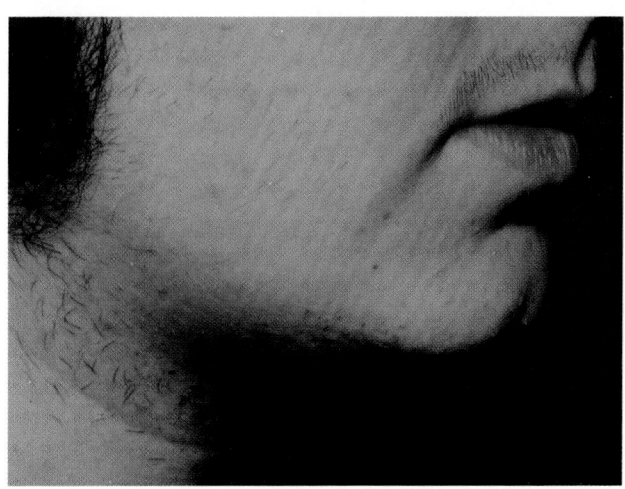

Leukonychia—White nails, either completely or in spots or patches under the nails (see page 1023).

Hirsutism—Excess hair. The condition normally develops over a few months (see page 1019).

Fungal Infections

Fungal infections are caused by microscopic plants that become parasites on your skin. Susceptibility to these infections is increased by poor hygiene, continually moist skin, or minor skin or nail injuries (see page 1012).

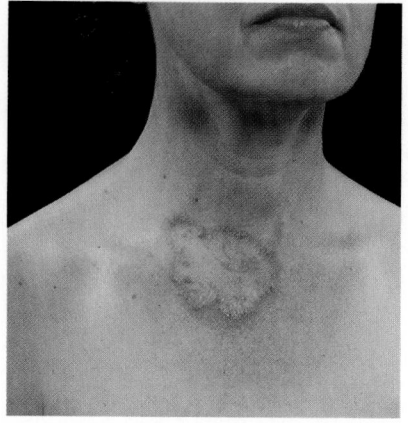

Ringworm (tinea corporis)—Itchy, red, scaly, slightly raised, expanding rings on the trunk, face, or groin or thigh fold. The ring grows outward as the infection spreads and the central area becomes less actively infected (see page 1013).

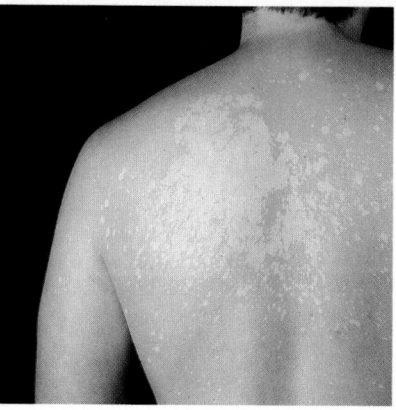

Tinea versicolor—Tissue-thin coating of fungus on your skin, characterized by small, slightly scaly, pale patches on the upper body and neck or face (see page 1013).

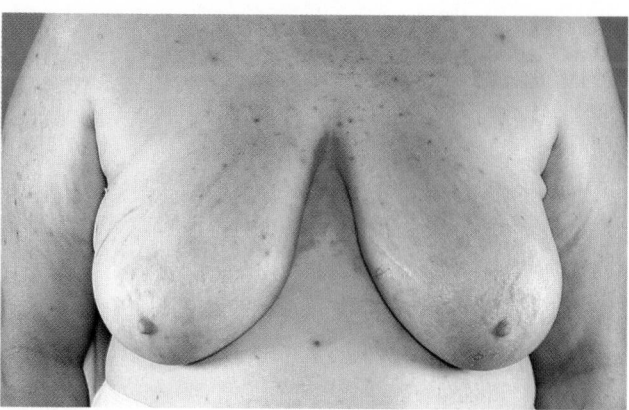

Intertrigo—Red, moist patches rimmed with small red bumps under the breasts, in armpits, navel, groin, or buttock or thigh fold, or between fingers or toes (see page 1012).

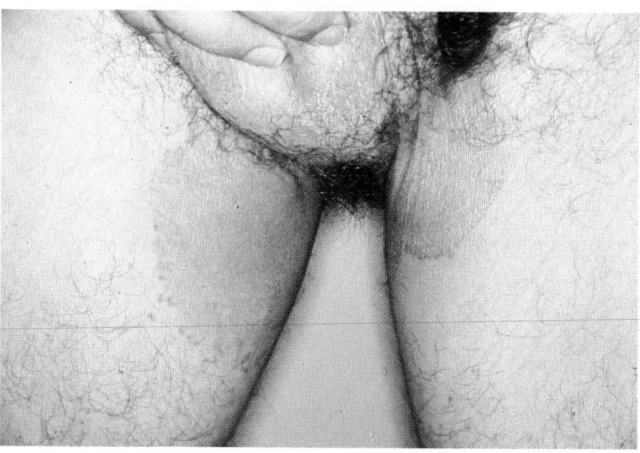

Jock itch (tinea cruris)—Red, moist, well-marked patches in the groin area (see page 1013).

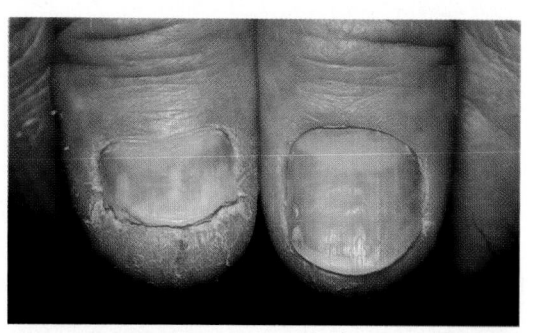

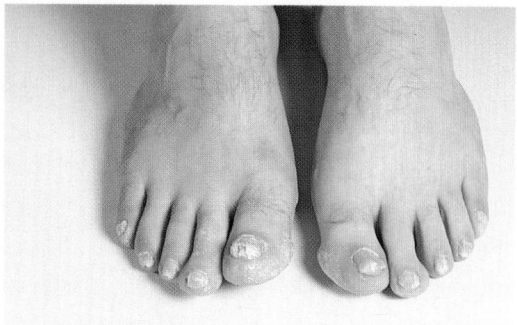

Onychomycosis—Fungal infection of the fingernails (top) or toenails (bottom) (see page 1022).

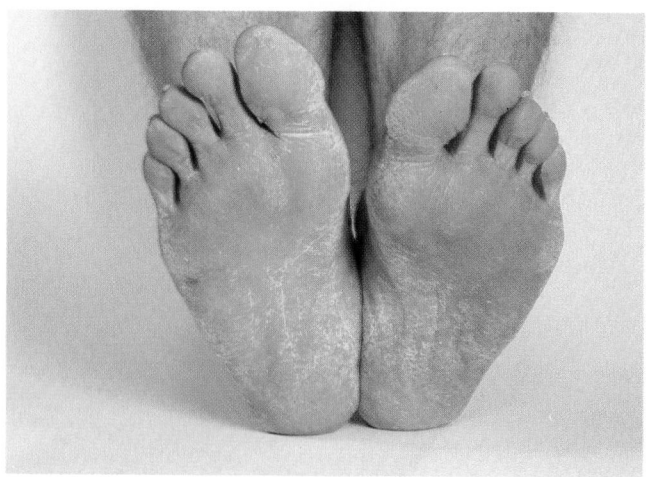

Athlete's foot (tinea pedis)—Itchy, red, soggy, flaking, and cracking skin between toes, or a few fluid-filled bumps on the side or sole of the foot. There also may be extreme dryness with small white scales on the side or sole of your foot or the palm of your hand (see page 1013).

Acne and Hives

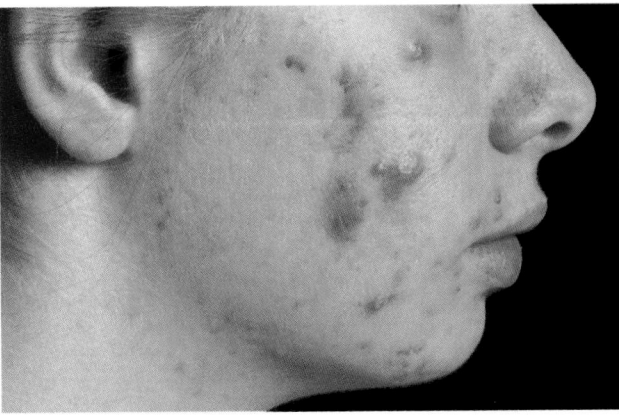

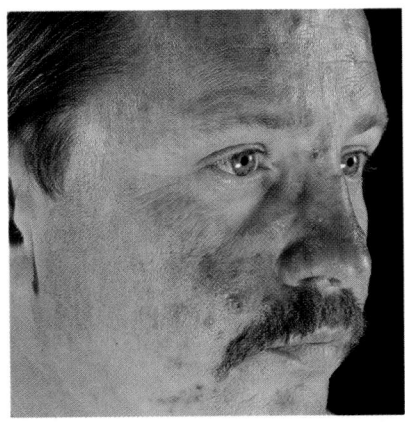

Cystic acne—Most severe form of acne. It results from hair follicles that are plugged by skin oils or dead cells from sebaceous glands. The resulting rupture within your skin may form boil-like infections (see page 990).

Acne rosacea—Chronic inflammation of the cheeks, nose, chin, forehead, or eyelids, with pimple-like pustules in the reddened area (see page 991).

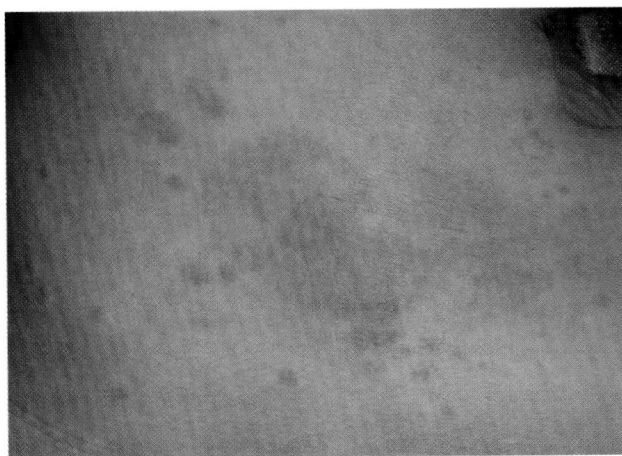

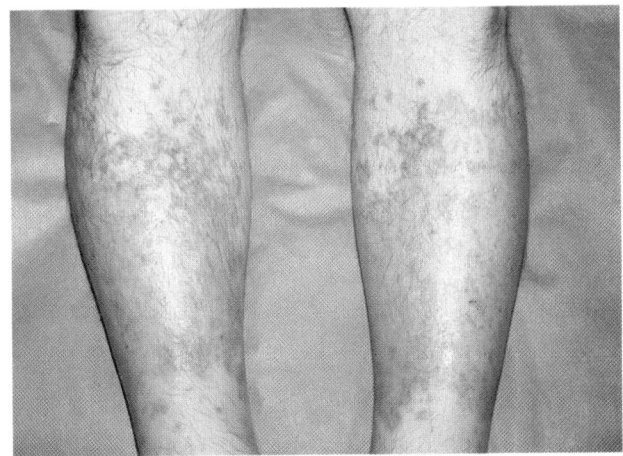

Hives (urticaria)—Acute hives (left) are characterized by raised, red, often itchy welts of various sizes that appear and disappear at random on the surface of the skin. If persistent, chronic hives (right) develop (see page 1038).

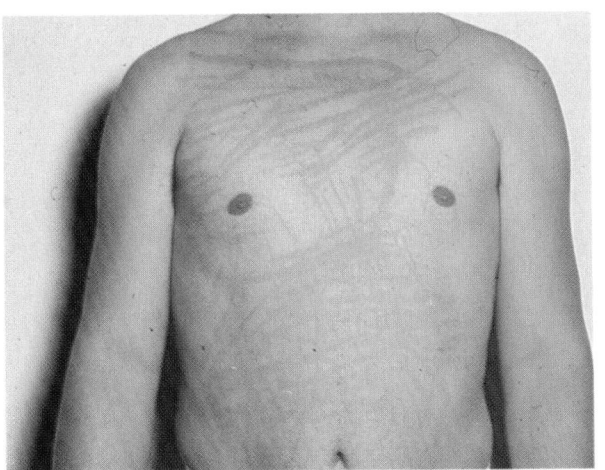

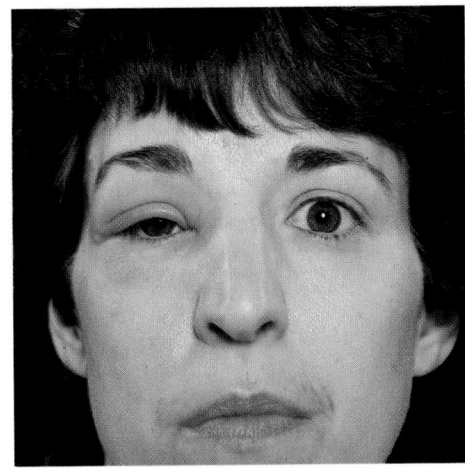

Dermographism—Welts that develop where the skin is scratched (see page 1039).

Angioedema—Large welts that develop below the surface of your skin, particularly on the eyes and lips, but also on the hands and feet and even in the throat (see page 1038).

Mouth (Oral) Disorders

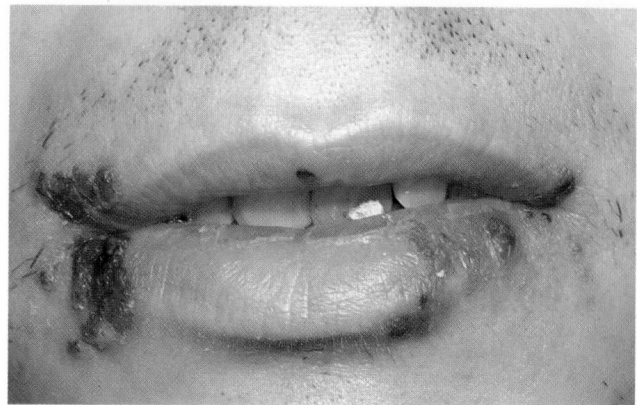

Cold sores (herpes simplex)—Often called fever blisters. They are single or clustered, small, fluid-filled blisters on a raised, red, painful area of the skin. The blisters form, break, and ooze; then a yellow crust forms and finally sloughs off to uncover pinkish, healing skin (see page 1010).

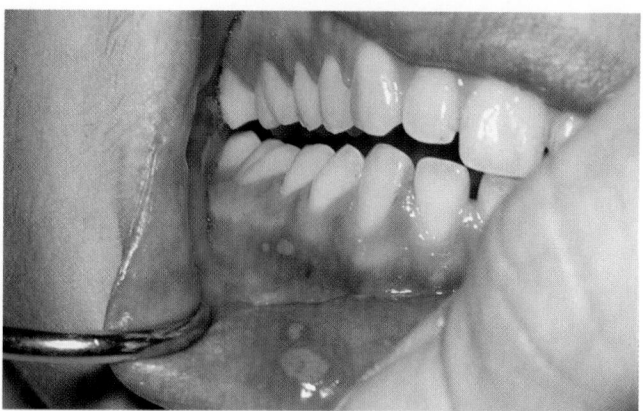

Canker sore (aphthous ulcer)—Occurs singly or in clusters on the inside surfaces of the cheeks or lips, on the tongue, at the base of the gums, or on the soft palate. It is a painful sore with a white or yellow center and a red border (see page 617).

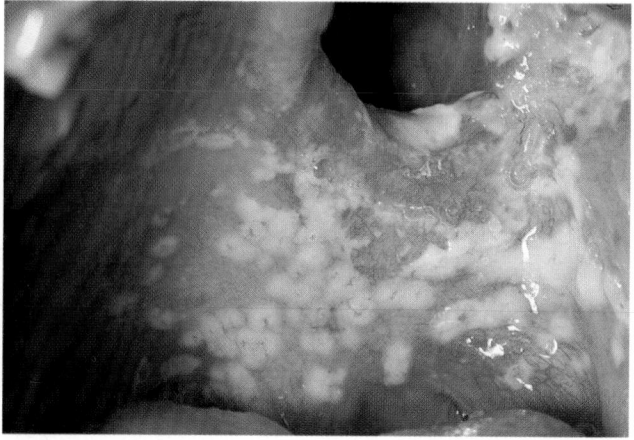

Oral thrush (candidiasis)—Slightly raised, creamy white, sore patches in your mouth or on your tongue. If the patches are brushed off, bleeding may result (see pages 16, 618, and 1013).

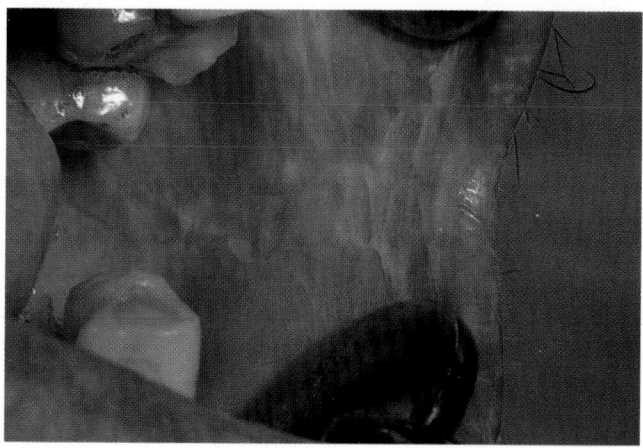

Oral lichen planus—Small, pale pimples that form a lacy network on the tongue or cheeks, or shiny, slightly raised patches on the tongue or cheeks (see pages 619 and 993).

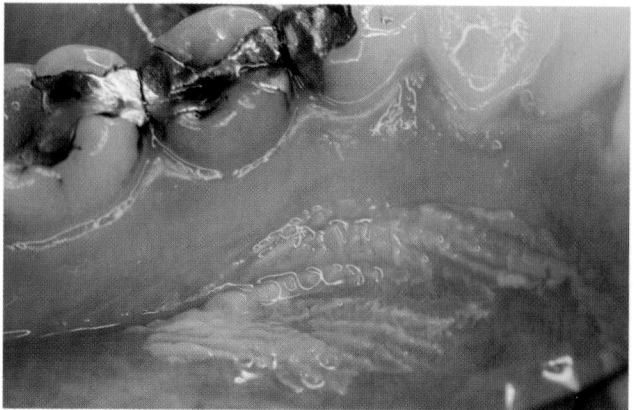

Leukoplakia—Thickened, hardened white patch on the cheek or tongue. If the patch develops in the mouth of a person who smokes or uses chewing tobacco, the condition is referred to as smoker's keratosis or snuff keratosis. This may be a precancerous lesion (see page 618).

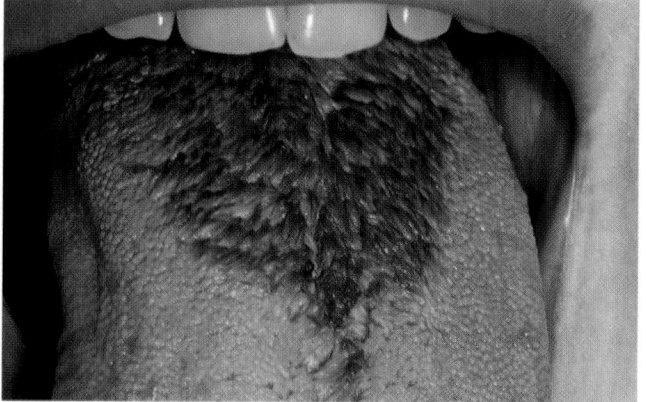

Black, hairy tongue—Hair-like projections that grow profusely on the tongue, giving it a hairy appearance. The tongue usually is not sore, but the appearance can be alarming. Growths can be removed by brushing gently with a toothbrush (see page 620).

Eye Disorders

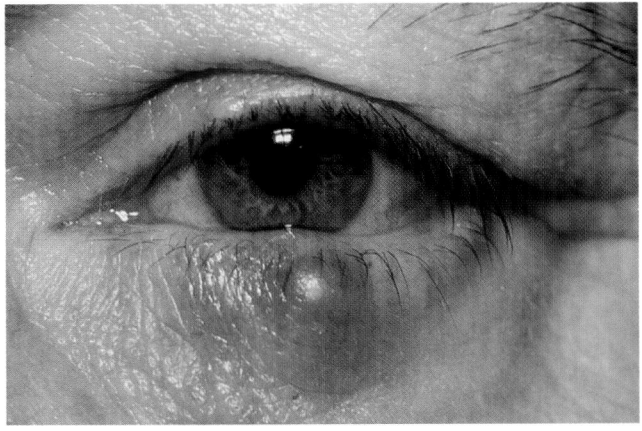

Sty (hordeolum)—Bacterial infection near the root (follicle) of an eye-lash. It is similar to a boil or pimple and is often painful (see page 536).

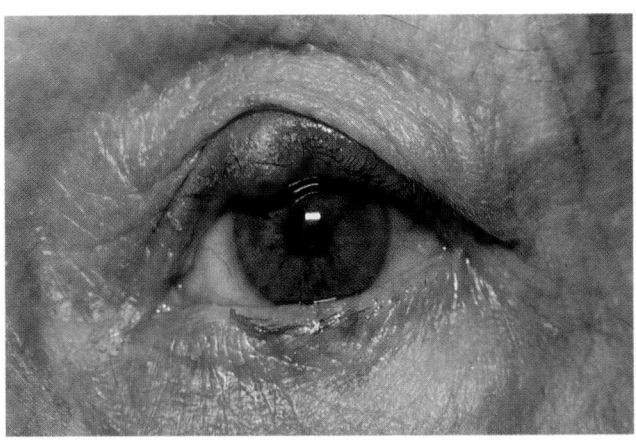

Chalazion—Painless swelling of the eyelid, resulting from blockage of one of the small glands that produce part of the tear layer (see page 536).

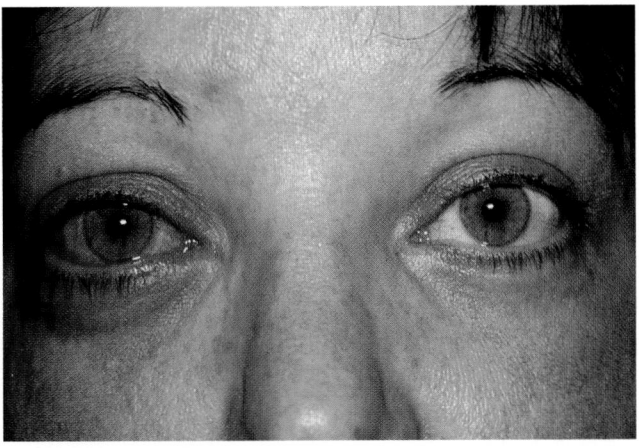

Conjunctivitis—Inflammation of the transparent membrane that lines the eyelid. It is characterized by redness and a gritty sensation in the eye, along with itching. Often, a discharge forms a crust during the night. If caused by a virus, this disorder is commonly known as pinkeye (see page 542).

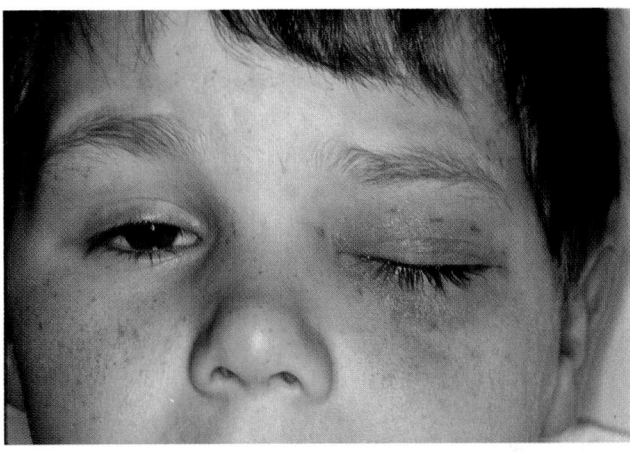

Orbital cellulitis—Swelling and redness of the eyelid, followed rapidly by pain and decreased vision. There may be displacement of the eye because of swelling. It requires prompt (emergency) treatment (see page 545).

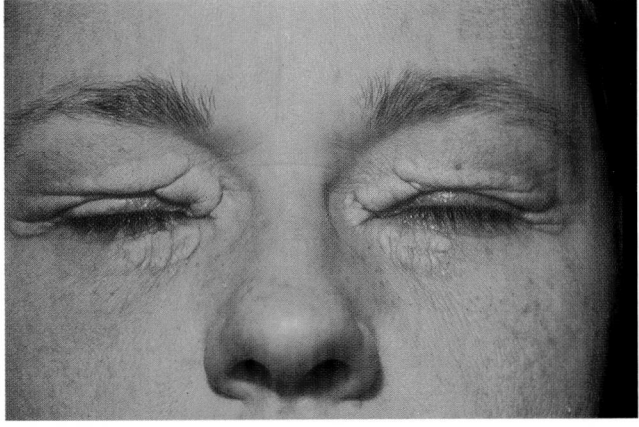

Xanthelasma—Soft, yellow, fatty, flat lesions that appear on the eyelids. The condition may be associated with elevated concentrations of cholesterol and triglycerides (see page 1001).

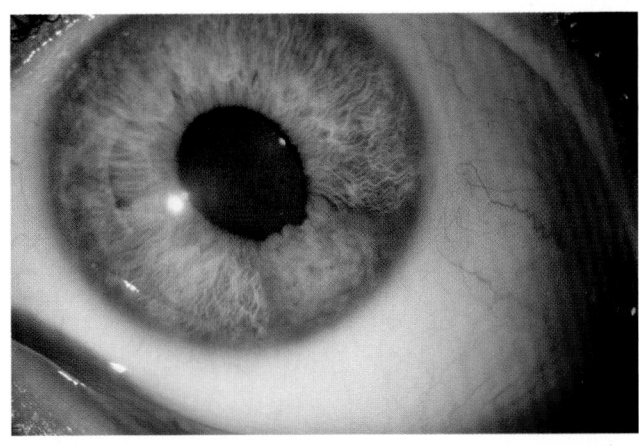

Iris melanoma—Development of a brown or black spot in the iris may suggest a melanoma, a cancer of the eye. If this occurs, see your ophthalmologist promptly (see page 546).

Skin Infections

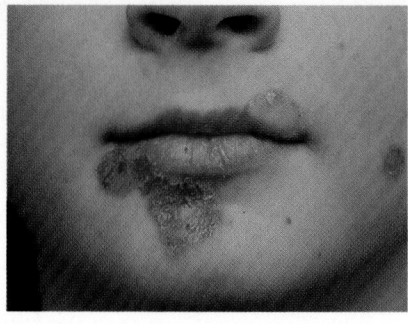

Impetigo—Fairly common superficial infection caused by bacteria (staphylococci, streptococci, or both) that usually invade at the site of a skin abrasion, scratch, or an insect bite. Infection starts with a red sore that blisters briefly and then oozes during the next few days to form a thick crust (see page 1007).

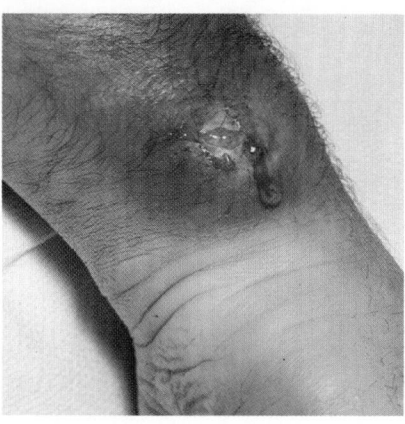

Carbuncle—Cluster of boils that form a connected area of infection under the skin. Swelling, redness, and pain may spread. It generally appears on your upper back or the nape of your neck (see page 1009).

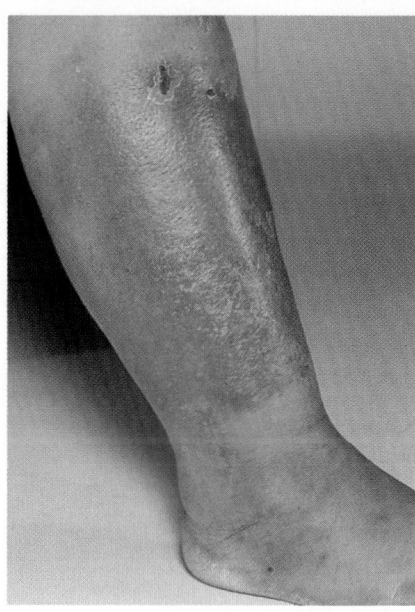

Cellulitis—This is generally caused by a bacterial infection. It is characterized by a painful area of hot, red, swollen skin (see page 1009).

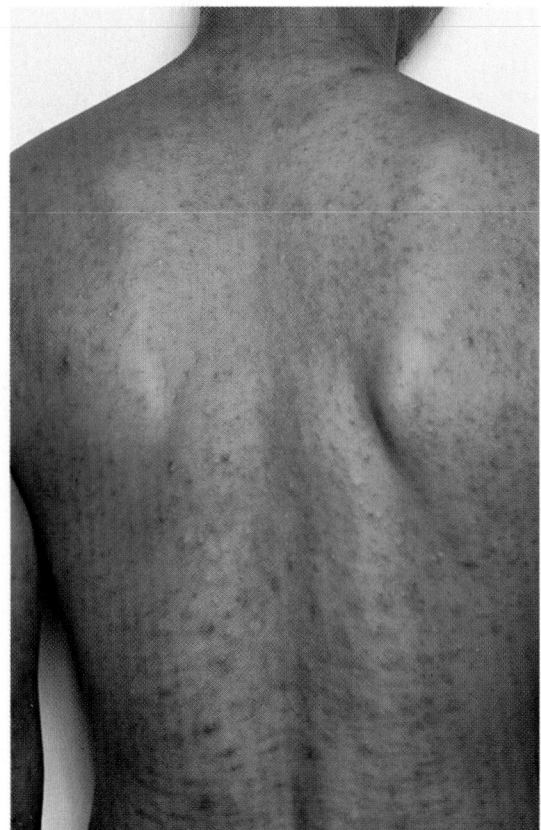

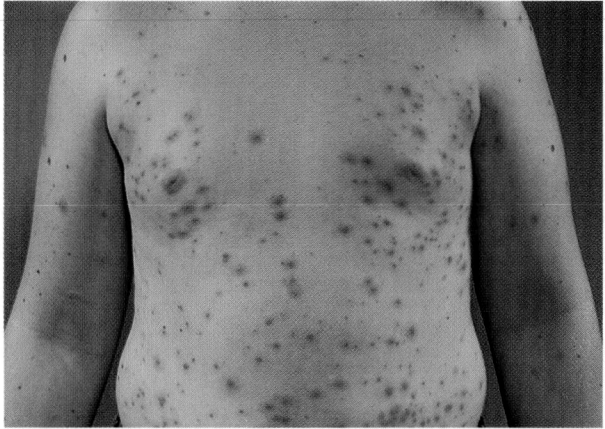

Folliculitis—Small, white-headed pimples around hair follicles. This is a superficial infection that generally is caused by bacteria or fungi. They can occur anywhere on your skin as a result of clothing friction, blockage of a hair follicle, or injury. Shaving the bearded area, neck, or underarms can aggravate this condition (see page 1007).

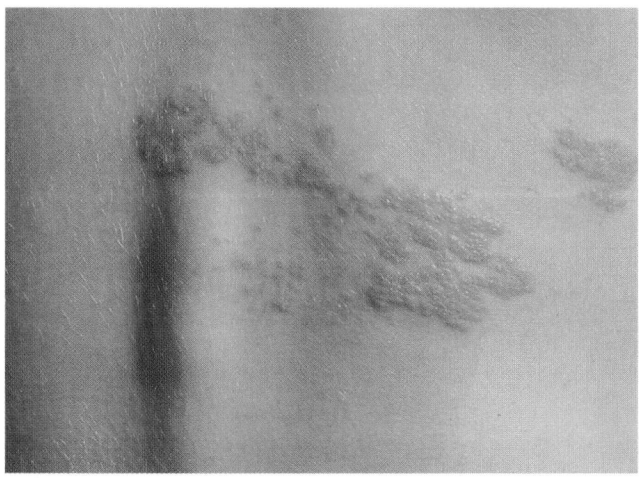

Shingles (herpes zoster)—Characterized by pain or a tingling sensation in a limited area of one side of your face or torso. A red rash follows, with small, fluid-filled blisters (see page 1011).

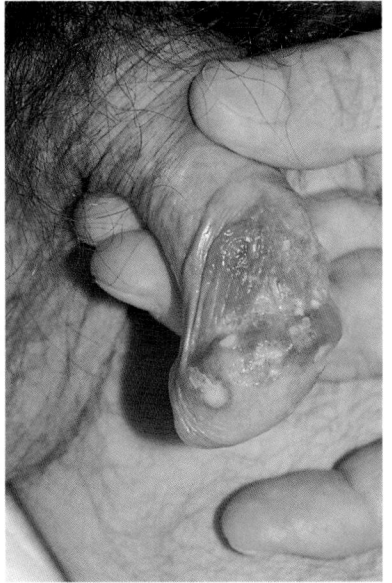

Genital herpes (herpes simplex type 2)—Lesion in the genital area, characterized by water blisters (vesicles) or open sores (ulcers). The ulcers begin as small, tender, red bumps and become water blisters within days. Pain or itching occurs. The blisters rupture, becoming ulcers that ooze or bleed. After 3 or 4 days, scabs form and the ulcers heal (see page 1090).

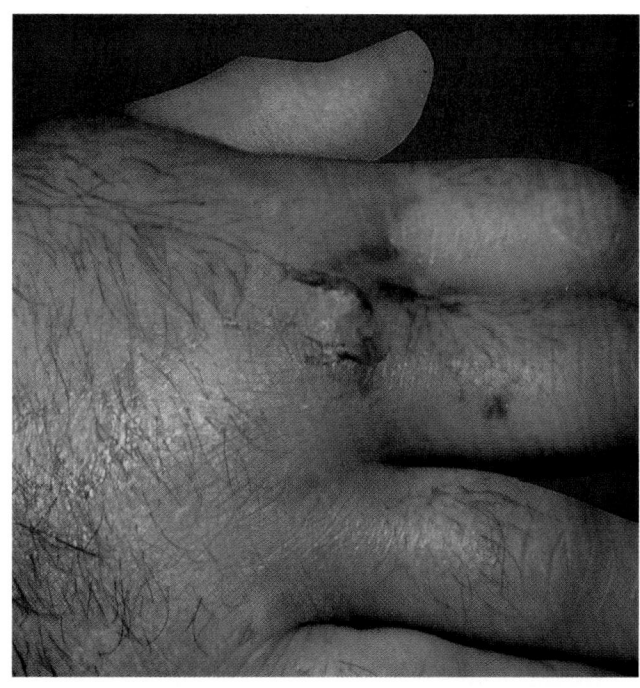

Human bite—Fight bites occur when, in the act of striking another person, the assailant cuts his or her hand or knuckles on the victim's teeth. Bacteria often enter the wound, causing infection. This injury requires prompt treatment (see pages 395 and 1015).

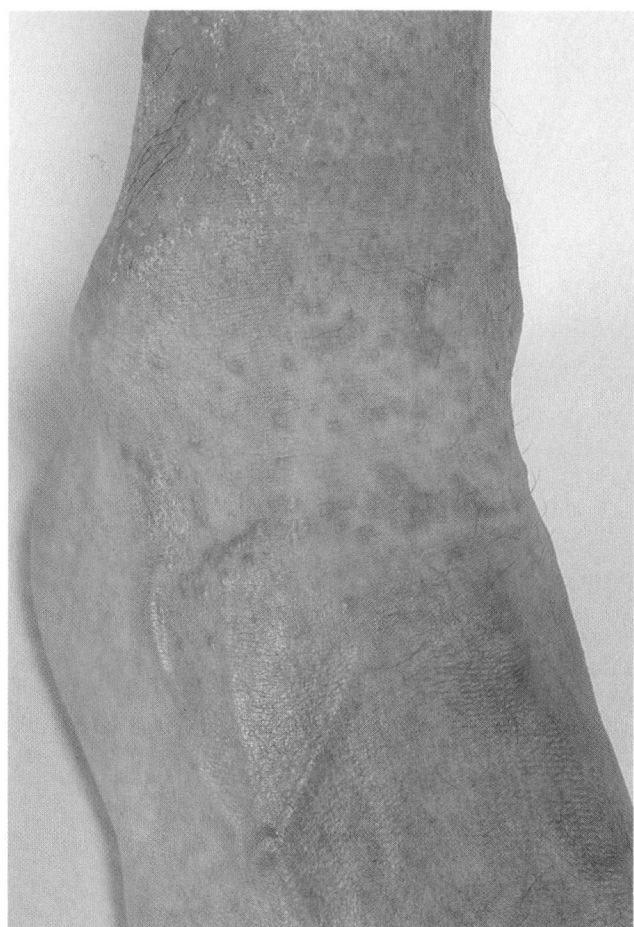

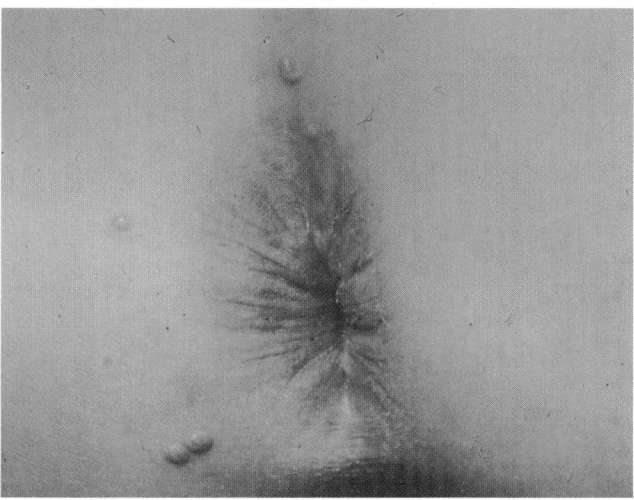

Molluscum contagiosum—A common viral infection of the skin, characterized by tiny, pearl-like projections with a core of white, cheesy matter. It is contagious by contact (see page 1012).

Portuguese man-of-war sting—Red, hive-like lesions in a line, along with stinging pain. It is caused by contact with toxic venom from a Portuguese man-of-war (see pages 399 and 1015).

Infestations and Bites

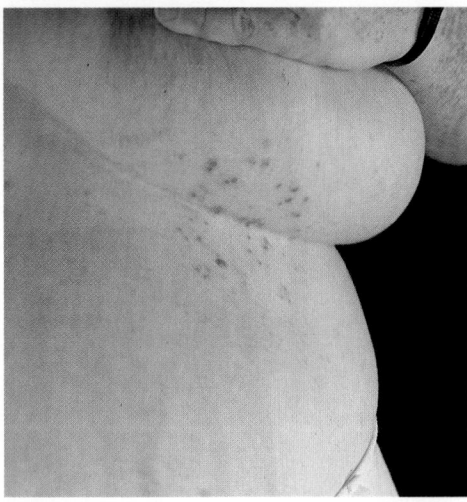

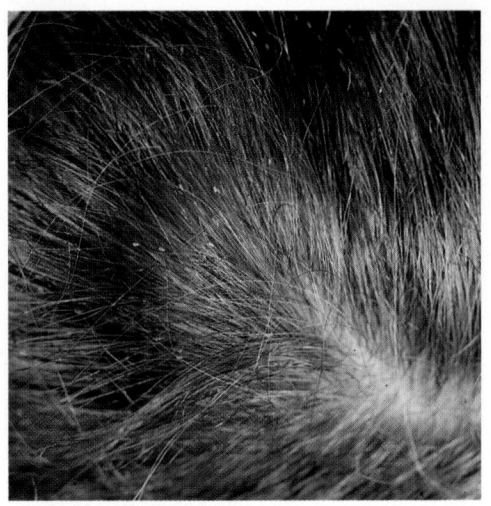

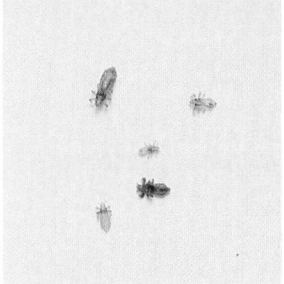

Lice—These tiny insects most frequently are transmitted by contact from person to person (see page 1085).

Scabies—Caused by tiny mites that burrow into your skin. The characteristic burrow looks like a thin, irregular pencil mark. Scabies causes severe itching (see page 1085).

Head lice—Found on the scalp and easiest to see at the nape of the neck and over the ears. Small nits (eggs) resembling tiny pussy-willow buds can be found on the hair shafts (see page 1085).

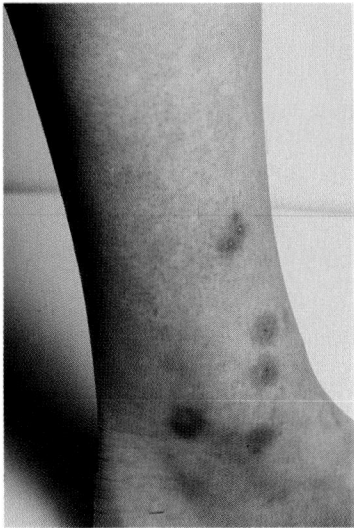

Chigger bite—Characterized by small red pimples and sometimes by hives. Intense itching is present at the site where the chigger inserts its feeding tube. Chiggers and ticks feed on human and animal blood (see page 1086).

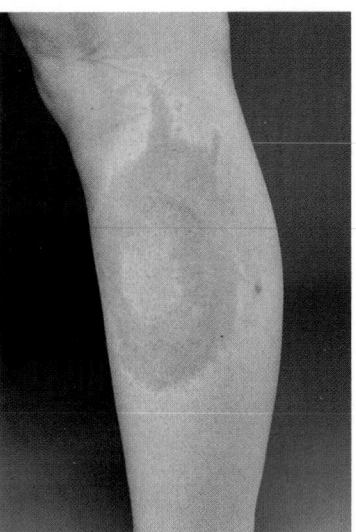

Lyme disease—Transmitted by a tick bite; results in a red rash that usually occurs at the site of the bite, followed by flu-like symptoms such as headache, chills, fever, body aches, and stiffness. The central portion of the rash clears as the rash spreads outward (see pages 396 and 1067).

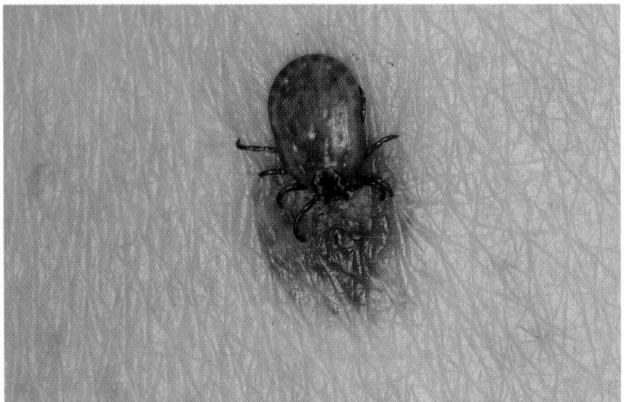

Tick bite—Small, hard, itchy lumps surrounded by a red halo (see pages 396 and 1087).

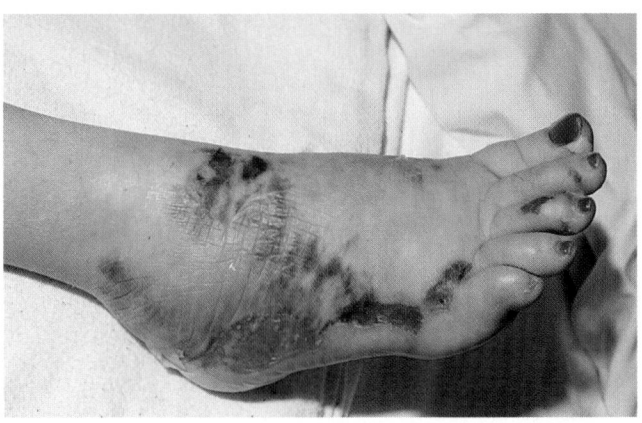

Spider bite (brown recluse)—Fluid-filled bump forms at the site of the bite, then sloughs off, sometimes leaving a large, deep, growing ulcer (see pages 396 and 1014).

Other Skin Diseases (Continued on page C-16)

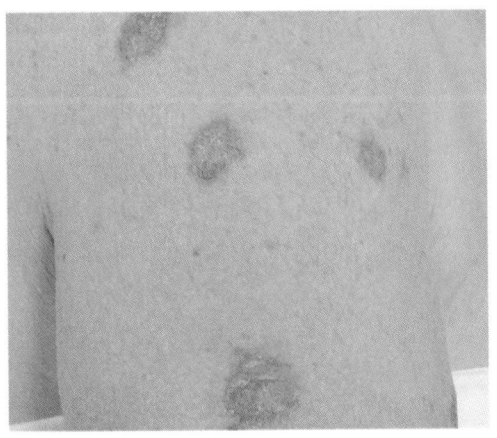

Nummular dermatitis—Inflammation of the skin in which the lesions are shaped like small coins (see Contact Dermatitis, page 987).

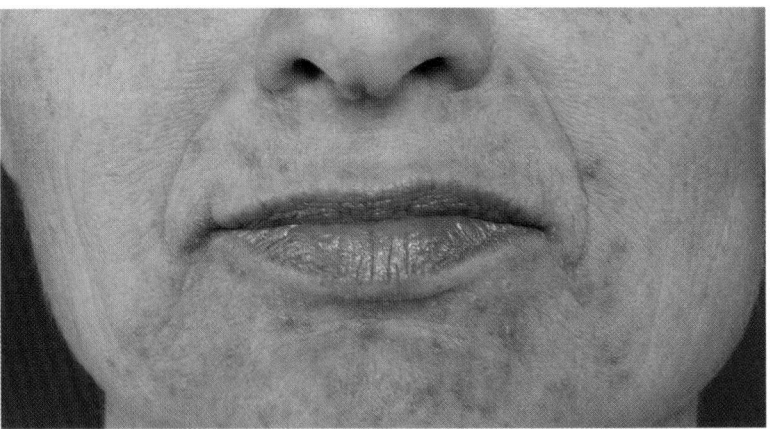

Perioral dermatitis—Inflammation of the skin around the mouth (see Contact Dermatitis, page 987).

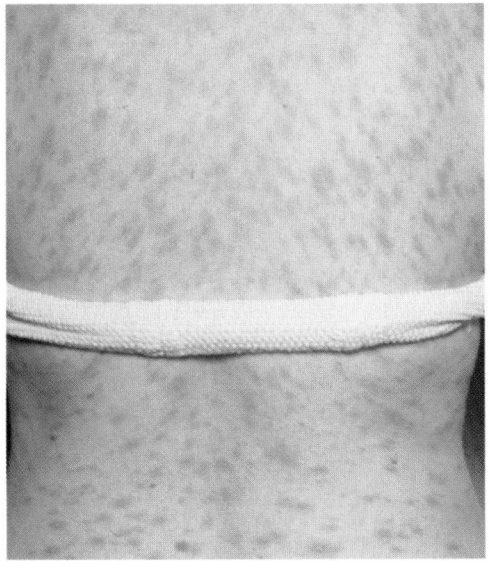

Pityriasis rosea—Common rash characterized by mild itching and red spots on the torso, upper arms, neck, and thighs. It frequently affects young people. A single, scaly, red patch on the torso may be the first sign. After several days, more spots may appear. It is probably caused by a virus. The rash disappears in 3 to 12 weeks (see page 993).

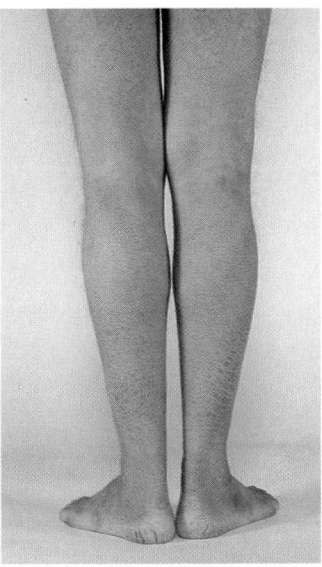

Ichthyosis—An inherited skin disorder in which the skin has a fish-scale appearance (see page 994).

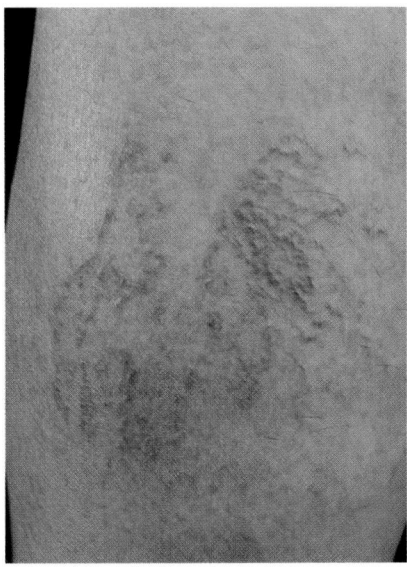

Spider veins—Collection of bluish veins seen through the skin of the leg (see page 1001).

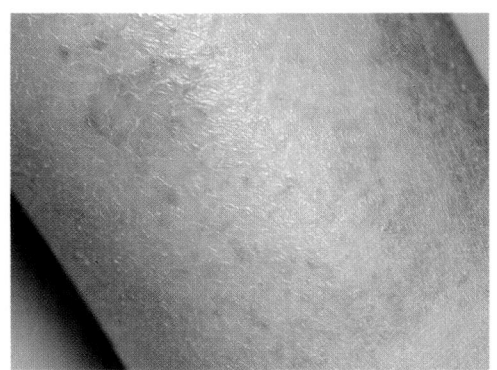

Dry skin (asteatosis)—Itchy, scaly skin. This common problem occurs particularly when air is low in humidity. The skin may become cracked. Round patches of irritated skin may develop. The most common sites are the lower legs, upper arms, sides, and thighs (see page 994).

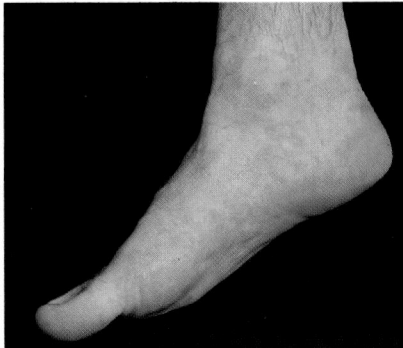

Drug rash—Skin changes may include redness, hives, blisters, and bleeding into the skin. Itching usually is present. It is caused by an allergic reaction to a medication (see page 996).

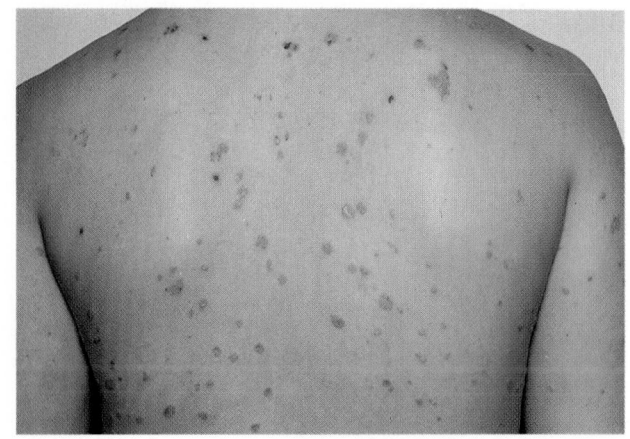

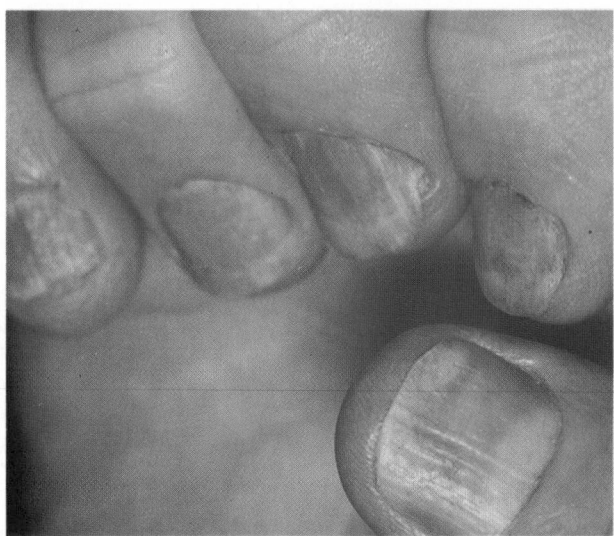

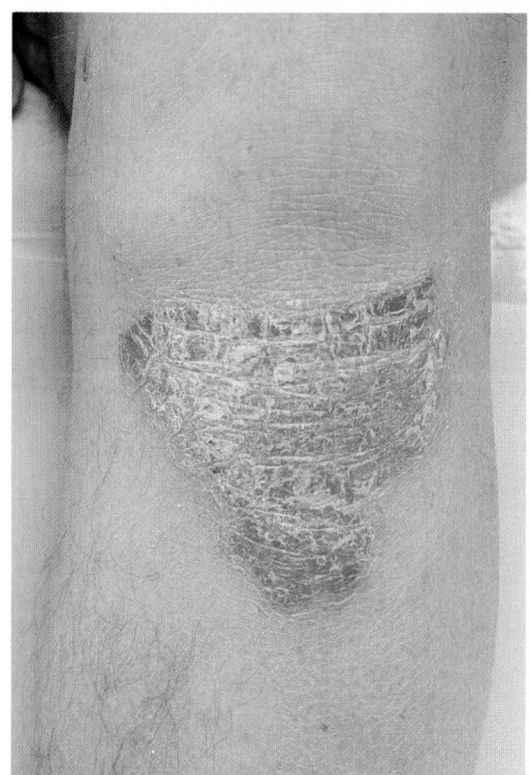

Psoriasis—Common skin disease characterized by flare-ups and partial remissions. Sometimes portions of the skin are covered with dry, red patches with silvery scales. These lesions may itch. Small, scaling dots may also be present. The most common sites are the trunk, knees, elbow, and scalp. Pits or ridges develop in the nails (see page 992).

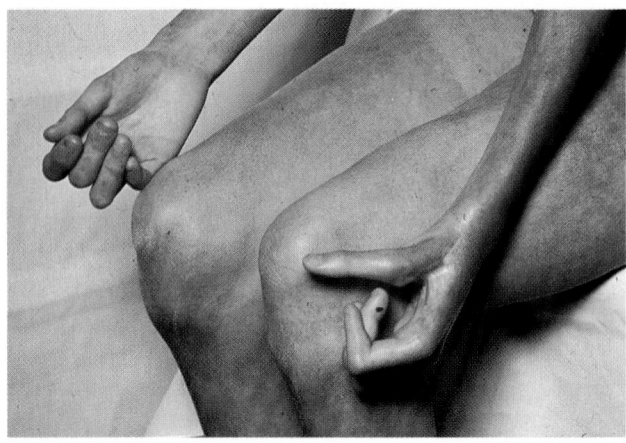

Scleroderma—Progressive systemic disorder with skin manifestations of thickening and tightening of the skin, especially on the arms, face, and hands, resulting in loss of flexibility (see page 919).

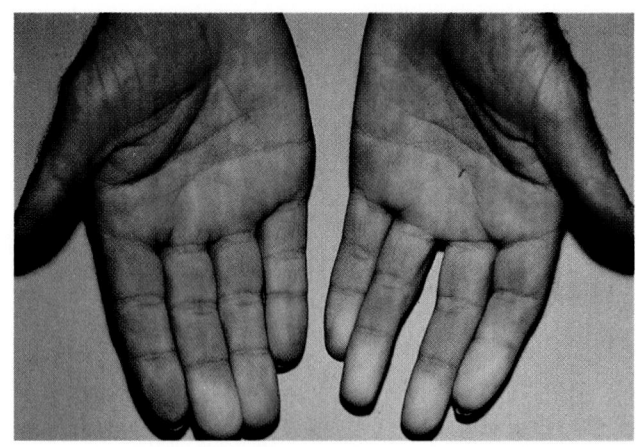

Raynaud's disease—A condition in which the fingers and toes turn white on exposure to cold, with an accompanying stinging pain. The skin may turn blue or red before it recovers (see page 697).

Boils and Carbuncles

Signs and Symptoms
- Swollen and tender nodule on your skin, usually pink or red
- Spreading area of swelling, redness, and pain in skin
- Fever or exhausted feeling

A boil (furuncle) is a local infection in one or more hair follicles and usually is caused by staphylococci. When there are multiple boils anywhere on the body, the condition is called furunculosis. In contrast, a carbuncle is a cluster of boils that forms a connected area of infection under the skin (see color photograph, page C-12). Contact with other parts of the body and other people spreads these infections easily.

Sometimes a boil will go away after the initial stage of itching or mild pain. More often, however, it grows rapidly over a few days; as pus collects within the lesion, pressure and pain increase. It comes to a head with a white or yellow center in the nodule and then bursts, drains, and heals. It may recur later near the same site and go through the same cycle.

Boils are very common, and most people get one at some time during their lifetime. A boil can occur anywhere on your skin but is most likely to appear on your face, neck, armpits, buttocks, or thighs.

Carbuncles commonly appear on the upper back and on the nape of your neck. They are less common than boils. Men are more prone to have them than women. Carbuncles develop slowly and may not reach your skin's surface to drain on their own.

Boils and carbuncles occur under various circumstances including poor hygiene, rundown physical condition, friction by clothing, and disorders including acne, dermatitis, diabetes mellitus, and pernicious anemia.

Diagnosis
The diagnosis is usually made by visual inspection of the affected area. Occasionally culture of the pus is necessary to determine the specific bacteria that caused the boil. Further tests of your blood and urine may be necessary if your physician suspects an underlying disorder.

How Serious Are Boils and Carbuncles?
A boil usually will burst within 2 weeks. Any carbuncle or boil that persists longer might spread the infection to your bloodstream or internal organs. Internal staphylococcal infections, which are life-threatening, often start from skin infections.

A boil or carbuncle on or near your nose, cheeks, forehead, or spine can spread even more rapidly to become a brain abscess or spinal abscess (see page 486). Prompt medical treatment can help prevent these serious complications.

A boil or carbuncle can produce permanent scarring, especially if it is improperly treated. The frequent occurrence of boils may indicate an underlying disorder that needs medical attention.

Treatment
Application of a warm tap-water compress to the boil for about 30 minutes every few hours will either cause it to regress and disappear or, more likely, to burst and drain much sooner. Never squeeze or lance your boil because you might spread the infection. Wash the infected area frequently with antibacterial soap, and prevent the drained matter from contacting other skin areas.

Your physician may prescribe oral antibiotic treatment for a carbuncle or boil that persists or is located on your face or spine. Surgical drainage is used for some boils and carbuncles.

Erysipelas and Cellulitis

Signs and Symptoms—Painful area of hot, red, swollen skin with lines or blisters

Cellulitis is an acute inflammation of the connective tissue in your skin that results from a bacterial infection (see color photograph, page C-12). It usually occurs with dermatitis, with a fungal infection, or after a skin injury and may be accompanied by a fever (see Wound Infections, page 1016).

Erysipelas is a severe streptococcal cellulitis in which the infected area is shiny and sharply defined. It is characterized by high fever and recurrences. Gangrene is a rare complication of these infections.

Blisters

Blisters develop when pressure or friction causes fluid to accumulate between the layers of your skin. If you feel a "hot spot" developing, stop what you're doing and cover the affected area with an adhesive bandage.

Thanks to the availability of antibiotics, blisters that become infected aren't usually a serious concern. But they are a common minor injury.

Don't puncture a blister unless it is painful or prevents you from walking or using one of your hands. Cover a small blister with an adhesive bandage, a large one with a porous, plastic-coated gauze pad that absorbs moisture and allows the wound to "breathe."

If you must open the blister, wash both your hands and the blister area with soap and warm water. Swab the blister with iodine or 70 percent alcohol. Puncture the blister at several points along the base with a sterile needle. Drain the fluid, but leave the overlying skin intact. Apply antibiotic ointment to the site and cover with a gauze pad. After a few days, use a tweezers to lift any dead skin and a scissors to cut it away. Reapply ointment and gauze, and check for signs of infection (redness or pus). See a physician if the blister becomes infected.

Treatment

After an examination, your physician may prescribe an antibiotic. This treatment usually stops the infection within a week. Elevating the infected area and applying hot, moist compresses to the site will help. If the infection spreads, you may require hospitalization for intravenous antibiotics and occasionally surgical treatment.

The pain may be sufficiently severe that your physician also may prescribe a medication for pain relief.

Lymphadenitis and Lymphangitis

Signs and Symptoms—Swollen areas of skin, sometimes with redness and pain

Lymphadenitis is an infection of lymph nodes by bacteria, viruses, fungi, or other disease-producing microorganisms; lymphangitis is a similar infection of the lymphatic channels. Pus-filled abscesses and cellulitis (see page 1009) also may occur.

Lymphangitis causes a throbbing pain in the area of the wound, malaise, a fever of 100 to 104 degrees Fahrenheit, loss of appetite, sweating, and chills. You may develop a red streak, running from the site of the infection up the extremity. Immediate treatment is essential. This infection can spread very rapidly—often in just a few hours—and may be fatal.

Diagnostic tests may include blood analyses and a lymph node culture or biopsy.

Treatment

Treatment varies, depending on the source of the infection. Antibiotic treatment—begun immediately—usually brings the disease under control in a few days, and you should recover completely. Also apply hot, moist compresses or a heating pad, elevating the area (if possible), and take aspirin. Abscesses may require drainage by your physician.

Cold Sores and Canker Sores

Signs and Symptoms
- Single or clustered, small, fluid-filled blisters on a raised, red, painful area of skin
- Painful sore inside your mouth, with a white or yellow center and red border

Cold sores, also called fever blisters, are very common infections (see color photograph, page C-10). They can appear anywhere on your body, but they are most likely to be on your gums and the outside of your mouth and lips, nose, cheeks, or fingers.

This infection, caused by the herpes simplex virus, is transmitted by contact with another person's active infection. Eating utensils, towels, and razors are other common sources. Type 1 herpes usually is responsible for fever blisters. Type 2 is responsible for genital herpes (see page 191).

Symptoms of your initial herpes infection may start as long as 20 days after exposure to the virus and may last for 7 to 10 days. The blisters form, break, and ooze; then a yellow crust forms and finally sloughs off to uncover pinkish, healing skin.

The virus reverts to a latent form within your nerve cells. However, it may emerge again as an active infection on or near the original site. You may experience an itch or heightened sensitivity at the site preceding each attack. Recurrences are generally milder than the initial infection and are triggered by menstruation, sun exposure, stress, or any illness with fever.

Canker sores that are not infectious last for 1 to 2 weeks (see color photograph, page C-10). In later stages of healing, they develop a gray membrane covering. Minor injuries, such as denture friction or biting the inside of your mouth, often precipitate development of a lesion.

Canker sores also commonly recur. They are probably a localized immune system reaction to unknown causes. These sores usually start between age 10 and 40 and may recur for years with one or more ulcers. Recurrences can be unpredictable or may be triggered by stress, fatigue, or food allergies. A tingling or burning sensation may precede an attack. Then a red spot or bump forms where an ulcer will appear. Severe attacks may have additional symptoms of fever, listlessness, and swollen glands. Women are more prone to develop canker sores than men. Sometimes there is a family history of the disease.

Diagnosis

Your physician will diagnose either disease by examining you. A culture of material from your sore or a blood test can confirm the presence of herpes simplex virus.

How Serious Are Cold Sores and Canker Sores?

Treatment often can alleviate cold sores. However, this infection can cause potentially serious complications. The infection can spread to your eye; this is the most frequent cause of corneal blindness in the United States.

If you have a cold sore, avoid contact with infants, anyone who has atopic dermatitis (see page 989), or those using an immune-system-suppression medication (such as persons with cancer or an organ transplant). Your virus can cause a life-threatening condition for these people.

Treatment

To reduce discomfort from a canker sore, avoid spicy and acidic foods. Apply ice to relieve the pain of a cold sore. Your physician may prescribe an antiviral medication called acyclovir for your cold sore.

Physicians usually recommend mouthwashes for recurring canker sores. For severe attacks, your physician may prescribe a solution containing an antibiotic or an antihistamine or suggest the use of a corticosteroid preparation applied locally or taken by mouth.

Shingles

Signs and Symptoms—Pain or tingling sensation in a limited area of one side of your body or face; a red rash follows, characterized by small, fluid-filled blisters

The same virus that causes chickenpox causes shingles (herpes zoster), a localized infection (see color photograph, page C-13). After you have had chickenpox, the virus may become dormant within your nerve cells. It can emerge years later as shingles.

For unknown reasons the symptoms occur in a sequence as the virus reactivates. The initial sensation is pain or tingling as the virus proliferates along one of the peripheral nerves that spreads outward from your spine. It affects only the area of your face or body served by that nerve. A rash appears 2 or 3 days later, after the virus reaches the nerve endings in your skin.

Over the next 3 to 5 days, the rash reaches its maximum extent. This can be a rectangular belt on one side of your body from your spine to your breastbone (*zoster* is Latin for "belt"), over an extremity, or on one side of your face or head. The blisters dry up in a few days, forming crusts that fall off 2 or 3 weeks after your initial symptoms.

Each year, about 300,000 Americans have a shingles infection. It can occur at any age but is most common after 50. Recurrence is possible and is more likely if you take a medication to suppress your immune system.

Because your immune system protects you from a new invasion by the virus that causes chickenpox, you cannot "catch" shingles from someone else if you've already had chickenpox. However, you can develop shingles if you have not had chickenpox and are exposed to someone with shingles.

Diagnosis

The diagnosis is based on the history of your symptoms and the characteristic appearance of the rash.

How Serious Is Shingles?

Shingles normally is not a serious condition, although you may have continuing pain for months or even years along the peripheral nerve involved. This agonizingly painful condition, called postherpetic neuralgia (PHN), occurs in half of the people who have had shingles and are older than 70.

Shingles damages nerve fibers. Their ability to send messages from your skin becomes confused and exaggerated. People with PHN often say they have multiple types of pain—sometimes at the same time.

When shingles affects a major nerve in your face, the trigeminal nerve, the rash can occur on your face and inside your mouth or eye. If you have shingles, any pain or rash in or near your eye requires prompt medical attention by an ophthalmologist, because an eye infection can lead to permanent eyesight damage.

Shingles can be debilitating if your immune system is weakened or if you have certain forms of cancer, including leukemia and Hodgkin's disease. Medications used after transplantation, for example, suppress your immune system and make you vulnerable to shingles.

Treatment

Early treatment of shingles is important, because prompt intervention can curtail the infection and possibly decrease your chances of persistent pain. See your physician as soon as symptoms occur.

To be most effective, therapy must begin at the first sign of the disease—preferably within 3 days of the onset of the disease. Aggressive treatment may prevent extensive damage to your nerves. It may help prevent a chronic pain pattern from forming in your central nervous system.

A three-pronged treatment approach includes high doses of an antiviral drug (acyclovir or ganciclovir) to reduce the duration and severity of symptoms, an anti-inflammatory drug to ease inflammation, and oral pain killers and injected anesthetics for severe pain.

You may obtain some relief by soaking your blistered areas with cool, wet compresses (aluminum acetate solution) and applying a soothing lotion. Analgesics such as aspirin may help alleviate the milder pain of PHN. Be sure to see an ophthalmologist if shingles may potentially involve your eye.

Molluscum Contagiosum

Signs and Symptoms—Tiny, pearl-like papules on the skin with a core of white, cheesy matter

Molluscum contagiosum is a relatively common viral infection of the skin (see color photograph, page C-13). Each small, globular papule characteristically has a small black dot on its summit. In children, nodules usually appear on the face, trunk, or limbs. The infection is contagious by contact. In adults, common sites are the genitals, abdomen, and inner thighs. It frequently is spread through sexual contact.

The firm nodules are often painless and disappear within a year. If the nodules and surrounding skin are injured, local spreading can occur.

Treatment

Left untreated, more lesions may occur as the virus sheds from lesions to normal skin. Your physician can remove the nodules by freezing, surgical scraping, or squeezing out the core matter.

Fungal Infections

Signs and Symptoms
- Itchy, red, soggy, flaking, and cracking skin between the toes
- Itchy, fluid-filled bumps on the sides or sole of your foot
- Extreme dryness with small, white scales on the sides or sole of your foot or the palm of your hand
- Itchy, red or grayish, scaling patches on the scalp, with partial baldness or broken hairs
- Itchy, red, scaly, slightly raised, expanding rings on the trunk, face, or groin/thigh fold
- Red, moist, well-marked patches, rimmed with small, red bumps in the armpits, navel, groin or buttock/thigh fold, under the breasts, or between fingers or toes
- Reddened areas with white patches inside the mouth or cracks at the mouth corner
- Small, slightly scaling, pale patches on the upper body, neck, or face

Fungal infections are caused by microscopic plants that become parasites on your skin. Your body hosts a great variety of microorganisms including mold- and yeast-like fungi. Some serve useful purposes, or cause no problems. Others can proliferate as infectious colonies.

Mold-like fungi called dermatophytes

cause athlete's foot, jock itch, and ringworm of the skin or scalp (see this page). These fungi live on dead tissues of your hair, nails, and the outer layer of your skin. Poor hygiene, continually moist skin, and minor skin or nail injuries increase your susceptibility to infection by these fungi.

Ringworm often affects children (see color photograph, page C-8). The characteristic rings may be irregular and can expand beyond the scalp. The ring grows outward as the infection spreads and the central area becomes less actively infected. This type of infection is very contagious and can be passed from shared hats, combs or brushes, and barber tools. It is also possible to be infected with scalp or skin ringworm from pets or domestic animals.

Some fungal infections are referred to as yeast or *Candida* infections. These ailments result from infection with a fungus of the genus *Candida*. Examples include diaper rash and oral infections, called oral thrush, which is common in babies (see color photographs, pages C-2 and C-10). Chafing can occur in folds of skin of overweight people. Genital infections (see page 1173) can be transmitted sexually.

Pregnancy, obesity, endocrine disorders such as diabetes mellitus, cancers such as leukemia, inherited or AIDS-produced immune system deficiencies, and use of certain medications (antibiotics effective against various organisms or large doses of adrenal corticosteroids) increase your susceptibility to a *Candida* infection.

Another type of yeast infection, tinea versicolor, appears as a tissue-thin coating of fungus on your skin (see color photograph, page C-8). The only symptoms are patches of discolored skin that slowly grow. Tinea versicolor is common among teenagers and young adults.

Diagnosis

Frequently, fungal infections cause quite specific skin changes. Thus, your physician may only need to examine your skin to make the diagnosis. At other times your physician will need to obtain material from the lesion for laboratory analysis.

How Serious Are Fungal Infections?

These infections are rarely life-threatening. They can range from mild to severe attacks and often persist or recur. Treatment is gen-erally successful, but may include long-term medication and continued use of preventive measures, particularly for infections in your nails.

A skin infection by *Candida* can spread through your bloodstream to internal organs. This is rare, but, if you have a fever, eye pain, visual disturbances, or symptoms of meningitis, prompt medical attention is necessary (see page 481). Although some people blame *Candida* infections for a wide variety of symptoms, including chronic fatigue syndrome (see page 1065), evidence for this is lacking.

Treatment

For athlete's foot, skin ringworm, and jock itch, apply over-the-counter antifungal agents (miconazole, clotrimazole, Whitfield's ointment, or Castellani paint). Your physician may prescribe an oral antifungal medication if one of these infections is chronic or severe, or for scalp ringworm. Antibiotics may be prescribed if a secondary bacterial infection develops.

To treat diaper rash in babies and chafing (intertrigo) infections in adults, apply over-the-counter antifungal agents and keep the area clean and dry, dusting it with antifungal powder. Oral thrush medications are available in lozenge or mouthwash form.

For severe or persistent *Candida* infections, your physician may prescribe an oral antifungal medication. Because there are potentially serious side effects from long-term oral use of antifungal medications, it's important that your physician supervise this treatment.

For tinea versicolor, frequent showering can help. Also apply sulfur medications (such as sodium thiosulfite or sodium hyposulfite) to your skin overnight for a month. An alternative medication is selenium sulfide, applied over a 5-day period.

Jock Itch and Athlete's Foot

Fungi that thrive in warm, moist areas cause jock itch and athlete's foot (see color photographs, page C-8). They are common in athletes as well as in people who are obese or who perspire a great deal. In both cases, the primary symptoms are itching and a rash.

Jock itch consists of itching in the groin and anal area; with athlete's foot there is itching, stinging, and burning on the soles of the feet, on the palms, and between the fingers and toes. Cracking of the skin and peeling may occur as well.

These infections are mildly contagious. Common means of transmission include contact in public showers and swimming areas, shared towels, or contaminated bath mats. Extreme dryness on your soles or palms is more likely to be associated with fungal infections of your nails (see page 1022).

Preventing or treating jock itch and athlete's foot requires good personal hygiene. To prevent jock itch, keep the area clean and dry, avoid chafing, and launder athletic supporters frequently. To treat it, dust the area with antifungal drying powders two or three times a day (no more or your irritation may become worse). Antifungal creams are available for use at bedtime.

Wearing sandals in a public shower or using foot troughs at the local pool entry may not prevent athlete's foot. The key to prevention is to keep your feet dry. Always dry them thoroughly after bathing. Antifungal powders also can help.

Avoid socks manufactured from synthetic fibers. Synthetic fibers do not absorb moisture very well. Instead, select socks made from cotton, wool, or a combination of these. And change your socks frequently. Wear well-ventilated shoes with leather soles, not shoes with synthetic uppers and hard rubber soles. Also, alternate daily among two or more pairs of shoes. Each pair then can dry completely and will absorb more moisture.

Insect Bites

Signs and Symptoms
- Itchy, red bumps
- Red, painful, ulcerating sore
- Local numbness or pins-and-needles sensation

Emergency Symptoms
- Swollen face, widespread numbness, muscle cramping, breathing difficulty, headache, nausea, or fever
- Coma

The injection of venom or other agents into your skin causes symptoms of insect bites. Most often the reaction is local and temporary. However, the venom can affect your entire body if you are hypersensitive to the venom or if it is exceptionally potent.

The bite of a black widow spider feels like a pinprick. Some people are not aware they've been bitten. At first, there may be only slight swelling and faint red marks in the area of the bite. Within a few hours, however, intense pain and stiffness begin. Other symptoms may include chills, fever, nausea, and severe abdominal pain. Generally, the pain lessens after a few hours but may return over the next 2 to 3 days.

Bites by the brown recluse (see color photograph, page C-14) and other spiders cause a mild stinging followed by local redness and intense pain within 8 hours. A fluid-filled bump forms at the site and then sloughs off, sometimes leaving a large, deep, growing ulcer. Your body reactions can vary from a mild fever and rash to nausea and listlessness.

Most ant bites cause only local redness and swelling. Fire ants, however, can produce many small, fluid-filled bumps that ulcerate like spider bites.

Other biting insects usually inject their chemicals as they feed on you. These insects include mosquitoes, fleas, flies, bedbugs, and chiggers.

Stings by bees, wasps, and hornets inject venom that causes immediate pain and rapidly growing red bumps. A sting will subside and turn itchy in a few hours, unless you have an allergic reaction (see Insect Sting Allergies, page 1051).

Diagnosis
Sometimes you can recognize an insect bite or sting easily, because you feel the sting when it happens. At other times, bites just seem to appear. If you have a severe reaction, knowing what bit you will help your physician determine the treatment.

How Serious Are Insect Bites?
Symptoms from a typical bite or sting generally last a few hours or days. However, if you are allergic to bee stings, or if you receive multiple stings, this can be life-threatening and requires emergency treatment. About 1 in 250 Americans is allergic to bee stings. These stings cause more deaths than snake bites. Poisonous spider bites are rarely fatal, but small children and the elderly are especially vulnerable.

Treatment
Mild insect bites are generally treated by applying ice cubes to decrease pain and over-the-counter hydrocortisone cream or calamine lotion to relieve itching or inflammation. Your physician may prescribe cor-

ticosteroid cream for more severe reactions.

Carefully remove bee stingers. More severe reactions may require immediate injections of antihistamine and an antispasm drug. If faintness, listlessness, or shortness of breath occurs, seek emergency medical care immediately. Your physician can prescribe an emergency medical kit for you to keep handy if you are hypersensitive to bee or hornet stings.

Persons with black widow spider bites may require hospitalization, where treatment includes hot soaks, intravenous infusion of calcium gluconate to relieve cramps, and injections of antivenin. Brown recluse spider bite treatment includes corticosteroid injections and surgical scraping of the ulcer.

Portuguese Man-of-War Stings

Signs and Symptoms
- Stinging and pain
- Red, hive-like lesions in a line
- Shortness of breath, nausea, stomach cramps, and emotional upset

The Portuguese man-of-war is a colony of free-floating individual organisms. Like the jellyfish, it is invertebrate (without a backbone). It is easy to recognize, on account of the highly characteristic blue or red bell-shaped body that floats at the surface of the water and ranges from less than 1 inch to more than a foot in width. A cluster of tentacles hangs beneath the body of the man-of-war. Most are short and frilly; however, one or more can be many feet long. These long fishing tentacles are responsible for the stings.

If you touch one of these tentacles it will whip around the contact area and inject a toxic venom into your skin. Because the venom (a neurotoxin) remains potent long after the man-of-war is dead, wading in shallow water or walking along the beach can be hazardous. The tentacles discharge their venom for long periods, even after they are separated from the main body of the man-of-war. The venom is carried into the victim by tiny barbs on the tentacles.

How Serious Are Man-of-War Stings?
Death from man-of-war stings is unusual, but stings can be painful. Common symptoms range from mild prickling to severe burning and numbness. A red line devel-

Human Bites

Animal bites are commonplace: about 1,000 people visit hospital emergency rooms each day for treatment of dog or other animal bites. Human bites are less common but represent an equally serious medical problem.

There are two kinds of human bites. A "true bite," like most animal bites, is the injury that results from flesh being caught between the teeth of the upper and lower jaws. "Fight bites" occur when, in the act of striking another person, an assailant cuts his or her knuckles on the victim's teeth (see color photograph, page C-13).

Such bites may seem superficial, but the cut (laceration) may extend below the skin, injuring tendons and joints. The human mouth also contains many bacteria, and the saliva that enters at the site of the puncture may cause serious infections. There is little risk of rabies, but there is danger of transmission of the hepatitis B virus.

You may fear embarrassment or even legal action if you go to the emergency room for treatment of a fight bite. However, remember that you risk a prolonged hospital stay, permanent joint stiffness, and even amputation if a serious infection is not promptly treated. Whether yours is a true bite or a fight bite, seek help before the risks become more serious.

ops on the area of the skin exposed to the tentacles. Sometimes a string of welts or blisters develops (see color photograph, page C-13).

Severe stings can lead to muscle cramping, fainting, coughing, vomiting, and difficulty breathing. In rare cases, a potentially fatal reaction (see Anaphylaxis, page 444) may occur.

Treatment
Here are practical tips for coping with man-of-war stings:

Get Out of the Water. The pain and cramps can be disabling and cause you to drown.

Deactivate the Stinging. Sprinkle the area with meat tenderizer, vinegar, salt, sugar, or even dry sand and gently rub this material into the wounds. This often offers quick relief.

Cleanse the Wound. After waiting 15 to 20 minutes, gently wash the area with sea water. Do not use fresh water and do not rub the skin, because either action could trigger discharge of more venom.

Remove the Stinging Tentacles. Apply a paste made of sea water and sand (or baking soda, talcum powder, or flour). Scrape the residue with a knife or other sharp object such as a clam shell. It is best to wear gloves or use a towel in removing the residue.

Apply Medication. You can use hydrocortisone cream (0.5 percent) to relieve redness and swelling. It is available without a prescription. A local anesthetic ointment (such as benzocaine) helps relieve pain, and a calamine-type lotion reduces itching. Mild analgesics such as aspirin and acetaminophen are often useful, but prescription pain killers may be necessary after severe stings.

Prevention. Extra clothing is your best protection from the man-of-war, particularly a wet suit or body stocking if you are swimming in waters where they live. Also, wear sneakers or plastic beach shoes while walking along the beach. And watch where you step.

Wound Infections

Signs and Symptoms
- Swelling, discoloration, and death of the surrounding tissue
- Hot, inflamed skin around a wound
- Elevated temperature

After an injury that causes a break in the skin or after an operation, various wound infections may occur. Among them is cellulitis (inflammation of the skin, see page 1009). Others can result in death or decay of tissues (gangrene).

Necrotizing Subcutaneous Infection
This is a severe infection caused by bacteria that infect the tissue through wounds. The primary symptoms are swelling, discoloration, and death of the surrounding tissue. The skin around the wound becomes hot, inflamed, tender, and red. If the infection worsens, the skin becomes discolored and gangrene may develop. Occasionally, this is referred to as an infection by "flesh-eating bacteria."

This infection most often is caused by aerobic bacteria (which require oxygen to live) or anaerobic bacteria (unable to live in the presence of oxygen). In treating it, your physician will select an antibiotic. To determine the correct antibiotic to prescribe, your physician will take a sample of pus for culture to identify the bacteria present. Your physician must often thoroughly open the wound, so that all infected tissue can be removed. One operation usually is not suf-ficient to remove all the dead tissue. It will frequently be necessary to perform a second operation. If the infection involves an arm or leg, amputation eventually may be necessary.

Gas Gangrene
Gangrene is death of the tissue. Gas gangrene results when a wound becomes infected by certain bacteria, usually *Clostridium*. This infection causes sudden pain and swelling around the wound, a moderate increase in temperature, a decrease in blood pressure, and a rapid heartbeat. Skin around the wound becomes pale due to fluid that builds up under it. A watery, foul-smelling, brownish red fluid is released later. The tissue changes from pale to dusky to highly discolored as the infection worsens. Left untreated, stupor, delirium, coma, and death result.

Treatment consists of penicillin given intravenously. Surgical removal of infected tissue is essential, and removal of surrounding tissue usually is necessary.

Cutaneous Abscess
Bacteria, usually occurring after a minor wound, causes this pus-filled sore on the skin. Sometimes the lymph glands in the area become swollen, and you may have a fever.

Treatment consists of opening the infected area, thoroughly cleaning and irrigating the wound with saline, and packing it with gauze for 24 to 48 hours to absorb the pus and discharge. Application of heat and, if possible, elevating the affected area help relieve the inflammation. Injection of antibiotics into a muscle or through a vein often is appropriate treatment for these infections.

Animal Bites
Cats and dogs cause most of the bite wounds seen in hospital emergency rooms. Cat bites are the most likely to cause a bacterial infection. If you are bitten by a cat or dog and have not had a tetanus shot recently, you may need a booster (see Tetanus, page 1070). You may also need rabies treatment (see Rabies, page 1070).

In all cases, prompt, thorough cleaning of the wound is essential. This often involves opening the wound and removing all areas of infected tissue. Also, soak your wound in warm water and, if possible, elevate and immobilize the affected part. You will probably receive an antibiotic.

Hair

Keratin, the same protein that makes up nails and the outer layer of skin, makes up hair. The part of the hair that rises out of your skin is the hair shaft or strand. An average head has about 100,000 of them.

Below your skin is the hair root, enclosed by a sac-like structure called the hair follicle. Tiny blood vessels at the base of the follicle provide nourishment. A nearby oil-producing gland keeps the hair shiny and somewhat waterproof.

Each strand consists of three layers. The outermost layer, or cuticle, is thin and colorless. The middle layer, or cortex, is the thickest. It determines your hair color and whether your hair is straight or curly.

Your hair color is due to melanin from your pigment cells. Blondes have few melanin granules in the cortex layer and brunettes have many. The innermost layer, or medulla, is nearly colorless and does not extend all the way to the tip of the hair shaft. Light reflected from the medulla creates the sheen and the variations in color tone.

Like skin cells, hair grows and is shed regularly. You normally lose 50 to 100 strands a day. The average rate of growth is about ½ inch a month. Each hair grows for 2 to 6 years and then rests. At any time, about 85 percent of your hair is growing and the other 15 percent is resting. After its rest period, the hair falls out and a new one starts to form.

Your hair says a lot about you. Getting it to make the statement you want may not be easy. Americans spend a great deal of time and money to curl, color, spike, slick, restore, or remove their hair. This section describes some of the problems you can have with your hair, as well as how to take proper care of it.

Female-Pattern Baldness

Signs and Symptoms
- General thinning of hair all over the head
- Moderate loss of hair on the crown or at your hairline

It is normal for a woman's hair to thin out gradually as she grows older. You might have as much hair at age 80 as you did at 18, but this would be unusual. The other extreme, extensive hair loss, is probably the result of inheriting, from both of your parents, genes that tend toward baldness. The hair loss in women is far less prominent than the usual male-pattern baldness.

The distribution of your hair is largely controlled by your endocrine system through a group of hormones known as androgens. Major changes in androgen production can have a significant effect on your hair. For example, you may find that during or after the hormonal changes of menopause, the hair on your head has definitely thinned out while your facial hair has grown more coarse.

Poor nutrition, pregnancy, internal or scalp disorders, hair damage, and medications can cause hair loss in women. When some substance or condition causes a transitory problem, you may experience a temporary hair loss (see page 1018).

Treatment
Your physician can diagnose female-pattern baldness by ruling out other causes for your hair loss. A dermatologist can advise you on various methods that might stop the hair loss or restore the hair that is lost. These methods, discussed in the section on making hair grow (see page 1019), include use of surface medications such as hormonal creams, irritants or sensitizers to promote hair growth, minoxidil treatments, and transplants.

You also may want to seek the advice of a hair-care expert in choosing a new hairstyle or perhaps a hairpiece that flatters you.

Male-Pattern Baldness

Signs and Symptoms
- Receding hairline
- Moderate to extensive loss of hair, especially on the crown

Male baldness usually begins with thinning at your hairline, followed by the appearance of a thinned or bald spot on the crown of your head. You also may find your hair is finer and does not grow as long as it once did. Common baldness accounts for 99 percent of hair loss in men and women. Unlike hair loss resulting from disease or other non-hereditary factors, hair loss due to common baldness is permanent.

Part of the explanation for this pattern is your inheritance, which is complex and not well understood. Baldness is also due to aging and is affected by hormones called androgens, a major determining factor for hair distribution in both sexes.

Your hair grows in a cycle, as described in the introduction to this section (see page 1017). At the end of its cycle, each resting hair falls out and a new hair normally forms in the root. In male-pattern baldness, the rate of growth and the intervals between periods of growth shorten. Thus, the periods of growth occur more often but more and more roots fail to produce new hair at the end of each cycle.

You may want to check with your physician to be sure that your hair loss is not the result of some medical problem (see Temporary Hair Loss, this page).

Treatment

Although there is no cure for common baldness, treatment may take one of two forms: surgical hair replacement or use of the prescription drug minoxidil. Both approaches are costly.

Although researchers continue to study and test minoxidil in combination with other medications, most experts concur that only about 30 percent of men who try it achieve new hair growth, and the drug's lifelong benefits have not been established. You must rub it into or spray it on your scalp twice daily and continue the treatment indefinitely. Any hair growth resulting from this treatment will cease if you stop using minoxidil.

Surgical hair replacement can give you back a head of your own hair. Available since the 1950s, this low-risk procedure involves removing tiny plugs (grafts) of your own hair-bearing skin (taken from the band of hair extending from above your ears around the back of your scalp) and transplanting them into tiny holes made in your scalp. During one session, your surgeon may transplant between 60 and 100 hair plugs, each about the diameter of a pencil eraser. Local anesthesia and mild sedatives minimize discomfort during the surgery. Hospitalization usually is unnecessary. You may need additional surgeries to fill the balding area.

Surgeons using newer micro- or mini-grafting techniques use smaller grafts, making it possible to fashion a more natural-looking hairline with few hairs in front and thicker clumps toward the back of your head. Your surgeon may implant 150 to 200 micro-grafts per surgical session. Large bald spots may still require several surgeries. This technique can also be effective when hair loss has caused diffuse thinning. Your surgeon will gradually transplant numerous tiny micro-grafts into small incisions that supplement existing hairs nearby.

Within a few days after your operation, tiny scabs form around each hair graft. When the scabs disappear, the donor hairs usually fall out. New hairs generally start to grow within a few months.

You may want to check with hair-care experts about hairpieces, weaving techniques, or changing your hairstyle. For some men, shorter hair minimizes the contrast produced by male-pattern baldness and creates a distinguished image. Schemes for growing hair are among the more common health-oriented scams. Evaluate any such proposal carefully.

Temporary Hair Loss

Signs and Symptoms
- Small bald patch(es) on the scalp
- General thinning of scalp hair
- Loss of scalp, eyebrow, and eyelash hair
- Complete loss of hair over the body

Gradual hair loss can occur for a wide variety of reasons including excessive hair styling treatments, tight hairstyles, compulsive abuse (twisting, rubbing, or pulling), skin diseases or infections, internal disorders, high fever, stress, poor nutrition (a crash diet or anorexia), use of birth control pills, and medical treatments such as with anticancer drugs.

Sudden hair loss most commonly is due to alopecia areata, a condition that occurs in 2 percent of the population. Alopecia areata starts abruptly with one or more circular bald patches, up to 3 inches across, that may overlap. These bald areas are smooth and painless (see color photograph, page C-7).

The cause of alopecia areata is unknown. Factors may include stress, family predisposition, and autoimmune reactions to your own hair follicles.

In 90 percent of the cases, the hair grows back within 6 to 24 months. The outcome is worse if the episode occurs early in life or if you lose all scalp hair in a single episode.

To diagnose alopecia areata, your physician will perform a complete medical history and examination. Tests may be necessary, if an underlying disorder might be the cause.

Treatment

Treatment will depend on curing or controlling any underlying condition, if one exists. Your physician may suggest various techniques to make your hair grow (see this page).

Hirsutism

Signs and Symptoms—Growth of hair in inappropriate locations (on the cheeks and upper lip for women, for example)

There is a paradox about hair. People generally regard an ample and healthy head of it as beautiful. But the presence of hair in inappropriate locations is not. Among women, for example, hair on the cheeks, upper lip, underarms, or legs is considered, by many women and men, to be unattractive.

The amounts of normal facial and body hair vary greatly from one person to another. Our society regards the norm to be almost no hair on the face, body, arms, or legs of women and only moderate body and extremity hair for men.

Many women develop considerable amounts of body and facial hair during puberty; in some cases, even faint mustaches appear. The normal secretion of androgen hormones produces many changes in a young girl's body, including hair growth in the pubic and armpit regions. Some women—mainly those of southern European or Middle-Eastern ancestry—develop noteworthy amounts of facial and body hair; others, typically of northern European extraction, do not.

In women, the amount of hair usually increases slowly with age, even past menopause. Similarly, men may develop considerable body hair as they age.

The presence of too much hair is called hirsutism. How much is too much is largely a matter of personal perception. Part of the solution to a cosmetic problem of excessive hair is the simple acceptance that the amount you have is right for you. On the other hand, if you have a sudden increase in hair (for example, over a period of a few months), consult your physician. There may be a medical cause.

Can Lost Hair Grow Again?

Even after your hair is lost, the roots usually remain alive. This suggests the possibility of new growth.

Cortisone tablets taken orally sometimes promote hair growth. Unfortunately, prolonged use can cause physical or mental side effects, and the new hair usually falls out when you discontinue the tablets. Other forms of cortisone are rubbed or injected into your scalp. Their effect is often temporary, and this treatment is practical and effective only for small areas.

Another method uses chemical irritants which are rubbed onto the scalp to cause chronic skin inflammation. Sometimes this makes hair grow. Some people apply allergen sensitizers to the scalp to stimulate hair growth. These methods require professional supervision and are time-consuming—but effective in some people.

Another approach uses minoxidil. This drug, developed to treat high blood pressure, had the unanticipated side effect of stimulating hair growth, sometimes in unwanted areas. For treating baldness, it is used as a topical lotion. The hair produced is usually fuzzy, the treatment is expensive, and the results vary.

The most successful method for treating male- and female-pattern baldness is hair transplantation. The dermatologist implants tiny plugs of skin, each containing about 10 hairs, into your scalp. These plugs are taken from a donor site, usually on the back or side of your head. Scars at the site are covered by the remaining hair. The transplanted hairs fall out in about 3 weeks, but new hairs are soon produced. Up to four transplantation sessions, at 4-month intervals, may be needed. This treatment also is expensive.

Your physician will consider the possibility of an adrenal or ovarian tumor (see pages 940 and 1189, respectively). Some drugs, such as the antiseizure medication phenytoin (Dilantin), may also cause growth of body hair. The eating disorder anorexia nervosa (see page 1102) often is associated with an increase in fine body hair. Sometimes hirsutism occurs for no known reason (see Hirsutism, page 940).

Treatment

If you worry about excessive facial or body hair for cosmetic reasons, you have several treatment options.

Plucking is the most common cosmetic method, if your problem is a few scattered hairs. There is always the possibility of an infection developing in the follicle. Wash the area first and dab on a little alcohol with a cotton ball. Use good tweezers to remove the hair by pulling it out in the direction it is growing.

Taking Proper Care of Your Hair

Each year, Americans spend millions of dollars on hair-care products and treatments. Unfortunately, some of these are not gentle enough or are used too frequently. The result is hair damage rather than hair care. Damaged hair stays damaged until it grows out and is cut off. This can take many months, because your hair grows only about ½ inch each month.

Your hair requires gentle handling. Wet hair is especially fragile, because it might become stretched. A natural-bristle brush is preferable to a synthetic one, because the synthetic material may cut your hair. Brush your hair gently from your scalp to disperse scalp oil over your hair. If you prefer a comb, use a wide-toothed comb to avoid injury to your hair.

Certain hairstyles and treatments can cause breakage or root damage. Avoid excessively tight braiding, buns, or ponytails, and do not roll your hair too tightly in curlers. Teasing and back combing should be done gently or not at all. Too much exposure to sun, wind, or swimming-pool chemicals will dry out your hair and cause it to knot.

The quality of your hair reflects in part the adequacy of your diet: Regular, well-rounded meals are best for you and your hair. Consuming extra protein or amino acid preparations will not promote hair growth. However, crash diets and eating disorders such as anorexia nervosa can damage hair dramatically. Claims made for the value of hair sample analysis have no validity and can be considered one of the many scams aimed at appealing to people concerned about their health.

Daily shampooing will not damage your hair, if you do it gently. The amount of washing your hair needs depends on the type of hair, the weather, your physical activity, and perhaps even your occupation.

For proper washing, wet your hair completely with warm water. Put the shampoo on with your hand and massage gently, using your fingertips instead of your nails as you work the lather outward from your scalp. Rinse thoroughly.

Buy shampoos tailored to your hair type—oily, dry, or normal. Protein shampoos do not penetrate your hair, but they do coat it, giving your hair more bulk. A protein shampoo acts as a shampoo and conditioner in one. Permanent-waved, straightened, or dyed hair needs low pH shampoos. Excessive flaking may require dandruff shampoos (see Dandruff, page 990). Follow your shampoo with a cream rinse or conditioner. These products lubricate your hair between washings and help minimize damage from brushing or combing. Those containing protein ingredients may also thicken your hair temporarily.

Towel dry by patting gently. Whenever possible, let your hair dry naturally in the air. If you must use a blower, use it on a low setting and leave your hair slightly damp. If you brush or comb your hair while it is wet, you pull out much more hair than you would by gently untangling it with your fingers and waiting until it is damp or dry before you carefully brush or comb it.

A styling gel or mousse can give your hair more body or thickness. They do not necessarily damage your hair, but you may experience extra dryness, especially at the hair ends.

Hair bleaches chemically alter the melanin granule in the middle layer of each hair strand. Despite careful treatment, persistent bleaching eventually damages even healthy, strong hair shafts, but it does not injure the roots from which future hair growth takes place.

Hair dyes work more like paint by covering hair strands with color or by mixing with the melanin granules without altering them. Dyes come in temporary form, which eventually wash out, and semi-permanent and permanent forms, which penetrate your hair. Before using one of the permanent forms, conduct a patch test to check for possible irritation. Permanent dyes require prior bleaching. Thus, the dying process does damage hair.

Curling is safest if you twist your hair into pin curls overnight. For safe curling of fine hair, wind slightly dampened hair around sponge rollers and let it air dry. Use of excessively hot rollers or curling irons may damage even coarse hair. Use these devices cautiously.

Permanent waving is safe for healthy hair, but you may find that it results in increased dryness and splitting. Straightening and permanent waving use the same chemical methods to change the properties of hair strands. The initial (waving) solution dissolves a chemical linkage in the hair. After the hair is arranged in its new, curly configuration, application of the second solution, the neutralizer, restores the linkage. Like other aggressive cosmetic treatments, permanent waving can be damaging when done to excess.

Plucking is a temporary solution. It does not make hair grow back darker or coarser. Check with your physician before plucking hair from a mole. Plucking causes rupture of the hair bulb and associated bleeding.

Shaving is another popular, but temporary, method. This can be very irritating to your skin if you do it haphazardly (see Proper Skin Care, page 986). Women commonly shave their underarms and lower legs, but shaving is also safe for facial hair. Shaving does not make your hair grow faster, darker, or coarser (more bristly).

The use of pumice and other abrasive agents is the oldest method of hair removal. This is slow and tedious, and the vigorous rubbing can irritate your skin. You may find it useful for scattered hairs, but it is not practical for large areas.

Bleaching is useful for large areas, such as forearms or thighs, to make unwanted hair less conspicuous. Use a product specially designed for this purpose, and follow the directions. Be sure to do the patch test on a small area to check for possible irritation.

Wax removal is popular among American women for removing hair on the upper lip, chin, and legs. Waxing can be painful and may irritate your skin. You should have it done by a trained cosmetician. As with plucking, infection of the hair follicles may occur. First, the cosmetician applies melted wax to the area, then, after it cools and sets, quickly strips it off in the direction of the hair growth. The results last longer than other temporary methods because the hair is pulled out below your skin's surface. New hairs generally appear after a month.

Depilatories are chemical agents that dissolve hair protein. You can buy them in foam, cream, or lotion form. Follow the directions, and test the product on a small area of your skin for possible irritation. Some women find depilatories inconvenient, because they must stay on for 10 to 15 minutes. Do not use these products on injured or inflamed skin.

Electrolysis is the most permanent method of hair removal. An electrologist inserts a very fine needle into each hair follicle, and a burst of electric current is delivered through the needle to destroy the hair root. The hair grows back about 30 percent of the time. Infections, scarring, or discoloration around the follicle may occur. It is wise to have the electrologist do a few hairs (perhaps six) and observe the results before embarking on an extensive program of hair removal. You may need several sessions because the maximum removal rate is about 100 hairs per visit. Electrolysis can be long, tedious, and expensive, but it might be a permanent solution to unwanted hair.

Fingernails and Toenails

Cells at the base of your nail beds produce your fingernails and toenails. Your nails are composed of laminated layers of a protein called keratin. Each nail grows toward the end of your finger or toe from a nail root that extends back into a groove of skin. Just in front of your nail root is your cuticle skin, which is attached to the nail surface and helps protect the new keratin cells that slowly emerge from below.

Your nails can give the first signal of an illness. They occasionally provide clues for diagnosis as well as information about your age and diet. They also assist you with the tasks of daily living, although you may not be conscious of how much you use them until an injury, infection, or other disorder limits your use of them. The following section describes the disorders that may develop in your nails and how to take proper care of your nails.

Paronychia

Signs and Symptoms—Red, swollen area on the skin next to a nail

Paronychia is a superficial infection of the skin around the nail. The most common cause of paronychia is either staphylococci or yeast (see color photograph, page C-7). It is usually the result of an injury, such as biting off a hangnail, or is caused by manipulating or pushing back the cuticle. *Para* means "alongside" and *onyx* means "nail" in Greek.

Care of Ingrown Toenails

Ingrown toenails usually occur on the big toe. They form when the edge of your nail curls and grows into the soft underlying tissue. They are caused by improper cutting of nails, by the way your nails grow (faster at the edge than at the center), and by pressure from ill-fitting shoes. Women who routinely wear pointed-toe, high-heeled shoes are especially likely to have this problem. If you have a slightly ingrown nail, pare off the excess nail and put tiny bits of sterile cotton under the affected edge to lift it up. Change the cotton daily until the pain and redness subside. If an infection develops (evidenced by severe pain and a discharge of pus), see your physician.

If you have a hangnail, do not attempt to pull it off. Pulling almost always rips into living tissue. Instead, clip it off neatly, leaving a slight angle outward. This may help prevent recurrence. Lubrication with hand lotion also can help prevent hangnails.

Healthy nails are smooth, without ridges or grooves. They are uniform in color and consistency and free of spots or discoloration. Remember that no nail-care product can give you healthy nails. The only way you can help your nails to look their best is to protect them from damage and irritants (chemicals and detergents), then clean and trim them regularly.

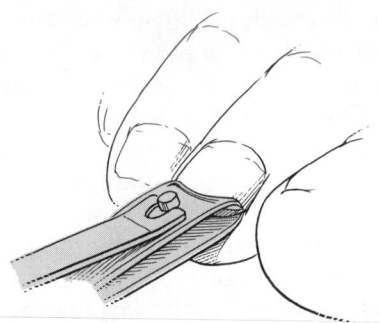

To avoid ingrown toenails, cut your nails straight across and not too short.

Bacterial paronychia usually is a sudden and painful infection. Superficial pus blisters may appear. Pressing the affected area can produce oozing pus.

Another form of paronychia is caused by fungal infections and is common among persons with diabetes mellitus and persons who have their hands in water for long periods of time. Fungal infections develop slowly but tend to persist. Sometimes both bacteria and fungi are present, causing greater swelling and pus.

An acute infection can extend around your nail and cuticle to invade beneath them in a painful abscess. Your cuticle becomes raised. The nail may become detached. Nail distortion or discoloration might occur. Although rare, the infection can penetrate into your finger and attack tendon tissue. Red lines along your skin are a signal that bacteria have entered your bloodstream. If this occurs, see your physician. The diagnosis may require a culture to determine which type of microorganism is causing your paronychia.

Treatment
Hot soaks will help decrease inflammation of the tissues. Follow these by topical application of an antibacterial agent (for bacterial infections) or 1 percent gentian violet solution if a fungal infection is present.

Fungal Infections of the Nails

Signs and Symptoms—Thickened, lusterless fingernails or toenails with discoloration or crumbling edges

Fungus spores may attach themselves to the dense bed of keratin cells that make up your nails. These microscopic plants can digest the keratin and live within it. The resulting infection, known as onychomycosis (tinea of the nails), can persist indefinitely (see color photograph, page C-8).

You can contract such infections in several ways, including walking barefoot in public places or as a complication of athlete's foot (see page 1013) or paronychia (see page 1021).

The associated fungal infection of the foot or hand can be mild and produce no inflammation, or it can be acute with blisters and painful swelling. Once the nails are involved, they may become thickened, detached, and shed, or the nail even may be destroyed. There is usually an accumulation of keratinous debris beneath the free edge of an infected nail.

Your physician's diagnostic tests may include scraping up some of the debris beneath the nail edge for microscopic examination to identify the fungus. The presence of a fungus will rule out other diseases of the nails.

Treatment
There are no good treatments for fungal infection of the nails. Solutions, creams, or ointments do not penetrate the nail, although they may help to control fungal infection of the surrounding skin. If you have a fungal infection that is disabling, or if the infection is excessively disfiguring, your physician may prescribe a systemic antifungal preparation. Sometimes it is difficult to tell whether these medications are effective. In addition, the nails grow so slowly that it takes 6 to 12 months to grow new nails free of infection.

Discoloration or Deformity of the Nails

Nails can be discolored or deformed in many ways. Minor injury is the most common cause. The black spot under your thumbnail after a hammer blow is blood. White, cloud-like marks on the tips are the result of minor trauma. A whitish discoloration of the nails of unknown cause is called leukonychia (see color photograph, page C-7). Splitting, peeling, or brittleness usually are signs of overexposure to strong soaps or chemicals. Tight or ill-fitting shoes can cause ingrown or thickened toenails. Proper care is important to prevent bacteria and other infectious organisms from gaining entry into tissues and possibly your bloodstream (see Taking Proper Care of Your Nails, this page).

Discoloration occurs with a number of ailments including fungal infections that can turn your nails yellow, gray, brown, or black. Injury, chemical exposure, or a reaction to medication also can cause an array of colors.

Internal disorders can deform your nails. Clubbing of your nails, a condition in which your fingers or toes thicken and the nails wrap around them, may indicate a problem in your lungs.

It is not unusual for your nails to be affected during an illness and to recover afterward. However, your nails grow slowly—about ⅛ inch a month for fingernails and about ¼ inch for toenails. Damage can be repaired only by the slow process of new growth. After your underlying disorder is under control or cured, your nails will gradually return to normal. But report any new changes in color or markings to your physician.

Once the drug is stopped, the fungus may return or the nails may remain permanently free of infection.

Taking Proper Care of Your Nails

Perhaps the single most important element in taking care of your nails is to avoid biting, picking, or injuring them. Even a minor cut alongside your nail can allow bacteria or fungi to enter and cause an infection. Because your nails grow slowly, an injured nail retains signs of its injury for several months.

Exposure to detergents and chemicals can weaken, split, and discolor your nails. To protect them, wear rubber or disposable plastic gloves with cotton liners. Between uses, turn rubber gloves inside-out to dry. This prevents microorganisms from growing in them.

Weekly trimming is important, because nails that are smooth and cared-for are less likely to become damaged. Use an emery board and sharp manicure scissors or clippers to trim your fingernails. If your nails are brittle or thick, trim them after bathing, when they are softer. Bevel the edges with the fine side of the emery board. If you prefer long nails, be careful to avoid accidental injury and accumulations of dirt under the edge. Although fashion encourages trimmed cuticles, avoid this practice. It can result in a point of entry for bacteria and fungi and thus promote infection.

Despite advertising claims, most polishes are identical chemically. They make your nails stronger only in the sense that the polish itself coats and thus protects the nail. If you polish your nails, apply several thin coats instead of one heavy one. Minimize use of nail-polish remover. It can weaken and dry your nails. Touch up chips with polish and apply new polish over old to avoid use of remover for as long as possible. Nail strengtheners can discolor or break your nails. Artificial nails may produce reactions beneath your nails. Cuticle removers are corrosive alkali-based products that destroy the naturally protective bands around your nails. There is no scientific evidence that gelatin capsules, calcium tablets, or other vitamin or protein products improve and strengthen your nails.

Trim your toenails straight across and not too short. You need to do this only about once a month, because toenails grow more slowly than fingernails. They also tend to be thicker, especially on your great toe, so the best time for a trim is after bathing.

Chapter 31

Allergies

Contents

Understanding Allergy, 1026

How Allergic Reactions Occur, 1028
Types of Allergens, 1029
Usual Kinds of Exposure, 1029
Latex Allergy, 1029

Discovering Causes, 1030
Testing for Allergens, 1031
Inappropriate Tests and Treatments, 1031
RAST, 1032

What Your Physician Can Do, 1032
Is the Condition a True Allergy? 1032
General Principles of Treatment, 1032
20th-Century Syndrome: Can You Be Allergic to Modern Times? 1033

Myths About Allergy, 1034
Allergies Are Psychosomatic, 1034
Antihistamines, 1034
Moving to Arizona Will Cure Allergies, 1035
Allergies Are All Sniffles and Scratches, But No One Ever Dies From Them, 1035
Short-Haired Pets Do Not Cause Allergies, 1035
You Can Catch Poison Ivy by Just Standing Near the Plant, 1035

Skin Allergies, 1035
Contact Dermatitis, 1036
Atopic Dermatitis, 1038
Hives and Angioedema, 1038
Allergy-Like Reactions to Heat, Cold, or Light, 1039

Respiratory Allergies, 1040
Hay Fever (Allergic Rhinitis), 1040
Nasal Polyps, 1041
Allergies to Mold, Dander, and Dust, 1042
Pollen, 1042
Cat Allergies, 1043
Asthma, 1044
Peak Flowmeter, 1045
Metered-Dose Inhaler, 1046
Asthma and Exercise, 1047

Allergies to Foods, Drugs, and Insect Stings, 1047
Food Allergies, 1048
Food Allergy vs. Food Intolerance, 1049
Drug Allergies, 1050
Insect Sting Allergies, 1051
Anaphylaxis, 1053

Understanding Allergy

Allergies are the result of a response by the body's immune system to agents it perceives as possibly dangerous. To understand allergies, it is important to have some idea about how the immune system works.

Your immune system's job is to protect your body from invaders that can harm it. An invader that activates your immune system is called an antigen. Antigens include harmful germs, viruses, and other foreign agents that can attack your body. Your immune system is vigilant in its search, recognition, and destruction of these antigens.

The key actors in the defense system are white blood cells known as lymphocytes, which are manufactured in enormous quantities in bone marrow. Some migrate to your thymus where they develop into specialized types of immune cells. Some lymphocytes also migrate from the bone marrow and thymus to your lymph nodes and other immune organs, including spleen, tonsils, adenoids, appendix, and small intestine. Other lymphocytes circulate throughout your blood and lymphatic vessels.

There are two major kinds of lymphocytes, the T cells and the B cells. Each type is responsible for a particular kind of response.

T cells are activated in the thymus gland. They attack antigens directly rather than by producing antibodies. They also can act in concert with B cells to destroy antigens.

The immunity the T cells provide is known as cell-mediated because the reaction between the antigen and the immune mechanism takes place on or within the cell. These cells respond to malignant growths and some viral and bacterial infections. They are important in the rejection of foreign tissue such as transplants. T cells make substances called lymphokines. These in turn can stimulate roaming scavenger cells called macrophages to engulf (phagocytize) bacteria.

B cells in contrast produce plasma cells; they in turn produce the antibodies that react with specific antigens. The reaction with antibodies circulating in the bloodstream neutralizes antigens by blocking them from entering cells or by making them susceptible to attack by macrophages. The immunity the plasma cells provide is called humoral, in reference to its location in the body's fluids.

The antibodies that B cells produce are made of a special kind of protein called immunoglobulin. There are five kinds of immunoglobulins (Igs): IgA, IgD, IgE, IgG, and IgM. Of these, IgE is most involved in allergic responses.

One characteristic that makes the immune

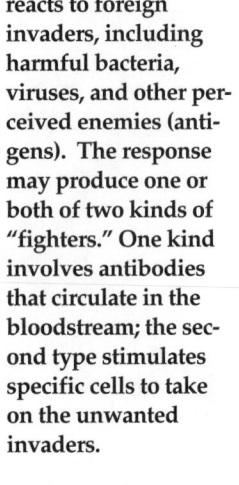

Your immune system reacts to foreign invaders, including harmful bacteria, viruses, and other perceived enemies (antigens). The response may produce one or both of two kinds of "fighters." One kind involves antibodies that circulate in the bloodstream; the second type stimulates specific cells to take on the unwanted invaders.

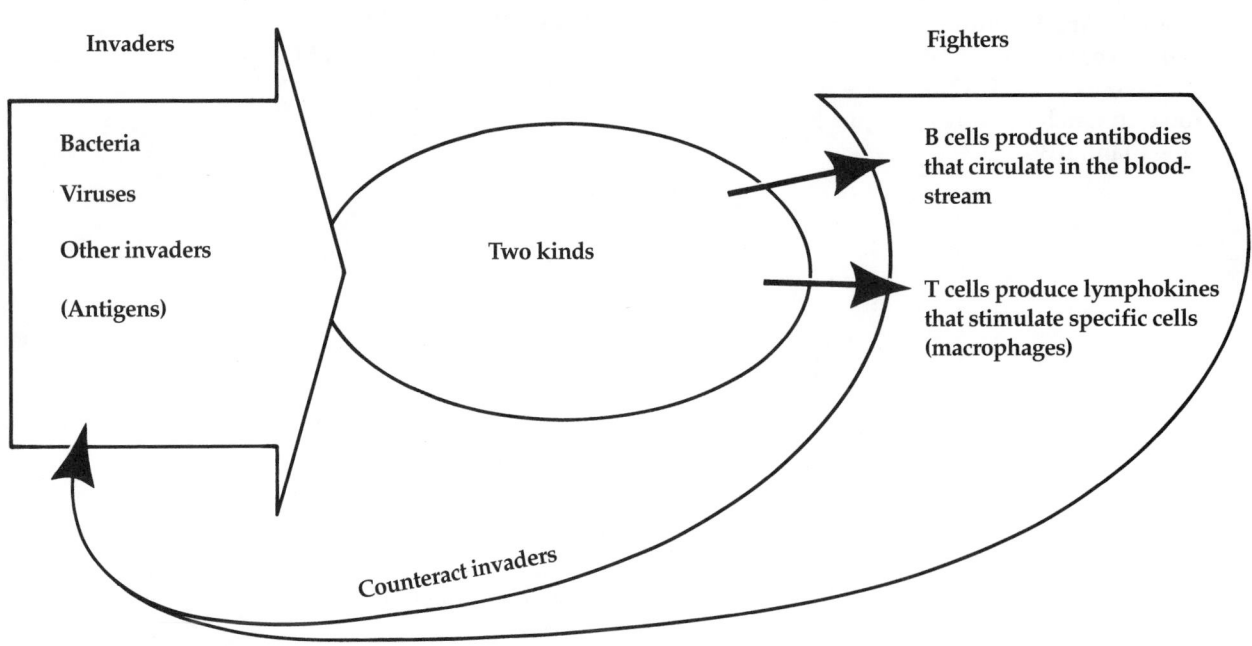

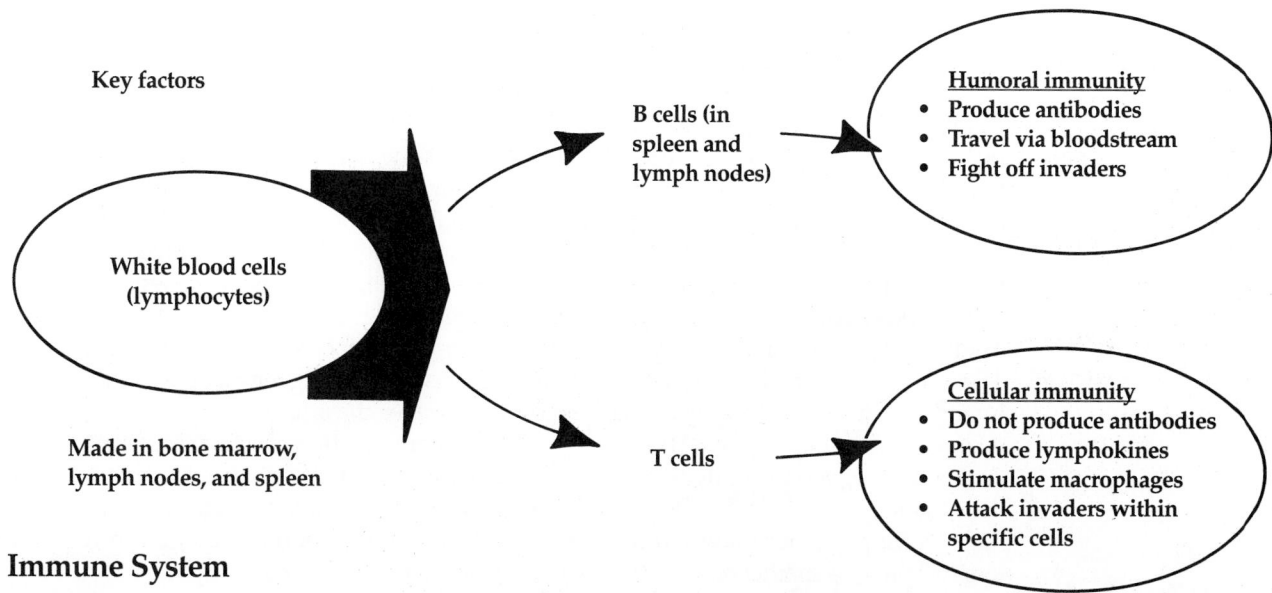

Immune System

White blood cells, known as lymphocytes, are of two major kinds: B cells and T cells. Both act in the short and long term to provide you with immune protection. In the short term, the B cells are responsible for humoral immunity and are activated in the lymph nodes and spleen to produce antibodies to fight off invaders in the bloodstream. The T cells from the thymus gland produce lymphokines, which stimulate macrophages to attack the invaders within specific cells.

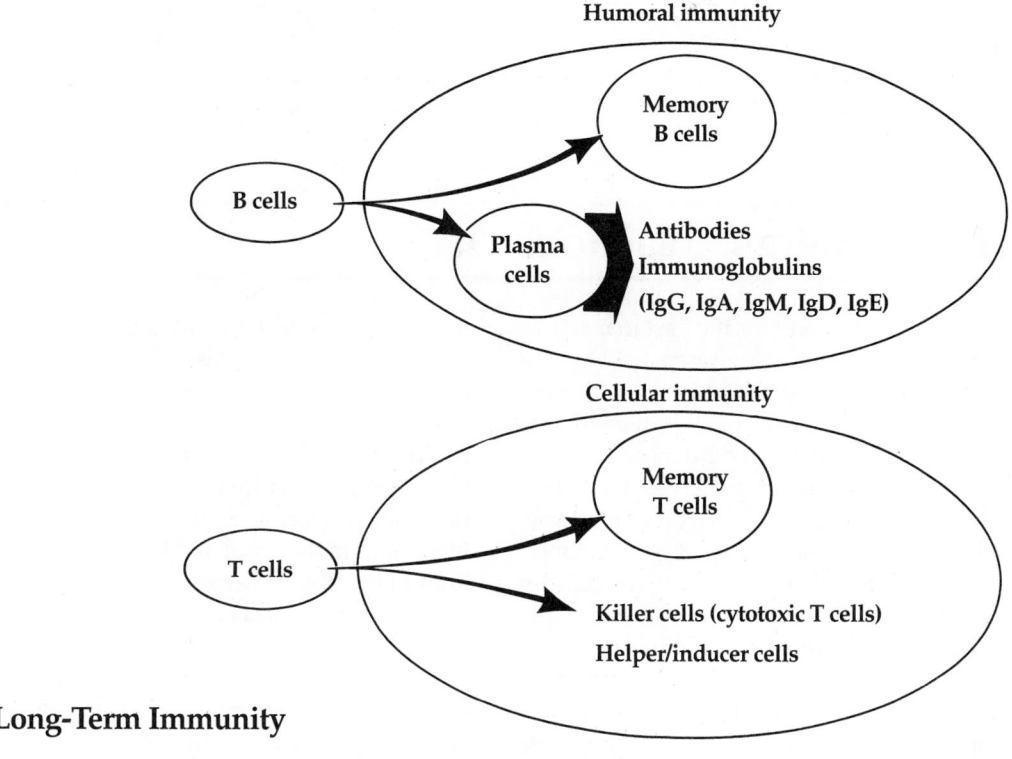

Long-Term Immunity

In the long term, the B cells and T cells "remember" (memory cells) the antigens they have done battle with, and they are prepared to act if the same invader (antigen) reappears.

system efficient is its memory capacity. Lymphocytes are "programmed to recognize" the chemical identity of invading antigens based on a previous encounter and then destroy them immediately on their reappearance. It is largely due to this memory part of immunity that we stay well.

Humans are born with natural immunity as a result of antibodies acquired from their mothers, but this immunity lasts only a few months before disappearing, to be replaced gradually by each infant's own immunity. The new immunity is acquired after the infant's own immune system has been exposed to a foreign agent. An example of such a developed immunity to a disease is the situation in chickenpox. Once you have had chickenpox, your body's immune system will prevent another bout of the disease, even though the virus that causes chickenpox may persist in your body for years (herpes zoster; see Shingles, page 1011).

Immune responses also develop when a very small amount of an antigen is intentionally introduced into the system in the form of a vaccine, such as for polio, diphtheria, tetanus, or measles. These antigens have been altered so that they cannot produce a full-scale infection of the disease, but they can produce an immune response. Thus, you may have mild muscle cramps and a low-grade fever for a few days after a vaccine has been injected. The most important result of the injection of this antigen is that it prepares the memory in certain lymphocytes, which then are ready to block a full-scale invasion, should one occur. The memory for many antigens generally is life-long.

The immune system does not attack everything foreign that enters the body. Most of the foods, drinks, and drugs that we ingest do not trigger an immune response. However, the immune system does respond to agents such as germs, viruses, and other invaders that cause harm. Occasionally, the immune system reacts to a harmless invader such as pollen or dander. It is this reaction, or rather overreaction, by your immune system that is known as an allergy. With an allergy, the response is to an otherwise harmless substance.

Many problems related to allergies can be handled by your primary care physician. Occasionally, however, you may be referred to an allergist, a specialist who deals with allergies. If your allergic problems are skin-related, consultation with a dermatologist may be necessary (see page 983).

How Allergic Reactions Occur

In most people, and for the vast majority of the time, the immune system works efficiently in protecting the body. In some people, however, it occasionally misreads the signals and responds to substances that actually are benign but are perceived as harmful antigens. Such reactions involve an interaction between a specific foreign substance, known as an allergen (an antigen that can stimulate antibody production), and a specific antibody (usually a protein).

When an allergen enters the system, it reacts with antibodies (IgE type) on the surface of basophils (a type of circulating white blood cell) or mast cells (a type of cell that lines the respiratory and gastrointestinal tracts and the skin). The basophils and mast cells then release histamine (a body chemical that can act as an irritating stimulant) and other harmful chemicals into the tissue to combat the allergen, which they perceive as dangerous.

The eosinophil, another circulating white blood cell, also is involved in the allergic reaction by increasing its numbers in the blood and in the nasal and bronchial secretions of the allergic person.

The result is a host of symptoms that vary in severity.

When histamine is released in the lungs, it causes secretion of mucus and narrowing and swelling of the lining of the airways. This leads to wheezing, coughing, and, sometimes, shortness of breath. When histamine is released in the nose and, rarely, the sinuses, it produces a runny nose, tearing eyes, and itching of the nose, throat, roof of the mouth, and eyes. In the skin, histamine produces hives and other rashes. When the digestive system is the site, stomach cramps and diarrhea may result. Occasionally, the entire system will be affected in a response known as anaphylactic shock, in which blood vessels dilate and air passages narrow, causing a slowing of the pulse, breathing difficulty, and other symptoms. Unconsciousness and occasionally death may result (see Anaphylaxis, page 1053).

Each allergen produces its own specific set of IgE antibodies. For this reason, a person may be sensitive to ragweed but not to mold allergens. It is possible for a person to have many different specific IgE antibodies, making him or her sensitive to many allergens. Indeed, it is not unusual for a person who is allergic to one substance to be allergic to one or two others.

The intensity of the allergic reaction varies widely. Some people have only mild sniffles during ragweed season; others react violently with an attack of asthma. The number of IgE antibodies present in the system controls the severity of symptoms: the more antibodies present, the stronger the reaction.

Types of Allergens

A surprising number of different things can cause allergic reactions. These include substances found outdoors, indoors, and in the foods we eat. Allergens may be present in certain medications, in parts of plants (such as pollen), in house dust, in animal dander, in molds, in fungi, in foods, and in insect venom. In these cases, it is a specific allergen that causes the body to overreact. However, some people can be sensitive to the chemical changes caused by exposure to heat or cold and by exercise.

Usual Kinds of Exposure

Those who are sensitive to certain allergens may be at risk of exposure daily because these allergens are common. Different allergens have different routes of entry into the body.

Exposure to the allergens of plants such as poison ivy, poison oak, and poison sumac occurs when a person merely brushes against the leaves. The allergic reaction usually occurs at the body site where the contact was made.

For instance, one commonly gets poison ivy as a result of brushing up against it accidentally while walking in a wooded area or handling it while gardening. The plant resin that causes the reaction is thus transferred to the skin, and a reaction subsequently occurs. The same reaction also may develop if the resin is deposited on clothing that then rubs against your skin.

Other contact reactions can be caused by prolonged exposure to certain metals such as nickel (used in costume jewelry) and chromium. People who are sensitive to certain cosmetics can develop rashes after exposure to nail polish, hair dyes, eye makeup, or lipstick. Health care workers and others tend to become allergic to latex after repeated exposures to gloves and other rubber articles.

Perhaps the most common exposure is by inhaling an offending allergen. Millions of people experience the effects of sensitivity to pollen as hay fever (although neither hay nor fever is involved). The medical term is allergic rhinitis. The respiratory system is affected when wind-borne pollen is inhaled. Exposure is inevitable during spring, summer, and autumn, the pollen-producing seasons.

During their reproductive cycle, molds release particles, which are borne in the air. When inhaled, they also can trigger a reaction in the respiratory system. A similar reaction can occur when a sensitive person inhales animal dander or house dust. These allergens tend to affect people more during the winter months, when more time is spent indoors.

In addition to these inhaled allergens, other materials in the air such as smoke, fumes, mists, and baby powder may cause allergic reactions in sensitive persons. Some hypersensitive people may react to the

---

Latex Allergy

If you're allergic to latex, it's possible that a trip to a restaurant may result in a reaction to the food you eat there. Exposure can occur when protein particles from latex join with cornstarch powder used on latex gloves that some food handlers wear. The protein can become airborne or be transferred to food or other objects. Simply rinsing the gloves before use, however, reduces the amount of surface allergen.

Most food handlers, though, don't use latex gloves. They wear "food-grade" plastic gloves, which don't transfer any particles to food. Just to be safe, check with the restaurant manager about the type of gloves used.

formaldehyde present in household products such as insulation, pressed board, permanent-press clothing, new furniture, and polishes.

For most people, the reaction to an inhaled allergen is characterized by cold-like symptoms—dripping nose, cough, and itchy, teary eyes. An asthma reaction can occur but is more rare. In this case, the airways in the lungs become swollen and a wheezing and a feeling of tightness in the chest are produced; often there also is production of thick mucus and a cough. During such a reaction, the affected person sometimes has difficulty breathing, and severe cases can be life-threatening.

Certain foods can cause an IgE response in very sensitive people. The foods found to be the cause in most reactions include milk, eggs, nuts, shellfish, fish, wheat, corn, berries, and legumes. In addition, certain materials used in the processing of foods cause allergic reactions; these include salicylates (found in all foods processed with cider or wine vinegar), tartrazine or Yellow Food Dye no. 5 (found in processed foods treated to enhance their color), sulfites (used to preserve fruits, vegetables, meats, and beverages such as wine), and gum arabic (used as a thickener in processed foods) (see Food Allergies, page 1048).

People can be allergic to certain drugs taken orally, intramuscularly, or intravenously. The most common offender by far is penicillin and its relatives, followed by other antibiotics, insulin, local anesthetics, and the contrast agents used in certain X-ray tests. Many people are sensitive to aspirin, even though the reaction it causes is not truly an allergic reaction. Rarely, an individual will react to aspirin by having a rash, hives, and aggravation of asthma. When this occurs, it may be life threatening. Almost any medicine has the potential to cause a reaction (see Drug Allergies, page 1050).

The bite or sting of insects can be responsible for exposure to an allergen for extremely sensitive people. In most people, the sting of a bee, wasp, or yellow jacket is uncomfortable for a couple of hours. However, in highly sensitive people, such a sting can trigger a systemic reaction (see Insect Sting Allergies, page 1051, and Anaphylaxis, page 1053).

In rare cases, people are sensitive (not allergic) to heat, cold, pressure, or light and sun rays; they have responses such as rashes, but these are not true allergic reactions (see Skin Allergies, page 1035). Just as rare is sensitivity to changes in the body that are caused by exercise. The responses usually are wheals and tiny hives. In some people, vigorous exercise may provoke the symptoms of asthma (see page 1047).

Discovering Causes

No one knows why some people become sensitive to certain substances such as plant resins, pollens, molds, house dust mites, foods, and drugs. Your physician will ask you a series of questions about your symptoms, your family's medical history, past medical problems, past and current emotional and social conditions, lifestyle (including work, eating, and recreation habits), and possible exposure to certain allergens. This interview is one of the most important sources of information useful in making a diagnosis.

One important clue in the medical history will be the answer to the question "Does either of your parents have allergies?" It is known that the tendency to develop allergies is inherited. People who have allergies frequently have a close relative who also has allergies or a hypersensitivity. However, they are not necessarily sensitive to the same allergens. You are less likely to inherit the sensitivity to a specific agent than you are to inherit the general tendency to develop sensitivities.

Other questions your physician asks will try to determine how various factors may cause an increased sensitivity to certain substances. Repeated or prolonged exposure to a specific substance might be responsible for a reaction—for example, a person who gardens in the spring and summer may experience an increase in hay fever symptoms. Such an observation is important because it suggests that the cause of the symptoms may be pollen or outdoor mold. As another example, the physician might ask for a list of all the foods eaten within the last 5 days to 2 weeks to determine if consumption of a certain food can be linked with the occurrence of the symptoms. The list of questions can be quite extensive.

Testing for Allergens

After the full medical history has been taken and affected areas of the lungs, skin, eyes, nose, and ears have been examined, the physician will select a testing method. The type of test to be used depends on the cause that is suspected.

Skin Test

The most commonly used test is the skin test, and several methods can be used. In the most common, a small amount of a suspected allergen is placed on the skin of either the forearm or the upper arm. Occasionally, skin on the back is used. The area is then pricked or scratched to introduce the allergen beneath the skin surface. Another common method is known as the intradermal method. It involves injecting a tiny amount of an allergen directly into the skin. With either method, the results are checked after 15 or 30 minutes.

If the skin at the test site is swollen and red, the test is considered to be positive for that allergen. In skin tests, several allergens are tested at the same time, as a means to eliminate possible allergens and because people often are sensitive to several agents.

If a skin test is positive, the person being tested is at higher risk for an allergic reaction if exposed to the allergen in its usual form. However, these tests are not foolproof: a person may test positive and yet not respond to the allergen in the course of everyday life. Also, a negative result does not rule out the possibility that the person is sensitive to that allergen. Skin tests must be interpreted cautiously. Tests with food allergens have the widest margin of error. This possibility of error on all tests is one reason why diagnosing allergies can be very difficult.

Skin tests are conducted for many forms

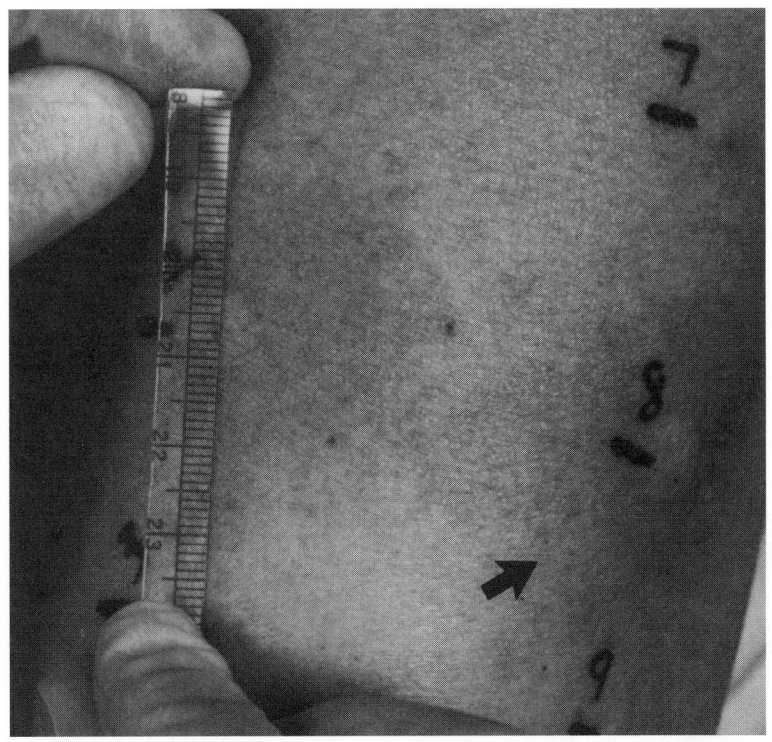

Skin test shows typical wheal and flare (arrow) allergic reaction to allergen introduced beneath the skin surface.

Inappropriate Tests and Treatments

If you think you may have food allergies, be wary of certain tests and treatments that have not proved valid. Do not accept cytotoxic testing, provocation and neutralization testing, or yeast hypersensitivity treatment.

Cytotoxic testing involves mixing extracts of foods in vials with samples of a person's white blood cells. Some people believe that if the cells change shape in any way, the individual is allergic to that food. Yet no proven correlation exists between this shape change and a food allergy.

In provocation and neutralization testing, the person is injected with a small amount of food extract to provoke symptoms. When symptoms occur, he or she is given "neutralizing" injections of the food on the theory that this will neutralize the effects of the first dose. This is an unproven test method.

Yeast hypersensitivity treatment is based on the theory that a yeast-like fungus called *Candida* is the cause of all allergies. People are told to remove from their diet all foods containing yeast and mold, including fruits, milk, refined carbohydrates (such as breads), and processed foods. Supposedly, this enables the body to correct the condition. No evidence, however, supports the notion that *Candida* has any relation to food allergies.

of allergies. They are particularly useful for respiratory allergies, penicillin allergy, latex allergy, and insect sting allergy. They may not be as useful for diagnosing food allergies. Drug allergies other than penicillin and closely related drugs cannot be diagnosed with a skin test.

Skin tests must be conducted carefully. If too much allergen is placed on the skin, a positive reaction will be produced even in persons who are not allergic. Also, in rare instances, an extremely sensitive person can have a full-scale anaphylactic reaction, requiring immediate treatment with an injection of adrenaline (see page 1053). The skin tests for airborne substances such as dust mites, animal dander, and pollens are the most reliable.

RAST

A laboratory test, the radioallergosorbent test (RAST), can reveal the causes of some allergies to inhaled substances. The RAST measures the amounts of specific IgE antibodies in a person's blood. In contrast to skin tests, RAST is more convenient and does not have even the slight risks of skin tests because all testing is done on a blood sample. Also, any antihistamine drugs the person may be taking to lessen allergic symptoms do not affect the test.

However, RAST is not as sensitive as skin tests and cannot test as many allergens. Additionally, results must come from a specialized laboratory and are not immediately available. RAST also may be considerably more expensive than skin tests.

What Your Physician Can Do

Is the Condition a True Allergy?

Because allergies often seem to have no explanation, a wide range of complaints are often blamed on them. However, allergic responses are fairly specific, even if the causes are often hard to pinpoint. A true allergy usually involves IgE antibodies of the immune system. During the allergic reaction, histamine is released into various tissues, which causes such symptoms as rashes and hives, respiratory discomfort including nasal congestion and asthma, and internal problems such as nausea and diarrhea.

Plants such as poison ivy, poison oak, and poison sumac react with the immune system's T lymphocytes. An itchy rash with blisters develops in sensitive people after contact with the resin of such plants.

Occasionally, people have reactions that may closely resemble an allergy but in fact are due to something other than an IgE immune response. Such reactions are particularly common in response to food. A food reaction can be caused by many factors other than an allergen. For instance, the food may be contaminated with toxin-producing bacteria, or the person may experience the effects of irritable bowel syndrome (see page 782), stress, or a food intolerance (such as lactose intolerance; see page 1049). The resulting symptoms, such as diarrhea and vomiting, may be confused with an allergy because they seem to happen whenever a person eats a particular food. The only way to assess the cause fully is to see a physician who can diagnose the problem and prescribe a suitable course of action.

Certain drug reactions commonly mimic allergic responses, although they do not involve the immune system. Aspirin can produce non-allergic reactions as well as reactions that resemble allergic reactions. The antibiotic ampicillin also may produce a non-allergic rash.

General Principles of Treatment

Effective methods of treatment for allergies involve several strategies. First, a proper diagnostic effort must be made to discover the true cause of your allergies. Your physician then must determine the best course of action to eliminate the problem or to alleviate the symptoms. The proper diagnostic effort includes evaluating your history and conducting tests such as skin tests, RAST, or an elimination trial for food allergies.

Avoidance

The best therapy for allergies is avoidance of the allergen. Avoiding a known allergen is fairly simple in the case of allergy to something like poison ivy, penicillin, or strawberries. However, it is not so simple for hay fever because these allergens are constantly in the air during certain months of the year or for allergy to house dust, which is present year-round even in the best-kept homes.

Medication

The basic drug treatment for most allergies is the administration of antihistamines. These drugs block the action of histamine, the substance that is largely responsible for the symptoms.

Many antihistamines are available in non-prescription preparations intended for relieving symptoms of colds. For many people who have respiratory allergies such as hay fever, mold, or house dust mite sensitivity, these drugs can control the nasal congestion, dripping nose, itchy eyes, dry throat, and cough. In more severe cases, and for hives, swelling of mucous membranes, or food allergies, antihistamines obtained by prescription are required.

The corticosteroid drugs (such as cortisone) are used for severe symptoms. These powerful anti-inflammatory drugs come in various forms for administration by injection, swallowing a pill, metered-dose inhaler, nasal spray, and topical application of a cream (see Corticosteroid Drugs, page 919). Available only by prescription, except for mild topical creams, these drugs can be very useful in treating allergies, but they have side effects that may need to be weighed against the seriousness of the symptoms. Generally, the side effects of nasal sprays and metered-dose inhalers are minimal. The corticosteroid-containing creams often used in treating contact dermatitis can cause skin problems in sensitive people and therefore should be used with care.

Cromolyn sodium is a non-corticosteroid drug that is prescribed in the treatment of some forms of allergies, particularly respiratory allergies. Use of this drug, in the form of a nasal spray and eyedrops, usually is begun in advance of the allergy season because the drug must be used for several weeks before its benefits become apparent. It helps to prevent severe symptoms in the nose and eyes when used daily.

The most severe allergic reaction is life-threatening anaphylaxis. In this situation, blood vessels are dilated and air passages in the lungs are constricted (sometimes causing

20th-Century Syndrome: Can You Be Allergic to Modern Times?

In most people, allergic reactions are the result of sensitivities to specific agents such as pollen, mold, and insect venom. Strong flower odors, exhaust fumes, ozone, cigarette smoke, and even temperature changes can affect sensitive people. However, some insist that they are allergic to all of these agents and more—almost everything in life. These people, more often women than men, experience dizziness, impaired concentration, headaches, and joint pain. Known as 20th-century syndrome in America and total allergy syndrome in Europe and Australia, this disorder is difficult to treat because it seems to be the result of emotional upheaval.

The symptoms are real, but the allergy is not.

20th-century syndrome does not come on suddenly. It usually emerges gradually, often after a traumatic event such as the death of a child or the loss of a job. As the symptoms increase, the person often becomes preoccupied with the problem. Frustrated that physicians can find no physical cause for the symptoms, the individual often sees dozens of physicians and other health practitioners before someone diagnoses the problem as allergy.

Unfortunately for the people who suffer from the syndrome, physicians known as clinical ecologists who are at the fringe of orthodox medicine prescribe treatments that are expensive, disruptive to patients' lives, and occasionally physically debilitating. Such treatments may require drastic measures such as quitting a job to move to the mountains, living in a home with no synthetic materials, eating only organic foods, drinking several quarts of water a day, and bathing with coconut oil. Despite these measures, rarely are the symptoms relieved permanently.

The best long-term treatment is psychiatric therapy to treat emotional stress. Unfortunately, people who suffer from 20th-century syndrome usually shun this treatment.

wheezing, low blood pressure, unconsciousness, and, occasionally, death). Treatment is injections of adrenaline (also known as epinephrine). This drug is used as an emergency medication most commonly for insect stings, drug allergies, and food allergies (see Anaphylaxis, page 1053).

Allergy Shots

Certain allergies, including those to pollens, molds, and insect poisons, often can be treated by immunotherapy (known as allergy shots). This form of therapy involves injecting very small amounts of known allergens to stimulate the body to produce a neutralizing antibody. Some allergists believe that neutralizing antibody blocks the interaction of IgE antibodies with the allergen. Other mechanisms also are probably involved. The treatment requires regular injections, often on a weekly basis, of increasing doses of the allergen until a maintenance dose is established. Then, injections of the maintenance dose are given monthly for up to several years.

Myths About Allergy

The causes of an allergy are not always readily apparent. Allergies often appear to be vague in origin and unpredictable in response. They are difficult to treat successfully. Therefore, it is not surprising that many misconceptions and myths have arisen about them.

Few people affected by allergies have escaped without hearing someone's notion of sage advice about what causes his or her allergies and how to cure them. Here are our comments on the most common myths about allergies.

Allergies Are Psychosomatic

Although some allergies affect the nose and sinuses, they are not "all in your head." Allergies are real; they are the result of a response by the immune system to specific

---

Antihistamines

When the immune system identifies an invader and produces IgE antibodies in response to it, the chemical histamine is released. Histamine is partly responsible for most allergic responses, including dripping nose, itchy eyes, dry throat, rashes and hives, asthma, anaphylactic shock, nausea, and diarrhea.

The drugs most widely used to combat the effects of histamines are known as antihistamines. Although very useful in treating the symptoms of various allergies, antihistamines do have side effects, some fewer than others. They can cause drowsiness, dryness of the nose and mouth, and blurred vision. Recently introduced prescription anti-histamines such as terfenadine (Seldane), astemizole (Hismanal), and loratidine (Claritin) have less tendency to cause drowsiness.

However, terfenadine and astemizole have been associated with serious heart rhythm disturbances in people with known or potential liver disease due to alcohol abuse, occupational exposure to liver toxins, drugs toxic to the liver, or other severe liver disease. People taking astemizole or terfenadine must avoid some other drugs, including the antibiotics erythromycin, troleandomycin, and clarithromycin and the oral anti-fungal drugs ketoconazole, itraconazole, fluconazole, and miconazole. Loratidine has not been reported to cause heart rhythm disturbances.

Because of the sleepiness that most antihistamines cause, avoid driving a car or operating heavy machinery when you are taking these drugs. Also avoid alcohol, which speeds the absorption of some antihistamines and also intensifies the drowsiness. Check with your physician before taking antihistamines. Antihistamines a physician prescribes may be stronger than those available over-the-counter, so follow instructions carefully. Sometimes the side effects can outweigh the benefits of antihistamines.

allergens. The symptoms may be affected by stress or emotions—science does not fully understand the relationship between body chemistry and emotions—but emotions do not cause the allergy.

Moving to Arizona Will Cure Allergies

For years, people who were bothered by seasonal allergies to pollens and molds thought that if they moved to the Southwest, where the foliage and climate are different from other regions, their allergies would disappear. Many enjoyed relief for a time but, although the desert is lacking in maple trees and ragweed, it does have other pollen-producing plants such as sagebrush, cottonwood, ash, and olive trees. People sensitive to some pollens and molds may develop allergies to the pollens and molds found in new environments. For example, people sensitive to ragweed may become sensitive to sagebrush pollen.

Allergies Are All Sniffles and Scratches, But No One Ever Dies From Them

Most allergic reactions do indeed mimic some of the symptoms of a head and chest cold. However, some allergic reactions can be very serious indeed. Highly sensitive people can enter a state of life-threatening shock as a result of being stung by a bee, wasp, hornet, or yellow jacket or the injection of penicillin. A person highly sensitive to certain foods can experience severe abdominal distress or shock after eating those foods. A rare form of hereditary angioedema can cause swelling of the throat that can block breathing. Although it is true that many allergies are merely an inconvenience, severe reactions must be taken seriously and treated promptly and properly.

Short-Haired Pets Do Not Cause Allergies

The length of an animal's fur does not determine whether the fur can be responsible for an allergy. In fact, the fur itself is not the culprit. The cause is the dander, the scales of skin that are constantly shed by all animals with hair or feathers. In addition, saliva and urine may cause a sensitivity. If you have allergies to furry pets, the only really safe pets are fish and reptiles.

You Can Catch Poison Ivy by Just Standing Near the Plant

The resin responsible for the sensitivity to poison ivy, poison oak, and poison sumac must actually touch the skin or clothing of a person to cause a reaction. The resin can be transferred from clothing to skin quite easily, which may explain why people who think they haven't touched the plants do have reactions. The irritating resins even can be carried in the smoke if the plant is burned.

Skin Allergies

Most Americans are susceptible to skin allergies or reactions at some time during their lives. The most common such sensitivity is to plants such as poison ivy, poison oak, or poison sumac. In susceptible individuals, contact with one of these plants produces an itchy, blistering rash. The swelling and itchy wheals of hives sometimes are caused by allergies. Another type of allergy causes swelling of tissues beneath the skin or in the throat (a condition called angioedema) for no apparent reason.

All of these discomforts are caused by histamines and other chemicals released into the skin or under the lining of the throat or bronchial passages as a result of an allergic response (see Understanding Allergy, page 1026). In the following pages, each of the common skin allergies, including dermatitis, hives, and angioedema, will be described.

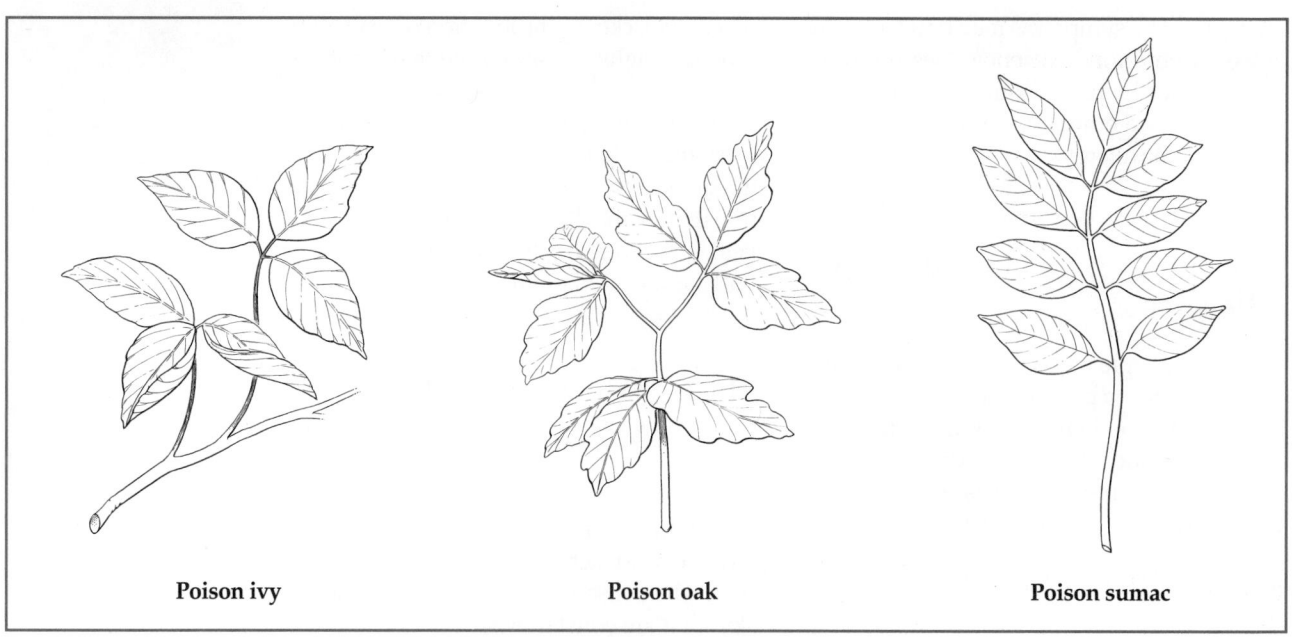

Poison ivy   Poison oak   Poison sumac

Contact Dermatitis

Signs and Symptoms
- Itchy rash consisting of small bumps, blisters, and general swelling
- Burning sensation of the eyes and mucous membranes

Each year, millions of people have a contact dermatitis, an irritation of the skin caused by direct contact with certain plants, cosmetics, chemicals, metals, or drugs. Contact dermatitis is a hypersensitivity produced by T cells, not by the more common IgE antibodies (see Understanding Allergy, page 1026). The most common irritants include the resins of poison ivy, poison oak, and poison sumac; the chemical para-phenylenediamine, which is used in hair and fur dyes, leather, and rubber and in printing; nickel compounds often used in jewelry; rubber compounds; ethylenediamine, a preservative used in creams and ophthalmic solutions; and dichromates, used in textile ink, paints, and leather processing.

"Leaves of three, let them be" is a familiar phrase for many people, and with good reason. Certain three-leaved plants, particularly poison ivy and poison oak, are probably the most common causes of contact dermatitis. Poison sumac, which has multiple leaves, is a common offender as well. Four of every five Americans become sensitive to these to some degree. Although the plants are different, the problem-causing substance is the same, an oily resin called urushiol.

A reaction occurs when a sensitive person comes in contact with a resin-containing plant (by brushing against the plant itself or against something, such as clothing or pet fur, that has brushed against it). It takes only a tiny amount of the resin to cause a reaction, but direct contact is essential. For this reason, poison ivy and other such rashes do not develop as a result of a person's being merely near the plant. Nor does the rash spread as a result of washing or scratching open rash blisters, because the resin is not present in blister fluid. However, it can be spread by accidentally rubbing the resin on other areas of the skin before all the resin is washed off. For example, the eyelids often become inflamed as a result of touching or rubbing the eyes with fingers or hands that have resin on them. Thorough bathing with soap after an exposure to one of these plants may prevent a reaction or lessen its severity.

Other plants also can cause contact dermatitis. These include heliotrope, found in the deserts of the Southwest; ragweed, both the leaves and the pollen; daisies; chrysanthemums; sagebrush; wormwood; celery; oranges; limes; and potatoes.

Certain chemicals and metals can cause rashes similar to poison ivy among persons who are particularly sensitive. Often, such sensitivities develop over a period of years of low-level exposure. These agents include the chemicals formaldehyde, chlorine, phenol (carbolic acid), and alcohols and metals such as nickel, chromium, mercury, and beryllium. Perhaps the most common reaction to metal occurs when costume jewelry containing nickel (watchbands, earrings, bracelets) comes into contact with sensitive skin over a prolonged period. An itchy, flaky, red patch develops over weeks or months (see color photograph, page C-3).

We most often think of exposure to chemicals as primarily an occupational hazard, but many such substances, particularly formaldehyde, are found in household products ranging from permanent-press clothing to dyes, polishes, plaster, paper, rugs, foam insulation, and the particle board used in home construction and furniture. Formaldehyde causes a burning sensation in the eyes and mucous membranes. Latex exposures commonly cause contact dermatitis and other reactions.

Some people are sensitive to allergens in eye makeup, hair dye, lipstick, and nail polish. Occasionally, perfumes, colognes, and antiperspirants also can cause skin reactions.

Diagnosis

A rash develops within 2 days after exposure. In very sensitive people it can develop as soon as a few hours. The affected area reddens and swells, and small itchy blisters and bumps form. The blisters first fill with clear fluid and then burst, revealing raw skin susceptible to bacteria and infection. The itching can range from minor to severe. The rash usually reaches its peak after about 5 days and is usually gone within 1 to 2 weeks.

Reactions to plants rarely develop on the soles, palms, and scalp. In the case of formaldehyde, a burning sensation of the eyes and linings of the nose, mouth, throat, or eyes (mucous membranes) develops.

How Serious Is Contact Dermatitis?

Contact dermatitis is an irritating condition that causes pain and discomfort, and the blisters can become infected. It can be temporarily debilitating, but it has no lasting effects.

Treatment

The itching of the contact dermatitis rash can be relieved by applying a paste made of baking soda or Epsom salts and water or using calamine lotion or nonprescription hydro-

cortisone creams. (Some people are sensitive to the agents in certain creams and lotions, which can aggravate the condition.) Do not apply alcohol because this tends to make the itching worse. Cover open blisters with sterile gauze to prevent infection. Creams and lotions do not help much when the blisters open, but they can be used again when the blisters close. Try not to scratch.

Severe cases or those in sensitive areas such as face, eyes, and the genital region should be treated by a physician, who may prescribe application of a cortisone ointment, use of an antihistamine, or taking a cortisone drug orally.

Prevention

Avoidance is the best way to prevent contact dermatitis. Allergens in household agents are not always easy to detect, but harmful plants are. Poison ivy is found in woodlands almost everywhere in the United States except California, where poison oak is found.

Learn to recognize offending plants, and avoid them or wear protective clothing when exposure seems likely. Poison ivy may be a low-growing plant, a bush, or a vine. Its leaves usually are glossy green in the summer and turn an attractive red, pink, or yellow in the autumn. They generally are elliptical in shape and grow in groups of three on a stem. Poison oak can grow as a low plant or bush. Its leaves, which resemble oak leaves, also grow three to a stem. Poison sumac may be a bush or a tree. It has two rows of leaflets, opposite each other, on each stem and a leaflet at the tip. The smooth edges of its leaves distinguish it from its harmless relative. Poison sumac tends to grow in marshy areas such as swamps and bogs.

If one of these poisonous plants grows in your yard, you can kill it with a herbicide. Pulling it out alone will not necessarily cure the problem because new growth can develop from the roots. Do not burn these plants because the resin can be carried in the smoke and cause internal as well as external reactions. Do not compost them either. Instead, dispose of them in a plastic bag.

Washing the harmful resin off the skin with soap within 5 or 10 minutes after exposure can avert an episode of contact dermatitis. Washing after this brief period will not always prevent a reaction but may help to contain it within a smaller area. Also remove carefully and wash clothes that have brushed against such resinous plants.

If your reactions are to household chemicals, take steps to decrease exposure. Wash all new permanent-press clothing several times before wearing, avoid insulating a home with formaldehyde foam, and apply a varnish to all particle board in the household to seal it. In the case of metal sensitivity, wear solid (not plated) gold and sterling silver jewelry. Cosmetics free of problem-causing ingredients are available. Avoid all latex articles if necessary.

Atopic Dermatitis

Signs and Symptoms—Extreme, persistent itching and thickening of the skin in patches

Atopic dermatitis, also known as eczema, generally occurs in babies and children, although it can occur at any time of life. About 70 percent of affected people have a family history of atopic dermatitis. Atopic dermatitis itself is not an allergy. However, about a third of the individuals who have it develop respiratory allergies such as hay fever and asthma (see Atopic Dermatitis, page 989, and color photograph of eczema, page C-2).

Diagnosis

Atopic dermatitis consists of patches of dry, extremely itchy, thickened skin. Characteristically, it affects the skin behind the knees and in the folds of the elbows. The itching is persistent, and it often drives the sufferers to frantic scratching. Babies and children who have it sweat more than normal, and they have dry skin and a greater than normal tendency to itch. Abrasion, heat, or stress can start these children scratching (see color photograph, page C-2).

Most infants with atopic dermatitis (about 3 percent of the population) are from families in which other members have allergy-related diseases such as hay fever or asthma. Children usually outgrow their atopic dermatitis by about age 6, although in some the improvement does not occur until puberty and in some it lasts into adulthood.

How Serious Is Atopic Dermatitis?

This form of eczema is irritating, but for most people it is a passing problem.

Treatment

Treatment for atopic dermatitis is primarily a matter of using creams, lotions, and antihistamines. The objective is to stop the intense itching because it causes scratching and thus more itching.

Keep the skin moist with creams and lotions. If the itching and scratching continue, your physician may prescribe antihistamines. Coal-tar ointments are often used when the condition has been present for months or years and the skin has become thickened and leather-like, a process known as lichenification. Corticosteroid creams and ointments are very useful in reducing the inflammation and itching.

Children should be bathed no more than three times a week, and these baths should be done rapidly with a mild neutral soap. Use of bath oil sometimes keeps the skin from drying too much. The fingernails should be kept short to decrease the damage caused by scratching.

Hives and Angioedema

Signs and Symptoms

Hives
- Raised red, often itchy, welts of various sizes that appear and disappear at random on the surface of the skin
- New welts develop where the skin is scratched (dermatographia)

Angioedema
- Large welts below the surface of the skin, particularly around the eyes and lips but also on the hands and feet, and in the throat

About one in five people experience hives at one time or another. The condition also is called urticaria (from the Latin *urtica*, for "nettle"). The lesions usually occur in batches rather than singly, and they may last a few minutes or for several days. Hives occur on the surface of the skin. Angioedema is a similar swelling that occurs beneath the skin (see color photograph, page C-9).

Hives and angioedema may result from the release of histamine and other chemicals into the bloodstream. The cause of the reaction often is unknown, although all sorts of substances have been found to cause hives, including foods, pollen, animal dander, drugs, latex, insect stings, infections, illness, cold, heat, light, and emotional distress. As with many allergies, there is a hereditary component to the development of hives and angioedema.

Foods that may cause problems in some sensitive people include berries, shellfish, fish, nuts, eggs, and milk. Penicillin and aspirin are known culprits. Pollen and animal dander are common inhalant agents.

Diagnosis

The primary symptom of hives and angioedema is a swelling of the skin into red welts. In the case of hives the swellings are often intensely itchy and appear on the surface of the skin. In angioedema, the swellings are deeper and appear primarily around the eyes and mouth, making them appear swollen. They also occur on the hands and feet, although less frequently.

In treating hives, your physician will begin by asking about your medical history. This may include asking you to create a detailed diary of exposure to possible irritants over a period of 2 weeks to a month. Because hives and angioedema can be caused by many different things and can be exacerbated by emotional conditions, it sometimes is impossible to determine the cause (see color photograph, page C-9).

How Serious Are Hives and Angioedema?

Hives and angioedema generally are harmless. They leave no lasting marks and sometimes are not even uncomfortable. However, there is one rare form, hereditary angioedema, that is more troublesome and can be dangerous. It is a disorder of a blood protein that is part of the immune system and may require special treatment. This reaction includes non-itchy swelling, possibly with painful abdominal cramping and diarrhea. When angioedema affects the throat or tongue, it causes the air passage to be blocked and can be life-threatening.

Treatment

Sometimes treatment is not needed. The standard treatment for hives and angioedema is antihistamines, but other drugs may be used, including adrenaline (epinephrine), terbutaline, and cimetidine. Occasionally, physicians prescribe a corticosteroid drug for oral use (see page 919). People who are allergic should avoid substances known to cause attacks.

Allergy-Like Reactions to Heat, Cold, or Light

Signs and Symptoms—A rash or swollen welts such as hives which appear as a result of exposure to heat, cold, sun, or rubbing

Emergency Symptoms—Muscle cramping, vomiting, and fainting as a result of immersion in cold water

One of the most puzzling of allergy-like reactions is that to physical stimuli such as pressure, heat, cold, light, and sunlight. Hives are the most common symptom. People who have this sort of response often have very sensitive skin. Sometimes, just the rubbing of a blunt object on the skin produces a swelling within a few minutes. In the condition called dermographia, when the skin is stroked lightly, as with a fingernail, it reddens almost immediately and a wheal develops where the skin was touched (see color photograph, page C-9).

Diagnosis

Physical allergy-like symptoms include tiny hives in response to vigorous exercise, a hot shower, or emotional stress; swelling of the hands and feet in response to pressure; and hives in response to rewarming of body parts that had been exposed to cold air. In testing for heat and cold reactions, your physician will take a complete history and conduct a test in which cold and hot objects are applied to the skin to see if a reaction occurs.

Treatment

The best method for treating hypersensitivity to heat and cold is to avoid them as much as possible. Wear warm clothing during cold weather. Take warm showers and baths rather than hot or cold ones. Avoid swimming or bathing in cold water if hives develop where your body is exposed to cold. Your physician may prescribe a strong antihistamine.

Prevent sun-induced hives by using sunscreens or avoiding sun exposure, especially if you are taking antibiotics, antihistamines, diuretics, antifungal agents, tranquilizers, and hypoglycemics. These drugs, as well as some perfumes, may cause such reactions if you are out in the sun.

Respiratory Allergies

Allergies of the respiratory tract often produce symptoms that are similar to those of a cold: congested head and chest, stuffy or runny nose, cough, and sneezes. Occasionally, wheezing also occurs with a respiratory allergy. In fact, allergies and colds are sometimes confused until one realizes that the symptoms of the allergic response last far longer than those of a cold, or they seem to appear (and disappear) with a suddenness uncharacteristic of the common cold.

For some people, such symptoms appear during a pollen season—spring, summer, or autumn. For others, the symptoms are manifested primarily in the winter when their home is closed to ventilation and house dust mites and molds are common. Still others experience symptoms when they enter a home in which a furred animal lives.

All respiratory allergies represent responses of the immune system to airborne allergens (see Understanding Allergy, page 1026). The following pages will discuss the common kinds of allergies to pollen, molds, dusts, and dander as well as asthma and nasal polyps.

Hay Fever (Allergic Rhinitis)

Signs and Symptoms
- Stuffy or runny nose
- Frequent sneezing
- Itchy eyes, nose, roof of mouth, or throat
- Cough

It's springtime. The air is sweet with the smell of fresh new flowers but you can't enjoy it because your head is stuffed up, your nose is sore, and your throat itches. Or it's autumn and the ragweed and other autumn plants are blooming and spreading their wind-blown pollen everywhere, including into your respiratory system—making your eyes teary, your head and nose congested, and the roof of your mouth itchy.

The sum of these symptoms is known as hay fever (technically, it is allergic rhinitis), although things other than hay usually cause the problem, and no fever is present.

No one knows why some people are more susceptible than others to the tiny airborne pollens of certain seasonal plants. In all likelihood a person's sensitivity is partly an inherited trait that affects the ability of the immune system to deal with potential invaders. Many believe that hay fever is a childhood disorder, something you grow out of by the time you reach adulthood. However, hay fever can develop at any time during life, and you can recover from it at any time. A person who has other allergies such as dermatitis or asthma or who has relatives with allergies is more likely to have hay fever.

People with hay fever react to specific allergens. Some are sensitive to only one or two substances; others are sensitive to many. When an allergic person inhales the pollen to which he or she is allergic, antibodies react with the pollen; this reaction causes histamine to be released. The histamine then causes the lining of the nose, sinuses, eyelids, and eyes to become inflamed. The sinuses may become congested, the nose runs, and the eyes, nose, throat, and roof of the mouth often itch. You may sneeze, sometimes violently and repeatedly—as many as 10 to 20 times in a row. Usually, attacks of the symptoms last about 15 to 20 minutes and happen several times a day. Many people find that their hay fever doesn't interfere with their lives in any substantial way. Every year at a certain time their noses are congested and they sneeze frequently for a couple of weeks.

Diagnosis
For many people, hay fever is a minor inconvenience at certain times of the year. If it is a significant interference in your life, a visit to an allergist is in order.

Your physician will begin by asking a series of questions to determine what sort of allergens cause congestion and how much they interfere with your normal habits. You may be asked to keep a diary to determine accurately when reactions occur most frequently. For instance, if your symptoms occur only in the spring, then you probably are allergic to pollens found only in the spring. If you have allergy attacks throughout the growing season, you may be allergic to several pollens.

Sometimes a series of skin tests may be used to determine which pollens you are most sensitive to. These include prick tests and occasionally a radioallergosorbent test (RAST) (see Testing for Allergens, page 1031).

Treatment

The most effective method for controlling the symptoms of hay fever is to avoid the allergens. During pollen season, stay indoors, especially on dry, windy days when pollen counts are high. Keep doors and windows closed. Air conditioning, particularly a filtered central system, also is helpful.

In mild cases of hay fever, relief often is provided by nonprescription antihistamines and decongestant tablets. However, antihistamines can produce drowsiness and a dryness of the throat and mouth that can cause as much discomfort as that of the hay fever. Antihistamines such as terfenadine, astemizole, or loratidine have less tendency to cause sleepiness (see Antihistamines, page 1034).

Avoid chronic use of over-the-counter nasal sprays and drops. Although they relieve symptoms at first, they can be addicting. After a number of weeks or months of daily use of these agents, the nose becomes increasingly congested and more frequent doses of the spray or drops are needed to clear it. The only way of resolving nose-drop addiction is to stop the use of the spray or drops and wait for the rebound congestion to subside. This usually takes a month or two.

If you are particularly bothered by hay fever, consult an allergist, who can determine what pollens you are allergic to and the best course of treatment. The allergist may prescribe an antihistamine that works well for you. Over-the-counter antihistamine tablets and eyedrops may give comfort. Your physician may prescribe a corticosteroid nasal spray in addition to other measures. Another useful drug is cromolyn, which is available as a nasal spray. You must use it for several weeks before you can expect to experience benefits. Levocabastine (Livostin) is a helpful prescription eyedrop.

The closest thing to a cure for hay fever is a series of immunizing injections (immunotherapy), which desensitize the system to allergens. In this series, increasing amounts of the offending allergen are given over time. Many people who undergo this therapy lose their sensitivity, usually within 2 years. However, the procedure is long and expensive and is not effective for 20 to 30 percent of patients.

Nasal Polyps

Signs and Symptoms
- Difficulty in breathing
- Difficulty in smelling odors

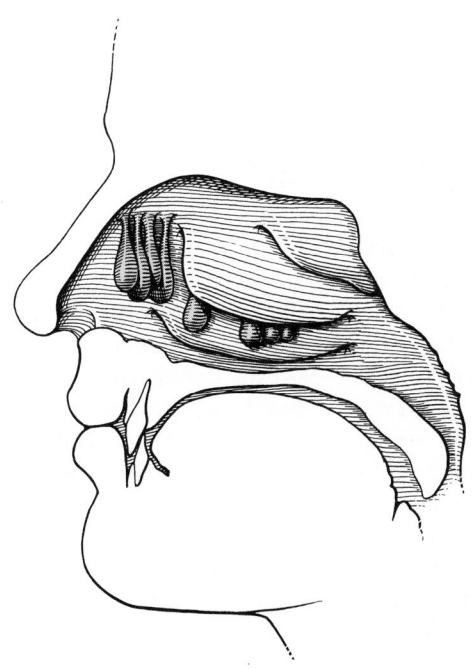

Pearl-like lumps in the lining of the nasal passage are called nasal polyps. If they cause breathing difficulty or recurrent sinus infections, these polyps can be removed in a simple surgical procedure.

When the mucous membrane that lines the inside of the nose swells and protrudes into the nasal passage, the swelling is known as a polyp. A polyp may appear singly or in clusters, making breathing or smelling odors difficult. Nasal polyps are caused by an overproduction of fluid in the mucous membrane, sometimes as a result of hay fever or some other nasal allergy. Often, no specific cause can be identified.

Diagnosis

If you notice that your nose never seems to clear, making it difficult to breathe through it or to smell odors, you may have nasal polyps. Headaches are a sign that a polyp may be blocking the opening between the nasal cavity and one of the sinuses.

Occasionally, you may be able to determine if you have polyps yourself. When you shine a light up your nostrils and examine them with a mirror, you may see pearl-like lumps. However, because polyps often are at the back of the nose, they are not seen easily.

Nasal polyps must be treated by a physician. To determine if polyps are present, your physician will use a nasal speculum, which looks like a pair of sugar tongs, to examine the inside of your nose.

How Serious Are Nasal Polyps?

Nasal polyps are an inconvenience but generally are not a serious threat to health. Sometimes they obstruct the drainage of the

Pollen

The pollens that are carried by bees from plant to plant are relatively harmless to humans because they are relatively large grains and have a waxy texture. However, those that the wind carries are lighter and smaller and do cause hay fever.

Wherever there are plants, there is pollen at some time of the year. Trees, both deciduous and evergreen, produce pollen in spring. Grasses and most flowers produce their pollen during June and July. Late-blooming plants such as ragweed produce pollen in early autumn. In warm climates with long growing seasons, pollen may be present in the air for 8 or 9 months of the year, whereas in climates with shorter growing seasons the pollen is present for less time.

The roadside plant ragweed heads the list of hay-fever-causing plants east of the Rocky Mountains. Other plant pollens that produce allergy less commonly include sagebrush, tumbleweed, redroot pigweed, spiny amaranth, burning bush, and English plantain.

Grass varieties that cause trouble include rye, timothy, redtop, Bermuda, orchard, sweet vernal, and bluegrasses. Most trees produce pollens that can cause problems, including maple, oak, ash, birch, poplar, elm, pecan, juniper, and cottonwood.

The amount of pollen in the air depends on the weather. Hot, dry breezes stir up pollen, whereas dampness washes the pollen to the ground. Most pollen particles are so small, often invisible, that they can be carried by the air into a house through open windows as well as through doors and screens. It does not take much pollen to produce a reaction, as little as 20 particles per cubic yard. Many plants can produce up to a million such particles. If kept well maintained, the filters in central air-conditioning systems may help remove pollen.

---

sinuses enough to cause recurring sinus infections and significant difficulty in breathing through the nose. Occasionally, there may be an association between use of aspirin and nasal polyps or between cystic fibrosis and nasal polyps (see page 720).

Treatment

Nasal polyps are removed surgically in an operation usually performed under local anesthesia. Polyps can reappear and may need to be removed as they develop.

Allergies to Mold, Dander, and Dust

Signs and Symptoms
- Stuffy, runny nose
- Frequent sneezing
- Itchy eyes, nose, roof of mouth, or throat
- Cough
- Wheezing

Not all hay fever (allergic rhinitis) (see page 1040) is caused by pollen. Identical reactions may occur from sensitivity to other inhaled allergens such as molds, animal dander, and the microscopic mites that live in house dust.

Some people experience an allergy attack when they enter an empty room. Others find that they have the symptoms of nasal allergy at random times all year long. Still others have the symptoms seasonally. All of these people may be reacting to airborne allergens other than common pollen.

Diagnosis

For most people, allergy to molds, dust, or animals is primarily an inconvenience. When it lasts only a few weeks each year it can be ignored or treated as the symptoms of a cold. Indeed, the symptoms are similar to those of a cold except that they last longer and the mucus discharge usually is clear. When the symptoms interfere with normal activities, a visit to an allergist is in order to determine the exact causes and a method of treatment.

When diagnosing inhalant allergies such as those to molds or dust, your allergist will ask a series of questions designed to determine how severe the reaction is, how often it occurs, whether it is year-round or seasonal, and the situations in which it occurs most frequently. You may be asked to keep a detailed diary for up to a month to determine frequency and possible causes. A series of skin tests may be used to identify the allergens to which you are most sensitive. The prick test is a common one. Occasionally, the radioallergosorbent test (RAST) also is used (see Testing for Allergens, page 1031).

Some people may be sensitive to more than one allergen; some or all of these may be responsible for their symptoms. Therefore it is difficult to pinpoint which allergens cause the most trouble.

How Serious Are These Allergies?

The cold-like symptoms of allergies are inconvenient and annoying but are not serious problems to general health.

Treatment

The most effective treatment for allergy to molds, dust, and animals is avoidance. This may be easier said than done because some allergens, particularly mold spores, are borne on the wind just like pollen. In those cases, staying indoors in an air-conditioned atmosphere is often the most useful preventive measure. When the allergen is dust, animal dander, or feathers, you can take steps to avoid some sources of irritation.

The medical treatment for allergies to molds, dust, and animals is often identical to that for allergic rhinitis. Nonprescription antihistamine tablets (see Antihistamines, page 1034) and decongestants relieve the symptoms for many people. When the reactions are severe or interfere with a person's life, a physician's care may be needed to provide a course of treatment. An allergist may prescribe antihistamine tablets, steroid or cromolyn nasal sprays to reduce the swelling of the mucous membrane of the nose, and levocabastine (Livostin) drops for eye irritation. Oral doses of steroids may be prescribed when reactions are severe (see Corticosteroid Drugs, page 919).

Drugs used to control allergic rhinitis have drawbacks. Many antihistamines cause drowsiness in most people, although they occasionally can have the reverse effect in others, causing them to be wakeful and nervous. The powerful anti-inflammatory steroids given by mouth also can induce a number of side effects when taken over a prolonged period.

As in allergic rhinitis, in other respiratory allergies the closest you can get to a cure is a course of desensitization. The allergens that cause the most trouble are diagnosed with skin tests. You will periodically be injected with small doses of the offending allergens. The doses are increased gradually as the body produces protective mechanisms to limit the release of histamine and other chemicals. Such therapy often is given on a weekly basis, and the course can run anywhere from 3 months to several years. After the main course is concluded, a course of maintenance shots begins, given every 2 to 6 weeks. This may last for several years.

Immunotherapy works well for many people, but it is not without a few problems.

Cat Allergies

Despite cats' ability to make more people scratch and sneeze than any other pet, feline fancy often wins over practicality. Of the 6 million Americans who are allergic to cats, about one-third keep a cat in their home. If you or someone you live with can't bear to get rid of your cat, follow these suggestions to help you live in your home more comfortably:

- Wash your cat once a week for several weeks to help reduce the amount of your cat's airborne allergen by 90 percent.
- Avoid carpets and upholstered furniture. Mop floors frequently and vacuum using a high-efficiency filter attachment.
- Use a high-efficiency particulate-arresting (HEPA) air cleaner to filter cat allergen in dust. The cleaner removes more than 99 percent of dust particles that pass through the filter.
- Keep your cat outside as much as possible and make your bedroom, especially the bed, and other rooms you spend a lot of time in off-limits.
- Increase ventilation to decrease allergen levels.

If you or someone in your home has asthma due to cat allergy, it is best to find your cat a new home. Continued exposure to cat allergen may lead to narrowing of the airways even after the exposure stops. After you find a new home for your cat, thoroughly clean your house. But remember, it can take weeks, even months, for allergens to disappear from carpeting and upholstered furniture.

It is expensive and inconvenient, carries risks of reactions, and doesn't work for everyone. Discuss the pros and cons with your primary care physician and your allergist.

Animals

Some people are allergic to the dander shed from the skin, fur, and feathers of animals and birds. The fur and feathers themselves are not the cause of year-round irritation. It is the scales shed from the skin that cause the allergy, along with the pet's saliva and urine. People allergic to pollens or molds may become allergic to animal dander as well. The only way to eliminate the problem is to avoid the source. This means not keeping pets. If you are sensitive to the tiny amounts of dander found in wool, avoid products made mostly with wool. Do not buy furniture or rugs made with animal hair.

Molds

Many allergy sufferers are sensitive to the spores of common molds that are carried by the air. Outdoor molds produce spores mostly in the summer and early autumn, although in warm climates they can be present all year. Indoor molds shed spores all year long, producing constant problems for sensitive people.

Molds thrive indoors in damp locations such as basements and bathrooms and in upholstered furniture and beds, rugs, stuffed animals, wood, books, and wallpaper. Outdoors they live in the soil and on compost or damp vegetation. Susceptible people react most noticeably when mowing grass, harvesting crops, or walking through tall grass and plants. Common offending molds include the indoor molds *Penicillium*, *Aspergillus*, *Mucor*, and *Rhizopus* and the outdoor molds *Alternaria* and *Hormodendrum*.

Mold spores are everywhere, so they cannot be eliminated. However, you can minimize the exposure. During the summer and autumn, keep doors and windows closed or use air-conditioning in your home, car, or office as much as possible. You can dry out a damp basement by using a dehumidifier. Be sure to clean the humidifer regularly so molds and other growths do not develop inside it.

Discard moldy or mildewed articles such as books, old shoes, and bedding. Wash wooden furniture with a weak solution of bleach and air it in the sun. Use synthetic fabrics for upholstery and bedding. Clean bathroom and basement walls with disinfectants. Instead of using wallpaper, paint walls with mold-proof paint.

Dust

Common house dust is a major cause of year-round suffering for sensitive people. House dust harbors all kinds of substances, including pollen, mold spores, fabric fibers, and detergents, but the primary cause of allergic reaction is microscopic insects called mites. Mites thrive during the summer, but most people's reactions are worse in the winter. This is probably due to the fact that the disintegrated fragments of the spider-like insects are more easily inhaled than the live animals. Disintegrated fibers from stuffing materials, mattresses, toys, furniture, blankets, carpets, and draperies also can be irritants.

The best way to deal with dust is to keep the house as clean as possible. This means not only vacuuming up visible dust frequently but also damp-mopping and dusting often. Wash scatter rugs and furniture covers weekly if possible. If you're the one cleaning, wear a dust mask. Avoid over-stuffed furniture and dust trappers such as bed ruffles, canopy beds, bunk beds, carpet, curtains, Venetian blinds, and upholstered furniture. Enclose pillows, mattresses, and box springs in allergen-proof coverings.

A central heating and air-conditioning system that filters and humidifies the air is a help. You can attach special air filters to the system. For limited areas, portable air purifiers are somewhat effective, but use one that does not produce ozone because it is a respiratory irritant.

Miscellaneous Irritants

Dozens of other substances can cause reactions among a very small percentage of people. These factors include smoke and fumes from industrial activities; tobacco smoke from cigarettes, cigars, and pipes; face and baby powder; latex; and powdered laundry detergents. People sensitive to respiratory allergens are more likely to be sensitive to other irritants.

Avoid irritating substances such as those involved in remodeling a room as much as possible—for example, paint and paint remover fumes or sawdust. Avoid smoking and exposure to smoke of all types, including smoke from cigarettes, wood fires, burning leaves, or rubbish. Use liquid laundry detergents. Do not use body or facial powders.

Asthma

Signs and Symptoms
- Wheezing
- Difficulty in breathing versus shortness of breath
- Painless tightness in the chest
- Coughing

Emergency Symptoms
- Extreme difficulty in breathing
- Bluish lips and nails
- Severe breathlessness
- Increased pulse rate
- Sweating
- Severe coughing

Asthma is characterized by periodic wheezing, chest tightness, coughing, and difficulty in breathing. Its cause is often unknown. Respiratory infections and exercise can aggravate the signs and symptoms of asthma, as can cold air, stress, and exposure to pollen, mold spores, animal dander, or house-dust mites. In adults, anti-inflammatory medications such as aspirin can aggravate asthma.

Approximately 10 percent of children and 5 percent of adults in the United States have asthma. It is usually an inherited condition and is not contagious. Asthma is the leading cause of chronic illness and school absenteeism in children. About half of the children who develop asthma do so before age 10.

Diagnosis

Difficulty in breathing or coughing episodes, sometimes producing mucus, are primary symptoms of asthma. The variable airflow obstruction in asthma results from an inflammation of the bronchial wall, tightening of the bronchial smooth muscle fibers, and increased production of mucus. Airflow through the swollen bronchial tubes is restricted, and a wheezing sound is produced when you inhale or exhale.

Symptoms of an asthma attack can occur within minutes after exposure to strenuous exercise or to an offending allergen. They may also be associated with a cold (respiratory infection) or may occur for no apparent reason.

Physicians use various tests to help diagnose asthma and its causes. A complete physical examination, breathing and allergy tests, and an X-ray examination may be needed. Your physician may also ask you to perform a breathing test at home to determine if there is a pattern to the attacks and thus narrow the list of possible causes (see Peak Flowmeter, this page).

How Serious Is Asthma?

Asthma attacks can vary from mild to life-threatening. Attacks can last minutes to hours or even days. A common cold can trigger an asthma attack, with symptoms of asthma outlasting those of the cold.

If you have asthma, you should be under the care of a physician because asthma attacks can be dangerous if airflow is severely obstructed. With professional help the attacks can be controlled and are seldom disabling or life-threatening.

Treatment

In addition to professional care, a sound understanding of asthma and self-help skills are of paramount importance to managing asthma. Easy-to-remember treatment fundamentals are provided here.

Peak Flowmeter

To help prevent or minimize a serious asthma attack, you can monitor your lung function on your own with a peak flowmeter. Like a thermometer or blood pressure cuff, a peak flowmeter gives an objective measure of your condition. This device is your "early warning system."

The peak flowmeter measures the peak amount of air you expel. A lower reading than usual may predict an asthma flare-up. Your physician may give you specific instructions on how to deal with low readings. If you need daily asthma therapy, use a peak flowmeter several times a day.

Several inexpensive models of peak flowmeters are available. To use the meter, follow these steps:

1. Connect the mouthpiece to the peak flowmeter.

2. Push the indicator to the bottom of the scale.

3. Take a deep breath and blow as hard and fast as possible with your lips tight around the mouthpiece.

4. Note the final position of the indicator. This is your peak flow rate.

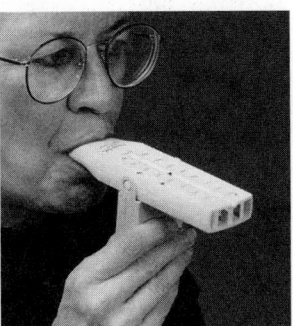

5. Slide the indicator back to the bottom of the scale and repeat the test two more times.

6. Record the highest reading of the three tests.

Activity
You may need to reexamine your activity levels and lifestyle. If you enjoy strenuous exercise, your regimen may need modification (see Asthma and Exercise, 1047).

Symptoms
Be alert to symptoms. Use a peak flowmeter to monitor your lung function regularly (see Peak Flowmeter, this page).

Trigger Control
Be aware of and try to avoid indoor and outdoor allergens and irritants. More than 2,000 indoor irritants can trigger an attack. Common triggers include tobacco smoke, house dust, and pets. Frequent outdoor triggers include pollen, mold, and cold air.

If you're allergic to pollen, use an air conditioner and keep windows closed during the pollen season. Install a high-efficiency

Metered-Dose Inhaler

One very useful aid in the treatment of asthma is the metered-dose inhaler (MDI). This device allows administration of medication into the lungs in specific amounts and is used for asthma medicines such as bronchodilators, cortisone, and cromolyn.

To take full advantage of the inhaler, you must use it properly. It takes a little practice to coordinate squeezing the device and inhaling through it. You may find that having a friend or family member observe as you practice the following steps will help you perfect your technique. The idea is to mix the medication with incoming air and pull this mixture into the lungs slowly.

1. Shake the inhaler well, perhaps 5 or 6 times.

2. Attach a spacer to the nozzle end of the inhaler. A spacer is a 4- to 8-inch-long tube that helps to distribute the medication evenly in the bronchial tubes. Many expensive commercial spacers are available, but any tube of similar size may be used effectively as a spacer.

3. Hold your head erect and sit up straight. Breathe in and out nor-

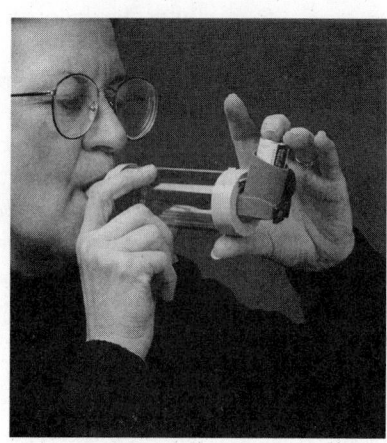

mally once, then stop for a moment. Do not try to push all the air from your lungs.

4. Close your mouth around the end of the spacer.

5. Squeeze the inhaler once, as you breathe in slowly. Keep inhaling even after finishing the squeeze. Continue inhaling for 5 to 7 seconds.

6. After inhaling, remove the spacer from your mouth and hold your breath for 10 seconds. Then, exhale through your nose.

7. If you need a second dose, breathe normally 4 or 5 times and repeat the sequence from step 1.

8. Gargle with water or brush your teeth after using a corticosteroid inhaler.

---

particulate-arresting (HEPA) filter on your furnace and maintain optimal humidity in your home. If you're allergic to house dust, attach a two-ply microfiltration bag or electrostatic filter to your vacuum cleaner.

Some adults with asthma experience severe attacks after taking nonsteroidal anti-inflammatory medications (NSAIDs), including aspirin or ibuprofen. You may need to avoid over-the-counter cold remedies and pain medications containing aspirin or ibuprofen. Foods with sulfites can also trigger an attack (see Sulfite Sensitivity, page 1049).

Health Care Team Partnership

Work closely with your physician. He or she is your partner in identifying causes of your asthma and in preventing or treating signs and symptoms.

Medications

Various medications are available and effective in controlling asthma. These are described here.

Preventers (Anti-Inflammatory Medications)

These drugs have replaced bronchodilators as mainstay medications. They are taken continuously to prevent attacks. Anti-inflammatory drugs reduce the number of inflammatory cells in airways and prevent blood vessels from leaking fluid into airway tissues. By reducing inflammation, they reduce spontaneous spasm of airway muscles. The most widely used anti-inflammatory medications include inhaled steroids, cromolyn sodium, and nedocromil sodium.

Inhaled steroids such as triamcinolone acetonide (Azmacort), beclomethasone dipropionate (Beclovent, Vanceril), and flunisolide (Aerobid) typically are used daily for moderate to severe disease. They help decrease the frequency of attacks and lower the dosage of an inhaled bronchodilator (beta agonist) needed to calm symptoms. Because inhalants deliver the medication directly to your airways, they cause fewer side effects than oral steroids (see Metered-Dose Inhaler, this page).

Other anti-inflammatory drugs include inhaled cromolyn sodium (Intal) and nedocromil sodium (Tilade). These can help prevent attacks in mild to moderate asthma when used daily. These drugs often are prescribed for children or young adults with asthma.

Relievers (Bronchodilators)
These medications open constricted airways and provide temporary relief during an attack. These include beta agonists, theophylline, and oral steroids.

Beta agonists are typically prescribed for mild, occasional symptoms. The more common drugs, such as albuterol (Proventil, Ventolin) and pirbuterol (Maxair), act quickly for use in acute attacks and before exercise or exposure to cold air. Prescribed "as needed," they relieve symptoms for up to 6 hours. Inhaled short-acting beta agonists don't correct underlying inflammation. Consequently, they aren't long-term solutions and can be easily overused.

Salmeterol (Serevent) is the longest-acting beta agonist inhalant. It relieves airway constriction for up to 12 hours and is often used to prevent symptoms, including nighttime attacks. Because salmeterol takes longer to act, it's not recommended for immediate relief during an attack. Beta agonists are also available as tablets but are not as speedy as inhalants.

You take *theophylline* as a pill to relieve nighttime symptoms. It's an older medication and is not as effective as a beta agonist, but it does last longer than the short-acting beta agonists.

Adults or children who have poorly controlled or severe asthma may need a short course, about 5 to 14 days, of an *oral steroid* such as prednisone.

Action Plan
With help from your physician, develop a written action plan for asthma control, including careful attention to all of the factors listed previously. Your plan should address your symptoms and medications, monitoring methods, and actions you should take in the event of acute symptoms. Follow the plan as long as it's effective. If you experience further difficulty, contact your physician for additional instructions.

With effective management, you can lead a normal, active, and healthy life.

What's Ahead?
As understanding of inflammation evolves, scientists hope to find new classes of drugs that interrupt the inflammatory process at key points. Researchers have discovered a gene associated with airway inflammation and constriction. Another gene, located on the same chromosome, is involved in allergic reactions. Ultimately, these discoveries may lead to gene therapy to prevent or treat asthma (see Color Guide to the Diagnosis and Treatment of Common Disorders, page 512).

Asthma and Exercise

In some people, asthma attacks are induced by exercise. This does not mean, however, that you need to eliminate exercise from your life. Although it may make breathing uncomfortable, regular exercise does not harm your lungs; rather it keeps your muscles in tone, which is important to your overall health.

The cause of an asthma attack after exercise is not known. Vigorous exercise is more likely to cause an asthma attack than is mild exercise. During cold weather, it is generally a good idea to exercise indoors because cold, dry air worsens the symptoms.

When you go out in cold weather, be sure to wear a soft scarf or a cold-air mask over your mouth and nose, even if you are just walking a short distance. You can purchase a cold-air mask at your local drugstore. Also, breathe through your nose so that your nose can warm, filter, and humidify the air that enters your lungs.

Taking medications to prevent asthma immediately before exercising also may help. Some of the medications that are effective are albuterol aerosol (Ventolin or Proventil) and, for some people, cromolyn aerosol (Intal) or nedocromil (Tilade). If you have asthma, be sure to talk to your physician about how to incorporate exercise into your lifestyle.

Allergies to Foods, Drugs, and Insect Stings

Allergies to foods, drugs, and insect stings may be the result of antibody responses to allergens that have come into contact with the internal systems of the body (see Understanding Allergy, page 1026). The symptoms may range from a simple rash to a systemic reaction involving the gastrointestinal tract and the respiratory and cardiovascular systems.

The symptoms may appear immediately after a specific food is eaten, a drug is administered, or a bee sting occurs. With some allergens, it may take several days, or even several weeks, for the reaction to develop.

Food Allergies

Signs and Symptoms
- Abdominal pain, diarrhea, nausea, or vomiting
- Fainting
- Hives, swelling beneath the skin (see page 1038), or eczema
- Swelling of the lips, eyes, face, tongue, and throat
- Nasal congestion
- Asthma

Emergency Symptoms
- Severe symptoms of the reactions listed above
- Anaphylaxis (see page 1053)

Few things are more distressing than a reaction to food because food represents something that nourishes and comforts. If you have experienced severe symptoms after eating, you may fear a recurrence. Perhaps this is why food allergies are the subject of widespread apprehension and misinformation.

Food allergies are specific responses of the immune system to a particular food or food component. The immune system produces vast numbers of antibodies to attack the food or food component, an occurrence that in turn releases histamine, which causes the symptoms.

Food allergies may be the most misunderstood of the allergies. Two out of five Americans believe they are allergic to specific foods. However, fewer than 1 percent have true food allergies. Most other discomforts do not involve release of histamine and should be termed food intolerances. Children have a higher percentage of food allergies than adults, but many of them grow out of these, often by around age 6. About 70 percent of food allergies develop in persons younger than 30.

Ninety percent of food allergies are caused by certain proteins in cow's milk, egg whites, peanuts, wheat, or soybeans. Other foods that can cause problems include berries, shellfish, corn, beans, and gum arabic (a thickener found in processed foods). Yellow Food Dye no. 5 may produce an allergic response (see Food Allergy vs. Food Intolerance, page 1049). Chocolate, long thought to be allergenic (particularly among children), is actually seldom a cause of allergy.

Diagnosis
Suppose you ate strawberries 2 days ago and now you have hives on your feet and hands. Yet you ate them a week ago and had no reaction. How could you be allergic to strawberries?

Most foods provoke an almost immediate reaction. For instance, if you eat something and within a few minutes your tongue and lips are swollen, it is easy to determine the cause. It is unusual for a food to cause a reaction that occurs more than 2 hours after eating.

To determine the cause of the problem, you may begin with a self-conducted elimination diet. Eliminate suspected foods from the diet for a week or two, then add them back to your diet one at a time. Such a method is not foolproof because psychological factors as well as physiologic factors come into play. If a person thinks he or she is sensitive to a food, this conviction well may play a part in triggering a response that may resemble but is probably not a true allergic reaction. If you've had a severe reaction, however, don't use this method.

Your physician will work through a number of diagnostic steps to help determine if you have a true food allergy. First, you will need to review the history of your symptoms, including when they occur, which foods cause problems, the amount of food needed to trigger symptoms, and whether you have a family history of allergies. Next, you may be asked to keep a detailed diary of everything you eat for several weeks, eating habits, symptoms, and medication use. Your physician also may conduct a physical examination.

A number of tests also are available to determine possible causes. The skin prick test signals activation of your immune system if you react to a small amount of food extract pricked into your skin. Negative skin tests are usually reliable, but positive skin tests are not because a test often can be positive for a substance that causes no reaction when it is eaten. A special approach is the double-blind challenge test. In this test, the person is given doses of suspected foods in disguised form so that neither the individual nor the physician knows what food is being administered. These results seem to be more

Food Allergy vs. Food Intolerance

Food allergy and food intolerance are frequently lumped together as a single condition. However, in a true allergic reaction the body releases histamine and other substances, which produce the gastrointestinal, respiratory, and skin symptoms associated with food allergies.

Food intolerance can produce somewhat similar symptoms, but the chemistry is quite different. No histamine is released. Common causes for a food intolerance include the absence of an enzyme that is needed to digest a specific food fully, irritable bowel syndrome, recurring stress, or food contaminated by a toxin. Such emotional and physical stresses can affect digestion and trigger adverse reactions.

Sometimes, no cause for particular problems is ever found. People claiming cures find a ready market. Untested theories abound, partly fueled by faddish self-help diet and nutrition books that label some foods as allergenic for conditions such as menstrual cramps, fatigue, nervousness, and hyperactivity and bed-wetting in children. Food plays no part in these—nor should cytotoxic testing, provocation and neutralization testing, or yeast hypersensitivity therapy, which are all unproven (see Inappropriate Tests and Treatments, page 1031).

One of the tricky aspects of diagnosing a food intolerance is that some people are allergic not to the food itself, such as peanuts, but to a substance or ingredient used in the preparation of the food. This is particularly true of foods containing lactose, wheat, monosodium glutamate, sulfites, salicylates, and possibly tartrazine.

Lactose Intolerance

As most people grow older, they are less able to tolerate lactose, a sugar found in milk. About 70 percent of the world's population—virtually everyone except Western Europeans and their descendants—are unable to process lactose efficiently after age 6. Even in infancy, 1 to 3 percent of all babies are lactose intolerant (see the discussion on lactose intolerance on page 772). Many people who are lactose intolerant can eat dairy products in which much of the lactose is already digested. These products include hard cheeses and cultured milk products such as yogurt and sour cream.

Wheat and Vegetable Intolerances

Intolerance to gluten, found primarily in wheat products, most commonly occurs in young children, who may or may not outgrow their sensitivity. Common vegetables that people are intolerant to include broccoli and peas, which produce intestinal gas, and mushrooms and wines, which produce indigestion and diarrhea.

Chinese Restaurant Syndrome

Monosodium glutamate (MSG), a commonly used flavor-enhancer, is thought to cause flushing, headache, and numbness about the mouth in susceptible people. Because many Chinese restaurants use MSG, these symptoms may occur after a susceptible person eats Chinese food; the reaction has come to be known as Chinese restaurant syndrome. MSG is also found in some seasoning mixtures and prepared foods.

Food Dye Sensitivity

Tartrazine, also known as Yellow Dye no. 5, is a food coloring used in foods, drugs, and cosmetics. It may produce allergic responses in some people who have asthma. Recent investigations question the role of tartrazine in these reactions. Foods colored yellow, orange, or yellow-green may contain tartrazine. Read all labels.

Sulfite Sensitivity

Sulfites are present in various foods, particularly wine, salads, fresh and dehydrated fruits, seafoods, potatoes, dehydrated soups, maraschino cherries, and some soft drinks. The sulfites help sanitize and preserve these foods. Although few people are sensitive to sulfites, about 4 to 8 percent of people with asthma are. If you are sensitive to sulfites and are eating away from home, ask whether sulfites have been added to the foods you may eat. Check food labels for the terms sodium bisulfite, potassium bisulfite, sodium sulfite, sulfur dioxide, and potassium metabisulfite.

Salicylate Sensitivity

Although very few people are sensitive to salicylates, they appear in many foods, especially fruits and their derivatives—vinegar, cider, and wine. If you are sensitive to salicylates, avoid any food prepared with them, including vinegar- and mayonnaise-based dressings, tartar sauce, and catsup; meats processed with vinegar such as corned beef; and pickles and other vegetables including avocado, corn, cucumbers, peppers, white potatoes, olives, and peppers. Beverages such as tea, root beer, fermented and distilled alcoholic beverages (except vodka) also have salicylates. In addition, avoid mint- and wintergreen-flavored foods.

conclusive, but this test is difficult and time-consuming.

In another test, immunoassays are used to check a sample of blood for antibodies specific to certain foods. This test is also more useful to exclude a food allergy than to diagnose one.

How Serious Are Food Allergies?

For most people, food allergies are uncomfortable, and often extremely so. Responses vary from minor sniffles and a cough to severe abdominal cramps, vomiting, and even anaphylactic shock. When a person reacts severely with an anaphylactic response—narrowed air passageways, rapid pulse, decrease in blood pressure, cardiovascular collapse, and shock—food allergies can be life-threatening.

Treatment

The only significant treatment for food allergy is avoidance of the food that causes the problem. For some people, eliminating certain foods from the diet is no hardship; for others who are allergic to foods common in the average diet it means living on a severely restricted diet that may make social eating difficult. When selecting substitute foods, people on restricted diets must be careful to choose foods that provide the necessary nutrients. They should avoid only those foods clearly shown to cause symptoms.

Emergency treatment is necessary when anaphylaxis develops. This includes an immediate injection of adrenaline (epinephrine) and a visit to the emergency room.

Sometimes it is not practical to avoid a food, particularly when that food is widely used. Occasionally, a reaction-causing food will not be detected. Also, some reactions may be irritating but not particularly dangerous or uncomfortable. If reaction to certain foods is a nuisance but not life-threatening, symptomatic relief may be considered. Your physician may prescribe antihistamines to relieve some symptoms. Skin reactions can be relieved with creams.

There are no ideal methods of treatment for food allergy, but people are not necessarily saddled with them for life. Children frequently grow out of their food allergies, often by age 6. Even adults may lose their sensitivities. Individuals of all ages lose sensitivities to milk, eggs, and soy products more quickly than to peanuts, walnuts, fish, and shellfish.

Drug Allergies

Signs and Symptoms
- Wheezing and difficulty in breathing
- Hives
- Generalized itching
- Rash
- Shock

Emergency Symptoms
- Anaphylaxis with severe swelling of eyes, lips, or tongue; swelling of the throat that causes difficulty in breathing; coughing or wheezing; hives; slurred speech; mental confusion; cramps; nausea and vomiting; anxiety; severe decrease in blood pressure resulting in unconsciousness (see page 1053)
- Severe asthma
- Obstruction of the throat by swelling

Almost any drug can cause an adverse reaction in someone. Reactions to most drugs are not common, but they can range from merely irritating to life-threatening. Some reactions are true allergic responses. (IgE antibodies are mobilized against the invading substance and histamine is released.) Others are side effects of a particular drug. Some are toxic effects of the drugs. Still others are reactions that are poorly understood or not understood at all. Your physician will determine the nature of the reactions you experience and what to do about them.

Penicillin and its relatives are responsible for many drug allergy reactions ranging from mild rashes to hives to immediate anaphylaxis. Most reactions are minor rashes. Only those who are extremely sensitive have the severe reaction of anaphylaxis. Many who are treated with another antibiotic, ampicillin, have a rash that is not an allergy.

Drugs that cause reactions include sulfas, barbiturates, anticonvulsants, insulin, and local anesthetics. In addition, contrast dyes that are injected into a person's blood vessels to help outline major organs in X-ray studies contain iodine and may cause an allergic reaction.

Almost a million Americans, primarily adults, have reactions to a common drug, aspirin. The response, hives, mimics the symptoms of a true allergy but has no immunologic basis. Almost a quarter of those who have chronic hives experience a worsening in their condition after they take aspirin. About 10 percent of those with asthma are sensitive to aspirin, too. In these persons, it can cause acute spasms of the bronchial tubes.

Diagnosis

A rash is the most common allergic reaction to drugs. Penicillins cause both a rash and hives and can be responsible for another reaction known as serum sickness. This reaction, which can take up to 3 weeks to develop, is characterized by fever, aching joints, swelling of the lymph glands, and rash. In very rare cases, penicillins, as well as streptomycin, insulin, and tetracycline, can cause anaphylactic shock.

Sensitivity to penicillin drugs can be diagnosed with a skin test. However, sensitivities to other drugs are not so easy to detect because for these the skin testing is ineffective or dangerous. That means that the physician must rely on the patient's memory about when and how certain drugs were taken, how much was taken, whether it was in combination with other drugs, how long after the dose the symptoms developed, and what other medications were being used at the time, including nonprescription items such as vitamins, laxatives, nose drops, cold remedies, and aspirin.

How Serious Is a Drug Allergy?

Severe reactions such as anaphylaxis or acute asthma are very serious because they can be life-threatening. Such reactions are rare. Most reactions are limited to rashes and hives. However, this does not mean that they can be ignored.

Treatment

The most common drug allergy reactions—rash, itching, and hives—are treated with antihistamines or, occasionally, steroid drugs (see Corticosteroid Drugs, page 919). Asthma reactions are treated with bronchodilators (see page 1047) and steroids. Anaphylaxis is treated with adrenaline injections (see page 1053).

Most drug allergies cannot be cured. The allergy to penicillin is an exception. In some cases, this sensitivity can be reduced enough so that the person can tolerate the drug. Small amounts of the drug are given in slowly increasing amounts. Sometimes antihistamines and steroids are given before and along with the penicillin doses to lessen the allergic reaction.

People who know they are allergic to certain drugs should avoid them. This means alerting their physicians of the sensitivity before treatment. It also may involve avoiding foods that may contain certain drugs. People sensitive to aspirin should avoid all aspirin-containing drugs.

Wear at all times an alert necklace or bracelet to indicate your allergy.

Insect Sting Allergies

Signs and Symptoms

- Hives
- Itchy eyes
- Constricted feeling of the throat and chest

Emergency Symptoms—Anaphylaxis with severe swelling of eyes, lips, or tongue; swelling of the throat that causes difficulty in breathing; coughing or wheezing; hives; slurred speech; mental confusion; cramps; nausea and vomiting; anxiety; severe decrease in blood pressure resulting in unconsciousness (see page 1053).

Most people consider the bite of a mosquito or the sting of a bee or wasp to be an irritation. The area may swell and itch or sting for several hours and then it returns to normal. However, perhaps as many as 1 to 2 percent of the population are extremely sensitive to insect venom, particularly that of

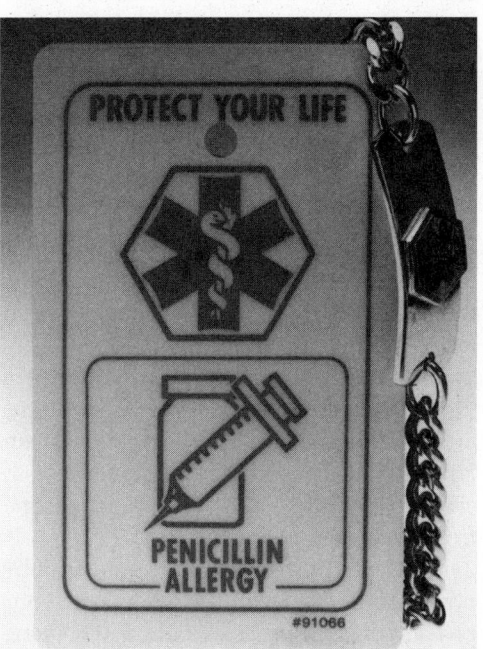

If you have a drug allergy, carry appropriate identification at all times.

insects such as bees, wasps, hornets, yellow jackets, and fire ants. Of these, yellow jackets are responsible for most of the reactions. Milder reactions that are not the allergy type can be caused by mosquitoes, ticks, biting flies, and some spiders.

The venom of most insects is composed of a number of chemicals. The toxic effects of the venom bother everyone by causing the redness, swelling, and itching at the site of the sting. In addition, in a sensitive person, an IgE antibody response occurs, thus releasing histamine into the system.

There is no one type of person likely to be allergic to insect stings. With some allergies, being sensitive to pollen or dust may predispose a person to being sensitive to other allergens. Such is not the case with insect sting allergies. People who work with bees often develop sensitivity as a result of multiple stings, but others can develop it at any time, after one or two stings or with the first one.

Diagnosis

Symptoms of insect sting allergy usually appear within a few minutes after the sting occurs. In people mildly sensitive to the venom, hives may develop and, in addition to the pain and intense itch around the site of the sting, the eyes may itch. Extremely sensitive people may have more serious symptoms such as severe hives and anaphylaxis, with constriction of the throat causing difficulty in breathing, abdominal and uterine cramps, nausea, vomiting, dizziness, severe drop in blood pressure, disorientation, and severe anxiety. They may also lapse into unconsciousness.

Severe reactions to insect stings can happen within 10 to 20 minutes, or they may not appear for several hours. Generally, the sooner the reaction begins, the more severe it will be. If a person exhibits any of the symptoms of a severe reaction, he or she should be treated immediately with adrenaline (epinephrine).

When the reaction is delayed, it often is in the form of serum sickness. The symptoms are fever, painful joints, hives, and swollen lymph glands. A person can experience both an immediate reaction and a delayed one from the same sting.

Diagnosis of the exact cause may not be possible immediately, but at some point your physician will ask questions about where the insect stung you, what it looked like, how it moved, what the sting looked like, and at what time of day and where the incident occurred. To confirm the diagnosis, your physician may perform skin tests several weeks after the incident.

How Serious Are Insect Sting Allergies?

Insect sting allergies are not to be taken lightly. The reactions can range from mild to life-threatening. A person who knows he or she is sensitive to stings should be under the care of a physician for any sting. Many people do not know they are highly sensitive, however, and their past experience is not always dependable because sensitivity can develop at any time.

Treatment

In the case of severe reactions, a physician or emergency medical team may perform cardiopulmonary resuscitation. Occasionally, if the throat is constricted enough to block passage of air, a tracheostomy will be performed and a tube will be inserted. An injection of adrenaline (epinephrine) will be administered. A strong dose of antihistamine can help decrease the severity of the reaction.

Corticosteroids, which act over a longer period of time than the emergency treatment with adrenaline, are often prescribed to reduce hives and other swelling (see Corticosteroid Drugs, page 919).

When the reaction is less severe, the person can help minimize the effects by keeping the venom as localized as possible: remove the stinger, and place a cold pack on the wound to keep swelling and itching down (see Insect Bites and Stings, page 395).

Once the diagnosis of insect sting allergy is made, there are a number of things you can do. For one, immunotherapy can be used to build your tolerance to the offending venom. Injections of small amounts of the venom will be administered every week until you can tolerate the amount of venom in a sting or bite. From then on, you will receive maintenance injections every 4 to 6 weeks for a 3- to 5-year period.

There are other things you can do, too. Begin by avoiding these kinds of insects as much as possible. Beekeepers should give up their hives. Avoid the things that attract these insects, too. Clothing with flowery prints or black, brown, or bright colors is attractive to certain insects, as are sweet perfumes, scented soaps, suntan lotions, and other cosmetics. White clothing does not interest bees and the insects related to them.

Wear shoes and long-sleeved shirts when you are outside. Wear close-fitting clothes that will not allow insects to fly inside them.

Avoid places where bees and other stinging insects are found. Orchards attract bees, as do flower gardens and fields or lawns containing clover. The food at picnics and outdoor concessions attracts wasps and bees.

If you feel in danger of being stung, act calm. Move away from the insect slowly and without sudden movement. Panicky flailing only agitates insects.

Extremely sensitive people can safeguard themselves by keeping an emergency kit containing antihistamine tablets and a syringe filled with adrenaline (epinephrine). Your physician can prescribe such a kit, to be used until you can reach a hospital. Wearing an alert bracelet or necklace or carrying an identification card will provide helpful information if an emergency team is summoned in the case of a severe reaction.

Anaphylaxis

Signs and Symptoms
- Constriction of airways, including swollen throat, resulting in breathing difficulty
- Shock associated with severe decrease in blood pressure
- Rapid pulse
- Cardiovascular collapse
- Hives and angioedema
- Nausea, vomiting, or diarrhea
- Dizziness, mental confusion, slurred speech, or extreme anxiety

Anaphylaxis is the most severe and frightening allergic response. Luckily, it is also the most infrequent, although each year several hundred Americans die from the reaction.

Anaphylaxis is an IgE antibody response to a large number of different antigens. The anaphylactic reaction is systemic, meaning that it is not limited to the site of the irritation. A mild reaction may cause only generalized hives and intense itching. A severe reaction is life-threatening because its most characteristic symptom is constriction of the air passageways in the bronchial tract or in the throat, or in both. It is often accompanied by shock—a situation in which there can be sudden decrease of blood pressure that causes a rapid pulse as well as weakness, paleness, mental confusion, unconsciousness, and cardiovascular collapse. These can cause death if not treated immediately.

Almost any allergen can cause the response, including insect venoms, pollens, latex, the horse serum used in a few vaccines, certain foods, drugs such as penicillin, aspirin, and insulin, and the contrast agents injected as part of some X-ray procedures. Some persons have anaphylactic reactions of unknown cause.

The anaphylactic response is quick, beginning seconds or minutes after an allergen is encountered. Anaphylaxis occurs more commonly after certain insect stings and bites and intravenous injection of certain drugs. Only rarely do pollens cause the anaphylactic response. Certain foods such as peanuts, true nuts, and shellfish also can cause fatal reactions.

A person who experiences a mild reaction may have a severe reaction with a subsequent exposure. A person also may become hypersensitive at any time, whether previously sensitized or not.

Treatment
The standard treatment for anaphylaxis is injection of adrenaline (epinephrine), which opens the airways and improves blood circulation. Cardiovascular resuscitation and emergency tracheostomy sometimes have to be performed as life-saving measures.

Chapter 32

Infectious Diseases

Contents

The Workings of Your Immune
System, 1056
    Enlargement of Lymph Nodes, 1057
    Antibacterial Agents, 1058
**Types of Infectious and Parasitic
  Agents, 1059**
    Antifungal Drugs, 1059
    Antiviral Drugs, 1060

Generalized Infections, 1060
HIV Infection and AIDS, 1060
    When a Loved One Has AIDS, 1063
Infectious Mononucleosis, 1064
    Chronic Fatigue Syndrome, 1065
Influenza, 1065
    Flu Shots, 1066
Lyme Disease, 1067
Cat Scratch Disease, 1067
Rocky Mountain Spotted Fever, 1068
Typhoid Fever, 1068
    Fever of Unknown Origin, 1069
Tetanus, 1070
Rabies, 1070

Common Contagious Diseases, 1071
Common Viral Colds, 1071
    How to Take a Temperature and How to
      Read a Thermometer, 1072
Measles, 1073
    The Dangers of Aspirin, 1073
German Measles, 1074
Roseola, 1074
Whooping Cough, 1075

Croup, 1076
Chickenpox, 1076
    Smallpox, 1077
Mumps, 1077
    Immunization Schedule for Normal,
      Healthy Infants and Children, 1078
Diphtheria, 1078
    Immunizations, 1079
Scarlet Fever, 1080

Parasitic Infestations, 1080
Malaria, 1080
Tapeworm, 1081
Trichinosis, 1082
Pinworms, 1082
Strongyloidosis, 1083
Ascariasis, 1083
Hookworm, 1084

Insect Infestations, 1085
Scabies, 1085
Lice, 1085
Fleas, 1086
Chiggers, 1086
Ticks, 1087

Sexually Transmitted Diseases, 1087
Gonorrhea, 1087
Chlamydial Infections, 1088
Syphilis, 1089
Genital Herpes, 1090
    Safe Sex, 1091
Venereal Warts, 1092

The Workings of Your Immune System

Your body has many mechanisms that defend you against infectious organisms (see Understanding Allergy, page 1026). Your skin and your gastrointestinal tract are the first lines of defense. If infectious organisms get past these barriers, the immune system takes up the challenge of eliminating any invaders.

There are two general categories of immune mechanisms: humoral and cell-mediated.

Humoral immunity is based on certain body proteins called antibodies, which are found dissolved in the blood and other body fluids. The antibodies are made by plasma cells, which are derived from certain white blood cells called B lymphocytes (or B cells). The antibodies are produced in response to exposure to a foreign substance. In birds, these plasma cells are derived from a particular structure called the bursa of Fabricius, hence the term B cell.

Any foreign substance that enters the body—such as by injection or through a wound—and causes the manufacture of antibodies is called an antigen. The antibody produced will "fit" the antigen much like a key fits a lock and neutralize that foreign substance or render it harmless. Antibodies are specific: each is effective against any antigen that caused its creation.

A good example of how antigens create antibodies to protect our bodies is the immunization for prevention of tetanus. Tetanus toxoid in a carefully determined amount is injected into the muscle. (A toxoid is a toxin that has been rendered harmless to your body but is still capable of producing immunity.) The body recognizes the tetanus toxoid and responds by creating antibodies that will neutralize the toxic substances produced by the tetanus organisms. Within a few weeks, these antibodies begin to circulate in the body's fluids and will persist in measurable amounts for many years.

Once the body has learned to produce a particular antibody, it can resume production of that antibody quite rapidly. Thus, if a person has had the initial series of immunization injections for tetanus, a single injection 5 to 10 years later (booster shot) can stimulate the appearance of protective amounts of antibodies in the blood within a few days.

Your immune system reacts to foreign invaders (antigens) such as infectious organisms. The immune response aims to neutralize or destroy the antigens, thus rendering them harmless. Antigens may activate B cells (lymphocytes), which primarily reside in blood, in lymph nodes along the gastrointestinal tract, and in bone marrow. In humoral immunity, B cells produce plasma cells, which, in turn, produce antibodies that neutralize antigens. In other situations, so-called memory B cells "remember" antigens and rapidly produce antibodies to inactivate them.

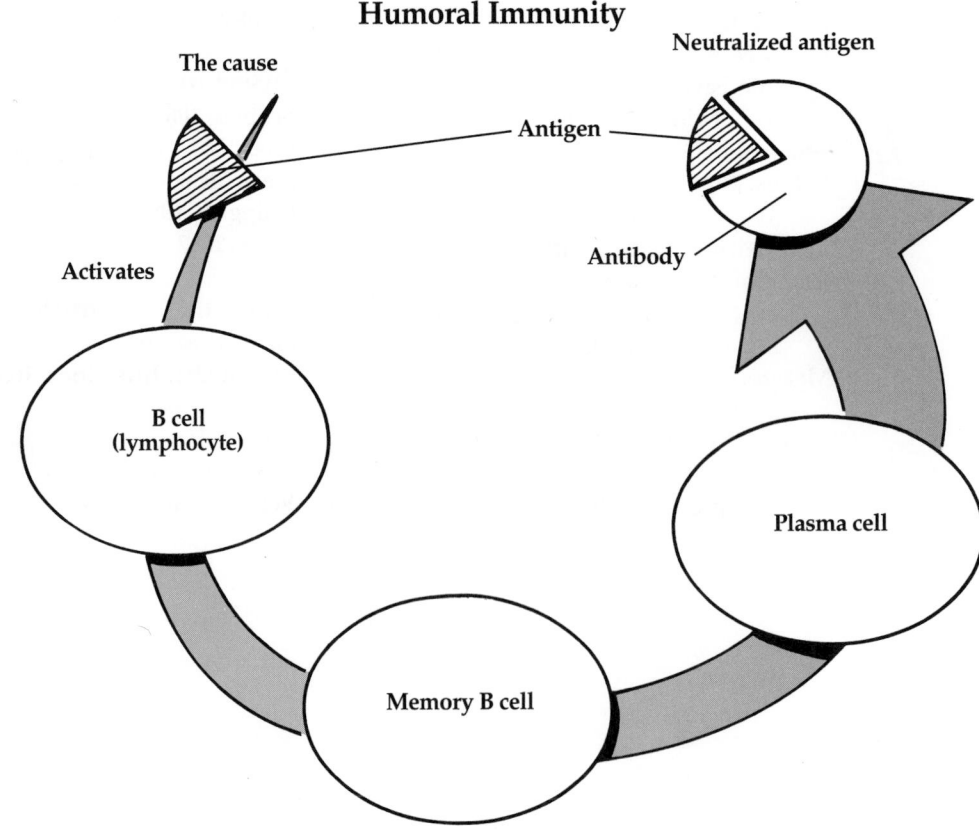

Humoral Immunity

The cause

Neutralized antigen

Antigen

Activates

Antibody

B cell (lymphocyte)

Plasma cell

Memory B cell

Cell-Mediated Immunity

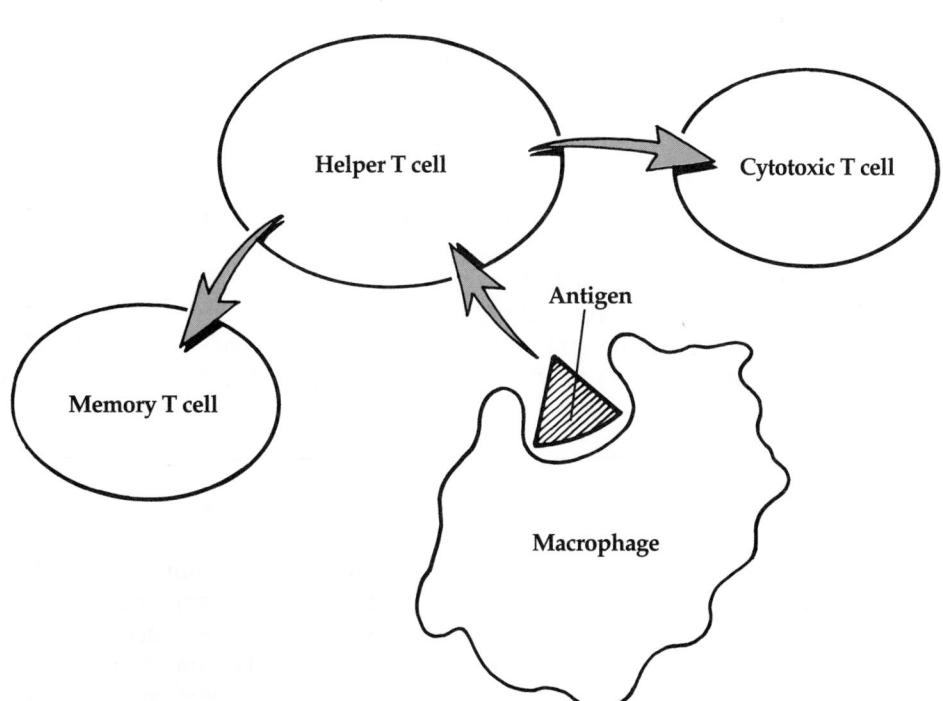

A second type of immune response is called cell-mediated immunity. In this type, foreign invaders (antigens) are engulfed (ingested) by macrophages, which process and present the antigens to T cells. The macrophages then activate the helper T cells, which aid in development of cytotoxic T cells (which kill antigens directly) and memory T cells (which stimulate an immune response on re-exposure to the same antigens).

Cell-mediated immunity is based on the actions of phagocytes and other white blood cells. Phagocytes are cells that can dissolve or engulf and destroy viruses, bacteria, fungi, and cells foreign to the body.

White blood cells that are involved in this defense are a type of lymphocyte called T cells because they are derived from the thymus gland. About 70 percent of the T cells are designated helper-inducer cells; the remaining 20 to 30 percent are cytotoxic cells. T cells play a central role in the regulation of the immune response.

The helper cells function to increase the number of cells (macrophages) that can engulf or dissolve foreign particles in response to an

Enlargement of Lymph Nodes

Lymph nodes function as sites of macrophage, T-cell, and B-cell contact with antigens as part of your immune response.

Enlargement of lymph nodes occurs as the result of an increase in the number of lymphocytes and macrophages needed to respond to foreign antigens. Lymph nodes also may enlarge because of infiltration of inflammatory cells involved in response to infections. They also become enlarged with increasing numbers of malignant lymphocytes or because there is infiltration of lymph nodes by metastatic malignant cells. An uncommon enlargement of lymph nodes occurs in certain lipid storage diseases.

It is not uncommon to feel small lymph nodes in the inguinal or groin area. In addition, smaller lymph nodes due to past infections may be present normally. If lymph nodes are newly enlarged and do not decrease in size over several weeks and there is no known source for enlargement such as a nearby infection, it may be prudent to seek further advice from your physician. Most of the time, enlarged lymph nodes in persons younger than 30 resolve in time. However, in persons older than 50, enlarged lymph nodes may suggest an underlying more serious disease.

Lymph nodes also occur in areas that are not palpable. Chronic hoarseness, coughing, wheezing, or unilateral enlargement or congestion of an extremity should be brought to the attention of your physician for further evaluation, because a potential cause is obstruction by lymph nodes. In addition, other diseases that affect the immune system such as rheumatoid arthritis, systemic lupus erythematosus (see page 918), and drug reactions may also result in enlarged lymph nodes. Occasionally, enlarged lymph nodes may be associated with enlargement of the spleen, because both have similar immune functions.

infection. Neutrophils, another type of white blood cell, also function in this fashion. They are greatly increased in number during infections such as pneumonia or appendicitis. The helper-inducer cells also facilitate the production of antibodies by stimulating growth and activity of B cells.

Lymphocytes are found in the bone marrow, in the spleen, circulating in the blood, and in the lymph nodes. The lymph nodes are collections of lymphocytes held together by connective or fibrous tissue. Some nodes are located in the neck, groin, and armpits, where they can be felt if they become firm and enlarged in the course of a disease. They often are mistakenly called lymph glands. Other lymph nodes are found in the abdomen and at the center of the lungs.

Lymph is a nearly colorless fluid that runs in channels in all parts of the body to and through the lymph nodes and, ultimately, into the bloodstream. The lymph nodes constitute a partial barrier to organisms that may be traveling in the lymph. For instance, if a virulent streptococcus bacterium penetrates the skin by way of a crack between the toes of a person with athlete's foot, it can multiply and travel up the leg in the lymph channels.

Antibacterial Agents

Before penicillin was discovered, very few medications were available to combat bacterial infections. Now, however, many antibacterial agents are available to treat infectious diseases, and more are continually being developed.

Most antibacterial agents are antibiotics (substances produced by microorganisms), but not all. Some are synthetic chemicals. All of the antibacterial agents may cause undesirable and sometimes serious effects, but this is uncommon.

Bacterial Specificity
Each antibiotic works against specific types of bacteria. Some affect only one or two kinds. Others affect many. When your physician first suspects you have an infectious disease, he or she may take samples of your blood, pus, urine, stool, or sputum to try to identify the organism and to determine how resistant or susceptible that particular strain will be to different antibiotics.

It usually takes at least 24 hours to get the results of these tests. Therefore, depending on the diagnosis, your physician may prescribe one of the antibiotics that attack a broad array of bacteria. Then, the culture results may suggest a change to a more appropriate antibiotic.

Topical Versus Oral Antibiotics
For certain localized infections of the eye, ear, or skin, antibiotics are applied topically as a solution or ointment. However, in most cases, antibiotics are given orally, intramuscularly, or intravenously. After an antibiotic (or any drug) is administered, it enters your bloodstream from your intestine (if taken orally), from muscles (if given intramuscularly), or directly (if given intravenously). Antibiotics are given intravenously or intramuscularly only if the infection is serious or the drug is not properly absorbed when taken orally.

Antibiotics at Work
Once absorbed into your bloodstream, the antibiotic circulates rapidly through your whole body. (It takes only about a minute for your heart to circulate all of the blood in your body.) However, the antibiotic will act only where it encounters particular bacteria. It does this either by killing the bacteria or by preventing them from multiplying, depending on the type of antibiotic and the dosage.

Kinds of Antibiotics
Some antibiotics such as the penicillins and cephalosporins kill bacteria by interfering with their ability to form cell walls, which ultimately causes their death. Most other antibacterial agents, including the aminoglycosides (such as gentamicin and streptomycin), the tetracyclines, the sulfonamides, and the macrolides (such as erythromycin), interfere with proteins and chemicals the bacteria need to multiply and survive. This allows your body's natural immune system to control and eliminate them.

Antibiotic Resistance
When bacteria are exposed to an antibiotic they may, over time, develop a resistance or tolerance to that antibiotic. This can happen quickly or slowly. The development of resistance does not change the appearance under the microscope or any other characteristic of that strain of bacteria. Whether or not a given strain of bacteria is resistant to an antibiotic can be determined only by sensitivity tests performed in the laboratory.

Because antibiotic resistance develops in the bacteria in our environment, some antibiotics have become less useful than they were in the past. Newer antibiotics are constantly being developed, but we can expect that they, too, will become less effective in a number of years. Infections that are acquired while a person is in a hospital are particularly likely to be caused by an antibiotic-resistant organism.

These channels carrying the infection may be seen beneath the skin as red streaks, sometimes incorrectly termed blood poisoning (also called lymphangitis, see page 1010). The lymph nodes in the groin of that leg become swollen and tender while keeping the infection in check at that level. In some diseases that cause multiplication and mobilization of lymphocytes and that involve the entire body, such as infectious mononucleosis, all of the lymph nodes and the spleen may become enlarged and can be felt by the physician during a physical examination.

Your immune system is a complex defense system for suppressing and eliminating infections. At the same time, infectious organisms have complex offense systems. The result is a constant battle between your body and infection—a battle your body usually wins, but not always.

Types of Infectious and Parasitic Agents

Agents that can invade your body live everywhere—in the air; on dust particles, food, and plants; on and in animals and humans; in soil and water; and on virtually every other surface. They range from microscopic organisms to larger parasites.

The vast majority of these organisms do not produce disease, but some do. This majority is usually kept under control by your immune system, but if your system becomes weakened or you encounter an organism to which you have not built up a resistance, illness results.

The basic types of organisms that cause infectious diseases are described below.

Bacteria

Bacteria are one-cell organisms that are visible only under a microscope. They appear as slender rods or groups of round cells, live without need for other organisms, and are able to live and multiply by subdivision. When infectious bacteria gain entry to your body, they multiply and may produce powerful chemicals, called toxins, that damage specific cells in the tissue they have invaded and cause you to become ill. A few of the more common groups of bacteria that cause disease are *Staphylococci*, *Streptococci*, *Chlamydia*, *Haemophilus*, *Gonococci*, and *Rickettsia*. Not all bacteria are harmful. Some bacteria that reside in our bodies (for example, our mouth or gut) are beneficial.

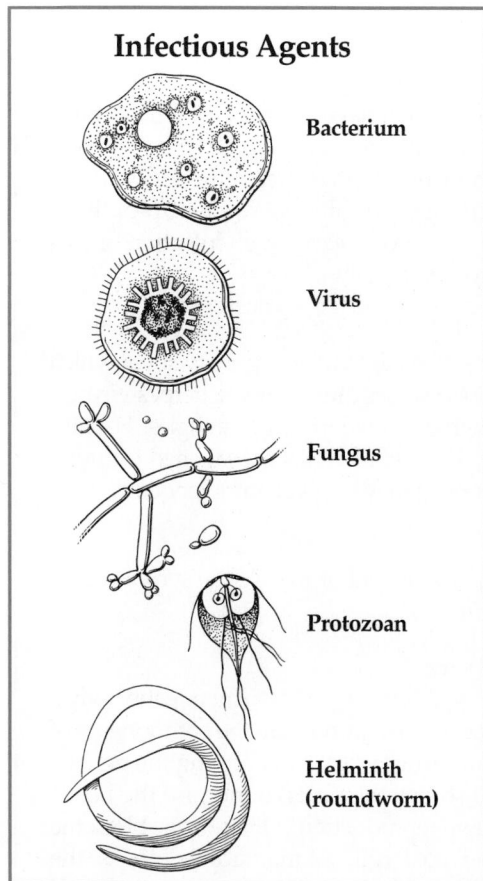

Infectious Agents

Bacterium

Virus

Fungus

Protozoan

Helminth
(roundworm)

Viruses

A virus is not able to reproduce on its own. In its simplest form, it is a capsule containing genetic material. When it invades your body, it enters some of your cells and takes them over, instructing these host cells to manufacture the parts it needs to multiply. In the process, the host cell eventually is destroyed. Polio, AIDS, and the common cold are among the many ailments caused by viruses.

Fungi

Molds, yeasts, and mushrooms all are types of fungi. Obviously, mushrooms are not

Antifungal Drugs

Infections caused by fungi, such as athlete's foot, jock itch, ringworm, and candidiasis, rarely heal without some drug therapy. There are several drugs that are effective in the treatment of fungal infections. Some should be applied only topically. Others may be taken orally or given as an injection.

Antifungal drugs act on the cell wall of the fungus, damaging it and allowing the contents of the cell to leak out, which kills the cell. When given topically, antifungal drugs rarely have adverse effects.

Antiviral Drugs

In the past 2 decades, drugs that have an effect on viruses have been introduced into medical practice. No drug completely eradicates a viral infection, but it can decrease the severity and duration of the infection. Viruses multiply extremely rapidly, so antiviral drugs must be given very early in an infection or as a preventive measure (prophylactically).

Acyclovir

The most commonly prescribed antiviral drug is acyclovir, which is used in the treatment of diseases caused by the herpes viruses, such as genital and oral herpes, chickenpox, and shingles. Usually, the drug is given orally. If the patient has a weakened immune system or a severe infection, it may be given intravenously.

Amantadine

This antiviral drug helps to prevent or to ease the symptoms of influenza (see page 1065).

How Antiviral Drugs Work

A virus cannot multiply on its own; it needs to invade the body's cells and cause the host cells to manufacture the components of the virus. Some antiviral drugs work by changing the genetic material of the host cell so that the virus cannot use the host's genetic material for its own reproduction. Other drugs block the enzyme activity of the host cell. Amantadine blocks the influenza virus from entering the host cell. However, antiviral drugs may have adverse side effects, so use caution.

infectious, but certain yeasts and molds can be. These single-cell organisms are slightly larger than bacteria. Of the thousands that are harmless or even helpful (yeast causes bread to rise), only about 100 cause disease. *Candida* is one example. It can produce thrush, an infection of the mouth and throat, in infants and in persons who have received antibiotics or have impaired immunity (see page 618).

Protozoa

Protozoa are single-cell organisms that may live within you as a parasite. Often these organisms spend part of their life cycle outside of humans, living in food, soil, water, or insects. The protozoa that cause malaria are an example. Many protozoa reside in the intestinal tract and are harmless, although some may cause disease.

Helminths

The word "helminth" comes from the Greek word *helmins*, meaning "worm." These are among the larger parasites. If they enter your body, they take up residence in your intestinal tract, lungs, liver, skin, or even brain, where they live off the nutrients in your body. The most common helminths are tapeworms and roundworms.

Generalized Infections

Among the challenges to your immune system are a wide range of diseases. Some are bacterial, some are viral, and still others have other causes.

In the following pages we discuss several of the most common infectious diseases, ranging from such familiar childhood ailments as measles and chickenpox to AIDS.

Note that in most cases in which an infectious disorder predominantly affects only one organ or body system (such as the heart, brain, or skin), the disease is discussed in the chapter devoted to that subject. The following diseases affect multiple systems of the body, hence the term "generalized infections."

HIV Infection and AIDS

Signs and Symptoms (HIV Infection)
- Persistent unexplained fatigue
- Soaking night sweats
- Shaking chills or fever higher than 100 degrees lasting for several weeks
- Unexplained weight loss of more than 10 percent of body weight in 1 to 2 months
- Unexplained swelling of lymph nodes which persists for more than 3 months
- Chronic diarrhea
- Persistent unexplained headaches
- Persistent dry cough and shortness of breath

- Persistent white spots or unusual blemishes on the tongue or in the mouth
- Persistent bruise-like blotches on or under the skin or inside the mouth, nose, or eyelids
- Difficulties with speech, memory, concentration, or coordination

AIDS (acquired immunodeficiency syndrome) is an immune deficient state caused by HIV (human immunodeficiency virus). This virus is believed to have entered the United States in the late 1970s, although it is not certain how HIV first infected humans. In the human population, its effects manifest as a progressive weakening of the immune system.

If your immune system is healthy, white blood cells and antibodies help to fight against microscopic germs to keep you free from disease. When a foreign organism enters your body, it is attacked and destroyed. This response is coordinated by T-cell lymphocytes (see The Workings of Your Immune System, page 1056).

When HIV enters your body, it cannot live on its own. It must take over another living cell to survive.

HIV attaches and enters the T-helper lymphocytes and incorporates its (HIV genes) genetic sequences into the host cells. HIV then replicates within the T-helper lymphocytes. HIV also infects macrophages, which are important HIV reservoir cells.

When the newly formed viruses burst out of the cell, they continue the cycle by infecting more T-helper lymphocytes. Your immune system tries to overcome this infection by producing antibodies and forming more helper cells. As these antibodies are being produced, you are considered to be in the process of "seroconversion." Most people who have seroconversion will have flu-like symptoms, which is known as acute HIV infection.

Once infected with HIV, most people have no symptoms and no indication that they are infected. However, from the point of exposure, infected individuals are able to transmit the virus to others.

Unfortunately, an HIV test is not accurate immediately after exposure, because it takes time for your body to produce an antibody response. The time between exposure to HIV and a positive HIV antibody test is called the "window period." This is the time it takes

an exposed individual to develop antibodies, usually 6 to 12 weeks, but it can take up to 6 months.

HIV continues to reproduce and eventually weakens your immune system to the point that opportunistic diseases (ones that your body would normally fight off) begin to affect you. Opportunistic diseases or a T-cell count less than 200 and a positive HIV antibody test are the deciding factors in the diagnosis of AIDS.

Unnamed until the early 1980s, AIDS is a worldwide pandemic. At the beginning of 1996, scientists estimated that more than 20 million people worldwide were infected with HIV and that more than 4.5 million people had AIDS. The World Health Organization estimates that by the year 2000, more than 40 million people worldwide will be HIV-positive. In the United States, it is estimated there are 1.5 million persons with HIV infection.

HIV crosses all cultures, all national borders, and all religions. You cannot tell by looking at an individual or by an individual's race, sex, or sexual orientation whether that person is HIV-positive. HIV can infect anyone. It does not discriminate.

How Do You Get AIDS?

For transmission to occur, three things must happen.

The Virus Must Exist

HIV must be present in certain secretions for transmission to occur during certain activities. If HIV is not present, it cannot be contracted.

HIV Must be Present in a Large Enough Concentration

Body fluids such as tears, sweat, and saliva do not carry significant amounts of HIV. Therefore, they are not considered to be modes of transmission.

The Virus Needs to Enter Your Bloodstream

Only when HIV is transmitted across normal barriers into the bloodstream does infection occur. You cannot contract HIV from casual contact such as hugging, kissing, or sharing household items. These activities do not provide a route for HIV to enter your bloodstream.

HIV can enter your body through four main body fluids: blood, semen (including pre-seminal fluid), vaginal fluids, and breast milk. The transmission can take place in several ways:

Sexual Contact. HIV can be contracted through sexual contact with an infected individual. This contact can be oral, anal, or vaginal between opposite-sex or same-sex partners.

One way to reduce the risk of transmission is to use a latex condom consistently and correctly during each sexual contact. It is important to remember that condoms are not perfect. They can help reduce but will not eliminate your risk of contracting HIV.

Absolute ways to prevent contracting HIV are abstinence from sexual intercourse and certainty that your sexual partner does not have an HIV infection. Also, decreasing the number of partners reduces your risk of infection.

Direct Blood Contact. Another method of transmission involves direct blood contact. The most common example of this method is the sharing of needles for any purpose (including drug use, steroid use, tattooing, and piercing).

Mother and Child. Transmission of HIV can occur between mother and child. This can happen when the baby is in the uterus, during the birth process, or during breast-feeding.

Blood Transfusion. Since 1985, federal law has mandated that all blood and blood products be tested for HIV antibodies. Currently, the risk of becoming infected through a blood transfusion is very low, about 1 in 250,000.

Health care providers who handle body fluids are at risk of becoming infected. However, the chance of contracting HIV while treating an infected patient is low. Annually, fewer than 3 of every 1,000 health care workers (less than 0.3 percent) who accidentally stick themselves with HIV-contaminated sharp instruments become HIV-positive themselves.

When learning about risks for contracting HIV and AIDS, it is just as important for you to know how HIV is not transmitted. HIV is not transmitted through casual contact such as hugging or kissing. It is not transmitted through contact with drinking fountains, public toilets, public phones, swimming pools, dishes, or insects.

Diagnosis

The HIV status of a person (HIV-positive or HIV-negative) can be determined only after testing the blood for antibodies to the virus. This test should be done between 3 and 6 months after the individual suspected he or she was exposed to HIV. This elapsed time is due to the "window period."

HIV-antibody tests involve a combination of procedures. Most blood is tested with the enzyme-linked imunosorbent assay (ELISA) screening test. If this detects HIV antibodies, the test is repeated. If the second ELISA also shows antibodies, another confirming test, known as the Western blot, is performed. This test is used to confirm the results of the ELISA. The combination of these methods makes testing for HIV antibodies nearly 100 percent accurate.

A T-helper cell count less than 200, or a diagnosis of an opportunistic disease in combination with a positive HIV test, is enough to diagnose AIDS. Some persons with a count less than 200 still do not look sick. However, the opportunistic diseases and low T-cell count are signs that the individual's immune system is beginning to fail.

The diagnosis of AIDS does not take place immediately after an individual becomes infected with HIV. In fact, the average time between exposure to HIV and the diagnosis of AIDS is typically between 10 and 12 years.

Some of the most common opportunistic diseases are *Pneumocystis carinii* pneumonia and Kaposi's sarcoma. *Pneumocystis carinii* is a microorganism that invades the lungs. Healthy persons normally can resist such an infection. However, in someone whose immune system is compromised, this infection multiplies in the lungs and leads to difficulty in breathing.

Kaposi's sarcoma is a rare cancer that also occurs in persons who have compromised immune systems. This usually manifests as red or purplish spots on the skin, lymph nodes, mouth, digestive tract, or lung tissues.

Before being tested for HIV or AIDS, one needs to consider the implications of a positive test. It is important to ask your physician whether testing is done on an anonymous or confidential basis. Confidential testing means that your results will be recorded, but no one can give them out without your permission (except where required by law). Anonymous testing means that your name is not recorded and only you can learn the results of your test. Regardless of which testing method you choose, you should choose a testing facility that offers counseling before and after testing and performs tests accurately.

When a Loved One Has AIDS

AIDS is a devastating and debilitating disease. Dealing with the effects and consequences of AIDS is difficult not only for the individual but also for his or her family and friends. Despite the advances being made with new medications, there is no cure for AIDS. The emotional and physical support of family and friends is vital in helping those with the disease to lead the most nearly normal life possible.

There are many things you can do and should know if you have a friend or relative who is stricken with AIDS. First and most important: know the facts (see page 1060)—many misconceptions exist about this disease.

Try to Be Nonjudgmental

Because the most common ways to contract AIDS are through high-risk sexual intercourse or via shared needles among intravenous drug users, hearing that a friend or relative has AIDS may cause conflicting emotions. If the person contracted the virus through high-risk behavior, and you disapprove of his or her lifestyle, you may be forced to confront that person's lifestyle for the first time. Realizing that someone you care about may die can bring out unresolved pain and problems between you. Especially because most AIDS patients are in the prime of their lives when the disease develops, the effects of the illness and the prospect of death are particularly hard to face.

Be Positive

Try to focus on the positive aspects of your relationship—who the individual is, why you care about him or her, and what you can do to help. Do not feel that you need to keep your feelings to yourself. Discuss them with the patient and others, including perhaps clergy, counselors, or members of support groups.

Do Not Go It Alone

You cannot care for an AIDS patient alone. It is important to establish a network of professionals, friends, and relatives who can provide help and support. Depending on his or her health, the patient should make as many of the personal decisions as possible.

It may be helpful to designate one or two people to serve as contacts for health care and other professionals, friends, and relatives who are concerned but not as involved in the day-to-day care of the individual. This person, or persons, also can look after the patient's business matters such as bills, insurance, and correspondence. You may want to consult an attorney about having one person assume power of attorney, with the right to make decisions on behalf of the patient if he or she is incapacitated (see How to Prepare an Advance Directive, page 1381).

A diagnosis of AIDS can have an effect on insurance, employment, education, and housing. So respect the person's right to privacy and let him or her decide who should know about the condition. Remember that the disease should not exclude someone from receiving care or services. The American Medical Association, other professional groups, federal law, and many state regulations state that you must not discriminate against AIDS patients.

Home Care

In providing home care, create an environment that is pleasant and comfortable. Maintain the person's personal hygiene. This is vital. Also, the individual should bathe regularly, especially if he or she suffers from fevers or night sweats. Hospital or home health care workers can teach you the rollover method for bathing a person and changing sheets without getting the person out of bed. Oral hygiene is also important. If a toothbrush causes bleeding, use a washcloth or sponge-tipped swab to clean the teeth and gums, or use a mouth rinse of warm salt water or dilute hydrogen peroxide.

Am I at Risk?

You cannot contract AIDS by coming into casual contact with a patient, but do avoid direct unprotected contact with the individual's blood, semen, vaginal secretions, or other secretions that contain blood, because these are infectious. Do not share razors, toothbrushes, or other items that may carry blood. Clothing, sheets, and towels that carry bodily secretions, vomit, or diarrhea should be removed and washed in hot, soapy water. If secretions with blood spill onto a hard surface, wash them off with a 1:10 solution of household bleach to kill the virus.

Wash your hands before and after any contact with the patient. When giving injections, cleaning the teeth, or washing the anal or genital areas, use disposable vinyl or latex gloves. If you handle feces, vomit, or urine, wear gloves. If the possibility exists that secretions may splash into your mouth or eyes, wear a mask and protective glasses. If you use needles and syringes as part of the person's care, use special (puncture-proof) containers to dispose of them and never bend, break, or recap a needle.

Remember that a person with AIDS needs your respect and affection and needs to carry on as normal a life as possible for as long as possible.

Treatment

It is important to choose a health care provider who is supportive and informed. Because there is no cure for HIV or AIDS, treatment will focus on controlling symptoms and prolonging life.

Your physician will monitor your immune system and assess your general health regularly to evaluate the development of your disease and to determine whether additional action is required. It is also important to practice good nutrition, hygiene, and general health. Probably one of the most crucial aspects of HIV and AIDS treatment is emotional support.

Medications

The three main categories of medications for HIV and AIDS are antiviral drugs, immune system boosters, and medications to help prevent or treat opportunistic infections.

Antiviral drugs are used in an attempt to interfere with the multiplication of HIV. These agents may prolong survival in people with symptomatic HIV infection. The earlier antiviral drugs—zidovudine (AZT), didanosine (DDI), zalcitabine (DDC), and stavudine (D4T)—acted by inhibiting replication of an HIV enzyme called reverse transcriptase.

A new class of medications is called "protease inhibitors" because they inhibit replication of HIV protease, a different enzyme. Examples include saquinavir (Invirase), ritonavir (Norvir), and indinavir (Crixivan). HIV protease is needed for formation and assembly of HIV proteins. The new drugs are taken in combination with reserve transcriptase inhibitors.

Immune boosters attempt to increase the immune system's ability to fight the virus. Often, drugs in this category are experimental and are available only through clinical trials (testing on a limited number of individuals through controlled laboratory studies). This form of treatment has not been very helpful, but it is an area of intense research.

Drugs for opportunistic infections are used because people with AIDS have a fairly predictable occurrence of opportunistic infections. Some of these serious infections can be prevented or treated with medications.

Vaccines

A vaccine for HIV and AIDS is being pursued. Unfortunately, certain characteristics of HIV make a vaccine difficult to develop.

HIV can hide in cells, it multiplies in great numbers, and it mutates rapidly (creates slightly different versions of itself).

Because a vaccine seems unlikely in the near future, the best way to fight HIV is through education, awareness, and avoiding behaviors that may transmit HIV. Learning the facts about HIV and AIDS is the best protection available.

Infectious Mononucleosis

Signs and Symptoms

- Fever
- Sore throat
- Loss of appetite
- Fatigue and weakness
- Sore muscles
- Swollen lymph nodes
- Pain on the upper left side of the abdomen

Infectious mononucleosis (mono) is also called Epstein-Barr virus infection after the herpes virus that causes the disease. This virus may affect anyone, but the infection most often occurs in people between the ages of 16 and 25, especially teenagers. It can occur as an epidemic or in single cases, and it is believed to be spread by infectious saliva. The incubation period for the disease is usually 7 to 14 days in children and adolescents. The incubation period is longer for adults. At times it may be 30 to 50 days.

Diagnosis

Infectious mononucleosis has a wide variety of symptoms. You may experience fever, sore throat, swollen lymph nodes, or, in some cases, enlargement of the spleen. Nausea, hepatitis, jaundice, headache, stiffness, chest pain, cough, tachycardia (rapid heartbeat), and arrhythmias also may be caused by the virus. Loss of appetite, muscle pain, fatigue, and weakness often are present, and some individuals have a red rash. This range of symptoms can make diagnosis difficult.

If mononucleosis is suspected, your physician may do a monospot test to verify the presence of the virus in your bloodstream.

How Serious Is Infectious Mononucleosis?

Mononucleosis is not a serious disease, except in rare cases in which the spleen becomes severely enlarged and ruptures or when other vital organs such as the brain or

Chronic Fatigue Syndrome

Recently, there has been a renewed interest in people who suffer chronically from fatigue, weakness, decreased ability to concentrate, and poor memory. In some of these cases, tests for the Epstein-Barr virus have been positive, leading some physicians to diagnose chronic infectious mononucleosis, but this has since been disproved.

Several things can produce fatigue, weakness, and loss of memory, including stress, an unidentified disease, or a psychological condition such as depression. Experts have developed the term chronic fatigue syndrome to designate this vague group of symptoms. (A syndrome is simply a constellation of symptoms.) No definite cause for the chronic fatigue syndrome has been found, although emotional and psychological factors may play a role. Usually, there is no evidence of underlying viral infection.

Certain criteria have been proposed that should be met before the diagnosis of chronic fatigue syndrome can be made. First, you must suffer from persistent or relapsing fatigue that lasts 6 or more consecutive months. All other known diseases, infections, or psychiatric illnesses that might cause these symptoms must be ruled out. Second, you must have four or more of the following criteria: 1) sore throat, 2) painful lymph nodes in the neck or armpits, 3) prolonged fatigue following previously tolerated exercise, 4) new generalized headaches, 5) unexplained muscle soreness, 6) pain that moves from one joint to another, without evidence of redness or swelling, 7) impaired memory and concentration, and 8) sleep disturbance.

For chronic fatigue syndrome, the symptoms are treated when possible and allowed to run their course.

The key question is whether these symptoms represent a new disease or are a collection of complaints without a clear cause.

Many physicians think chronic fatigue syndrome is not a new disease. Many people who claimed to have symptoms of fatigue underwent tests that showed they had been exposed to the Epstein-Barr virus. However, further analysis has shown that many people exposed to the Epstein-Barr virus are free of symptoms of chronic fatigue syndrome. And not all those who do say they have symptoms have been exposed to the virus.

The chronic fatigue syndrome is just that—a syndrome (constellation) of symptoms. In most cases, there is no serious underlying disease causing it.

---

heart are infected. Persons with infectious mononucleosis do need support and understanding because even though most of the symptoms are not severely debilitating in themselves, the disease may cause prolonged fatigue and weakness. In most cases, the fever, swollen lymph nodes, and enlargement of the spleen disappear after 10 days. However, it may take 2 to 3 months before you feel completely back to normal.

Treatment

There is no specific antiviral treatment for infectious mononucleosis. Bed rest is the primary recommendation. Generally, do not expect to return to your normal routine for at least 2 to 3 weeks. Your physician may ask you to avoid contact sports for several months. Drinking plenty of water and fruit juices helps to relieve the fever and sore throat and keeps you from becoming dehydrated. Aspirin and, for a sore throat, gargling (one-half teaspoon of salt in a glass of warm water) several times a day are suggested.

The sore throat of infectious mononucleosis occasionally is aggravated by a streptococcal infection, which requires treatment with an antibiotic.

See your physician immediately if you experience sudden sharp pains in the left upper side of your abdomen. This could mean a rapidly enlarging or even ruptured spleen. This is rare, but if a rupture should occur, emergency surgery may be required.

Influenza

Signs and Symptoms
- Fever and chills
- Sore throat
- Cough
- Muscular aches and pains
- Fatigue and weakness
- Nasal congestion

Like the common cold, influenza—or flu, as it is commonly called—is primarily spread between people indoors, especially at schools, nursing homes, and other places where large numbers of people gather. Outbreaks usually occur in the winter and early spring. Unfortunately, many viral diseases that are not influenza also are called flu, which causes considerable confusion.

There are three types of influenza viruses. All of them are spread from person to person by inhalation of infected droplets from the air. Type A usually is responsible for the large influenza epidemics. Types B and C are not as widespread: type B causes smaller, more localized outbreaks, and type C is less common and usually causes only a mild illness.

Types B and C are fairly stable viruses. Type A is constantly changing, with new strains appearing regularly. This results in a new epidemic every few years, and the disease arises in a number of areas concurrently. Every 10 to 40 years, influenza breaks out as a pandemic, affecting people all over the world.

Diagnosis

Influenza usually comes on suddenly, causing fever (usually of 101 to 102 degrees Fahrenheit, but sometimes reaching 106 degrees Fahrenheit), chills, muscular aches and pains, weakness, malaise, nasal congestion, flushed face, dry cough, and sore throat. All of the symptoms are similar to those of the common cold but usually are more severe. Influenza typically develops after an incubation period of 1 to 4 days, and the fever may last for 3 to 5 days, although it can last as little as 1 day or as long as a week.

Diagnosing influenza with complete certainty is difficult because it is similar to many mild illnesses that are accompanied by a fever. If your physician suspects influenza, he or she may be able to isolate the virus from throat washings or may do a blood test to look for antibodies to the virus. These tests are mainly of value to public health officials, who can better advise the public if they know the character and extent of the disease in a community.

How Serious Is Influenza?

Influenza itself generally is not dangerous and usually lasts only for 1 day to a week. However, complications can follow influenza, such as acute sinusitis, bronchitis, and pneumonia. Pneumococcal pneumonia is the most common complication; staphylococcal pneumonia is also serious and can lead to death. Elderly people and people with weakened immune systems or severe medical disorders, such as chronic heart or lung diseases, are at a greater risk and should be vaccinated (see Flu Shots, this page).

Treatment

There is no specific treatment for influenza. Bed rest is important, as are proper nutrition and drinking lots of liquids. Inhaling steam or taking a sedative cough medicine may temporarily relieve the cough, and analgesics help to decrease the fever and muscle soreness. The antiviral drug amantadine, which is taken orally, may be helpful in relieving the signs and symptoms of influenza A. Anti-

---

Flu Shots

Each year, a flu vaccine is recommended by the Centers for Disease Control based on a prediction as to which strain of influenza virus will be prevalent. We highly recommend immunization for people with impaired immune systems or with serious illnesses such as chronic heart or kidney disease, lung disease or impaired ability to breathe (including heavy smokers), cystic fibrosis, chronic anemia (such as sickle cell anemia), or severe diabetes. Elderly people, especially those older than 65, also should be vaccinated. Health care workers, police officers and fire fighters, and others on whom public safety depends should receive immunization.

The vaccine is given as one injection into the upper arm in the early fall, just before the flu season begins. Children may sometimes receive the vaccine in two separate injections, 1 to 2 weeks apart. In subsequent years, only a booster shot each fall is needed. If you are subsequently exposed to the flu, the shot does not guarantee that you will not get the disease, but most likely you will have only a mild illness. Because the virus changes so rapidly, however, protection is not permanent, and you must get a new vaccination each season.

The vaccine may cause some soreness at the site where the shot is given. A very small percentage of people run a slight fever and have minor muscular aches beginning 6 to 24 hours after immunization. These discomforts may last for a day or two, but severe reactions are rare. However, people who are sensitive to eggs and egg products may experience a severe allergic reaction, and they probably should not be immunized. If you are pregnant, wait until after your third month before being vaccinated.

biotics do not provide relief and should be used only to treat the complications caused by bacterial infection.

Prevention

The primary way to prevent influenza is by use of influenza vaccine each fall. Amantadine hydrochloride is also effective at greatly decreasing the risk of infection. However, if used for prevention, it must be started before or immediately after exposure to the influenza A virus. It usually is prescribed only for persons at risk for a severe case of the disease or complications. Note that amantadine protects against only influenza A, but the vaccine protects against both the A and the B influenza strains. Neither prevents other types of viral diseases.

Lyme Disease

Signs and Symptoms
- Characteristic red rash at the site of a tick bite
- Headache
- Chills and fever
- Body aches
- Joint inflammation and arthritis

Named after a large outbreak among children in Lyme, Connecticut, this disease is caused by an organism (spirochete) that is transmitted by a certain type of tick. From May to October, the tick is found throughout the United States, especially on the east and west coasts and in Wisconsin and Minnesota.

Diagnosis
Lyme disease is difficult to diagnose because it mimics various other diseases. A characteristic red rash usually occurs at the site of the tick bite, followed by flu-like symptoms such as headache, chills, fever, and body aches and stiffness (see color photograph, page C-14). However, the bite may go entirely unnoticed. A few weeks to months later, facial paralysis, joint inflammation, various neurologic symptoms, and sometimes heart palpitations and heart block (see page 672) may occur.

Your physician may do a blood test to look for antibodies to the organism. However, the test is not always conclusive.

How Serious Is Lyme Disease?
If caught in its early stages, the disease can be eliminated with use of antibiotics. If not treated early, complications involving the joints, heart, and brain can occur.

Treatment

Medication
Therapy consists of antibiotics. Aspirin helps to relieve joint inflammation.

Prevention
When walking in wooded or grassy areas, wear shoes, long pants tucked into socks, and long-sleeved shirts. Check yourself and your pets often for ticks. If you find any, remove them immediately by using a tweezers. Do not yank or crush the tick, but pull carefully and steadily.

Cat Scratch Disease

Signs and Symptoms
- Enlarged lymph nodes
- Low-grade fever
- Skin papule or pustule
- Fatigue
- Headache
- Sore throat

Cat scratch disease (CSD) is thought to be caused by the bacterial organism *Rochalimaea henselae*. Almost all people affected with this disease have a history of exposure to cats, and most will also have experienced a cat scratch or bite. The disease is believed to be transmitted directly after a scratch, bite, or lick, usually from a kitten. Generally, the cat shows no evidence of disease.

A primary skin papule or pustule may form 3 to 10 days from the time of scratch or contact. Enlarged, tender lymph nodes de-

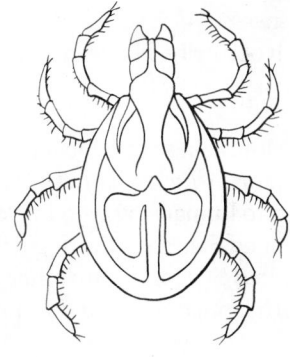

The *Ixodes scapularis* tick carries the Lyme disease bacterium.

velop 2 to 3 weeks after contact with a cat. Node enlargement may persist for 2 to 4 months, or occasionally longer. Approximately one-third of affected individuals have enlarged lymph nodes involving several sites. The disease occurs in both children and adults.

Diagnosis

The diagnosis of CSD is suggested by enlarged lymph nodes that develop 2 to 3 weeks after contact with a cat. The presence of a papule or pustule at the site of a scratch or bite strengthens the diagnosis. A cat scratch antigen skin test is positive in most affected individuals. However, the skin test only reflects previous exposure to the causative agent.

How Serious Is Cat Scratch Disease?

Long-term complications are uncommon. Enlarged lymph nodes, however, may persist for a number of months or even years. A single episode of CSD appears to confer lifelong immunity.

Treatment

If a pustule at the site of a bite begins to break down or is quite tender, needle aspiration by a physician may be considered to relieve pain and hasten recovery. In addition, application of moist soaks may improve drainage and shorten the duration of tender lymph nodes. Most of the time, the symptoms resolve without specific treatment. If the disease is widespread, your physician may consider using antibiotics.

Rocky Mountain Spotted Fever

Signs and Symptoms

- Chills and fever
- Severe headache
- Widespread aches and pains
- Restlessness
- Red rash occurring between days 2 and 6 of fever

Rocky Mountain spotted fever is caused by the organism *Rickettsia rickettsii* and is transmitted to humans by wood ticks in the western United States, by the dog tick in the eastern United States, and by other ticks in the southern United States and Central and South America. In the United States, it occurs primarily during the late spring and early summer and is most common in the eastern part of the country.

Diagnosis

Three to 10 days after being bitten by an infected tick, you experience nausea, headache, loss of appetite, and a sore throat. As the disease develops, fever, chills, tenderness and soreness in the bones and muscles, restlessness, insomnia, abdominal pain, and vomiting occur. You may have a cough and, possibly, delirium, lethargy, and stupor. Between the second and sixth days of the fever, a red rash appears on your wrists and ankles and spreads up your arms and legs to your chest. Your physician may do a blood test in an attempt to establish the diagnosis or may stain a specimen of the rash to search for the presence of the causative organism.

How Serious Is Rocky Mountain Spotted Fever?

In mild cases and when treated promptly, Rocky Mountain spotted fever is fairly benign. Even without treatment, mild cases will disappear after 2 weeks. However, in severe cases, the disease can be serious or even fatal, especially in elderly people.

Treatment

Medication

If antibiotics are given early, they usually eliminate the fever quickly. Prompt treatment is important because the disease may progress rapidly.

Typhoid Fever

Signs and Symptoms

- Fever
- Headache
- Weakness and fatigue
- Sore throat
- Cough
- Diarrhea

Emergency Symptoms

- Sudden drop in temperature
- Shock characterized by decrease in urination, light-headed feeling particularly on standing up, lethargy, and change in level of consciousness

Typhoid fever is caused by the bacterium *Salmonella typhi*. It is contracted by consuming contaminated food or fluids. It is rare in developed countries, but it can be acquired overseas in underdeveloped countries. The bacteria penetrate the wall of the small intestine and cause inflammation of the lymph nodes and the spleen. Chronic carriers are possible sources of the disease. These are people who carry typhoid bacteria in their intestinal tract for years but have no symptoms. In developing countries with poor sanitary conditions and unsafe water supplies, epidemics of typhoid fever may occur.

Diagnosis

Although it may come on suddenly with chills and fever, especially in children, the disease usually develops slowly. It begins with headache, cough, weakness and fatigue, generalized aches, and sore throat. Vomiting, constipation or diarrhea, and abdominal pain are often present as well. There is fever that usually is highest in the evening.

If typhoid fever is untreated, the second stage sets in after 7 to 10 days. The individual becomes extremely ill. The fever becomes continuous, and the patient develops diarrhea the consistency and color of pea soup, or severe constipation. In severe cases, the person may fall into the "typhoid state," lying motionless with eyes half-closed and appearing wasted and exhausted. After about the second week, a rash may appear on the chest and back. It disappears in 3 to 4 days.

If there are no complications, the person begins to improve slowly. Abdominal symptoms disappear gradually and the fever falls in steps, becoming normal after another week to 10 days. However, the disease can recur at any time up to 2 weeks after the fever has subsided.

About a third of patients have complications. Intestinal bleeding, usually during the third week, is manifested by a sudden decrease in blood pressure, increase in pulse, and signs of shock followed by blood in the stool. Perforation of the intestine also may occur in the third week and cause an increase in body temperature and pulse, rigidity, and abdominal pain and tenderness. Other, rarer, complications include pneumonia, psychosis, meningitis, and infection of the bladder, kidney, or spine (called typhoid spine).

To diagnose typhoid fever, your physician will take samples of your blood, urine, and stool, and the laboratory will attempt to grow the organism from these samples.

How Serious Is Typhoid Fever?

Untreated, typhoid fever is very serious. Even when treated, a small number of people who have it may not survive. Elderly people and people who are already debilitated are especially vulnerable. In children, the disease usually is milder. When complications develop, the outlook is poor. A few patients become chronic carriers who can be completely asymptomatic.

Treatment

Because the person can easily become malnourished and dehydrated, ingestion of fluids plus a high-calorie, nonbulky diet is important. At times, administration of fluids through a vein (intravenous feeding) is necessary. Because the bacteria are present in the stool and urine, care must be taken to avoid unprotected contact with contaminated clothing and bedding.

Medication

Your physician will prescribe an antibiotic to which the organism is sensitive. The choice depends on the strain of the bacteria.

Fever of Unknown Origin

Fever is the most common body reaction to an infection—but a fever does not necessarily signify that you have an infection. A fever can develop as one of the symptoms of some noninfectious diseases, and sometimes it is not possible to identify the cause. If you have recurrent temperatures greater than 100.5 degrees Fahrenheit for more than 3 weeks and there is no obvious cause, even after extensive evaluation, the diagnosis may be "fever of unknown origin."

Some of the tests your physician may use to try to identify the cause of your fever are blood tests, frequent physical examinations, and X-ray examinations. In some cases, a biopsy of your arteries, lymph nodes, bone marrow, liver, or muscles may be necessary.

Sometimes, a medication can cause an adverse reaction, resulting in a fever. If you stop taking the medication, the fever usually disappears within a week.

It is not always possible to determine why you have a fever, but through persistence the cause usually can be identified, and your physician can prescribe an appropriate treatment.

Prevention

Currently there are two types of typhoid vaccines, an oral form and an injection form. The oral vaccine is given as four capsules taken every other day. The injection vaccine is given as a single dose. Both the vaccines are less than 100 percent effective. People who plan to live or to travel in an area where the disease is prevalent, or who may have been exposed during an epidemic outbreak, should be immunized. Proper environmental hygiene is important, and carriers must never be allowed to work as food handlers.

Tetanus

Signs and Symptoms
- Stiffness of the jaw, neck, and other muscles
- Irritability
- Spasms of the jaw and neck muscles
- Painful convulsions

Tetanus, also known as lockjaw, is caused by bacteria whose spores are found in soil. If the spores enter a deep wound with low oxygen content, they germinate and produce a toxin, tetanospasmin, which interferes with the nerves controlling your muscles. The incubation period from the time of the injury until symptoms appear is 5 days to 3 weeks (average, 8 to 12 days).

Diagnosis
Although some affected persons may experience only pain and tingling at the wound site and some spasms in nearby muscles, most have stiffness of the jaw and of the neck, difficulty swallowing, and irritability. Spasms of the jaw or facial muscles follow, progressing to spasms and rigidity of the neck, abdominal, and back muscles. Finally, painful convulsions caused by minor stimuli affect the respiratory muscles so that the individual is unable to breathe. The person is usually awake and alert throughout the disease.

How Serious Is Tetanus?
If muscle spasms develop early, chances of recovery are poor. Tetanus is serious, often leading to death, especially in small children and elderly people. For this reason, prevention is the best treatment.

Treatment
Consult your physician immediately if you incur a wound that is contaminated with soil, particularly if it is deep. If you have had a series of tetanus shots previously and more than 5 years have passed since your last booster shot, your physician probably will give you a booster shot of the vaccine tetanus toxoid. Your body will quickly manufacture the needed antibodies to protect you against tetanus. Treatment with antibiotics and opening and cleaning of the wound also may be necessary.

If you acquire tetanus, hospitalization will be required, most likely in an intensive care unit.

Prevention

Active immunization is vital for everyone. It is usually given to children as part of the DTP shot (see page 1079), with booster shots every 10 years, or at the time of a major injury if it has been more than 5 years since your last booster.

Rabies

Signs and Symptoms
- Pain and then tingling at the site of an animal bite
- Skin sensitivity
- Excessive drooling of saliva
- Inability to swallow liquids
- Rage alternating with calm
- Convulsions and paralysis leading to death

Rabies is caused by a virus that affects the brain. It is transmitted to humans by saliva from the bite of an infected animal. Dogs and cats may be infected, and many bats, skunks, and foxes are infected; rodents are unlikely to be. The incubation period from the time of the bite until symptoms appear is usually 3 to 7 weeks but can range from 10 days to 2 years.

Diagnosis
Left untreated, rabies begins with pain followed by tingling at the site of an animal bite. The person is extremely sensitive to temperature changes and air currents and tends to choke whenever he or she tries to swallow liquids. Restlessness, muscle spasms, rage and extreme excitability, and excessive drooling are also present. Finally, convulsions and paralysis ensue.

How Serious Is Rabies?

Rabies is almost always fatal. Death due to heart or respiratory failure and paralysis usually occurs within 7 to 25 days after symptoms appear.

Treatment

If you are bitten by a dog, cat, or farm animal, the animal should be caught, confined, and observed by a veterinarian for a week to 10 days. If bitten by a wild animal, the animal should be killed, if possible, and the brain tested for rabies. Wild raccoons, skunks, bats, coyotes, wolves, and foxes generally are presumed to have rabies.

Your physician must decide whether or not to treat for rabies. Treatment consists of administration of a passive antibody (half directly to the wound and half injected into a muscle) and a vaccine, given as five injections, one on your first visit along with the antibody, and then again 3, 7, 14, and 28 days after the first shot.

Common Contagious Diseases

Many of the most familiar diseases of childhood—chickenpox, measles, mumps—are highly infectious ailments that can be passed easily from person to person. Although many of these ailments are taken for granted as a part of childhood, others, like dreaded polio, are very serious indeed. Still others are likely to be harmless in children but can be serious in adults—for example, German measles in pregnant women or chickenpox in adults.

Ordinarily, the diagnosis of these common diseases is made on the basis of their characteristic symptoms and signs and to some extent on the presence of other cases in the community. Blood tests to confirm the diagnosis are usually unnecessary. Occasionally, such tests are done to help public health authorities determine the nature and extent of a disease in a community.

Today, immunizations make it possible to avoid altogether certain of these problems. In the following pages, we discuss the common contagious disorders and review appropriate procedures and schedules for immunizations.

Common Viral Colds

Signs and Symptoms

- Watery, runny nose, progressing to nasal congestion
- Sneezing
- Watery eyes
- Sore throat
- Cough
- Slight fever that may be accompanied by shivering, body aches, and chills
- Headache
- Overall malaise

Everyone experiences a cold now and then. In fact, perhaps as many as half of all short-term illnesses are colds or other acute viral respiratory illnesses, which include croup (see page 1076), pharyngitis (see page 592), laryngitis (see page 595), acute bronchitis (see page 702), and some types of pneumonia (see page 704).

Colds are most common in children. They usually have their first cold during their first year of life and are especially susceptible to them until about age 6, when their immunities seem to be established (see Common and Recurrent Colds, page 86).

As we get older, we tend to be less susceptible to colds, but statistics suggest that three or four colds per year per person is typical.

Most colds are caused by a virus. The common cold is not the result of one specific virus. More than 200 different viral strains cause acute respiratory illnesses. These include the rhinoviruses, the group most often associated with the so-called common cold. Most colds primarily affect the nose and throat, although the same viruses can cause bronchitis in the lungs and laryngitis in the larynx. More serious bacterial infections of the throat, ears, and lungs can follow a viral cold.

Colds are spread primarily by two routes. First, direct contact with infected secretions is the most effective method. Shaking hands with a person who has been blowing his or her nose or coughing into his or her hand is a common way of coming in contact with that person's virus. Second, open sneezing and coughing also spread the virus into the air to be inhaled by others, but this is a less efficient method of transfer.

Myths and popular wisdom about catching colds abound: if you get wet in a rainstorm or go out with wet hair, you surely will catch a cold; if you are exposed to cold air, you will come down with one; fatigue and

lack of sleep are sure causes of colds. However, none of these have been proved in clinical studies to affect the risk of becoming infected with a cold virus.

Colds do have a seasonal bias. More people have colds during fall, winter, and spring than during summer.

Diagnosis

The general symptoms of a cold are fairly standard and include congestion of the head and nose, cough, sneezing, hoarseness, and watery eyes. Because so many different viruses cause colds, the symptoms can vary considerably. For instance, you may have a

---

How to Take a Temperature and How to Read a Thermometer

Normally, your temperature shows a definite pattern: low in the morning, gradually increasing during the day, and reaching its maximum during late afternoon or evening. Ordinarily, body temperature varies by 1 to 2 degrees Fahrenheit over the course of the day, usually not exceeding 99.9 degrees Fahrenheit.

Thus, the mark at 98.6 degrees Fahrenheit (37 degrees centigrade) on your thermometer is only a general guide. Readings somewhat above this are not necessarily abnormal. Increased body temperature does not become dangerous until it goes above 105 degrees Fahrenheit.

Ordinarily, your body controls its temperature to be within the range from 97 degrees Fahrenheit in the morning to 99 in the evening. When fever is present, the mechanisms that control body temperature are simply set a few degrees higher—for example, 102 degrees Fahrenheit instead of the normal 97 to 99. When a fever begins, you feel chilly and may shiver. You may be more comfortable wrapped in a blanket or huddled with a heating pad because this will help your body gain heat and reach the new set point. Then, when your temperature reaches the new set point (for example, 102 degrees Fahrenheit), you will no longer feel cold

and will stop shivering.

If whatever caused the fever disappears or if you take acetaminophen, the set point will return toward the normal range and you will feel warm. Therefore, you will seek cooler surroundings and will perspire profusely, both of which tend to dissipate body heat.

There are several ways to take your temperature. Oral and rectal thermometers are essentially glass tubes containing a column of mercury. As the mercury expands, in response to the heat from your body, it moves up the column.

An oral thermometer has a long, slender bulb at one end containing mercury and is used in the mouth or under the armpit. A rectal thermometer has a shorter, stubby bulb of mercury at one end and is used in the rectum, usually in children. Electronic and temperature strip thermometers are also available, but the latter are generally less accurate. When you are purchasing a thermometer, look for one with a column that is easy to see and with degree markings that are easy to read.

Before taking a temperature, make sure that the top of the mercury column is down near the bulb. Hold the thermometer firmly at the end away from the mercury bulb

and shake it with several abrupt downward flicks of your wrist. Then, wash the thermometer in cold water. To read the thermometer, hold it near the light and rotate it slowly until you see the silver column of mercury.

In adults and children 7 years or older, the temperature is taken orally by inserting the bulb end of the thermometer under the tongue and having the patient close his or her mouth. After 1 minute, you can remove the thermometer and read it.

In children younger than 7, the temperature can be taken by placing an oral thermometer in the armpit and having the child cross his or her arms across the chest. After 3 minutes, remove the thermometer, read the temperature, and add 1 degree Fahrenheit to convert to oral temperature. You also can use a rectal thermometer in young children. Insert the bulb end of the thermometer a short way into the child's rectum, while holding the child down with your arm, if necessary. After 1 or 2 minutes, remove the thermometer, read the temperature, and subtract 1 degree Fahrenheit to convert to oral temperature.

After taking a temperature, rinse a mercury thermometer in cold water or alcohol.

mild fever and chills during one cold but not during another. In one, the cough may be more troublesome than the runny nose.

Onset of a cold usually comes within 1 to 2 days after exposure and may be signaled at first by an itching or sore throat, increasing congestion of the nose, or mild body aches or headache. A watery, runny nose is often the first major symptom. After a while, the discharge becomes thick and yellowish green.

A normally healthy person has no need to see a physician for a cold. However, if it lasts for more than 10 days to 2 weeks, see your physician to make sure that no secondary bacterial infection of the lungs, larynx, trachea, sinuses, or ear has set in. If you have a history of any such infections, consult your physician without delay.

How Serious Is a Cold?

Colds are general nuisances that for the most part must just be waited out. Occasionally, however, a more serious secondary bacterial respiratory infection can follow a cold and must be treated aggressively by a physician.

Treatment

Because a cold is a viral infection, antibiotics are not needed. The cold usually lasts 3 to 4 days, but may last up to 10 to 14 days. Therefore, treating a cold is largely a matter of patience.

Self-Help

There are measures you can take to help you feel better. Rest at home if you feel tired, are drowsy from medications, or have a bad cough. Staying at home also helps avoid infecting others. Remain in a warm (not hot) room in which the air is moistened by a humidifier or vaporizer. Drink lots of fluids (to loosen the mucus). Adults can take aspirin for aches and pains. Children should use acetaminophen instead.

Nonprescription cold remedies, decongestants, and cough syrups may help to relieve some of the symptoms, but they will not cure the cold or make it any shorter in duration. Many people find cough drops useful to keep their throat lubricated. However, they can upset the stomach after a while, so consider sucking hard candy instead.

A sore throat can be relieved by gargling with warm salty water several times a day or by using a nonprescription topical anesthetic to relieve throat discomfort. Be careful not to use nasal sprays or drops for more than a few days because they can become addicting.

Some people ask their physicians for antibiotics to fight a cold. Unless there is a bacterial infection present, antibiotics are of no use.

Measles

Signs and Symptoms

- Fever
- Cough, sneezing
- Inflamed eyes (conjunctivitis)
- Sore throat
- Tiny white spots on the lining of the cheek
- Rash

Measles, also known as rubeola, is a common childhood illness, although adults also are susceptible. The virus that causes the disorder is transmitted by inhalation of infecting droplets such as from a sneeze. Measles is most contagious before the rash appears, making it difficult to avoid the disease. Until the rash disappears, you still can pass it on to others. Once you have had measles, you are permanently immune and will not contract the disease again.

Diagnosis

Measles begins as a fever, often as high as 104 to 105 degrees Fahrenheit, with a persistent cough, sneezing, inflamed eyes (conjunctivitis), and sore throat. After about 4 days, a

---

The Dangers of Aspirin

Aspirin is an effective drug for treating a wide range of symptoms and disorders. We think of it as mild and harmless, but in certain cases, it can be very dangerous. The notable risks are described here.

In Children

Do not give aspirin to children who have a fever. Aspirin seems to be related, in some unknown way, to the very serious condition Reye's syndrome (see page 484).

In Adults

Aspirin may cause minor bleeding from the stomach, so it should be used only when necessary. If your stools appear black and tarry, you may have gastrointestinal bleeding. Discuss your aspirin use with your physician. He or she may recommend a coated aspirin or an aspirin substitute such as acetaminophen.

red, blotchy rash appears on the face and behind the ears. The rash spreads to the chest and back and, finally, to the arms and legs. By the time it reaches the arms and legs, it has begun to fade from the face (see color photograph, page C-1).

The symptoms usually appear 10 to 14 days after exposure to the virus. The diagnosis ordinarily is made on the basis of the characteristic rash and the small white spots on the inside lining of the cheek.

Occasionally, your physician may obtain a blood sample to test for the presence of antibodies to the virus, but this is usually done only as a part of a public health survey to define the nature and extent of an epidemic.

How Serious Is Measles?

Normally, the infection lasts for 10 days to 2 weeks, and the person recovers completely. In a small number of cases, pneumonia may develop early in the course of the illness, or complications may arise immediately after appearance of the rash. Encephalitis, which causes vomiting, convulsions, coma, and brain disorders, or a bacterial infection (such as pneumonia) may develop.

Treatment

Medication
Acetaminophen and a sedative cough medicine may be taken. Remain isolated until a week after the rash disappears and stay in bed until the fever disappears. If a bacterial infection develops, your physician may prescribe an antibiotic.

Prevention
The measles vaccine is effective and is usually given as a combined measles/mumps/rubella (MMR) inoculation. Physicians recommend that the MMR vaccine be given to children between 12 and 15 months of age, and again between 4 and 6 years of age (before entering school).

German Measles

Signs and Symptoms
- Rash
- Mild fever

German measles (rubella) is only moderately infectious. It is transmitted by inhalation of droplets of moisture that are carrying the virus. The incubation period is 2 to 3 weeks, and the affected person is contagious for 1 week before the rash appears.

Diagnosis

The symptoms of the disease usually are mild and sometimes are hardly noticed. They may include mild fever, enlarged lymph nodes, and a fine, pink rash that appears on the face, the trunk, and then the arms and legs (see color photograph, page C-1). The rash usually disappears in 3 to 5 days, lasting no more than 1 day on each part of the body. In many cases, the rash does not even occur. Your physician may take a blood sample to check for antibodies to the virus.

How Serious Is Rubella?

In itself, rubella is a mild infection. Once you have had the disease, you usually are permanently immune. However, if a woman is pregnant when she contracts rubella, the consequences for her unborn child may be severe. The child may have one or more of various problems, including growth retardation, cataracts, rashes, deafness, congenital heart defects, and defects of other organs. The highest risk to the fetus is during the first trimester, but exposure during the second trimester is also dangerous.

Treatment

The infection is allowed to run its course, although taking acetaminophen may help to relieve symptoms. Treatment of a child who was exposed to the disease while in the mother's uterus, particularly in the first trimester, depends on his or her problems and often requires years of medical and surgical care. If you contract rubella while you are pregnant, the risk of congenital deformities should be discussed with your physician.

Prevention
Usually, a combined measles/mumps/rubella vaccination is given. Live weakened (attenuated) vaccine should be given to all girls before they begin menstruating. If a woman is given the vaccine, she must be cautioned to practice birth control or abstinence for at least 3 months after vaccination.

Roseola

Signs and Symptoms
- High fever

- Swollen lymph nodes in the neck
- Rash on trunk and neck

Roseola is caused by human herpes virus 6. The route of transmission is probably through the respiratory system. The viral infection usually affects young children, but can occasionally affect adults. The infection is usually not serious, but occasionally complications may occur.

Diagnosis

The primary symptom is a sudden, high fever (to 104 degrees Fahrenheit) in a child 6 months to 3 years old. The child may be irritable, and his or her lymph nodes become swollen. Convulsions can be caused by the high fever (see page 69). As the fever goes down, a rash appears on the trunk and neck and may last a few hours to a few days (see color photograph, page C-1).

Roseola is usually diagnosed by the symptoms and can be confirmed by an antibody test in the blood.

Treatment

Treatment consists of acetaminophen and application of tepid sponges to bring the fever down. The convulsions usually are brief if they occur, but your physician may prescribe anticonvulsant medication.

Whooping Cough

Signs and Symptoms
- Sneezing and nasal congestion
- Tearing
- Loss of appetite
- Malaise
- A hacking cough, often followed by explosive coughs that end in a high-pitched whoop

Emergency Symptoms—Difficulty breathing and blue lips

Whooping cough gets its name from the high-pitched "whooping" sound characteristic of the disease. It is also known as pertussis, after the bacterium that causes it, *Bordetella pertussis*.

Whooping cough primarily occurs in infants younger than 2 years and is contracted by inhaling infected airborne droplets, often from an adult with a mild case of the disease. The disease is most contagious early, but it can be transmitted until the infection is completely cleared.

Diagnosis

Diagnosing whooping cough in its initial stages is difficult because the symptoms are similar to those of a common cold. After 10 days to 2 weeks, the characteristic whooping cough may develop. The person has spasms of rapid, consecutive coughs followed by a strained, hurried, deep inhalation with a high-pitched whooping sound.

Coughing attacks can be set off by several stimuli, such as fright, anger, crying, and sneezing. The person may cough up large amounts of thick phlegm, and vomiting is common. About 4 weeks after the coughing attacks begin, the symptoms gradually disappear.

How Serious Is Whooping Cough?

With antibiotic therapy, most children recover from whooping cough without incident. However, whooping cough can lead to pneumonia with subsequent damage to the lungs. Asphyxia (lack of oxygen) may lead to brain damage in some very severe cases. If a child's lips turn blue, this means that the child is having difficulty breathing and should receive emergency care.

Treatment

The child should be given small meals frequently and plenty of fluids.

Medication

Antibiotics are given. In life-threatening cases, corticosteroids may be given for several days. Cough medicines provide little benefit.

Prevention

Whooping cough is uncommon in the United States because of the widespread immunization (vaccination) of children. In other countries in which immunization against whooping cough has lagged, the consequences have been disastrous, with deaths occurring from the reemergence of whooping cough.

There are some risks from the vaccine, and your physician can discuss these with you. Immunizations are generally given as a combination of vaccines against diphtheria, tetanus, and whooping cough (pertussis), known as the DTP vaccine. No connection has been found between the DTP vaccine and sudden infant death syndrome.

Croup

Signs and Symptoms
- Loud, brassy cough
- Difficulty breathing

Emergency Symptoms
- Drooling or great difficulty swallowing
- Inability to bend the neck forward
- Unconsciousness
- Blue or dusky lips
- High-pitched noises when inhaling
- Worsening cough
- Increasing difficulty breathing
- Heart rate exceeding 160 beats per minute

Croup is an infection of the voice box (larynx), windpipe (trachea), and bronchial tubes that usually is caused by a virus. It occurs most often in children between the ages of 3 months and 5 years. Boys are more likely than girls to get croup. An upper respiratory illness of several days' duration usually precedes the symptoms of croup.

Because of a narrowing of the airway, a child with croup has a tight, brassy cough that may resemble the barking of a seal. The child's voice usually is hoarse. It is difficult for the child to inhale. Agitation and crying make the breathing difficulties worse. The child usually is more comfortable sitting up than lying down.

Croup typically lasts 3 to 4 days. During that time it may go from mild to severe several times. Usually the condition worsens at night and improves in the morning.

Treatment
Because almost all cases are caused by certain respiratory viruses, antibiotics are not used in treatment.

Most children with croup can be cared for at home. Warm, moist air seems to relieve some of the airway swelling and ease the cough. Run the hot water in your shower for 10 minutes with the bathroom door closed. Once the room looks like a steam bath, take your child into the bathroom for at least 10 minutes. Other methods of creating humidity include using a humidifier in the child's room (not a hot vaporizer). Fill the humidifier with warm water and have the child put his or her face in the mist and breathe deeply through the mouth. A wet washcloth placed loosely over the nose and mouth or taking the child out in the fresh air for a few minutes also may relieve symptoms.

A child with croup is often frightened and crying, which worsens the problem, so try to both reassure and distract him or her with a cuddle, a book, or a favorite game.

If your child has croup, encourage him or her to drink clear, warm fluids, which may help loosen thickened secretions. During the illness, it is a good idea to sleep in the same room with your child, so you will be alert to any worsening of his or her condition. And do not let anyone smoke in the house, because cigarette smoke can make croup worse.

Occasionally, croup may cause complete obstruction of the airway. This is an emergency situation that usually occurs over the course of several hours and can be fatal if the child does not receive immediate medical care. To guard against this dangerous complication, be alert for the emergency symptoms described above. If you notice any of these symptoms or if your child seems to be getting worse, call your child's physician or get emergency help.

Chickenpox

Signs and Symptoms
- Fever
- Weakness
- Red, itchy rash

Chickenpox, also known as varicella, occurs primarily in children, although adults who are not immune can contract it. It is contagious and is spread by breathing in infected respiratory droplets or by unprotected direct contact with the rash when it has ruptured. In persons who have had chickenpox, the virus can cause shingles later in life (see page 1011).

Diagnosis
The best-known symptom of chickenpox is the itchy, red rash that breaks out on the face, scalp, chest, back, and, to a lesser extent, arms and legs (see color photograph, page C-1). The rash usually appears about 2 weeks after exposure to the virus and begins as superficial spots.

The spots quickly fill with a clear fluid, rupture, and turn crusty. These then slough off in a week or two. The rash continues to break out for the first 1 to 5 days, so spots at various stages of development may be present at the same time. Fever and malaise, mild in children and more severe in adults, also develop.

How Serious Is Chickenpox?

In children, chickenpox is a mild disease, but in adults it is more serious. In adults, pneumonia may develop, which can lead to death, although this is rare. In persons with suppressed immune systems, such as children with leukemia or kidney transplants, the disease is very serious. Although uncommon, encephalitis may occur, but recovery usually is complete.

If a pregnant woman contracts chickenpox during the first or second trimester, there is a small risk that her child will be born with a congenital malformation. When a pregnant woman contracts the disease within 5 days of delivery, there is a high risk of the newborn having serious disease. The child should be immunized immediately with varicella-zoster immune globulin (VZIG).

Chickenpox seldom lasts for more than 2 weeks, from the appearance of the first rash to the disappearance of the last one. A secondary infection of the ruptured rash by bacteria may cause high fever and skin scarring.

Treatment

To prevent spreading of the disease, isolate the person with chickenpox until the rash crusts. Keep the skin clean by frequent baths or, once the fever has subsided, showers. Cool, wet compresses or tepid water baths may help to relieve itching. Complications are treated according to their symptoms. A secondary bacterial pneumonia is treated with antibiotics.

Medication

Occasionally antihistamines are used to help relieve the itching. Acyclovir is used for severe varicella infections involving the lungs or the brain and in persons with a depressed immune system. Routine use of acyclovir for all children with chickenpox probably is not necessary.

Prevention

If your baby is between 12 and 18 months of age, ask your physician if your child should receive a dose of a newly available chickenpox vaccine. Healthy children older than 13, and adults who have no history of chickenpox and have never been immunized against the disease, should also consider receiving the vaccine, two doses 4 to 8 weeks apart.

Persons with suppressed immune systems and who are not immune to chicken-

---

Smallpox

The eradication of smallpox is a success story of modern medicine. Smallpox was once a highly infectious viral disease that would spread in epidemics, causing death in up to 40 percent of its victims. The disease caused severe headache, fever, and a red, blistering rash that often left scars.

At the end of the 18th century, Edward Jenner, an English physician, discovered that inoculation with cowpox virus, which is usually harmless, prevented smallpox. Campaigns were launched in the United States and Europe to inoculate people against smallpox. However, as late as 1967, when the World Health Organization (WHO) launched a global campaign to eliminate this disease, outbreaks still occurred regularly in many countries.

After 10 years of effort, this international campaign was successful and the disease was eradicated. Smallpox vaccination is no longer necessary.

---

pox should receive varicella-zoster immune globulin (VZIG) after being exposed to chickenpox.

Mumps

Signs and Symptoms

- Swollen, painful salivary glands
- Fever
- Weakness and fatigue
- Inflammation of the pancreas, testicles, ovaries, or brain

Mumps is a childhood disease, but it can occur in adults. Its clinical name is epidemic parotitis. Mumps is caused by a virus and spread by inhalation of infected droplets. The affected person becomes contagious 1 day before the symptoms appear, is most contagious for another 3 days, and then becomes less contagious as the swelling goes down.

Diagnosis

The symptoms of mumps usually appear 2 to 3 weeks after the virus infection begins. The primary—and best known—symptom is swollen, painful salivary glands, causing the cheeks to puff out (see color photograph, page C-1). In small children, fever is usually slight. If the affected person experiences headaches and becomes lethargic, inflammation of the brain and its lining (meningoencephalitis) may be present. Pain in the upper abdomen, nausea, and vomiting may indicate inflammation of the pancreas. Lower abdominal pain in women may mean inflammation of the ovaries. This is often difficult to diagnose.

In about a quarter of the men who contract mumps, inflammation of the testicles (orchitis) (see page 1201) develops. Your physician can confirm this diagnosis by identifying the mumps virus in your saliva or by finding an increase in mumps antibodies in your blood. However, this sort of testing is rarely necessary.

How Serious Is Mumps?

Mumps makes you uncomfortable, but it usually is not a serious disease and rarely lasts more than 2 weeks. In some cases, however, encephalitis may develop, which is a serious complication of mumps and can lead to neurologic symptoms and, rarely, death. Orchitis is uncomfortable and occasionally causes sterility.

Treatment

There is no specific treatment for mumps. Your physician may advise bed rest until the fever disappears. Isolation to prevent the spread of the disease also may be appropriate. For most of the complications that may arise, treatment depends on the symptoms. Occasionally, an analgesic such as acetaminophen may be advised.

Prevention

The live virus vaccine against mumps is safe and effective and should be given to all children more than 1 year old. It may be given by itself or combined with other vaccines. Use of this vaccine has greatly decreased the incidence of mumps in the United States.

Diphtheria

Signs and Symptoms
- Sore throat and hoarseness
- Nasal discharge
- Malaise and fever
- Thick gray membrane covering the throat and tonsils
- Rapid pulse

Diphtheria is an acute infection caused by the bacterium *Corynebacterium diphtheriae*. It usually attacks the respiratory tract. Infection occurs by inhalation of airborne droplets exhaled by a person with the disease or by a carrier who has no symptoms. The organism also can infect skin wounds or any mucous membrane. The disease is now rare in the United States.

Diagnosis

After an incubation period of 2 days to a week, a mild sore throat, fever, and malaise develop. Your physician will look for a gray membrane covering your throat and tonsils.

How Serious Is Diphtheria?

With proper treatment, the prognosis is good if no complications develop. However, the gray diphtheria membrane can be dangerous because it may obstruct breathing. In addition, the disease may cause a serious heart infection called myocarditis (see page 687).

In some cases, the bacteria may affect the cranial nerves, causing nasal speech, regurgitation of food, and inability to swallow. This is seldom fatal, unless paralysis of the respiratory muscles develops. If the person survives these complications, recovery is slow but complete.

Treatment

A person with diphtheria should be isolated, kept at bed rest for 10 to 14 days, and fed a liquid to soft diet.

Medication

Administration of diphtheria antitoxin is essential. Antibiotics are given to eradicate the infection and the carrier state.

Immunization Schedule for Normal, Healthy Infants and Children

Age	Vaccine
0-1 month	Hepatitis B
2 months	DTP (diphtheria/tetanus/pertussis)
	OPV (oral polio virus)
	Hib (*Haemophilus* B)
2-4 months	Hepatitis B
4 months	DTP, OPV, Hib
6 months	DTP, OPV, Hib
6-18 months	Hepatitis B*
12-15 months	MMR (measles/mumps/rubella), Hib
12-18 months	DTP, varicella
4-6 years	DTP, OPV, MMR (before entering school)
14-16 years	Td (tetanus booster shot every 10 years)

*Children who have not completed the hepatitis B vaccine series in infancy should receive it before adolescence (11 to 16 years of age).

Immunizations

In the United States, nearly all children are vaccinated by age 4 or 5 years because they must be immunized before they are allowed to enter school. Some parents put off vaccination until their child reaches school age. This puts the child at needless risk of contracting potentially severe diseases.

For most vaccines, immunization should begin when a child reaches age 2 to 3 months. Immunization with live vaccines—for polio, measles, mumps, and rubella—should be completed by the time the child reaches 18 months of age.

The available vaccines and the ages when they should be given are described below. Note: Manufacturers' dose and age recommendations can vary.

Diphtheria

This vaccine usually is given in combination with tetanus and pertussis (whooping cough) vaccines (DTP shot). The immunization should be started when the child reaches 2 months of age and is given as a series of 5 shots. Children older than 12 years and adults should receive tetanus/diphtheria toxoid, adult type. A booster shot should be given every 10 years.

Whooping Cough (Pertussis)

Immunization is begun between 1 and 3 months of age, usually in combination with tetanus and diphtheria. A few children may have a reaction to the shot, in which case no further injections should be given. The vaccine generally should not be given to children older than 6 years.

Tetanus

Tetanus toxoid usually is given to children in a series of 5 shots, in combination with diphtheria and pertussis immunization. It is given at ages 2, 4, and 6 months, again at 18 months, and before the child enters school. A tetanus/diphtheria booster is given every 10 years.

Polio

Poliomyelitis vaccine generally is given orally as a live vaccine at ages 2 and 4 months and at 18 months (and 6 months if polio is prevalent in the area). Although further vaccination is not essential, a final dose has been recommended just before the child enters school (between 4 and 6 years of age).

Measles

A live weakened measles vaccine routinely is given to healthy children at about 15 months of age, usually in combination with mumps and rubella vaccines. If it is likely that a child will be exposed to measles before that age, he or she should be vaccinated earlier, but a second shot may be necessary at age 15 months because the child may not have developed antibodies to the virus after the first vaccination. If the immunization schedule is missed, older children and adults can be safely inoculated with the live vaccine. Children who have leukemia or some other severe debilitating illness or are receiving radiation, corticosteroid, or antimetabolite therapy should not be vaccinated.

Mumps

Mumps vaccine is given in one dose, usually in combination with the measles and rubella vaccines. It should not be given to children younger than 1 year.

Rubella

Usually this vaccine is given at age 15 months, in combination with measles and mumps vaccines. Although rubella is not a particularly serious disease, if a woman is exposed to rubella while she is pregnant, there may be dire consequences for her unborn child in the form of severe birth defects. Therefore, live weakened (attenuated) vaccine should be given to all girls before they begin menstruating. If a woman is given the vaccine, she must avoid pregnancy for at least 3 months thereafter.

Haemophilus Type B

Immunization with the *Haemophilus influenzae* type B conjugate vaccine is recommended for all children. It is given at 2, 4, 6, and 12 to 18 months. This vaccine has significantly reduced severe *Haemophilus* infections in young children.

Hepatitis A

A safe and effective vaccine is available for people at high risk for hepatitis A or travelers to countries with a high rate of infection with hepatitis A. This vaccine also is being considered for universal use in children. Persons younger than 18 years receive a three-injection series of vaccine; those older than 18 receive two injections.

Hepatitis B

A vaccine is available for people who are at risk of contracting the disease and are not immune (see page 802). It is also now recommended that children be immunized against hepatitis B during the first month of life, at 2 to 4 months, and again at 6 to 18 months.

Rabies

If you are bitten by a rabid animal, you must receive a vaccine, given as five injections on separate days (the first day and 3, 7, 14, and 28 days later), along with a passive antibody given on the first day. Failure to get the shots can be fatal (see page 1070). If you are traveling to an area where rabies is common (India, parts of South America), consider pre-exposure prophylactic treatment.

Pneumonia

There is a vaccine that gives protection against pneumococcal pneumonia (see page 704). The primary vaccination is very safe. However, because it may increase adverse side effects, repeat or booster shots are not recommended for everyone. Only those who are at increased risk for pneumococcal infections (such as previous removal of spleen or receipt of a transplanted organ) should have them. Also, very young children may not be protected by the current vaccine, but newer pneumococcal vaccines are being tested.

Chickenpox (Varicella)

A vaccine for the prevention of chickenpox (varicella) is available and should be considered for children between ages 12 and 18 months. Unvaccinated children older than 18 months who have not had chickenpox should also be considered for vaccination. Children younger than 13 years receive one dose of vaccine. Those older than 13 receive two doses given 4 to 8 weeks apart.

Prevention

Immunization (vaccination), ordinarily carried out in infancy, is by injection of a combination of vaccines that includes whooping cough (pertussis) and tetanus (see pages 1075 and 1070). The vaccine is very effective. A booster shot every 10 years is appropriate, especially if you travel to an area where diphtheria is common.

Scarlet Fever

Signs and Symptoms

- Sore throat
- Fever
- Chills
- Rash on neck and chest

Scarlet fever was once a common, serious childhood illness but now is quite rare. Caused by a specific type of streptococcal bacteria, scarlet fever usually begins suddenly with sore throat, fever, and chills. The bacteria produce a specific type of toxin (erythrogenic toxin) that causes a rash. Within 12 to 36 hours, the rash appears on the neck and chest but not on the face. Then it spreads over the body. The rash has a sandpaper consistency (see color photograph, page C-1). Often, the area of greatest involvement is above the armpits and the groin. The tongue becomes swollen and bright red.

The rash usually disappears after 3 days, and the fever disappears. The tongue may be swollen for somewhat longer, but recovery usually is uneventful.

Treatment

Your physician probably will prescribe penicillin or another antibiotic for a minimum of 10 days. Drink plenty of liquids, get bed rest, and use acetaminophen to help relieve the symptoms.

Parasitic Infestations

Parasites range from the microscopic, single-celled organisms called protozoa to larger parasites called helminths (from the Greek word *helmins,* meaning "worm"). Protozoa often spend part of their life cycle outside of humans, living in food, soil, water, or insects. The protozoan that causes malaria is a well-known example. Protozoa are always present in your body but are kept under control by your immune system.

Tapeworms and roundworms are the most common types of helminths, the larger parasites. If they enter your body, they take up residence in your intestinal tract, lungs, liver, skin, or even brain, where they live off the nutrients available at those sites.

Malaria

Signs and Symptoms

- Sequential chills, fever, and sweating
- Headache
- Muscle pains
- Anemia

Malaria is spread primarily by the female *Anopheles* mosquito, although it also may be transmitted by contaminated blood transfusions and by sharing of needles among intravenous drug users. The disease is found primarily in the rural areas of tropical and subtropical countries. Worldwide, more than 200 million people have malaria. In the United States, about 1,000 cases are reported each year, primarily among people returning from areas where this genus of mosquito thrives.

The female mosquito becomes infected with the malarial parasite when it bites a human who has malaria and ingests blood containing the protozoa. After developing in the mosquito, the parasite is then transmitted to other humans by subsequent bites of the mosquito. In the human, the parasite migrates to the liver. After developing further, the parasite enters the bloodstream and infects red blood cells. In these cells they multiply and, 48 to 72 hours later, depending on the species, cause the red blood cells to rupture, releasing a new generation of parasites.

Diagnosis

The symptoms of malaria relate closely to the parasite's life cycle. After an incubation period of anywhere from 8 days to 8 months, chills begin, lasting 15 minutes to an hour, which correspond to the rupture of the red blood cells and to the increase in body temperature. Headache, vomiting, and nausea also may occur.

Body temperature remains high for several hours, and then a sweating stage begins as body temperature falls. The cycle may recur every 48 or 72 hours, depending on the species of protozoan.

If you experience any of these symptoms within a year of traveling to an area where malaria is present, see your physician immediately. The usual diagnostic test is examination of a blood smear.

How Serious Is Malaria?

Left untreated, malaria can be fatal. The disease may end after 6 to 8 months, but it can persist for up to 3 years or even longer with certain species.

Treatment

Prevention and Medication

There is no vaccine, as yet, against malaria, but effective preventive medications are available. In most countries of the world where malaria exists, resistance has developed to chloroquine. If you will be traveling

in malaria-prone areas, your health care provider may prescribe mefloquine instead. Review your itinerary with your physician to plan the most effective preventive measures. You should start taking either of these medications 1 week before you leave home, and continue to take the medication while you are traveling and for 4 weeks after leaving the malaria area. Discuss with your physician possible adverse reactions to mefloquine. Also, be sure to review your past and current medical history for any contraindications to taking the medicine.

Take precautions in a malaria-prone area to avoid being bitten by mosquitoes. Sleep under mosquito netting, stay in buildings with screens on doors and windows, stay indoors between dusk and dawn (times when the mosquito feeds), and wear mosquito repellent.

Because malaria infection often is initially thought to be a flu-like illness or some other viral disease, be wary if you develop an illness with fever within 12 months after traveling to a malaria area. Tell your physician about your trip. A blood test can determine if you have the disease.

Both malaria and the drugs that prevent it may cause miscarriage or stillbirth in pregnant women.

Tapeworm

Signs and Symptoms

- Presence of eggs in stool or worm segments in clothing, bedding, or stool
- Hunger, dizziness, fatigue
- Loss of appetite and weight
- Vomiting
- Irritability

The tapeworms usually found in humans represent only six species. The beef tapeworm (the largest, up to 75 feet in length), fish tapeworm, and pork tapeworm usually are acquired by eating infected raw or undercooked beef, fish, or pork, respectively. The dwarf tapeworm is transmitted directly from one person to another. The rodent tapeworm (common in rats) is transmitted by accidentally swallowing infected rat fleas, beetles, or cockroaches, usually after they have gotten into cereals or other stored foods. The dog tapeworm is typically found in children who come into close contact with infested dogs or cats and have swallowed infected fleas or lice.

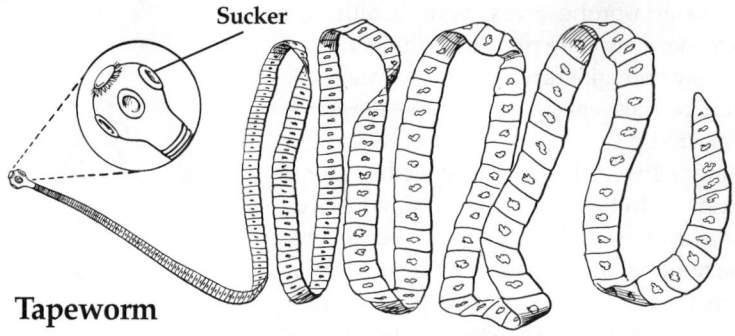

Sucker

Tapeworm

Diagnosis

Tapeworms usually cause few symptoms. The beef, pork, and fish tapeworms may cause hunger, dizziness, and fatigue. The three smaller tapeworms may cause loss of appetite, weight loss, vomiting, and irritability (especially in children). In severe cases, nausea, diarrhea, and abdominal pain may be present. Tapeworms are usually discovered when eggs are found in the stool or worm segments are found in the stool, bedding, or clothing. Your physician will make the diagnosis by obtaining segments and examining them under the microscope.

How Serious Is a Tapeworm Infestation?

The presence of tapeworms in the intestine usually is not a serious situation. However, certain types of tapeworms can penetrate the intestinal wall and spread to various internal organs. The resulting condition then may become very serious.

Treatment

Medication

Many drugs are available to treat tapeworm. The worm in the intestine usually begins to disintegrate and is passed out of the body within 24 to 48 hours after start of treatment. It is generally assumed that the worm has been eliminated if no segments reappear after 3 to 5 months.

Trichinosis

Signs and Symptoms

- Diarrhea and cramps
- Malaise
- Fever
- Muscle pain and tenderness
- Swelling of the face

Trichinella spiralis lives in the intestines of most carnivores, including marine animals.

The female worm releases larvae that enter muscles and form cysts. When the infected muscle is eaten, the cysts develop into a new generation of worms. Humans usually get trichinosis from eating infected raw or undercooked pork or pork products or from eating beef that has been ground in a contaminated meat grinder or mixed with infected pork. The incidence of infection has been greatly decreased by public health measures, but meat from wild animals, especially bear, is one continuing source of infection.

Diagnosis

Two to 12 days after eating infected meat, you may experience diarrhea, abdominal cramps, and malaise lasting 1 to 7 days, although some people may have no symptoms at all. When the muscles are invaded by the larvae, muscle pain and tenderness, fever, swelling of the face, weakness, sensitivity to light, and conjunctivitis may be present and usually last about 6 weeks.

To diagnose trichinosis, your physician probably will do a blood test and possibly a muscle biopsy to detect the larvae.

How Serious Is Trichinosis?

Except in severe cases, when it can be fatal, trichinosis is not serious and usually resolves on its own.

Treatment

In most cases, treatment is not necessary. During the initial stage, a medication may be prescribed.

Prevention

Trichinosis is easily prevented by thoroughly cooking meat or freezing it at 5 degrees Fahrenheit for 3 weeks.

Pinworms

Signs and Symptoms

- Severe itching of the anal area at night
- Insomnia, irritability, restlessness
- Vague gastrointestinal symptoms

Humans are the only host of the pinworm, which lives in the lower intestine. At night, the female worm migrates out through the anus, lays large numbers of eggs, and dies. After a few hours, the eggs can be spread to other individuals or can reinfect the host if they are transferred to the mouth by contaminated food, drinks, or hands. After the eggs are swallowed, they hatch in the small intestine and migrate down to the lower intestine. The entire cycle takes 3 to 4 weeks, and eggs are viable for up to 2 to 3 weeks. Pinworm occurs more frequently in children than in adults.

Diagnosis

The primary symptom is severe itching around the anus, particularly at night, although some patients may experience no noticeable symptoms. Pinworm is diagnosed by identifying eggs taken from the anal area. The most reliable method is to apply a short piece of cellophane tape to the itching area and then spread it on a slide for microscopic examination. The examination must be done in the morning before the affected person has defecated or bathed.

How Serious Is Pinworm Infestation?

The infection is annoying, but it is not serious and is easily cured. However, reinfection is common.

Treatment

Persons with symptoms, and often other members of the household as well, should be treated. In addition, affected persons should avoid scratching and should take special care to keep their fingernails clean, to wash their hands after defecating, and to wash the bedding to help prevent the spread or recurrence of the infection.

Medication

Appropriate medications are available and are very effective. One example is mebendazole (Vermox).

Strongyloidosis

Signs and Symptoms

- Small, sometimes itchy skin lesions
- Diarrhea, sometimes alternating with constipation
- Abdominal pain
- Flatulence

Strongyloidosis comes from the scientific name of the small worm *Strongyloides stercoralis*, which causes the disease. Also known as threadworm, it is found in many tropical and subtropical areas, although strongyloidosis sometimes occurs in temperate areas,

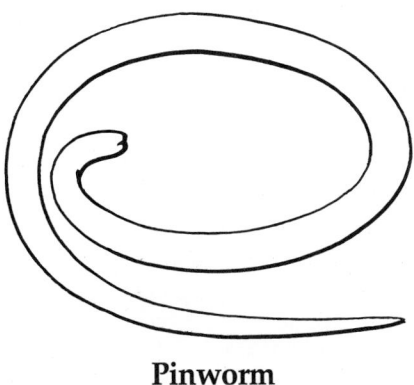

Pinworm

including the United States. It is common in overcrowded, unsanitary conditions such as mental institutions and jails.

Diagnosis

The first sign of infestation is small, red, and sometimes itchy lesions caused by the larvae entering the skin. The larvae travel through the bloodstream to the lungs, from which they rise to the throat and are swallowed. They then inhabit the intestine and cause diarrhea (sometimes alternating with constipation), abdominal pain, and flatulence.

The abdominal pain is similar to the dull, burning cramp caused by an ulcer. Nausea, vomiting, and loss of appetite also may occur. In severe cases with diarrhea, the stool contains blood and mucus. While they are in the lungs, the worms may cause a dry cough, irritation of the throat, or a low-grade fever, wheezing, difficulty breathing, and bronchitis. Determining the cause of the disease is difficult because of the wide variety of symptoms, but finding the larvae in the feces or duodenal fluid confirms the diagnosis.

Unless the infection is an overwhelming one, most persons recover completely once the worms are eliminated.

Treatment

Medications are available to treat strongyloidosis.

Ascariasis

Signs and Symptoms

- Vomiting, accompanied by stomach pain and bloating
- Wheezing, coughing, or difficulty in breathing

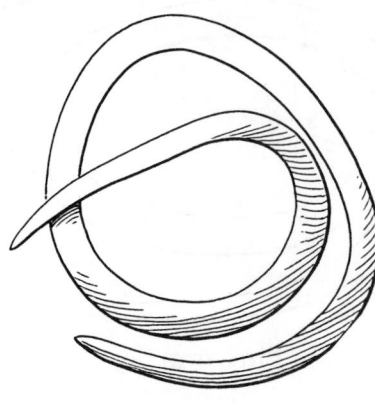

Ascaris lumbricoides

Ascaris lumbricoides is the largest of the roundworms and also is the most common intestinal worm. It is found wherever human feces are used as fertilizer or standards of hygiene are poor. The worm only affects humans, and infestation is most severe in children. The eggs are found in the soil and enter humans who consume contaminated food or drink. After migrating to the lungs, the larvae eventually take up residence in the small intestine, where they develop into an adult form that lives for a year or more. In the lungs, they cause wheezing, cough, and difficulty breathing and can cause permanent damage. In the intestine, the worms cause vomiting, upper abdominal discomfort, distention, and occasionally a bowel obstruction (see page 793).

Treatment
Treatment consists of taking antiparasitic drugs.

Hookworm

Signs and Symptoms
- Dry cough
- Difficulty breathing
- Low-grade fever
- Weakness and fatigue
- Loss of appetite
- Diarrhea
- Ulcer-like abdominal pain
- Pallor

Hookworm is widespread in tropical and subtropical areas. The larva lives in damp

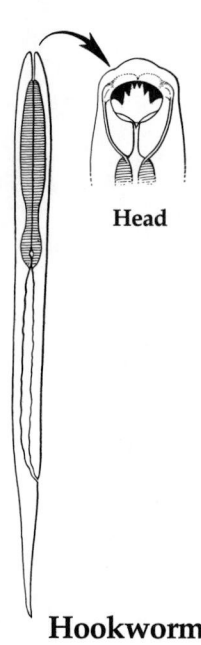

Head

Hookworm

soil until it penetrates the skin between the toes, whereupon it travels in the bloodstream to the lungs. Then, it rises to the mouth, is swallowed, and attaches to the lining of the small intestine, where it develops into a half-inch-long adult worm. The disease may affect anyone, but children are particularly susceptible to severe infestations.

Diagnosis
At the spot where they enter the skin, the larvae cause an itchy rash called ground itch. When in the lungs, they provoke a dry cough, wheezing, difficulty breathing, a low-grade fever, and sputum tinged with blood. Two weeks after entering the skin, they reach the intestine.

You may experience no symptoms, but in people with serious infestations or without adequate iron intake, the worms can cause a loss of appetite, diarrhea (usually with stool containing blood), abdominal pain, weakness and fatigue, pallor, and possibly anemia. Finding eggs in the feces confirms the diagnosis.

How Serious Is Hookworm Infestation?
Because the worms do not reproduce in humans, they simply die and disappear in 1 year or in 3 to 5 years, depending on the species. People with mild or severe cases usually recover completely if they are treated adequately and are not reinfected.

Treatment
If you have no intestinal symptoms, treatment is unnecessary. The worms eventually will be passed out of your system. If you have a serious infestation, antiparasitic medication is necessary. A diet high in protein, vitamins, and iron supplements prevents malnutrition and anemia until the infestation is eradicated.

Medication
Several types of medications may be prescribed. However, certain of them should not be used by pregnant women, so if you are pregnant, be sure your physician is aware of your condition.

Prevention
Toilet facilities that prevent contamination of the soil will break the cycle of infection. Also, always wear shoes when in contaminated areas. They afford good protection.

Insect Infestations

Some infestations are caused by small insects that attach themselves to your skin and feed off your blood. In the United States, these organisms are annoying but most do not cause dangerous illness. However, some insects do transmit viruses or bacteria that can cause serious illness in humans.

Scabies

Signs and Symptoms
- Itching at night
- Thin, pencil-like lines on your skin

In scabies, tiny mites, almost impossible to see without a magnifying glass, cause severe itching (see color photograph, page C-14). Usually the itching is worse at night. Found worldwide among all groups of people and at all ages, they often infest an entire family. Scabies are spread by close physical contact and, less often, by sharing clothing or bed sheets with an infested person. Canine scabies can be transmitted from dogs to humans.

Diagnosis
Scabies prefer to burrow into certain areas of the skin, such as between your fingers, in your armpits, around your waist, along the insides of your wrists, on the back of your elbows, on your ankles and soles of the feet, around the breasts and genitals, and on your buttocks. They form a characteristic burrow that looks like a thin, irregular pencil mark.

Your physician will look for such a burrow and will remove the mite located at the end of one to confirm the diagnosis. Although not serious, scabies are very annoying.

Treatment

Medication
Treatment involves eliminating the infestation. Several creams and lotions are available and are usually applied all over the body, from the neck down, and left on for 8 to 10 hours. Two medications commonly used are 5 percent permethrin (Elimite) cream or lindane (Kwell). Your physician will prescribe the appropriate medication. Because of the high rate of infestation, it may be appropriate that all family members and sexual partners be treated, even if no infestation is apparent.

Lice

Signs and Symptoms
- Intense itching
- Lice on the scalp, body, clothing, or pubic or other body hair
- Nits on hair shafts

Lice are tiny parasitic insects. Head lice (*Pediculus humanus capitus*) often are spread among schoolchildren by contact, clothing, or hairbrushes. Body lice (*Pediculus humanus corporis*) are generally spread through clothing or bedding.

Pubic lice (*Phthirus pubis*, commonly referred to as "crabs") can be spread by sexual contact, clothing, bedding, or even toilet seats.

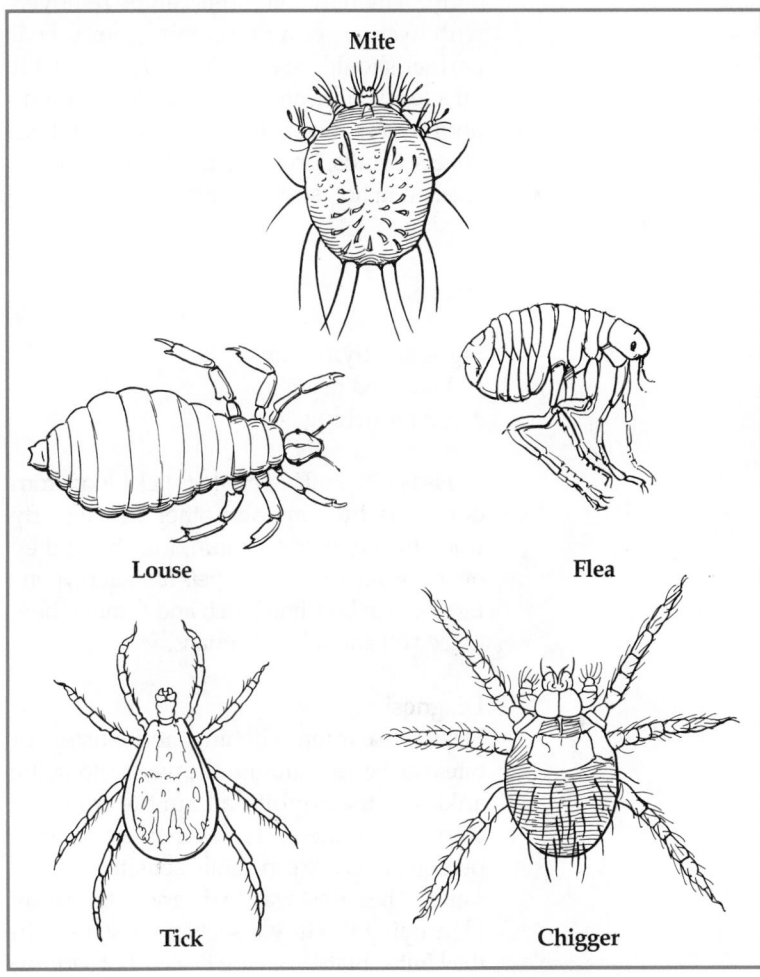

Mite

Louse

Flea

Tick

Chigger

Diagnosis

The first sign is intense itching. With body lice, some people have hives and others have abrasions from scratching. Head lice are found on the scalp and are easiest to see at the nape of the neck and over the ears. Small nits (eggs) that resemble tiny pussy willow buds can be found on the hair shafts. Body lice are difficult to find on the body because they burrow into the skin, but they usually can be detected in the seams of underwear. Pubic lice are found on the skin and hair of the pubic area (see color photograph, page C-14).

Lice do not cause a serious medical problem. However, they can be annoying and are easily spread.

Treatment

Medication

Several lotions and shampoos, both prescription and over-the-counter, are available. Examples include lindane (Kwell) and 1 percent permethrin (Nix) solution. Apply the product to all infected and hairy parts of the body. Any remaining nits can be removed with tweezers or a fine comb. Your sexual partner should be examined and treated if infected. Children should be kept at home until at least one treatment has been applied. Sheets, combs, brushes, and hats should be washed in hot, soapy water.

Fleas

Signs and Symptoms
- Localized rash
- Severe itching

Fleas are small insects that suck blood from dogs, cats, humans, and other animals. By using their tremendous jumping ability, they often spread from family pets to their owners. Eggs laid in bedding hatch and remain there to feed off animals or humans.

Diagnosis

Fleas cause intense itching, and clusters of bites can be seen around the waist, along the ankles, in the armpits, and in the crooks of elbows and knees. Hives may develop in persons who are especially sensitive to flea saliva. The surest way to diagnose fleas is by identifying the tiny insects themselves. In the United States, having fleas is not serious, and normally you do not need to see your physician if you have them. But they are very annoying and should be eliminated.

Treatment

Calamine lotion may help to relieve the itching, but the problem will continue until the fleas are eliminated. Persistent treatment of animals and their living areas is necessary. Once fleas are established, their elimination is difficult, and just putting a flea collar on your pet is not sufficient.

Various flea insecticides are available. Spray one of these on your pet's bedding, as well as on your own, if you suspect that fleas have become established there. Furniture and carpeting also should be sprayed. Home foggers help eliminate the insects; however, be careful to remove other pets, such as birds and fish, because they are very sensitive to these insecticides. If you have a heavy infestation of fleas, or your own treatments are not effective, you may have to call in a professional exterminator.

Chiggers

Signs and Symptoms
- Intense itching
- Pimple-like bumps or hives

Chiggers, also known as red bugs or harvest mites, are the larvae of a type of mite. In the United States, they are found primarily in the South, although they can be found as far north as Canada. Chiggers live in areas of tall grass or brush and on the edges of woods. Farmers, hunters, hikers, and others who spend a lot of time in the woods are most likely to become infested.

Diagnosis

The larvae prefer warm, moist places and usually take up residence around your waist, on your ankles, in the crooks of your elbows and armpits, in the groin area, and wherever clothing is tight. The small red insects attach themselves to the skin and insert a feeding tube to reach a source of blood, causing small red pimples and sometimes hives. Several hours after they have inserted their feeding tube, there is intense itching at the site.

Chiggers remain in the same spot for 1 to 4 days and then drop off, full of blood. The best way to diagnose an infestation of chiggers is by identifying the mite itself. They can be found in the center of pimples that have not yet been scratched. In the United States, chiggers do not cause any diseases but are very annoying because of the intense itching (see color photograph, page C-14).

Treatment

Medication
Treatment is aimed at relieving the itching. Your physician may prescribe an antihistamine, and corticosteroid creams or lotions can be applied directly to the pimples.

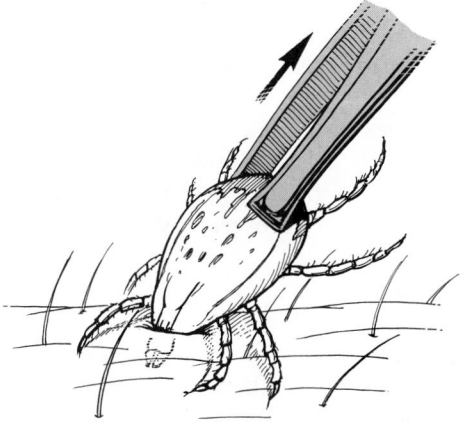

To remove a tick, use tweezers to pull the tick gently (slowly and steadily).

Ticks

Signs and Symptoms
- Itching
- Presence of ticks
- Small, hard lumps surrounded by a red circle

Ticks are small, flat insects that feed on blood. They live in tall grasses, brush, and wooded areas and attach to animals or persons passing by. After walking through such areas, check for ticks. They often lodge in hair, around ankles, and in the genital area.

Diagnosis
Ticks are most easily identified and removed before they attach themselves to the skin. Once embedded, they cause a small, hard, itchy lump surrounded by a red halo. Some ticks produce toxins that paralyze the nerves of the leg. The paralysis moves from the site of the tick up toward the trunk (see color photograph, page C-14).

How Serious Is a Tick Infestation?
Tick infestation can be serious because ticks may be carriers of Lyme disease (see page 1067) or Rocky Mountain spotted fever (see page 1068).

A condition called tick paralysis, which can resemble poliomyelitis, may occur after a tick has fed on the person for several days. It can be very serious but, if the tick is removed, the symptoms usually disappear.

Treatment
Do not scratch a tick bite. If you do, the body of the insect may break off, leaving the head embedded in your skin. Treatment consists of gently (slowly and steadily) removing the tick using tweezers.

Particularly in areas where Rocky Mountain spotted fever is known to be present, never detach a tick from a pet with your bare hands, because infection may result.

Sexually Transmitted Diseases

Bacteria and viruses transmitted by sexual contact can cause various infections. Gonorrhea, chlamydial infection, and syphilis are bacterial in origin. Herpes and venereal warts are viral infections. These infections will be discussed in the following pages. Many other diseases that often are sexually transmitted, such as hepatitis (see page 801) and AIDS (see page 1060), are discussed elsewhere in this book.

Gonorrhea

Signs and Symptoms
- Thick, pus-like discharge from the urethra
- Burning, frequent urination

Gonorrhea is caused by the bacterium *Neisseria gonorrhoeae* and is a common communicable disease. In the United States, almost 500, 000 cases are reported each year.

It is most common in persons 15 to 29 years old and is contracted through sexual contact. It occurs in both men and women; women may have no symptoms, at least not for several weeks or months.

Homosexual men also may have no symptoms, especially when the infection affects the pharynx or rectum.

Diagnosis

In men, the first symptoms of gonorrhea generally appear between 2 days and 2 weeks after exposure to the bacteria. First, there is a tingling sensation in the urethra (the passageway that carries urine from the bladder to the outside of the body). A few hours later, urination becomes painful, and a milky discharge is noted. As the infection progresses, urethral pain becomes more pronounced and large amounts of creamy, pus-like discharge are produced.

In women, symptoms may not appear for 1 to 3 weeks. The infection usually affects the cervix and reproductive organs but can involve the urethra. In some women, gonorrhea causes frequent, urgent, and painful urination along with a pus-like discharge from the vagina or urethra. In most women, however, the only symptoms are a slight increase in vaginal discharge and some inflammation, which may be evident only on physical examination. These symptoms are so mild that many women do not realize they have the infection. Often, the only suggestion that a woman may have gonorrhea is that men known to have had sexual contact with her have developed the disease.

In both sexes, rectal gonorrhea may result from anal intercourse with an infected person or from the infection spreading from the genital area. It may cause some discomfort in the anal area and rectal discharge, but in many cases no symptoms are present. Oral sex can produce pharyngeal gonorrhea with a sore throat, pain on swallowing, and redness of the throat and tonsils. Again, many persons so affected have no symptoms. If the infection spreads to the eye, it can cause a red, inflamed eye (conjunctivitis).

To confirm a diagnosis of gonorrhea, your physician will take specimens of the discharge or infected tissue for culture. This must be done before antibiotic therapy is begun. The symptoms of gonorrhea are similar to those of a number of other sexually transmitted diseases, including nongonococcal urethritis (see page 1174) and cervicitis or vaginitis caused by *Chlamydia*, *Candida*, or other organisms (see page 1173). Often, several different infectious bacteria will be present; all must be treated. Blood tests for syphilis should be performed on all persons who have gonorrhea.

How Serious Is Gonorrhea?

Gonorrhea is an acute infection that can become chronic if not treated. In men, gonorrhea may lead to epididymitis (see page 1198). In women, it can spread to the uterus and fallopian tubes, causing pelvic inflammatory disease, which may result in scarring of the tubes and infertility (see page 1187). Gonorrhea also can spread through the bloodstream to cause infection in other parts of the body. Fever, rash, and joint pain and stiffness are possible results. These complications can cause permanent damage. If treated adequately, gonorrheal infections usually can be cured. However, more and more strains of gonococci are appearing that are resistant to some types of antibiotic treatment. It is important that all sexual partners be examined, appropriate specimens cultured, and all infections treated.

Treatment

Because gonorrhea is contagious, it is important that you abstain from sexual contact until your infection is completely eliminated. General therapy for complications in men consists of hot sitz baths, bed rest, cold packs, and immobilization if epididymitis is present. In women, infection of the fallopian tubes requires bed rest and possibly surgical treatment if this does not clear. Follow-up culture of infected sites is recommended.

Medication

Your physician will prescribe appropriate antibiotics. Analgesics also may be prescribed for relief of pain.

Chlamydial Infections

Signs and Symptoms
- Painful urination
- Vaginal discharge in women
- Urethral discharge in men

Another genital infection in men and women is caused by the bacterium *Chlamydia trachomatis*. This organism is transmitted by either vaginal or anal sex.

Touching your eye with a hand that is moistened with infectious secretions can cause an eye infection, and a mother can pass the infection to her child during delivery, causing pneumonia. *Chlamydia trachomatis* is the most common cause of blindness worldwide. It causes serious eye infections in children in many developing areas, including India, Africa, and the Middle East.

Diagnosis

Diagnosis of a genital chlamydial infection can be difficult because in many cases, especially in women, there may be minimal or no symptoms. When symptoms are present, they are very similar to those of gonorrhea.

In men, chlamydial infection may cause a burning sensation during urination and a discharge from the urethra. The symptoms are milder than in gonorrhea and may appear 1 to 3 weeks after exposure to the bacteria. Women may experience burning urination, a thin vaginal discharge, or lower abdominal pain, but many must rely on having their sexual partners inform them that they have the disease.

Tests for chlamydial infection involve identifying the bacteria in secretions from the cervix (in women) or from urethral or seminal fluid (in men). Identification is made by staining the bacteria (monoclonal antibody test).

How Serious Is Chlamydial Infection?

It was once thought that chlamydial infections affected only men; women were simply carriers. However, it now is known that chlamydial infections can be serious both in men, causing inflammation of the urethra and epididymis, and in women, causing urethral infection and inflammation of the cervix and other pelvic organs. If you engage in anal sex, this organism may cause inflammation of the rectum. Conjunctivitis may occur during the first 2 weeks after birth, or chlamydial pneumonia may develop in the newborn.

Treatment

If the presence of a chlamydial infection is confirmed, or even highly suspected, all sexual partners must be treated, even though they may not have symptoms. Otherwise, they will pass the disease back and forth between them.

Medication

Antibiotics generally are prescribed for chlamydial infections. The infection should disappear within 1 to 2 weeks. If it does not,

check again with your physician. He or she may use the results of cultures to determine treatment response.

Prevention

Having only a stable, monogamous sexual relationship with an uninfected partner is the surest way of avoiding the disease. Using a condom during sexual intercourse probably decreases the risk of chlamydial infection.

Syphilis

Signs and Symptoms

Primary
- Painless sores on genitals, rectum, tongue, or lips
- Enlarged lymph nodes in the groin

Secondary
- Rash over any area of the body, but especially on the palms of the hands and soles of the feet
- Mouth sores
- Fever
- Headache
- Soreness and aching in the bones and joints

Syphilis is a complex disease caused by the spirochete (a type of bacterium) *Treponema pallidum*. Although once very prevalent, it has become very uncommon among heterosexual persons compared with gonorrheal and chlamydial infections. However, recently the incidence has increased, especially in poor, urban areas of the United States and in persons with AIDS (see page 1060). Usually transmitted by sexual contact, the organism gains entrance to the body through minor cuts or abrasions in the skin or mucous membranes. It also can be transmitted by infected blood and from a mother to her unborn child during pregnancy.

Diagnosis

Syphilis has three stages. In the primary stage, painless sores appear on the genitals, the genital area, the rectum (particularly in male homosexuals), or the mouth at 10 days to 6 weeks after exposure. Generally, these lesions are painless. Pain does occur if the sore becomes infected secondarily with other bacteria. Your physician will also look for swollen lymph nodes in the groin area.

Whenever possible, a rapid diagnosis can be made by microscopic examination of a discharge from open sores. A blood test is also available to test for the presence of the bacteria.

The second stage begins anywhere from a week to 6 months after the first stage. A red rash may appear on any surface of the body, including the palms of the hands and the soles of the feet. Lesions sometimes appear on the lips, mouth, throat, genitals, and anus. During this stage, the lesions on the skin and mucous membranes are extremely infectious. You also may have flu-like symptoms—headache and aching in the bones and joints.

An intermediate period is called latent syphilis, during which no symptoms are present. During this time, syphilis is diagnosed by special blood tests. However, if the disease has not been treated adequately, the bacteria continue to spread throughout the body, and there may be a relapse.

The last stage, known as tertiary syphilis, includes widespread infection, which is often serious. By this time, the bacteria have spread throughout the body and may affect any of the internal organs, including bones, heart, and brain. Examination of the spinal fluid may be necessary to determine whether the brain is involved.

How Serious Is Syphilis?

Syphilis can be completely cured if the diagnosis is made early and the infection is treated appropriately. However, if it is not treated, the disease can lead to death. If a woman contracts the disease while she is pregnant, it can be transmitted to her unborn child, causing deformities or death of the child.

Treatment

In both the primary and the secondary stages of syphilis, antibiotic therapy is all that is necessary. However, the disease is very contagious during these two stages, especially the secondary. Do not engage in sexual contact until at least two follow-up blood tests indicate that your infection has been eliminated. There is no vaccine against syphilis. Follow-up blood tests are required at regular intervals for at least 1 year to monitor treatment.

Medication

Penicillin is extremely effective in treating the early stages of syphilis and fairly effective in the late stages. For persons who are sensitive to penicillin, another antibiotic drug will be prescribed.

Genital Herpes

Signs and Symptoms

- Pain or itching in the genital area (women) or on the penis (men)
- Water blisters (vesicles) or open sores (ulcers)

Herpes is caused by the herpes simplex virus (HSV) and may affect the genital area (usually HSV-2) or the mouth and lips (usually HSV-1, see page 1010). Genital herpes is transmitted by vaginal or anal sex. The virus enters the body through tiny cuts in the skin or mucous membranes. It can infect the eyes by contact with a contaminated finger. It affects both men and women.

Diagnosis

The initial symptom of HSV-2 is pain or itching of the skin around the genital area. This stage is known as the prodromal period and begins 2 to 7 days after exposure to the virus. Anywhere from a few hours to several days after the prodromal stage, sores begin to appear. In women they erupt in the vaginal area, external genitals, buttocks, and anus. In men, they are on the penis, scrotum, buttocks, anus, and thighs. Sores may be present but invisible inside the cervix (women) or urethra (men) (see color photograph, page C-13).

While the ulcers are present, it may be painful to urinate. The ulcers begin as small, tender, red bumps and become watery blisters within a few days. They then rupture, becoming ulcers that ooze or bleed. After 3 to 4 days, scabs form and the ulcers heal. You may experience pain and tenderness in the genital area until the infection clears. During the first outbreak, you may experience flu-like symptoms—headache and fever—as well as swollen lymph nodes in the groin.

Your physician can confirm the diagnosis by culturing the water blisters or early ulcers. A thorough examination for other sexually related diseases is important. Often at least one other sexually transmitted disease is present in addition to herpes.

How Serious Is Genital Herpes?

There is no cure or vaccine for herpes at present. The virus remains dormant in the infected areas and periodically reactivates, causing symptoms. The disease is very contagious whenever sores are present.

Herpes generally does not cause any other serious permanent complications besides the

Safe Sex

Sexually transmitted disease (STD) is on the increase in the United States among heterosexual people and among homosexual people with the HIV virus.

Some may be offended by an open discussion of "safe sex," but it is important that you understand what behaviors put you and your family and friends at risk of contracting disease. All of us must take responsibility for protecting ourselves and our partners.

Most STDs are treatable, but HIV has no cure, and death will eventually occur in most cases. Therefore, education about this disease is especially vital.

Although HIV can be spread through shared use of contaminated needles or, rarely, through blood transfusion, it usually is transmitted by sexual contact. The virus is present in semen and vaginal secretions and enters a person's body through small tears in the vaginal or rectal tissues that can develop during sexual activity. Transmission of the virus occurs only after intimate contact with infected blood, semen, or vaginal secretions.

STDs such as chlamydial infections, gonorrhea, herpes, venereal warts, and syphilis also are highly contagious during sexual exposure. Many of them can be spread through only one sexual contact. However, none of these infections is spread through casual contact such as handshaking, talking, sitting on a toilet seat, or living in the same house with an infected person. The microorganisms that cause STDs, including HIV, all die quickly once they are outside the body.

The only sure way of preventing STDs and AIDS is through sexual abstinence or a relationship with only one uninfected person. If you have several sexual partners, either heterosexual or homosexual, you place yourself at high risk of contracting disease. And at present, no vaccine is available to prevent any of the STDs.

Although condoms do not completely eliminate the risk, correct and consistent use of a latex condom and avoidance of certain sexual practices can decrease the risk of contracting AIDS as well as other STDs.

The condom, also known as a prophylactic or rubber, is a thin sheath that covers the erect penis. When used correctly, a latex condom can help prevent pregnancy and decrease the chance of contracting most STDs, including AIDS.

Condoms can be purchased over the counter at any drugstore and are available in various thicknesses, colors, and shapes. They may be lubricated or unlubricated, have a plain end or a reservoir end, and have a smooth (the most common), ribbed, or corrugated texture. Usually the cost ranges from 50 cents to a dollar each. The condom package should mention STD protection. One should always check the expiration date on the package to be certain the condom is not expired.

Condoms sometimes are made of animal membrane; however, experts believe that the pores in such natural "skin" condoms may allow HIV to pass through. The use of latex condoms is recommended.

About a third of the condoms now sold in the United States are bought by women. Condoms should be stored at room temperature until needed. The condom can be placed on the erect penis as a part of the initial foreplay. A man who objects to a condom may be less opposed to wearing one if his partner puts it on for him. To be effective, the condom must be undamaged, applied to the erect penis before any genital contact, and remain intact and snugly in place until it is removed on completion of sexual activity. The use of extra lubrication (even with lubricated condoms) can help prevent the condom from breaking. Use only water-based lubricants. Oil-based lubricants can cause a

condom to break down.

A new female condom is available. it can help reduce the risk of contracting an STD. The availability of this female condom gives women more control over their personal health. Most forms of female-directed contraception (for example, the pill, the diaphragm) do not provide protection against STDs, although studies indicate that use of the spermicide nonoxynol-9 does decrease the frequency of gonorrhea and chlamydial infections. Using spermicide in conjunction with a diaphragm also may help kill bacteria.

Different sexual practices carry different degrees of risk of contracting HIV. Receptive (passive) anal intercourse is the riskiest because this may damage the anal and rectal membranes and allow the AIDS virus to enter the bloodstream. The passive partner is at much higher risk of contracting the AIDS virus than is the active partner, although gonorrhea and syphilis can be acquired from the passive partner's rectum. Most studies have focused on male homosexuals, but heterosexual anal sex carries similar risks.

Heterosexual vaginal intercourse, particularly with multiple partners, carries a risk of contracting HIV. The virus is believed to be transmitted more easily from the man to the woman than vice versa. This type of sex is how most other STDs are transmitted.

Oral/genital sex is also a possible means of transmission of HIV, gonorrhea, herpes, syphilis, and other STDs. Inserting the penis in the mouth (fellatio) with ejaculation and swallowing of semen is the most common cause of throat gonorrhea. Oral contact with the clitoris and vaginal opening (cunnilingus) is a frequent method of transmission of the herpes virus. Activities that involve only skin to skin contact such as hugging, massage, and mutual masturbation, with no exposure to body fluids, rarely spread disease.

sores. Newborn infants can become infected as they pass through the birth canal of mothers with open sores, which may result in brain damage, blindness, or death. This infection is more common in infants of mothers who are having their first outbreak of active herpes infection at the time of delivery. The incidence of herpes infection in the newborn is increasing as the incidence of genital herpes in women increases.

Treatment
Topical treatment consists of keeping the sores clean and dry.

Medication
During the initial outbreak, the antiviral drug acyclovir in oral form helps speed up healing. This initial treatment does not prevent recurrences. However, if recurrences are frequent, oral acyclovir treatment can be taken daily to suppress the herpes virus.

Prevention
Herpes is very contagious when the sores are present. Abstain from sexual contact until they are completely healed. Using a condom during sexual intercourse probably reduces the risk of acquiring the infection. A monogamous sexual relationship with an uninfected partner is the surest way of avoiding the disease.

Venereal Warts

Signs and Symptoms—Warty growths on the genitals

Venereal warts (also called genital warts) are caused by the human papillomavirus (HPV). This virus causes warts on the skin. Venereal warts affect both men and women and are easily transmitted through sexual contact. Persons with an impaired immune system and pregnant women are more susceptible.

Diagnosis
Venereal warts are very similar to common skin warts in appearance. They may develop from 3 weeks to 3 months after exposure to the virus. In men, they usually appear near the tip of the penis and sometimes on the shaft or on the scrotum. In women, they may appear on the vaginal lips, inside the vagina, on the cervix, or around the anus. HPV can also cause cervical lesions. Your physician generally will be able to diagnose venereal warts by physical examination.

How Serious Are Venereal Warts?
Venereal warts generally are not a serious condition, although they are contagious. However, women with cervical lesions caused by HPV have a higher risk of cervical cancer. Women with these lesions should have a Papanicolaou (Pap) smear each year (see page 1181).

Treatment
Treatment of both partners and removal of all the warts are important. Medications applied directly to the warts may be helpful. A surgical procedure involving freezing of tissues (cryosurgery) is often used.

Lasers are now used to remove large venereal warts, as is electrodesiccation (drying the tissue by the use of electrical current), followed by removal of the wart at its base. These treatments may require local or general anesthesia

Chapter 33

Mental Health

Contents

What Is Mental Health? 1095
Definitions, 1095

Normal Development, 1096
Adjusting to Adolescence, 1096
Adjusting to Adulthood, 1097
Adjusting to Aging, 1097

Problems in Childhood, 1097
Bedwetting (Enuresis), 1098
Encopresis, 1098
Learning Disorder, 1099
Obesity, 1099
Mental Retardation, 1099
Infantile Autism, 1100

Problems in Adolescence, 1101
Adolescent Depression, 1101
Teenage Suicide, 1101
Anorexia Nervosa, 1102
Bulimia Nervosa, 1102
Drug and Alcohol Abuse, 1102
Victim of Violence, 1103

Problems in the Elderly, 1103
Depression in the Elderly, 1103
How to Help Someone Who Is
Depressed, 1104
Paranoid Reactions in the Elderly, 1104
Sleep Disorders in the Elderly, 1104

Personality Problems, 1105
Paranoid Personality Disorder, 1105
Schizoid Personality Disorder, 1105
Schizotypal Personality Disorder, 1106
Antisocial Personality Disorder, 1106
Borderline Personality Disorder, 1106
Histrionic Personality Disorder, 1107
Narcissistic Personality Disorder, 1107
Psychotherapy, 1107

Avoidant Personality Disorder, 1108
Dependent Personality Disorder, 1108
Obsessive-Compulsive Personality
Disorder, 1108
Passive-Aggressive Personality
Disorder, 1109

Grief Responses, 1109
The Grief Process, 1109
Absent Grief Reaction, 1110
When Your Friend Is Grieving, 1111

Sleep Disorders, 1112
Insomnia, 1112
What Is Normal Sleep? 1112
Sleep Apnea, 1114
Snoring, 1114
Narcolepsy, 1114
Restless Legs (Nocturnal Jerking
Movements), 1115
Sleep Clinics, 1115
Naps—Bane or Boon for a Good Night's
Sleep? 1116
Nightmares and Night Terrors, 1116
Sleepwalking, 1116
Bruxism, 1117
Dreams—What and Why? 1117
Shift Disorders, 1117

Anxiety Disorders, 1118
Anxiety Reactions, 1118
What's That Knot in My Stomach? 1118
Panic Attacks, 1119
Hyperventilation, 1119
Phobias, 1119
Antianxiety Medications, 1120
Relaxation Techniques, 1121
Obsessive-Compulsive Disorder, 1121
Post-Traumatic Stress Disorder, 1121

Depression and Mood
Disorders, 1122
Situational Depression, 1122
 Prozac, 1123
Major Depressive Disorder, 1123
Manic-Depressive Illness, 1125
 Warning Signs of Potential Suicide, 1125
Seasonal Affective Disorder, 1126

Thought Disorders, 1127
Schizophrenia, 1127
Brief Reactive Psychosis, 1128
Alcohol- or Drug-Induced Psychosis, 1129

Addictive Behavior, 1129
Alcohol Dependency, 1129
Compulsive Gambling, 1130
Caffeine Addiction, 1131

Drug Dependency, 1131
Central Nervous System Depressants, 1131
Central Nervous System Stimulants, 1132
 Detoxification, 1133
Opioids, 1133
 Hallucinogens, 1134
Marijuana and Cannabis Compounds, 1134

Psychosomatic Illness, 1135
Conversion Disorder, 1135
Somatization Disorder, 1135
Hypochondriasis, 1135
 Chronic Pain Centers, 1136
Chronic Pain Disorders, 1136
 Minnesota Multiphasic Personality
 Inventory (MMPI), 1137

What Is Mental Health?

Defining mental health is difficult—professionals have debated this for generations. Mental health describes the ability to cope with life's transitions, traumatic experiences, and losses in a way that allows your personality to remain intact and even contributes to emotional growth.

If you are mentally healthy, instead of attempting to repress all conflicts and distress, you learn to accept them, to understand them, and to cope with your reactions to them, so that life can go on.

Thus, a definition of mental health to some degree is bound by culture and circumstances. Different cultures have different ways of coping with stress. For example, in one country the death of a close relative may be received with wailing, while in another the ability to carry on without an obvious display of emotion is considered appropriate and healthy. Behavior that is considered highly erratic in one culture may be perfectly acceptable in another.

Within the bounds of everyday life, however, there are certain traits that are characteristic of mental health. The ability to function may be the most obvious.

If you are mentally healthy, you can sustain relationships with family and friends and carry out your responsibilities in the workplace and at home. Such responsibilities may vary—holding down a steady job, caring for children, or some other activity—but the common denominator for mentally healthy people is the ability to meet these responsibilities with some semblance of harmony with loved ones and society (see Controlling Stress, page 307).

If you are healthy, you also have a realistic perception of the motivations of others. Although not always accurate, these perceptions do not involve bizarre delusions such as imagining that the mailman is planning to hurl a Molotov cocktail at your front door. Unlike a psychotic person, the theoretically "healthy person" has normal thought processes that are essentially logical and reasonable. You can converse with others in a reasoned and rational way. Ideas proceed in a rational manner from one to the next, rather than jumping helter-skelter.

Definitions

In our society, anxiety and lack of self-esteem may be the two biggest obstacles to achieving mental health. Anxiety may be a symptom of unresolved or stressful conflict. At times, anxiety may be evident in actual physical symptoms. Your lack of self-esteem may be the result of failing to live up to expectations. In addition, complaints of fatigue, insomnia, and poor concentration are common and may be clues to an underlying depressive disorder.

The term "personality" suggests characteristic ways of thinking, behaving, and reacting to your surroundings. A person who habitually uses inappropriate or stereotyped ways of coping with the environment has a personality disorder.

Psychosis is a condition in which thinking processes are disordered by delusions, hallucinations, or both. Schizophrenia is an example.

The term "dementia" describes a progressive and incapacitating deterioration of mental capability that results from organic brain disease. Brain tissue function may deteriorate to the extent that social interactions and occupational performance are affected. Probably the most striking feature of dementia is memory loss, although depression or anxiety may also occur. Alzheimer's disease is a familiar and frequently discussed example. Dementia usually is irreversible.

Because dementia generally is the result of organic brain disorders, it is discussed in Chapter 19, Your Brain and Nervous System (see page 457).

Even when your physician suspects a psychiatric disorder, he or she should give due consideration to the possibility that the symptoms and signs may be the result of a medical disease. Your physician should eliminate the possibility of an underlying medical condition with appropriate laboratory and radiologic tests; only then is a psychiatric diagnosis appropriate.

Your primary care physician can treat many common psychiatric disorders. In some situations, you may need a referral to a mental health specialist, such as a psychiatrist or psychologist.

A psychiatrist is a physician who completed a 4-year course of study in a recognized medical school and 4 years of postgraduate training (residency) in the specialty of psychiatry. Most psychiatrists are certified as specialists in psychiatry by the American Board of Psychiatry and Neurology. Some psychiatrists subspecialize in subjects such as child and adolescent psychiatry, geriatric psychiatry, addiction psychiatry, or forensic psychiatry. Because psychiatrists are physicians and trained in the use of drugs, they may prescribe medications.

A psychologist is trained in dealing with emotional issues. Psychologists have an advanced degree, plus specialized training. They perform psychometric evaluations of patients, use psychotherapy, and sometimes use relaxation techniques. Psychologists do not prescribe medications or do physical examinations on their patients. Many are involved in psychological research, and some specialize in helping certain types of patients such as those with physical or sexual impairments.

A psychoanalyst is a psychiatrist or psychologist who has had special training in the practice of psychoanalysis, which is a form of psychotherapy. Psychoanalysis is a highly specialized type of therapy.

If you are suspected of having a psychiatric disorder, you may receive a referral to a psychiatrist or psychologist. This mental health professional will conduct a mental status examination to evaluate your thinking patterns. In an attempt to gain some insight into your illness, he or she will evaluate your orientation, level of awareness, thought, attention, and judgment.

The psychiatrist or psychologist will evaluate your emotional state and behavior and determine whether there is any evidence of perception disorders such as hallucinations or disorders of memory.

We introduce the term "nervous breakdown" only to discard it. Sometimes people use the term to describe a serious mental illness in a person who is unable to deal with the stresses and strains of ordinary life. However, the term is not specific, and thus is not helpful in defining a mental health problem and making recommendations for treatment.

This chapter discusses a host of common psychiatric problems. Some of the ailments are true diseases or disorders; others may be matters of personal adjustment to a life-change or specific event.

Normal Development

Mental health is not the absence of conflict—it is the ability to cope with it. As we progress through life, most of us encounter certain predictable patterns of conflict. Being able to recognize these as such, rather than assuming that our difficulties are unique, can be very reassuring.

For centuries, as far back as the ancient Hindus, people have recognized various stages of life. For example, Shakespeare referred to the "seven ages of man." Contemporary psychologists speak of a predictable pattern of adjustments that we make as we pass from infancy and childhood through the teenage years on to adulthood and into old age.

Adjusting to Adolescence

Interest in sexuality is a hallmark of the teenage years, a period when puberty turns a child's body into that of an adult. But, contrary to popular belief, the teenager is rapidly maturing in many other aspects of life as well.

The adolescent's most important question is "Who am I?" The effort to answer it usually points away from parents and toward the peer group. The quest for personal identity and separation from family may involve acting "cool," experimenting with smoking, drinking, or sex, and wearing unusual or sexually suggestive clothing. This process of breaking away can be frustrating to parents, but it is an essential part of an adolescent's attempt to take responsibility for his or her own behavior and direction.

We can view the adjustment to adolescence as a three-stage process. During early adolescence (ages 12 to 15), the theme is separation. The intense ties to parents and siblings characteristic of childhood dissolve, and the adolescent frequently becomes increasingly anxious and emotionally fragile.

He or she may express the emotional upheaval with behavior that is often termed "acting out"—dressing like a rock star, writing graffiti, or losing interest in school achievement.

Middle adolescence (ages 16 to 18) is a time of coming to terms with sexual identity and relationships with the opposite sex. For many teenagers this means being recognized as a "real man" or a "real woman," often through provocative dress and behavior. By late adolescence (ages 18 to 20), the young person resolves the separation problem and becomes preoccupied with establishing his or her adult identity, particularly in terms of career. Although adolescence is a time of turmoil and rebellion for many people, the majority of teenagers pass through this phase of life relatively smoothly (see Teenage Years, page 137).

Adjusting to Adulthood

During young adulthood—from the early 20s to the early or middle 40s—men and women face critical decisions and choices. Most enter into a career, select a mate, and establish a family. This means giving up the free time we enjoyed as children and adolescents in order to get on with the business of life.

For most young adults, this is a period when intimacy and isolation are the major emotional issues. The emotional disorders of this time typically reflect anguish or protest against failures at intimacy.

The onset of middle adulthood—mid-life or middle age—begins in the fifth decade of life. In mid-life, it is normal to look back at the road we did not take, to review past successes and failures, satisfactions and disappointments, and to evaluate them in the context of youthful dreams and aspirations. If you are childless, you may need to come to terms with the family that you might have had. If you are a parent whose children are leaving home, you face the "empty nest." By mid-life we begin to recognize our own limitations as well as our own mortality.

At this stage it is also not uncommon to feel trapped—by financial burdens, by social and professional roles, and even by chronology, as the generation caught between the responsibilities for aging parents and those for children. At mid-life you may try to cope by trying to escape or repress negative feelings. Or you may begin to turn outward toward the rest of society and feel ready to "make a contribution" to others (see Young Adulthood, page 161, and Middle Years, page 219).

Adjusting to Aging

The decline most people experience in physical health during old age greatly affects emotional adjustment. At least three of every four people older than 65 have at least one chronic physical disorder; 1 of 10 finds it difficult to move about away from home. By this age, less than 20 percent of men—and even fewer women—are still in the workforce. Major losses, such as the death of a spouse, occur, and one-fourth of people older than 65 live alone. Fifteen percent of people older than 65 have either a functional or an organic brain disorder, such as Alzheimer's disease, and 5 percent are in nursing homes.

As a result of such limitations, when you are older you may feel isolated, lack social contacts, and lose out on intellectual stimulation. All of these tend to contribute to a decrease in mental capacities (see Later Years, page 231).

Problems in Childhood

Despite its image as a carefree time of life, childhood is far from easy. Many children experience emotional difficulties of one sort or another as they deal with a wide range of issues, including self-control, learning to socialize with peers, and separation from parents.

As a result, if you are a parent, you may become easily alarmed, wondering whether every nightmare is an indication of phobia or every hectic day is a sure sign of hyperactivity. For the most part, however, physicians diagnose serious emotional problems on the basis of a long-term pattern of symptoms and not the occasional wet bed or playground fight.

In the pages that follow are some of the more common childhood problems that have mental or psychiatric origins (see also School Phobias, page 133).

Bedwetting (Enuresis)

Signs and Symptoms—Involuntary voiding of urine at least twice a month by a child at least 5 years old

"Mommy, I wet my bed." Virtually every parent hears those words at one time or another, and many young children do have "accidents" during the night now and then.

However, true bedwetting (enuresis) is the involuntary voiding of urine at least twice a month in a child age 5 or older. Usually it does not indicate an emotional problem. Children vary markedly in the age at which they are physiologically ready to stop wetting.

If your child has never been totally dry for a year, the condition is known as primary enuresis. Eighty percent of children who wet their beds suffer from primary enuresis. Your child may start wetting again after having been dry for at least a year. This is called secondary enuresis. It often develops temporarily in reaction to a stressful change in your child's environment—birth of a sibling, the first week of school, or your departure on a trip, for example.

Enuresis is much more common in boys than in girls. Your child may urinate during the first third of the night and remember nothing of the occurrence. Although in 1 percent of the cases enuresis continues into adulthood, most children are continent by adolescence. Aside from wet pajamas, enuresis itself causes no direct impairment of your child's life, but social ostracism by peers (at sleep-overs and camp, for example) and anger and rejection by parents can damage self-esteem.

Treatment
Limiting your child's intake of liquids before bedtime is one way to make it easier for him or her to stay dry. Getting the child up to go to the bathroom at night also may help. Behavior modification techniques often are effective in eliminating enuresis. For example, you may want to use wall charts with gold stars awarded for dry nights to inspire your child to work toward token rewards and favorite treats.

Behavior modification devices with an alarm to awaken your child may help, if your child is motivated to stop wetting. Your physician may prescribe and monitor the use of a medication, such as imipramine, if the problem persists.

In the case of secondary enuresis, your child should be examined to rule out any organic problems—for example, infection, seizure disorder, or diabetes. Should the problem appear to be a reaction to stress, psychotherapy or family therapy may be helpful.

Although having to change bed linens repeatedly because of the bedwetting can be exasperating, it is important to express support rather than anger to your child, in order to enlist cooperation and avoid further loss of self-esteem.

Encopresis

Signs and Symptoms—Repeated passage of feces (stool) into inappropriate places (other than the toilet or potty) by a child at least 4 years old

Encopresis is repeated defecation in inappropriate places, such as underwear or the floor. By definition, the diagnosis of encopresis is made only after your child is 4. It does not include instances of stool incontinence with an organic cause. Encopresis is 5 times more common in boys than in girls. Twenty-five percent of children with encopresis also have enuresis (see this page).

Usually, the stools are hard and painful, because your child holds back for long periods. Because the constipation makes defecation painful, your child may resist having a bowel movement. Use of stool softeners and suppositories can help the dilated rectum resume its normal size.

How Serious Is Encopresis?
Sometimes the condition develops in association with psychosocial stress, such as entering school or the birth of a sibling. But the condition may be part of a passive-aggressive relationship with parents, especially if deliberate smearing is evident. If your child feels ashamed, he or she may try to avoid potentially embarrassing situations such as attending camp.

Treatment
Your physician may recommend establishment of regular routines for sitting your child on the toilet, consuming a high-fiber diet,

and sometimes using stool softeners. Behavior modification techniques—such as a system of rewards for stools your child successfully passes into the toilet—are often helpful. Never shame or punish your child. You may need to use suppositories and enemas to relieve severe retention and impaction, but do not use them repeatedly.

Family therapy also helps you examine an overall pattern of oppositional behavior. You may learn greater respect for your child's individuality, and your child can learn more direct ways to express anger.

Learning Disorder

If your child has a learning disorder, he or she will show inadequate development of a specific academic skill. This is not the result of a demonstrable physical or neurologic disorder, mental retardation, or insufficient educational opportunities. Usually your child will have difficulty with one particular academic skill—reading, arithmetic, language, or speech. (For a comprehensive discussion of learning disorders, see page 129.)

Obesity

Signs and Symptoms—Weight greater than normal by 20 percent or more

We become obese, which is defined as overweight by 20 percent or more of normal body weight, by consuming more calories than our bodies can use. Excess calories stored as fat produce the excess body weight.

There is evidence that early feeding patterns may play a major role in a cultural rather than genetic transmission of obesity from one generation to the next. Many people say that today's American children are notably less physically fit than their counterparts in previous generations. They are less active and engage in considerably less exercise, which markedly decreases their caloric needs. Another cause may be the nature of foods they eat—fast foods, snack foods, and sweets, children's perennial favorites, are extremely high in calories.

How Serious Is Obesity?

Various estimates place the frequency of obesity in children between 16 and 33 percent. Eighty percent of children who are obese between the ages of 10 and 13 will be obese when they are adults. Because these children tend to be less popular with peers and do less well at sports, they frequently have a poor self-image.

Treatment

If your child is obese, you may find it helpful to keep a diary of everything he or she eats for a week and of all physical activities. An examination by a physician who knows your child's history can help determine an appropriate weight.

If weight gain can be kept in check while your child continues to grow in height, the obesity gradually corrects itself. This is easiest to achieve with moderate changes in eating and activity patterns, such as avoiding second helpings and limiting snacks to fruits and vegetables. These changes probably will produce a healthier and longer-lasting result than will a drastic or rigidly planned diet (see page 113).

Mental Retardation

Signs and Symptoms

- Score of 72 or below on an individually administered intelligence test
- Slow development of language and motor skills
- Social and emotional immaturity
- Poor school performance in most or all subjects

Mental retardation may be due to inborn chromosomal or metabolic abnormalities such as Down syndrome (see page 44) or phenylketonuria (PKU; see page 8). Prenatal rubella, toxoplasmosis, and heavy alcohol drinking during pregnancy are also possible causes.

Children may develop mild mental deficiencies in economically or socially deprived situations in which they lack adequate language models, are chronically understimulated, or have environments that are unstructured and unpredictable. Another possible cause is severe head trauma.

A person who scores 72 or below on one of the individually administered intelligence tests (for example, the Wechsler or Stanford-Binet) may be diagnosed as mentally retarded. A physician, psychiatrist, clinical psychologist, audiologist, and speech pathologist may all be involved in the evaluation process.

Limitations in the mental capacity of developmentally disabled individuals may range from mild to profound. Mild retardation may not be recognized until a child begins school and is compared with other students. A person with profound retardation may require special care and almost total supervision from early in life.

Some developmentally disabled people have mental limitations that are apparent only by behavior in certain situations. A developmentally disabled person may have difficulty interacting with others due to a lack of social skills or an inability to effectively communicate, and may be vulnerable to the influence of strangers.

Treatment

A child diagnosed with mental retardation may attend "mainstream" classes and specialized skill training classes conducted by special education teachers. Depending on the level of disability, care providers may be effective in helping the developmentally disabled individual to manage personal needs. Adults with this disability may profit from special occupational or vocational training and may perform competently in supervised work situations.

Supervised living services are available for people with mild or moderate retardation who can live on their own. A care provider may visit weekly, daily, or several times a day, depending on need, to provide skills training, assist with medications or appointments, or just to chat. Facilities are also available for those requiring more supervision and care (see Group Homes for the Developmentally Disabled and Mentally Ill, page 1328).

When mental retardation appears to have environmental causes, preschool training (in programs such as Head Start) may offset some of the cultural deprivation (see Mental Retardation, page 1099).

Infantile Autism

Signs and Symptoms
- Appearance of living in his or her own world
- Bizarre reactions to people and objects in the environment
- Poor communication
- Aversion to cuddling, and even abhorrence of physical contact
- Virtually total lack of social interaction

Infantile autism (now often called pervasive developmental disorder) is one of the most severe mental illnesses of childhood. An autistic child is extremely unresponsive to other people. He or she communicates very poorly, does not cuddle, and may even seem to be repulsed by physical contact. Autistic children fail to seek comfort when distressed, do not imitate adults normally (for example, don't "wave bye-bye"), and have virtually no social interaction.

An autistic child may exhibit stereotyped body movements (hand-flicking or -twisting, spinning, head-banging), is fascinated by parts of objects (say, spinning the wheels on a toy car), gets very upset over even the slightest change in his or her environment (movement of furniture or objects, for example), and is unreasonably insistent on routines.

Autism usually appears before your child is 30 months old. Your autistic child often may not speak or may only mimic sounds made by others, has difficulty naming objects, and makes bizarre facial expressions and gestures. Occasionally, an autistic child will have an extraordinary talent, similar to the case of the adult "idiot savant."

We do not know how the disorder develops, although maternal rubella (see page 1074), PKU (see Phenylketonuria, page 8), encephalitis (see page 482), or meningitis (see page 481) may predispose a child to it. It is 50 times more common in siblings of autistic children than it is in the general population. It occurs 3 to 4 times more frequently in boys than in girls.

Not all children who display some autistic behaviors have infantile autism. Reliable diagnosis of this disorder requires the skills of an expert in child psychiatry or child psychology.

Treatment

It is very difficult to treat this disorder. The most effective treatments use a combination of special education, behavioral therapy, and medication. Many autistic children function at a subnormal intellectual level. Others are intellectually bright and perform well in school subjects but have severe social adjustment problems. Not all children with autism are severely incapacitated. Some have a mild form of autism (Asperger's syndrome) that produces social awkwardness, but they function in school and eventually may become gainfully employed.

Problems in Adolescence

Adolescence is a time of tumultuous changes in a child's physical and emotional makeup. Many observers have called the adolescent "a child in an adult's body."

Frequently adolescents are unreasonably critical of their appearance. "I hate my nose!" "Don't I look fat in these pants?" Nearly every adolescent finds something disagreeable about the way he or she looks. These comments often reflect concerns about self-image. Sometimes, such statements are obvious bids for reassurance; the child wants to hear that he or she is worthy of love.

In some cases, however, there is a hidden message. For example, if you have recently divorced, your child may be saying that he or she believes the divorce happened because there is something wrong with him or her. The most constructive course of action is to ask why he or she feels that way. Often, it is not necessary to do any more than provide a willing ear.

An adolescent's difficulties center not only on his or her intense self-awareness and sexuality but also on the often traumatic and uneven journey from being a dependent child to becoming a young adult who is beginning to separate from parents. In the following pages, we discuss problems adolescents face.

exhibits many of the previously listed signs and symptoms may be depressed.

Parents need to be alert and take steps to be sure the adolescent is evaluated by a physician to rule out physical illness. A child psychiatrist may be consulted to confirm that the adolescent is depressed. If untreated, depression may last for months. Severe teenage depression is serious, because it may lead to suicide, the third leading cause of adolescent death.

Sometimes depression is an obvious reaction to a disturbing event such as the death of a relative, the break-up with a close friend, failure at school, or a move to a new environment. Often there is no apparent cause. Such depressions tend to run in families (see page 1023).

Treatment

Adolescent depression is treated with a combination of antidepressant medications and psychotherapy (see page 1107). Psychotherapy alone is effective for milder forms of depression; medication is necessary for severe depression. If there is a risk of suicide, it may be necessary to treat the adolescent in a hospital psychiatric unit.

Adolescent Depression

Signs and Symptoms

- Depressed or irritable mood most of the day, nearly every day
- Marked loss of interest in nearly all activities
- Changes in appetite and weight (usually a loss of appetite leading to weight loss; sometimes increased eating)
- Trouble sleeping at night or excessive daytime sleeping
- Daily fatigue or energy loss
- Continued feelings of worthlessness or inappropriate guilt
- Trouble concentrating or indecisiveness, nearly every day
- Recurrent thoughts of death or suicide

Few teenagers look cheerful most of the time. Many sleep for hours on end when offered the opportunity. But a teenager who

Teenage Suicide

We live in a society in which the family structure is radically changing, and teenagers have enormous difficulties coping with the highly emotional issues of separation and identity. They may also feel unwanted by their families or have trouble in school, which leads to feelings of failure. Pregnancy and trouble with the law can be overwhelming to a teenager.

Teenagers who attempt suicide may want to escape a life that seems intolerable or attempt to "punish" their parents, whom they perceive as uncaring or unfair. Your suicidal teenager may not know how to deal with pain and a feeling of failure. We often associate family loss with teenage suicide—a divorce or a parent's death, for example. Depression and psychosis also may be involved. Some teenage suicide is accidental, resulting from drug abuse or from deviant sexual practices.

If your teenager threatens suicide, take him or her seriously. (For further information, see Warning Signs of Potential Suicide, page 1125.) Psychotherapy can help the suicidal teenager, especially by focusing on how to deal with loss or anger (see page 1107).

Anorexia Nervosa

Signs and Symptoms
- Unrealistic fear of becoming fat
- Excessive dieting and exercise
- Significant weight loss or failure to gain weight during a period of growth
- Refusal to maintain a normal body weight
- Absence of menstrual periods
- Preoccupation with food, calories, and food preparation

Many teenagers diet for a few days or weeks. Those who go on to develop anorexia nervosa persist to the point of emaciation, despite warnings from their family and friends.

This disorder occurs almost exclusively in adolescent girls and young adult women, although males account for a few cases (less than 10 percent). Typically, an adolescent girl who is normal in weight, or somewhat overweight, begins to eliminate snack foods and high-calorie foods from her diet. She begins to skip meals, and her food restriction becomes increasingly stringent. Often, dieting is accompanied by frantic exercise.

She may take great interest in reading recipes, counting calories, preparing food, and baking for her family. She may encourage others to eat, whereas she avoids eating. This food restriction results in progressive loss of body fat. When the adolescent induces vomiting and inappropriately uses laxatives and diuretics to speed weight loss, even more serious physical changes result.

We don't know the specific cause of anorexia nervosa. Multiple factors play a role. Some individuals seem to have a biologic predisposition that becomes apparent at the time of puberty. Individual psychological factors, such as a fear of sexuality, may play a role, as may family pressures and conflicts. Society's emphasis on extreme thinness encourages excessive dieting.

When the problem is identified early, treatment can prevent progression of the illness, and complete recovery is possible. However, the illness can be severe and last for several years. In extreme cases, death may result.

Treatment
In most instances, psychotherapy, diet counseling, and counseling for the parents are recommended while the adolescent with anorexia nervosa remains at home. When weight loss is out of control and dangerous practices such as vomiting and abuse of laxatives and diuretics have caused physical harm, hospitalization for more intensive treatment becomes necessary.

Bulimia Nervosa

Signs and Symptoms
- Recurrent episodes of binge eating
- Self-induced vomiting or laxative abuse
- Weight within fairly normal range
- Fear of becoming fat

Often called the "binge and purge" disorder, bulimia nervosa involves the consumption of excessive amounts of food—usually high-calorie sweets—in a short time. The gorging may continue until a feeling of fullness or a stomachache interrupts. Because the individual fears gaining weight, self-induced vomiting (the most common form of purging) and abuse of laxatives occur.

This disorder most frequently affects late adolescent and young adult women.

Unlike persons with anorexia nervosa, women who binge and purge usually realize that their eating is abnormal. They often become depressed after binges.

Bulimia nervosa is serious, because the habit is disruptive to work and social life. Purging can have very serious health consequences by depleting the body of water and potassium, and it can even result in death.

Treatment
The keys to treating bulimia include educating the person about the consequences of bingeing and purging, and establishing healthful eating habits. This is best done by a psychiatrist and dietitian experienced in the treatment of eating disorders. Antidepressant medications sometimes may reduce the urge to binge-eat. Psychotherapy may also help by dealing with associated adjustment problems. When bingeing and purging are out of control and there are physical complications, hospitalization for more intensive treatment may be necessary

Drug and Alcohol Abuse

The abuse of drugs, both legal and illegal, is alarmingly common among adolescents.

Depending on the drug and on the teenager, it may be merely experimentation or a serious addiction.

For information on the symptoms and treatment of drug abuse, see Medications and Drug Abuse, page 335, and Drug Dependency, page 1131.

Victim of Violence

Signs and Symptoms
- Multiple bruises
- Multiple old fractures
- Unexplained injuries
- Pain in the genital area
- Sudden changes in behavior
- Loss of appetite
- Problems in school
- Abdominal pain

It often is hard for teenagers to discuss violence, particularly violence directed at themselves. This is especially true in cases of physical or sexual abuse by a relative, friend, or other trusted figure. Often, the victim is afraid to report the problem, fearing adult retaliation and also fearing the loss of the adult's love. If you notice that an adolescent has unexplained injuries or pain, or exhibits sudden changes in behavior, seek professional help. Several resources in your community can provide information and support: your physician, a school counselor, crisis hotlines in your community, hospital emergency rooms, rape crisis centers, domestic violence programs, and shelters for battered women and children.

Treatment
Sometimes an adolescent will confide in a trusted adult—a teacher, a relative, or a member of the clergy, for example. To secure the adolescent's protection from further harm, the first step is to report the abuse to your local child protection agency or the child's physician. The case will then be investigated by law enforcement officials or social workers, who will determine the child's degree of risk and plan accordingly for his or her safety.

If the adolescent has suffered a major trauma (such as violence, sexual or physical abuse, or rape), psychotherapy and, in the case of incest, family therapy can help the young person cope with the reality of the situation and restore his or her self-esteem.

Problems in the Elderly

Just as children and young people struggle to adjust to the changes that occur in their bodies and in their lives, so do elderly people. Physical or mental changes in older people may result in a loss of mobility, sexual problems, or a general feeling of being unable to cope. Changes in circumstances may produce isolation or loneliness. As we age, we often experience greater difficulty in facing and dealing with changes. Some of the following problems are common among elderly people.

Depression in the Elderly

Signs and Symptoms
- Loss of interest or pleasure in usual activities
- Feeling sad or "blue"
- Poor appetite and weight loss
- Sleep disturbance
- Loss of energy and fatigue
- Difficulty in concentrating, or memory loss

In an older person, depression can be difficult to recognize. Often, a depressed elderly person does not fit the typical profile of a depressed person, a person who is supposed to be generally sad and tearful. Elderly people who are depressed occasionally may complain of fatigue, weakness, insomnia, poor appetite, restless anxiety, poor concentration, or lack of interest in sex. In rare cases, however, a depressed older person may become so withdrawn that he or she has difficulty understanding even simple requests (see Vascular Dementia, page 471). It's more common for a person with mild to moderate dementia (such as Alzheimer's disease, see page 470) to have coexisting major depression. At times, physicians find it difficult to diagnose depression in elderly people.

There are various causes of depression among aging people. These include loneliness (especially after loss of a spouse), chronic illness and pain, difficulty getting around or even performing simple tasks, frustration over memory loss, and lack of a sense of purpose in the absence of a job or a family to worry about. Sometimes depression may actually be a sign of a medical illness (such as hypothyroidism; see page 948). Your physician can rule out medical disorders with symptoms that mimic depression. Many medications can contribute to depression in elderly people. Often, no cause for depression is found (see page 1123). Evidence of a biochemical explanation of this disorder is not yet conclusive.

Treatment

If a medication causes or contributes to the depression, it may be gradually withdrawn under careful supervision. Depression among the elderly can often be alleviated through nonmedical means: participation in group activities that provide companionship and regular outings; regular visits from young people ("adoptive grandparent" programs); and, in the case of relatively healthy retirees, performing volunteer work in the community.

More serious forms of depression may require further evaluation and treatment under the careful supervision of a physician. Treatment may include the use of antidepressant drugs and electroconvulsive therapy (see page 1124).

Paranoid Reactions in the Elderly

Signs and Symptoms—Delusions that last for months or longer and involve real-life situations such as being followed, being poisoned, having a disease, or being deceived by a spouse

Paranoid symptoms and delusions occur occasionally in elderly people, at times in those who are hard of hearing. Typically, the first symptom of paranoia will be that the older person becomes highly suspicious of a member of the family or a friend. These symptoms may be a sign of depression or early dementia (see page 471). The correct diagnosis must be made before therapy can begin.

Treatment

Antipsychotic drugs such as haloperidol (Haldol) or respiridone (Resperdol) often can help, although these medications must be used with caution in a supervised setting.

Sleep Disorders in the Elderly

Signs and Symptoms

- Confusing days and nights (day/night reversal)
- Prolonged delay in falling asleep
- Frequent nocturnal awakening

Sleep disturbance is a common problem among elderly people and is worse in those with psychiatric disorders. At best, sleep in old age is "not what it used to be." It takes longer to fall asleep than it used to. Older people sleep less soundly and they frequently wake up during the night. Generally, elderly people also need less sleep.

There are two potential causes of sleep disturbance among aging people. First, they may be in pain, often from such common ailments as arthritis. Second, the individual may not be getting enough activity during the day. And sleeping through the night until morning may be difficult in institutions, where bedtime may be scheduled as early as 7 p.m.

How to Help Someone Who Is Depressed

The most important thing you can do for a depressed person is to help him or her get appropriate professional help. When depression is diagnosed and treatment has begun, encourage the individual to continue with treatment until it concludes. It may take several weeks for the benefits of antidepressant medication to become obvious.

During this time, offer emotional support. Engage the person in conversation and listen carefully. Allow the individual to express his or her feelings, but point out realities and offer hope.

Do not expect the depressed individual to "snap out of it." Don't accuse him or her of laziness or feigned illness. Remember, depression is an illness that requires both time and appropriate treatment before healing can occur.

Never ignore remarks about suicide. Always report such remarks to the physician treating the individual.

If you are caring for the depressed person, ask for help when you need it. Trying to deal with a depressed person alone can be exhausting and make you feel helpless. You may need to investigate the home health care option (see page 1319).

Other possible causes include medical problems such as congestive heart failure (see page 659), esophageal reflux (see page 742), frequent urination, anxiety, depression, excessive use of stimulants (coffee in the evening, for example), or alcohol or drug use. An aging person with frequent sleep disturbances not only exhausts his or her caretakers and family but also tires himself or herself out.

Treatment

When a person is not sleeping well because of pain, aspirin or acetaminophen may help when sleeping pills do not. A moderate exercise program, a quiet, comfortable bed, and a drink of warm milk at bedtime can improve the sleep pattern. When there are no identifiable physical or psychological causes, occasional use of a short-acting benzodiazepine or a sedating antidepressant can help. These should not be used on a regular basis. Benzodiazepine drugs can be habit-forming; antidepressant medications are not. All possible causes for the sleeplessness should be explored before using these drugs. (For a general discussion of sleep disorders, see page 1112.)

Personality Problems

Although there are many types of personality disorders, they all reflect an inability to accept the demands and limitations of the outside world. These disorders may regularly interfere with your behavior and with your interactions with family or persons at work or play.

Before the diagnosis of a personality disorder is conclusive, physicians must rule out medical and neurologic changes that can mimic personality disorders. Often, people with personality disorders have had emotional problems during childhood.

Only about one in five people with personality disorders seeks psychiatric help and treatment. The majority experience long-standing difficulties in marriage, in maintaining stable employment, and in friendships.

If you have a personality disorder, you may not recognize the reasons for your problems. You may tend to blame others for your own actions or thoughts. Treatment generally consists of psychotherapy (see page 1107), although occasionally medication can help. The key to therapy is establishing a trusting relationship.

Paranoid Personality Disorder

Signs and Symptoms
* Suspicious of and overly sensitive to perceived injuries, slights, and tricks by others
* Frequent blaming of others

* Secretive
* Lack of humor or insight
* Exaggerated sense of own importance

If you have this disorder you may be overly worried that others are "out to get you." Because you may spend a great deal of energy looking for hidden, sinister meanings behind the behavior of others, you may be easily offended. People with this disorder show a limited range of emotions and may appear cold and humorless. They easily become hostile.

Treatment

Treatment is difficult, although psychotherapy (see page 1107) may be of help.

Schizoid Personality Disorder

Signs and Symptoms
* Aloofness and emotional coldness
* Lack of close friendships
* Isolation
* Lack of energy
* Indifference to praise from or criticism by others

People with schizoid personality disorder appear to have little need for other people and are usually loners. If you have this disorder, you may live in nearly total social isolation, lacking any close friendships and remaining aloof from everyone you encounter.

Treatment

Treatment of schizoid personality disorder is difficult. In some cases, however, psychotherapy (see page 1107) may be beneficial.

Schizotypal Personality Disorder

Signs and Symptoms
- Disordered or irrational thinking
- Odd speech (vague or metaphoric)
- Inappropriate ideas of reference (attributing unusual significance to neutral events)
- Suspiciousness

Persons with schizotypal personality disorder show many similarities to schizophrenics (see Schizophrenia, page 1127) in their odd ways of thinking, perceiving the world, and speaking, but their symptoms are not sufficiently pervasive or strong to warrant a diagnosis of schizophrenia. Although they are often socially isolated, the difficulties these persons have are primarily in understanding (cognition) and not interpersonal (as with the schizoid personality).

Treatment

There is no known cure for schizotypal personality disorder. Psychotherapy (see page 1107) may be beneficial in certain cases.

Antisocial Personality Disorder

Signs and Symptoms
- Lack of concern regarding society's rules and expectations
- Repeated violation of the rights of others
- Unlawful behavior
- Lack of regard for truth
- In parents, neglect or abuse of child or children
- Physical aggression, including spouse abuse
- Lack of remorse

If you have an antisocial personality disorder, you show a lack of concern for the expectations and rules of the society in which you live and repeatedly violate the rights of others. The popular term for an individual with this disorder is sociopath.

Although the diagnosis is limited to persons older than 18, it requires a history of antisocial behavior. Before age 15, these individuals often display a pattern of lying, trouble with the law, truancy, delinquency, and substance abuse and may have run away from home. As adults, people with this disorder often commit acts that are against the law, fail to live up to the requirements of a job or financial or parenting responsibilities, and are reckless in personal behavior (driving while intoxicated, for example). They are unable to sustain long-term relationships with one sexual partner, frequently abuse alcohol or drugs, and are aggressive and irritable.

Antisocial personality disorder is not just a medical term for criminality; it describes a long-standing disorder that usually lands those who have it not in a psychiatrist's office but in court or prison.

Suicide, alcoholism, vagrancy, and social isolation are common among those commonly called sociopaths, but what is remarkable is their apparent lack of anxiety or depression in situations in which such emotions might be expected. Despite all their run-ins with the law, they can present a charming and strikingly normal facade.

Treatment

There is no simple or widely effective method of treating the sociopath.

Borderline Personality Disorder

Signs and Symptoms
- Chronic difficulty in maintaining a positive self-image
- Moodiness
- Interpersonal problems
- Impulsive, often damaging behavior (such as suicide attempts)

If you have borderline personality disorder, you may think of it as having "stable instability." You may have chronic problems such as moodiness, sudden anger, sad or fearful periods, or feeling empty inside. Despite the fact that you may not get along well with others, you usually do not like to be alone. You may tend to characterize others as either "all good" or "all bad" as a defense mechanism.

Treatment

Treatment of borderline personality disorder is difficult and often unsuccessful. In certain cases, psychotherapy (see this page) may be helpful.

Histrionic Personality Disorder

Signs and Symptoms
- Relationships that appear very intense but are in fact superficial
- Highly dramatic and engaging manner, emotions expressed in an exaggerated way
- Self-centered
- Constantly seeking attention and praise
- Sexualization of relationships
- Low tolerance of frustration

This problem usually makes for stormy and ungratifying interpersonal relationships. It is diagnosed much more frequently in women than in men, and it seems to run in families. The behavior might be a combination of learned and inherited characteristics.

Treatment
There is no widely effective method of treating histrionic personality disorder. In some cases, however, psychotherapy (see this page) can have a beneficial effect.

Narcissistic Personality Disorder

Signs and Symptoms
- Exaggerated sense of own importance, power, and talents
- Seeks admiration
- Indifferent to emotions and needs of others
- Difficulty in coping with rejection

Psychotherapy

Psychotherapy is a method of treating emotional problems. The therapist and the patient seek to develop a supportive working relationship. In the sanctuary of the office, the therapist encourages you to feel comfortable discussing your problems and conflicts and to feel optimistic that therapy can help. The therapist may interpret your problems and suggest different ways to cope with them.

There are dozens of different kinds of therapy. Basically, however, they fall into two categories.

In one category are the psychodynamic therapies. These therapies seek to help you understand better the psychological forces that motivate your actions, with the goal that these insights reveal possibilities for change. Psychoanalysis is one well-known example of this kind of therapy, although in recent years it has been used only rarely.

In the second category are the behavior therapies. As the name implies, they deal not with inner feelings and motivations, but use specific techniques to change behavioral symptoms. Therapy to create a dislike for smoking is an example of behavior therapy.

Psychotherapy cannot change the world around you. Therapy sessions will not eliminate job stress or financial problems or change the personality of a difficult spouse. What it can do, however, is help you learn to cope more effectively with your environment, evaluate your priorities and your responses to stress, and understand and accept yourself as you are.

In practice, most therapies involve a mixture of self-exploration by the patient and supportive-directive work by the therapist. Psychodynamic therapy may be one-on-one between you and a therapist, or it may take place in a group setting.

Psychodynamic therapy usually is a combination of discussion, explanation, relaxation, exploration, and support. It attempts to make connections between your internal experiences and your responses to life events. Psychodrama is a unique form of group therapy. It may last for only a few sessions that deal with a specific problem, or it may be long-term and open-ended.

Broadly speaking, behavior therapy covers a group of related methods and techniques, all based on learning theory. Rather than assuming that the problem that brings you to the therapist's office is symptomatic of an underlying psychological disorder, behavior therapists work on the problem behavior itself. They concentrate on helping you learn to change your response to a particular problem situation.

To achieve this, they most frequently use classic conditioning principles—the basis for Pavlov's famous experiment with dogs. For example, through systematic desensitization, which is repeated exposure to a situation or stimulus that frightens or upsets you, you can learn to conquer a phobia or an anxiety state.

Other methods of behavior therapy include anxiety management training, social skills training, and assertiveness training.

The narcissistic person has an inflated sense of his or her own uniqueness, importance, and gifts. When rejected, he or she displays excessive anger or shame and has trouble viewing others realistically, characterizing them as "perfect" or "worthless," with very little in between.

Treatment
There is no known cure for narcissistic personality disorder, although psychotherapy (see page 1107) may be effective for certain people.

Avoidant Personality Disorder

Signs and Symptoms
- Exaggerated worry over being rejected or humiliated, resulting in avoidance of close ties with other people
- Low self-esteem

Avoidant people are preoccupied with their own shortcomings, and consequently fear rejection. This causes them to withdraw from other people. They often do seem to wish for intimacy, however, despite their lack of close ties.

Treatment
Treating avoidant personality disorder is difficult, and there is no known cure. In certain cases, however, psychotherapy (see page 1107) may be beneficial.

Dependent Personality Disorder

Signs and Symptoms
- Views self as inept or helpless
- Avoids personal responsibility and allows others to assume it for important life decisions and daily choices
- Chronically unable to meet the ordinary demands of life, but not mentally retarded

If you are dependent, you permit others to make simple daily choices and major life decisions for you. You may allow others to take over the important aspects of your life. You see yourself as inadequate and, in order to avoid taking responsibility, willingly subordinate your own desires and needs to those of other people.

Treatment
There is no known cure for dependent personality disorder, but psychotherapy (see page 1107) may be appropriate.

Obsessive-Compulsive Personality Disorder

Signs and Symptoms
- Pervasive pattern of perfectionism and inflexibility
- Symptoms begin by early childhood

The term obsessive-compulsive personality disorder (sometimes shortened to compulsive personality disorder) describes individuals who tend to be preoccupied with detail, rules, and procedures. Often these individuals insist on things being done a specific way. Sometimes they are ineffective because of their indecisiveness. Obsessive-compulsive individuals place a higher value on work and possessions than on interpersonal relationships. They often have difficulty expressing warm, emotional feelings toward others and are sometimes perceived as being aloof, cold, or indifferent.

The following features may be present:

1. So bent on perfection that it becomes very difficult to complete a task

2. Preoccupied with details—rules, regulations, lists, and schedules, often losing sight of the point of an activity

3. Wanting to control situations, unreasonably insistent that everyone "do it my way," and unwilling to delegate tasks because of the belief that no one else can do them correctly

4. Overzealous devotion to work in preference to leisure activities and friendships (workaholism)—without apparent financial necessity

5. Markedly indecisive because of worry about priorities

6. Highly moralistic and inflexible about moral and ethical questions, without a basis in cultural or religious identification

7. Displays affection only in restricted ways

8. Is stingy with time, money, or gifts, even when the stinginess offers no personal gain

9. Is a "pack rat," unable to throw anything away, no matter how worthless the object may be

Treatment
There is no specific treatment for this personality disorder.

Passive-Aggressive Personality Disorder

Signs and Symptoms
- Procrastinates
- Sulky, irritable, or argumentative behavior
- Tends to work slowly or deliberately do a bad job on tasks that he or she does not really want to do
- Protests (unrealistically) that everyone is making unreasonable demands
- "Forgets" obligations
- Believes that he or she is doing a much better job than others think he or she is
- Resents useful suggestions from others on how to be more productive
- Fails to do his or her share of the work, thereby obstructing others' efforts
- Unreasonably criticizes or scorns people in positions of authority

If you exhibit a pervasive pattern of passive resistance to demands for adequate performance, both in social circumstances and in the workplace, you may have a passive-aggressive personality disorder. It begins in early adulthood and occurs in various contexts.

People with this disorder resent responsibility in both work and social spheres. They show this resentment through the signs and symptoms listed above rather than openly expressed anger, and they use procrastination, inefficiency, and "forgetfulness" to avoid fulfilling their obligations. Rather than take responsibility for their own actions, they tend to blame and manipulate others.

Treatment
Professional counseling may help identify and change the destructive patterns of passive-aggressive behavior.

Grief Responses

The word "grief" refers to our subjective feelings and emotions after the loss of a loved one (usually through death, but also after the dissolution of a relationship). We call the collective processes by which we resolve grief mourning.

The Grief Process

Grieving is the emotional and physical response to a loss, the process of coming to terms with it and letting go. Grieving takes a long time, and it is hard work. It is a private journey that is different for everyone.

When you lose a loved one, whether through death or the dissolution of a relationship, your life will never be the same because you will never again be the same person. This is not to say that all the changes will be negative. You'll grow and stretch in ways you never dreamed possible. Intro-spection, developing new coping styles, questioning values and lifestyle, and grieving all help you find inner strength and resiliency. You'll emerge a more caring and compassionate human being.

Signs and Symptoms
- Tightness or pain in chest and throat
- Sleep disturbances ranging from insomnia to a desire to sleep all the time
- Weight loss or gain
- Inability to concentrate
- Disorientation
- Headaches or other physical complaints
- Withdrawal from social activities
- Lack of interest in normal routines such as cooking, shopping, or personal hygiene
- Sighing
- Anger, resentment, bitterness
- Irritability
- Sexual difficulties
- Mood swings

Your responses to loss will depend on many factors. For example, if the deceased suffered from a chronic disease, his or her death may seem like a blessing; and the time spent in what is known as anticipatory grief, or mourning before the actual loss, can diminish the impact of death. The death of a young child, however, is likely to leave a parent grief-stricken no matter how much anticipatory grief has taken place.

The public behavior of a grieving person is greatly affected by family style and cultural influences. In some cultures, weeping and wailing are the norm; in others, a "stiff upper lip" is required.

Tranquilizers or antidepressant drugs usually are not appropriate, nor is alcohol. You must work through your feelings, not mask them. There is no treatment for grief, other than time.

Our society expects you to be over your grief in about a year, after you've passed through the events of a full calendar year without the presence of your loved one. Signs and symptoms, however, often persist much longer. Even though you may never get over the loss entirely, after healthy grieving you can return to a normal life.

Grief is different for each person, but enough similarities exist that it is often divided into stages. These have no set timeline or even sequence. You might skip a stage, remain for a while in one, or experience several at once.

Absent Grief Reaction

Although our culture tends to praise people who appear serene in the face of great pain, refusing to deal with the reality of a loss—or being unable to face it—can be unhealthy.

Grief that is not expressed openly comes out in other ways. Often, signs of an absent grief reaction only show up over time. The bereaved person may seem oddly euphoric. He or she may begin to experience persisting physical symptoms similar to those the deceased had. Or his or her behavior may become unaccountably erratic on the anniversary of the loss or on occasions of significance to the departed, such as a birthday or favorite holiday.

The grief may be displaced onto another loss that seems trifling by comparison or onto the problems of another person.

Dealing with grief is essential. If your loved one is avoiding it, encourage that person to seek counseling.

Stages of Grief

Denial and Protest

For the first days or weeks you may have trouble believing that the person really died. Your mind may seem fuzzy and you may have trouble concentrating; you may hear only half of what people say to you. You may not function well.

Despair

The pain of new grief is so raw that you may feel it physically. You may have recurrent dreams about the person, or hear the person's voice.

Anger is common, but it can be hard to find an appropriate target for it. This might make you strike out at those around you. Medical staff are a common target, as are family and friends, the world in general, or even yourself.

Express your anger rather than let it turn inward. Talk it out with someone or unleash it in physically constructive ways like exercise or gardening.

Grieving is also a time of searching for answers. Why me? Why this person? Some question their faith. Others become preoccupied with the details of the accident or illness.

Depression

This longest of the grief phases might last for months. You may have difficulty sleeping or you might want to sleep all the time. You may lose the motivation to perform even ordinary daily activities at home, while doing anything outside your home can be nearly impossible.

It helps to frame your days with simple routines to keep some semblance of balance. Try to care for yourself in rudimentary ways like looking nice each day, eating healthful foods, and getting some exercise even if all you do is walk around the block.

Social withdrawal is common during this time if you feel detached from the community or embarrassed that you'll cry in public. You might need to stay close to home and restrict your social life to people you feel emotionally safe with.

Resolution and Acceptance

For a long time, maybe many months, you have been working through your grief, but it's still not over. The final stage is just beginning.

Slowly the sun begins to shine. Your

energy level picks up, you feel more comfortable in social situations, you can talk about the person without falling apart, and you can enjoy yourself without feeling guilty. You will still have bad days, but you will rebound more quickly.

Resolution means accepting that you will live the rest of your life without the person. It means accepting the new person you have become through the growth of grieving. Resolution comes in its own time; it takes courage to go through the process and learn to live again.

Finding Support

We live in a death-denying society that doesn't allow enough time or give enough support for grieving. The grief process can take years, but some people will expect you to be back to normal in a month or two. It's important to find people who will be supportive.

No one should grieve alone. More than at any other time of your life, you need to surround yourself with people who can listen to you, reflect with you, care for you, hold you, cry with you, remember with you.

Family and Friends

When a death occurs in a family, every member is affected. Most families and friends draw together to share their grief and let their strong ties support them. Sometimes, though, even close family members let you down. They might lack the capacity to understand the depth of your loss, be afraid to let themselves try, or think they have to keep up a brave front. Then you may need to turn elsewhere for support.

Support Groups

You can be helped by being with others who have had a similar loss. Many hospitals and communities offer organized support groups where people can share their experiences, problems, feelings, and fears. Their members are willing to listen to you long after others think you "should be over it."

Helping Yourself

Finding support means reaching out to others. Much of your grief work, however, must be done alone, and tools are available to help you. Search the library for books and articles that deal with grief. They will make you aware that you are not alone, that others have faced similar losses and have survived. Their words can help you move forward. You can try expressing your own feelings in a diary or journal or by writing poems or stories. What's important is that you deal with your grief, not run from it.

Professional Help

If you are having difficulty coping despite all your efforts, it may be time to consult a professional. Social workers, clergy, psychologists, and psychiatrists are specially trained to help people work through grief. You can ask for referrals from physicians, nurses, social workers, religious organizations, organized support groups, or your funeral director.

If your relationship with the deceased was ambivalent—one of you was excessively dependent, for instance, or you were married to an alcoholic—resolving your grief may be more difficult. A professional can help you focus on both the positive and the negative aspects of your relationship with the person for whom you grieve.

When Your Friend Is Grieving

If someone you know is mourning, you can help ease the pain. Stay in touch, and arrange to stop and offer your condolences as soon as it's convenient. Sometimes it's best to wait until after the memorial service. You may not have the opportunity to say more than a word or two of greeting and affection at the memorial service. Sometimes you don't even need to say anything; a quick hug or squeeze of the hand can simply show you care. Remember, it's not the words but your expression of concern that's important.

Offer your help and support. People's needs vary after a funeral. If you're a close friend or relative, you may help with the day-to-day household management, shopping, cooking, child care, telephone answering, and greeting visitors. Encourage the bereaved person to eat, sleep, and groom to help him or her avoid becoming depressed. When you visit your friend, listen. Allow your friend to express feelings honestly, and be prepared to share the pain and accept anger if it comes out.

Keep your friend involved in routine activities. You may invite the bereaved person to spend some time in your home or accompany you on an outing. You may want to encourage your friend to join a support group for survivors that many hospitals, clinics, and local mental health organizations offer.

Sleep Disorders

Many people report problems with sleep. It is important to realize that our sleep patterns change as we go through life.

All sleep is not the same. By measuring brain waves, sleep researchers have identified several different stages of sleep which recur at fairly regular cycles throughout a night's sleep. We progress from wakefulness to drowsiness to moderate sleep to deep, restorative sleep. The amount of deep sleep decreases with age. Dream sleep, or rapid-eye-movement (REM) sleep, occurs 1 to 2 hours after you fall asleep. The first REM sleep period is the shortest. You may experience several longer REM sleep periods as the night progresses. During REM sleep, our eyes move rapidly behind our closed lids.

REM sleep cannot be truly called light or deep sleep; it is a different kind of sleep. It is the stage when most dreaming occurs and it is characterized by irregular breathing and different heart rates compared to the other sleep stages. REM sleep also is characterized by penile erections in males.

During REM sleep, your brain waves, as displayed by an electroencephalograph (EEG; see page 1344), suggest faster electrical activity at lower amplitude than at other stages of sleep, which makes the waves superficially similar to those of wakefulness. REM sleep is not absolutely vital for life.

Your brain undergoes a number of changes during sleep. During REM sleep your brain consumes increased amounts of oxygen and has increased blood flow. People awakened during REM sleep may recall vivid dreams. During a normal night's sleep there are four or five REM-sleep periods; they occur about once every 90 minutes as part of the sleep cycle and total about 1½ hours.

Sleep disorders are of various kinds and may be the result of physical conditions, stress, or other factors.

Insomnia

Signs and Symptoms
- Inability to sleep enough at night
- Difficulty falling asleep
- Night awakening in an adult
- Daytime fatigue

What Is Normal Sleep?

"Sleep" is the word we use to define both a biological state and a behavioral state in which we are quiet and relatively unresponsive to external stimuli. Sleep is regular, recurring, and easily reversible (unlike a coma, for example). Most people spend about one-third of their life in the state of unconsciousness that is sleep, about 7½ hours a night for a middle-aged adult.

When we do not get enough sleep, we may feel less alert and vigorous—or confused and fatigued. Lack of sleep affects not only your energy level but also your mental and social functioning. Sleep deprivation over prolonged periods causes psychological disturbances in normal persons. In fact, going long periods without adequate sleep is so well-recognized as disorienting and demoralizing that forced sleep deprivation is a widely used brainwashing technique.

Sleep patterns vary considerably according to age. The newborn infant may spend as much as half of its total sleeping time in dream sleep, or rapid eye movement (REM) sleep, and may sleep five or six times a day. Infants fall into REM sleep immediately, whereas adults must pass through other stages of sleep first.

Some researchers suggest that the frequency of REM sleep in newborns may reflect a need for stimulation from within, to allow the central nervous system to mature in an orderly fashion.

Others suggest that REM sleep has a role in processing new information, which is acquired at a very high rate in childhood. As the child grows, the sleeping habits become more organized: frequent, unpredictable periods of sleep give way to two naps in the daytime, gradually decreasing to one and then to the adult pattern of one long nocturnal period with no daytime nap.

In later years, however, many people seem to return to frequent daytime naps and sleep less at night. These patterns vary with individuals, depending on neurologic development and other factors, but the overall progression has been identified as the norm through the human life span.

We define insomnia simply as the inability to get "enough" sleep. A person with insomnia may complain that he or she "didn't sleep a wink," although in fact there usually was some sleep.

An occasional individual claims to hardly sleep at all and yet actually does sleep for 4 or more hours a night. What may be happening is frequent awakenings, leading to the perception of no sleep. In older people, the pattern of sleeping less and awakening more often at night seems to be common and is not insomnia.

The causes of insomnia are many and varied. A change in your environment, such as a new work schedule or jet lag, can cause difficulty in sleeping. Drinking excessive amounts of coffee, tea, or cola drinks can cause insomnia. If you are especially sensitive to caffeine, even a cup or two during the day can keep you awake at night. The use of other stimulants (amphetamines, methylphenidate) also contributes to insomnia.

Although a drink or two of an alcoholic beverage seems to help some people relax enough to fall asleep, even moderate amounts of alcohol can distort normal sleeping patterns. The ability to fall asleep may be increased, but sleep is poor later during the night as the blood alcohol level decreases. The use of certain medications can cause insomnia. Many of the psychoactive drugs—such as the antidepressants and benzodiazepines—actively interfere with the sleep cycle, particularly with prolonged use.

Insomnia may be caused by another medical condition such as pain, allergies, and sleep apnea (see page 1114), restless legs syndrome (see page 1115), drug abuse or withdrawal, or endocrine abnormalities like Cushing's syndrome (see page 937) and hyperthyroidism (see page 947).

Psychological factors can affect your sleep. Insomnia may be a symptom of a transient problem or of a long-term underlying disorder. Sometimes people go through periods of sleeplessness because of temporary anxiety—over an upcoming job interview or examination, for example. In middle-aged and older people, depression may result in insomnia, particularly during the early morning hours. Chronic anxiety, reflecting fears, can cause sleep-onset insomnia. People who tend to have nightmares may find themselves awakening suddenly while in REM sleep.

Sleeping patterns are highly individual, and techniques that help you sleep may not help someone else. The first thing to consider when you are suffering from insomnia is how to make simple changes in your bedtime routine that will help you sleep. Here are a few suggestions to help you sleep better: reduce the amount of time you spend in bed to allow you to sleep more deeply when you do finally sleep. If worries keep you awake, attempt to deal with them early in the evening. Write them down and identify solutions. If a bedside clock keeps you awake at night, put it in a dresser drawer or under the bed. Avoid caffeine (cola, tea, cocoa, and coffee) after your evening meal. Shun tobacco, because nicotine can cause shallow sleeping and sleeplessness.

Examples of changes that may help you feel sleepy include restricting your bedtime reading and television viewing to light topics that are not emotionally upsetting—for example, no horror stories. It's best to establish a stable time for going to bed and getting up each day. Avoid strenuous exercise or emotional upset in the period immediately preceding bedtime. Taking a warm bath or drinking a cup of warm milk may help you relax. Exercise during the day may help your body feel fatigued enough to need rest at bedtime. Even though you may be tired from your sleepless nights, avoid napping during the day, so that you can reestablish a pattern of sleeping at night. Habitual daytime naps may be a cause of insomnia. Try to deal with your worries and concerns by making plans early in the evening. If you do not have time for physical exertion during the day, take a walk 5 to 6 hours before bedtime, but do not do anything too strenuous or you probably will have trouble dropping off to sleep.

Most importantly, relax. Some people work too hard at getting to sleep. Let nature take over. If sleep doesn't come naturally, read a book, listen to music, or watch television to get your mind off your sleeping difficulties.

Treatment

If you are unable to reestablish a sleeping pattern by using a home remedy, it is a good idea to have a careful medical evaluation, because there are many potential causes of insomnia. If an underlying psychological problem is contributing to insomnia, it may be helpful to discuss it with a mental health professional.

Be cautious about the use of sleeping pills. If you are awake at night because of pain from a medical or surgical condition, your doctor may recommend that you use a sleeping medication for a short time along with an analgesic such as aspirin or acetaminophen. Sleeping pills (also known as sedatives or hypnotics) not only lose their effectiveness after 4 to 6 months but also may disturb your sleeping pattern and thus contribute to insomnia.

Sleep Apnea

Signs and Symptoms
- Excessive daytime sleepiness
- Extremely loud snoring
- Observed episodes of breathing stoppage during sleep
- Morning headache

Sleep apnea (from the Greek *a pnein*, "without breathing") is a disorder in which there are recurrent episodes of breathing stoppage during sleep. An obstruction to the movement of air in the upper respiratory passages causes sleep apnea.

At night you may snore very loudly, and in the daytime you may be very sleepy if you have sleep apnea. You may wake up with a headache.

In sleep apnea, the muscles in the walls of your throat (pharynx) relax so that the walls collapse on themselves. The flow of air is obstructed or nearly so. After 10 to 30 seconds or more of no exchange of air, you arouse toward a lighter level of sleep, the muscles regain their normal tone (tenseness), the obstruction is relieved, and you breathe.

The obstruction to breathing prevents you from ever reaching deep or restorative sleep, so you feel as if you had been without sleep, even though you have slept all night.

In adults, obesity is a contributing factor, and weight reduction often gives some relief. Some persons who are of normal weight or moderately overweight may experience sleep apnea. This diagnosis can be suspected from their excessive daytime sleepiness and their pattern of snoring—periods during which breathing ceases, followed by deep gasps and then the resumption of breathing. Studies in a sleep laboratory (see page 1115) can confirm the diagnosis.

More than half of all cases of sleep apnea are diagnosed in people age 40 years or older. Sleep apnea is a major contributor to daytime drowsiness; 30 to 60 percent of people with severe daytime sleepiness have sleep apnea.

Treatment
Weight reduction is very important and often gives substantial relief. However, many obese persons find it difficult to adhere to a schedule of reduced-calorie eating, plus exercise—even with the promise of some relief from distressing symptoms.

Sleep disorder specialists sometimes help you learn to use a machine that delivers air through a mask placed over your nose at a pressure somewhat greater than that of the surrounding air. This is called continuous positive airway pressure (CPAP). The air pressure is just enough to open your upper airway passages—preventing apnea and snoring. This machine may be very helpful.

Surgical procedures to increase the size of the throat are only partially effective.

Narcolepsy

Signs and Symptoms
- Abnormal tendency to sleep during the day
- Desire to sleep longer than the usual 7 to 8 hours
- Episodic attacks of REM sleep during the day that may cause attacks of muscle paralysis
- Feeling of paralysis on going to sleep or waking up
- Dream-like hallucinations

Snoring

Snoring is very common. Some studies have shown that up to 50 percent of adult males snore. Some snorers have sleep apnea, but many do not. However, snoring may be very disruptive to your partner's sleep. Recent research has shown that snoring itself may disrupt nighttime sleep and cause you to be sleepy during the day. If snoring is disturbing your sleep or there is a possibility of sleep apnea, a sleep study may be necessary. Treatment of snoring is much the same as treatment of sleep apnea (see this page) except that laser surgery is now being used at some centers. The surgeon removes the uvula and soft palate with the expectation that snoring lessens or goes away. We don't know the long-term effectiveness of laser surgery of the palate.

Narcolepsy (from the Greek *narke*, meaning "stupor") is popularly known as sleeping sickness. It is the abnormal tendency to sleep during the day. If you have narcolepsy, you experience episodes of uncontrollable sleepiness. You then sleep briefly and awaken refreshed, only to become sleepy again within an hour or so. These sleep attacks occur after meals, but they may also occur during active times—for example, while you are driving a car, having a conversation, or making love.

Possible aggravating factors include environmental causes, such as alternating work weeks (that is, working nights one week and days the next). It is likely that narcolepsy represents a neurologic problem of sleep-wake mechanisms in the brain.

Diagnosis

Although daytime sleepiness is a symptom of both sleep apnea and narcolepsy, there is an important observable difference. Unlike the person with sleep apnea, the person with narcolepsy has brief sleep attacks and feels refreshed on awakening. Many cases of narcolepsy are associated with cataplexy. This consists of attacks of paralysis of various muscles, at times provoked by laughter or other emotions. When such an attack occurs, the person will experience weakening of the knees, the jaw will drop, and the person even may fall to the floor. During awakening after a night's sleep, the person with narcolepsy may be unable to move for a few minutes, a condition called sleep paralysis. Many also have hallucinations that seem like dreams.

Narcolepsy is usually diagnosed between the ages of 15 and 25. Often, the clue is difficulty in staying awake in class. Men and women are affected in equal numbers.

Treatment

To prevent sudden sleep attacks, plan naps so that your body will feel rested when you need to be awake. Allow plenty of time for sleep at night. Forced naps—say, one to four of them for 10 minutes or so each—when you are really feeling drowsy can enable you to function normally without medication. Because you may be especially sleepy after a meal, eat light meals during the day and avoid a heavy meal just before an important activity. Moderate amounts of caffeine—especially coffee, tea, or cola drinks—may help you stay awake.

Adjusting to living with narcolepsy and coping with the emotional problems your illness may be causing in your workplace and relationships will help enormously.

Medication

Medical treatment of narcolepsy includes stimulant pills such as dextroamphetamine and methylphenidate. If you have cataplexy, your physician may prescribe an antidepressant medication to suppress the attacks of REM sleep.

Restless Legs (Nocturnal Jerking Movements)

Signs and Symptoms

- Unpleasant creeping sensations deep inside the calves and occasionally in the feet, thighs, or arms while awake, especially while lying down
- Irresistible urge to move the legs
- Possible worsening of symptoms during times of stress

Restless legs syndrome is a condition in which your legs feel extremely uncomfortable unless you move them. This discomfort commonly begins shortly after you go to bed. Often, you feel as if you want to get out of bed and walk or move your legs. Such activity briefly relieves the symptoms, but they return. These symptoms usually last for an hour or more. Myoclonus (from the Greek *myo*, for "muscle," and *klonos*, for "violent motion") is the name given to these contractions. They should not be confused with leg cramps (see page 871).

With restless legs syndrome, you may feel creeping sensations deep inside your calves while you are awake (especially when lying

Sleep Clinics

Many hospitals and medical centers operate sleep clinics to diagnose sleep disorders. You enter the unit during the early evening hours and spend the night in a comfortable bed. Electrocardiographic (ECG, or heart monitor, see page 1343) and electroencephalographic (EEG, brain monitor, see page 1344) recordings are often used throughout the night. In addition, your breathing is monitored.

In men who have problems with impotence, the occurrence and duration of nocturnal erections also can be monitored.

The results of these studies often allow the specialist in sleep disorders to identify the problem and offer appropriate treatment.

Naps—Bane or Boon for a Good Night's Sleep?

Should you follow that irresistible urge to take a snooze during the day?

It depends. One of five people who do nap feels energized and clearheaded and sleeps well at night. The others sleep poorly at night.

A slight drop in your body temperature indicates that the urge for a mid-day snooze (usually between 1 and 4 p.m.) is built into your body's biologic clock. Americans usually ignore the urge, while other cultures incorporate it into their lifestyles.

The "Naptitude" Test

To discover how naps affect your energy level and quality of nighttime rest, take a daily nap for a week. The next week, don't nap. Keep a sleep log, recording when you go to bed at night, how long it takes you to fall asleep, how many times you awaken during the night, how many total hours you sleep, and how you feel in the morning. Also record how you feel after the midday snoozes. After two weeks, judge whether naps work for you.

Napping Tips

Keep it short to avoid interfering with your nighttime sleep—half an hour is ideal. Take your nap mid-afternoon, if possible. If you can't nap, just lie down and rest. But set the alarm, just in case.

down). Occasionally, it similarly affects your feet, thighs, or arms. They feel unpleasant but not painful.

These disorders are not dangerous, although they can be uncomfortable and disruptive to sleep.

Periodic jerking movements (nocturnal myoclonus) may occur while you sleep. They may awaken you and disturb your nighttime sleep. The jerking may also disturb your bed partner.

Treatment

We see these related disorders mostly in middle-aged and older people, and they seem to get worse during times of stress. Muscle relaxation techniques can help, as can a warm bath before bed. In some cases, your physician may prescribe a medication such as clonazepam or a combination of levodopa and carbidopa (Sinemet).

Nightmares and Night Terrors

Signs and Symptoms

- Nightmares: unpleasant or frightening dreams that take place during REM or dreaming sleep
- Night terrors: screaming and arousal from sleep, with no memory of a frightening dream except perhaps a frightening image

A nightmare is a dream from which you may awaken in fright. Especially when they recur, nightmares may suggest a psychological disturbance or stress brought on by a difficult situation. However, perfectly normal people have nightmares from time to time.

Night terrors are usually disorders of childhood. They are common between ages 3 and 5 and happen much less often after that. During deep sleep the child may wake up screaming, terrified, and unable to explain what happened or to be comforted or fully awakened. Although the terror may last for 10 or 20 minutes, the child generally will be unable to remember the episode the next morning. Night terrors may be more frightening to the parent than the child.

Night terrors usually happen during the first third of the night, while nightmares frequently occur near morning. Night terrors appear far more terrifying than nightmares, but the affected person will not be able to remember what happened, aside from a frightening image. However, you may remember a nightmare vividly.

Night terrors seem to run in families. In adults they can get worse with the use of alcohol, and emotional tension can make them more likely to occur. Usually, adults who frequently have nightmares or night terrors are experiencing considerable conflict and stress in their waking lives.

Treatment

Children usually outgrow night terrors. In adults often there is no specific treatment for nightmares, but psychotherapy (see page 1107) may help.

Sleepwalking

Signs and Symptoms

- Walking or other activities (opening closet doors, going to the bathroom, driving) during sleep
- Activity usually occurs during the first third of the night
- Duration is typically a few minutes to half an hour

- Confusion or disorientation on awakening is characteristic

Sleepwalking describes not only walking but other activities performed during sleep—rearranging furniture, dressing or undressing, and even getting into a car and driving. It usually occurs during the first third of the night and can be very brief or can go on as long as half an hour.

The sleepwalker's eyes are open, the facial expression is blank or dazed, and he or she will be confused or disoriented if awakened. Many people believe that sleepwalkers do not get hurt during their "travels." However, this is a misconception; sleepwalkers are commonly injured by tripping or losing their balance.

Sleepwalking occurs at various ages. However, young children, who often sit up in bed and appear to be awake, rarely leave the bed and actually walk. Sleepwalking occurs most frequently between the ages of 6 and 12. Psychological factors, including fatigue and prior sleep loss, probably cause sleepwalking in children. With adults, there may be personality disturbance as well as anxiety or conflict. Sleepwalking also seems to run in families.

Treatment

There is no specific treatment for sleepwalking. To prevent injury, however, it is a good idea to make the room and house safe for the sleepwalker: avoid leaving objects the sleepwalker can trip on, electrical cords, or small furniture in the middle of the bedroom. Block the top of a staircase with a gate. It may be helpful to avoid use of alcohol and other central nervous system depressants.

Medication

If your physician considers medication necessary, short-acting tranquilizers such as benzodiazepines may be helpful. Psychotherapy and relaxation training may also help.

Bruxism

Signs and Symptoms—Grinding, gnashing, or clenching of the teeth during sleep

Bruxism is grinding or clenching of your teeth during sleep. About 15 percent of normal people report this. Sometimes it can be

---

Dreams—What and Why?

Dreaming is mental activity that occurs as you sleep. We don't know the exact cause, but dreams may help you sort out your impressions, ideas, and feelings. They may be a clue to what concerns you when you're awake.

We believe that dreams occur only during periods of rapid eye movement (REM) sleep. These periods of "deep" sleep generally last about 20 minutes per episode and occur 4 or 5 times a night. If you are aroused during REM sleep, you may vividly recall your dreams, but if you're aroused after the dream is over, you may remember nothing.

We don't know why some people say they dream in color, while others say they don't.

We study changes in brain activity that accompany dreaming with an electroencephalogram (EEG). This machine records minute electrical impulses produced by your brain's activity.

---

so violent that your teeth become damaged. Often, it is so loud that you cannot duplicate the sound while awake. Your bed partner is often awakened. Bruxism usually seems to occur in the early part of the night.

Treatment

Sometimes bruxism is caused by a problem in occlusion (the way the upper and lower teeth fit together when your jaws are closed). However, psychological factors usually are involved. People with bruxism seem to be especially anxious. They are often tense and appear to be suppressing anger. Bruxism often gets worse after alcohol intake. Psychotherapy, alcohol abstinence, and adjustment of your bite may help. A dentist can create a plastic guard to wear during sleep to prevent further damage to the teeth if this is warranted.

Shift Disorders

Some people have a sleep disorder caused by rotations in their work shifts. They may be chronically tired and have insomnia (see page 1112). In general, if you routinely work at night, your bedroom should be as quiet as possible for sleep during the day. It is better to remain "shifted" on the days you're not working. However, for many people, this is not possible. Avoid use of sleeping pills.

Anxiety Disorders

Ours has been called the age of anxiety. Anxiety is a common emotion and, in its mild form, may be helpful in adapting to stressful situations. It is widespread but often hard to explain.

Although in popular speech the word "anxiety" may mean no more than worry or concern, in medicine we define it specifically as a painful or apprehensive uneasiness about some impending or anticipated ill fortune. It is an emotional reaction that manifests itself in various physical symptoms of different degrees of intensity.

Anxiety Reactions

Signs and Symptoms
- Tension over or terror about a danger whose source is often unrecognized
- Rapid heartbeat or respiration
- Tremor
- Gastrointestinal distress
- Motor tension (trembling, muscle aches, restlessness, inability to relax)
- Perspiring
- Dry mouth
- Dizziness
- Impatience and irritability, insomnia, or difficulty in concentrating
- With generalized anxiety disorder, persistent anxiety for at least a month without any specific phobia or panic attack
- Possible drug abuse to avoid symptoms

Anxiety, in the field of mental health, refers to tension or terror about an unidentified danger. This differs from fear, for which there is a specific, recognizable cause.

Anxiety and fear are normal emotions: the fight-or-flight response is natural in the face of danger or stress. The symptoms—quickened heart rate, increased blood pressure and muscle tension, and increased awareness—represent an almost involuntary response marked by several physical reactions that are the result of an increased flow of catecholamines (chemicals in your blood that include epinephrine and that stimulate your sympathetic nervous system).

The fight-or-flight reaction gives you the extra strength you need to overcome or escape from a dangerous situation. An important characteristic of anxiety, however, is that you cannot always determine exactly what that dangerous situation is.

Diagnosis
The signs of anxiety are similar to those of fear—your heart begins to pound faster, you breathe rapidly, you may tremble, and your stomach becomes upset. Unlike ordinary fear, however, with anxiety you may not know exactly what it is that has you so distressed, or the apparent source of anxiety may seem minor compared with the intensity of your emotional reaction.

Fear is a reaction to an understandable, identifiable, current danger; anxiety is a conscious reaction to an unconscious stimulus. Anxiety also can be the first noticeable sign of depression or full-blown psychosis. Anxiety may be a response to a specific stress, in which case it may be termed situational anxiety; it also can be a generalized feeling of uneasiness called free-floating anxiety.

The generalized anxiety disorder features persistent anxiety for at least a month, without any specific phobia or panic attack. Your symptoms may include muscle tension, trembling, muscle aches, inability to relax, restlessness, sweating, palpitations, rapid breathing and pulse, dry mouth, dizziness, nausea, stomach pain, apprehension, impatience, irritability, insomnia, difficulty concentrating, and fatigue on awakening.

Anxiety can be associated with physical illness. Sometimes people try to avoid anxiety by abusing drugs such as alcohol, barbit-

---

What's That Knot in My Stomach?

Just as stress or anxiety can bring on a tension headache, it can also cause tension in your stomach. Smooth muscles in the lining of your stomach and intestine may suddenly contract, giving you the feeling of a "knot" much like a muscle cramp in your leg.

While this may cause discomfort or pain, it isn't serious. As your anxiety lessens, the feeling usually goes away. If the knot is persistent or intense, or if you also have nausea, vomiting, diarrhea, or difficulty swallowing, see your physician. These symptoms could indicate a more serious problem such as an ulcer, a hernia, or a tumor.

urates, and anti-anxiety agents and even may become dependent on a medication. Occasionally, these drugs contribute to the anxiety state. Anxiety disorders sometimes can be traced back to childhood fears, stresses, or losses that are reactivated later in life.

Treatment

Treatment may include antianxiety medications (such as benzodiazepines), psychotherapy (see page 1107) to help you understand the conflicts that are producing the anxiety, and behavior therapy (see page 1121) to teach relaxation techniques. Do not try to resolve your anxiety by using antianxiety medications for a long time, because there is a risk of dependency and addiction. Short-term use with the smallest dose that is effective is safer (see Controlling Stress, page 307).

Panic Attacks

Signs and Symptoms

- Feelings of fear or extreme tension and a sense of impending doom
- Shortness of breath
- Palpitations, chest pain or discomfort, or feelings of choking or smothering
- Dizziness or unsteadiness
- Sense of unreality
- Tingling in your extremities (hands or feet); hot and cold flashes; inexplicable perspiration
- Trembling
- Fear of losing your mind, dying, or losing control
- Nausea, vomiting, or diarrhea

A panic attack is an unexplained and unprovoked fight-or-flight response. Your body displays the normal physical reaction to a life-threatening situation or extreme physical exertion, but there is no apparent stimulus. All of a sudden you are panting, your heart is pounding, your head is swimming, and your palms are damp.

Panic disorders tend to run in families, and many researchers believe that biochemical factors may play a crucial role in this condition. It is a fairly common disorder. Because so many of the symptoms of a panic attack resemble those of an organic disorder, people often fail to recognize them and visit physicians in the mistaken belief that they have cardiac or respiratory problems.

Hyperventilation

Hyperventilation (from the Greek *hyper*, meaning "over" or "above," and the Latin *ventus* for "wind") is breathing too heavily with, paradoxically, a sensation of not being able to get enough air. A common occurrence during anxiety, it causes various symptoms including faintness and a tingling sensation in various parts of the body. This is why you may feel faint on hearing very bad news or at other traumatic life moments.

When you breathe quickly, an imbalance of gases is created in your blood, and this causes the symptoms. Because you are anxious, you often are not even aware that you are breathing too quickly.

Because hyperventilation is so often associated with or provoked by anxiety, it is occasionally treated with tranquilizers. However, such medication is unnecessary in most cases.

Hyperventilation can be relieved by a homespun remedy you might recognize as the traditional cure for hiccups. Simply hold your breath or try breathing into and out of a paper bag so that the exhaled carbon dioxide is reinhaled. This will help to restore the proper balance of blood gases and thus relieve the accompanying sensation.

Treatment

Medication

In most cases, one of the family of drugs called the tricyclic antidepressants will relieve the problem of panic attacks. Many victims of this disorder also live in a constant state of fear of the attacks themselves, and brief treatment with antianxiety drugs may be helpful.

Other Therapies

Psychotherapy (see page 1107) can help uncover the underlying causes, but behavior therapy, and relaxation therapy in particular (see page 1121), may be useful in eliminating the symptoms.

Phobias

Signs and Symptoms

- Persistent, irrational fear of a specific object, activity, or situation
- Compelling desire to avoid what you fear
- Impaired ability to function at normal tasks

A phobia (from the Greek *phobos*, "fear" or "flight") is a persistent, irrational fear of something—either an object, such as an insect, or a situation, such as being in crowds. This produces a compelling desire to avoid

Antianxiety Medications

Treating anxiety with drugs has come a long way since barbiturates were widely used for this purpose. Today, physicians use a family of drugs called anxiolytics to relieve the symptoms of anxiety. Most of these anxiety-fighting drugs are from a family called the benzodiazepines. Examples include lorazepam (Ativan), diazepam (Valium), alprazolam (Xanax), and chlordiazepoxide (Librium).

Like barbiturates, anxiolytics are sedatives and central muscle relaxants. And, also like the barbiturates, they are addictive. What makes them an improvement over barbiturates, however, is that they depress your respiratory system less and therefore are less risky with suicidal patients.

Anxiolytics are widely prescribed for various disorders, including anxiety disorders and phobias. If you have an anxiety disorder or a related syndrome (such as hypochondriasis), you may have sudden attacks of intense fear as well as shortness of breath, pain and pressure in the head and chest, sweating, and numbness of the fingers and toes. You may also experience insomnia, depression, phobias, obsessions, compulsions, and other problems and may be likely to abuse alcohol and sleeping pills.

Anxiolytics usually are administered orally. Potential side effects of these medications include drowsiness, ataxia (inability to coordinate voluntary muscle movements), and confusion. It is important not to drive or attempt to operate heavy machinery while using them. Using alcohol while being treated with anxiolytics is especially dangerous. In older or extremely agitated people, low doses of anxiolytics may cause transient states of excitement, in which case use of the drug should be discontinued. When you no longer need therapy, it is important that you discontinue use of the anxiolytic drug gradually, because otherwise restlessness, insomnia, nightmares, and even seizures can occur. You must use anxiolytic drugs cautiously if you have or have had alcohol dependency.

the feared object or situation.

If you have a phobia, you may be unable to control your emotions. You may try to avoid the object of your phobia at virtually all costs, even though you may understand that your fear is excessive or unrealistic.

Diagnosis

If the phobia causes no major disturbance in your life, it is not considered a disorder. When the fear impairs your ability to function at normal tasks, however, it needs to be diagnosed and treated.

One example is agoraphobia, fear of being in public places. Nearly a million people in this country, 85 percent of them women, suffer from agoraphobia, which usually begins between the ages of 18 and 35 and is usually associated with panic disorder. Another common example is claustrophobia (from the Latin *claustrum*, an "enclosed place"), the irrational fear of being in a confined or crowded place. Morbid fear of heights is acrophobia (from the Greek *akros*, "high").

Some degree of discomfort in any of these situations may be perfectly normal under certain circumstances, but when the fear becomes irrational and uncontrollable to the extent that it affects your normal social interactions and daily life, it is considered a phobia. The fear is usually experienced not only at the time you face the object of the phobia but also when you anticipate encountering it (anticipatory anxiety). Phobias may be a part of anxiety or panic attacks.

Treatment

According to psychoanalytic theory, phobias do not represent a reaction to real danger, but are an underlying fear or hidden conflict within the affected person. His or her fears of forbidden sexual or aggressive impulses—of danger from within—are transposed onto some external object—for example, snakes. This is a defense mechanism known as displacement.

For this reason, psychotherapy (see page 1107) to uncover the original meanings of the fears and to help you learn to cope with them can be helpful. But behavior therapy (see page 1121) also can be quite successful for phobias. One widely used approach is systematic desensitization, which repeatedly exposes you to the frightening stimulus until your fear diminishes. For example, you may begin by thinking about snakes and then go on to looking at pictures of them and, finally, see some live ones. Antidepressant drug therapy may help some patients who have a phobic disorder.

Relaxation Techniques

Although relaxation techniques resemble meditative and contemplative methods that have been part of Eastern and Western religious practices for centuries, Edmund Jacobson introduced them as psychotherapeutic relaxation training in the 1920s to teach hypertensive people to relax.

There are many different approaches to relaxation therapy. In progressive muscle relaxation, you learn to focus on each muscle. First, you tense a muscle and hold that tension for 5 or 10 seconds until you can easily identify the muscle or muscle group involved by slight discomfort. Then, you slowly release the muscle, repeating the procedure with various muscle groups so that you become familiar with the sensation of relaxing your entire body. A biofeedback machine may monitor muscle tension levels during the training sessions.

In other relaxation therapies the approach differs. In autogenic training, you concentrate on self-suggestions of warmth and heaviness in your limbs. Hypnosis involves having the hypnotist provide suggestions of relaxation and mental calm. Biofeedback is a method of relieving symptoms of distress by relaxing your muscles. We use it to reduce stress and, as a part of systematic desensitization, to treat phobic anxiety. It involves monitoring of one of your physiologic systems—heart, respiration, or skin resistance—so that you can become more aware of your own body's stress and thus control it.

The various methods of meditation—such as Zen, yoga, or transcendental meditation—are based on using mental repetition of a neutral word or symbol in a quiet, comfortable environment.

The ideal setting for relaxation training is a quiet room where you can rest comfortably on the floor or in a reclining chair or bed. You need to feel relatively at ease but not tired. An instructor can be a great help in directing your attention toward your inner self. You will learn to concentrate and to relax at the same time—and be able to do it yourself at home. You may listen to a tape, although live training may be more effective. Eventually, you learn to relax without verbal cues from another person.

Obsessive-Compulsive Disorder

Signs and Symptoms
- Recurrent persistent ideas, thoughts, or impulses that are experienced involuntarily and appear to be senseless
- Repetitive behavior that is performed regularly, even though it appears senseless

Individuals with an obsessive-compulsive disorder experience recurrent obsessions (persistent thoughts) or compulsions (persistent behaviors) or both that are perceived as being senseless and repugnant. Obsessions include thoughts of violence, fears of contamination, fears of becoming infected, and doubt. Examples of compulsions include repeatedly checking the doors to make sure they are locked, repeatedly washing your hands, and counting steps while you walk. The obsessions and compulsions do not always occur at the same time in the same person. The disorder seems to be slightly more common in women than men. This disorder generally begins in late adolescence or young adulthood; it rarely occurs in children. At times, the disorder is accompanied by depression or anxiety.

If you have an obsessive-compulsive disorder, you may do virtually everything in a meticulous, precise, orderly fashion. When the compulsive need is not fulfilled, you may experience overwhelming anxiety.

Treatment
Therapy is helpful at times. Your physician may advise antidepressants or other drug therapy.

Post-Traumatic Stress Disorder

Signs and Symptoms
- Persistent reexperiencing of a traumatic event in intrusive recollections, distressing dreams, hallucinations, distress at anniversaries of the trauma, and avoidance of thoughts, feelings, and activities associated with the trauma
- Feeling of detachment or estrangement from others, inability to have loving feelings
- Markedly diminished interest in significant activities
- In young children, developmental regression in such areas as toilet training and language
- Sense of a foreshortened future, no hope of family life, career, or living to old age

- Increased arousal (not present before the trauma), with at least two of the following: trouble sleeping, anger, difficulty concentrating, exaggerated startle response, and physiologic reaction to situations that remind the person of the traumatic event

Post-traumatic stress disorder occurs among survivors of events that are generally acknowledged to be traumatic—rape, war, torture, earthquake, or death camps. A physical trauma is often involved, but there is always a characteristic psychological component: the person has lived through a period in which he or she was faced with intense fear, helplessness, loss of control, and the threat of annihilation.

Very young and very old people who experience major traumas seem to be especially susceptible to post-traumatic stress, presumably because young children have inadequately developed coping mechanisms and elderly people may be overly rigid and have fewer social supports.

Your symptoms may appear immediately after the event or be delayed by 6 months or more. You may feel a sense of estrangement from other people and of difficulty enjoying activities that were previously pleasurable—particularly those associated with intimacy, such as sexual contact.

Flashbacks are one aspect of post-traumatic stress disorder in victims of major life traumas—an automobile accident, an airplane crash, a wartime experience, kidnapping or hostage situation, or physical assault—in which the original experience was one of intense fear and utter loss of control. The flashback is a vivid sense of reliving the experience, and you may perceive it as real.

Treatment

Medication
Minor tranquilizers such as diazepam (Valium) and chlordiazepoxide (Librium) can decrease the symptoms of anxiety.

Other Therapies
Behavioral techniques, especially relaxation therapy and progressive desensitization, may help to decrease symptoms such as anxiety and phobia. Psychotherapy (see page 1107) can provide support and, in severe cases, the insight and relief you need to cope with your reaction to the original trauma.

Depression and Mood Disorders

There are various kinds of depression, and they have some symptoms in common. These symptoms may include withdrawal from usual activities, disturbed sleep, loss of appetite, inability to concentrate or to make decisions, decreased energy level, feelings of worthlessness and guilt, and even thoughts of suicide and death. When your depression is mild, changes in your environment may lead to some improvement, but not when your depression is severe.

There also are age-associated features. In early childhood, separation anxiety is a common factor. In early adolescence, negative and antisocial behavior may occur. Older boys and girls exhibit sexual acting out, truancy, and running away. In elderly people, pseudodementia—depression that is evident primarily as a loss of intellectual functioning—must be carefully differentiated from the true dementia caused by organic mental disorder.

This section deals with various kinds of depression and the treatment options that are available to you. In addition, it discusses the warning signs of potential suicide, a complication of any serious depression.

Situational Depression

Signs and Symptoms
- Sense of helplessness and gloom
- Grief
- Loss of self-esteem
- Feeling that life is meaningless
- Anxiety or worry
- Irritability
- Retreat from relationships with others

Also known as adjustment disorder with depressed mood, situational depression is a prolonged episode of "the blues" that may occur after a disappointment or loss or during mid-life.

Situational depression is not the same as normal grieving after the death of a loved one, illness, or other misfortune, although it may be triggered by such an event.

Depression also may be a side effect of certain medications, particularly in a person who tends toward depression.

Treatment

Situational depression may decrease when the problem that triggered it fades. However, you may become so depressed that there is a risk of suicide. Consequently, it is important to provide emotional support.

At first, when you are acutely depressed, psychotherapy can provide that support while antidepressant medication helps to relieve the symptoms. Then, when the symptoms improve, psychotherapy can help you understand why the depression occurred: Are there solutions to your external life problems that might prove less stressful? Did the episode that triggered the depression recall a childhood conflict long buried in your unconscious? Do you have low self-esteem, view the situation as hopeless, or feel uncomfortable expressing negative feelings such as hostility or anger? Would a change of scenery or routine be helpful?

A professional may recommend one of several different types of therapy in the case of depression. Cognitive therapy can help you view your situation differently by identifying and testing self-defeating ways of thinking about it (negative cognitions). For example, if you tend to be pessimistic you are likely to suffer from feelings of hopelessness. If you expect failure, you may be apathetic and unwilling to exert yourself. Once the therapist has helped you to identify these thinking patterns, you can develop new approaches to the situation.

Family therapy can help you improve your marriage or family life or both, so that the depression does not adversely affect other family members and the family members do not contribute further to your depression.

Major Depressive Disorder

Signs and Symptoms
- Change in physical demeanor—either a noticeable slowing down or "dragging," or a discernible speeding up or agitation
- Distinct quality to the depressed mood (different from the feeling one has after the death of a loved one)
- Lack of response to environmental changes

Prozac

Since its approval by the Food and Drug Administration in 1987, Prozac (fluoxetine) has become the most frequently prescribed drug for treating serious depression and obsessive-compulsive disorder. Prozac belongs to a class of antidepressants called selective serotonin re-uptake inhibitors (SSRIs). SSRIs act on serotonin, the neurotransmitter (a chemical) in the brain that helps brain cells (neurons) send and receive messages.

SSRIs work by making more serotonin available between neurons, perhaps helping transmit messages more easily. Serotonin is thought to play a crucial role in mood states, especially depression.

If you take Prozac for depression it will usually lift your mood. If you take Prozac for an anxiety-related condition you may become calmer. If you do not respond to Prozac, your physician may try another SSRI, such as sertraline (Zoloft) or paroxetine (Paxil).

The advantage of SSRIs over other antidepressants is that they are not habit-forming. Short-term side effects, if they occur, seem to be mild. Side effects might include insomnia or a change in sleep patterns, anxiety and restlessness (similar to a caffeine effect), mild digestive problems or loss of appetite, sexual problems including increased desire, and occasionally rashes. So far, there is no evidence of any long-term side effects.

Several years ago, a report linked Prozac to suicide. More recent studies have shown that the risk of encouraging suicidal tendencies is quite low. SSRIs usually reduce the risk of self-harmful behaviors in people with serious depression.

If you feel a little "blue," but are not suffering from true depression, you should not take Prozac. The notion that an SSRI will give you a sense of euphoria if you are psychologically well is false.

(day/night, sun/rain, leisure/work)
- Loss of interest in activities usually enjoyed, including sex
- Fatigue or loss of energy
- Poor appetite and attendant weight loss
- Insomnia or hypersomnia
- Self-reproach or inappropriate guilt
- Suicidal behavior
- Sometimes, hallucinations or delusions
- No apparent "trigger" (precipitating event)

A major depressive disorder, sometimes called endogenous depression, is not merely sadness or grief but is a genuine psychiatric illness that affects both your mind and your body. If you are depressed, you tend to retreat from human relationships, have trouble functioning in society and using your talents, be unable to enjoy life, and even feel suicidal.

Stricken with much more desperate feelings than merely the "blues" or being "down in the dumps," you may become incapacitated, be unable to hold a steady job, derive no pleasure from your life, and have difficulty interacting with others. Sometimes, although not always, you may have psychotic symptoms such as hallucinations or delusions. By and large, however, the physical symptoms of depression—a characteristic hollowness around your eyes, uninflected speech, and a slowed gait—are the signs of depression.

Depression is more common among women than among men. Because it is both debilitating and associated with suicidal tendencies, a major depressive disorder is considered serious. But this type of depression, even in its most severe form, occasionally is self-limited. It may run its course and terminate without treatment within 6 months to a year. Meanwhile, however, your existence may be almost intolerable, and suicide is a great temptation.

Treatment

Because depression is so common, many therapies have been developed to treat it. At first, treatment of a major depression often includes hospitalization, especially if you threaten suicide or display suicidal behavior.

The various types of therapy have some characteristics in common. Virtually all therapeutic situations operate on the assumption that you can change, that you can learn to cope better with life traumas and inner struggles. If you are depressed, you usually visit the psychiatrist because you believe that there is hope for relief.

Psychotherapy

Psychotherapy is used, often in conjunction with medication, to help you understand the sources of your depression and to find other ways of coping with inner conflicts.

Cognitive therapy is a short-term psychotherapy developed to treat both depression and anxiety. The idea is that self-defeating patterns of thinking make us feel depressed because our negative thoughts influence our feelings. In cognitive therapy, you may be asked to write down your negative thoughts. The therapist then helps you identify the distortions in them and suggests constructive alternatives.

Antidepressive Medications

Medications to treat depression come in three main types: the tricyclic antidepressants (TCAs), selective serotonin re-uptake inhibitors (SSRIs), and the monoamine oxidase inhibitors (MAOIs).

Antidepressants are more helpful when your depression has isolated episodes that seem to have a life of their own rather than in chronic or situational depression. Imipramine (Tofranil) and amitriptyline (Elavil) are the most frequently used tricyclic antidepressants, but the SSRIs are the most common type of antidepressant medication used today. Examples are fluoxetine (Prozac), sertraline (Zoloft), and paroxetine (Paxil). However, no medications deal with the intrapsychic and interpersonal issues that may have contributed to your depression. For this reason, the most effective treatment may be to use both medication and psychotherapy.

Electroconvulsive (Shock) Therapy

In the movies, electroconvulsive therapy (ECT) has been depicted as repressive and cruel, but most psychiatrists consider it one of the most effective and humane treatments for depression. It is used primarily for major depressive episodes.

Unlike antidepressants, ECT works quickly (often within a few days) and is more likely to be decisively helpful when the problem is serious. Physicians do not know exactly how it works, but it may alter the rate at which brain chemicals, called catecholamines, affect your central nervous system cells.

Before undergoing ECT, you are anesthetized with a barbiturate and a muscle relaxant. Side effects commonly include temporary memory loss, headaches, and muscle aches. Nonetheless, ECT remains the most effective treatment available for major depression. Its risks are significantly lower than the risks of untreated severe depression (which include suicide). ECT can be safely used in most medically ill and elderly patients.

Manic-Depressive Illness

Signs and Symptoms
- Alternating pattern of emotional highs (characterized by high-spirited behavior) and emotional lows or depressions
- The manic and major depression episodes may alternate rapidly every few days

- Symptoms of depression are prominent and last for a full day or more

Mental health professionals refer to manic-depressive illness as bipolar disorder. It is characterized by recurring periods of mental illness in which episodes of excitement and hyperactivity (mania) either occur alone or alternate with periods of depression.

Everyone has moods, but extreme and unpredictable mood swings from highly excited euphoria to the darkest depths of despair and depression characterize bipolar disorder. In most people, mood changes are a response to events in the environment but, when elation or depression occurs without relation to the circumstances, this is manic-depressive illness.

Warning Signs of Potential Suicide

Too often, family and associates are shocked at a suicide, saying things like, "I had no idea; he seemed so happy." In fact, your behavior may not match descriptions of these warning signs precisely but, related to your normal personality, changes may be evident.

When you or someone you know displays warning signs of potential suicide, it is important to keep a close watch (to see that the opportunity for suicide does not arise) and to seek professional help as soon as possible. Begin by calling your local suicide hotline or a local psychiatrist or psychologist.

A person who is contemplating taking his or her own life may show one or more signs (see below). However, it is important to keep in mind that these warning signs are only guidelines. There is no one type of suicidal person.

Signs

Withdrawal
You are unwilling to communicate and appear to have an overwhelming urge to be alone. You are withdrawing into a shell. Trouble at work can be a symptom of a with-

drawal from the workplace, just as poor grades can signal a retreat from school. Rejection of forms of recreation you usually consider pleasurable may also be a warning sign.

Moodiness
Although we all have our ups and downs, when the shifts are drastic—an emotional "high" one day followed by being "down in the dumps" the next—there is cause for alarm. Sudden, inexplicable calm after a spell of gloom is a danger sign; it may indicate that you may have decided on suicide as the solution to the problem.

Life Crisis or Trauma
If you are deeply depressed, divorce, death, or an accident can trigger a suicide attempt. The loss of self-esteem that may occur after loss of a job or a financial setback may produce suicidal thinking.

Personality Change
The wallflower turns into the life of the party, or vice versa. Or there might be a change in attitude toward personal appearance or a change in energy level.

Threat
You may state outright that you want to commit suicide, saying things like "I wish I'd never been born," or "You're going to be better off when I'm gone." The popular assumption that people who threaten suicide never really do it is not true.

Gift-Giving
You may begin to "bequeath" your most cherished belongings to friends and loved ones.

Depression
You appear to be physically depressed and may be unable to function socially or in the workplace.

Aggression
The suicidal urge may be manifested in your sudden participation in dangerous activities such as high-speed driving or unsafe sex.

The risk that the suicide actually will be completed is greater in older men, in people who have lost a spouse (by divorce or death), in alcoholics, in those with a history of previous suicide attempts, or in those with a family history of suicide.

Your feelings may become so intense that they take over completely, and you lose contact with the real world. The manic phase usually is the episode that may require the person to be hospitalized. During the manic episode, you may feel very "high" or irritable. Euphoria may not be obvious to those who do not know you well, but friends and loved ones will come to recognize it as unusual or as typical of the manic phase. Your speech and thoughts seem to run at high speed, so fast that it is difficult to understand them. Your speech may become so laden with puns, jokes, and plays on words that, after a while, it makes little sense.

The self-esteem of an individual with manic-depressive illness may soar, often to the point of delusions of grandeur. In fact, you are likely to be hyperactive, eager to take on far more activities than you can reasonably handle. Should such activities be thwarted, however, irritability may result. You may have an inability to judge the consequences of your actions, manifested in shopping sprees, self-destructive sexual activity, unwise business decisions, or reckless driving. You may change moods frequently, alternately laughing and crying, and there may be fleeting delusions or hallucinations.

If untreated, the manic episode may last for weeks, during which you are physically restless, highly talkative, likely to sleep less, and easily distracted.

During the depressed phase (which is the more frequent form of the illness), you appear depressed for most of the day, nearly every day. You lose interest and pleasure in nearly all activities, may lose or gain a great deal of weight, and usually have a change in sleeping patterns. You may be fatigued, suffer from feelings of worthlessness, and have trouble concentrating. You may withdraw completely, speaking only rarely. Often, there are recurrent thoughts of death and suicide. If untreated, the depressive phase may last for months.

Often, two or more complete cycles (a manic episode and a major depression that follow each other with no period of remission) will occur within a year. This situation may be called rapid cycling and seems to be more chronic than other types of bipolar disorder. Although major depression is more common in women, bipolar disorder is equally common in men and women. About 1 percent of the adult population have had this disease.

The disorder usually appears between the ages of 15 and 25. It occurs much more often in immediate relatives of people with bipolar disorder than in the general population.

Treatment

Medication

Tranquilizing drugs help control the manic phase. Antidepressant drugs can treat the depression episodes. Lithium carbonate is the standard treatment for manic episodes, and the regular use of this drug may prevent uncontrolled mood swings. Certain anticonvulsant drugs such as carbamazepine (Tegretol) can be helpful in persons who cannot tolerate lithium carbonate.

Other Therapies

In severe cases, electroconvulsive therapy may be necessary (see page 1124). It is always important to be aware that the danger of suicide is present. When you appear to have suicidal tendencies, it is important for those closest to you to express a caring attitude (see Warning Signs of Potential Suicide, page 1125). In these cases, however, you will probably need to be hospitalized.

Hospitalization also is necessary if you are in a depressed phase and regress so much that you are unable to take care of personal needs at home. Likewise, if your physician prescribes electroconvulsive therapy or expects the antidepressant medication to have severe side effects, it may be appropriate to admit you to the hospital. However, considering how severe the depressed phase often is in bipolar disorder, it is surprising how frequently outpatient treatment is successful.

During the depressed phase, psychotherapy usually serves only as a means of emotional support. The therapist will explain the illness to those closest to you, establish a rapport with you, and foster a sense of hope and planning for the future. You may receive a structured daily program, and the therapist will determine the risk of suicide and intervene when necessary.

Seasonal Affective Disorder

Signs and Symptoms
- Depression caused by a specific season of the year, most often winter
- Headaches, irritability, low energy level
- Crying spells

Seasonal affective disorder (SAD) is an extreme form of the "winter blahs." True forms of this disorder are unusual; most people with "cabin fever" do not have SAD.

If you do have it, you tend to sleep a great deal in the winter. You may gain a great deal of weight because you gorge on carbohydrates. Low on energy and highly irritable, you get many headaches, feel very stressed, and may have crying spells. The cause of SAD is not yet known, but it may be linked to your body's biologic clock, which controls temperature and hormone production. It usually begins in adolescents or young adults and is more common among women than men. Some people outgrow it, but it may last a lifetime.

Treatment
A recent innovation in the treatment of SAD uses fluorescent bulbs for light therapy. Patients may read, but not sleep, for several hours a day in front of specially designed, bright lights. The symptoms usually subside within a few days, but they reappear if therapy is stopped. Researchers are investigating the use of full-spectrum light bulbs to extend the hours of sunlight artificially.

Thought Disorders

A psychosis is an impairment of thinking in which your interpretation of reality and of daily events is severely abnormal. Psychosis is actually a symptom of a disordered brain; there is substantial evidence that chemical abnormalities cause the problem.

Schizophrenia

Signs and Symptoms
- Two or more of the following for at least 1 week: delusions, prominent hallucinations for much of the day, incoherence, lack of or inappropriate display of emotions, bizarre delusions (such as talking with Martians)
- Problems or decreased ability to function in work, in social interactions, and with personal hygiene
- Continuous signs for at least 6 months
- No evidence of an organic cause

Schizophrenia is the most common and destructive of the psychoses. It may be difficult to treat, and it is the most likely to be permanent. If you have schizophrenia, you withdraw from the people and activities in the world around you and retreat into a world of delusions and fantasies.

If you have schizophrenia you are unable to sustain self-initiated, goal-directed activity and have delusions that are often multiple, fragmented, or bizarre—that you are being persecuted, or that the FBI wants to kill you.

There may be a loosening of associations, with your conversation jumping from one idea to a completely unrelated one. Or you may chatter away and yet fail to convey any information. Speech is vague, very abstract, or repetitive. You may play with language, making up new words that seem highly important but make no sense to anyone else.

Hallucinations are common, and you are especially likely to hear voices, although you should not confuse schizophrenia with cases of multiple personality. If you have schizophrenia, your face tends to be expressionless and your voice a monotone. Your normal sense of self has been lost. You are likely to be socially withdrawn. Conversely, you may be clingy and intrusive with strangers. There is a marked lack of response to the surrounding environment. You may appear very rigid or in a stupor or may display inappropriate excitement through odd mannerisms and grimacing. Pacing and rocking are common. The schizophrenic may have a disheveled, bewildered appearance and may dress or groom eccentrically.

Schizophrenia usually appears during adolescence or early adulthood, although it may begin in middle or late adult life. The cause is not known, although many believe it is an inherited disorder. There is some evidence that genetic influences combine with environmental ones.

Schizophrenia seems to be equally common in both sexes. Once the signs appear, it is uncommon for you to return to the level of functioning achieved before the disorder began. Usually, there are acute periods of schizophrenic behavior with residual impairment between episodes.

There are different types of schizophrenia: the catatonic type (which may involve stupor or mutism, or rapid alternation between the extremes of excitement and stupor); disorganized schizophrenia (when you are incoherent and either expressionless or display inappropriate emotions); and paranoid schizophrenia (characterized by a preoccupation with one or more systematized delusions, such as the belief that you are a famous individual, or with frequent auditory hallucinations related to a single theme).

Treatment

Because there are more theories about schizophrenia than about virtually any other mental disorder, there also are many treatments. Generally, persons with acute or severe episodes of schizophrenia are treated in the hospital.

Your physician may prescribe antipsychotic drugs, such as one of the phenothiazines, to decrease excitement and agitated depression and to improve your thought processes. Your physician may use electroconvulsive therapy (ECT) in the hospital in an acute case. Antipsychotic drugs usually produce an improvement and allow you to be released from the hospital. However, if you fail to continue to take the medication, the symptoms invariably return.

These antipsychotic drugs appear to act by blocking the chemical receptors in your brain that normally link via dopamine, a chemical nerve messenger. Although they are very effective, they do cause a range of side effects: dry mouth, sensitization of your skin to sunlight, constipation, loss of bladder control, blurred vision, orthostatic hypotension (feeling of faintness on rising quickly from chair or bed), or tremor.

Supportive psychotherapy (see page 1107) may help you to return to a more normal, less withdrawn life.

Brief Reactive Psychosis

Signs and Symptoms
- Disordered thinking or delusions (false beliefs)—anything from thinking that your dead grandmother is alive to believing that all restaurant food is poisoned—that you will not give up even in the face of logical argument
- Disorders of perception (especially hallucinations)
- Language disorders (conversation that makes no sense or wanders)
- Disturbance of affect (the emotion you appear to express is either not consistent with what you are thinking or shifts much more rapidly than normal)
- Symptoms last at least a few days but no more than a month

If you suddenly display psychotic symptoms for at least a few hours but not more than a month and eventually return to your previous level of functioning, the diagnosis is brief reactive psychosis.

The symptoms often appear after an extremely stressful event such as the loss of a loved one or combat duty. You go through turmoil, experiencing a rapid fluctuation of emotions or overwhelming confusion. You may be aware of your symptoms, or they may be obvious to others from your conversation.

Behavior and dress may be bizarre, and you may adopt peculiar postures. You may frequently scream or, alternatively, become mute. Speech may be foolish, often involving the repetition of nonsense phrases. There may be passing hallucinations or delusions, and you may be disoriented and have trouble remembering things.

This disorder usually appears during adolescence or in the early adult years. Often, the symptoms will subside in a day or two. Afterward, you may continue to feel a loss of self-esteem or be mildly depressed for a while.

Treatment

Medication
Treatment involves use of drugs often referred to as major tranquilizers, such as chlorpromazine (Thorazine) or haloperidol (Haldol), which are antipsychotics. They do not really induce tranquillity, but instead they decrease or completely eliminate psychotic symptoms and behavior.

Other Therapies
Psychotherapy (see page 1107) is also helpful in providing support and helping the person to cope with the emotional trauma from which the psychosis originated.

Alcohol- or Drug-Induced Psychosis

Signs and Symptoms

- Delirium
- Aggression, hostility, or violent behavior
- "Bad trip" or fearful mental disorientation (panic, delusions, hallucinations) after use of a hallucinogenic drug
- Behavior resembling schizophrenia after use of certain combinations (such as alcohol and barbiturates) or overdoses of drugs (such as sleeping pills or antidepressants)

This disorder is known technically as psychoactive substance-induced organic mental disorder. It is a psychosis caused by the use of certain drugs (particularly hallucinogens or amphetamines), by overdose of common drugs, or by alcohol abuse or untreated withdrawal.

You may display all or many of the symptoms of acute psychosis or schizophrenia—disorientation, violence, visual hallucinations (see pages 1128 and 1127). Often, the delirium is so similar to psychosis that the only way to be certain that it has been caused by chemical means is through laboratory tests.

Overdoses of cocaine or amphetamines are two major causes.

Even people who are usually calm and controlled may become aggressive and violently hostile. Untreated withdrawal from these drugs or from alcohol may cause delirium, seizures, or terrifying hallucinations. Even some drugs used for medical reasons may cause psychosis-like behavior after you take an overdose of them. These include over-the-counter sleeping pills and antihistamines as well as antidepressants and drugs used for Parkinson's disease.

A psychotic reaction, popularly known as a "bad trip," to hallucinogenic drugs such as LSD or PCP (angel dust) and occasionally marijuana or hashish, is a frightening, disorienting mental reaction. You experience panic, anxiety, and a feeling of disorientation. Your fear of "losing your mind" is often accompanied by delusions and hallucinations.

Treatment

For your own safety, you need to be isolated in a safe, quiet environment and accompanied by someone who will provide reassurance if you are on a "bad trip." It may be necessary to treat you with an antipsychotic drug such as haloperidol to bring you back to reality.

Addictive Behavior

Although the word "addiction" tends to bring drugs to mind, you can be addicted to a wide variety of substances and practices, from coffee or tobacco to compulsive gambling. However, the term "addictive behavior" also refers to psychological dependencies such as overeating.

The main characteristic of addictive behavior is that you feel a compelling need to engage in the particular activity or to use the addictive substance without deriving pleasure or gain from it.

"The main point," wrote Dostoevsky, a compulsive gambler, "is the game itself. I swear it is not greed for money, although I am sorely in need of money."

In this section we discuss the type of behavior that accompanies the use of alcohol and other addictive behaviors. We also consider the use and misuse of substances such as alcohol and tobacco. Drug dependency is discussed in a later section (see page 1131).

Alcohol Dependency

Signs and Symptoms

- Repeated declarations that you have resolved to give up drinking altogether, with denials that you have a drinking problem
- Feeling of guilt about drinking
- Tendency to drink too much
- Desire to continue drinking after friends say you have had enough
- Irritation when family or friends comment on your drinking
- Arguments about drinking

- Inability to remember the previous evening's activities on awakening, with assurance from companions you did not pass out (black out)
- Regret over things done or said while drinking
- Efforts to avoid family or friends while drinking
- Financial problems
- Inability to meet demands of a steady job
- Eating irregularly while drinking
- Being arrested for driving while under the influence of alcohol or having a car accident after drinking
- "The shakes" on awakening, which disappear after "a little drink"
- Steady drinking for several days at a time
- Delusions or hallucinations after periods of drinking
- Loss of memory and concentration

Alcoholism is a chronic and often progressive disease characterized by periods of preoccupation with alcohol, impaired control over alcohol intake, and repetitive use of alcohol, despite the known risk of adverse consequences related to drinking. In this context, alcoholism is alcohol dependence. (See Alcohol Abuse and Alcoholism, page 325.)

Often, you begin to become dependent on alcohol after discovering that having a few drinks helps to relieve stress from family problems, difficulties at work, or social isolation. Despite occasional hangovers and the fact that this relief is only temporary, you gradually fall into the pattern of drinking whenever you feel tense. Unfortunately, the more an alcohol-dependent person drinks, the less tension he or she can tolerate without alcohol.

The actual number of drinks is not the critical issue, because some people can easily become intoxicated after very few. The diagnosis of alcohol dependency is made when you have difficulty getting through the day without regular alcohol consumption. We are not yet certain of the cause of alcoholism, although it does seem to run in families and there is some evidence pointing to a genetic predisposition. Alcoholism tends to be underdiagnosed because one classic trait of alcoholics is that they deny their dependency.

Approximately 7 million Americans abuse alcohol and 11 million are alcoholics. Alcoholism is more common among men than women (although the prevalence among women is increasing) and among the urban poor and minority groups.

Treatment

In treating alcoholism, a fundamental principle is "Once an alcoholic, always an alcoholic." Most research indicates that an alcoholic is unable to become a normal social drinker. Consequently, treatment aims to eliminate alcohol totally from your routine. You must never take another drink. Alcoholics Anonymous (AA) is the most effective treatment program known. It provides group support, a 12-step abstinence program with a spiritual base, and gentle confrontation of the various ways in which alcoholics deny their illness. In conjunction with AA, aversive therapy may discourage drinking: the drug disulfiram (Antabuse) blocks the normal oxidation of alcohol so that acetaldehyde accumulates in the bloodstream and causes unpleasant symptoms such as rapid pulse and vomiting.

You may need psychotherapy (see page 1107) to help restore your self-esteem and establish new patterns of healthy behavior (see Alcohol Abuse and Alcoholism, page 325).

Compulsive Gambling

Signs and Symptoms

- Gambling gradually proceeds from occasional to habitual, with higher and higher stakes risked and other interests—family, and sometimes work—neglected
- Craving for the painful but pleasurable tension derived from risk of gambling
- Feeling guilty when you lose money and trying to keep the loss a secret
- Lying to conceal losses
- Continuing to gamble, whether winning or losing, until the place closes or you have no money left
- Resorting to unlawful activities (larceny, fraud, embezzlement) in order to afford the habit and pay debts

Gambling (pathologic gambling) tends to be a more common compulsion among men than among women. It often goes hand-in-hand with excessive drinking. It is serious to the extent that it disrupts your personal life and may cause financial ruin.

Treatment

Treatment includes psychotherapy (individual and group) (see page 1107) and support groups such as Gamblers Anonymous.

Caffeine Addiction

Signs and Symptoms
- Anxiety manifestations
- Muscle twitching and sensory disturbances such as ringing in your ears or flashing of lights
- Heart palpitations
- Gastrointestinal pain or diarrhea
- Periods of inexhaustibility
- Insomnia
- Withdrawal symptoms if daily intake is interrupted: headache, drowsiness and lethargy, irritability, nervousness, vague depression, or occasional yawning
- Depression
- In women, may contribute to breast tenderness

If you are addicted to coffee, you easily recognize a "caffeine high": your heart pounds, you are jumpy, and you may have gastric distress. When you try to give up coffee, you get a headache and often feel drowsy. Caffeine is found not only in coffee but also in chocolate and cola drinks.

Treatment
You can cure your caffeine addiction by discontinuing or decreasing your intake. When you are thirsty, drink decaffeinated beverages or water. Symptoms should begin clearing up in 4 to 10 days.

Drug Dependency

Dependence on drugs, whether prescription or illegal, is dangerous because of its long-term physical effects, its disruptive effect on family and work, and the risks associated with sudden withdrawal. Sometimes people maintain a dependence on a prescription drug by collecting prescriptions from various unsuspecting physicians. Illegal drugs are hazardous not only by their nature but also because of the risk of contamination with other dangerous substances. In most cases, help is essential, whether in the form of support groups, drug-free residential communities, or day-care centers. (See Medications and Drug Abuse, page 335.)

Central Nervous System Depressants

Signs and Symptoms
- Drowsiness or coma
- Slurred speech
- Lack of coordination
- Memory impairment
- Confusion
- Tremor or decreased muscle tone
- Agitation
- Paranoia
- Inappropriate display of emotions

Central nervous system depressants, also known as downers, include prescription drugs such as sedatives, hypnotics, and anti-anxiety agents. The effects of their use resemble those of drunkenness but without alcohol consumption. Aside from the difficulties these drugs usually cause in your family and work lives, there is also a danger of death from an overdose.

Glue
Young children may sniff glue, which is a central nervous system depressant, when they are as young as age 6 or 7. They sniff the glue directly from the tube or in plastic bags or from smears on pieces of cloth. At first a few sniffs may give a "high," but the child develops a tolerance in a matter of weeks or months. Chronic users may have to use several tubes before achieving the desired effect. The initial symptoms are similar to those of alcoholic inebriation, including slurred speech, dizziness, breakdown of inhibitions, drowsiness, and amnesia. The child may have hallucinations, lose weight, and occasionally lose consciousness.

Barbiturates
Most people begin taking barbiturates for relief from unbearable tension, anxiety, or

inadequacy. Middle-aged people may obtain the drug from their physicians in response to complaints of nervousness or trouble sleeping. They may be chronically intoxicated for years without anyone around them realizing it, until their ability to work becomes impaired or they begin to exhibit signs such as slurred speech. Teenagers or young adults may ingest barbiturates to "get high."

Barbiturates, especially the short-acting kind such as secobarbital, produce psychological dependence as well as physical dependence after 1 or 2 months of taking doses above the recommended therapeutic level. The most commonly available on the black market are secobarbital (reds, red devils), phenobarbital (yellows), and a combination of secobarbital and amobarbital (reds and blues, rainbows). Some young adults take barbiturates intravenously.

Benzodiazepines

Physicians often prescribe drugs of the benzodiazepine group—chlordiazepoxide (Librium), diazepam (Valium), alprazolam (Xanax), and lorazipam (Ativan)—to control anxiety and to control the symptoms of alcohol withdrawal. These are frequently abused, particularly by persons who obtain prescriptions from multiple physicians, and they can cause marked central nervous system effects.

Treatment

A child with a glue-sniffing habit should see a child psychologist. Treatment of addiction to barbiturates or benzodiazepines includes getting you to withdraw from the drug safely—withdrawal symptoms can range from mild (such as anxiety, weakness, profuse sweating, and insomnia) to seizures—and preventing you from starting again. The latter usually is achieved with the help of drug support groups (see also Detoxification, page 1133).

Central Nervous System Stimulants

Signs and Symptoms
- Agitation
- Rapid speech
- Irritability
- Difficulty concentrating
- Debilitating cycle of "runs" (heavy use for several days a week) and "crashes" (let-

downs when you are forced to stop using the drug because of agitation, paranoia, and malnutrition)
- Nasal congestion (with cocaine)

The most widely used central nervous system stimulants are amphetamines and cocaine. Amphetamines (also known as uppers) produce an extraordinarily high degree of psychological dependence that amounts to a compulsion. Abusers develop a high degree of tolerance to the euphoric effects. The effects last for several hours. There is less physical dependence in the sense of a biochemical or physiologic need and, therefore, less of a withdrawal syndrome of the kind found in alcohol or heroin addiction.

Some people view cocaine as a safe "recreational" drug. In reality, cocaine is far more dangerous than we once thought. Cocaine generally is taken by sniffing (snorting), although users are smoking it in a crystalline form (crack) with increasing frequency. Occasionally, users inject it through a vein. The drug is rapidly absorbed, and its effects begin quickly, with initial stimulation and mood enhancement.

Cocaine triggers a release of the hormones epinephrine and norepinephrine from your sympathetic nervous system. These hormones stimulate your heart to pump faster and more powerfully. Also, your blood pressure and body temperature increase, you become more alert, and your appetite diminishes. These reactions result in the rush of euphoria, the illusion of control, and heightened sexual drive commonly associated with using cocaine.

Even a single modest dose of cocaine can kill you. Injecting or smoking crack can be more dangerous because a greater amount of the drug goes into your bloodstream. Cocaine can overwork your heart, forcing it to beat too fast and too powerfully. As your heart tires, it may beat irregularly or stop. Cocaine also can induce coronary artery spasm, a sudden narrowing of the arteries leading to your heart. Such spasms can cause a blood clot to form, even in otherwise normal arteries. If the spasm or clot completely blocks the flow of blood to your heart, it can cause a heart attack, dangerous heartbeat irregularities, or sudden death.

Thus, cocaine can kill you quickly, even if your heart is perfectly healthy. The size of the dose is not important. Superbly conditioned athletes have succumbed to the potent and variable effects of cocaine after a single modest dose.

The chronic use of cocaine can disrupt eating and sleeping habits and can produce psychological disturbances such as irritability and disturbed concentration. After the euphoria of cocaine subsides, you often feel irritable or may have an acute anxiety reaction along with occasional hallucinations. The craving for cocaine can become overwhelming. When smoked as crack, cocaine is almost instantly addictive.

Treatment

If you withdraw from amphetamines, you may experience a depression so severe that you become suicidal. Withdrawal also commonly produces extreme lethargy, fatigue, anxiety, and terrifying nightmares. The amphetamine psychosis is generally self-limiting, however, and treatment usually requires little more than supportive measures. You may receive psychotherapy (see page 1107), but your dependence on the drug often interferes with its effectiveness. Drug support groups with multi-step abstinence programs may help.

Treatment of a cocaine overdose is a medical emergency. You may require hospitalization in an intensive care unit for monitoring of your blood pressure and heart rhythm and for treatment of seizures if they occur.

Treatment of chronic cocaine abuse often requires the combined efforts of the family physician and mental health professionals. Individual and group psychotherapy (see page 1107) are often useful.

Opioids

Signs and Symptoms
- Depression, often of an agitated type
- Anxiety symptoms
- Impulsiveness
- Fear of failure
- Low self-esteem, hopelessness, and aggression
- Limited coping strategies and low frustration tolerance
- Need for immediate gratification
- Friends who are drug users

Opium (Greek for "juice") is produced from the milky discharge from the unripe seed capsules of the poppy plant. Opioids include opiates (substances naturally produced from opium), such as heroin and morphine, and synthetic substances that have morphine-like action. Physicians may prescribe them as pain relievers, anesthetics, or cough suppressants (such as codeine and methadone).

Users usually inject heroin, an illegal drug. Because addicts tend to be indifferent to hygiene when using syringes, infections of the skin and systemic organs are common, especially tuberculosis and low-level chronic hepatitis without jaundice. By sharing needles, people transmit viruses like hepatitis B and HIV. Both are common among intravenous drug users.

In recent years there has been a steady increase in the number of opiate addicts from middle-class homes.

Treatment
We once believed that addiction to these narcotic drugs was easily acquired and hard to break. A follow-up study of drug users among Vietnam veterans, however, found that most of the men who used narcotics extensively in Vietnam stopped when they came home and had not begun again. Treatment involves safe withdrawal from the addiction (often with the use of methadone) and supportive psychotherapy (see page 1107) to help in the return to a productive life.

Detoxification

If you become intoxicated with alcohol or any other drug, it may be necessary to carry out a process called detoxification. The chronic alcoholic is in danger of seizures or delirium tremens (DTs) or even death if detoxification is not carried out systematically. Similarly, if you have been using drugs such as benzodiazepine or barbiturates, you risk having seizures. Whether the intoxicating drug agent is alcohol, an opioid such as heroin, a barbiturate, or a tranquilizer, you are likely to be very uncomfortable for a number of days after you begin the withdrawal from the addictive substance.

Detoxification includes supportive measures—for example, sometimes the amount of intoxicant used is decreased slowly. If you are addicted to a drug of the benzodiazepine family, it is important to decrease amounts gradually to avoid the risk of seizures. Detoxification often requires a week or more of treatment, ideally in a hospital. Once you have safely finished detoxification, you should enter a program of reeducation about drug use. These programs often last several weeks and are usually done on an outpatient basis.

Hallucinogens

In the 1960s, people, many of them young, conducted various "experiments" on the effects of hallucinogenic drugs on their consciousness. Recreational use of such powerful chemicals as LSD and PCP has waxed and waned in recent years, but the hazardous practice is still commonplace.

Drugs

LSD (lysergic acid diethylamide) is not addictive. However, it does produce profound changes in mood and thought processes that may result in hallucinations and a state resembling acute psychosis. Unusually brilliant and intense perceptions may accompany the other effects. With a "bad trip," acute panic reaction or psychotic symptoms may occur; suicide attempts also have been known to occur. In addition, rapid heart rate, hypertension, and tremors are often noted.

PCP (phencyclidine) sometimes is described as a dissociative anesthetic. It is used widely by veterinarians to immobilize large animals briefly. Some people either smoke it or inject it or use it to adulterate LSD, amphetamines, or cocaine sold on the street. The most common street preparation is angel dust, a white granular powder containing the drug at 50 to 100 percent strength.

In low doses (5 mg), PCP produces excitement, incoordination, and absence of sensation (analgesia). In high doses it can cause drooling (hypersalivation), vomiting, stupor, or coma.

PCP overdose symptoms often resemble those of an acute schizophrenic reaction. Chronic use of PCP causes insomnia, anorexia, and severe changes in behavior, including chronic schizophrenia. When there is acute psychosis associated with PCP, the person is at high risk for suicide or violence toward others.

Dealing With the Effects

Usually, the psychotic effects of LSD wear off in 12 to 18 hours, and psychiatric help is unnecessary. It is essential to protect you so that you cannot physically harm yourself (or others). Companionship and reassurance are essential. Disturbing recurrences of symptoms may appear even months later. Abrupt abstinence from LSD does not produce withdrawal symptoms, although you may need supportive reassurance from a mental health professional after a panic episode that may follow the use of LSD.

If you take an overdose of PCP, prompt use of life-support measures in a hospital intensive care unit is critical to treating coma, convulsions, and breathing difficulties. A PCP overdose can cause death.

Marijuana and Cannabis Compounds

Signs and Symptoms
- Introversion
- Lack of drive
- Poor judgment
- Disorientation
- Agitation
- Delirium

People make marijuana cigarettes from the leaves and flowers of the plant. They make hashish from the concentrated resin of the same plant, *Cannabis sativa*. Your body absorbs the psychoactive substance in these drugs, delta-9-tetrahydrocannabinol (THC), more rapidly from marijuana smoke than after orally ingesting cannabis compounds.

If you are acutely intoxicated with marijuana or hashish, you feel relaxed and euphoric, an effect similar to mild or moderate drunkenness. Your thinking usually is impaired, and these compounds affect your concentration and perceptual and psychomotor functions. Marijuana can bring on severe emotional disorders in persons who are emotionally unstable.

If you become a chronic marijuana abuser, you may lose interest in everyday events of life and socially desirable goals. You devote more and more of your time to buying and using the drug.

Chronic users may have an increased heart rate, redness of eyes (conjunctival injection), and decrease in lung function. They develop tolerance and need to smoke more frequently to obtain the euphoria.

Treatment

If you are habitually abusing these substances, psychotherapy may help develop self-esteem, provide support, and point the way toward a more productive and satisfying pattern of living.

Withdrawal symptoms from chronic use of marijuana include sweating, tremors, nausea, vomiting, diarrhea, irritability, and difficulty in sleeping (see page 342).

Psychosomatic Illness

Only in the 20th century has there been a comprehensive scientific attempt to understand the complex relationship between psychiatric health and physical health. In the past, such links were usually superstitious ones: for example, people said that a person who contracted a crippling illness had incurred the anger of the gods. The term psychosomatic (from the Greek *psyche*, meaning "soul," and *soma*, meaning "body") was coined in the 19th century.

Psychosomatic illnesses, called somatoform disorders by most health professionals, are those that may begin at a time of crisis in your life, show a time relationship with stressful situations, and clear up when the situation changes for the better or you learn to adapt.

Physical symptoms caused by emotional factors characterize these disorders. The disorder usually affects only one organ system, such as the skin or gastrointestinal tract. The symptoms often resemble those that normally accompany emotional upset, but in psychosomatic disorders they are more intense and last for a sustained period.

Conversion Disorder

Signs and Symptoms
- Physical problem suggesting a physical disorder
- Link between the appearance of the symptom and a psychosocial stress
- No awareness of intentionally producing the symptom
- Although pain or sexual dysfunction may exist, the symptom is not limited to these problems

When a physical problem that appears to have an organic cause but really is an expression of a psychological conflict or need occurs, we call this a conversion disorder, formerly known as hysterical neurosis. The classic examples are paralysis, seizure, and blindness, but vomiting and false pregnancy also can be conversion symptoms. Usually, the disorder enables you to keep the internal conflict out of conscious awareness, to avoid a particularly disliked activity, or to receive support from others that might not otherwise be forthcoming. This disorder usually appears in adolescence or early adulthood.

Treatment
Because there generally is a correlation between the appearance of a conversion disorder and a stressful situation, the problem usually will clear up when the situation improves or you adapt. Psychotherapy (see page 1107) and hypnosis have been successfull treatments of this disorder.

Somatization Disorder

Signs and Symptoms
- History of many physical complaints or a belief that you are sickly
- Various symptoms for which your physician finds no organic cause and for which you take prescription medicine, visit a physician, or make lifestyle changes

In somatization disorder you may have many physical complaints that last for several years and have no physical basis found by a physician. You may be vague or highly dramatic about the complaints. The problems usually are gastrointestinal, sexual, pain-related, cardiopulmonary, or neurologic (such as numbness and tingling).

The symptoms usually begin in adolescence and the disorder is more common among females.

Treatment
Through psychotherapy (see page 1107), it may be possible to determine the psychological motivation for the disorder.

In stressful situations, we tend to suppress our emotions, particularly aggressive ones, and this may lead to the formation of psychosomatic symptoms. As a result, although the physical symptoms need to be treated, supportive psychotherapy may be of enormous help.

Hypochondriasis

Signs and Symptoms
- Preoccupation with fear of illness or supposed illness
- No apparent physical disorder that can account for the physical signs or sensations
- Disturbance lasts at least 6 months

Chronic Pain Centers

In 1976, a survey found 17 pain clinics in the United States. At present, there are between 500 and 1,000.

In these centers, physicians and therapists representing various specialties work with you toward the goal of pain control. This team approach is essential because with chronic pain it is unlikely that any one technique will work. The professionals in an interdisciplinary center treat not only the pain itself but also the disruption it usually causes within a marriage and family as a result of your disability, loss of income, depression, and anxiety. A chronic pain center may treat people as inpatients or outpatients.

Because there is no licensing procedure, it is important to investigate carefully before enrolling at a pain clinic. In most cases, an interdisciplinary pain-treatment program is the most likely to produce results.

- Belief of illness is not of delusional intensity—that is, you can accept the possibility that you may not in fact have a serious disease

Hypochondriasis is an obsessive preoccupation with supposed ill health in which you interpret physical signs or sensations as evidence of physical illness. Your physician can find no physical disorder on thorough physical evaluation, but you continue to have an unwarranted fear of disease.

You may interpret a change in heart rate, perspiration, or gastrointestinal pain as evidence of a serious disease. Or you may become preoccupied with a specific organ—for example, worrying that you have heart disease. There usually is a considerable amount of "doctor-shopping," during which you visit a series of physicians and are disappointed when they tell you that all is well.

Often, you give the impression of relishing the misery of the imagined ailment while bemoaning its consequences; you usually are overdemanding of physicians and unappreciative of their help. The symptoms rarely fit any pattern known to medicine.

Unlike Munchausen's syndrome (factitious disorder), in which you fabricate a physical illness or self-inflict injury in order to gratify an inordinate need for attention, if you are a hypochondriac, you genuinely believe that you are physically ill.

Treatment

As with all somatoform disorders, once your physician makes a diagnosis (which includes eliminating genuine organic causes for your complaint), psychotherapy (see page 1107) can often be helpful in helping you to work through the conflicts that underlie the disorder.

Chronic Pain Disorders

Signs and Symptoms

- Preoccupation with pain for at least 6 months
- No physical disorder or effects of injury to account for the pain, or a complaint of pain or resulting social or occupational impairment grossly in excess of what your physician expects from the physical findings

Chronic pain disorder (somatoform pain disorder) is preoccupation with pain without physical findings adequate to explain the pain or its intensity. (This disorder should not be confused with chronic pain that does have a physical basis, such as chronic pain associated with arthritis.) Your pain may be inconsistent with the anatomy of the nervous system or may mimic a known disease entity (as in angina or sciatica) without any apparent organic cause being revealed by extensive diagnostic evaluation.

There may be evidence that psychological factors are contributing to the pain, especially if the pain is clearly associated with an environmental stimulus that seems to be related to a psychological conflict or need. Sometimes the pain seems to enable you to avoid some disagreeable activity or to get support from family, friends, or professionals that otherwise might not be available. But there do not always seem to be psychological factors. In somatoform pain disorder there is no physical explanation to account for the pain—for example, the tension headaches caused by muscle spasm.

This disorder is serious because of its effect on your daily life. Typically, you become incapacitated, quit working, go from physician to physician, use too many pain-killers without relief, and basically assume the role of an invalid. As a result, you will likely be depressed.

In this disorder, which usually begins

between ages 30 and 50, the pain typically appears suddenly and worsens severely over a few weeks or months. There is some evidence that people with this disorder tend to be close biologic relatives of people with more painful injuries and illnesses, depression, or alcohol dependence. Somatoform pain disorder is diagnosed almost twice as frequently in females as in males. The problem is especially difficult when pain without apparent cause occurs after an industrial accident and there is a claim for compensation.

Treatment

As with other somatoform disorders, organic causes need to be eliminated. In compensation cases, quick resolution yields the best chance for relief.

Pain management centers help you deal

Minnesota Multiphasic Personality Inventory (MMPI)

This is an objective personality test consisting of more than 500 standard true-or-false questions that can provide a description of your overall personality profile. When used correctly, it reveals a great deal about your grasp of reality, impulse control, depression, guilt, major defenses, and symptoms due to psychological problems. Commercial computer services offer fairly sophisticated interpretations of the MMPI.

with chronic pain. Such centers usually provide drug withdrawal, teach better living habits and biofeedback, and provide relaxation and physical therapy and group psychotherapy (see Chronic Pain Centers, page 1136).

Chapter 34

Women's Health

Contents

Female Organs, 1140
Gynecologic Organs, 1140
Pelvic Examination, 1141
Selecting a Gynecologist, 1142
Breasts, 1142

Menses and Menstrual Disorders, 1143
Puberty and Menarche, 1143
Normal Menstrual Cycle, 1144
Menstrual Care, 1145
Toxic Shock Syndrome, 1145
Oral Contraceptives, 1146
Premenstrual Syndrome, 1147
Mittelschmerz, 1148
Painful Menses, 1148
Absence of Periods, 1148
Infrequent Periods, 1149
Sports and Menses, 1150
Heavy Periods, 1150
Dilatation and Curettage, 1151
Dysfunctional Uterine Bleeding, 1152
Menopause, 1153
Postmenopausal Bleeding, 1155
Primary Ovarian Failure, 1155
Abnormalities of the Hypothalamus, Thyroid,
Pituitary, Adrenal Glands, and Ovaries, 1156

Problems of the Breast, 1157
Normal Breast, 1157
Premenstrual Tenderness and Swelling, 1158
Lumps in the Breast, 1158
Breast Self-Examination, 1160
Breast Infections, 1160
Nipple Problems, 1161
Yeast Infections, 1161
Galactorrhea, 1162
Breastfeeding, 1162
Intraductal Papilloma, 1163
Cancers of the Breast, 1163
Stereotaxic Breast Biopsy, 1164
Mammograms, 1165
Surgery for Breast Cancer, 1166
Swelling After Mastectomy, 1168

Vaginal and Vulvar Disorders, 1168
Developmental Disorders, 1169
Vulvitis, 1170
Atrophic Vulvar Dystrophy, 1170

Pruritus Vulvae, 1170
Vaginal Hygiene, 1171
Genital Warts, 1171
Bartholin's Gland Abscess, 1172
Sebaceous Cysts, 1172
Cancer of the Vulva, 1172
Pubic Lice, 1173
Vaginitis, 1173
Atrophic Vaginitis, 1174
Vaginal Cysts, 1174
Nonspecific Urethritis, 1174
Loss of Pelvic Support, 1175
Vaginal Pain, 1175
Exercises for Incontinence, 1176
Vaginal Cancer, 1176

Cervix, Uterus, and Fallopian Tube
Disorders, 1177
Developmental Disorders, 1178
Cervical Polyps, 1178
Cervicitis, 1179
Nabothian Cyst, 1179
Cervical Dysplasia, 1179
Cancer of the Cervix, 1180
Pap Smear, 1181
Fibroids, 1182
Endometrial Polyps, 1182
Endometrial Hyperplasia, 1183
Cancer of the Uterus, 1183
Hysterectomy, 1184
Hydatidiform Mole, 1185
Endometriosis, 1185
Adenomyosis, 1186
Pelvic Inflammatory Disease, 1187
Pelvic Pain, 1187

Ovarian Disorders, 1189
Ovarian Cysts and Benign Tumors, 1189
Cancer of the Ovary, 1190
Polycystic Ovarian Syndrome, 1191

Bladder and Urethral Disorders, 1192
Chronic Urethritis, 1192
Honeymoon Cystitis, 1192
Urine Incontinence and Other Urine Loss
Problems, 1193
Interstitial Cystitis, 1193
Irritable Bladder, 1193

Female Organs

Gynecologic Organs

Gynecologic organs are those associated with childbearing, including the ovaries, fallopian tubes, and uterus. The term "gynecology" means the study of women—from the Greek words *gyne*, meaning "woman," and *logos*, meaning "study."

Your two ovaries are located about 4 or 5 inches below your waist, midway in your pelvic cavity. Each is only about the size of an almond. At birth, your ovaries are already stocked with a lifetime supply of roughly 1 million ova, or eggs. Between puberty and menopause, the ovaries generally release one egg each month, at the midpoint of the menstrual cycle. They also produce the female sex hormones estrogen and progesterone.

Between each ovary and your uterus lies one of your fallopian tubes. Each of these tubes is the thickness of a lead pencil and contains a passageway no wider than a needle. Each is approximately 4 inches long and is connected to your uterus. The uterus, shaped like an upside-down pear, is about 2.5 inches long in a nonpregnant woman.

The walls of your uterus are thick and made up primarily of powerful muscles that contract during childbirth to push the baby out. The narrow neck of your uterus is called the cervix, and it also has thick walls. Ordinarily, the opening of the cervix is exceedingly small—big enough for menstrual fluids to pass through but not large enough that a tampon, for example, could

accidentally be thrust up into it. During childbirth, the cervical opening expands to allow passage of the baby.

Your cervix extends into your vagina, which is a muscular tube about 5 inches long. Most of the time the walls of your vagina touch, but they can expand to accommodate something as small as a tampon or as large as a full-term baby. Cells in your vaginal walls secrete lubricants. In girls, the hymen—a thin membrane—partly blocks the opening of the vaginal canal. It often remains intact until first sexual intercourse. In rare cases, a physician has to make an incision in the hymen before a girl can menstruate.

The opening to your vagina is shielded by external genitals. The whole area is called the vulva. It consists of the mons pubis, the labia, the clitoris, and the opening (vestibule) of your vagina. The mons pubis is the pad of fatty tissue at the base of your abdomen that becomes covered with hair at puberty. The labia are double folds of tissue that extend downward on either side of your vagina; the outer folds are the labia majora and the inner folds are the labia minora (*labium* is the Latin word for "lip"). Where the labia meet, near the front of the body, they cover a small protrusion, which is the tip of the clitoris. During sexual arousal, your clitoris, like the male penis, becomes erect. Important glands, called Bartholin's glands, are located in the vestibule of your vagina; the substances they secrete lubricate your vaginal opening.

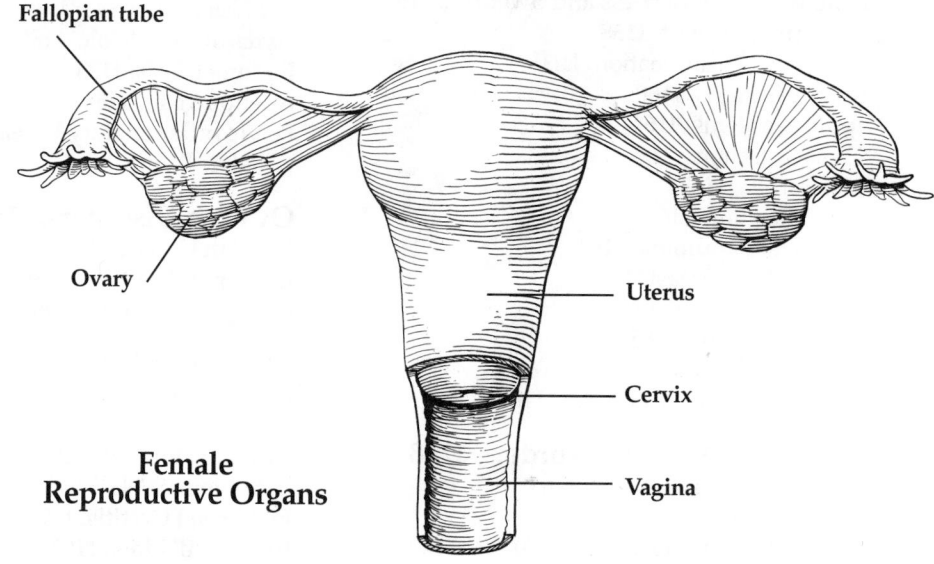

Fallopian tube

Ovary

Uterus

Cervix

Vagina

Female Reproductive Organs

Between the clitoris and your vagina is another, smaller opening, the entrance to your urethra. The urethra is a passageway, about 1.5 inches long, that leads to your bladder, where urine is stored. Your bladder is located between your pubic bone and your uterus. Both males and females have a bladder and urethra; however, men and women develop different urinary problems, or sometimes the same problem affects them differently. Consequently, this chapter will also cover women's urinary disorders (see page 1192).

Pelvic Examination

A pelvic examination is a simple procedure that can be done by your gynecologist or family physician. You will be asked to lie flat on your back on an examining table with your knees bent. Usually, your heels rest in metal supports called stirrups. The physician first examines your external genitals to make sure they look normal—no sores, discolorations, or swellings, for example. The internal examination is next. To see the inner walls of the vagina and the cervix, the physician inserts an instrument called a speculum to hold the vaginal walls apart and then shines a light inside to look for lesions, inflammation, signs of abnormal discharge, or anything else that is unusual. Generally, the next step is to take a sample of cells from the cervix. This is done, with the speculum in place, by scraping the cervix gently with a small spatula, brush, or cotton swab. The sample is sent to a laboratory for a Pap test (see page 1181), which is used to screen for cancer of the cervix, or for other tests.

Your physician cannot see your internal organs such as your uterus and ovaries, but can examine them by touch (palpation) after removing the speculum. To do this, your physician inserts two lubricated, gloved fingers into your vagina. By pressing down on your abdomen with the other hand while maneuvering the fingers inside your vagina, he or she can locate your uterus, ovaries, and other organs, judge their size, and confirm that they are in the proper position. By exploring the contours of these organs, your physician sometimes can detect tumors or cysts.

To palpate the same organs from a different angle, and to examine your rectum, your physician also may insert a finger into your

rectum and manipulate that finger, together with one or more fingers, in your vagina.

As the physician palpates your internal organs, you may feel somewhat uncomfortable. However, the experience should not be painful; if you do experience pain or tender-

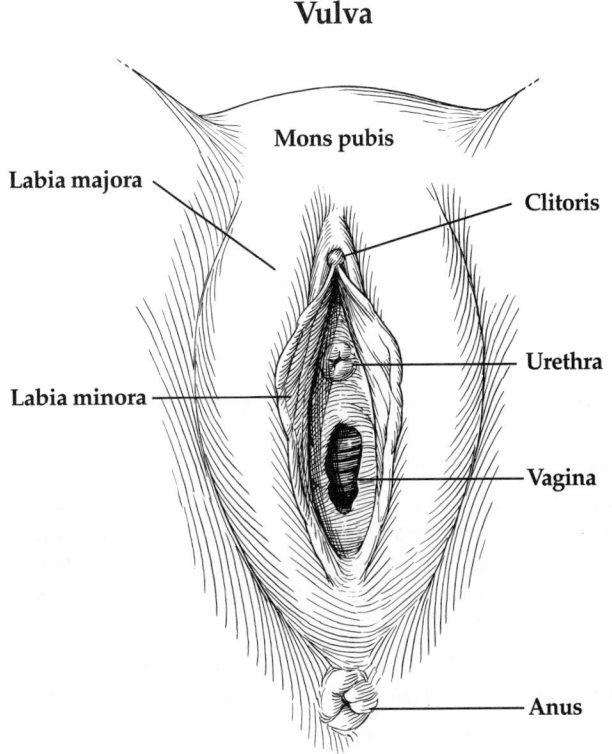

Vulva

Mons pubis
Labia majora
Clitoris
Urethra
Labia minora
Vagina
Anus

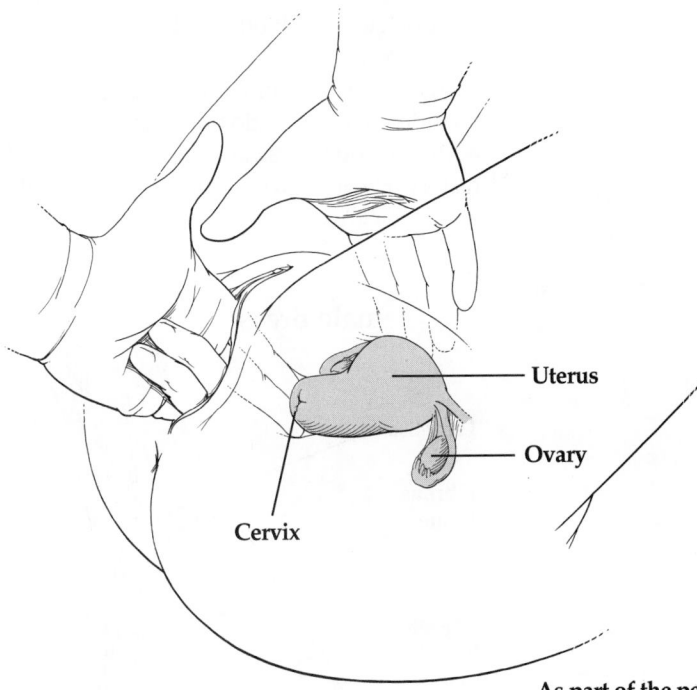

Uterus
Ovary
Cervix

As part of the pelvic examination, your physician will insert two gloved fingers inside your vagina. While simultaneously pressing down on your abdomen, he or she can examine your uterus, ovaries, and other organs.

Selecting a Gynecologist

Gynecologists are physicians who are trained to treat disorders that affect a woman's reproductive system. You might consult a gynecologist for menstrual problems (problems with your periods) and problems affecting your breasts; for cancer that develops in any of your reproductive organs; for treatment of infertility or sexually transmitted diseases; for difficulties during menopause (change of life); and for advice on birth control, abortion, or sexual problems. Because gynecologists also are trained as obstetricians, many handle pregnancy and childbirth. Many women choose to use a gynecologist as their primary care physician during their reproductive years.

In some areas of the country, gynecologists are not available. In these areas, general practitioners, family practitioners, internists, or nurse practitioners can provide routine gynecologic care. Another alternative is the certified nurse-midwife (CNM), a nurse who has had specialized training. CNMs deliver babies under some circumstances and provide well-woman care, including routine breast examinations and pelvic examinations with Papanicolaou (Pap) smears (see pages 1160 and 1181). They always work with one or more physicians who are available for consultations and in emergencies.

You may not need a gynecologist for routine care, but might consult one for serious conditions. To select a gynecologist, you can ask another physician to recommend someone, or you can call a local hospital for suggestions.

During your first visit to the gynecologist, you will be looking for answers to important questions. Is the physician willing to take time to explain things in language you can understand? Will he or she readily answer questions over the telephone? Most of all, are you comfortable with this person? If you are not, you will want to consult other gynecologists before making a final choice.

---

ness, say so immediately. There will be less discomfort if you can relax the muscles in your pelvic area. It often helps to take slow, deep breaths.

A routine gynecologic checkup generally includes an examination of your breasts. In addition, your physician will take a medical history. He or she will want to know the date of your last menstrual period, unless you are too young to menstruate. You will generally be asked about past pregnancies, childbirths, and abortions and about what form of birth control you are using, if any. You usually will be weighed and have your blood pressure measured, and you may be asked for urine and blood samples for laboratory analysis.

The American College of Obstetricians and Gynecologists recommends that you have an initial pelvic examination at age 18, earlier if you are sexually active.

Breasts

For the most part, your breasts consist of fat and connective tissue that protect a network of milk-producing glands and blood vessels. During lactation, these glands secrete milk into a system of ducts that eventually come together just behind the nipple. Your breasts are attached to the muscles of your chest wall (the pectoral muscles) by connective tissue.

Your nipples are made of erectile tissue. Some are constantly erect and protruding, some are inverted (turn inward), and others are normally flat but become erect when it is cold, when something brushes against them, or during sexual arousal. All three types of nipples are perfectly normal.

Encircling your nipple is the areola, a ring of tissue the same color as your nipple.

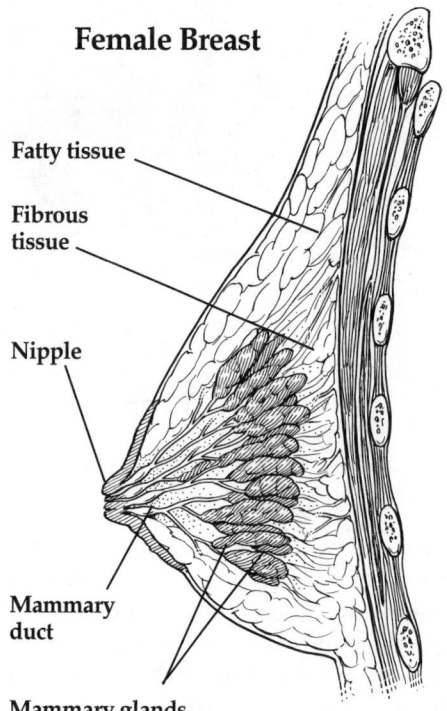

Female Breast

Fatty tissue

Fibrous tissue

Nipple

Mammary duct

Mammary glands

Oil glands in your areola lubricate your nipple during breastfeeding; in some women, these glands are visible as small bumps. Many normal women have hairs growing at the edges of the areola. There is no reason to remove them. In some women who take birth control pills, the number of hairs increases.

Some women are self-conscious about their breasts: they think that their breasts are too small or too large, or they are concerned because one is larger than the other. Actually, size makes no difference either in sexual responsiveness or in ability to nurse a baby. Women who have small breasts are as responsive as women with large breasts, and they can feed an infant just as successfully. Furthermore, it is normal and usual for your two breasts to be somewhat different in size and shape. For some reason, it is common for the right breast to be smaller than the left.

Menses and Menstrual Disorders

Puberty and Menarche

Puberty begins when a girl is about 8 years old. Her pituitary gland begins to secrete two key hormones in increasing amounts: follicle-stimulating hormone and luteinizing hormone. These hormones travel via the bloodstream to the ovaries, where they trigger growth and change.

At birth, your ovaries actually contain all the ova (eggs) they will ever have. However, the eggs remain almost dormant until stimulated by a surge of pituitary hormones. Then the ova begin to enlarge and to develop additional layers of outer cells, and these cells start to produce another hormone called estrogen. During childhood, a girl's body produces estrogen in very small quantities, but at puberty her estrogen level increases about 20-fold. Meanwhile, the ovaries themselves grow in size as the ova develop, and other internal reproductive organs also grow and mature.

Soon there are external signs of change. The girl's breasts begin to bud as estrogen induces the development of milk ducts. One breast may start to grow before the other does, and the two may develop at different rates; usually, they become approximately equal in size. Next, the girl develops pubic hair and, later, underarm hair. She experiences a growth spurt, and as her hips and breasts become more rounded, she begins to look more like a woman.

Approximately 2 years after a girl's breasts begin to bud, she generally reaches menarche; that is, she menstruates for the first time. Menarche marks the beginning of her reproductive life, and menopause (the cessation of ovarian functioning) will mark the end of it. The term "menarche" is derived from the ancient words for "month"—*men*—and "beginning"—*arche*. Males have no counterpart for menarche, which marks a dramatic change in a female's biologic status. A girl's attitude toward menstruation, and her feelings about what it means to be a woman, may be influenced by the way her family and friends respond to her first menses.

Menarche typically happens after age 9 years and before 16 years. On the average, American girls begin menstruating at 13 years, which is earlier than previous generations of American women began. For the past 100 years, the average age at menarche in the United States has been dropping at the rate of 3 or 4 months every decade. Medical experts believe this has happened because girls today are better nourished. Apparently, before hormonal changes can begin, a girl either must have reached a critical body weight, around 106 pounds, or must have reached that weight and also must have a specific amount of body fat and body water. At any rate, girls who are overweight usually have their first menstrual period earlier than those who are not. However, girls who are very athletic, are malnourished, or have a chronic, debilitating disease generally begin menstruating later.

If a girl's breasts begin to bud before she is 8 years old or if she has her first period before age 9 years, we recommend that you consult a physician. This rare condition is called precocious puberty. It has several possible causes. Premature sexual development can be a symptom of something serious (see Sexual Precocity, page 135), but it is usually treatable.

It is also a good idea to consult a physician if a girl has no breast development by age 14 years or has not begun to menstruate by the time she is 16 years old—especially if she is concerned about it.

For the first few years after menarche, it is normal for a girl's menstrual cycle to be irregular and for her to skip a cycle altogether at times. Her ovaries probably are not releasing an ovum every single month. However, it is wise to recognize that a young woman may become pregnant even before her first period, because the first egg may be released before menstruation begins.

In medical terms, puberty ends only after menstruation is established and regular.

Normal Menstrual Cycle

Your menstrual cycle begins on the first day of flow of one menstrual period and ends on the first day of flow of the next. The release of an egg (ovum), a single cell barely visible to the naked eye, occurs approximately in the middle of the normal menstrual cycle. Normally, only one ovary releases an egg each month, in random order.

Each month, even as you menstruate, several follicles have begun to develop in one of your ovaries, and your next cycle is under way. These follicles are tiny sacs, each containing a single immature egg. After a week or so, one follicle begins to outgrow the others, which then shrink to normal size. Meanwhile, your ovaries secrete more and more estrogen, much of it produced by the outer cells of that single, dominant follicle. The estrogen acts on the endometrium (the lining of the uterus), causing it to grow and thicken. A day or two before ovulation, estrogen levels peak; they then start to decrease, and the dominant follicle begins to produce tiny amounts of the hormone progesterone. The follicle swells, ruptures, and releases the egg. Other events include a slight increase in body temperature and a change in secretions from the glands in your cervix.

After it is released from the follicle, the egg floats into your fallopian tube and begins a journey to your uterus that generally takes about 6 days. While the egg is in transit, a sperm may fertilize it. Fertilization generally takes place within 24 hours after ovulation,

before the egg has traveled more than a third of the way down the tube.

Even as the egg drifts toward your uterus, its empty follicle in your ovary changes. Once again, the follicle enlarges rapidly—at this stage, it is called the corpus luteum—and it begins to secrete large quantities of progesterone and estrogen. Under the impact of these hormones, your endometrium continues to develop. Its glands secrete substances and release nutrients; its blood supply increases, as do the number of tiny blood vessels in the tissue. By the end of your menstrual cycle, the uterine lining has doubled in thickness, and large amounts of nutrients have been stored there, ready to nourish a fertilized egg.

If pregnancy occurs and a fertilized egg implants itself in your endometrium, hormones secreted by the corpus luteum will help to sustain it. If that does not happen, the egg disintegrates or leaves your body in vaginal secretions, usually even before menstruation begins. Meanwhile, within about 2 weeks after ovulation, the corpus luteum begins to shrink, and levels of both estrogen and progesterone decrease. Your uterus starts to shed its lining, and menstrual bleeding, known as menses, begins.

Menstrual flow actually consists not only of blood but also of vaginal and cervical secretions and tissue sloughed from the lining of your uterus. By the fourth or fifth day of your period, the endometrium has become thin, but the process of rebuilding it has already begun.

On the average, a menstrual cycle is 28 days long, although cycles normally range anywhere from 23 to 35 days long. If your cycle does not fall within this range, it may still be completely normal, although extremely long or extremely short cycles are sometimes associated with infertility. On the average, the menstrual period itself lasts 4 days; periods as short as 2 days or as long as 7 are not unusual.

At some point in your life, your period will likely become temporarily irregular for no obvious reason. You may skip a period or have one that is much longer, shorter, or heavier than normal. Sometimes this change simply reflects your age: menstrual periods are apt to last longer both at menarche and as you approach menopause. However, at other times, stress may play a role. Your monthly cycle is regulated by hormones ultimately controlled by your hypothalamus, an area at the base of your brain that acts as a kind of thermostat for your whole system. Your hypothalamus in turn interacts with your pituitary gland, some of whose hormones regulate the hormone action of your ovary, which affects your uterus. Given the complexity of your system and the fact that both physical and mental stress can affect your hypothalamus, it is remarkable that women's cycles are as regular as they are.

The sections that follow suggest specific guidelines to help you distinguish ordinary menstrual irregularity from times when you need to consult a physician. Many of the disorders, such as amenorrhea and dysmenorrhea, have similar names. They incorporate two Greek words, *men*, meaning "month," because menses are a monthly occurrence, and *rhoia*, meaning "flow."

Toxic Shock Syndrome

Signs and Symptoms
- Sudden fever of 102° Fahrenheit or higher
- Vomiting or diarrhea
- Dizziness, a feeling of weakness, fainting, disorientation
- A rash resembling a sunburn, particularly on your palms and the soles of your feet

Toxic shock syndrome (TSS) is a rare but potentially dangerous disorder that has been associated most often with the use of tampons and occasionally with the use of contraceptive sponges, especially by women younger than 30.

In the early 1980s, there was a small epidemic of TSS, for the most part involving young, menstruating women who had been using a particular brand of super-absorbent tampons. Researchers reported that TSS seemed to be caused by toxins, or poisons, produced by a type of bacteria called *Staphylococcus aureus*. These bacteria often are present in the body and cause no problems. Some researchers theorized that when women left super-absorbent tampons in place for a long time, the tampons could become a breeding ground for these bacteria. Others suggested that the super-absorbent fibers in the tampons scratched the surface of the vagina, and thus made it possible for the bacteria or their toxins to enter the bloodstream.

The brand of tampons associated with the original TSS epidemic was taken off the market. Since then, the number of cases of

---

Menstrual Care

In the past, menstruating women used cloths to catch their menstrual flow, rinsing them out and reusing them. Today, commercially made sanitary napkins are available, as are tampons and menstrual sponges that women insert into the vagina to absorb menstrual fluids.

Boxes of napkins and tampons are often labeled "regular" or "super." These terms refer to the product's ability to absorb, rather than to its physical size. Because there are no common standards, and one brand's "regular" may be as absorbent as another brand's "super," you will have to find out by trial and error what works for you. Because of the risk of toxic shock syndrome (see this page), many physicians now advise women to alternate tampons with napkins, not to leave tampons in place for very long, and to use napkins at night.

An inexpensive alternative to napkins and tampons is the menstrual sponge. It is a natural sponge you wear internally, rinse out, and reuse. Menstrual sponges have not been sterilized, nor have tampons. The same precautions apply to sponges as to tampons: do not leave them in place for too long, and use a pad at night.

If you have been using a napkin or tampon that is scented or deodorized, your vagina or vulva may begin to itch or become irritated during your period. Some women are allergic to the chemicals used in these products. Menstrual fluid is actually odorless until it comes into contact with bacteria and air. In general, if you bathe often and change napkins, tampons, or sponges often, you will not have a problem with odor.

From a health point of view, it is not harmful to have intercourse while you are menstruating. Some women use a diaphragm, lubricated with contraceptive jelly, to block menstrual flow temporarily.

TSS has declined, despite the fact that today most tampons contain some super-absorbent fiber. In recent years, there have been a few cases of TSS in women who had been wearing a diaphragm or a contraceptive sponge. However, 25 to 30 percent of those who develop TSS today are not young, menstruating women, but are older women, men, or even children; often, it strikes soon after an operation.

Diagnosis
Call your physician immediately if you experience the above symptoms, especially if you are menstruating or have just finished menstruating and have been using tampons. (Even before you call, remove the tampon.) Tell your physician what your symptoms are, how long you have had them, and when your period started.

Other possible symptoms include a head-

Oral Contraceptives

Oral contraceptives are highly effective: their failure rate is less than 1 percent. Today's birth control pills are very different from the original formulation because manufacturers have reduced the dose of female hormones. When oral contraceptives contained high levels of estrogen, they caused heart and circulatory disorders in some women. You still face some risks if you take the newer, low-dose pills; but the danger is now slight, especially if you are younger than 30 years. Smoking may increase these risks.

Two types of oral contraceptives are available. The combination pill, which contains both estrogen and progestin, has only one-tenth as much estrogen as the original birth control pill and half as much progestin. The so-called mini-pill, which has only progestin, is also low-dose. The result of these changes is that it is now statistically safer to take the pill than it is not to use birth control at all, because the death rate associated with normal pregnancy or elective abortion is higher than that associated with taking the pill. The newer pills with the newer progestagens have fewer side effects, such as headache and depression, than previous formulations.

The Pill Is Not for Everyone

Some women should not use oral contraceptives. You should not be taking the combination pill if you have a history of strokes, blood clots, high blood pressure, severe diabetes, or breast or uterine cancer, or if you have active liver disease or sickle cell disease. In addition, because studies show that the risks associated with oral contraceptives increase with smoking and to a lesser extent age, physicians generally recommend that all women who smoke should stop taking the pill once they are older than 35.

Side Effects

Because there is still some small risk that the pill will cause a stroke, there are danger signs to watch for if you are taking it. If you are having more headaches than usual, or if you feel faint or begin to have speech difficulties, call a physician. These effects are not a cause for concern with the low-dose pills. Also, be sure you discuss your use of oral contraception with your physician before any surgery.

Oral contraceptives also have other, less serious, side effects. You may sometimes bleed slightly between menstrual periods, or you may not menstruate at all, especially when you first start to take the pill. There are dozens of birth control pills on the market, and usually your physician can eliminate these problems by prescribing a different brand. Some women menstruate regularly while they are taking the pill but stop having periods after they discontinue using it. This effect is almost always temporary. Roughly 5 percent of women who use oral contraceptives develop some increase in blood pressure after about 5 years. In most cases, their blood pressure returns to normal if they stop taking the pill.

Other possible side effects include nausea, breast tenderness, fluid retention, depression, and nervousness. In addition, you may gain a little weight, either because of water retention or because the pill has increased your appetite and you are eating more.

Drug Interactions

If you are getting a new prescription of any kind, remember to tell the physician that you are taking the pill, because it can interact with other drugs such as some anticonvulsants and antibiotics.

Good News

Not all side effects are harmful, and oral contraceptives have some beneficial effects that are a welcome bonus. While you are taking the pill, you are less likely to have heavy menstrual bleeding or severe cramps or to develop breast lumps, iron-deficiency anemia, ovarian cysts, ovarian cancer, or rheumatoid arthritis. Your periods should be regular, light, and predictable. Young women taking the pill also seem to have lower rates of uterine cancer than other women. Furthermore, there is no convincing evidence that women who take the pill develop breast cancer or any other type of malignancy more often than women who don't. (For information on other birth control methods, see page 170.)

ache, sore throat, aching muscles, and bloodshot eyes. The rash may appear on various parts of your body, including the palms of your hands and the soles of your feet; after a week or so, the skin on your hands and feet generally begins to peel.

How Serious Is TSS?

TSS symptoms develop suddenly, and the disease is actually fatal in about 3 percent of all cases. It can cause blood pressure to plummet, and if that happens, you may go into shock. Kidney failure also results in some cases.

Treatment

If you develop a serious case of TSS, you will need antibiotics. Because *Staphylococcus aureus* organisms can be resistant to penicillin and ampicillin, you may need some other type of medication. If your blood pressure begins to drop, you will have to be hospitalized and given medication to stabilize it and fluids to prevent dehydration.

Prevention
You can reduce your chances of getting TSS if you change your tampons at least every eight hours. Women who are known to have problems with *Staphylococcus aureus* infections should not wear tampons at all.

TSS tends to recur—up to 30 percent of persons who have had it once get it again, although subsequent attacks are not usually as serious. Women who have had TSS should not use tampons at all.

Premenstrual Syndrome

Signs and Symptoms—A predictable pattern of physical and emotional changes that occur just before menstruation

Physical changes may include bloating, fluid retention, weight gain, breast soreness, abdominal swelling, clumsiness, aching, swollen hands and feet, fatigue, nausea, vomiting, diarrhea, constipation, headaches, skin problems, or respiratory problems.

Emotional changes may include depression, irritability, anxiety, tension, mood swings, difficulty in concentrating, or lethargy.

For 2 to 5 percent of women, premenstrual syndrome (PMS) is a severe problem. Many others experience it to a moderate or mild degree. The symptoms can develop any time after the midpoint in your menstrual cycle, and they disappear soon after your period starts. They tend to wax and wane from month to month, and they are more apt to trouble women in their 20s and 30s.

No one really knows what causes PMS. It is undoubtedly related to cyclic changes in hormone levels, because symptoms disappear during pregnancy and after menopause. Stress can aggravate the problem, but it is not the sole cause. Occasionally, some women with severe PMS may have an undiagnosed depression, though depression alone does not explain all the symptoms of PMS. Some people have unfairly blamed PMS at times for symptoms arising out of emotional states.

Diagnosis
A physician will attribute a particular symptom to PMS only if it is part of a predictable premenstrual pattern. Hence, your physician may ask you to keep a record for several menstrual cycles before you come in for a consultation. On a calendar or in a diary, you record all symptoms, along with the day you first noticed them and the day they disappeared. Note, too, the day your period began.

How Serious Is PMS?
PMS can be hard to tolerate but, because it does not reflect any harmful underlying disorder, it is not considered serious. There is no cure for it except menopause—although it usually disappears of its own accord before that. However, some of the symptoms of PMS can be treated by a physician.

Treatment

Medication
Each of the medications currently used to treat PMS actually fails to help most women; yet, because individual reactions differ, each does help some women.

To reduce water retention and bloating, a physician can prescribe a diuretic. It is easy to become dependent on diuretics and to search for ever stronger agents because of the perceived distress from swelling. You can try oral contraceptives (see page 1146), although they aggravate symptoms about as often as they relieve them. For severe irritability, tranquilizers may help, although they pose their own risk. Vitamin B_6 supplements have been used widely, but there is no evidence that they are effective, and large doses of this vitamin are dangerous.

Nutrition and Exercise
By avoiding salt in the last few days before your period, you can reduce bloating and fluid retention. If you also avoid caffeine, you may feel less irritable and tense and have less of a problem with breast soreness. Many women say that regular exercise helps, because it provides an emotional lift at a time when they need one.

Women who have only mild PMS sometimes find that just recording their symptoms for a few months is all the help they need. Once it is clear that their problems are predictable and short-lived, PMS is easier to tolerate.

Mittelschmerz

Signs and Symptoms
- Pain in the lower abdomen at the time of ovulation
- Sometimes slight vaginal bleeding accompanying the pain

Mittelschmerz (a German word meaning "middle pain") occurs at the midpoint in the menstrual cycle, at the time of ovulation. Typically, the pain is a dull ache that lasts anywhere from a few minutes to a few hours; it may or may not be accompanied by minimal bleeding.

We don't know the cause. According to one theory, when an ovarian follicle ruptures and releases an egg, fluid from the follicle may escape into your abdominal cavity and cause irritation. The rapid drop in estrogen that occurs at the time of ovulation may cause bleeding.

The timing and location of the pain usually serve to identify mittelschmerz. On rare occasions, the pain is severe enough to resemble appendicitis (see page 772). It does not seem to indicate any underlying disorder.

Treatment

Medication
You can take a mild analgesic such as aspirin or acetaminophen to ease the pain.

Painful Menses

Signs and Symptoms
- Pain in the lower abdomen during menstruation, possibly extending to the hips, lower back, or thighs
- Nausea, vomiting, diarrhea, or general aching during menstruation

It is normal to have mild abdominal cramps on the first day or two of your period—more than half of all women do. However, 10 percent experience such severe pain that they cannot manage their normal routine unless they take medication.

The problem is called primary dysmenorrhea if the pain is not a symptom of some underlying gynecologic disorder but is an exaggeration of normal processes. (The prefix *dys* means "difficult," *men* signifies "month," and *rhoia* means "a flow.") Medical experts believe that primary dysmenorrhea is caused by excessive levels of prostaglandins, substances that make the uterus contract.

When a gynecologic disorder causes painful menstruation, it is known as secondary dysmenorrhea. In general, we suspect a secondary cause when the pain lasts longer than the first 1 to 3 days of the menstrual period, occurs between periods with or without bleeding, occurs a few days before your period begins, and is accompanied by spotting or by gushing of blood. The underlying cause could be fibroids (see page 1182), adenomyosis (see page 1186), a sexually transmitted disease (see page 1087), endometriosis (see page 1185), pelvic inflammatory disease (see page 1187), or an ovarian cyst or tumor (see page 1189).

Diagnosis
Your physician's first concern is to check for the underlying disorders that cause secondary dysmenorrhea. You will have a pelvic examination (see page 1141) and perhaps blood tests and a urinalysis. The physician may use ultrasound to get a picture of your internal organs (see page 1335) or laparoscopy (see page 1346) for a direct look.

How Serious Is Dysmenorrhea?
Primary dysmenorrhea is painful but not harmful. It is more common during adolescence, and it is apt to ease or disappear altogether by the time you are in your mid-20s or once you have had a baby. Secondary dysmenorrhea is more serious, but most of the underlying disorders that produce it are treatable.

Treatment

Medication
For primary dysmenorrhea, your physician may prescribe an analgesic drug. Medications such as ibuprofen, mefenamic acid, naproxen, and indomethacin work for about 80 percent of the women who take them. Oral contraceptives and aspirin also may relieve the discomfort.

For secondary dysmenorrhea, the treatment varies with the underlying cause.

Absence of Periods

Signs and Symptoms
- In young girls: menstruation has not yet begun at age 16 (primary amenorrhea)

- In adult women who are not pregnant: absence of menstruation for 6 months or longer (secondary amenorrhea)

If you reach the age of 16 years without ever menstruating, the chances are that you are developing normally but a little later than most girls. If you are very athletic or if you are quite thin, menarche could be delayed (see page 1150). However, because there is a small possibility that you have a hormonal abnormality, consult a physician, especially if other sexual changes are also delayed—if your breasts and pubic hair have not yet begun to grow, for example. Failure to menstruate also is called amenorrhea, a word that combines the Greek negative prefix *a-* (the equivalent of the English un-) with *men*, for "month," and *rhoia*, meaning "flow." If you have never menstruated, the condition is called primary amenorrhea.

If you have been menstruating for years and suddenly you miss one or several periods, you have secondary amenorrhea. There are several possible explanations for this. You might be pregnant, perhaps you lost a lot of weight rather quickly or have been exercising a lot (see page 1150), or you may have been under stress. Very obese women sometimes fail to menstruate. You also may be taking a medication that suppresses menses as a side effect. If you just quit taking oral contraceptives, you may not have a period for several months. In addition, breastfeeding can delay menstruation, and if you are reaching the age of menopause (see page 1153), it would be normal to begin skipping periods.

Secondary amenorrhea due to such causes is quite common. More serious problems, such as tumors or disorders of the pituitary gland, also can cause amenorrhea, but they are rare (see Pituitary Gland Disorders, page 941). Failure to resume menstruation after childbirth, particularly if lactation does not take place either, may mean that the pituitary gland failed either partly or completely at the time of delivery, a condition called postpartum pituitary necrosis.

If you have been menstruating regularly and your period is more than 2 weeks late, you may want to perform a home pregnancy test or see your health care provider to find out whether you are pregnant. However, if you are sure you could not be pregnant and you have no other symptoms, there is no harm in waiting for 6 to 9 months before consulting a physician. Keep in mind, though, that even though you are not menstruating, you could still become pregnant if you do not take precautions.

Diagnosis

Whether you have primary or secondary amenorrhea, your physician may do a pelvic examination (see page 1141). He or she will check to see whether your vaginal walls seem moist and otherwise normal and will examine your cervical mucus, looking for signs that your ovaries are producing normal amounts of estrogen. Another way to determine your estrogen status is to have you take progesterone for a few days, and then wait to see whether you bleed from your vagina. Bleeding indicates that estrogen is not the problem, and your physician may want to check whether you have polycystic ovaries (see page 1191). If you do not bleed despite taking progesterone, your ovaries are probably secreting little or no estrogen and you may not be ovulating. Several disorders can suppress ovulation; blood tests and X-rays can help your physician determine the cause.

How Serious Is Amenorrhea?

Amenorrhea is seldom a sign that anything is seriously wrong. However, if you are not menstruating, you may find it difficult to become pregnant. If you do become pregnant, your physician will probably refer you to a specialist in infertility.

Treatment

Medication
Your physician may prescribe various types of hormones to see whether your ovaries are functioning normally.

Provided no underlying disorder is causing your amenorrhea, treatment is generally unnecessary. However, because women who are not menstruating seem susceptible to osteoporosis (see page 894), your physician may suggest that you take estrogen and a calcium supplement.

If an underlying disorder is to blame for either primary or secondary amenorrhea, your physician will prescribe an appropriate medication.

Infrequent Periods

Signs and Symptoms—Fewer menstrual periods than the usual 11 to 13 per year

Sports and Menses

Female ballet dancers, female joggers, and women who are involved in vigorous sports frequently find that they skip menstrual periods or stop menstruating altogether. This is more likely to happen if you are young, especially if your cycle is generally irregular. In fact, teenagers who train heavily are often in their late teens before they actually have their first menstrual period.

Medical experts believe that several factors are involved, including stress and perhaps the ratio of fat cells in your body to other cells (going on a crash diet and losing a lot of weight very rapidly also can interfere with menstruation). In both cases, you stop menstruating because your ovaries do not produce estrogen in the cyclic manner that causes the uterine lining to thicken and then shed (see page 1144).

If you reduce your exercise schedule or gain weight, you probably will begin to menstruate again. If that does not work—or if you do not want to exercise less or gain weight—your physician may suggest that you take estrogen in low doses. There is a good reason for this recommendation. If you are not producing normal amounts of estrogen you may be susceptible to osteoporosis (see page 894), a thinning of the bones that can make fractures more likely in later years.

Be aware, however, that you cannot simply forget about birth control just because your reproductive system seems to have shut down. You could ovulate at any time and be at risk for pregnancy.

Some women ovulate and menstruate normally but less often than most. This is called oligomenorrhea, a term that combines three Greek words: *oligo*, which means "few," *men*, for "month," and *rhoia*, for "flow."

It is normal to menstruate less frequently as you approach menopause. However, some women have infrequent menses all their adult lives—no one knows exactly why. Occasionally, a woman not nearing menopause begins to menstruate infrequently and at the same time develops acne and an unusual amount of hair on her face and body; the problem may be an excess of androgen, produced either by her adrenal gland or by a tumor of the ovary (see Adrenal Gland Disorders, page 937, and Idiopathic Hirsutism, page 940).

Diagnosis

Your physician will take a careful history, do a pelvic examination (see page 1141), and is likely to order blood and urine tests to measure levels of various hormones.

How Serious Is Oligomenorrhea?

In most cases oligomenorrhea presents no danger to your health and requires no treatment. However, if you menstruate infrequently and find you cannot become pregnant, you may need to see a specialist in infertility.

Treatment

Medication

If the cause of your oligomenorrhea is that your ovaries are producing too little estrogen, your physician may prescribe an estrogen to compensate. This treatment will restore normal menstruation and help prevent osteoporosis (see page 894).

If the cause of your problem is too much androgen, treatment will be dictated by findings concerning the underlying causes (see Adrenal Gland Disorders, page 937).

Heavy Periods

Signs and Symptoms

- Menstrual periods that last longer than 7 days
- Periods in which bleeding is unusually heavy

Heavy periods are common, especially in young women who are not yet ovulating regularly and in older women approaching menopause. However, any woman at any time in her reproductive life may experience heavy menstrual bleeding; some women have heavy periods almost every cycle. Menorrhagia, the medical term for heavy periods, is derived from the Greek words *men*, meaning "month," and *rhegnynai*, meaning "to burst forth." The disorder also is known as hypermenorrhea.

Often, heavy periods reflect some spontaneous disturbance of the hormone cycle. However, they also can be caused by fibroids (see page 1182), pelvic infection (see page 1187), or, rarely, endometriosis (see page 1185). An intrauterine device (IUD) used for birth control also can cause menorrhagia; when that happens, the IUD often has to be removed.

If your heavy period is a one-time occurrence and it arrives late, you could be having a miscarriage. Call a physician immediately. If the miscarriage is incomplete, you may need to have dilatation and curettage (D and C)—a minor operation in which the physician gently scrapes out the uterus (see page 1151)—

Dilatation and Curettage

Dilatation and curettage—generally referred to as a D and C—is a minor surgical procedure in which your physician first dilates your cervix and then inserts a thin, spoon-shaped instrument (curette) to scrape the lining of your uterus.

The opening to your cervix is normally tiny and tight. To dilate it during a D and C, a physician may insert a series of tapering rods, each thicker than the previous one, or stretch it with other types of instruments.

The traditional D and C involves scraping your uterine lining with a curette, a long, thin, spoon-shaped instrument. However, today physicians sometimes use vacuum aspiration—low-pressure suction—to remove endometrial tissue.

Your physician may use a D and C to diagnose a problem. If you have been menstruating too often or very heavily, your physician may be able to determine the cause by examining uterine scrapings under a microscope (see Heavy Periods, page 1150, and Dysfunctional Uterine Bleeding, page 1152). Sometimes the D and C itself cures the problem, temporarily or permanently. In addition, a D and C can help diagnose uterine fibroids (see page 1182), endometrial polyps (see page 1182), uterine cancer (see page 1183), and cervical cancer (see page 1180).

In addition to diagnosing certain problems, D and C can also be used to treat them. Your physician may remove endometrial polyps that protrude through your cervix during a D and C, and, very occasionally, scrape away fibroids, although this usually requires a major operation.

In addition, if you have had a miscarriage or an incomplete abortion, you may need to have the remaining uterine lining or products of conception scraped or suctioned away to prevent infection. Although the D and C used to be the standard method for early abortion, vacuum aspiration has largely replaced it (see page 199).

D and C can be done in a physician's office with a local anesthetic. However, sometimes physicians prefer to do the procedure in a hospital and use a general anesthetic; then your pelvic muscles relax completely and a more thorough examination is possible.

If you have a D and C done in a hospital, you generally can go home the same day or the next day. You may experience some vaginal bleeding for a few days afterward and may have some cramps or back pain, but you usually can resume normal activities almost immediately. However, you should not have sex or use tampons for a few weeks, until your cervix is once again normal and your endometrium is healed completely.

Although a D and C is a minor procedure, no operation is entirely without risk. In rare cases, infection or hemorrhage develops, your uterus or surrounding organs are perforated during the procedure, or complications develop due to the anesthesia.

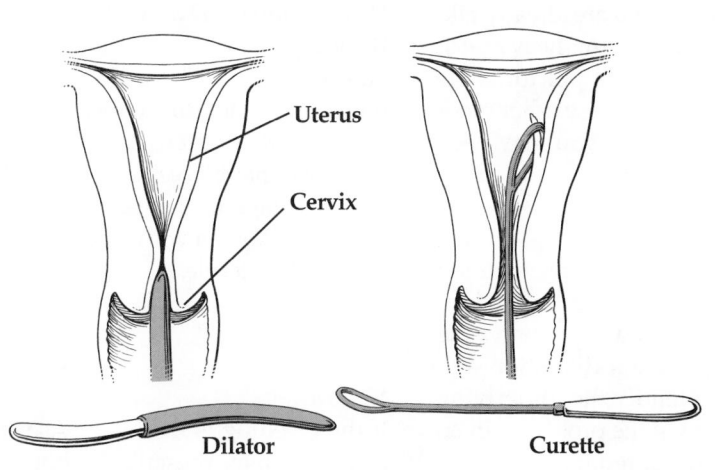

To perform a dilatation and curettage (D and C), your physician will start by using a series of surgical instruments called dilators. These tapering rods are used to open (dilate) the cervix. After dilation, your physician inserts another instrument, called a curette, which is used to scrape a small amount of tissue from the wall of the uterus.

or perhaps a simple suction procedure.

You probably do not need medical help if you have a single heavy period that is not late and you have no reason to think you were pregnant. In that case, simply reduce your activity until the bleeding eases. If it does not stop within 24 hours, call your physician.

If you have several heavy periods, see a physician to make sure that you are not developing iron-deficiency anemia from the loss of blood and that you have no underlying disorder.

Diagnosis

Your physician will do a pelvic examination (see page 1141) to check for abnormalities of your uterus. Your physician may also do a Pap test (see page 1181) and a biopsy of your cervix (see page 1332) or your endometrium. In addition, you might have a blood test to make sure you are not anemic and to check for signs of other problems that could be causing the heavy bleeding. If you are anemic, your physician will evaluate other sources of blood loss.

How Serious Is Menorrhagia?

Menorrhagia is inconvenient, and it can be distressing. However, there is rarely any serious underlying disorder, although you do have to be careful not to become anemic.

Treatment

Medication

If you are young and your uterus is in normal condition, the physician will probably prescribe estrogen or progesterone or both, often in the form of birth control pills, to reduce the bleeding. If you are already taking the pill and are still having heavy periods, or you cannot take the pill for some reason, your physician may use other medications. If you are anemic, you may need iron tablets.

Surgery

If you are older or if you are a young woman but after a few months on medication you are still having heavy periods, your physician may schedule a dilatation and curettage to try to identify the underlying disorder that is causing the problem. Even if the dilatation and curettage (see page 1151) does not establish the cause, it often stops the heavy bleeding. As a last resort, if other means fail, your physician may recommend a hysterectomy.

Dysfunctional Uterine Bleeding

Signs and Symptoms—Vaginal bleeding that occurs at irregular intervals and is unpredictable in amount or duration

Dysfunctional uterine bleeding is usually painless. The term itself means a benign cause of irregular bleeding. It happens most often in girls who have just begun to menstruate, in women approaching menopause, or as a consequence of stress or illness. In most cases, the uterine lining has overdeveloped because the ovaries are not producing hormones in the normal way.

When dysfunctional uterine bleeding is not due to life stage or stress, the underlying cause may be polycystic ovarian disease (see page 1191). Less frequently, the problem is an estrogen-producing ovarian tumor or abnormal estrogen metabolism due to liver disease. However, if you have been taking a medication that contains estrogen, that could be to blame.

Diagnosis

Your physician will want to take a careful menstrual history and do a pelvic examination (see page 1141) to make sure the source of the bleeding is actually your uterus and not your bladder, vagina, or cervix. Your physician also will try to determine whether an ectopic pregnancy or an early miscarriage could cause the bleeding.

How Serious Is Dysfunctional Uterine Bleeding?

Your physician will treat bleeding that continues and is not due to menarche or menopause. Medication can usually control dysfunctional bleeding; if not, a dilatation and curettage (see page 1151) generally is effective. Women with chronic bleeding are frequently infertile.

Treatment

Medication

If the bleeding is moderately severe, your physician may prescribe a short course of oral contraceptives containing a relatively high dose of estrogen. If the problem is severe, you may require hospitalization, bed rest, and injections of estrogen or progesterone. After this treatment, you may need iron replacement if you have become anemic, and you may take oral contraceptives for several months to prevent a recurrence.

Surgery

If hormone therapy fails to control the bleeding, your physician may recommend an endometrial biopsy or a dilatation and curettage to determine the cause of bleeding. In fact, the dilatation and curettage sometimes solves the problem.

Menopause

Signs and Symptoms

- Hot flashes: a sudden reddening of the face associated with a feeling of warmth
- Painful intercourse, due to a gradual thinning of vaginal tissues and lessening of lubrication
- Nervousness, depression, irritability, insomnia
- Much later, back pain and brittle bones due to osteoporosis
- No signs or symptoms

Menopause is a natural stage of life (see page 1144). In the simplest terms, it is a transition from the time when you menstruated and could have children to the time when you no longer experience the monthly menstrual flow and can no longer become pregnant. In technical terms, it happens when the ovaries no longer produce enough estrogen to properly stimulate the lining of your uterus and vagina.

Menopause comes naturally to most women at some time between ages 40 and 55 years. Once you are in mid-life, you will suspect you are approaching menopause when your periods become irregular and unpredictable. You may menstruate more often or less often; you may skip some periods altogether; you may have shorter periods or longer and heavier ones. Perhaps one-third of all women experience no such irregularities—one day they simply stop menstruating. However, for most women, menopause is a gradual process that takes anywhere from several months to several years as the ovaries produce less and less estrogen. Estrogen is still produced elsewhere in your body, but the total amount available decreases dramatically around the time of menopause. Finally, the amount of estrogen is so low that it can no longer stimulate your endometrium to proliferate and grow, at which point you reach menopause.

Medically, the word menopause simply means the permanent end of menstruation. It is derived from the Greek words for "month" (*men*) and "cessation" (*pausis*). Literally, menopause occurs when you menstruate for the last time, though in popular use the word generally refers to a period of several years, from your first menstrual irregularities to the time when your body has adjusted completely to hormonal changes.

Although girls in this country have been reaching menarche at younger ages than previous generations did, the onset of menopause has been occurring somewhat later in life. It is not unusual now for a woman to be menstruating in her mid-50s. However, the median age at the last menstruation is 50 to 51 years. Because a woman's life expectancy may be almost 80 years, about a third of her life is likely to occur after menopause.

The dramatic decrease in estrogen levels that leads to menopause is responsible for hot flashes and vaginal changes. Hot flashes happen when blood vessels dilate. Some women experience very mild flashes (or flushes, as they are also called), but others are extremely uncomfortable during flashes. If you are in the latter group, you may wake up drenched with perspiration many times in the course of a night. During the day, you may feel conspicuous and embarrassed when flashes strike, because you feel your face heat up and you begin to perspire. It helps to remember that most of the time the flashes produce only a slight change in skin color and go unnoticed by others.

To some degree, all women experience gradual vaginal changes during menopause. A thinning of vaginal tissues and a lessening of lubrication may mean that intercourse becomes painful. If sex does become uncomfortable, a water-soluble lubricating jelly should solve the problem. Another result of vaginal changes and a parallel thinning of tissues in the urinary tract is that you may become more susceptible to both vaginal and urinary infections.

Osteoporosis can be a more serious problem. It is a disorder common in old age in which your bones become porous and brittle (see Bone Diseases, page 894).

A small percentage of women develop emotional problems during menopause that seem to be linked to hormonal changes. However, the connection is difficult to prove or disprove, because mid-life can be a difficult time for both women and men—children leave home, a spouse may die, parents may be in poor health or may die. Any of these changes can trigger the kind of depression and anxiety that sometimes are attributed to menopause.

However, menopause also can affect your physical and mental health in positive ways. For instance, if you have migraine headaches or endometriosis, the symptoms may disappear after menopause, and fibroids usually shrink (see pages 1185 and 1182). In addition, you no longer need to worry about becoming pregnant. Often, relationships can be enhanced by fewer family demands.

Diagnosis

You may want to see a physician to get relief from hot flashes and other concerns of menopause or because you have skipped a period and want to be sure you are not pregnant. In these cases, your physician will also probably take a history, do a pelvic examination, and—if appropriate—do a pregnancy test.

Because you may still be ovulating, your physician undoubtedly will advise you to continue to use birth control for a time even after you appear to have stopped menstruating.

How Serious Are the Concerns Associated With Menopause?

Most menopausal problems are not considered serious, because they do no harm and they are self-limiting. If you do nothing about them, they will go away of their own accord within a couple of months or a couple of years. However, associated problems such as osteoporosis and arteriosclerotic heart disease can be debilitating and potentially fatal (see Osteoporosis, page 894).

Treatment

Medication

Estrogen replacement therapy can relieve hot flashes and halt the thinning of vaginal tissue temporarily; it also may delay the progression of osteoporosis.

Estrogen replacement therapy was popular during the 1970s, until researchers linked it to a slightly increased risk of cancer of the lining of the uterus (endometrial cancer). Today, the treatment has changed. It generally involves the lowest effective dose of estrogen (for example, 0.625 milligram of Premarin daily) combined with progestin, because studies show that adding progestin reduces the risk of endometrial cancer. Typically, estrogen replacement therapy involves taking tablets of estrogen for the first 11 to 15 days of every month and then taking estrogen and progestin together for about 10 days. Then you stop taking both medications and have vaginal bleeding for several days. Women who take this therapy to relieve hot flashes and vaginal problems generally continue to do so for many years. Some physicians now use progestin during

the first 10 to 12 days of the month rather than mid-month to the end. Some physicians use continuous therapy (daily progestin and Premarin). You can discuss the options with your physician.

Some medical experts would like to see estrogen therapy more widely used to prevent osteoporosis. Others urge caution because of the potential dangers involved. Many physicians think that you should seriously consider estrogen replacement therapy if you are especially at risk for developing osteoporosis. You are at risk if you are small-boned or thin, smoke, drink alcohol, or come from northern European stock, especially if someone in your immediate family, such as your mother or an aunt, has had osteoporosis.

Most physicians strongly recommend estrogen replacement therapy for women who went through menopause prematurely. Menopause is considered premature if you stopped menstruating before the age of 40 years, either naturally or because your ovaries were surgically removed (see Hysterectomy, page 1184).

Estrogen replacement has a beneficial effect in the prevention of cardiovascular disease by increasing your HDL cholesterol and reducing your LDL cholesterol (see page 639). If you already have coronary artery disease, estrogen can reduce your risk of a heart attack.

While you are taking estrogen, be sure to have a mammogram yearly (see page 1165). Each year you should also have a gynecologic examination that includes a Pap smear.

Physicians occasionally may use megestrol acetate as an alternative treatment for hot flashes. This medication can reduce the frequency and severity of hot flashes.

For the emotional problems that sometimes occur during mid-life, treatment depends on your specific symptoms. Possible treatments include antidepressants for severe depression, occasional use of sleeping pills for temporary insomnia, and psychotherapy when it is appropriate. Estrogen replacement is sometimes effective for relieving emotional problems.

Nutrition and Exercise

To prevent osteoporosis, you need a diet rich in sources of calcium, such as milk and some green vegetables. A woman should have at least 1,000 milligrams of calcium a day. Most physicians who prescribe estrogen replacement therapy to prevent osteoporosis also advise their patients to take calcium, either in pills or in their diet. In addition, they suggest regular exercise, because there is evidence that weight-bearing exercise, such as walking and jogging, can slow bone loss. Exercise also may yield a feeling of well-being (see page 894).

Postmenopausal Bleeding

Signs and Symptoms—Vaginal bleeding that occurs a year or more after your final menstrual period

If you suddenly begin to bleed unexpectedly from your vagina after menopause, there are many possible explanations. You may have developed a vaginal infection, or you might occasionally bleed a bit after intercourse or from douching, just because the walls of your vagina are thinner and more fragile (see page 1153).

Estrogen and progestin, taken as medications, can cause bleeding. Because cancer of the endometrium (see page 1183) also can be a cause of bleeding, you should see a physician as soon as possible.

Diagnosis
Your physician will do a pelvic examination (see page 1141). His or her first concern will be to establish the source of the blood because it could be from almost anywhere in your reproductive tract, including your uterus and its lower part, your cervix, or your vagina. It could even be coming from your urinary tract or rectum.

If it appears that you are bleeding from your vagina, your physician will probably want to do a Pap smear (see page 1181), an endometrial biopsy, and perhaps a vaginal ultrasound test. If any of the tests are abnormal, your physician may do a cervical biopsy or a uterine dilatation and curettage (or both) to further evaluate the source of bleeding. Both are minor surgical procedures. During a cervical biopsy, a small piece of tissue is cut from your cervix; in a dilatation and curettage, your physician will scrape the inner walls of your uterus (see page 1151). If a uterine cancer or other abnormality is found, a hysterectomy will be done.

Sometimes, even after exhaustive study, a physician cannot find any explanation for an episode of postmenopausal bleeding. If the bleeding never recurs, there is no reason for concern, but if it happens again, you will need to be reexamined.

How Serious Is Postmenopausal Bleeding?
It can be trivial, or extremely serious, or anything in between, depending on what causes the bleeding.

Treatment
Treatment depends on the underlying disorder. For example, if the tissue lining your vagina has become fragile, your physician may prescribe a vaginal cream or suppository that contains estrogen. Physicians generally treat vaginal infections with antibiotics. If you have cancer, you may need an operation, radiation, chemotherapy, or some combination of these treatments.

Primary Ovarian Failure

Signs and Symptoms
- First menstrual period has not occurred by age 16
- Breasts and pubic hair may not have developed
- Genitals may not look normal

Because of chromosome abnormalities, some girls are born without all the usual internal or external organs of their sex. Sometimes this is noticeable at birth, but often the first clue is that the girl does not begin menstruating at puberty. She may or may not develop breasts and pubic hair, depending on the nature of her genetic problem.

One-third of the girls who fail to menstruate have a disorder called gonadal dysgenesis (abnormal ovaries). There are several different types of gonadal dysgenesis, but the most common—it occurs in 1 of every 2,500 female newborn babies—is Turner's syndrome. A teenage girl with Turner's syndrome is very short, her body is childlike in appearance, her breasts have not developed, and she has little or no pubic or underarm hair. Her internal reproductive organs are also childlike, and her ovaries are simply streaks of fiber with no follicles or ova; these are known as streak gonads.

Complete testicular feminization is another congenital problem that may result in a failure to menstruate. At puberty, the girl develops breasts but little or no pubic or underarm hair. Her genitals appear to be normal, but her vagina is short and she has no cervix; some girls have no vagina at all. She has no uterus, ovaries, or fallopian tubes; instead, somewhere in her abdominal cavity, she has undescended testicles. She is generally feminine in her behavior and outlook. The undescended testicles are slightly at risk as a site for cancer.

Diagnosis

When girls reach their late teens without menstruating, most often they are simply late in developing (see page 1148). However, if a physician has reason to think congenital problems might be involved, these problems will be checked, because hormone treatment can make a great difference in many such cases. The physician will do a pelvic examination (see page 1141) and may order blood tests to measure circulating hormones. Because the physician will want to know exactly which chromosomes are abnormal, chromosome studies are often helpful.

A physician also can learn more about the status of the ovaries by prescribing a course of the female sex hormone progesterone. If the ovaries are producing estrogen, a course of progesterone will induce bleeding from the uterus; this is called withdrawal bleeding. This bleeding also implies that the uterus has an endometrium (lining) that can be stimulated.

How Serious Is Primary Ovarian Failure?

It can be serious because of the risk of cancer. In some cases of primary ovarian failure, enough of the ovary is normal for the girl to menstruate occasionally and eventually to conceive, but most often she never menstruates and is infertile. However, if she is treated at puberty with female sex hormones, she will develop breasts and all the usual secondary sex characteristics. This will also protect her to a considerable extent from developing osteoporosis.

Treatment

Medication

Physicians generally prescribe estrogen and progesterone to develop and maintain secondary sex characteristics.

Surgery

Specialists advise removal of any testicular tissue if the chromosome abnormality that produced them is the sort (testicular feminization) that predisposes them to cancer. Surgery also can correct the appearance of

external genitals that are sexually ambiguous or even create a vagina that will be functional for purposes of intercourse but not reproduction.

Abnormalities of the Hypothalamus, Thyroid, Pituitary, Adrenal Glands, and Ovaries

Signs and Symptoms—Disruption of menstrual periods

A complex cascade of hormones governs the menstrual cycle. The hypothalamus, which is a part of your brain, sends chemicals called releasing factors directly to your pituitary gland; your pituitary then releases pituitary hormones (called gonadotropins), which travel through your bloodstream to your ovaries, where they cause ovarian follicles to produce estrogen and progesterone (for more details, see Pituitary Gland Disorders, page 941). Estrogen and progesterone prepare your uterus for a possible pregnancy. Things can go wrong at any stage in this process.

Menstrual irregularity may have various causes: problems in the hypothalamus, a part of your brain that can be affected by illness; drug abuse; a drastic loss of weight; or stress. More rarely, your hypothalamus develops a disorder such as a tumor or infection that affects menstruation.

If your pituitary gland stops producing its hormones, your ovaries are the first organs to be affected. When a young girl fails to develop sexually, it may be either because her pituitary is not producing enough gonadotropins or because of ovarian failure (see page 1155). Sometimes the pituitary produces too much of the hormone prolactin, either in reaction to certain drugs, such as tranquilizers and oral contraceptives, or—very rarely—because of a pituitary tumor. Prolactin helps prevent pregnancy while a woman is breastfeeding; released in excess at other times, it can prevent ovulation and menstruation (see Galactorrhea, page 1162).

Sometimes, your ovaries themselves develop cysts or tumors and fail to release their hormones in normal amounts (see page 1189). Your menstrual cycle also can be disrupted by disorders of your thyroid gland (see Thyroid Disorders, page 945). If your thyroid is overactive, you may stop menstruating or have scanty periods; if it is underactive, menstruation can be prolonged and heavy and you also may lose interest in sex. Changes in your adrenal glands also can cause changes in menstrual patterns, which medication may correct.

Diagnosis

Your physician will want to do a general physical examination and a pelvic examination (see page 1141). Blood tests can measure the levels of various hormones circulating in your blood. If pituitary hormones seem to be present in normal amounts, for example, but you show signs of estrogen deprivation, such as a thinning of the vaginal walls, the problem may be with your ovaries. Blood tests can identify adrenal problems, or scans can check for tumors. Your physician can use a laparoscope, a thin, tube-like instrument equipped with a light (see page 1346), to look for ovarian cysts.

How Serious Are These Abnormalities?

Some abnormalities, such as malignant tumors, are serious. Others are not—for example, menstrual irregularity that is simply a reaction to stress or to tranquilizers that you have been taking.

Treatment

Medication

The treatment used depends on the underlying problem. If your body is not producing a hormone in the normal way, you often can receive it as a medication—estrogen, for example, or a thyroid hormone for hypothyroidism.

Surgery

If the basic disorder is a tumor, you will probably need surgery or radiation.

Problems of the Breast

Normal Breast

From the time a woman reaches puberty until after menopause, her breasts change continually as her hormones fluctuate. At puberty, when your body begins to produce estrogen in quantity, your breasts rapidly develop both stroma—a framework of connective tissue—and a system of glands and ducts. However, it is the fat cells that are deposited at the same time that provide the bulk of your breast tissue.

From puberty on, your breasts change every month, growing larger over the course of your menstrual cycle. During the first half of the cycle, your ovaries release estrogen, which causes new cells to grow in glands, ducts, and other breast tissue, and more blood flows to your breasts. During the second half of the cycle, glands in your breasts are bombarded with progesterone as well as estrogen, and they begin to secrete substances that are the precursors of breast milk. If you do not become pregnant, your hormone levels decrease, your body absorbs both the secretions and the new cells, and the blood supply to your breasts diminishes.

Some women's breasts become painfully engorged toward the end of their menstrual cycles (see Premenstrual Tenderness and Swelling, page 1158). Others have cysts in their breasts that enlarge at that time (see page 1158). Birth control pills also can cause breast tenderness and swelling as side effects, although these are not problems for most women who take them.

During pregnancy, your breasts enlarge considerably—together, they may gain as much as a pound. Your duct system, stimulated by hormones produced by the placenta and the pituitary gland, grows and branches. More cells are laid down in the stroma, and fat cells are added. Your nipple and areola are apt to grow larger and, in light-skinned women, to become darker; these changes are often permanent.

Once a baby is born, other hormones affect your breasts. Milk production is regulated by prolactin, which is produced by your pituitary gland. When your baby is weaned and breast stimulation ends, prolactin production eases off, the flow of breast milk ceases, and eventually your breasts return to their normal size and condition.

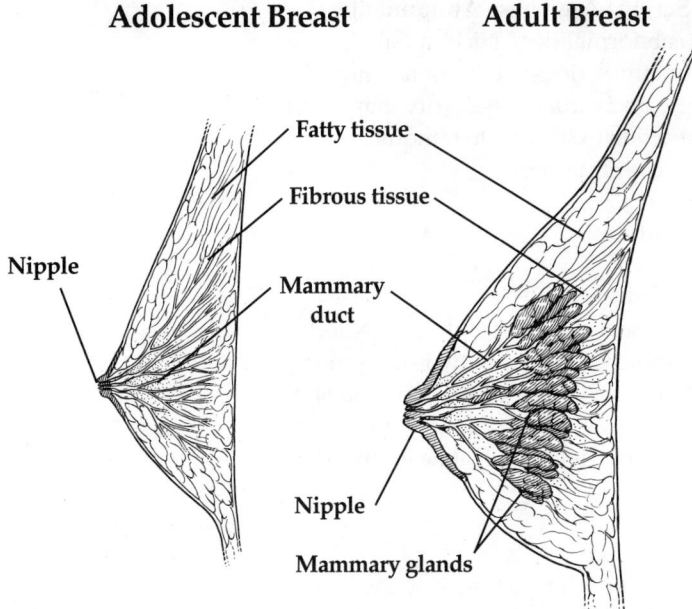

Adolescent Breast   **Adult Breast**

Fatty tissue

Fibrous tissue

Nipple

Mammary
duct

Nipple

Mammary glands

During puberty, the
normal breast rapidly
develops fibrous tissue
(stroma). The adult
breast has more fatty
tissue. The breast
changes in response to
monthly variations in
hormone levels.

At menopause, the breast changes that
accompanied your menstrual cycle cease.
Some problems, such as cystic breast lumps,
diminish or disappear. However, the likelihood of breast cancer increases. Diagnosing
it early makes a big difference. For that reason, examine your breasts once a month at
every age, but especially after menopause
(see Breast Self-Examination, page 1160). At
age 40, begin having mammography (see
page 1165), and after age 50, have an annual
mammogram.

Premenstrual Tenderness and Swelling

Signs and Symptoms—Breasts that are
swollen and painful just before menstrual
periods

Just as your uterine lining thickens each
month in preparation for a possible pregnancy, over the course of the month your
breasts develop new cells in their glands and
ducts to prepare for breastfeeding (see page
1162). Thus, in the week or so before you
menstruate, your breasts enlarge. For some
women the change is extreme and uncomfortable.

Breast engorgement is one of the symptoms of premenstrual syndrome (see page
1147). No one knows exactly what causes
this syndrome, but it may be related to hormonal changes that take place toward the
end of your menstrual cycle.

Diagnosis

Your physician may ask you to keep a record
of all your premenstrual symptoms for a few
months, noting particularly the day on
which your breasts become uncomfortable,
the day your discomfort ends, and the day
your period starts. Although it can be
painful, premenstrual breast tenderness is
not considered serious.

Treatment

Medication

Your physician may prescribe a diuretic. It
can be taken for the last 10 days before the
onset of your period or for 1 or 2 days before
your symptoms usually appear.

Self-Help

You may feel more comfortable if you cut
down on salt intake at the end of your cycle,
because salt causes tissues to retain more
fluid, which makes engorgement worse.
Some women find that it also helps to avoid
caffeine, sugar, and alcohol. A comfortable
brassiere, worn 24 hours a day, may help too.

Lumps in the Breast

Signs and Symptoms
- One or more lumps in your breasts, which
  may or may not be painful
- A greenish or straw-colored discharge
  may be expressed from your nipples

The vast majority of breast lumps are not
malignant. Nevertheless, some are, so if you
find a lump, call your physician. If it is late
in your menstrual cycle, you may prefer to
wait a few days, because the lump may disappear after menstruation, which would
indicate that it is a harmless cyst.

Cysts are produced by a benign condition
called fibroglandular changes. (It is also
sometimes called fibrocystic changes, chronic
cystic mastitis, mammary dysplasia, or
benign breast disease.) A cyst is a fluid-filled
sac that tends to get bigger toward the end of
your menstrual cycle, when your body is
retaining more fluid. Some cysts are very
tiny, but others can be as large as a hen's egg.
If pressed, the large ones may change shape
slightly, and they can be moved about a bit
under the skin.

No one knows what causes cysts. Because
they generally disappear after menopause,

ovarian hormones are probably involved. You are most likely to develop fibrocystic changes between the ages of 25 and 50 years, with one lump or several located in both breasts.

Breast lumps that are not cysts and are not cancer are most likely to be fibroadenomas (or adenofibromas), benign tumors that most often are found in young women. A fibroadenoma has a firm, smooth, rubbery feeling and a well-defined shape. It can be moved about under the skin.

There are also other types of lumps. An infection can produce a lump (see page 1160), as can severe injury. A lump could also be a lipoma—a tumor of the fatty tissues. It may be an intraductal papilloma (see page 1163), especially if it is blocking a duct, which would cause a cyst. None of these conditions are malignant.

Diagnosis

Your physician's chief concern will be to make sure the lumps in your breast are not cancer. If you have a single lump that feels like a cyst, your physician may try to aspirate its fluid contents by using a thin needle. This can be done in the physician's office or under the guidance of ultrasound, and you may not even need a local anesthetic. If the fluid can be aspirated, the lump will disappear, an indication that it was a cyst. The fluid can be sent to a laboratory to be analyzed for signs of malignancy if it is bloody or appears abnormal.

If a lump does not feel like a cyst, or if your physician is unable to draw out any fluid, your physician may recommend a mammogram, a special breast X-ray (see page 1165). Ultrasonography is often useful (see page 1335). A lump that refuses to yield fluid may still be a cyst.

If ultrasonography shows a solid area rather than a hollow cyst, the next step is a biopsy to remove some or all of the lump and examine it under a microscope. A needle biopsy, which removes a very small core of tissue, can be done in your physician's office with local anesthesia. A stereotaxic biopsy, performed by radiologists with local anesthesia in an outpatient setting, is an important newer method of obtaining tissue for microscopic examination. A surgical biopsy, removing the whole lump, is another way to determine the nature of the lump. A surgical biopsy is done in a hospital, with either local or general anesthesia.

Normal Breast　　**Breast With Cysts**

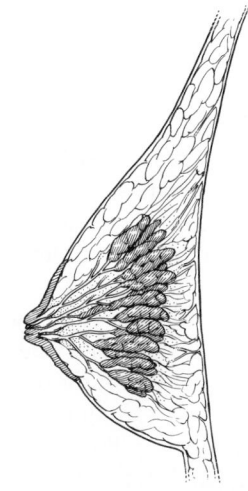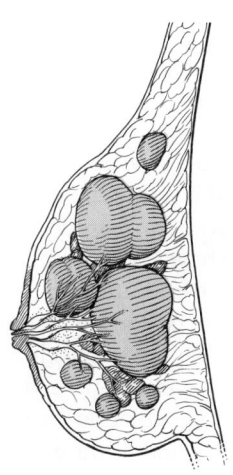

How Serious Are Breast Lumps?

If they are not malignant, they are not harmful beyond occasional discomfort. According to some recent studies, if you have fibrocystic changes you are not more likely to develop breast cancer than anyone else. (Older studies suggested a slightly increased risk.) However, women with lumpy breasts may have more trouble detecting a malignant tumor, should one develop.

Treatment

Medication

Many women prefer to take mild analgesics, such as aspirin or ibuprofen, and otherwise tolerate the discomfort. Good breast support with a well-fitted bra, worn even at night, is also effective. Danazol and bromocriptine relieve breast pain for many women, but both can have unpleasant side effects and are expensive. Some women say vitamin E helps, but there is no solid evidence that it works.

Surgery

Your physician may aspirate cysts to ensure that they are simple cysts or to relieve pain; otherwise, they need not be removed or treated unless they recur or enlarge after aspiration. Fibroadenomas and other benign tumors may be left, or they can be removed if they are large or uncomfortable.

Nutrition

If you smoke or if you drink caffeinated substances, you may want to cut down or quit altogether. Although the evidence is inconclusive, some women have reported that their lumps subsided after they stopped smoking or gave up caffeine.

Breast Self-Examination

Although 75 percent of all breast lumps are benign, some are not. Thus, regular self-examination can save your life, because breast cancer is curable if it is caught early.

Examine your breasts once a month. If you have not yet reached menopause, the best time is a few days after your period ends, because your breasts are less likely to be tender or swollen then. If you are no longer menstruating, pick a day of the month and do the examination regularly on that day.

Stand in front of a mirror. With your arms at your sides, look at the skin on your breasts for any sign of puckering, for dimples, or for changes in the size or shape of your breasts. If your nipples are not normally inverted, look to see whether they are now pushed in. Rest your hands on your hips, then place them behind your head; in each position, check for the same signs.

Next, step into the shower and, once your breasts are wet and soapy, place your left hand behind your head and examine your left breast with your right hand. Think of your breast as the face of a clock, and place your right hand at 12 o'clock, at the top of the breast. Hold your hand flat, fingertips pressed together, and make a tiny circling motion, feeling for lumps. Move your hand to 1 o'clock, to 2 o'clock, and so on. Once you return to 12, slide your fingertips closer to your nipple and repeat the motions you just went through, going around the clock in a circle within the first circle; then make an even smaller circle. Continue until you have checked the tissue under

your nipple; look for discharge from your nipple at that time. Finish by examining the area adjacent to your breast, below your armpit, because it also contains breast tissue. Repeat the whole procedure using your left hand on your right breast.

In addition, examine your breasts while you are lying on your back. Again look for nipple discharge. To examine your right breast, put a pillow under your right shoulder and place your right hand under your head. To examine your left breast, place the pillow under your left shoulder and your left hand under your head.

If your breasts are normally lumpy because of fibrocystic changes (see Lumps in the Breast, page 1158), you will want to make a note of how many lumps you have, where they are located, and their approximate size. Then, with each self-examination, you can check for changes.

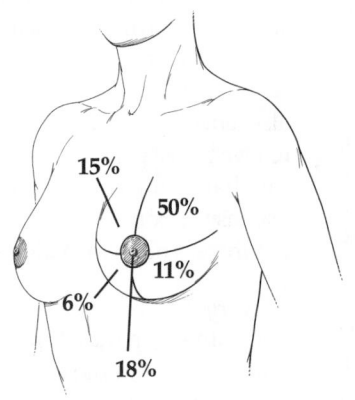

Cancer develops more frequently in some areas of the breast than others.

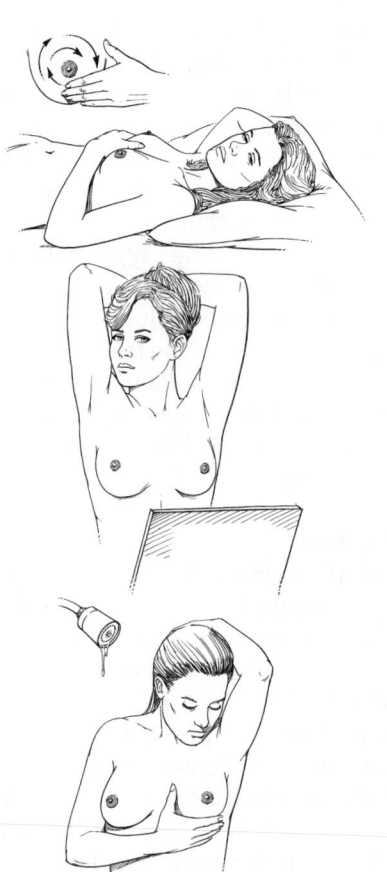

Use your eyes and hands to search for lumps, thickened areas, or swelling in your breasts. While lying and standing, a circular massaging motion is appropriate (see top and bottom illustrations). Both are necessary for a complete exam. Soap and water during a shower can facilitate the procedure. At center: Looking in a mirror also can help. Elevate your arms and look for changes in the natural symmetry of both breasts. Also note any unusual discharge from your nipples.

Breast Infections

Signs and Symptoms
- A red, tender, painful swelling or lump in your breast
- Swelling of the nearby glands in your armpit
- Fever (rare)

Breast infections, sometimes called mastitis, are not uncommon in women who are nursing a baby or who recently have stopped breastfeeding. Such infections are caused by bacteria that enter your breast. If the infection is severe, it can become an abscess. Surrounding tissues protect themselves by secreting a substance that hardens into a kind of wall around the infection, and pus collects inside.

Diagnosis

In a woman who is breastfeeding, the symptoms listed above strongly suggest an infection. However, breast infections occasionally do develop in women who have not been breastfeeding. Because the symptoms are similar to those of a rare form of cancer, in such cases the physician will want to test carefully to rule out malignancy. This testing may include a mammogram, ultrasound, a needle biopsy, or a surgical biopsy (see pages 1164 and 1165).

How Serious Are Breast Infections?

Breast infections usually respond quickly to antibiotics. If they do not and an abscess forms, it can be drained.

Treatment

Prevention

If you are breastfeeding, keep your nipples clean and dry between feedings and do not wear clothing that irritates them.

Medication

Your physician will prescribe an antibiotic and perhaps an analgesic for pain and fever. If you are breastfeeding, continue breastfeeding. These drugs should have no harmful effects on either your milk supply or the baby. Getting adequate rest and increasing your intake of fluids also can help.

Surgery

Usually, the antibiotic is sufficient. If it is not, the abscess can be drained. Your physician may aspirate it with a needle or make a small incision at the edge of your areola to let the pus out. The incision leaves a minimal scar.

Nipple Problems

Signs and Symptoms

- Discharge from your nipple
- Nipple that is inverted, as if pulled in from below (only if newly inverted)
- Lumps in your areola (the area surrounding your nipple)
- Scaling of your nipple

It is always wise to pay attention to changes in your nipples. Although most often the

---

Yeast Infections

Yeast (*Candida*) is a fungal organism that may infect your nipples and breasts. You may experience pain in your nipple or breast, even when your baby is correctly positioned at your breast and sucking properly. The pain can be in one nipple or breast or in both.

Nipple symptoms include red, itchy, flaky skin on the nipple or areola. Cracked nipples that don't heal are suspect.

Symptoms in your breast may include a burning, throbbing pain during or after feeding sessions. Your baby may have no symptoms or may have thrush (see page 16) or a diaper rash.

Yeast outbreaks can occur after antibiotic treatment. See your health care provider for diagnosis and treatment.

---

cause is benign, it could be cancer.

If whitish or greenish fluid leaks from your nipples, it is probably breast milk, especially if it comes from both nipples (see Breastfeeding, page 215, and Galactorrhea, page 1162). If the fluid is greenish or straw-colored, it may be due to fibrocystic changes (see page 1158). A discharge that is dark red or black contains blood and may indicate a tiny, benign tumor growing in a milk duct (see page 1163), although breast cancer is a remote possibility.

Indented or retracted nipples are normal if you have had them since puberty. Later in life, if a previously normal nipple develops an indentation, it can be a sign of cancer.

Lumps in your areola are generally cysts, formed because oil glands have become blocked. If an infection develops, a cyst may become a boil.

Scaling of a nipple is usually due to benign changes. If it persists, a biopsy may be necessary to exclude an underlying cancer.

Diagnosis

If you have nipple discharge, your physician will want to examine your breasts and may get a sample of the discharge for laboratory analysis. To be sure no malignancy is involved, he or she may do other tests. For a newly retracted nipple or a bloody discharge, tests for cancer are definitely in order (see page 1163). Your physician's physical examination will likely identify a cyst or boil.

How Serious Are Nipple Problems?

Nipple discharge and retracted nipples are serious only when they are evidence of cancer. Cysts can be ignored unless they become infected, in which case antibiotics usually will solve the problem. If nipple scaling persists, see your physician.

Treatment

For boils, your physician probably will prescribe an antibiotic. Whether or not surgery is necessary depends on the underlying problem.

Galactorrhea

Signs and Symptoms

- Whitish or greenish discharge from your nipples, usually from both breasts
- May be accompanied by amenorrhea (missed menstrual period, see page 1148)

Normally, you produce breast milk only

Breastfeeding

Many women decide to breastfeed not only for the health benefit to their babies but also to optimize bonding. Breast milk is a substance of great biologic complexity. It provides your baby with unique protection against infections and allergies and stimulates the development of his or her immune system.

Colostrum is the sticky yellowish fluid secreted by the breast for the first several days after birth. Colostrum contains many hormones and antibodies that are of benefit to your baby. Then, after 3 to 5 days, your pituitary gland directs your breasts to produce mature milk, which contains essential nutrients. Your baby's suckling and removal of milk from your breasts subsequently sustain your milk production.

The flow of your breast milk is controlled by your let-down reflex. When your baby suckles, your nipples respond by sending sensory impulses to your brain. Your pituitary gland releases hormones (principally oxytocin) that travel in your bloodstream. When the hormones reach your breasts, they cause the cells surrounding your alveoli (the cavities where milk is produced) to contract, expressing milk into the ducts. Initially, this process may take several minutes. Once breastfeeding is established, the let-down reflex is easily triggered; often just the sound of the baby crying stimulates it.

Breastfeeding should be enjoyable for both you and your baby, but expect some temporary nipple tenderness as you begin. Don't expect pain. Pain is a sign that something is wrong. Make sure your baby's mouth is centered on the nipple area. Nipple damage can be avoided by properly positioning your baby at your breast.

You may experience a plugged milk duct when you breastfeed, or you may develop a breast lump that is hot and painful. For relief, try heat, rest, massage, and prolonged, frequent nursing.

Mastitis is a breast infection usually caused by bacteria on the skin. Symptoms may include fever, flu-like symptoms, and a painful, reddened area on the surface of your breast. For relief, increase fluids and rest and apply heat to the affected area. Also, notify your physician, who may prescribe antibiotic therapy.

Breastfeeding is recommended for your baby's first year. Weaning should be a gradual process (see page 216). Abrupt weaning can be difficult for you and your baby and can result in engorged breasts. Solid food, started at about 6 months, begins the gradual weaning process. Breast pumps can be used intermittently to allow for a normal lifestyle.

Prolactin, the hormone that helps prepare your breasts for breastfeeding, also offers some protection from pregnancy. However, it is wise not to rely on it for birth control. You may ovulate while breastfeeding even if you do not menstruate.

Nonlactating Breast   Lactating Breast

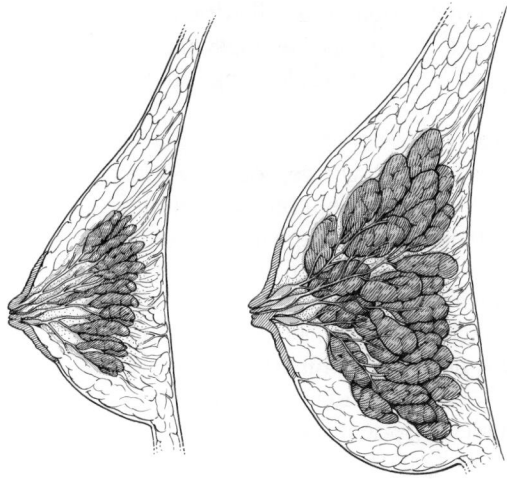

If you breastfeed, the system of ducts and glands within your breast expands as milk is produced (lactation).

after giving birth and perhaps for a few days before. If your nipples leak milk at other times, you have an unusual condition called galactorrhea (from the Greek words *gala*, for "milk," and *rhoia*, for "flow").

Galactorrhea is something of a mystery. Researchers report that in about 50 percent of the cases a cause cannot be found, and in 25 percent of the cases it is due to a type of pituitary tumor called a prolactinoma, which is usually benign but secretes prolactin, the hormone that regulates your production of breast milk (see Prolactinoma, page 942). In the remaining 25 percent of cases, galactorrhea has various causes—for instance, it can be a symptom of hypothyroidism or a side effect of a medication. Drugs that can cause galactorrhea include methyldopa (a medicine used for high blood pressure), phenothiazines (a category of tranquilizers), several types of antidepressants, and dextroamphetamine.

Diagnosis

Your physician will examine your breasts and the fluid they are producing to make sure it is not the bloody discharge that occasionally is associated with breast cancer (see this page). Your medical history will reveal whether the galactorrhea could be a side effect of some drug. If it is not, your physician will probably test for hypothyroidism (see page 948) and may want blood tests to check your prolactin level and a CT scan (a type of X-ray, see page 1334) of the hypothalamus and pituitary.

How Serious Is Galactorrhea?

Galactorrhea is no threat to your health unless it is caused by a pituitary tumor. Such tumors grow slowly and some eventually stabilize. They often can be treated successfully with medication; if that fails, your physician may use surgery or radiation.

Treatment

Medication
For hypothyroidism, thyroxine is prescribed. If you have a pituitary tumor or tests find no explanation for your galactorrhea, your physician may prescribe bromocriptine, which can shrink a tumor and reduce prolactin levels. Bromocriptine often cures galactorrhea even if it is of unknown origin.

Surgery
For a large pituitary tumor, surgery may be

necessary. Because such tumors tend to recur, you may need long-term treatment with bromocriptine or a course of radiation.

Intraductal Papilloma

Signs and Symptoms
- Watery or bloody discharge from your nipple
- A very small lump beneath your nipple

Intraductal papillomas are tiny, benign tumors that grow within the milk ducts of your breast at the point where they reach your nipple. Relatively uncommon, these tumors are often too small to feel.

Diagnosis
Your physician will go through the usual diagnostic procedure for breast lumps (see page 1158) to make sure you do not have breast cancer. He or she will apply gentle pressure in the areolar area to try to identify the duct containing the papilloma so that the duct can be excised with the tumor. Intraductal papillomas are benign but should be removed, because that is the only way to be sure the lump is a papilloma rather than a cancer.

Treatment

Surgery
If there is a palpable lump, a surgeon can remove it. When no lump is present, careful follow-up is necessary, including regular mammograms.

Cancers of the Breast

Signs and Symptoms
- A lump or thickening in your breast, which may not be painful or even tender
- Clear or bloody discharge from a nipple
- Retracted nipple
- A change in the contours of your breasts—one may be higher than the other, for example
- Any flattening or indentation of the skin of your breast
- Redness or pitting of your skin, like the skin of an orange

One of every nine women will develop breast cancer at some point in her life. Although the disease often can be treated

Breast cancer spreads (metastasizes) through your lymph system (shown here) and through your bloodstream.

successfully if it is caught early, breast cancer still kills more women than any other cancer except lung cancer.

Scientists do not know what causes breast cancer. However, studies have identified certain factors that make it more likely for a woman to develop the disease. You have a significantly higher risk than most women if your mother or sister had breast cancer, especially if she developed it while young or in both breasts. Your risk is somewhat increased if you have never had children or if you were older than 35 when you had your first child. Having cancer in one breast increases your chances of developing it in the other one. The risk of breast cancer also rises with age. Most cancers, however, develop in women who have no identifiable risk factors.

There is very little you can do to modify most of these risk factors. However, you can be alert for the symptoms listed above and be screened for breast cancer so a malignant tumor can be caught in its early stages. If you

are between 20 and 40 years old, have a physician examine you at least once every 3 years; if you are older than 40 years, have an examination once a year. Many cancer experts believe that women, particularly women who have risk factors for breast cancer, should have mammography every year or two (see page 1165), beginning in their 40s. Women older than 50 years should have mammography annually. Screening for breast cancer saves lives by discovering the cancer at an earlier and potentially curable stage.

Diagnosis

Your physician will examine your breasts carefully. He or she may also squeeze your nipple area gently to see whether there is any discharge and will feel your armpits for signs that your lymph nodes might be involved, because breast cancer can spread through the lymph system.

A mammogram is the next step. A suspicious lesion may correspond to a palpable lump. The mammogram may also reveal a suspicious area that does not correspond to a palpable lesion. Physicians cannot detect all breast cancers on a mammogram. As many as 10 percent go undetected.

If you have a breast lump that can be felt or is identified on a mammogram, your physician or radiologist may also obtain an ultrasound scan (see page 1335) to see if the lesion appears cystic (filled with fluid). Your physician may use a thin needle to try to draw fluid from it. The fluid can be analyzed for malignant cells. In addition, if the lump disappears after the fluid is withdrawn, the chances are that it is simply a cyst and of no concern (see Lumps in the Breast, page 1158).

A surgical biopsy, usually removing the entire lump, is the only way to be absolutely certain whether a lump is malignant. Your physician probably will advise such a biopsy if fluid cannot be drawn from the lump, if the lump does not collapse after the fluid has been drawn out, if the lump recurs, or if the fluid contains blood or malignant cells. Your physician may use a wire to localize an abnormality that is visible on a mammogram but not detectable to the touch.

You may have a needle biopsy of a particularly accessible lump in your physician's office with local anesthesia. Your physician probably will do a surgical biopsy in a hospital with local or general anesthesia. The surgeon removes the entire lump for microscopic and biochemical examination by the

Stereotaxic Breast Biopsy

In this new, nonsurgical procedure, your physician uses mammograms taken from different angles to calculate the exact location of a suspicious area. A computer then aligns a needle with the area, allowing a radiologist to remove a small amount of tissue.

Stereotaxic biopsy takes about 30 to 45 minutes under local anesthesia. It doesn't leave a scar, costs about one-third that of a surgical biopsy, and may be as accurate.

Mammograms

A mammogram is a special breast X-ray that can detect tumors so small that your physician cannot feel them. Mammography saves lives by identifying breast cancer at a stage when it is potentially still curable. However, the test is not infallible. Occasionally it fails to show a tumor, and at other times it indicates a problem when there is none. Screening by mammography is best combined with regular breast examinations done by your physician and with self-examination (see page 1160).

There is controversy within the medical profession about the age at which you should begin to have regular mammograms. Young women rarely develop breast cancer, and, in any case, their breasts are often so dense that they do not X-ray well.

Most medical experts agree that women younger than 35 who are not in a high-risk category need not have mammograms, and that women older than 50 should have them annually. Controversy has

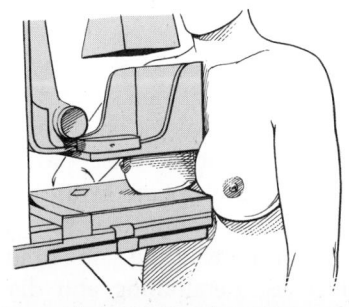

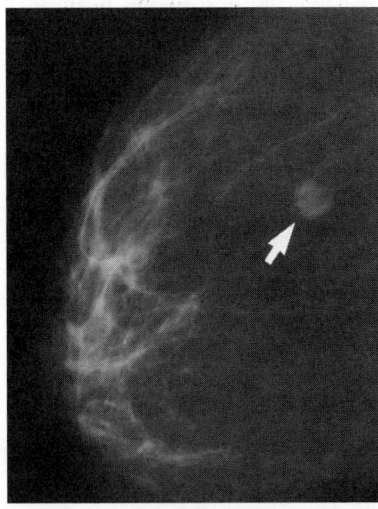

Arrow shows a breast cancer on a mammogram. Mammograms are produced by a special X-ray device (top) that can detect tumors before you or your physician can feel them.

centered on whether screening is necessary for women in their 40s and on whether a woman should have a baseline mammogram (to establish a norm for her breasts) at age 35. Recent studies indicate that regular mammograms do save lives among women in their 40s, but the value of the baseline X-ray remains questionable.

Today, this seems to be the best advice:

- If you are younger than 40, you do not need mammography unless you develop a problem or are in a high-risk category (for instance, if you have a family history of breast cancer).
- If you are between 40 and 49 and have a family history of breast cancer, have a mammogram once a year.
- If you are between 40 and 49, have no symptoms or self-found lumps, and have no family history of breast cancer, discuss your particular situation with your doctor.
- After the age of 50, have a mammogram annually.

pathologist. If the results are positive, the lump is malignant; if not, you will be told that it is benign. In more than 70 percent of biopsies, the lump is benign.

Researchers have recently identified the gene responsible for some types of breast cancer. This may bring physicians a step closer to earlier diagnosis of individuals at risk.

How Serious Is Breast Cancer?

Breast cancer itself is not lethal. The disease kills by metastasizing—that is, by spreading through your lymph system or bloodstream to other parts of your body. Thus, if breast cancer is caught early, while confined to your duct, while the tumor is small, and before malignant cells have spread to neighboring lymph nodes, there is a 90 to 95 percent chance of a cure. With the greater use of mammography, we can detect breast cancer at an earlier stage. Seventy-five percent of all women diagnosed with breast cancer are cured.

Treatment

Surgery

Surgery is the initial treatment for breast cancer (see Surgery for Breast Cancer, page 1166). Today, we often combine surgery with radiation therapy, hormone therapy, or chemotherapy.

In virtually every operation for breast cancer, your surgeon removes some lymph nodes from your armpit. Tests will look for signs of malignancy. The presence or absence of a malignant tumor in the lymph glands of your armpit is most important for planning treatment after the operation.

Radiation

If you elect and are a candidate for a breast conservation approach (lumpectomy), breast radiation is necessary. Occasionally, if you have had a mastectomy, radiation to your chest wall may be necessary after surgery to kill any cancer cells that may have escaped surgical removal. If the breast cancer has

Surgery for Breast Cancer

In many cases, routine mammography and heightened awareness among women and their physicians have contributed to earlier diagnosis of breast cancer. When discovered at its earliest stage, breast cancer is highly curable.

Surgery for breast cancer begins with confirmation of the abnormalities detected by your physical examination or mammogram. Your surgeon will obtain a tissue biopsy for microscopic examination and to determine hormone markers on tumor cells. Depending on the size, location, and mammographic appearance of the abnormality, this biopsy can take the form of a needle biopsy (core biopsy) or an open biopsy (requiring a small incision). More than 70% of all biopsies are benign.

If breast cancer is diagnosed, you and your physician must make a decision about your surgical options for treating the cancer. Your physician's advice will be based in part on the size of your tumor, its location, the type of cancer, and whether the malignancy seems to have spread or not. A discussion of the surgical options follows.

Radical Mastectomy

Radical mastectomy involves removing your entire breast, including a portion of skin containing your nipple and areola, as well as your underlying chest wall muscles. Your physician will also remove extensive lymph nodes underneath your armpit (axilla) to attempt to halt the spread of cancer. This operation, commonly performed until 20 years ago, is disfiguring and results in significant arm swelling (lymphedema) and diminished arm mobility. Surgeons seldom perform this today, except for large, locally advanced tumors invading large segments of your chest wall (pectoral) muscles.

Modified Radical Mastectomy

As physicians gained further insight into the biologic behavior of breast cancer, it became apparent that less radical operations are just as effective at treating the primary tumor and are, at the same time, much less debilitating and disfiguring. A modified radical mastectomy is similar to the old radical mastectomy, but your chest wall muscles are spared and many fewer lymph nodes are removed. Maintaining your chest wall (pectoralis) muscles facilitates prosthetic reconstruction, if you want this. We now know that cancer that has spread to your armpit (axillary) lymph nodes is more aggressive and will require additional treatment such as hormonal therapy or chemotherapy and possibly radiation to the area of your armpit. However, removing numerous lymph nodes (as compared to only 10 to 15 nodes) does not reduce your risk of death from breast cancer.

Breast Conservation Therapy

More recent investigations show that we can obtain cure rates similar to those of modified radical mastectomy by removing the tumor itself along with a small rim of normal breast tissue, if you then follow this treatment (lumpectomy, wide local excision) with a 4- to 6-week course of radiation to the lumpectomy site and the remaining breast tissue. Your physician will sample armpit (axillary) nodes through a separate small armpit incision, for the reasons previously outlined. This type of surgery is best suited for small breast cancers.

Simple Mastectomy

This operation is similar to modified radical mastectomy. However, in this procedure your surgeon intentionally does not remove your armpit (axillary) lymph nodes. This operation is most appropriate when your cancer is in multiple sites within your breast

Modified Radical Mastectomy

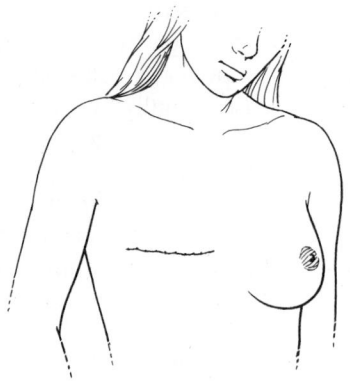

In a modified radical mastectomy your entire breast is removed, along with lymph nodes from your adjacent armpit. Chest muscles remain intact.

Breast Conservation Therapy

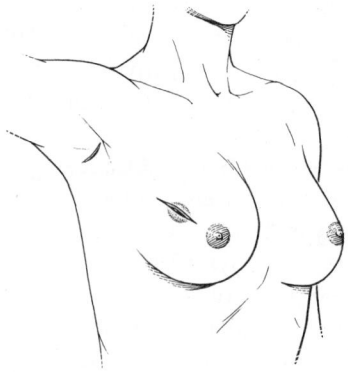

Breast conservation therapy preserves your breast following a lumpectomy and axillary node sampling, by radiating remaining breast tissue.

but not extending beyond the ducts themselves (carcinoma in situ). Here the risk of your cancer spreading to your lymph nodes is negligible. Some women elect to have a prophylactic (preventive) simple mastectomy because they are in a high risk group for developing breast cancer.

Subcutaneous Mastectomy
Your surgeon removes only your breast tissue, sparing your skin, nipple, areola, chest wall muscles, and lymph nodes. This is not a breast cancer operation and is primarily performed by plastic surgeons as a preventive (prophylactic) measure in persons at high risk for this disease. Surgeons couple this operation with the submuscular placement of an artificial breast prosthesis to reestablish your breast contour. Although this greatly reduces your risk of developing breast cancer, the risk is not zero, because some breast tissue remains attached to your overlying nipple. This region, however, is quite easy to examine on a regular basis.

Palliative Surgery
Lumpectomy alone, without radiation or subsequent mastectomy, may be appropriate if you have widespread cancer that has gone beyond the confines of your breast and armpit (bone, brain, liver). This procedure will at least confirm the diagnosis, provide tissue for laboratory analysis (hormone receptor studies), and may provide some degree of tumor control. When tumors are large and ulcerating, destroying your overlying skin, a simple mastectomy may provide relief from pain, infection, and bleeding, although such advanced tumors are generally incurable.

Breast Reconstruction
Today, many women undergoing mastectomy have breast reconstruction. Although controversy exists about the safety of prosthetic silicone implants, the FDA still approves the use of saline (saltwater)-filled silicone implants in post-mastectomy patients. Tens of thousands of women have had excellent results from such procedures with high satisfaction rates. If you are reluctant to have a prosthetic implant but still desire reconstruction, your surgeon may obtain excellent results shaping mounds from skin, fat, and muscle taken from your abdominal wall or chest. This is a much more formidable operation and is not possible for everyone. You can have either type of reconstruction at the time of your mastectomy or as a delayed procedure, depending on your and your physician's preference. In any case, it is not a good idea to use your own nipple for reconstruction following a mastectomy for cancer, as it may serve as a site for cancer recurrence. Plastic surgeons can readily reconstruct and pigment (tattoo) a new nipple and areola. Reconstruction does not interfere with chemotherapy or hormone therapy, nor does it hide recurrences or increase the likelihood that your cancer will recur.

Conclusion
It is important that you and your physician thoroughly discuss the options available for removing your cancer and reconstructing your breast. To help you make the best decisions, check out available reading materials, and if you are at all uncomfortable, request another opinion.

If you have had breast cancer surgery, several self-help groups can help you. Ask your physician to contact Reach to Recovery, a program of the American Cancer Society. Volunteers will visit you in the hospital to give you practical advice (exercises, bra prosthesis, etc.) and moral support.

Breast Reconstruction

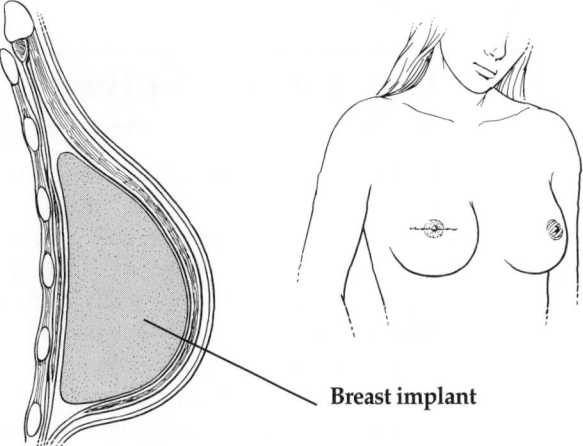

Breast implant

In breast reconstruction, your physician places a breast implant beneath your chest wall muscles. Your physician also can reconstruct your areola and nipple.

Swelling After Mastectomy

Most swelling associated with a mastectomy occurs in the first year after surgery. Be sure to check with your physician right away if you have swelling.

During surgery your physician removed breast tissue and, to see if the cancer had spread, lymph nodes in your armpit. The lymph nodes act as filters for fluid that normally "leaks" from blood vessels and cells. This fluid then travels through lymph channels to reenter your bloodstream. Removing the nodes can disrupt lymph drainage from your arm and cause swelling. In time, many of the lymph channels may re-form, and the swelling may diminish.

But it's important to check out any swelling, as it can also result from kidney or heart disease, an infection, or a return of the breast cancer.

spread to your bone, your physician may use radiation to relieve pain.

Hormone Therapy

After your surgery, your cancer specialist (oncologist) will determine whether you would benefit from additional therapy to prevent the growth of any breast cancer cells that might have spread but are undetectable. Some cancers respond to treatment with hormones—usually drugs that counteract estrogen. Physicians frequently use tamoxifen in this setting.

If your breast cancer recurs, your physician may use hormone therapy. Hormone therapy can stop a tumor from growing or actually cause it to shrink; it can give you a partial or complete remission. If one hormone stops working, another may help. In this way, physicians can frequently stall the disease for years. When hormones are no longer effective, your physician may try another approach, usually chemotherapy.

Chemotherapy

The anticancer drugs given in chemotherapy are more toxic than hormones but are beneficial for certain individuals with breast cancer. After your initial surgery, your oncologist will determine whether you will benefit from chemotherapy. The purpose of chemotherapy is to try to kill any breast cancer cells that might have spread outside your breast.

If your breast cancer has recurred, chemotherapy may stop tumor growth or cause shrinkage. This can slow the progress of your disease and relieve symptoms. Chemotherapy has unpleasant side effects: lowering of your white blood cell count, thus increasing the risk of infection; hair loss; nausea; and increase in fatigue. Physicians use various drugs in different combinations, depending on your prior treatment, overall health, and risk of side effects.

Vaginal and Vulvar Disorders

Your vagina is the passageway that connects your uterus to your external genitals. It is about 5 inches long and its walls are lined with strong muscles. Most of the time your vagina is so narrow that the walls touch, but it can expand dramatically. The neck of your uterus, the cervix, extends into your vagina at the upper end. In young girls, the other (outer) end is partially blocked by a thin membrane called the hymen. It is rare for a hymen to close off the vagina altogether. The membrane is sometimes semicircular and covers just part of your vaginal opening, or if it is circular it generally has at least one hole in it.

The area of the external genitals is called the vulva (see page 1141). They include the mons pubis, a pad of fatty tissue at the base of your abdomen that is covered with hair after puberty, and the lip-like folds of tissue—the labia majora and, inside them, the labia minora—that shield your vagina and urethra. Just behind the mons pubis, where the labia come together, is your clitoris, a small protrusion that becomes distended during sexual arousal. Your urethra, the tiny opening just behind your clitoris, leads to your bladder, where urine is stored. Behind your urethra is your vagina. Various glands located in your vulva and your vagina lubricate the area.

Developmental Disorders

Signs and Symptoms

- Little or no vagina, or a very short vagina and no cervix
- Genitals in a female that somewhat resemble male genitals

At the moment of conception, the embryo acquires either male (XY) or female (XX) chromosomes. For the next 40 days, males and females are indistinguishable. Then, if the fetus has a Y chromosome, testicles will develop. If a Y chromosome is not present and two X chromosomes are present, ovaries will develop. These organs secrete male or female hormones, respectively, and, in response, the fetus develops either a female or a male urogenital tract.

Something can go wrong at any stage. For instance, in a female fetus, an internal duct called the mullerian duct develops into fallopian tubes, a uterus, and the upper portion of the vagina. If something interferes with this process, the baby may be born without a vagina, with one that is very short, or perhaps without a uterus. This condition is known as mullerian agenesis. Because most of the abnormalities are internal, and as long as the child has a vaginal opening, there may be no sign of the problem until she reaches puberty and fails to menstruate.

A girl born with little or no vagina also could have the condition called complete testicular feminization (also called androgen resistance syndrome). She has no cervix, uterus, or ovaries but instead has testicles—often internally. She was genetically programmed to be a male but has abnormal androgen receptors; thus, before birth, male hormones were not able to connect with those receptors in the usual way to produce male genitals. At puberty, she develops breasts but little or no pubic or underarm hair. However, she is apt to be completely feminine in her attitudes and identity.

Sometimes a female is born with genitals that seem sexually ambiguous. She may have an unusually large clitoris, almost like a tiny penis, or the labia majora may be partially fused together and look a bit like a male scrotum. The most common cause for ambiguous genitals is congenital adrenal hyperplasia (see page 941), sometimes called pseudohermaphroditism. In such cases, the body does not produce enough of certain enzymes at a crucial time in fetal life. A female born with this condition is usually normal internally.

When a baby is born with ambiguous genitals, you should consult a specialist immediately. The child will be "assigned" a sex, depending on the chromosomes and what the genitals and internal organs are like; early surgery can then alter the genitals, if necessary. If the genital ambiguity is due to congenital adrenal hyperplasia, fetal shock (addisonian crisis) might develop unless your physician is on the alert to prevent it (see page 941).

Diagnosis

Your physician will do a physical examination and take a family history, because developmental disorders often (but not always) run in families. Laboratory tests done on blood or skin cells can establish which chromosomes caused the condition, and this information can have a bearing on how the problem is treated. Laboratory tests also can identify abnormality of androgen receptors.

How Serious Are Developmental Disorders?

Most girls who have mullerian agenesis are infertile, but some have a normal or near-normal uterus and ovaries and can conceive and give birth if a surgeon creates an artificial vagina. Girls with congenital adrenal hyperplasia actually have normal internal organs; if the abnormalities in the vulva are surgically corrected and the girls are given proper medication, they, too, can have children. Girls with testicular feminization are invariably infertile, but they have a normal appearance except for scanty body hair.

Treatment

Medication

For congenital adrenal hyperplasia, physicians usually prescribe glucocorticoids (cortisone-related steroids) to allow breasts to develop and menstruation to occur. For testicular feminization, the doctor ordinarily removes the testicles because of the risk of malignancy; estrogens are given at puberty to create and sustain secondary sex characteristics such as breasts.

Surgery

For girls born without a normal vagina, surgeons can create an artificial one. This is generally done if there is a chance that the girl can have children, but it also allows sexual activity. In cases of testicular feminization, the testicles usually are removed, because there is a risk that they will become cancerous.

Vulvitis

Signs and Symptoms

- Swelling of your vulva, with redness and itching
- Blisters that may ooze or crust over
- Skin of your vulva may thicken and turn whitish when the condition is chronic

Vulvitis is an inflammation of your external genitals, or vulva. (The Greek suffix *itis* means "inflammation.") It can be caused by an allergic reaction to a vaginal spray, to the detergent with which you wash your underwear, or to a medication, or it could be simply from poor hygiene. The inflammation also may be caused by a bacterial, viral, or fungal infection (see page 1173) or be cancer (page 1172).

Diagnosis

Your physician will do a pelvic examination (see page 1141) and may also order blood tests, a urinalysis, and other laboratory tests. If a sexually transmitted disease could be involved, your physician may test you for that. If the inflammation persists, you may need to have a biopsy to make sure there is no malignancy; this is apt to be an office procedure done with a local anesthetic. Except when it is caused by cancer, vulvitis is seldom serious.

Treatment

Medication

The medication your physician will use depends on the cause of the problem. Whatever the cause, a cortisone cream usually will relieve the itching.

Self-Help

Keep the area clean and dry; wear loose, absorbent clothing and cotton underpants. If the vulvitis consistently occurs after you use a spray or deodorant, contact your physician. The cause of the vulvitis may be an allergy. Bear in mind that an allergic reaction usually takes several days to develop (see Skin Allergies, page 1035).

Atrophic Vulvar Dystrophy

Signs and Symptoms

- Dry, itchy, reddened areas in your vulva
- Later, these areas may turn white or develop blisters
- Some areas turn white and thicken
- Skin becomes papery or shiny; clitoris and vaginal opening may shrink

Dystrophy is a kind of degeneration of tissue; the word is derived from the Greek words for "bad" (*dys*) and "nourishment" (*trophe*). It is more likely to occur in women who are past menopause. The term "lichen sclerosus et atrophicus" is sometimes used for this condition. This condition may involve the skin around your rectum and vulva. Malignancy may develop in the affected skin. Leukoplakia (whitish areas) may require biopsy.

Diagnosis

To make sure you do not have cancer, your physician may do a vulvar biopsy (cut out a small piece of tissue to be analyzed). For this procedure, your physician usually will use either a local or general anesthetic. During a physical examination, your physician also will check for signs of an underlying infection. Except when cancerous, vulvar dystrophy is not serious.

Treatment

Medication

Treatment depends on the source of the problem; however, a cortisone or testosterone cream generally will relieve symptoms.

It is important to have periodic examinations to identify potentially malignant changes, if they should develop.

Pruritus Vulvae

Signs and Symptoms—Intense itching, burning, or irritation in your genital area

Pruritus means itching (the Latin word for "to itch" is *prurire*). When your vulva itches, possible explanations include seborrheic dermatitis (see page 989), an allergy (see page 1035), an infection (see page 1173), or occasionally some systemic disease. Before puberty and after menopause, your vulva may itch and become irritated for no dis-

Vaginal Hygiene

Washing your genitals once a day with a mild soap and water is sufficient. In a normal woman, douches and feminine hygiene sprays are unnecessary, and at times they can be harmful.

Normally, your vagina is self-cleansing. Your vaginal walls produce their own fluid, which carries away dead cells and organisms as it flows downward. This healthy discharge is either clear or milky, although it is yellowish when it dries. It is somewhat slippery and has a mild, not unpleasant odor. It increases in amount at about the time you ovulate and during sexual arousal. If you have a copious vaginal discharge that is a different color or that has a strong smell, you probably have a vaginal infection (see page 1173) and should see a physician.

Some commercial douches also contain irritating chemicals. In addition, they can change your normally acidic vaginal environment, a condition that discourages the growth of yeasts and other organisms that can cause infections. In fact, your doctor may prescribe dilute vinegar douches to help maintain normal acidity as well as for their cleaning action. Douching also can wash away the plug of mucus that normally covers your cervix and prevents infectious organisms from getting into your uterus.

Despite all these negative effects, there are some problems for which your physician may advise douching. If so, be sure to hang the douche bag no more than 2 feet above your hips to reduce the fluid pressure; otherwise, vaginal organisms may be forced up into your uterus, where they can cause an infection.

The bacteria and yeasts that cause vaginal infections tend to thrive in hot, moist conditions. For that reason, it is a good idea to wear cotton underpants or synthetic underpants with a cotton crotch and to avoid tight panty hose. Tight, nylon underpants and hose trap heat and moisture in the genital area. One last point: always wipe from front to back to avoid contaminating your vagina with bacteria from a bowel movement.

---

cernible reason; the problem may be an inadequate amount of estrogen.

Diagnosis

Laboratory tests done on samples of vaginal discharge or vaginal tissue or colposcopy (examination with an instrument that provides a magnified view of the surface of the vagina, see page 1346) can generally identify infections. The source of an allergy may be obvious; if not, tests can be done. Pruritus vulvae is not serious. However, if you develop patches of whitened skin in your vulva, see your physician.

Treatment

Self-Help

If the itching is not accompanied by discharge or other symptoms, you can wait a couple of weeks before calling a physician while you try to solve the problem yourself. Stop using feminine hygiene sprays or other products that could be irritating your vulva. Wear cotton underpants, avoid panty hose, and bathe the area once a day with unscented soap.

Medication

A physician can prescribe a corticosteroid cream to help relieve your symptoms. Otherwise, medication depends on the underlying cause of the problem. If your physician identifies an infection called condyloma, caused by human papillomavirus, there are several choices of medications for treatment.

Surgery

If whitened skin (leukoplakia) develops in your vulva, your physician may suggest a minor surgical procedure to remove it. If your doctor finds an infection caused by the human papillomavirus, you may need further treatment.

Genital Warts

Signs and Symptoms

- Tiny pink or red swellings in your genital area that grow quickly
- Several warts close together can take on a cauliflower shape

Genital warts (also known as venereal

warts or condyloma acuminata) are common. They are caused by the papillomavirus, and usually you get them from direct sexual contact with someone who has them. The incubation period is 1 to 6 months. These warts can grow on your vulva, the walls of your vagina, your cervix, or your perineum (the area between the external genitals and anus). Sometimes they occur during pregnancy, possibly due to changes in the immune system.

Diagnosis

Your physician usually can diagnose genital warts by their appearance. However, because other sexually transmitted infections, such as gonorrhea or syphilis (see page 1087), also can occur as a result of the sexual exposure that caused the warts, you may need other tests to rule these out and perhaps a biopsy to rule out cancer (see page 1332).

How Serious Are Genital Warts?

By themselves, genital warts are mainly a nuisance, because they have a tendency to recur. However, they also have been associated with cancer of the cervix and of the rectum. If you have had genital warts, be sure to have a Pap smear annually (see page 1181).

Treatment

If you have an ongoing infection, your physician will treat that, because the warts may disappear when the infection does. Otherwise, your physician may paint the warts a few times with a chemical that often clears them up (do not use over-the-counter wart paints).

If medication does not work or if the warts recur, you may require treatment with electric cautery, a laser beam, or possible surgical removal.

Bartholin's Gland Abscess

Signs and Symptoms—A hot, tender, swollen lump just inside the vagina

Bartholin's glands—named for Danish anatomist Casper Bartholin—are located at the entrance to your vagina, one on each side. They can become infected, sometimes as a result of gonorrhea. At first, the infection may ooze pus, but if the opening to your gland becomes blocked, an abscess results.

Diagnosis

Your physician will look for symptoms of a vaginal infection (see page 1173) and will order laboratory tests.

How Serious Is Bartholin's Gland Abscess?

The abscess itself generally responds to treatment, although sometimes a benign Bartholin's cyst forms afterward and may need to be removed surgically. Gonorrhea is dangerous and can leave you sterile unless it is treated.

Treatment

Your physician may lance and drain the abcess.

Sebaceous Cysts

Signs and Symptoms

• A soft, smooth lump in the skin of the vulva, sometimes with a tiny dark dot in the center

Sebaceous glands, just beneath the surface of your skin, produce an oily substance that keeps skin supple. If the opening of a sebaceous gland is obstructed, a fluid-filled cyst may develop. Such cysts are painless and common, but they are prone to infection. An infected cyst may burst and drain, only to recur because the sac of the cyst remains.

Physicians identify sebaceous cysts by the way they look. They are harmless and most people simply ignore them.

Treatment

If a cyst becomes infected, your physician can prescribe an antibiotic. A cyst that is bothersome can be removed surgically as an outpatient operation with a local anesthetic.

Cancer of the Vulva

Signs and Symptoms

• A small, hard, itchy lump in the skin of your vulva
• Vulvar ulcer with raised edges; may bleed or seep fluid

Cancer of the vulva is rare. It accounts for just 3 to 4 percent of all tumors of the female reproductive organs. It is more common after menopause.

To diagnose a suspicious lump in your vulva, your physician removes a tiny piece of tissue for laboratory analysis. Cancer of the vulva generally grows very slowly, and early treatment means a complete cure.

Treatment

Surgery
Usually, a vulvectomy is necessary: the surgeon removes the tumor, surrounding skin, and perhaps lymph glands in your groin and the skin between your lymph glands and the tumor. The type of cancer and size of the tumor determine how much tissue must be removed. You may also need radiation therapy.

Pubic Lice

Signs and Symptoms
- Grayish insects the size of a pinhead in pubic hair
- Tiny white particles clinging to the hair (the eggs of the lice)
- Severe itching

You can catch pubic lice by having intercourse with someone who has them or, rarely, from clothing or bedding. Sometimes the lice—which also may be found in hair on other parts of your body—produce no symptoms. Then again, you may have itching and a slight, bluish rash. Pubic lice often are called crabs because they hang on with crab-like claws. The problem is also known as pediculosis pubis (the Greek word for louse is *pediculus*).

Treatment

Medication
Your physician may suggest an over-the-counter medication such as RID (pyrethrins with piperonyl butoxide) or may prescribe lindane (Kwell; gamma benzene hexachloride). Lindane is more potent and sometimes causes allergic reactions. It should not be used by pregnant women or infants. You may need to apply these medications again a week later, and your sexual partner also should be treated. If you have crabs in your eyelashes or eyebrows, do not use RID or Kwell, because they can damage your eyes; use an ophthalmic ointment (physostigmine) instead.

To keep from becoming reinfested, dry-clean your clothing, sheets, blankets, and towels or wash them in very hot water.

Wash enough for day-to-day living. Set everything else aside for 2 weeks where it will not come into contact with human beings. This interval is time for the louse eggs to hatch and the lice to die of starvation. Treat infested mattresses the same way.

Vaginitis

Signs and Symptoms
- Unusual discharge from your vagina
- Itching, irritation
- Pain during intercourse
- Pain in your lower abdomen
- Vaginal bleeding

If you have some of the symptoms listed above, you may have a vaginal infection (vaginitis), which is common and treatable, or a sexually transmitted disease, which is more serious but is also treatable. It is possible to have either disorder and have no symptoms. We discuss sexually transmitted diseases on pages 157 and 1087.

Vaginitis is an inflammation of your vagina, usually caused by an infection. A vaginal infection can be sexually transmitted, but you may catch it in other ways. However, as with a sexually transmitted disease, you should tell your sexual partner that you have an infection and that he may need treatment. Do not have intercourse until your symptoms have disappeared.

There are three common kinds of vaginitis: trichomoniasis, yeast infections, and nonspecific vaginitis.

Trichomoniasis
This is caused by a parasite. You may have no symptoms at all, or you may develop a smelly, greenish yellow, sometimes frothy, discharge. Most of the time you get trichomoniasis through intercourse.

Yeast Infections
A fungus causes yeast infections. The main symptom is itchiness, but you also may have a white discharge that resembles cottage cheese. You are more likely to develop a yeast infection if you are pregnant or have diabetes, if you are taking antibiotics, corticosteroid medications, or the pill, or if you have an iron deficiency.

Nonspecific Vaginitis
We generally call this type bacterial vaginosis.

Several different organisms probably cause it, including *Gardnerella vaginalis*. Many women have no symptoms at all, but others develop a white or grayish, fishy-smelling discharge that coats the vaginal walls.

Diagnosis

Your physician makes a diagnosis by taking a history, doing a pelvic examination (see page 1141), and identifying the organisms responsible through laboratory analysis of samples of discharge or tissue scrapings. Sometimes blood tests may also help.

How Serious Is Vaginitis?

Vaginitis is common and, because it tends to recur, annoying.

Treatment

Medication

Physicians usually treat trichomonal vaginitis with metronidazole tablets and yeast infections with antifungal creams or suppositories. For nonspecific vaginitis (bacterial vaginosis), your doctor may prescribe metronidazole or clindamycin.

Atrophic Vaginitis

Signs and Symptoms

- Soreness, burning, or itching in your vagina
- Slight bleeding after intercourse
- Painful intercourse
- Thin, watery vaginal discharge

Atrophic vaginitis is an inflammation of your vagina caused by degeneration of the vaginal tissue. (Atrophic combines the Greek word *trophe*, for "nourishment," with the negative prefix *a*.) The problem is most likely to develop after menopause, although it can occur during breastfeeding. In both situations, your estrogen production decreases, and the walls of your vagina may become drier, thinner, and less elastic and may bleed easily.

A pelvic examination (see page 1141) may be all that is necessary to diagnose the problem, although your physician may order laboratory tests if it appears that you may have a vaginal infection. Atrophic vaginitis is likely to be little more than a discomfort, but it can interfere with your sex life.

Treatment

Medication

In breastfeeding women, the problem is temporary. If you have passed menopause, your physician may recommend estrogen replacement therapy (see page 1154), or you can apply estrogen directly to your vagina as a cream or suppository. These are not cures but provide a kind of daily maintenance.

If the primary problem is painful intercourse, use of a water-soluble lubricant may help. Regular sexual activity actually improves circulation in your vagina and helps keep your tissues supple.

Vaginal Cysts

Signs and Symptoms

- Small swellings in the walls of your vagina
- A lump that bulges out of your vaginal opening

Several types of benign cysts can develop in your vagina. The most common are inclusion cysts and Gartner duct cysts. Inclusion cysts are caused by trauma—after operation or childbirth, for example, your vaginal walls may not heal to perfect smoothness. Gartner duct cysts are vestiges of a duct that serves a purpose before birth and then disappears. Sometimes a Gartner cyst enlarges enough to poke through your vaginal opening.

If a physician has reason to suspect cancer, he or she may biopsy the cyst. However, your physician can identify most cysts during a pelvic examination.

Treatment

Surgery

You may elect to ignore a vaginal cyst. If it causes discomfort, however, your doctor can surgically remove a cyst. If the cyst is small enough, your doctor can remove it in the office with local anesthesia.

Nonspecific Urethritis

Signs and Symptoms

- Frequent urination accompanied by a stinging or burning sensation
- Lower abdominal pain
- Occasional thin vaginal discharge

Nonspecific urethritis is an inflammation of your urethra (see page 1088) that is sometimes caused by *Chlamydia*. It also may be caused by a bacterium called *Ureaplasma urealyticum*. The symptoms occur within 10 to 20 days after exposure. However, most women have no symptoms at all. However, if the disease is untreated, complications such as pelvic inflammatory disease (an infection of the fallopian tubes, ovaries, uterus, or cervix) can develop later. Men are more likely to have symptoms. Therefore, if your sex partner develops urethritis you should be checked; his infection could be due to *Ureaplasma*, *Chlamydia*, or some other sexually transmitted disease.

Diagnosis

Your physician makes a diagnosis by taking a history and doing a pelvic examination (see page 1141) to rule out any other contributing cause and then identifies the responsible organisms using a urethral swab.

How Serious Is Nonspecific Urethritis?

Generally, this disease is more annoying than serious, particularly if it is recognized and treated early.

Treatment

Antibiotics are the standard treatment for nonspecific urethritis.

Loss of Pelvic Support

Signs and Symptoms

- A bulge in the walls of your vagina
- A feeling of fullness and discomfort when you bear down internally, sometimes with backache
- Stress incontinence (when you laugh or cough, you leak urine)
- Difficulty in passing urine or defecating
- A sensation of bearing down or of pelvic pressure when lifting or when you are on your feet for a long time

The organs that fill your lower abdomen—such as your bladder, uterus, and small intestine—are supported by your pelvic floor, a sheet of muscles and ligaments. These muscles also help close off your urethra where it leaves your bladder. They can become stretched or slack as a result of childbirth or aging or because of a hereditary weakness.

Vaginal Pain

When vaginal pain occurs during intercourse, it is called dyspareunia (from the Greek prefix *dys*, meaning "something bad or difficult," and *pareunos*, meaning "lying beside"). The most frequent causes are a vaginal infection (see page 1173) or herpes. The symptoms are vaginal soreness or persistent or recurrent pain during intercourse. Sometimes your vagina may simply be irritated by a douche, feminine hygiene spray, or contraceptive cream or jelly.

Dyspareunia also can result from bladder problems such as cystitis or urethritis (see pages 1193 and 1192). If intercourse causes deep internal pain, you may have endometriosis (see page 1185) or tears in the ligaments that support your uterus (see Loss of Pelvic Support, this page), or you could have some other disorder of your cervix, uterus, fallopian tubes, or ovaries.

If you are breastfeeding or are past menopause, your vaginal tissues may have thinned because you are producing less estrogen (see page 1153). An episiotomy from a recent delivery (see page 210) may have scarred your vagina. Sometimes if you are tense during intercourse, your vagina may not become sufficiently lubricated. Some women also have a problem called vaginismus—involuntary contractions of muscles at the opening to the vagina. Vaginal cancer is very rare, but it, too, could be the source of your pain (see page 1176).

To determine the causes of vaginal pain, your physician will do a pelvic examination (see page 1141) and may order blood tests, a urinalysis, or other laboratory tests. Treatment depends on what is causing your pain.

When that happens, some of your internal organs may prolapse—that is, they may sink lower in your body. As a result, you may have any of the symptoms listed above or none at all. Prolapse is more likely to develop in elderly women and in those who have given birth to several children.

Sometimes your uterus droops downward into your vagina. In extreme cases, your cervix may actually protrude from your vaginal opening. When either your bladder (cystocele) or your urethra prolapses, they produce a bulge in the front wall of your vagina. A bulge in the back wall may mean that either your small intestine or your lower rectum (rectocele) has prolapsed. When that happens, bowel movements may become difficult.

Diagnosis

The telltale bulges in your vaginal wall usually make prolapses easy to diagnose during a pelvic examination (see page 1141).

Exercises for Incontinence

If you urinate involuntarily at times (stress incontinence), the muscles of your pelvic floor may have become weakened as you grew older. By investing a few minutes a day in simple exercises that can be done anywhere, you may be able to regain bladder control.

The muscles that control your bladder are those surrounding your anus and vagina; they are called the pubococcygeal muscles. In the 1950s, Dr. A.M. Kegel developed an exercise regimen to strengthen them.

Begin by contracting your anal sphincter, as you would to prevent a bowel movement or stop urine flow. Relax, and then repeat the contraction. Do this 20 or 30 times. Repeat the exercise several times a day. As the tone in your pubococcygeal muscles gradually improves, you should have better bladder control; as a bonus, many women find that they also are more sexually responsive.

How Serious Is Loss of Pelvic Support?

Minor prolapses are common, especially in elderly women. As long as yours is minor and you are not feeling too uncomfortable, there is no rush to treat the problem. Exercise and weight loss may resolve it. However, when your bladder or urethra slips, sometimes urine is trapped in your bladder for long periods, creating a breeding ground for bacteria. Thus, you may have repeated urinary tract infections, and a surgical repair may be the best solution. A prolapsed lower rectum does not generally require operation unless the bulge is large or symptoms are troublesome.

Treatment

Self-Help

Simple exercises (called Kegel exercises) are sometimes the only treatment you need (see Exercises for Incontinence, this page). Other possible remedies include going on a diet if you are overweight and eating high-fiber foods (they will help you move your bowels without straining).

If these measures are not enough, your physician can fit you with a vaginal pessary, a rubber device that fits around your cervix and helps to prop up prolapsed organs. You will have to remove it regularly to clean it.

Surgery

If an operation is necessary, you can have a procedure called a vaginal repair. A surgeon elevates your prolapsed organ, or organs, back into place and tightens the muscles and ligaments of your pelvic floor. Surgery for a symptomatic prolapsed uterus would include a vaginal hysterectomy (see page 1184).

As an alternative, your physician may consider collagen injections as an option to surgery. Under local anesthetic or intravenous sedation, collagen is injected through a cystoscope into the lining of your urethra. This procedure adds bulk to the tissues of your urethra, helping to close the gap that allowed leakage of urine.

Vaginal Cancer

Signs and Symptoms

- Watery discharge from your vagina
- Bleeding after intercourse or a pelvic examination
- Pain during intercourse
- A frequent or urgent need to urinate or painful bowel movements

**Normal Position
of Uterus**

Prolapsed Uterus

If muscles that form your pelvic floor weaken, your uterus may drop lower (prolapse) into your vagina (see arrow) until your cervix protrudes from your vaginal opening (not shown)

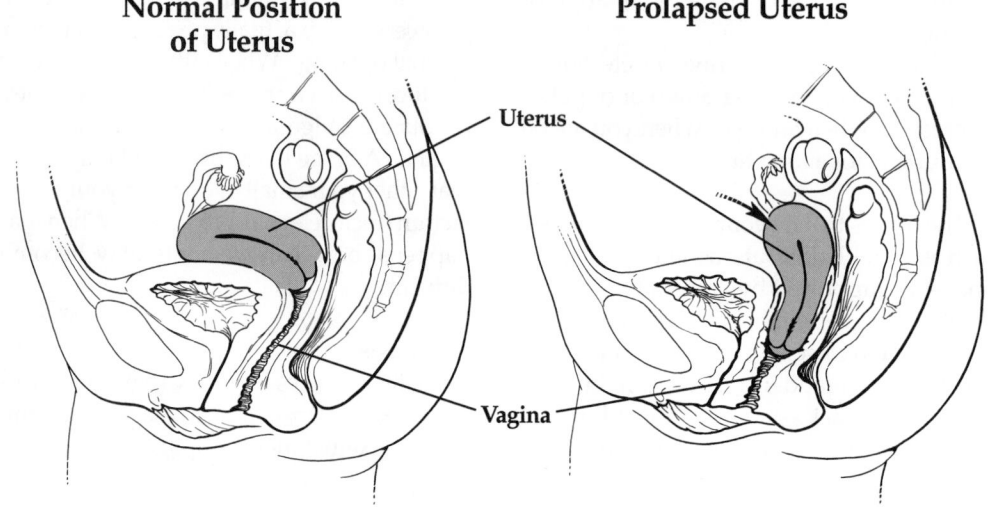

Uterus

Vagina

Vaginal cancer is extremely rare. Of all the different types of cancer that can develop in a woman's reproductive organs, only about 1 percent are cancers of the vagina. They are most likely to occur in women between the ages of 45 and 65 years, and 95 percent of them are slow-growing squamous cell tumors. They often extend to your bladder or rectum, causing painful defecation or a frequent, urgent need to urinate.

In recent years, a different type of vaginal cancer, called clear cell adenocarcinoma, has been diagnosed in very young women born to mothers who took diethylstilbestrol (DES) during pregnancy. Beginning in the 1940s, doctors often prescribed DES, a synthetic estrogen, for women who seemed in danger of miscarrying. By 1971, it was clear that DES produced a birth defect in which a type of glandular tissue normally found in the cervical canal was incorporated into the vaginal walls. This condition is called vaginal adenosis, and many so-called DES daughters have it. If you have vaginal adenosis, you do not need treatment, but must be watched, because this condition can lead to clear cell adenocarcinoma. The worst-case estimate is that 1 in 700 DES daughters will get this cancer; some experts predict it will be only 1 in 7,000. The peak years for vulnerability are between the ages of 15 and 22 years. DES daughters also may have a higher than normal chance of developing cervical cancer (see page 1180).

Fortunately, physicians have not prescribed DES for 25 years. However, if you are a DES daughter, contact a gynecologist, both because of the risk of vaginal cancer and because DES can cause other, less serious problems. Afterward, you should have regular checkups. Clear cell adenocarcinomas are fast-growing and in the early stages sometimes produce no symptoms. However, with regular checkups, your physician can spot and treat the problem early.

Diagnosis

Sometimes a Pap test (see page 1181) is the first clue pointing to a vaginal cancer. When a vaginal cancer is in such an early stage that the physician cannot see or feel it, a colposcopic exam (see page 1346) is helpful. During this examination your physician may paint your cervix and the walls of your vagina with an iodine solution (Schiller's test); normal tissue stains dark brown, but malignant cells do not stain. Because adenosis and some other benign conditions also fail to stain, Schiller's is not a definitive test for cancer, but it does show the physician which area to biopsy. Colposcopy also may identify the source of abnormal cells.

If you are a DES daughter, your pelvic examinations should include a careful inspection of your cervix and vagina, with a Pap smear not only of your cervix but of your vaginal walls.

How Serious Are Vaginal Cancers?

They are rare but can be deadly: overall, the 5-year survival rate without recurrence is about 30 percent. The statistics are somewhat more encouraging for clear cell adenocarcinoma—the survival rate is 80 to 85 percent.

Treatment

Surgery

The extent of the operation depends on where the cancer is located, how far it extends, and your age and condition. If the malignancy is localized in the upper third of your vagina, the surgeon probably will remove your uterus and that part of your vagina. He or she will probably also remove some pelvic lymph nodes to find out whether the cancer has spread to your lymph system. Otherwise you may have less extensive surgery with radiation therapy afterward. Plastic surgery can often reconstruct the missing section of your vagina.

Cervix, Uterus, and Fallopian Tube Disorders

Your uterus, or womb, is the organ that shelters the fetus when you are pregnant. Except during pregnancy, it is about 2.5 inches long. Powerful muscles in the thick walls of your uterus contract during childbirth to expel your baby. Your uterus is shaped like an upside-down pear. The narrower end, the cervix, extends into your vagina, and your cervix, too, has thick walls. Its opening is ordinarily very tiny.

Two thin tubes, called the fallopian tubes, are connected to your uterus, one on each side of its broad top. Each tube is about 4 inches long and about the thickness of a lead pencil, with an inner channel that is needle-thin. Each tube extends from the interior of your uterus to a place close to your ovary. Once a month, one of the ovaries releases an egg which travels down your fallopian tube to your uterus.

Developmental Disorders

Signs and Symptoms
- Failure to begin menstruating at puberty
- Inability to conceive or carry a pregnancy to term

Because of genetic problems or because something goes wrong during prenatal life, some women are born with abnormalities of the cervix, uterus, or fallopian tubes. These can range from an almost total absence of female reproductive organs (see page 1169) to minor discrepancies that nevertheless make it difficult to conceive or carry a pregnancy to term.

Some women born to mothers who took a synthetic estrogen called diethylstilbestrol (DES) during their pregnancies have an abnormal cervix or a uterus that is T-shaped rather than the usual pear shape. During pregnancy, your cervix may be too weak to support your fetus, or your uterus may not expand enough. DES daughters are more likely to miscarry than most women. Although these congenital abnormalities are not life-threatening, they are distressing to women who want children.

Diagnosis
If your physician suspects a developmental disorder in your uterus or fallopian tubes, he or she may order a type of X-ray called a hysterosalpingogram (also known as a utero-tubogram, see page 1346). Because soft tissues cannot be seen on an X-ray, this procedure uses a special dye that does register on the film. The dye is injected into your uterus and travels up your fallopian tubes and into your abdominal cavity, where your body absorbs it. While the dye is spreading, a radiologist takes a series of X-rays. The procedure can be somewhat uncomfortable, especially if your physician uses pressure to force the dye through the tubes; you may be given a local anesthetic, injected into your cervix, or an oral medication to help you relax. Your physician probably will want to do the hysterosalpingogram during the first half of your menstrual cycle, before ovulation, to avoid any risk that a fertilized egg might be exposed to radiation, which could lead to birth defects.

Two other procedures allow a physician to examine your ovaries, fallopian tubes, and uterus. Your physician may use vaginal ultrasound or laparoscopy to evaluate these areas. Laparoscopy (see page 1346) allows direct visualization of your internal genitals. Laparoscopy requires either intravenous sedation or general anesthesia in a hospital setting.

Treatment

Surgery
Surgeons sometimes can correct a cervix that is unable to sustain a pregnancy to term and fix certain structural problems of your uterus. However, infertility specialists usually try to rule out every other possible cause before they consider surgery, even if your uterus does not look completely normal.

Cervical Polyps

Signs and Symptoms
- Bleeding after intercourse, between periods, or after menopause
- Unusually heavy periods
- Heavy, watery, bloody discharge from your vagina
- Crampy pelvic pain

If you have these symptoms, see a physician immediately, because they could be due either to harmless cervical polyps or to cervical cancer (see page 1180). Polyps sometimes cause no symptoms at all and your physician may find them during a routine pelvic examination.

Cervical polyps are growths, rather like grapes, that generally protrude from the mouth of your cervix. You may have a single polyp or a cluster. They are common and often occur during pregnancy because of hormonal changes. They also may appear after your cervix has been injured.

They are rarely cancerous, and a small one may not even produce symptoms. However, large polyps can cause bleeding or make it difficult for you to become pregnant, so you may want to have them removed.

Diagnosis

Because polyps are very occasionally malignant, your physician will probably do a Pap test (see page 1181) and perhaps a biopsy (see page 1332), removing a sample of tissue for laboratory analysis.

Treatment

Surgery

Your physician can remove a single polyp in a brief office procedure with local anesthesia. If you have many large polyps, you may have to be hospitalized for the operation. If the polyps recur—which rarely happens—you may need dilatation and curettage (see page 1151) to remove them permanently; in this minor surgical procedure, the surgeon gently scrapes the lining of your uterus.

Cervicitis

Signs and Symptoms
- Vaginal discharge that is clear, grayish, or yellow
- Pain during intercourse
- Frequent, urgent need to urinate; painful urination
- Burning or itching in your genital area
- Bleeding after intercourse

Cervicitis is an inflammation of your cervix (the Greek suffix *itis* means "inflammation"). It can be caused by a local infection, especially if your cervix is damaged during childbirth. However, cervicitis is also a symptom of vaginal infections, of various sexually transmitted diseases (see page 1087), and of pelvic inflammatory disease (see page 1187).

Diagnosis

During a pelvic examination (see page 1141), your physician swabs your cervix to get a tissue sample and sends this sample to a laboratory to identify the organism responsible. Your physician also may do a Pap test (see page 1181) to rule out cervical cancer. You may also have colposcopy (see page 1346).

Treatment

Your physician will prescribe the antibiotic or sulfa drug that is most effective against the organisms involved. In severe cases, your physician may cauterize your cervix with cryosurgery (application of extreme cold) or with an electrically heated instrument in an office procedure.

Nabothian Cyst

Signs and Symptoms—A fluid-filled lump on your cervix, noted during a pelvic examination

A nabothian cyst (named for Martin Naboth, a German anatomist) occurs when a mucus gland on your cervix becomes obstructed, either because new tissue grows over it, usually after childbirth, or—in an elderly woman—because thinning cervical tissue has trapped natural secretions.

Generally, your physician diagnoses a nabothian cyst during a pelvic examination (see page 1141). A nabothian cyst rarely requires treatment.

Treatment

Surgery

If necessary, your physician can remove the cyst by cauterizing it or through cryosurgery (application of extreme cold). This is an office procedure and seldom requires even local anesthesia.

Cervical Dysplasia

Sometimes a Pap test (see page 1181) shows a type of cell that is considered to be precancerous. The condition is called dysplasia (*dys* is the Greek prefix meaning "bad," and *plasis* means "molding"). Cervical dysplasia can be mild, moderate, or severe. Mild dysplasia often disappears of its own accord. However, if it does not, it can be the first step in a process that will lead to cancer some years later.

Dysplasia most often is found in women between the ages of 25 and 35, but it can occur at any age from the teen years on. It has been linked to sexually transmitted diseases caused by viruses, and it is more apt to occur in women who have many sex partners or who began to have intercourse before they were 18.

Diagnosis

If your Pap smear reveals dysplasia, you will

need to have a colposcopy and biopsy (see page 1346). You probably can have this done in your physician's office. A colposcope is an instrument equipped with a magnifying lens and a light. Your physician uses it to examine your cervix while doing a biopsy—removing a bit of your cervix to send for laboratory analysis. You may or may not need a local anesthetic for this. If results are negative, you will need to return for another Pap test in 4 to 6 months.

Occasionally, your physician may remove a piece of tissue using a thin wire loop and carefully controlled electrical current. This is called a loop electrosurgical excisional procedure (LEEP).

How Serious Is Cervical Dysplasia?

It may simply disappear. If it does not, treatment will take care of it.

Treatment

Surgery

Physicians usually treat cervical dysplasia by cauterization, LEEP, or laser surgery.

Cauterization destroys the abnormal tissue. You may have this done in a physician's office or in a hospital on an outpatient basis. Usually, anesthesia is unnecessary.

In laser surgery, a high-energy beam of light burns away the dysplasia. There is little or no damage to surrounding tissue, and the area heals quickly. This is usually an outpatient hospital or office procedure.

For extensive dysplasia, you may have a cone biopsy. A cone-shaped slice of your cervix is removed and analyzed. This surgical procedure requires general anesthesia in a hospital. You will have to rest at home for a few days afterward. If the analysis shows that your surgeon excised all the abnormal tissue, you may need no further treatment.

Conization decreases cervical mucus, which might increase your tendency to miscarry. If you become pregnant and you have had a cone biopsy, tell your physician about it.

After you are treated for dysplasia, your physician will recommend periodic reevaluations.

Cancer of the Cervix

Signs and Symptoms

- Bleeding from your vagina after intercourse, between periods, or after menopause
- Watery, bloody discharge from your vagina; it may be heavy and smelly
- In later stages, a dull backache and general poor health

Cervical cancer is one of the more common cancers that affect female reproductive organs. It is most likely to occur when you are between the ages of 30 and 55.

You are more likely than most women to develop cervical cancer if you have had a sexually transmitted viral infection, such as genital warts; if you began having sex before you were 18 years old; or if you have had many sex partners.

Diagnosis

Your physician will do a Pap test (see page 1181) and probably a colposcopy and biopsy (see pages 1346 and 1332). A colposcope is an instrument with a magnifying lens that permits a close look at your cervix. For a biopsy, your physician removes a fragment of tissue from your cervix for a laboratory analysis; this is the only way to determine whether tissue is malignant.

If the biopsy shows that you do have cancer, your physician may do a conization and a dilatation and curettage, gently scraping your uterine lining for tissue samples (see page 1151) to find out whether the cancer has spread to your uterus. Then he or she will determine the stage of the disease on the basis of the extent of the tumor. This "staging" of the cancer is the key to determining how extensive your treatment must be. Treatment may require a radical hysterectomy or radiation therapy or both.

How Serious Is Cancer of the Cervix?

Cervical cancer is serious if it has spread beyond the uterus. Invasive cancer of the cervix is the cause of death in about 3 percent of American women who die of cancer.

Treatment

Surgery

Your physician probably will do a radical hysterectomy for an invasive cancer that involves a large part of your cervix and extends into your uterus. The surgeon removes your uterus (including the cervix), upper vagina, some surrounding tissue and lymph nodes, and the fallopian tubes, but may leave one or both ovaries in place in a young woman. You may have radiation therapy afterward. If a biopsy of the nodes shows that the cancer has already spread, you also may have chemotherapy.

Radiation

For cervical cancer, the cure rates for surgery and radiation are nearly identical. Among women with localized cancer (confined to the cervix) treated with radiation, 75 to 90 percent survive for at least 5 years; among those with cancer that has spread beyond the cervix, the 5-year survival rate is about 45 to 55 percent. Radiation treatments often involve both radiation delivered by a machine and internal radiation from radioactive material implanted in your uterus or in the upper part of your vagina and left there for several days while you remain in the hospital. The implanting is done under general anesthesia.

Radiation has some distressing side effects, although not everyone experiences them. They can include diarrhea, rectal bleeding, and fatigue. For a few months afterward, you may have trouble retaining urine. If you did not have a hysterectomy, the radiation treatments probably will disrupt your menstrual cycle and they may give you symptoms of menopause, such as hot flashes, if you have not yet passed menopause. Radiation therapy also can cause some narrowing and shortening of your vagina. However, using a lubricating jelly just before intercourse generally solves the problem.

You will need regular checkups and tests for at least 5 years after treatment for cervical cancer.

Pap Smear

Since the early 1940s, the death rate of women with cervical cancer has decreased by 70 percent, largely because so many women have Pap smear screening. Although it is not infallible, this test detects 95 percent of cervical cancers and—what is more important—detects them at a stage when they cannot yet be seen with the naked eye but can be treated and almost invariably cured.

Occasionally, the Pap smear will identify an endometrial or ovarian cancer.

You will have a Pap smear, named for G.N. Papanicolaou, its developer, during a pelvic examination (see page 1141). At most, it causes slight discomfort. Using a wooden spatula, brush, or cotton swab, your physician gently scrapes the entire surface of your cervix to gather cells and also takes a cell sample from inside your cervical canal by inserting a brush. The cells are sent to a laboratory for microscopic analysis.

A negative result means that your cervix is normal; a positive result indicates the presence of abnormal cells. A positive result does not prove that you have cancer or even dysplasia (see page 1179), a precancerous condition. However, it usually means you should have further evaluation, such as colposcopic examination and biopsy.

You should have your first Pap smear at age 18, or earlier if you start having intercourse. At 1-year intervals, you should have your second and third Pap smears. If three Pap smears have normal results, you can have Pap smears done thereafter at longer intervals agreed on by you and your physician, unless you are in a high-risk group, in which case you should be tested once a year. Women most at risk are those who began having intercourse before they were 18, who have had multiple sex partners, or who have had a sexually transmitted disease.

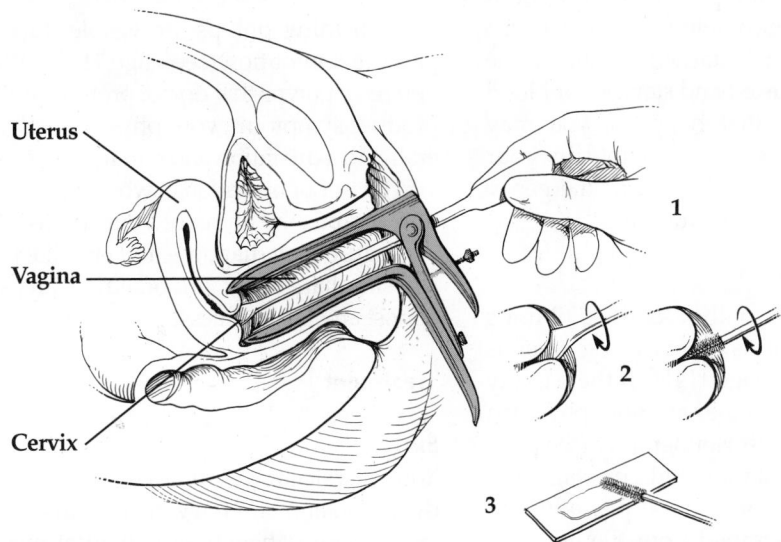

Uterus

Vagina

Cervix

1

2

3

With speculum in place, your physician rotates a wooden spatula and then a brush to remove a sample of cells (1 and 2). The cells are smeared onto a glass slide (3) for examination under a microscope.

Fibroids

Signs and Symptoms
- Heavy or prolonged menstrual periods
- Pain or pressure in your lower abdomen or lower back

Emergency Symptoms—Sudden, sharp pain low in your abdomen

A fibroid is a benign tumor that develops within your uterine wall or is attached to it. Although you may have a single fibroid, you are more likely to have several of them. They can be as small as a pea or as large as a grapefruit. Most women who have them have no symptoms. (Fibroids also are called leiomyomas, myomas, or fibromyomas.)

Normally, fibroids grow slowly. However, they respond to increased levels of estrogen, which allows them to expand rapidly during pregnancy or if you are taking oral contraceptives or estrogen replacement therapy. After menopause, these tumors usually shrink and often disappear completely.

Fibroids rarely become malignant, and most cause few problems. They also are extremely common—about 20 percent of women older than 35 years have them. Nevertheless, if you have fibroids, have regular checkups to make sure they do not grow too large. If your periods become very heavy, you could develop iron-deficiency anemia. Fibroids can make conception difficult, and if you are pregnant, they could cause a miscarriage or interfere with delivery. Sometimes, a fibroid attached to your uterine wall becomes twisted and starved for blood and oxygen. If that happens, you may suddenly feel a sharp pain low in your abdomen, and you will need an emergency operation to remove the tumor.

Diagnosis
Your physician usually identifies fibroids when he or she feels them during a pelvic examination (see page 1141). If there is any question about what they are, your physician will order CT or ultrasonography (see page 1335) or do a dilatation and curettage (see page 1151), a minor surgical procedure in which tissue is scraped from the lining of your uterus.

Treatment
If you have no symptoms, treatment may be unnecessary. If you have symptoms and are not planning to have children, your physician probably will recommend a hysterectomy—removal of your uterus (see page 1184). As an alternative, a surgeon can simply remove the fibroids. However, this procedure, called a myomectomy, is also a major operation and has a higher rate of complications than a hysterectomy. In about 10 percent of cases, the fibroids return.

Endometrial Polyps

Signs and Symptoms
- Spotting between menstrual periods, especially after intercourse or douching
- Pelvic cramps
- Heavy or prolonged periods

Endometrial polyps are small, soft growths in the lining of your uterus (the endometrium). They are almost never malignant, and they occur most often at about the time of menopause. You may have one or a cluster of them.

Usually, endometrial polyps will produce no symptoms. However, polyps may protrude into your vagina, causing cramps as they expand the opening of your cervix. If protruding polyps become twisted and lose their blood supply, they can become infected. Polyps often occur together with endometrial hyperplasia (see page 1183) or solid growths called fibroids (see this page).

Protruding polyps are visible during a pelvic examination (see page 1141). When you have polyps that do not protrude and do produce symptoms, your physician will generally do a dilatation and curettage (see page 1151), a minor operation in which your physician scrapes the lining of your uterus. This procedure may diagnose and cure the problem simultaneously. Endometrial polyps are almost always harmless.

Treatment

Surgery
Your physician can remove polyps during dilatation and curettage, usually in a hospital on an outpatient basis with local anesthesia. After removing them, your physician will want the polyps analyzed to be sure they are not malignant. On occasion, they may recur.

Endometrial Hyperplasia

Signs and Symptoms
- Bleeding between menstrual periods
- Heavy or prolonged menstrual periods

Endometrial hyperplasia occurs when your uterine lining—the endometrium—grows too thick. Teenagers and women approaching menopause are most apt to have this problem.

It is easy to treat, but it must be distinguished from a precancerous condition called adenomatous hyperplasia.

Diagnosis
If your physician suspects endometrial hyperplasia, he or she will want to do an endometrial biopsy and will remove a small sample of your endometrium for laboratory analysis. The discomfort this office procedure causes resembles menstrual cramps.

Treatment
If you are young, taking birth control pills for a few months often will solve the problem. If oral contraceptives fail or if you are an older woman, you should have a dilatation and curettage (see page 1151), a procedure in which tissue samples are scraped from your uterine lining. If laboratory analysis of the tissue shows precancerous cells, you probably will have to have a hysterectomy (see page 1184). Although you could try hormone therapy instead, you run the risk that cancer will develop later.

Cancer of the Uterus

Signs and Symptoms
- Vaginal bleeding after menopause
- Before menopause, heavy periods or bleeding between periods
- A pink, watery discharge from your vagina

Cancer of the uterus also is called endometrial cancer, because it starts in the endometrium, the lining of your uterus. It is one of the most common—and most curable—of the cancers that afflict American women, if it is detected early. It most often occurs after menopause, in women between the ages of 50 and 70.

Obesity predisposes you to endometrial cancer. Furthermore, it makes treatment (operation and irradiation) difficult.

Today, estrogen replacement therapy uses lower doses of estrogen, combined for part of the month with progestin. Thus, if you are taking appropriate estrogen replacement therapy, you have no greater risk of uterine cancer than the population at large. However, estrogen taken alone for menopausal symptoms may cause bleeding. Thus, bleeding caused by endometrial cancer may be mistakenly attributed to the estrogen, and the diagnosis will be delayed.

Women who are at high risk for uterine cancer include those who have never given birth to a child, those who were still menstruating at age 52, and those with a history of infertility or irregular periods. Women who have been taking birth control pills have a decreased risk of endometrial cancer.

Diagnosis
In its earliest stage, uterine cancer produces no symptoms. Pap smears (see page 1181) detect it in less than half the cases, and it is not noticeable during a pelvic examination (see page 1141). The first clue often is vaginal bleeding.

If you develop symptoms, your physician can do an endometrial biopsy. In this office procedure, your physician removes a small piece of tissue from your uterine lining for laboratory analysis; usually, you do not need anesthesia. If you do have uterine cancer, the biopsy detects it most of the time. Alternatively, a dilatation and curettage (D and C) can be done (see page 1151).

If you have cancer, and there is reason to think it may have spread beyond the uterus, your physician will do a series of tests to locate any secondary tumors.

How Serious Is Uterine Cancer?
It is usually slow-growing and is apt to be localized when it is discovered. Thus, most

Endometrial cancer is a common disorder that develops in the lining of your uterus (endometrium). It usually is curable if diagnosed early.

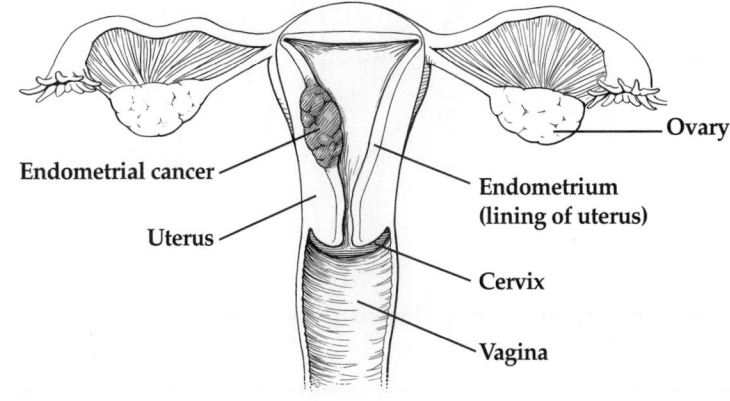

Endometrial cancer — Ovary — Endometrium (lining of uterus) — Uterus — Cervix — Vagina

women who have it can be cured. When it is diagnosed early, the 5-year survival rate is 88 percent; even when it has already spread to adjacent tissue, the rate is 75 percent. Rarely, the tumor is a faster-growing, deadlier type, and results are not as good.

Treatment

Surgery

Most physicians will recommend a hysterectomy (see this page), the removal of your uterus. Your fallopian tubes and ovaries also will be removed, because the cancer tends to spread to those organs.

Radiation

If the cancer already has extended beyond your uterus, you may have radiation therapy after the operation. Sometimes, radiation is used instead of surgery. It may be deep X-ray therapy delivered by a machine or a radioactive implant inserted in your uterus or vagina while you are under general anesthesia. Your

---

Hysterectomy

A hysterectomy is the removal of your uterus. (The Greek word *hystera* means "womb"; *ektome* means "incision.") You may need a hysterectomy if you develop cancer of the uterus; if you have severe endometriosis (see page 1185), fibroids (see page 1182), or pelvic adhesions which bind your uterus to neighboring organs; if you have severe and uncontrollable bleeding; or if your uterus has dropped down and is protruding from your vagina. Physicians also perform hysterectomies for other reasons.

Hysterectomies are not all alike. A partial hysterectomy leaves your cervix and the base of your uterus intact. In a total hysterectomy, the entire uterus, including the cervix, is removed. A total hysterectomy with bilateral salpingo-oophorectomy is removal of your uterus, cervix, fallopian tubes (*salpingo*), and both ovaries (*oophor*), whereas a radical hysterectomy extends even further and also includes removal of the upper part of your vagina and some lymph nodes. The condition that makes the hysterectomy necessary determines how much your surgeon will remove.

In doing a hysterectomy, the surgeon most often makes an incision in your lower abdomen, either horizontally just above the pubic hair or vertically from your navel to the hairline. However, sometimes your surgeon will perform a vaginal hysterectomy. This is done through an incision made at the top of your vagina. Either operation takes 1 to 2 hours under general anesthesia. If you have a large ovarian or uterine tumor or cancer, your surgeon will use the abdominal approach. Many surgeons prefer it, in any case, because it gives them a better look at various pelvic organs. They usually use the vaginal approach to manage uterine prolapse.

Although some surgeons routinely advise removal of the ovaries to prevent ovarian cancer in women older than 40, this is a controversial issue. On the one hand, ovarian cancer is deadly. It has a cure rate of only 10 to 20 percent. On the other hand, cancer of the ovaries is uncommon.

If you have a hysterectomy, you probably will remain in the hospital for about 4 days. Possible complications include pelvic infections, kidney and bladder infections, and hemorrhage. After you get home, you will have to forgo tub baths and douches, driving the car, and lifting heavy objects for a time, and for 6 to 8 weeks you must forgo sex and active sports.

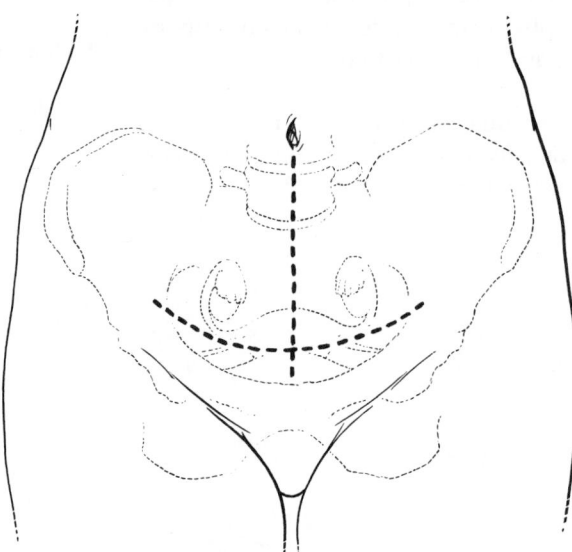

In performing an abdominal hysterectomy, your surgeon may elect either a horizontal or a vertical incision.

physician will leave the radioactive implant in place for a few days, and you will be hospitalized for the duration. Your treatment may require a combination of these methods.

Medication

If the cancer has metastasized (spread) to other parts of your body, progestin can often stop it from growing, sometimes for 2 to 3 years or even longer. Your physician also may use other anticancer medications.

Hydatidiform Mole

Signs and Symptoms
- During pregnancy, your uterus grows much faster than it should
- Vaginal bleeding, severe nausea and vomiting, no fetal movement
- Passage of grape-like tissue from your vagina
- High blood pressure

A rare benign growth called hydatidiform mole sometimes develops at the beginning of pregnancy from tissue surrounding the fertilized egg that would normally produce a placenta. In such cases, the fetus dies. (If placental tissue is left in your uterus after childbirth or a miscarriage, a mole also can develop, sometimes years later.)

If you have the symptoms listed above, see a physician as soon as possible. It is essential to remove the tumor. It grows quickly and can become large. In addition, although more than 80 percent of such moles are benign, 15 percent develop into a condition called invasive mole. This mole—still benign—reaches so deeply into your uterine wall that it can cause a hemorrhage and other serious problems. A choriocarcinoma, a fast-growing malignant tumor that soon spreads to other parts of the body, follows 2 to 3 percent of hydatidiform moles.

Hydatidiform moles are more common in older women. One occurs in about every 2,000 gestations in the United States and more often in other parts of the world.

Diagnosis
To make sure you are not experiencing some other complication of pregnancy in which your fetus is normal, your physician probably will use ultrasonography. Because hydatidiform moles produce quantities of human chorionic gonadotropin, a hormone that can be detected in urine or blood, your physician may order a urine or blood test.

How Serious Are Hydatidiform Moles?
A noninvasive mole can be removed easily, and invasive moles and malignant tumors also are treatable. In fact, even for choriocarcinoma, the overall cure rate is 75 to 85 percent.

Treatment

Surgery
Your physician can remove the mole, usually by suction, in a procedure similar to dilatation and curettage (see page 1151). Afterward, your physician will monitor your levels of human chorionic gonadotropin, which should return to normal. If they do not, you may have developed either an invasive mole or choriocarcinoma.

Your physician may recommend removal of your uterus (see Hysterectomy, page 1184), but he or she is more likely to suggest chemotherapy.

Chemotherapy
For both invasive moles and choriocarcinoma, chemotherapy provides good results. Furthermore, you can still have a child afterward, and you avoid a major operation.

Endometriosis

Signs and Symptoms
- Painful menstruation—pain may begin before and extend several days after a period
- Occasional heavy periods
- Sharp pain deep in your pelvis during intercourse
- Infertility
- Pain when straining to have a bowel movement

Endometriosis occurs when bits of your endometrium (the tissue that lines your uterus) somehow escape your uterus and become implanted on other pelvic organs. Some experts believe the implants occur due to menstrual flow that backs up into the fallopian tubes and spills into the pelvic cavity. Most often, the implants develop on the outside of the ovaries, fallopian tubes, or the uterus or its supporting ligaments.

These mislocated cells imitate the menstrual cycle (see page 1144), first thickening and then bleeding as menstruation begins. Because the implants are embedded within other tissue, there is nowhere for the blood to go. They form blood blisters, irritating the surrounding tissue, which may create a cyst to encapsulate the blister. The cyst, in turn, may become a scar or an adhesion (abnormal tissue that binds organs together). Scars and adhesions on your ovaries or fallopian tubes can prevent pregnancy.

Experts estimate that 10 to 15 percent of American women of childbearing age have endometriosis. Most have no symptoms and require no treatment, but for some this is a progressive disease that becomes more painful and debilitating over time. Endometriosis, which may occasionally run in families, is most likely to occur between the ages of 25 and 40 in women who have not had children.

Menopause usually cures mild or moderate endometriosis. However, estrogen replacement therapy may reactivate it.

Diagnosis

Although physicians often can feel patches of endometriosis during a pelvic examination, laparoscopy is the only way to confirm the finding. It is important to be certain, because ovarian cancer produces similar symptoms, and the hormones usually prescribed to treat endometriosis can make cancer grow faster. A laparoscope is a slim instrument equipped with a light. It is inserted into your abdomen through a small incision, and your physician looks through it to see your pelvic organs. Laparoscopy is a minor procedure done with local or general anesthesia, often on an outpatient basis (see page 1346).

How Serious Is Endometriosis?

Endometrial implants are rarely malignant, but they are frequently associated with infertility. Although the symptoms may wax and wane, they often get worse with time.

Treatment

Pregnancy

If you have endometriosis in an early stage, your physician may suggest that you become pregnant soon if you want to have children, because it may become more difficult to conceive later on. During pregnancy, endometriosis implants generally shrink and the symptoms may disappear. However, if you have endometriosis you are more likely than most to have a pregnancy outside of your uterus (ectopic pregnancy) (see page 199).

Medication

Birth control pills may relieve the symptoms. If that treatment is not sufficient, various hormones can stop menstruation completely for a time. Your physician may prescribe danazol (a testosterone derivative) or a gonadotropin-releasing hormone agonist. It sometimes actually shrinks implants; after 6 months on medication and then withdrawal of the drug, some women do conceive.

Surgery

If drugs fail, your physician can remove the implants surgically or destroy them with electrocautery, although some surgeons believe that laser surgery, done during laparoscopy, is less likely to produce scars and adhesions. Unfortunately, recurrences are common. If nothing else works and the pain is severe, it may be necessary to remove your uterus and ovaries (see Hysterectomy, page 1184).

Adenomyosis

Signs and Symptoms

- Menstrual cramps that last throughout a period; they get worse as you grow older
- Prolonged, excessive menstrual bleeding

In adenomyosis, some of the endometrial tissue that lines your uterus begins to grow within its muscular walls. This is most likely to happen late in your childbearing years and after you have had children. Many women who have adenomyosis have no symptoms.

During a pelvic examination (see page 1141), your physician generally finds that your uterus is enlarged and tender. That fact, and the symptoms listed above, indicate adenomyosis, which is generally harmless but can be painful.

Treatment

If you are nearing menopause, your physician may prescribe painkillers and suggest no other treatment because the problem generally disappears when menstruation ends. If your pain is severe or menopause is years away, your physician may suggest that your uterus be removed (see Hysterectomy, page 1184).

Pelvic Inflammatory Disease

Signs and Symptoms
- Severe pain and tenderness in your lower abdomen, perhaps with fever and vomiting (acute disease)
- Mild, recurrent pain in your lower abdomen, perhaps with backache, irregular menstrual periods
- Infertility (chronic disease)
- Pain during intercourse
- Periods that start early or are heavy
- Copious, foul-smelling vaginal discharge

Emergency Symptoms—Severe pain low in your abdomen; nausea, vomiting, and signs of shock, such as faintness

Strictly speaking, pelvic inflammatory disease (PID) is an infection of your fallopian tubes (salpingitis). However, infections of the ovaries, uterus, and cervix also have come to be called PID.

Usually, you acquire the organisms responsible for PID through sexual intercourse. Salpingitis develops in almost 15 percent of women with gonorrhea. However, other bacteria also can cause PID, and the infection can sometimes be traced to childbirth or to procedures such as an endometrial biopsy or dilatation and curettage. Every year, about 1 million American women develop PID. Some have no symptoms and are never diagnosed; some develop a low-level, chronic infection; and others have an acute attack.

If you use a diaphragm or if your partner uses a condom, you are somewhat protected from PID. If you use an intrauterine device (IUD), you are more likely to develop the disorder. You are most vulnerable to infection during menstruation. If you have PID, your sexual partner should seek treatment too, even if he has no symptoms. If he has an infection, he may reinfect you.

Pelvic Pain

Any time you have a pain in your pelvic region that lasts more than a few hours, that recurs, or that is accompanied by other symptoms such as fever or vaginal bleeding, see a physician. Your physician will ask many questions about the pain. Such information is important for diagnosis. Significant distinctions include whether it is acute (like the onslaught of pain and fever that sometimes marks the beginning of pelvic inflammatory disease) or chronic (meaning that it has been with you for a while) and, if it is chronic, whether it is episodic (it comes and goes) or continuous. Your physician will ask whether the pain is associated with your menstrual periods, bowel or bladder habits, intercourse, or physical activity.

Acute Pain
Pelvic Infection
If you develop severe pain in your lower abdomen a few days after a menstrual period, perhaps accompanied by fever or vomiting, you may have acute pelvic inflammatory disease (see this page). The pain often starts in the middle of your abdomen and gradually moves lower down and to both sides, a sign that the infection has spread from your uterus into your fallopian tubes.

Your abdomen will be tender when your physician presses it. You may have a smelly discharge from your vagina or vaginal bleeding. If you suddenly develop signs of shock, such as cold, clammy skin, rapid breathing, or an irregular heartbeat, get medical help immediately: an abscess, caused by the infection, may have perforated or you may be hemorrhaging internally.

Complications of Early Pregnancy
During the first trimester of pregnancy, pain in your lower abdomen or back may mean you are having a miscarriage (see page 197). The pain may be dull and constant, or sharp and intermittent. You may have spotting or heavy bleeding from your vagina. Call a physician immediately. If the pain is severe enough and the bleeding heavy enough, the fetus may be dead. You may need dilatation and curettage (see page 1151) to prevent infection.

Ectopic Pregnancy
If you develop a sudden, constant, severe pain in your lower abdomen, especially if it is located only on one side and is followed by vaginal bleeding, you may have an ectopic pregnancy. That means a fertilized egg is developing in one of your ovaries or fallopian tubes rather than in your uterus. If you faint soon after the pain strikes, you are probably in shock because the tube has ruptured. You will need emergency treatment (see Ectopic Pregnancy, page 199).

Nongynecologic Causes
Your reproductive organs do not cause all acute abdominal pain. Appendicitis, for example, often begins as a sudden, intense pain in

the general vicinity of your navel, then changes to pain in the lower right side of your abdomen (see page 772). Diverticulitis and bladder infections cause pain in your lower abdomen. When the pain of diverticulitis is intense, it may feel like a belt around your body (see page 781). Gallstones can cause attacks of severe pain, starting in your upper abdomen and extending toward your right shoulder blade (see page 812).

Episodic Pain

Dyspareunia

Dyspareunia is the name for pain that occurs only, or primarily, during intercourse. It has several possible causes. If you are breastfeeding or are past menopause, your body is no longer producing estrogen in the same quantities, and your vaginal tissue may have become thinner and more fragile (see page 1153). Also, an allergic reaction may have irritated the walls of your vagina or you may have vaginal cysts (see page 1172), a vaginal infection, or a sexually transmitted disease such as herpes or genital warts (see page 1092). If you recently had a baby, the discomfort could be due to scars from an episiotomy (see page 210).

The problem also could be a bladder infection (see page 842). It could be loss of pelvic support (see page 1175). If pain occurs only when your partner thrusts deeply, the cause probably lies in your uterus or beyond: it could be pelvic inflammatory disease (see page 1187), an ectopic pregnancy (see page 199), endometriosis (see page 1185), or cysts or a tumor in your ovaries (see page 1189). Finally, if none of the above conditions explain your pain, you may have vaginismus—for psychological reasons, during intercourse your vagina produces little lubrication and your vaginal muscles go into spasms.

Midcycle Pelvic Pain

You may experience pain in your lower abdomen at midcycle, when you ovulate. Called mittelschmerz (see page 1148), the pain is typically a dull ache that can last a few minutes or a few hours.

Dysmenorrhea

Excess prostaglandins produced by the endometrium (see page 1148) may cause severe pain during menstruation. Or the problem may be temporary, a result of giving up oral contraceptives or of using an intrauterine device. However, if you also have a fever and have had a heavy, unpleasant discharge between menstrual periods, you may have a vaginal or pelvic infection (see page 1187).

Chronic Pain

Endometriosis or Adenomyosis

Pain in your lower abdomen that begins a little before a menstrual period starts, continues throughout your period, and actually gets worse right afterward may be due to endometriosis (see page 1185) or adenomyosis (see page 1186). In either case, the pain often accompanies heavy menstrual flow. In endometriosis, the kind of tissue that normally lines your uterus becomes implanted on other pelvic organs such as your ovaries and fallopian tubes. In adenomyosis, that same tissue begins to grow inside the walls of your uterus.

Chronic Salpingitis

If you have had pelvic inflammatory disease (see page 1187), especially if you have had recurring bouts of it, you may develop chronic pain in your pelvis. It generally gets worse during menstruation and during intercourse.

Pelvic Pain Syndrome

You may notice considerable pelvic discomfort every month during the 7 to 10 days before you menstruate. The pain is worse when you sit or stand and better when you lie down; your lower back and legs also may ache. Intercourse may be painful, and normal vaginal discharge may be increased. You may have symptoms associated with premenstrual syndrome (see page 1147), such as headaches, insomnia, and fatigue. The cause may be congestion due to the increase in blood flow to your uterus just before menstruation.

Nongynecologic Causes

Chronic pelvic pain also can originate with nonreproductive organs in your urinary and intestinal tracts. A bladder infection (see page 842) sometimes causes a gnawing pain just above your pubic bone when you urinate; you also may note a burning sensation in the urethra. Other symptoms are a frequent, urgent need to urinate and occasionally blood in your urine. Irritable or spastic colon produces a crampy abdominal pain, often accompanied by nausea, vomiting, diarrhea, or constipation. If abdominal pain accompanies a distended abdomen and follows several days of constipation, you may have a blockage of your intestine.

Diagnosis

During a pelvic examination (see page 1141), your physician will use a cotton swab to take samples from your vagina and cervix. Your physician will send them to a laboratory for analysis to determine what organism is causing the infection. If there is any question about the diagnosis, or about how widespread the infection is, your physician can do a laparoscopy. He or she will insert a thin, lighted instrument through a small incision in your abdomen and view your pelvic organs. You are likely to have this hospital procedure as an outpatient with local or general anesthesia.

How Serious Is PID?

If you do not seek treatment, PID can be serious. An abscess may develop on your fallopian tubes or ovaries, creating a surgical emergency if it perforates. If your tubes or ovaries become damaged or scarred, you may be unable to conceive. PID also can lead to peritonitis, an inflammation of the membrane that lines your abdominal cavity. Peritonitis is always serious and needs intensive treatment with antibiotics. In rare cases, if bacteria invade your bloodstream, PID can lead to blood poisoning (septicemia) and inflammation and infection of your joints.

PID can have severe long-term consequences; they include chronic pelvic pain due to adhesions, lingering infection, and ectopic pregnancy, in which the fetus grows outside your uterus, usually in one of your fallopian tubes.

Treatment

Medication

A physician rarely waits for the results of laboratory tests before giving medication. Thus, to begin with, your physician may prescribe a combination of antibiotics; you may receive a different medication once your laboratory results are known. Your physician also may prescribe a painkiller and will recommend bed rest. You may even be hospitalized for a short time if you have a severe case or if it fails to respond quickly to medication. PID recurs in about 15 to 25 percent of cases.

Surgery

Surgery is rarely necessary. However, if an abscess ruptures or threatens to rupture, your physician may drain or remove it. If it is removed, a fallopian tube or an ovary or both may also be removed.

Ovarian Disorders

Each of your two ovaries is about the size of an almond. They are located in your abdomen, above and to the side of your uterus and about 4 to 5 inches below your waist. At birth, a female has roughly 1 million undeveloped eggs (ova) stored in her ovaries, each housed in its own follicle. Every month, from the time of puberty until menopause, one ovum grows until rupture of its follicle releases it. The ovum moves downward through your fallopian tube to your uterus.

Your ovaries also produce the female sex hormones estrogen and progesterone, which regulate your menstrual cycle. During the first half of the cycle, your ovaries secrete estrogen. Most of it is manufactured by the outer cells of the single follicle where the ovum is growing. Estrogen causes your uterine lining to thicken in order to receive a fertilized egg.

Just before ovulation, the same follicle begins to produce tiny amounts of progesterone. After the egg is released, the follicle expands rapidly—at this stage it is called the corpus luteum—and steps up production of both progesterone and estrogen. These hormones act together to complete the development of your uterine lining. If pregnancy occurs, hormones secreted by the corpus luteum help to sustain the pregnancy. If it does not occur, the corpus luteum begins to shrink, and levels of estrogen and progesterone decrease. As a result, your uterus will shed its lining, resulting in menstruation.

Ovarian Cysts and Benign Tumors

Signs and Symptoms

- Usually no symptoms
- Dull ache in your abdomen or a sense of pressure or fullness
- Pain during intercourse
- Delayed, irregular, or painful menstrual periods
- Firm, painless swelling of your lower abdomen
- Abrupt onset of sharp pain in your lower abdomen

Emergency Symptoms—Sudden, severe abdominal pain with fever and perhaps vomiting

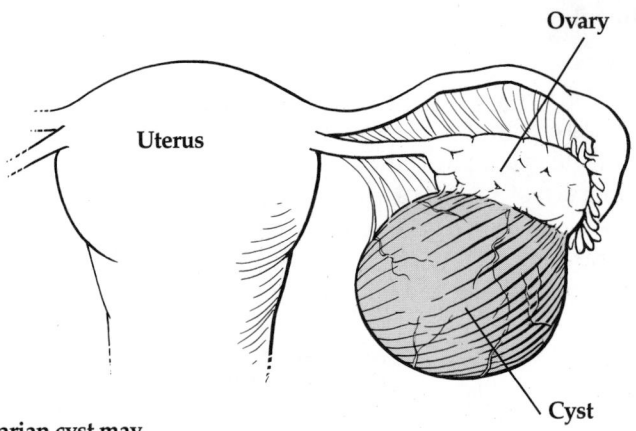

An ovarian cyst may be detected during a routine pelvic examination.

Most ovarian cysts are harmless and disappear of their own accord. Other types of cysts should be taken as a warning. Often, they are benign themselves and do not even cause symptoms—your physician finds them during a routine pelvic examination. However, women who develop such cysts between the ages of 50 and 70 have a higher risk of ovarian cancer and should have regular pelvic examinations.

A cyst is a sac, often filled with fluid; a tumor is a solid lump. Benign tumors do not invade neighboring tissue or spread to other parts of the body the way malignant tumors do. However, if a benign tumor or ovarian cyst is large, it can cause abdominal discomfort. In some cases, it may interfere with your production of ovarian hormones and result in irregular bleeding from your vagina or an increase in body hair. If a large tumor or cyst presses on your bladder, you may need to urinate more frequently because its capacity is diminished.

If a tumor or cyst becomes twisted, you may experience spasmodic pain. Sudden or sharp pain may mean a cyst has ruptured. The twisting or rupture of a cyst may increase the likelihood of an infection. If you have severe abdominal pain, fever, and vomiting, or if you have symptoms of shock such as cold, clammy skin and rapid breathing, get help immediately.

Diagnosis

If your physician finds something that feels like an ovarian cyst or tumor during a pelvic examination (see page 1141), he or she may order an ultrasound examination and perhaps a laparoscopy to confirm the diagnosis. For laparoscopy, a minor surgical procedure, your physician uses a slim, lighted instrument inserted into your abdomen through a small incision to see your ovaries (see page 1346).

Treatment

If you have a cyst and no symptoms and are younger than 40, you can wait through two or three menstrual cycles to see if it goes away. If it does not, your physician may prescribe hormones or remove it surgically.

Surgery

If a cyst causes problems or does not regress or disappear in two or three menstrual cycles, you may need an operation or other procedure. Sometimes, your physician can drain the cyst through a laparoscope, but more often it requires surgical removal in a hospital. If you are older than 40 and the cyst is larger than 2 inches in diameter or if you are postmenopausal, your physician may remove the cyst surgically. Your physician also will remove tumors. If a cyst or tumor is not too large, your ovary can be left intact.

Cancer of the Ovary

Signs and Symptoms
- Usually, no symptoms initially
- Vague abdominal discomfort and mild indigestion
- Swollen abdomen and pain in your lower abdomen (late stage of the disease)

Ovarian cancer can be deadly. In its early stages, it produces few noticeable symptoms, and frequently it is discovered during a routine pelvic examination. If undiscovered, it eventually causes symptoms, and the tumor may produce fluid that causes your abdomen to swell. Seventy to 80 percent of the time, the disease has already advanced when it is diagnosed.

Ovarian cancer generally develops after menopause. If you have never been pregnant or have had trouble conceiving, you are somewhat more likely to get cancer of the ovaries. Conversely, you are less likely to get it if you have had several children or have taken birth control pills. However, in either case, an annual pelvic examination still is important, because early diagnosis and treatment give you the best chance for a cure.

Diagnosis

If a pelvic examination (see page 1141) reveals a growth on an ovary, your physician will order an ultrasound test or a CT scan to evaluate the growth. Three out of four ovarian tumors are not malignant.

How Serious Is Cancer of the Ovary?

When detected early, ovarian cancer's 5-year survival rate is 60 to 80 percent. However, the survival rate is only 30 to 40 percent overall, because this type of malignancy is seldom found soon enough. Nevertheless, with aggressive surgery and chemotherapy, women with advanced ovarian cancer are now surviving longer than before such treatment was used.

Treatment

Surgery

If you are a young woman who wants to preserve the option to have children and your tumor is discovered early, your surgeon may remove only the involved ovary and its fallopian tube. However, the most common type of tumor often occurs in both ovaries. If that is the case, or if the disease already has begun to spread, your surgeon will remove both ovaries and also your uterus, fallopian tubes, nearby lymph glands, and a fold of tissue known as the omentum, because ovarian cancer often spreads to the omentum. In addition, your surgeon will take many samples of tissue and fluid from your abdomen to examine for cancer cells.

Chemotherapy

The oncologist (cancer specialist) will probably treat you with a combination of several drugs. After chemotherapy, a tumor usually shrinks. However, 12 to 18 months later, it often begins to grow again. Because it is then resistant to the original drugs, your oncologist will use a different combination of drugs in the second course of chemotherapy.

Radiation

In rare instances radiation therapy may also be advised.

Polycystic Ovarian Syndrome

Signs and Symptoms

- Unpredictable menstrual periods, or failure to menstruate
- Infertility
- An unusual amount of facial hair

This is a disease of young women. Most who get it never had a normal menstrual rhythm in their teens and eventually may stop menstruating altogether (some never start). Their faces can be rather hairy and they may be overweight. Menses occurs without cramping. Most of the time, they do not ovulate. For reasons we do not understand, their ovarian follicles develop but form cysts instead of releasing an egg; eventually, each ovary is a mass of small cysts.

An advanced form of polycystic ovarian syndrome is known as the Stein-Leventhal syndrome. It causes infertility, but is often treatable.

Diagnosis

During a pelvic examination (see page 1141), your physician generally can feel that your ovaries are enlarged. Blood tests will reveal a typical pattern of hormones present in abnormal amounts.

Treatment

Medication

If you do not want to become pregnant, your physician may prescribe birth control pills or long-acting progestins such as medroxyprogesterone to suppress ovulation and forestall any possible precancerous changes in the lining of your uterus. If you want to conceive, you may be given a fertility drug. Clomiphene induces ovulation in most women, but less than half will eventually conceive. If clomiphene does not work, your physician may consider giving you gonadotropins.

Surgery

If, despite medication, you fail to conceive, sometimes a laparoscopic operation can be done on the wall of your ovary, which may improve your chances of conceiving.

Polycystic ovarian syndrome is a disorder involving irregular menstrual periods and occasionally an excess of facial and body hair. The ovaries develop cysts and fail to release eggs.

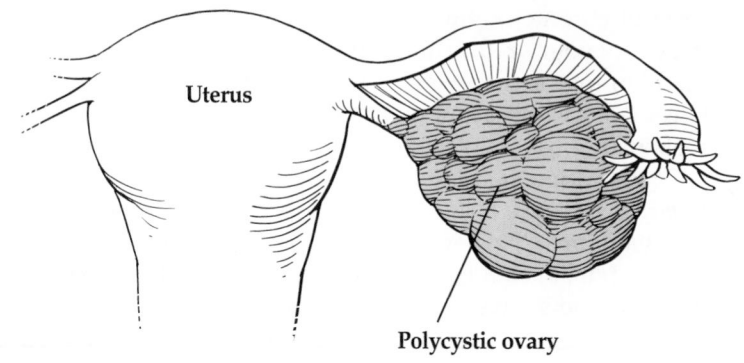

Uterus

Polycystic ovary

Bladder and Urethral Disorders

Your bladder lies between your pubic bone and your uterus. It is the sac where urine is stored after it has been produced by your kidneys. Your bladder has stretchable, muscular walls that expand as it fills with urine. When those walls contract, the urine is squeezed out into your urethra, a thin tube about 1.5 inches long. The opening to your urethra is located between your clitoris and your vagina (see page 1141).

Both males and females have a bladder and urethra, but these organs are somewhat different in each sex. For that reason, different problems can develop, and some disorders are more likely to develop in women than in men. For example, because a woman's urethra is close to both her vagina and her anus, which often harbor bacteria, and is shorter than the male's urethra, infections of the bladder (cystitis) and urethra (urethritis) are more common in women. In addition, some older women experience urinary problems, such as incontinence, when the muscles of the pelvic floor, which support the bladder and other internal organs, weaken and allow those organs to sag lower in the body.

This section covers urinary tract problems common to women. For other urinary disorders, see page 825.

Chronic Urethritis

Signs and Symptoms
- Discomfort on urination, which persists or recurs
- Frequent urination

Sometimes your urethra may remain irritated and inflamed over weeks or months, with or without evidence of a bacterial infection. When this happens, you feel the need to urinate frequently, and urinating is uncomfortable. As your chronically inflamed urethra has undergone periods of healing, it has gradually narrowed.

Inflammation that extends into the bottom of your bladder is called trigonitis. Your doctor uses a lighted, tubular instrument (see Cystoscopy, page 849) that can be inserted into your bladder to diagnose trigonitis.

Honeymoon Cystitis

You may develop symptoms of cystitis (see page 842), such as frequent, painful urination, almost every time you have intercourse. The symptoms generally last for a day or two and then disappear, only to recur the next time you have sex. The problem is sometimes called honeymoon cystitis, although it is actually a form of chronic urethritis—it is generally your urethra, not your bladder, that is inflamed. (The Greek suffix *itis* means "an inflammation.")

Usually, an infection, often *Chlamydia* (see page 1088), causes the symptoms. However, if you soak in bubble bath or use feminine hygiene sprays or douches,

these can irritate your urethra. Or, your urethra may be bruised by sexual activity, thus the term "honeymoon cystitis."

If bath oils, sprays, or douches cause the problem, you can simply stop using them, and the symptoms should disappear. Otherwise, see a physician. Your physician will ask for a urine sample and test it for bacteria. If you do have an infection, antibiotics generally will clear it up. However, sometimes laboratory tests fail to find any microorganisms that could be responsible; and some women, even after treatment with an antibiotic, continue to have symptoms whenever they have intercourse. In such cases, your physician may

suggest preventive measures. You may need to take an antibiotic, such as a low dose of nitrofurantoin or trimethoprim-sulfamethoxazole (Bactrim or Septra) every time you have sex.

You can do other things to make honeymoon cystitis less likely. Wash your genital and anal areas daily with mild soap and water. Before you have sex, be sure your partner's hands and penis are clean. After intercourse, empty your bladder immediately to flush bacteria out of your urethra. Use a water-soluble lubricant during intercourse to make penetration easier and bruising less likely; do not use petroleum jelly because it is not water-soluble.

Treatment

Medication
Your physician may prescribe antibiotics or sulfa drugs if there is evidence of actual infection. Other treatments—for instance, stretching (dilating) your urethra with an instrument—may help.

Urine Incontinence and Other Urine Loss Problems

Signs and Symptoms
- Involuntary urination
- Small amounts of urine escape under pressure—for instance, when you cough or sneeze

If you find that you need to urinate so suddenly and urgently that you cannot hold back, you have urgency incontinence. You may have a low-grade urinary infection. If you lose control only a little bit, and only when you cough, sneeze, laugh, or lift something, it is stress incontinence. It generally is due to weakening of the muscles of the pelvic floor that support your bladder and close off the top of your urethra. Those muscles can deteriorate because of childbirth, being overweight, or aging (see page 1175). Disorders such as Alzheimer's disease (see page 470) and spinal cord injury also can cause incontinence.

Tests may include a urine sample for laboratory analysis and culture, and cystoscopy or urodynamic studies or both.

Treatment

Medication
Your physician will treat bladder infections with antibiotics (see page 1058). Sometimes using estrogen cream in your vagina will reduce urethral irritation.

Surgery
For stress incontinence, surgery can tighten your pelvic floor muscles, or your physician can fit you with a pessary (a device that encircles the cervix) to wear in your vagina during the day to support your pelvic organs.

Self-Help
You can strengthen pelvic muscles with simple exercise (see Exercises for Incontinence, page 1176).

Interstitial Cystitis

Signs and Symptoms—Painful and frequent urination

Interstitial cystitis is an inflammation of your bladder wall. This uncommon condition almost always affects only women in their childbearing years. Although the exact cause is unknown, we do know that it is not the result of infection or cancer.

Diagnosis
A urologist diagnoses interstitial cystitis by visually examining your bladder lining through an instrument called a cystoscope.

Treatment
Although pain medications provide relief for some people, there is no specific treatment for interstitial cystitis. If symptoms are severe, a urologist may administer medication directly to your bladder wall through a cystoscope. At best, however, these approaches only make your symptoms more tolerable. But it's important to remember that the condition does not indicate a more serious underlying disease and that the initial symptoms rarely worsen and, in some instances, abate with time.

Irritable Bladder

Signs and Symptoms
- Sudden and sometimes uncontrollable urge to urinate
- Frequent need to urinate during the night

You may have an irritable bladder—one that contracts uncontrollably at times—if you often need to urinate so suddenly and urgently that you do not always make it to the bathroom. The problem is fairly common. Sometimes an infection is to blame, but often the cause is unclear, although your bladder may be chronically inflamed. This disorder can be distressing, but it is not dangerous. It should be distinguished from an inflamed bladder.

Diagnosis
Your physician will want a urine specimen for laboratory analysis. You may have a special kind of X-ray taken while you are urinating (a voiding cystogram). Cystoscopy is another possibility (see page 849); this is a procedure

in which a lighted instrument is inserted through your urethra into your bladder.

Treatment

Medication

Physicians use antibiotics to treat infections. Drugs such as imipramine can relax the muscles that make your bladder contract. Other medications can reduce the activity of the nerves that control the contraction.

Self-Help

When irritable bladder is not due to an infection, it may be treated through bladder training techniques.

Chapter 35

Men's Health

Contents

Male Genital Organs, 1196

Problems Related to the Testicles
and Scrotum, 1197
Testicular Torsion, 1197
Testicular Failure, 1198
  Injury to the Testicles, 1198
Epididymitis, 1198
Scrotal Masses, 1199
Hydrocele, 1200
  Self-Examination of the Testicles, 1200
Varicocele, 1201
Orchitis, 1201
Undescended Testicle, 1202
Cancer of the Testicle, 1202

Penis, Urethra, and Bladder, 1203
Cystitis, 1203
Penile Warts, 1204
Urethritis, 1204
  Noninfectious Urethral Discharge, 1205

Urethral Stricture, 1205
Balanitis, 1205
  Hygiene for Men, 1205
  Sexually Transmitted Diseases in
    Men, 1206
Curvature of the Penis, 1206
  Priapism, 1206
Paraphimosis, 1206
Cancer of the Penis, 1206
Urinary Incontinence, 1207
  Urinary Tract Infections in Men, 1208

Disorders of the Prostate Gland, 1209
Enlarged Prostate, 1209
  Transurethral Resection of the
    Prostate, 1210
Acute Prostatitis, 1210
Chronic Prostatitis, 1211
Cancer of the Prostate, 1211

Sexual Problems of Men, 1212

Male Genital Organs

In terms of function, the main purpose of the male genital organs is to produce sperm cells and transport them to the female reproductive system. As with the female genital organs (see Women's Health, page 1139), there is some overlap between the genital system and the urinary system, with some of the same organs being used in each. The link is so close that a genital system disorder frequently causes symptoms in the urinary system, and vice versa. A urologist is a physician who deals with both the genital and urinary organs in men; urologists also deal with urinary tract problems in women.

The main male genital organs are the penis, the testicles, the vas deferens (the duct through which the sperm passes), the seminal vesicles, and the prostate gland.

The penis is a sexual organ and also transports urine. The urethra, which runs the length of the penis through its center, carries urine during voiding and semen during ejaculation. There are many blood vessels in the penis, and these are involved in producing an erection. During sexual arousal, these vessels supply blood to three cylindrical, sponge-like structures that run parallel to the urethra along the length of the penis. As these structures fill with blood, the penis expands, straightens, and stiffens.

The testicles (or testes) are two oval organs about 2 inches long. They are contained in a pouch of skin, called the scrotum, which hangs below the abdomen and behind the penis. In each testicle there is a tightly packed mass of coiled tubes surrounded by a protective capsule. At puberty the testicles begin to produce the sperm cells that are used in reproduction. This process continues throughout life. In addition to producing sperm cells, the testicles secrete the male hormone testosterone, which plays an important role in the development and maintenance of the typical masculine physical characteristics (such as facial hair, greater muscle mass and strength, and a deeper voice).

Sperm production must take place at a temperature that is lower than the temperature within the body. This is made possible by the testicles' location outside the abdominal cavity.

The sperm cells that are constantly being produced within each testicle are transported through the epididymis (the cord-like structure at the top and rear of the testicles) and the vas deferens and then stored in the seminal vesicles. The mixture of the sperm cells with the fluids formed by the seminal vesicles and the prostate gland forms the semen that is ejaculated during sexual activity. Although sperm cells make up only a small portion of the semen, a single ejaculation contains as many as 500 million sperm. After sexual intercourse, one of these cells may reach and fertilize an egg in the female (see page 167).

The prostate gland contributes fluids to the semen. Among other things, these fluids appear to increase the ability of the sperm to survive within the vagina. As a man ages, the prostate gland frequently enlarges. Sometimes this causes the gland to press against the urethra. This pressure makes urination more difficult and may require surgical correction (described on page 1209).

Male Genital Organs

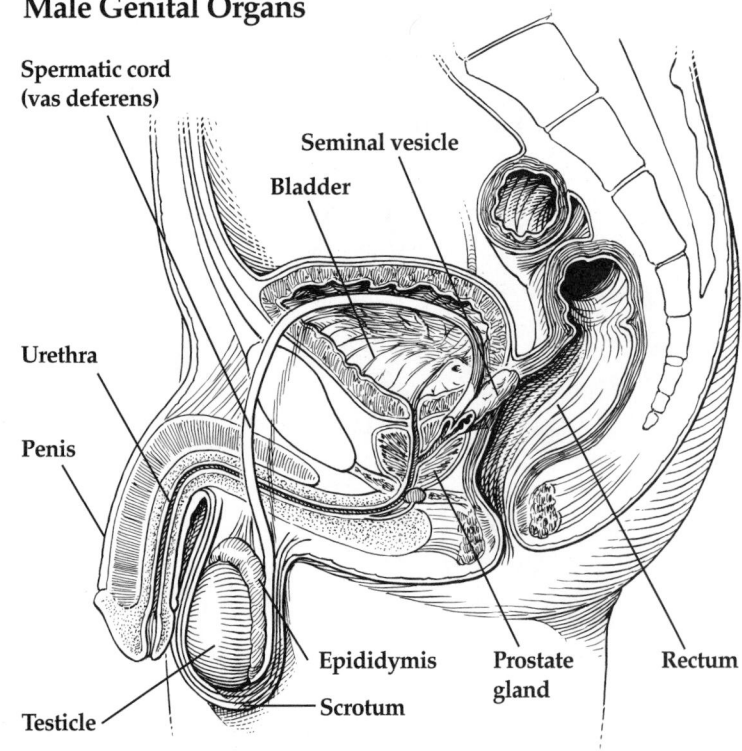

Spermatic cord (vas deferens)

Seminal vesicle

Bladder

Urethra

Penis

Epididymis

Scrotum

Prostate gland

Rectum

Testicle

Problems Related to the Testicles and Scrotum

The testicles (testes) play two important roles: they produce the sperm cells used in reproduction, and they secrete hormones (for example, testosterone) that play a key role in male body development. Their location in the scrotum, a pouch outside the pelvic area, keeps them at a temperature lower than that within the abdominal cavity, which is required for adequate sperm production.

The relatively exposed location of the testicles and scrotum does make them prone to injuries. But it also makes it easy to examine them for potentially life-threatening problems such as cancer.

This section covers the main problems that can occur in the testicles themselves, in the epididymis (the cord-like structure near the top of the testicles) and vas deferens (sperm transport tubes), and in the spermatic cords (which suspend the testicles) within the scrotum. Self-examination of the testicles also is described.

Testicular Torsion

Signs and Symptoms
- Sudden, generally severe, pain in one testicle
- Elevation of one testicle within the scrotum
- Nausea and vomiting
- Sensation of faintness
- Swelling
- Fever

Emergency Symptoms—Sudden, severe testicular pain that arises spontaneously or after strenuous physical activity

Each testicle is suspended within the scrotum on a spermatic cord, which contains the blood vessels that supply that testicle. In testicular torsion, the testicle twists on its spermatic cord, cutting off the blood supply to the testicle. Testicular torsion sometimes occurs without any apparent cause, even during sleep. At other times, it happens after strenuous physical activity.

Testicular torsion is uncommon, but it can occur at any age. It usually occurs in young children, although it also may occur around the time of puberty or, rarely, in babies.

Diagnosis
Testicular torsion causes severe local pain, often accompanied by nausea, faintness, and vomiting, with no precipitating physical injury to suggest testicular torsion. However, these same symptoms can also be caused by inflammation within the scrotum and by a tumor. The symptoms of testicular torsion and epididymitis (see page 1198) are similar. One way to distinguish between the two ailments is to lift the painful testicle while standing; with torsion, the testicle will probably hurt more as a result; with epididymitis, it will probably hurt less. To help differentiate testicular torsion from other conditions affecting the scrotum, a testicular ultrasound examination will often be ordered by your physician.

In some cases, a surgical procedure may be necessary to establish the diagnosis and to correct the testicular torsion.

How Serious Is Testicular Torsion?
Severe pain in a testicle requires immediate medical attention. If the torsion is not corrected within a few hours—often by an operation—the testicle will be damaged from a lack of blood supply and will have to be removed from the scrotum.

It is uncommon for the twisted cord to untwist without medical intervention.

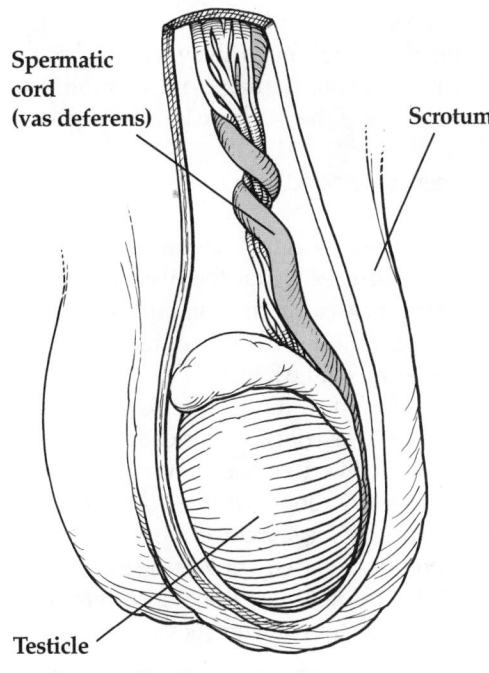

Spermatic cord (vas deferens)

Scrotum

Testicle

In testicular torsion, the testicle twists on its spermatic cord, cutting off the blood supply and producing sudden, severe pain.

Treatment

Surgery
Testicular torsion requires prompt corrective surgery to return the testicle to its normal position and to anchor it in place. In addition, the testicle on the other side is often anchored in place as a precaution to prevent possible torsion of that testicle in the future.

Other Therapies
Sometimes it is possible for the physician to manipulate the twisted testicle carefully and to return it to its normal position. In this case, an operation later probably will be desirable anyway, to secure the testicle in its normal position and thus prevent a recurrence.

Testicular Failure

Signs and Symptoms
- Infertility
- Possible lack of sexual drive
- Delay of puberty or of development of male characteristics, in some cases

---

Injury to the Testicles

The male genital organs are not located inside the abdomen; therefore, they are prone to injury. Pain caused by a blow to the testicles is severe. Fortunately, however, lasting injury to the testicles is rare. The sponginess of their tissues and the flexibility of their location enable them to absorb considerable shock without permanent harm.

If your testicles have been injured by a blunt object or in a fall and the pain and swelling of the scrotum go away within about an hour, there probably is no serious damage. If the scrotum remains swollen or is bruised, or if the pain persists, seek medical care promptly.

If your scrotum has been penetrated by a sharp object, seek emergency care.

The same precautions apply in the case of babies and children. Persistent pain, swelling, or bruises signal the need to see a physician promptly. A young male can become infertile from an untreated testicular injury even though he has not reached the age of sexual maturity at the time of the injury.

There are many causes of pain in the testicles other than injury. Most of these causes are described in this chapter. The important thing to remember is this: if severe pain persists, see a physician or go to an emergency room. Untreated testicular injury or other conditions affecting the testicles can have serious complications such as blood clots, infertility, or even loss of a testicle. (Loss of a single testicle does not cause impotence, infertility, or loss of sex drive or other male characteristics.)

The term "testicular failure" refers to the inability of the testicles to produce sperm or, in some cases, to produce male hormones. The causes of such failure include chromosome abnormalities present before birth, problems affecting sexual maturation, and damage to mature, normally developed testicles caused by disease, drugs, or injury. Testicular failure is uncommon.

Diagnosis
Testicular failure is one of many possible causes of infertility. To establish the cause of infertility, the physician must interview and examine both sexual partners and also perform blood, urine, and semen tests (see Health Issues of Partners, page 1213). The diagnosis will depend on the results of such tests.

In cases of slowed or absent sexual maturation, the diagnosis will be by interview, physical examination, and appropriate related tests.

How Serious Is Testicular Failure?
Testicular failure is neither life-threatening nor the first stage in some degenerative process. Instead, its seriousness relates to the symptoms themselves—infertility, possible lack of sex drive, or delayed sexual maturation.

Treatment

Medication
Restoration of a normal sex drive or continuity of normal sexual development often can be achieved by the administration of male hormones. However, fertility rarely can be restored.

Epididymitis

Signs and Symptoms
- Pain in the scrotum, generally severe, which develops gradually over several hours or days
- Fever
- Swelling

At the top and rear of each testicle is a coiled tube that transports sperm to the vas deferens. This tube is the epididymis. Epididymitis is inflammation of this structure. The swollen area will feel hot and sausage-shaped to the touch. Epididymitis usually is caused by bacteria. Sometimes it can arise from unknown causes.

Diagnosis

Pain in the testicles that develops over several hours and is accompanied by fever suggests epididymitis. Usually, only one testicle is affected. The physician may take a urine sample and a sample of prostate gland secretions in an attempt to identify the infecting organism.

How Serious Is Epididymitis?

Epididymitis usually is an acute ailment that can be corrected with medication, without any damage to the genital organs. Occasionally, chronic epididymitis develops. This rarely requires surgical treatment.

Treatment

Medication

Antibiotics are prescribed to combat epididymitis that is of bacterial origin. Because your sex partner may be infected with the same bacteria, similar treatment of your partner may be necessary.

Other Therapies

Treatment for epididymitis also includes bed rest, application of ice packs to the scrotum, elevating the scrotum, and use of pain medication.

Scrotal Masses

Signs and Symptoms

- Lump or swelling in the scrotum
- Possible local pain or tenderness

Scrotal masses have various causes. These include tumors, cysts and other inflammations, physical injury, and inguinal hernia.

The tumors may be either benign or malignant. Tumors growing within the testicles themselves most often are malignant (cancerous); those located elsewhere within the scrotum are usually benign (noncancerous). Cancer of the testicles is discussed later in this chapter.

A common type of painless, benign cyst is a spermatic cyst, or spermatocele. It grows adjacent to the epididymis near the top of a testicle. Hydrocele and varicocele, described later in this chapter (see pages 1200 and 1201, respectively), also are painless, benign sources of scrotal swelling. Hematocele is a scrotal mass caused by physical injury, and it consists of an accumulation of blood.

With an inguinal hernia, a portion of the intestine may drop into the scrotum and cause it to bulge.

Diagnosis

Every scrotal mass should be evaluated by a physician. If the mass is a tumor, it could be malignant. The tumor must be removed surgically before an accurate diagnosis can be made. Blood tests and a painless ultrasound examination (see page 1335) help to distinguish the many harmless causes of scrotal masses from tumors.

How Serious Are Scrotal Masses?

Malignant tumors are serious. If detected before the cancer spreads (see Self-Examination of the Testicles, page 1200), they usually can be treated effectively.

Treatment

Surgery

If you have a testicular tumor, surgical removal of the tumor is necessary. Testicular cancer requires surgical removal of the entire testicle and possibly additional treatment as well.

Inguinal hernias generally require surgery (see Inguinal Hernias, page 822). Other causes of scrotal masses usually do not require any treatment.

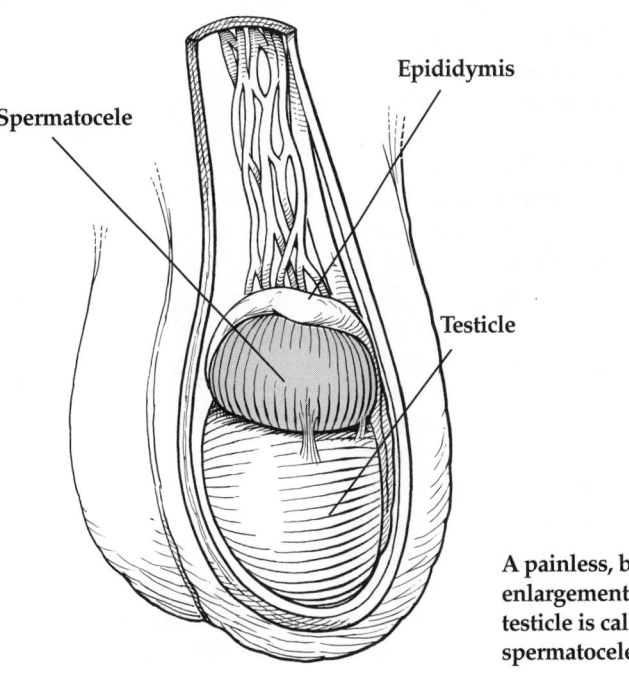

A painless, benign enlargement atop the testicle is called a spermatocele.

Hydrocele

Signs and Symptoms—Soft, usually painless, swelling in the scrotum

The term hydrocele comes from the Greek *hydro* for "water" and *cele* for "tumor." A testicular hydrocele is a collection of watery fluid in the sheath that holds the testicle. Normally, this sheath contains just enough fluid to lubricate the testicle. The larger amount, which makes the hydrocele, develops either because the body produces too much fluid or because it does not absorb enough fluid. Hydroceles are a common cause of scrotal swelling and may occur with one or both testicles. Hydroceles may occur at any age but are most common in older men.

Diagnosis

To help differentiate a hydrocele from a tumor or other source of swelling, the physician will carefully feel the swollen area and probably will hold a light to the scrotum. If the swelling is a hydrocele, the light will shine through it. A painless ultrasound examination also may be performed.

How Serious Is a Hydrocele?

A hydrocele is not serious. Treatment is usually not required unless the scrotum is so swollen that it is uncomfortable.

Treatment

Surgery

If discomfort persists in the scrotum, surgery may be necessary. Also, the fluid can be drawn off (aspirated) with a needle and syringe. This procedure is simple but, because the fluid usually will accumulate again, it is seldom done. In addition, needle aspiration is potentially hazardous because of possible introduction of infection. Thus, aspiration should be used only in patients for whom surgery has too high a risk.

Self-Examination of the Testicles

Cancer of the testicles is a potential killer—but, if detected early, it can usually be cured.

A simple examination that takes only a minute or two can detect a growth in the testicles in its early stages. Like the breast self-examination for women, self-examination of the testicles is easy and important, and it may turn out to be life-saving. Because cancer of the testicles occurs more often in younger men than in older men, monthly self-examination of the testicles should begin at high-school age.

Perform the examination after a shower or warm bath, when the skin of the scrotum is loose and relaxed. Examine one testicle at a time. Grasp the testicle and roll it gently between your thumb and forefinger. As you do so, feel for any lump on the surface of the testicle. Also, notice if the testicle is enlarged, hardened, or otherwise different from how it was at the last examination. (A small firm area near the rear of the testicle is a normal part of the testicle; the cord leading upward from the top of the testicle is also a normal part of the scrotum and is not a growth.)

If you feel a lump on a testicle or any change in the testicle, this does not necessarily mean that you have cancer. But visit your physician soon to find out.

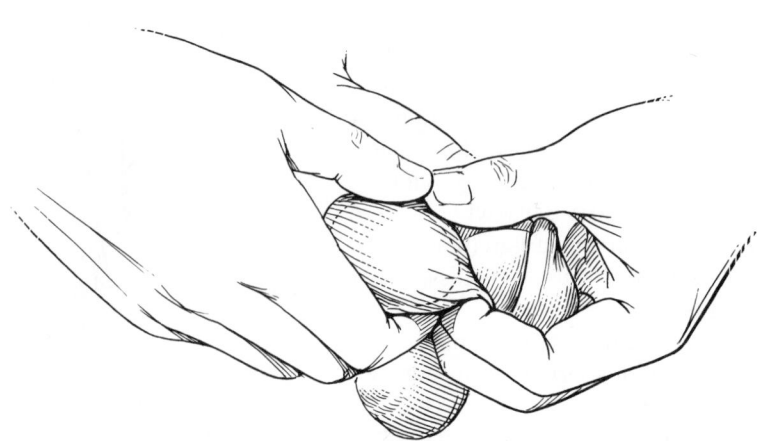

A regular self-examination of the testicles can identify dangerous growths early—in time for a cure. Grasp and roll the testicle between your thumb and forefinger, feeling for lumps, swelling, hardness, or other changes.

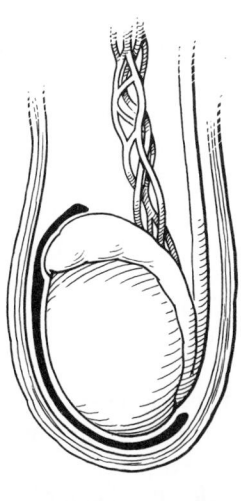

Normal testicle

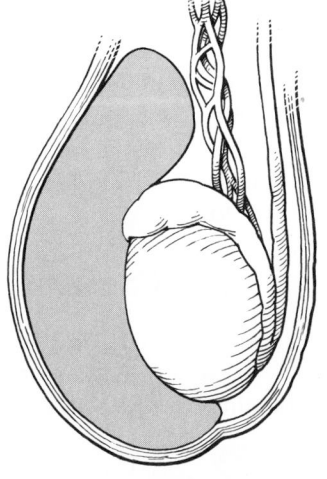

Hydrocele

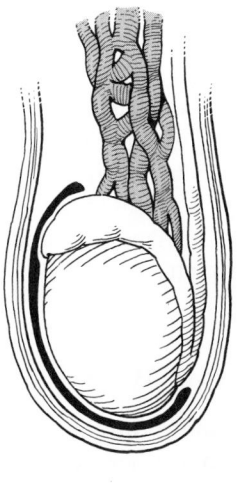

Varicocele

A hydrocele is a harmless but abnormal accumulation of watery fluid within the scrotum. The condition usually requires no treatment. A varicocele is a swelling within the scrotum due to varicose (enlarged) veins. To prevent infertility, this condition may require treatment.

Varicocele

Signs and Symptoms—Swelling in the scrotum, usually on the left side. The swelling is painless, and the area feels like a bag of worms. This sensation may nearly disappear when you lie down

A varicocele is a swelling in the scrotum caused by varicose (enlarged) veins. The blood backs up in the veins leading from the testicles because of a problem with valves located inside the veins.

Diagnosis
Your physician will carefully feel the swollen scrotum and may hold a light to the swollen area. If the problem is a varicocele, the light will not shine through the blood in the veins. A painless ultrasound examination also may be done.

How Serious Is a Varicocele?
The varicocele itself is not a serious disorder. The problem is that the backed-up blood in the testicles can contribute to infertility. If this is the case, surgical tying off (ligation) of the varicocele improves the chances of restoring fertility.

Treatment

Surgery
When infertility is evident and a varicocele exists, surgery to ligate the varicocele may be advisable. This procedure often can be done on an outpatient basis. Unless a varicocele is associated with infertility, surgical ligation is rarely necessary.

Orchitis

Signs and Symptoms
- Pain in the scrotum
- Swelling, generally on one side of the scrotum only
- A feeling of weight in the scrotum

Orchitis is an inflammation of the testicle, often due to a bacterial infection or the mumps virus. Orchitis may also occur in association with infection of the prostate or the epididymis. Many diseases that are much less common may have orchitis among their manifestations.

Diagnosis
Your physician will carefully feel the swelling in your scrotum. Because the symptoms of orchitis are similar to those of epididymitis (see page 1198) and other conditions affecting the testicles, your physician also may take a urine sample and perform other tests to identify associated infections.

How Serious Is Orchitis?
Orchitis can permanently damage one or both testicles. This could result in diminished size of the testicle and infertility.

Treatment

Medication

Orchitis associated with bacterial infections is treated with antibiotics. However, orchitis associated with viral infections such as mumps is treated only by conservative means such as rest and medications to relieve pain.

Undescended Testicle

Signs and Symptoms—Scrotum contains one (or no) rather than two testicles

Before birth, the testicles develop inside the male infant's abdomen. Usually, they move down into their permanent place in the scrotum 1 month before birth. A small percentage of male infants are born with one or both testicles undescended.

In most of these babies, the testicles will descend into the scrotum during the first few years of life, without any medical intervention. In some cases, however, medication or surgery may be necessary. A testicle that remains undescended by age 5 may not be able to make sperm later in life.

There are less common causes that may require extensive study for diagnosis. Sometimes, both testicles are present but one is smaller than normal.

Diagnosis

Your physician can confirm the absence or the stunted development of a testicle by feeling the scrotum. Other tests may be required before determining the appropriate action for correcting the condition.

How Serious Is Undescended Testicle?

The absence of a testicle is not serious. In the case of infants or young children, the condition often corrects itself or can be corrected with medication or surgery. After age 5, however, the situation can lead to a non-functional testicle. Even after it descends, or after surgical correction, a testicle that was undescended will be more vulnerable to cancer than a normal testicle.

Treatment

Medication

Hormones often are given to induce an undescended testicle to descend into the scrotum.

Surgery

For testicles that do not descend early in life or in response to hormones, surgery is required to prevent loss of function to the testicle and to lessen later vulnerability to testicular cancer. The best age for the treatment is 12 to 18 months.

Cancer of the Testicle

Signs and Symptoms
- A lump or swelling in a testicle
- A heavy feeling in a testicle (sometimes)

Cancer of the testicle often begins in the cells that produce sperm. The cancer first is noticed as a hard lump on the testicle. This lump usually is not painful to the touch. In the early stages, there are no other symptoms. Most men discover the tumor themselves (see Self-Examination of the Testicles, page 1200). The earlier this discovery is made, the better. Usually, the cancer affects only one testicle.

Testicular cancer is more common in younger men, particularly between ages 15 and 35, and it is more common in white men than in black men. If one or both testicles are undescended at birth, the risk of cancer in either testicle later in life is greater. If detected and treated early, testicular cancer often can be cured.

Diagnosis

A self-examination can detect the presence of a possible growth or tumor within the scrotum. Begin regular self-examination of your testicles in your teen years (see page 156). Regardless of whether or not pain is associated with the growth, if you discover such a lump, visit your physician without delay. An ultrasound examination may be performed to aid in the diagnosis.

A tumor in the testicle is almost always malignant (cancerous), but examination by a physician is required to determine if in fact a tumor is present. Other conditions affecting the testicles and scrotum can produce a lump that feels quite similar (see Epididymitis, page 1198; Scrotal Masses, page 1199; Hydrocele, page 1200; Varicocele, page 1201; and Orchitis, page 1201), and some of them are harmless.

If you do have a tumor in a testicle, surgical removal of the testicle is necessary. If the tumor is malignant, blood tests, X-rays, and other tests may be necessary to determine if the cancer has spread to other parts of the body.

How Serious Is Cancer of the Testicle?

The most common type of testicular cancer, seminoma, can be cured in nearly all cases if it is discovered and treated early. When all types of testicular cancer are considered, including cancers discovered at a late stage, about 90 percent of men with this condition will live for 5 years or more after treatment.

Treatment

Surgery

Surgical removal of the affected testicle is necessary. This does not imply any loss of virility because the remaining healthy testicle can maintain the body's normal sexual and hormone-production functions. If both testicles are lost, infertility will result. However, male hormones given by injection about every 3 weeks will maintain essentially normal sexual function.

Cancer of Testicle

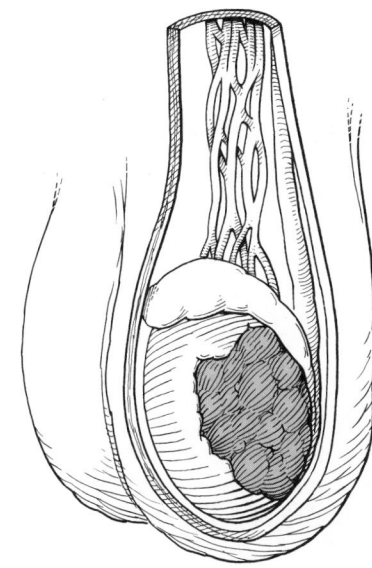

A painless lump in the testicle may indicate cancer. Consult your physician immediately. The earlier it is treated, the greater your chance of cure.

Other Therapies

Radiation therapy and chemotherapy may be used to prevent the spread of cancer to other parts of the body or to combat it if spread has begun.

Penis, Urethra, and Bladder

The penis functions both as a sexual organ and to transport urine. Each function sometimes can be affected by infections and other problems. The urethra, a tube that runs the length of the penis through the center, transports semen and urine.

Urine originates in the kidneys (see page 826) and is conveyed by the ureters to the bladder, a storage pouch within the abdomen, before it is excreted from the body through the urethra. Although the distance from the bladder to the outside is much longer in men than it is in women, infecting organisms sometimes can travel the entire length of the male urethra into the bladder.

Cystitis

Signs and Symptoms

- Painful urination (a burning or itching feeling)
- Frequent or urgent need to urinate
- Cloudy, smelly, bloody urine (sometimes)
- Lower abdominal pain (sometimes)
- Slight fever (sometimes)

Cystitis is an inflammation of the bladder, usually the result of an infection. The term comes from the Greek word *cyst* for "bladder." Rarely, the inflammation is caused by something other than an infection, such as in interstitial cystitis. Because of the length of the urethra in men, when men develop cystitis it often is caused by some problem, such as an enlarged prostate, that has interfered with the emptying of the bladder.

Cystitis is uncommon in men. Although it is easy to treat, the underlying problem must be treated as well to avoid recurrence.

Diagnosis

A physician will diagnose cystitis based on the description of the symptoms and on tests. Cultures of the urine may be needed to identify the bacteria that may be causing the infection. Other tests may include analysis of urine, cystoscopy (visualization of the urethra and bladder with a special viewing device, see page 849), and a special type of X-ray called an intravenous pyelogram (IVP, see page 829).

How Serious Is Cystitis?

Cystitis is not serious if it is treated promptly and properly. If the cystitis and the underlying cause are not treated, however, the cystitis can become chronic or recurrent.

Treatment

Medication

Antibiotics are given to combat the organism that causes the cystitis. Additional medications, or surgery, may be required to correct an associated underlying problem.

Penile Warts

Signs and Symptoms
- Warts on the shaft or head of the penis
- No visible lesions

Warts on the penis are similar to warts found elsewhere on the body. All warts, including penile warts, are caused by a virus. This means that warts are contagious. Warts in the genital area can be transmitted to or received from one's partner during sexual activity. Consequently, if you have penile warts, both you and your sexual partner may require treatment.

Diagnosis

Penile warts are diagnosed on the basis of their appearance. Sometimes a growth on the penis may look like a wart but in reality be a symptom of a sexually transmitted disease or a malignant tumor. If your physician suspects one of these other problems, tests will be performed to establish a diagnosis and to permit planning of effective treatment.

Warts that are not visible may become apparent after application of an acetic acid (vinegar) solution. This procedure may be done if your sex partner has changes suggesting that the virus has been transmitted. The changes may be revealed during a gynecologic examination or Pap test (see page 1141).

How Serious Are Penile Warts?

Penile warts should be treated because they can spread to a sexual partner and can also proliferate on your penis. Women are at increased risk for cervical cancer when exposed to penile warts. If your sex partner has an abnormal Pap test, you should be evaluated for penile warts even if signs or symptoms are not readily apparent. If you have these warts, you and your partner will both need treatment to prevent a recurrence that could lead to cervical cancer in your partner.

Treatment

Medication

Your physician will require a preparation (such as tincture of podophyllum resin) to apply to the warts in order to remove them. (Do not purchase over-the-counter wart paints yourself and apply them to the penis because they are designed for skin that is less sensitive than the skin of the penis.) Sometimes, more involved treatment is necessary to remove the warts, such as freezing, laser surgery, or destruction by an electrical current.

Urethritis

Signs and Symptoms
- Burning pain when urinating or ejaculating
- Need to urinate frequently
- Discharge from the penis

Urethritis is an inflammation of the urethra, the duct in the penis through which urine and semen pass. It often is caused by a sexually transmitted disease, particularly gonorrhea or chlamydiosis (see page 1087). Sometimes the cause is unknown. The discharge that often is associated with urethritis can vary in color from clear to yellow and can vary in consistency from thin to thick. Urethritis generally is easy to cure. The affected person's sexual partner probably should be treated as well. Urethritis is sometimes associated with a form of arthritis called Reiter's syndrome (see page 913).

Diagnosis

Pain during urination and a discharge from the penis are reasons to visit a physician. Your urine and the discharge fluid will be tested to identify the infecting organism.

How Serious Is Urethritis?

In most cases of urethritis the infection goes away after treatment. Sometimes, repeated treatments are necessary. In a small number of cases, the urethritis resists treatment and urethral stricture, epididymitis, prostatitis, or other complications will occur.

Treatment

Medication
Antibiotics are given to treat urethritis. Your sexual partner may also require treatment.

Urethral Stricture

Signs and Symptoms
- Slow, weak urine stream
- Dribbling

Urethral stricture is a narrowing of the urethra (the narrow tube through the penis that transports urine and semen) to such a degree that the passage of urine is impeded. This is a rare condition. There are various causes of urethral stricture, including injury to the penis or disease that produces scar tissue, which gradually shrinks and narrows the urethral passage. In extreme instances, the passage can even become blocked. Urethral stricture may become evident a number of years after an acute episode of gonorrhea.

Diagnosis
Consult your physician if you have difficulty or pain in urinating. A number of infections and conditions other than urethral stricture can be responsible. Your physician will examine your penis and may perform various tests, including examination of the urethra with a thin, flexible instrument called a cystoscope (see page 849).

How Serious Is Urethral Stricture?
To restore the ability to urinate normally and painlessly, the urethral stricture must be treated. Usually, the first approach is to stretch the urethra by dilating it with a thin instrument (called a sound) that is inserted into the urethra. Local anesthesia is used. This treatment must be repeated a number of times. If the passageway does not remain adequate after repeated dilations, a surgical procedure may be necessary.

The severity of the stricture usually is monitored by using the cystoscope. If a surgical procedure is performed, it is done with special instruments through the cystoscope.

Noninfectious Urethral Discharge

This rare but disconcerting condition may occur in men who abruptly cease normal sexual activity, perhaps due to the illness of their partner or to some other reason not related to the man's own health. A man with noninfectious urethral discharge may observe spots on his undershorts or a urethral discharge during bowel movements.

The discharge is merely the passage of normal prostatic fluid. It will cease over time or on resumption of his usual sexual patterns.

Balanitis

Signs and Symptoms—Irritation and redness of the end of the penis

Balanitis is an inflammation of the tip (glans) of the penis. Balanitis is a fairly common genital ailment. It is more frequent in uncircumcised males, particularly if the foreskin is narrowed so that it cannot be pulled back easily.

There are various types of balanitis. The underlying causes include urinary tract infection, irritation from clothing that rubs against the penis or from chemicals used in cleaning or manufacturing the clothing, and reaction to contraceptive creams. Men with diabetes are especially prone to balanitis as a result of the high sugar content of their urine. Yeast infection also is a common cause.

Diagnosis
If you have a penis irritation that does not go away in a day or two, visit your physician or a urologist. Your physician will examine your penis and may perform tests to rule out other, more serious, types of infection. If bal-

---

Hygiene for Men

Wash your penis and scrotum the same way you wash other parts of your body: with soap and water every day. If your penis is uncircumcised, don't forget to pull back the foreskin and clean the head of the penis beneath it. These basic hygienic practices will help keep the genitals clean and free from minor infections.

Look for signs of disease as you clean. Possible trouble signs include sores or growths. If you find any, visit a physician (see Self-Examination of the Testicles, page 1200).

Washing will not prevent acquiring a sexually transmitted disease, however. For suggestions on avoiding venereal disease, see Sexually Transmitted Diseases in Men, page 1206.

Sexually Transmitted Diseases in Men

Sexually transmitted diseases can have tragic consequences. Such diseases are transmitted by contact with an infected person through vaginal intercourse, anal intercourse, or oral sexual activity. In the case of AIDS (acquired immunodeficiency syndrome), possible routes of transmission are infected semen, saliva, and blood, particularly blood on hypodermic needles shared by infected drug addicts. Symptoms do not develop immediately after invasion by the organism, and the course and consequences of the disease vary with the disease itself (see Sexually Transmitted Diseases, page 1087, and AIDS, page 1060).

Wearing a condom during sexual activity offers much protection against acquiring or passing along a sexually transmitted disease. However, use of condoms does not offer foolproof protection. The only certain way to avoid disease is to engage in sexual activity only with a trusted, noninfected partner.

anitis is diagnosed, your physician probably will analyze your urine to see if you have diabetes.

Treatment

The principal treatment for balanitis is cleanliness (see Hygiene for Men, page 1205). In an uncircumcised man whose foreskin cannot be easily retracted, circumcision may be needed to prevent or relieve balanitis. Use of antibiotics or antifungal agents may be required to cure bacterial or yeast infections.

Curvature of the Penis

Signs and Symptoms—Painful (sometimes) bend in the penis that develops during an erection and makes sexual intercourse difficult or impossible

Curvature of the penis, also known as Peyronie's disease after the French physician who first described it, mainly affects men ages 40 to 60. Scar tissue (plaque) forms inside the penis. The scar tissue is dense and firm and will not fill with blood during an erection. This causes the penis to curve toward the side of the scar. Why the scar tissue forms is not understood.

Diagnosis

If you have curvature of the penis, you can feel the plaque that causes it as a ridge running along the penis beneath the skin.

How Serious Is Curvature of the Penis?

The symptoms often are mild and do not always grow worse with time. In many cases, the disease goes away on its own, but this may require several years. The best approach is to give the condition a chance to improve on its own. If it does not, consult a urologist.

Priapism

This very rare condition occurs as a result of some type of spinal cord disorder, of leukemia, or of inflammation of the urethra. It is a sustained, often painful, erection that occurs without sexual stimulation.

In priapism, the penile shaft is firm but the head (glans) of the penis is soft. The penis becomes filled with blood as during a normal erection, but the blood does not drain out and the erection does not go away as it normally would after sexual activity or stimulation ceases. The name priapism derives from the Latin name for a male fertility god in classical mythology, Priapus.

If you have a painful erection that does not go away, seek medical help. Prompt treatment is necessary to preserve the ability of your penis to have a normal erection. Your physician will examine the penis and perform tests to determine the underlying cause.

Paraphimosis

Signs and Symptoms

- Painful swelling in the end of an uncircumcised penis
- Retracted foreskin that cannot be pulled back over the head of the penis to cover it

Emergency Symptoms—Severe swelling in the end of an uncircumcised penis

Paraphimosis occurs when the foreskin is pulled back and cannot be returned over the head (glans) of the penis. Consult a urologist or an emergency room physician immediately. Surgical treatment by circumcision or partial circumcision will probably be necessary to release the foreskin. If treatment is prompt, permanent damage to the penis generally can be avoided.

Cancer of the Penis

Signs and Symptoms

- Painless sore on the penis—an ulcer, a nodule, or a wart-like sore
- Other types of painless sores or warts on the penis

Cancer of the penis is rare. When it occurs, it most often affects uncircumcised males. In its early stages, small, painless growths occur on the penis, usually near its end. Without surgical removal and tests, these growths may be indistinguishable from penile warts. As the malignant growth progresses, there may be pain and bleeding.

Diagnosis

Any growth on the penis is a good reason to see a urologist promptly. Through examination and possible surgical removal and tests of the growth, your physician can determine whether the growth is malignant. If it is found to be malignant, more tests will be necessary to see whether the cancer has spread to other parts of your body and to plan the best treatment to combat spread.

How Serious Is Cancer of the Penis?

As with any other form of cancer, cancer of the penis can be life-threatening. The earlier it is detected and treated, the better the chances are for curing it.

Treatment

Surgery

Removal of the malignant growth, and possibly of adjacent portions of the penis, will be required. If a large portion of the penis must be removed, as with an advanced cancer, often a portion can be left that is sufficient for sexual activity and urination.

Other Therapies

Radiation therapy and chemotherapy may be used to prevent or to combat the spread of the disease to other parts of the body.

Urinary Incontinence

Signs and Symptoms—Inability to control urination some or all of the time

Urinary incontinence—the inability to keep urine in your body until you decide to release it—can have several causes. The muscular and neural systems that control the retention or release of urine are complex, and they can be affected by illness, medications, urinary tract infections, prostate gland problems, or an operation on the urinary tract.

In children, problems of bed-wetting are common (see page 1098). After puberty, how-ever, urinary incontinence is rare until the later decades of life. It is estimated that a third or more of elderly people who are hospitalized or who live in long-term-care facilities are incontinent. Among older persons living at home, the percentage is much smaller, around 10 percent. Urinary incontinence is more frequent in women than in men.

In many cases, bladder control can be regained by treating the underlying cause, by use of drugs, or by modifying daily habits. If urinary incontinence persists, special aids are also available to help manage the problem.

Diagnosis

Your physician will ask questions about the medications you take, operations you have undergone, and infections that you may have experienced. Your penis, rectum, and abdominal area will be examined, and a urine specimen will be taken for analysis. Sometimes, a painless ultrasound examination, a special X-ray called an intravenous pyelogram (IVP, see page 829), or cystoscopic examination (see page 849) may be required.

How Serious Is Urinary Incontinence?

Your physician will want to determine the cause of the leakage to rule out underlying disorders that may require treatment. People with urinary incontinence often withdraw socially. This is unfortunate. Normal daily hygiene and appropriate use and changing of pads or diapers generally will prevent offensive odors. Treatments are available, and there are ways to live with the problem if it persists.

Other risks include infectious reactions to urine on the skin or to the catheters sometimes used to control incontinence.

Treatment

Self-Help

Your physician may advise specific exercises to strengthen the pelvic area or bladder training techniques to regain control of urination. Often, a simple adjustment in daily routine—such as altering the times that you take medication or the hours you sleep—can make the difference. With some people, remembering to go to the bathroom is difficult, and use of an alarm can help. It is also handy to have a urinal nearby if the bathroom is distant or if handicaps make getting there in time a problem.

When incontinence cannot be eliminated,

special aids can help. Absorbent undergarments are available that neutralize the odor of urine and keep the skin fairly dry. Devices can be used to catch the urine, such as a type of condom that fits over the penis and drains urine through a tube into a plastic bag. There is also a type of foam rubber clamp that can be worn around the penis, which occasionally is helpful. For more difficult cases, a catheter is placed through the penis to the bladder, to drain the urine to an external plastic bag (the plastic bags are emptied and cleaned or changed as needed).

Medication
Your physician may prescribe medications to combat incontinence.

Surgery
The underlying cause of the incontinence, such as prostate gland problems, sometimes requires surgical correction (see page 1210). In some types of incontinence problems, your urologist may recommend a surgically implanted artificial sphincter, which allows you to control its open (voiding) and closed (continent) settings.

Urinary Tract Infections in Men

Although urinary tract infections (UTIs) are more common in women, they do affect men. The classic symptom is difficulty in urinating or a painful sensation when you urinate. Even when you feel the urge, you can't pass urine freely, or you release only a small amount. The urge quickly returns.

Most UTIs aren't dangerous if you get proper care. But if you also have pain in your abdomen or back, chills, fever, or vomiting, your kidneys may be infected. A kidney infection is a serious medical condition requiring prompt treatment and, perhaps, hospitalization.

The most common cause of UTIs is the *Escherichia coli* (*E. coli*) bacterium. It resides in your intestinal tract and may migrate through your lymph system to your bladder. Inflammation of the bladder (cystitis) can result from infection with *E. coli*. Other factors can also promote UTIs in men:

- Prostate problems—Your prostate gland is walnut-sized and situated below your bladder, surrounding your urethra. A UTI can occur if your prostate gland enlarges and constricts your urethra, preventing your bladder from emptying completely. Leftover urine can create a breeding ground for bacteria. Enlargement of the prostate gland is a normal part of aging, but infection is not. Your prostate gland secretes proteins into your seminal fluid. These proteins have an antibacterial property. Little or no production of these proteins by your prostate can make you more susceptible to infection.

- Invasive medical procedures—a urinary catheter can introduce bacteria, especially if the catheter stays in place for several days. Infection-causing bacteria also may be introduced when a catheter is first inserted.

- Narrowed urethra—Frequent inflammation of your urethra (urethritis) can scar and narrow your urethra. This is called a urethral stricture. In years past, physicians believed strictures usually were caused by recurrent bouts with a sexually transmitted disease, such as gonorrhea. Today, strictures are more commonly associated with catheters or use of instruments used to explore or treat urologic problems.

- Dehydration—An inadequate intake of fluids can lead to stagnant (concentrated) urine. Hot weather can lead to dehydration.

Your physician can diagnose a UTI from symptoms and tests, including urinalysis and a urine culture. Don't "push" fluids before a test. Fluids can dilute your urine sample and reduce the accuracy of tests.

Your physician will prescribe a broad-spectrum antibiotic or a sulfa-type drug. Symptoms usually subside after several days, but be sure to take all your prescribed medication.

Disorders of the Prostate Gland

The prostate gland is located within the pelvis, beneath the bladder. It surrounds the urethra, the tube through which urine passes. This gland plays an important function in reproduction by contributing fluids to the semen. Among other things, these fluids appear to improve the survival of ejaculated sperm within the vagina. As men age, it is common for the prostate gland to enlarge and thus interfere with urination. Other prostate problems covered in this section include infections (prostatitis) and cancer.

Enlarged Prostate

Signs and Symptoms
- Need to urinate frequently
- Difficulty in starting the stream
- Decreased strength and force of urine stream
- Inability to sleep through the night without getting up to urinate
- Dribbling after the end of urination

Emergency Symptom—Complete inability to urinate

The prostate gland, present only in males, has an important sexual function: contributing fluids to the semen used to transport sperm. As a normal result of aging, the prostate gland often enlarges, starting in the late 40s. Because it surrounds the urethra, growth of the prostate can restrict the flow of urine through the urethra during urination.

If the enlargement is sufficient, the restriction can lead to the symptoms described above.

An enlargement of the prostate gland that is noncancerous is also called benign prostatic hyperplasia. Four of every five men develop benign enlargement of the prostate by age 80. It is estimated that 25 to 30 percent of men in the United States will need to have some type of procedure on their prostate to correct symptoms during their lifetime. The word "benign" distinguishes this condition from cancerous growth of the prostate, which can also occur (see Cancer of the Prostate, page 1211). The word "hyperplasia" means an increase in size.

The symptoms of an enlarged prostate vary in severity from slight to nearly complete inability to urinate. Men are usually annoyed by the symptoms, and in some cases they are alarmed by them. As the enlargement continues, the symptoms usually worsen, often gradually. However, this condition can be readily corrected by surgery, generally without complications.

Diagnosis
Your physician may ask you to fill out a prostate symptoms score questionnaire to grade the seriousness of your symptoms. Your physician can examine your prostate by inserting a gloved finger well into the rectum and feeling the gland with it. A urine test may be performed. A blood test to check for kidney function may also be performed. The urine flow may be measured with an electronic flowmeter. A prostate-specific antigen

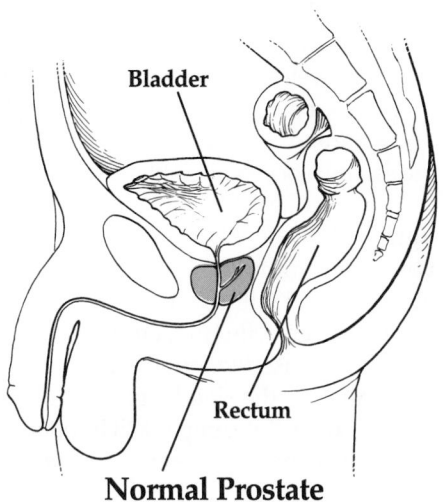

Normal Prostate

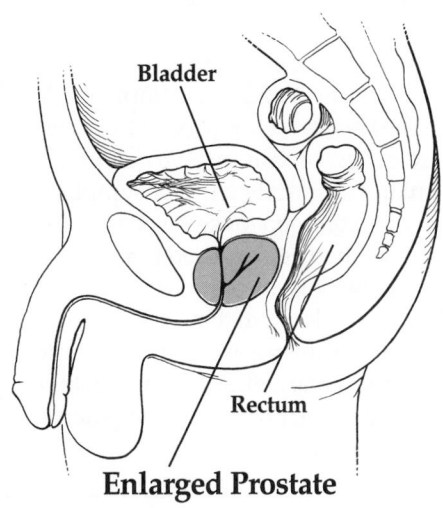

Enlarged Prostate

An enlarged prostate can produce difficulty in urination because the flow of urine is restricted.

(PSA) blood test will often be done as well to rule out the possibility that cancer of the prostate is contributing to your symptoms. Sometimes the bladder may be examined with a cystoscope (see page 849).

How Serious Is an Enlarged Prostate?

If your symptoms are mild, then it might be reasonable to only observe. If you have moderate to severe symptoms, you should be evaluated by a urologist. He or she may give you the options of either watchful waiting or surgical intervention, or new types of medical therapy for an enlarged prostate may be discussed.

Treatment

Your urologist may recommend medical treatment for benign enlargement of the prostate as a first consideration. Medicines that shrink the prostate gland or improve the flow of urine by relaxing tissues in the area of the prostate gland are available. Medications called alpha-blockers, such as terazosin and doxazocin, are sometimes used. Another drug call finasteride, which affects the male hormones inside the prostate, can also be used. Often, individuals are treated with medical therapy before surgery is recommended.

Surgical treatment can decrease the size of the prostate gland, or it can remove it and thus eliminate the condition. Today, the most common surgical procedure is transurethral resection of the prostate (TURP), which is performed without any incision in the abdomen. Sometimes, however, because of the size of the gland, surgical removal of the prostate through the abdomen is necessary.

Urologists are evaluating new surgical techniques that are safe, easy to perform, associated with a short hospital stay and recovery, and may have fewer side effects. These techniques include transurethral incision of the prostate (a less invasive procedure than TURP), prostatic stents, and microwave and laser therapy. You may want to discuss these options with your urologist.

Acute Prostatitis

Signs and Symptoms

- Sudden moderate to high fever
- Chills
- Frequent and difficult urination
- Urgent need to urinate
- Pain in the lower back and in the area between the rectum and the testicles
- Pain or a burning sensation while urinating
- Blood in the urine (sometimes)

Acute prostatitis is a sudden infection of the prostate gland). A portion of the prostate, or all of it, will be inflamed. Acute prostatitis often leads to bladder inflammation (cystitis) as well (see page 1203). It requires prompt treatment. Abscesses can develop in the prostate and, in extreme cases, the flow of urine can be blocked altogether.

Diagnosis

If you have symptoms of acute prostatitis, visit a physician without delay. Your physician will examine your prostate gland with a gloved finger inserted into your rectum. In acute prostatitis, the gland will be extremely tender. Also, a urine sample will be obtained for the tests needed to identify the bacteria causing the infection.

Transurethral Resection of the Prostate

The surgical procedure now chosen by most urologists to decrease the size of an enlarged prostate is transurethral resection of the prostate (TURP). The word "transurethral" refers to the fact that the procedure is done via the urethra, the tube that transports the urine from the bladder through the penis. The patient is anesthetized, generally with a spinal anesthetic but sometimes with a general anesthetic. Then, a thin tube called a resectoscope or operating cystoscope is carefully inserted into the urethra and manipulated so that its end, where the electric cutting device is located, enters the prostate.

This device is equipped with a miniature telescope. While viewing the urinary tract through the telescope, the urologist controls the cutting device and carefully removes small pieces of the enlarged part of the prostate gland. In effect, the urologist cores out a channel for an unhindered flow of urine.

After the operation, the resectoscope is removed and a catheter is inserted through the urethra into the bladder, where it remains for a day or two so that the bladder can empty while the enlarged channel heals. The hospital stay is about 3 to 4 days.

Transurethral prostate resection usually relieves all of the symptoms caused by the enlarged prostate without complications. After prostate surgery, it is common for some or all of the semen to enter the bladder rather than be ejaculated through the penis during sexual activity (known as retrograde ejaculation, described on page 1229). There is no harm in this—the semen is then voided with the urine—but it can impair fertility. In some cases the prostate again becomes enlarged, requiring another operation. In rare cases, prostate surgery can lead to impotence or to complete inability to control urination.

How Serious Is Acute Prostatitis?

Untreated acute prostatitis can lead to abscesses of the prostate or complete retention of urine. Acute prostatitis generally can be corrected with antibiotics. In severe cases, hospitalization may be necessary. Although acute prostatitis is generally cured, in some cases chronic prostatitis follows.

Treatment

Medication

Antibiotics, given by mouth or intravenously, are used to treat acute prostatitis.

Chronic Prostatitis

Signs and Symptoms
- Urination is frequent and there is burning with passage
- Urgent need to urinate
- Pain in the pelvis and genital area
- Painful ejaculation

Chronic prostatitis (chronic means long-lasting or recurring) is an infection of the prostate gland. In some cases chronic prostatitis follows acute prostatitis. The symptoms generally are milder than those of acute prostatitis. This ailment may or may not be associated with other urinary tract infections.

Diagnosis

If you have the symptoms of chronic prostatitis, visit your physician, who will examine your prostate gland with a gloved finger inserted into the rectum. A urine sample will be taken for tests to identify the infecting organism. Other tests also may be required.

How Serious Is Chronic Prostatitis?

Chronic prostatitis affects men to different degrees. The symptoms can range from discomfort to pain. Chronic prostatitis sometimes is due to bacteria that can cause, or have spread from, other urinary tract infections, which should be eliminated.

Treatment

Self-Help

Hot sitz baths sometimes provide relief from the symptoms of chronic prostatitis. Massage of the prostate formerly was a frequent means of treatment but is less commonly used today.

Medication

Antibiotics are often given to treat chronic prostatitis. Sometimes pain medications or medications to reduce the inflammation are used to relieve symptoms.

Cancer of the Prostate

Signs and Symptoms
- Decreased strength of urine stream
- Difficulty starting to urinate
- Hip or back pain
- Blood in the urine

Cancer of the prostate gland is common—it ranks third among the types of cancer that kill American men. Its symptoms also overlap with those of benign (noncancerous) prostate gland enlargement, a very common condition among middle-aged and older men, which means that prostate cancer may be mistaken for benign prostate enlargement, giving the disease time to spread.

Prostate cancer is most frequent in men ages 60 to 80. It is more common in black men than it is in white men. Its cause is unknown. The prostate enlargement that is common as men get older does not lead to prostate cancer.

If detected early, cancer of the prostate can be cured. It can be detected early, before it causes symptoms, by digital rectal examination, a routine procedure in which the physician inserts a gloved finger into the rectum and feels the prostate gland. This examination should be performed during the regular checkup in men 40 or older.

Once the symptoms of prostate cancer begin to appear, cure is less likely. This is why the regular digital examination is so important.

Although there remains controversy as to the benefits of screening, both the American Urological Association and the American Cancer Society recommend a yearly digital rectal examination and serum prostate-specific antigen (PSA) testing on every man 50 or older. These tests should begin at age 40 for men with a strong family history of prostate cancer or for black men.

Diagnosis

Prostate cancer is best found by the digital rectal examination and prostate-specific antigen (PSA) blood test performed during the regular checkup. If a hard lump is present on the gland, other tests, such as X-rays and blood and urine analyses, are performed. An ultrasound examination of the prostate is often done to evaluate the gland for the presence of suspicious areas that are hard to palpate with the digital examination. In addition, the ultrasound helps guide the biopsy needle, in which a small portion of the prostate gland is removed for examination under a microscope to determine if it is malignant. This sample is often taken with a needle inserted through the skin between the scrotum and the rectum or through the surface of the rectum itself.

If the sample proves malignant, more tests will be required to determine whether the cancer has spread to other parts of the body and to plan a treatment program.

Sometimes the presence of cancer will not be apparent on digital examination and the diagnosis of cancer will be established only on microscopic examination of the tissue removed during the course of operation.

Cancer of the prostate tends to spread to the bones, and occasionally the diagnosis is made in the course of investigating progressive back pain. Bone scans are often used to determine whether the malignancy has spread to the skeleton.

How Serious Is Cancer of the Prostate?

If found early, cancer of the prostate can be cured by surgery or radiation therapy. If the cancer has spread outside the prostate, treatment is then directed primarily at slowing the progress of the disease and relieving symptoms. Prostate cancer grows very slowly, and even when the disease is metastatic (has spread beyond the prostate), individuals can live for many years with proper treatment. You will generally be monitored by an oncologist who has special expertise in dealing with metastatic prostate cancer.

Treatment

If the prostate cancer is found early and there is no sign of spread outside the prostate to the bone or lymph nodes, the cancer can often be cured by surgical removal of the prostate or by radiation therapy. If the disease has spread, hormonal therapy may be recommended. Male hormones promote the growth of prostate cancer. Elimination of male hormone can be accomplished by surgically removing the testicles (orchiectomy) or by giving monthly injections of a medication (such as leuprolide or goserelin acetate). These agents prevent your body from producing male hormones. Side effects of hormonal therapy may include impotence, hot flashes, and weight gain. The benefit of retarding the growth of cancer outweighs these side effects. Female sex hormones were used in the past but are generally not used now.

Sexual Problems of Men

These problems include difficulties in achieving an erection, ejaculating too soon, and other problems associated with erection and ejaculation. Male sexual problems range in seriousness from quite minor to some that may be very damaging to one's self-image or sex life. Fortunately, effective treatment is available.

The cause of and the solution to such sexual problems frequently involve the sexual partner as well (see Health Issues of Partners, page 1213).

Chapter 36

Health Issues of Partners

Contents

Normal Reproduction, 1214

Infertility, 1215
Magnitude of the Problem, 1215
Evaluation, 1215
Causes, 1217
Therapy, 1218
    Ethical Considerations in Fertility
    Therapy, 1220

**Sexuality and Sexual
Dysfunction, 1221**
Desire Disorders in Women, 1222
Sensation Disorders in Women, 1222
Orgasm Disorders in Women, 1223
    Loss of Sexual Desire in Women, 1225

Impotence, 1225
Erection Abnormalities, 1227
Blood in the Semen, 1228
Premature Ejaculation, 1228
Retrogade Ejaculation, 1229
    Loss of Sexual Desire in Men, 1229

Sexual Crises, 1230
Rape, 1230
    Rape Prevention Tips, 1231
Physical Abuse, 1231
    Information for Women in Abusive
    Relationships, 1233
Sexual Abuse of Adolescents, 1233

Normal Reproduction

In normal reproduction, the sperm (the male reproductive cell) fuses with the egg (the female reproductive cell). Genetic information contained in the two parent cells mixes. From this fused cell, an embryo begins to develop; 9 months later, after the embryo has undergone incredible development within the uterus of the mother, a baby is born. To understand the workings and the problems of the reproductive systems, we must understand the steps that must occur for successful fertilization.

Sperm cells are produced by the male's testicles under the influence of hormones. From the testicles, the sperm travel through several internal organs before they reach the penis. These organs include the prostate gland and the seminal vesicles, which secrete fluids that create a healthy environment in which the sperm can live. The mixture of these fluids and the sperm, known as semen, is stored in the seminal vesicles until ejaculation.

During sexual intercourse, semen is ejaculated from the penis into the vagina. Although sperm are only a small portion of semen, a single ejaculation can contain from a quarter billion to 1 billion sperm. Each sperm cell has a long whip-like tail that propels it toward the egg. Although many sperm are produced, only about 200 or fewer sperm reach the area of the egg in the fallopian tube.

In the female, eggs are produced by the

Sperm

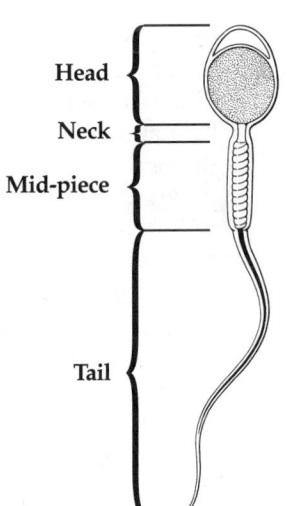

Head

Neck

Mid-piece

Tail

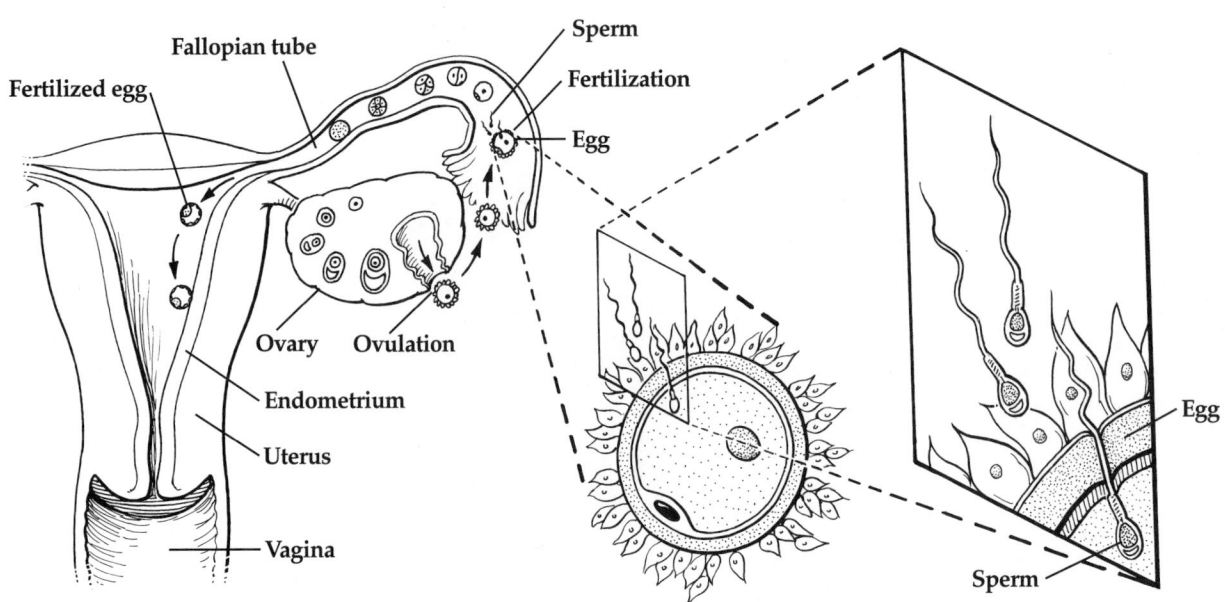

During each menstrual cycle, an egg is released by one of the ovaries. This is called ovulation. The egg travels into the fallopian tube. If fertilization is to occur, sperm ejaculated into the vagina must swim up through the uterus and into the fallopian tube, where one sperm penetrates the egg (see insets). The fertilized egg travels into the uterus, where it imbeds itself in the lining of the uterus (endometrium).

two ovaries. Before birth, every female has a supply of egg cells in each ovary. Before girls reach sexual maturity, most of their eggs are lost through attrition rather than through ovulation. Once menses begins, one of the ovaries releases one, and occasionally more, of these eggs each month.

Once released, the egg must travel a short distance from the ovary to the entrance of a fallopian tube, which joins an ovary and the uterus (womb) and is used to transport the egg. The egg travels slowly, requiring several days to travel through the fallopian tube. If a sperm cell is able to "swim" successfully from the point in the vagina where it left the penis all the way up through the uterus and into the fallopian tube, fertilization can occur.

Once a single sperm successfully penetrates the egg, its membrane changes to prevent additional sperm from entering the egg. The fertilized egg then slowly continues its passage down the fallopian tube for several more days, dividing and growing as it travels. The fertilized egg rapidly advances through the lower portion of the tube and then remains in the uterine cavity for another 3 to 4 days before implanting in the wall of the uterus. The embryo, or fetus, will develop from this point until birth (or miscarriage). (For further discussion of the function and malfunction of the reproductive organs, see pages 163, 167, 1140, and 1196.)

Infertility

Infertility is a common problem in partners. Fortunately, major advances have been made in recent decades, and the problem of infertility can be solved in many cases. This section outlines the methods used in the evaluation of infertility, the major causes of it, and the various options for treating it. The section concludes with ethical considerations of fertility therapy.

Problems of infertility can include problems with the sperm, problems with the egg, or difficulties encountered in their union. Abnormal function of the fallopian tube or uterus, infections, and immunologic and other factors may also cause infertility. Infertility problems also can result from sexual dysfunction, which is discussed later in this chapter. To physicians, the term infertility usually means the inability to become pregnant after 1 year of frequent sexual intercourse without using any contraception. For many couples, the odds are not as good as they might be (for example, more than a year might be required before pregnancy occurs), but infertility can be overcome.

Note that infertility is not the same thing as sterility, which means the inability to conceive a child under any circumstances. With infertility, the possibility of conceiving a child has by no means been ruled out. To many people and their physicians, the diagnosis of infertility may best be regarded as a challenge.

Magnitude of the Problem

Ten to 15 percent of couples are infertile (according to the definition given above). Of these couples, the man is the infertile partner in about 30 percent of cases and contributes to the infertility problem in an additional 20 percent of cases; the woman is infertile 50 to 70 percent of the time. In both men and women, various factors can account for infertility.

Evaluation

If you and your partner are unable to achieve conception within a reasonable time and would like to do so, seek help. The woman's gynecologist, the man's urologist, or the family physician can determine whether there is a fertility problem that requires a specialist or clinic that treats infertility problems.

Forty percent of infertile couples have more than one cause of their infertility. Thus, your physician will usually begin a comprehensive infertility examination of both partners. Usually the only diagnostic test for the male is semen analysis.

Before embarking on infertility tests, a couple should be aware that a certain amount of commitment is required. The physician or clinic will need to determine exactly what your sexual habits are and, moreover, may make recommendations about how you may need to change those habits. The tests and periods of trial and error may extend over several months. Evaluation is expensive and in some cases entails operations and uncomfortable procedures, and the expenses may not be reimbursable by many medical plans. Finally, there is no guarantee, even after all the tests and counseling, that conception will occur.

However, for couples eager to have their own child, such evaluation is the route to take. It may result in a successful pregnancy.

Tests for the Man

For a man to be fertile, his testicles must produce enough sperm, the sperm must be able to reach the seminal vesicles, and the sperm must be ejaculated effectively into the woman's vagina. Tests for the man attempt to determine whether any of these steps are impeded.

The first step is a general physical examination. This includes examination of the genitals and questions concerning your medical history, illnesses or disabilities, medications, and sexual habits.

Your physician may ask for a specimen of ejaculated semen. This is generally obtained by masturbating, or interrupting intercourse, and ejaculating the semen into a clean container. Your physician will provide instructions. Such a specimen may be required more than once.

The semen is then analyzed by a laboratory, and the quantity, color, and presence of infections or blood are noted. Principally, however, the analysis is of the sperm themselves. The laboratory will determine the concentration of sperm present in the ejaculate, their shape, and their motility (activity).

Other tests also are required sometimes, such as a blood test to determine the level of testosterone or other hormones.

Tests for the Woman

For a woman to be fertile, her ovaries must release healthy eggs regularly and her reproductive tract must allow the eggs and sperm unobstructed passage for a possible union in the fallopian tubes.

A general physical examination is the first step. This includes an ordinary gynecologic examination (see page 1141). Your physician will ask many questions concerning your health history, illnesses, medications, menstrual cycle, and sexual habits.

Specific fertility tests follow. A useful test is the cervical mucus test. This test is performed at about the time when ovulation should occur, and at a time between 2 and 16 hours after intercourse. Your physician will take a tiny sample of the mucus lining your cervix, which is the lower portion of the uterus where it meets the vagina. The procedure is painless. The sample is examined under a microscope to determine how well sperm penetrate and survive.

Endometrial biopsy, another test, can help to determine whether and when ovulation is occurring and whether the lining of the uterus is hormonally prepared. In this test, the physician takes a small sample of tissue from the uterine lining shortly before the beginning of the menstrual period.

A blood test is sometimes performed to determine the levels of hormones involved in successful ovulation and, sometimes, to look for infections.

Basal body temperature charting is rarely used today in fertility clinics because it poorly indicates the time of ovulation.

Once one or more of these tests have been performed, your physician will know whether ovulation occurs and whether sperm can survive in the female's reproductive tract. If no problems have been uncovered, additional information may be needed.

Hysteroscopy is a procedure in which a small instrument is used to examine the interior of the cervix and uterus for irregularities that might lead to infertility. This test sometimes is done under general anesthesia.

Hysterosalpingography is a test that also is used to evaluate the condition of the uterus as well as the fallopian tubes. A fluid is injected into the uterus and an X-ray is obtained to determine whether the fluid progresses out of the uterus and up the fallopian tubes. Blockages or problems often can be located, and these may be corrected with medications or operation.

Another test is laparoscopy; it involves a brief operation, with either local or general anesthesia, to insert a thin viewing device into the abdomen and pelvis to examine the fallopian tubes, ovaries, and uterus. A small incision is made beneath the navel, and a needle is inserted into the abdominal cavity. A small quantity of gas (usually carbon dioxide) is pumped into the abdomen to create a space for entry of a laparoscope, a thin, illuminated telescope.

The most common problem identified at

laparoscopy is endometriosis (see pages 1185, 1188, and 1346). Through the laparoscope, your physician can also spot blockages or irregularities of the fallopian tubes and uterus; often, a dye is injected into the cervical canal and through the uterus and fallopian tubes to determine whether they are open. At the end of the procedure, the gas and laparoscope are drawn out and the incision is closed. The test may help to identify blockages or other problems that could be corrected surgically. This can be done either in the hospital or on an outpatient basis.

These are the primary types of tests used to determine the possible causes of female infertility. Not everyone needs to undergo all, or even many, of the tests before the cause is found. Which tests are used and their sequence depend on discussion and agreement between you and the physician or clinic involved.

In up to 20 percent of infertile women, regardless of which tests are used, no cause can be found.

Causes

The cause of infertility can involve the man, the woman, or both. The physical examinations and tests discussed above should help your physician or clinic to pinpoint the cause.

Sometimes the problem is not really one of infertility but a more general sexual problem. For example, an impotent man might be fertile if he could obtain an erection to have intercourse. Similarly, premature ejaculation, before the penis is very far into the vagina, greatly lessens the chances of a sperm meeting the egg. These and other general sexual problems are discussed in the section Sexuality and Sexual Dysfunction (see page 1221).

Aside from such basic mechanical problems, the prime cause of infertility in a man is likely to be a problem with the sperm. Azoospermia is the complete absence of sperm in the semen, generally due to a disorder of the testicles or a blockage in the passage leading from the testicles. In oligospermia, sperm are present in the semen but not in enough quantity to fertilize an egg readily. The causes of these and other disorders of the sperm include problems with the testicles, hormone disorders, and infections.

An important cause of male infertility is varicocele (see page 1201), a problem of vari-

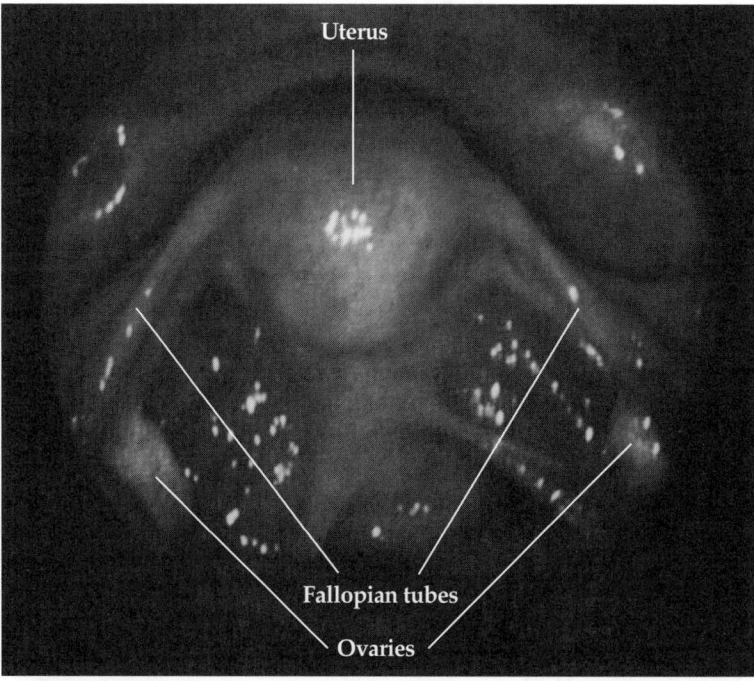

By using a laparoscope, your physician can visualize your uterus and other pelvic organs.

cose changes in veins surrounding the testicle, which can sometimes be corrected surgically. The varicosities prevent normal cooling of the testicles and thereby raise the testicular temperature—a factor that impairs sperm production. Several other problems with the testicles also can be responsible for infertility.

Hormone disorders often can be identified by a blood test, and these sometimes can be treated. Sexually transmitted diseases or other infections can block the passageways through which sperm travel, or they can injure sperm (impairing their ability to reach the egg) or kill them. Injuries also can affect sperm production. Mumps (and other infections) sometimes can cause an inflammation of one or both testicles (orchitis) that can permanently impair or prevent sperm production in the affected testicle (see page 1201).

In some men, sperm production is perfectly normal but the sperm are ejaculated into the bladder rather than out the penis (see Retrograde Ejaculation, page 1229).

In women, the failure to release an egg each menstrual cycle, called anovulation, is responsible for infertility problems in up to 15 percent of cases. It can be caused by various factors. If menstruation does not occur or occurs only occasionally, there may be a problem with the way the uterus or ovaries developed. Even if a woman has normal periods, however, she still can have impaired ovulation.

Hyperprolactinemia, a condition in which the blood contains an excess amount of the hormone prolactin, can cause anovulation. The hypothalamus, a part of the brain, produces hormones that normally stimulate a woman's pituitary gland, which in turn triggers the release of an egg. If the hypothalamus does not secrete the hormones, no egg is released. Additional causes of anovulation include chronic debilitating diseases such as uncontrolled diabetes or thyroid disease.

When ovulation is normal, the problem lies elsewhere. Abnormalities of the fallopian tubes are the problem, or part of the problem, as often as a third of the time. Tumors or irregularities in the formation of the fallopian tubes can block passage of the egg. In a condition called endometriosis, some of the tissue that lines the uterus and is shed each month during the menstrual period is present in the abdomen somewhere outside the uterus. This tissue can interfere with the passage of released eggs to or through the fallopian tubes, causing infertility (see page 1185).

Sometimes, ovulation occurs normally and the egg passes successfully through the fallopian tubes, only to encounter other problems. These include luteal-phase defects, in which something (frequently a hormonal abnormality) interferes with the further development of the egg once it has been released, or the endometrium (lining of the uterus) is not prepared to nourish the fertilized egg.

Uterine factors are sometimes a cause of infertility. These include an irregular shape of the uterus or tumors (see page 1178). A retroverted or retroflexed uterus is almost never a cause of infertility. Surgical correction may or may not restore fertility. Similarly, cervical factors can be responsible for infertility; these include cervix irregularities or growths that block the sperm or problems with the cervical mucus which damage the sperm or impede its passage.

Immunologic factors also can be responsible. A few women are allergic to sperm, and their bodies produce antibodies that kill sperm before a sperm can penetrate an egg.

Similarly, some men produce antibodies that are meant to fight an infection but inadvertently attack sperm instead. Treatment of the infection may eradicate this problem.

In men as well as women, numerous diseases that can affect the genitourinary tract can cause infertility. These include the sexually transmitted diseases (see page 1087).

Pelvic inflammatory disease is caused by sexually transmitted diseases such as gonorrhea, chlamydial infection, and vaginitis and, less commonly, by tuberculosis and anaerobic streptococcal infection (see page 1187). These diseases can cause problems, depending on the amount of fallopian tube inflammation and the amount of irritation at the end of the tube and around the ovary. Even with severe pelvic inflammatory disease with known tubal and ovarian involvement, aggressive treatment with antibiotics and conservative operation allow subsequent fertility in 25 to 30 percent of cases.

Therapy

The numerous treatments for infertility depend on the cause. Recent developments in therapy have increased the number of once-infertile couples who can achieve pregnancy.

Some causes of infertility cannot be corrected. However, even then, various means of insemination or embryo transfer may be possible so that the woman can still become pregnant.

This section divides infertility therapy into two categories: 1) restoring or bringing about fertility, and 2) assisted reproductive technology (ART).

Therapy to Restore Fertility

Sperm survive in the female reproductive tract for up to 72 hours, and an egg can be fertilized for up to 24 hours. Therefore, by having intercourse every 2 to 3 days at mid-cycle, couples can effectively eliminate faulty timing as a contributing factor to infertility. This is particularly effective in couples with impaired fertility rather than infertility—for example, when the man has oligospermia (see page 1217).

General sexual problems, such as impotence or premature ejaculation, also can be treated to improve fertility. These problems and their treatment are discussed in the section Sexuality and Sexual Dysfunction (see page 1221).

When the source of infertility lies in the man's sperm (or lack of it), restoring or initiating fertility is sometimes possible. For example, varicocele, a common source of problems with the sperm, can be corrected surgically, and in some instances this also will restore fertility. Problems with the testicles, prostate gland, seminal vesicles, and urethra also can be treated (see Men's Health, page 1195).

When sperm production is impaired because of damage to the sperm-producing areas of the testicle, drug treatment has been of little use. In extremely rare instances when sperm production is impaired because of a pituitary gland problem, the use of human chorionic gonadotropin or human pituitary gonadotropin has been helpful. When infections hamper sperm production, block the transport of sperm, or damage or kill the sperm, treatment of the infection often restores fertility. This is particularly true of sexually transmitted diseases, and both partners must be treated.

In the woman, treatment also depends on the results of the examination and tests. Treating any infection or underlying illness is, as usual, the first step. If the fertility problem is related to anovulation (failure to release an egg), your physician can attempt to bring about ovulation. Generally, clomiphene citrate, human menotropin gonadotropins, or gonadotropin-releasing hormones with or without human chorionic gonadotropin are administered.

Blockages, tumors, or other problems in the fallopian tubes usually are repaired surgically. Microsurgical techniques permit delicate operations on the fallopian tubes. Surgical repair offers a 30 percent chance of pregnancy.

Endometriosis (see page 1185) can be a cause of infertility. Although hormones (birth control pills) are effective for treating endometriosis and relieving pain, they have not been useful in treating infertility. If you have endometriosis, an attempt to eradicate it will be made during laparoscopy. Your physician will then treat you with superovulation therapy or in vitro fertilization (see below). These options are effective in treating endometriosis-related infertility.

Assisted Reproductive Technology (ART)

Other medical advances also enable many couples to have their own biologic child. Assisted reproductive technology (ART) helps the woman of an infertile couple become pregnant. The ART health care team includes physicians, psychologists, embryologists, laboratory technicians, nurses, and allied health professionals who work together to help infertile couples.

In vitro fertilization (IVF) is the most commonly used technique of ART. It involves retrieving mature eggs from the woman, fertilizing them with sperm in a dish in a laboratory, and implanting the fertilized eggs in the uterus two days later. Other forms of ART include zygote intrafallopian transfer (ZIFT), in which a zygote (fused egg) is placed into a fallopian tube the day after removal. The zygote moves naturally down the tube and into the uterus. With gamete intrafallopian transfer (GIFT), unfertilized eggs and sperm are placed directly into a fallopian tube. The eggs are fertilized while in the fallopian tube, and the fertilized eggs move naturally down the tube and into the uterus.

The success of these different techniques is comparable. Individual circumstances may make one or the other preferable. Some programs have more success with GIFT than with IVF. Considerable differences exist between program techniques, patient back-

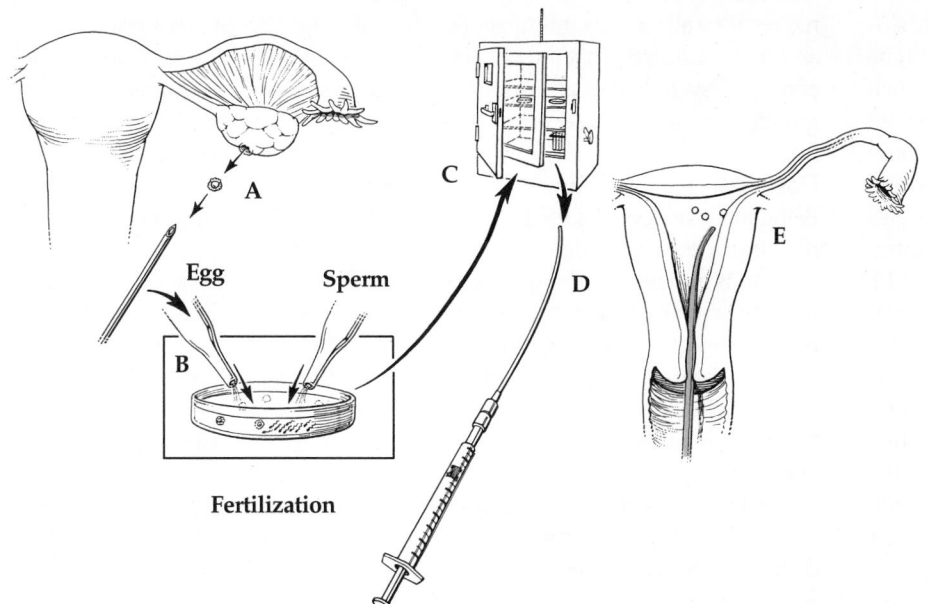

Egg   Sperm

Fertilization

For in vitro fertilization, the physician uses a needle to remove eggs from the ovary (A). The eggs and sperm from a donor are combined in a Petri dish (B) and placed in an incubator (C). If fertilization occurs, the fertilized ova are retrieved and transferred by means of a cannula (D) to the uterus (E).

grounds, and the way that success rates are measured. Because IVF, ZIFT, and GIFT have not been compared in the same series of patients, it is not possible to say that one technique yields a higher pregnancy rate than the other.

The process for IVF begins with a woman taking fertility drugs to stimulate her ovaries to produce more eggs than usual. About one week before your period (before hormones start the process of egg stimulation), you may receive an injection of a medication that reduces the hormones that promote the development of eggs in the ovary. To see if the drug has reduced egg development, a vaginal ultrasound test and blood test are performed after about 10 days. If egg development has not been reduced, the drug therapy may be continued for another week or two.

When the function of the ovaries has been temporarily stopped, you will receive hormone injections for about 7 days to stimulate the development of ovarian follicles (fluid-filled sacs in which the eggs mature). More blood tests and another vaginal ultrasound test will be done to determine follicle growth. It is important to monitor follicle growth so that mature eggs are retrieved.

After the appropriate degree of ovarian stimulation is reached, another hormone, called human chorionic gonadotropin (hCG), is injected to help the eggs mature and to trigger ovulation. Eggs are retrieved 34 to 38 hours after the hCG injection, or shortly before ovulation (egg release) would normally occur.

It usually takes 20 to 50 minutes to retrieve the eggs. Medication is administered through an intravenous (IV) line to help keep you comfortable and relaxed throughout the procedure. Using transvaginal ultrasound (see page 1335), your physician guides a needle through the vagina to the ovary. In general, eggs are recovered from about 80 percent of the mature follicles seen on ultrasound. After

---

Ethical Considerations in Fertility Therapy

Determining the cause of infertility and treating it are demanding tasks both for the partners and for the physician or clinic. Much energy is required over a protracted period. New techniques are being developed constantly, and physicians are pleased to be able to use them for a couple's benefit.

Measure Your Own Attitudes
It is important for a couple considering fertility therapy to examine their own attitudes toward such therapy. Just because something can be done doesn't mean that it should be done. Attitudes toward conception vary greatly. Some couples believe that if having sexual intercourse does not produce a child, then they should accept the situation; this may be their religious or ethical position. Conversely, some couples are so eager to have their biologic child that they believe that to achieve that end no tests are too prolonged, no therapy too complicated, and no expense, procedure, or hardship too great.

Most couples find themselves somewhere between these two positions. Fertility clinics, and physicians who specialize in fertility problems, often are prepared to discuss ethical issues with you. They can help you to define or discover your own attitudes. These discussions should include what can realistically be expected. Even though medical science has provided many new techniques, they all have their limitations and rates of success that are not 100 percent. Psychologists and support groups also are available.

Don't Take It Personally
Being infertile does not mean that a man is any less masculine or that a woman is any less feminine. Infertility does not make anyone incomplete or defective. It has nothing to do with attractiveness or sexual prowess. Moreover, it is not a negative comment on a couple's relationship.

Medically speaking, infertility is simply the existence of some obstacle in the long and exceedingly complex chain of events that lead to pregnancy. It should not be viewed as a tragedy.

Consider the Ethical Questions
When fertilization is not possible through sexual intercourse but only through other methods such as artificial insemination, some couples believe that a line has been crossed and ethical considerations are raised.

A significant distinction for many people is donor sperm or donor eggs from someone other than the partner. Using sperm or eggs from a stranger raises many ethical issues: Who was he or she? (Most sperm banks ensure anonymity.) Does the donor have any rights concerning the child? Might future court decisions award donors visitation rights?

In the end, only you and your partner can answer such questions or address such issues. But the time to consider your ethical positions on fertility therapy is before pregnancy occurs as a result of such therapy.

being removed from the follicles, the fluid that contains the eggs is immediately taken to the embryology laboratory. The eggs are put in a special solution and placed in an incubator. The amount of time the eggs are in the incubator depends on their maturity. When mature, the eggs are inseminated (mixed with the sperm). Usually about 80 percent of the eggs are fertilized when male factor infertility is not present. The eggs are checked 24 hours after they are retrieved. Fertilization can be confirmed at this time.

If you have IVF, the embryos are transferred to the uterus 2 days after fertilization is confirmed. (With ZIFT and GIFT, zygotes and gametes are placed in a fallopian tube.) Embryo transfer is a brief procedure that is also performed in a procedure room. A soft, flexible catheter (cannula) is threaded through the cervix and into the uterus. Six embryos are usually transferred. The number depends on the quality of the embryos and other factors. Extra embryos can be cryopreserved (frozen) and used at a later time. If conception does not occur following the embryo transfer, or if you want more children, the frozen embryos may be used at a later date. This means you will not have to repeat the ovarian stimulation and retrieval process.

You need to stay in bed for the 2 days following the embryo transfer procedure. A pregnancy test is usually done 2 weeks after the procedure.

The overall national success rate for IVF is about 20 percent. Many programs exceed a 40 percent chance of success within one cycle. This is now recommended more often as first-line therapy. IVF is the treatment of choice if both fallopian tubes are blocked. It also is used widely for a number of other conditions such as endometriosis, unexplained infertility, cervical factor infertility, male factor infertility, and ovulation disorders.

ART works best when the woman has a healthy uterus, responds well to fertility drugs, ovulates naturally, or uses donor eggs and the man has healthy sperm or donor sperm are available. There is a lower success rate in women older than 40, women faced with early menopause who no longer produce as many eggs, and women with untreated conditions of the uterus such as scar tissue or some uterine fibroids and polyps. The success rate is also lower in men with low sperm counts, low sperm motility, or abnormal sperm function.

The risks associated with ART involve the medications and the procedure used to remove the eggs. These risks include hemorrhage, infection, damage to adjacent organs, and an overstimulation of ovaries, which causes ovarian enlargement and abdominal discomfort. In addition, there is an increased chance of multiple pregnancy. However, research shows that there is no higher risk of genetic abnormalities in the child conceived with ART.

Other ART techniques include electro-ejaculation, which uses an electric stimulus to bring about ejaculation so that semen can be obtained. This procedure can be used in men with spinal cord injury who cannot otherwise achieve ejaculation.

Aspiration techniques include removing sperm from parts of the male reproductive tract such as the epididymis, vas deferens, or testicle.

A new technique is called intracytoplasmic sperm injection. This involves a micromanipulation (microscopic technique) in which a single sperm is injected directly into an egg to achieve fertilization. Fertilization rates are comparable to those achieved with standard insemination. This has been especially helpful in couples who have previously failed to achieve fertilization with standard techniques and in men with low sperm concentrations.

Sexuality and Sexual Dysfunction

Sexual dysfunction simply means problems or obstacles encountered in the course of sexual intercourse. The problems can be experienced by either the man or the woman. It is rare, however, for only one of the partners to be affected; for example, premature ejaculation, a problem in the man, will likely lead to sexual satisfaction problems for the woman.

This section first discusses problems that can occur in the woman: desire disorders, sensation disorders, and orgasm disorders. Because these problems are not always easy to distinguish, read all three sections if you suspect you have one of these dysfunctions.

The second part of this section covers problems in the man: impotence, erection abnormalities, and premature ejaculation. The solution to sexual problems in either partner, as will be seen, often entails the understanding and cooperation of both partners.

Desire Disorders in Women

Signs and Symptoms

- Diminished or absent sexual desire
- Insufficient sexual desire to sustain interest in sexual activity

Sexual desire is an interest in having sexual activity with a partner. Sometimes sexual activity, including orgasm, may take place even though the desire for it is lessened or nonexistent.

How much desire is "too little" is, of course, a personal judgment that will differ from woman to woman. If you wish you had more sexual desire, then you probably are experiencing too little.

On average, men desire sexual relations more often than women; the fact that your partner desires sex more frequently than you do does not necessarily mean that you have a desire problem. Instead, it suggests a disparity in desire between the two of you. In such cases, counseling is sometimes in order; it generally results in a compromise and better understanding on the part of both partners.

In the female (as in the male), sexual desire can stem from various sources, including the senses of sight, touch, hearing, and smell, and from thoughts and emotions. The attractiveness of a partner and the nature of the relationship with the partner can figure heavily in the presence or absence of sexual desire. Desire lessens somewhat during the later years of life.

It is important to realize that diminished or absent sexual desire during one sexual encounter or another is not a sign of a problem. This may happen to any woman. It is perfectly normal and is generally transient. Diminished or absent desire that persists over time, however, can create problems for a woman's self-image and damage the sexual life of both partners.

Causes can be nonphysical, physical, or both. Among nonphysical causes, discord with one's partner is common, as is depres-

sion. Physical causes include various illnesses, hormonal imbalances, and side effects of medications. When desire disorders persist, treatment is usually possible.

Diagnosis

Although a physician is not needed to diagnose a desire disorder (you will be able to recognize this yourself), he or she can be helpful in separating it from other possible problems and in suggesting treatment. Your physician will ask questions concerning your relationship with your partner, your physical condition, and your history of illnesses. Your physician will also ask about your medications because some drugs such as antidepressants and antihypertensives may diminish sexual desire.

How Serious Are Desire Disorders?

In and of themselves, desire disorders are not harmful. Most, in fact, are merely passing events in a marriage or relationship. A persisting desire disorder, however, can have a negative effect on the sex lives of both partners and can damage the self-image of both.

Treatment

If a physical illness is present, your physician will treat the illness. Similarly, your physician may replace or eliminate medications that you take to determine whether they have an impact.

Most commonly, however, the cause is nonphysical. Your physician may suggest counseling of one or both partners with a therapist or may offer some guidelines or specific programs to follow to increase desire.

Sensation Disorders in Women

Signs and Symptoms

- Diminished or nonexistent sexual excitement during sexual activity
- A dry, rather than lubricated, vagina during sexual intercourse, despite ample opportunity for sexual stimulation during foreplay
- Sometimes, painful intercourse

There is a fine distinction between desire disorders (see this page) and sensation disorders. With a sensation disorder, the desire for sexual activity is present but pleasurable sensations are not obtained from such activity. In other words, you would like to have sex, but when you do your body does not seem to cooperate and usually shows this by failing to secrete enough vaginal lubrication. The sexual act does not excite you as it should.

As with other sexual problems, the first thing to realize is that an occurrence or two does not mean that you have a problem. A sensation disorder has to persist for it to be a problem at all.

The causes of a sensation disorder are varied. Nonphysical causes predominate; they include anger or hostility toward the partner, depression, and stress. To appreciate the sensations involved during sexual activity, one has to be able to focus on them, and anything that interferes with this can be at the root of the problem.

Lack of stimulation by the partner also can be a cause. Sufficient foreplay is important; failing to respond to a partner who does not provide as much foreplay as you want is not a sensation disorder at all—it is a normal reaction to inadequate sexual stimulation. The same applies during the sexual act itself: a sensation disorder is present only if ample attention is paid to your sexual needs without resulting in excitation.

A physical sensation disorder is dyspareunia (painful intercourse). Several physical ailments affecting the genital area can be responsible for this condition, including vaginal irritations, infections, growths, and reactions to devices or substances used for contraception.

The absence of sufficient vaginal lubrication due to a lack of ample foreplay or desire also can, of course, cause painful intercourse. After menopause, the mucus lining of the vagina generally becomes somewhat thinner and drier, and previously pleasurable intercourse may become painful.

Diagnosis

If you suspect that you have a sensation disorder, discuss this with your physician. Your physician will ask questions concerning your physical health, the medications you take, your relationship with your partner, and your experiences during sexual intercourse.

If intercourse is painful, a pelvic examination will be necessary (see page 1141). Your physician also will ask questions to help pinpoint when you experience the pain and where in the vagina; for example, if deep thrusts hurt, your physician may suspect a problem such as endometriosis.

How Serious Are Sensation Disorders?

A persisting sensation disorder can damage your sex life, taking the pleasure out of sex. It also can cause problems for your partner, who knows that he is not satisfying you. Beyond these consequences, however, physical damage does not generally result from a sensation disorder. If an inflammation, growth, or injury is present, however, continued intercourse can aggravate the condition.

Treatment

If you have an illness that causes a sensation disorder as a secondary effect, your physician will treat it. The medications you are taking or the contraceptives you are using may be altered or eliminated to determine whether they affect your sexual responsiveness. In addition, vaginal lubricants can be used during intercourse to alleviate a common source of pain.

In some cases, however, treatment will be directed toward nonphysical causes, and counseling may be necessary. The counseling may include recommending specific measures to help you and your partner achieve the pleasurable sensations normally associated with sexual activity.

If an underlying problem in the relationship between you and your partner is the cause of the sensation disorder, marital counseling or other forms of therapy may be advised.

Orgasm Disorders in Women

Signs and Symptoms—Failure to attain orgasm during sexual activity

Some women never attain orgasm and yet have pleasurable sexual experiences, some obtain orgasm only part of the time, and others have orgasm every time they have intercourse. It is a change in these patterns leading to dissatisfaction with sexual activity that warrants evaluation.

Orgasm disorders are closely related to sensation disorders (see page 1222). In general, if you do not experience ample pleasurable sensations from sexual activity, you will not experience orgasm either. In some cases of orgasm disorder, a woman does experience orgasm but has to work unreasonably hard or long to attain it.

Orgasm is a complex event, involving sexual desire and sexual stimulation. Foreplay and sexual intercourse itself must reasonably approximate the needs of the particular woman in terms of the way it is done and how long it lasts. Communicating these needs to a responsive partner will relieve many orgasm disorders.

It is also important to realize that a large percentage of women—estimates range from a third to two-thirds of all women—require stimulation of the clitoris to reach an orgasm. Do not assume that you have an orgasm disorder until your partner or you have thoroughly experimented with direct stimulation of the clitoris before, during, or after intercourse and you find you still cannot attain orgasm.

Causes can be nonphysical, physical, or both. A common physical cause is simply that intercourse hurts. Physicians refer to this as dyspareunia. Disorders in the female genitourinary tract, such as minor injuries or abrasions and infections, or reactions to contraceptive creams or devices can cause painful intercourse, as can a lack of ample vaginal lubrication. Sometimes dyspareunia is experienced after menopause, when the vaginal lining becomes somewhat drier and thinner; use of lubricants can overcome this condition. Endometriosis also can be a cause of dyspareunia (see page 1185).

Nonphysical causes can include problems in the relationship with the partner, depression, anger, or other factors that affect the ability to focus on pleasurable sexual sensations. A few women inhibit their orgasm out of fear of "letting go" or losing control, perhaps believing that this implies dependence on the partner.

Diagnosis

You, rather than your physician, are the one who knows you are not experiencing orgasms. It is helpful to discuss the problem with your physician, however, so that he or she can determine the cause and suggest the appropriate course of action to take to regain (or initiate) the ability to have orgasms.

Your physician will ask questions concerning your physical health, the medications you take and the contraceptives you use, your relationship with your partner, and your experiences during sexual intercourse. If intercourse is painful, your physician will perform a pelvic examination.

How Serious Are Orgasm Disorders?

A persisting orgasm disorder can render your sex life unsatisfying or less satisfying than it might be. This is its most serious consequence. However, some women who do not experience orgasms often enjoy foreplay and sexual stimulation during intercourse a great deal and do not think that they are missing anything by not having an orgasm. This is a judgment a woman must make on her own.

Physical consequences of orgasm disorders themselves are rare. If an inflammation or injury is present, however, continued intercourse can aggravate the condition, and it should be treated.

Some women find the inability to have orgasms damaging to their self-image, although this need not be the case. The problem usually can be corrected; when it cannot, a woman is not rendered any less feminine, in any way "incomplete," or unable to enjoy sexual activity with her partner.

Also, your partner may be disturbed by your orgasm disorder, feeling that he fails to satisfy you. Reassurance concerning your enjoyment of the act even in the absence of orgasm can be helpful.

Treatment

If you have an illness or injury that causes an orgasm disorder, your physician will treat it. The medications you take or the contraceptives you use may be altered or eliminated to

Vulva

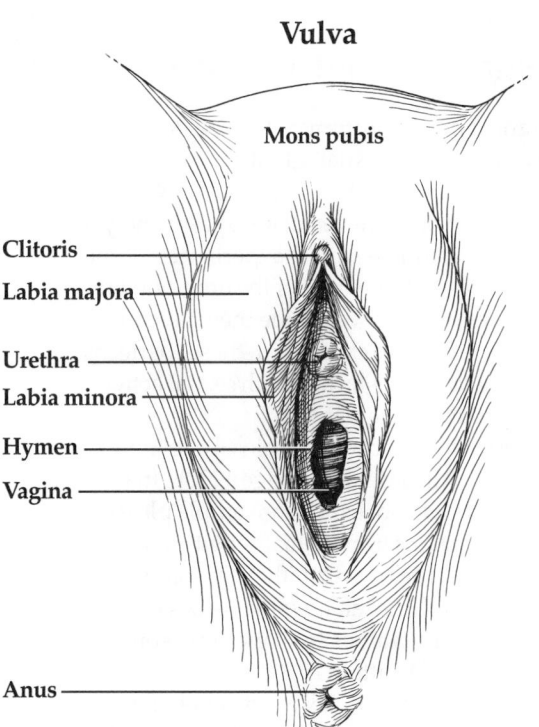

Mons pubis

Clitoris

Labia majora

Urethra

Labia minora

Hymen

Vagina

Anus

Loss of Sexual Desire in Women

It is normal for a woman to experience sexual desire from puberty until well beyond menopause. Diminished sexual desire or a loss of desire altogether is generally due to some specific problem or situation. The most common cause in a woman is day-to-day discord with her partner. This is present, to one degree or another, in about three of four cases that are discussed with physicians.

The second most common cause of desire problems is inadequate stimulation by the partner. A man who focuses merely on satisfying himself can rarely satisfy a woman. A well-intentioned, considerate partner may satisfy a woman and himself simultaneously.

Sometimes a woman fails to discover her potential in sexual relationships because of inadequate knowledge of her anatomy, of the importance of timing during the sex act, or of the need to communicate her needs to her partner. Gradually, as a consequence of bland or unsatisfying sexual experiences, she can sometimes lose interest. Worse, such an absence of desire is sometimes reinforced by the "common wisdom," from an earlier era, that it is unseemly for a woman to experience desire, to experience very much desire, or to continue experiencing it after childbearing years; such attitudes are as wrong today as they were then.

Physical problems are sometimes the cause of a loss of desire. The presence of some disease or disability can diminish desire, and many medications also suppress feelings of sexual desire as a side effect.

Loss of desire generally can be reversed. A physician can guide you to a therapist who can help resolve problems with your partner. Your therapist also can suggest measures to help you regain sexual desire. In the case of a physical problem, your physician can treat the particular ailment or can suggest substitute medications that do not suppress desire.

---

determine whether they affect your responsiveness.

In most cases, treatment will be directed toward nonphysical causes and will involve suggestions or counseling. Experimenting with clitoral stimulation before, during, and after intercourse may solve the problem. Your physician may suggest counseling, which may include specific measures to help you and your partner regain the pleasurable sensations associated with sexual activity. The use of vaginal lubricants also may be helpful.

Your physician also may suggest a set of simple exercises (known as Kegel exercises, see page 1176) that can help you develop the muscles in the outer third of the vagina that are involved in pleasurable sensations. These same muscles also help control the flow of urine.

If an underlying problem in the relationship between you and your partner is a possible cause of your inability to experience orgasm, marital counseling or another form of therapy may be advised.

Impotence

Signs and Symptoms—Inability of the penis to become erect or to stay erect

Impotence is a persistent inability to obtain an erection or to keep it long enough for sexual intercourse. The name comes from the Latin word *impotentia*, which means "lack of strength."

It is important to realize that an occasional episode of impotence happens to most men, is perfectly normal, and is nothing to worry about. When it proves to be a pattern or a persistent problem, however, impotence can be a detriment to a man's self-image as well as to his sexual life. Fortunately, impotence often can be cured.

A first step toward curing impotence is to understand how an erection occurs. The penis has two cylindrical, sponge-like structures that run along its length parallel to the urethra (the tube that carries semen and urine). When a man is sexually aroused, nerve impulses cause the blood flow to the cylinders to increase to about 7 times the normal amount. This sudden influx of blood expands the sponge-like structures and thus straightens and stiffens the penis, producing an erection. Continued sexual arousal or excitation maintains the higher rate of blood flow, keeping the erection. After ejaculation, or when the sexual excitation passes, the excess blood drains out of the spongy tissue and the penis returns to its nonerect size and shape.

Note that three important steps take place

to produce the erection. The first step is sexual arousal, which men obtain from the senses of sight, touch, hearing, and smell and from thoughts. The second step is communication of the sexual excitation by the body's nervous system from the brain to the penis. The third step is a relaxing action of the blood vessels that supply the penis, allowing more blood to flow into the shafts that produce the erection. If something affects any of these three factors—arousal, nervous system response, or vascular system response—or the delicate balance among them, impotence can result.

Diminished sexual desire or even loss of sexual desire is not the same thing as impotence (see Loss of Sexual Desire in Men, page 1229). Impotence refers to the inability to have an erection and to use the penis for sexual activity when desire and opportunity are present.

Impotence affects about 10 million American men. It affects more older men than younger men—nearly 20 percent of men are impotent at age 60 years and more

Spongy erectile tissue

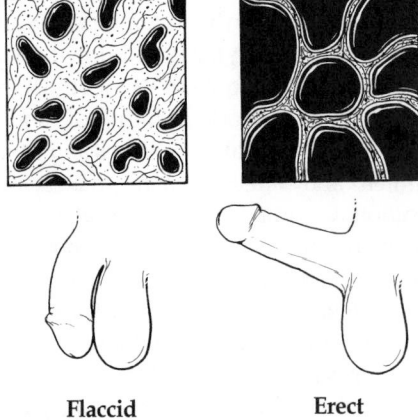

In an erection, two cylindrical, sponge-like erectile structures become engorged with blood. After orgasm, excess blood drains from the spongy tissue, leaving the penis flaccid.

Flaccid   **Erect**

than 70 percent are impotent at age 80 years. However, impotence is by no means an inevitable consequence of aging, and treatment in older men is often as effective as it is in younger men.

Nonphysical causes may account for impotence. The most common nonphysical cause is stress or anxiety. If a man cannot relax and focus on the sexual situation, or if he is overwhelmed or confused by circumstances, it is difficult for the three-stage erection process to take place. This happens to almost every man at some time.

Impotence is also an occasional side effect of psychological problems such as depression. Negative feelings toward the sexual partner—or expressed by the sexual partner—such as resentment, hostility, or lack of interest also can be a factor in impotence.

The important thing is not to assume that an episode of impotence means that you have a permanent problem and should expect it to happen again during the next sexual encounter. Because thought processes are so important in erection, such a negative assumption can, in some cases, bring the problem about. The best thing to do if you experience an episode of impotence is to forget it and expect a more successful experience at another time. Such an episode is not a lasting comment on a man's virility or masculinity.

It is important too for the man experiencing transient or persisting impotence to remember his sexual partner. To a greater or lesser degree, a woman may consider an erection as a comment on her desirability; lack of an erection may communicate undesirability to the partner, and reassurance is helpful. A woman's self-image can be damaged by her partner's impotence, but this can be avoided if the man makes it clear that she attracts him or if the woman herself realizes that impotence is only rarely caused by lack of interest.

Physical causes account for many of the cases of impotence. These include (from the most to the least frequent) diabetic neuropathy, cardiovascular disorders, prescription medicines, operation for cancer of the prostate, fractures that injure the spinal cord, multiple sclerosis, hormone disorders, and alcoholism and other forms of drug abuse.

The physical and nonphysical causes of impotence interact. For example, a minor physical problem that slows sexual response may cause anxiety about attaining an erection, and the anxiety worsens the impotence.

Diagnosis

If episodes of impotence keep occurring, consult your physician. Your physician will ask questions about how the impotence developed, medications that you take, physical ailments, and factors such as stress.

If your physician suspects mainly nonphysical causes, he or she may ask whether you obtain erections during masturbation, with a partner, or while you sleep. Most men experience many erections (without remembering them) during sleep. A simple test—wrapping a special perforated tape around the penis before sleeping—can confirm whether you have nocturnal erections. If the tape is separated in the morning, your penis was erect at some point during the night. Tests of this type confirm nonphysical causes.

If your physician suspects that physical causes are involved, other tests, such as angiography to determine the adequacy of the arterial circulation of the genital organs, neurologic evaluation to exclude neuropathy, and measurements of the male hormone level in the blood, may be performed. Prescription drugs may be eliminated or replaced one at a time to see whether they are responsible.

How Serious Is Impotence?

Impotence can be cured. Depending on the cause of impotence, various treatments can be considered.

Treatment

Psychological Therapy

If nonphysical causes are entirely responsible, your physician may suggest visiting a psychiatrist, psychologist, or sex therapist, either alone or with your partner.

Medication

In some patients with hormone deficiencies, hormones can be given. No hormones should be given, however, unless your physician has documented that your hormone levels are low and the cause of the low hormones has been well established. No patient with a history of prostate cancer should receive male hormone shots or pills.

Penile Injections

In many men, impotence is caused by a decrease in the blood supply to the penis. In others there is an abnormality of the nerve supply of the penis. An ideal therapeutic solution in these patients may be injecting the penis with medication that increases blood flow. Candidates for this treatment undergo a test dose of this medication in their physician's office and then are taught how to use it on their own.

Vacuum Constriction Device

This device is used to induce engorgement of the penis, which increases its rigidity. After the penis is engorged, a rubber constricting band is placed around the penis, prolonging the erection. Many persons find these devices very satisfactory. They do not involve surgery, are reasonably priced, and are available at most drugstores. However, they do require a physician's prescription for purchase.

Surgery

Surgery can be performed either to revascularize the penis in certain patients with vascular insufficiency or to implant a penile prosthesis. Types of penile implants range from a semirigid rod type to an inflatable type. The attributes of each type of penile implant are best described by your physician.

Erection Abnormalities

Signs and Symptoms

- Inability of the penis to become or stay erect
- A painful (sometimes) bend in the penis during an erection
- A prolonged, painful erection

An erection is a prerequisite for intercourse and most other sexual activity. Problems with erection, of whatever type, can hamper sexual activity. The three main kinds of erectile abnormalities are impotence, Peyronie's disease, and priapism.

The first abnormality, impotence, was discussed on page 1225. The second type of erection abnormality is Peyronie's disease (curvature of the erect penis). This is less common than impotence. It affects men mainly between the ages of 40 and 60 years, can make sexual intercourse difficult or impossible, and is caused by scar tissue that forms inside the penis for reasons that are unknown. It is not related to any infection, tumor, contagious disease, or sexual practice. Most cases of Peyronie's disease disappear spontaneously within 1 to 3 years after onset. If the degree of curvature precludes inter-

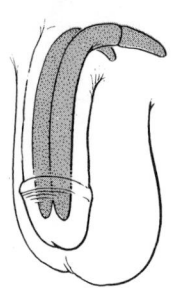

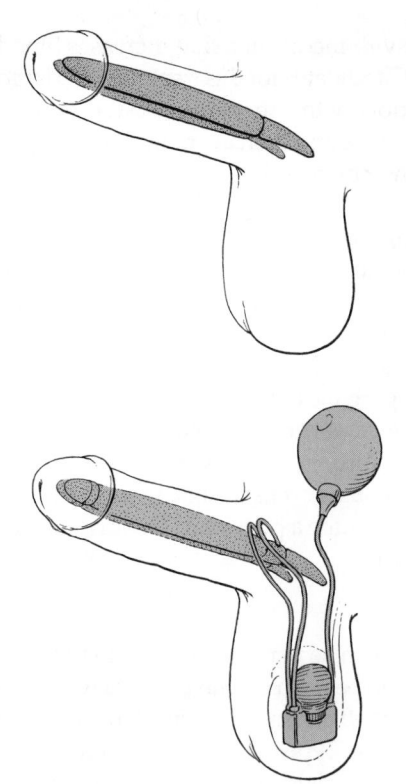

In men who are incapable of attaining erection, special devices may be implanted surgically. Among the varieties of implants in use today are semirigid implants that maintain a firmness at all times but allow the penis to be tucked close to the body when not in use for intercourse (top drawings), and an inflatable device that uses fluid reservoirs and a pump you operate mechanically to produce erection (right).

course (it usually does not), surgical procedures can correct this deformity (see Curvature of the Penis, page 1206).

Priapism, the third type of erectile abnormality, is a prolonged, painful erection of the penis with no associated sexual excitement. (The name is derived from the Latin name for a male fertility god in classical mythology, Priapus.) In its effect, priapism is the opposite of impotence. This is a rare, potentially dangerous condition that requires prompt medical treatment (see Priapism, page 1206).

Blood in the Semen

Signs and Symptoms—Blood in the semen

Blood in the semen (hematospermia) alarms many men but seldom should. Hematospermia is sometimes known as hemospermia. The color of the semen ranges from pink to red. If you or your partner sees blood in your ejaculated semen but you have no other symptoms, you probably do not have any physical disorder.

To make sure, however, visit your physician and have a thorough physical examination of your genital area, including your prostate and testicles. If your physician finds nothing wrong, further tests usually are unnecessary. You may or may not notice

bloody semen again; but, in any case, it is not cause for alarm.

The source of the blood in hematospermia is not clear. It probably comes from the vessels lining the seminal vesicles and may be the result of some harmless inflammation.

Premature Ejaculation

Signs and Symptoms—Ejaculation during foreplay with a sexual partner, or at a point during intercourse too soon to satisfy the partner

The only thing wrong with premature ejaculation is its timing—too soon, before either partner has had an opportunity to enjoy the sexual act fully. In rare cases, merely touching a woman is enough to bring about ejaculation. More commonly, ejaculation occurs when the penis first enters the vagina or very shortly after it enters the vagina.

Premature ejaculation is a common sexual problem, especially for young men. The cause is rarely physical, and treatment that involves the partner's help is almost always successful.

Premature ejaculation can be recognized without a physician's aid and is not serious. However, it has a detrimental effect on the sex life of both partners—a responsive female partner does not have time to attain orgasm, and the male partner experiences orgasm but after so little sexual activity as to deprive him of much of the pleasure involved. On occasion, men become so frustrated at premature ejaculations that they become impotent. Such anxiety is unnecessary because the solution is simple.

Treatment
Premature ejaculation can be treated with the "squeeze" technique. The method works as follows.

Begin sexual activity as usual, including penile stimulation, until you feel almost ready to ejaculate. Then have your partner squeeze the end of the penis, at the point where the glans joins the shaft, for a period of several seconds. After the squeeze is released, wait for about half a minute, and then go back to foreplay. You will notice that squeezing the penis causes it to become less erect but that when sexual stimulation is resumed it soon regains full erection.

If you again feel that you are about to ejaculate, have your partner repeat the squeeze process. By repeating this as many times as necessary, you can reach the point of entering your partner without having ejaculated. After a few practice sessions, the feeling of knowing how to delay ejaculation will become a habit without the squeeze technique and you will continue through successful intercourse.

Retrograde Ejaculation

Signs and Symptoms—Little or no semen is ejaculated from the penis during a sexual climax

Retrograde ejaculation is a fairly unusual, and harmless, phenomenon in which, rather than emerging from the end of the penis, the semen enters the bladder during orgasm. The word retrograde in the name refers to the backward direction of the semen.

Retrograde ejaculation may be distinguished from absence of ejaculation by voiding through a red-colored cloth immediately after intercourse or masturbation. When retrograde ejaculation occurs, the cloth acts as a strainer to trap the seminal discharge, which will appear on the red cloth. With absence of ejaculation, no seminal discharge will appear on the cloth.

Absence of ejaculation usually is due to a functional inability to achieve orgasm. Sexual counseling should be considered. In certain instances, absence of ejaculation may be due to injury of the seminal vesicles or some types of genitourinary surgery.

Various conditions can cause retrograde ejaculation, including diabetes, prostate surgery, urethral surgery, and use of mood-altering or antihypertensive drugs. It is most likely to occur among men who have diabetes.

Diagnosis

You will notice the symptom of retrograde ejaculation. A physician can confirm the diagnosis by tests such as a test of your urine after ejaculation to see if it contains a large quantity of sperm.

How Serious Is Retrograde Ejaculation?

Retrograde ejaculation is harmless. Semen that enters the bladder is simply expelled with the urine during urination. However, retrograde ejaculation does prevent fertility if no semen at all goes out the penis or diminishes fertility if a decreased quantity of semen emerges.

Treatment

Medication

If the retrograde ejaculation is caused by drugs that you are taking, use of the drugs can be stopped or you can switch to others in an effort to restore normal ejaculation.

Retrograde ejaculation may also be corrected by certain prescription drugs such as ephedrine, adrenaline, or Ornade (a combination of chlorpheniramine and phenylpropanolamine). Infertility due to retrograde ejaculation sometimes can be reversed by artificial insemination with sperm obtained by catheterization immediately after intercourse.

Loss of Sexual Desire in Men

Men can have various problems with their erections and with ejaculation that complicate sexual activity. But what about when the urge to have sex itself goes away?

A complete absence of sexual desire is unusual, but lessened sexual desire is not. After about age 60, most men experience somewhat diminished sexual desire, although this varies greatly from one man to another.

The first cause to consider is a physical ailment. Illnesses that cause persistent pain, weakness, or fatigue are prone to lessen sexual desire, as are emotional factors such as depression, anger toward your partner, and stress. Apathy or lack of enthusiasm from your partner also can lead to dampened desire.

In addition to the physical and nonphysical causes of loss of desire, medications taken to combat these disorders can also reduce sexual desire. When this is the case, substitute medications generally can be found.

In many men, loss of desire may occur because of inadequate communication of arousal needs between partners and poor timing of the act of intercourse. It is also important to realize that impotence usually does not imply a lack of desire but is a problem that your physician can treat.

Loss of desire often can be cured. If you experience a persisting loss of sexual desire, do not assume that this is the natural course of events. Seek help from your physician. Changes in medication, counseling, or other forms of therapy may be in order.

Sexual Crises

The problems described thus far in the chapter—although inconvenient or even dismaying—for the most part are not emergencies. The rest of this chapter addresses true crisis situations: rape, physical abuse, and sexual abuse of adolescents.

The section on rape is addressed to the adult or teenager who has been raped and needs to know where to turn or to the concerned friend or parent who wants to help. The section on physical abuse concerns bodily harm inflicted by one partner on another, regardless of whether or not sexual activity is involved. The section on sexual abuse of adolescents offers practical advice on where victims can seek help.

Although females are the prime victims of all three types of crimes, males are also sometimes victims.

Rape

Signs and Symptoms—Forced sexual intercourse, oral sexual activity, or anal intercourse

Lack of consent is the factor that differentiates rape from acceptable sexual activity: rape is forced on you, sometimes by violence or threats of violence and sometimes by deception.

People of all ages, from infancy through old age, can be rape victims. The rapist can be a stranger, but in about half of cases the rapist is known to the victim. About half of the instances of rape occur in the victim's own home. Rapists are often members of the extended family. In 90 percent of cases, the rapist is of the same race as the victim. In some instances, a woman's rapist is her husband.

Although rape of a man is more rare than rape of a woman, men can be the victims of rape, by other men or by women. They suffer the same types of mental damage and require the same care as women.

Regardless of the identities of the victim and the rapist, rape is psychologically and sometimes physically devastating. Rape is a crime, although it is one of the most difficult crimes to prosecute successfully. The recognition that forced sexual activity by one's own spouse can constitute rape is fairly recent and even more difficult to prosecute successfully. Nevertheless, if you have been raped, once you have sought the help that you need, you should also report the crime to the police.

Most rapes are planned by the rapist and are not the result of impulse—although the victim may be picked on impulse. The rapist is often not after sexual pleasure but needs an outlet to express anger and aggression.

Many techniques can be used to avoid becoming a rape victim (see Rape Prevention Tips, page 1231). If you are attacked by a potential rapist, how to resist—or whether to resist at all—depends on the individual and the circumstances. One technique is to stall for time, in the hope that someone may come along and help. Some women have avoided rape by saying they have a sexually transmitted disease. Resistance possibilities that are more active include the use of any self-defense techniques you are proficient at, such as screaming, breaking a window, or kicking the attacker forcefully in the testicles to disable him long enough to enable you to escape.

However, if you think you will be harmed if you resist, or if resistance does not work, submit. It is preferable to being killed or seriously injured. Note that as far as later prosecution goes, rape is a crime regardless of whether you resist or submit.

If you have been raped, you should seek immediate medical care at a rape treatment center at a major hospital, from your regular physician, or from a hospital emergency room (see page 428). If you are not certain where to go, look in the telephone book under "Rape" for the number of a local rape hotline, which can provide advice on a physician to see and other help, including personal support and legal advice. Do not bathe or douche before you are examined by a physician.

The physician who examines you has several jobs. First and foremost is treating any injuries and providing psychological support; second, obtaining evidence that can be used to prosecute the rapist. Taking evidence involves asking you to describe the rape. In addition, the physician will examine you for sexually transmitted disease and for the presence of semen, blood, or other materials from the rapist that could be used as evidence.

Rape Prevention Tips

Like most crimes, sexual assault cannot always be prevented, but you can take steps to reduce your risks. Some examples follow.

Sexual Limits

How friendly is too friendly? This is a judgment call—one that you must make whenever you are alone with a man. Always remember that you have the right (but not the obligation) to establish limits and that it is okay to change those limits as required by the circumstances. When it comes to sexual intercourse, you should never feel pressured.

Communication

Make your limitations known to the other person. Avoid sending any messages (verbal or nonverbal) that could be misleading.

Know Yourself

Pay attention to your emotions. Do not let circumstances override your good judgment. If it seems as though you are being pressured, then you are being pressured, and it is time to say "Good-by."

Be Observant

Sometimes you can anticipate circumstances that can lead to rape. For example, avoid eye contact with an individual who stares at you. If someone seems to enjoy sitting or standing too close to you, move aside. If an individual is blocking your way, walk in another direction (confidently, avoiding eye contact). Avoid people who speak or act as though they know you intimately when they do not.

Assert Yourself

If someone grabs or pushes you or disregards your negative response to any physical or verbal act, tell the individual, in a firm tone of voice, to "bug off." The language may seem unrefined or rude, but in circumstances such as this you may need to be uncharacteristically direct. Always remember that it is okay to become angry. Also, it is important to react quickly with your negative response. If assertiveness is a problem for you, consider an assertiveness training course. Such courses are available in most communities.

How Serious Is Rape?

A rape victim has endured a terrible experience. In most cases, the physical consequences are not long-lasting, and in fact there may not be any at all. Wounds and scratches heal; if there is a possibility of sexually transmitted disease or pregnancy, medications can be given.

The emotional and psychological consequences are often harder to deal with. Women may become unreasonably fearful (as opposed to rationally cautious) as a result of having been raped, may become depressed, or may have trouble with existing or future relationships with men. Sometimes women wrongly assume that they are to blame for the rape or for not resisting effectively.

Even if a woman manages to avoid all of these pitfalls, explaining what happened to the physician, to the police, and to family and friends is an ordeal. If the rapist is caught, recounting the experience in court can be another ordeal.

However, lasting emotional and psychological consequences of having been raped can be avoided or overcome through counseling with someone who is trained in helping rape victims.

Treatment

Your physician will treat any physical injuries. He or she can also refer you to a rape crisis center or community organization that will provide counseling and other support.

If there is a possibility of pregnancy as a result of the rape, the physician may give you a drug known as diethylstilbestrol (DES), which may prevent pregnancy. Medications can be prescribed to reduce the risk of acquiring a sexually transmitted disease. A follow-up examination and tests are generally necessary after several weeks to determine whether pregnancy has occurred or if a sexually transmitted disease has been acquired.

Sympathetic counseling is a cornerstone of effective rape treatment.

Physical Abuse

Signs and Symptoms

- Deliberate abuse of your body by another
- Deliberate abuse of your body by another in connection with sexual activity

If someone is attacked and beaten on the street, an obvious crime of violence has been committed, and the first place to which most of us would turn is the police or a hospital. If you have been injured by a stranger, seek such help without delay.

Our principal concern here, however, is physical abuse that can be fully as damaging but occurs in a more "seemingly normal" situation—generally the home. The person inflicting the abuse can be a husband, wife, companion, relative, or someone else known to the victim. (Rape, a particular form of physical abuse, is discussed on page 1230; the sexual abuse of adolescents is discussed on page 1233.)

Some cultures, primarily in the past, held that a man had the right to beat his wife if he was so inclined and that she should put up with it. This attitude is no longer acceptable, but remnants of it can still be encountered. It should be clear in your mind that it is wrong if your spouse, friend, or someone else abuses your body. You do not have to put up with it; battering is a crime and help is available.

The most common pattern of physical abuse is spouse abuse. The person inflicting the abuse has psychological problems that are unlikely to simply go away on their own. In many cases, the beatings will continue for years, as long as what is left of the relationship lasts or until the spouse dies.

Husbands are also the victims of physical abuse by wives. Friends, lovers, and relatives are the victims of abuse by other friends, lovers, or relatives. Regardless of the combination, abuse is wrong and the victim is entitled to help and protection.

One type of physical abuse is connected with sexual activity. A relatively small number of people, of either sex, experience heightened sexual response when pain or humiliation is associated with the activity. For example, a sexual sadist may obtain sexual pleasure by inflicting harm on his or her partner. A sexual masochist receives sexual pleasure by experiencing such pain. Both sadism and masochism run the gamut from minor or even feigned pain to torture and even murder.

Some aggression during sexual activity is perfectly normal and it does not imply that either partner is a sadist, masochist, or potential sex offender. Probably the clearest dividing line between the acceptable and the unacceptable for most people is pain: when something hurts, you avoid it or stop it. If a partner expects your participation in some activity that hurts you and you do not enjoy it, then that activity is physical abuse.

In other words, physical abuse can be connected or not connected with sexual activity. The result for the victim in either case is the same—physical and mental suffering, often prolonged because of repeated episodes.

Diagnosis

Someone's deliberate infliction of harm to your body, regardless of whether or not sexual activity is involved, constitutes physical abuse. See a physician or go to a hospital emergency room for treatment of the physical injuries.

Equally important is ensuring that the abuse stops. Your physician or hospital personnel can refer you to persons who can provide sympathetic counseling and intervention. Many communities have organizations that provide safe shelter for battered women who fear reprisals or greater abuse.

The police also can be helpful, but they are equipped to respond to emergency situations and not to solve long-term problems. For example, a woman may call the police to get her husband to stop beating her, or the neighbors may call. The husband will be reprimanded and possibly jailed, but the situation generally will be repeated in the future. Your physician, social workers, hospital emergency personnel, or counselors on spouse-abuse hotlines are more able to set you on the right track toward solving the problem permanently.

How Serious Is Physical Abuse?

Severe physical injuries, including death, can result. Even minor injuries that accumulate over time can be debilitating. The emotional and psychological damage inflicted by abuse can be just as devastating as the physical damage.

Treatment

Cuts, broken bones, and other physical injuries will require medical care, including operation for severe injuries. Your physician or a hospital emergency room can provide such care. Counseling is necessary to help you avoid further abuse; a physician, nurse, social worker, or worker for a spouse-abuse hotline can put you in touch with organizations or individuals who provide such counseling. They can also help you seek safe shelter if you are in imminent danger.

For emotional rehabilitation after abuse, a psychiatrist, psychologist, or social worker can be helpful.

Information for Women in Abusive Relationships

More than 90 percent of abused adults are women, according to The American College of Obstetricians and Gynecologists. Abuse can include battering and physical assault, sexual assault, and psychological abuse, such as making you do degrading or humiliating things, threatening to harm you or your children, damaging valued possessions, hurting pets, or exerting too much control over your life.

Who Is at Risk for an Abusive Relationship?

If you have already experienced family violence, sexual assault or incest, or physical abuse from a male partner, you have a higher risk of being in an abusive relationship. The following are signs that you may be involved in an unhealthy relationship:

- Your partner frightens you with threats of violence or by throwing things when he is angry
- Your partner says it's your fault if he hits you
- Your partner promises that it won't happen again, but it does

What Should a Woman Do If Her Partner Is Abusive?

- Tell someone. Let someone know about your situation so you can contact that person in case you need to leave suddenly.
- Ensure your safety. Plan to leave quickly. Pack a suitcase and leave it with a friend or neighbor. Keep important documents handy so you can take them with you. Know where you will go and how you'll get there at any time of day.

Signs of Impending Danger

- Your partner talks about using or has access to a weapon, especially a gun

- He extends his threats to children, other family members, or pets
- He sexually assaults you
- He shows little guilt and remorse after a violent episode

If you recognize these or other signs of impending danger, get away before a violent incident occurs.

If You Cannot Escape Violence

- Call your physician or go to an emergency room if you are hurt, even if you think your injuries are minor. Keep a copy of the medical records in case you decide to file charges.
- Call the police.

You will eventually have to face difficult decisions about the future. Many resources are available to help you with the important choices of whether to try to improve your relationship or to break away from your partner permanently.

If you decide to help the abusing partner seek care for his or her behavior problems, your physician, a marriage counselor, or a social worker should be able to provide referral for such care.

Sexual Abuse of Adolescents

Signs and Symptoms—Forced sexual activity or sexual contact against your will

This section is addressed to the adolescent who believes that he or she has been abused sexually. In addition, a parent who suspects that the teenager is being abused by another adult, sibling, or friend can read this to determine how the problem can be handled.

"Abuse" is anything that is done to your body without your consent or approval. Sexual abuse includes sexual intercourse without consent (which is rape), forced oral sexual contact, forced anal intercourse, or any other activity involving unwilling exposure of your body or unwilling contact with someone else's body. (For more about rape, see page 1230.) Sexual abuse can happen to people of either sex, and it is against the law.

The sexual abuser can be a parent, brother or sister, friend, acquaintance, or unknown adult or teenager. Abuse happening within the family also is wrong. For example, a father does not have the right to sexually molest his daughter, even if the mother knows about it and does nothing. Seek help.

There are two ways to deal with sexual abuse. The best way—unfortunately, it is not always possible—is to prevent the abuse from happening. Prevention methods include not associating with persons likely to inflict abuse; taking safety precautions about being out at night; locking doors; saying "no"; resisting physically; and trying to get away. If someone threatens you with a weapon or overwhelming force, however, physical resistance may only result in worse abuse, injury, or death.

The second method is making sure that physical abuse does not happen again. If you are abused sexually, tell your parents and the police, who will advise you on how to prevent its happening again. If a parent is the one inflicting the abuse, go straight to a physician, a hospital emergency room, the police, your clergy, or a relative you can trust. Physicians are required by law in all states to report cases of child abuse (which includes adolescent sexual abuse) to the proper authorities.

In addition, many communities have groups that offer free emergency counseling to child-abuse victims and rape victims. Experienced, sympathetic counselors can give you confidential advice on the next step to take.

Sometimes adolescents—particularly younger adolescents—are in doubt about exactly to whom their body belongs. It is simple: you need only remember that your body belongs only to you. If someone is abusing it, seek help from relatives, a teacher, a social worker, a counselor, the police, or a physician to see that the abuse stops.

Diagnosis

See your physician or go to a hospital emergency room to discuss sexual abuse. If you do not know what physician to go to or if you are not near a hospital, ask a reliable adult for advice or phone a child-abuse hotline.

A physician can help you to recover physically and emotionally from the experience and can help to ensure that it does not happen again. In addition, a physician can note physical evidence of abuse or rape for possible use in legal prosecution of the abuser (see Sexual Assault and Sexual Abuse, page 428).

How Serious Is Sexual Abuse in Adolescents?

Most sexual abuse in adolescents does not leave lasting physical injuries. The body can recover from the wounds and fractures. You also can recover from the emotional effects of abuse. However, if the abuse continues, it can damage your ability to form normal, trusting relationships with people. Continued abuse also increases the possibility of serious physical harm.

For the person inflicting the sexual abuse, it is very serious: he or she is committing a crime.

Treatment

A physician can treat physical injuries caused by the abuse. He or she also may refer you for counseling with social workers or other professionals so that you can express your feelings about the abuse. Talking about it with someone who understands can help you to work through the emotional problems that the abuse causes.

If the abuse is occurring within the home and if social workers believe that the abuse will continue there, they will find you a new home or foster-care environment where you can live in safety.

Part V

Modern Medical Care

Health care is becoming increasingly complex. These chapters summarize key issues and offer specific recommendations that will enable you to better understand and deal with problems such as selecting a health care provider, coping with cancer, understanding medications and medical tests, arranging care for an elderly parent, and dealing with death.

Contents

37 Understanding and Using the Health Care System . . 1237
38 The Modern Pharmacy 1271
39 Understanding Your Medications 1281
40 Cancer 1289
41 Dealing With Death 1309
42 Home Care and Elder Care 1319
43 Medical Tests 1329

Chapter 37

Understanding and Using the Health Care System

Contents

The Health Care System Today, 1238
Advance of Technology, 1238
Health Care in Evolution, 1238
Health Care of the Future, 1240

Health Care Providers, 1241
Training the M.D., 1241
    Medical Specialties, 1242
Nurses, 1243
Other Health Care Professionals and Skilled
    Workers, 1244
Alternative Medicine, 1244

Your Personal Physician, 1245
Finding a Personal Physician, 1246
    Getting the Most From a Visit to Your
        Physician, 1246
Second Opinions, 1247

Communication Between You and Your
Physician, 1247
Your Expectations and Responsibilities, 1247
Advance Directives, 1248
When to Change Physicians, 1249

Your Medical Examination, 1249
How Often Should I Consult My
    Physician? 1250
    How to Gather a Family History, 1251
Physical Examination, 1251
Laboratory Tests, 1252

Understanding the Specialties, 1252

Reasonable Expectations From Medical
Care, 1253

Health Care Facilities, 1254
Office-Based Practices, 1254
Hospital Outpatient Departments, 1254
Freestanding Emergency Centers, 1254
Neighborhood and Primary Health Care
    Centers, 1255

Nursing Homes, 1255
Hospices, 1255
Mental Health Facilities, 1256
Maternal and Child Care, 1257
Rehabilitation Centers, 1257

Your Hospital Stay, 1258
    Bedside Communication: 10 Questions for
        Your Physician, 1258
Entering the Hospital, 1258
During Your Stay, 1259
    Hospital Visits, 1259
Leaving the Hospital, 1260

Surgery, 1260
Presurgical Evaluation, 1260
Anesthesia, 1260
Your Operation, 1262
Postoperative Recovery, 1262
Ambulatory Surgery, 1262

How to Pay Your Medical Bills, 1263
Medicare Supplemental Insurance, 1264
Diagnostic-Related Groups (DRGs), 1265
    Was Your Hospital Stay Too Short? 1265
Conventional Health Insurance, 1265
Health Maintenance Organizations, 1266
Preferred Provider Organizations, 1267
    Utilization Review Boards, 1267

Malpractice and Lawsuits, 1267
Bringing a Malpractice Suit, 1268
Informed Consent, 1268

Quackery, 1268
Dangers of Quack Medicines, 1269
Identifying Fraudulent Medical "Cures," 1269
Thwarting Quackery, 1270

Health Headlines, 1270
    What Makes News? 1270

The Health Care System Today

The American health care system may be the finest in the world. Our medical schools and teaching hospitals, the level of training offered to physicians and nurses, and highly advanced medical technology attract some of the finest students, both American and foreign. American medical institutions, both public and private, lead the world's research.

In the following pages we consider our system as it functions today. We discuss the training medical professionals receive, the economics of health care, and the range of facilities available to suit the varied needs of you and your family.

Advance of Technology

Consider the long-established tradition of the visit to your physician's office. At first glance this may seem unchanged from the way it was 50 years ago: your physician determines your blood pressure, listens to your chest with a stethoscope, and thumps your knees with a little rubber hammer. Yet, thanks to technologic advances, much has changed.

Now, your physician may have an on-site electrocardiograph machine or other test equipment. When your physician suspects certain health problems, he or she can choose from among various diagnostic tests and prescribe from a wide range of new and older medications. Some of the newest medications are the products of genetic engineering techniques—unknown only a few years ago.

Now, physicians perform many operations, such as reattaching nerves and blood vessels of severed limbs, aided by microscopes. Microsurgery was unavailable a few years ago. Heart surgery, done with various newly developed methods, saves lives of people who formerly would have died. Organ transplantations have become commonplace. Many Americans have undergone successful cataract surgery on an outpatient basis.

Technology also helps us avoid operations. Now, physicians can break up kidney stones by directing sound waves at them (see Kidney Stone Lithotripsy, page 846). Arthroscopic surgery helps avoid major surgery and lengthy rehabilitation for knee injuries (see Arthroscopy, page 878). If you have already had a heart attack, you can take new drugs that help lower the risk of further heart attacks and avoid cardiovascular surgery.

We are making strides in prolonging life and preventing disease, even with problems for which scientists have not yet found a cure, such as many forms of cancer and AIDS. Chemotherapy and irradiation have enabled us to make progress in cancer treatment. Genetic engineering has produced new forms of treatment. Research continues at an intense pace, bringing greater understanding of our immune system.

The advance of medical technology, with the associated progress in surgical techniques, instrumentation, and materials, has produced positive results. You may know someone who is alive today thanks to a pacemaker, a CT scan that revealed a suspected problem early enough for it to be corrected, or a medication that keeps a serious condition under control. The introduction of a complex new machine, technique, or medication brings with it the need to learn about its full range of benefits and its most cost-effective use.

Many of today's physicians stress the importance of patient education, counseling persons on lifestyle changes and offering support and understanding as well as a willingness to undertake heroic technologic measures when appropriate.

To the medical researcher, this is an exciting time. Many barriers seem about to tumble. Almost daily, scientists learn more about cancer, Alzheimer's disease, AIDS, and other serious human afflictions. We have barely tapped the potential of biotechnology and genetic engineering. The future of these and other areas in medical technology holds promise for us all.

Health Care in Evolution

The American health care system has many parts (most of which we describe in this chapter). It may be hard to realize that the one-physician rural clinic and the large teaching hospital staffed with specialists belong to the same system, but they do. And recent trends have affected all parts of the system.

One trend is specialization. Before World

War II, most people had a family physician who was a general practitioner. Today, general practitioners are rare, and the physician who provides your basic care is more likely to be a specialist in internal medicine or in family medicine. Most American medical school graduates go on to train in one of the 24 approved medical specialties (see Medical Specialties, page 1242).

Most graduates go into private practice, either alone (solo practice) or with a group of physicians (group practice). In private practice, the physician cares for you in his or her office or in a hospital setting. Payment comes directly from you or from insurance or government-funded programs. Nonprivate work in the fields of anesthesiology, pathology, radiology, or emergency room care may take the form of salaried employment in government public health posts, medical schools, research and teaching positions (although many physicians on medical school faculties are permitted to practice on a part-time basis), or hospitals.

Another trend is the changing nature of medical practice. Before World War II, most general practitioners were solo practitioners. They often made house calls. Although some of us still receive our medical care this way, physicians today are likely to be part of a group practice, a health maintenance organization (HMO), or a clinic rather than in a solo practice. The costs, to physicians, of practicing medicine have increased, and the new clinical and group arrangements are one way to meet these overhead costs. Such arrangements also offer physicians an opportunity to work in a more medically stimulating environment, benefiting from the experience of other physicians and sharing facilities, equipment, staff, and expertise.

Another change from recent years is that health care now is much more complex. There used to be just the physician and the hospital. Although these remain the cornerstones of the health care system, the traditional idea of the physician has changed to include many different specialized physicians and health care specialists such as nurse-practitioners and physician assistants. In addition to hospitals, you may receive care in clinics, HMOs, neighborhood health centers, freestanding emergency centers, nursing homes, and hospices, all of which we discuss in this chapter.

A key force in the continual evolution of health care delivery systems is financial; another is the spread of specialization. The numerous medical advances make this field of knowledge much more complicated than it used to be. It was once possible for a physician to be familiar with the whole range of medicine and to keep up with the new developments published in technical journals. Now there is too much to learn. With the explosion of new technology, medications, and other options for treatment, it is a formidable challenge for your physician to remain current, even in his or her own specialty.

It is important to find one physician—a general practitioner, internist, pediatrician, or family medicine specialist—to take on the overall responsibility for your care and the care of your family. Sometimes, this "primary care physician" actually is a team of physicians. Thus, one physician (or team) will be familiar with your medical history and problems. You call on this person (or team) with your health concerns and for routine checkups. When necessary, your primary care physician or team will refer you to a specialist and keep track of what that specialist recommends.

You can find such a physician or team in private practice, in a group practice, in an HMO, or in one of various types of clinics (these facilities are described later in the chapter). It is well worth your trouble to seek out such a physician or team to handle your general care. Your health will benefit.

Another change in the health care system is how the costs of medical services are paid. Previously, people who were able paid for their own medical care, and physicians and hospitals could afford to charge little or nothing to those unable to pay. This approach has changed significantly, due both to greater costs produced by scientific technologic advances and to increased regulation of fees by Medicare and insurance companies. The federally funded Medicare program for elderly people and the Medicaid program (funded by federal and state governments) for people with low incomes has lessened but not solved the problems of lower-income groups. In addition, conventional group insurance programs, funded jointly by employers and employees, are much more common.

Having more sources of funding for medical care has led to increased numbers of patients seeking the help of physicians and health care facilities. Thus, more medical care reaches those who need it, whether or not they can afford it. If you can afford to pay insurance premiums, you now have options, such as whether to join an HMO for prepaid care or to remain under the care of physicians that you individually select.

Despite expanded funding for medical care, many people today do not receive adequate care. Medicare does not pay all medical expenses for elderly people, nor does Medicaid for poor people. As a result, many people forgo care. A century ago, many Americans visited a physician only in an emergency; this situation is still true, as you can see in many hospital emergency rooms. Perhaps the greatest tragedy is the number of children born in poverty to mothers who did not receive proper prenatal care. Many of these children will not receive appropriate medical attention during their childhood.

We face two major problems: 1) providing access to medical care for everyone, and 2) controlling cost. Although health insurance, federal funds, and community welfare services pay a substantial portion of the bills for most people, there are some who fall through the cracks and, because they cannot pay, may not seek medical care until they are seriously ill.

Striking a balance between providing good medical care and lowering costs or at least restraining further increases is a difficult challenge. It raises fundamental questions.

Should we discourage further development of health care techniques because of potential costs? True, some useful techniques are extremely expensive. However, other advances, such as polio immunization, are relatively inexpensive to apply and can avoid the alternative of providing treatment to those who, without immunization, would have become ill with polio.

How much can we restrict the use of tests and treatments without significantly impairing the quality of medical care? The need for cost containment further complicates ethical considerations in life-and-death decisions, which advances in technology make more complex. There is no easy solution to the cost-versus-care issue.

The challenges remain formidable. The more you know about who the participants are and how the system works, the better your chances are of seeking and finding appropriate, affordable, and quality care for you and your family.

Health Care of the Future

As we look to the future of health care in the United States, the status quo is not a realistic option. Mayo Clinic supports health care reforms, including the goal of universal health insurance coverage for all Americans. Changes in two areas could dramatically improve the American system. First, we need to correct access problems in the current system. Second, we need to create a competitive atmosphere that rewards the delivery of high-quality care at a reasonable price.

We believe these changes would encourage universal insurance coverage and reduce costs. Consensus appears to be forming around several changes. Insurance reforms should include portability (your health insurance should remain in effect when you change jobs), a movement toward community rating, a ban on exclusions for preexisting conditions, and a requirement for insurers to cover all applicants. Low-income Americans should receive sliding-scale subsidies to help purchase insurance, through either a tax credit or a voucher system. All certified health plans should be required to offer a defined, minimum standard benefit package.

It's important not to underestimate the desire of individuals for freedom of choice in matters of health care, as they define it. We should establish voluntary purchasing pools to allow small businesses and individuals to join in purchasing insurance at community rates. The pools would serve as information clearinghouses to enable consumers to compare price and quality of plans, although they would not be regulatory bodies, have price control authority, or be allowed to limit the number of plans marketed (including fee-for-service options).

It's important to retain employer involvement in providing health insurance; it is a vital force driving the current innovation in service delivery and quality of care. Employers should not relinquish this role to purchasing pools or health alliances.

All parts of the health care system should equitably share the costs of societal benefits provided by academic medical centers, including costs of research, education, and unreimbursed care (which will remain a need under any plan). This concept is critical to the survival of these essential programs, because a market-based system will hold little incentive for insurers or health plans to pay the additional costs. The tax-exempt status for centers that provide these societal benefits should also be continued.

Health plans and providers should have uniform data collection requirements, focused on the minimal data necessary to allow consumers (employers and individuals) to make informed choices of health insurance plans and providers, based on the price and quality of the care delivered. Nonessential data collection adds to costs without adding value. Standardization of billing and claims information forms and elimination of unnecessary micromanagement by government or alliances will significantly reduce paperwork and administrative hassles.

Meaningful legal reforms can reduce the practice of defensive medicine and its asso-ciated costs. Limiting tax subsidies for any health insurance to the average cost of a standard benefit package not only will generate revenue to help pay for subsidies to low-income Americans but also will remove an incentive to provide nonessential coverage at taxpayers' expense.

Even though the current U.S. health system is flawed and needs reform, we must make every effort not to make it worse. We should avoid regulatory health alliances and limits on patient choice of plans or the number of plans offered, including fee-for-service plans. We also recommend avoiding price controls or financing health care with further cuts in the rates of Medicare payments.

Health Care Providers

When you seek health care, you must interact with physicians, nurses, and other health care professionals. This section describes the diverse kinds of physicians, beginning with the various training regimens and including an explanation of when and why specialization occurs. Then we consider nurses, including some of the newer roles that they assume. We also include a brief description of allied health care professionals.

Training the M.D.

The physician, or medical doctor (M.D.), is ultimately responsible for delivering health care. Although the system could not function without nurses or other professionals, final responsibility for your care falls on your physician.

Becoming a physician requires, first, an undergraduate college degree. Medical school follows, with its 4-year curriculum. The first 2 years of medical school traditionally focus on the scientific foundations of medicine, including courses in human anatomy, physiology, genetics, biochemistry, microbiology, molecular biology, pharmacology, and behavior, along with an introduction to patient care, which is the focus of the third and fourth years of medical school. While continuing classwork, the medical student works with physicians in treating patients. The main areas of medicine covered during the third and fourth years are internal medicine, surgery, pediatrics, obstetrics and gynecology, family medicine, and psychiatry.

After successfully completing a 4-year medical school program, the student receives the M.D. (Doctor of Medicine) degree. To obtain a state license to practice medicine, however, the physician must pursue graduate training in a hospital or other health care facility. Years ago, a physician spent the first year after receiving the M.D. degree in an internship that provided experience in the common areas of medicine.

Today, the physician usually begins a residency program in family medicine, internal medicine, or some other specialty right away. At the end of 1 year of such training and experience, the physician may take an examination to obtain a state license to practice medicine as a general practitioner. Today it is uncommon for physicians to actually start their practice at this point.

Physicians must annually renew the state license to practice. A state licensing board not only examines the credentials of and gives examinations to physicians wanting to practice in that state but also hears reports of inappropriate or unprofessional behavior by

Medical Specialties

The American Board of Medical Specialties governs the primary specialties. In addition to the specialties, many subspecialties have boards that operate within the authority of one or another of the primary boards. Therefore, if your physician is a gastroenterologist, for example, he or she initially received board certification in internal medicine, and then received subspecialty certification in gastroenterology. The various specialty and subspecialty boards are listed here.

Specialties
Allergy and Immunology
Anesthesiology
Colon and Rectal Surgery
Dermatology
Emergency Medicine
Family Practice
Internal Medicine
Medical Genetics
Neurological Surgery
Nuclear Medicine
Obstetrics and Gynecology
Ophthalmology
Orthopedic Surgery
Otolaryngology
Pathology
Pediatrics
Physical Medicine and Rehabilitation
Plastic Surgery
Preventive Medicine
Psychiatry and Neurology
Radiology
Surgery
Thoracic Surgery
Urology

Subspecialties
Addiction Psychiatry
Adolescent Medicine
Blood Banking and Transfusion Medicine
Cardiac Electrophysiology
Cardiovascular Disease
Chemical Pathology
Child and Adolescent Psychiatry
Clinical and Laboratory Dermatological
 Immunology
Clinical and Laboratory Immunology
Clinical Neurophysiology
Critical Care Medicine
Cytopathology
Dermatopathology
Endocrinology, Diabetes, and Metabolism

Forensic Pathology
Forensic Psychiatry
Gastroenterology
General Vascular Surgery
Geriatric Medicine
Geriatric Psychiatry
Gynecologic Oncology
Hand Surgery
Hematology
Immunopathology
Infectious Disease
Maternal and Fetal Medicine
Medical Microbiology
Medical Oncology
Medical Toxicology
Neonatal-Perinatal Medicine
Nephrology
Neuropathology
Nuclear Radiology
Otology and Neurotology
Pain Management
Pediatric Cardiology
Pediatric Critical Care Medicine
Pediatric Emergency Medicine
Pediatric Endocrinology
Pediatric Gastroenterology
Pediatric Hematology-Oncology
Pediatric Infectious Diseases
Pediatric Nephrology
Pediatric Otolaryngology
Pediatric Pathology
Pediatric Pulmonology
Pediatric Radiology
Pediatric Rheumatology
Pediatric Surgery
Pulmonary Disease
Reproductive Endocrinology
Rheumatology
Sports Medicine
Surgery of the Hand
Surgical Critical Care
Undersea Medicine

physicians. When necessary, the board may revoke a physician's license. A physician who moves from one state to another must obtain a license in the state to which he or she is moving. Often this can be done by reciprocity—that is, the second state recognizes the credentials from the first state. However, some states insist that the physician take all of the qualifying examinations.

Most physicians now continue their graduate education (residency) beyond the first year. They work as residents at a hospital or health care facility for another 2 to 6 years or longer, gaining knowledge and experience in their medical specialty. Then they have the option of being examined for possible certification by the board in charge of their particular specialty (there are 24 of these). Many specialties are broadly based. For example, the fields of family medicine, internal medicine, general surgery, and pediatrics encompass a wide range of problems. Some physicians choose to go into medical research or teaching, in addition to or in place of a clinical practice of medicine.

Why do physicians put in all those years of specialty training—in addition to 4 years of college and 4 years of medical school—in order to specialize? Perhaps they desire to master a discipline. Medicine is such a broad and complex field that one physician reasonably can expect to grasp only a portion of it (a specialty) and to apply it in any depth.

Once the physician enters practice, his or her education is by no means over. Physicians continue their postgraduate education, by means of brief intensive courses, to keep up with developments in their fields. Some states require physicians to obtain a specified amount of continuing education to keep their licenses. Medical boards that govern particular specialties also have continuing education requirements, which may be more stringent than those of the states. In addition to formalized postgraduate courses, the main ways that physicians attempt to keep abreast of the medical information explosion are through reading medical journals and attending conferences.

Nurses

As a consumer in the health care system, you may deal with nurses more frequently than physicians, especially in hospitals, where nurses provide much of the care.

Like your physician, nurses want to help you get well. The nurse observes symptoms and listens to you describe them. He or she helps carry out the treatment plan and evaluate the results. The nurse often provides information for you and your family on managing health care problems at home.

When both a physician and a nurse treat your health problem, the nurse plays a supporting and assisting role. Frequently, there also is a slight difference in the nurse's focus, with the physician concentrating on your medical problem and the nurse focusing more on how you react to and deal with the problem and its accompanying symptoms and discomforts.

The initials R.N. after a person's name mean Registered Nurse. To be an R.N., a person must complete a course of study and pass a licensing examination in the state where he or she intends to practice. Some nurses have postgraduate degrees.

The initials L.P.N. mean Licensed Practical Nurse. The L.P.N. course of study is shorter and less academically oriented than that of the R.N. The L.P.N. generally provides services under the guidance of an R.N.

Although most nurses are generalists, some specialize. In hospitals or clinics, some nurses work in a particular area of care such as cardiology, pediatrics, or psychiatry. Other specialized types of nurses include the nurse-anesthetist, nurse-clinician, nurse-educator, nurse-midwife, and nurse-practitioner. A nurse-practitioner performs the same basic tasks as a physician, examining and treating patients, frequently in a setting where physicians are scarce or unavailable. However, they cannot write prescriptions.

Most nurses work in hospitals. Some nurses work in clinics, in physicians' offices, for home-care agencies, or in private practice (especially nurse-practitioners and nurse-midwives). Nurses' aides have little or no formal instruction but have learned their skills by working under the supervision of R.N.s and L.P.N.s. They provide many valuable services in the hospital setting.

From the beginning of the nursing profession in the 1800s, nurses have focused on educating others about sound health practices. The goal of health education is to improve health and prevent complications, provide you with knowledge you need to make informed decisions, allay fears and anxieties, and promote good health. Nurses also conduct research and publish their results in respected journals, in addition to keeping abreast of new developments in nursing and medicine and attending professional conferences.

Other Health Care Professionals and Skilled Workers

In addition to physicians and nurses, many other people are vital to delivering effective health care. Other types of health care professionals and skilled workers are listed here, together with a description of what they do:

- Attendants and orderlies provide various basic services such as transporting patients and helping nurses in health care facilities.
- Audiologists are specialists in the science of hearing. They evaluate hearing defects and assist in correcting them.
- Dental hygienists clean teeth, take dental X-rays, and perform other preventive dental services.
- Emergency medical technicians (EMTs) offer emergency care, including life support, and transport sick and injured people to medical facilities.
- Exercise physiologists scientifically evaluate the effects of exercise on body function and make recommendations for healthful exercise.
- Home health aides help homebound people with dressing, grooming, and eating and perform simple nursing tasks such as changing bandages (see Home Health Care, page 1322).
- Laboratory technicians perform tests and analyses on your blood, urine, and other substances to help in diagnosing your condition and monitoring your progress.
- Medical records personnel keep patient files up to date and accessible.
- Midwives assist in prenatal care, attend women in labor, and assist in the delivery of babies.
- Nurses' aides carry out nonspecialized basic tasks in health care facilities, such as feeding and bathing patients and making beds.
- Occupational therapists help you, if you are injured or disabled, regain your ability to carry out everyday tasks, including recommending possible physical modifications of your home.

- Opticians grind and fit your eyeglass lenses and contact lenses.
- Optometrists test your vision and prescribe eyeglasses.
- Pharmacists formulate and dispense medicines according to your physicians' prescriptions.
- Physical therapists help you, if you are injured or disabled, regain lost physical functions, using techniques such as exercise, massage, and ultrasound.
- Physicians' assistants examine patients, diagnose some health problems, and suggest a course of treatment, under your physician's supervision.
- Podiatrists treat injuries and other problems of your feet.
- Psychologists diagnose and treat mental health problems, using primarily counseling, testing, and therapy.
- Radiology technicians help take and develop X-rays, CT scans, and other types of tests based on radiation.
- Recreational therapists use group activities including music and games to help withdrawn, depressed, and other patients improve communication or behavior patterns.
- Registered dietitians help specify and modify foods to address your specific health conditions.
- Respiratory therapists use respirators and other devices to improve your breathing ability and capacity.
- Social workers provide counseling about health-related and other problems and help you obtain financing, care after your hospital dismissal, and other needed services.
- Speech therapists treat disorders and injuries that affect your ability to speak, such as helping a child overcome a lisp or an adult regain speaking skills after a stroke.

Alternative Medicine

We know that about one-third of all Americans use a type of alternative medicine at some time. Alternative medicine is a blanket term used to describe several interventions not taught widely in American medical schools or generally used in U.S. hospitals. Some of these alternative approaches come to the U.S. from foreign cultures.

Alternative medicine includes a wide variety of unconventional therapies, some administered by physicians. Most people who use alternative medicine still visit their physician, but they neglect to discuss their use of alternative approaches with the physician. This holding back of information can cause problems if the caregivers use treatments that are not compatible. Most insurance does not cover alternative therapies, or covers them only partially.

Categories of alternative medicine include aromatherapy (you inhale, bathe in, or have "essential oils" distilled from plants and herbs massaged into your skin); folk remedies; ayurveda (disease is an imbalance of movement, structure, and metabolism, and it is treated with herbs, diet, meditation, and yoga); macrobiotics and other lifestyle diets; megavitamin therapy; spiritual healing; crystal ther-

apy; relaxation therapy; guided imagery (a trained therapist or audiotape helps you relax and visualize positive outcomes); hypnosis; chiropractic (contending that your spine is key to your health, usually treatment is with direct spinal manipulation); energy healing; herbal medicine (using plants or plant-based substances to treat a wide range of illnesses and enhance physical functions); and homeopathy (stimulating your body's defenses with tiny doses of substances that would cause disease symptoms in larger amounts).

In some cases, the lines between alternative medicine and traditional medicine are becoming fuzzy, as some physicians adopt some alternative techniques in their practices. You must be cautious, however, because most of the alternatives are unproven and some are even risky or downright dangerous.

Your Personal Physician

Knowledge of illness and the ability to treat it are growing rapidly. In fact, you should no longer expect a single physician to know everything about the thousands of identified ailments, common and uncommon. As a result, specialties and subspecialties try to manage this explosion of knowledge.

One result of the increasing specialization is that some people believe they can get the best care by seeing a specialist for whatever part of their body is bothering them. They may visit a gastroenterologist for a perceived intestinal problem, or a rheumatologist or orthopedist for joint problems, and so on. Also, people are much more mobile today than they were in the past. You are not typical if you spend your entire life in the same town (and under the long-term care of the same physician). As a result of these two trends, you may no longer have one person you would describe as your personal physician.

Yet, you still can find a personal physician. He or she is someone you trust, have confidence in, and feel comfortable with. In some situations, more than one physician will serve as your personal physician. This may occur in a group or HMO setting (see Health

Maintenance Organizations, page 1266) in which you may see different physicians but where all of your medical records remain together for easy access and review.

It is important to have a physician who can advise you candidly when your personal life and habits affect your health. Your personal physician can care for you better if he or she is knowledgeable about the health of other family members and knows of diseases that occur with high frequency in your family. Your physician should also know about sources of tension in your workplace or at home that may affect your health.

A good personal physician will help you obtain specialty consultations when you need them and make sure that one treatment does not conflict with another. This role is particularly important when you have long-term or multiple health problems that require consultation with specialists. Your personal (primary care) physician is generally responsible for coordinating and overseeing your preventive care, treatment when a problem arises, and rehabilitation after treatment.

In medicine today, this physician is usually a specialist in family practice, internal medicine (for adults), or pediatrics (see Medical Specialties, page 1242). Family practice has been in existence as a specialty of its own, with board certification, since 1970. To be certified in family practice, a physician must complete 3 years of advanced training in family medicine. He or she will have some training in almost every aspect of medicine, including obstetrics and pediatrics. An internist is a physician who diagnoses and treats medical diseases of adults. He or she also can deal with nearly every health problem you might have. Pediatricians diagnose and treat medical diseases of children.

After medical school, a personal (primary care) physician enters a training program in his or her chosen specialty, which generally lasts 3 years. After finishing a specialty training program, a physician may choose to obtain further training in a subspecialty. For example, someone trained in the specialty of internal medicine may obtain further training in the subspecialty of cardiology (study of heart disorders). Occasionally, a physician with subspecialty training may still serve as your personal physician (see Understanding the Specialties, page 1252).

In addition to such educational and training experiences, your physician should also care for you as a person.

Finding a Personal Physician

The first step in finding a personal physician is to gather a list of names. Don't worry about how long your list is at this stage—you can narrow it down later.

Before you move into a new community, ask your current physician for recommendations. You can also obtain names from various other sources. One good place to start is your local or county medical society, which should be able to provide you with a list of physicians in your area. Consumer affairs groups may have information or may even have a guidebook on local physicians.

Your local hospital is another possible source of names, as are the Yellow Pages of your telephone book (look for internists, pediatricians, and general or family practitioners). Your local library has several directories, including the American Medical Directory, that list physicians. This directory has information about every physician who belongs to the American Medical Association, including their address, age, education (undergraduate and medical), certifications as specialists, and specialty associations they belong to.

Ask your friends and colleagues for recommendations. Inquire about availability and promptness for returning telephone calls if you have a medical question. In the same way, no matter where you obtain names, consider accessibility. Include only those physicians whose offices are located within or near your community and are reasonably accessible from your home or workplace.

Call the office of each physician on your list. You will probably speak to a receptionist or medical assistant. Introduce yourself and tell him or her you are looking for a personal physician.

Take note of the receptionist's tone. Is it warm, friendly, concerned? Does this individual answer your questions directly?

Ask what hospital the physician uses, what the fee schedules are for checkups and office visits, and what the physician's office hours are. Does the receptionist give you directions to the office? How accessible is it?

Inquire about coverage for emergency situations that occur outside normal office hours. Ask how much time the physician allots for appointments. Your physician should allow at least a half hour for a routine initial examination; subsequent appointments should last at least 10 minutes. If you have particular religious or other strong feelings that may affect the care you seek, inquire about the physician's willingness to accommodate these concerns.

Getting the Most From a Visit to Your Physician

Here are a few tips for benefiting the most from your visit to the physician. If you arrive on time, your visit should not be hurried. Know your own and your family's medical history; it's important that you be prepared to discuss your own previous medical conditions and those of blood-related family members with your physician.

Bring all medications you're taking in their original containers, so that your physician can see the types and dosages of the drugs you're taking. Answer your physician's questions accurately and completely, but don't speculate on your diagnosis. Be sure to speak up if you have questions or doubts about your diagnosis or treatment or about a medication, including its benefits, side effects, or the amount of time it takes for it to work.

Second Opinions

Given the various treatments and technologies available today—and their frequently high cost—many people seek a second opinion before proceeding with many treatments. In fact, some health insurance agencies insist that you obtain a second opinion before you have certain surgical procedures.

Either you or your physician can initiate the decision to get a second opinion. A good physician who is uncertain about a diagnosis will have no reservations about referring you to a specialist. In fact, the physician may be glad to have another trained professional confirm the diagnosis. Second opinions also may be useful when the diagnosis is clear but the choice of treatments is less so; for many diseases there are several significantly different treatments available. Therefore, if a diagnosis is very serious; if the treatment your physician advises is risky, experimental, or controversial; or if major surgery appears necessary, a second opinion may be in your best interest.

Don't feel that you need to be secretive about requesting a second opinion. Tell your physician that you would like a second opinion just to review the diagnosis or the appropriateness of the procedure. Remember, your physician's principal concern is to ensure your continued good health.

Communication Between You and Your Physician

Traditionally, many people accepted a physician's advice without question. Today, however, we know that this system of one-way communication does not benefit either you or your physician. Better care results when you actively participate in your medical care.

The best medical care results from a partnership between you and your physician. To make an accurate diagnosis, your physician needs information only you can provide. In the same way, many treatments require that you help your physician—and yourself—by following his or her instructions precisely. (When treatments fail, the cause is frequently the patient's failure to follow the physician's instructions precisely.)

You will receive the best health care if you work with your physician to determine which treatment is best for you. Ask questions. Understand what your health care providers are doing and why. Understand clearly what to expect from your disorder and its treatment.

Feel free to contact your physician to discuss unexpected events, discomforts, or other problems. Your confidence both in your physician's abilities and in his or her openness in listening to your concerns and observations is essential to proper physician-patient communication. You need to be willing to listen and be guided by the advice your physician provides.

Your Expectations and Responsibilities

Becoming a partner with your physician in maintaining your health is not always easy. This partnership becomes most important when you or a loved one is sick—yet, in times of illness your feelings of fear and helplessness can make communication more difficult.

As a patient, you have certain expectations and responsibilities. For example, expect the following:

1. Information: as much information as you want about your illness

2. Time: a reasonable amount of time to ask questions and discuss concerns

3. Cost estimates: information on how much your care will cost

4. Reasonable access to your physician: don't expect to see your physician at any time day or night, but you should be able to consult your physician as your medical condition dictates and as your physician's schedule permits

5. Emergency contacts: knowing where care is available in an emergency if you cannot reach your own physician

6. Timely appointments: seeing your physician within a reasonable time of your scheduled appointment, except in unusual circumstances

7. Changes in physicians: ability to change physicians at your discretion and expect that your medical information will be promptly forwarded to your new physician

8. Confidentiality: that your condition and your medical records are your business and your physician's; if you consult a specialist, he or she may need to review your records; for some conditions (such as certain infectious diseases), the law requires your physician to notify public health authorities; your physician's office should not release your records to insurance companies, employers, or others without your approval

9. Decision-making ability: participating in decisions about your care, based on your knowledge of your illness

It is your responsibility to inform your physician of all information that might relate to your illness. Information that initially may seem completely unrelated—concerning your medical history, family, home and work situations—may have a direct and sometimes crucial impact on your current problem.

Be on time for office appointments; if you must cancel, do so at least 24 hours in advance. As a courtesy to your physician (whose schedule may be busy) and to gain maximum benefit from your appointment, plan what you will ask. Ask your physician for an explanation if you don't understand something.

When your physician prescribes a treatment, follow it accurately. If you can't, let your physician know. He or she may suggest that you try an alternative treatment. Be patient—often a treatment takes time to have an effect, but inform your physician promptly of any adverse effects, worsening symptoms, or complications.

Advance Directives

Today, many people want a voice in determining the treatment they are to receive if they become terminally ill and are unable to communicate their wishes. Advance directives offer this capability. These legal documents spell out the types of medical treatments and life-sustaining measures you do and don't want. They also allow for someone you've appointed to make medical decisions on your behalf. They become active only if you lose your mental competence or suffer an injury or disease that impairs your ability to communicate.

As part of the admission process, federal law requires hospitals, nursing homes, hospices, and home health care agencies to ask every person older than 18 if he or she has an advance directive. That information is documented in your record. The hospital also must give you written information about your right, under state law, to accept or reject medical treatment. Whether or not you have an advance directive, federal law requires the hospital to provide you the same treatment options.

Two common types of advance directives are living wills and durable powers of attorney for health care.

Living Will

Living wills are written in general language because no one can anticipate all possible circumstances. They can follow a general guideline or be specific. For example, your living will might prohibit heroic procedures, but then your physician has to make certain distinctions: Is the use of a respirator a heroic measure? What about a blood transfusion? As new technologies are developed and yesterday's heroic treatments become routine, the problem becomes increasingly complicated.

To draft a living will, it is useful but not essential to get help from an attorney. It is also important to realize that all living wills have limitations because few of us can predict our way of death. You might consider stating in your living will your wish that extraordinary technologic procedures not be used when your condition is terminal. But at what point is a condition to be considered terminal? In some states, the "terminal" condition is clearly defined, but in general this remains a subject of considerable debate.

A living will may seem to you to be an appropriate step, but by itself it carries only moral force in stating your preferences. To give legal authority to living wills, most states have passed statutes, often called natural death acts. In these states, the statutes interpret the extent of the authority and the legal force of the living will.

The statutes are not uniform among states.

Each state's law has unique characteristics. To ensure that your living will conforms to your state's requirements and will have the intended effect, be familiar with the appropriate laws in your state. Some states have laws that include forms you must use for this purpose.

Once you've created a living will, review and update it often. Medical technology and your views and wishes are subject to change. It's also important to know that you have the option to revoke your living will or other advance directive at any time.

Durable Power of Attorney for Health Care

In addition to a living will, you may want to consider a document invoking a durable power of attorney for health care. This document identifies the person you've selected to make health-related decisions for you should you become incapacitated, and it gives this person legal authority to act on your behalf.

Usually the person is a trusted friend or relative. A proxy helps ensure that your wishes aren't misinterpreted or ignored. Also, your proxy can respond specifically to the unique questions that your condition may create.

The combination of a durable power of attorney for health care and a living will provides maximum personal participation in the face of many medical situations that require difficult decisions. Discuss these decisions with your family so that your wishes are well understood.

(For examples of forms used to designate a durable power of attorney for health care or to state your wishes with a living will, see page 1382.)

When to Change Physicians

A good physician will welcome your taking an active role in your health care. If your physician puts you off and resents your reasonable questions, consider changing physicians.

Like other professionals, physicians provide services. But a physician's services are unique and involve an intimacy that relationships with other service providers don't. Building these relationships takes time. It's essential that you and your physician have confidence and trust in one another. Select your physician carefully. Get to know him or her. Avoid jumping from physician to physician. If something annoys you, or if a misunderstanding arises, discuss it.

Sometimes a patient and physician are basically incompatible. Do you feel you can't trust your physician? Are you uncomfortable talking about personal aspects of your life or illness? Is your physician condescending or brusque? Do you think he or she isn't always straightforward and honest with you? Do you often believe that you aren't getting your physician's complete attention? Are you rushed during appointments? Is your physician unavailable, or is after-hours coverage inadequate? Are your philosophies and lifestyles incompatible? Does your physician fail to follow through on problems when they arise?

If the answer to all or many of these questions is "yes," you may need to change physicians.

If you decide to change, let your former physician know why. Although it is easier simply to leave, give your physician an opportunity to hear why the physician-patient relationship failed. Also, be sure to have a summary of your medical records forwarded to your new physician.

Your Medical Examination

Generally, you need a thorough medical examination at least every few years—more frequently if you have a specific health problem that requires continuing care (see How Often Should I Consult My Physician? page 1250). A physician is less able to provide you with optimal care if he or she sees you only when you are sick.

Before heading to your physician for a checkup, think about what you want to discuss. This may save you from forgetting a question you want to ask. Prepare a written list summarizing symptoms that concern you, medications you are taking, and questions. Such a list should not be extensive; just jot down five or six items that you don't want to forget.

Think about your symptoms before you see your physician. For example, if you have a specific medical complaint such as abdominal discomfort, tell your physician what it feels like, how intense it is, how long it lasts, where it occurs, how far it spreads from its beginning point, what precipitates the pain, what makes it better, what makes it worse, whether it occurs with any other symptoms, and how often it occurs.

If this is your first visit to a new physician for a general examination, he or she should obtain your complete medical history. Be prepared to give a description of illnesses experienced by your parents, siblings, and grandparents (see How to Gather a Family History, page 1251). Inform your physician of prior illnesses, hospitalizations, accidents, operations, or allergies. You will be asked a long list of questions reviewing each of your body's systems. Your physician should take detailed notes of any past problems.

How Often Should I Consult My Physician?

The answer to this question varies, depending on whom you ask. Consult your physician if you have pain or other symptoms. However, the absence of disagreeable symptoms does not necessarily guarantee that you are in good health.

In the early stages, many diseases, including diabetes, high blood pressure, and some forms of cancer, are asymptomatic (without symptoms) but are detectable and treatable when found early. A periodic medical examination aims to diagnose treatable, asymptomatic diseases and to correct modifiable disease risk factors. These goals imply a comprehensive physical examination and laboratory evaluation (see Physical Examination, page 1251).

How often should you have a medical examination? All of us have different needs. Nevertheless, some guidelines may be useful to you in discussing this issue with your physician. The guidelines given here are for people who have no symptoms of disease.

Regular Physical Examinations
The interval between examinations depends on your age. If you are between ages 18 and 30, every 5 or 6 years is appropriate, perhaps at ages 18 and 24. After age 30, every 3 years

is probably a better frequency. Between ages 40 and 60, an every-other-year schedule is sensible; after age 60, have a checkup annually.

Self-Examination
Self-examinations are also important. Men should begin regular self-examination of the testicles in their teens (see Self-Examination of the Testicles, page 1200). Women of child-bearing age or older should examine their breasts monthly (see Breast Self-Examination, page 1160).

In addition to periodic health checkups and self-examinations, specific studies can help keep you healthy. These guidelines aid you in discussing them with your physician.

Annual Pelvic Examination and Pap Smear
Women should schedule these tests annually from the time they become sexually active (see Pelvic Examination, page 1141, and Pap Smear, page 1181).

Mammography
If you are younger than 40, you probably do not need mammography unless you develop a problem or are in a high-risk category (for instance, if you have a family history of breast cancer). If you are between 40 and 49, have no symptoms or lumps, and have no family history of breast cancer, have mammography done to determine a "baseline" (a test to determine what is normal for you). Then have the test every 2 years. After the age of 50, have mammography annually.

Digital Rectal Examination
You should have this with each general comprehensive physical examination (see page B-5).

Proctosigmoidoscopy
In the absence of any family history of colon cancer, this examination (which involves insertion of an instrument into your rectum) should be done initially at age 45, and every 3 to 5 years thereafter (see page 791). Also, an annual stool blood test may increase your chance for early detection of colorectal cancer (see page 790).

Blood Lipid Measurements
You should have blood cholesterol, HDL cholesterol, and triglyceride tests as early as possible (preteen years, for example), partic-

ularly if there is a family history of athero-sclerosis. If test results are within normal limits, you should have these tests repeated at least every 5 years (see What Do Measurements of Blood Fats Mean? page 640).

Chest X-Ray

There is debate about when you should have a chest X-ray. In the absence of any heart or lung disease, it may not be necessary before age 40. It is reasonable to have a baseline chest X-ray at approximately age 40 and thereafter to have the test only when your physician recommends it.

Glaucoma Screening

You should have this brief, painless eye examination at age 40, and as your physician recommends.

Resting Electrocardiography

Before age 40, have a baseline test; subsequently have the test as your physician recommends.

Blood Pressure Measurement

Have your blood pressure taken at every physical examination, more often if your physician advises.

Physical Examination

Your physician will supply you with a dressing gown and ask you to undress, so that he or she can perform a physical examination. If you want complete, quality care, you must tell your physician all the details of your health history and allow him or her to examine your entire body. Your physician will perform this examination with professionalism, humanity, and respect for you.

Physical examinations may vary slightly, but the basic elements of a thorough examination are the same. Your height, weight, and blood pressure are usually checked. Your physician will record your heart rate and will listen to your heart closely with a stethoscope, ideally while you are lying down and while you are sitting up. Your physician will also use the stethoscope to listen for any abnormal sounds in your lungs and abdomen. Your physician will examine your eyes, ears, nose, throat, and the skin on your face. Your physician will check the extent of your visual field (that is, your side vision).

How to Gather a Family History

In preparation for your medical examination, gather information about any childhood illnesses, accidents, or operations. You should offer additional information about other members of your family and their illnesses.

Obviously, it is important for your physician to know about any genetic diseases in your family (Huntington's disease and sickle cell anemia are two examples). Parents pass these ailments to their children, although not to every child in each generation.

Similarly, many common diseases have apparent familial links. For example, if your father has heart disease, it does not necessarily mean you also will have heart disease. But your physician should know about the history of this illness in your family, so that he or she can watch for symptoms early and recommend preventive measures that may reduce other controllable risk factors (see page 638).

To assemble a family history, make a list of any chronic diseases affecting your parents, grandparents, brothers, sisters, children, and even aunts and uncles. Keep track of whether they are on your mother's or father's side of the family. Such diseases include high blood pressure; cancers of the breast, uterus, and colon; diabetes; arthritis; Alzheimer's disease; allergies; emphysema; heart disease; and kidney disease. Also record any unusual diseases, even those that you don't believe are hereditary.

Note any twins born in your family or documented miscarriages. Finally, note whether any immediate relatives died at a young age from an illness. Provide this information to your primary physician for your medical record.

Your physician will carefully palpate your abdomen to check for enlargement of your liver, spleen, or aorta or any other abnormalities. You may walk a few steps, so that your physician can observe any abnormalities of gait or balance. Your physician will feel for pulsations of arteries in your neck, groin, knees, and feet. Your neck, armpits, and groin will be examined for the presence of swollen lymph nodes. Your physician will tap your knees and ankles with a small rubber hammer to check your reflexes.

For women, the examination may include a breast and pelvic examination, including a Papanicolaou, or Pap, smear (see Pelvic Examination, page 1141, and Pap Smear, page 1181). These can be part of your regular physical examination. Both men and women should have a rectal examination, and men should have their prostate gland palpated. Your physician may request samples of your urine or blood for testing.

The examination should proceed smoothly,

without interruption, and should be thorough and methodical. The steps in the examination probably will not be limited to those mentioned above, especially if your physician suspects a problem that requires further examination, questioning, or testing.

Your physician will ask if you have questions and have you amplify any points on which you have information, such as any scars, sensitive areas, or family traits.

At the end of the examination, your physician will forthrightly discuss any significant findings. Review the important points with your physician to make sure you understand them.

Laboratory Tests

Your physician will probably request laboratory tests in conjunction with your physical examination. These include a urinalysis, an X-ray of your chest, and blood tests. Electrocardiography may also be done, particularly if you are older than 40.

There are two categories of blood tests. The hematology group tests measure the number of white and red blood cells and the number of platelets. Your hemoglobin concentration is measured, and the varieties of white cells are enumerated. All this is done in an automated procedure. Figures reflect the average size and hemoglobin content of red blood cells. The hematology group tests are done to find any evidence of the different kinds of anemia, leukemia, and other disorders of your blood-forming system.

The second category of blood tests consists of several chemistry measurements—blood sugar and other substances, enzymes that reflect liver and kidney function, electrolytes, and blood fat concentrations, such as cholesterol and triglycerides. Your physician will obtain measurements of other substances in your blood if the physical examination or your symptoms suggest the likelihood of particular diseases or disorders.

Because doing such routine tests if you have no symptoms of illness and no abnormal findings in your physical examination only occasionally reveals a previously unsuspected illness, some people argue that in the interest of cost-containment you can forgo them. Most people, however, want and value the reassurance of normal laboratory tests. Furthermore, having an electrocardiogram and a good-quality chest X-ray on file may be very useful in the future for comparisons, particularly if you develop new symptoms and have questionable findings on an electrocardiogram or chest X-ray at a later time.

When your test results are complete, your physician will discuss them with you. If the initial tests suggest some type of abnormality, your physician may recommend further testing.

Understanding the Specialties

Your primary care physician should provide you with general health care on a regular basis. However, at times your personal physician may be uncertain about a diagnosis or about the best treatment for your symptoms. In such circumstances, you, your physician, or both of you may want a second opinion, a situation that does not necessarily reflect on your physician's competence.

Consulting another physician, one with special training, is appropriate in the following circumstances:

1. If you have a rare disease or an unusual manifestation of a common disease

2. If you need a special procedure or operation

3. If you are not responding to therapy

4. If your disease is progressing especially rapidly or new complications are developing

Your physician, you, or your insurance

company may request the second opinion. Many insurance companies now insist on second opinions before they will agree to pay for certain procedures.

A wide variety of specialists are experts in particular organ systems and diseases. Often, areas of expertise overlap. For instance, if you have been diagnosed as having lung cancer, you may see a lung (pulmonary) specialist, a cancer specialist (oncologist), a radiotherapist (who will supervise radiation therapy), and a thoracic surgeon. All are medical doctors.

Do not be surprised if different physicians recommend slightly different treatments. Remember, medicine is not an exact science. Different physicians—each highly qualified and experienced—may favor different choices from among the therapies available for the same disease. All treatments may be reasonable, but each will have advantages and disadvantages. So keep in mind that a specialist's opinion is just an opinion. Your primary care physician can help you determine which treatment is best for you.

Finding a specialist for your disease can be as simple as obtaining the names of several physicians from your personal physician and making an appointment with one of them; often your physician or the nurse will contact the specialist, brief the second physician about your case, and schedule an appointment for you. Or you can locate a specialist on your own, much the same as you would look for a primary care physician (see Your Personal Physician, page 1245). If you live in a rural area or have an especially rare or complex medical problem, you may have to go to a major teaching hospital to find an appropriate specialist.

Before you see the specialist, put together a short list of your questions. The specialist is likely to ask you about your medical history again and may repeat some of the tests you have already undergone. Nevertheless, make sure that a copy of your medical records reaches the specialist. And feel free to ask how much the consultation will cost. For a listing of the various specialties and subspecialties, see page 1242.

Reasonable Expectations From Medical Care

What can you reasonably expect from medical care? The answer to that question is complicated and subjective. A range of factors, including your health at any given moment and your experience with medicine, affects your hopes, worries, and health concerns. To further complicate matters, the rapidly escalating cost of health care raises questions about how much you are willing—or able—to pay for health care.

People are living longer, mainly because science has conquered many acute and infectious diseases that once struck people down at a relatively early age. In recent years, mortality rates for most cancers have not changed dramatically, but death rates have declined for many common causes of death, including heart disease, stroke, diabetes, and peptic ulcer. The infant death rate, on average, has also declined—although there remains a significant difference in death rates for infants of mothers with little or no prenatal care and

poor access to the health care system.

Developments in medical research have enabled us to accurately predict, detect, diagnose, and treat countless diseases. As people live longer, chronic diseases occupy more of your physician's time. An increased emphasis on preventive medicine is spurring lifestyle changes by Americans which also may result in lower disease and death rates.

Remember that, despite remarkable advances, modern medicine does not have all the answers. However, an effective partnership with your physician can relieve many medical concerns and discomforts. We can prevent or more effectively treat many diseases that caused early death years ago. We can diagnose many serious disorders earlier, when treatments are much more effective. And, for incurable disorders, we have increasingly more effective means of relieving pain and of prolonging or ensuring a better quality of life.

Health Care Facilities

The American health care system offers health care to its medical consumers in many settings. Most health care takes place in the outpatient or office setting or in the hospital.

Most hospitals are general or comprehensive, although many will lack some services such as neurologic surgery or emergency room care. In addition, some specialized hospitals offer only a limited category of services. For example, some hospitals restrict care and operations to diseases of the eye, orthopedics, obstetrics, or other specialties.

Recently, more types of facilities serve health consumers. These facilities are a response to experimentation with new means of delivering health care and cutting costs.

This section describes various types of health care facilities other than hospitals. We discuss specialized facilities such as mental health centers, nursing homes, hospices, hospital outpatient departments, office practices, freestanding emergency centers, neighborhood health centers, and rehabilitation centers.

Office-Based Practices

The three main types of office-based medical practice are solo practice, group practice, and health maintenance organization (HMO). In solo practice, a physician works alone rather than with partners or in a clinic. Some general practitioners, internists, and other specialists practice privately. A nurse or assistant may help your physician with the workload. When you are under the care of a physician in solo practice, he or she is on call for emergency advice 24 hours a day. When your physician is on vacation or ill, he or she will provide you with the name of someone to consult if necessary during the interim.

A group practice can include two or more physicians. They share the 24-hour-a-day care burden as well as the office and personnel expenses. In addition, it is helpful when your physician can consult with a colleague about some cases. For you, the patient, the main difference between group practice and single-physician practice is that you may already know the replacement physician when yours is on vacation or sick. Some groups include various specialists, another advantage if you need them. Larger groups also may have clinical support facilities such as on-site laboratories.

The bill for care in solo or group practices is paid by conventional medical insurance, Medicare or Medicaid, or the patients themselves.

The HMO is another type of group practice (see Health Maintenance Organizations, page 1267).

If you need hospital care, a solo, group-practice, or HMO physician will send you to the hospital with which he or she is affiliated.

Hospital Outpatient Departments

Hospital outpatient departments offer health services by appointment or on a walk-in basis. Services can include the full range of the hospital's facilities and staff—physicians, nurses, laboratories, operating rooms, recovery rooms—but you leave the same day that you come in, without occupying a hospital bed overnight.

Recently, the proportion of hospital services offered on an outpatient basis has increased greatly. Physicians routinely perform many operations that recently involved a hospital stay—such as hernia repair, breast biopsy, cataract removal, and operations on children—on an outpatient basis.

The main advantage (to you, your insurer, or both) of outpatient care is lower cost. Another is that you can spend any recovery period necessary (from an operation, for example) in your own home.

Freestanding Emergency Centers

Freestanding emergency centers (sometimes called "urgicenters" because they treat urgent cases) are like a hospital's emergency room without the hospital attached. Freestanding emergency centers do not have the extensive resources of a hospital emergency room. They generally are private, profit-making facilities and may not provide the level of follow-up attention that a hospital or your physician would provide.

Freestanding emergency centers provide

treatment on a drop-in basis, like hospital emergency rooms, but typically with shorter waits. They usually restrict care to minor emergencies that do not require hospitalization, such as closing and suturing wounds or treating a high fever.

Many medical procedures performed in freestanding emergency centers could easily be done in your physician's office or clinic, but these centers are open for more hours (some never close) and do not require an appointment. The care at these centers generally costs more than care in a physician's office or clinic, but less than in a hospital emergency room.

Freestanding emergency centers vary in the quality of care they provide. Therefore, before using one (and, if possible, before an emergency), ask your physician for an opinion concerning the quality of care and whether the center can transfer severely ill or injured patients to a hospital when necessary.

Neighborhood and Primary Health Care Centers

A neighborhood health care center or primary health care center offers clinical care by appointment or on a drop-in basis. These government-supported centers, which originated in the 1960s, provide medical care in either rural or urban areas that do not have enough (or any) physicians and hospitals. Payment is by Medicaid, Medicare, conventional insurance, or directly by the person needing care (sometimes on a sliding-fee scale based on ability to pay). Some centers offer care to migrant farm workers as well as to residents of the area.

The services offered by neighborhood or primary health care centers vary, depending on the size of the facility and other types of health care services that the area offers. In general, they offer the kinds of medical care and procedures commonly available in a clinic or hospital outpatient department. Unfortunately, many of the centers closed in recent years for lack of funding.

Nursing Homes

Nursing homes offer care and supervision for people requiring help with such daily activities as eating, dressing, bathing, or toileting. Most nursing homes also offer ongoing skilled nursing and medical attention. Residents are typically elderly.

Admission to a nursing home is no longer considered the "last stop." Now, your physician may recommend a stay in a nursing home during your recovery from a stroke, hip fracture, or illness. And with the increasing emphasis on shorter hospital stays for medical or surgical problems, nursing homes can be a "transition" to the next level of care. People often leave nursing homes to return to independent living arrangements.

There are two main types of nursing homes: skilled-care homes and intermediate-care homes. A skilled-care home offers 24-hour nursing services as well as restorative, physical, occupational, and other therapies. An intermediate-care home offers fewer of these intensive nursing and rehabilitative services. Both types of homes provide supervision and help with daily activities. Most nursing homes are or are becoming skilled-care homes.

Most nursing homes are for-profit businesses. These homes should provide as pleasant an atmosphere as possible for their occupants (see Selecting a Good Home, page 247).

A hospital discharge planner, private care manager, or social worker may recommend nursing homes that do not have prohibitively long waiting lists and can advise you on financing nursing home care. Medicare, Medicaid, private health insurance, the Veterans Administration, trade unions, or fraternal organizations may offer financial assistance.

If you do not require constant or extensive care and help, a nursing home may not be the place to go. The various alternative forms of care available if you need just a little help or nursing attention include home care (see page 1319), adult day care, day hospitals, and medical day care. Other options include retirement communities and special housing designed for elderly people. Before you decide on a nursing home, see When Is a Nursing Home Appropriate? (page 247).

Hospices

A hospice program provides care for people who are terminally ill and for their families. Some hospices are small, independent programs, and others are part of a hospital. The hospice movement began in Europe and has recently expanded in this country.

Hospices are based on the philosophy that if you have no medical hope of recovery, you should be as comfortable as possible. If you are terminally ill, a hospital's normal routine, with its busy atmosphere, numerous interruptions, and focus on getting better, is probably irrelevant and disturbing.

A hospice addresses the two biggest fears that most dying people have—the fear of pain and the fear of being alone. The hospice staff administers appropriate pain relief, provides nursing care, and offers plenty of reassurance. The staff and your family see to it that you are not alone during this last and important phase of your life.

You must request admission to a hospice program. Your physician can assist you with this process. Sometimes hospice care is provided at home, unless you become too ill; care then may continue in an institution. Ideally, you will have the same caregivers in both settings.

After your death, caregivers in your hospice program also may help your family manage their bereavement.

Medicare and other types of insurance provide coverage for some hospice care (see page 1264).

Mental Health Facilities

You can receive mental health services in various settings. Services may begin with your primary care physician, who can evaluate, may treat, or who may refer you to a specialist. In a sudden crisis situation, use the hospital emergency room. For problems that require less-immediate attention, you or your primary physician can gain access to psychiatrists and psychologists in three main settings.

The first is in a private, office-based practice. The cost of visiting a psychiatrist or psychologist in private practice can be high, but sometimes insurance may cover part of the cost.

The second setting is the community-based mental health clinic, with a staff of mental health professionals. Community-based centers generally receive some type of government support. It will cost you less than visiting a professional in private practice. Some clinics set your fee on a sliding scale based on your ability to pay.

Ideally, community-based centers devote a portion of their efforts to caring for and supervising mentally ill persons living in group homes. The introduction of antipsychotic medications in the past few decades has enabled state mental hospitals to dismiss many people to live in communities. In addition, states have abandoned many such hospitals in the interest of economy. Unfortunately, group homes cannot care for some people who are severely disabled. If people fail to take the prescribed antipsychotic medication, their condition may deteriorate, and they may become homeless.

The third major place where you can find psychiatrists and psychologists is a hospital-run mental health clinic or outpatient department. Not all hospitals provide outpatient mental health services.

Some mental and emotional problems require long-term care that is possible only within a residential institution. Every state and many large cities and counties have some type of residential mental health facility. Usually, your physician must recommend your admission to a residential facility and your family must consent.

The quality of care in residential institutions varies greatly. Some are overwhelmed with more patients than the staff can reasonably care for and the facilities can handle. Visit a facility before you try to admit someone, and if anything about it disturbs you, discuss alternatives with your physician.

Private residential mental health facilities, if available, tend to offer a better staff-to-patient ratio. They may have a waiting list, and they tend to be substantially more expensive.

Homes are available for mentally retarded and mentally ill people. These facilities provide a safe learning environment, personal care, activities, and social interaction. They focus on providing skills that promote independence, such as community involvement and social skills. Most residents participate in supervised employment.

The trained staff work under the direction and supervision of registered nurses, dietitians, psychologists, physical therapists, occupational therapists, and speech therapists.

Many adult care centers and nursing homes also admit patients with mental problems.

For people with long-term but minor mental health problems, home care may be a viable alternative to residence in a group home (see Home Health Care, page 1322).

Maternal and Child Care

Many community health centers have maternal and child care programs that provide care both before and after your baby is born. Funding for these programs comes from federal and other government sources, and thus the care may be provided without charge to you if your income is below a specified level.

Care should begin early, during your second month of pregnancy, and should continue at regular intervals through the remainder of your pregnancy. We cannot overemphasize the importance of sound nutrition and good health habits during the prenatal period. Prenatal medical care and good nutrition greatly decrease the infant mortality rate as well as problems associated with pregnancy and childbirth. The result is a healthier baby and mother (see Concerns During Pregnancy, page 175).

The infant, and later the child, should continue to receive appropriate medical attention, including immunizations, nutrition counseling, and help with health problems that arise.

Rehabilitation Centers

The focus of rehabilitation is on your regaining some or all of the physical abilities that you lose through injury, illness, or disease.

For example, if you are a runner and injure an Achilles tendon, physical therapy with ultrasound may help speed the tendon's natural healing process and your ability to return to running. The physical therapist also can recommend specific exercises to help avoid the problem's recurrence.

If you have a stroke, physical and occupational therapy help restore use of muscles affected by the stroke, and speech therapy may help restore lost speech capacity if the stroke affected your brain's speech center.

Services

Various specialized types of therapists provide rehabilitation care. Generally, if you need rehabilitation, your physician will refer you to a therapist who may also monitor the course of your recovery.

Physical therapists help restore your use of muscles and parts of your body with heat, cold, massage, whirlpool baths, ultrasound, and other techniques as well as restorative exercises. Occupational therapists help to restore your ability to carry out daily functions, including adjusting to disabilities, (using devices such as wheelchairs) and modifying your home environment. Speech therapists use special techniques to help correct speech disorders or restore speech you lose through a stroke or other injury. Inhalation therapists use respirators and other breathing aids to help restore or support your breathing capacity. Audiologists help diagnose hearing loss and recommend aids for hearing. Registered dietitians provide advice on your diet to recover from, or avoid, particular types of problems. Physiatrists and other physicians coordinate the efforts of other members of the team. Usually, team members periodically hold conferences (often once a week) to discuss your progress and make decisions regarding your care.

Settings

You can obtain rehabilitation services in various settings. Many hospitals offer rehabilitation services on an outpatient basis. Rehabilitation services may or may not be separated within the hospital into a specific department, but most hospitals are good sources for therapists who can help with your rehabilitation.

You can also find sports medicine clinics, freestanding or as departments of hospitals, across the country. The physicians and therapists at such clinics help not only injured athletes but also other people who need to regain or improve the use of limbs and muscles.

Skilled-care nursing homes frequently provide physical and occupational therapy and sometimes other forms of therapy such as speech therapy. If you have had a stroke or serious illness, your physician may recommend that you spend some time recovering at a nursing home before you return to your home. During such a stay, you and your medical team can focus on your rehabilitation, if the nursing home offers skilled medical care rather than merely custodial care. Evaluate nursing homes (see Nursing Homes, page 1255) and their ability to provide rehabilitation services before selecting one.

You also can find physical therapists, occupational therapists, speech therapists, and other types of therapists in clinical practice, in private office-based practice, and in some health maintenance organizations.

Therapists can make home visits if you

cannot leave your home conveniently. Many community-based as well as profit-making home health service agencies offer rehabilitation therapy (see Home Health Care, page 1322).

How do you find a therapist if you need one? If you are hospitalized, the medical team in the hospital—in particular, the dismissal planner—advises you on follow-up therapy for rehabilitation. If you have not been hospitalized but believe you need rehabilitation therapy, seek your physician's opinion and recommendations on where you can obtain the care you need.

If you need rehabilitation, many organizations will provide advice and help. These include Rehabilitation International, the National Rehabilitation Association, the Easter Seal Society, the National Amputation Foundation, the Disabled American Veterans Association, and numerous organizations concerned with specific types of disabilities and illnesses (such as blindness, hearing impairment, cancer, and arthritis).

Within limits, many types of insurance cover some therapy for rehabilitation purposes.

Your Hospital Stay

Suppose your physician has decided to admit you to the hospital. Going to a hospital 150 years ago was strictly a last-resort measure. Today, however, a hospital stay is rarely a final event.

In the hospital, skilled teams of physicians, nurses, technicians, therapists, dietitians, and support staff work together to provide care for you in a setting of high-technology medical equipment that can perform a vast array of medical tests and procedures. Still, staying at a hospital can be a frightening prospect—it means that you are sick enough, or need a procedure that is serious enough, to require a stay in the highly sophisticated environment of a hospital.

Entering the Hospital

What should you bring with you? You do not need to bring much—clothing for the trip home, slippers, reading or other material to pass the time, a minimal amount of cash, and basic toiletries. Also, bring a form of identification, insurance information, any medical records, any medications you take, and whatever else your physician suggests you may need. The hospital will supply you with a hospital gown (you may want your own pajamas), meals, and most of the other services you require.

Once you get to the hospital, your first stop will probably be the admitting office. You will meet with an admitting officer to review your medical history, financial information, insurance forms, and the hospital's fees and to obtain a room assignment.

Many hospitals provide you with a plastic card they use for billing purposes. They will place an identification bracelet on your

---

Bedside Communication: 10 Questions for Your Physician

If you must be hospitalized, ask your physician the questions listed here. They will help communication and enhance your satisfaction with your care.

1. What do my symptoms mean?

2. Do the medications have any side effects?

3. What is this test for?

4. What risks does my treatment involve?

5. Do I have any options other than the treatment you've prescribed?

6. How do the benefits of my treatment compare with the risks?

7. What emotional reactions should I expect from my illness?

8. How long will I stay in the hospital?

9. Do I need to limit my activities at home?

10. What symptoms warrant a call to you once I return home?

wrist. The bracelet lists your name, age, hospital identification number, any allergies you have, and perhaps other information. It is important to wear this bracelet throughout your stay.

If you enter the hospital as an emergency patient, the entry procedure may be somewhat different. An admitting officer probably will obtain the necessary information from a family member or, if you are well enough, will visit you in your room.

During Your Stay

After you are admitted, you will be escorted to your room. You will meet members of the nursing staff who are responsible for your daily care. If you have questions during your hospital stay, contact your nurse or physician.

If you are unhappy with some aspect of your care, discuss the situation with your nurse or physician. If you are not satisfied that your complaint is resolved, check to see if the hospital has a patient representative or advocate. These people help clear up such problems.

Every hospital has specific routines and policies regarding visiting hours, patient meals, services, and other practical aspects of day-to-day life in the hospital. Usually, the policies, procedures, and services of hospitals are described in printed literature that you receive on admission. These policies may vary, depending on which unit of the hospital you are in. For instance, visiting hours will be different for an intensive care unit than for a general care unit.

Utilization review boards constantly review the reasons for admitting you to the hospital. If it appears that you could receive

---

Hospital Visits

Your hospital visit to a friend or relative may help move the person toward recovery. It's hard to do an exact analysis and produce statistical findings, but many physicians can tell you about visits from friends and relatives that proved to be strong medicine for some of their patients.

Unfortunately, many people feel ill at ease in a hospital setting and are reluctant to call on a recuperating patient. However, knowing a bit of the basic etiquette of the circumstances may make the situation seem easier and more natural for you.

The basic guidelines given here may help you feel more comfortable visiting a sick friend.

Phone Ahead
Let the person know you are coming. Hospitals have routines that should not be interrupted—tests or physician rounds in the mornings, for example. Perhaps your friend or relative relishes a nap at 3:00 p.m. or simply is not ready for vis-

itors. Set up a convenient time for both of you.

Do not interrupt at mealtime—it's difficult to eat comfortably and talk too.

Keep the Visit Brief
The person you are visiting is ill or recuperating, and resting is part of recovery. Talking and visiting may be draining, so 10 or 20 minutes is probably the ideal length for a visit.

Obey Hospital Regulations
Stop and check in at the nurses' station on the way to the person's room. Visit during scheduled visiting hours.

If you are bringing plants or foods, check with the nurses first; the person may be on a special diet and certain hospital units do not allow plants.

Do not interfere with care—if a nurse or physician arrives, ask whether you should leave.

Sit Down, Listen
Pull up a chair (do not sit on the

bed), and try to be at eye level with the person. Never probe about what is wrong or what is going to happen: let the patient tell you whatever he or she feels comfortable sharing. Keep your personal hospital experiences to yourself. Let the patient talk at his or her own pace and steer the conversation.

Express Your Feelings
Do not hesitate to express affection. You can express a lot with a sincere hug, pat on the arm, or squeeze of the hand.

Commonsense Rules
Even if it is not forbidden (it usually is), do not smoke. Never offer medications—that is the job of the physician and hospital personnel.

Check first before you bring children—they can often lift spirits, but they may not be welcome. If youngsters do accompany you, keep your visit short.

If you are ill, stay home: the person in the hospital does not need to be exposed to another ailment.

the care you need in a nonhospital setting, the board may refuse to authorize your admission, and you may be responsible for all or a portion of your hospital bill. Hospitals maintain a system of surveillance to help avoid these situations. Your physician will discuss this with you if the nurses and physicians responsible for surveillance think that your hospitalization is not justified or that you have remained in the hospital longer than necessary.

Leaving the Hospital

Once your physician determines that you are well enough to leave, the hospital will dismiss you. Before you leave, plan for your dismissal. This planning involves making arrangements for any home medical care you need, determining what follow-up appointments you should have, and teaching you how and when to take your medications and do other procedures relating to your illness.

Surgery

You and your physician have discussed your illness. You have reviewed all the alternative treatments and their risks and benefits and have decided that the best course of action involves surgery.

For most people, entering the hospital for an operation is a frightening prospect. However, taking an active role in your care and making sure you understand the process may go far toward relieving your anxieties. Understanding what is going on helps reduce the fear factor in most situations.

Be particular about whom you choose to perform your operation. Usually your primary physician will recommend a surgeon who has extensive experience with the operation you will undergo. Also, choose a good facility, one that is well equipped and adequately staffed. During the operation, a team of professionals is responsible for bringing you through it safely. This team consists of your surgeon, an anesthesiologist, nurses, and, sometimes, physicians-in-training who assist with the operation. Your personal physician may also attend. You need to feel confident that each member of your team is highly skilled.

Presurgical Evaluation

Before you have an operation, your physician should review your medical history in detail and uncover any medical conditions, reactions, or allergies that may affect the outcome. As much as possible, existing medical problems will be corrected before an operation. At most hospitals, the anesthesiologist will conduct his or her own evaluation and has the right to refuse to administer anesthetics if the risks outweigh the risks of no surgery.

Be sure to inform your physician of all medications you are taking, including diuretics, aspirin, and even seemingly insignificant over-the-counter medications. These are easy medications to overlook, because they are used so commonly; but they can have a significant effect on your recovery. For example, aspirin can interfere with your blood's ability to clot. This could increase the risk of excessive bleeding during or after your operation.

As part of your presurgical evaluation, you may undergo several laboratory tests, particularly if you are older than 40 years or have other medical problems. These tests may include electrocardiography to evaluate your heart and a chest X-ray. Often, you will have blood tests.

If you have a history of a diseased valve in your heart, you may receive antibiotics as a preventive measure before such operations as dental extractions, hemorrhoid operations, or other procedures that may involve tissue contact with bacteria (see Infective Endocarditis: Protection and Prevention, page 679).

Anesthesia

The development of anesthesia, which reduces or eliminates pain, has made it possible for physicians to practice modern surgery. Various anesthetic techniques are available.

In most instances, the anesthesiologist will visit you before your operation. He or she will review any pertinent medical problems with you and ask some additional questions. The anesthesiologist may ask you whether any family members have had adverse reactions to anesthetics, because there are several inherited disorders that can cause severe reactions to certain anesthetics.

The anesthesiologist will recommend a type of anesthetic on the basis of your physical and emotional status and the operation being done. For most operations it is imperative that you avoid solid foods within at least 8 to 10 hours before you receive an anesthetic. This precaution helps to prevent you from aspirating stomach contents into your lungs during or after the surgery. You will be given instructions as to when to stop taking clear liquids before the procedure.

The three main categories of anesthesia are local, regional, and general.

Local Anesthesia

Local anesthesia is generally the safest. The physician injects the anesthetic into your skin at or near the site of the operation. The injection numbs the area to pain and any other sensation, usually for a relatively short time.

You remain conscious during the operation. Local anesthesia is used for localized operations or for certain other more extensive operations in patients for whom general or regional anesthesia is too risky.

Sometimes if you have an operation while you are under local anesthesia, you will have a catheter in one of your veins (usually in an arm) so that you can receive fluids intravenously. This also provides access to give sedatives and other medications. You may receive a solution that helps prevent dehydration. For other types of anesthesia, you will always have an intravenous line.

Regional Anesthesia

Regional anesthesia is similar to local anesthesia in that you remain conscious. However, in most instances you are also sedated. There are four main types of regional anesthesia: spinal, epidural, caudal, and major nerve block.

The main advantages of regional anesthesia are that it is useful for more extensive procedures than local anesthesia and that it affects only the region of your body that is anesthetized. Therefore, it has little effect on other areas of your body, such as your heart, lungs, and brain. Regional anesthesia also can provide excellent relief of pain after your operation.

Spinal anesthesia may be used for operations below the navel, such as hernia repair; rectal, bladder, prostate, and pelvic operations; and operations on your legs and hips. Your physician injects the anesthetic through a small needle into the fluid-filled space surrounding your spinal cord. You receive the injection, which generally is painless, while you are lying on your side or sitting. Side effects, such as nausea and vomiting, breathing difficulties, light-headedness, or pain, occur infrequently during the operation and usually are easy to manage. After the operation, you may have some minor discomfort at the site of the injection. Headaches, which may last for several days, occur only rarely and can be treated effectively.

Physicians use epidural and caudal anesthesia for many of the same procedures for which spinal anesthesia is effective. An injection is given just outside the sac that contains your spinal fluid. The advantage of the technique is that the physician can place a small catheter to allow easy reinjection during longer operations and for treatment of pain for several days after the operation. Injections of narcotics (such as morphine) through these catheters provide excellent pain relief with few side effects.

Anesthesiologists use regional nerve blocks most commonly in your arms but can use them in almost any area of your body. Your physician places a small needle into the area through which a major nerve passes. Often you will feel a sensation of a mild electric shock in the region of this nerve, such as in your finger. This tells the anesthesiologist that the needle is in the correct place. The physician then injects a local anesthetic drug through this needle and the intended area of your body becomes numb and immobile. Side effects, such as minor pain during the operation, are rare, and persistent numb areas or tingling, lasting several days or longer, is extremely rare.

General Anesthesia

An anesthesiologist administers general anesthetics either by inhalation or by intravenous injection. These drugs circulate in your bloodstream to all areas of your body, including your brain, and cause loss of consciousness.

Because general anesthetics affect all areas

of your body, such as the heart and lungs, side effects are more common. However, most of these side effects are temporary and easily managed by the anesthesiologist or nurse anesthetist who is with you throughout your operation.

All general anesthetics depress your breathing and alter the function of your heart, and they may affect your blood pressure. To prevent problems, an anesthesiologist or nurse anesthetist continually monitors your blood pressure, heart rate and rhythm, breathing, and temperature. In most instances, a breathing tube is placed to ensure adequate breathing.

Other side effects that may occur after general anesthesia, such as nausea and vomiting, sore throat, muscle pain, and other aches and pains, usually are brief or easily treated. More serious complications, such as heart attack, kidney damage, and stroke, are extremely rare. They almost never occur in the absence of preexisting conditions. Proper screening and treatment of any serious medical illnesses in advance of the procedure, as well as careful monitoring of your vital signs during the operation, greatly reduce all of these risks.

Your Operation

In most cases, hospital staff will bring you to the operating room on a rolling table and then transfer and position you comfortably on the operating table. During the operation, your surgical team may rotate or tilt the table to provide complete access to the site of your operation.

Your medical team will take great care to avoid an infection. They will shave and disinfect the area involved in your surgery. You may have an initial shaving before you come to the operating room. All instruments and supplies are sterile, and the team wears gowns and masks. Team members monitor your blood pressure, heart rate, and breathing carefully throughout the operation and after the procedure. Intravenous fluids slowly enter a vein to maintain normal levels of water in your body and to serve as an avenue for giving drugs, if necessary, during your operation. If you are going to have a general anesthetic, either intravenously or by inhalation, the anesthetist provides for your respiratory needs.

Postoperative Recovery

After your operation, you will stay in the recovery room until you wake up and your vital signs are stable. It is important that hospital staff closely monitor you throughout your recovery period. Specially trained personnel will be with you during your postoperative recovery and will pay special attention to adjustment of medication, pain control, and your respiratory effort.

After some major operations, such as complicated neurologic or cardiac procedures, you will be moved to an intensive care unit (ICU). This area has complex monitoring equipment, mechanical devices to assist breathing, and resuscitation equipment, all maintained by a highly trained staff of physicians and nurses. You will receive fluids and blood through an intravenous tube in your arm. If you had surgery on your intestines, you probably will have a tube exiting from your nose to drain intestinal secretions and swallowed air. The tube is removed as soon as your intestines resume their normal functions.

Once you have recovered sufficiently and no longer require the close monitoring and sophisticated life-support systems of the ICU, you will move to a general nursing unit. The staff will encourage you to do deep-breathing exercises and to walk, both of which assist in your recovery. Besides providing for your care, your nurse also will educate you on any special care you must have after you leave the hospital. Finally, when you are well enough to go home, your physician will dismiss you.

After dismissal you probably will come back to the hospital or your physician's office for follow-up examinations. Your physician will advise you on when and how quickly you can resume normal activities.

Ambulatory Surgery

Ambulatory surgery, same-day surgery, and outpatient surgery are all terms for the same concept. Given the high cost of staying overnight at a hospital and increasing pressure to keep costs down, same-day surgery has become increasingly common.

Physicians perform many surgical procedures on an outpatient basis. Generally this means you come to the facility, have the operation, and leave on the same day. A family member or friend should come with you.

You can have same-day surgery at either an outpatient (or ambulatory) clinic within a hospital or at a freestanding "surgicenter." The advantage of an ambulatory center at a hospital is that it's easier to deal with complications if they arise, whereas a surgicenter may be some distance from a hospital.

Some of the surgical procedures done on an outpatient basis are simple hernia repairs, tissue biopsies, abortions, D and Cs (dilatation and curettage), vasectomies, and some cosmetic procedures.

The initial steps are not much different from those for inpatient procedures (see page 1260). A physician or nurse will take your medical history and tell you what to expect. Tell your physician or nurse if you have diabetes. An identification band may be placed on your wrist.

If you are having an anesthetic, you must not eat or drink anything for 8 to 10 hours before the operation, unless your physician instructs you otherwise. You will receive instructions on the use of clear liquids (water, apple juice, grape juice, or soft drinks—but no milk) before your operation.

In addition, if you receive an anesthetic, do not drive yourself home afterward. Have a family member or friend drive for you.

Leave your jewelry and valuables home or give them to the person accompanying you. Wear comfortable clothing that is easy to remove, and do not wear makeup or nail polish. If you wear contact lenses, hearing aids, glasses, false teeth, or a removable bridge, make sure you bring along a case to put them in. The center will provide you with a hospital gown and slippers.

After the operation, a nurse will give you instructions on how to care for yourself at home and arrange for future appointments if needed.

How to Pay Your Medical Bills

In the United States, physicians and hospitals usually bill for individual services rendered—so much per office visit, a certain amount per day of stay in a hospital, a certain fee for a particular laboratory test. This fee-for-service arrangement can become expensive, especially if you receive a lot of services—with an operation, for example. Most of us cannot pay extensive medical expenses on short notice.

If you have extensive health problems, medical expenses will be less of a burden for you if they are added together for everyone and then averaged out. This is the philosophy behind health maintenance organizations (HMOs; see page 1266), conventional group insurance policies (both of which are described below), and government-aided insurance supported by tax dollars. Within a large group, many people may need a few hundred dollars of medical care each year, some may not see a physician in 10 years, and an occasional person may incur hospital and surgical fees of a quarter million dollars. Care offered as a group plan would charge each of these people the same or nearly the same fee.

This type of averaged coverage for costs of medical care is offered to Americans in four main ways: conventional insurance, Medicare, Medicaid, and prepaid health plans. With Medicare and Medicaid, the government assumes a major share of the costs.

Medicare is available to all Americans age 65 or older, to some handicapped persons, and to certain persons with kidney disease who qualify under the end-stage renal disease program (see Chronic Kidney Failure, page 854). The federal government supports Medicare through taxes and covers some, but by no means all, medical care. You must first pay a deductible amount, which varies each time the government modifies Medicare provisions, before Medicare payment begins. For expenses Medicare covers, you receive reimbursement for a large percentage but not the total cost. You then must pay the remainder from your personal resources, through privately purchased major medical plans, or by Medicaid. Part A of Medicare is basic hospital insurance that starts automatically when you receive Social Security benefits at age 65, after you are entitled to Social Security disability benefits for 2 years, or if you have end-stage kidney disease. Part A pays on a sliding scale, depending on how much care you receive in the following categories: hospital care, skilled nursing care, skilled home health care, and hospice care for terminally ill people. Part B is a voluntary medical insurance that is deducted from your Social Security check. After you pay the $100 deductible, Medicare pays 80 percent of allowed charges from physicians and surgeons, outpatient hospital services, medically necessary home health care, and additional services such as tests, dressings, and physical therapy.

Medicaid is also a government-supported program administered by the state, with funds coming from both state and federal governments. The coverage is for people whose incomes fall below a particular level, regardless of their age. Persons with Medicaid coverage have few or no out-of-pocket expenses. The specific coverage of Medicaid varies a good deal from state to state, however, and both Medicare and Medicaid are subject to constant revision.

Your local Social Security Administration office can supply details on current Medicare coverage. For Medicaid information, contact your local welfare agency, social services agency, or Social Security Administration office.

Medicare Supplemental Insurance

Legislators designed Medicare in the 1960s to ensure that older Americans could receive medical care without the threat of exhausting their life savings. Medicare covers many, but not all, health care needs of older Americans. Yet even as Medicare benefits have grown, it's becoming increasingly difficult for recipients to pay their total medical bills. Even though Medicare covers "reasonable" costs for "necessary" care, it can leave you with significant expenses. In response, insurance companies designed policies that help bridge the gap between Medicare coverage and the amount of your medical bill.

If you want this supplemental insurance, shop carefully, because annual premiums vary widely in price. If you travel or live outside the United States, consider a supplemental policy with international coverage. But don't pay a premium for minor benefits like discount coupons for over-the-counter medications. Ask your financial adviser for an impartial opinion as you review costs and benefits of several policies. Do not believe anyone who claims that a Medicare supplement is a government-sponsored program. Federal and state governments don't sell or service supplemental insurance policies. Ask for proof that a company is licensed by your state to sell such insurance, and don't let a salesperson pressure you to make a decision.

If you do sign up for a policy, don't pay in cash. Write a check, money order, or bank draft payable to the insurance company, not to the agent or any other individual. Find out how easy it is to file claims and how quickly and accurately they're processed. A single comprehensive policy costs less and is easier to work with than several overlapping policies. Remember that if you want to switch policies, the new plan may impose a waiting period (usually 30 days) before coverage begins.

Check for "preexisting" exclusions, and don't let the advertising phrase "No medical exam required" mislead you. Many policies wait 6 months before covering conditions for which you received prior medical advice or treatment. Know your maximum benefits. Most policies limit payment for a condition or the number of days of care you receive. Some policies pay less than Medicare or nothing at all for treatment in a physician's office or hospital outpatient service.

Check your right to renew. Policies with automatic or guaranteed renewal offer extra protection. Although your premiums may rise, the company can't cancel your policy. Beware of companies that renew your coverage on an individual basis. Most policies cannot be canceled because of claims you make or disputes you may have with the company.

Remember that supplements fill only the gaps within Medicare's coverage, such as the charges you're responsible for beyond the Medicare allotment (called the "allowed charge") and a deductible that you pay before Medicare coverage begins. Medicare doesn't cover the full cost of medical services in several areas. Non-allowed services include dentures, hearing aids, or custodial nursing care, although it does cover some aspects of skilled nursing care and home health care. Be sure to complete the application carefully, or a company may deny coverage for any unlisted conditions or cancel your policy.

Additional options for closing the Medicare gap include HMOs, in which you pre-pay a fixed amount for your care. Other options exist through your employer. If you are retired, your former employer may provide Medicare supplemental insurance. If you work past age 65, your employer must provide you the same benefits that younger workers receive, making Medicare your secondary coverage. You may find religious and fraternal group insurance that is less costly than individual policies to members after age 65. And remember that insurance against specific diseases is not a Medicare supplement.

Diagnostic-Related Groups (DRGs)

For decades, hospitals have recorded patients' diagnoses, courses of treatment, and costs of hospitalization. To aid the federal government in its efforts to contain hospital costs, researchers carefully examined a multitude of hospital records. On the basis of their findings, they arrived at a series of formulas, called Diagnostic-Related Groups (DRGs), that attempt to determine the average length of time necessary to treat any illness you may have and the cost of treating that illness in the hospital. Medicare reimburses hospitals at a set rate for each DRG, regardless of how long you stay in the hospital.

If your physician determines that you need hospitalization and you are covered by Medicare, a hospital representative is notified of your diagnosis and proposed testing and treatment plan. The hospital representative (usually a physician or a nurse) determines whether the diagnosis and plan warrant hospitalization under the DRG guidelines. Medicare will deny payment for admissions judged unwarranted. Your hospital generally receives a lump-sum payment based on your diagnosis, regardless of your length of stay. The hospital cannot charge Medicare beneficiaries more than the amount Medicare allows for the admission or for any more hospital days than are "usual" for your condition. If your physician or the hospital fails to follow DRG guidelines, they may be penalized.

Use of DRGs by the Medicare system has decreased the number of days you're likely to stay in the hospital recuperating when acute care isn't absolutely necessary. You will have tests on an outpatient basis for which you may have previously been admitted to the hospital.

Physicians and administrators have con-

Was Your Hospital Stay Too Short?

If your last hospital stay seemed to be cut too short, you probably experienced a consequence of the Diagnostic-Related Groups (DRGs). Hospitals must now evaluate your need for continued 24-hour medical care on the basis of strict criteria. If you have questions or concerns about your hospitalization, contact your hospital's administrative office or DRG specialist, if one is available.

cerns about the DRG system. Although DRGs offer a proven way to help limit costs associated with health care, it's important that the system be flexible enough to ensure that you receive the most up-to-date care when you need it. Physicians are also concerned that the DRG system may penalize "teaching" hospitals, where patients with more complicated conditions frequently go, making it difficult to provide care within the DRG rates. And, because Medicare's hospital reimbursement rates for DRGs have not kept pace with inflation, hospitals are under extreme financial pressure and must "cost-shift" to private insurance companies to recoup the costs of providing service.

Conventional Health Insurance

Most large employers offer some type of health coverage plan for their employees. The choice is typically conventional group insurance, some form of preferred provider network, and joining a health maintenance organization (see page 1266). Depending on the employer and the coverage offered, you may pay for a portion of the insurance coverage as a payroll deduction, and the employer pays for the remainder as a "benefit." Some policies offer coverage for spouses and dependents at rates that are higher than coverage for a single person.

If you leave your job and want to continue that policy's coverage on your own, you can do that through your former employer if new coverage is unavailable elsewhere, although at greatly increased rates. It may be cheaper to obtain new coverage as a member of another group. Various organizations to which you belong may offer you group insurance policies if you are self-employed or unemployed.

In conventional insurance, the insurance company generally reimburses you for medical expenses arising from illness or injury, including costs of surgery, hospital stays, some prescriptions, and some types of rehabilitation therapy. Most plans also cover maternity expenses. There is generally a waiting period between the date when your coverage under the policy starts and when maternity benefits or coverage for treatment of long-term illnesses takes effect.

You may not always be reimbursed for visits to your physician for regular checkups. However, if you have a particular problem to discuss with your physician during your visit, your insurance company may cover it.

Before your reimbursement begins, there generally is a deductible amount that you must pay first ($200 or $500 per year are typical deductibles). Insurance often reimburses expenses beyond that in large part (such as 80 percent) rather than fully.

Insurers reimburse you for major expenses, such as surgery and hospital stays, up to a point that the insurer determines is usual, customary, and reasonable. For example, if your surgeon charges $3,000 for an operation, and the insurer determines that the maximum reasonable charge for that particular operation is $2,000, the insurer will pay the lesser amount or a percentage of it. You must pay the remaining amount privately or with additional insurance coverage such as major medical insurance. Employers and group plans frequently offer major medical insurance in addition to their basic policy. You also can purchase it privately.

You should understand one thing about conventional insurance: there is no "standard" insurance. Even insurance plans that have paid the hospital bills of generations of Americans, such as Blue Cross/Blue Shield, offer different levels or degrees of coverage according to the specific policy that the employer or other group asked the company to write. The coverage varies greatly.

Your policy will explain what your coverage includes. Many companies summarize the coverage in a pamphlet or summary plan description, but you will get more precise details by looking at the actual policy or contacting a knowledgeable representative of the insurance company or the insurance plan's administrator at your job.

All insurance policies have caps (limits) on what they will pay. For example, a policy might pay for up to 3 months of hospitalization (but no more), 100 home visits a year from a registered nurse, or $1,000,000 in total benefits over a lifetime. It is a good idea to determine what these caps are before disaster strikes. Insurance agents can advise you on additional insurance that you can purchase to cover costs above the specified caps.

You may not realize that your medical expenses may be covered by private insurance policies. Workers' compensation applies to injuries you sustain on your job, and automobile insurance may cover medical expenses arising from car accidents. Homeowners' policies often contain some liability coverage for visitors who are injured. Athletic associations frequently cover injuries sustained by athletes during sporting events.

Health Maintenance Organizations

Health maintenance organizations (HMOs) offer medical coverage in a way that is fundamentally different from conventional insurance. An HMO is a group of providers including physicians, nurses, and other health care specialists. You become a member of an HMO for a fixed monthly fee.

The system works this way. When you or a family member wants a regular medical checkup, you visit a physician associated with the HMO. If you become ill, sustain an injury, or need surgery, the HMO will provide and pay for the medical services you need, either at its own facilities or at an affiliated hospital. Emergency services are usually covered wherever they are provided, but there may be an emergency room out-of-pocket expense.

The idea behind HMOs is that they attempt to offer more complete medical coverage, ranging from preventive physical examinations that conventional insurance usually does not cover to serious problems that conventional insurance usually does cover.

Many employers will pay some or all of your cost of belonging to an HMO, as an alternative to paying for some or all of your coverage under a group insurance policy. It is also possible to join an HMO as an individual or as a member of an interest group (a union, professional association, or the like) to which you belong.

There are drawbacks to HMOs. At most HMOs, you can visit only the HMO's own physicians or those to whom the HMO refers you. Thus, you are not free to choose a physician who is not a member of the HMO. If you need treatment or hospitalization for a serious illness such as cancer, the HMO may not pay for the specialists or hospital that you would have chosen.

Keep in mind that, as with any health insurance program, the coverage is never truly total. HMO policies frequently contain exclusions (particular types of medical care that are not covered, such as vision and hearing problems) and caps (maximums on the amount that will be spent). Read descriptions of HMO coverage carefully or ask a knowledgeable HMO administrator.

However, there are advantages to HMO care. These include coverage that is usually more complete than with conventional insurance, ready access to a physician as well as other health care professionals at a location that has your medical history file on hand, and no financial penalty for visiting a physician for a minor problem or a checkup.

Preferred Provider Organizations

Preferred provider organizations (PPOs) represent yet another attempt to deliver medical care at a lower cost. A PPO is a network of physicians and hospitals designated by a particular self-insured business or insurance company to provide medical services. The physicians agree, in negotiations with the business or insurance company, to offer medical services at fees that are lower than the going rate in exchange for a steady supply of patients.

A PPO is not a health care organization like an HMO. It is merely a modification of the stipulations of some conventional insurance policies to favor certain physicians and hospitals. Your physicians submit bills for each service rendered, in the same way as

Utilization Review Boards

Just as an auditor goes over a firm's financial ledgers to look for irregularities, a utilization review board has the task of determining whether hospital care is justified. Since the introduction of Medicare in 1966, utilization review boards have sprung into existence across the country. Currently, the government, private insurance companies, and HMOs all use utilization review boards.

Utilization review boards focus on the care offered to you as an individual patient as well as on overall patterns of care over time. Case by case, the boards check to see that the services rendered were medically necessary and that they could be provided only in the hospital setting. Utilization review boards are alert to any evidence of abuse of hospital services.

Utilization review can take place at various times, such as before you enter the hospital, on admission, during dismissal planning, or before settling insurance claims. The second opinion program that your insurance policy may require before an operation is approved is a form of utilization review.

Sometimes utilization review boards monitor the quality as well as the costs of care. Quality and cost are not necessarily in conflict: poor-quality care may make additional, subsequent care necessary, subjecting you to repeated procedures and incurring added costs.

The operation of the utilization review boards lowers costs by shortening hospital stays but adds to the administrative costs of health care.

any physician in private practice does.

Some insurance companies and businesses offer you inducements to use a PPO physician. For example, the insurance company may pay the full cost of care rather than a percentage of the cost or may waive the deductible.

The intent is to lower costs—for the insurance company, the employer paying part of the bill for insurance coverage, and you, the insured person who pays the remainder. The utilization review board is a control mechanism incorporated into all PPOs.

Malpractice and Lawsuits

Malpractice occurs when your physician is negligent. In other words, your physician fails to exercise the care and professional skill usually exercised by the ordinary physician under similar circumstances, causing you injury.

The number of malpractice cases brought to court in the United States has increased in recent years. One result is that rates of malpractice insurance for physicians have spiraled upward. An expensive malpractice suit, settlement, or judgment increases the cost of malpractice insurance for all physicians, not just the one being sued. This is an important factor in the high cost of medical care today.

Bringing a Malpractice Suit

If you suffer long-term injury that you believe is due to negligence on the part of your physician, you have the right to bring a malpractice suit. If you die, a survivor can file a suit.

The first step in bringing a malpractice suit is consulting with an attorney, who will gather the medical records and history and then submit them to an expert physician to determine whether there is a valid case. Because the opinions of physicians may differ, the lawyer may get a second or even a third opinion. The physician's lawyer will usually obtain a statement from the patient describing the events that led to the damages.

Even after you have a lawyer and file suit, the outcome is by no means ensured. Many people settle out of court before a judge and jury ever hear one word of the evidence. Yet, despite headlines about enormous malpractice judgments, most cases that go to trial are resolved in favor of the physician.

If the defending physician feels strongly that he or she followed standard medical practices, the case may go to trial. In most cases, the court will require the plaintiff to call an expert witness (that is, another physician who is qualified to testify about the case).

A responsible lawyer will consider a case seriously and in detail before deciding whether to bring a claim. And a patient or surviving family of a patient should consider seriously whether they want to go through the trauma and expense of a court trial.

Better communication between you and your physician could prevent many malpractice suits. All too often, it is miscommunication between you and your physician or your incomplete understanding of the proceedings that results in the pain, expense, and other hardships associated with a malpractice suit.

Informed Consent

Few procedures or treatments in medicine are entirely risk-free. To make sure patients know of these risks beforehand, the medical profession adopted a rule called informed consent. This requires physicians to explain to you certain significant risks involved in a particular treatment. Depending on the situation, informed consent may require your physician to explain to you the diagnosis, the nature of the treatment, any risks or side effects involved, the consequences of not receiving the particular treatment, and any alternative treatments that are available. Sometimes you will be asked to sign a form stating that your physician gave you this information. It's a good idea for both you and your physician to include a member of your family in the discussion.

You have the ultimate control of your body and the right to refuse a particular treatment. However, if you have a psychiatric illness, if you are a minor, or if you are under the influence of medication, illegal drugs, or alcohol, you may not be able to give your consent.

Quackery

The ancestor of today's medical quack sold "life-saving elixirs" from the back of a horse-drawn wagon. The so-called magical potions of yesteryear may have faded into history, but medical quackery—defined as the promotion for a profit of medical schemes or remedies known to be useless or unproven—still is alive and well.

Each year, one of every four Americans will use quack medical treatments. We spend a total of at least $25 billion for these treatments. At best, the drugs, devices, and lifestyles are worthless; at worst, they lead to physical harm and even death.

So why is quackery so successful? Its success lies in the fact that it takes advantage of a basic human vulnerability—the yearning for a quick cure, whether for cancer, AIDS, arthritis, obesity, male baldness, or other human complaints, simple or serious. Oddly, medical quackery knows no educational boundaries; in fact, recent studies show that if you have a college education, you are actually more likely to use unproven treatments than are those with less formal education.

You are more likely to use fraudulent medical cures if you are isolated and lack the support of family and friends. You may have absolute faith in the written word, believing that if something is published, it must be true. Disease, or the fear of disease, may result in a frantic willingness to try anything. Because medicine has no cure for many problems, you may turn to quack remedies as a last hope.

Dangers of Quack Medicines

Instead of offering hope, fraudulent medical treatments can provide a threat. Besides being useless, sometimes they are actually dangerous. They may consist of medications that are harmless when taken in moderation but harmful when taken in doses prescribed by the quack. Another potential risk is that manufacturers of quack drugs often do not produce their products under the strict quality control measures required of legitimate drug companies. These drugs also may contain substances that, although safe by themselves, become harmful when mixed or taken in combination with certain foods, drink, or other drugs that you may be taking.

Quack medicines also can be dangerous to your financial well-being. The American Medical Association estimates that most victims of fraudulent medical treatments spend $500 to $1,000 annually. Of the estimated $25 billion spent on quack medicine each year, some $5 billion is spent on ineffective treatments for cancer. People older than 65, many on fixed incomes, spend at least $10 billion annually. Often those who spend the most on quack medicines can least afford to.

Another risk of quack remedies is that if you trust the miraculous promises of the quack, you may be losing precious time while you pursue a nonexistent cure instead of an actual one. Some cancers and other diseases respond well to medical therapy, especially if detected and treated early.

Quack medicine promoters may play on your emotions. You may think it's your fault that you have a disease or fail to recover. This feeling of guilt may affect your loved ones also, causing them to pursue quack

remedies as a cure. Finally, fraudulent promoters may try to generate anxiety to sell solutions to medical problems you do not really have.

One classic ploy used by purveyors of quackery is the testimonial. In fact, someone you know may even have tried a quack medicine and found it to work. However, this does not mean the medicine produced the "cure."

Many chronic or incurable diseases wax and wane. Symptoms sometimes will disappear, only to recur later. If you happen to be taking a quack medicine at a time when symptoms disappear, you may believe that the quack remedy was the cause. Also, the placebo effect is a well-documented medical phenomenon. Placebos have no active ingredients, but if you believe in the cure, scientists hypothesize that certain chemicals in your brain may be activated that actually cause your symptoms to diminish. However, quack medical treatments can make for expensive placebos.

Identifying Fraudulent Medical "Cures"

Identifying quack medicine is not always easy. Although most fraudulent promoters are simply looking for a quick buck or personal fame, some are sincere people who are misled. Some have fake degrees from mail-order "diploma mills." Others have actual degrees but no longer follow the high standards of their field. Others proclaim themselves to be "doctors"—even though their degrees are not in medicine but are in some other, often unrelated, field. Promoters often cloak their advertising in official-sounding, scientific language.

Watch out for promotions that describe medical treatments with adjectives such as "secret," "proven," "miracle," "foreign," "breakthrough," and "overnight." Also beware of glowing testimonials from happy patients. Quacks tend to claim they are fighting against a conspiracy of established physicians who are unwilling to acknowledge new treatments. They claim their products provide a complete cure for various problems without any side effects.

Quacks often make the offer sound safe, with money-back guarantees. Finally, they often exert pressure, claiming that this is a "limited offer," available for only a short time. Medical quackery can range from mail-order advertisements for "quick-loss" diets to sophisticated promotions you see on television.

Thwarting Quackery

Three federal institutions—the Food and Drug Administration, the Federal Trade Commission, and the U.S. Postal Service (which can take action against anyone who uses the mail to promote fraud)—work to prevent quackery. However, the large volume of fraudulent promotions overwhelms the small enforcement staffs and limited budgets designated for fighting quackery. And it often takes a long time to stop a determined quack.

The best ally you have in avoiding quackery, therefore, is yourself. If someone pressures you to spend money for a "quick cure," resist it. Beware of vague, dramatic claims. Find out exactly what the treatment is supposed to do and what evidence exists to prove it is effective. Ask your physician, pharmacist, or registered dietitian for advice, and ask if your medical insurance will help pay for the treatment. Get other, independent opinions from local health organizations or consumer groups.

Finally, remember that if it sounds too good to be true, it probably is.

Health Headlines

How can you sort notable, accurate health news from nonsense? It seems that every time you open a newspaper, turn on the TV, or read a magazine, you find contradictory or confusing health information. But there are ways you can sift through health news and glean the nuggets that really may make a difference in your life.

First, know the source of the information. Does the article or news report attribute the information to a respected publication, organization, or medical professional? Look beyond the statistics. When reports use statistics such as "a 30 percent increase" or phrases such as "higher risk," take a closer look at the exact numbers. Find out what they compare. If the report deals with a condition that occurs infrequently, "higher" may still mean "very low."

Scrutinize the results. Does the information show a direct cause and effect between two factors? Or is it merely an association? For example, someone could argue there's an association between matches and lung cancer, because matches light the tobacco that causes lung cancer. But lighted matches don't cause lung cancer. It typically takes years of consecutive studies to prove cause and effect. The results of one study usually aren't enough proof. Be quick to question, slow to change. If new information conflicts with conventional wisdom or how you're living, regard it warily. Results of one study usually don't warrant lifestyle changes. Always consider a study one small piece of the big picture. Most of the time, simply rely on your common sense. If health news makes you question your treatment, medication, or diet, ask your physician whether the report applies to you.

What Makes News?

The media often report the most interesting and intriguing news. This sometimes gives you a distorted view of health issues.

In 1992, the Center for Media and Public Affairs published a review of more than 1,000 news reports spanning 20 years. The review showed how scientists and the media (major television networks, news magazines, leading national newspapers) can have differing views on health issues.

Scientists agreed with the media's reporting of tobacco as one of the top three environmental risks of cancer. The scientists also identified diet and sunlight among the top three. But the media most often reported about food additives and chemicals—putting diet and sunlight 12th and 13th on their list.

Chapter 38

The Modern Pharmacy

Contents

Medications and You, 1272
Medication Guidelines, 1272
    Medications: Some Basic Dos and
    Don'ts, 1273
Medication Classifications, 1274
Administering Medication, 1274

Adverse Drug Reactions, 1275
    Your Home Medicine Chest, 1276
Food and Drug Interactions, 1277
Keep a Medicine Calendar, 1278
Your Medication Family Index, 1278

Medications and You

The modern pharmacy does not offer magical cures for all or even most diseases and disorders. However, today's medicine chest does contain an ever-increasing variety of tablets, capsules, lozenges, syrups, suppositories, powders, topical solutions, creams, gels, and other preparations. Many of these products do serve to relieve, calm, soothe, relax, and, yes, even help cure us of some of our aches, pains, and other complaints.

That is not to say, however, that all of these drugs are without risks. In fact, thousands of Americans are hospitalized each year because of adverse reactions to drugs or inappropriate use of medicines. In some cases, the problem is the result of a drug sensitivity or allergy; in others, especially the elderly, the interaction of multiple drugs can lead to uncomfortable or dangerous side effects. In still other instances, the problem results from known and predictable side effects of certain drugs, but such side effects occur infrequently enough that the efficacy of the drug outweighs such potential dangers (see Adverse Drug Reactions, page 1275).

Medication Guidelines

No matter what your age or condition, there are fundamental rules to follow when taking medications. These are described here.

Tell Your Physician About All Aspects of Your Health

Whether your physician is treating you for a cold or for cancer, he or she needs to know your medical history. In particular, inform your physician about any chronic disease you have (especially heart disease, hypertension, or glaucoma), whether you are taking prescription medications, and whether you are allergic to certain drugs. In such instances, a prescription that for most people is entirely safe could be life-threatening.

Advise your physician of any over-the-counter (OTC) drugs you are taking, including laxatives or antacids; aspirin or acetaminophen; cough, cold, or hay fever medicines; or mineral or vitamin supplements. Nonprescription drugs can be potent, and some can cause serious reactions when mixed with prescription drugs. For some people a proper dose of OTC drugs may need to be less than the amount recommended on the label, especially in elderly and very young people.

Tell your physician if you are or are planning to become pregnant. Numerous drugs can cross the placenta to your unborn fetus; some can result in birth defects. Your physician may change your medications if you are pregnant or breastfeeding to avoid affecting your fetus or child.

Tell your physician how much alcohol you consume. Be accurate: do not underestimate your consumption.

Follow Instructions

If your prescription says "Take three times a day after meals," do not take the medication twice or four times a day.

Anyone who uses more than the recommended dosage is in danger of an overdose. The "more is better" theory does not apply to drugs. If you miss a dose, do not double the next dose. If you have questions, call your pharmacist.

Read the label carefully. Make sure the instructions are clear. For example, if your prescription label directs you to take your medicine "four times a day," it could mean that you should take the medication with every meal and at bedtime. Or, it could mean that you should take it at precise 6-hour intervals around the clock. If you have questions, ask your physician or pharmacist to clarify exactly when you are to take your medicine.

If the bottle says a liquid preparation is to be shaken before you take it, shake it. If you are to take a drug before, with, or after a meal, do as instructed. Failure to follow such instructions can result in inadequate amounts of the drug in your body or unwanted side effects. Follow all instructions, not just those you find convenient.

Never increase the number of tablets or capsules you are taking without first consulting your physician; in the same way, do not stop taking a drug just because your symptoms seem to lessen. Take your medication for the entire length of time prescribed, even if symptoms for which you are using the drug have disappeared. Talk to your physician before discontinuing use of the drug.

If you are taking numerous medications on a daily basis, keep a record of what you take (see Keep a Medicine Calendar, page 1278).

Never take medications in the dark. This is a potentially dangerous practice. It can lead you to take the wrong medication or the wrong quantity. A missed dose of one drug or too much of another can be hazardous to your health.

Inform Your Physician of Side Effects
Discuss any side effects with your physician immediately. If the drug makes you nauseous, if you experience headache, dizziness, blurred vision, ringing in your ears, or shortness of breath, or if you develop hives, consult your physician immediately. It may be a reaction to the medication (see Side Effects, page 337).

Be Familiar With Your Medications
Remember names of medications you are taking. Read labels carefully. Ask your physician or pharmacist how the drug works. Make a special effort to understand their explanation.

Ask your physician or pharmacist about potential side effects, about any dietary restrictions you should follow, whether you should avoid alcohol while taking the drug, or if there are other concerns of which you should be aware. If you get a prescription refilled and it appears different from what you had been taking, ask your pharmacist why.

Have Prescriptions Filled at One Pharmacy
This can help you avoid problems with drug interactions. Your pharmacist is trained to know how drugs work and interact. By dispensing each of the prescription drugs you purchase, your pharmacist can help monitor the mix of medications, even if they are prescribed by different physicians. He or she also can advise you when to take your medicines and how to take or use them properly. Your pharmacist also may alert you to possible side effects and tell you what to do in case of an adverse reaction. Your pharmacist can also help you select OTC drugs that won't interfere with your prescription drugs.

Store and Dispose of Medications Properly
Keep medicines out of the reach of children; do not save old medications past their expiration date (see Your Home Medicine Chest, page 1276).

Do not share prescription medications with others: the purpose of controlling the

---

Medications: Some Basic Dos and Don'ts

Do store medicines properly. Most require a dry, secure place at room temperature and out of direct sunlight. Some drugs need refrigeration. A bathroom cabinet is a poor place to store medications because of temperature and moisture variations.

Do keep drugs out of a child's reach. When visiting people with children, make sure your purse doesn't contain pills.

Do discard outdated medications—prescription and over-the-counter. Old medicine can lose its potency and sometimes become toxic.

Don't lend or share prescription drugs. What helps you might harm others.

Don't fall into the more-is-better trap. Take the prescribed amount of your medicine. Taking more, or less, can result in serious problems.

Don't take a medication in the dark. You may take the wrong pill or the wrong amount.

---

availability of prescription drugs is to ensure that appropriate medications are given to people who can tolerate, need, and will be helped by them. A well-intentioned friend or relative with leftover pills is a poor substitute for a physician who is familiar with your medical history and general health.

Avoid Mixing Drugs and Alcohol
Use of many drugs along with alcohol can cause harmful interactions. In particular, sedatives and tranquilizers pose a danger. Discuss your consumption of alcohol with your physician. Ask whether there are risks of interactions with medicines prescribed for your use. (See Addiction to Tranquilizers, page 340, and Addiction to Analgesics, page 341.)

Keep Medicines in Original Containers
Keep all medications in their original, labeled prescription containers with caps on tightly. Never mix medications in the same container. Prescription containers are designed to protect medications from light and moisture. If you have a problem with the size of a container, ask your pharmacist to split the supply into multiple containers. If you have trouble opening a container with a safety cap, ask your pharmacist for a nonsafety cap for your medication.

Keep Phone Numbers Handy
Keep the names and telephone numbers of your physician, pharmacist, nearest poison control center, and rescue squad on or near your phone (see page 438).

Medication Classifications

Mastering the complexities of the modern pharmacy is not necessary for the average consumer. However, a working familiarity with basic facts about drugs you take can help you use today's medicines as safely and effectively as possible.

Over-the-Counter Versus Prescription Drugs

Over-the-counter (OTC) drugs are those you can purchase without a prescription. Examples are aspirin, many cough medicines and cold remedies, and innumerable other drugs offered to help you deal with ailments ranging from rashes to constipation to menstrual discomfort.

Prescription drugs may be purchased only from a licensed pharmacy and require a written prescription. They include a wide range of medications, from powerful painkillers to anticancer medications to familiar antibiotics such as penicillin.

Is It a Generic or a Brand Name Drug?

When a drug is discovered or produced in a laboratory, it is first given a generic name, a name designated by a committee of drug experts and approved by governmental agencies. This name identifies the drug as unique and distinguishes it from all others. The generic name is nonproprietary (that is, it is not owned by one company or individual).

When the drug is first approved to be sold to the public, it is usually given another name, a brand name, by the original manufacturer.

In general, the Food and Drug Administration (FDA) licenses a manufacturer to sell a given drug for a fixed period. During that time, the manufacturer owns the exclusive (proprietary) right to sell that medication and attempts to establish the drug in the marketplace under its own brand name.

Typically, the brand name of a drug is shorter and easier to pronounce and remember than the generic name. Examples are brand name drugs such as Librium, Tylenol, Valium, and Dilantin.

After the patent rights expire, the drug becomes public property. The initial manufacturer continues to own exclusive rights to the brand name it established, but other drug companies can manufacture and market the drug under its generic or their own brand name. Some drugs (for example, tetracycline

and prednisone) are sold primarily under generic names. More often, drugs are sold under both generic and various brand names.

One example is the pain reliever acetaminophen: it is sold as a generic drug (acetaminophen) and under the brand names Tylenol, Anacin-3, Datril, and Panadol, among others. To complicate matters further, both generic and brand name drugs may be sold as combination drugs, in which two or more medications are blended and sold under brand or generic names.

The expiration of the proprietary license to manufacture a drug means that other makers can enter the marketplace, and, in many cases, the resulting competition lowers the price of the drug.

Price is usually the principal advantage of purchasing a generic rather than a brand name drug. However, some physicians believe that manufacturing standards for generic drugs may be less than those of the brand name drugs originally produced. The FDA must approve the sale of all medications—brand name or generic.

Your physician, working with your pharmacist, is your best guide in selecting the right drug—and the right form (brand name or generic)—for your disorders. If cost is a concern and generic versions of a drug you are taking on a maintenance basis are available, discuss the matter with both your physician and your pharmacist.

By law, pharmacists may fill prescriptions with generic medicine instead of the brand name drug specified by the physician. But generic and brand name drugs are not always equally effective for everyone. Switching to a generic or another brand name medication could affect your health. For example, small variations in blood levels of drugs such as digoxin or warfarin can alter its effectiveness.

If you or your physician want to be sure the drug dispensed is a brand name product, be sure your physician includes the words "dispense as written" on the prescription form (or similar words, depending on your state's regulations).

Administering Medication

Oral Medications

When you swallow a capsule or tablet, it travels down your esophagus to your stomach and, eventually, to your intestines, where the medication is absorbed by your bloodstream and distributed throughout your body. That is the route it is supposed to take.

Occasionally, oral medications stick to the inner lining of the esophagus. If the medication dissolves there, it can cause irritation, sometimes leading to vomiting or chest pains.

Here are ways to help ensure that your medications make it to their destination:

- Drink at least half a glass of water when taking a pill. Sip a little water first to lubricate your esophagus. Swallow the pill with a mouthful of water; then drink the rest to wash the medication down.
- Stand up or sit up straight when taking a pill. Remain upright for at least a minute and a half after you swallow it.
- Consider an alternative form of your medicine. If you have problems swallowing medications, consult your physician or pharmacist. Your medication may be available in a form that is easier to swallow, such as a liquid.
- If a pill sticks in your esophagus, eat a soft, bulky food such as a banana. The bulk of the banana passing down your esophagus may carry the pill with it.

Other Medications
Other forms of delivery also can be difficult. Use the following techniques to simplify self-administration of ointments, drops, suppositories, and douches.

Eye Ointment
Wash your hands first—always. Then lie down or sit with your head tilted back. Draw the lower eyelid down, look upward, and place approximately a half-inch bead of the ointment along the inside margin of your eyelid. Do not touch your eye or eyelid with the tube. Close your eye, then gently remove any excess ointment from your eyelashes with a tissue.

Eyedrops
Position yourself in the same way as for administering eye ointment. Wash your hands, tilt your head back, draw the lower eyelid down, and look upward. Place the drops in the pocket formed between your lower eyelid and eye. Avoid putting drops directly on the cornea, and do not touch the dropper itself to your eye. Close your eye, then gently remove any excess solution from the eyelashes or lid with a tissue.

Nose Drops
Lie down or sit with your head tilted back. Check the tip of the dropper to be sure it is not chipped or cracked. Breathing through your mouth, place the prescribed number of drops in your nose. Do not touch the sides of your nasal openings with the dropper. Remain reclined or seated with your head tilted for several minutes so the medication can spread through your nasal cavity.

Ear Drops
Check the tip of the dropper to be sure it is not chipped or cracked. Tilt your head so that the affected ear is angled upward. Straighten the ear canal to receive the medicine by drawing your earlobe down and back. Then deliver the prescribed number of drops into your ear, avoiding touching your ear canal with the dropper.

Suppositories
For a rectal suppository, wear rubber or plastic gloves. If you have hemorrhoids, coat the suppository well with petroleum jelly. Lie on your side and insert the suppository, pointed end first, high into the rectum. Push the bottom of the suppository sideways to be sure that some portion of it touches the bowel wall. If you have trouble retaining the suppository, you may not have inserted it high enough. You also may find it helpful to hold your buttocks together for a short while after inserting the suppository.

Douches
Use a thoroughly cleaned and rinsed syringe (unless the douche is of the disposable type, in which case use each fresh syringe and bag only once). Using slightly warm (tepid) water, fill the bag with the solution. Administer the douche while lying or sitting. If lying, draw your knees up and raise your hips. Insert the syringe into the vagina. After douching, cleanse or dispose of the douching equipment.

Adverse Drug Reactions

Adverse drug reactions can occur for many reasons. Some are the result of an overdose: intentionally or accidentally, people may take too much of a drug and their systems react. Other reactions are the result of kidney or liver disease, which makes individuals more susceptible to certain kinds of drug toxicity.

Your Home Medicine Chest

Having a designated area—whether it is a medicine cabinet, beside your bed, or a corner of a kitchen cupboard—can help you keep medications you need to take organized and easy to find. A medicine chest also can help keep your medicines safely out of the reach of children.

Where Should It Be?

Most bathrooms have built-in medicine cabinets; yet bathing and showering areas, because of humidity produced by hot water, are less-than-perfect locations for storing drugs. Your refrigerator is also an inappropriate storage area for most drugs. A locked cabinet in your kitchen or bedroom may be an optimal place.

Be Concerned for Children

Regardless of location, your medicine cabinet should keep prescription and nonprescription drugs safely away from the reach of children. Even if visits from youngsters are rare, take care to keep drugs out of their reach. Also, buy childproof packages, especially if you have young children, grandchildren, or very young guests.

Be especially careful to properly store medications you take daily. Never take storage for granted.

Remember that it is easy to absent-mindedly leave medications on a kitchen counter or bedside table where a toddler may find their bright colors irresistible.

If you have drugs that must be refrigerated, put them on a high shelf that is well out of the reach of children.

Discard Outdated Drugs

Flush unused, outdated prescription drugs down the toilet. Medicine deteriorates over time. If you develop the same health problem you had several years ago, do not resume taking leftover medicine. Instead, consult your physician and get a new prescription.

Keep medicines in their original containers, otherwise you or members of your family may get confused. Taking the wrong medicines or inappropriate combinations of medicines can be dangerous. If the label gets separated from a medicine container and there is any doubt as to its contents, discard the medicine immediately.

What Should It Contain?

In addition to whatever prescription or over-the-counter drugs your physician recommends for your use,

there are other key items a well-equipped medicine chest should have on hand, such as the following:

- Pain relievers: aspirin or, for children, aspirin substitutes such as acetaminophen
- Syrup of ipecac: a liquid used to promote vomiting and used in certain kinds of poisoning emergencies (see Handling Poisoning Emergencies, page 438)—do not use unless so instructed by your physician or a Poison Control Center.
- Bandages: adhesive strip bandages, adhesive tape and sterile gauze pads, elastic bandages, and surgical bandages (Steri-Strips)
- Tools, including scissors to cut bandages and tweezers to remove splinters
- A thermometer (include a rectal-type thermometer if you have an infant)
- Absorbent cotton and rubbing alcohol
- Over-the-counter pharmaceuticals, including antidiarrheal medication, antacids, cough syrup, calamine or other mild lotion for itching, a sunscreen to prevent sunburn, and skin creams or lotions to treat sunburn.

Depending on several factors, including your body weight, health, and age, most drugs on the market are safe and are associated with only minor or rare potential complications. When prescribing a drug for your use, your physician may alert you to possible side effects. Your pharmacist, too, will counsel you on how to take the drug and also about its risks. In the case of over-the-counter drugs, the packaging in which the medications are sold frequently offers warnings regarding side effects.

In the case of many prescription drugs, a complete list of potential side effects can be frightening. However, few drugs on the market today produce significant side effects

in more than a small fraction of persons who take them. Elderly people are more likely to experience side effects (see Medication Misuse in the Elderly, page 340). Sometimes a side effect can be eliminated simply by reducing the dosage of another drug or by reorganizing the sequence in which you take medications.

Among the serious potential side effects are drug allergies, anaphylactic reactions, and the complications of multiple drug use.

Drug Allergy

Allergic reactions to most drugs are uncommon. Sometimes the effects of an adverse drug reaction are mistaken for a drug allergy.

Follow your physician's directions carefully when taking a medication. If unusual symptoms develop, consult your physician or pharmacist immediately.

Rash is the most common allergic drug reaction. More serious reactions may include wheezing and difficulty in breathing, an itching sensation over your entire body, and even shock (see Shock, page 441).

Penicillin and related drugs are responsible for many allergic reactions to drugs. The reactions range from mild rashes to hives to immediate anaphylaxis (see this page). Most people who develop reactions have minor rashes, and only those who are extremely sensitive have the more serious reaction of anaphylaxis.

If you know you are allergic to certain drugs—avoid them. This means alerting your physician or dentist to your sensitivity before treatment. People sensitive to aspirin should avoid all aspirin-containing drugs.

Wear a medical alert necklace or bracelet indicating your allergy, or carry a card that provides this information (see Drug Allergies, page 1050).

Anaphylaxis

Anaphylaxis is the most dangerous of allergic responses; it is also the least common.

An anaphylactic reaction may cause only generalized hives and intense itching, but a severe reaction can be life-threatening. The most characteristic symptom is a constriction of the passageways in the bronchial tree or throat or both which causes difficulty in breathing.

Shock—a sudden decrease of blood pressure that causes rapid pulse, weakness, paleness, mental confusion, nausea and vomiting, unconsciousness, and cardiovascular collapse—also may occur. Shock can cause death if not treated promptly.

In sensitive people, drugs such as penicillin, aspirin, insulin, and the contrast injection agents used in some X-ray studies can result in anaphylaxis in a matter of minutes or even seconds.

The standard treatment for anaphylaxis is an injection of epinephrine (adrenaline), which opens the airways and blood vessels. Cardiopulmonary resuscitation (CPR) and emergency tracheostomy (making an opening in the windpipe) sometimes have to be performed as lifesaving measures (see Anaphylaxis, page 444, and Cardiopulmonary Resuscitation, page 408).

Hazards of Multiple-Drug Use

A drug that is entirely safe when taken on its own can become a health hazard if taken in combination with another drug or several other drugs.

As you age, changes occur in your body that put you at greater risk for problems with medication. For example, the proportion of your body that is made up of water and lean muscle tissue decreases while the percentage of fat increases. Therefore, drugs that your body stores in fat tissue (called fat-soluble drugs) can accumulate to higher levels as you grow older. Also, as you age your liver and kidneys become less efficient at breaking down and eliminating drugs, so medications remain in your body longer. A buildup of drugs can result, with potentially dangerous side effects.

If you have several illnesses, each new symptom may result in a visit to your physician—and a new prescription. Too often, physicians give prescriptions without regard to medicines already being consumed. Beware of this.

With multiple drug use, it is hardly surprising that people often become confused and take too little or too much of one or more drugs, or experience unwanted side effects from drug interactions.

You may need assistance in following drug therapies, especially if you have multiple diseases that require the correct use of several medicines each day.

Review the schedule of all of your medicines with your physician or pharmacist, particularly if a new medicine is added, to determine whether the schedule can be simplified (see Keep a Medicine Calendar, page 1278).

Food and Drug Interactions

The drugs you take and the foods you eat are both processed and absorbed by your upper gastrointestinal tract. Thus, it should come as no surprise that certain foods and certain drugs, when taken in combination, can have results that differ from results you might experience if you were to consume the same substances on separate occasions.

Sometimes a combination can be beneficial. At other times, the interactions with food can be dangerous. In any case, your physician and pharmacist should anticipate such potential problems and give you specific instructions on how and when to take your drugs.

A few general guidelines and explanations also may help:

- Follow all instructions. Listen to your physician or pharmacist. Read the label too. If the instructions are to take your medication with a meal, do so.
- Drink at least half a glass of water when taking a medication. This helps ensure that the pill goes down. It also can aid absorption and may eliminate or decrease potential stomach irritation.
- Instructions to take a drug on an empty stomach mean you should take it at least 1 hour before or 2 to 3 hours after eating.
- In the absence of other instructions, take the drug at a time when you are most likely to remember to take it.
- Take the drug at the same time each day. If you vary your routine from one day to the next, the effects of the medication can change.
- Do not drink tea, coffee, or other hot beverages with your medications. Hot temperatures destroy the effectiveness of many drugs.
- Beware of alcohol interactions: if the medication is labeled (or your physician or pharmacist warns you) "Do not take with alcohol"—then do not. Alcohol has potentially lethal interactions when taken with certain prescription medications, but even some over-the-counter medications can make you especially drowsy when combined with alcoholic beverages.
- Never play pharmacist. Do not open, crush, or dissolve tablets or capsules without checking first with your physician or pharmacist. If you find a liquid medication difficult to take because of a disagreeable taste, mix it with juice or applesauce—but do not mix more than one dose at a time— and take all of it immediately. If the drug/food mixture is left around, someone else might take it.

Keep a Medicine Calendar

Ask your primary care physician or pharmacist to help you work out a medicine calendar. This is a master schedule of drugs you take and when they are to be taken.

If you have concerns or questions, take along all medicines you currently are using. This might include medicines prescribed by other physicians and over-the-counter medications you take for minor ailments (such as antacids; constipation remedies; cough syrups; hay fever, cold, and cough remedies; and even mineral and vitamin supplements).

Together with your physician or pharmacist, develop a medicine calendar by identifying each drug and assigning regular consumption times and dosages for each.

The effort required in preparing your calendar will help make your physician or pharmacist more aware of the drugs you take and may eliminate unnecessary drugs or reduce the frequency or dosage of others. As a result, you are less likely to experience unwanted drug interactions.

Your physician or pharmacist also may be able to simplify the drug-taking process: certain medicines can be taken together, perhaps just before or after meals. By consolidating and organizing the ritual of taking your medicines, your physician or pharmacist will ensure that the correct dose and timing are achieved to make the medication most effective.

Your Medication Family Index

Here are some of the categories into which most of the commonly prescribed medications are divided. Use this index in conjunction with the medication directory (see page 1281) to identify the nature and function of drugs you are taking.

Anabolic steroids: drugs closely related to natural hormones of the male and that mimic their effects. These drugs are used in treating various skeletal and growth disorders and certain types of anemia. Athletes sometimes use anabolic steroids to build up body tissue—a practice that is unhealthy, unwise, and illegal.

Analgesics: pain-relieving drugs. These drugs are generally divided into two categories: narcotic and nonnarcotic pain-relieving drugs. Narcotic analgesics, most of which are derived from opium, are used for relief of severe pain. Nonnarcotic analgesics are used to relieve mild pain. Some also reduce inflammation. See Anti-inflammatory agents.

Androgens: hormones that stimulate the production of male sexual characteristics.

Angiotensin-converting enzyme (ACE) inhibitors: drugs that block the formation of a natural body chemical and relax blood vessels, thereby reducing blood pressure. They are also used to treat congestive heart failure.

Antacids: drugs used for relief of symptoms of indigestion or disorders caused by excess acid. These medications work by neutralizing stomach acids.

Antialcoholic drugs: drugs used in the treatment of alcoholism. When alcohol is consumed in conjunction with antialcoholic drugs such as disulfiram, the result is flushing, headache, chest pain, nausea, weakness, and repeated vomiting.

Antianxiety agents: also called anxiolytics, sedatives, or tranquilizers, these drugs relax muscles, reduce tension, relieve anxiety, and may be used to treat insomnia. The largest family of antianxiety drugs is the benzodiazepines.

Antiarrhythmics: medications used to control unwanted variations in heart rhythms. Digitalis is one antiarrhythmic drug; certain recent varieties are classified as beta-adrenergic blockers or calcium channel blocking drugs. See Calcium channel blockers.

Antiasthmatics: drugs used in the treatment of asthma. These medications work by dilating (expanding) airways in the lungs.

Antibacterials: see Antibiotics.

Antibiotics: drugs used to fight bacterial infection. Penicillin is a naturally occurring variety, but synthetic antibiotics include cephalosporins.

Anticancer drugs: see Cytotoxic drugs.

Anticoagulants: drugs prescribed to prevent blood from clotting (some are called "blood thinners").

Anticonvulsants: drugs used to prevent seizures.

Antidepressants: mood-lifting drugs. The major categories of antidepressants are the tricyclics, selective serotonin reuptake inhibitors (SSRIs), and monoamine oxidase inhibitors (MAOIs).

Antidiabetic agents: drugs used in the treatment of diabetes. Antidiabetic drugs are used to restore the body's ability to use sugar normally. Insulin is one variety; it usually is used in people whose bodies produce little or no natural insulin. Insulin is administered by subcutaneous injections. Other antidiabetic drugs, called hypoglycemic drugs, are given orally.

Antidiarrheals: drugs used to relieve diarrhea.

Antiemetics: medications used to treat nausea and vomiting.

Antiepileptics: see Anticonvulsants.

Antifungals: drugs used to treat infections caused by fungi.

Antiglaucoma agents: medications used to treat glaucoma. These drugs act to reduce pressure in the eye.

Antihistamines: drugs used to treat allergies, asthma, nausea, motion sickness, nasal congestion, coughing, and itching.

Antihypertensives: medications prescribed to reduce high blood pressure (hypertension). Antihypertensives also are classified as belonging to one of several drug families according to the way they work. The subdivisions include drugs that increase the rate at which your body eliminates urine and salt (see Diuretics), drugs that block many of the effects of epinephrine (adrenaline) in your body (see Beta-adrenergic blockers), drugs that block the entry of calcium into the walls of your small arteries (see Calcium channel blockers), and drugs that block formation of a natural body chemical and dilate small arteries (see Angiotensin-converting enzyme inhibitors). The calcium channel blockers and the angiotensin-converting enzyme inhibitors both cause the walls of your small arteries to dilate.

Anti-infectives: drugs used to fight infection.

Anti-inflammatory agents: drugs used to reduce inflammation. Inflammation results in an increased blood flow, which in turn produces swelling, redness, pain, and heat. One of the body's defense mechanisms, inflammation occurs in response to infection, injury, and certain chronic diseases such as rheumatoid arthritis. Aspirin and corticosteroids are anti-inflammatory drugs.

Antiparkinsonians: drugs used to treat the trembling, rigidity, or other symptoms of Parkinson's disease.

Antipruritics: drugs used to reduce itching.

Antipsychotic agents: drugs used to treat a type of psychiatric disorder.

Antipyretics: fever-reducing drugs. These drugs, including aspirin and acetaminophen, directly affect the temperature-regulating center in the brain, the hypothalamus.

Antispasmodics: drugs used to relieve involuntary muscle spasms such as may occur in the gastrointestinal tract or urinary bladder.

Antivirals: drugs used to treat viral infections.

Anxiolytics: see Antianxiety agents.

Benzodiazepines: see Antianxiety agents.

Beta-adrenergic blockers: also known as beta blockers. They work by blocking the stimulating effect of epinephrine (adrenaline) on your heart. They also are effective for reducing blood pressure.

Bronchodilators: drugs that open (dilate) the main airways (bronchi) in your lungs. They are used primarily to treat asthma.

Calcium channel blockers: also known as calcium blockers. They function by blocking entry of the mineral calcium into your cells. They are effective for reducing blood pressure and in reducing the work of the heart.

Cholesterol-reducing agents: drugs used to lower blood cholesterol concentrations.

Corticosteroids: used principally as anti-inflammatory drugs (see Anti-inflammatory agents). Various corticosteroid drugs are used to treat arthritis, asthma, bursitis, certain skin diseases, adrenal gland insufficiency, thyroiditis, some cancers, and other disorders.

Cough suppressants: often called antitussives. They are used to suppress coughs.

Cytotoxic drugs: anticancer drugs. This is a broad category of drugs used to treat various cancers.

Decongestants: drugs used to relieve nasal congestion. They work by constricting blood vessels in your nose, which serves to reduce swelling. They are used to treat nasal swelling related to allergies and the common cold.

Digitalis preparations: a group of heart drugs. They are used to treat heart failure by stimulating the heart to increase the force of its contractions. They also are effective for treating atrial fibrillation, a heart rhythm abnormality.

Diuretics: also called water pills, these drugs increase the volume of urine and salt released by the kidneys. Most often, diuretics are used to treat hypertension and congestive heart failure.

Estrogen hormones: female sex hormones that stimulate and maintain female sex characteristics. Estrogens are used to treat menstrual and menopausal disorders and also are used as oral contraceptives.

Expectorants: drugs that stimulate the expulsion of mucus or phlegm from the lungs or throat. They often are one of several ingredients in cough medications.

Fever-reducing drugs: see Antipyretics.

Gout medications: drugs used to treat gouty arthritis. These drugs work to decrease the amount of uric acid in the body, either by limiting its production or by promoting its excretion.

Heart rhythm regulators: see Antiarrhythmics.

Histamine H$_2$ blockers: drugs used to treat ulcers and related disorders in which there is excess stomach acid. These medications work to inhibit the secretion of gastric acid.

Hypnotics: sleeping medications. Benzodiazepines are the most common type of hypnotic drug.

Hypoglycemics: see Antidiabetic agents.

Immunosuppressants: drugs that impair the workings of the body's immune system. They may be used to treat disorders such as rheumatoid arthritis, ulcerative colitis, and some cancers and to prevent the body's rejection of transplanted organs.

Laxatives: constipation drugs. A range of laxatives are available that work to increase the action (motility) of the intestines or to stimulate the addition of water to the stool to increase its bulk and ease of passage.

Male sex hormones: see Androgens.

Monoamine oxidase inhibitors (MAOIs): see Antidepressants.

Motility agents: Drugs used to increase the movement of food through the gastrointestinal tract.

Muscle relaxants: drugs used to relax muscles. They are used to treat muscle spasms associated with injury of muscles, bones, and joints.

Nitrates: heart drugs. They may increase blood flow through the coronary arteries and often are used in patients with angina.

Nonsteroidal anti-inflammatory drugs (NSAIDs): see Analgesics and Anti-inflammatory agents.

Penicillin: see Antibiotics.

Phenothiazines: drugs used for their antipsychotic effect. Occasionally they are used to control vomiting.

Salicylates: see Analgesics and Anti-inflammatory agents.

Sedatives: see Antianxiety agents and Hypnotics.

Sulfa drugs: see Antibiotics.

Tetracyclines: see Antibiotics.

Tranquilizers: see Antianxiety agents and Antipsychotic agents.

Vasodilators: heart drugs. These medications stimulate the arteries of the heart to enlarge (dilate). They often are used to treat angina pectoris or lower blood pressure.

Xanthines: drugs used to dilate bronchial passageways.

Chapter 39

Understanding Your Medications

Contents

This chapter contains a listing of common prescription and over-the-counter medications.

Dictionary of Common Medications

Thousands of medications are available in pharmacies from coast to coast. We discuss many of these preparations elsewhere in this book, generally in conjunction with specific diseases.

Scientists are continually at work developing new drugs. Pharmaceutical manufacturers constantly compete to be first in marketing effective new preparations. As a result, new products are released almost daily.

Because of this continuous advance in knowledge and the changing nature of the marketplace, a chapter such as this would require many hundreds of pages to be complete. Our purpose is more modest.

In these pages, you will find entries for medications we know to be commonly prescribed or recommended by physicians nationwide. We include generic and brand names. The list is not comprehensive and does not represent an endorsement of any product or company.

A generic name is the name given to a drug when it is first developed. This name identifies the medication as being unique from all others. In this chapter, generic names are shown in **boldface** type. In *italic* type, we list some of the brand names

under which certain generic medications are sold. The brand name is the proprietary name assigned to the drug by each manufacturer (see Medication Classifications, page 1274). Unless the drug listed is identified as a nonprescription (over-the-counter) drug by the letters OTC, it is available only by prescription.

In Your Medication Family Index (see page 1278), we list principal categories into which most of the commonly prescribed medications are divided. For example, you will find ANALGESIC, the category (painkiller) in which acetaminophen belongs. Acetaminophen is the generic name. Many brands are available.

In taking any medication, it is important to follow instructions and to take precautions regarding proper dosage, storage, and administration of the drug (see The Modern Pharmacy, page 1271, for specific advice). Be alert for side effects. Side effects usually are minor but sometimes can be serious. Should such symptoms as dizziness, nausea, abdominal discomfort, or other untoward reactions occur, consult your physician or pharmacist immediately (see Adverse Drug Reactions, page 1275).

Accupril: Brand name of the antihypertensive quinapril.

Acetaminophen With Codeine: A compound analgesic.

Acetaminophen: An analgesic-antipyretic. OTC.

Acetylsalicylic Acid: The chemical name for aspirin. OTC.

Actifed: Brand name of the combination containing triprolidine and pseudoephedrine, for treatment of allergy or colds. OTC.

Acyclovir: An antiviral.

Adalat: Brand name of nifedipine, a heart medication.

Advil: Brand name of the analgesic and anti-inflammatory ibuprofen 200 mg. OTC.

Afrin: Brand name of the nasal decongestant oxymetazoline. OTC.

Albuterol: A bronchodilator.

Aleve: Brand name of the analgesic naproxen sodium 220 mg. OTC.

Alprazolam: An antianxiety drug.

Altace: Brand name of the antihypertensive ramipril.

Aluminum and Magnesium Hydroxide: An antacid product. OTC.

Ambien: Brand name of the hypnotic and sedative zolpidem.

Amitriptyline: An antidepressant.

Amlodipine: An antihypertensive.

Amoxicillin: An antibiotic.

Amoxicillin/Clavulanic Acid: An antibiotic combination product.

Amoxil: Brand name of the antibiotic amoxicillin.

Ansaid: Brand name of the analgesic and anti-inflammatory flurbiprofen.

Aspirin: An analgesic, antipyretic, and anti-inflammatory. Also known as acetylsalicylic acid. OTC.

Astemizole: An antihistamine.

Atenolol: An antihypertensive and heart drug.

Ativan: Brand name of the antianxiety drug lorazepam.

Atrovent: Brand name of the bronchodilator ipratropium.

Attapulgite: An antidiarrheal. OTC.

Augmentin: Brand name of the antibiotic combination amoxicillin/clavulanic acid.

Axid: Brand name of the histamine-blocker anti-ulcer drug nizatidine.

Azithromycin: An antibiotic.

Azmacort: Brand name of the corticosteroid drug triamcinolone.

Bactroban: Brand name for the topical antibiotic mupirocin.

Beclomethasone: A corticosteroid.

Beconase AQ: Brand name of the corticosteroid beclomethasone.

Benadryl: Brand name of the antihistamine diphenhydramine. OTC.

Benazepril: An antihypertensive.

Benzoyl Peroxide: An antiacne drug. OTC.

Biaxin: Brand name of the antibiotic clarithromycin.

Bisacodyl: A laxative. OTC.

Brompheniramine: An antihistamine. OTC.

Brompheniramine/Phenylpropanolamine: A combination drug used in treating allergies and colds. OTC.

Bumetanide: A diuretic and antihypertensive.

Bumex: Brand name of the diuretic and antihypertensive bumetanide.

BuSpar: Brand name of the antianxiety drug buspirone.

Buspirone: An antianxiety drug.

Butalbital/Codeine: A migraine analgesic combination.

Calan: Brand name of the antihypertensive verapamil.

Capoten: Brand name of the antihypertensive and heart drug captopril.

Captopril: An antihypertensive and heart drug.

Carafate: Brand name of sucralfate, which protects the lining of the stomach.

Carbamazepine: An anticonvulsant.

Cardizem: Brand name of the heart drug diltiazem.

Cardura: Brand name of the heart drug doxazosin.

Ceclor: Brand name of the antibiotic cefaclor.

Cefaclor: An antibiotic.

Cefadroxil: An antibiotic.

Cefixime: An antibiotic.

Cefprozil: An antibiotic.

Ceftin: Brand name of the antibiotic cefuroxime.

Cefuroxime: An antibiotic.

Cefzil: Brand name of the antibiotic cefprozil.

Cephalexin: An antibiotic.

Children's Motrin: Brand name of the pediatric analgesic and anti-inflammatory ibuprofen.

Chlorhexidine: A drug used to treat gingivitis.

Chlorpheniramine: An antihistamine. OTC.

Chlor-Trimeton: Brand name of the antihistamine chlorpheniramine. OTC.

Cimetidine: A histamine-blocker anti-ulcer drug.

Cipro: Brand name of the antibiotic ciprofloxacin.

Ciprofloxacin: An antibiotic.

Cisapride: A drug that prevents nighttime heartburn.

Clarithromycin: An antibiotic.

Claritin: Brand name of the antihistamine loratidine.

Clearasil: Brand name of the antiacne drug benzoyl peroxide. OTC.

Clemastine/Phenylpropanolamine: An allergy or cold treatment. OTC.

Clonazepam: An anticonvulsant.

Clotrimazole/Betamethasone: An antifungal combination.

Colace: Brand name of the stool softener docusate. OTC.

Compazine: Brand name of the antinausea drug prochlorperazine.

Coumadin: Brand name of the anticoagulant warfarin.

Cromolyn: An antiallergy drug.

Cyclobenzaprine: An antispasmodic.

Darvocet-N: Brand name of the analgesic combination propoxyphene and acetaminophen.

Daypro: Brand name of the analgesic and anti-inflammatory oxaprozin.

Delsym: Brand name of dextromethorphan, used in treating coughs associated with the common cold. OTC.

Deltasone: Brand name of the corticosteroid prednisone.

Demulen: Brand name of the oral contraceptive combination ethynodiol/ethinyl estradiol.

Depakote: Brand name of the anticonvulsant divalproex.

Desogen: Brand name of the oral contraceptive combination desogestrel/ethinyl estradiol.

Desogestrel/Ethinyl Estradiol: An oral contraceptive combination.

Dexbrompheniramine/Pseudoephedrine: A combination used in treating allergies and colds. OTC.

Dextromethorphan: A cough suppressant. OTC.

Dextromethorphan/Guaifenesin: An expectorant and cough suppressant combination. OTC.

DiaβBeta: Brand name of the hypoglycemic (antidiabetic) drug glyburide.

Diazepam: An antianxiety drug.

Diclofenac: An analgesic and anti-inflammatory drug.

Dicyclomine: An antispasmodic.

Digoxin: A heart drug.

Dilacor XR: Brand name of the heart drug diltiazem.

Dilantin: Brand name of the anticonvulsant phenytoin.

Diltiazem: A heart drug.

Dimetapp: Brand name of the antihistamine and decongestant combination brompheniramine and phenylpropanolamine. OTC.

Diphenhydramine: An antihistamine. OTC.

Divalproex: An anticonvulsant.

Docusate: A stool softener. OTC.

Doxazosin: A heart drug.

Doxepin: An antidepressant.

Drixoral: Brand name of the combination containing dexbrompheniramine and pseudoephedrine, for the treatment of allergy or cold. OTC.

Dulcolax: Brand name of the laxative bisacodyl. OTC.

Duricef: Brand name of the antibiotic cefadroxil.

Dyazide: Brand name of the antihypertensive and diuretic combination triamterene/hydrochlorothiazide.

DynaCirc: Brand name of the heart drug isradipine.

EES: Brand name of the antibiotic erythromycin.

Elavil: Brand name of the antidepressant amitriptyline.

Elocon: Brand name of the topical corticosteroid mometasone.

E-Mycin: Brand name of the antibiotic erythromycin.

Enalapril: An antihypertensive and heart drug.

Endep: Brand name of the antidepressant amitriptyline.

Entex LA: Brand name of the decongestant and expectorant combination phenylpropanolamine/guaifenesin.

Ery-Tab: Brand name of the antibiotic erythromycin.

Erythromycin: An antibiotic.

Estrace: Brand name of the estrogen hormone estradiol.

Estraderm: Brand name of the topical preparation of estrogen (applied as a patch).

Estrogen: Generic name for female sex hormone.

Estropipate: An estrogen hormone.

Ethinyl Estradiol/Levonorgestrel: An oral contraceptive combination.

Ethynodiol/Ethinyl Estradiol: An oral contraceptive combination.

Etodolac: An analgesic and anti-inflammatory.

Famotidine: A histamine-blocker ulcer drug.

Ferrous Sulfate: An iron supplement.

Fiorinal With Codeine: Brand name of the migraine analgesic combination butalbital, codeine, caffeine, and aspirin.

Floxin: Brand name of the antibiotic ofloxacin.

Fluoxetine: An antidepressant.

Flurbiprofen: An analgesic and anti-inflammatory.

Furosemide: A diuretic.

Gemfibrozil: An antilipidemic (cholesterol-reducing).

Glipizide: A hypoglycemic (antidiabetic) drug.

Glucotrol: Brand name of the hypoglycemic (antidiabetic) drug glipizide.

Glyburide: A hypoglycemic (antidiabetic) drug.

Glynase: Brand name of the hypoglycemic (antidiabetic) drug glyburide.

Guaifenesin: An expectorant. OTC.

Hismanal: Brand name of the antihistamine astemizole.

Hydrochlorothiazide: An antihypertensive and diuretic.

Hydrocodone With Acetaminophen: A compound analgesic.

Hydrocortisone Cream: A corticosteroid used topically. OTC for up to 1 percent. Prescription at higher strengths.

Hytrin: Brand name of the antihypertensive terazosin.

Ibuprofen: An analgesic and anti-inflammatory. Strength of 200 mg is OTC.

Imitrex: Brand name of sumatriptan, used to treat migraine attacks.

Imodium: Brand name of the antidiarrheal loperamide. OTC for tablets and liquid preparations.

Indapamide: An antihypertensive and diuretic.

Inderal: Brand name of the antiarrhythmia heart drug propranolol.

Intal: Brand name of the antiallergy drug cromolyn.

Ipratropium: A bronchodilator.

Isosorbide Dinitrate: A heart (antianginal) drug.

K-Dur: Brand name of a potassium supplement.

Kaopectate: Brand name of the antidiarrheal attapulgite. OTC.

Ketoconazole: An antifungal.

Ketorolac: An analgesic and anti-inflammatory.

Klonopin: Brand name of the anticonvulsant drug clonazepam.

Klor-Con: Brand name of a potassium supplement.

Lanoxin: Brand name of the heart drug digoxin.

Lasix: Brand name of the diuretic and antihypertensive furosemide.

Levodopa/Carbidopa: An antiparkinsonism combination drug.

Levonorgestrel/Ethinyl Estradiol: An oral contraceptive combination.

Levothyroxine Sodium: Thyroid hormone.

Levoxine: Brand name of the thyroid hormone levothyroxine sodium.

Lisinopril: An antihypertensive and heart drug

Lodine: Brand name of the analgesic and anti-inflammatory etodolac.

Loestrin: Brand name of the oral contraceptive combination norethindrone/ethinyl estradiol.

Lo/Ovral: Brand name of the oral contraceptive combination drug norgestrel/ethinyl estradiol.

Loperamide: An antidiarrheal. OTC for tablets and liquid preparations.

Lopressor: Brand name of the antihypertensive and heart drug metoprolol.

Lorabid: Brand name of the antibiotic loracarbef.

Loracarbef: An antibiotic.

Loratidine: An antihistamine.

Lorazepam: An antianxiety drug.

Lortab: Brand name of the analgesic combination hydrocodone/acetaminophen.

Lotensin: Brand name of the antihypertensive benazepril.

Lotrisone: Brand name of the topical antifungal combination clotrimazole and betamethasone.

Lovastatin: An antilipidemic (cholesterol-reducing).

Lozol: Brand name of the antihypertensive and diuretic indapamide.

Maalox: Brand name of an antacid product containing aluminum and magnesium hydroxide. OTC.

Macrobid: Brand name of the antibiotic nitrofurantoin macrocrystals.

Magnesium Hydroxide: An antacid. OTC.

Maxzide: Brand name of the antihypertensive and diuretic combination triamterene/hydrochlorothiazide.

Meclizine: An antinausea and motion sickness drug. OTC (in some preparations).

Medroxyprogesterone: Progesterone hormone.

Metamucil: Brand name of the bulk-forming laxative psyllium. OTC.

Methylphenidate: An amphetamine-like drug.

Metoprolol: An antihypertensive and heart drug.

Mevacor: Brand name of the antilipidemic (cholesterol-reducing) drug lovastatin.

Micro-K: Brand name of a potassium supplement.

Micronase: Brand name of the hypoglycemic (antidiabetic) drug glyburide.

Milk of Magnesia: An antacid, magnesium hydroxide. OTC.

Mometasone: A topical corticosteroid.

Mupirocin: An external antibiotic.

Mylanta: Brand name of an antacid and anti-gas product containing aluminum and magnesium hydroxide plus simethicone. OTC.

Nabumetone: An analgesic and anti-inflammatory.

Naldecon: Brand name of the allergy and cold combination drug phenylephrine/phenylpropanolamine/phenyltoloxamine/chlorpheniramine. OTC.

Naprosyn: Brand name of the analgesic and anti-inflammatory naproxen.

Naproxen: An analgesic and anti-inflammatory drug.

Nasacort: Brand name of the corticosteroid triamcinolone.

Nifedipine: A heart drug.

Nitro-Dur: Brand name of the heart drug nitroglycerin.

Nitrofurantoin Macrocrystals: An antibiotic.

Nitroglycerin: A heart (antianginal) drug.

Nitrostat: Brand name of the heart drug nitroglycerin.

Nizatidine: A histamine-blocker anti-ulcer drug.

Nizoral: Brand name of the antifungal ketoconazole.

Nolvadex: Brand name of the anticancer drug tamoxifen.

Norethindrone/Ethinyl Estradiol: A contraceptive combination drug.

Norgestrel/Ethinyl Estradiol: A contraceptive combination drug.

Nortriptyline: An antidepressant.

Norvasc: Brand name of the antihypertensive amlodipine.

Nystatin: An antifungal.

Ofloxacin: An antibiotic.

Ogen: Brand name of the estrogen hormone estropipate.

Omeprazole: An acid-secretion blocker anti-ulcer drug.

Orasone: Brand name of the corticosteroid prednisone.

Ortho-Cept: Brand name of the oral contraceptive combination desogestrel/ethinyl estradiol.

Ortho-Novum: Brand name of the oral contraceptive combination norethindrone/ethinyl estradiol.

Oxaprozin: An analgesic and anti-inflammatory.

Oxy 5 & 10: Brand name of the antiacne drug benzoyl peroxide. OTC.

Oxycodone/Acetaminophen: An analgesic combination.

Oxymetazoline: A nasal decongestant drug.

Paroxetine: An antidepressant.

Paxil: Brand name of the antidepressant paroxetine.

PCE: Brand name of the antibiotic erythromycin.

Penicillin V: An antibiotic.

Pentoxifylline: A drug used to improve blood flow.

Pepcid: Brand name of the histamine-blocker anti-ulcer drug famotidine.

Peridex: Brand name of the drug chlorhexidine, used to treat gingivitis.

Phenergan: Brand name of the antihistamine promethazine.

Phenylephrine/Phenylpropanolamine/Phenyltoloxamine/Chlorpheniramine: A combination used in treating allergies and colds. OTC.

Phenylpropanolamine/Guaifenesin: A decongestant and expectorant combination.

Phenytoin: An anticonvulsant.

Potassium Chloride: A potassium supplement.

Pravachol: Brand name of the antilipidemic (cholesterol-reducing) pravastatin.

Pravastatin: An antilipidemic (cholesterol-reducing).

Prednisone: A corticosteroid.

Premarin: Brand name of the oral or vaginal female hormone estrogen.

Prilosec: Brand name of the acid-secretion blocker anti-ulcer drug omeprazole.

Prinivil: Brand name of the antihypertensive and heart drug lisinopril.

Procardia: Brand name of the heart drug nifedipine.

Prochlorperazine: An antinausea drug.

Promethazine: An antihistamine.

Propoxyphene With Acetaminophen: A compound analgesic drug.

Propranolol: An antiarrhythmia heart drug.

Propulsid: Brand name of the drug cisapride that prevents nighttime heartburn.

Proventil: Brand name of the bronchodilator albuterol.

Provera: Brand name of the progesterone hormone medroxyprogesterone.

Prozac: Brand name of the antidepressant fluoxetine.

Pseudoephedrine: A decongestant. OTC.

Psyllium: A bulk-forming laxative. OTC.

Quinapril: An antihypertensive.

Ramipril: An antihypertensive.

Ranitidine: A histamine-blocker anti-ulcer drug.

Relafen: Brand name of the analgesic and anti-inflammatory nabumetone.

Retin-A: Brand name of the antiacne drug tretinoin.

Ritalin: Brand name of the amphetamine-like drug methylphenidate.

Robitussin: Brand name of the expectorant guaifenesin. OTC.

Robitussin-DM: Brand name of the expectorant and cough suppressant combination dextromethorphan/guaifenesin. OTC.

Roxicet: Brand name of the analgesic combination oxycodone and acetaminophen.

Seldane: Brand name of the antihistamine drug terfenadine.

Seldane-D: Brand name of the antihistamine/decongestant combination terfenadine/pseudoephedrine.

Selenium: A dandruff treatment. OTC.

Selsun Blue: Brand name of the dandruff treatment selenium. OTC.

Sertraline: An antidepressant.

Simethicone: An antigas (antiflatulent) product. OTC.

Simvastatin: An antilipidemic (cholesterol-reducing).

Sinemet: Brand name of the antiparkinsonism combination levodopa/carbidopa.

Slo-Bid: Brand name of the bronchodilator theophylline.

Sucralfate: A drug that has protective properties for the lining of the stomach.

Sudafed: Brand name of the decongestant pseudoephedrine. OTC.

Sumatriptan: A drug used to treat migraine attacks.

Sumycin: Brand name of the antibiotic tetracycline.

Suprax: Brand name of the antibiotic cefixime.

Synthroid: Brand name of the thyroid hormone levothyroxine sodium.

Tagamet: Brand name of the histamine-blocker anti-ulcer drug cimetidine.

Tamoxifen: An anticancer drug.

Tavist-D: Brand name of the allergy and cold combination treatment clemastine/phenylpropanolamine. OTC.

Tegretol: Brand name of the anticonvulsant drug carbamazepine.

Tenormin: Brand name of the antihypertensive and heart drug atenolol.

Terazol: Brand name of the antifungal terconazole.

Terazosin: An antihypertensive.

Terconazole: An antifungal.

Terfenadine: An antihistamine.

Terfenadine/Pseudoephedrine: An antihistamine/decongestant.

Tetracycline: An antibiotic.

Theo-Dur: Brand name of the bronchodilator theophylline.

Theophylline: A bronchodilator.

Thyroid: Thyroid hormone.

Timolol: An antihypertensive and antiglaucoma drug.

Timoptic: Brand name of the antihypertensive and antiglaucoma drug timolol.

Tinactin: Brand name of the topical antifungal agent tolnaftate. OTC.

Tolnaftate: A topical antifungal. OTC.

Toradol: Brand name of the analgesic and anti-inflammatory ketorolac.

Trental: Brand name of pentoxifylline, used to improve blood flow.

Tretinoin: An antiacne drug.

Triamcinolone: A corticosteroid.

Triamterene/Hydrochlorothiazide: An antihypertensive and diuretic combination.

Tri-Levlen: Brand name of the oral contraceptive combination levonorgestrel/ethinyl estradiol.

Trimethoprim/Sulfamethoxazole: An antibiotic combination.

Trimox: Brand name of the antibiotic amoxicillin.

Triphasil: Brand name of the oral contraceptive combination levonorgestrel/ ethinyl estradiol.

Triprolidine/Pseudoephedrine: An allergy or cold treatment. OTC.

Tylenol With Codeine: Brand name of the analgesic combination acetaminophen with codeine.

Valium: Brand name of the antianxiety drug diazepam.

Vancenase AQ: Brand name of the corticosteroid beclomethasone.

Vanceril: Brand name of the corticosteroid beclomethasone.

Vasotec: Brand name of the antihypertensive and heart drug enalapril.

Veetids: Brand name of the drug penicillin V.

Ventolin: Brand name of the drug albuterol.

Verapamil: An antihypertensive.

Verelan: Brand name of the antihypertensive verapamil.

Vicodin: Brand name of the analgesic combination hydrocodone/acetaminophen.

Voltaren: Brand name of the analgesic and anti-inflammatory diclofenac.

Warfarin: An anticoagulant.

Xanax: Brand name of the antianxiety drug alprazolam.

Zantac: Brand name of the histamine blocker anti-ulcer drug ranitidine.

Zestril: Brand name of the antihypertensive and heart drug lisinopril.

Zithromax: Brand name of the antibiotic azithromycin.

Zocor: Brand name of the antilipidemic (cholesterol-reducing) drug simvastatin.

Zoloft: Brand name of the antidepressant sertraline.

Zolpidem: A hypnotic and sedative.

Zovirax: Brand name of the antiviral acyclovir.

Chapter 40

Cancer

Contents

Understanding Cancer, 1290

The Biology of Cancer, 1291
A Genetic Disease, 1291
Cancer Diagnosis, 1293
  Cancer Warning Signs, 1293
Cancer Screening, 1293
  Cancer Prevention, 1294
Cancer Clusters in Populations, 1296

Living With Cancer, 1296
Cancer Treatment, 1297
New Methods to Fight Cancer, 1299
Choosing a Physician and a Place for
  Cancer Treatment, 1299

Cancer Facilities, 1300
Cancer Centers Supported by the National
  Cancer Institute, 1301
Nutrition and Cancer, 1303
Cancer Pain, 1303

Cancer Rehabilitation, 1304
Hospices, 1305
  Coping With Survival, 1306

Cancer in Children, 1307
How to Deal With Cancer in Your
  Child, 1307

Understanding Cancer

It is estimated that more than 10 million Americans alive today have had cancer, and 7 million were diagnosed with cancer 5 or more years ago. Most of these 7 million can be considered cured.

There are more than 100 different types of cancer. Some cancers can affect just one organ, and others are more generalized. In each of its types, however, cancer always consists of uncontrolled growth and spread of abnormal cells.

Many people have a fear of cancer, perhaps because to them it is an incurable disease. The facts do not support this idea. About 544,000 Americans, or 4 of every 10 people who are found to have cancer this year, will be cured (cured is defined as being free of any evidence of the disease for 5 years or more). These cured individuals will have the same life expectancy as others of the same age and sex who have never had cancer. In addition, they can anticipate leading meaningful and productive lives.

Despite such impressive statistics, cancer remains a serious disease. Annually, cancer is diagnosed in almost 1.4 million persons (excluding non-melanoma skin cancer). Cancer causes more than 500,000 deaths each year, and nearly one of every four deaths in the United States is from cancer.

Why cancer develops in some people who are exposed to potentially cancer-causing agents but not in others is not fully known. But we do know that most cancers develop slowly. It may be 5 to 40 years after exposure to a cancer-causing agent before there is any evidence of the disease. Cancer of the lung, for example, may not appear until 25 years or more after sustained exposure to tobacco smoke. This long delay between exposure and development of the disease may partly explain why so many people ignore the warnings associated with smoking (see Tobacco, page 315).

Cancer Incidence and Deaths by Site and Sex—1995 Estimates

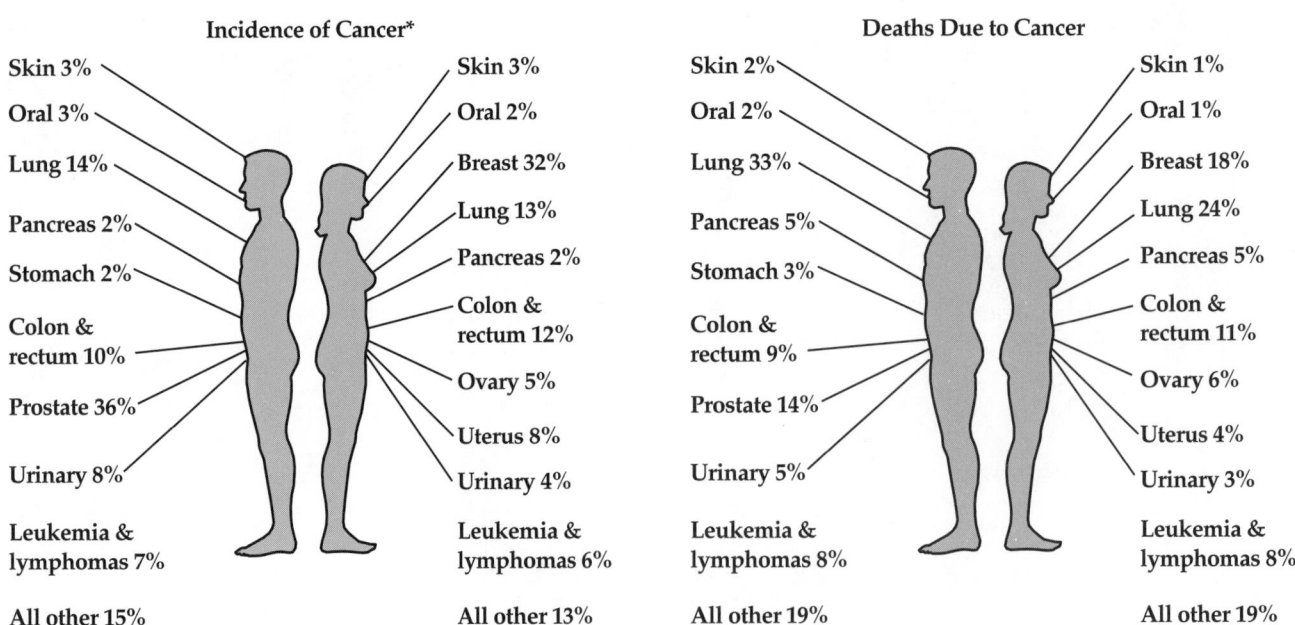

Incidence of Cancer*

Skin 3%
Oral 3%
Lung 14%
Pancreas 2%
Stomach 2%
Colon & rectum 10%
Prostate 36%
Urinary 8%
Leukemia & lymphomas 7%
All other 15%

Skin 3%
Oral 2%
Breast 32%
Lung 13%
Pancreas 2%
Colon & rectum 12%
Ovary 5%
Uterus 8%
Urinary 4%
Leukemia & lymphomas 6%
All other 13%

Deaths Due to Cancer

Skin 2%
Oral 2%
Lung 33%
Pancreas 5%
Stomach 3%
Colon & rectum 9%
Prostate 14%
Urinary 5%
Leukemia & lymphomas 8%
All other 19%

Skin 1%
Oral 1%
Breast 18%
Lung 24%
Pancreas 5%
Colon & rectum 11%
Ovary 6%
Uterus 4%
Urinary 3%
Leukemia & lymphomas 8%
All other 19%

*Excluding basal and squamous cell skin cancers and in situ carcinomas, except bladder.
By permission of the American Cancer Society.

The Biology of Cancer

A biomedical revolution is under way that is advancing knowledge of the causes of cancer, yielding new and more effective treatments for cancers, and inspiring greater hope for prevention of cancers in the future. This revolution is built on scientific investigation of the basic processes that cause cancer.

Your body is a living, growing system that contains billions of individual cells. These cells carry out all of your body's functions, such as metabolism, transportation, excretion, reproduction, and locomotion.

Your body grows and develops as a result of increases in numbers of new cells and their changes into different types of tissue. New cells are created through the process of cell division (mitosis). Different types of cells are created by an accompanying process called cell differentiation (differentiation is the process by which cells acquire a specialized function). Cell division results in the normal pattern of human growth; cell differentiation makes possible the normal, orderly pattern of growth and development.

Unlike normal cells, cancer cells lack the controls that stop, or "switch off," growth. They divide without restraint, displacing neighboring normal cells by crowding them out and affecting their normal function and growth by competing with them for available nutrients. These uncontrolled cells can grow into a mass called a tumor and invade and destroy nearby normal tissue. They also can migrate in a process called "metastasis," spreading via the blood or lymph system to other parts of the body. It is important to note that not all cells that have rapid or uncontrolled growth are cancer cells. Cells may amass as benign tumors, which do not invade or destroy surrounding tissues.

Although science has yet to understand the processes by which all cells grow, divide, communicate, and differentiate, much has been learned about what goes on within the nucleus of a cell to further our understanding of how normal cells are activated or altered into cancerous cells in both inherited and non-inherited forms of cancer.

A Genetic Disease

Your body contains 60 trillion cells. The information that determines the growth and activities of cells is contained in your genes. Within the nucleus of each cell reside 46 chromosomes—half from your mother and half from your father. In 1944, scientists discovered that the chief component of chromosomes is the chemical deoxyribonucleic acid (DNA), which determines everything from the color of your eyes to risk factors for cancer and other diseases.

In 1953, scientists learned that chromosomes are made of long, double-stranded sequences of DNA arranged in what is known as the double helix. Encoded within DNA are instructions or "blueprints"—the basis of heredity—which include the sequence of chemical components for the manufacture of the proteins that control how cells work. These instructions for making proteins use only four chemicals: adenine (A), thymine (T), guanine (G), and cytosine (C). A specific sequence or triplet of three of the four letters instructs the protein-making machinery. The entire sequence of combinations makes a gene.

Our entire collection of genes, called the human genome, consists of 50,000 to 100,000 individual genes. Scientists from around the world are working together to transcribe and translate this language of heredity with the goal of mapping and then cross-referencing genes associated with diseases.

All genes are under some form of control. Cells selectively express certain genes in response to stress, injury, infections, hormones, growth factors, and many other external stimuli. Control (regulatory) genes may cause a gene to express its gene product (protein) continuously, such as an enzyme required for cellular metabolism. For others, the control genes will adjust gene expression to respond to a physiologic need of the body, such as for insulin. Regulation of gene expression is an important area of study for scientists.

What goes awry to produce cancer cells? Cancer is caused by factors that are external (chemicals, radiation, and viruses) and internal (hormones, immune and metabolic conditions, and inherited mutations). Some of these factors are avoidable; others are not. Scientists have identified many of the controllable risk factors that increase our chances of getting cancer (see Cancer Prevention, page 1294). A complex mix of these factors, acting together or in some cascade of events, promotes cancer cell growth.

When the genetic programming of a normal cell is disrupted, its malignant potential is released. All of us carry this malignant potential within us in normal genes known as proto-oncogenes. Products of these genes perform useful functions, such as regulating cell division and cell differentiation. These functions, however, may be compromised with aging or by exposure to cancer-causing (carcinogenic) agents. When this happens, they may be activated to become oncogenes (*oncos*, from the Greek for "mass" or "tumor"), coordinating the conversion of normal cells to cancer cells.

During the past 2 decades, great advances have been made in understanding how genes are activated or inactivated. This progress is due in great part to the development in 1973 of recombinant DNA technology, which allows the DNA from a different organism to be "spliced" or recombined to form a "new" piece of DNA in the laboratory.

This gene-splicing technology has made it possible for scientists to further study and confirm that multiple mechanisms or agents may be involved in activating an oncogene. For example, proto-oncogenes may be fused, rearranged, or relocated from their normal location in a cell's DNA, causing a disruption in the genetic coding sequences. Until these "broken" chromosomes are fully understood, the exact way in which oncogenes transform normal cells into cancer cells will remain a mystery.

Geneticists have long suspected that altered chromosomes play a role in the genesis of tumors. It was research on a family of tumor viruses—known as retroviruses—that led investigators to specific cancer genes in humans, and to begin to explore whether chromosome rearrangement may be one way to activate proto-oncogenes. The identification of this activated group of genes, collectively known as oncogenes, was a quantum leap in cancer research. Such discoveries are due in part to the 1983 discovery of polymerase chain reaction (PCR), a laboratory method by which a small fragment of DNA can be quickly reproduced (amplified) millions of times. The development of this technology helped lead to the identification of the first genetic marker for cystic fibrosis, and it is continuing to aid scientists in the search for specific cancer genes.

In addition to oncogenes, tumor suppressor genes are known to play a role in cancer development, particularly in inherited cancers. Tumor suppressor genes, which were discovered in 1986, are normally protective, acting to prevent the unregulated growth of cancer cells and the cancer-inducing effect of activated oncogenes. If one of these tumor-suppressing genes is absent or its protein product is unable to work properly, the cancer-producing action of an undetected oncogene may not be completely suppressed and a tumor may develop.

Research must continue if we are to understand how transformed or mutated cells are able to bypass the body's immune response without being recognized or attacked. One theory suggests that the proteins made under the direction of oncogenes, produced in vastly larger amounts than normal, cause the cells to grow abnormally and to send messages different from what they should send. Hence, these signals confuse and evade the body's immune response.

Such progress in our understanding of the cancer process can be attributed largely to the recombinant DNA technology of the 1970s. Before this technology was available, it was difficult to study the genetics of human disease. Today, scientists in the laboratory can isolate and manipulate the action of individual cancer-causing genes—a process called genetic engineering—creating models of human disease and pinpointing genes that are solely responsible for specific types of cancer. Genetic engineering opened the doors for scientists to correct impaired immune systems using biologic response modifiers, natural substances that mesh with the body's own immune defenses in response to cancer. Biologic response modifiers, including growth factors that stimulate cells of the immune system, hold the hope that emerging forms of immunotherapy can enhance the body's own disease-fighting system to control cancer. Such approaches are aimed at developing gene therapies that target specific genetic defects.

A major roadblock in treating cancer with immunotherapy was finding a way to deliver the body's own antibodies or anticancer drugs to the site of the cancer. Again, genetic engineering made possible monoclonal antibodies, disease-fighting cells produced by genetically fusing cancer cells with normal cells. Monoclonal antibodies are designed to tag and locate cancer cells and to deliver antibodies or drugs to a specific site with great precision. The potential of these immunologic "bullets" in diagnosing and treating cancer continues to be studied.

For the first time in history, the strategies to conquer cancers are available. The oncogene hypothesis, the discovery of tumor suppressors, and the application of recombinant DNA techniques to study cancers and develop more effective and precisely targeted drugs are a few of the advances revolutionizing our understanding and treatment of cancer. As the human genome is mapped, we will also learn if we are predisposed to cancer. The future holds the promise of applying emerging scientific information to the early diagnosis and treatment of cancer, and ultimately to the prevention of this complex disease.

Cancer Diagnosis

The best diagnosis of cancer is an early diagnosis. The earlier the cancer is detected, the greater the chances it can be treated before it spreads to other tissues or organs in the body. With the cancer screening procedures available today, many cancers can now be detected early enough to be cured.

Every diagnosis of cancer attempts to identify the type and location of the cancer. Each type of cancer has its own characteristic rate of growth, tendency to spread, and particular set of target tissues or organs to which it is likely to spread.

Identifying the kind of cancer enables your physician to anticipate how it is likely to behave and to plan appropriate treatment procedures. The diagnosis also involves determining the extent to which the cancer has already spread (staging). Finally, your physician needs to assess how the malignancy may have affected or will affect your health.

Among other things, these determinations will guide your physician as to the type of treatment suited to your cancer. You should not be alarmed if the diagnosis and "staging" of the disease require several days or weeks. An accurate diagnosis, on which your entire therapy program will be based, usually requires laboratory study of a tissue sample (biopsy), X-rays, and other laboratory procedures.

Cancer Warning Signs

According to the American Cancer Society, if you have any of these seven warning signs, consult your physician immediately:

- Change in bowel or bladder habits
- Sore that does not heal
- Unusual bleeding or discharge
- Thickening or lump in a breast or elsewhere in your body
- Indigestion or swallowing difficulty
- Obvious change in a wart or mole
- Nagging cough or hoarseness

Cancer Screening

Screening tests vary in complexity and cost. Most of the widely used tests are designed to discover common forms of cancer in persons at highest risk.

Cancer screening tests must be practical. This means that the test should detect the cancer early enough that the chances for a full recovery are still high.

Safety is also important. The test itself should not pose a dangerous health hazard. Twenty years ago, the mammography procedure used to detect breast cancer had a relatively high radiation exposure and itself may have been a factor in cancer development. Today, however, mammography exposes women to only small amounts of radiation, so the examination is much safer.

Periodic screening tests for cancer do not have the same preventive value in all cases and all types of cancer. With lung cancer, for example, frequent X-rays of the chest or analysis of sputum will not significantly improve your chances of surviving a bout with lung cancer, especially if you smoke. Although early detection is important, the cure rate with lung cancer is still less than 15 percent. Consequently, if you smoke or are exposed to chemicals in your home or work environment, see your physician about the advisability of screening for lung cancer. But even more crucial than watching for indications of the disease is exercising all options available to you that will reduce your exposure to the potential carcinogens. Quitting smoking is one such strategy.

Other cancers can be detected early enough that survival rates significantly improve. The cancer screening tests described here are part of a cancer prevention program

Cancer Prevention

There are no guarantees—yet taking precautions to avoid cancer risk factors makes good sense. Try to follow the guidelines given here.

Tobacco Use
In a word, don't. Smoking is responsible for almost 90 percent of all deaths from lung cancer and for about 30 percent of all cancer deaths (see Tobacco, page 315). Use of smokeless tobacco puts you at increased risk of cancer of the mouth, larynx, throat, or esophagus (see the Risks of Chewing Tobacco, page 319).

Sun Exposure
Recent research points to the sun as the chief villain in almost all of the half-million annual cases of non-melanoma skin cancer. Limit your exposure to the sun, especially if you are light-skinned. Use a sun blocker, too (see How to Avoid Sunburn, page 997).

Alcohol
Be reasonable in your consumption of alcohol. Heavy drinkers are at increased risk of oral cancer and cancers of the larynx, throat, esophagus, or liver (see Alcohol Abuse and Alcoholism, page 325).

Menopause Treatments
The use of estrogen by women for treating the symptoms of menopause and preventing osteoporosis poses certain risks for endometrial cancer. Weigh carefully the benefits and risks of estrogen replacement therapy when discussing its use with your physician (see Menopause, page 1153).

Radiation Exposure
Excessive exposure to ionizing (X-ray) radiation poses an increased risk of cancer (see Radiation and Your Health, page 376). Most medical X-rays are adjusted to deliver the lowest dose possible without sacrificing the quality of the image and without subjecting you to excess radiation.

There may be a potential risk with radon in your home (see The Radon Risk, page 378).

Industrial Exposure
Exposure to nickel, chromate, asbestos, vinyl chloride, and certain other industrial agents increases the risk of certain cancers.

Nutrition
What you eat may have an effect on your cancer risk. Diets high in fats or salt-cured, smoked, or nitrite-cured foods may be potentially hazardous, but foods rich in vitamins A and C or high in fiber may help lower your risk for certain cancers (see Nutrition and Cancer Protection, page 280).

---

recommended by the American Cancer Society.

Breast Cancer
Warning signs: Any lump or thickening in the breast or bleeding or discharge from the nipple.

Cancer risk factors: Breast cancer most often occurs in women older than 50; in women who have never had children, had their first child after age 30, have never breastfed, are more than 40 percent over their ideal weight, or who reached sexual maturity late or had a late menopause; and in women from families in which there is a history of premenopausal breast cancer in mother or sisters.

Checkup guidelines: Every woman should examine her breasts carefully and expertly once a month (see Breast Self-Examination, page 1160).

In addition, women between the ages of 20 and 40 should have their breasts examined by a physician every 3 years; women older than 40 should have this examination every year. If you are between 35 and 39, consider having a baseline mammogram. If you are between 40 and 49, have no symptoms or lumps, and have no family history of breast cancer, have a mammogram every 1 to 2 years (see page 1165). After age 50, have a mammogram annually. If you have a family history of breast cancer, have a mammogram annually starting at age 40.

Cervical Cancer
Warning signs: Abnormal vaginal bleeding.

Cancer risk factors: Having had genital herpes or genital wart infections; having had sexual intercourse shortly after reaching puberty; or having many sexual partners.

Checkup guidelines: Women older than 18 or women younger than 18 who are sexually active should have a Pap test (see page 1181) and pelvic examination annually. Your physician may decide that after three or more consecutive satisfactory normal annual examinations, the Pap test can be performed less frequently.

Colorectal Cancer
Warning signs: Any rectal bleeding or long-term change in your bowel habits.

Cancer risk factors: History of colorectal polyps (see page 786) or of colorectal cancer in a family member or chronic ulcerative colitis (see page 777).

Checkup guidelines: Men and women older than 40 should have a digital rectal examination annually. Moreover, in the absence of a family history of colon cancer, men and women should have an initial sigmoidoscopic examination at age 45 and every 3 to 5 years thereafter (see page 791). A stool test for blood each year (see page 790) is usually recommended, even though the findings are not foolproof.

Endometrial Cancer

Warning signs: Abnormal vaginal bleeding.

Cancer risk factors: History of infertility or failure to ovulate; late onset of menopause or prolonged estrogen therapy after menopause; obesity; heavy smoking.

Checkup guidelines: On reaching menopause, women who have had a history of infertility, obesity, failure to ovulate, abnormal uterine bleeding, or estrogen therapy should have an endometrial biopsy (see page 1183).

Lung Cancer

Warning signs: Nagging cough, coughing up blood; persistent attacks of pneumonia or bronchitis; chest pain.

Cancer risk factors: Heavy smoking and exposure to environmental pollutants, particularly asbestos (see Asbestosis, page 728).

Checkup guidelines: Every person older than 40 should have a baseline chest X-ray. Subsequent chest X-rays should be done at the discretion of your physician.

Oral Cancer

Warning signs: Any change of color in your mouth or sore in your mouth that fails to heal.

Cancer risk factors: Most common in men older than 45, heavy smokers, and users of smokeless (chewing) tobacco, especially when coupled with heavy use of alcohol (see page 599).

Checkup guidelines: If you have a sore that fails to heal, see your physician or dentist.

Prostate Cancer

Warning signs: Difficulty in urination; persistent pain in the lower back, pelvis, or upper thighs; blood in the urine.

Cancer risk factors: Most common among men older than 70.

Checkup guidelines: If you are older than 40, you should have a digital rectal examination at the time of your periodic medical examination (see page 1211). The PSA (prostate-specific antigen) blood test and the ultrasound examination of the prostate to detect prostate cancer are not yet established as routine tests.

Skin Cancer

Warning signs: A small lesion with an irregular border and red, white, blue, or blue-black spots on trunk or limbs; shiny, firm bump or lesions from pearl to black anywhere on the skin; dark lesions on palms, soles, tips of fingers and toes; large brownish spot with darker speckles on skin exposed to sun; red-purple spots anywhere on the skin; purple-brown or dark blue nodules on toes or leg; pearly or waxy bump on face, ear, or neck; flat, flesh-colored or brown scar-like lesion on chest or back; firm, red nodule or flat lesion with scaly or crusted surface on face, ears, neck, hands, or arms; change in a mole or any sore that fails to heal (see Skin Cancers, page 1004).

Cancer risk factors: Fair skin, blue eyes, or red hair in men and women; severe sunburn in childhood; family history of birthmarks or moles (dysplastic nevus syndrome).

Checkup guidelines: If you have any skin lesion that has the warning signs listed here, see your physician.

Testicular Cancer

Warning signs: Any lump on the testicle or change in its size.

Cancer risk factors: Strikes younger men more often than older men (uncommon after age 40); undescended testicles (see page 1202).

Checkup guidelines: Men of all ages, starting in late teenage years, should examine their testicles monthly (see Self-Examination of the Testicles, page 1200).

Throat Cancer

Warning signs: Hoarseness.

Cancer risk factors: Heavy smoking, particularly when coupled with substantial use of alcohol.

Checkup guidelines: Examination by a throat specialist in the event of a change in the character of your speech lasting more than a few weeks, or annually if you are a heavy smoker.

Urinary Tract and Bladder Cancer

Warning signs: Blood in the urine; back pain; loss of weight and appetite; persistent fever; anemia.

Cancer risk factors: Most common in men older than 50; heavy smokers; history of chronic urinary tract infections.

Checkup guidelines: The routine urinalysis performed during your complete physical examination will reveal if there is any blood in your urine (hematuria). If hematuria is found, your physician may do a cystoscopic examination and a biopsy if abnormal tissue is found (see page 849). Your physician also may obtain an X-ray of your kidney (see Kidney X-Ray, page 829).

Cancer Clusters in Populations

At times, cancer seems to occur more frequently in certain groups or in certain geographic locations. Such clusters of cancer suggest that some factor in the environment may be responsible.

A well-demonstrated example is the occurrence of a particular lung tumor (mesothelioma) among industrial workers exposed to asbestos. This tumor occurs at a much greater frequency in asbestos-exposed persons who also smoke (see Asbestosis, page 728). Another example is the high frequency of cancer of the stomach in Japan, although no single environmental factor has been identified with certainty to explain the Japanese susceptibility to this tumor.

Occasionally, data collected by public health facilities will show an increased frequency of a disease in a certain community. A search then begins for an explanation. Most often, such clusters are explained by the laws of chance or by changes in medical referral patterns; for example, a new specialist moving into a community may have cases referred to him or her. This may appear to be an increase in specific disease when, in fact, these patients have been present for some time in the community.

The mathematical expression of the laws of chance tells us not only that most communities or groups of people of similar age and background will have about the same frequency of various diseases but also that, from time to time, there will be a concentration of one disease or another in certain groups of people. This statistical phenomenon might be compared to dealing a hand of cards. Usually the cards in a hand will be fairly evenly distributed among the four suits, but you also can expect that now and then you will be dealt a hand composed almost entirely of one suit. Mathematicians can calculate the exact odds that such an event will occur.

It is important to separate the clusters of cancer that are merely statistical from those that are caused by environmental factors. Quite properly, much attention and concern are being expressed these days about exposure to substances that have been shown to produce cancers in laboratory animals. However, it is also important to remember that scientific proof that a cluster of cancers is in fact a consequence of exposure to potentially toxic substances known to be present in a given community depends on careful statistical comparison of the exposed group of persons with people known to have little or no exposure.

Living With Cancer

More frequently than ever before, cancer can be cured. The probability of a complete cure and extended survival is continually improving because of our growing knowledge and understanding of cancer. As a result, new therapies that selectively kill cancer cells are steadily being developed. These therapies are not only more effective but also safer.

The management of pain also has been greatly improved over the years to the point that most pain, even that of terminally ill cancer patients, can be controlled. There are additional therapies that can help you cope with treatment and its effects. In the following pages, we describe the treatments now available, how to go about getting appropriate care, and other key issues in living and dealing with cancer and its treatment.

Cancer Treatment

No two cancer treatment regimens are the same; each person with cancer is unique. But the basic therapeutic options that are available to most persons with cancer are similar: surgery, radiation therapy, and chemotherapy.

Why one form of treatment is more appropriate than another in a given person depends on the individual diagnosis, the stage to which the disease has developed, and other factors such as the person's age, sex, general health, and, in women, menopausal status.

A critical part of the diagnosis is determination of whether the cancer has spread. A diagnostic process called staging determines what other tissues or organs may have been invaded by the tumor. Staging not only helps your physician plan the treatment but also evaluates the likelihood of its success or failure. For example, your physician may learn whether a localized treatment such as surgery or radiation therapy would be sufficient or whether a systemic form of treatment such as chemotherapy will be needed to kill cancer cells that have spread to other parts of your body.

Surgery

Surgery has long been the foundation of cancer treatment. The goals of surgery can vary. It can be done to determine whether or not the growth is malignant, to remove a cancerous growth from the body, or to learn if malignant cells have spread to other parts of the body.

Sometimes surgery is directed primarily toward relief of obstruction, for example, of the bile ducts or the intestine. At other times, when it is not possible to remove all of the cancerous growth, the surgeon will remove as much as possible (a debulking procedure) in order to make chemotherapy or radiation more effective.

Surgery is most successful if the cancer has not spread. Sometimes, however, cancer cells that break off from the site where the cancer first appeared (the primary tumor) may travel through blood or lymph vessels to other sites within the body to form secondary tumors. In these instances, the cancer is said to have metastasized. If cells spread before the primary growth is removed, cancer may recur at other locations, even after the primary tumor has been excised.

If the cancer is widespread, surgery is unlikely to cure it. Occasionally, a single secondary tumor appears after removal of the primary cancer and, in some cases, the surgical removal of this single lesion makes a cure possible. This situation may occur in cancer of the colon or testicles, among others. The secondary tumor, in most circumstances, is located in the lung, liver, or brain.

Radiation Therapy

By careful aiming and regulation of dose, high-energy radiation can be used to destroy cancer cells. Radiation therapy (also referred to as radiotherapy, X-ray therapy, cobalt treatment, or irradiation) is either part of the treatment or the only treatment for about half of all patients. This form of treatment is effective only for the cancer cells within the area receiving the radiation (the field).

Radiation may be used before surgery to shrink a cancerous tumor, after surgery to stop growth of any remaining cancer cells, or alone or with anticancer drugs to destroy a malignant tumor. It is particularly effective when used to treat certain types of localized cancers such as malignant tumors of the lymph nodes or vocal cords.

Like surgery, however, radiation usually is not curative if the cancer cells have spread throughout the body or outside the area of radiation. It can be used even if a cure is not probable because it can shrink tumors, which decreases the pressure and pain they cause, or it can stop their bleeding.

Generally, radiation produces less physical disfigurement than radical surgery does, but it may produce troublesome side effects. These side effects are related to the damage X-rays do to normal tissue. You may have to cope with irritated or thickened skin, swallowing difficulties, dry mouth, nausea, diarrhea, hair loss, and a loss of energy. How serious and extensive these side effects become depends on where and how much radiation is used.

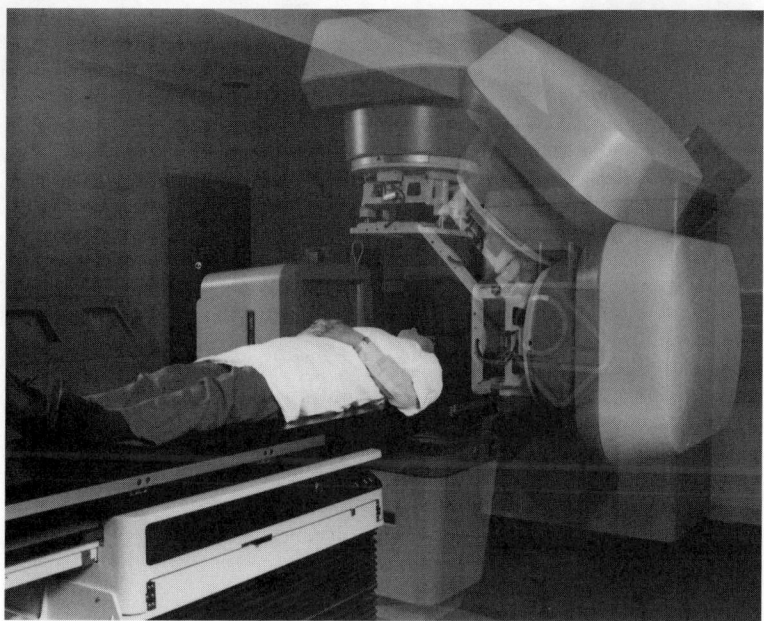

Radiation therapy can be used to effectively destroy cancer cells. During treatment, this device slowly rotates to deliver radiation more effectively.

Chemotherapy

Chemotherapy is the use of medication to treat cancer. For some types of malignancy, such as Hodgkin's disease (see Lymphomas, page 968), leukemia in children (see Leukemias, page 964), or cancer of the testicles (see page 1202), chemotherapy may produce a cure even when the cancer is widespread. In other cases in which the cancer is not curable, chemotherapy can relieve symptoms and enhance the quality of life for a patient.

Cancer chemotherapy does not always mean the use of only a single drug. Combination chemotherapy consists of giving a group of drugs that work together to kill cancer cells. If anticancer drugs are used in an attempt to destroy any cancer cells that may remain after surgery or radiation therapy, it is referred to as adjuvant chemotherapy. Adjuvant chemotherapy (the Latin *adjuvans* means "aiding") is a preventive measure commonly used for cancer, such as breast cancer that has spread into the lymph nodes of the armpit and was discovered at the time of initial surgery. For some cancers, such as those arising from the head and neck area, chemotherapy may be given "up front," meaning before surgery or radiation therapy. This concept is called "neoadjuvant therapy."

Anticancer drugs can affect normal tissue cells as well. The normal cells most likely to be affected are those that divide rapidly, such as in the bone marrow, gastrointestinal tract, reproductive system, and hair follicles.

These cells usually recover shortly after the treatment.

Depending on the specific drugs used, chemotherapy can produce various side effects similar to those of radiation therapy. These toxic reactions include loss of hair, sores in the mouth, difficulty swallowing (esophagitis), dry mouth, nausea, vomiting, diarrhea, bleeding, and infection. Less common problems include damage to the heart, liver, lungs, kidneys, or nerves (which may result in numbness or tingling of the hands or feet).

In general, these effects of chemotherapy and radiation are reversible. Coping with effects of treatment is a focus of health care providers.

Immunotherapy

The body's immune system (see The Workings of the Immune System, page 1056) acts as a surveillance system to guard against the presence of what it interprets to be foreign substances. For example, the immune response to the presence of an organ that was transplanted from an unrelated donor might be rejection of the organ.

Cancer cells also are seen as foreign. For years, researchers have been trying to find ways to enhance the body's natural immune reaction toward cancer cells. When used as a method of treatment, this technique is called immunotherapy.

Immunotherapy might involve the use of biologic agents, known as lymphokines, that normally are produced by immunologically oriented cells. The best documented immunotherapeutic agents are interferons and interleukin-2.

Until recently, the results of immunotherapy against cancer were disappointing, but researchers recently have had success controlling a few types of cancer with one type of interferon, interferon-alpha. Specifically, interferon often produces remarkable improvement in people with a rare cancer known as hairy cell leukemia. It also provides limited benefit against certain types of lymph system cancer. Unfortunately, interferon therapy produces little or no improvement against the major cancer killers that arise in the lung, breast, and digestive tract.

We are learning more about how the immune system recognizes and attacks malignant cells. This major field of cancer research eventually may lead to effective immunotherapy techniques against many types of cancer.

New Methods to Fight Cancer

Cancer treatment is constantly evolving. Some of these methods are now accepted therapy, and others are under investigation and are experimental. Physicians often combine these approaches with chemotherapy and radiation.

Colony-Stimulating Factors
Because chemotherapy may impair your bone marrow, which makes white blood cells, you become more vulnerable to infection. Colony-stimulating factors encourage production of white blood cells. This lets you tolerate higher doses of chemotherapy, improving your chance for remission or cure while decreasing the chance for infection.

T Cells
T cells recognize and attack cancer cells. Researchers hope to remove T cells from the body, stimulate growth, and return them in large numbers to fight cancer. Someday, vaccines may be available to promote growth of T cells.

Tumor Necrosis Factors
These proteins destroy tumor cells. Your body produces small amounts naturally. Researchers are looking at ways to make larger amounts.

Monoclonal Antibodies
Antibodies are natural proteins that spot and attack "foreign" substances, including cancer cells. Monoclonal antibodies made in a laboratory can focus on specific types of cancer. By attaching themselves to tumor cells, they may help deliver medications and radiation to fight cancer.

Lasers
High-intensity light shows potential for treating cancers of the skin, trachea, lungs, esophagus, stomach, colon, rectum, and anus.

Gene Therapy
Many tumors grow because normal genes go awry, changing healthy cells into cancerous cells. Genes that help fight cancer can also fail to work properly. With gene therapy, physicians hope to replace defective genes and encourage the growth of healthy genes.

Hyperthermia
Since the early 1800s, physicians have known that heat can harm some tumors. Researchers now are evaluating hyperthermia to treat cancer of the breast, lymph nodes, skin, eyes, and cervix. Still, the value of hyperthermia has yet to be established.

Choosing a Physician and a Place for Cancer Treatment

The choice of physician and hospital, as well as all decisions about your diagnosis, treatment, and rehabilitation, should be shared. With the complexity involved in all these decisions, they are too important to be left to any one person, including you.

If you suspect that you have cancer or cancer has been diagnosed, the best policy is to share your fears and concerns with family members and loved ones. People who know and care about you can be helpful in sharing the pain and responsibility of making critical decisions.

Never relinquish your responsibility for your health out of a feeling of helplessness. No situation need ever be beyond your control. You always have the option to ask questions, change your mind, and express your fears to everyone involved. You may not be able to change the diagnosis—but you can and should be the decision-maker regarding your care and treatment.

Physicians
The American Cancer Society (ACS) recommends that a team be formed to help you during this period. This team includes not only yourself, your family, and loved ones but also a variety of medical professionals, primarily physicians and other health professionals trained to deal with one or another aspect of your illness: radiotherapists, surgeons, and medical oncologists (cancer specialists) as well as dietitians, physical therapists, and others. To coordinate the diagnostic and therapeutic efforts that may be considered, it is recommended that you appoint what the ACS calls a physician adviser or primary care physician.

The physician adviser may be your personal family physician or a specialist who is directing the overall treatment of the cancer.

What is important to understand is that the physician you select for this role should be qualified to advise you on the entire process—diagnosis, treatment, and rehabilitation. Moreover, he or she should be available and willing to provide long-term, continuing care.

If for any reason you are not comfortable in your relationship with your physician, tell him or her what bothers you. If you remain dissatisfied with any aspect of your care, get a second opinion from another physician (see Second Opinions, page 1247). Do this as soon as possible because it is more difficult to start over once a physician begins the treatment.

This is also the time to talk about your primary care physician's willingness to involve other physicians in your treatment. Questions like these need not be difficult to ask or answer. Your physician should be happy to answer intelligent and thoughtful questions because this suggests the prospect of an open and frank relationship. If, on the other hand, this does not occur, look elsewhere.

Cancer Centers

Your physician adviser will conduct some of the initial diagnostic tests, such as a Pap smear or biopsy. If the diagnosis requires tests for which this physician's office is not equipped, you may be referred to a specialist at a medical center.

Depending on the type of cancer and the treatment you require, you may find yourself spending a substantial amount of time at a medical center specializing in the treatment of cancer. Your physician adviser will help you locate and evaluate an appropriate center. Another source of information is the American College of Surgeons. A rule of thumb is the greater the number of beds in the hospital (perhaps 500 or more), the more likely it will have experience in treating cancer.

Usually, a hospital directly connected to or affiliated with a medical school offers a broader range and higher quality of care because these institutions draw prominent clinicians, researchers, and educators for their medical facilities and teaching staff. Teaching hospitals (those in which residents are trained, although there may be no medical school directly affiliated with the hospital) also often are good facilities, although their services are usually not as extensive as those found in a hospital/medical school tandem.

Your illness may require you to go to more than one medical center. One center may provide the diagnosis, another may conduct the treatment based on the diagnosis, and a third may provide the rehabilitation.

Most large or community medical centers are equipped to treat cancer cases that do not require a high degree of specialization. However, if you need complicated or experimental treatment, or if physicians at your local hospital are inexperienced in treating your specific type of cancer, you might be referred to a specialized cancer center.

In teaching hospitals (hospitals with residents), there often are carefully organized trials of treatments in progress. Some of these trials compare new modes of therapy with the best currently available treatment. Other trials study new agents or approaches in a non-comparative manner. If you are offered a chance to enter one of these trials, you must be given a frank and comprehensive description of the risks and possible benefits. While such clinical trials are clearly experimental, the careful application of these therapies, whether new or old, generally will provide some of the most promising treatments currently available.

Cancer Facilities

The National Cancer Institute (NCI) has designated 41 medical centers throughout the United States as Comprehensive and Clinical Cancer Centers. These centers provide leadership in cancer research. They develop programs involving scientists and physicians from many fields.

In addition to providing state-of-the-art diagnosis and treatment of cancer, these cancer centers conduct interdisciplinary programs in basic clinical research, cancer control, and education.

Comprehensive and Clinical Cancer Centers offer the most extensive range of cancer treatment found in the United States, including therapies that are still considered investigational. When you call to make an appointment at a specific center, you may want to ask whether it has a designation from the National Cancer Institute. If not, learn if it has an approved cancer program sponsored by the American College of Surgeons. These are programs that have met specific requirements and standards for the treatment of malignant disease.

Cancer Centers Supported by the National Cancer Institute

The National Cancer Institute supports several cancer centers throughout the country that develop and investigate new methods of cancer diagnosis and treatment. Information about referral procedures, treatment costs, and services available to patients can be obtained from the cancer centers listed here:

Alabama
Comprehensive Cancer Center
University of Alabama at Birmingham
1824 Sixth Avenue South, Room 237
Birmingham, AL 35293-3300

Arizona
Arizona Cancer Center
The University of Arizona
1501 North Campbell Avenue
Tucson, AZ 85724

California
City of Hope Cancer Research Center and
  Beckman Research Institute
Needleman Building, Room 102
1500 East Duarte Road
Duarte, CA 91010

USC Norris Comprehensive Cancer Center
University of Southern California
1441 Eastlake Avenue
Los Angeles, CA 90033-0800

Jonsson Comprehensive Cancer Center
University of California at Los Angeles
Factor Building, Room 8-684
10833 Le Conte Avenue
Los Angeles, CA 90095-1781

UCI Cancer Center
University of California at Irvine
101 The City Drive
Building 23, Rt. 81
Orange, CA 92668

UCSD Cancer Center
200 West Arbor Drive
San Diego, CA 92103-8421

Colorado
University of Colorado Cancer Center
University of Colorado Health Science Center
4200 East Ninth Avenue, Box B188
Denver, CO 80262

Connecticut
Comprehensive Cancer Center
Yale University School of Medicine
333 Cedar Street, Box 208028
New Haven, CT 06520-8028

District of Columbia
Lombardi Cancer Research Center
Georgetown University Medical Center
3800 Reservoir Road, NW
Washington, DC 20007

Florida
Sylvester Comprehensive Cancer Center
University of Miami Medical School
P. O. Box 016960 (D72)
Miami, FL 33101

Illinois
University of Chicago Cancer Research
  Center
5841 South Maryland Avenue, MC1140
Chicago, IL 60637-1470

Lurie Cancer Center
Northwestern University
303 East Chicago Avenue, Olson 8250
Chicago, IL 60611

Maryland
The Johns Hopkins Oncology Center
600 North Wolfe Street, Room 157
Baltimore, MD 21287-8943

Massachusetts
Dana-Farber Cancer Institute
44 Binney Street, Room 1828
Boston, MA 02115

Michigan
Comprehensive Cancer Center
University of Michigan
102 Observatory
Ann Arbor, MI 48109-0724

Barbara Ann Karmanos Cancer Institute
Wayne State University
110 East Warren Avenue
Detroit, MI 48201-1379

Minnesota
Mayo Cancer Center
Mayo Foundation
Mayo Building, East 12
200 First Street SW
Rochester, MN 55905

New Hampshire
Norris Cotton Cancer Center
Dartmouth-Hitchcock Medical Center
One Medical Center Drive, Hinman Box 7920
Lebanon, NH 03756-0001

New York
Cancer Research Center
Albert Einstein College of Medicine
Chanin Building, Room 330
1300 Morris Park Avenue
Bronx, NY 10461

Roswell Park Cancer Institute
Elm and Carlton Streets
Buffalo, NY 14263-0001

Memorial Sloan-Kettering Cancer Center
1275 York Avenue
New York, NY 10021

Columbia-Presbyterian Cancer Center
Columbia University
701 West 168th Street, Room 1509
New York, NY 10032

Kaplan Cancer Center
New York University Medical Center
550 First Avenue
New York, NY 10016

University of Rochester Cancer Center
601 Elmwood Avenue, Box 704
Rochester, NY 14642

North Carolina
UNC Lineberger Comprehensive Cancer
  Center
UNC School of Medicine, CB-7295
102 West Drive
Chapel Hill, NC 27599-7295

Duke Comprehensive Cancer Center
Duke University Medical Center
Box 3843
Durham, NC 27710

Comprehensive Cancer Center
Wake Forest University
Bowman Gray School of Medicine
Medical Center Boulevard
Winston-Salem, NC 27157-1082

Ohio
Cancer Research Center
Case Western Reserve University
11100 Euclid Avenue, Wearn 151
Cleveland, OH 44106-5065

Arthur G. James Cancer Hospital
Ohio State University
300 West Tenth Avenue, Suite 521
Columbus, OH 43210-1240

Pennsylvania
Fox Chase Cancer Center
7701 Burholme Avenue
Philadelphia, PA 19111

University of Pennsylvania Cancer Center
Sixth Floor Penn Tower
3400 Spruce Street
Philadelphia, PA 19104-4283

University of Pittsburgh Cancer Institute
200 Meyran Avenue
Pittsburgh, PA 15213-3305

Tennessee
St. Jude Children's Research Hospital
332 North Lauderdale
Memphis, TN 38105-2794

Vanderbilt Cancer Center
Vanderbilt University
649 Medical Research Building II
Nashville, TN 37232-6838

Texas
M.D. Anderson Cancer Center
University of Texas
1515 Holcombe Boulevard, Box 91
Houston, TX 77030

San Antonio Cancer Institute
8122 Datapoint Drive, Suite 600
San Antonio, TX 78229

Utah
Huntsman Cancer Institute
University of Utah
Building 533, Suite 7410
Salt Lake City, UT 84112

Vermont
Vermont Cancer Center
University of Vermont
One South Prospect Street
Burlington, VT 05401-3498

Virginia
Cancer Center
University of Virginia, Health Sciences
  Center
Hospital Box 334
Charlottesville, VA 22908

Massey Cancer Center
Medical College of Virginia/VCU
P.O. Box 980037
Richmond, VA 23298-0230

Washington
Fred Hutchinson Cancer Research Center
1124 Columbia Street, LY301
Seattle, WA 98104

Wisconsin
Comprehensive Cancer Center
600 Highland Avenue, Room K4/614
Madison, WI 53792-0001

For additional information about cancer, write:
Office of Cancer Communications
National Cancer Institute
Bethesda, MD 20892

Or call the toll-free telephone number of the Cancer Information Service:
1-800-4-CANCER.

Nutrition and Cancer

A person who has cancer and is in sound nutritional shape is better able to tolerate the side effects of chemotherapy, radiation, and surgery. Furthermore, good nutrition improves the sense of well-being, enhances tissue function and repair, and improves the immune function of the person with cancer. However, common and difficult problems often associated with cancer have been weight loss and malnutrition. When advanced (severe), this is sometimes called cancer cachexia.

Many factors can contribute to weight loss. The disease or its treatment can decrease appetite and food intake (anorexia) or interfere with the consumption, digestion, absorption, or utilization of food by your body.

Many cancers affect the nutritional status adversely even before the diagnosis or treatment. Depending on the type of cancer, malnutrition may result from anorexia, obstruction (blockage) by a tumor that impairs food intake or digestion, malabsorption of nutrients in the gastrointestinal tract, or disturbances in fluid balance due to vomiting and diarrhea.

Often, a person with cancer who experiences severe anorexia simply cannot eat in spite of his or her understanding that nourishment is required. For various reasons, many people with cancer are either unable to taste their food or experience changes in taste. It is not uncommon for them to find that they often feel full after eating only a few bites of food.

The radiation, surgery, and chemotherapy used as treatment for cancer may cause symptoms, such as nausea, alterations in taste and smell, sore mouth, diarrhea, anorexia, or difficulty in swallowing, that predispose people to nutritional problems. The treatment also may increase the body's need for calories and protein to rebuild damaged tissues.

Recent advances in the subject of nutrition have been very helpful in the management of cancer cachexia. Today, in most cases, weight loss is not considered an inevitable consequence of cancer. There are many simple, constructive steps that you can take to improve intake and ensure maintenance of your body weight. In addition, new feeding techniques such as tube feedings, intravenous feedings, and improved oral supplements have been developed that enable almost everyone, even those with complicated nutritional problems, to improve their nutritional status. Clinical trials have documented the value of a medication called megestrol acetate, a pill taken several times each day, to increase weight in a person with cancer. The medication is also available as syrup.

Your physician, often in consultation with a dietitian who is especially knowledgeable about cancer and nutrition, can offer you further advice concerning nutrition.

Clinical studies have shown that a sound nutritional state can improve a person's chance of undergoing successful treatment and withstanding the rigors of cancer, but no conclusive evidence exists to indicate that decreased or excessive amounts of any nutrient have a beneficial role in the treatment of cancer. (See Nutrition and the Cancer Patient, page 281, and Nutrition and Cancer Protection, page 280.)

Cancer Pain

Cancer does not always cause pain. More than half of all persons with cancer do not experience exceptional pain; often the pain is moderate and far less intense than that experienced in some forms of arthritis or nerve disorders. In general, pain relief can be achieved by tumor control with surgery, radiation therapy, or chemotherapy.

Some persons with cancer do have episodes of more severe pain; in general, the more advanced the cancer, the greater likelihood of some periods of severe pain.

When cancer pain that is not relieved initially by cancer treatment does occur, there are many other ways of obtaining relief.

Through a combination of pain-relieving drugs and non-drug methods, most people with cancer can function as well as the other symptoms of the disease will permit. As a result, one of the primary goals of cancer treatment is to decrease pain with as few side effects as possible.

Causes of Pain

Cancer pain depends on the type of cancer and the stage of the disease. Cancer pain can be dull, aching, sharp, constant, intermittent, mild, moderate, or severe. It may be caused by pressure of the tumor on a nerve, poor circulation because of blocked blood vessels, blocked organ in the body, bone fractures, infection, or side effects from surgery. Emotional responses to the cancer, such as anxiety, depression, or feelings of hopelessness, can make the pain seem worse.

Pharmacologic Relief of Pain

The principal treatment for cancer is pain-relieving drugs (analgesics). Although many drugs are used to treat cancer pain, most fall into two categories: non-narcotics and narcotics.

Non-narcotics include aspirin, acetaminophen, and nonsteroidal anti-inflammatory drugs (NSAIDs). Many patients fear that aspirin is not strong enough to treat their pain. Yet, aspirin can be highly effective and provide the same amount of pain relief as many of the more powerful painkillers. In combination with codeine or meperidine (Demerol), aspirin can effectively control mild to moderate pain.

Most NSAIDs are prescription drugs. The benefits of these agents are that they are slightly more potent and more convenient to take than aspirin and they require fewer pills per day.

Antidepressants, anticonvulsants, and steroids are other non-narcotic agents that may help relieve cancer pain.

Narcotics, such as morphine and codeine, are the more powerful painkillers used to treat moderate to severe pain. Many cancer patients fear addiction will occur if they take narcotics as part of their cancer treatment.

This fear is largely unfounded.

When used under proper medical control, the chance for addiction to narcotics is very small. Besides, if a narcotic is needed to relieve severe pain for a long period of time, the comfort it provides is often more important than any possibility of an addiction.

Sometimes tranquilizers are used in combination with analgesics. The tranquilizers offer no relief of the pain, but they may help you tolerate the discomfort and can be an integral part of treatment.

In some cases, larger doses of narcotics or tranquilizers can cause confusion or delirium. This may limit their usefulness. Although most narcotics are typically administered by oral route or injection, one type of narcotic (fentanyl) can be administered by a patch applied to the skin. This patch is about the size of a credit card and is usually changed about every 72 hours. In some patients, this is a very convenient and effective way of providing durable pain relief.

In addition to medications, your physician may recommend one or more non-drug treatments for cancer pain relief.

Radiation therapy delivered to a selected site, such as a bone involved with cancer, can shrink the tumor and lessen or eliminate the pain.

Nerve pathways that carry pain impulses to the brain can be blocked either by the injection of certain substances into or around the nerve or by surgery. These procedures have risks and some are considered experimental. However, for those who cannot tolerate the side effects of other pain medications, these methods can be helpful. For some cancers, such as pancreatic cancers, these procedures have become almost routine.

Your physician also may suggest some behavioral modification methods, in combination with other pain-relief methods, to help decrease your anxiety and build your confidence in coping with pain. These methods include hypnosis, biofeedback, breathing and relaxation exercises, massage, transcutaneous electrical nerve stimulation (TENS) (see page 480), and hot or cold packs.

Cancer Rehabilitation

Rehabilitation, a significant part of the treatment of cancer, is often planned before the treatment begins. The choice of your treatment may dictate the scope and nature of your rehabilitation.

Whatever form the rehabilitation takes,

the goal is always the same—to restore you to as normal a lifestyle as possible. This might mean job retraining, homemaker services, an exercise program, or learning to use a prosthesis. Such wide-ranging skills and services usually call for a team approach. Depending on need, you may see a number of health-care professionals besides your primary physician. These include physical medicine physician specialists (physiatrists), social workers, physical therapists, and occupational therapists.

Some of the more common rehabilitation efforts involve a speech therapist or speech pathologist who can help with retraining for speech after a surgical procedure on the larynx or mouth (see page 598); an enterostomal therapist who instructs in the use of the artificial opening, made as a result of either colon or bladder surgery, for eliminating body wastes (see Colostomy and Ileostomy, page 777, and Bladder Cancer, page 848); or a physical or occupational therapist to help in learning how to use an artificial limb. The initial stage of the rehabilitation can be started in the hospital, or all of the rehabilitation may be offered in the home or in an outpatient center.

Do not be discouraged if you find your initial efforts difficult and the results disappointing. Progress may come slowly and the work may be hard. But do not give up and withdraw from the rehabilitation program that has been designed for you. Follow your therapist's instructions. If you have problems, do not hesitate to discuss them with your therapist, physiatrist, or physician advisor.

To help during this transition in your life, there are many volunteer support groups made up primarily of patients who have recovered from cancer. Their desire is to help the person with cancer through the usually difficult period of adjustment during and after treatment. One of the best known is the Reach to Recovery program of the American Cancer Society for women recovering from breast cancer. If you inform your physician that you would like to talk with someone from this group, a volunteer will pay a visit while you are still in the hospital. Two other volunteer cancer support groups are the Ostomy Rehabilitation Program for people with abdominal stomas and the Laryngectomee Club for those who lose their natural voice because of cancer surgery.

Older people may find returning to normal life especially difficult; many youngsters do too. These behaviors, which may involve depression or a refusal to try to adjust, can place added stress on the other members of the family. CanSurmount is an organization devoted to the support and care of those recovering and their families during this period. I CAN COPE is another volunteer group that advises the patient and family on cancer therapy, treatment side effects, nutrition issues, and other topics of interest.

You can learn the whereabouts of the nearest chapter of these or other such support groups by calling the American Cancer Society (ACS) in your area. The ACS also can help you with problems of transportation and home-care items and with contacting community groups such as Community Mental Health and Family Services.

It is important to understand that this is a time in your life when you must learn to accept help. Going it alone is probably unwise and may be impossible. You can benefit greatly from allowing people who have themselves recovered from cancer to advise and support you.

Hospices

The word "hospice" comes from the Latin word for guest; it is the root that forms the words hospital, hospitality, and hostel. Hospice conveys a sense of caring and shelter.

In the Middle Ages, the hospice was a way station for travelers. Today, hospice has another meaning. A hospice is a program—sometimes within the confines of a medical center or based in a person's home—that offers a coordinated, interdisciplinary program of care and services for terminally ill people and their families.

Team Approach

At the heart of the hospice approach is the team. Hospice workers, who include physicians, nurses, social workers, and clergy, provide an integration of various skills to help both the dying person and the family. Physicians and nurses provide medical services; social workers can assist with psychosocial support for the person and family and help with financial planning, insurance, and funeral arrangements; clergy offer spiritual counseling for both the dying person and his or her family; and volunteers help the hospice staff with clerical assistance and the person and family with their daily needs

Coping With Survival

In many ways, surviving cancer is a process. It begins the minute cancer affects your life and continues after treatment is completed.

Traditionally, a survivor is someone in whom there's no evidence of active disease after treatment is completed, a determination often made after an average of 5 years.

Despite the relief of winning cancer's physical battle, the end of treatment also means emotional challenges. Recovery may take a different way of thinking about yourself and relating to others. Here are some ways to help you adjust to the change from "patient" to "survivor."

As you leave behind the health care professionals who have supported you, turn to your family and friends and talk about your adjustment to life as a cancer sur-

vivor. Joining an organized support group may also help.

You may wonder how to tell the difference between normal health problems and a relapse of cancer. Change your focus to staying healthy. Exercise regularly, eat well, and get enough rest. If you have health concerns, discuss them with your physician.

During cancer treatment, relationships with friends and family centered on your illness. Learning to re-focus those relationships on health and a future together takes a new way of thinking. Expect reclaiming your place in your family and circle of friends to be challenging for everybody. Tell others how you feel and openly address their fears or questions. A counselor can help if you want an impartial moderator.

Many of the old stigmas associated with cancer still exist. Remind friends and coworkers that cancer isn't contagious and that research shows cancer survivors are just as productive as other workers.

If you experience difficulties in switching or obtaining new health insurance, find out if your state provides health insurance for people who are difficult to insure. Look into group insurance options through professional, fraternal, or political organizations.

Adjusting to life after cancer treatment means putting away old fears and uncertainties. And it means facing new ones. As you and others adapt to these changes, you may start feeling completely recovered.

(for example, transportation, meal preparation, looking after the one who is ill).

In this setting, the entire staff concerned with delivery of care meets frequently. Everyone's opinion counts, especially that of the patient. The goal is to allow the person to live his or her last days in comfort and to adequately prepare for death. The care offered to the family does not suddenly stop at the person's death—the hospice team continues to provide care for the family in the form of bereavement services.

Palliative Care

The hospice concept is not a resignation to death, as many people believe. Hospice care neither hastens nor postpones death. Rather, the hospice program emphasizes quality of life, with the focus on symptom control and psychosocial counseling rather than reversal of the disease process.

Planning the care involves educating the terminally ill patient and his or her family. In some cases, the individual with the terminal ailment can decide what medications to take and when. Careful consideration is given to all options, and a decision is made in conjunction with the hospice team.

Patient and Family

In the hospice system, patients are not passive recipients of medical care nor are the families mere bystanders. The person receiving hospice care is encouraged to make decisions about his or her treatment, relationships with other people, personal business, and preferences about burial and memorial services.

One goal of hospice care is to treat the entire unit of care—that is, the terminally ill person and the family. Efforts of the team are directed to supporting the family and its needs, as well as those of the terminally ill person. Family members may assume an active role as caregivers. They may learn to administer drugs. They also come to understand what to expect when a loved one is at the point of death.

Types of Hospices

There now are many hospices across the United States. The services are offered in a range of formats. In some instances, hospice care is offered at home but in coordination with a program at a local hospital; in some communities, there are independent hospices with no formal ties to any medical institution. Some hospitals also have rooms designated for hospice care.

Whatever the details of a particular hospice's organization, the emphasis in most programs is on home care, with short-term in-hospital care when necessary. What distinguishes the hospice is the nature of the care: the goal is to affirm life yet to accept death as a normal process. Through personalized service and a caring community of people, hospice caregivers aim to help the dying person and his or her family to prepare for a death that is inevitable.

Hospice care is covered by Medicare and many private insurance plans and, in many states, by Medical Assistance. To find what hospice services are available in your region, contact: National Hospice Organization, 1901 North Moore Street, Suite 901, Arlington, VA 22209. (For general information and referrals, call 1-800-658-8898.)

Cancer in Children

Cancer is rare in children. In addition, the most progress has been made—and the chances of cure are highest—in cancers that affect children. Only 25 years ago, almost all children with cancer died of it, usually within a year. Modern treatment now makes prolonged survival and cures not only possible but also likely with most kinds of childhood cancer. At least 70 percent of all American children with cancer now survive.

Still, many types of cancer are life-threatening, especially if they are not detected early and treated properly. Cancer remains responsible for more deaths than any other type of disease in school-age and preschool children (only accidents claim more lives in these age groups).

The most common childhood cancer is leukemia (see Leukemias, page 964). With new treatments, the outlook for children with this disease has brightened considerably in recent years. The other major class of childhood cancers are brain tumors (see page 492). Other cancers that occur in children are Wilms' tumor (a tumor of the kidney, see page 847), bone cancer (see Bone Tumors, page 899), soft tissue sarcomas (see page 888), and lymphomas (see page 968).

The causes of these cancers remain unknown. However, some agents such as certain chemicals and viruses are thought to trigger some cancers by altering the genetic material of normal cells. Cancer is not contagious. We all have oncogenes (see The Biology of Cancer, page 1291), the genes that can activate cells to become cancerous. It is not yet clear what turns them on or off.

It is important to choose carefully where to have your child treated for cancer. With the help of your child's physician, seek out a center where the staff is experienced at providing the latest advances in treatment for children with cancer. The center and its staff also should offer the emotional support that the entire family needs (see Cancer Facilities, page 1300).

A team of specialists in childhood cancer is necessary to deliver the best treatment. This therapy is complex and often requires a combination of surgery, chemotherapy, and radiation. People with the needed expertise are usually gathered only in cancer centers, children's hospitals, or large medical centers.

Such centers are often affiliated with major medical schools. Perhaps you live far from the nearest center. If so, it is usually sufficient for your child's care to be planned, started, and directed from there. In close cooperation with a cancer center staff, a local physician may be able to provide some of the treatment and interim tests. This kind of arrangement minimizes the cost and the change in location for the child and family.

Both you and your child's health-care team should prepare your child thoroughly for all the new experiences involved in these treatments. Be truthful with your child. Be supportive. Reassure your child that everybody is trying to make him or her better. Make sure that your physicians and nurses help answer all of your child's health-related questions.

How to Deal With Cancer in Your Child

Especially when it involves your child, a diagnosis of cancer often causes feelings of despair. However, modern treatment offers the hope in most children of prolonged survival and cure. With the increasing survival rates, there is a better understanding of the emotional needs of children who live with cancer and of their families.

Having a child with cancer can be very stressful for the strongest of families. Because of this, pediatric cancer teams are available to help you. They generally consist of physicians, nurses, social workers, and clergy who are trained to help families with these difficult emotions. The team provides comprehensive care that supports the entire family throughout the course of the disease. Mental health professionals are available to assist you in anticipating difficult times and in formulating a plan to cope in a psychologically healthy way. Psychosocial support mechanisms can provide guidance related to important issues such as maintaining normal family relationships, school issues, and financial burdens.

It is important to support and console your child, but it is also critical to maintain as much normalcy as possible in his or her life. Keeping schedules, rules, and previous expectations in place as appropriate conveys a message that you trust your child's ability to cope with difficulty and that, as a parent, you will help him or her prepare for a long future.

School plays a critical role in your child's life. It is important to communicate closely with school personnel to establish behavioral and academic expectations that incur normalcy. Most schools are able to provide individualized instruction if this is required during periods of intense treatment.

Although it is natural to focus on the immediate needs of your child, it is important to save time and energy for your well children too. Siblings can be very supportive to their ill brother or sister but must know their own special place in the family is secure.

Economic stress is not unusual for families with a seriously ill child. Financial burdens not only include the cost of treatment but also may involve increased travel, lodging, and child-care expenses. Incomes may be affected by disrupted work schedules. Your treatment team understands this and often can make suggestions about services that are available to lessen the strain.

The diagnosis of cancer in your child can call into question philosophical and religious beliefs. It can cause parents to feel frightened, angry, and guilty. It is important to understand that these reactions, even though intense, are normal. Members of your treatment team—physicians, nurses, social workers, and clergy—are available to support you and your family during this difficult time. In spite of the difficulties, many families develop closer, more supportive and trusting relationships as a result.

Chapter 41

Dealing With Death

Contents

Dying and Death, 1310

Terminal Illness, 1310
Should the Dying Person Be Told? 1310
The Act of Dying, 1311
Approaching Death, 1311
Role of the Chaplain or Clergy, 1311
Making Decisions, 1312

Death, 1314
The Formalities of Death, 1314
  Organ Donation, 1315
Autopsies, 1315
Bereavement, 1316
Children and Death, 1317

Dying and Death

Whether death is embraced as a part of life or viewed as a tragic loss, dealing with it rarely is easy.

The circumstances of death have a great deal to do with how we react. For most of us, the sudden and shocking death of a child is quite different from the final end to the pain of a long illness.

Because death challenges our understanding of the mystery of life, it always will be held in awe. New discoveries in science raise expectations for cures and medical miracles. As a consequence of these and other factors, when death occurs we often are more surprised than understanding and accepting of the event. Perhaps, if we can come to understand the medical and legal facts of death we may have less fear and be able to deal more immediately with the reality of death.

It is important to realize that death is quite different from dying. Death is an end point, the event in which life ceases. But dying is an essential part of the life process. For many dying persons, life's experiences still have significant meaning and importance.

Terminal Illness

Death is inevitable. But it appears in many different guises. Sometimes it is sudden and comes without warning; at other times, it marches relentlessly into a person's life.

With a terminal illness, the dying person, his or her physician, and perhaps a circle of family and friends are given time to prepare for death. They can discuss with family members issues such as nutritional support, continuation of medical treatments, and resuscitation. The dying person can make clear his or her choice as to whether an autopsy is to be performed, organs are to be donated, or the body is to be given to science, as well as review the details of funeral or burial arrangements or any business that affects a legal will.

As fearful as the reality of dying may be to many persons, the dying person usually reaches some level of acceptance. However, for the families, prolonged terminal illness brings out complicated and painful emotional reactions. In some instances, the bereaved may choose to ignore their loved one's inevitable death or to avoid any talk of it, even with the dying person. Such silence from friends and family may add to the ordeal of the terminally ill person.

Although the time of dying may be traumatic for everyone involved, it is also a time to come to terms with the passing of a life. Dying can be an occasion filled with moments of grateful remembrance and hope-filled meaning.

Should the Dying Person Be Told?

Most dying people can and should be told of their impending death. In general, dying persons want to be informed of the reality of their situations. In most cases, a properly informed person is fortified, not undermined.

Dying people often dread potential abandonment, humiliation, and loneliness at the end of their lives. They believe their personal relationships will suffer during this time and they will not be treated as normal human beings.

These concerns are reinforced if the dying person is deprived of the right to dignity and an opportunity to talk about the natural fears of, and wonderment about, death.

The person who is terminally ill may find it easier to talk to someone who is not a relative. Most hospitals have a supportive care program with trained staff members who can make it easier for the dying person and his or her family to get through this difficult time. In some instances, the psychiatric social worker or hospital chaplain can be of help when needed to make it easier for the person and family members to talk about their attitudes toward death. Once the terrible silence is broken, both the person and his or her family have the opportunity to talk about the future of family members.

The Act of Dying

Pain, both physical and emotional, is usually the principal fear of a dying person. The good news is that today the available methods of pain control make it possible to provide relief, with a minimum of side effects to compromise the comfort or dignity of the dying person.

Many large hospitals operate pain clinics or hospice programs (see Hospices, page 1255) that are staffed by teams of specialists. Most physical pain can be successfully controlled with effective painkilling drugs. Biofeedback and relaxation therapy often alleviate the sensation of pain. These approaches alone, however, cannot always relieve all of the pain, particularly the profound psychological pain of someone who is dying (see Cancer Pain, page 1303).

Dying has been characterized as a five-stage process. The initial stage is denial and isolation; anger and resentment follow as the second stage. The third stage involves an attempt to "bargain" and perhaps postpone the inevitable. A period of depression and an accompanying sense of loss follow as the fourth. Finally, at the fifth stage the dying person is able to accept the reality of impending death.

Most terminally ill people are shocked when told that they are dying. First they express disbelief. When they reach the second stage, the point at which they no longer can deny the fact of their approaching death, their bafflement may be replaced by anger. At this stage, anger and resentment may be directed toward anyone and everyone, including those helping and loving them. They often feel as if they have been cruelly robbed of the rest of their lives.

Frequently, the third stage prompts a profound question: "Why me?" At this point, the person attempts to negotiate or postpone what is inevitable. Often the person tries to bargain with God or fate; usually the desired "deal" involves a period of time without pain and discomfort. If eventually the person can surmount the denial, anger, and futile bargaining, depression may set in.

Once the depression lifts, the final stage of this process of dying often is acceptance. The acceptance does not necessarily bring happiness or even understanding. Rather, the acceptance on the part of the dying person involves an understanding that he or she can die in the manner he or she wishes.

Not everyone goes through these stages in the same manner. Some may skip a stage, others may experience two or three at the same time, and some may experience them out of order. But ultimate acceptance of one's impending death often involves these steps.

Approaching Death

The experience of dying can be strongly influenced by the behavior and attitudes of those who care for the dying person, especially loved ones. For example, dying people frequently demand they not be left alone. They fear not only the moment of death with its uncertainties but also that they might be abandoned.

Offering consolation and reassurance at these moments is difficult but necessary. Many dying people are made less fearful when comforted in the values of their faith traditions. There is comfort in being assured that most people near death don't feel pain.

There are various signs that the moment of death may be near. The dying person may become fidgety or restless and have difficulty breathing. A physician may provide medications to make the person more comfortable in such circumstances. In some cases, especially if the dying person is able, breathing can be eased if he or she can be placed in a sitting position or allowed to lie on one side with a pillow under the head.

Even though the dying person may not be able to communicate, he or she often can hear much of what is being said. Despite any sense of powerlessness you may feel, your very presence can be all the comfort the dying person seeks. Simply hold the person's hand. Physical contact at this time can be comforting. If you don't know what to say, remember that silence can be golden.

Role of the Chaplain or Clergy

The hospital chaplain or a representative of your own faith can be an invaluable resource to you.

In most hospitals, chaplains are unit-based. They work with all the patients and family members in a particular area of the hospital, regardless of religious beliefs or faith practices.

Chaplains become familiar with medical procedures and recurring concerns and questions of people admitted to a particular unit.

The chaplain's most important role is simply to provide support and act as an advocate or liaison. The hospital environment can create feelings of dependence and helplessness. A person in the hospital may feel alienated from family and friends. He or she may be unwilling to share feelings of guilt or anxiety. The chaplain can bridge communication between family members or between the patient and the medical staff.

On entering the hospital, you can request that a chaplain be involved in your care. Your chaplain will be part of your health care team and will work with your physician, nurses, therapists, and social workers. Your chaplain can also put you in touch with a clergy member of your own faith. In most hospitals, a chaplain is available to patients and family members 24 hours a day.

When terminal illness is diagnosed, people often ask questions such as "Why is this happening to me?" and "Did I do something to cause this?" A chaplain can help you explore your support systems, coping mechanisms, values, and religious beliefs to find answers to the questions you might have about suffering and dying.

Chaplains are trained in dealing with important decisions such as maintaining or discontinuing life-sustaining measures and donation of organs. If you have specific convictions that relate to your health care, your chaplain can serve as a mediator between faith and scientific communities. But most often the chaplain's role is to offer support as patient and family members make decisions. A chaplain may also provide comfort in the traditional role of offering you the chance to share in the formal rituals of your church.

Making Decisions

With the advent of modern drugs, surgical techniques, and life-sustaining technologies, medicine can prolong the lives and ease the pain of seriously ill people. In this age of extraordinary life-support capabilities, physical death due to the natural failure of the heart or lungs sometimes can be postponed until life-prolonging measures are withdrawn.

Recent legal decisions support the rights of people, and in particular those who have had a prolonged illness, to live their final days as they choose. These court decisions reflect society's evolving perspective that dying involves the whole person—not only physical but also emotional and spiritual aspects. Whenever possible, the choice of whether or not to proceed with extraordinary measures should be a matter for the dying person to decide.

Advance Directives

One of the most important conversations you can have with your physician is a frank talk about how you would wish to be treated if you can no longer communicate.

Advance directives, including living wills and documents granting durable power of attorney for health care, are legal documents that go into effect if you are no longer able to make decisions about your health care.

Advance directives may simply state your values and beliefs, or may give specific information about the types of medical care and life-sustaining measures you do or don't want implemented.

Your physician can talk to you about creating advance directives. The physician, hospital staff, or business office can help you find resources explaining your state's laws and forms to get you started. (For more information on advance directives, see page 1248. For examples of forms used to designate a durable power of attorney for health care or to state your wishes with a living will, see page 1381.)

Discontinuing, Withholding, or Limiting Treatment

You need not—and should not—wait until you are terminally ill to participate in decisions made about the treatment you are to receive. And your wishes should be communicated to all caregivers.

A serious illness may reach a point at which further treatment may just prolong the process of dying. At this point, you and your family, with help from your physician and perhaps a clergy member, may agree to stop further treatment except to ease pain and provide comfort. You and your family also may decide not to carry out cardiopulmonary resuscitation.

Decisions that involve highly sensitive ethical matters may bring out differences of opinion among family members. Intentionally removing life-support systems may not present a dilemma for someone who sees the choice only in terms of death with dignity. For another relative, removing life-support systems would violate deep beliefs about the preservation of life.

The correct course of action is not always obvious. Discussions in the family may grow heated and give rise to yet more questions. This is why it's best to communicate your feelings early and clearly to those whom you entrust with decisions about care at the end of life.

Laws regarding living wills often include a disclaimer specifying that the law's intent is not to authorize euthanasia or assisted suicide. The Council on Ethical and Judicial Affairs of the American Medical Association has made it very clear that "euthanasia" is a euphemism for the intentional killing of a person and that this is not part of the practice of medicine, whether or not there is such a request from the patient. The Council statement further notes that the intentional termination of the life of one human being by another (so-called mercy killing) is contrary to public policy, medical tradition, and the most fundamental measures of human value and worth.

The American College of Physicians draws a firm line between not starting or withdrawing life-sustaining interventions and euthanasia or assisted suicide. Medical killing would involve the administration of a lethal agent (such as a deliberate overdose of morphine) to a person with the clear intention of causing immediate death. Although a mentally competent person may refuse medical therapies and the physician must comply with this refusal, the physician should never intentionally and directly cause death or assist a patient to commit suicide. This type of euthanasia remains illegal in most of the United States. Even if legalized, according to the American College of Physicians, such an action would violate the ethical standards of medical practice.

The boundary between euthanasia (an act of willfully ending a life) and death with dignity will not always be clear. Some treatments have a double effect. On one hand, the primary effect of a narcotic such as morphine is to relieve pain, but, on the other hand, an inescapable secondary effect is depression of the ability to breathe, which can lead to death.

Life-supporting medical technology is a double-edged sword. Its use has permitted physicians to resuscitate patients who might not have survived several decades ago. But this new ability brings with it complicated moral problems never encountered before. For physicians, one of the biggest challenges is to continue to keep the dying person and members of the family informed of potential "heroic measures." For most people, the challenge is to discover, often by discussion with their physician, the personal impact of life-sustaining treatments. It is the well-informed patient who is most likely to make wise decisions about medical treatment.

"Do Not Resuscitate" Orders

The directive "do not resuscitate" (DNR) means that cardiopulmonary resuscitation (CPR) is not to be done when the person's heart stops or the person stops breathing.

CPR is intended to be used when the threat of death occurs suddenly and unexpectedly in an apparently healthy person. It is rarely if ever appropriate in a patient with a terminal, irreversible illness when death is expected at any time. Furthermore, CPR is rarely effective for elderly persons outside the hospital, when it's difficult to determine when their hearts stopped or they stopped breathing.

The initials DNR are usually prominently displayed on the charts of patients in hospitals or nursing homes when it has been decided that CPR is not to be used. The decision to place DNR on the chart is made by the patient and the physician; if the patient is not competent, it is made by the relatives and the physician. Sometimes the decision is part of a living will (see page 1248).

The decision as to whether or not to use CPR shouldn't have to be made in an emergency situation. This is the reason for making the decision early and making everyone who might be involved aware of it. Placing DNR on a patient's chart does not imply that any lesser quality of care will be given.

In addition to deciding about the use of CPR, questions regarding use of other life-sustaining measures such as antibiotics, kidney dialysis, blood transfusions, and respirators (aids to breathing) will arise in the care of the person with a terminal illness. It is best that discussions of such measures be carried out before the patient has lost his or her decision-making capacity and before a medical crisis has occurred.

Another issue is whether to use artificial feeding, usually by means of a tube through the nose into the stomach, to treat an otherwise healthy person who becomes permanently unconscious. There are several difficult questions: Is an unconscious person completely unaware of his or her surroundings? If feedings are discontinued, will the person experience thirst and hunger? Is withdrawal of such feeding for an otherwise nonterminally ill person a form of euthanasia?

Euthanasia includes a practice sometimes referred to as assisted suicide in which one person furnishes the means for another person to end his or her life. This can imply tacit encouragement for the person to proceed with the suicide. But euthanasia is not the same as withholding treatment that might be lifesaving. An example might be the decision not to use antibiotics when pneumonia develops in a terminally ill person. The decision to accept or reject medical treatment is an appropriate ethical and legal action.

Many difficult decisions are made in the care of a terminally ill person. In making such decisions, unique factors must be weighed. Although there are no rules, general principles of ethical behavior for physicians are formulated and revised from time to time by authoritative sources such as the American Medical Association and the American College of Physicians.

Death

Of late we have developed the capacity to keep people alive in circumstances in which it was not possible in years past. Consequently, these new life-sustaining technologies have virtually transformed our definitions of death.

Only a few years ago, anyone who had lost consciousness, was unable to breathe, and had no heartbeat was considered to be dead. Today, however, in some instances life-support systems can revive such a person and, in part, continue to support or to replace some of these necessary functions. Physicians now are often able to maintain heart or lung function even when the entire brain ceases to function. This remarkable ability to sustain life brings with it certain ethical, legal, and medical problems.

Most states recognize that a person is legally dead when there is either irreversible cessation of circulation and respiration or irreversible cessation and function of the entire brain including the brainstem (which controls breathing).

The Formalities of Death

Death is a legal event that calls for several formalities. Before a funeral can take place, you must secure a medical death certificate that shows the cause of death and formally registers the death. In some instances, the death may have to be investigated by the medical examiner or the coroner, and an autopsy may be ordered An autopsy provides more information about a person's illness; it may be required by law if the death resulted from an accident, is unexpected and unexplained, or is a suspected homicide or suicide (see Autopsies, page 1315). After these matters are resolved, the family usually works with a funeral home on any final arrangements.

The death certificate is a legal document that certifies the cause of death. It is completed by a licensed physician who usually has been in attendance at the time of death. If the physician has examined or treated the patient regularly or shortly prior to death, he or she generally is not obliged to examine the body before signing the certificate.

Sometimes, deaths must be investigated by the medical examiner or coroner. He or she will establish the cause of death and sign the certificate rather than the family physician or the physician in attendance.

The funeral director can be helpful in making virtually all of your other decisions concerning the funeral and burial arrangements. You may even want to make these arrangements before or during the time of the terminal illness.

First, the funeral director will come to the home or hospital to remove the body and take it to the funeral home. Later, members of the family will meet with the funeral director (usually at the funeral home) to discuss arrangements. Family members should make it quite clear how elaborate or simple the funeral will be and how the details are to be handled. Because these are emotionally difficult times and funeral arrangements can be expensive, you may want to seek help in making these decisions from someone who is not personally involved, such as a member of the clergy, a close friend, or an attorney.

Funeral and burial decisions include the type and location of the funeral service and the final disposition of the remains (that is, burial or cremation). If the body is to be donated to research, the funeral director will deliver the body to the designated institution.

Funeral ceremonies can be held at the funeral home or a place of worship or both. If the family has religious affiliation, the funeral director can recommend a member of the clergy or appropriate authority. In addition to the funeral service, there is often a brief ceremony at the grave site.

Fees and terms of payment are made with the funeral director at the time funeral arrangements are made. Usually, payment is not required in advance, but these expenses become the first legal obligation of the estate of the deceased.

After the funeral, a probate judge will designate the executor or personal representative of the estate. This is often a member of the family, the family attorney, or a close friend. The executor is responsible for the financial affairs of the deceased, which may include the funeral expenses.

After all payments are made, any remaining assets are distributed according to the deceased's will or the laws of the state in which the person lived. Specific procedures may vary from state to state.

Autopsies

"Autopsy" comes from Greek words meaning "to see with one's own eyes." It is a detailed examination of the body to determine the cause of death. It is performed by a medical specialist, a pathologist, who reports findings to the attending physician. On request, the attending physician will discuss findings with the family.

In the 1940s, an autopsy was performed after about half of all hospital deaths; but autopsies now occur only 10 to 15 percent of the time. Some physicians believe modern diagnostic measures performed during the life of the patient establish the cause of death so well that autopsy is superfluous. Others think that today's sophisticated technology

---

Organ Donation

As a result of technologic advances, livers, corneas, hearts, kidneys, and other organs and tissues now can be transplanted. However, these operations are possible only when the needed organs are donated.

If you're willing to donate organs for use after your death, register as a designated organ donor. You can do this either by executing a living will or, in some states, by having a notation added to your driver's license. In some cases, the pain of an impending death may be eased by arranging for an organ donation that saves the life of another person—or even, in some cases, several persons.

Organ transplantation is less common at hospitals outside major medical centers. However, all hospitals are required by law to inform relatives of potential donors about the United Network for Organ Sharing (UNOS), established in 1984 by the National Organ Transplantation Act. UNOS maintains an extensive computer network to ensure equitable distribution of donated organs.

If you would like to become an organ donor, discuss the procedure for UNOS registration with your physician or a local hospital administrator.

---

has replaced autopsy as a way to help educate young physicians on understanding how a disease affects the human body. In many cases, families are reluctant to permit an autopsy. They believe the procedure is degrading or that the deceased has "suffered enough."

All of these factors add up to a marked decline in autopsies. This is unfortunate because they still play an important role.

Benefits to the Surviving Family Members

Hereditary Disorders
Autopsy may reveal conditions that affect children and siblings. For example, if polycystic kidney disease (see page 831) is found, close relatives of childbearing age may want genetic counseling before they have children.

Emotional Security
Family members may feel they could have prevented the death. In the case of a fatal heart attack, they might berate themselves for not insisting their loved one take it easier. An autopsy may reveal that the person had a preexisting heart condition that could have taken his or her life at any time.

Insurance Settlements
Knowing the cause of death can help resolve disputes that affect the benefits survivors

receive. If a person with a heart problem dies from a fall, insurance benefits may vary depending on whether death was accidental or the result of the heart ailment.

Benefits to Medical Science

Much of what we know about diseases, including statistical information, was discovered and confirmed through autopsies.

Advances in medical knowledge depend in part on study of human tissue removed at autopsy. Pathologic observations truly have taught us a great deal about human disease. For example, such data helped to confirm the association between cigarette smoking and lung cancer.

Autopsies discovered the nature and character of hyperparathyroidism (see page 950) and viral hepatitis (see page 801), and the effects of toxic chemicals and other industrial hazards on the lungs.

Quality Assurance

Physicians use autopsy data to assess their accuracy in diagnosis and treatment. Autopsy findings also help measure the overall quality of care in a hospital and community.

Vital Statistics

The causes of death keep changing. Deaths from infectious diseases are less common today, but degenerative illness takes a greater toll. Public health officials use information from autopsies to monitor these trends. Death statistics influence government spending for health care, the enactment of safety standards, and the design of medical equipment.

Emerging Illness

Early medical understanding of AIDS, legionnaires' disease, and toxic shock syndrome all came from autopsy studies.

Arranging for an Autopsy

Autopsies usually are required by state or local law when death results from an accident, is unexpected or unexplained, or is a suspected homicide or suicide. Otherwise, autopsies require the permission of the next of kin.

Read the consent form carefully. When you sign the consent form, you can authorize only a limited autopsy that restricts the procedure to specific parts of the body. However, this limits the amount of useful information and often leaves questions unanswered. The procedure is usually handled discreetly and in a confidential manner. Consent forms generally permit removal of internal organs and tissue.

There are many misconceptions about autopsy and tissue removal. For example, a properly done autopsy will not disfigure the body; at an open-casket funeral service observers won't be able to tell an autopsy was performed. Autopsy does not interfere with embalming of the body, nor need it delay the funeral. Also, the majority of religious faiths allow autopsy.

In most instances, when you grant permission for an elective autopsy, the bill will be paid by the hospital. Medicare won't pay for the procedure. When death occurs outside a hospital and family members request an autopsy, they usually must pay for it.

If you want an autopsy performed after your death, make a provision in your advance directive (see page 1248) that refers to this elective procedure. Then be sure to notify your loved ones of the provision. Knowing your preference will spare your loved ones the burden of decision making during a time of grief.

We believe physicians should recommend autopsies more often and survivors should request them more frequently. Without the data gained from autopsies, family members may have to cope with lingering questions that might have been answered. Furthermore, valuable information is lost on the possible cause and effectiveness of treatment of many diseases, especially cancer and heart disease. Through autopsy findings, the dead can help the living.

Bereavement

We experience many losses throughout our lives, and the longer we live, the more losses we suffer. Bereavement is your response to a loss. It usually refers to subjective feelings after the loss of a loved one, usually through death, but also after the dissolution of a relationship. Our ability to adapt to the stress of these losses in our lives often influences our health.

When grief disrupts our daily routines, our health can be negatively affected. Grief and the loneliness of loss can contribute to depression, excessive use of alcohol, and even suicide.

The death of a loved one is never easy to accept, and a sudden loss can be especially distressing. However, a long, terminal illness before the death can be emotionally, physically, and financially draining. To protect yourself from a grief-related illness, take care of your health. Monitor any medical problems you had before the loss and seek professional help if new symptoms develop.

Although there are cultural norms for mourning, there is no single right way to grieve, nor is there a fixed timetable for coping with grief. Some people may seem to return to normal emotions and activities within a month, but bereavement more often is measured in years rather than weeks or months.

During your bereavement, seek help from clergy, friends, and counselors. And remember, it is entirely appropriate—and essential for both your mental and your physical health—to express your emotions. Healthy mourning is the process that helps us accept our losses so we can go on with our lives. Suppressing your emotions through excess activity, work, alcohol, or drugs may prolong the mourning process.

People cope with their grief in different ways. This can be explained partly by differences in cultural heritage. Some people grieve openly, others privately. And it is not always evident someone is grieving. Nevertheless, grief needs to be expressed or processed so it can be healed. If it's not, symptoms such as erratic behavior or failing health may appear (see Grief Responses, page 1109).

Children and Death

Children are often overlooked in times of grief. But death is a crisis that should be shared by everyone in the family. Children may experience a silence and secrecy that isolate them from the rest of the family and deny them the opportunity to grieve with other family members.

Telling a child that a parent is going to die, or that the child is dying, is difficult for everyone, including physicians and nurses. At the same time, children have a right to know about anything that affects them or their families. Not telling them is a breach of trust and, in truth, most children, like adults, have a sort of sixth sense that alerts them when something is wrong.

Why They Need to Know

Children can sense when a parent is seriously ill, but young children in particular usually can't interpret their suspicions. If left alone with his or her suspicions, the small child may somehow feel responsible for the illness or death of a parent. They need help integrating their observations into day-to-day reality.

When told the truth in a language they can understand, most children have a remarkable capacity for dealing with truth. Even the weight of very sad truths is preferable to the anxiety of too much uncertainty. If you talk with them, they won't feel cut off from that part of the family that "knows." In turn, you won't need to be so secretive. You may even find your young children can be a comfort to you and others. Instead of burdening them with the darkness of unspoken fears, discussing the issue of death and loss with them permits them to live more freely.

Your local library and bookstore are good resources for books that explain death and dying in terms young children can understand.

When and From Whom?

When should children be told? The simple answer is, as soon as possible. Children should be told about their loved one's health status immediately after the initial diagnosis. Keep them informed as treatment progresses and tell them how it is affecting the person's health. Any change in appearance or disposition should not go unexplained. Children of different ages should probably be told individually; but after the initial disclosure, efforts should be made to make it a shared experience among all the children.

It is generally best for a parent or both parents together to tell the child or children. And your tears are not to be disguised. On the contrary, they give permission for your child to cry and to grieve with you. If you aren't available or are unable to tell the child, ask a friend or relative who is close to your child. Finally, the task can be left to a nurse or physician. However, a young child may consider them strangers whose word is subject to disbelief.

How Much Information?

Children need to be told as much as they can understand. There is no single "right" way to tell children about death. They should be told what has happened and what will happen. Parents should be guided by their own styles and what they feel comfortable in discussing. At all times children should be told that no matter what the outcome they will always be loved. They should be encouraged to ask questions, and these questions should be answered simply. Their fears may keep them from asking questions, so encourage them by asking them how they feel. At no time should you lie, make promises you may not be able to keep, or be afraid to say, "I don't know."

How Will They Respond?

Young children fear being separated from their parents. Being left in the care of strangers may suggest they've been abandoned. During this period, discipline can be difficult because they may need to seek attention. If you suspend the normal rules of conduct, it may be alarming to them. It's more appropriate to reassure children of your love while expecting the same cooperation and good behavior from them. As the children come to learn what is happening, they should be assured that nothing they said or did, including any possible bad behavior, caused the illness or death.

Very young children (younger than 3 years) believe everything is possible; there are no limits to their parents' powers. To preschoolers, death is still reversible; nothing is final. School-age children younger than 9 usually understand that death is a biologic event rather than someone appearing or disappearing in a supernatural form. But it is only at about age 9 that they're able to grasp death as the final, irreversible end of human life.

School-age children can become overly concerned about details and misjudge their significance. Guard against overwhelming them with specific data. Teachers and school counselors can be helpful in weighing the gravity and meaning of the information the children have learned from you.

After the Death of a Parent

The death of a parent is a powerful event in the life of a child. Many children are able to resume a normal lifestyle in a matter of weeks. Others suffer the effects of an unhealed wound throughout their childhood and adult lives. Why one child is able to deal with the death of a parent and another is not depends in part on how the child is told and how the rest of the family accepts the loss.

Children initially may deny the reality of the death, express anger, or act out in rebellion. They also may repress any feelings associated with the loss. Children should be encouraged to share their emotional experience to whatever degree they can. Allow their friends to come into the home during the time of mourning. Their friends can be a comfort, and the friends' knowing about the death can deepen the reality of the loss for the child.

Keep in mind that children have a remarkable capacity for adjustment. The changes they see in themselves, in the world around them, and in those who surround them constitute an endless string of events to be absorbed. Whether the news is bad or good, children usually succeed in working their way through life's events—even those that seem unfair and unreasonable, like the death of a beloved parent.

Chapter 42

Home Care and Elder Care

Contents

Home Health Services, 1320
Sources of Help, 1320
  Choosing an Agency, 1321
Reimbursement for Services, 1321
Equipment Needs, 1322

Home Health Care, 1322
Selecting a Location, 1323
Medications, 1323
Making the Bed, 1323
Mealtimes, 1323
Bathing, 1324

Bedpans and Bed Urinals, 1324
Bedsores, 1325
Vomiting, 1325
Returning to Independence, 1325

Rehabilitation Programs, 1326

Adult Day Care, 1327

Independent Living Centers, 1328
  Group Homes for the Developmentally
  Disabled and Mentally Ill, 1328

Home Health Services

For many people, the best place to get well is at home. During illness or recuperation from an injury, the sophisticated medical facilities and specialized professional staff of a hospital often are unnecessary. Similarly, services provided by a nursing home are not needed. As you recover from most illnesses or injuries, your own home is the most comfortable place to be.

Another major advantage of care at home is that it may be less costly. When given the choice, people tend to feel better, eat better, and get well quicker at home. In the following pages, the whys and wherefores of home care are introduced. The types of home health services that are available to assist with home care are described. Also covered are vocational rehabilitation programs, adult day care, and independent living centers.

Sources of Help

Skilled medical, nursing, and rehabilitation services may be available right in your home by outside organizations. These kinds of assistance are known collectively as home health services. Many organizations in the United States provide home health services, including several private companies such as the Visiting Nurse Association (which began in the 19th century), hospitals, nursing homes, community social service agencies, and city and county health departments.

Services available to you depend on your needs and the particular program or programs that exist in your area. Agencies that offer skilled nursing care can provide a nursing service to monitor your health status, give injections, change bandages, and perform other nursing tasks. Sometimes various forms of therapy are also available in the home, including physical, occupational, speech, hearing, and respiratory therapies. Most agencies provide social workers and some even have dental care, laboratory testing, and pharmacy services. Meals and housekeeping services may be available.

Home-care agencies that offer such skilled nursing, therapeutic, and supplemental services do so under the direction of your physician. A medically trained case worker or case manager may be responsible for coordinating the care provided to you or the individual in need of the help.

Many organizations offer supportive rather than skilled services. With these, a home aide regularly spends time in the home, perhaps every day, although in some cases alternate days or even once a week is sufficient. The aide may help with basic tasks such as bathing, dressing, shopping, cooking, eating, and doing housekeeping chores. A home aide also can handle certain simple nursing tasks, such as taking a temperature. For many people, help with some everyday activities can make it possible to continue living independently at home rather than in a nursing home. Some home health aides will move in with you, although they are not widely available.

Since the 1960s, a home service that has improved the lives of countless elderly people is Meals on Wheels. Local Meals on Wheels services often are administered through senior citizens centers. In many communities, this service delivers one hot, nutritional meal a day at a low cost, either 5 or 7 days a week. Meals on Wheels is a great help to people who find it difficult to prepare a balanced meal. Some communities also have other nutrition services such as group dining for the elderly.

To find out which services are available where you live, ask a hospital dismissal planner, a social worker, your local or county health department, senior citizens center, or your physician. In addition, churches, synagogues, welfare departments, and charitable organizations such as the United Way often can provide information on services available. You can also look in the Yellow Pages under "Nurses" or "Home Health Agencies."

If you live in an area that has multiple home care alternatives, compare the services offered. Important points to consider are whether your insurer approves payment to the agency, whether the services match your present and future needs, the amount of medical or skilled supervision that the agency offers, which hours a day or week are covered, and whether replacement aides are available to fill in when regularly assigned individuals cannot come. Speak with people who have actually used the service to get their opinions.

Medicare, Medicaid, private insurance, and other programs often pay for home health services, although usually with limitations (see Reimbursement for Services, this page). A prescreening evaluation may be required.

Reimbursement for Services

Home health services are paid for in five main ways: by Medicare, Medicaid, insurance carriers, health maintenance organizations, or the person being cared for (or the family), sometimes on a sliding-fee scale.

Understand Your Coverage
The sources listed here may provide partial or total reimbursement for home health services. However, determining exactly what coverage a particular source offers may not be easy.

Begin by reading the insurance policy (not merely a brochure summarizing the benefits). Then speak to a knowledgeable person in the organization. Persist until you are able to determine exactly what the benefits are. Home health services may be referred to under a different name or under a broader category, so even if it appears at first that home care services are not covered, be sure you read the fine print or have it explained to you.

Regardless of the type of coverage, there will be limits, as with any insurance policy. In the case of home health services, limits usually are placed on the types of services (for example, skilled nursing), the length of visits (the number of hours), and the number of visits (for example, per week, per year, or for the life of the policy).

Medicare
Medicare covers people age 65 years or older as well as some disabled people. Medicare pays for some, but not all, home health services. Visits by nurses or by physical, speech, or other therapists may be covered. The services of someone to help with chores around the house and with bathing and dressing generally are not covered. However, personal care services such as bathing and dressing can be covered by Medicare if skilled services such as nursing, speech, or other therapy are being provided. For more information, contact your social worker, your local Social Security Administration office, or senior citizens center.

Choosing an Agency

If you are considering contracting the services of a home health care agency, here are 10 important questions you should ask:

1. Is the agency certified by Medicare or Medicaid?

2. What services does the agency offer?

3. What are the costs of various services?

4. What is the professional training of the nursing staff? (Does the agency employ registered nurses and licensed practical nurses? Who is the nursing supervisor?)

5. How many hours of training do homemaker or home health aides receive?

6. What geographic area does the agency serve?

7. What are the agency's operating hours? (Does it provide care on weekends? Is 24-hour care available?)

8. Who assumes responsibility for care given?

9. Are agency employees insured and bonded?

10. Will the agency maintain communication with your physician?

Medicaid
Medicaid covers people of all ages with low incomes, but coverage varies from state to state. Some home health services may be covered in your state but, again, inquire at your local social services or Social Security Administration office.

Private Insurance Carriers
Private insurance policies may pay for some home health services. Find out from the person who handles benefits at your place of employment, from your insurance agent, or directly from the insurance company.

Other Sources
In addition to the medical insurance your company provides or that you buy for yourself, do not overlook two other possible sources of reimbursement: automobile insurance policies (if you were injured in an automobile accident) and workers' compensation insurance (if you were injured on the job).

Health Maintenance Organizations

Health maintenance organizations (HMOs) generally offer some home care on a limited basis. Coverage will vary depending on the rules of the particular organization. Ask an administrator at your HMO (see page 1266).

Direct Payment

Home health services can be paid for directly. Most nonprofit and government-aided home health care organizations, when their costs are not completely covered by the sources mentioned above, bill for their services on a sliding-fee scale based on ability to pay. For-profit private agencies generally do not use a sliding-fee scale.

Equipment Needs

If you are cared for at home, you may require or benefit from special equipment, such as a wheelchair, walker, or even a hospital bed.

This is often called "durable medical equipment." Some drugstores and medical supply houses rent, sell, and service such items.

For expensive equipment, renting is a money-saving alternative because the need for the equipment may be temporary. Drugstores and medical supply houses often stock a range of other sickroom supplies useful in home care.

Alternatively, the American Cancer Society, the Arthritis Foundation, the Easter Seal Society, the American Diabetes Association, and other comparable organizations sometimes are able to lend medical and nursing equipment.

Talk to your physical therapist, hospital dismissal planner, social worker, or physician; they may be aware of wholesale distributors or other sources of these goods at reasonable prices. Do not hesitate to shop around. Even if you are buying only medication, the monthly costs can be high, and the retail price may vary greatly.

Home Health Care

At some point, everyone needs home care. For most of us, a childhood illness meant staying home and being nursed back to health. As adults with a minor illness such as the flu or a cold, we recover at home. Home care for a more serious or prolonged condition is essentially a variation on the same, familiar theme.

The home health care industry is a growing one, due to many factors. Medical insurance reimbursements are tighter. Increasing numbers of people with AIDS require long-term care. People age 85 or older are the fastest-growing age group in America today, and the average person in this group has three major chronic health problems for which he or she will eventually need health care services.

Hospitals dismiss patients sooner and treat more people on an outpatient basis. This means that some people who are recovering from accidents, from opera-

tions, from illnesses such as cancer, heart attacks, or strokes, or from chronic conditions such as diabetes must recover at home. The requirements of the person being cared for vary with his or her daily activities, the available services, and the other caregivers in the household. Most often, total responsibility falls on the shoulders of one person; sometimes the burden is simply too much for the health and well-being of that individual.

To meet these varied needs, home health care agencies employ people with a wide range of skills. Their services range from help with bathing and dressing to temporary, round-the-clock assistance. In addition, certain developments and retirement communities provide assisted-care living, transitional care, and respite care. What you choose depends on your needs; home care should lie within the limits of a family's physical, emotional, and financial resources.

Selecting a Location

Locate the room used for home health care on the ground floor, ideally near a bathroom. The reasons are safety and to save the person requiring home care the risk (and energy drain) of having to negotiate stairs. In addition, the caregiver is saved the time and trouble of trips up and down the stairs many times a day.

If possible, move the person's bed into the new room. Sometimes a small thing such as sleeping in one's own bed offers a psychological lift. If falling out of bed is a possibility, add a guardrail. If a special bed is required, a hospital bed may be available from a medical supply store or drugstore.

Unless the person being cared for has serious disabilities, not only the bedroom but also other rooms may need some changes. A recliner or other comfortable chair should be available. It may be necessary to try out several to find one that suits the physical abilities of the individual.

Arrange the bedroom and the parts of the house where the person will spend the most time for maximal comfort and convenience. A bedside table or the type of table that fits over the bed is a must.

Because a person's quality of life and recovery are linked to one's sense of well-being, a feeling of independence should be provided. If the person values familiar objects, place them in the room, ideally in their usual places. Items of convenience— remote control for the television, a telephone, books and magazines, tissues, a wastebasket—should be within reach of the person whose mobility is limited. Some items might be kept in a bedside caddy that fastens onto the side of the bed.

At the same time, make sure that the bed, table, and other areas are easily accessible to caregivers. Remove objects that can be readily tripped over, such as throw rugs or unnecessary furniture.

Alternatively, encouraging mobility may be a part of the recovery process. Do not make life too easy for the person who should be gaining strength and independence. One way to encourage someone to get out of a bed that has been rendered perhaps too comfortable is to locate some items of interest—such as magazines, the television, or the recliner—across the room or in a different room.

Medications

One of the main functions of a nurse in a hospital is to give the correct medications at the proper times. At home, this becomes the responsibility of the caregiver.

Make sure that medicines are given exactly as the physician prescribes, in both dose and frequency. Know medications by their dosage (usually in milligrams) as well as by their color and shape. Always be alert to the possibility of side effects. Ask the physician which side effects to watch for. Sometimes multiple medications interact in ways a physician did not anticipate. If the person you are caring for develops unexpected, new, or worsening symptoms, call the physician. Use a medication dispenser (available in pharmacies) to properly administer medications. A home health care nurse can help you set up a system.

Making the Bed

If the person spends a great deal of time in bed, change the sheets, covers, and pillowcases frequently. If the person is in bed all the time, make the bed every morning and evening. Tuck in the sheets. Cotton sheets are preferable to synthetic sheets because they absorb moisture.

An old mattress that slopes to the side can present a hazard for falling while getting in and out of bed. Replace it with a firmer new one or put a bed board beneath it.

The person probably will prefer more than one pillow, arranged so that the head and shoulders are supported. Occasionally turning the pillows over provides a thoughtful touch of comfort. To prevent the development of sores, change the person's position frequently—back, and side-to-side—and place pillows between the knees.

Use props and wedges to help someone sit up in bed. Place a cushion between the feet and the board at the foot of the bed to prevent discomfort from pressure in the raised or sitting position.

Mealtimes

Meals are a social activity and a key source of pleasure for someone who must spend a great deal of time in bed. Follow diet instructions given by the physician, nutritional therapist, or nurse. Vary the diet as much as possible, and include foods the person especially enjoys. Enhance the pleasure of mealtime with appropriate treats, careful food preparation, and attractive presentation. Eat with the person to add a sense of "normalcy" to the meal.

Many people confined to their beds can still feed themselves from a tray beside the bed or from an over-the-bed table. Use bendable straws for the beverages. If the person cannot eat alone and needs to use a spoon, you may find that pureed and finely cut foods are the easiest for you or another caregiver to serve and for the sick person to eat. Test foods to be sure that they are not too hot. To keep them warm, use insulated dishes or single-serving vacuum containers.

If the person you're caring for cannot or will not eat the food, or loses weight, report these problems to the physician or visiting nurse.

Bathing

Bathing presents a special challenge in home care. Bathing is a personal activity that people generally prefer doing alone. To help retain as much privacy as possible, helpful bathing products may be rented or purchased.

Often all that is required is a tub bench (a special seat that runs across the bathtub) or a grabrail mounted on the wall near the tub. With such aids, the person with impaired balance or limited mobility may be able to get safely in and out of the tub or shower alone. Place a nonslip rubber mat or adhesive strips on the tub bottom; make sure that there is no towel or mat on the floor that the person can slip on. Help with bathing can be a valuable service from a home care professional.

In considering bathroom safety, remember that another bathroom danger is burns. Disabled people may find themselves trapped in a running bath or shower, unable to move away from water that has suddenly turned scalding hot (or, for that matter, icy cold). The temperature of the hot water can be adjusted at the hot water tank. Set the temperature no higher than is necessary for washing dishes or clothes. Faucets are available (and are required by law in new construction in some states) that automatically turn off when the water exceeds a preset temperature.

Put a bell or cordless intercom in the bathroom so the person can summon help if necessary.

The person who is unable to leave the bed to bathe can have a sponge bath. The following suggestions may make the task easier, and may help prevent sores:

1. Place a disposable or rubber pad under the person.

2. Uncover and wash a small part of the body at a time, to avoid chilling. Start at the top (head) and work to the bottom (feet).

3. Use comfortably warm water. Place a towel between the part of the body being washed and the bed.

4. Use soap sparingly, mainly on the face, under the arms, and for the genital area. Remember, soap is an irritant if it is not rinsed off.

5. When drying, pat with the towel rather than rubbing. (Rubbing can encourage bedsores.) Take special care to dry skin folds and, in women, beneath the breasts.

Bedpans and Bed Urinals

The person unable to leave the bed requires a bedpan or (for men) bed urinal. A few simple considerations can make their use a little easier.

Keep the pan or urinal in a warm and easily accessible place; a cold container can be a disagreeable shock.

When positioning the pan for use, maneuver it under the buttocks. If the person cannot sit, roll him or her to the side, slide the pan under (pressing it down into the mattress as far as possible), and roll the person back.

Privacy is as important—perhaps more so—to the bed-bound person as to the rest of us, so provide as much as possible. Leave the room or draw a curtain while the person is actually using the bedpan. Be patient, making sure to allow the person enough time.

Many people are able to get up out of bed but are unable to make the trip to the bathroom, particularly if the bathroom is a long walk or a flight of stairs away. In such cases, a commode may be the solution. A commode is simply a chair with a toilet-like attachment under the bottom, which can be removed for easy cleaning. After use, immediately empty. An apparatus designed to assist in lifting a person to reach the commode is available.

If the person can reach the bathroom, the toilet may require some modification for safe use. A grabrail on the wall near the toilet, or freestanding rails on either side of the toilet, can be installed. If the toilet is too low, special seats that raise the height are available.

Bedsores

Bedsores, also known as pressure sores or decubitus ulcers, sometimes develop on weight-bearing parts of the body, especially where the bones are near the skin (in particular, the hips, shoulder blades, elbows, base of the spine, knees, ankles, and heels). In some individuals, just a few hours of constant pressure can be enough to initiate a bedsore.

A bedsore begins as a reddened, sensitive patch of skin and progresses to a sore or ulcer. It may or may not be painful. Treatment of a bedsore requires the attention of a nurse or physician, and healing may take a long time. Prevention is therefore the best approach.

Prevent bedsores by frequent repositioning. Encourage the bedridden person to move regularly to keep pressure from building on one spot. If the person cannot move alone, help him or her. Change position at least every 2 hours. Use pillows or foam wedges to shift the load of a heavy or paralyzed individual.

Splints placed at pressure points are also helpful. Special anatomically shaped cushions, such as those used in wheelchairs, can be placed in the bed to distribute weight more evenly and keep pressure from building in one spot. Also helpful are synthetic sheepskin bed pads, air mattresses, and "egg-crate" pads (foam padding resembling the cardboard packaging in which eggs are traditionally sold). Specially designed pads for heels and elbows are also available. You can rent bed cradles from medical supply stores; these raise the weight of covers off the body and create a tent-like structure.

Changes in bedding, drying thoroughly after baths, a balanced diet, and exercise are important for avoiding bedsores. Even the bed-bound person can exercise; if the person cannot do it alone, then movement of the joints by others will help prevent bedsores.

Vomiting

If the person is liable to vomit, keep a bowl within easy reach. Some people can handle vomiting on their own and prefer to be left alone until they are done. Others feel comforted with someone nearby. In either case, offer water to rinse out the person's mouth afterward, and sponge off his or her face.

Avoid solid food after a vomiting episode. Encourage liquids to replace lost body fluids. The nurse or physician can advise on which liquids are best. Tea, diluted fruit juice, water, chicken broth, and gelatin are among the liquids most easily tolerated. If the vomiting is a new symptom, inform your physician.

Returning to Independence

Home care is not static. Whether the care at home follows dismissal from a hospital or the occurrence of an illness or disability that is treated at home from the start, the ultimate aim of convalescence is a return to one's former status.

Convalescence presents special challenges for the caregiver. There are common pitfalls to avoid. For example, avoid becoming so bound up in the job of delivering care or coordinating home health services that you forget the ultimate goal: a return to independence.

Sometimes the person being cared for becomes needlessly accustomed to being waited on. This pattern can prolong care beyond what the condition warrants. The ill or injured person—whether child or adult, male or female—can consciously or unconsciously perpetuate the period of care. A return to normal activities can be retarded or even put off altogether.

If you are the patient, do not confine yourself to bed. Getting out of bed and moving about is an important aspect of home care unless your physician recommends otherwise. When you remain confined to bed, your unused muscles weaken and bone loss accelerates (see Osteoporosis, page 894). The longer the time spent in bed, the more difficult it becomes to regain mobility. Moreover, some potentially fatal infections and conditions, such as pneumonia (see page 704), thrombophlebitis (see page 694), and pulmonary embolism (see page 734), are more likely to develop in persons who are confined to bed.

Approach getting up for the first few times carefully and gradually. Your blood pressure and balance need to adjust. Sit on the edge of the bed a few minutes before trying to stand up. Standing or even sitting up the first few times may make you feel dizzy and weak. Next, take a short, slow trip from your bed to a recliner or chair. Have someone assist you if you are unsteady. As your strength increases and you regain the ability to move about, the trips can become longer, with less assistance required.

A physical or occupational therapist (or both) can be useful during convalescence. Physical therapists recommend exercises aimed at specific disabilities as well as at general recovery. They also might offer massage, ultrasound therapy, and other healing treatments. Occupational therapists help you relearn particular skills useful in daily living, how to use prostheses or mechanical devices, and how to make modifications in your home environment to promote independence.

Other types of therapists can help you recover from a specific illness. If you have had a stroke (see Stroke, page 461), a speech therapist may help you regain language skills. Arrangements can be made for a home program. Talk to the coordinating home health service organization or individual. Therapists are also available in clinics, hospital outpatient departments, and private practice.

The recovery period is a dynamic time. As people come a few steps nearer to independence, they may become harder to handle. Some are eager to resume normal activities all at once, thinking they are completely recovered when in fact they are only on the way to recovery. Others are disappointed at their rate of recovery or at the discovery that they are not well "all at once." These attitudes can lead to relapses, setbacks, and depression. The physician, therapist, or visiting nurse can help inform both caregiver and patient as to what degree of recovery might be reasonably expected within a particular time. As a caregiver, your responsibilities involve more than helping the person's body or mind to recover its health. You also need to take an active role in helping the patient recover self-confidence and good spirits, an equally important but less quantifiable task.

Rehabilitation Programs

Specialized programs exist for rehabilitation after certain acute illnesses. Depending on the type and severity of the illness or injury, rehabilitation may involve more than one step. If you have had a stroke, for example, rehabilitation may begin with physical and speech therapy soon after the stroke. If you have lost a limb through injury or cancer, physical therapists will help you learn how to use an artificial limb.

A second step may involve the services of another type of specialist, the occupational therapist. The word "occupation" in the title is misleading because occupational therapy is not aimed solely at helping carry out a particular job but at regaining the ability to handle everyday tasks. The occupational therapist visits your home and takes careful stock of what you can and cannot do and of barriers and obstacles to everyday tasks in your home. The therapist might suggest rearranging furniture, adding a wheelchair ramp, and the like. Aids to bathing and grooming may be recommended. The occupational therapist promotes a return to one's previous lifestyle.

In addition, an occupational therapist tries to identify, and if necessary reawaken, an interest in hobbies or going places or whatever might help rekindle optimism and an active interest in life—which is vital to regaining or maintaining health. Educating caregivers about when to help and when to let someone do things alone is another function.

A specialized step beyond physical and occupational therapy is vocational rehabilitation. Various organizations promote a return to the workforce for people with a disability or illness that does not affect their ability to work but might make them appear to others (or, initially, to themselves) as less than able. Vocational rehabilitation programs offer specific job training to overcome a handicap. Many such programs will help with job placements.

For more on Rehabilitation Centers, see page 1257.

Adult Day Care

An important consideration of home care is the person providing the care. Caring for an injured or disabled person over a long period can be extremely taxing. In a large family in which some family members spend significant amounts of time at home and can share the caregiving responsibility, the burden will be felt the least. But if care is being provided by one person, who may have a job, be in poor health, or in any case have his or her own life to lead, home care can be an unacceptable burden.

Adult day care can offer an alternative. It is a service whereby someone who cannot be left alone is looked after in a supervised setting during the day. Adult day care is suitable for the person who is disabled, is recuperating, or requires help performing everyday activities and who is able to leave the home. Depending on the program, people can attend for part of the day for one, two, or more days a week. Transportation to and from the day-care center often can be arranged.

At the day-care center, the person has an opportunity to be with other people, adding a sense of normalcy and stimulation to his or her life. Activities both with groups and individually are often encouraged. A midday meal is served. Some centers arrange formal activities.

A variant of the adult day-care center is the medical day-care center. Here, medical and nursing attention are provided in addition to the supervision, social activities, and meals. The person can visit the facility on an as-needed basis for some particular medical procedure, nursing care, or a type of therapy that is required. Such a visit might be necessary once or twice a week or every day.

Medical day care is often located in a hospital or a skilled nursing home, but the person returns home every night. (Alternatively, certain nursing homes admit elderly people on a temporary basis. If you are caring for someone in your home or theirs, this option allows you to take a vacation or recover from fatigue or illness.)

Some communities offer day care specifically aimed at individuals with cognitive impairment disorders such as Alzheimer's disease (see page 470). Such centers offer psychological services as well as supervision and activities.

The advantage of adult or medical day care is an easing of the burden for the caregiver. It provides a chance to work, run errands, pursue interests, or simply relax. In addition, skilled medical, nursing, or mental health services may be available that cannot be so readily obtained at home.

The person requiring care may also benefit from a change of scene and caregivers. Alternatively, however, the person may find the day-care center a dreary and unpleasant place to spend time. Check the facility yourself for your impression of the quality of care and the atmosphere.

Your hospital dismissal planner, physician, visiting nurse, or social worker should be able to tell you whether your community has facilities for adult day care. Adult day care may be offered by community health centers, psychiatric facilities, the Salvation Army, and other service organizations. (For further discussions of other alternatives, see page 245.)

Independent Living Centers

Alternatives to home care can be less restrictive and more conducive to an independent, healthy life. Independent living centers are one such alternative. These are specially designed for people who can function basically on their own but may need a little help.

An independent living center contains separate living quarters for each person, couple, or family. The center offers some services that are shared by all—usually meal preparation and monitoring. Meals are typically served in a common area that doubles as, or is near to, a central room for socialization and meetings. If residents want to, they can prepare their own meals in their own kitchens. Monitoring is handled in various ways, such as an alarm in each apartment that is connected to a control desk or nursing station that may be able to offer paramedical assistance.

The living center may incorporate elements of assistance into its architectural design, such as guardrails in bathrooms and in common hallways, wheelchair ramps, conveniently located kitchen cupboards, and easy-to-use appliance controls.

Some apartment buildings are designed for the needs of elderly people. Payment often is on a rental basis. If you are interested, apply early because there often is a waiting list. Although this type of center does not offer nursing care, residents can arrange for such care from the various home health service agencies that are available through the center or from other community sources.

Continuing-care retirement communities (CCRCs) are an increasingly popular option that links residential quarters to nutrition, social, and health care services. CCRCs are common in areas with large populations of retired people, such as Florida and Arizona, but can be found throughout the country. The living standards offered, and the costs, vary greatly. Most of the good ones are expensive, but prices range widely. Advance payments of $25,000 to $150,000, plus a monthly fee of $400 to $1,000, are not uncommon. Varied payment plans are available. Some centers receive government funding and charge rent to residents on a sliding-fee scale based on the ability to pay. As a rule, this type of center has a lengthy waiting list and demands a significant amount of independence. While most offer assisted-care living and some have full-service nursing homes, often you must be in good health to get in. (For more about CCRCs, see page 246.)

Another type of living alternative is offered by nonmedical residential institutions. Accommodations range from independent apartments at one extreme to shared rooms at the other. In addition to providing meals and monitoring, such institutions offer help with personal care, housekeeping, and shopping. Some offer continuous personal and nursing care, and there is little if any distinction between these institutions and nursing homes.

Foster homes also offer what amounts to home care in a group setting. Often these are called "board-and-care" homes. Residents may, for example, have their own rooms but share common areas for meals and socializing. Nursing care, continuous or intermittent, may be offered in a foster home.

Group Homes for the Developmentally Disabled and Mentally Ill

People with mental or emotional handicaps present a special challenge in home care. For example, a young developmentally disabled man who is a rational, cheerful, capable person may need a little help with some daily activities.

Ideally, these individuals are cared for at home in a family setting in which one or more family members are at home rather than at work. "Cared for" may even be a misnomer: for example, the young man described above may need only someone to tell him when it is time to wash his hair and to suggest activities when he is bored. This is neither intensive nor continuous care, nor is it always burdensome.

Group homes for the developmentally disabled and mentally ill offer such care when there is no family to provide it. In the best of these homes, the environment is like a home. Residents have some independence in their living arrangements, such as their own rooms with their personal belongings, but aides help them carry out grooming and daily activities, while mental health professionals help in the treatment of, or rehabilitation from, their mental problems. Some group homes are a type of foster care in which all the residents have mental rather than physical problems. Others are similar to the typical nursing home or foster home, which has a population of people with both physical and mental difficulties.

Chapter 43

Medical Tests

Contents

Kinds of Diagnostic Tests, 1330

Blood Tests, 1330
Complete Blood Cell Count (CBC), 1330
Blood Chemistry Group, 1330
Lipids, 1331
Sedimentation Rate, 1331
Coagulation Tests, 1331
Drug Tests, 1331
Enzyme Tests, 1331
    A Note on Test Results, 1331
Thyroid Studies, 1331
Arterial Blood Gas Analysis, 1332

Biopsies, 1332
Bone Marrow Aspiration and Biopsy, 1332
Liver Biopsy, 1333

Endoscopic Tests, 1333
Laryngoscopy, 1333

Body Scans, 1334
CT Scanning, 1334
Magnetic Resonance Imaging, 1334
Ultrasonography, 1335
    Pelvic Ultrasonography in Pregnancy, 1335
    Perspectives on Radiologic
      Examinations, 1335

Radionuclide (Nuclear) Scans, 1336
Bone Scan, 1336
Lung Scan, 1336
Liver Scan, 1336
Radioactive Iodine Uptake Test and
  Thyroid Scan, 1337
Tumor Imaging, 1337
Scanning for Infections, 1338

Heart (Cardiac) Scans, 1339

Heart Catheterization, 1340

Special X-Ray Procedures, 1341
Arthrography, 1341
Cerebral Arteriography, 1341
Kidney X-Ray, 1341
Bile and Pancreatic Duct X-Rays, 1341
Myelography, 1341

Other Examinations, 1342
Fluorescein Angiography, 1342
Echocardiography, 1342
Ophthalmoscopy, 1342
Impedance Plethysmography and
  Venography, 1342

Electrical Tests, 1343
Electrocardiography (ECG), 1343
Exercise Tolerance Test, 1344
Electroencephalography (EEG), 1344
Electromyography (EMG), 1344

Microbiologic Tests, 1345
Throat Culture, 1345
Synovial Fluid Analysis, 1345
Cerebrospinal Fluid Analysis, 1345

Reproductive and Urologic
Tests, 1346
Hysterosalpingography, 1346
Colposcopy, 1346
Laparoscopy in Women, 1346
    Home Medical Testing Kits, 1347
Cystoscopy, 1347
Urine Tests, 1347

Kinds of Diagnostic Tests

To reach a diagnosis, your physician requires information. Your medical history, the symptoms you report, and the physical examination he or she conducts are ways your physician obtains this information.

In addition, your physician will order diagnostic tests to obtain more information about you. In the pages that follow, we describe various medical tests—blood tests, tissue sample tests (biopsies), imaging tests (in which X-ray or other technologies are used to create an image of an area within your body)—and other tests as well.

The diverse kinds of diagnostic tests can be divided into two broad categories: invasive and noninvasive.

Invasive tests require direct "invasion" of the interior of your body; noninvasive tests are done outside your body. Invasive tests are performed to get a better view of your internal organs or to remove tissue (biopsy) for study. Noninvasive tests measure function or produce an indirect view of the inside of your body, as in many X-ray procedures.

The value of diagnostic testing depends on factors such as need, what can be reasonably discovered, and risks posed, if any. Before undergoing any test, understand the procedure, risks, possible alternatives, and anticipated benefits.

Blood Tests

Blood tests are used to rule out or to help diagnose disease. Routine blood tests can detect the possible presence of a wide variety of conditions, including various types of anemia, infections, and leukemia, to name only a few.

The drawing of a small amount of blood into a vial usually takes only a few seconds and can be done in a laboratory, in your physician's office, or in a hospital. Special preparations are not necessary. (Some tests require overnight fasting; others require no fasting at all. Follow your physician's instructions.)

Blood can be drawn from many sites. If only a drop or two is necessary, the blood usually is drawn from a fingertip and is placed in a small container called a capillary pipette.

If more than a drop of blood is required, the person drawing the blood will select a vein, cleanse the skin over it with alcohol, and then gently insert a thin needle. Blood will pass through the needle into an attached sterile syringe or vacuum container. Then the needle is withdrawn and the puncture wound is wiped again with an antiseptic.

In most routine examinations, blood testing includes a complete blood cell count (CBC), a chemistry group, and blood lipids. Literally hundreds of other blood tests can be obtained. Common ones include thyroid studies (to determine the output of the thyroid gland) and coagulation studies (to determine the rate at which the blood thickens or clots). Your physician will choose the most appropriate tests for you.

Below we describe in more detail some of the principal types of blood tests.

Complete Blood Cell Count (CBC)

The CBC is the most common blood test. It usually is part of a complete health checkup. The term "count" refers to the counting of each type of blood cell in a given volume of your blood.

The CBC measures the amount of hemoglobin, the percentage of the sample that is composed of red blood cells (hematocrit), the number and kinds of white blood cells, and the number of platelets. Like routine urinalysis, this test can signal the possible presence of a wide variety of conditions, including various types of anemia, infections, and leukemia.

Blood Chemistry Group

Often automated, the blood chemistry group tests may include an analysis of electrolytes (sodium, potassium, chloride, and phosphorus), tests for glucose (blood sugar), a series of liver function tests (including measurement of bilirubin), and tests for uric acid, creatinine (a kidney function test), and albumin (a major protein in the blood). Sometimes, different combinations of tests are used.

Lipids

Another common blood test is for lipids. This test measures the blood level of fats including total cholesterol, high-density lipoprotein (HDL) cholesterol, and triglycerides, all of which are related to risk of coronary artery disease (see What Do Measurements of Blood Fats Mean? page 640).

Sedimentation Rate

This blood test, also called erythrocyte sedimentation rate (ESR), determines the rate at which red blood cells settle to the bottom of a tube. If the cells settle faster than normal, this can suggest an infection, anemia, inflammation, rheumatoid arthritis, rheumatic fever, or one of several types of cancer.

Coagulation Tests

Coagulation tests detect abnormal levels of substances in your blood that control the speed at which your blood clots. For example, tests of the partial thromboplastin time (PTT) and prothrombin time (PT) can help identify blood-clotting diseases and liver diseases and are commonly used in monitoring patients taking blood-thinning medications (anticoagulants).

Drug Tests

It often is helpful to know the amount of a drug in the blood (in general or at a specific time), such as the heart drug digoxin (Lanoxin). Tests of drug levels (there are many) can reveal such information precisely.

Enzyme Tests

Your blood can be tested for levels of enzymes that may indicate damage to certain organs

---

A Note on Test Results

To be of value, test results must be accurate. How can accuracy be checked?

To help ensure dependability of blood tests, for example, solutions with known amounts of the substance being sought are interspersed with blood samples being analyzed. Another check on accuracy is the periodic testing of unknown samples prepared by other laboratories. In both cases, the results provide a way to judge accuracy (or inaccuracy) of testing procedures. Even with these precautions, however, errors can occur.

All variations in test results are not to be blamed on laboratory error. For instance, the amounts of the substances in your blood can vary from day to day or even from hour to hour. Also, some substances in your blood can interfere with test procedures and lead to false results.

There may be only a small difference between normal and abnormal results. Normal values for a substance in the blood usually are established by analyzing blood from a group of people who are in good health. The range of normal is commonly set by selecting values that will include 95 percent of the results of tests done on these healthy people. The line between normal and abnormal is set in an arbitrary manner—thus, there usually is overlap between test results that suggest disease and those that do not.

If a laboratory measures 15 or 20 different substances in your blood, there is a good chance that one or more of these results will be outside the normal range. If the apparently abnormal tests are repeated, they are likely to give results within the normal range. But a deviation from the normal range due to early or minimal disease will continue to be found on repeated testing. Sometimes, repeated testing is necessary to determine whether a marginal test result is the result of disease.

---

such as the liver, pancreas, or heart. For example, certain enzymes are normally found in large amounts within liver cells, but in small amounts in the blood. Large amounts in the blood may indicate liver disease.

Other enzymes ordinarily found in the heart may leak into the blood from damaged heart cells after a heart attack (myocardial infarction). If you experience chest pain, a test for these enzymes may be done.

Thyroid Studies

These tests measure blood levels of certain hormones including thyroxine, thyroid-stimulating hormone, and others. Such studies are useful in distinguishing among the possible causes of thyroid disorders.

Arterial Blood Gas Analysis

This test measures the acidity (pH) of your blood and the amount of oxygen and carbon dioxide dissolved in it. The procedure differs substantially from a standard blood test.

The skin over the artery to be punctured is cleaned with an antiseptic, and a local anesthetic is injected. (An artery is chosen, rather than a vein, because the blood sample must be freshly oxygenated from the heart and lungs.) The selected artery, usually in the wrist, is punctured with a sterile needle attached to a disposable syringe. The interior of the syringe is oil-coated to prevent room air from contaminating the blood sample. The physician or technician draws a sample of blood and then removes the needle from the artery. The blood sample is transferred from the syringe into sterile tubes that are placed in a blood gas analyzer.

After the blood sample has been drawn, you will be asked to apply pressure to the puncture site and rest quietly for 15 minutes before resuming normal activities.

Biopsies

A biopsy is the removal of a sample of tissue for study, usually under a microscope. Biopsies are necessary to rule out disease or to confirm diagnoses such as cancer. The sample can be removed with a needle, with a knife (sometimes through a surgical incision), or by a special device inserted through an endoscope (an instrument gently inserted into a natural opening in the body).

Most samples are treated chemically and sliced into very thin sections. These sections are placed on glass slides, stained (to enhance contrast), and studied under a microscope by a pathologist (a person who specializes in changes in body tissue) or a hematologist (a specialist in blood and blood-forming tissues), or both.

Some samples can be interpreted almost immediately by a pathologist. This procedure (which was developed at Mayo Clinic) is called frozen section and can be useful in diagnosing cancer within minutes after the sample is obtained.

Virtually all of the fiberoptic instruments used in examining the trachea (windpipe), lungs, and upper and lower gastrointestinal tract also can be used to obtain tissue from the body. These instruments include bronchoscopes, colonoscopes, proctosigmoidoscopes, and esophagogastroduodenoscopes. Rigid instruments (such as cystoscopes) are also used to perform biopsies.

Bone Marrow Aspiration and Biopsy

A needle can be used to obtain material from your bone marrow for study. This needle rests in a slender sleeve of metal (stylet) that cuts a tiny channel for the needle to pass through. The needle is sharp enough and strong enough to penetrate the thin bone of the breast (sternum) or the back of the pelvic bone for aspiration (sucking up, like a vacuum cleaner) of the bone marrow into a syringe. In infants, bone marrow is often obtained from the tibia (lower bone of the leg).

Bone marrow aspiration is used in the diagnosis of a wide variety of disorders of the blood or blood-forming organs, including anemia, leukemia, and lymphoma. Bone marrow aspiration also is used to evaluate the effectiveness of chemotherapy on malignancies involving the bone marrow. The test takes a few minutes and usually can be performed in a physician's office, a laboratory, or a hospital.

You will receive a local anesthetic at the site from which the bone marrow sample is to be taken. After the skin is sterilized with an antiseptic, a health care professional will insert the aspirating needle into the spongy marrow-filled bone of your pelvic bone or breastbone. Less than a teaspoon of marrow will be withdrawn.

You will feel some pressure as the biopsy needle is inserted, and there will be a dull, deep pain when the marrow is removed. But the pain will be only momentary. The needle then is removed, a bandage is placed on the wound, and the specimen is immediately prepared for microscopic examination.

Bone marrow aspiration differs slightly from a bone marrow biopsy. In a biopsy, a small solid core of marrow tissue is removed intact. Aside from that, the procedures are essentially the same and often are performed at the same time.

After the procedure, the puncture site may be tender and bruised for several days. The principal risk is bleeding from the puncture site, but this is rare.

Liver Biopsy

This safe and relatively simple procedure is used in the diagnosis of liver diseases such as cirrhosis, hepatitis, and cancer. It also may be used to determine the effects of drugs on the liver. The test may be performed on an outpatient basis or in a hospital.

You may be asked to refrain from eating or drinking for several hours before the test. Before the test starts, you will disrobe and put on an examination gown.

During the procedure you will be asked to lie absolutely still on an examining table. The area where the biopsy needle is to be inserted (between or under the right ribs) will be cleansed and anesthetized. Then you will be asked to inhale deeply and to hold your breath as the needle is gently inserted through the skin and into the liver.

When the needle has reached the liver, it is rotated and then removed. This takes only a few seconds. The tissue specimen captured by the needle is placed in a sterile container and sent to a pathology laboratory for study.

After the procedure, a dressing will be placed on the tiny wound. For the next 3 to 4 hours, bed rest is recommended. Your pulse and blood pressure will be taken periodically. If light-headedness occurs, particularly when you stand up after the initial observation period of 3 to 4 hours, consult your physician. He or she will want to rule out bleeding after the biopsy. Occasionally, a mild, non-aspirin-containing analgesic is given.

Endoscopic Tests

An endoscope is an instrument used to examine the interior of a hollow organ or cavity. It consists of either a flexible or a rigid hollow tube connected to an optical system that allows the person directing the tube to see tissues at the far end of the tube.

The endoscope has become indispensable for diagnosing a wide range of ailments in many different specialties. To the pulmonary (lung) specialist, the endoscope (known as a bronchoscope) is the key piece of equipment for examining the trachea and bronchial tree. It is used to help locate tumors, constrictions, secretions, and bleeding sites in the bronchial tubes and to diagnose lung cancer, tuberculosis, and other pulmonary diseases (see Bronchoscopy, page 726).

The gastroenterologist, who is concerned with the stomach, intestines, and other digestive organs, also uses an endoscope. Gastrointestinal procedures include gastroscopy (which provides a direct view of your esophagus, stomach, and duodenum), sigmoidoscopy (for examining your rectum and sigmoid portion of your large intestine), and colonoscopy (for examining the lining of your colon from the anus to the junction of your small and large intestines) (see Upper Gastrointestinal Endoscopy, page 760; Colonoscopy, page 788; and Screening for Colon Cancer, page 790).

Other specialties use endoscopes to look at joints (see Arthroscopy, page 878), the bladder (see Cystoscopy, page 849), and other organs.

Laryngoscopy

This procedure gives your physician a direct view into your larynx (voice box). Problems such as a tumor, a foreign object, or nerve injury are often diagnosed in this fashion. This procedure usually is performed in the physician's office. No preparation is required.

A local anesthetic may be sprayed into your nose and throat to decrease discomfort. Then a fiberoptic endoscope is inserted into your nose and carefully threaded down your throat into your larynx. The light and the lens system of the endoscope make it possible for your physician to view your larynx and, usually, to diagnose or rule out a health problem. A rigid laryngoscope also is commonly used. This is inserted through the mouth.

There are no serious risks with this procedure, although you may experience some temporary soreness in your nose and throat and cough up a small quantity of blood if a biopsy is required.

Body Scans

The X-ray examination is not new—it has been used for viewing structures such as bones, heart, and lungs for more than a century. Breast X-rays (see Mammograms, page 1165), dental X-rays (see page 369), barium X-rays of the esophagus, stomach, and intestine (see page 762), and other such examinations use traditional technology. Examination of many internal organs has improved dramatically in the past decade with the advent of computerized scanning equipment. The three types of scanning most commonly available are computed tomography (CT), magnetic resonance imaging (MRI), and ultrasonography.

CT, MRI, and ultrasonography are similar in that they provide detailed cross-sectional images of the inside of the body—like slices through a loaf of bread. However, they use different methods for producing their images: CT uses a very thin X-ray beam, MRI uses a magnetic field and radio waves, and ultrasound uses high-frequency sound waves. CT, MRI, and ultrasound are safe, painless procedures that are usually done on an outpatient basis.

CT Scanning

A CT scan creates a more detailed image of your internal organs than a conventional X-ray. The scanner sends a narrow X-ray beam through your body and detects the beam as it leaves your body. Computer analysis of changes in the X-ray beam caused by your body tissues creates an image showing many soft-tissue structures and organs not seen on a standard X-ray. (See CT and MRI Scans, page 494.)

You will be asked to lie flat on a movable table. It is guided into the center of the CT scanner, which resembles an enormous doughnut. You will need to lie still, holding your breath as directed while scans are performed. A "dye" (contrast medium) is often injected through a vein to improve the contrast of the image. This liquid contains iodine, so before the test begins you will be asked if you are allergic to iodine. If your abdomen is being scanned, you will be asked to drink an oral contrast medium prior to your scan.

Magnetic Resonance Imaging

This imaging technique uses magnetic fields and radio waves to generate cross-sectional pictures of the head and body. These images display internal anatomy with remarkable clarity. Because the images demonstrate tissue properties that are different from those evaluated with other imaging methods, they can provide unique diagnostic information. (See CT and MRI Scans, page 494.)

There is no known risk associated with MRI, although for safety reasons examinations are usually not performed on patients with cardiac pacemakers and other implanted metallic devices.

There are many different types of MRI examinations. In some cases, a special type of contrast material will be injected into a vein to enhance certain tissues in the images. After the examination is complete, the images will be interpreted by a diagnostic radiologist.

Ultrasonography

Ultrasonography, also known as sonography, uses a wand-like device (transducer) to send and receive high-frequency (inaudible to the human ear) sound waves (ultrasound) through your body. After the sound waves pass through tissue and are reflected back, they are transformed by a computer into a moving image that is displayed on a video screen and photographed for analysis.

In recent years, the role of ultrasonography in medical care has expanded substantially. This safe procedure is used to examine organs in the abdomen (including the gallbladder, liver, pancreas, kidneys, spleen, and aorta), pelvis (including the uterus, ovaries, prostate), neck (thyroid and parathyroid gland), testicles, and breast. The examination is also valuable during pregnancy for viewing the fetus in the uterus (see this page). In addition, ultrasonography allows the physician to evaluate your arteries and veins. For example, narrowing of the carotid arteries, which can lead to stroke, is detectable by ultrasound.

Radiologists also use ultrasound and CT to carefully guide minimal invasive procedures such as drainage of infection by small catheters (tubes) and thin-needle biopsy of tumors. These procedures are often performed on an outpatient basis.

Pelvic Ultrasonography in Pregnancy

This painless procedure allows your physician to see the fetus inside your uterus without exposing you or your fetus to X-rays. The ultrasound procedure will not have any effect on the fetus. The image, known as a sonogram, reveals many important aspects of pregnancy, including the position, size, and gestational age of the fetus; multiple pregnancy; and location of the placenta. In early pregnancy, ultrasonography is used to distinguish between normal pregnancy in the uterus and pregnancies that occur elsewhere, such as in the fallopian tubes (tubal pregnancy).

The procedure takes about 15 minutes and is often performed on an outpatient basis. If you are at an early stage in your pregnancy, you may be asked to drink several glasses of water about an hour before this examination. (For best results, your bladder must be full.) In later stages of pregnancy, ingestion of water is not needed because the uterus and fetus enlarge and are seen well without a full urinary bladder.

You will be asked to disrobe and wear a special gown. A gel will be applied to your abdomen, and then the transducer, a wand-like device, will be gently pressed against this lubricated area. If your physician considers it necessary, another transducer may be placed in the vagina to allow for a much closer view of the early pregnancy. The transducer sends high-frequency sound waves into the body and receives the sound waves reflected by the tissues. A computer translates the reflected sound waves into a moving image, which is analyzed by your physician. These pictures are photographed for later analysis.

Perspectives on Radiologic Examinations

Safety
Every plant, animal, and human being living on this planet is exposed to radiation every day. Most of this radiation comes from natural sources, including outer space, the earth, and even your own body. Less than 15 percent of this radiation is produced by medical examinations.

Radiologic examinations are safe. The amount of radiation used for routine X-ray examinations is low and has been reduced dramatically over the years, thanks to improvements in technology. No radiation remains after an X-ray examination. You actually receive less radiation from a chest X-ray than you would receive from cosmic radiation while flying from New York to Los Angeles.

Costs
Because diagnostic radiology uses sensitive and complex equipment, you might think that the radiologic portion of health care costs is large. In fact, diagnostic radiology represents only 3.5 percent of health care costs. Consider how much higher health care costs would be without the accurate diagnostic and treatment-guiding information that radiology provides.

Benefits
Diagnostic radiologic examinations promote better health care and can decrease health care costs by:

- Detecting disease early, often at a curable stage
- Frequently establishing the diagnosis
- Providing reassurance when examination results are normal
- Decreasing the need for exploratory surgery
- Providing a detailed "map" if surgery is necessary
- Guiding procedures accurately and safely (needle biopsy, infection drainage, angioplasty, etc.)
- Painlessly monitoring the progress of treatment

Radionuclide (Nuclear) Scans

This imaging process uses small amounts of radioactive tracers (radioisotopes) that are attached to various substances (radiopharmaceuticals). The preparations are introduced into the body by injection, inhalation, or swallowing. Then a special detector called a gamma camera produces pictures of the radioisotopes in internal organs, permitting your physician to examine the size, shape, and function of the organs. The images also can help to distinguish between normal and abnormal tissue. This scanning procedure is somewhat the reverse of a traditional X-ray. Instead of the X-rays coming from outside the body, the radiation source is inside the body.

The radiopharmaceuticals are generally cleared rapidly from your body within several hours to a few days. To some extent, the radioactive material will initially be distributed throughout your body. Therefore, this type of scanning will not be used if you are pregnant or if you are breastfeeding—unless the information needed is vitally important and cannot be obtained in another way. If you are breastfeeding or think you may be pregnant, inform your physician of this before any radioisotope study begins.

Bone Scan

This procedure is useful in diagnosing cancer, infection, or the cause of unexplained bone pain, such as a subtle or hidden bone fracture. Bone scanning can be performed in an outpatient or hospital setting.

You receive an injection of a special radiopharmaceutical preparation (a technetium-99m methylene diphosphonate compound). Then you wait several hours while the material is absorbed in your bones and the balance eliminated by your kidneys. During that time you will drink several glasses of water, and you will need to urinate frequently to help remove the unabsorbed material from your system. You can then leave the laboratory if you wish until the scans (pictures) are to be taken, approximately 3 hours after the injection.

For the scanning, you lie still on a table. A special gamma camera records pictures of the pattern of localization (attachment to the surface) of the radiopharmaceutical to your bones. An uneven distribution of the radiopharmaceutical may indicate a problem. Areas of increased accumulation of radiopharmaceutical are called "hot spots." A bone fracture or arthritis will show up as hot spots.

After the procedure, special care is not required.

Lung Scan

Lung scanning (also called VQ scanning) most commonly is used to determine if there is a blood clot in a lung (pulmonary embolism). The entire procedure takes about 45 minutes and can be performed in a hospital or an outpatient facility.

You inhale a small amount of radiopharmaceutical, and pictures of the airflow into the lungs are taken with a gamma camera. Following this, a small amount of a different radiopharmaceutical is injected into a vein in your arm, and pictures of the lung blood flow are taken in several different positions. The lung blood flow and airflow images are compared by the physician interpreting the study.

After the procedure, special care is not required.

Liver Scan

A liver scan is performed to determine the size, shape, and function of the liver. It can detect the presence of cysts, abscesses, or tumors in the liver as well as evidence of cancer that may have spread into or arise from the liver. The procedure also can reveal the damage done to the liver by hepatitis, cirrhosis, or abdominal injury. A liver scan takes about 30 minutes. It can be performed in a hospital or an outpatient facility.

You may be asked to partially disrobe for the procedure, in which a radioactive material is first injected into a vein in your arm. Then, while you are lying down, you will be asked to move into different positions while a special gamma camera records images of the radiopharmaceutical that has been taken up (localized) in your liver.

After the procedure, special care is not required.

Radioactive Iodine Uptake Test and Thyroid Scan

The iodine uptake test and the thyroid scan are two methods for measuring the size, structure, and function of the thyroid gland. They are valuable in the diagnosis of an over-functioning thyroid gland (hyperthyroidism) and an underfunctioning thyroid gland (hypothyroidism). They also are used to evaluate thyroid nodules. Both tests can be done on an outpatient basis or in a hospital. Depending on the purpose of the test, you may be asked to temporarily discontinue any thyroid medication you may be taking.

Iodine Uptake Test

For the iodine uptake test, you swallow a very small amount of radioiodine in a capsule or in liquid form. You return 6 or 24 hours later, or at both times, to measure the ability of your thyroid gland to concentrate the iodine. (Your thyroid gland uses iodine to make thyroid hormone.) For the measurement, you will lie on your back on a table with your head stretched backward. A counting instrument is placed over your neck to measure the iodine taken up by the thyroid gland.

Thyroid Scan

The thyroid scan is slightly different in that it produces an actual image of your thyroid gland. This study requires an injection (or possibly swallowing) of the radiopharmaceutical preparation. The gamma camera detects the radioisotope that has collected in your thyroid gland and then produces an image on the screen. The image can be interpreted on the screen or photographed for interpretation by your physician.

After the procedure, special care is not required.

Tumor Imaging

There are an increasing number of new radionuclide imaging studies using radiopharmaceuticals that localize in tumors. The tumor imaging agents include radiolabeled peptides (small proteins), radiolabeled monoclonal antibodies (larger proteins),

positron emitting molecules for positron emission tomography (PET scanning), and other radiopharmaceuticals taken up by tumors. Many of these are useful for imaging certain types of tumors.

Each radiopharmaceutical binds to the tumor because of a unique property allowing binding to the surface of the tumor cell or uptake into the tumor cell differently than in normal cells. These imaging studies have great potential, but currently most are undergoing clinical evaluation, and many are just being incorporated into cancer screening or evaluation of patients after cancer treatment.

All of the agents listed below are radioisotopes or have a radioisotope attached that can be imaged with special cameras to identify sites of tumor involvement. Each different type of scan may require a different preparation, which you should discuss with your physician.

Peptides

Indium-111 pentetreotide (also called OctreoScan) is a small protein. It binds to tumors that have a particular protein on the surface of the cell called somatostatin receptor. This radiopharmaceutical can identify the location of certain tumors of the pancreas (islet cell tumors), uncommon abdominal tumors (carcinoid tumors), certain lung cancers (small cell), and certain thyroid tumors (medullary thyroid carcinoma). In addition, the usefulness of this imaging in other types of tumors is being studied.

Scanning multiple areas of the body with a gamma camera generally begins at 4 to 6 hours after injection of the radiopharmaceutical into an arm vein and is repeated the next day. No special preparation is required, but laxatives may be given before the study to improve the imaging.

Monoclonal Antibodies

Indium-111 satumomab pendetide (also called OncoScint) is a monoclonal antibody (a larger protein) labeled with indium-111 as a radiotracer. The radiopharmaceutical binds to a specific protein on the tumor cell surface of colon (large bowel) cancers, rectal cancers, and ovarian cancers. Images are generally obtained 48 to 128 hours after injection of the radiopharmaceutical, and frequently imaging is done on more than 1 day.

Other monoclonal antibodies should be

available in the future for imaging other types of tumors.

Tumor-Specific Radioisotopes

Iodine-131 scanning is done after complete or partial surgical removal of the thyroid for thyroid cancer. The iodine is taken by mouth as a liquid or in a capsule, and scans of the neck or whole body are obtained with a gamma camera 24 or 48 hours later, or at both times.

The scan is done to check for any remaining or recurrent thyroid cancer. The imaging study requires you to discontinue your thyroid medications prior to the scan. Ask your physician about how and when you should stop taking your thyroid medications and about any special dietary restrictions. After the procedure, no special care is required.

Gallium-67 imaging is used to scan several different types of tumors, most commonly lymphoma (cancer of the lymphatic glands), including Hodgkin's disease (one type of lymphoma). Thallium-201 and technetium-99m sestamibi, which have been approved for heart scans, are now also being evaluated as tumor-imaging agents.

Positron Emission Tomography (PET Scan)

Many of the molecules normally found in the human body can be synthesized to include a positron-emitting radioisotope (special type of radioactive tracer) in the molecule or in a very similar molecule (analogue). This makes it possible to take pictures of the distribution of molecules such as glucose (a form of sugar found in the body), water, and many other molecules naturally found in our bodies.

Fluorine-18 fluorodeoxyglucose (also called FDG) is an example of a positron-emitting molecule that is taken up by certain body organs and tumors because it is very similar to glucose. It is most useful for identifying certain tumors when other procedures such as CT scans or MRI scans cannot determine if a possible abnormality seen is normal or represents the presence of a tumor. Additionally, FDG can image the heart and brain for diagnosing problems other than tumors.

PET scans require special cameras, and imaging is done shortly after the radiopharmaceutical is injected into a vein in the arm. After the procedure, special care is not required.

Scanning for Infections

Two types of studies use radiopharmaceutical preparations to look for infections: the gallium scan and the indium-labeled white blood cell scan. The procedures are similar but are used for different clinical problems.

A special gamma camera records the location of the radiopharmaceutical. Images of abnormal tissues are quite different from those of normal tissues, allowing your physician to detect possible sites of infection (see Radionuclide [Nuclear] Scans, page 1336).

Gallium Scanning

This procedure uses a radiopharmaceutical (gallium-67) that is given intravenously and then collects (localizes) in abnormal tissues such as sites of infection or inflammation and in certain tumors.

After you receive an injection of the radiopharmaceutical, you can leave. You will return for imaging at various times, beginning as soon as 6 hours later, but more often 24 or 48 hours later. In the meantime, you may be directed to take a laxative to help remove the unbound gallium from your bowel.

A special gamma camera will record several images over your abdomen, chest, or other areas where an infection may be suspected. The scanning procedure takes about 1 to 1½ hours.

You may be asked to return on 1 or more subsequent days to record more pictures of the gallium location. This procedure may suggest to your physician locations in your body that require examination by means of other techniques such as ultrasonography, CT, or some other X-ray procedure (see Body Scans, page 1334).

After the procedure, special care is not necessary.

Indium-Labeled White Blood Cell Scanning

This procedure uses a sample of your own white blood cells, which are removed, labeled with a radiopharmaceutical (tracer), and then returned to your bloodstream. These specially marked white blood cells will collect at sites of active infection or inflammation.

Your physician might ask you to discontinue any antibiotics you may be taking before this test.

First, blood is drawn from a vein in your arm. In a laboratory, the white blood cells in the sample are separated from other components of the blood, including the red blood cells. Then a small amount of radioisotope is added to the white blood cells and binds to them. Two or 3 hours later, these labeled white blood cells are returned to your body by injection into a vein in your arm.

Images (approximately 6) are taken with a gamma camera at 24 hours after the injection of your labeled white blood cells. The pictures show where the labeled white blood cells have collected. Imaging may take 1 or 2 hours and usually is performed in a hospital or outpatient facility.

After the procedure is finished, special care is not necessary.

Heart (Cardiac) Scans

There are two important radionuclide procedures available for imaging the heart: myocardial perfusion imaging (pictures of the cardiac muscle blood flow) and radionuclide angiography (images of the cardiac muscle contraction). The procedures give different information about your heart and are performed using different radiopharmaceuticals.

In both tests, a special gamma camera detects the location or motion of the radiopharmaceutical within the heart and records multiple images. The image of an abnormal heart may be quite different from that of a normal one, which aids in evaluating the function of the heart and in diagnosing the cause of heart problems.

Myocardial Perfusion Imaging (Cardiac Muscle Blood Flow)

A myocardial perfusion scan can show areas of cardiac muscle damage (myocardial infarction) or areas of muscle not getting enough blood (myocardial ischemia) that may decrease the ability of the heart to pump blood or may result in a myocardial infarction (commonly called a heart attack). Thallium or other, newer radiopharmaceuticals (labeled with the radioisotope technetium-99m) are taken up in the myocardium (muscle) of the heart, following injection into an arm vein prior to imaging.

The study is usually performed both at rest and with stress. The stress study (which increases blood flow in the blood vessels of the heart) is done either with exercise or with short-acting medications (pharmacologic stress). When the pharmacologic stress study is done, the medication is administered by injection into an arm vein. Whether you use exercise or pharmacologic stress for the scan may depend on your ability to exercise on a treadmill or which stress test may better evaluate your specific problem. Each type of test may require a different preparation, so discuss with your physician whether you should eat, avoid caffeine, or stop taking any medications prior to the study.

During the study, electrocardiogram (ECG) leads are placed on your chest (see Electrocardiography, page 1343). Electrocardiogram and blood pressure readings are taken while you exercise on a treadmill or while the pharmacologic stress medication is being injected. Just before the end of your workout or the end of the medication injection, the radiopharmaceutical that localizes in your heart muscle will be injected into a vein in your arm.

A special gamma camera records multiple images of your heart while you lie on a table. The imaging at rest is done either before or after the stress imaging for comparison. Completion of each set of images requires 45 minutes to 1 hour. The procedures are performed in a hospital or outpatient facility.

Special care or precautions are unnecessary after the procedure is complete.

Radionuclide Angiography (MUGA Scan)

This procedure can reveal how effectively your heart is functioning. It can be done either at rest or during exercise, or in both circumstances.

You will receive an injection of a chemical (stannous pyrophosphate) into an arm vein. A short time later, a small amount of your blood is drawn into a syringe containing a small amount of the radioisotope technetium-99m. The blood with the stannous pyrophosphate and technetium-99m are mixed and allowed to remain together for 10 minutes, during which time your red blood cells absorb the radioisotope. These labeled red blood cells are injected back into your blood and circulate through your heart.

The scanning procedure itself requires 1 hour or less and is performed in a hospital or outpatient facility. During the scanning, an electrocardiogram will be recorded from ECG leads attached to your chest. A special gamma camera is placed over your heart in several positions to image your heart function.

The efficiency of the heart muscle contractions is measured along with the size of the heart chambers. These images can be made while you are at rest or while you pedal a bicycle, either upright or lying down.

Once the procedure is finished, special care or precautions are unnecessary.

Heart Catheterization

Heart catheterization refers to any procedure where catheters (hollow tubes) are placed in the heart to obtain specific information about cardiac anatomy or function. Cardiac catheterization can provide physicians with information about the degree of narrowing or leakage of a heart valve, the pumping performance of the heart muscle, and the pressures inside the cardiac chambers and lungs. Congenital heart defects can also be detected and quantified. By far the most common reason for performing heart catheterization today is to determine the presence, location, and severity of narrowings in the coronary arteries (see Scans and Coronary Angiogram, page 656).

Heart catheterizations are performed in specialized laboratories that contain sophisticated X-ray and pressure-monitoring equipment. Most catheterization laboratories are located in large, specialized hospitals, although in recent years mobile catheterization laboratories have been developed that allow the procedure to be performed in smaller communities. In most cases, nonemergency catheterization can be performed on an outpatient basis.

In preparation for a heart catheterization procedure, you should not eat any food or drink any liquids for at least 8 hours before the procedure. You will disrobe and wear a gown during the test.

Before the catheterization procedure begins, you will receive a mild sedative, but you will remain conscious during the procedure. Electrocardiographic leads will be placed on your chest so that your physician can monitor the action of your heart throughout the test. An intravenous line is also placed in one of your arm veins so that fluids and medications, if needed, can be administered.

An artery or vein in your groin, or occasionally in your arm, is selected for insertion of the catheter that is to be gently guided into your heart or other area. The insertion site is cleansed with an antiseptic and draped in a sterile fashion. A local anesthetic is injected into the skin and deeper tissues. There should be no further pain after this. A 4- to 5-inch sheath is inserted into the blood vessel to help prevent bleeding and to allow the exchange of catheters during the procedure if necessary.

When the catheter is in place, pressure measurements are obtained, and a contrast medium (dye) is delivered through the catheter to visualize your heart chambers or coronary arteries. At these times, you may be asked to take deep breaths or to hold your breath. These breathing maneuvers improve the quality of the X-ray pictures. Your physician may ask you to dissolve a nitroglycerin tablet under your tongue to dilate your blood vessels prior to injecting the contrast medium. Results of the catheterization are monitored on a television screen during the test and recorded on film for later study.

When the physician has collected the necessary information, the catheter is removed and the examination is complete. You will then be taken to a recovery room, where the sheath is removed.

For the first 20 to 30 minutes after removal of the sheath, direct pressure is placed on the catheter insertion site. You will be kept in bed for several hours to periodically check your vital signs and the insertion site for soreness, swelling, or blood loss. If needed, you will also be given pain medication.

Although this is a common procedure, serious complications are associated with it.

For example, if the catheter loosens an existing blood clot or cholesterol deposit within an artery, a stroke or heart attack can occur. In people with poor kidney function, the contrast medium can cause further kidney damage. Bleeding from the arterial insertion site can also occur. Still, the risk of serious complications (such as stroke, heart attack, or even death) is low, approximately 1 in 1,000. The risks are lowest in young, healthy people and highest in older people with serious medical problems.

Special X-Ray Procedures

Arthrography

An arthrogram is an X-ray of a joint, especially a knee, ankle, or shoulder. The test is used to detect suspected tears in cartilage and other joint abnormalities. It takes less than an hour and is performed with X-ray guidance. It can be done in an outpatient setting or a hospital.

You will be given a local anesthetic, and then a liquid contrast medium (dye) will be injected into the joint to enhance the clarity of the pictures that are to be made. (If your physician chooses to draw fluid from the joint for other studies, he or she will do this before administering the contrast medium.) You may be asked to move the joint to help distribute the dye throughout the area. The joint then will be examined with a fluoroscope, and X-rays will be made.

After the procedure, rest the joint for at least a day, or as long as your physician recommends, before resuming normal activity. You may experience some swelling or discomfort in the joint. This should pass in 1 to 2 days. If it does not, see your physician (see Arthroscopy, page 878). Your physician may need additional X-ray procedures or imaging studies such as an MRI scan (see page 1334) for further diagnosis.

Cerebral Arteriography

Cerebral arteriography is performed by injecting a contrast medium (dye) into a major artery leading to the brain. The dye spreads to other areas of the brain (see Cerebral Arteriography, page 464).

Kidney X-Ray

This procedure, which also is called intravenous pyelography (IVP) or excretory urography, provides images of the kidneys and lower urinary tract (see The Kidney X-Ray, page 829). If your physician suspects an abnormality, this may be the first radiologic test done. Generally there are no side effects. An ultrasound or CT scan may be needed to provide more detailed information.

Bile and Pancreatic Duct X-Rays

X-ray examination of the bile and pancreatic ducts can identify gallstones, narrowings (strictures), cancer of the pancreas or bile duct, or other abnormalities. Contrast medium (dye) is injected into the bile and pancreatic ducts through an endoscope (see pages 815 and 816).

Myelography

Myelography is an X-ray examination of the space around the spinal cord. A lumbar puncture (also called a spinal tap) is done, and a radiopaque dye (contrast medium) is injected into the space around the spinal cord. X-rays are then made to show the configuration of the space around the spinal cord and whether it is distorted by the presence of a slipped disc (herniated intervertebral disc), spinal cord tumor, an abnormal collection of blood vessels, or other disorders (see Myelography, page 510).

Other Examinations

Fluorescein Angiography

Fluorescein angiography (or eye angiography) produces photographs of blood vessels in the eye to evaluate eye disorders including retinopathy, tumors, and circulatory or inflammatory disorders of the eye. The test takes about 30 minutes and can be performed in a physician's office or in an ophthalmologic photography laboratory.

A technician or physician places drops in your eyes to dilate your pupils. After the pupils have dilated, you may be asked to loosen any constricting clothing around your neck before being positioned at the camera.

Fluorescein dye is then injected into a vein in your hand or arm. After the dye has moved to your eyes, several photographs are made in rapid sequence. Another series of photographs are taken several minutes later.

After the procedure, some discoloration, soreness, or swelling may appear at the site of the puncture, although this is unusual. Your vision may be blurred from the eyedrops for the rest of the day. In addition, your skin and urine may appear slightly discolored for 1 or 2 days after the procedure.

Echocardiography

This procedure uses a device that detects sound reflected from the beating heart and creates an image from which the size, shape, and motion of the heart can be determined (see The Echocardiogram: Images Made With Sound, page 683).

Ophthalmoscopy

This examination permits your physician to see the back of your eye (the fundus) to examine your retina, optic disc, and the network of tiny vessels that supply your eye with blood. This is an important part of every complete physical examination because the fundus can reveal useful information about your general health. The fundus is the only place in your body where veins and arteries can be observed directly, without an invasive procedure.

If you have high blood pressure, changes in these vessels can indicate the severity of your problem (see High Blood Pressure, page 647). Early clues to circulatory disturbances in your brain may appear in the vessels at the back of your eye. Specifically, particles of cholesterol-containing material or crystalline plaques may be a clue to atherosclerosis (see Atherosclerosis: What Is It? page 636). Changes in these blood vessels also can suggest complications of diabetes.

Part of this procedure also includes examining your optic nerve. This nerve, which looks like a cream-colored disc, gathers together all the nerve fibers from the retina to transmit visual images to your brain. This disc is actually an extension of your brain. When a person has a disease that causes increased pressure in the skull, such as a brain tumor or meningitis, the optic disc may appear blurred or swollen.

Although eye specialists include this procedure as part of a complete eye evaluation, the more limited test (often called a funduscopic examination) frequently is performed by family physicians, internists, and neurologists. The examination takes only a few minutes.

Your physician may place 1 or 2 drops of medicine into your eyes to dilate your pupils. This may cause blurring of your close vision for a time. Your physician may then dim the room light and, as you pick a point to stare at, he or she will shine a light from the ophthalmoscope into each eye and look through the pupil to the fundus.

This is a painless procedure. However, if you receive eyedrops, your eyes may be sensitive to light for several hours afterward because your pupils are dilated. Do not drive until your pupils have readjusted to bright light and your vision is no longer blurred.

Impedance Plethysmography and Venography

These procedures are used to detect blood clots in deep veins of your body, particularly in your legs. Detection of blood clots is important because clots can lead to a pulmonary embolism (see page 734).

Impedance Plethysmography

This procedure generally takes between 30 and 45 minutes and can be performed in a laboratory, a physician's office, or a hospital.

No special preparation is necessary. You probably will be asked to undress and wear a special gown. Electrodes are attached above the calf of your leg and a blood pressure cuff is wrapped around your thigh and inflated as if your blood pressure is to be taken on your thigh. A machine records the electrode's readings both when the cuff is inflated and when it is deflated. If the size of your leg does not change normally during and after inflation of the cuff, a blood clot may be present within your leg.

Venography

Venography often is performed after impedance plethysmography suggests that a blood clot may be present. Sometimes it is the only procedure performed to diagnose blood clots. This is an X-ray procedure that produces images of the veins in the legs and feet. It takes between 45 minutes and 1 hour and can be performed in a laboratory, a physician's office, or a hospital.

You may have to fast for 4 hours prior to the procedure, and you probably will be asked to undress and wear a special gown. A local anesthetic is injected into the area where a liquid contrast medium (dye) will be injected to enhance the clarity of the X-ray pictures. The site for this injection is a large vein in your foot or ankle. As the contrast medium is injected, you may feel a warming or mild burning sensation in your leg. Your veins can then be observed by means of an X-ray procedure called fluoroscopy. The X-rays are recorded for further study.

At some point during the test, you may be asked to flex your calf muscles or push your foot against the physician's or technician's hand to help direct more blood into the veins of your leg. A tourniquet is often placed around the leg to force the contrast medium into the deeper veins.

After the procedure, your pulse, blood pressure, and temperature will be checked. You will be observed for swelling, soreness, redness, bleeding, or infection due to the puncture. You may experience a sensation of nausea or mild light-headedness or have a mild headache for a few hours. If these symptoms persist, inform your physician.

Electrical Tests

Your body generates electrical currents as you go about your normal activities. Scientists have detected electrical activity in the brain, muscles, heart, and other organs and tissue and have devised unique ways of recording this activity. Studying these recordings can reveal abnormalities that can be used to diagnose disorders.

Electrocardiography (ECG)

This test measures the pattern of electrical impulses generated in your heart. It can help identify damage to the heart muscle, irregular rhythms, enlargement (hypertrophy) of a chamber of your heart, or damage caused by a heart attack. It also can measure the effectiveness of a pacemaker. Electrocardio-

graphy, which records the electrical forces produced during each heartbeat, has become one of the most common cardiac diagnostic tests. The procedure takes only a few minutes, is painless, and can be performed routinely in a physician's office.

Generally, no special preparations are necessary. After you have undressed from the waist up, you lie on a comfortable bed or examining table and relax. Electrodes are attached to your wrists, ankles, and chest. During the procedure, breathe normally but do not move or talk because any disturbance may distort test results.

After the procedure, the electrodes are removed, and you can resume normal activities (see Twenty-Four-Hour Cardiac Monitoring and Event Recording, page 671).

Exercise Tolerance Test

This test reveals the efficiency and function of the heart under stress (see The Exercise Tolerance Test, page 655).

Electroencephalography (EEG)

Electroencephalography measures the waves of electrical activity produced by the brain. Often, it is used in diagnosing and managing seizure disorders. If you are awake when the recording is made, the test takes about 30 minutes. (Some EEG tests are done while you sleep.) Most often, the test is performed in a hospital, but it can be done in a laboratory or physician's office.

If you are taking antiseizure medications, continue taking them unless otherwise instructed by your physician. Tell the person performing the test about any medicines you are taking. Because electrodes will be attached to your scalp, shampoo your hair before the test to help remove any hair spray, tonic, or oil.

As many as 16 to 30 small electrodes will be attached to your scalp with paste or an elastic cap as you relax on your back in a bed or reclining chair. The test is painless, but you must remain motionless. Periodically you may be asked to breathe deeply and steadily for 3 minutes or to stare at a patterned board. Alternatively, a light may be flashed in your eyes. These actions stimulate the brain. The electrical impulses from your brain are detected by the electrodes and sent on to the electroencephalography machine, which records the impulses (brain waves) on a continuously moving paper sheet.

If the test is to be a sleep electroencephalogram, you should stay awake the night before or get very little sleep. To help you fall asleep, you may be given a sedative before this test begins.

After the test, the paste used to attach the electrodes to your scalp may be washed off with ordinary shampoo.

Electromyography (EMG)

Electromyography measures the tiny electrical discharges produced in muscles. A variation of this test, the nerve conduction study, can measure the speed at which nerves carry electrical signals.

Electromyography is used to help diagnose muscle or nerve disorders such as muscular dystrophy (see page 888) and amyotrophic lateral sclerosis (see page 477) and some problems involving the spinal cord. A nerve conduction test, also referred to as electroneurography, is often used to diagnose peripheral nerve disorders, including carpal tunnel syndrome.

Electromyography usually is performed on an outpatient basis. It takes about an hour to complete. If many muscles are studied, however, the test takes longer.

Tell your physician or the technician conducting the test the names of any medicines you have taken in the previous 2 days. You will be asked to disrobe and wear a gown.

In electromyography, a thin-needle electrode is gently inserted into each muscle to be studied. You may feel a brief, sharp pain each time this needle is inserted but, because nothing is injected through it, this pain usually is less than that from a typical hypodermic injection.

A fine wire leads from the needle to an electronic instrument that detects electrical currents in your muscle. The patterns of electrical activity are recorded when the muscle is at rest and as you voluntarily tighten it. These patterns are viewed on a screen and may be recorded on film for further analysis.

Nerve conduction tests are performed in somewhat the same manner, except that needles are not used. Two small, disc-like recording electrodes are taped to your skin directly above the nerve to be studied or above a muscle connected to that nerve. Then a small instrument with metal prongs applies a mild shock over the nerve. This electrical signal moves down the nerve, passing under the disc-like electrodes. By comparing the recording of the signal at each electrode site and calculating the time it takes to travel between them, the speed of conduction along the nerve is easily determined. The nature of the signal from the nerve or muscle also helps to determine whether nerve or muscle fibers have been damaged by disease. Large nerves normally conduct signals at a speed (velocity) of about 110 miles an hour. In some nerve disorders, this conduction time is dramatically slower.

Microbiologic Tests

Any body fluid or tissue can be cultured if the presence of a microorganism is suspected. (A culture is the growing of a microorganism in a laboratory for study.) All cultures require enough time for the organism to grow to sufficient numbers to be identified. Some cultures, such as those for tuberculosis or fungi, sometimes require months. Once there are sufficient organisms in the culture, the infecting agent can be identified and its susceptibility to various antibodies can be evaluated.

Most cultures are obtained to identify a bacterium that may be causing an infection. Cultures also are obtained for the diagnosis of tuberculosis or a fungal infection. It also is possible to culture some viruses.

Throat Culture

This is a common microbiologic test in cases of pharyngitis, an inflammation or infection of the throat caused by various bacteria, viruses, or fungi.

If you have a sore throat, especially if accompanied by fever, swollen glands, or pus (exudate) in your throat, your sore throat may be caused by *Streptococcus* bacteria. This infection is commonly called strep throat. Because inadequate treatment of this type of sore throat can lead to rheumatic fever or acute glomerulonephritis (see page 836), be sure to have a throat culture.

Obtaining a specimen for a throat culture takes only a few seconds and is most often done in a laboratory or a physician's office.

Using a tongue depressor to permit a clear view through your mouth, your nurse or physician will look for redness and pus on your tonsils or on the back of your throat. If a throat culture is needed, a sterile swab will be rubbed over the back of your throat to obtain a sample of the secretions there. The swab is sent to a laboratory for analysis.

Some physicians use a rapid streptococcal test, which gives a fast diagnosis when it is positive. Because these rapid tests do not detect all sore throats caused by *Streptococcus*, a negative rapid test needs to be confirmed by throat culture.

Synovial Fluid Analysis

This test examines the lubricating (synovial) fluid secreted by the synovial membranes, which line joints in your body. The test is useful in the diagnosis of some types of arthritis (primarily those caused by infection, gout, or pseudogout). Obtaining the sample for the test takes about half an hour or less and usually is done in a physician's office or hospital.

No special preparations are necessary. The skin over the joint is cleaned with an antiseptic. Usually, a local or topical anesthetic is applied. Using a thin needle, your physician withdraws a sample of fluid for analysis, including culture of the fluid if infection is a possible diagnosis, and for examination for crystals to diagnose gout or pseudogout. If needed, medication (usually a corticosteroid preparation) can be injected into the joint space through this needle after the specimen is taken.

After the test, there often is slight pain at the puncture site, but this is brief. Discomfort also may occur when the needle penetrates the joint lining, but this also is relatively mild and brief. After the procedure is complete, the antiseptic is washed off and a small bandage is applied. If cortisone was injected, the joint space may be slightly uncomfortable for several hours, but then will feel better.

Avoid excessive use of the joint for a few days, even though the pain and swelling may diminish. If pain worsens or if the joint becomes red and warm, contact your physician immediately. He or she may want to examine the area to make sure there is no infection, although this is very uncommon.

Cerebrospinal Fluid Analysis

For this test, a small amount of cerebrospinal fluid is removed from your spinal column by lumbar puncture (spinal tap) for analysis. Analysis of this fluid can help in the diagnosis of meningitis, hemorrhage around the brain and spinal cord, tumors, syphilis, infections of the central nervous system, or noninflammatory conditions of the central nervous system. The procedure can be conducted on an outpatient basis in a hospital, in a laboratory, or in a physician's office and requires only a few minutes (see Lumbar Puncture, page 485).

Reproductive and Urologic Tests

The functions of the reproductive and urologic organs require diverse, specialized tests that aid in examination of these organs and in the diagnosis of their disorders.

Hysterosalpingography

In this test, X-ray pictures of the interior of the uterus and fallopian tubes are obtained. The pictures are used to evaluate infertility in women by detecting abnormalities in the fallopian tubes such as adhesions, obstructions, injuries, or the presence of foreign objects. Also, irregularities of the inner contour of the uterus can be visualized. The test takes about 30 minutes and can be performed in a laboratory, in a physician's office, or in a hospital.

You will disrobe and wear a gown. Once you lie down on the examining table and place your feet in the stirrups, an instrument called a speculum is carefully inserted into your vagina. A hook-like instrument (tenaculum) is used to hold your cervix in place.

A liquid contrast medium (dye) is then gently injected through a small tube into the uterus and fallopian tubes. There may be slight discomfort when the contrast medium reaches your uterus. If the tubes are blocked, the point of obstruction will be visible on the viewing screen of an X-ray device (fluoroscope). You may be asked to change positions occasionally to obtain better X-rays.

After the test, you may feel cramps, nausea, or dizziness, but these symptoms will pass. You also may have a bloody vaginal discharge.

Colposcopy

This procedure often is the first test done after a Pap smear gives abnormal results (see Pap Smear, page 1181). The colposcope (a modified binocular set) provides a magnified view of the cervix, vagina, and vulva and is used to determine the location of any cancerous or precancerous lesion present in these areas. The test takes about 15 minutes and is done in a physician's office.

Advise your physician of any medications you are taking. You will disrobe and wear a gown. On the examining table, you place your feet in the stirrups and then a speculum is inserted into your vagina. If any suspected lesion is found with the colposcope, a biopsy is done to confirm the severity. Any minor bleeding that may occur will be stopped before the procedure is completed.

Laparoscopy in Women

This procedure provides direct visual examination of your reproductive organs. It is used to detect endometriosis, ectopic pregnancy, pelvic inflammatory disease, cancer, or potential causes of pelvic pain or infertility. The procedure usually is done in a hospital on an outpatient basis and takes from ½ to 2 hours to complete.

Do not eat or drink for 12 hours before the procedure. You will disrobe and wear a gown. Once you receive an anesthetic (either a general or a local), a small incision will be made in your abdomen and a needle will be inserted to inflate your abdomen with a gas (carbon dioxide). Then the laparoscope, a long metal tube with a lens and tiny light source on one end, is inserted to examine the interior of your abdomen.

The anesthetic makes this procedure virtually painless. A special dye may be injected through the cervix into the uterine cavity to check for obstructions in the fallopian tubes. Surgical procedures that can be performed through the laparoscope include tubal ligation (female sterilization), cutting of adhe-

Home Medical Testing Kits

Your pharmacy or drugstore has a selection of kits that can be used to perform medical tests at home, without the involvement of a physician or health care professional. However, it is important to be aware of the disadvantages of using these kits. The types of kits available at present include the following:

1. Pregnancy tests to determine whether you are pregnant

2. Ovulation prediction tests to help determine the best time for intercourse that may lead to conception

3. Sugar tests, of either urine or blood, to determine whether diabetes is present

4. Other urine tests, such as for excess protein (which may signal a kidney problem)

5. Tests to detect hidden blood in the stool, which may indicate a tumor in the colon

Like most tests in a medical laboratory, home tests use urine, blood, or stool. Some of the kits are relatively inexpensive. The containers, test strips, and other paraphernalia contained in the kit are thrown away after use. Some kits contain enough supplies to perform the test more than once.

The advantages of doing a test with a kit are convenience and a reduced cost over having a medical laboratory perform the test. However, there are several disadvantages.

First, there is the risk of simply doing the test wrong—and therefore getting a misleading result. The instructions contained in the kit have to be followed exactly or the test will not work properly. A physician or health care professional in a medical laboratory is less likely to make a mistake because he or she has more expertise and experience and better equipment.

Second, medical tests do not always work right. This is true for tests done at home and for tests performed in a medical laboratory. A certain percentage of tests have results that suggest that something is true when it is not (false-positive). For example, a false-positive test result would indicate that you do have hidden blood in the stool when in fact you do not, or that you are pregnant when you are not.

Alternatively, a certain percentage of test results indicate that something is not true when it is (false-negative). For example, a false-negative test result would indicate that your blood glucose concentration is normal when it is not, or that you are not pregnant when you are. A physician is in a better position to judge false-negative and false-positive test results based on other medical evidence, training, and experience.

Third, you may interpret the result incorrectly. Changes in the results of the test, such as the color, may be confusing.

Finally, after performing the test, it is often very difficult to decide what to do next. For example, if you are certain there is blood in your stool but the test indicates otherwise, should you still see your physician?

In fact, it is often necessary to see your physician or have the test repeated by a medical laboratory no matter what the result, so you end up duplicating the expense. Use these home testing kits with caution: they are not a substitute for appropriate medical care, especially when you think you may be at risk of a serious medical condition.

---

sions, removal of an ovary, removal of some types of fibroids, and, sometimes, assisting in removal of your uterus (hysterectomy). Once the abdominal gas is expelled and the laparoscope removed, stitches are used to close the small incision.

If you received a general anesthetic, your vital signs will be checked for the next 4 hours. Any pain in your abdomen should disappear within 2 days.

Cystoscopy

Cystoscopy provides the opportunity to view your bladder and urethra. It is used to diagnose urinary tract disorders that produce symptoms such as painful urination, slowness of the urinary stream, incomplete emptying, dribbling and leakage of urine, and blood in the urine (see Cystoscopy, page 849).

Urine Tests

A routine urinalysis is a part of most comprehensive health examinations. Urinalysis includes tests for glucose (sugar), protein, bilirubin, and ketones in the urine. None of these substances are present normally, so their presence usually indicates a disease process.

The urine sediment also is examined under the microscope for the presence of white and red blood cells and debris. Detection of these substances may indicate the presence of an infection, tumor, or a disorder of the kidneys, ureter, or bladder, and further testing may be required.

Besides the routine urinalysis, there are many other specific tests that can be done on the urine. Most of these involve the detection of abnormal substances produced by your body or cultures if an infection is suspected. Urine can be analyzed for the presence of many drugs, including illicit drugs. Some of these tests can be done on a routine sample of urine; others require careful timing or even collection of the sample under sterile conditions.

In some instances, you will be asked to obtain a clean-catch urine collection. In this situation, you will be asked to void several ounces of urine into a toilet before collecting the sample of urine for analysis.

Appendices

Look here for information on how to convert a Fahrenheit temperature reading to centigrade, for concise definitions of common and uncommon medical terms, or for names, addresses, and telephone numbers of organizations that offer health information. You'll also find practical guidance on how to prepare a living will and a durable power of attorney for health care.

Contents

I   Conversion Tables (Weights and Measures). 1351

II Understanding Medical Terms. 1355

III Where to Go for More Information. 1373

IV How to Prepare an Advance Directive. 1381

Appendix I

Conversion Tables (Weights and Measures)

Contents

Linear Measurements, 1352

Sample Conversions for Metric Heights and Weights, 1352

Volume, 1353

Weight, 1353
Sample Conversion From Metric Weight, 1353

Temperature, 1354
  Centigrade (Celsius) to Fahrenheit, 1354
  Fahrenheit to Centigrade (Celsius), 1354

Household Measures, 1354

Linear Measurements

Millimeters, Centimeters, Meters, and Kilometers		Inches, Feet, Yards, and Miles
1.0 millimeter (mm)	=	0.04 inch (in)
1.0 centimeter (cm) = 10 mm	=	0.39 in
2.54 cm	=	1.0 in
30.48 cm	=	1.0 foot (ft) = 12 in
0.9144 meter (m)	=	1.0 yard (yd) = 3 ft
1.0 m = 100 cm	=	39.37 in
1.0 kilometer (km) = 1,000 m	=	0.622 mile (mi)
1.609 km	=	1.0 mi = 5,280 ft

Sample Conversions for Metric Heights and Weights

Height			Weight	
Centimeters	Feet	Inches (approx)	Kilograms	Pounds
15	0	6	1	2.2
30	1	0	5	11
45	1	6	10	22
60	1	11½	15	33
75	2	5½	20	44
90	2	11	25	55
105	3	5	30	66
115	3	9	35	77
120	3	11	40	88
125	4	1	45	99
130	4	3	50	110
135	4	5	55	121
140	4	7	60	132
145	4	9	65	143
150	4	11	70	154
155	5	1	75	165
160	5	3	80	176
165	5	5	85	187
170	5	7	90	198
175	5	9	95	209
180	5	11	100	220
185	6	1	105	231
190	6	3	110	242
195	6	5	115	253
200	6	7	120	264
205	6	9	125	275
210	6	11	130	286
215	7	1		

Volume

Milliliters and Liters		Ounces, Quarts, and Cubic Inches
1.0 milliliter (mL)	=	0.034 fluid ounce (fl oz)
16.3866 mL	=	1.0 cubic inch (in^3)
16.3866 mL	=	0.558 fl oz
29.57 mL	=	1.0 ounce (fl oz) = 1.8047 in^3
0.9463 liter (L)	=	1.0 quart (qt) = 32.0 fl oz
1.0 L = 1,000 mL	=	1.057 qt

Weight

Milligrams, Grams, and Kilograms		Grains, Ounces, and Pounds
1.0 milligram (mg)	=	0.015 grain (gr)
64.8 mg	=	1.0 gr
1.0 gram (g)	=	15.0 gr
1.0 g	=	0.035 ounce (oz)
31.1 g	=	1.0 oz
453.59 g	=	1.0 pound (lb) = 16 oz
1.0 kilogram (kg) = 1,000 g	=	2.2 lb

Sample Conversion From Metric Weight

Symbol	When You Know	Multiply by	To Find
g	grams	0.035	ounces (oz)
kg	kilograms	2.2	pounds (lb)

Temperature

Centigrade (Celsius) to Fahrenheit

Multiply centigrade degrees by 9/5 and add 32 to the result.

(Example: 25°C x 9/5 = 45 + 32 = 77°F)

Fahrenheit to Centigrade (Celsius)

Subtract 32 from Fahrenheit degrees and multiply the result by 5/9.

(Example: 77°F – 32 = 45 x 5/9 = 25°C)

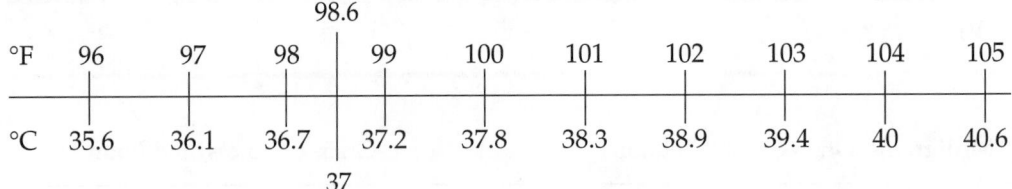

Household Measures

1 teaspoon	=	⅛ fluid ounce
3 teaspoons	=	1 tablespoon
1 tablespoon	=	½ fluid ounce
16 tablespoons (wet)	=	1 cup
12 tablespoons (dry)	=	1 cup
1 cup	=	8 fluid ounces
1 pint	=	2 cups or 16 fl oz

Note: Household measures are imprecise. For example, a household teaspoon is defined as containing between 3 and 5 milliliters. Thus, *never* substitute household equivalents for more precise dosages prescribed by your physician.

Appendix II

Understanding Medical Terms

Contents

Easy-to-understand explanations of the words your health care provider may use.

Glossary

The language of medicine is rich with specialized words. This wealth of vocabulary is a mixed blessing. Your physician can use precise terminology to describe conditions and symptoms to his or her colleagues. Yet in some cases, that same terminology can be confusing, worrisome, or incomprehensible to the uninitiated listener.

In the text of this book, we have tried to use language familiar to the layperson whenever possible to enhance the readability and utility of the book. In most cases, when a medical term is introduced, we define it first and then put the term in parentheses.

However, for those instances in which terms are confusing or unclear, we have assembled the glossary that follows. In it you will find a wide range of commonly used medical terms.

Given limitations of space, we have not incorporated the names of all or even most ailments discussed in the book; those are defined in entries devoted to them in the text and can be found by using the index at the back of this book. Similarly, you can find drug terms in The Modern Pharmacy (see page 1271) and terms that describe testing procedures in Medical Tests (see page 1329).

Abortion: The ending of a pregnancy by expulsion or extraction of the fetus from the womb before it is viable, usually before the 20th week of gestation.

Abrasion: A spot rubbed bare of skin or mucous membrane; or, the normal wearing of tooth enamel by chewing.

Abscess: A localized formation of pus in a cavity caused by the disintegration or displacement of tissue due to bacterial infection.

Acute: Term used to describe disorders or symptoms that occur abruptly or disorders or symptoms that run a short course; opposite of chronic.

Addiction: Physical or emotional (or both) dependence on a substance (most often alcohol or another drug), usually requiring increasing amounts to achieve the same effect.

Adhesion: A union of two surfaces, as in a wound healing.

Adrenal glands: Endocrine glands that produce a range of hormones, including epinephrine (adrenaline), norepinephrine, and the corticosteroid hormones.

Adrenaline: See Epinephrine.

Aerobic: Requiring the presence of oxygen. Aerobic exercise, for example, is vigorous, requiring increased oxygen consumption. See Anaerobic.

Afterbirth: The placenta and membranes discharged from the uterus after childbirth.

Albumin: A protein found widely in animal and plant tissues; its presence in the urine is one sign of kidney disease.

Aldosterone: Adrenal hormone that affects the body's handling of sodium, chloride, and potassium.

Allergen: Any substance that produces an allergic reaction. Common allergens include animal fur, house dust mites, pollen, and certain foods.

Allergy: An exaggerated reaction to a substance or condition produced by the release of histamine or histamine-like substances in affected cells. Symptoms may include rashes, nasal congestion, asthma, and occasionally shock. See Histamine.

Alveoli: Microscopic air sacs in the lungs where gases are exchanged; or, tooth socket.

Amanita mushrooms: Group of mushrooms, most of which are highly poisonous when eaten.

Ambulatory: Able to walk.

Amino acid: A component of protein, containing nitrogen. The body produces many amino acids; those it needs but cannot synthesize are known as essential amino acids and must be obtained through the diet.

Amnesia: Loss of memory.

Amniotic fluid: The protective liquid surrounding the fetus in the womb.

Amputation: The act of cutting off or removing a limb or other body part.

Anaerobic: Able to live without oxygen, as certain bacteria; or, a type of exercise in which short, vigorous bursts of activity requiring little additional oxygen are performed. See Aerobic.

Anaphylaxis: An immediate and sometimes life-threatening allergic hypersensitivity reaction. Symptoms can include shock, breathing difficulty, itching and hives, convulsions, and coma. See Shock.

Androgen: A hormone such as testosterone and androsterone responsible for the development of male characteristics. Produced in the testicles in the male; also found in small amounts in females.

Anemia: Condition characterized by a reduced number of red blood cells, amount of hemoglobin, or amount of blood.

Anesthesia: Partial or complete loss of feeling or sensation sometimes accompanied by loss of consciousness. Local anesthesia is confined to a particular region of the body. General anesthesia includes the whole body.

Aneurysm: The localized enlargement of a blood vessel, usually an artery, to form a bulge or sac.

Angina pectoris: Episodic pain in the chest due to a temporary inadequacy of the blood supply to the heart.

Angioedema: Allergic swelling of the mucous membranes, tissues beneath the skin, or an internal organ.

Anorexia: Loss of appetite, often due to depression, fever, illness, widespread cancer, or addiction to alcohol or drugs.

Anorexia nervosa: Loss of appetite caused by an emotional disturbance; it most often affects young women between 12 and 21 years old and can result in severe loss of weight and even death.

Antibody: Protein of the immune system that counteracts or eliminates foreign substances known as antigens.

Antidote: Substance that neutralizes the effects of a poison.

Antigen: Substance foreign to the body that causes antibodies to form.

Anus: Outlet of the rectum, through which fecal waste passes.

Aorta: Largest artery in the body; it carries blood from the heart's left ventricle and distributes it throughout the body.

Aphasia: Loss of the ability to speak or to understand speech because of brain injury.

Aplastic: Arrested development of a tissue or an organ.

Apnea: Temporary cessation of breathing.

Aqueous humor: Transparent fluid within the anterior and posterior chambers of the eye.

Areola: Circular, pigmented area around the nipple of the breast.

Arrhythmia: Irregular heartbeat.

Arteriole: Tiny artery that joins a larger artery to a capillary.

Arteriosclerosis: Condition in which the walls of arteries become hard and thick, sometimes interfering with blood circulation.

Artery: Blood vessel that carries blood from the heart to other tissues of the body.

Arthroplasty: Surgical replacement or repair of a joint.

Asphyxia: Suffocation due to insufficient oxygen intake.

Aspiration: Removal of fluids by suction from cavities such as the nose, throat, or lungs; or, the inhalation into the lungs of fluids, such as water in drowning or stomach contents in vomiting.

Asthma: Condition characterized by congestion in bronchial tubes, causing wheezing, coughing, and difficulty breathing.

Asymptomatic: Without symptoms.

Ataxia: Incoordination of voluntary muscle movements.

Atherosclerosis: Condition in which fatty deposits accumulate in the lining of the arteries, resulting in smaller, less flexible pathways for the blood.

Atresia: Congenital absence of an opening in the body.

Atria: Cavities or chambers such as the upper chambers of the heart, which receive blood from veins and pass the blood to the ventricles. (Singular form is atrium.)

Atrophy: Wasting of tissue or organ due to disease or lack of use.

Aura: Sensation felt before the onset of a convulsion or migraine headache.

Autoimmune response: Reaction of the body against one or some of its own tissues that are perceived as foreign substances, resulting in production of antibodies against that tissue.

Autonomic nervous system: Portion of the nervous system that regulates involuntary body functions.

Autopsy: Examination of tissues and organs of the body after death.

Avulsion: Forced tearing away of a body part or structure such as a limb or tooth.

Bacteria: Single-celled microorganisms, some of which cause disease and some of which are beneficial to biologic processes.

B cell: Lymphocyte of the bone marrow that works as part of the immune system by producing antibodies to fight infection.

Benign: Term meaning essentially harmless; not progressive or recurrent.

Bicuspid: One of four teeth in the adult mouth having two points, located between the canine and molar.

Bile: Bitter-tasting fluid produced by the

liver and temporarily stored in the gall-bladder before discharge into the small intestine. In the small bowel the bile facilitates the digestion of fats.

Bilirubin: Orange or yellowish pigment in bile that is the result of breakdown of hemoglobin. An excess of bilirubin produces jaundice.

Biofeedback: Behavior-training program that teaches a person how to control autonomic reactions such as heart rate, blood pressure, skin temperature, and muscular tension.

Bladder: Membranous sac that holds secretions, most commonly the sac that collects urine before its elimination.

Blood pressure: Constant force placed on the walls of the arteries. See Diastole and Systole.

Bone marrow: Soft material found inside bone cavities that is the site of formation of blood cells.

Bowel: Small or large intestine. The small intestine is sometimes called the small bowel.

Brain stem: Portion of the brain that connects the hemispheres with the spinal cord. Consists of medulla oblongata, pons, and midbrain.

Brand-name drug: A drug carrying a trademark name designated by its manufacturer.

Bronchi: The two main breathing tubes leading from the trachea to the lungs.

Bronchiole: One of the subdivisions of a bronchus or bronchial tube.

Bruise: Injury in which blood vessels beneath the skin are broken and blood escapes to produce a discolored area.

Bursa: Fluid-filled sac near or involving a joint or bony prominence that helps to reduce friction between a tendon or bone or between bone and skin during movement.

Cachexia: Malnutrition and wasting due to illness.

Calcitonin: A hormone produced by the thyroid gland that affects the amount of calcium in the blood.

Calculus: Accumulation of mineral salts in various parts of the body or on the teeth which resembles stone.

Callus: Area of thickened skin.

Calorie: The amount of heat needed to raise the temperature of 1 gram of water by 1 degree centigrade.

Cancer: General term for various illnesses characterized by abnormal growth of cells, forming malignant tumors that can develop in various parts of the body. See Malignant and Benign.

Canine: One of four teeth found between the molars and incisors; also known as eye teeth.

Capillaries: Minute blood vessels connecting the smallest arteries to the smallest veins.

Carbohydrate: A group of compounds composed of starches or sugars and found primarily in breads and cereals and in fruits and vegetables.

Carcinogen: Potential cancer-causing agent.

Cardiac: Pertaining to the heart.

Cardiac arrest: Sudden stopping of circulation by cessation of the heartbeat.

Cardiopulmonary: Pertaining to the heart and lung.

Cardiopulmonary resuscitation (CPR): Technique for reviving a person whose heart and breathing have stopped and who is unconscious.

Cardiovascular: Pertaining to the heart and blood vessels.

Caries: Decay of tooth or bone due to bacteria; also known as cavities.

Carotid artery: Principal artery of neck; carries blood to head and brain.

Cartilage: Dense, white connective tissue located in the joints, nose, and ear.

Cataract: Opacity of the eye lens that obstructs vision.

Catheter: Small, flexible tube that may be inserted into various parts of the body to inject or remove liquid.

Cerebellum: Portion of the brain responsible for balance and coordination.

Cerebrovascular: Pertaining to the blood vessels of the brain.

Cerebrum: Largest portion of the brain, containing the two hemispheres; responsible for speech, memory, vision, personality, and muscle control in certain parts of your body.

Cervix: The neck of an organ, such as the neck of the uterus.

Cesarean section: Surgical removal of a baby from the womb through an incision in the abdomen and wall of the uterus.

Chemotherapy: Treatment of disease by using chemicals that have a direct effect on the disease-causing organism or disease cells; widely used in the treatment of cancer.

Cholesterol: Fat-like substance synthesized in the liver and found in the blood, brain, liver, and bile and as deposits in the walls of blood vessels. Essential to the production of sex hormones. Found in foods of animal sources and thought to contribute to heart disease when eaten in large quantities over a long period of time.

Choroid: Membrane of the eye between the sclera (white) and the retina; together with the iris and ciliary body it makes up the uvea.

Chromosome: One of 46 rod-shaped structures in the nucleus of each cell that carries information regarding heredity.

Chronic: Term used to describe long-lasting diseases or conditions.

Chyme: Mixture of partly digested food and digestive secretions found in the stomach.

Cilia: Eyelashes; or, other smaller hair-like projections lining the bronchi and upper respiratory tract.

Claudication: Pain in muscles during exercise, produced by inadequate arterial blood flow.

Clinical: Pertaining to information gathered from working with patients, as distinct from laboratory findings.

Clitoris: Small, erectile organ of the external female genitals.

Coagulate: To solidify or change from a liquid to a semisolid, as when blood clots.

Cochlea: Snail-shaped tube of the inner ear that is the receptor for hearing.

Cognitive: Pertaining to the mental process of thought, including perception, reasoning, intuition, and memory.

Coitus: Sexual intercourse between a man and woman in which the man inserts his penis into the woman's vagina.

Colic: Pain in abdomen produced by intermittent spasm of the intestines. In infants, it may be manifested by episodes of crying, with a distended abdomen and the legs drawn up to the chest.

Collagen: Fibrous protein found in connective tissues such as skin, ligaments, and cartilage.

Colon: The large intestine extending from the small intestine to the anus. It is responsible for extracting water from undigested food and storing the waste, which is eliminated in bowel movements.

Colorectal: Pertaining to the colon and rectum.

Colostrum: The thin, lemon-colored liquid produced by a mother's breasts in the first day or so after giving birth. Its antibodies are beneficial to the infant.

Coma: An abnormal state of deep unconsciousness due to illness or accident.

Conception: Fertilization of an egg by a sperm.

Concussion: Temporary disturbance of brain function due to a blow to the head.

Congenital: Term used to describe something present at birth, especially an abnormality.

Congestion: The presence of excessive blood or fluid, such as mucus, in an organ or tissue.

Conjunctiva: Transparent membrane that lines the eyelid and covers the front of the eyeball (except for the cornea).

Constipation: The difficult passage of hard, dry stools.

Contracture: Permanent tightness or shortening of a muscle due to disease.

Contrast agent: A liquid substance (dye) opaque to X-rays that is taken into the gastrointestinal tract or injected into a blood vessel or into the fluid-filled space around the spinal cord to permit X-ray visualization of structures of the body that could not otherwise be seen by X-ray.

Contusion: Bruise.

Convulsion: A sudden attack usually characterized by loss of consciousness and severe, sustained, rhythmic contractions of some or all voluntary muscles. Convulsions are most often a manifestation of a seizure disorder (epilepsy).

Cornea: Transparent part of the eye through which the iris and pupil may be seen.

Coronary: Pertaining to arteries that supply blood to the heart.

Corticosteroids: Hormones produced by the cortex of the adrenal glands; also, a class of such hormones used as medications.

Cranium: Portion of the skull that houses the brain.

Creatinine: Substance excreted in the urine. Excretion rate can be used to evaluate kidney function.

Curettage: Scraping of a cavity, such as the uterus.

Cuspid: Tooth with one point, located between the incisors and bicuspids toward the front of the mouth, sometimes called the canine tooth.

Cyanosis: Bluish discoloration of the skin due to a lack of oxygen in the blood.

Cyst: A closed sac or cavity filled with a fluid, gas, or semisolid substance.

Debility: A state of physical weakness.

Dehydration: The result of excessive loss of body fluids or inadequate fluid consumption.

Delirium: A state of mental confusion, sometimes characterized by disordered speech and often accompanied by hallucinations.

Delusion: Belief held despite evidence as to its falsehood.

Dementia: Mental deterioration due to organic causes.

Dentin: The tissue of a tooth beneath the enamel and enclosing the pulp cavity.

Deoxyribonucleic acid (DNA): A substance found in the nucleus of cells that carries hereditary information.

Depression: A feeling of extreme sadness and discouragement. Symptoms also may include disruption of sleeping and eating patterns and lack of energy.

Dermatitis: Inflammation of the skin, often characterized by itching and redness.

Dermis: The layer of skin beneath the epidermis.

Detoxification: Process of cleansing the body of a drug such as alcohol.

Dextrose (glucose): A simple sugar that is found in the blood; a main component of honey and corn syrup.

Diabetes mellitus: A disorder characterized by high levels of glucose in the blood. Diabetes mellitus may be caused by a failure of the pancreas to produce sufficient insulin or by resistance of the body to the action of insulin.

Diagnosis: Identification of a disease or disorder by a physician.

Dialysis: Technique of removing waste and toxins from the blood, used primarily when the kidneys fail or in cases of overdose of a drug.

Diaphragm: Muscle that separates the abdomen from the chest; or, a rubber or plastic device that fits over the cervix to help prevent conception.

Diastole: Period during the heart cycle in which the muscle relaxes, followed by contraction (systole). In a blood pressure reading, the lower number is the diastolic measurement.

Digit: A finger or toe.

Dilate: To expand or open an organ such as the pupil of the eye or a passageway such as an artery.

Disc: A plate-like structure such as the cartilage cushion found between each vertebra.

Dislocation: Displacement of a bone from its normal position at a joint.

Dominant: A mode of inheritance in which a gene from only one parent is required for a trait to appear in an offspring. See Recessive.

Duodenum: The part of the small intestine closest to the stomach.

Dura mater: The tough outer membrane covering the spinal cord and brain.

Dysplasia: Abnormal development of tissue.

Ect-, Ecto-: Prefixes meaning outside.

Ectopic: Abnormal placement, such as a pregnancy that occurs outside the uterus (tubal pregnancy).

Eczema: Acute or chronic inflammatory condition of the skin characterized by itching and scaling.

Edema: Swelling of body tissues due to excessive fluid.

Effusion: Accumulation of fluid in body cavities or between tissues.

Ejaculation: Ejection of semen during male orgasm.

Embolism: Obstruction of a blood vessel by a blood clot, air bubble, fat deposit, or other foreign substance.

Embryo: The human organism from the time of implantation in the uterus to the end of the second month after conception.

Emetic: Substance that induces vomiting.

Emission: Discharge of fluid.

En-, Endo-: Prefixes meaning inside or within.

Endocardium: The thin, inner membrane that lines the cavities of the heart. See Epicardium and Myocardium

Endoscope: An illuminated optical instrument used to visualize the inside of a hollow organ or cavity.

Enema: Introduction of fluid into the rectum and colon to induce a bowel movement to empty those structures.

Enzyme: A complex protein present in digestive juices or within cells that acts as a catalyst for chemical reactions.

Epicardium: The thin, exterior membrane that covers the heart muscle. See Endocardium and Myocardium.

Epidermis: Outermost layer of the skin.

Epiglottis: Flap of cartilage that covers the larynx.

Epilepsy: See Seizure.

Epinephrine and Norepinephrine: Naturally occurring hormones that increase heart rate and blood pressure and affect other body functions.

Erection: Swelling and stiffening of the penis, characteristic of sexual arousal.

Erythema: Area of reddened skin due to dilatation of capillaries beneath the skin.

Erythrocytes: Red blood cells; they transport oxygen.

Esophagus: The muscular tube that connects the throat with the stomach.

Estrogen: Hormone produced primarily in

women that contributes to the development of female secondary sex characteristics and cyclic changes such as menstruation and pregnancy. Oral replacement doses of estrogen are often used to lessen the effects of menopause. The hormone is also produced in small quantities in men.

Ethanol: Grain or ethyl alcohol.

Eustachian tube: Tube connecting the middle ear to the pharynx.

Faint: To lose consciousness briefly as a result of insufficient blood to the brain.

Fallopian tube: One of two tubes, located on each side of a woman's uterus, that convey the egg from the ovary to the cavity of the uterus.

False labor: Irregular pains and contractions that give a pregnant woman the illusion that labor has begun.

Fats: A group of organic compounds that are composed of fatty acids. Fats are either saturated or unsaturated. Unsaturated fats are classified further as either monounsaturated or polyunsaturated.

Febrile: Feverish.

Feces: Body waste such as food residue discharged from the bowels.

Femur: Thighbone.

Fertility: The ability to conceive or to cause conception.

Fertilization: Process of conception in which a sperm penetrates an ovum, usually in the fallopian tube.

Fetus: Name given to fertilized ovum from the second month of pregnancy to delivery.

Fiber: Food substance that resists chemical digestion and passes through the system essentially unchanged. Fiber adds bulk to the diet and aids in the removal of feces.

Fibrillation: Quivering or uncontrollable contraction of muscles. When it occurs in the cardiac muscle it causes an irregular heartbeat.

Fibroid: Common term for fibroma, a benign tumor of connective and muscular tissue, usually of the uterus.

Fibula: The smaller of two bones that run from the knee to the ankle.

Flatulence: Excessive gas in the stomach and intestine.

Fluoride: Element found in nature. Adequate consumption of fluoride helps prevent tooth decay and possibly strengthens bone.

Follicle: Small tubular gland or sac in the skin or ovary; or, an aggregation of cells in a lymph node.

Fontanelle: A soft spot atop an infant's head where the bones of the skull have yet to join.

Forceps: Surgical instrument, resembling pincers, that is used for grasping or compressing tissue.

Fracture: To break or crack a bone; or, a break or a crack in a bone.

Fructose: A sugar found in fruit, corn syrup, and honey.

Fungus: Organism of plant origin that lacks chlorophyll; some fungi can cause irritation or disease.

Gallbladder: Sac located under the liver. It stores bile secreted from the liver and releases it into the small intestine during digestion.

Gamma globulin: A protein found in the blood that helps fight infection.

Ganglion: Mass of nerve tissue made up mostly of nerve cell bodies. Also, a cystic tumor in a tendon sheath.

Gangrene: Death of body tissue, usually due to a lack of blood supply; the tissue shrinks and turns black.

Gastric: Pertaining to the stomach.

Gastrointestinal tract: The stomach and intestines.

Gene: Structure within a chromosome that is responsible for inheritance of a particular characteristic.

Generalized: Overall, not limited to one area of the body.

Generic drug: The non-trademark name of a drug.

Genetic engineering: Manufacture, alteration, or repair of genetic material by artificial means.

Genitals: Reproductive organs.

Geriatrics: The branch of medicine that specializes in the care of problems related to aging.

Germ: A microorganism; some may cause disease.

Gestation: The period of time from conception to birth.

Gigantism: Disorder caused by an overproduction of growth hormone by the pituitary gland. It results in excessive body height and size. Also known as giantism.

Gland: Any organ or tissue that releases a substance to be used elsewhere in the body; endocrine glands release hormones directly into the bloodstream.

Globulin: A category of blood proteins of which antibodies are formed.

Globus: A sensation of a lump in your throat in the absence of a physical abnormality; may be related to stress.

Glomeruli: Microscopic clusters of blood vessels in the kidneys, responsible for filtering waste from the blood.

Glucagon: Pancreatic hormone that releases the body's stored sugar (glycogen) from the liver into the blood.

Glucose: Blood sugar, also known as dextrose.

Gluten: Plant proteins found in grains such as wheat, rye, oats, and barley.

Glycogen: Stored form of sugar (glucose) in the liver.

Goiter: Enlargement of the thyroid gland.

Gonads: See Ovaries and Testicles.

Grand mal: Generalized convulsion accompanied by loss of consciousness.

Granulocytes: White blood cells (leukocytes), manufactured in the bone marrow, that contain granules. They digest and destroy bacteria.

Groin: Lower abdominal area where the trunk and thigh meet.

Halitosis: Bad breath.

Hallucination: A false perception with no basis in reality; may be seen, heard, or smelled.

Hamstrings: Muscles at the back of the thigh. The tendons of the hamstring muscles can be felt at the back of the knee.

Handicapped: Impaired physically or mentally so that normal activities are interfered with.

Heart attack: Descriptive term for a myocardial infarction: a painful, and sometimes fatal, incident caused by the blockage of one or more of the coronary arteries resulting in sudden interruption of blood to a part of the heart.

Heartburn: A burning sensation beneath the breastbone (sternum) resulting from regurgitation of gastric juices (reflux) from the stomach into the esophagus.

Heart murmur: An abnormal sound heard during the normal heartbeat. The condition can be benign or a sign of a diseased heart valve or other heart abnormality.

Hemangioma: Benign tumor of dilated blood vessels.

Hematemesis: Vomiting of blood.

Hematoma: Blood-filled swelling beneath the skin or in an organ, due to injury to a blood vessel.

Hematuria: Blood or blood clots in the urine.

Hemiplegia: Paralysis of one side of the body.

Hemodialysis: Mechanical removal of chemical waste from the blood.

Hemoglobin: A pigmented protein that contains iron and is found in the red blood cells. Hemoglobin transports oxygen to body tissues.

Hemoptysis: Coughing or spitting up of blood that comes from bleeding in the larynx, trachea, or lungs.

Hemorrhage: Bleeding (internal or external) caused by damage to a blood vessel.

Hemorrhoid: Swollen vein in and around the anus that may bleed.

Hepatic: Pertaining to the liver.

Heredity: Transmission of genetic traits from parent to child.

Hernia: Protrusion of an organ or structure into surrounding tissues. Commonly called a rupture.

Hiccup: Involuntary spasm of the diaphragm, followed quickly by shutting of the glottis, resulting in a sharp, sudden intake of breath.

High blood pressure: See Hypertension.

Hirsutism: Excessive growth of body or facial hair.

Histamine: Body chemical present in tissue that, when released, stimulates production of gastric juices for digestion; or, the active agent of allergic reactions that result when excessive amounts of histamine are released to combat a perceived invader. The site affected becomes swollen and congested, resulting in hives (skin), asthma (lining of the bronchial passages), or hay fever (lining of the nose).

Hives: Eruption of itchy red and white wheals on the skin as a result of excessive histamine release within the skin.

Hormone: A substance (secreted by an endocrine gland) that is carried through the bloodstream to various organs of the body, where it serves to regulate various body functions.

Humerus: Bone of the upper arm.

Humoral: Pertaining to body fluids.

Hydrogenation: Process of changing an unsaturated fat to a more solid, saturated one.

Hymen: Membrane partially covering opening to the vagina.

Hymenoptera: Order of insects that includes bees, wasps, and ants.

Hyper-: Prefix meaning excessive or increased.

Hyperactivity: Condition of disturbed behavior characterized by constant overactivity, distractibility, impulsiveness, inability to concentrate, and aggressiveness.

Hyperglycemia: Condition in which an excess of sugar (glucose) is present in the bloodstream.

Hyperplasia: Excessive growth of tissues in an organ, causing increased size.

Hypertension: Condition in which the blood is pumped through the body under abnormally high pressure; also known as high blood pressure.

Hypo-: Prefix meaning inadequate or insufficient.

Hypochondria: Excessive concern about health.

Hypoglycemia: Condition in which the sugar (glucose) in the bloodstream falls below normal amounts.

Hypotension: Low blood pressure.

Hypothalamus: A portion of the brain; partly responsible for basic functions such as appetite, sleep, body temperature, and procreation.

Hypoxia: Decreased concentration of oxygen in the blood.

Iatrogenic disease: Disorder or disease resulting as a side effect of a prescribed treatment.

Idiopathic: Pertaining to a condition or disease of unknown cause.

Ileum: Lower portion of the small intestine.

Ilium: The upper portion of the hipbone.

Immobilize: To make a limb or part immovable in order to aid healing.

Immunity: State of being resistant to a disease, particularly an infectious one.

Immunization: Introduction of antigens into the body in very small quantities in order to stimulate the development of immunity.

Immunoglobulin: A protein that can act as an antibody.

Impacted: Pressed firmly together so as to be immovable.

Impotence: Inability of a man to achieve or keep an erection and engage in sexual intercourse.

Incision: A cut made with a knife.

Incisors: The eight front teeth, four in the upper jaw and four in the lower jaw.

Incontinence: Inability to control release of urine or feces.

Indigestion: Incomplete or abnormal digestion.

Infarct: An area of tissue that dies because of blockage of its blood supply.

Infection: Condition in which the body or a part of it is invaded by a microorganism such as a bacterium or virus.

Infectious: Ability to transmit or cause a disease.

Infertility: Inability to reproduce.

Inflammation: Body tissue's reaction to injury from infection, physical injury, or irritation, resulting in swelling, pain, heat, and redness.

Inguinal: Pertaining to the groin area where the trunk and legs meet.

Inoperable: Unsuitable for treatment by surgery.

Insemination: Insertion of semen into the vagina; may result in fertilization of an egg.

Insomnia: Inability to sleep.

Insulin: Pancreatic hormone that enables the body to regulate the amount of sugar (glucose) in the bloodstream. (See Diabetes mellitus.)

Intestines: Portion of the digestive tract extending from stomach to anus and responsible for much of the absorption of nutrients. See Colon, Duodenum, Ileum, and Jejunum.

Intolerance: Inability to tolerate pain, a drug therapy, or substances such as glucose and lactose.

Intracranial: Within the skull.

Intravenous: Within or into a vein.

Intrinsic factor: A substance found in the gastric juices that allows for the absorption of vitamin B_{12} from the intestine.

Involuntary: Cannot be controlled through will.

Iris: The round, colored membrane of the eye surrounding the pupil, which serves to control the amount of light reaching the retina.

Ischemia: Deficiency of blood within an organ or part of an organ. Often refers to the situation in which an artery is narrowed or blocked by spasm or atherosclerosis and cannot deliver sufficient blood to the organ it supplies.

Isotope: One of a number of chemical elements that have similar structures but not identical weights. Some isotopes are radioactive.

-itis: Suffix meaning inflammation.

Jaundice: A yellowing of the skin produced by blockage of the bile passages or by the liver's inability to metabolize bilirubin.

Jejunum: The portion of the small intestine located between the duodenum and ileum.

Joint: The point of juncture between two or more bones where movement occurs.

Jugular veins: The two veins on the sides of the neck that carry blood from the brain and head to the heart.

Keloid: Abnormally thick scar that can form after surgery or injury.

Keratin: Protein found in hair, nails, and the outer layers of skin.

Ketoacidosis: Sometimes fatal complication of insulin-dependent diabetes that results from too little insulin. It can cause loss of consciousness (diabetic coma).

Kidneys: The two bean-shaped organs located in the back portion of the upper abdomen, one on each side of the spine. Responsible for the formation and excretion of urine and regulation of the water, electrolyte, and acid-base content of blood.

Kyphosis: Excessive curvature of the spine, resulting in humpback, hunchback, or rounding of the shoulders. May result from diseases such as osteoarthritis or rheumatoid arthritis, osteoporosis, or rickets, from conditions such as compression fracture, or from a congenital abnormality.

Labia: Two sets of lip-like genital organs in women. The labia majora are two folds of skin and fatty tissue that protect the vulva; the labia minora are smaller folds inside the labia majora.

Labor: Process of muscle contraction by which a baby is born.

Labyrinth: Portion of the inner ear responsible for balance.

Laceration: Flesh wound caused by tearing.

Lacrimal gland: Gland of the eye that secretes tears.

Lactation: Process of production and secretion of milk from the breasts.

Lactose: Sugar found naturally in milk.

Larynx: Structure of the voice box, composed of cartilage housing the vocal cords and the muscles and ligaments used to produce sound.

Lens: Transparent structure in the eye that focuses light to form an image on the back of the retina.

Lesion: Area of tissue either injured (as in a wound, abscess, or sore) or altered (as in a tumor, mole, or cyst).

Leukocytes: White blood cells; they fight infection.

Libido: Sexual drive.

Ligament: Strong fibrous connective tissue resembling a band or sheet that connects a bone to another bone.

Ligature: Filament (synthetic or natural) for tying off blood vessels during surgery to keep them from bleeding. The procedure itself is called ligation.

Lipid: Descriptive term for a fat or fat-like substance found in the blood, such as cholesterol.

Liposuction: Process of removing fat deposits from beneath the skin by using a suction device.

Lithiasis: Formation of calculi deposits such as gallstones and kidney stones.

Liver: Largest internal organ in the body. It is the site of many metabolic functions, including secreting bile, neutralizing poisons, synthesizing proteins, and storing glycogen and certain minerals and vitamins.

Localized: Limited to a discrete area, as in an infection or disease. See Generalized and Systemic.

Lordosis: Exaggerated curvature of the lower portion of the spine, causing swayback.

Lumbar: Pertaining to the lower back.

Lungs: The two cone-shaped spongy organs of respiration located around the bronchial tree. The lungs bring air and blood into close contact so that oxygen can be added to the blood and carbon dioxide can be removed.

Lymph: Clear fluid present in lymphatic vessels.

Lymph node: Small round structures found throughout the body that produce lymphocytes and monocytes, that help protect the body from invasion by bacteria or other organisms.

Lymphocytes: Disease-fighting white blood cells made in the lymph nodes and distributed throughout the body by way of the lymphatic fluid and blood.

Maceration: Softening of tissue by soaking in liquid.

Macrophage: Cells found throughout the body, particularly in the spleen, that have the ability to ingest other substances such as worn-out red blood cells; also important in the immune response.

Malabsorption: Inadequate absorption of nutrients from the small intestine. Symptoms of malabsorption syndrome include loose fatty stools, diarrhea, weight loss, weakness, and anemia.

Malaise: General feeling of illness, discomfort, and uneasiness, often a sign of infection.

Malignant: Term used to describe cancerous tumors that can grow uncontrollably and spread (metastasize).

Malnutrition: Deficiency of nourishment in the body due to lack of healthful food or improper digestion and distribution of nutrients.

Malpresentation: Abnormal position of the fetus during labor, making normal delivery difficult or impossible.

Mammary gland: Compound gland of the breast that secretes milk.

Mandible: Lower jaw.

Mania: Mental disorder characterized by an intense feeling of elation and excitability, often accompanied by increased activity.

Masticate: Chew.

Mastoid process: Round, honeycombed bone mass located behind the ear.

Maxilla: Upper jaw.

Meconium stool: The newborn's first bowel movement, composed of intestinal secretions and amniotic fluid, usually dark green.

Medulla: Center of an organ, gland, or bone.

Melanin: Pigment that provides dark color to hair, skin, and choroid of the eye.

Membrane: Thin, soft layer of tissue that lines, separates, or covers organs or structures.

Meninges: The membranes that cover the spinal cord and brain.

Menopause: The gradual cessation of menstruation, at the end of which a woman is no longer able to reproduce.

Menstruation: Monthly shedding of blood and tissue from the lining of the uterus.

Mesentery: Fold in the abdominal lining that connects the intestine to the back of the abdominal wall and contains the arteries and veins that supply the intestines.

Metabolism: The process by which food is transformed, energy is derived, and tissues are broken down into waste products.

Metastasis: Spreading of a disease from one part of the body to another, usually by movement of cells (as in cancer) or bacteria through the lymph or blood system.

Microbes: One-celled organisms such as bacteria, many of which cause disease.

Micturition: Urination.

Miosis: Abnormal pupil contraction, often a sign of disease or disorder.

Miscarriage: Premature, spontaneous termination of a pregnancy (spontaneous abortion).

Mitosis: Type of cell division in which the new cells have the same number of chromosomes as the parent cell.

Mitral valve: Heart valve that allows oxygenated blood to move into the left ventricle from the left atrium and prevents the reverse flow.

Molars: The grinding or chewing teeth, located at the back of both jaws.

Mono-: Prefix meaning one.

Motility: Ability to move.

Mucous membrane: Thin, moist membrane that lines passages and cavities that are in contact with air, such as nose, mouth, and eyes.

Muscle: Tissue that produces movement by its ability to contract.

Musculoskeletal: Pertaining to the muscles and the skeleton.

Myalgia: Muscle tenderness or pain.

Myelin: White, fat-like substance that forms a sheath around some nerves.

Myocardium: The heart muscle. See Endocardium and Epicardium.

Myopathy: Any disease of the muscle.

Narcosis: A state of stupor often induced by drugs or other agents.

Nares: Nostrils.

Natal: Pertaining to birth.

Nausea: Sensation of stomach sickness, often followed by vomiting.

Necrosis: Death of areas of tissue surrounded by healthy tissue.

Neonatal: Pertaining to a newborn up to 4 weeks old.

Neoplasm: New and abnormal growth.

Nephritis: Inflammation of the kidney.

Nephron: A structure of the kidney in which blood is filtered to remove waste and form urine.

Nerve: Bundle of fibers that connect the brain and spinal cord with various parts of the body and through which impulses pass.

Neuralgia: Sharp pain along the course of a nerve.

Neuron: A nerve cell.

Neuropathy: Any nerve disease.

Neurotransmitter: Nerve cell chemicals that act as messengers in the brain and nervous system.

Node: Small, round or egg-shaped tissue or structure.

Nonsteroidal anti-inflammatory drugs (NSAIDs): Medications, used to reduce inflammation, that are not cortisone-based.

Norepinephrine (sometimes called **Noradrenaline**): See Epinephrine.

Nucleus: Center portion of all cells, except red blood cells, essential for cell growth, nourishment, and reproduction.

Obesity: Abnormal body weight, usually defined as more than 20 percent above average for age, height, and bone structure.

Occipital: Pertaining to the back of the head.

Occlusion: Closure of a passage such as ducts or blood vessels; in dentistry, the alignment of upper and lower teeth when the jaws are closed.

Occult: Undetectable without magnification.

Ocular: Pertaining to the eye.

Olfactory: Pertaining to the sense of smell.

-oma: Suffix meaning tumor.

Oncogenes: Genes present in normal cells that, upon exposure to cancer-inducing viruses, lead to development of tumors.

Optic nerve: Nerve that carries visual impulses from the retina to the brain, where they are interpreted.

Orbit: Eye socket.

Orgasm: Climax of sexual intercourse or stimulation of sexual organs. In the man, it is associated with the ejaculation of sperm; in the woman, with contractions of the vagina.

-osis: Suffix meaning diseased state.

Osseous: Pertaining to bones.

Osteopathy: Any bone disease; or, a school of medicine that specializes in treatments that enable the body to heal itself.

Ovaries: Gonadal glands in the female that produce eggs (ova) for reproduction and the female sex hormones, estrogen and progesterone.

Over-the-counter: Medications sold without a prescription.

Ovulation: Monthly discharging of an egg (ovum) from an ovary. It occurs approximately 14 days before the onset of the next menstrual period.

Ovum: The female reproductive cell (egg) that is capable of developing into an embryo, a fetus, and then a baby after fertilization by a sperm.

Oxytocin: Pituitary hormone in women that stimulates the release of breast milk.

Pacemaker: A group of cells, known as the sinoatrial node, that are located in the atrium of the heart and serve to regulate the rate and rhythm of the heart. Also, an artificial cardiac pacemaker is an electrical device used to simulate the natural process by generating electrical impulses. An artificial pacemaker can be placed outside or inside the chest.

Palate: The hard roof of the mouth.

Palpate: To feel or examine by touch.

Palpitation: Rapid or throbbing sensation felt as a result of a fluttering or rapid, forceful beating of the heart.

Palsy: Paralysis; loss of sensation or ability to move or control movement.

Pancreas: Gland that produces enzymes essential to the digestion of food. The islets of Langerhans within the pancreas secrete insulin into the blood.

Papilla: A nipple-like protuberance.

Paralysis: The inability to move a part of the body. Partial paralysis is known as paresis.

Paranoia: Mental disorder characterized by suspicion, delusions of persecution, and jealousy.

Paraplegia: Loss of movement and sensation below the waist, including the legs.

Parasite: An organism that lives on or within another organism at the expense of the host.

Parathyroid glands: Endocrine glands located beneath the thyroid gland that regulate the level of calcium in the blood.

Parenteral: Methods of administering medication, fluid, or nutrition other than swallowing, including intravenous, subcutaneous, or intramuscular.

Paroxysm: A sudden attack, such as a spasm or convulsion; or recurrence of symptoms of a disease.

Patella: Kneecap.

Pathogen: Disease-producing microorganism.

Pathology: Study of the cause and nature of a disease.

Pectoral: Pertaining to the chest.

Pelvis: Basin-shaped bone structure connecting the spine with the legs.

Penis: Male organ for urination and copulation.

Pepsin: The main enzyme in the digestive juices of the stomach.

Peptic: Pertaining to digestion or the enzyme pepsin.

Percussion: A method of examination by tapping the fingertips over various areas of the body to determine position, size, and consistency of a structure beneath the skin.

Perforation: Process of making a hole, or the hole itself.

Pericardium: Membranous sac enclosing the heart.

Perineum: External area between the vulva and anus in a woman or between the scrotum and anus in a man.

Periodontal: Pertaining to the area immediately around a tooth.

Periosteum: Leather-like tissue that encases bone.

Peristalsis: Wave-like contraction of muscles, particularly in the digestive system, that forces food or food residue through the digestive tract.

Peritoneum: Membrane lining the abdominal cavity.

Peritonitis: Inflammation or infection of the peritoneum.

Pernicious: Destructive, sometimes fatal. Pernicious anemia is a particular form of anemia caused by inability to absorb vitamin B_{12} from the intestinal tract.

Perspiration: Sweat, the salty fluid excreted from the sweat glands of the skin.

Petechiae: Small subcutaneous hemorrhages that appear in the skin and mucous membranes. Also, the red spots caused by flea bites.

Petit mal: Mild form of epileptic attack, characterized by a blank stare and temporary cessation of activity.

Pharmacology: Study of drugs and their effects on living beings.

Pharynx: Upper portion of the throat; the passageway for air from the nose to the larynx and for food from the mouth to the esophagus.

Phlegm: Thick mucus, especially from the sinuses or respiratory tract.

Phobia: Persistent, irrational fear.

Pigment: Coloring matter.

Pineal body: Small, cone-shaped gland in the brain, the function of which is unclear.

Pinna: Exterior part of the ear, the portion that is easily visible.

Pituitary gland: An endocrine gland that produces a range of hormones to help control the body's long-term growth, day-to-day functioning, and reproductive capabilities; sometimes called the "master gland."

Placebo: Substance given for psychological benefit or as part of a clinical research study; it has no specific pharmacologic activity against illness.

Placenta: Spongy uterine structure developed during pregnancy through which the fetus takes nourishment and discards waste via the umbilical cord. The placenta is shed after delivery, when it is known as the afterbirth.

Plague: Term previously used to describe any deadly contagious epidemic disease. Now used primarily to describe infection by *Yersinia pestis* (bubonic or pneumonic plague).

Plaque: A film or deposit of bacteria and other material on the surface of a tooth that may lead to tooth decay or periodontal disease.

Plasma: Fluid part of the blood and lymph.

Platelet: Colorless round or oval microscopic-sized disc found in the blood. Also known as thrombocytes, platelets are necessary for the clotting of blood.

Pleura: The membrane that covers both lungs and lines the chest cavity.

Poly-: Prefix meaning multiple; more than normal.

Polyp: A usually benign tumor, often with a stem, found commonly in the nose, uterus, and colon.

Postpartum: Pertaining to the time after childbirth.

Prepuce: The foreskin over the glans of the penis.

Primary care physician: Physician responsible for providing or coordinating a person's general health care.

Progesterone: Female sex hormone responsible for, among other things, the thickening of the uterine lining to prepare for conception and implantation.

Prognosis: Prediction of the course and outcome of a disease.

Prolactin: Pituitary hormone that stimulates the breasts to produce milk.

Prolapse: Displacement of an organ or a structure, such as the uterus or bladder, by dropping down or protruding.

Prophylaxis: Prevention of disease or its spread by following certain rules or taking specific precautions.

Prostaglandins: A group of extremely active substances found in many parts of the body that affect many organs. Certain prostaglandins have a role in stimulating the uterine contractions of labor.

Prostate gland: Gland located at the base of the bladder in men.

Prosthesis: An artificial substitute for a missing body part, such as an arm or leg.

Protein: One of many complex nitrogen-containing compounds, composed of amino acids; essential for the growth and repair of tissue.

Prothrombin: A chemical substance found in circulating blood that interacts with calcium salts to form thrombin, a step in the process of blood clotting.

Pruritus: Itching.

Psychogenic: Originating in the mind; also pertaining to the development of the mind.

Psychomotor: Pertaining to voluntary physical movement.

Psychosis: Mental disturbance of serious magnitude that is characterized by loss of contact with reality. Delusions and hallucinations are often present.

Psychosomatic: Pertaining to the relationship of the mind and body. Psychosomatic illnesses are those in which a physical disorder is caused or aggravated by emotional factors.

Ptosis: Drooping, as of an eyelid.

Ptyalin: An enzyme found in saliva that helps to break down starch into sugars.

Puberty: Period of rapid change in boys and girls during which secondary sex characteristics mature. In girls (usually between 9 and 16 years) it is marked by menarche (the beginning of menstruation), and in boys (between 13 and 15 years) it is marked by discharge of semen and deepening of the voice.

Pulmonary: Pertaining to the lungs.

Pupil: The circular opening in the center of the iris through which light passes to the retina. The size of the opening diminishes in bright light and enlarges in dim light.

Purpura: A condition characterized by hemorrhages of tiny blood vessels causing patches on the skin or on mucous membranes. The patches begin as red and then change to purple and then brownish yellow before disappearing.

Purulent: Forming or containing pus.

Pus: Thick, whitish yellow fluid containing leukocytes (white blood cells) and bacteria, formed at the site of certain kinds of infections.

Pylorus: Lower opening of the stomach into the duodenum.

Pyrexia: Fever.

Quadriplegia: Complete paralysis of all limbs.

Radiation therapy: The use of high-energy penetrating waves to treat disease. Sources of radiation used in radiation therapy include X-ray, cobalt, and radium.

Radius: Smaller of the two bones in the lower arm; it connects to the base of the thumb.

Radon: A radioactive gas found in nature that is the byproduct of disintegrating radium.

Rash: Eruption on the skin, usually temporary.

Recessive: A mode of inheritance in which a gene that causes a trait must be present from both parents for the trait to become manifest in an offspring. See Dominant.

Rectum: The lowest portion of the large intestine. Stores stool until it is emptied.

Reflex: An involuntary response to a stimulus.

Reflux: Backflow or regurgitation.

Refractory: Stubborn, as in a condition that resists treatment or a nerve or muscle that resists stimulation.

Rejection: Refusal to accept, as with a transplanted organ.

Relapse: Recurrence of disease or symptoms after apparent recovery.

Remission: Abatement of symptoms.

REM sleep: The period of sleep known as rapid eye movement sleep, when dreaming seems to occur and the eyes move cyclically even though closed.

Renal: Pertaining to the kidneys.

Resection: Partial surgical removal of an organ or tissue.

Respiration: Breathing.

Resuscitation: Restoration of breathing or heartbeat after apparent death.

Retina: Light-sensitive layer of tissue located at the back of the eye that is composed of rods and cones, and transmits nerve impulses to the brain.

Retinopathy: Abnormality of the retina that may cause deterioration of eyesight.

Rhinovirus: A large subgroup of viruses (probably more than 100) that cause the common cold.

Risk factors: Factors including chemical, physiological, behavioral, psychological, genetic, or environmental that increase chances of a disease developing.

Rods: Long, slender bodies within the retina that perceive faint light; also, rod-shaped bacteria.

Root canal: Cavity in the root of the tooth that contains nerves.

Roughage: Indigestible fiber of fruits, vegetables, and cereals that aids in the evacuation of waste.

Rupture: Tearing or bursting of tissue or an organ.

Sacroiliac joint: The juncture between the sacrum and the ilium. Not a true joint because there is no movement at this point.

Sacrum: Triangular bone at the base of the spine just above the coccyx. Composed of five fused vertebrae, it is a part of the bony pelvis.

Saline: Salt (sodium chloride) solution.

Saliva: Fluid, secreted by the salivary and mucous glands of the mouth, that moistens food and begins the process of digestion.

Scapula: Shoulder blade.

Sciatic nerve: Largest nerve in the body, it is formed by the motor and sensory nerves to and from the legs and feet. It emerges from the base of the spinal cord as a number of roots and then passes through the pelvis and down the back of the thigh.

Sclera: The fibrous outer membrane of the eye, extending from the optic nerve to the cornea.

Sclerosis: Hardening or thickening of an organ or tissue, usually due to abnormal or excessive growth of fibrous tissue.

Scrotum: Skin sac in a male that holds the testicles.

Sebaceous glands: Oil glands of the skin.

Sebum: Fatty substance secreted by sebaceous glands to lubricate the skin.

Secretion: The process of producing materials by glands; also, the substance produced.

Seizure: A sudden attack often including convulsions; this symptom, if recurrent, often is referred to as a seizure disorder or as epilepsy.

Semen: Thick, whitish fluid containing reproductive cells (spermatozoa) and other fluids, discharged through the male urethra at ejaculation.

Seminal vesicles: Sac-like structures in the male, located behind the bladder, which secrete fluid that is part of the composition of semen.

Senescence: Process of aging.

Sepsis: State of being infected with disease-causing microorganisms in the bloodstream, usually with an accompanying fever.

Septicemia: Presence of disease-causing bacteria in the blood; also known as blood poisoning.

Septum: A wall dividing two cavities or compartments.

Serum: Watery fluid left after coagulation of the blood to form a clot. Serum containing antibodies to a specific disease may be injected into a person to give temporary resistance to that disease; this is called passive immunity. See Vaccine.

Shock: Clinical condition in which the body reacts to injury or severe pain by dilation or relaxation of blood vessels, producing what can be called circulatory failure. Symptoms include rapid pulse, very low blood pressure, pallor, cold, clammy skin, and sometimes unconsciousness.

Shunt: A passage that diverts blood flow from one main route to another. Often constructed artificially.

Side effects: Unwanted changes produced by medication or other treatment, ranging from trivial and transient (minor headache or dry mouth) to more serious (asthma, gastrointestinal bleeding).

Sinuses: Empty spaces or cavities within bone structure; most commonly, the several sets of cavities adjacent to and connected to the nose by small openings.

Somatostatin: Hormone that helps regulate the body's production and release of the pancreatic hormones insulin and glucagon. It is also found in other tissues of the body, where it may have other functions.

Spasm: Involuntary movement produced by a muscular contraction.

Speculum: Device used to examine body canals such as the nose or vagina.

Spermatozoa: Male cells that, upon combining with a female egg, result in fertilization. Produced by the testicles and transmitted within semen. Also referred to as sperm.

Spermicide: Birth control agent used to kill sperm cells by contact.

Sphincter: Circular muscles at an orifice that, upon contraction, close the opening. The body has several sphincter muscles, including those at the anus, bladder, and opening to the stomach from the esophagus.

Sphygmomanometer: Device used to measure blood pressure.

Spinal canal: The cavity that contains the spinal cord and is protected by vertebrae of the backbone.

Spinal column: The bony assemblage of vertebrae that enclose and protect the spinal cord.

Spinal cord: Lengthy, cord-like bundle of nerves that link nerves of the trunk and extremities with the brain.

Spleen: Organ located to the left and just in front of the stomach that stores and at times manufactures blood cells.

Sprain: Joint injury in which ligament damage is sustained.

Sputum: The fluid produced upon coughing. If certain disorders or infections are suspected, the sputum may be examined in a laboratory.

Staging: The process of categorizing the extent and spread of a disease such as cancer for the purpose of planning treatment.

Stenosis: The abnormal narrowing or closure of an opening or passageway in the body.

Sterilization: The process by which all microorganisms (bacteria, viruses, and parasites) are removed from a substance, as in the sterilization of surgical instruments to prevent infection. Or, the process, usually surgical, of rendering a man or woman incapable of reproduction.

Sternum: The breastbone, in the upper central portion of the chest and abutted by the ends of the clavicle and the ribs.

Steroids: See Corticosteroids.

Stillborn: A fetus dead at birth.

Stomach: The sac-like organ to which food is delivered by the esophagus. After the food is processed mechanically by a churning action and chemically with gastric acids, it passes from the stomach to the small intestine.

Stool: Body waste, such as food residue, evacuated from the bowels.

Strain: Muscular injury produced by abuse or overuse of a muscle.

Striae: Streaks or stripes.

Stroke: A condition produced by a blood clot that lodges in an artery and blocks the flow of blood to a portion of the brain, producing symptoms ranging from paralysis of limbs and loss of speech to unconsciousness and death. Less commonly, a stroke may be the result of bleeding into the substance of the brain.

Stupor: A state of reduced consciousness in which responsiveness and feeling are lessened.

Subacute: Term used to distinguish the intermediate duration of a disease that is neither chronic (long-lasting) nor characteristically of brief duration (acute).

Subcutaneous: Beneath the skin.

Sucrose: The simple sugar processed from sugarcane and sugar beets.

Sunblock: Over-the-counter preparation applied to the skin to limit damage from the rays of the sun.

Suppository: Pharmaceutical preparation in a solid form, intended to be inserted into an organ such as the rectum or vagina.

Suppuration: The formation and discharge of pus from an injury or infection.

Suture: The process of joining two surfaces by stitching; or, the surgical stitch itself.

Synapse: The junction between two nerve cells (neurons).

Syncope: Fainting.

Syndrome: A collection of signs and symptoms that characterize an ailment.

Synovial fluid: The clear, fluid lubricant found in a joint.

Systemic: Affecting or pertaining to the entire body rather than one of its parts.

Systole: The portion of the heart cycle during which the heart muscle is contracting.

Tachycardia: Abnormally rapid heart rate (more than 100 beats per minute).

Tartar: Plaque deposits on the teeth that lead to tooth decay.

T cell: A type of white blood cell (lymphocyte) that acts as a part of the body's immune system.

Tendon: Cord-like tissue that connects muscles to bones.

Testicles (testes): Gonadal glands in the male that produce sperm (spermatozoa) for reproduction and the male sex hormone testosterone.

Testosterone: Male sex hormone produced by the testicles.

Thoracic: Having to do with the chest (thorax).

Thorax: The portion of the body below the neck and above the diaphragm; the chest.

Thrombin: An enzyme that is part of the process of blood coagulation.

Thrombocyte: Blood platelet, essential to the clotting process.

Thrombus: A blood clot.

Thymus: A gland located in the upper chest that produces T cells, essential to developing the body's immune response.

Thyroid gland: Endocrine gland that helps control the body's rate of function and contributes to maintaining a balance between the calcium in the blood and in the bones through production of the hormones thyroxine and calcitonin.

Thyroxine: Thyroid hormone that controls the pace of chemical activity (metabolism) in the body.

Tibia: The larger of the two bones in the lower leg; the shinbone.

Tic: An involuntary muscle spasm, usually of the face, head, neck, or shoulder; a twitch.

Tissue: A collection of similar cells that, taken together, form a body structure.

Tonsils: Two masses of lymph tissues, located on either side of the back of the throat, that help filter out unwanted bacteria.

Topical: Pertaining to a certain surface area of the body.

Tourniquet: A device that is tightened over an extremity to stop bleeding.

Toxemia: A condition in which toxins circulate throughout the body via the blood.

Toxic: Poisonous.

Toxin: A poisonous compound.

Toxoid: A biological toxin treated so that it is no longer dangerous but, upon injection into the body, will induce antibodies to form. An example is tetanus toxoid.

Trachea: The tube that connects the throat (pharynx) to the bronchial tubes in the lungs. Sometimes called the windpipe.

Traction: Mechanical pulling on a body part, used in treating certain fractures and dislocations.

Transfusion: Delivery of blood or a blood component into the bloodstream via injection.

Transplantation: The surgical movement of an organ or tissue from one position (or person) to another.

Trauma: An injury such as a burn, wound, or broken bone.

Tremor: An involuntary quaking; tremor can result from disease, a nervous disorder, the side effect of a medication, or some other cause.

Triceps: Muscle in the arm that, upon contraction, extends the arm at the elbow.

Tricuspid valve: Heart valve between the right atrium and the right ventricle.

Trigeminal nerve: The nerve that delivers sensory stimuli to the brain from the face, teeth, and tongue.

Triglyceride: A form of fat that the body makes from sugar, alcohol, or excess calories.

Tubule: A small tube or canal, especially in the kidneys.

Tumor: Abnormal growth of tissue. The tumor may be malignant (cancerous) or benign (noncancerous).

Tympanic membrane: The eardrum.

Ulcer: An open sore on the skin or a mucous membrane.

Ulna: Larger of the two bones in the lower arm.

Ultrasound: Sound waves of a frequency beyond human hearing which change in velocity depending on the density of the body part or other object being studied. A device that can collect echoes and form an image for diagnostic purposes.

Umbilicus: The scar formed by removal of the umbilical cord from the newborn following birth; the navel.

Urea: Principal waste product in the urine; a nitrogen-containing product of protein metabolism. Its concentration in blood may be used as a measure of kidney function.

Ureter: The tube that delivers urine from the kidney to the bladder.

Urethra: Tube draining the bladder to outside the body; in the male, this canal is also the passage for semen.

Uric acid: A waste by-product of metabolism. When too little is excreted or too much is produced, the buildup can lead to the development of gout.

Urination: Act of voiding fluid wastes (urine).

Urine: Fluid waste produced in the kidneys, stored in the bladder, and released through the urethra.

Urticaria: See Hives.

Uterus: Female organ that during normal pregnancy contains the embryo and fetus. Located in the lower abdomen, the uterus is a pear-shaped, muscular organ also known as the womb.

Uvea: Layer of the eye beneath the sclera, consisting of the iris, ciliary body, and choroid. The visible pigments in the eye are seen in the uvea.

Uvula: Tissue hanging from the back of the soft palate.

Vaccination: Injection of a vaccine to create immunity to a specific disease.

Vaccine: Weakened or killed infectious microorganisms or other substances introduced into the body to stimulate immunity and provide protection against certain infectious diseases.

Vagina: The canal (birth canal) connecting the external female genitals with the uterus.

Vagus nerve: Nerve that serves the esophagus, larynx, stomach, intestines, lungs, and heart.

Varicose veins: Distended or twisted veins.

Vascular: Pertaining to blood vessels; includes veins and arteries.

Vas deferens: Duct that transports sperm from the testicles to the urethra.

Vein: Blood vessel that carries blood back to the heart.

Venous: Pertaining to the veins.

Ventricle: One of two lower chambers of the heart; or, any small cavity.

Venule: Small vein.

Verruca: A wart.

Vertebra: One of the 33 bony sections that make up the spine.

Vertigo: Dizziness.

Vesicle: A small sac containing fluid.

Viral: Pertaining to or caused by a virus.

Virulent: Highly infectious or harmful.

Virus: Tiny organism that causes disease; viruses range from minor (the common cold) to deadly (AIDS).

Viscera: The internal organs, in particular those located within the abdominal cavity.

Vital signs: Rate of breathing, heart rate, body temperature, and blood pressure.

Vitamins: Organic substances that are found in small amounts in food and are essential for most chemical processes in the body.

Vitreous humor: Gelatinous substance found within the eye.

Vocal cords: Small folds in the cavity of the larynx (voice box) that are involved in the production of sound.

Vomit: The ejection of partially digested matter from the stomach through the mouth; or, the material itself (emesis).

Vulva: External female genitals, including the clitoris and labia.

Wart: Harmless growth on the skin, produced by a virus.

Wen: Cyst that develops in a sebaceous gland.

Withdrawal: The state experienced when addicting medications, illegal drugs, or alcohol are withdrawn. Symptoms may be physiological or psychological or both.

Womb: The female organ in which the fetus develops. See Uterus.

X-ray: Electromagnetic wave that penetrates most solid matter and will produce an image on film upon emerging from the body part or other object being studied. Also called roentgen ray.

Zygote: The egg after it is fertilized by a sperm.

Appendix III

Where to Go for More Information

Contents

A listing of organizations that provide facts on a wide range of diseases and health conditions.

Health Information Sources

It's been said that we live in an Information Age. Never before have Americans been bombarded with so much data, including sometimes seemingly conflicting information on how to stay healthy, cope with illness, control health care costs, and deal with an increasingly complex health care system.

This book is devoted to providing answers to a wide range of health and medical issues. But no single volume can address all of the questions and issues that may interest you and other readers now and in the future.

What follows is a sampling of some of the many organizations offering health information that may be helpful. We intend neither to promote nor endorse these organizations.

Acoustic Neuroma Association
PO Box 12402
Atlanta, GA 30355
(404) 237-8023

Aerobics and Fitness Foundation Association
15250 Ventura Boulevard
Suite 200
Sherman Oaks, CA 91403
(800) 446-4322

Agency for Health Care Policy and Research
PO Box 8547
Silver Spring, MD 20907
(800) 358-9295

Al-Anon Family Group Headquarters
1372 Broadway
New York, NY 10018
(800) 356-9996

Alcohol, Drug Abuse, and Mental Health Administration
5600 Fischers Lane
Parklawn Bldg, Room 12-105
Rockville, MD 20857
(301) 443-3783

Alcoholics Anonymous
475 Riverside Drive
11th Floor
New York, NY 10115
(212) 870-3400
(check local listings nationwide)

Alexander Graham Bell Association for the Deaf, Inc.
3417 Volta Place NW
Washington, DC 20007-2778
(202) 337-5220

Alzheimer's Association
919 N. Michigan Avenue
Suite 1000
Chicago, IL 60611-1676
(800) 272-3900

Alzheimer's Disease Education and Referral Center
PO Box 8250
Silver Spring, MD 20907-8250
(800) 822-2762

American Academy of Allergy and Immunology
611 E. Wells Street
Milwaukee, WI 53202
(800) 822-2762

American Academy of Dermatology
PO Box 681069
Schaumburg, IL 60168
(mail only)

American Academy of Family Physicians
8880 Ward Parkway
Kansas City, MO 64114-2797
(800) 274-2237

American Academy of Implant Prosthodontics
5555 Peachtree-Dunwoody Road NE
Atlanta, GA 30342
(404) 847-9200

American Academy of Ophthalmology
Inquiry Clerk
655 Beach Street
San Francisco, CA 94109-1336
(mail only)

American Academy of Orthopaedic Surgeons
6330 N. River Road
Rosemount, IL 60018
(708) 823-7186

American Academy of Otolaryngology—Head and Neck Surgery
One Prince Street
Alexandria, VA 22314
(703) 836-4444

American Association of Endodontists
211 E. Chicago Avenue
Chicago, IL 60611-1676
(800) 272-3900

American Association of Kidney Patients
100 S. Ashley Drive
Suite 280
Tampa, FL 33602
(800) 749-2257

American Association of Neurological Surgeons
22 S. Washington Street
Park Ridge, IL 60068
(708) 692-9500

American Board of Medical Specialties Public Education Program
(800) 776-2378

American Board of Oral Pathology
PO Box 25915
Tampa, FL 33622-5915
(813) 286-2444

American Board of Orthodontics
401 N. Lindbergh Boulevard
Suite 308
St. Louis, MO 63105
(314) 432-6130

American Board of Periodontology
University of Maryland
Baltimore College of Dental Surgery
666 W. Baltimore Street
Room 3-C-08
Baltimore, MD 21201
(410) 706-2432

American Brain Tumor Association
2720 River Road
Des Plaines, IL 60618
(800) 886-2282

American Cancer Society
1599 Clifton Road NE
Atlanta, GA 30329
(800) ACS-2345

**American Chronic Pain
Association, Inc.**
PO Box 850
Rocklin, CA 95677
(916) 632-0922

American College of Cardiology
9111 Old Georgetown Road
Bethesda, MD 20814-1699
(800) 253-4636

**American College of Emergency
Physicians**
1111 19th Street NW
Suite 650
Washington, DC 20036
(800) 320-0610

**American College of Obstetricians
and Gynecologists**
Resource Center
409 12th Street SW
Washington, DC 20024-2188
(202) 638-5577

American College of Radiology
1891 Preston White Drive
Reston, VA 22091
(mail only)

American College of Surgeons
55 E. Erie
Chicago, IL 60611
(312) 664-4050

American Council of the Blind
1155 15th Street NW
Suite 720
Washington, DC 20005
(800) 424-8666

American Dental Association
211 E. Chicago Avenue
Chicago, IL 60611
(312) 440-2500

American Diabetes Association
1660 Duke Street
Alexandria, VA 22314
(800) 342-2383

American Dietetic Association
Nutrition Information Hotline
216 W. Jackson Boulevard
Chicago, IL 60606
(800) 366-1655

**American Foundation for Urologic
Disease**
300 W. Pratt Street
Suite 401
Baltimore, MD 21201
(800) 242-2383

American Geriatrics Society
770 Lexington Avenue
Suite 300
New York, NY 10021
(212) 308-1414

American Health Foundation
320 E. 43rd Street
New York, NY 10017
(212) 953-1900

**American Hearing Research
Foundation**
55 E. Washington Street
Suite 2022
Chicago, IL 60602
(312) 726-9670

American Heart Association
7272 Greenville Avenue
Dallas, TX 75231
(800) AHA-USA-1

American Hospital Association
One N. Franklin
Chicago, IL 60601
(312) 422-3000

American Lung Association
(800) LUNG-USA

American Lupus Society
260 Maple Court
Suite 123
Ventura, CA 93003
(800) 331-1802

**American Occupational Therapy
Association, Inc.**
4720 Montgomery Lane
PO Box 31220
Bethesda, MD 20814-1220
(301) 652-2682

American Paralysis Association
500 Morris Avenue
Springfield, NJ 07081
(800) 225-0292

**American Parkinson's Disease
Association**
1250 Hylan Boulevard
Staten Island, NY 10305
(800) 223-2732

American Psychiatric Association
Division of Public Affairs
1400 K Street NW
Suite 501
Washington, DC 20005
(202) 682-6220

**American Self-Help Group
Clearinghouse**
Northwest Covenant Medical
Center
25 Pocono Road
Denville, NJ 07834
(201) 625-7101

**American Social Health
Association HealthLine**
PO Box 13827
Research Triangle Park, NC 27709
(800) 972-8500

**American Society for Reproductive
Medicine**
1209 Montgomery Highway
Birmingham, AL 35216
(205) 978-5000

**American Speech-Language-
Hearing Association**
Director of Media Branch
10801 Rockville Pike
Rockville, MD 20852
(800) 638-8255

American Tinnitus Association
PO Box 5
Portland, OR 97207
(503) 248-9985

American Trauma Society
8903 Presidential Parkway
Suite 512
Upper Marlboro, MD 20772-2656
(800) 556-7890

Amyotrophic Lateral Sclerosis Association
21021 Ventura Boulevard
Suite 321
Woodland Hills, CA 91364
(800) 782-4747

Ankylosing Spondylitis Association of America
PO Box 5872
Sherman Oaks, CA 91413
(800) 777-8189

Associated Services for the Blind
919 Walnut Street
Philadelphia, PA 19107
(215) 627-0600

Association for Macular Diseases, Inc.
210 E. 64th Street
New York, NY 10021
(212) 605-3719

Asthma and Allergy Foundation of America
1125 15th Street NW
Suite 502
Washington, DC 20005
(800) 7-ASTHMA

Benign Essential Blepharospasm Research Foundation, Inc.
PO Box 12468
Beaumont, TX 77726-2468
(409) 832-0788

Better Hearing Institute
PO Box 1840
Washington, DC 20013
(800) EAR-WELL

Cancer Care, Inc.
1800 Avenue of the Americas
New York, NY 10036
(212) 221-3300
(800) 813-HOPE

*For hearing impaired

Cancer Information Service Program of the National Cancer Institute
(800) 4-CANCER

Centers for Disease Control
PO Box 13827
Research Triangle Park, NC 27709
National AIDS Hotline
(800) 342-2437
(800) 344-7432 (Spanish)
*(800) 243-7889 (TTY)
National Sexually Transmitted Diseases Hotline
(800) 227-8922

Centers for Disease Control and Prevention
Office on Smoking and Health
4770 Buford Highway NE
Mail Stop K-50
Atlanta, GA 30341
(800) CDC-1311

Centers for Disease Control and Prevention
Public Inquiries
1600 Clifton Road NE
Bldg. 1, SSB249
MS A 34
Atlanta, GA 30333
(404) 639-3534

Centers for Nutrition Policy and Promotion
1120 20th Street NW
Suite 200
North Lobby
Washington, DC 20036
(202) 418-2312

Clearinghouse on Child Abuse and Neglect Information
PO Box 1182
Washington, DC 20013
(800) 394-3366

Clearinghouse on Disability Information
Office of Special Education and Rehabilitative Services
Switzer Bldg., Room 3132
Washington, DC 20202-2524
(202) 205-8241

Consumer Health Information Resource Institute
300 E. Pink Hill Road
Independence, MO 64111
(816) 228-4595

Consumer Information Center
Consumer Information Catalogue
Pueblo, CO 81009
(719) 948-4000

Crohn's and Colitis Foundation of America
386 Park Avenue South
17th Floor
New York, NY 10016
(800) 343-3637

Cystic Fibrosis Foundation
6931 Arlington Road
Bethesda, MD 20814
(800) FIGHT-CF

Depression and Related Affective Disorders Association
Johns Hopkins Hospital
600 N. Wolfe Street
Meyer 3-181
Baltimore, MD 21287-7381
(410) 955-4647

Digestive Disease National Coalition
711 Second Street NE
Suite 200
Washington, DC 20002
(202) 544-7497

EnviroHealth
2605 Meridian Parkway
Suite 115
Durham, NC 27713
(800) 643-4794

Epilepsy Foundation of America
4351 Garden City Drive
Landover, MD 20785
(800) EFA-1000

Eye Bank Association of America
1001 Connecticut Avenue NW
Suite 601
Washington, DC 20036
(202) 775-4999

Food and Consumer Service
3101 Park Center Drive
Alexandria, VA 22302
(703) 305-2000

Food and Drug Administration
Office of Consumer Affairs
5600 Fischers Lane
Rockville, MD 20857
(301) 443-3170

Foundation Fighting Blindness
1401 Mt. Royal Avenue
Baltimore, MD 21217
(800) 683-5555
*(800) 683-5551 (TTY)

Foundation for Hospice and Home Care
320 A Street NE
Washington, DC 20002
(202) 547-6586

Gamblers Anonymous
PO Box 17173
Los Angeles, CA 90017
(213) 386-8789

Gastro-Intestinal Research Foundation
70 E. Lake Street
Suite 1015
Chicago, IL 60601
(312) 332-1350

Guiding Eyes for the Blind, Inc.
611 Granite Springs Road
Yorktown Heights, NY 10598
(800) 942-0149

Guillain-Barré Syndrome Foundation International
PO Box 262
Wynnewood, PA 19096
(610) 667-0131

Health Resources and Services Administration
5600 Fischers Lane
Parklawn Bldg., Room 14-45
Rockville, MD 20857
(301) 443-3376

Hearing Aid Helpline
20361 Middlebelt Road
Livonia, MI 48152
(800) 521-5247

Herpes Resource Center
PO Box 13827
Research Triangle Park, NC 27709
(800) 230-6039

Hospice Education Institute
Hospicelink
190 Westbrook Road
Suite 2
Essex, CT 06426
(800) 331-1620

Huntington's Disease Society of America
140 West 22nd Street
6th Floor
New York, NY 10011
(800) 345-HDSA

Intestinal Disease Foundation, Inc.
1323 Forbes Avenue
Suite 200
Pittsburgh, PA 15219
(412) 261-5888

Juvenile Diabetes Foundation International
Public Relations Department
432 Park Avenue South
New York, NY 10016
(800) JDF-CURE

Leukemia Society of America
600 Third Avenue
New York, NY 10016
(800) 955-4LSA

Lighthouse National Center for Vision and Aging
111 E. 59th Street
New York, NY 10022
(800) 334-5497

Living Bank
PO Box 6725
Houston, TX 77265
(800) 528-2971

Lupus Foundation of America, Inc.
1323 Forbes Avenue
Suite 200
Pittsburgh, PA 15219
(800) 800-5776

March of Dimes Birth Defects Foundation
1275 Mamaroneck Avenue
White Plains, NY 10605
(914) 428-7100

Mended Hearts
7272 Greenville Avenue
Dallas, TX 75231-4596
(214) 706-1442

Myasthenia Gravis Foundation National Office
222 South Riverside Plaza
Chicago, IL 60606
(800) 541-5454

National Alliance of Breast Cancer Organizations
9 E. 37th Street
10th Floor
New York, NY 10016
(212) 719-0154

National Alopecia Areata Foundation
710 C Street
Suite 11
San Rafael, CA 94901
(415) 456-4644

National Aphasia Association
PO Box 1887
Murray Hill Station
New York, NY 10156-0611
(800) 922-4NAA

National Arthritis, Musculo-skeletal and Skin Diseases
Information Clearinghouse
PO Box AMS
9000 Rockville Pike
Bethesda, MD 20892
(301) 495-4484

National Association for Home Care
519 C Street NE
Washington, DC 20002
(202) 547-7424

National Association for Music Therapy
8455 Colesville Road
Suite 930
Silver Spring, MD 20910
(301) 589-3300

National Association for Visually Handicapped
22 W. 21st Street
6th Floor
New York, NY 10010
(212) 889-3141

National Association of the Deaf
814 Thayer Avenue
Silver Spring, MD 20910-4500
(301) 587-1788 Voice
*(301) 587-1789 TTY

National Ataxia Foundation
15500 Wayzata Boulevard
Suite 750
Wayzata, MN 55391
(612) 473-7666

*For hearing impaired

National Brain Tumor Foundation
785 Market Street
Suite 1600
San Francisco, CA 94103
(800) 934-CURE

National Cancer Institute
Public Inquiries
Bldg. 31, Room 10A-18
9000 Rockville Pike
Bethesda, MD 20892
(800) 422-6237

National Center for Human Genome Research
Bldg. 31, Room B1C-35
9000 Rockville Pike
Bethesda, MD 20892
(301) 402-0911

National Chronic Pain Outreach Association, Inc.
7979 Old Georgetown Road
Suite 100
Bethesda, MD 20814
(301) 652-4948

National Clearinghouse for Alcohol and Drug Information
PO Box 2345
Rockville, MD 20847-2345
(800) 729-6686

National Coalition for Cancer Survivorship
1010 Wayne Avenue
5th Floor
Silver Spring, MD 20910
(301) 650-8868

National Council of Senior Citizens
1331 F Street NW
Washington, DC 20004-1171
(202) 347-8800

National Council on Alcoholism and Drug Dependence
12 W. 21st Street
New York, NY 10010
(800) 622-2255

National Depressive and Manic-Depressive Association
730 N. Franklin
Suite 501
Chicago, IL 60610
(800) 82-NDMDA

National Diabetes Information Clearinghouse
1 Information Way
Bethesda, MD 20892-3560
(mail only)

National Digestive Diseases Information Clearinghouse
2 Information Way
Bethesda, MD 20892-3570
(mail only)

National Down Syndrome Society
666 Broadway
8th Floor
New York, NY 10012-2317
(800) 221-4602

National Easter Seal Society
230 West Monroe
Suite 1800
Chicago IL 60606
(312) 726-6200

National Eye Institute
2020 Vision Place
Bethesda, MD 20892-3655
(301) 496-5248

National Federation of the Blind
1800 Johnson Street
Baltimore, MD 21230
(410) 659-9314

National Federation of the Blind
Diabetics Division
811 Cherry Street
Suite 309
Columbia, MO 65201
(314) 875-8911

National Headache Foundation
5252 N. Western Avenue
Chicago, IL 60625
(800) 843-2256

National Health Information Referral Center
PO Box 1133
Washington, DC 20013-1133
(mail only)

National Heart, Lung, and Blood Institute Information Center
PO Box 30105
Bethesda, MD 20824-0105
(800) 575-WELL (recording only)

National Hemophilia Foundation
110 Greene Street
Room 303
New York, NY 10012
(800) 42-HANDI

National Herpes Hotline
PO Box 13827
Research Triangle Park, NC 27709
(919) 361-8488

National Information Center on Deafness
Gallaudet University
800 Florida Avenue NE
Washington, DC 20002
(202) 651-5051

National Institute for Occupational Safety and Health
4676 Columbia Parkway
Cincinnati, OH 45226
(800) 356-4674

National Institute of Alcohol Abuse and Alcoholism
600 Executive Boulevard
Willco Bldg.
Rockville, MD 20852
(301) 443-3860

National Institute of Allergy and Infectious Diseases
Bldg 31, Room 7A-50
9000 Rockville Pike
Bethesda, MD 20892
(301) 496-5717

National Institute of Arthritis and Musculoskeletal and Skin Diseases
Bldg. 31, Room 4C-05
9000 Rockville Pike
Bethesda, MD 20892
(301) 496-8188

National Institute of Child Health and Human Development
Bldg. 31, Room 2A-34
9000 Rockville Pike
Bethesda, MD 20892
(301) 496-5133

National Institute of Dental Research
Bldg. 31, Room 2C-35
9000 Rockville Pike
Bethesda, MD 20892
(301) 496-4261

National Institute of Diabetes and Digestive and Kidney Diseases
Bldg. 31, Room 9A-04
9000 Rockville Pike
Bethesda, MD 20892
(301) 496-3583

National Institute of Environmental Health Sciences
PO Box 12233
Research Triangle Park, NC 27709
(919) 541-3345

National Institute of General Medical Sciences
Bldg. 45, Room 3AS-43
9000 Rockville Pike
Bethesda, MD 20892
(301) 496-7301

National Institute of Mental Health Public Inquiries
5600 Fischers Lane
Room 7C-02
Rockville, MD 20857
(301) 443-4513
(800) 421-4211 (Depression)
(800) 64-PANIC (Panic Disorder)

National Institute on Aging
Bldg. 31, Room 5C-27
9000 Rockville Pike
Bethesda, MD 20892
(301) 496-1752

National Institute on Deafness and Other Communicative Disorders
Bldg. 31, Room 3C-35
9000 Rockville Pike
Bethesda, MD 20892
(301) 496-7243

National Institute on Drug Abuse
Parklawn Bldg., 10A-39
Rockville, MD 20857
(301) 443-1124

National Jewish Center for Immunology and Respiratory Medicine
1400 Jackson Street
Denver, CO 80206
(800) 222-LUNG

National Kidney Foundation
30 E. 33rd Street
New York, NY 10016
(800) 622-9010

National Kidney and Urologic Diseases Information Clearinghouse
3 Information Way
Bethesda, MD 20892-3580
(mail only)

National Library of Medicine
Bldg. 38, Room 2S-10
9000 Rockville Pike
Bethesda, MD 20892
(301) 496-6308

National Mental Health Association
1021 Prince Street
Alexandria, VA 22314-2971
(800) 969-NMHA

National Neurofibromatosis Foundation
95 Pine Street
16th Floor
New York, NY 10005
(800) 323-7938

National Organization for Rare Disorders
PO Box 8923
New Fairfield, CT 06812
(800) 999-6673

National Osteoporosis Foundation
1150 17th Street NW
Suite 500
Washington, DC 20036-4603
(800) 223-9994

National Parkinson Foundation
1501 NW 9th Avenue
Miami, FL 33136
(800) 327-4545

National Psoriasis Foundation
6600 SW 92nd Avenue
Suite 300
Portland, OR 97223
(800) 723-9166

National Rehabilitation Information Center
8455 Colesville Road
Suite 935
Silver Spring, MD 20910
(800) 34-NARIC

National Resource Center on Homelessness and Mental Illness
Policy Research Associates
262 Delaware Avenue
Delmar, NY 12054
(800) 444-7415

National Sleep Foundation
1367 Connecticut Avenue NW
Suite 200
Washington, DC 20036
(mail only)

National Society for Patient Representation and Consumer Affairs
One N. Franklin
Chicago, IL 60601
(312) 422-3999

National Spinal Cord Injury Association
545 Cummings Avenue
Suite 29
Cambridge, MA 02138
(800) 962-9629

National Spinal Cord Injury Hotline
2201 Argonne Drive
Baltimore, MD 21218
(800) 526-3456

National Stroke Association
8480 East Orchard Road
Suite 1000
Englewood, CO 80110-5015
(800) 787-6537

National Sudden Infant Death Syndrome Resource Center
8201 Greensboro Drive
Suite 600
McLean, VA 22102
(703) 821-8955

National Tuberous Sclerosis Association
8000 Corporate Drive
Suite 120
Landover, MD 20785
(800) 225-6872

Neurological Institute
PO Box 5801
Bethesda, MD 20824
(301) 496-5751

Office of Alternative Medicine
EPS, Room 450
9000 Rockville Pike
Bethesda, MD 20892
(301) 496-7498

Office of Research for Women's Health
Bldg. 1, Room 201
9000 Rockville Pike
Bethesda, MD 20892
(301) 496-1770

Paget Foundation
200 Varick Street
Suite 1004
New York, NY 10014-4810
(800) 23-PAGET

Parkinson's Disease Foundation
710 W. 168th Street
New York, NY 10032
(800) 457-6676

President's Council on Physical Fitness and Sports
701 Pennsylvania Avenue NW
Suite 250
Washington, DC 20004
(202) 272-3421

Prevent Blindness America
500 East Remington Road
Schaumburg, IL 60173
(800) 331-2020

Public Health Service
Office of Communications
Room 728-H
200 Independence Avenue SW
Washington, DC 20201
(202) 690-6867

Sickle Cell Disease Association of America, Inc.
200 Corporate Point
Suite 495
Culver City, CA 90230
(800) 421-8453

Sjögren's Syndrome Foundation
333 North Broadway
Jericho, NY 11753
(516) 933-6365

Skin Cancer Foundation
Box 561
New York, NY 10156
(800) SKIN-490

Spina Bifida Association of America
4590 MacArthur Boulevard NW
Suite 250
Washington, DC 20007
(800) 621-3141

Stuttering Foundation of America
3100 Walnut Grove Road
Suite 603
PO Box 11749
Memphis, TN 38111-0749
(800) 992-9392

Thyroid Foundation of America, Inc.
Ruth Sleeper Hall
RSL 350
Boston, MA 02114
(800) 832-8321

Tourette Syndrome Association
42-40 Bell Boulevard
Bayside, NY 11361-2820
(718) 224-2999

Transplant Recipients International Organization
1735 I Street NW
Suite 917
Washington, DC 20006
(800) TRIO-386

United Ostomy Association
36 Executive Park
Suite 120
Irvine, CA 92714
(800) 826-0826

United Scleroderma Foundation
PO Box 399
Watsonville, CA 95007-0399
(800) 722-HOPE

US TOO International (Prostate Cancer Survivor Support Groups)
930 North York Road
Suite 50
Hinsdale, IL 60521-2993

VISION Foundation, Inc.
818 Mt. Auburn Street
Watertown, MA 02172
(617) 926-4232

Visiting Nurse Association of America
3801 E. Florida Avenue
Suite 900
Denver, CO 80210
(303) 753-0218

Women's Sports Foundation
Eisenhower Park
East Meadow, NY 11554
(800) 227-3988

World Health Organization
2 UN Plaza
Suite DC2-0970
New York, NY 10017
(212) 963-3952

Y-ME
National Organization for Breast Cancer Information and Support
212 W. Van Buren
4th Floor
Chicago, IL 60607
(800) 221-2141
(312) 986-8228 (24 hours)

Appendix IV

How to Prepare an Advance Directive

Contents

Look here to find examples of legal documents that go into effect if you are no longer able to make decisions about your health care.

Examples of Advance Directives

Advance directives, including living wills and documents granting durable power of attorney for health care, are legal documents that go into effect if you are no longer able to make decisions about your health care. Advance directives may simply state your values and beliefs or may give specific information about the types of medical care and life-sustaining measures you do or don't want implemented (See Advance Directives, pages 1248 and 1312).

The use of advance directives is controlled by laws in the individual states. A document accepted in one state may not be accepted in another state. However, many states do allow a person to use a form that was prepared in another state.

Before preparing an advance directive, ask your health care provider if a particular form or procedure is required for the state in which the health care provider resides.

The following documents are examples of forms used in two states (Florida and Minnesota) to designate a durable power of attorney for health care and two forms for living wills. Notice that Florida law suggests, but does not require, a specific form. Minnesota law does not have a required form for designation of a durable power of attorney for health care but does have a required form for a living will.

These forms are examples only. In deciding to prepare an advance directive, consult your health care provider, religious adviser, and family or friends. Community organizations, such as senior citizens centers or public libraries, may also have information.

A lawyer is not needed to prepare an advance directive, although consulting with one may be useful to answer questions about the status of a state's law on advance directives.

After preparing an advance directive, give copies to your health care providers, the health care agent or agents designated in your document, and selected family members. Keep your copy of the document in an easy-to-reach place, and make sure that selected members of your family or friends know how to find it or have a copy of it.

Review the document every year or when your family situation or health condition changes. You want to be sure that the document continues to express your wishes about your health care.

Under Florida law, the following form may but need not be used to designate a health care surrogate (durable power of attorney for health care).

DESIGNATION OF HEALTH CARE SURROGATE

Name: _____
            (Last)   (First)   (Middle Initial)

In the event that I have been determined to be incapacitated to provide informed consent for medical treatment and surgical and diagnostic procedures, I wish to designate as my surrogate for health care decisions:

Name: _____
Address: _____
_____
Zip Code: _____
Phone: _____

I fully understand that this designation will permit my designee to make health care decisions and to provide, withhold, or withdraw consent on my behalf; to apply for public benefits to defray the cost of health care; and to authorize my admission to or transfer from a health care facility.

Additional instructions (optional): _____
_____
_____
_____

I further affirm that this designation is not being made as a condition of treatment or admission to a health care facility. I will notify and send a copy of this document to the following persons other than my surrogate, so they may know who my surrogate is.

Name: _____
Name: _____

Signed: _____
Date: _____

Witnesses: 1. _____
              2. _____

Under Florida law the following form may but need not be used to prepare a living will.

LIVING WILL

Declaration made this _____ day of _____, 19_____. I, _____, willfully and voluntarily make known my desire that my dying not be artificially prolonged under the circumstances set forth below, and I do hereby declare:

If at any time I have a terminal condition and if my attending or treating physician and another consulting physician have determined that there is no medical probability of my recovery from such condition, I direct that life-prolonging procedures be withheld or withdrawn when the application of such procedures would serve only to prolong artificially the process of dying, and that I be permitted to die naturally with only the administration of medication or the performance of any medical procedure deemed necessary to provide me with comfort care or to alleviate pain.

It is my intention that this declaration be honored by my family and physician as the final expression of my legal right to refuse medical or surgical treatment and to accept the consequences for such refusal.

In the event that I have been determined to be unable to provide express and informed consent regarding the withholding, withdrawal, or continuation of life-prolonging procedures, I wish to designate, as my surrogate to carry out the provisions of this declaration:

Name: _____

Address: _____

Zip Code: _____

Phone: _____

I understand the full import of this declaration, and I am emotionally and mentally competent to make this declaration.

Additional Instructions (optional): _____

_____

_____

Signed: _____

Witness: _____

Address: _____

Phone: _____

Witness: _____

Address: _____

Phone: _____

Under Minnesota law the following form may but need not be used to prepare a durable power of attorney for health care.

DURABLE POWER OF ATTORNEY FOR HEALTH CARE

I appoint_____ as my agent (my attorney in fact) to make any health care decision for me when, in the judgment of my attending physician, I am unable to make or communicate the decision myself and my agent consents to make or communicate the decision on my behalf.

My agent has the power to make any health care decision for me. This power includes the power to give consent, to refuse consent, or to withdraw consent to any care, treatment, service, or procedure to maintain, diagnose, or treat my physical or mental condition, including giving me food or water by artificial means. My agent has the power, where consistent with the laws of this state, to make a health care decision to withhold or stop health care necessary to keep me alive. It is my intention that my agent or any alternative agent has a personal obligation to me to make health care decisions for me consistent with my expressed wishes. I understand, however, that my agent or any alternative agent has no legal duty to act.

My agent and any alternative agents have consented to act as my agent. My agent and any alternative agents have been notified that they will be nominated as a guardian or conservator for me.

My agent must act consistently with my desires as stated in this document or as otherwise made known by me to my agent.

My agent has the same right as I would have to receive, review, and obtain copies of my medical records and to consent to disclosure of those records.

Optional Provisions:

I hereby designate the following alternative agent(s) acting individually in the order listed to act if the above named agent is unable, unavailable, or unwilling to serve:_____
_____
_____
_____

I hereby give the following specific instruction to my agent or any alternative agents:____
_____
_____
_____

I hereby make the following limitations on the right of my agent or any alternative agents to receive, review, obtain copies of, and consent to the disclosure of my medical records:____
_____
_____
_____

I hereby impose the following limitations on the right of my agent or any alternative agents to act as guardian or conservator for purposes of section 525.544:_____
_____
_____
_____

IN WITNESS WHEREOF, I have signed or acknowledged before me this _____ day of
_____, 19_____.

_____
(Signature of Principal)

STATE OF MINNESOTA
COUNTY OF_____

The foregoing instrument was signed or acknowledged before me this_____day of
_____, 19_____, by the principal named above. I am not the agent or alternative agent
in this instrument.

_____
(Signature of Notary Public)

or

I certify that I am at least 18 years of age and that in my presence on the date appearing
above, the principal signed or acknowledged the signing of this instrument. I am not named
as agent or alternative agent in the instrument. If I am a health care provider or an employee
of a health care provider providing direct care to the principal on the date appearing above, I
have so noted below.

_____   _____
Witness Signature   Witness Signature

_____   _____
Address   Address

Health Care Provider?   Health Care Provider?
  Yes____   No____   Yes____   No____

Under Minnesota law the following form, or one substantially in the same form, must be used to prepare a living will:

HEALTH CARE LIVING WILL

Notice:

This is an important legal document. Before signing this document, you should know these important facts:

(a)   This document gives your health care providers, or your designated proxy, the power and guidance to make health care decisions according to your wishes when you are in a terminal condition and cannot do so. This document may include what kind of treatment you want or do not want and under what circumstances you want these decisions to be made. You may state whether you want or do not want to receive any treatment.

(b)   If you name a proxy in this document, and that person agrees to serve as your proxy, that person has a duty to act consistently with your wishes. If the proxy does not know your wishes, the proxy has the duty to act in your best interests. If you do not name a proxy, your health care providers have a duty to act consistently with your instructions or tell you that they are unwilling to do so.

(c)   This document will remain valid and in effect until and unless you amend or revoke it. Review this document periodically to make sure it continues to reflect your preferences. You may amend or revoke the living will at any time by notifying your health care providers.

(d)   Your named proxy has the same right as you have to examine your medical records and to consent to their disclosure for purposes related to your health care or insurance unless you limit this right in this document.

(e)   If there is anything in this document that you do not understand, you should ask for professional help to have it explained to you.

TO MY FAMILY, DOCTORS, AND ALL THOSE CONCERNED WITH MY CARE:

I, _____, born on _____(birth-date), being an adult of sound mind, willfully and voluntarily make this statement as a directive to be followed if I am in a terminal condition and become unable to participate in decisions regarding my health care. I understand that my health care providers are legally bound to act consistently with my wishes, within the limits of reasonable medical practice and other applicable law. I also understand that I have the right to make medical and health care decisions for myself as long as I am able to do so and to revoke this living will at any time.

(1)   The following are my feelings and wishes regarding my health care (you may state the circumstances under which this living will applies): _____
_____
_____
_____

(2)   I particularly want to have all appropriate health care that will help in the following ways (you may give instructions for care you do want): _____
_____
_____
_____

(3)   I particularly do not want the following (you may list specific treatment you do not want in certain circumstances): _____
_____
_____
_____

(4) I particularly want to have the following kinds of life-sustaining treatment if I am diagnosed to have a terminal condition (you may want to list the specific types of life-sustaining treatments that you do want if you have a terminal condition): _____

_____

_____

_____

(5) I particularly do not want the following kinds of life-sustaining treatment if I am diagnosed to have a terminal condition (you may want to list the specific types of life-sustaining treatments that you do not want if you have a terminal condition): _____

_____

_____

_____

(6) I recognize that if I reject artificially administered sustenance, then I may die of dehydration or malnutrition rather than from my illness or injury. The following are my feelings and wishes regarding artificially administered sustenance should I have a terminal condition (you may want to indicate whether you wish to receive food and fluids given to you in some other way than by mouth if you have a terminal condition): _____

_____

_____

_____

(7) Thoughts I feel are relevant to my instructions. (You may, but need not, give your religious beliefs, philosophy, or other personal values that you feel are important. You may also state preferences concerning the location of your care.): _____

_____

_____

_____

(8) Proxy Designation. (If you wish, you may name someone to see that your wishes are carried out, but you do not have to do this. You may also name a proxy without including specific instructions regarding your care. If you name a proxy, you should discuss your wishes with that person.)

If I become unable to communicate my instructions, I designate the following person(s) to act on my behalf consistently with my instructions, if any, as stated in this document. Unless I write instructions that limit my proxy's authority, my proxy has full power and authority to make health care decisions for me. If a guardian or conservator of the person is to be appointed for me, I nominate my proxy named in this document to act as guardian or conservator of my person.

Name: _____

Address: _____

Phone Number: _____

Relationship (If any): _____

If the person I have named above refuses or is unable or unavailable to act on my behalf, or if I revoke that person's authority to act as my proxy, I authorize the following person to do so:

Name: _____

Address: _____

Phone Number: _____

Relationship (If any): _____

I understand that I have the right to revoke the appointment of the persons named above to act on my behalf at any time by communicating that decision to the proxy or my health care provider.

(9) Organ Donation After Death. (If you wish, you may indicate whether you want to be an organ donor upon your death.) Initial the statement which expresses your wish:

_____ In the event of my death, I would like to donate my organs. I understand that to become an organ donor, I must be declared brain dead. My organ function may be maintained artificially on a breathing machine (i.e., artificial ventilation), so that my organs can be removed.

Limitations or special wishes (If any): _____
_____

I understand that, upon my death, my next of kin may be asked permission for donation. Therefore, it is in my best interests to inform my next of kin about my decision ahead of time and ask them to honor my request.

I (have) (have not) agreed in another document or on another form to donate some or all of my organs when I die.

_____ I do not wish to become an organ donor upon my death.

Date: _____
Signed:_____
State of: _____
County of:_____

Subscribed, sworn to, and acknowledged before me by _____ on this _____ day of _____ , 19____.

_____
NOTARY PUBLIC

or

(Sign and date here in the presence of two adult witnesses, neither of whom is entitled to any part of your estate under a will or by operation of law, and neither of whom is your proxy.)

I certify that the declarant voluntarily signed this living will in my presence and that the declarant is personally known to me. I am not named as a proxy by the living will, and to the best of my knowledge, I am not entitled to any part of the estate of the declarant under a will or by operation of law.

Witness: _____Address: _____

Witness: _____Address: _____

Reminder: Keep the signed original with your personal papers. Give signed copies to your doctors, family, and proxy.

Index

A

AA (Alcoholics Anonymous), 334, 1130
AARP (American Association of Retired
  Persons), 235
abdominal pain, 435-36
  from appendicitis, 436
  bowel obstruction, 436
  from diverticulitis, 436
  from gallstones, 435
  from gastroenteritis, 435
  from pancreatitis, 435
  from peptic ulcers, 435, 753-57
  recurrent, 120
  in school-age children, 120
abdominal wounds, first aid for, 401
abortions:
  D and C for, 1151
  elective, 199
  in first trimester of pregnancy, 199
  spontaneous, 197-98
  therapeutic, 199
abrasions, corneal, 452
abscesses:
  anorectal, 798
  in Bartholin's glands, 1172
  cutaneous, 1016
  dental, 433
  epidural, 486-88
  of liver, 810-12
  of lungs, 708-10
  peritonsillar, 595-96
  in teeth, 607-8
absence seizures, 497
abuse:
  of elderly, 234
  physical, 1231-33
  of preschool children, 110
  sexual, see sexual abuse
abuse, substance, see alcohol abuse; drug
  abuse
accidents, 119, 160
  automobile, 160
accommodative esotropia, 66
Accutane (isotretinoin), 186
ACE inhibitors, 652, 660, 1279
acetaminophen, 1279
achalasia, 745-46
Achilles tendinitis, 874
acid poisoning, 439
acne, 990-91, C-9
  in infants, 69
  rosacea, C-9
  in teenagers, 158
acoustic neuromas, 584
acoustic trauma, 582
acquired immune deficiency syndrome,
    see AIDS
acral lentiginous melanomas, 1006, C-6

acrochordons, 1002, C-4
acrocyanosis, 697
acromegaly, 898, 942
ACS (American Cancer Society), 280-81,
  1299
actinic keratoses, 1002, C-4
acute conditions, see specific topics
acyclovir, 1060
ADA (American Diabetes Association),
    284, 285, 932
addictions, 1129-31
  to alcohol, see alcoholism, alcoholics
  to caffeine, 1131
  to drugs, see drug dependence, drug
    addiction
  to gambling, 1130
  to nicotine, 316; see also smoking
  to nose drops, 587
Addison, Thomas, 938
Addison's disease, 938-39
  dehydration in, 443
  hypovolemic shock in, 443
  nutrition and, 939
adenine, B-8
adenocarcinomas, renal, 847
adenofibromas, 1159
adenoidectomies, 593
adenomas, pituitary, 943
adenomatous goiters, 946
adenomyosis, 1186
  pelvic pain in, 1188
ADH (antidiuretic hormone), 945
Administration on Aging, U.S., 245
adolescents, see teenagers
adrenal gland disorders, 443, 937-41, 1156-57
  Addison's disease, 443, 938-39
  congenital adrenal hyperplasia, 9, 941,
    1169
  Cushing's syndrome, 937-38
  menses and menstrual disorders
    related to, 1156-57
adrenal gland tumors, 939
  aldosteronomas, 940-41
  Conn's syndrome, 940-41
  hirsutism in, 940, 1019-21, C-7
  pheochromocytomas, 939
adrenal hyperplasia, congenital, 9, 941, 1169
adrenaline (epinephrine), 924, 929
  for anaphylaxis, 398, 445, 1053, 1277
adrenarche, 135
adrenocortical hypofunction, 938-39
adult day-care, 246, 1327
adulthood, adjusting to, 1097
adults:
  aspirin as dangerous for, 1073
  evaluating fitness of, 295-96
  hypopituitarism in, 944
  middle-aged, see middle years
  thermometers used on, 424

young, see young adults
advance directives, 1248-49, 1312, 1381-89
advertising, for tobacco, 317
aerobic exercise, 290-91
  in cardiovascular fitness, 644-47
  for elderly, 236-37
  low-impact, 196
age:
  in abnormal blood fat levels, 642
  as chronic glaucoma risk factor, 551
  hearing loss and, 579-81
  as heart and blood-vessel disorders
    risk factor, 644
  as pregnancy risk factor, 194
age spots, 227-28, 244
aggression, 1125
aging, 232-37
  adjusting to, 1097
  baldness and, 227
  of bones, 226
  of cardiovascular system, 225
  of digestive system, 225-26
  hair and, 227
  of joints, 226-27
  loss of independence in, 234-35
  menopause and, 228
  in middle years, 224-30
  physical changes of, 233-34
  process of, 232-37
  of skin, 227-28
  statistics about, 232-33
  success in, 235-36
agnogenic myeloid metaplasia, 972-73
agranulocytosis, 974
Agriculture Department, U.S., 183, 258, 281
AIDS (acquired immune deficiency syn-
    drome), 1060-64
  emergency symptoms of, 488
  home care for victims of, 1063
  intestinal malabsorption problems in, 771
  nervous system and, 488
  in pregnancy, 193
  risk factors of, 1063
  safe sex and, 1091
  signs and symptoms of, 1060-61
  transmission of, 1061-62
  treatment of, 488, 1064
Ainsworth, Mary B., 36
air, asbestos in, 729
air pollution, 373-75, 732
  from chlorofluorocarbons, 373-74
  from cigarette smoke, 374
  from formaldehyde, 374
  indoor, 374-75
  from industrial and power plants, 373
  from motor vehicle exhaust, 373
  occupationally related lung disease
    from, 728-34
  taking action on, 375

air-puff tonometers, 553
AITP (autoimmune thrombocytopenic purpura), 978-79
Al-Anon, 334
Alateen, 334
alcohol:
    black coffee and, 329
    in body, 326-27, 329
    calories in, 279, 327
    cancer and, 329, 1294
    cardiovascular system affected by, 328-29
    dependence on, see alcoholism, alcoholics
    ethyl, 326-27
    excessive and frequent consumption of, 330-31
    excuses for consumption of, 331
    gastrointestinal tract affected by, 328
    heart muscle disease and, 686
    hypothermia and, 329
    increased tolerance to, 329-30
    interaction with tranquilizers, 340
    intoxication with, 327, 429-30
    mixing drugs with, 340, 1273
    in pregnancy, 195, 328
    preoccupation with, 330
    solitary consumption of, 331
    symptomatic use of, 331
    teenagers' use of, 152, 153, 332, 1102-3
    understanding of, 326-34
    withdrawal from, 330, 333, 429-30
    in workplace, 359
alcohol abuse, 325-34
    brain and nervous system and, 328
    cardiovascular system and, 328-29
    gastrointestinal system and, 328
    in middle years, 221
    sexual functioning and, 329
    short- and long-term effects of, 327-29
alcoholic heart disease, 686
alcoholic hepatitis, 803
alcohol-induced cirrhosis, 805
alcohol-induced psychosis, 1129
alcohol intoxication, 327
    emergency treatment of, 429-30
Alcoholics Anonymous (AA), 334, 1130
alcoholism, alcoholics, 326, 1129-30
    acceptance of, 333
    complete abstinence in treatment of, 333, 1130
    continuing support in treatment of, 334
    denial in, 329
    detoxification with withdrawal in treatment of, 333
    dietary risks of, 286
    drugs in treatment of, 334
    in elderly, 329
    families of, 332
    help for, 331-32
    intervention on behalf of, 331-32
    myths about, 329
    neurologic complications in, 328
    penetrating protective shell of, 331
    psychiatric and psychological treatment of, 334
    recognition of, 329-31
    recovery programs for, 334, 1130
    screening tests for, 330
    support groups for, 334, 1130
    treatment of, 332-34, 1130
aldosteronomas, 940-41

alkali poisoning, 439
alkaline reflux gastritis, 756
allergens:
    avoidance of, 1033
    testing for, 1030-32
    types of, 1029
    usual exposures to, 1029-30
allergic alveolitis, 731
allergic angiitis, 921
allergic rhinitis (hay fever), 1029, 1040-41
allergies, 1025-53
    allergy shots for, 1034
    anaphylaxis and, 1053
    angioedema in, 415, 1038-39
    to animals, 1035, 1042-44
    asthma, see asthma
    atopic dermatitis, 14-15, 989, 1038, C-2
    avoidance in treatment of, 1033
    to cats, 1043
    contact dermatitis, see contact dermatitis
    discovering causes of, 1030-32
    to drugs, 439, 1030, 1050-51, 1276-77
    to food, see food allergies
    hay fever, 1029, 1040-41
    to heat and cold, 1039
    hives, 415, 994, 1038-39, C-9
    inappropriate tests for, 1031
    to insect bites, 1030, 1051-53
    to latex, 1029
    medication for, 1033-34
    to mold and dust, 1042-44
    myths about, 1034-35
    nasal polyps, 1041-42
    physical location as cause of, 1035
    to poison ivy, 1035
    to pollen, 1042
    as psychosomatic, 1034-35
    RAST (radioallergosorbent test) for, 1032
    reactions in, 1028-30
    respiratory, see respiratory allergies
    seriousness of, 1035
    skin, see skin allergies
    skin tests for, 1031-32
    treatment of, 1032-34
    20th century syndrome, 374, 1033
    understanding of, 1026-28
allogeneic bone marrow transplants, 967
alopecia areata, 1018-19, C-7
alpha₁-antitrypsin deficiency, 807
alpha-fetoprotein analysis, 180-81
alpha-thalassemia, 962-63
Alport's syndrome, 833
ALS (amyotrophic lateral sclerosis), 477
alternative medicine, 1244-45
altitude, exercise and, 305
altitude disorders, 417-18
alveolitis, allergic, 731
Alzheimer's disease, 470-71
AMA (American Medical Association), Medical Directory of, 1246
amantadine, 1060
amblyopia, 534-36
    corrective measures for, 535-36
    early recognition of, 534-35
    in infants, 65
    nonsurgical treatment of, 536
    optical approaches to, 536
    in preschool children, 90
ambulatory surgery, 1262-63
amenorrhea, 1149
American Association of Retired Persons (AARP), 235

American Board of Psychiatry and Neurology, 1096
American Cancer Society (ACS), 280-81, 1299
American College of Emergency Physicians, 391
American College of Obstetricians and Gynecologists, 1142, 1223
American College of Physicians and Surgeons, 1300, 1313
American College of Sports Medicine, 305
American Diabetes Association (ADA), 284, 285, 932
American Express, 380
American Foundation for the Blind, 239
American Heart Association, 679
American Lung Association, 374
American Medical Association (AMA), 1246
American Red Cross, 391
amniocentesis, 181
amphetamines, 1129, 1132
amputations, 879-80
    in arterial embolism, 693
    in arteriosclerosis of the extremities, 691-92
    in Buerger's disease, 698
    in frostbite, 698
    traumatic, 450-51
amyloidosis, 771-72, 974-75
amyotrophic lateral sclerosis (ALS), 477
anabolic steroids, 345-46, 1278
anaerobic exercise, 290-91
    in cardiovascular fitness, 645
anal fissures, 796-97
anal fistulas, 796-97
analgesic nephropathy, 835
analgesics, 1278
    dependence on, 341, 346
    narcotic, 346, 431, 1278
anal itch, 796
anal pain, 798
anaphylaxis, 444-45, 1029, 1033-34, 1053
    in reaction to medication, 1277
    treatment of, 1053
anastomosis, ileo-anal, 780
androgen resistance syndrome, 1169
androgens, 1278
anemias, 956-82
    aplastic, 963
    of chronic disease, 963
    Cooley's, 963
    folic acid deficiency, 959-60
    G6PD deficiency, 962
    hemolytic, 956, 962
    iron-deficiency, 121-22, 159, 275, 957-58, 1151
    pernicious, 958-59
    in pregnancy, 188
    from rare hemoglobin diseases, 961
    sickle cell disease, 833-34, 960-62
    sideroblastic, 963
    thalassemia, 962-63
anesthesia, 1260-62
    epidural, 211-12
    general, 1261-62
    local, 1261
    regional, 1261
    spinal, 211-12
aneurysms, aortic, 693-94, B-2
angiitis, allergic, 921
angina pectoris, 657-59, B-3
    exercise for, 658

angiodysplasia of colon, 794
angioedema, 415, 1038-39, C-9
  first aid for, 415
angiofibromas, juvenile, 589
angiography:
  in diagnosis of coronary artery disease,
    656, 1339-40
  fluorescein, 1342
  radionuclide, 656, 1339-40
angiomas, cherry, 1002, C-4
angioplasty, coronary, 666, B-3
angiotensin-converting enzyme inhibitors,
  652, 660, 1279
  in treating hypertension, 652
angle tumors, 584
animal bites, 394-95
  emergency treatment of, 394-95
  infections caused by, 394-95, 1016
  minor, 394
  risk of rabies in, 395
  serious, 394
animals, respiratory allergies to, 1035,
  1042-44
ankylosing spondylitis, 913, 914
annular pancreas, 822
anorectal abscesses, 798
anorectal disorders, 795-800
  abscesses, 798
  anal itch, 796
  anal pain, 798
  fecal incontinence, 799-800
  hemorrhoids, 188, 795-96, 797
  imperforate anus, 57
  proctitis, 797, 798-99
anorexia nervosa, 152, 1102
anovulation, 1217, 1218
Antabuse (disulfiram), 334, 1279
ant bites, 1014
antacids, 260, 1279
antenatal testing, see prenatal tests
antepartum hemorrhage, 205
anthracosis, 730-31
antialcoholic drugs, 1279
antianxiety agents, 1120, 1279
antiarrhythmics, 1279
antiasthmatics, 1279
antibacterial agents, 1058
antibiotic-associated diarrhea, 769-70
antibiotics, 1279
  topically vs. orally administered, 1058
  for ulcers, 754
antibodies, 1056
  monoclonal, 1299, 1337-38
antibody reactions, 981
anticoagulants, 1279
anticonvulsants, 1279
antidepressants, 1123, 1124, 1279
antidiabetic agents, 1279
antidiarrheals, 1279
antidiuretic hormone (ADH), 941, 945
antiemetics, 1279
antifungal drugs, 1059, 1279
antigens, 1026-28
antiglaucoma agents, 1279
antihistamines, 1279
  in allergy treatment, 1033, 1034
  for coughs, 703
antihypertension medications, 642, 651-52,
  1279
anti-infectives, 1279
anti-inflammatory agents, 1279
antioxidant nutrients, 265-66

antiparkinsonians, 1279
antipruritics, 1279
antipsychotic agents, 1279
antipyretics, 1279
antisocial personality disorder, 1106
antispasmodics, 1279
antiviral drugs, 1060, 1279
anus:
  imperforate, 57
  see also anorectal disorders
anxiety, anxiety disorders, 1095, 1118-22
  antianxiety medications for, 1120, 1123,
    1279
  anxiety reactions, 1118-19
  biofeedback for, 1121
  hyperventilation in, 1119
  knot in stomach, 1118
  during menopause, 1153
  obsessive-compulsive disorder, 1108-9,
    1121
  panic attacks, 151, 1119
  phobias, 91-92, 133-34, 1119-20
  post-traumatic stress disorder, 1121-22
  in teenagers, 151
aorta, coarctation of, 52
aortic aneurysms, 693-94, B-2
aortic regurgitation, 685
aortic stenosis, 53, 683-85
aortic valve problems, 53, 682-85
Apgar test, 6
  areas assessed by, 6
aphthous ulcers, 617, C-10
aplastic anemia, 963
apocrine glands, 985
appendicitis, 436, 772-73
appetite:
  of newborns, 10, 14
  of preschool children, 85
  weight control and, 278
  see also feeding
applanation tonometers, 553
arms, fractures of, 447-48
aromatherapy, 1245
arrhythmias, 663, 669-72
ART (assisted reproductive technology),
  1219-21
arterial bleeding, 399
arterial blood gas analyses, 1332
arterial embolisms, 692-93
arterial occlusions, acute, 850-51
  pain in, 437
arteriography, cerebral, 464, 1341
arteriosclerosis of extremities, 690-92
  risk factors for, 691
arteritis, cranial, 565-66, 921
arthritis:
  at base of thumb, 885-86
  crystal-induced, 916
  gonococcal, 915
  infectious, 914-15
  inflammatory, 913-14
  of inflammatory bowel disease, 913
  juvenile rheumatoid, 911-13
  in middle years, 226-27
  psoriatic, 913
  rheumatic fever, 915
  rheumatoid, 909-11
  sexual function and, 230
  staphylococcal, 915
  tuberculous, 915
  viral, 915
  wear-and-tear, 908

arthrography, 1341
arthroscopy, 878
artificial cardiac pacemakers, 675
artificial limbs, 879
artificial speech aids, 598
artificial tears, 538
asbestos:
  in air, 729
  in drinking water, 372
  removal of, from buildings, 729
asbestosis, 728-30
ascariasis, 1083-84
ascites, 808
ASD (atrial septal defect), 52
aspergillosis, 712
aspiration pneumonia, 704
aspirin, 1279
  dangers of, 1073
  in preventing heart attacks, 663
  in treating abnormal blood fat levels, 642
assisted reproductive technology (ART),
  1219-21
asteatosis, 244, 994, C-15
asthma, 720, 1044-47
  cardiac, 661
  exercise and, 1047
  first aid for, 413
  MDIs (metered-dose inhalers) for, 1046
  occupational, 731
  peak flowmeters and, 1045
  in pregnancy, 190
  severe, 413
astigmatism, 527-28
atelectasis, 723
atherectomy, 667
atherosclerosis, 467, 636-37
  in diabetes mellitus, 929-30
  sexual function and, 230
atherosclerotic plaque, B-3
athletes:
  anabolic steroids used by, 345-46
  beta blockers used by, 346
  beta$_2$-agonists used by, 346
  carbohydrate loading by, 275-76
  corticosteroids used by, 347
  diuretics used by, 347
  drinking water for, 274-75
  drug abuse by, 345-47
  growth hormone used by, 347
  high-protein diets for, 276
  iron-deficiency anemia in, 275
  narcotic analgesics used by, 346
  normal eating for, 274-75
  pregame meals for, 276
  psychomotor stimulant drugs used by,
    346
  special diets for, 141, 275-76
  sympathomimetic amines used by, 346
  water-weight diets for, 276
  see also sports
athlete's foot, 1013-14, C-8
atonic cerebral palsy, 55
atopic dermatitis, 14-15, 989, 1038, C-2
ATP (autoimmune thrombocytopenic
  purpura), 978-79
atrial fibrillation and flutter, 670
atrial heartbeat, ectopic, 669-70
atrial septal defect (ASD), 52
atrophic vaginitis, 1174
atrophic vulvar dystrophy, 1170
atropine, 676
attention deficit disorder, 132-33

autism, infantile, 108, 1100
autoimmune thrombocytopenic purpura
    (AITP; ATP), 978-79
autologous bone marrow transplants,
    967-68
automobile accidents, 160
autonomic nervous system, 459
autopsies, 1315-16
    arranging for, 1316
    emerging illnesses identified by, 1316
    for emotional security, 1315
    hereditary disorders revealed by, 1315
    for insurance settlements, 1315-16
    for medical research, 1316
    for quality assurance, 1316
    for vital statistics, 1316
autosomal genes, 42-43
avoidant personality disorder, 1108
avulsions (loss of teeth), 624
ayurveda, 1245
azoospermia, 1217

B

babies, healthy, 5-9
    bowel movements of, 7-8
    crying of, 8
    feeding of, 7
    growth and development of, 6-8
    hearing of, 7
    language of, 7, 62
    personality and behavior in, 30-37
    posture and motor capabilities of, 7-8,
        61-62
    sleeping of, 8
    vision of, 7
    weights of, 5
    see also infants; newborns
Babinski reflex, 460
baby blues, 216-17
back, 899-907
    corsets for, 904
    injuries to, 303-4, 448
    posture and, 902-3
    protection of, 303-4, 901-3
    see also spinal cord, disorders of
backaches, B-1
    from exercise, 304
    from muscle strains and spasms, 900-904
    in pregnancy, 187-88
    sciatica and, 905, B-1
    self-help for, 903-4
    weight loss and, 304, 902
bacterial digestive system disorders,
    767-68
bacterial overgrowth, 771
bad breath, 620
bad trips, 1129
bagassosis, 731
Baker, William Morrant, 909
Baker's cyst, 909
baking soda, 368
balanitis, 1205-6
baldness:
    female-pattern, 1017
    male-pattern, 1017-18
    in middle years, 227
    temporary, 1018-19
    treatment of, 1017, 1018, 1019
balloon angioplasty, B-3
ballooning (aneurysm), B-2
barber's itch, 1007

barbiturates, dependence on, 1131-32
barium X-rays, 762-63
barotitis media, 574
barotrauma, 574
Barrett's esophagus, 744
barrier methods of contraception, 172-73
Bartholin, Casper, 1172
Bartholin's gland, 1140
    abscesses, 1172
basal cell cancer, 1005, C-6
basal metabolic rate, 947
baseball finger, 874
basements, safety in, 355
bathing:
    home care and, 1324
    after ileostomies or colostomies, 778
    of newborns, 27-28
    preventing dry skin in, 994
bathrooms, safety in, 240, 354
bathtubs, baby, 27
batteries, swallowing of, 427
B cells, 1026-27, 1056
bed urinals, 1324-25
bedding, SIDS and, 70
bedpans, 1324-25
bedrooms, safety in, 240, 354
beds:
    making of, 1323
    smoking in, 351
bedsores, 1325
bedtime, fussiness at, 37
bedwetting (enuresis), 89, 1098
bee stings, 396
behavior, see psychosocial development of
    personality and behavior
behavior emergencies, 429-32
    hyperventilation, 431-32, 1119
    sudden personality changes, 430
    suicidal thoughts, 431
Bell, Sylvia, 36
Bell's palsy, 493-95
bends, 417-18
benign prostatic hyperplasia (BPH), 1209,
    B-5
benzodiazepines, dependence on, 1132
bereavement, see grief responses
Berger's disease, 838
beta-adrenergic blockers, 1280
    for heart attacks, 664
    for heart rate and rhythm disorders,
        676
    for hypertension, 652
beta-thalassemia, 963
beta$_2$-agonists, 346
bicipital tendinitis, 917
bicycles, bicycling:
    accidents with, 160
    cross-country, 299-300
    exercise with, 299-300, 357
    for fitness, 299-300
    mountain, 299
    racing, 299
    safety in, 357
    selection of, 299-300
    stationary, 299
bifocal contact lenses, 529
bifocals, 529
bile duct:
    choledochal cysts in, 817-18
    X-rays of, 815, 816, 1341
bile duct cancer, 815
bile duct obstructions, 814-17

    in bile duct cancer, 815
    endoscopic treatment of, 817
    hemobilia as cause of, 814
    in PSC (primary sclerosing cholangitis),
        814-15
    trauma as cause of, 814
biliary atresia, 56
biliary cirrhosis, 806
bilirubin, 13, 800
"binge and purge" disorder (bulimia
    nervosa), 152, 1102-3
biofeedback, 1121
biopsies:
    bone marrow aspirations and, 1332-33
    of liver, 807, 1333
bipolar disorder, 1125-26
birth, see delivery
birth control, see contraception
birth control pills, 1146
    for men, 166
    side effects of, 172
    for women, 171-72
birth control shots, 173
birth defects, see genetic disorders
birth injuries:
    caput succedaneum, 21
    cephalhematomas, 21
    dislocation of nasal septum, 22
    facial nerve palsies, 22
    fractured collarbones, 22
birthing rooms, 208
birthmarks, 1002
    cavernous hemangiomas, 16, C-2
    hemangiomas, 15-16, 1002, C-2
    milia, 15, 69, C-2
    on newborns, 15-16
    port-wine stains, 16, C-2
    salmon patches, 15
    strawberry hemangiomas, 15-16, C-2
bites and stings, 394-99
    by animals, 394-95, 1016
    avoidance of, 360
    by bees, 396
    emergency treatment of, 394-95, 396
    by fire ants, 396
    by hornets, 396
    by humans, 395, 1015, C-13
    infections caused by, 395, 1014-15
    by insects, see insect bites and stings
    by jellyfish, 398-99
    mild, 396
    poisonous, 397
    by Portuguese man-of-war, 398-99,
        1015-16, C-13
    risk of rabies in, 395
    by scorpions, 396
    serious, 395
    by snakes, 398
    by spiders, 396, 1014, C-14
    by ticks, 396, 398, 1087, C-14
    by wasps, 396
    by yellow jackets, 396
bitewings, 369
black eye, 533
black lung disease, 730-31
blackheads, 990
blackouts:
    in alcoholics, 331
    see also fainting spells
black widow spiders, 396
bladder cancer, 848-50
    screening for, 1296

bladder disorders, 1192-94
    chronic urethritis, 1192-93
    cystitis, 94-95, 159, 436, 842, 1192, 1193,
        1203-4
    irritable bladder, 1192-93
    in men, 1203-4, 1207-8
    trauma in, 835-36
    urinary incontinence, *see* incontinence,
        urinary
bladder stones, 845-47
blastocysts, 176
bleeding (hemorrhaging):
    from abdominal wounds, 401
    antepartum, 205
    arterial, 399
    from body openings, 401-2
    from bruises, 401
    capillary, 399
    cerebral, 433, 461-62, 564
    from cuts, 401
    from D and C, 1151
    emergencies, 399-403
    epidural, 468-69
    esophageal, 808
    extradural, 468-69
    in eyes, 452, 544
    in fractures, 447
    in gastrointestinal tract, 759-61
    internal, 402
    in minor wounds, 392
    from nose, 403, 586-87
    postmenopausal, 1155
    postpartum, 214
    in pregnancy, 178
    from punctures, 401
    rectal, 403, 797
    severe, 400
    shock and, 441-43
    from soft tissue injuries, 401
    stopping of, 400
    subarachnoid, 433, 462
    subconjunctival, 544
    subdural, 466-68
    tourniquets for, 450
    in traumatic amputations, 450-51
    from uterus, 1152
    from vagina, 49, 134-35, 403, 1151
    venous, 399
bleeding disorders, 975-79
    DIC (disseminated intravascular
        coagulation), 977-78
    hemophilia, 975-77
    thrombocytopenia, 978-79
    von Willebrand's disease, 977
blepharitis, 539-40
blindness:
    cataracts as cause of, 35
    color, 548-50
    in newborns, 35-36
    night, 561-62
    in retinopathy, 35
    see also vision disorders
blink reflex, 4, 34
blisters, 1010
    avoidance of, 360
    fever, 1010, C-10
blood:
    coughing of, 402
    in semen, 1228
    transfusions of, 981
    understanding of, 954-56
    in urine, 403, 832

vomiting of, 12, 402
blood chemistry group tests, 1330-31
blood disorders, 953-82
    acute lymphocytic leukemia, 966-67
    acute nonlymphocytic leukemia, 965-66
    agnogenic myeloid metaplasia, 972-73
    agranulocytosis, 974
    amyloidosis, 771-72, 974-75
    anemia of chronic disease, 963
    aplastic anemia, 963
    bone marrow growth disorders, 971-95
    bone marrow transplants for, 967-68
    chronic lymphocytic leukemia, 966
    chronic myelogenous leukemia, 964-65
    enlarged spleen, 954
    folic acid deficiency anemia, 959-60
    granulocytopenia, 974
    G6PD deficiency, 962
    hemolytic anemias, 956, 962
    Hodgkin's disease, 969-70
    iron-deficiency anemia, 121-22, 159,
        275, 957-58
    leukemias, 964-68
    lymphomas, 968-71
    monoclonal gammopathy of undeter-
        mined significance, 973
    multiple myeloma, 973-74
    non-Hodgkin's lymphoma, 970-71
    pernicious anemia, 958-59
    polycythemia vera, 971-72
    porphyrias, 961
    rare hemoglobin diseases, 961
    sickle cell disease, 833-34, 960-62
    sideroblastic anemia, 963
    thalassemia, 962-63
blood fat, 643-44
    age and, 642
    diet and, 641
    measurement of, 640
    treatment of, 642
blood groups, 980
blood lipid measurements, 1250-51, 1331
blood pressure:
    classifications of, 648
    high, *see* hypertension
    low, 650
    measurement of, 649, 652, 1251
    normal, 648
blood pressure drugs, 642, 651-52, 1279
blood sugar:
    concentration, refraction problems
        caused by, 527
    control of, 527
blood tests, 657, 1330-32
    arterial blood gas analyses, 1332
    blood chemistry group, 1330-31
    CBCs, 955, 1330
    coagulation, 1331
    in diagnosing coronary artery disease,
        657
    for enzymes, 1331
    for lipids, 1250-51, 1331
    for presence of drugs, 1331
    results of, 1331
    sedimentation rate, 1331
    thyroid studies, 1331
blood transfusions, 979-82
    adverse reactions to, 981-82
    antibody reactions to, 981
    of coagulation factor concentrate, 981
    communicable diseases spread by, 981
    of cryoprecipitate, 980-81

donation procedure in, 979-81
    of fresh-frozen plasma, 980
    of granulocytes, 981
    with own blood, 982
    of platelets, 981
    of red blood cells, 980
    synthetic substitutes in, 982
    types of, 980-81
blood vessels, 633-35, A-8
    disorders of, *see* heart and blood
        vessels, disorders of
    system of, 634-35
bloody show, 207
Blount's disease, 97
boat safety, 361
body openings, first aid for bleeding from,
    401-2
body scans, 1334-35
    CT, 494, 1334
    MRI, 494, 1334
    ultrasonography, 180, 683, 1335
boils, 1009
bonding, 6, 31-32
bone marrow aspirations, biopsies and,
    1332-33
bone marrow growth disorders, 971-75
    agnogenic myeloid metaplasia, 972-73
    amyloidosis, 771-72, 974-75
    multiple myelomas, 973-74
    polycythemia vera, 971-72
bone marrow transplants, 967-68
    allogeneic, 967
    autologous, 967-68
    process of, 968
    risks of, 968
    syngeneic, 967
bone scans, 1336
bones, 226, 862, A-4
bones, disorders of, 894-99
    acromegaly and, 898
    cancer of, 889
    common problems, 863-66
    dislocations, *see* dislocations
    endocrine system and, 898
    fibromyalgia, 883
    fibrous dysplasia, 898
    fractures, *see* fractures
    gigantism and, 898
    heel pain, 874-76
    hyperparathyroidism and, 898
    hypopituitarism, 898, 943-44
    nursemaid's dislocation, 866
    osteomalacia, 896-97
    osteomyelitis, 899
    osteoporosis, *see* osteoporosis
    Paget's disease of bone, 897-98
    rickets, 833, 896-97
    shin splints, 870-71
    tumors, 899
    see also musculoskeletal system, dis-
        orders of
borage, 355
borderline personality disorder, 1106-7
bottle-feeding, 39-40
    bottle care and, 41
    breastfeeding vs., 40
    techniques for, 39-40
botulism, 268-69, 441, 488-89
bowel:
    vascular problems of, 816
    see also colon
bowel habits:

in colon cancer screening, 790
of newborns, 7-8
bowel obstruction, 436
bowlegs, 97
boys, teenage:
    sexual changes in, 139-40
    see also teenagers
BPD (bronchopulmonary dysplasia), 20
BPH (benign prostatic hyperplasia), 1209,
    B-5
BPPV (benign paroxysmal positional ver-
    tigo), 584-85
braces, support, 879
brain and nervous system, 457-60, A-10
    short- and long-term effects of alcohol
        abuse on, 328
    workings of, 458-60
brain and nervous system, disorders of,
    461-517
    in AIDS, 488
    ALS (amyotrophic lateral sclerosis), 477
    Alzheimer's disease, 470-71
    Bell's palsy, 493-95
    botulism, 268-69, 441, 488-89
    brain attack, 461
    brain cancer, 492-93
    brain injuries, 490-91
    brain tumors, 492-93
    cerebral palsy, 54-55, 478-79
    cervical spondylosis, 509
    Charcot-Marie-Tooth disease, 513-14
    chronic, 469-81
    cluster headaches, 505-6
    concussions, 451, 490-91
    dementia, 470, 471-72, 473, 1095
    encephalitis, 482-84
    epidural abscesses, 486-88
    essential tremor, 475
    extradural hemorrhage, 468-69
    febrile seizures, 69, 70, 120-21, 497-98
    Friedreich's ataxia, 478
    grand mal seizures, 496-97
    Guillain-Barré syndrome, 513
    headaches, see headaches
    Huntington's chorea, 477-78
    hydrocephalus, 54, 489-90
    infections, 481-89
    meningitis, 382, 433, 481-82
    migraine headaches, 120, 159, 432-33,
        502-4
    MS (multiple sclerosis), 475-77
    myasthenia gravis, 479-81
    myelomeningocele, 514
    neuralgias, 514-15
    neuroblastomas, 493
    Parkinson's disease, 472-74
    of peripheral nervous system, 506,
        509-16
    peripheral neuropathies, 509-11
    petit mal seizures, 497
    physical therapy in rehabilitation for,
        480
    poliomyelitis, 382, 485-86, 1079
    post-polio syndrome, 487
    Reye's syndrome, 484
    seizures, see seizures
    spinal stenosis, 516-17
    of spine, see spinal cord, disorders of
    stroke and vascular disorders, see
        strokes and vascular disorders
    structural, 53-54, 489-95
    subdural hemorrhage, 466-68

syringomyelia, 514
temporal lobe seizures, 498-99
tension-type headaches, 501-2
TIA (transient ischemic attack), 463-66
tic disorders, 475
torticollis, 479
trigeminal neuralgia, 515-16
brainstem, 458
breads, see grains
breast cancer, 169, 1163-68, B-4
    breast conservation therapy for, 1166
    chemotherapy for, 1168
    hormone therapy for, 1168
    mammograms in identification of, 169,
        1165, 1250
    palliative surgery for, 1167
    radiation therapy for, 1165-68
    screening for, 1294
    surgery for, 1166-67
breast conservation therapy, 1166
breast disease, benign, 1158
breast problems, 1157-68
    benign breast disease, 1158
    blocked milk ducts, 216
    cysts, 1158-59
    engorgement, 216
    enlargement in newborn, 50
    galactorrhea, 1162-63
    infections, 1160-61
    infectious mastitis, 216, 1160-61
    intraductal papillomas, 1163
    lumps, 1158-59, B-4
    nipples, 39, 49-50, 216, 1161-62
    after pregnancy, 216
    premenstrual tenderness and swelling,
        1158
    in school-age children, 134
    stereotaxic breast biopsy and, 1164
    yeast infections, 1161
breastfeeding, 1162
    bottle-feeding vs., 40
    of newborns, 6, 39-41
    nutrition in, 39-41
    after pregnancy, 215-16
    techniques for, 39
    weaning from, 216
breasts:
    development of, 1143-44
    normal, 1142-43, 1157-58
    post-surgical reconstruction of, 1167
    self-examination of, 169, 1160, B-4
breath, bad, 620
breath, holding of, 92
breathing:
    changes in, 85
    deep, 717
    diaphragmatic, 717
    of preschool children, 85
    pursed-lip, 717
    relaxed, 313
    shallow, 20
breathing emergencies, 406-14
    clearing obstructed airways in, 406-8
    coughing vs. choking in, 406
    CPR in, 408-13
    in croup, epiglottitis, or bronchitis, 413
    Heimlich maneuver for, 407
    in infants, 63
    in newborns, 9
    recognizing obstructed airways in,
        406-7
    severe asthma attacks, 413

breech presentation, 209
bronchiectasis, 708
    postural drainage for, 709
bronchiolitis, 701-2
bronchitis, 413
    acute, 702
    chronic, 714-15
    industrial, 733
bronchodilators, 1280
bronchopulmonary dysplasia (BPD), 20
bronchoscopy, 726
bronze diabetes, 958
brown lung, 731-33
brown recluse spiders, 396, C-14
bruises:
    first aid for, 401
    of thighs, 872
brushing teeth, 101, 366-67
bruxism, 1117
Buerger, Leo, 698
Buerger's disease, 698
bulimia nervosa, 152, 1102-3
bumper pads, 28
bunions, 891-92
burning feet, 890
burns, 403-5
    chemical, 404-5, 531-33
    classifications of, 403-4
    electrical, 404
    first aid for, 403-5
    first-degree, 403
    major, 405
    minor, 405
    preschool children and, 99
    second-degree, 404
    third-degree, 404
bursa of Fabricius, 1056
bursitis, 917-18
    popliteal, 909
butter, margarine vs., 254
bypass surgery, B-3
byssinosis, 731-33

C

caffeine:
    addiction to, 1131
    benefits of, 273
    in diet, 273-74
    drawbacks of, 273
    health and, 273-74
    in pregnancy, 185, 186, 194
    to sober up after drinking, 329
CAH (congenital adrenal hyperplasia), 9,
    941, 1169
calcitonin, 945-47, 950
calcium, 255
    foods rich in, 267
    for nutrition and weight control in
        pregnancy, 184
    osteoporosis and, 266-67
calcium channel blockers, 1280
    for heart attacks, 664
    for heart rate and rhythm disorders,
        676
    for hypertension, 652
calcium kidney stones, 286, 844
calculus, 365, 367-68
calendar method of contraception, 171
calf stretches, 293
calluses, 890-91
calories, 255-56

in alcoholic beverages, 279, 327
daily weight control deficit in, 277
in exercise, 301
for newborns, 38
for nutrition and weight control in
    pregnancy, 183
in school lunches, 123
camping, safety in, 360-61
Campylobacter, 767
campylodactyly, 45
cancer, 1289-1308
of adrenal gland, 939
alcohol and, 329, 1294
antioxidants in delay of, 266
basal cell, 1005, C-6
of bile duct, 815
biology of, 1291-96
of bladder, 848-50, 1296
of bones, 899
of brain, 492-93
of breasts, 169, 1163-68, 1250, 1294, B-4
of cervix, 1180-81, 1294
chemotherapy for, 1168, 1185, 1191, 1298
in children, 966-67, 1307-8
choosing physicians and places for
    treatment of, 1299-1300
of colon, 789-91, 1250, 1294-95
colorectal, 789-91, 1294-95
coping with survival of, 1306
diagnosis of, 1293
of endometrium, 1183-84, 1295
of esophagus, 750
of eyelids, 558
of eyes, 546
as genetic disease, 1291-93
immunotherapy for, 1298-99
industrial exposures and, 373, 1294
of islet cells, 757-58, 936
Kaposi's sarcoma, 1006, C-6
of kidneys, 847-48
of liver, 808-9
living with, 1296-1304
of lungs, 723-27, 1295
malignant melanomas, 1005-6, C-6
medullary thyroid, 946
menopause treatments and, 1294
of mouth, 621-22, 1295
of muscles, 888
new treatments for, 1299
nutrition and, 280-83, 373, 1294, 1303
of orbits, 558
of ovaries, 1190-91
pain in, 1303-4
of pancreas, 820-21, 936
of penis, 1206-7
in population clusters, 1296
of prostate, 1211-12, 1295, B-5
radiation exposure and, 1294
radiation therapy for, *see* radiation
    therapy
rectal, 789-91, 1294-95
rehabilitation in treatment of, 1304-7
of salivary duct, 623
screening for, 1293-96
sexual function and, 230
of skin, 244, 1004-6, 1295, C-6
of small intestine, 779-81
smoking and, 1294
of spinal cord, 508-9
squamous cell, 1005, C-6
sun exposure and, 373, 1294
surgery for, 1297

of testicles, 1202-3, 1295
of throat, 599-600, 1295-96
of thyroid, 946
transitional cell, 847
upper gastrointestinal endoscopy for,
    761
of ureter, 847-48
of urinary tract, 1296
of uterus, 1183-85
of vagina, 1176-77
of vulva, 1172-73
warning signs of, 1293
cancer centers, 1300-3
clinical, 1301-3
comprehensive, 1301-3
selection of, 1300
cancer patients:
hospices in rehabilitation of, 1305-7
nutrition and, 280-83
palliative care in rehabilitation of, 1306
team approach in rehabilitation of,
    1305-6
cancer prevention, 373, 1294
diet and, 280-81, 373
industrial exposure and, 373
passive smoking and, 373
sun exposure and, 373
Candida, 1031
Candida esophagitis, 744
candidiasis, C-2, C-10
canker sores, 617, 1010-11, C-10
cannabis compounds, dependence on, 1134
CAPD (continuous ambulatory peritoneal
    dialysis), 857
caput succedaneum, 21
car safety, 356-57
avoiding distractions in, 357
car maintenance in, 357
car seats for, 23-24, 72-73, 356
CO (carbon monoxide) poisoning and,
    376
defensive driving for, 356-57
impaired driving and, 357
for preschool children, 100
seat belts for, 356
weather conditions in, 357
car seats, 356
for infants, 72-73
for newborns, 23-24
carbohydrates, 253
in diabetics' diets, 284-85
loading, 275-76
for newborns, 38
for nutrition and weight control in
    pregnancy, 184
tooth decay related to intake of, 608
carbon monoxide (CO) poisoning, 376, 419
emergency treatment of, 419
carbuncles, 1009, C-12
carcinoid syndrome, 774
carcinomas, renal cell, 847
cardiac arrest, 674-76
cardiac arrhythmias, 669-72
as result of heart attack, 663
cardiac asthma, 661
cardiac cycle, 634
cardiac death, sudden, 674-76
cardiac monitoring, twenty-four-hour, 671
cardiac muscle blood flow, 1339
cardiac pacemakers, artificial, 675
cardiac rehabilitation, 668
cardiac scans, 1339-40

cardiac tamponade, 689
cardiogenic shock, 443-44
cardiomyopathies, 686-87
congestive, 686
dilated, 686
hypertrophic, 686
restrictive, 686
cardiopulmonary resuscitation (CPR), 391,
    408-13, 664
absence of pulse in, 410
alternating pumping and breathing in,
    411
breathing for victim in, 410
checking for breathing in, 409
checking for pulse in, 410
on children, 411
clearing airway in, 409
continuing breathing in, 410
delivering two slow breaths in, 409-10
hand positioning in, 411
head tilt/chin lift in, 409
on infants, 412
locking elbows in, 411
modified jaw thrust in, 409
positioning victim for, 409
pumping heart in, 411
restoring circulation in, 410-11
summoning assistance in, 409
two-person, 411
cardiovascular fitness, 644-47
aerobic exercise for, 644-47
anaerobic exercise in, 645
extensiveness of workouts for, 645-46
frequency of workouts for, 646
ideal exercise for, 646-47
measuring pulse in, 645
starting of, 647
walking for, 297-98, 647
warm-ups and cool-downs in, 292-94,
    647, 867
cardiovascular system:
anabolic steroids and, 345
in middle years, 225
short- and long-term effects of alcohol
    abuse on, 328-29
see also heart and blood vessels, dis-
    orders of
carotid endarterectomy, 467
carpal tunnel syndrome, 884-85
casts, 865
cat allergies, 1043
cat scratch disease, 1067-68
cataracts, 553-56, 558
antioxidants in delay of, 266
in newborns, 35
secondary, 558
surgery for, 554-56, 558
cautery, 587
cavernous hemangiomas, 16, C-2
CBCs (complete blood cell counts), 955,
    1330
CCPD (continuous cyclic peritoneal
    dialysis), 857
CCRCs (continuing-care retirement
    communities), 246
CCUs (coronary care units), 662
celiac sprue, 770-71
gluten-free diet for, 285
cell-mediated mechanisms, 1026, 1057-59
cells, B-8
cellulitis, 1009-10, C-12
orbital, 452-53, 545-46, C-11

Center for Media and Public Affairs, 1270
Centers for Disease Control, 305, 1066
central auditory disorders:
    in infants, 65
    in newborns, 35
    in preschool children, 107
central nervous system, 458-60
central nervous system, disorders of:
    AIDS and, 488
    botulism and, 488-89
    cerebral palsy, 54-55, 478-79
    Down syndrome, 44
    encephalitis, 482-84
    epidural abscesses, 486-88
    hydrocephalus, 54, 489-90
    meningitis, 382, 433, 481-82
    in newborns, 53-55
    poliomyelitis, 382, 485-86, 1079
    Reye's syndrome, 484
    spina bifida occulta, 53-54
central nervous system depressants,
        dependence on, 1131-32
central nervous system stimulants, depen-
        dence on, 1132-33
central retinal artery occlusion, 452
cephalhematomas, 21
cerclage, 203
cereals, see grains
cerebellum, 458
cerebral arteriography, 464, 1341
cerebral hemorrhages, 461-62, 564
    head pain in, 433
cerebral palsy, 54-55, 478-79
    atonic, 55
    extrapyramidal (athetotic), 55
    in newborns, 54-55
    spastic, 55
cerebrospinal fluid, 459
    analyses of, 1345-46
cerebrovascular disease, see strokes and
        vascular diseases
cerebrum, 458
cervical cancer, 1180-81
    Pap smears in detection of, 1181
    radiation therapy for, 1181
    screening for, 1294
cervical caps, 173
cervical dysplasia, 1179-80
cervical polyps, 1178-79
cervical spondylosis, 509
cervicitis, 1179
cervix, 1140-41
cervix, disorders of, 1177-81
    cancer, 1180-81, 1294
    cervicitis, 1179
    developmental, 1178
    dysplasia, 1179-80
    nabothian cysts, 1179
    polyps, 1178-79
cervix, incompetent, 203
cesarean sections, 212-13
    complications in, 213
    necessity of, 212
    pregnancy after, 213
    procedure in, 212-13
    recovery from, 213
Chagas disease, 792
chalazion, C-11
chaparral, 355
chaplains, 1311-12
Charcot-Marie-Tooth disease, 513-14
Charcot's joint, 931

charley horse, 871-72
checkups, 1249-52
    for eyes, 524
    laboratory tests and, 1252
    neurologic, 460
    pelvic examinations in, 1141-42, 1250
    in preventing tooth decay, 603-4
    for school-age children, 118
    for teenagers, 156-57
chelating drugs, 637
chemical burns, 404-5, 531-33
chemical peel, 999
chemicals:
    in eyes, 405, 531-33
    lawn, 375
    multiple sensitivities to, 374
chemotherapy:
    for breast cancer, 1168
    for cancer, 1168, 1191, 1298
    for hydatidiform moles, 1185
    for ovarian cancer, 1191
cherry angiomas, 1002, C-4
chest pains, 433-35
    chest wall, 434
    in heart attacks, 434
    in pneumonia with pleurisy, 434-35
    in pulmonary embolisms, 434
chest percussion, 709
chest X-rays, 1251
    in diagnosing coronary artery disease,
        657
chewing tobacco:
    risks of, 319-20
    see also smoking
chickenpox (varicella), 1076-77, 1080, C-1
    contagiousness of, 102
    in pregnancy, 191
chiggers, 1086-87, C-14
child abuse:
    of preschool children, 110
    sexual, see sexual abuse
child care facilities, 1257
childbirth, see delivery
childhood diseases, 102, 118, C-1
    see also specific diseases
childhood leukemia, 966-67
children:
    aspirin as dangerous for, 1073
    CPR (cardiopulmonary resuscitation)
        on, 412
    death and, 1317-18
    evaluating fitness of, 295
    exercise for, 295
    handicapped, 110-12
    immunization schedule for, 1078
    preschool, see preschool children
    safety at play for, 99-100, 353
    safety on farm for, 360
    school-age, see school-age children
    using thermometers on, 424
    see also infants; newborns
children, problems of, 1097-1100
    cancer, 966-67, 1307-8
    choking, 408
    clubfoot, 46, 912
    congenital dislocation of hip, 46, 912
    ear tubes in treatment of, 576
    encopresis, 89, 1098-99
    enuresis, 89, 1098
    fevers, 425
    hypopituitarism, 943-44
    infantile autism, 108, 1100

joint disorders, 912
    Legg-Calvé-Perthes disease, 912
    mental retardation, 108-9, 1099-1100
    obesity, 113-14, 123-24, 1099
    Osgood-Schlatter disease, 159, 912
    slipped capital femoral epiphysis, 912
    sun exposure, 362
    swallowing foreign objects, 427
    see also learning problems
Chinese restaurant syndrome, 1049
chiropractic, 1245
chlamydial infections, 1088-89
    in pregnancy, 193
chloasma patches, 995, C-7
chlorofluorocarbons, air pollution from,
        373-74
choking, 406-14
    coughing vs., 406
    obstructed airways as cause of, 406-8
    preschool children and, 100
    universal signal for, 406
choledochal cysts, 817-18
cholera:
    hypovolemic shock in, 443
    vaccination against, 383
cholesteatoma, 577
cholesterol, 122, 254
    HDL, 254, 639, 640, 644
    LDL, 254, 266, 639, 640-42
    measuring levels of, 639, 640
    as risk factor in heart and blood vessel
        disorders, 639-43
cholesterol-reducing agents, 1280
cholestyramine, 642
chondromalacia, 876
chordee, 48
choriocarcinomas, 1185
chorionic villus sampling, 181
choroiditis, 560-61
Christmas disease, 976
chromosome abnormalities, 43
chromosomes, B-8
chronic diseases:
    anemias of, 963
    in preschool children, 83
    special diets for, 284-86
    see also specific conditions
chronic fatigue syndrome, 1065
chronic obstructive pulmonary disease
        (COPD), 714, 715-20
chronic pain centers, 1136
chronic pain disorders, 1136-37
Churg-Strauss disease, 921
cigar smoke, see smoking
cigarettes:
    low-yield, 318-19
    see also smoking
circulatory problems, 690-98
    acrocyanosis, 697
    aortic aneurysms, 693-94, B-2
    arterial embolisms, 692-93
    arteriosclerosis of extremities, 690-92
    Buerger's disease, 698
    deep-vein thrombosis, 695
    dry gangrene, 692
    frostbite, 416-17, 698
    gangrene of extremities, 692
    lymphedema, 695
    Raynaud's disease, 697-98, C-16
    Raynaud's phenomenon, 697
    superficial thrombophlebitis, 694
    support stockings for, 696

thrombophlebitis, 437, 694-95
varicose veins, 188, 695-97
wet gangrene, 692
circumcision, 7
cirrhosis, 804-8
alcohol-induced, 805
ascites in, 808
cryptogenic, 805-6
esophageal bleeding in, 808
hepatic encephalopathy in, 808
portal hypertension in, 807
primary biliary, 806
secondary biliary, 806
spontaneous bacterial peritonitis in, 808
claudication, intermittent, 690-92, 871
cleaning products, 352
cleft lip, 51
cleft palate, 51
clergy, 1311-12
clicks, ventricular, 634
clitoris, 1140-41
enlargement of, 49
Clostridium perfringens, food poisoning
from, 268
clothing:
for infants, 73-74
for newborns, 23
clubfoot, 46, 912
clubhand, 45
coagulation factor concentrate, transfusions
of, 981
coagulation tests, 1331
coal worker's pneumoconiosis, 730-31
coarctation of aorta, 52
cobalt treatment, *see* radiation therapy
cocaine, 152, 343, 1129, 1132-33
coccidioidomycosis, 713
cochlear implants, 580
coitus interruptus, 165-66
cold sores, 1010-11, C-10
cold weather:
exercise in, 304-5
safety in, 362
skin allergies to, 1039
colds, common viral, 1071-73
in preschool children, 86-87
recurrent, 86-87
self-help for, 1073
colestipol, 642
colic, 9, 11, 36
excessive crying due to, 9, 11-12
treatment of, 12
colitis:
ischemic, 794
ulcerative, 777-79
collagen diseases, *see* immunologic
rheumatic disorders
collagen injections, 999
collarbones, fractures of, 22
colobomas, 560
colon, 740
angiodysplasia of, 794
barium X-rays of, 762-63
cancer of, 789-91, 1250, 1294-95
giant, 792
polyps in, 786-89, 797
spastic, 782
see also intestines, disorders of
colon cancer, 789-91, 1294-95
screening for, 790, 1250
colon polyps, 786-89, 797
colonoscopies, 788

colony-stimulating factors, 1299
color blindness, 548-50
colorectal cancer, 789-91
screening for, 790, 1294-95
colostomies, 777-78
colostrum, 6
colposcopy, 1346
coltsfoot, 355
coma:
hyperosmolar, 423, 926, 929-30
hypoglycemic, 926, 927-28
myxedema, 949
combination skin, 986
comfrey, 355
communicable diseases, *see* contagious
diseases, common
communicating:
with hearing-impaired people, 579
with physicians, 1247-49, 1258, 1272
see also language; speech
community-acquired pneumonia, 704
community services:
adult day-care, 246, 1327
day respite care programs, 246
for elderly, 245-48
home health care, 246
nursing homes, 247-48, 1255
nutrition services, 247
respite care programs, 246
complete blood cell counts (CBCs), 955,
1330
comprehensive cancer centers, 1301-3
compulsive personality disorder, 1108-9,
1121
computed tomography (CT) scanning,
494, 1334
concussions, 451, 490-91
condoms, 165
condyloma acuminata (genital warts),
1092, 1171-72
conflicts:
in family, 310
marital, 310
in workplace, 310
confusion, fevers accompanied by, 424
congenital adrenal hyperplasia (CAH), 9,
941, 1169
congenital defects, *see* genetic disorders
congenital dislocation of hip, 46, 912
congenital gastrointestinal tract disorders,
see gastrointestinal tract disorders,
congenital
congenital heart disorders, *see* heart disorders, congenital
congenital kidney disorders, 827-31
anatomic abnormalities, 827-30
dropped kidney, 828
duplication of kidney, 828
floating kidney, 828
horseshoe kidney, 828
hydronephrosis, 829-30
medullary sponge kidney, 830
multicystic dysplasia, 829
solitary kidney, 827
ureteral pelvic junction obstruction,
828
vesicoureteral reflux, 830-31
congenital lobar emphysema, 58
congenital nephrotic syndrome, 833
congenital obstruction of nasolacrimal
duct, 50-51
congenital pancreatic abnormalities, 822

annular pancreas, 822
pancreas divisum, 822
congestive cardiomyopathy, 686
congestive heart failure, 659-60, 663
diet for, 660
as result of heart attack, 663
conjunctivitis, 542-43, C-11
acute, 453
contagiousness of, 102
connective tissue diseases, *see* immunologic rheumatic disorders
Conn's syndrome, 940-41
constipation:
causes of, 784
chronic, 784-85
in elderly, 241
feeding problems due to, 41-42
in infants, 67
laxatives for, 784-85
in newborns, 13
in pregnancy, 187
in preschool children, 87
constrictive pericarditis, 689
contact dermatitis, 987-88, 1036-38, C-2, C-3
first aid for, 415
severe, 415
contact lenses:
bifocal, 529
candidates for, 528
caring for, 530
after cataract surgery, 556
combination, 529
disposable soft, 529
extended-wear soft, 529
fitting of, 529
gas-permeable hard, 529
hard, 529
problems with, 529-30
soft, 529
contagious diseases, common, 1071-80
blood transfusions in spread of, 981
chickenpox, 102, 191, 1076-77, 1080, C-1
common viral colds, 86-87, 1071-73
croup, 413, 1076
diarrhea, *see* diarrhea
diphtheria, 226, 382, 1078-80
German measles, 191, 1074, 1079, C-1
immunizations against, *see* immunizations
measles, 1073-74, 1079, C-1
mumps, 1077-78, 1079, C-1
roseola, 1074-75, C-1
scarlet fever, 1080, C-1
whooping cough, 382, 1075, 1079
continuing-care retirement communities
(CCRCs), 246
continuous ambulatory peritoneal dialysis
(CAPD), 857
continuous cyclic peritoneal dialysis
(CCPD), 857
contraception:
barrier methods, 172-73
birth control pills, 166, 171-72, 1146
birth control shots, 173-74
calendar method, 171
cervical caps, 173
coitus interruptus, 165-66
condoms, 165
diaphragms, 172-73
implants, 173
IUDs (intrauterine devices), 172
for men, 165-67

mucothermal method, 171
mucus inspection method, 171
natural family planning, 171
after pregnancy, 218
teenagers' use of, 148-49
temperature method, 171
vaginal sponges, 173
convalescence:
from extradural hemorrhages, 469
from subdural hemorrhages, 468
conversion disorder, 1135
conversion tables, 1351-54
convulsions, see seizures
cool-downs, 294, 867
in cardiovascular fitness, 647
Cooley's anemia, 963
CO (carbon monoxide) poisoning, 376, 419
emergency treatment of, 419
COPD (chronic obstructive pulmonary
disease), 714, 715-20
corneal abrasions, 452
corneal injury, 546-47
corneal problems, 546-47
infections, 547
transplantation in, 548
ulcers, 547
vitamin A deficiency in, 547
corns, 890-91
coronary angioplasty, 666, B-3
coronary artery bypass surgery, 665, B-3
coronary artery disease, 654-68, B-3
angina pectoris, 657-59
aspirin in prevention of, 664
beta-adrenergic blockers for, 664
blood tests in diagnosis of, 657
calcium channel blockers for, 664
cardiac arrhythmias, 663, 669-72
cardiac rehabilitation for, 668
CCUs (coronary care units) in, 662
chest X-rays in diagnosis of, 657
congestive heart failure, 659-60, 663
coronary angioplasty for, 666, B-3
coronary artery bypass surgery for, 665,
B-3
death from, 663
in diabetes mellitus, 643, 929-30
diagnostic tests for, 654-57, 1343-44
diet after, 668
ECGs for, 654, 655-57, 1343
exercise after, 668
exercise tolerance tests in diagnosis of,
655
nitrates for, 664
pain killers for, 664
pulmonary edema, 660-61
radionuclide angiograms in diagnosis
of, 656, 1339-40
stopping smoking after, 668
stress after, 668
thallium exercise scans in diagnosis of,
656
weight control after, 668
see also heart attacks
coronary care units (CCUs), 662
cor pulmonale, 735
corsets, 904
corticosteroids, 1280
abuse of, 347
in allergy treatment, 1033
for joint disorders, 919
cortisol, 929
cosmetic surgery, 228

candidates for, 228
danger in, 228
for eyelids, 541
healing after, 228
procedure in, 228
costochondritis, 434, 883-84
coughing:
of blood, 402
choking vs., 406
coughs:
antihistamines for, 703
causes of, 703
controlled, 717
expectorants for, 1280
in minor illnesses, 394
suppressants for, 1280
treatment of, 703
Council on Post-Secondary Accreditation,
252
CPR, see cardiopulmonary resuscitation
crabs (pubic lice), 1173
crack cocaine, 152, 343
cradle cap, 14, 68, C-2
cramps, 871-72
cranial arteritis, 921
eye disorders and, 565-66
craniopharyngiomas, 943
cretinism, 949
cribs, selection of, 28
Crigler-Najjar syndrome, 812
Crohn's disease, 774-77
cromolyn sodium, 1033
cross-country bicycles, 299-300
cross-country ski machines, 299
crossed eyes, 66, 90
croup, 1076
breathing difficulty due to, 413
crying:
colic as cause of, 9, 11-12
excessive, 9, 11-12, 63
in infant behavior, 36
by infants, 63
by newborns, 7, 8, 9
reasons for, 11
cryoprecipitate, transfusions of, 980-81
cryptococcosis, 712-13
cryptogenic cirrhosis, 805-6
Cryptosporidium, 769
crystal-induced arthritis, 916
CT (computed tomography) scanning,
494, 1334
curvature of penis, 1206, 1227-28
Cushing, Harvey, 937
Cushing's syndrome, 937-38, 942
cuts, first aid for bleeding from, 401
cystic acne, 990, C-9
cystic fibrosis, 720-21
postural drainage for, 709
cystic mastitis, chronic, 1158
cystine kidney stones, 844
cystinuria, 832-33
cystitis, 94-95, 159, 842, 1192, 1203-4
interstitial, 842, 1193
in men, 1203-4
pelvic pain from, 436
cystoscopy, 849, 1347
cysts:
Baker's, 909
in breasts, 1158-59, B-4
choledochal, 817-18
in ears, 571
in kidneys, 847

nabothian, 1179
ovarian, 436, 1189-90
popliteal, 876
sebaceous, 990, 1172
spermatic, 1199
in vagina, 1174
in vulva, 1172
cytomegalovirus, 193, 767
cytosine, B-8
cytotoxic drugs, 1280
cytotoxic testing, 1031

D

D and C (dilatation and curettage), 1151,
1152
dairy products, 113, 262
dander, respiratory allergies to, 1035,
1042-44
dandruff, 990
day care:
for adults, 246, 1327
for preschool children, 101-2
day respite care programs, 246
deafness:
hereditary, 578
see also hearing disorders
death and dying, 1309-18
act of, 1311
advance directives and, 1248-49, 1312,
1381-89
approaching, 1311
autopsies and, 1315-16
being informed of, 1310
bereavement and, 1316-17
children and, 1317-18
clergy and chaplains and, 1311-12
discontinuing, withholding, or limiting
treatment in, 1312-13
formalities of, 1314-15
from heart attack, 663
intrauterine, 206
making decisions about, 1312-14
organ donation and, 1315
of parents, 221, 1318
of spouses, 221-22
by suicide, see suicides
of teenagers, 154-55
terminal illness and, 1310-14
decompression sickness, 417-18
decongestants, 1280
deep-breathing exercises, 717
deep-vein thrombosis, 695
defibrillators, internal cardioverter-, 672
degenerative joint disease, 906, 908
dehydration:
in addisonian crises, 443
in cholera, 443
emergency treatment of, 443
from excessive use of diuretics, 443
in gastroenteritis, 443
in infants, 63
shock and, 443
delirium tremens (DTs), 330
delivery (birth):
abnormal fetal positions in, 209-10
breech presentation in, 209
by cesarean section, 212-13
electronic fetal monitoring in, 210
epidural anesthesia in, 211-12
episiotomies in, 210-11

fetal blood sampling in, 210
  by forceps, 211
  and induction of labor, 210
  labor and, 207-14
  local anesthetics in, 211
  narcotics in, 211
  newborns immediately after, 5-6
  occiput posterior in, 210
  pain relief in, 211-12
  postpartum hemorrhage and, 214
  procedures encountered in, 210-11
  prolonged labor and, 208
  retained placenta and, 214
  spinal anesthesia in, 211-12
  transverse presentation in, 209
  by vacuum extraction, 211
dementia, 470, 471-72, 1095
  tests for, 473
dental and oral disorders, 602-29, C-10
  abscesses, 433
  acute glossitis, 619
  avulsion, 624
  broken jaw, 623-24
  canker sores, 617, 1010-11, C-10
  dentures in, 626-29
  developmental, 614-17
  discolored teeth, 614-15
  discolored tongue, 621
  dislocated jaw, 623-24
  facial and mandibular trauma and
      fracture, 623-25
  geographic tongue, 620
  gingivitis, 364-65, 610-11, 612-13
  gingivostomatitis, 618
  hairy tongue, 620-21, C-10
  halitosis, 620
  head pain in, 433
  impacted teeth, 614
  infections and diseases of mouth,
      617-22
  leukoplakia, 618-19, C-10
  misshapen teeth, 614-15
  oral cancer, 621-22, 1295
  oral lichen planus, 619, C-10
  oral thrush, 618, C-10
  orthodontic treatment of, 615-17
  partial dentures in, 626
  periodontal disease, 364-65, 609-13
  periodontitis, 611-12
  prosthodontic treatment of, 626-29
  salivary duct stones, 623
  salivary duct tumors, 623
  salivary gland disorders, 622-23
  salivary gland infections, 622
  temporomandibular joint problems,
      624-25
  tongue disorders, 619-21
  trench mouth, 612-13
  see also tooth decay
dental procedures, heart valve disorders
    and, 679
dental X-rays, 369
dentists:
  checkups with, 603-4
  pediatric, 604
  for preschool children, 101
  specialties of, 604
dentures, 626-29
  fitting of, 626-27
  partial, 626
  problems with, 627-29
  proper care of, 627

deoxyribonucleic acid (DNA), B-8
dependent personality disorder, 1108
depression:
  adolescent, 154-55, 1101
  antidepressants and, 1123, 1124, 1279
  in elderly, 243-44, 1103-4
  endogenous, 1124-25
  helping someone with, 1104
  in middle years, 223-24
  during menopause, 228-29, 1153
  postpartum, 216-18
  Prozac and, 1123
  as sign of potential suicide, 1125
  see also mood disorders
dermabrasion, 999
dermatitis:
  atopic, 14-15, 989, 1038, C-2
  contact, 415, 987-88, 1036-38, C-2, C-3
  diaper, C-2
  neuro-, 988-89, C-3
  nickel, C-3
  nummular, C-15
  overtreatment, 990
  perioral, C-15
  seborrheic, 989, 990, B-2, C-3
  stasis, 989, C-3
dermatomyositis, 920-21
dermographism, C-9
DES (diethylstilbestrol), 1177
desire disorders, 1222, 1225, 1229
desserts, 122
detergent worker's lung, 731
detoxification:
  for alcoholism, 333
  for drug dependence, 1133
development of personality and behavior,
      see psychosocial development of
      personality and behavior
developmental disorders of cervix, uterus,
      and fallopian tubes, 1178
developmental disorders of mouth and
      teeth, 614-17
  impacted teeth, 614
  misshapen and discolored teeth, 614-15
  orthodontic treatment of, 615-17
developmental disorders of vagina and
      vulva, 49, 1169-70
developmental dysplasia of the hip, 912
diabetes:
  bronze, 958
  in pregnancy (gestational), 21, 189
diabetes insipidus, 944-45
diabetes mellitus, 925-31
  atherosclerosis in, 929-30
  Charcot's joint and, 931
  as chronic glaucoma risk factor, 551
  coronary heart disease in, 643, 929-30
  diagnosis of, 927
  emergency symptoms of, 926
  exercise and, 932-33
  eye disorders and, 562-63, 930
  foot problems and, 930, 931
  gastroparesis in, 772
  glucose self-monitoring in, 933
  in heart and blood vessel disorders,
      643, 929-30
  hyperosmolar coma in, 423, 926, 929-30
  hypertension in, 929-30
  hypoglycemic coma in, 926, 927-28
  insulin-dependent (IDDM) (juvenile-
      onset; type I), 926-27
  insulin for, 933-34

insulin reaction in, 422-23, 926, 927-28
  ketoacidosis in, 423, 926, 928-29
  kidney disease and, 930
  medication for, 933-35
  nephropathy in, 838-39, 930
  neuropathy and, 930
  newborns and, 21
  non-insulin-dependent (NIDDM)
      (adult-onset; type II), 926-27
  nutrition and, 284-85, 932
  oral hypoglycemic agents for, 934-35
  prevention of, 936
  reactive hypoglycemia and, 929
  retinopathy in, 558, 562-63, 930
  seriousness of, 927
  sexual function and, 230
  signs and symptoms of, 925-27
  stable, 926
  third nerve palsy, 563
  treatment of, 931-36
  vision problems in, 930
diabetic emergencies, 422-23
  hyperosmolar comas, 423, 926, 929-30
  insulin reaction, 422-23
  ketoacidosis, 423, 926, 928-29
diabetics' diets, 284-85, 932
  fats and carbohydrates in, 284-85
diagnostic-related groups (DRGs), 1265
dialysis:
  for acute kidney failure, 857
  continuous ambulatory peritoneal, 857
  continuous cyclic peritoneal, 857
  for kidney failure, 856-57
  peritoneal, 857
diaper rash, 14, C-2
  disposable diapers and, 29
  infants and, 68
diapers:
  cloth, 28-29
  dermatitis from, C-2
  disposable, 28-29, 74
  for infants, 74
  for newborns, 28-29
  for preschool children, 98
diaphragm (muscle):
  breathing and, 717
  herniated, 57-58
  hiccups and, 745
diaphragms (contraceptive device), 172-73
diarrhea:
  antibiotic-associated, 769-70
  contagiousness of, 102
  cytomegalovirus-induced, 767
  feeding problems and, 41
  in infants, 63, 66-67
  in minor illnesses, 394
  in newborns, 10, 13
  peptic ulcer surgery and, 756
  in preschool children, 85, 87-88
  traveler's, 269, 383-85
diazinon, 375
DIC (disseminated intravascular coagula-
      tion), 977-78
dicumarol, 186
Dietary Guidelines for Americans, 258-62
dietetic food labels, 263-64
diethylstilbestrol (DES), 1177
diets:
  acne and, 991
  antioxidants in, 265-66
  for athletes, 141, 275-76
  balanced, 113

basic components of food in, 253-56
blood fat levels and, 641
caffeine in, 185, 186, 194, 273-74, 329, 1131
calcium in, 184, 255, 266-67
cancer prevention and, 280-81, 373
carbohydrate loading in, 275-76
for celiac sprue, 285
for chronic diseases, 284-86
for chronic pancreatitis, 820
for diabetics, 284-85, 932
disease and, 280-86
exercise and, 278-80
fiber in, 123, 256, 288, 783
fiber supplements in, 784
food fads in, 286-88
gluten-free, 285
healthful, 252-80
and heart and blood vessel disorders, 280, 639-43, 653, 660, 668
high-protein, 276
ideal, 252-58
iron-deficiency anemia and, 275
iron in, 958
for kidney failure, 286
for kidney stones, 286
for liver disease, 286
old-age, 241
as pregnancy risk factor, 194
prudent, 259-61
salt and hypertension in, 283-84, 653
for school-age children, 121
SIDS (sudden infant death syndrome) and, 69
special, 275-76, 285-86, 932
for teeth of preschool children, 101
traveler's diarrhea and, 384-85
in treatment of hypertension, 283-84, 653
vegetarian, 276-77
water-weight, 276
see also food; nutrition; weight control
diffuse spasm, 746
digestive system, A-7
in middle years, 225-26
workings of, 739-41
see also gastrointestinal tract
digestive system, disorders of, 741-824
achalasia, 745-46
acute hepatitis A, 801
acute hepatitis B, 801
acute pancreatitis, 818-19
acute viral gastroenteritis, 766-67
acute viral hepatitis, 801-8
AIDS and, 771
alcohol-induced cirrhosis, 805
alcoholic hepatitis, 803
alpha$_1$-antitrypsin deficiency, 807
amyloidosis and, 771-72, 974-75
anal fissures and fistulas, 796-97
anal itch, 796
anal pain, 798
angiodysplasia of colon, 794
annular pancreas, 822
anorectal abscesses, 798
anorectal disorders, 57, 188, 795-800
antibiotic-associated diarrhea, 769-70
appendicitis, 436, 772-73
bacterial, 767-68
bacterial overgrowth, 771
Barrett's esophagus, 744
bile duct cancer, 815
bile duct obstructions, 814-17

Campylobacter, 767
Candida esophagitis, 744
carcinoid syndrome, 774
celiac sprue, 285, 770-71
choledochal cysts, 817-18
chronic constipation, 784-85
chronic hepatitis, 804
chronic pancreatitis, 819-20
cirrhosis, 804-8
colon cancer, 789-91, 1250, 1294-95
colon polyps, 786-89, 797
colonoscopies in, 788
colostomies in, 777-78
congenital pancreatic abnormalities, 822
Crigler-Najjar syndrome, 812
Crohn's disease, 774-77
cryptogenic cirrhosis, 805-6
Cryptosporidium, 769
cytomegalovirus, 193, 767
diabetic intestinal disorders, 772
diffuse spasm, 746
diverticulosis and diverticulitis, 436, 781-82
drug-induced, 758-59
drug-induced hepatitis, 803
Dubin-Johnson hyperbilirubinemia, 812
duodenal ulcers, 753-54
enlarged liver, 809-10
Entamoeba histolytica, 768-69
eosinophilic gastroenteritis, 764
Escherichia coli, 268, 768
esophageal rupture, 751
esophageal stricture, 748-49
esophageal tumors, 750
esophageal varices, 750-51
esophagitis, 744-45, 760-61
familial Mediterranean fever, 793
fecal impaction, 786
fecal incontinence, 799-800
femoral hernias, 823-24
and fiber in diet, 783
food poisoning, 267-70, 440-41, 488-89, 769
foreign bodies in esophagus, 749
gallstones, 435, 812-14
gastric ulcers, 754-55
gastritis, 758
gastrointestinal tract bleeding, 759-61
gastrointestinal tract infections, 766-69
gastrostomies in, 747
genetic liver problems, 811-12
Giardia lamblia, 768
Gilbert's syndrome, 811-12
heartburn, 187, 435, 742-44
hemochromatosis and, 806-7
hemorrhoids, 188, 795-96, 797
hepatitis A, 269, 382, 801, 1079
hepatitis B, 192-93, 382, 801, 1079
hepatitis C, 801-2
hernias, 743, 822-24
herpes simplex esophagitis, 744
hiatal hernias, 743
hiccups, 745
idiopathic intestinal pseudo-obstruction, 774
ileostomies in, 777-78
incisional hernias, 824
indigestion, 752-53
inguinal hernias, 822-23
intestinal gas, 260, 785-86
intestinal malabsorption problems, 770-72

intestinal obstruction, 793-94
intussusception, 773-74
irritable bowel syndrome, 782-84
ischemic colitis, 794
lactose intolerance, 772, 1049
laparoscopic surgery and, 817
liver abscesses, 810-12
liver tumors, 808-9
malignant pancreatic tumors, 820-21
Meckel's diverticulum, 773
megacolon, 57, 791-92
Ménétrier's disease, 764
mesenteric ischemia, 794
nontropical sprue, 770-71
Norwalk virus, 767
pancreas divisum, 822
parasitic, 768-69
paraumbilical hernias, 824
peptic ulcers, 435, 753-57, 760-61
peritonitis, 792
pharyngeal diverticula, 746-47
pharyngeal paralysis, 747-48
pill-induced esophagitis, 745
primary biliary cirrhosis, 806
primary intestinal pseudo-obstruction, 774
proctitis, 797, 798-99
protein-losing enteropathy, 774
PSC (primary sclerosing cholangitis), 814-15
radiation esophagitis, 744
rectal cancer, 789-91
rotavirus, 766-67
Salmonella, 268, 767-68
scleroderma and, 771
scleroderma of esophagus, 744
secondary biliary cirrhosis, 806
Shigella, 768
short-bowel syndrome, 772
small intestine tumors, 779-81
of stomach, 751-64
stomach dilation, 764
stomach tumors, 761-64
swallowing problems, 745-48, 760-61
toxic hepatitis, 803
tropical sprue, 771
ulcerative colitis, 777-79
upper gastrointestinal endoscopy in, 760-61
vascular problems of bowel, 794
Whipple's disease, 771
Wilson's disease, 807
Zollinger-Ellison syndrome, 757-58, 936
see also esophageal problems; intestines, disorders of; liver disease; pancreatic diseases
digital rectal examinations, 1250, B-5
digitalis, 1280
for heart rate and rhythm disorders, 676
Dilantin, 186
dilated cardiomyopathy, 686
dilatation and curettage (D and C), 1151
diphtheria, 1078-80
vaccination against, 226, 382, 1079
diplegia, 55
disease prevention:
diet in, 280-81, 283-84
for infants, 74-75
for newborns, 29-30
for preschool children, 98
dishpan hands, C-3
dislocations, 449, 866

of hip, congenital, 46, 912
immobilization of, 866
of jaw, 623-24
of nasal septum, 22
nursemaid's, 866
rehabilitation for, 866
disseminated intravascular coagulation
(DIC), 977-78
disulfiram (Antabuse), 334, 1279
diuretics, 186, 1280
abuse of, 347
excessive use of, 443
for hypertension, 651
diverticula, pharyngeal, 746-47
diverticular disease, 797
diverticulitis, 436, 781-82
diverticulosis, 781-82
diverticulum, Meckel's, 773
divorces, 221
dizziness, 584-85
DNA (deoxyribonucleic acid), B-8
DNR (do not resuscitate) orders, 1313-14
dominant genes, 42
Doppler, office, 179-80
double vision, 535
douches, administration of, 1275
Down syndrome, 44
downers, 431, 1131
dreams, 1117
DRGs (diagnostic-related groups), 1265
driving:
defensive, 357
impaired, 357
drool rashes, 69
drowning:
near, 418
preschool children and, 99
drug abuse:
with anabolic steroids, 345-46
with analgesics, 341, 346
with beta blockers, 346
with beta$_2$-agonists, 346
with cocaine, 152, 343
with corticosteroids, 347
definitions related to, 337
with diuretics, 347
drug use vs., 336-37
with growth hormone, 347
with hallucinogens, 343-44
illegal drugs and, 342-45
with inhalants, 344
with marijuana, 342-43
meaning of, 337
medications and, 335-47
in middle years, 221
mixing drugs and alcohol in, 340
multiple drug use in, 340
with narcotic analgesics, 346
with opiates, 344-45
with PCP (phencyclidine), 344
in pregnancy, 336
with psychomotor stimulant drugs, 346
recognition of, 347-49
sports and, 345-47
with sympathomimetic amines, 346
by teenagers, 152-53, 338, 1102-3
with tranquilizers, 340-41
drug allergies, 439, 1030, 1050-51, 1276-77
emergency symptoms of, 1050
drug dependence, drug addiction, 1131-34
on analgesics, 341, 346
on barbiturates, 1131-32

on benzodiazepines, 1132
on cannabis compounds, 1134
on central nervous system depressants,
1131-32
on central nervous system stimulants,
1132-33
definition of, 337, 341
detoxification for, 1133
on glue, 1131
on hallucinogens, 1134
on marijuana, 152, 342-43, 1134
on opioids, 1133
recognition of, 347-49
of teenagers, 152-53, 338, 1102-3
on tranquilizers, 340-41
drug-induced hepatitis, 803
drug-induced psychosis, 1129
drug-induced stomach problems, 758-59
drug intoxication, acute, 429-31
emergency treatment of, 431
from illegal drugs, 430-31
from legal drugs, 430
from mind-altering drugs, 430-31
from narcotics, 431
from uppers and downers, 431
withdrawal from, 431
drug rashes, 996, C-15
drug tests, 1331
drug withdrawal, 431
in newborns, 22
drugs, illegal:
abuse and dependence on, 342-45
intoxication from, 430-31
mind-altering, 430-31
narcotics, see narcotics
in pregnancy, 195
uppers and downers, 431, 1132
in workplace, 359
drugs, therapeutic, 1271-80
for abnormal blood fat levels, 642
for Achilles tendinitis, 874
for acne, 991
for acute ear infection, 575
for acute lymphocytic leukemia, 967
for acute nonlymphocytic leukemia,
965-66
for acute painful shoulder, 917
for acute pancreatitis, 819
for acute prostatitis, 1211
for Addison's disease, 938-39
administering to children, 120
administration of, 120, 1274-75
adverse reactions to, 1275-77
for AIDS, 1064
with alcohol, 340, 1273
for alcoholism, 334
in allergy treatment, 1033-34
for Alzheimer's disease, 471
for amenorrhea, 1149
for amyloidosis, 975
for amyotrophic lateral sclerosis, 477
anal itch in reaction to, 796
anaphylactic reactions to, 1277
for angina pectoris, 658-59
antifungal, 1059, 1279
antiviral, 1060, 1279
for arterial embolisms, 693
for arteriosclerosis of extremities, 691-92
for atrophic vaginitis, 1174
for atrophic vulvar dystrophy, 1170
for backaches, 904
for baseball finger, 874

basic dos and don'ts of, 1273
becoming familiar with, 1273
for bile duct obstructions, 817
birth defects caused by, 186
for blepharitis, 540
for breast infections, 1161
for brief reactive psychosis, 1128
for bronchiectasis, 708
for cancer pain, 1304
for cardiomyopathy, 687
for carpal tunnel syndrome, 884
for cerebral palsy, 479
for cervical spondylosis, 509
for chickenpox, 1077
for chiggers, 1087
for chlamydial infections, 1088-89
for chronic bronchitis, 715
for chronic ear infection, 576
for chronic lymphocytic leukemia, 966
for chronic myelogenous leukemia,
964-65
for chronic pancreatitis, 820
for chronic prostatitis, 1211
for chronic urethritis, 1193
classifications of, 1274, 1278-80
for coccidioidomycosis, 713
and communicating with physicians
about all aspects of health, 1272
for congestive heart failure, 660
for conjunctivitis, 543
for costochondritis, 883-84
for Crohn's disease, 776
for cryptococcosis, 712-13
curbing costs with, 245
for Cushing's syndrome, 937-38
for cystic fibrosis, 721
for cystitis, 1204
for depression, 1123, 1124, 1279
for dermatomyositis, 920-21
for developmental disorders of vagina
and vulva, 1169
for diabetes insipidus, 944-45
for diabetes mellitus, 933-35
dictionary of, 1282-88
for diphtheria, 1078
directory of, 1281-88
for dislocations, 866
douches, 1275
drug abuse and, 335-47
for dysfunctional uterine bleeding, 1152
ear drops, 1275
for elderly, 244-45, 340
for encephalitis, 483
for endometriosis, 1186
for epididymitis, 1199
for epidural abscesses, 487-88
establishing dosages of, 340
eye ointment, 1275
eyedrops, 538, 1275
for febrile seizures, 497-98
for fibromyalgia, 883
filling prescriptions for, 1273
for folic acid anemia, 960
following instructions for use of,
1272-73
food interactions with, 1277-78
for fractures, 865
for galactorrhea, 1162-63
for gastritis, 758
generic vs. brand name, 1274
for genital herpes, 1092
for genital warts, 1172

for gonorrhea, 1088
gout and, 916, 1280
for grand mal seizures, 496
for heart attacks, 664
for heart rate and rhythm disorders, 676
for heel pain, 876
for hemolytic anemias, 962
for hemophilia, 976-77
for histoplasmosis, 712
for Hodgkin's disease, 970
for home care, 1323
for hookworm, 1084
for Huntington's chorea, 478
for hypertension, 642, 651-52, 1279
for hyperthyroidism, 948
for hypopituitarism, 944
for hypothyroidism, 949
for impotence, 1227
for indigestion, 752-53
for infective endocarditis, 679-80
interactions of, 245
intoxication from, 430-31
for iron-deficiency anemia, 958
for irritable bladder, 1194
for kidney stones, 845
for laryngitis, 599
for legionnaires' disease, 707
for lice, 1085-86
list of families of, 1278-80
for loss of limbs, 880
for lumps in breasts, 1159
for lung abscesses, 708-10
for Lyme disease, 1067
for major depressive disorder, 1124
for malaria, 1080-81
for manic-depressive illness, 1126
for measles, 1074
medicine calendars for, 1278
for Meniere's disease, 583
for meningitis, 482
for menopause, 1154
for menorrhagia, 1152
for mitral valve problems, 681
for mitral valve prolapse, 682
for mittelschmerz, 1148
for multiple myelomas, 973-74
multiple use of, 245, 340, 1277
for muscle cramps, 872
for myasthenia gravis, 481
for narcolepsy, 1115
for neuralgias, 514-15
for non-Hodgkin's lymphomas, 970
nose drops, 587, 1275
for oligomenorrhea, 1150
oral contraceptive interaction with, 1146
for orchitis, 1202
original containers of, 1273
for osteoarthritis, 909
for osteomalacia, 897
for osteoporosis, 896
OTC vs. prescription, 1274
for otosclerosis, 579
outdated, 1276
for Paget's disease of bone, 897-98
for painful menses, 1148
for panic attacks, 1119
for Parkinson's disease, 474
for penile warts, 1204
for peptic ulcers, 754, 755
for pericarditis, 689
for pernicious anemia, 959
for petit mal seizures, 497

for PID (pelvic inflammatory disease), 1189
pill-box strategy for, 244-45
pills, 1274-75
for pinworms, 1082-83
for pleurisy and pleural effusions, 711
for PMS (premenstrual syndrome), 1147
for pneumonia, 705
poisoning from, 439-40
as poisons, 352
for polycystic ovarian syndrome, 1191
for polycythemia vera, 972
for polymyositis, 920-21
for post-traumatic stress disorder, 1121-22
in pregnancy, 185-86
for premenstrual tenderness and swelling of breasts, 1158
for primary ovarian failure, 1156
for proctitis, 799
for pruritus vulvae, 1170-71
for psoriasis, 993
for pubic lice, 1173
for pulled muscles, 868
for pulmonary edema, 660-61
for pulmonary embolisms, 734
quack-prescribed, 1269-70
for Raynaud's disease, 697-98, C-16
for reflex sympathetic dystrophy syndrome, 887
for retrograde ejaculation, 1229
for Reye's syndrome, 484
for rheumatoid arthritis, 910-11
for rickets, 897
for Rocky Mountain spotted fever, 1068
for runner's knee, 873
for sarcoidosis, 721
for scabies, 1085
for scleroderma, 920
sexual function and, 230
for shin splints, 870-71
for sickle cell disease, 961
side effects of, 337, 340, 652, 1273
for sinusitis, 591
for Sjögren's syndrome, 920
skin rashes from, 996
for sleepwalking, 1117
for spinal cord trauma, 507
for spinal stenosis, 516-17
for sprains, 870
for STDs, 158, 1088, 1089, 1090, 1092
for stomach tumors, 764
storage and disposal of, 1273
for strokes, 463, 565, 663
for strongyloidosis, 1083
for subdural hemorrhage, 468
for sunburn, 997
for syphilis, 1090
for systemic lupus erythematosus, 918
for tapeworms, 1081-82
for TB (tuberculosis), 706
for temporal lobe seizures, 499
for tendinitis, 882
for tennis elbow, 873
for tenosynovitis, 882
for tension-type headaches, 502
for testicular failure, 1198
for thrombocytopenia, 979
for thrombophlebitis, 695
for TIA (transient ischemic attack), 466
for tic disorders, 475
for tonsillitis, 594

for traumatic injury to bladder and urethra, 836
for travel, 384
for typhoid fever, 1069
for ulcerative colitis, 779
for undescended testicles, 1202
for urethritis, 1205
for urine loss problems, 1193, 1208
for uterine cancer, 1185
for vaginitis, 1174
for vesicoureteral reflux, 830
for vulvitis, 1170
for whooping cough, 1075
workings of, 336-37
in workplace, 359
see also specific medications
dry eyes, 538-39
dry gangrene, 692
dry skin, 986, 994, C-15
DTs (delirium tremens), 330
Dubin-Johnson hyperbilirubinemia, 812
Duchenne's muscular dystrophy, 888
ductus arteriosus, 52
dumping syndrome, 756
duodenal ulcers, 753-54
Dupuytren's contracture, 886-87
durable powers of attorney for health care, 1249, 1383, 1385-86
dust, 358-59
   respiratory allergies to, 1042-44
dwarfism (dysplasia), 46, 925
dysfunctional uterine bleeding, 1152
dyslexia (specific reading disability), 131-32
dysmenorrhea (painful menses):
   primary, 1148
   secondary, 1148
   in teenagers, 159
dyspareunia (painful intercourse), 170, 1188
dyspepsia (indigestion), 752-53
dysplasia:
   bronchopulmonary, 20
   cervical, 1179-80
   fibrous, 898
   of the hip, developmental, 912
   mammary, 1158
   multicystic, 829
dysplasia (dwarfism), 46

E

ear drops, administration of, 1275
ear infections:
   acute, 574-75
   chronic, 575-76
ear pain, acute, head pain in, 433
eardrums, ruptured or perforated, 572
earmuffs, 573
earplugs, 573
ears:
   anatomy of, 568
   newborn care of, 25
   protection of, 358, 573
   protruding, 585
ears, disorders of, 570-86
   acoustic neuromas, 584
   acoustic trauma, 582
   acute ear infection, 574-75
   age-related hearing loss, 579-81
   barotrauma, 574
   benign cysts and tumors, 571
   benign paroxysmal positional vertigo, 584-85

cholesteatoma, 577
chronic ear infection, 575-76
    ear tubes in treatment of, 576
    emergency treatment of, 426-27
    foreign objects in ears, 426-27, 571-72
    hereditary deafness, 578
    labyrinthitis, 583-84
    mastoiditis, 577-78
    Meniere's disease, 582-83
    noise and sound levels in, 573
    occupational hearing loss, 572-74
    otosclerosis, 578-79
    protruding ears, 585
    ruptured or perforated eardrums, 572
    swimmer's ear, 570-71
    tinnitus, 582
    wax blockage, 585-86
eccrine glands, 985
ECG (electrocardiography), 654, 655-57,
        671, 1251, 1343
    resting, 1251
echocardiography, 634, 683, 1342
eclampsia, 204-5
ECT (electroconvulsive therapy), 1124-25
ecthyma, 1007
ectopic atrial heartbeat, 669-70
ectopic pregnancy, 199-200, 436, 1187
    pelvic pain in, 1187
    ruptured, 436
ectropion, 541-42
eczema, 1038, C-3
    infantile, 14-15, 989, C-2
    seborrheic, 14, 68, C-2
edema (swelling):
    in pregnancy, 189
    pulmonary, 660-61
edetate disodium (EDTA), 637
EDTA (edetate disodium), 637
Education Department, U.S., 252
EEG (electroencephalography), 1344
eggs:
    in balanced diet for preschool children,
        113
    proper handling of, 273
ejaculation:
    premature, 1228-29
    retrograde, 1229
elastosis, solar, 998-1000
elder care, see home care and elder care
Elder Care Locator, 245
elderly, 231-48
    abuse of, 234
    adult day-care for, 246
    alcoholism in, 329
    community services for, 245-48
    constipation in, 241
    day respite care programs for, 246
    depression in, 243-44, 1103-4
    drugs and, 244-45, 340
    drugs and alcohol mixed by, 340
    establishing dosages and monitoring
        side effects of drugs in, 340
    exercise programs for, 236-37, 296
    failing eyesight in, 238-39
    falling by, 240
    financial security in, 236
    forgetfulness in, 237-38
    foster care homes for, 247
    hearing loss in, 242-43, 579-81
    home health care for, 246; see also home
        care and elder care
    impaired mobility in, 239-40

    incontinence in, 240-41
    loss of independence in, 234-35
    multiple drug use by, 245, 340
    nursing homes for, 247-48, 1255
    nutrition of, 241
    nutrition services for, 247
    paranoia in, 1104
    physical changes in, 233-34
    respite care programs for, 246
    in retirement communities, 246
    sexual desire in, 242
    skin cancer in, 244
    skin problems in, 244
    sleep disorders in, 1104-5
    sleep patterns of, 233
    special problems of, 237-45
    specific drug problems of, 340
    support of pelvic organs in, 244, 1175-76
    voice changes in, 243
electrical burns, 404
electrical injuries, 418
    emergency treatment of, 418
    getting person away from electricity in,
        419
    shock in, 418
electrical tests, 1343-44
    ECG, 654, 655-57, 671, 1251, 1343
    EEG, 1344
    EMG, 1344
    exercise tolerance, 655, 1344
electrocardiography (ECG), 654, 655-57,
        671, 1251, 1343
    resting, 1251
electroconvulsive (shock) therapy (ECT),
        1124-25
electroencephalography (EEG), 1344
electromyography (EMG), 1344
electronic fetal monitoring, 210
electronic fetal nonstress and stress tests,
        182
electronic monitoring, SIDS and, 71
electronic sphygmomanometers, 649
electrophysiologic testing, 673
embolisms:
    arterial, 692-93
    pulmonary, 434, 734-35
embolus, 461
emergencies, 389-453
    abdominal pain, 435-36
    acute arterial occlusion, 437
    acute conjunctivitis, 453
    acute ear pain, 433
    acute glaucoma, 452, 550-51
    acute iritis, 453
    acute joint pain, 437
    acute venous obstruction, 437
    alcohol intoxication, 429-30
    altitude disorders, 417-18
    anaphylaxis, 444-45
    appendicitis, 436
    arm fractures, 447-48
    behavioral, 429-32
    bleeding, 399-403
    blood in eye, 452, 544
    botulism, 441
    bowel obstruction, 436
    breathing, 9, 63, 406-14
    burns, 403-5
    central retinal artery occlusions, 452
    cerebral hemorrhages, 433
    chest pains, 433-34
    CO (carbon monoxide) poisoning, 419

    common sense in, 391-94
    concussions, 451
    corneal abrasions, 452
    cystitis, 436
    decompression sickness, 417-18
    definition of, 392
    dehydration, 443
    dental abscesses, 433
    diabetic, 422-23
    diabetic ketoacidosis, 423, 926, 928-29
    dislocations, 449
    diverticulitis, 436
    electrical injuries, 418
    environmental, 414-19
    eye injuries, 452-53, 544
    eyelid laceration, 452
    fainting spells, 420
    fevers, 423-25
    follow-up treatment of, 391-92
    food allergies, 441
    food poisoning, 440-41
    foreign bodies in ears, 426-27, 571-72
    foreign bodies in eyes, 425-26, 531
    foreign bodies in nose, 427
    fractures, 445-49
    frostbite, 416-17
    gallstones, 435
    gastroenteritis, 435, 440-41
    genitourinary, 428-29, 1197-98
    head pains, 432-33
    head trauma, 451-52
    heart attacks, 434
    heart-related shock, 443-44
    heat cramps, 416
    heat exhaustion, 415-16
    heat stress, 414-16
    heatstroke, 414-15
    hip fractures, 448-49
    hyperosmolar coma, 423, 926, 929-30
    hypertensive crises, 422
    hypothermia, 416
    inhaled foreign objects, 427
    insulin reaction, 422-23
    intoxication, 429-31
    intracranial hematomas, 451
    kidney stones, 436
    leg fractures, 448
    limb fractures, 445-48
    medication poisoning, 439-40
    meningitis, 433
    migraine headaches, 432-33
    near drowning, 418
    orbital cellulitis, 452-53, 545, C-11
    ovarian cysts, 436
    pain, 432-37
    pain in extremities, 436-37
    pancreatitis, 435
    pelvic fractures, 448-49
    pelvic pain, 436
    perforated peptic ulcers, 435
    pneumonia with pleurisy, 434-35
    poisoning, 437-41
    poisonous plants, 440
    pulmonary embolisms, 434
    pyelonephritis, 436
    retinal detachment, 452
    ruptured ectopic pregnancy, 436
    seizures, 421
    septic shock, 444
    sexual abuse, 428
    sexual assault, 428
    shock, 441-45

skin, 415
skull fractures, 451
smoke inhalation, 419
spinal injuries, 448
sprains, 449
strokes, 421-22
subarachnoid hemorrhages, 433
sudden personality changes, 430
sunburn, 414
swallowed foreign objects, 427
testicular torsion, 428
thrombophlebitis, 437
tooth avulsion, 453
toxic shock syndrome, 445
trauma, 445-53
trauma to external genitals, 428-29
traumatic amputations, 450-51
ureteral stones, 436
warning signs of, 391
emergency centers, freestanding, 1254-55
emergency rooms, 391
EMG (electromyography), 1344
emotional needs, 36
emphysema, 715-20
congenital lobar, 58
smoking and, 715-16, 718, 719
empyema, 710-11
encephalitis, 482-84
encephalopathy, hepatic, 808
encopresis, 89, 1098-99
endarterectomy, 467
endocrine system, 924-52, A-11
endocrine system, disorders of, 925-52
acromegaly, 898, 942
Addison's disease, 443, 938-39
adenomatous goiters, 946
adrenal gland disorders, 9, 443, 937-41,
1156-57, 1169
adrenal gland tumors, 939-41
aldosteronomas, 940-41
atherosclerosis in, 929-30
bones and, 898
chronic pancreatitis, 819-20
congenital adrenal hyperplasia, 9, 941,
1169
coronary artery disease in, 929-30
Cushing's syndrome, 937-38
diabetes insipidus, 944-45
diabetes mellitus, see diabetes mellitus
gastrinomas, 757-58, 936
gigantism, 898, 942
glucagonomas, 936
glucose self-monitoring in, 933
goiters, 946, 947
Graves' disease, 563-64, 946, 947
hirsutism, 940, 1019-21, C-7
hyperfunctioning thyroid nodules, 947
hyperosmolar coma, 423, 926, 929-30
hyperparathyroidism, 898, 950-51
hypertension in, 929-30
hyperthyroidism, 9, 947-48
hypoglycemic coma, 926, 927-28
hypoparathyroidism, 951-52
hypopituitarism, 898, 943-44
hypothyroidism, 9, 948-50
insulin reaction in, 422-23, 926-28
insulinomas, 936
islet cell tumors of pancreas, 757-58, 936
ketoacidosis, 423, 926, 928-29
lymphocytic thyroiditis, 946
medullary thyroid cancer, 946
menses and menstrual disorders

related to, 1156-57
nonfunctioning pituitary tumors, 943
parathyroid disorders, 898, 950-52
pheochromocytomas, 939
pituitary gland disorders, 898, 941-45,
1156-57
pituitary gland tumors, 898, 942-44, 1163
prolactinomas, 942-43, 1163
simple goiter, 946
subacute thyroiditis, 946
thyroid cancer, 946
thyroid disorders, 945-50, 1156-57
vision problems in, 562-63, 930
see also pancreatic disorders
endocrine system, workings of, 924-25
endodontists, 604
endogenous depression, 1124-25
endometrial cancer, 1183-84
screening for, 1295
endometrial hyperplasia, 1183
endometrial polyps, 1182
endometriosis, 1185-86
pelvic pain in, 1188
in pregnancy, 1186
endoscopic retrograde cholangiopancreatography (ERCP), 816
endoscopic tests, 1333-34
for bile duct obstructions, 817
laryngoscopy, 1333-34
end-stage renal disease, 855-57
kidney transplantation for, 857-58
endurance exercise, 295
engorgement, 216
Entamoeba histolytica, 768-69
enteropathy, protein-losing, 774
entropion, 541-42
enuresis (bedwetting), 89, 1098
environment, 371-78
air pollution and, 373-75, 726, 732
allergies and, 374
cancer prevention and, 373
contaminated fish and, 269-70
CO (carbon monoxide) poisoning and,
376
drinking water and, 372
indoor pollution and, 374-75
radiation and, 376-78
environmental emergencies, 414-19
altitude disorders, 417
CO (carbon monoxide) poisoning, 419
decompression sickness, 417
electrical injuries, 418
frostbite, 416-17
heat cramps, 416
heat exhaustion, 415-16
heat stress, 414-16
heatstroke, 414-15
hypothermia, 416
near drowning, 418
smoke inhalation, 419
sunburn, 414
Environmental Protection Agency (EPA),
270, 372, 375
enzyme tests, 1331
eosinophilic gastroenteritis, 764
eosinophils, 1028
EPA (Environmental Protection Agency),
270, 372, 375
epidemic parotitis, see mumps
epididymis, 164, 1196, 1197
epididymitis, 1198-99
epidural abscesses, 486-88

epidural anesthesia, 211-12
epidural hemorrhages, 468-69
epiglottitis, 413, 594-95
epilepsy:
in pregnancy, 190
seizures in, see seizures
epinephrine (adrenaline), 924, 929
for anaphylaxis, 398, 445, 1053, 1277
epiphysitis, 159
episcleritis, 543-44
episiotomies, 210-11
episodic pelvic pain, 1188
Epstein-Barr virus, 158-59, 1064-65
Epstein pearls, 50
ERCP (endoscopic retrograde cholangiopancreatography), 816
erection abnormalities, 1227-28
erysipelas, 1009-10
erythema toxicum, 16
erythrocyte sedimentation rate (ESR), 1331
erythromycin, 5
Escherichia coli, 268, 768
esophageal cancer, 1188
esophageal motility studies, 746
esophageal problems, 741-51
achalasia, 745-46
atresia in newborns, 56
Barrett's esophagus, 744
bleeding in cirrhosis, 808
Candida esophagitis, 744
diffuse spasm, 746
esophageal cancer, 750
esophagitis, 744-45, 760-61
foreign bodies, 749
heartburn, 187, 435, 742-44
herpes simplex esophagitis, 744
hiatal hernias, 743
hiccups, 745
pharyngeal diverticula, 746-47
pharyngeal paralysis, 747-48
pill-induced esophagitis, 745
radiation esophagitis, 744
rupture, 751
scleroderma, 744
stricture, 748-49
swallowing problems, 745-48, 760-61
tumors, 750
esophageal reflux (heartburn), 187, 435,
742-44
esophageal speech, 598
esophageal varices, 750-51
esophagitis, 760
Candida, 744
herpes simplex, 744
pill-induced, 745
radiation, 744
upper gastrointestinal endoscopy for,
760-61
esophagogastroduodenoscopy, 760-61
esophagus, 739
barium X-rays of, 750, 762-63
esotropia, accommodative, 66
ESR (erythrocyte sedimentation rate), 1331
essential tremor, 475
estrogen, 228, 1143, 1144, 1150, 1152, 1153,
1156, 1157, 1168, 1189, 1280
in birth control pills, 171, 1146
deprivation, 1157
estrogen replacement therapy, 1154
ethyl alcohol (ethanol), 326-27
examinations, see checkups
excretory urography, 829, 1341

exercise, 289-306
    for adults, 295-96
    aerobic, 196, 236-37, 290-91, 644-47
    anaerobic, 290-91, 645
    for angina pectoris, 658
    asthma and, 1047
    avoiding injuries in, 302-4
    back in, 304
    benefits of, 290-91
    bicycling for, 299-300, 357
    calf stretches in, 293
    calories used in, 301
    cardiovascular, *see* cardiovascular fitness
    for children, 295
    in cold weather, 304-5
    after colostomies, 778
    common forms of, 297-302
    cool-downs in, 294, 647, 867
    for coping with stress, 313-14
    cross-country cycling as, 299-300
    deep-breathing, 717
    diabetes mellitus and, 932-33
    duration in, 292-94
    elements of, 292-94
    endurance, 295
    extensiveness of, 645-46
    fitness and, 289-306
    fitness evaluation and, 295-96
    flexibility, 295
    frequency of, 292, 646
    getting started with, 294
    hamstring stretches in, 293
    after heart attacks, 296, 668
    for hemophilia, 976
    at high altitude, 305
    in hot weather, 304
    ideal, 646-47
    identifying goals for, 294-95
    after ileostomies, 778
    for incontinence, 1176
    intensity in, 292
    machines for, 299
    measuring pulse after, 645
    menopause and, 1154-55
    motivation for, 279, 305
    for osteoarthritis, 908
    osteoporosis and, 895
    pacing in, 867
    perceived exertion scales for, 295, 646
    for PMS (premenstrual syndrome), 1147
    posture in, 303
    pregnancy and, 195-96, 296
    in rehabilitation for chronic neurologic
        problems, 480
    for rheumatoid arthritis, 910
    rules for, 291
    selection of, 646-47
    staying active and, 305-6
    strengthening, 294
    stretches in, 292, 293
    thigh stretches in, 293
    in treatment of hypertension, 653
    walking for, 297-98, 647
    warm-ups for, 292-94, 647, 867
    weight control and, 278-80
    weight training for, 300-302
exercise programs, 290-91
    for bicycling, 299-300
    for disabled, 296
    for elderly, 236-37, 296
    heart rate targets in, 296
    for jogging, 298

    for obese adults, 296
exercise tolerance tests, 655, 1344
exostoses, 571
expectorants, 1280
extradural hemorrhages, 468-69
extremities:
    acute venous obstruction in, 437
    arteriosclerosis of, 690-92
    gangrene of, 692
    of infants, 10
    pain in, 436-37
eye angiography, 1342
eye emergencies, 452-53
    acute conjunctivitis, 453
    acute glaucoma, 452, 550-51
    acute iritis, 453
    blood in eye, 452, 544
    central retinal artery occlusion, 452
    corneal abrasions, 452
    eyelid laceration, 452
    foreign bodies, 425-26, 531
    hyphema, 533
    orbital cellulitis, 452-53, 545-46, C-11
    retinal detachment, 452, 557-59
eye examinations, 524
eye experts, types of, 522
eye ointment, administration of, 1275
eyedrops, 538, 1275
    administration of, 1275
eyeglasses, 239
eyelid disorders, 536-42
    blepharitis, 539-40
    cancer, 558
    chalazion, C-11
    cosmetic surgery for, 541
    drooping eyelids, 540-42
    dry eyes, 538-39
    ectropion, 541-42
    entropion, 541-42
    eyedrops for, 538, 1275
    infections of tear ducts, 539
    itchy eyelids, 539
    lacerations, 452
    laser therapy for, 558
    lumps, 536-37
    orbital cellulitis, 452-53, 545-46, C-11
    sties, 536-37, C-11
    tearing problems, 537-39
    tumors, 558
    twitchy eyelids, 540
    watering eyes, 538-39
    xanthelasmas, 1001, C-11
eyelids, drooping, 540-42
eyes, 519-66
    anatomy of, 520-22
    contact lenses for, 528-30, 556
    grease and chemical hazards to, 405,
        531-33
    makeup hazardous to, 532
    and mechanism of sight, 522
    newborn care of, 25
    of newborns, 5
    protection of, 358, 532
    sports risks to, 532
    sunglasses for, 532
    workplace risks to, 358, 532
eyes, disorders of, 542-66, C-11
    acute glaucoma, 452, 550-51
    amblyopia, 65, 90, 534-36
    astigmatism, 527-28
    blood sugar concentration as cause of,
        527

    cancer, 546
    cataracts, 35, 266, 553-56, 558
    chemical damage, 405, 531-33
    choroiditis, 560-61
    chronic glaucoma, 551-53
    colobomas, 560
    color blindness, 548-50
    conjunctivitis, 102, 453, 542-43, C-11
    corneal infections, 547
    corneal injury, 546-47
    corneal problems, 546-47
    corneal transplantation in, 548
    corneal ulcers, 547
    corrective measures for, 535-36
    cranial arteritis and, 565-66
    diabetes mellitus and, 562-63, 930
    diabetic retinopathy, 558, 562-63, 930
    double vision, 535
    early recognition of, 534-35
    episcleritis, 543-44
    failing eyesight, 238-39
    farsightedness, 525-26
    floaters, 561
    foreign bodies, 425-26, 531
    glaucoma, 452, 550-53, 558, 1251
    Graves' disease and, 563-64
    hemorrhages, 452, 544
    hereditary, 526
    hypertension and, 564
    infections, 29, 539, 547
    iritis, 453, 544
    laser therapy for, 558
    macular degeneration, 556-57
    melanomas, 546, C-11
    nearsightedness, 523-25
    optic neuritis, 560
    optic neuropathy, 560
    orbital cellulitis, 452-53, 545-46, C-11
    presbyopia, 526-27
    radial keratotomy for, 525
    refraction problems, 522-28
    retinal detachment, 452, 557-59
    retinal vessel occlusion, 559-60
    retinitis pigmentosa, 561-62
    retinoblastomas, 545-46
    scleritis, 543-44
    spots, 561
    strabismus, 65-66, 90, 534-36
    subconjunctival hemorrhage, 544
    in systemic diseases, 562-66
    third nerve palsy, 563
    uveitis, 544
    visual, 548-62
    vitamin A deficiency in, 547
    as warning signs of strokes, 564-65
    see also blindness; vision disorders
eyes, trauma to, 531-33
    black eyes from, 533
    chemical burns, 532
    from foreign bodies, 425-26, 531
    hyphema from, 533

F

facelifts, 228
    see also cosmetic surgery
facial and mandibular trauma and fracture,
    623-25
    avulsion, 624
    temporomandibular joint problems,
        624-25
facial nerve palsies, 22, 493-95

facial tics, 475
fainting spells (syncope), 420, 674
    first aid for, 420
    while lying down, 420
    while seated, 420
    taking it easy after, 420
fallen arches, 892
falling:
    by elderly, 240
    by preschool children, 92, 100
fallopian tubes, 168, 1140, 1144, 1214-15
fallopian tubes, disorders of:
    developmental, 1178
    PID (pelvic inflammatory disease),
        168-69, 1187-89
false labor, 208
familial colonic polyposis, 787
familial Mediterranean fever, 793
familial tremor, 475
family history:
    as chronic glaucoma risk factor, 551
    in colon cancer screening, 790
    gathering of, 1251
    for genetic evaluation, 43-44
family life:
    of alcoholics, 332
    conflicts in, 310
    divorces in, 221
    hospices and, 1306
    loss of parents in, 221, 1318
    loss of spouse in, 221-22
    in middle years, 220-22
    parenting in, 220-21
    stress in, 310
family planning, 170-74
    natural, 171
    see also contraception
family practice, 1246
farmer's lung, 733
farms:
    operating machinery on, 359-60
    pesticides, fuels, and fire risks on, 360
    safety on, 359-60
farsightedness (hyperopia), 66, 525-26
fasting, 288
fat, body, 257
fatigue syndrome, chronic, 1065
fats, 253-54
    in butter vs. margarine, 254
    in diabetics' diets, 284
    for newborns, 38
    for nutrition and weight control in
        pregnancy, 184
    as risk factor in heart and blood vessel
        disorders, 639-43
    for school-age children, 122
    in school lunches, 123
FDA (Food and Drug Administration),
    271, 355, 477, 1274
fears, see phobias
febrile seizures, 120-21, 497-98
    in infants, 69, 70
fecal impaction, 786
fecal incontinence, 799-800
feeding:
    bottle care and, 41
    of infants, 78-80
    of newborns, 7, 39-42
    see also appetite; diets; mealtimes
feeding problems:
    constipation and, 41-42
    diarrhea and, 41

failure to gain weight, 42
    falling asleep as cause of, 41
    in infants, 79-80
    in newborns, 40-42
    overfeeding, 41, 80
    regurgitation and vomiting due to,
        41, 80
    undereating, 41
    underfeeding, 41, 80
feeding schedules:
    for breastfed infants, 39
    infant behavior and, 36
    for newborns, 39
feet, problems of, 889-94
    abnormalities, 45-46
    arteriosclerosis and, 691
    bunions, 891-92
    burning feet, 890
    calluses, 890-91
    corns, 890-91
    diabetes and, 930, 931
    flatfeet, 95-96, 892
    hammer toe, 892-93
    ingrown toenails, 893, 1022
    in-toeing, 45
    mallet toe, 892-93
    metatarsalgia, 889
    Morton's neuroma, 890
    out-toeing, 45
    and shopping for shoes, 890
    stasis dermatitis, 989, C-3
    tired feet, 892
    ulcers, 893-94
female-pattern baldness, 1017
female pseudohermaphroditism, 49
fertility, see infertility
fertility therapy, 1218-21
    ethical considerations in, 1220
fertilization, 176
fetal activity, monitoring of, 181-82
fetal blood sampling, 210
fetal monitoring, electronic, 210
fetal nonstress and stress tests, electronic,
    182
fetal positions, 7
    abnormal, 209-10
    breech presentation, 209
    occiput anterior, 209
    occiput posterior, 210
    transverse presentation, 209
fever blisters, 1010, C-10
fevers:
    definition of, 423-24
    high, 424
    in infants, 62-63
    in minor illnesses, 393-94
    in newborns, 9, 10-11, 424
    in preschool children, 85
    prolonged, 424
    seizures without, 70
    seriousness of, 10-11
    with severe headache, stiff neck, severe
        swelling of throat, or mental
        confusion, 424
    treatment of, 425
    unexplained, 424, 1069
fiber, 288
    adequate, 783
    benefits of, 256, 783
    disadvantages of, 783
    in school lunches, 123

fiber supplements, 784
fibrillation:
    atrial, 670
    ventricular, 672
fibroadenomas, 1159
fibrocystic changes, 1158
fibroglandular changes, 1158
fibroids, 1182
fibromyalgia, 883
fibromyomas, 1182
fibroplasia, retrolental, 35
fibrosis, idiopathic pulmonary, 722
fibrositis, 883
fibrous dysplasia, 898
fighting, 105
fight-or-flight response, 308
fillings, 606-7
financial security, 236
finger sweeps, 407
fingernails, 1021-23
    healthy, 985
    of newborns, 25
    proper care of, 1023
fingernails, disorders of, 1021-23
    deformation, 1023
    discoloration, 1023
    fungal infections, 1022-23
    leukonychia, C-7
    paronychia, 1021-22, C-7
fingers:
    baseball, 874
    sucking of, 106
    syndactyly of, 45
fire ant stings, 396
fire safety, 350-51, 357-58
fireworks, 351
first aid, 389-453
    for abdominal wounds, 401
    for alcohol intoxication, 429-30
    for altitude disorders, 417-18
    for anaphylaxis, 444-45
    for angioedema, 415
    for animal bites, 394
    basic supplies for, 392
    for bleeding emergencies, 399-403
    for bleeding from body openings, 401-2
    for bleeding from wounds and injuries,
        399-403
    for blood in urine, 403
    for breathing emergencies, 9, 63, 406-14
    for bruises, 401
    for burns, 403-5
    for CO (carbon monoxide) poisoning,
        419
    for chemicals in eyes, 405
    for contact dermatitis, 415
    for coughing of blood, 402
    CPR (cardiopulmonary resuscitation)
        in, 391, 408-13
    for cuts, 401
    for decompression sickness, 417-18
    for dehydration, 443
    for diabetic ketoacidosis, 423
    for dislocations, 449
    for drug intoxication, 430-31
    for electrical injury, 418
    for eye emergencies, 452-53
    for fainting spells, 420
    for fevers, 425
    for foreign bodies in ears, 426-27
    for foreign bodies in eyes, 425-26
    for foreign bodies in nose, 427

for fractures, 445-49
for frostbite, 416-17
for head trauma, 451-52
for heart-related shock, 443-44
for heat cramps, 416
for heat exhaustion, 415-16
for heatstroke, 414-15
for human bites, 395
for hyperosmolar coma, 423
for hypertensive crises, 422
for hyperventilation, 431-32
for hypothermia, 416
for inhaled foreign objects, 427
for insulin reaction, 422-23, 928
for internal bleeding, 402
for jellyfish stings, 398-99
for major burns, 405
for mild sunburn, 414
for minor bites, 394
for minor burns at home, 405
for minor illnesses, 393-94
for minor wounds, 392
for near drowning, 418
for nosebleeds, 403
for poisoning, 437-41
for poisoning from medications, 439-40
for poisoning from plants, 440
for poisonous stings, 397-98
for punctures, 401
for rectal bleeding, 403
after seizures, 421
in seizures, 421
for septic shock, 444
for severe asthma attacks, 413
for severe sunburn, 414
for shock, 418, 441-45
for skin emergencies, 415
for smoke inhalation, 419
for snake bites, 398
for soft tissue injuries, 401
for sprains, 449
for strokes, 421-22
for testicular torsion, 428
for tick bites, 396
for tooth avulsion, 453
for trauma, 428-29, 445-53
for trauma to external genitals, 428-29
for traumatic amputations, 450-51
for vaginal bleeding, 403
for vomiting of blood, 402
first aid kits, 392
first-degree burns, 403
fish, contaminated, food poisoning from,
    269-70
fish-scale disease, 994
fissures, anal, 796-97
fistulas, anal, 796-97
flatfeet, 95-96, 892
flatus (intestinal gas), 260, 785-86
fleas, 1086
flexibility exercise, 295
floaters, 561
floating kidney, 828
flossing, technique in, 366-67
flowmeters, peak, 1045
flu, see influenza
fluorescein angiography, 1342
fluoride:
    preschool children and, 101
    tooth decay and, 101, 370, 608-9
fluoxetine, 1123
flutters, atrial, 670

fluvastatin, 642
focal and segmental glomerulosclerosis,
    838
folic acid deficiency anemia, 959-60
follicle-stimulating hormone (FSH), 167
folliculitis, 1007, C-12
fontanelles (soft spots):
    in infants, 63
    in newborns, 26
food:
    basic components of, 253-56
    caffeine in, 185, 186, 194, 273-74, 329,
        1131
    calcium-rich, 267
    daily guide to, 261-62
    drug interactions with, 1277-78
    high-fiber, 783
    intestinal gas caused by, 785-86
    irradiation of, 271-72
    moldy, 273
    myths about, 288
    naturally occurring intoxicants in, 270
    of nursing homes, 247-48
    pesticide contamination of, 268
    processing of, 271-72
    proper handling of, 272-73
    see also diets
food allergies, 441, 1048-50
    emergency symptoms of, 1048
    food intolerance vs., 1049
Food and Drug Administration (FDA),
    271, 355, 477, 1274
food fads, 286-88
Food Guide Pyramid, 261-62
food intolerance:
    Chinese restaurant syndrome in, 1049
    food allergy vs., 1049
    to food dyes, 1049
    to lactose, 772, 1049
    to sulfites, 1049
    to wheat and vegetables, 1049
food labels, 263-64
    definition of terms on, 264
food poisoning, 440-41
    botulism, 268-69, 441, 488-89
    from Clostridium perfringens, 268
    from contaminated fish, 269-70
    gastroenteritis in, 440
    hepatitis A from, 269
    infectious, 267-70
    prevention of, 769
    from Salmonella, 268
    from Staphylococcus aureus, 268
    traveler's diarrhea and, 269
    treatment of, 769
food safety, 267-71
    at picnics, 269
footwear, posture and, 903
forceps deliveries, 211
foreign bodies:
    in ears, 426-27, 571-72
    in esophagus, 749
    in eyes, 425-26, 531
    in nose, 427
    swallowed, 90, 427
forgetfulness, in elderly, 237-38
formaldehyde, indoor pollution from, 374
foster care homes, 247
fractures, 445-49, 863-65
    of arms, 447-48
    casts for, 865
    of collarbone, 22

complete, 446
compound, 446
facial, 623-25
first aid for, 445-49
of hips, 448-49
immobilization of, 865
impacted, 446
of jaw, 623-24
of legs, 448
of limbs, 445-48
mandibular, 623-25
pathologic, 446
of pelvis, 448-49
recognition of, 446
rehabilitation for, 865
shock in, 447
simple, 446
of skull, 451
splints for, 865
traction for, 865
free weights, 301
freestanding emergency centers, 1254-55
fresh-frozen plasma, 980
Friedreich's ataxia, 478
frostbite, 416-17, 698
    emergency treatment of, 417
    prevention of, 417
    warming process for, 417
fruits, 261
    examples of servings of, 262
    for preschool children, 113
    for school-age children, 122
FSH (follicle-stimulating hormone), 167
fuels:
    farm safety and, 360
    nephropathy from, 835
fumes, 358-59
    occupationally related lung disease
        from, 732
fungal diseases of lungs, 711-13
    aspergillosis, 712
    coccidioidomycosis, 713
    cryptococcosis, 712-13
    histoplasmosis, 711-12
fungal infections of nails, 1022-23
fungal infections of skin, 1012-14, C-2, C-8
fungi, 1059-60, C-8
funnel chest, 46-47
furuncles, 1009

G

gag reflex, 4, 34
galactorrhea, 1162-63
galactosemia, screening for, 8
gallbladder, 741, 817
gallium scanning, 1338
gallstones, 812-14
    abdominal pain from, 435
    dissolution of, 813
    surgery for, 813, B-7
gambling, compulsive, 1130
ganglion, 886
gangrene:
    dry, 692
    of extremities, 692
    gas, 1016
    wet, 692
garage, safety in, 355
garden products, 352
Gardner's syndrome, 787
Gartner duct cysts, 1174

gas, intestinal (flatus), 260, 785-86
gas gangrene, infections caused by, 1016
gas-permeable hard contact lenses, 529
   caring for, 530
gases, 358-59
   occupationally related lung disease
      from, 726, 731-34
gastric ulcers, 754-55
gastrinomas (Zollinger-Ellison syndrome),
   757-58, 936
gastritis, 758
   alkaline reflux, 756
gastroenteritis, 440-41
   abdominal pain from, 435
   bacterial, 767-68
   eosinophilic, 764
   viral, 766-67
gastrointestinal surgery, heart valve disorders and, 679
gastrointestinal tract:
   short- and long-term effects of alcohol
      abuse on, 328
   see also digestive system
gastrointestinal tract, infections of, 766-69
   acute viral gastroenteritis, 766-67
   antibiotic-associated diarrhea, 769-70
   bacterial, 767-68
   Campylobacter, 767
   Cryptosporidium, 769
   cytomegalovirus, 193, 767
   emergency symptoms of, 766
   Entamoeba histolytica, 768-69
   Escherichia coli, 268, 768
   food poisoning, see food poisoning
   Giardia lamblia, 768
   Norwalk virus, 767
   parasitic, 768-69
   rotavirus, 766-67
   Salmonella, 268, 767-68
   Shigella, 768
   viral, 766-67
   see also intestines, disorders of; stomach
      problems
gastrointestinal tract bleeding, 759-61
   upper gastrointestinal endoscopy for,
      761
gastrointestinal tract disorders, congenital,
   55-58
   biliary atresia, 56
   diaphragmatic hernias, 57-58
   esophageal atresia, 56
   gastroschisis, 58
   Hirschsprung's disease, 57, 792
   imperforate anus, 57
   intestinal atresia, 57
   omphalocele, 58
   pyloric stenosis, 55-56
gastroparesis, diabetic, 772
gastroschisis, 58
gastroscopy, 760-61
gastrostomies, 747
gemfibrozil, 642
gender:
   as risk factor in heart and blood vessel
      disorders, 644
   see also men; women
gene therapy, 1299, B-8
generic drugs, brand name drugs vs., 1274
genetic amniocentesis, 181
genetic disorders, 42-51, B-8
   abnormal feet, 45-46
   abnormal hands, 44-45

campylodactyly, 45
cancer, 1291-93
clubfoot, 46, 912
clubhand, 45
congenital dislocation of hip, 46, 912
drugs as cause of, 186
dwarfism, 46
extra toes, 46
hypospadias, 48-49
in-toeing and out-toeing, 45
polydactyly, 45
radiation as cause of, 194
single mutant gene disorders, 42-43
of skeleton, 46
syndactyly of fingers, 45
syndactyly of toes, 45-46
genetic evaluations, 43-44
genetic liver problems, 811-12
   Crigler-Najjar syndrome, 812
   Dubin-Johnson hyperbilirubinemia, 812
   Gilbert's syndrome, 811-12
genetics, 42-43
genital herpes, 1090-92, C-13
   in pregnancy, 191
genital warts, 1092, 1171-72
   in women, 1171-72
genitals, see sexual organs
genitourinary emergencies, 428-29
   sexual abuse, 428
   sexual assault, 428
   testicular torsion, 428-29, 1197-98
   trauma to external genitals, 428-29
geographic tongue, 620
German measles (rubella), 1074, C-1
   in pregnancy, 52, 191
   vaccination against, 1079
germanium, 355
gestational diabetes, 21, 189
giant cell arteritis, 565-66
giant colon, 792
Giardia lamblia, 768
gigantism, 898, 925, 942
Gilbert's syndrome, 811-12
gingivitis, 364-65, 610-11
   necrotizing ulcerative, 612-13
gingivostomatitis, 618
girls, school-age:
   adrenarche in, 135
   breast abnormalities in, 134
   genital infections in, 136
   vaginal bleeding in, 134-35
girls, teenage:
   sexual changes in, 140
   see also teenagers
glaucoma, 550-53, 558
   acute, 452, 550-51
   chronic, 551-53
   laser therapy for, 558
   open-angle, 551
   screening for, 1251
   testing for, 553
globus hystericus, 593
globus sensation, 593
globus syndrome, 593
glomerulonephritis:
   acute, 836-38
   chronic, 838-40
   hemolytic-uremic syndrome, 838
   Henoch-Schönlein purpura, 837-38
   membranous, 838
   mesangial proliferative, 838
   secondary to other diseases, 839

glomerulosclerosis, focal and segmental,
   838
glossitis, acute, 619
glucagon, 925, 929
glucagonomas, 936
glucose self-monitoring, 933
glucose-6-phosphate dehydrogenase
   (G6PD), 956
   deficiency of, 962
glue, dependence on, 1131
gluten-free diets, 285
goiter, 946
   adenomatous, 946
   in Graves' disease, 946
   hyperfunctioning nodular, 947
   in lymphocytic thyroiditis, 946
   in medullary thyroid cancer, 946
   simple, 946
   in subacute thyroiditis, 946
   in thyroid cancer, 946
gonadal dysgenesis, 1155
gonadotropins, 1156
gonococcal arthritis, 915
gonorrhea, 1087-88
   in pregnancy, 193
Goodpasture's syndrome, 722-23
gout, 916
   joint pain from, 437
   medications for, 916, 1280
   nutrition and, 916
grains, 261
   examples of servings of, 262
   fiber in, 288
   for preschool children, 113
   for school-age children, 122
grand mal seizures, 496-97
granulocytes, transfusions of, 981
granulocytopenia, 974
granulomas, umbilical, 30
granulomatosis, 921
grasp, palmar, 33
grasp reflex, 33
Graves' disease, 563-64
   eye problems associated with, 563-64
   goiters in, 946
   in hyperthyroidism, 946, 947
graying hair, 227
grease, protecting eyes from, 532
green bile, vomiting of, 13
grief responses, 1109-11
   absence of, 1110
   for death of loved ones, 1316-17
   helping someone with, 1111
   stages in, 1110-11
   support groups and, 1111
grinding of teeth, 1117
group B streptococci, 193
group homes, 1328
growing pains, 119-20
growth and development:
   of infants, 60-62
   intellectual, 142
   milestones in, 60-62
   motor, 7-8, 61-62
   of newborns, 6-8
   of 1-year-olds, 82-83
   of 2-year-olds, 83
   of 3-year-olds, 83-84
   of 4-year-olds, 84
   of 5-year-olds, 84
   of preschool children, 82-84
   of school-age children, 116-17

of teenagers, 139
verbal, 62
growth disorders, 83
growth hormone, 929
abuse of, 347
for hypopituitarism, 944
G6PD (glucose-6-phosphate dehydrogenase), 956
deficiency of, 962
guanine, B-8
guided imagery, 1245
Guillain-Barré syndrome, 513
gum disease, 364-65, 610-13
gun safety, 356
gynecologic evaluations, 1141-42, 1250
gynecologic organs, 1140-41
gynecologists, selection of, 1142
gynecomastia, 139

H

hair, 1017-21, C-7
alopecia areata and, 1018-19, C-7
graying of, 227
healthy, 984
in middle years, 227
of newborns, 5
proper care of, 1020
thinning of, 227
hair disorders, 1017-21
baldness, 227, 1017-19
hirsutism, 940, 1019-21, C-7
temporary hair loss, 1018-19
hairiness, 940, 1019-21, C-7
hairy tongue, 620-21, C-10
halitosis, 620
hallucinogens:
abuse of, 343-44
dependence on, 1134
hammer toe, 892-93
hamstring stretches, 293
hand washing, handling food and, 272
handicapped children, care of, 110-12
hands, abnormal, 44-45
hangnails, 1022
hardening of arteries, see atherosclerosis
harvest mites (chiggers), 1086-87, C-14
hay fever (allergic rhinitis), 1029, 1040-41
hCG (human chorionic gonadotropin), 198
HDL cholesterol, 254, 639, 640, 644
head:
CT and MRI scans of, 494
see also skull
head lice, 102, C-14
head pain, 432-33
in acute ear pain, 433
in cerebral hemorrhages, 433
in dental abscesses, 433
in meningitis, 433
in subarachnoid hemorrhages, 433
head trauma, 451-52
concussions, 451, 490-91
intracranial hematomas, 451
skull fractures, 451
headaches, 499-506
assessment of, 500
cluster, 505-6
fevers accompanied by, 424
migraine, 120, 159, 432-33, 502-4
recurrent, 120
in school-age children, 120
tension-type, 501-2

Health and Human Services Department, U.S., 183, 281, 555
health care centers:
neighborhood, 1255
primary, 1255
health care system, 1237-70
alternative medicine and, 1244-45
ambulatory surgery in, 1262-63
anesthesia in, 1260-62
changing physicians in, 1249
child care in, 1257
communication between patients and physicians in, 1247-49, 1258, 1272
conventional health insurance in, 1265-66
current state of, 1238-41
evolution of, 1238-40
expectations and responsibilities of patients in, 1247-48
facilities of, 1254-58
freestanding emergency centers in, 1254-55
future of, 1240-41
general anesthesia in, 1261-62
health care providers in, 1241-45
HMOs in, 1266-67, 1322
hospices in, 1255-56, 1305-7
hospital admittance and, 1258-59
hospital dismissal and, 1260
hospital outpatient departments in, 1254
hospital stays in, 1258-60
hospital visits and, 1259
informed consent and, 1268
laboratory tests in, 1252
lawsuits in, 1267-68
list of professionals in, 1244
local anesthesia in, 1261
malpractice in, 1267-68
maternal care in, 1257
M.D. training in, 1241-43
medical examinations in, see checkups
mental health facilities in, 1256
neighborhood health-care centers in, 1255
nurses in, 5, 1243-44
nursing homes in, 247-48, 1255
office-based practices in, 1254
paying medical bills in, 1263-67
personal physician in, 1245-47
physicians in, see physicians
postoperative recovery in, 1262
PPOs (preferred provider organizations) in, 1267
presurgical evaluation in, 1260
primary health-care centers in, 1255
quackery in, 1268-70
reasonable expectations from, 1253
regional anesthesia in, 1261
rehabilitation centers in, 1257-58
second opinions in, 1247
selecting personal physicians in, 1246, 1299-1300
surgery in, see surgery
technologic advances in, 1238
utilization review boards in, 1267
health insurance:
autopsies and, 1315-16
future of, 1240
home care and, 1321-22
medical supplemental insurance, 1264-65

paying medical bills with, 1263-67
health maintenance organizations (HMOs), 1266-67
home care and, 1322
hearing, sense of, A-14
development of, 65
in infants, 64-65
in newborns, 7, 34-35
hearing aids, 243
cochlear implants, 580
hearing loss and, 579-81
for otosclerosis, 579
hearing disorders:
age-related, 579-81
in central auditory disorders, 35, 65, 107
conductive, 34-35, 64, 107
in elderly, 242-43, 579-81
hereditary deafness, 578
in infants, 64-65
mixed, 35, 64-65, 107
occupational, 572-74
in preschool children, 106-7
recreational risks and, 573
sensorineural, 35, 64, 107, 573
in teenagers, 160
see also ears, disorders of
hearing-impaired people, communicating with, 579
hearing tests, 573
heart, 631-98, A-8
cardiac cycle of, 634
clicks of, 634
donation of, 688
healthy, 633-35
parts of, 633
heart and blood vessels, disorders of, 647-98
acrocyanosis, 697
acute arterial occlusion, 437, 850-51
acute pericarditis, 689
age as risk factor in, 644
alcoholic heart disease, 686
allergic angiitis, 921
angina pectoris, 657-59
angiotensin-converting enzyme for, 652
antioxidants in delay of, 266
aortic aneurysms, 693-94, B-2
aortic regurgitation, 685
aortic stenosis, 53, 683-85
aortic valve problems, 53, 682-85
arterial embolisms, 692-93
arteriosclerosis of extremities, 690-92
artificial cardiac pacemakers for, 675
aspirin in prevention of, 663
atherosclerosis, 230, 467, 636-37, 929-30
atrial fibrillation and flutter, 670
atrial septal defect, 52
beta-adrenergic blockers for, 652, 664, 676
blood fat levels and, 640, 643-44
blood tests for, 657
Buerger's disease, 698
calcium channel blockers for, 652, 664, 676
cardiac arrhythmias, 663, 669-72
cardiac rehabilitation for, 668
cardiac tamponade, 689
cardiomyopathy, 686-87
CCUs (coronary care units) in, 662
chelation therapy for, 637
chest X-rays for, 657

cholesterol as risk factor in, 639-43
coarctation of aorta, 52
congenital heart disorders, 51-53, 635, 683-85
congestive heart failure, 659-60, 663
constrictive pericarditis, 689
controllable risk factors in, 638-39
coronary angioplasty for, 666
coronary artery bypass surgery for, 665, B-3
cor pulmonale, 735
cranial arteritis, 565-66, 921
death from, 663
deep-vein thrombosis, 695
diabetes mellitus as risk factor in, 643, 929-30
diet and, 280, 639-43, 653, 660, 668
dietary fats as risk factor in, 639-43
digitalis for, 676
dilated cardiomyopathy, 686
diuretics for, 651
dry gangrene, 692
ECGs for, 654, 655-57, 671, 1343
echocardiograms for, 634, 683, 1342
ectopic atrial heartbeat, 669-70
electrophysiologic testing for, 673
enlarged heart, B-2
establishing drug therapy for, 652
exercise and, 296, 653, 668
exercise tolerance tests for, 655
fainting spells in, 420, 674
frostbite, 416-17, 698
gangrene of extremities, 692
gender as risk factor in, 644
granulomatosis, 921
heart arrhythmias, 663, 669-72
heart block, 672-74
heart-lung transplantation in, 736
of heart muscle, 686-89
of heart rate and rhythm, 663, 669-76
heart transplantation in, 688
heart valve valvuloplasty for, 681
heredity as risk factor in, 644
hypersensitivity vasculitis, 921
hypertension, see hypertension
hypertensive heart disease, 650
hypertrophic cardiomyopathy, 686
hypotension, 650
infective endocarditis, 678-80
internal cardioverter-defibrillators and, 672
kidney disease resulting from, 650-51
kidneys and, 850-52
lifestyle as risk factor in, 643-44
living with risks of, 635-44
lung-related, 734-36
lymphedema, 695
malignant hypertension, 852
mitral valve prolapse, 682
mitral valve regurgitation, 680
mitral valve stenosis, 680
murmurs, 16, 634
myocarditis, 687
nitrates for, 664
obesity as risk factor in, 643
pain killers for, 664
paroxysmal atrial tachycardia, 671-72
patent ductus arteriosus, 52
pericarditis, 687-89
of pericardium, 686, 687-89
polyarteritis, 921
postural hypotension, 650

pulmonary edema, 660-61
pulmonary embolism, 434, 734-35
pulmonary stenosis, 53
pulmonary valve problems, 685
radionuclide angiograms for, 656, 1339-40
radionuclide scans for, 656
Raynaud's disease, 697-98, C-16
renal artery stenosis, 851
renal vein thrombosis, 852
restrictive cardiomyopathy, 686
rheumatic fever, 677-78
salt restriction for, 283-84, 653
sick sinus syndrome, 670
smoking as risk factor in, 639
stopping smoking after, 668
stress after, 668
sudden cardiac death, 674-76
superficial thrombophlebitis, 694
tetralogy of Fallot, 53
thallium exercise scans for, 656
thrombophlebitis, 437, 694-95
transposition of great vessels, 53
tricuspid valve problems, 685
twenty-four-hour cardiac monitoring in, 671
uncontrollable risk factors in, 644
varicose veins, 188, 695-97
vasculitis, 921
ventricular septal defect, 52
ventricular tachycardia and fibrillation, 672
weight control after, 668
wet gangrene, 692
see also circulatory problems; coronary artery disease; heart attacks; heart valve disorders; strokes and vascular disorders
heart arrhythmias, 663, 669-72
atrial fibrillation and flutter, 670
ectopic atrial heartbeat, 669-70
internal cardioverter-defibrillators and, 672
paroxysmal atrial tachycardia, 671-72
ventricular tachycardia and fibrillation, 672
heart attacks, 661-68
aspirin in prevention of, 663
beta-adrenergic blockers for, 664
calcium channel blockers for, 664
cardiac arrhythmias resulting from, 663
cardiac rehabilitation for, 668
CCUs (coronary care units) in, 662
chest pains in, 434
complications in, 663
congestive heart failure resulting from, 663
coronary angioplasty for, 666
coronary artery bypass surgery for, 665, B-3
CPR (cardiopulmonary resuscitation) for, 664
death from, 663
diagnosis of, 662
diet after, 668
emergency signs and symptoms of, 661
exercise after, 296, 668
medication for, 664
nitrates for, 664
pain killers for, 664
recovery from, 664
seriousness of, 662-63
sexual activity after, 229, 667

signs and symptoms of, 434
stopping smoking after, 668
stress after, 668
symptoms of, 662
treatment of, 664
weight control after, 668
heartbeat:
ectopic atrial, 669-70
listening to, 634
heart block, 672-74
heartburn, 435, 742-44
in pregnancy, 187
heart catheterization, 1340-41
heart disease:
alcoholic, 686
diet and, 280
hypertensive, 650
in pregnancy, 190
sexual function and, 230
heart disorders, congenital, 635
aortic stenosis, 53, 683-85
atrial septal defect, 52
coarctation of aorta, 52
in newborns, 51-53
patent ductus arteriosus, 52
pulmonary stenosis, 53
tetralogy of Fallot, 53
transposition of great vessels, 53
ventricular septal defect, 52
heart failure, congestive, 659-60, 663
heart-lung transplantation, 736
heart murmurs, 634
innocent, 16
heart muscle, diseases of, 686-89
alcohol consumption and, 687
alcoholic heart disease, 686
cardiomyopathy, 686-87
dilated cardiomyopathy, 686
hypertrophic cardiomyopathy, 686
myocarditis, 687
restrictive cardiomyopathy, 686
heart rate and rhythm disorders, 669-76
arrhythmias, 663, 669-72
artificial cardiac pacemakers for, 675
atrial fibrillation and flutter, 670
calcium channel blockers for, 676
ectopic atrial heartbeat, 669-70
fainting spells in, 674
heart block, 672-74
paroxysmal atrial tachycardia, 671-72
twenty-four-hour cardiac monitoring in, 671
ventricular tachycardia and fibrillation, 672
heart rate targets, 296
heart-related shock, 443-44
emergency treatment of, 444
heart scans, 656, 1339-40
heart valve disorders, 677-85
aortic regurgitation, 685
aortic stenosis, 53, 683-85
aortic valve problems, 53, 682-85
dental procedures and, 679
infective endocarditis, 679
lung and skin infections and, 679
mitral valve prolapse, 682
mitral valve regurgitation, 680
mitral valve stenosis, 680
oral or respiratory surgery and, 679
pulmonary valve problems, 685
rheumatic fever, 677-78
tricuspid valve problems, 685

urologic or gastrointestinal surgery and, 679
valve repairs in, 684
valve replacements in, 684
valvuloplasties for, 681
heat, skin allergies to, 1039
heat collapse, 415-16
heat cramps, emergency treatment of, 416
heat exhaustion, emergency treatment of, 415-16
heat rashes, 69
heat stress, 414-16
heatstroke, 414-15
    emergency treatment of, 414-15
heavy metals, 372
heel pain, 874-76
height tables, 259
Heimlich maneuver, 407
    on obese people, 407
    on pregnant women, 407
    self-administration of, 407
helminths, 1060
hemangiomas, 15-16, 1002, C-2
    cavernous, 16, C-2
    strawberry, 15-16, C-2
hematemesis, 402
hematoceles, 1199
hematomas, intracranial, 451
hematospermia, 1228
hematuria, 403, 832
    benign, 832
    nonfamilial benign, 832
hemiplegia, 55
hemobilia, bile duct obstructions due to, 814
hemochromatosis, 806-7, 958
hemodialysis, 856-57
hemoglobin status, 955
hemoglobinopathies, 961
hemolytic anemias, 956, 962
hemolytic-uremic syndrome, 838
hemophilia, 975-77
    vascular, 977
hemoptysis, 402
hemorrhagic stroke, 462
hemorrhaging, see bleeding
hemorrhoids, 795-96, 797
    in pregnancy, 188
Henoch-Schönlein purpura, 837-38
hepatic encephalopathy, 808
hepatitis:
    acute viral, 801-8
    alcoholic, 803
    chronic, 804
    drug-induced, 803
    toxic, 803
    vaccination for, 802
hepatitis A:
    acute, 801
    from food poisoning, 269
    vaccination against, 382, 1079
hepatitis B:
    acute, 801
    in pregnancy, 192-93
    vaccination against, 382, 1079
hepatitis C, 801-2
hepatomegaly, 809-10
herbal medicine, 1245
herbal supplements, 355
hereditary disorders:
    autopsies and, 1315
    deafness as, 578
    of eyes, 526

and heart and blood vessel disorders, 644
    obesity as, 124, 288
hermaphroditism, 49
hernias, 822-24
    diaphragmatic, 57-58
    femoral, 823-24
    hiatal, 743
    incisional, 824
    inguinal, 822-23, 1199
    paraumbilical, 824
    umbilical, 17
herniated discs, 904-6, B-1
heroin, 1133
herpes, genital, 191, 1090-92, C-13
herpes simplex, C-10
    esophagitis, 744
herpes zoster, 1011, C-13
hiccups, 745
high blood pressure, see hypertension
high-fiber foods, 783
high-protein diets, 276
hiking, safety in, 360-61
hip:
    congenital dislocation of, 46, 912
    fractures of, 448-49
Hirschsprung's disease, 57, 792
hirsutism, 940, 1019-21, C-7
histamine, 1028-29
histamine H$_2$ blockers, 1280
histoplasmosis, 711-12
histrionic personality disorder, 1107
HIV (human immunodeficiency virus), 488, 1061
hives (urticaria), 415, 994, 1038-39, C-9
HMOs (health maintenance organizations), 1266-67
    home care and, 1322
Hodgkin's disease, 969-70
Holter monitors, 671
home:
    avoiding falls in, 240
    checklist for safety in, 353-55
    child-proofing of, 352-53
    CO (carbon monoxide) contamination in, 376
    fire prevention in, 350-51
    fireworks in, 351
    food safety in, 267-71
    gun safety in, 356
    infants in, 352-53
    medicine chests in, 1276
    preschool children in, 99-100
    radon in, 378
    safety outside of, 356-62
    treating minor burns at, 405
home care and elder care, 1319-28
    adult day-care in, 1327
    for AIDS victims, 1063
    bathing and, 1324
    bedpans and bed urinals in, 1325
    bedsores and, 1325
    choosing agency for, 1321
    for elderly, 246
    equipment needs for, 1322
    help for, 1320-21
    HMOs and, 1322
    independent living centers as alternatives to, 1328
    insurance coverage for, 1321-22
    making beds in, 1324-25
    mealtimes in, 1323-24

Medicaid and, 1321
    medical testing kits for, 1347
    Medicare and, 1321
    medications for, 1323
    oxygen supplies for, 718
    private insurance carriers and, 1321
    rehabilitation programs in, 1326-27
    reimbursements for, 1321-22
    returning to independence in, 1325-26
    selecting location for, 1323
    services for, 1320-22
    vomiting and, 1325
homeopathy, 1245
homosexuality, 149
honeymoon cystitis, 842, 1192
hookworm, 1084
hordeolum, 536-37, C-11
hormonal disorders, 83, 1217
hormone therapy:
    for hypopituitarism, 944
    for males, 164, 944, 1212
    for thyroid disorders, 946
    for women, 944, 1152, 1154, 1168, 1169
hormones, see specific hormones
hornet stings, 396
horseshoe kidney, 828
hospices, 1255-56
    palliative care in, 1306
    patients and families in, 1306
    team approach in, 1305-6
    in treatment of cancer, 1305-7
    types of, 1306-7
hospital-acquired pneumonia, 704
hospitals:
    admittance to, 1258-59
    dismissal from, 1260
    length of stay in, 1265
    outpatient departments of, 1254
    school-age children and, 128-29
    stays in, 1258-60
    visiting patients in, 1259
hot tubs, 195
hot weather, exercise in, 304
hotel fire safety, 357-58
household products, 374
human bites, 395, C-13
    emergency treatment of, 395
    infections from, 1015
human chorionic gonadotropin (hCG), 198
human immunodeficiency virus (HIV), 488, 1061
humidifier lung, 731
humoral mechanisms, 1056
Huntington, George, 477
Huntington's chorea, 477-78
hydatidiform moles, 1185
hydramnios, 202-3
hydrocele, 49, 1200
hydrocephalus, 489-90
    in newborns, 54
hydrocortisone, 944
hydronephrosis, congenital, 829-30
hygiene:
    anal itch due to, 796
    dental, 363-70
    for infants, 71-75
    for men, 1205
    oral, 617
    for school-age children, 118
    for vagina, 1171
hyperactivity, 133
hyperbilirubinemia, 812

hyperfunctioning nodular goiters, 947
hyperfunctioning thyroid nodules, 947
hypernephromas, 847-48
hyperopia (farsightedness), 66, 525-26
hyperosmolar coma, 423, 926, 929-30
    first aid for, 423
hyperparathyroidism, 898, 950-51
hyperprolactinemia, 1217
hypersensitivity vasculitis, 921
hypertension (high blood pressure),
        647-53, B-2
    angiotensin-converting enzyme
        inhibitors for, 652
    beta-adrenergic blockers for, 652
    calcium channel blockers for, 652
    causes of, 648-50
    complications of, 650-51
    in diabetes mellitus, 929-30
    diet and, 283-84, 653
    diuretics for, 651
    drug treatments of, 642, 651-52, 1279
    exercise for, 653
    eye disorders and, 564
    in heart and blood vessel disorders,
        638-39
    hypertensive heart disease due to, 650
    isolated systolic, 651
    kidney disease due to, 650-51
    malignant, 852
    portal, 807
    in pregnancy, 189-90
    salt intake and, 283-84, 653
    self-help for, 653
    strokes due to, 650
hypertensive crises, 422
hypertensive heart disease, 650
hyperthermia, 1299
hyperthyroidism, 947-48
    adenomatous goiters, 946
    emergency symptoms of, 947
    goiters and, 946
    Graves' disease in, 946, 947
    hyperfunctioning thyroid nodules in,
        947
    lymphocytic thyroiditis, 946
    medullary thyroid cancer, 946
    nutrition and, 948
    simple goiters, 946
    subacute thyroiditis, 946
    thyroid cancer and, 946
hypertrophic cardiomyopathy, 686
hypertrophic scarring, 1003
hyperventilation:
    in anxiety disorders, 1119
    treatment of, 431-32
hyphema, 533
hypnotics, 1280
hypocalcemia, 951
hypochondriasis, 1135-36
hypofunction, adrenocortical, 938-39
hypoglycemia:
    insulin reaction and, 927-28
    in peptic ulcer surgery, 756
    reactive, 929
hypoglycemic agents, oral, 934-35
hypoglycemic coma, 926, 927-28
hypoparathyroidism, 951-52
hypopituitarism, 898, 943-44
    emergency symptoms of, 944
    growth hormone for, 944
hypospadias, 48-49
hypotension (low blood pressure), 650

postural, 650
hypothalamus, 458, 1144-45
hypothalamus disorders, menses and
        menstrual disorders related to,
        1156-57, 1218
hypothermia, 416
    alcohol and, 329
    emergency treatment of, 416
hypothyroidism, 948-50
    cretinism caused by, 949
    emergency symptoms of, 948
    myxedema coma in, 949
    nutrition and, 949-50
    screening newborns for, 9
hypovolemic shock, 441-43
    in Addisonian crises, 443
    in cholera, 443
    emergency treatment of, 441-43
    in excessive use of diuretics, 443
    in gastroenteritis, 443
hysterectomies, 229-30, 1184
hysterical neurosis, 1135
hysterosalpingography, 1346

I

IAMAT (International Association for
        Medical Assistance to Travelers),
        380
ichthyosis, 994, C-15
IDDM (insulin-dependent diabetes melli-
        tus), 926-27
idiot savants, 108
IgA nephropathy, 838
ileo-anal anastomosis, 780
ileostomies, 777-78
immobilization:
    for baseball finger, 874
    for dislocations, 866
    for fractures, 865
immune system, A-16
    antibacterial agents and, 1058
    cell-mediated mechanisms of, 1026,
        1057-59
    humoral mechanisms of, 1056
    infectious agents and, 1059-60
    parasitic agents and, 1059-60
    workings of, 1056-59
immunizations:
    for chickenpox, 1080
    for cholera, 383
    for diphtheria, 226, 382, 1079
    for German measles, 1079
    for hepatitis, 802
    for hepatitis A, 382, 1079
    for hepatitis B, 382, 1079
    for influenza, 226, 382, 1066
    for influenza type B, 1079
    for malaria, 382-83
    for measles, 1074, 1079
    for meningococcal meningitis, 382
    for mumps, 1079
    for pertussis, 382, 1079
    for plague, 383
    for pneumococcal pneumonia, 226, 382
    for pneumonia, 382, 1080
    for polio, 382, 1079
    for rabies, 382, 1079
    scheduling of, 156, 226, 1078
    for school-age children, 118
    for smallpox, 383

for tetanus, 226, 382, 393, 1079
for travel, 380-83
for typhoid, 383
for yellow fever, 383
immunologic rheumatic disorders, 918-22
    allergic angiitis, 921
    cranial arteritis, 565-66, 921
    dermatomyositis, 920-21
    enlargement of lymph nodes, 1057
    granulomatosis, 921
    hypersensitivity vasculitis, 921
    polyarteritis, 921
    polymyalgia rheumatica, 922
    polymyositis, 920-21
    scleroderma, 771, 919-20
    Sjögren's syndrome, 920
    systemic lupus erythematosus, 918-19
    vasculitis, 921
immunosuppressants, 1280
immunotherapy, 1298-99
impacted fractures, 446
impacted teeth, 614
impaired mobility, 239-40
impedance plethysmography, 1342-43
imperforate anus, 57
impetigo, 1007, C-12
implants, contraceptive, 173
impotence, 1225-27
    in middle years, 229, 230
    psychotherapy for, 1227
inclusion cysts, 1174
incompetent cervix, 203
incontinence, fecal, 799-800
incontinence, urinary, 1207-8
    in elderly, 240-41
    exercises for, 1176
    medication for, 1193, 1208
    in men, 1207-8
    self-help for, 1207-8
    in women, 1193
independence, loss of, 234-35
independent living centers, 1328
indigestion (dyspepsia), 752-53
indium-labeled white blood cell scanning,
        1338-39
indoor pollution, 374-75
industrial bronchitis, 733
industrial exposures:
    air pollution and, 373
    cancer and, 373, 1294
    occupationally related lung disease
        and, 728-34
infant carriers, 24
infantile autism, 108, 1100
infantile eczema, 14-15, 989, 1038, C-2
infantile lobar emphysema, 58
infants, 59-80
    acne in, 69
    amblyopia in, 65
    breathing problems of, 63
    car seats for, 72-73
    central auditory disorders in, 65
    clothing for, 73-74
    common concerns about, 62-71
    conductive hearing loss in, 64
    constant crying by, 63
    constipation in, 41-42, 67
    CPR (cardiopulmonary resuscitation)
        on, 412
    cradle cap of, 14, 68, C-2
    dehydration in, 63
    of diabetic mothers, 21

diaper care for, 74
diaper rash of, 68
diarrhea in, 41, 63, 66-67
drool rashes of, 69
drug withdrawal by, 22
febrile seizures in, 69, 70
feeding problems of, 79-80
feeding recommendations for, 78-79
fevers of, 62-63
in first year, 60-62
fontanelles of, 63
general care and hygiene for, 71-75
hearing loss in, 64-65
hearing of, 64
heat rashes of, 69
home safety for, 352-53
immunization schedule for, 1078
jumpers for, 73
language of, 7, 62, 93
lead poisoning in, 71
milestones for, 60-62
milia in, 15, 69, C-2
mixed hearing loss in, 64
motor development in, 61-62
normal developmental milestones in, 75-76
normal growth and development of, 60-62
nutrition of, 78-80
objects swallowed by, 90
overfeeding of, 41, 80
personality and behavior in, 36-37, 75-78
pneumothorax in, 20-21
preventing spread of disease to, 74-75
rashes of, 68-69
reflexes and responses of, 32-34
regurgitation by, 63, 67-68, 80
safety for, 26-28, 71-72, 352-53
seizures in, 69, 70
sensorineural hearing loss in, 64
sibling relationships of, 77-78
SIDS (sudden infant death syndrome) in, 69-71
signs of illness in, 62-63
sleep patterns of, 61
sleeping problems of, 61, 77
spitting up by, 12, 41
strabismus in, 65-66
swings for, 73
toys for, 73
trimming nails of, 25
underfeeding of, 41, 80
verbal development in, 7, 62
vision of, 65-66
vomiting by, 63, 67-68, 80
walkers for, 73
weight gain by, 42, 63-64
see also babies, healthy; newborns
infarctions, myocardial, *see* heart attacks
infections:
agents of, 1059-60
of breasts, 1160-61
and enlargement of lymph nodes, 1057
gallium scanning for, 1338
genital, 136
indium-labeled white blood cell scanning for, 1338-39
jaundice in, 13
of joints, 437
necrotizing subcutaneous, 1016
radionuclide scans for, 1338-39
of urinary tract, 94-95, 159, 841-43, 1208

yeast, 1161, 1173
infections and diseases of the mouth, 617-22
acute glossitis, 619
canker sores, 617, 1010-11, C-10
discolored tongue, 621
geographic tongue, 620
gingivostomatitis, 618
hairy tongue, 620-21, C-10
halitosis, 620
leukoplakia, 618-19, C-10
oral cancer, 621-22, 1295
oral lichen planus, 619, C-10
oral thrush, 618, C-10
salivary duct stones, 623
salivary duct tumors, 623
salivary gland infections, 622
tongue disorders, 619-21
infections of the central nervous system, 481-89
AIDS and, 488
botulism and, 488-89
encephalitis, 482-84
epidural abscesses, 486-88
meningitis, 382, 433, 481-82
poliomyelitis, 382, 485-86, 1079
Reye's syndrome, 484
infections of the eyes, 29, 539
in cornea, 547
infections of the gastrointestinal tract, 766-69
acute viral gastroenteritis, 766-67
antibiotic-related diarrhea, 769-70
bacterial, 767-68
Campylobacter, 767
Cryptosporidium, 769
cytomegalovirus, 193, 767
emergency symptoms of, 766
Entamoeba histolytica, 768-69
Escherichia coli, 268, 768
food poisoning, *see* food poisoning
Giardia lamblia, 768
Norwalk virus, 767
parasitic, 768-69
rotavirus, 766-67
Salmonella, 268, 767-68
Shigella, 768
viral, 766-67
infections of the respiratory system, 701-11
acute bronchitis, 702
aspiration pneumonia, 704
bronchiectasis, 708, 709
bronchiolitis, 701-2
community-acquired pneumonia, 704
cystic fibrosis, 709, 720-21
empyema, 710-11
hospital-acquired pneumonia, 704
legionnaires' disease, 707
pneumonia, *see* pneumonia
TB (tuberculosis), 705-7
infections of the skin, 1007-16, C-12, C-13
from animal bites, 394-95, 1016
athlete's foot, 1013-14, C-8
boils, 1009
canker sores, 617, 1010-11, C-10
carbuncles, 1009, C-12
cellulitis, 1009-10, C-12
cold sores, 1010-11, C-10
cutaneous abscesses, 1016
erysipelas, 1009-10
folliculitis, 1007, C-12
fungal, 1012-14, C-2, C-8

from gas gangrene, 1016
from human bites, 395, 1015, C-13
impetigo, 1007, C-12
from insect bites, 1014-15
intertrigo, C-8
jock itch, 1013-14, C-8
lymphadenitis, 1010
lymphangitis, 1010
molluscum contagiosum, 1012, C-13
necrotizing subcutaneous, 1016
onychomycosis, C-8
from Portuguese man-of-war stings, 398-99, 1015-16, C-13
ringworm, C-8
shingles, 1011-12, C-13
tinea versicolor, C-8
from wounds, 1016
infectious arthritis, 914-15
infectious diseases, 1055-92
acyclovir for, 1060
AIDS, *see* AIDS
amantadine for, 1060
antibacterial agents and, 1058
antibiotics for, 1058, 1279
antifungal drugs for, 1059, 1279
antiviral drugs for, 1060, 1279
ascariasis, 1083-84
cat scratch disease, 1067-68
cell-mediated mechanisms and, 1026, 1057-59
chickenpox, 102, 191, 1076-77, 1080, C-1
from chiggers, 1086-87, C-14
chlamydial, 193, 1088-89
chronic fatigue syndrome, 1065
common contagious, 1071-80
common viral colds, 86-87, 1071-73
croup, 413, 1076
cystitis, 94-95, 159, 436, 842, 1192, 1193, 1203-4
diphtheria, 226, 382, 1078-80
fevers of unknown origin, 1069
from fleas, 1086
genital herpes, 191, 1090-92, C-13
genital warts, 1092, 1171-72
German measles, 191, 1074, 1079, C-1
gonorrhea, 193, 1087-88
hookworm, 1084
humoral mechanisms and, 1056
immune system and, 1056-59
immunizations against, *see* immunizations
infectious agents and, 1059-60
infectious mononucleosis, 158-59, 1064-65
influenza, 226, 382, 1065-67, 1079
insect infestations, 1085-87
from lice, 102, 1085-86, 1173, C-14
Lyme disease, 396, 915, 1067, C-14
malaria, 382-83, 1080-81
measles, 1073-74, 1079, C-1
mumps, 1077-78, 1079, C-1
parasitic infestations, 1080-84
pertussis, 382, 1075, 1079
pinworms, 1082-83
in pregnancy, 191-93
preventing spread of, 74-75
rabies, 382, 395, 1070-71, 1079
Rocky Mountain spotted fever, 1068
roseola, 1074-75, C-1
safe sex and, 1091
from scabies, 1085, C-14
scarlet fever, 1080, C-1

in school-age children, 118
sexually transmitted, *see* sexually transmitted diseases
smallpox, 383, 1077
strongyloidosis, 1083
syphilis, 193, 1089-90
tapeworm, 1081-82
tetanus, 226, 382, 393, 1070, 1079
from ticks, 396, 398, 1087, C-14
trichinosis, 1082
typhoid fever, 383, 1068-70
urethritis, 842-43, 1174-75, 1192-93, 1204-5
whooping cough, 382, 1075, 1079
infectious food poisoning, 267-70
infectious kidney disorders, 841-42
infectious mastitis, 216, 1160-61
infectious mononucleosis, 1064-65
in teenagers, 158-59
infective endocarditis, 678-80
infertility, 1215-21
assisted reproductive technology in, 1219-21
causes of, 1217-18
evaluation of, 1215-17
tests for, 1216-17
therapy for, 1218-21
infestations, *see* insect infestations; parasitic infestations
inflammatory arthritis, 911-13
inflammatory bowel disease, 774-79
arthritis of, 913
inflammatory kidney disorders, 836-41
influenza (flu), 1065-67
vaccination against, 226, 382, 1066
influenza type B, vaccination against, 1079
information sources, 1373-80
informed consent, 1268
ingrown toenails, 893
care for, 1022
inhalants, 344-45
inhaled foreign objects, 427
injuries:
Achilles tendinitis, 874
arthroscopy for, 878
in athletic activities, 160, 302-4, 867, 870
to back, 303-4, 448
baseball finger, 874
in birth, *see* birth injuries
to bladder, 835-36
to bones, 863-66
to brain, 490-91
to cornea, 546-47
dislocations, 449, 623-24, 866
electrical, 418
in exercise, avoiding of, 302-4
first aid for bleeding from, 399-403
fractures, *see* fractures
heel pain in, 874-76
of kidneys, 95, 834-35
to knees, 876-77
loose bodies in knees, 877
meniscal tears in knees, 876
muscle cramps, 871-72
to musculoskeletal system, 863-79
nursemaid's dislocation, 866
pulled muscles, 868-69
runner's knee, 873
of school-age children, 119
severed tendons, 867-68
shin splints, 870-71
shock and, 418
of soft tissue, 401

to spine, 448
sprains, 449, 869-70
tennis elbow, 872-73
to testicles, 1198
thigh bruises, 872
to ureters, 834-35
to urethra, 835-36
in-line skating, 160
insect bites and stings, 395-98, 1051-53, C-14
allergic reactions to, 1030, 1051-53
by bees, 396
emergency symptoms of, 1051
emergency treatment of, 396-98
by fire ants, 396
by hornets, 396
mild, 396
poisonous, 397-98
by scorpions, 396
skin infections from, 1014-15
by spiders, 396, 1014, C-14
by ticks, 396, 398, 1087, C-14
treatment of, 396-98, 1052-53
by wasps, 396
by yellow jackets, 396
insect infestations, 1085-87, C-14
chiggers, 1086-87, C-14
fleas, 1086
lice, 102, 1085-86, 1173, C-14
scabies, 1085, C-14
ticks, 396, 398, 1087, C-14
insomnia, 1112-14
during menopause, 1153
insulin, 924, 1279
in diabetes mellitus, 925-28, 932-35
insulin reaction, 422-23, 926
first aid for, 422-23, 928
hypoglycemia and, 927-28
insulinomas, 936
insurance:
travel protection, 380
see also health insurance
intellectual growth and development, 142
intermittent claudication, 690-92, 871
internal cardioverter-defibrillators, 672
internal mammary artery bypass graft, B-3
International Association for Medical Assistance to Travelers (IAMAT), 380
interpersonal conflicts, stress in, 310
interstitial cystitis, 842, 1193
interstitial lung disease, 721-23
Goodpasture's syndrome, 722-23
idiopathic pulmonary fibrosis, 722
pulmonary alveolar proteinosis, 722
interstitial nephritis, acute, 836
intertrigo, C-8
intestinal atresia (obstruction), 57, 793-94
intestinal gas, 260, 785-86
intestinal lymphangiectasia, 774
intestinal pseudo-obstruction, primary or idiopathic, 774
intestines, *see* bowel; colon; large intestine; small intestine
intestines, disorders of, 765-94
acute viral gastroenteritis, 766-67
in AIDS, 771
amyloidosis, 771-72, 974-75
angiodysplasia of colon, 794
antibiotic-associated diarrhea, 769-70
appendicitis, 436, 772-73
atresia (obstruction), 57, 793-94
bacterial, 767-68
bacterial overgrowth, 771

Campylobacter, 767
carcinoid syndrome, 774
celiac sprue, 285, 770-71
chronic constipation, 784-85
colon cancer, 789-91, 1250, 1294-95
colon polyps, 786-89, 797
colonoscopies in, 788
colostomies in, 777-78
congenital, *see* gastrointestinal tract disorders, congenital
Crohn's disease, 774-77
Cryptosporidium, 769
diabetic, 772
diverticulosis and diverticulitis, 436, 781-82
Entamoeba histolytica, 768-69
Escherichia coli, 268, 768
familial Mediterranean fever, 793
fecal impaction, 786
and fiber in diet, 783
food poisoning, 267-70, 440-41, 488-89, 769
gastrointestinal tract infections, 766-69
Giardia lamblia, 768
idiopathic intestinal pseudo-obstruction, 774
ileostomies in, 777-78
intestinal gas, 260, 785-86
intestinal obstruction, 793-94
intussusception, 773-74
irritable bowel syndrome, 782-84
ischemic colitis, 794
lactose intolerance, 772, 1049
malabsorption, 770-72
Meckel's diverticulum, 773
megacolon, 57, 791-92
mesenteric ischemia, 794
nontropical sprue, 770-71
Norwalk virus, 767
parasitic, 768-69
peritonitis, 792
primary intestinal pseudo-obstruction, 774
protein-losing enteropathy, 774
rectal cancer, 789-91
rotavirus, 766-67
Salmonella, 268, 767-68
scleroderma, 771
Shigella, 768
short-bowel syndrome, 772
small intestine tumors, 779-81
treatment of, 769
tropical sprue, 771
ulcerative colitis, 777-79
vascular problems of bowel, 794
Whipple's disease, 771
in-toeing, 45
intoxication:
from alcohol, 327, 429-30
from illegal drugs, 430-31
from legal drugs, 430
from mind-altering drugs, 430-31
from narcotics, 431
from uppers and downers, 431
intracranial hematomas, 451
intraductal papillomas, 1163
intraocular lens implants, 556
intrauterine death, 206
intrauterine devices (IUDs), 172
intrauterine growth, retardation of, 179
intravenous pyelography (IVP), 829, 1341
intussusception, 773-74

invasive moles, 1185
in vitro fertilization (IVF), 1219-21
iodine:
    deficiencies, 946, 949-50
    radioactive, 948
    uptake tests, 1337
iris melanoma, 546, C-11
iritis, 544
    acute, 453
iron, 288, 958
iron-deficiency anemia, 957-58
    in athletes, 275
    from heavy periods, 1151
    in school-age children, 121-22
    in teenagers, 159
irradiation, *see* radiation therapy
irradiation, food, 271-72
irritable bladder, 1192-93
irritable bowel syndrome, 782-84
ischemia, 461
    mesenteric, 794
    renal, 853
ischemic colitis, 794
ischemic strokes, 564
ISH (isolated systolic hypertension), 651
islet cell tumors:
    gastrinomas, 757-58, 936
    glucagonomas, 936
    insulinomas, 936
isolated systolic hypertension (ISH), 651
isotretinoin (Accutane), 186
itching (pruritus), 995
    anal, 796
    causes of, 995
    in eyelids, 539
    jock itch, 1013-14, C-8
    in pregnancy, 190
    of vulva, 1170-71
IUDs (intrauterine devices), 172
IVF (in vitro fertilization), 1219-21
IVP (intravenous pyelography), 829, 1341

J

jammed finger, 874
jaundice, 800
    in newborns, 10, 13-14
    physiologic, 13
    as result of infection, 13
jaw:
    dislocation of, 623-24
    fractures of, 623-24
jellyfish stings, 398-99
    emergency treatment of, 401
Jenner, Edward, 1077
jet lag, prevention of, 385-86
job conflicts, stress in, 310
jock itch, 1013-14, C-8
jogging, program for, 298
joints, 862
    in middle years, 226-27
joints, disorders of, 907-18, B-6
    acute painful shoulder, 917
    ankylosing spondylitis, 913, 914
    arthritis of inflammatory bowel
        disease, 913
    Baker's cyst, 909
    bursitis, 917-18
    of childhood, 912
    clubfoot, 46, 912
    congenital dislocation of hip, 46, 912

corticosteroid drugs for, 919
degenerative joint disease, 906, 908
gonococcal arthritis, 915
gout, 437, 916, 1280
infections, 437
infectious arthritis, 915
inflammatory arthritis, 913-14
joint replacement in, 911
juvenile rheumatoid arthritis, 911-13
Legg-Calvé-Perthes disease, 912
Lyme disease, 396, 915, 1067, C-14
Osgood-Schlatter disease, 159, 912
osteoarthritis, 509, 906, 907-9, B-1
pain in, 437
psoriatic arthritis, 913
Reiter's syndrome, 913-14
rheumatic fever arthritis, 915
rheumatoid arthritis, 909-11
slipped capital femoral epiphysis, 912
staphylococcal arthritis, 915
temporomandibular, 624-25
tuberculous arthritis, 915
viral arthritis, 915
jumpers, 73
juvenile angiofibromas, 589
juvenile papillomas, 597
juvenile rheumatoid arthritis, 911-13

K

Kaposi's sarcoma, 1006, C-6
Kegel, A. M., 1176
keloids, 1003, C-5
keratoses, C-10
    actinic, 1002, C-4
    seborrheic, 1002, C-4
keratotomy, radial, 525
ketoacidosis, 926, 928-29
    first aid for, 423
kidney failure, 852-58, B-2
    acute, 853-54
    CAPD (continuous ambulatory peri-
        toneal dialysis) for, 857
    chronic, 854-55
    dialysis treatments of, 856-57
    end-stage renal disease, 855-57
    hemodialysis for, 856-57
    nephrotoxic agents as cause of, 853
    peritoneal dialysis for, 857
    renal ischemia as cause of, 853
    special diets for, 286
kidney injuries, 95, 834-35
    acute uric acid nephropathy, 835
    analgesic nephropathy, 835
    lead nephropathy, 835
    nephropathy from solvents and fuels,
        835
    toxic, 835
kidney stones, 843-45
    calcium, 286, 844
    cystine, 844
    lithotripsy for, 846
    nutrition and, 845
    pelvic pain from, 436
    special diets for, 286
    struvite, 844
    uric acid, 844
kidneys:
    transplantation of, 857-58
    workings of, 826-27
    X-rays of, 829, 1341
kidneys, cancer of, 847-48

renal cell carcinomas, 847
transitional cell, 847
Wilms' tumor, 847
kidneys, disorders of, 825-58
    acute arterial occlusion in, 850-51
    acute glomerulonephritis, 836-38
    acute interstitial nephritis, 836
    acute kidney failure, 853-54
    acute pyelonephritis, 841-42
    Alport's syndrome, 833
    anatomic abnormalities, 827-30
    blood vessel problems, 850-52
    cancer, *see* kidneys, cancer of
    chronic glomerulonephritis, 838-40
    chronic kidney failure, 854-55
    congenital, 827-31
    congenital hydronephrosis, 829
    congenital nephrotic syndrome, 833
    congenital ureteral pelvic junction
        obstruction, 828
    cystinuria, 832-33
    cysts, 847
    diabetes and, 930
    diabetic nephropathy, 838-39, 930
    dropped kidney, 828
    duplication of kidney, 828
    end-stage renal disease, 855-57
    floating kidney, 828
    focal and segmental glomeruloscler-
        osis, 838
    hematuria in, 832
    hemolytic-uremic syndrome, 838
    Henoch-Schönlein purpura, 837-38
    horseshoe kidney, 828
    hydronephrosis, 829-30
    hypertension as cause of, 650-51
    IgA nephropathy, 838
    infectious, 841-42
    inflammatory, 836-41
    inherited, 831-34
    injuries to, *see* kidney injuries
    interstitial cystitis, 842, 1193
    kidney failure, *see* kidney failure
    kidney stones, *see* kidney stones
    malignant hypertension, 852
    medullary sponge kidney, 830
    membranous glomerulonephritis, 838
    mesangial proliferative glomerulo-
        nephritis, 838
    multicystic dysplasia, 829
    nephrotic syndrome, 840-41
    polycystic kidney disease, 831-32
    renal artery stenosis, 851
    renal tubular acidosis, 833
    renal tubule defects, 833
    renal vein thrombosis, 852
    sickle cell disease, 833-34, 960-62
    solitary kidney, 827
    ureteral pelvic junction obstruction,
        828
    vesicoureteral reflux, 830-31
    vitamin D-resistant hypophosphatemic
        rickets, 833
kitchens, safety in, 240, 353-54
knee injuries, 876-77
    loose bodies in, 877
    meniscal tears in, 876
    pain and, 876
    support braces for, 879
    swelling, 877
knock-knees, 96-97
Koop, C. Everett, 252

L

labia, 1140
labor:
  abnormal fetal positions in, 209-10
  beginning of, 207
  breech presentation in, 209
  delivery and, 207-14
  duration, 207-8
  electronic fetal monitoring in, 210
  epidural anesthesia in, 211-12
  episiotomies in, 210-11
  false, 208
  fetal blood sampling in, 210
  induction of, 210
  local anesthetics in, 211
  narcotics in, 211
  occiput posterior in, 210
  pain relief in, 211-12
  postpartum hemorrhage and, 214
  premature, 201-2
  procedures encountered in, 210-11
  prolonged, 208
  retained placenta and, 214
  spinal anesthesia in, 211-12
  three stages of, 207-8
  transverse presentation in, 209
laboratory tests, 1252
  see also medical tests
labyrinthitis, 583-84
lactation, nutrition and, 215-16
lactose intolerance, 772, 1049
language:
  of infants, 7, 62, 93
  of newborns, 7
  of preschool children, 92-94, 107
  of school-age children, 132
  stuttering and, 93
  see also communicating; speech
lanugo, 5
laparoscopic surgery, 817, B-7
laparoscopy, 174, 1157, 1346-47
large intestine, 740
  angiodysplasia of, 794
  barium X-rays of, 762-63
  disorders of, see intestines, disorders of
laryngectomies, voice aids after, 598
laryngitis, 595-99
laryngoscopy, 1333-34
laser therapy:
  for diabetic retinopathy, 558
  in eye diseases, 558
  for glaucoma, 558
  for macular degeneration, 558
  for orbital and eyelid tumors, 558
  in retinal reattachment, 558
  for secondary cataracts, 558
lasers, 1004, 1299
latex allergy, 1029
lawn chemicals, 375
lawsuits, 1267-68
laxatives, 1280
  abuse of, 785
  for constipation, 784-85
  kinds of, 785
lazy eye, 65, 90
LDL cholesterol, 254, 266, 639, 640-42
lead nephropathy, 835
lead poisoning, 71
learning problems:
  attention deficit disorder, 132-33
  disorders, 129, 1099

dyslexia, 131-32
  hearing disorders as cause of, 106-7
  hyperactivity, 133
  in preschool children, 106-8
  in school-age children, 129-34
  school phobia, 133-34
  speech disorders as cause of, 107
  vision problems as cause of, 108
Legg-Calvé-Perthes disease, 912
legionnaires' disease, 707
legs:
  fractures of, 448
  restless, 1115-16
  spider veins in, 1001, C-15
leiomyomas, 1182
lenses, corrective:
  after cataract surgery, 556
  for nearsightedness, 525
  see also contact lenses
lens implants, intraocular, 556
lentigines, senile, 1003, C-4
lentigo maligna melanomas, 1006, C-6
lethargy:
  in newborns, 10
  in preschool children, 85
leukemias, 964-68
  acute lymphocytic, 966-67
  acute nonlymphocytic, 965-66
  bone marrow transplants for, 967-68
  chronic lymphocytic, 966
  chronic myelogenous, 964-65
leukocytes (white blood cells), 955
leukonychia, C-7
leukoplakia, 597, 618-19, C-10
LH (luteinizing hormone), 167
lice, 1085-86
  head, 102, C-14
  pubic, 1173
licensed practical nurse (L.P.N.), 1243
lichen planus, 993
  oral, 619, C-10
lichen sclerosus et atrophicus, 1170
lichen simplex chronicus, 988-89
lifestyles:
  crises in, 1125
  healthful, 119
  as risk factor in heart and blood vessel
    disorders, 643-44
  in treating indigestion, 753
lifting, protecting back in, 303-4, 901-2
lightning, safety and, 361-62
limbs:
  absence or loss of, 450-51, 879-80
  amputation of, 450-51, 691-92, 693, 698,
    879-80
  artificial, 879
  fractures of, 445-48
  reattachment of, 880
lipids, blood tests for, 1250-51, 1331
lipoproteins:
  HDL, 254, 639, 640, 644
  LDL, 254, 266, 639, 640-42
lithiasis, renal, see kidney stones
lithotripsy, 846
Little League elbow, 872
liver, 741
  anabolic steroids and, 345
liver abscesses, 810-12
liver biopsies, 807, 1333
liver disease, 800-818
  acute viral hepatitis, 801-8
  alcoholic hepatitis, 803

alcohol-induced cirrhosis, 805
alpha$_1$-antitrypsin deficiency, 807
cancer, 808-9
chronic hepatitis, 804
cirrhosis, 804-8
Crigler-Najjar syndrome, 812
cryptogenic cirrhosis, 805-6
Dubin-Johnson hyperbilirubinemia, 812
enlarged liver, 809-10
genetic, 811-12
Gilbert's syndrome, 811-12
hemochromatosis, 806-7, 958
hepatitis A, 269, 382, 801, 1079
hepatitis B, 192-93, 382, 1079
hepatitis C, 801-2
primary biliary cirrhosis, 806
secondary biliary cirrhosis, 806
special diets for, 286
toxic and drug-induced hepatitis, 803
Wilson's disease, 807
liver scans, 1336-37
liver spots, 227-28, 244, 1003, C-4
liver transplantation, 811
liver tumors, 808-9
living rooms, safety in, 354
living wills, 1248-49, 1312, 1384, 1387-89
lobar emphysema, congenital, 58
lockjaw, 393, 1070
Lou Gehrig's disease, 477
lovastatin, 642
low blood pressure (hypotension), 650
  postural, 650
L.P.N. (licensed practical nurse), 1243
LSD (lysergic acid diethylamide), 343-44,
    1129, 1134
lumbar puncture (spinal tap), 485, 510
lumbar stenosis, 906
lump in throat, 593
lumpectomies, 1166, B-4
lumps:
  in breasts, 1158-59, B-4
  on body, 1293
  on eyelids, 536-37
lung cancer, 724-27, 729-30
  bronchoscopy for, 726
  lung removal for, 727
  screening for, 1295
  smoking and, 725
lung scans, 1336
lungs, A-8, A-9
  normal functioning of, 700-1
lungs, disorders of, 701-36
  abscesses, 708-10
  acute bronchitis, 702
  allergic alveolitis, 731
  asbestosis, 728-30
  aspergillosis, 712
  aspiration pneumonia, 704
  asthma, see asthma
  atelectasis, 723
  breathing techniques for, 717
  bronchiectasis, 708, 709
  bronchiolitis, 701-2
  bronchitis, 413, 702, 714-15, 733
  bronchoscopy for, 726
  byssinosis, 731-33
  cardiovascular system and, 734-36
  chest percussion for, 709
  chronic, 714-27
  chronic bronchitis, 714-15
  coccidioidomycosis, 713
  community-acquired pneumonia, 704

controlled coughs for, 717
cor pulmonale and, 735
cryptococcosis, 712-13
cystic fibrosis, 709, 720-21
emphysema, 58, 715-20
empyema, 710-11
farmer's lung, 733
fungal, 711-13
Goodpasture's syndrome, 722-23
heart-lung transplantation in, 736
heart valve disorders and, 679
histoplasmosis, 711-12
home oxygen supplies for, 718
hospital-acquired pneumonia, 704
idiopathic pulmonary fibrosis, 722
industrial bronchitis, 733
interstitial lung disease, 721-23
legionnaires' disease, 707
lung cancer, *see* lung cancer
occupational asthma, 731
occupationally related, 728-34
pleurisy and pleural effusions, 434-35, 711
pneumoconiosis, 730-31
pneumonia, *see* pneumonia
pneumothorax, 20-21, 723-24
postural drainage for, 709
pulmonary alveolar proteinosis, 722
pulmonary embolisms and, 434, 734-35
respiratory infections, 701-11
sarcoidosis, 721
silicosis, 730-31
silo-filler's disease, 733-34
TB (tuberculosis), 705-7
lupus (systemic lupus erythematosus),
    918-19
luteinizing hormone (LH), 167
Lyme disease, 396, 915, 1067, C-14
lymph, 955
lymph nodes, enlargement of, 1057
lymphadenitis, 1010
lymphangiectasia, intestinal, 774
lymphangitis, 1010
lymphedema, 695
lymphocytes, 1026-28
lymphocytic leukemias:
    acute, 966-67
    chronic, 966
lymphocytic thyroiditis, 946
lymphomas, 968-71
    Hodgkin's disease, 969-70
    non-Hodgkin's, 970-71
lysergic acid diethylamide (LSD), 343-44,
    1129, 1134

M

macular degeneration, 556-57
    laser therapy for, 558
magazines, health news in, 1270
magnetic resonance imaging (MRI), 1334
    of head, 494
magnifiers, 239
ma huang, 355
major depressive disorder, 1123-25
    antidepressive medications for, 1124
    ECT (electroconvulsive therapy) for,
        1124-25
    psychotherapy for, 1124
makeup, hazards to eyes from, 532
malabsorption problems, intestinal, 770-72
    in AIDS, 771
    amyloidosis, 771-72, 974-75

bacterial overgrowth, 771
celiac sprue, 285, 770-71
lactose intolerance, 772, 1049
nontropical sprue, 770-71
in peptic ulcer surgery, 756
scleroderma, 771
short-bowel syndrome, 772
tropical sprue, 771
Whipple's disease, 771
malaria, 1080-81
    prevention of, 382-83
male birth control pills, 166
male-pattern baldness, 1017-18
male pseudohermaphroditism, 49
malignant hypertension, 852
malignant melanomas, 1005-6, C-6
malignant pancreatic tumors, 820-21, 936
mallet finger, 874
mallet toe, 892-93
malnutrition, 83
    see also nutrition
malpractice suits, 1267-68
    bringing of, 1268
    informed consent and, 1268
mammary dysplasia, 1158
mammography, 169, 1165, 1250
manic-depressive illness, 1125-26
maple bark stripper's disease, 731
margarine, butter vs., 254
marijuana, 152
    abuse of, 342-43
    dependence on, 342-43, 1134
    emphysema and, 719
marital conflicts, stress in, 310
mastectomies:
    modified radical, 1166, B-4
    radical, 1166
    simple, 1166-67
    subcutaneous, 1167
    swelling after, 1168
mastitis:
    chronic cystic, 1158
    infectious, 216, 1160-61
mastoiditis, 577-78
masturbation, 149
maternal care facilities, 1257
mattresses for newborns, 28
M.D. (medical doctor), *see* physicians
MDIs (metered-dose inhalers), 1046
meals, pregame, 276
Meals on Wheels, 247
mealtimes, in home care, 1323-24
measles, 1073-74, C-1
    vaccination against, 1074, 1079
meats, 262
    Escherichia coli in, 268
    examples of servings of, 262
    for preschool children, 113
    proper handling of, 272
    for school-age children, 122
Meckel's diverticulum, 773
media, 1270
Medicaid, home care and, 1321
medical bills, payment of, 1263-67
    with conventional health insurance,
        1265-66
    diagnostic-related groups and, 1265
    with HMOs, 1266-67
    medical supplemental insurance and,
        1264-65
    with PPOs (preferred provider organi-
        zations), 1267

utilization review boards and, 1267
medical doctor (M.D.), *see* physicians
medical histories, 603-4
medical records, 381
medical research and science, autopsies
    and, 1316
medical supplemental insurance, 1264-65
medical terms, list of, 1355-72
medical testing kits, 1347
medical tests, 1329-48
    arterial blood gas analyses, 1332
    arthrography, 1341
    bile duct X-rays, 815, 816, 1341
    biopsies, 807, 1332-33
    blood chemistry group, 1330-31
    body scans, 494, 1334-35
    bone marrow aspirations, 1332-33
    bone scans, 1336
    CBCs (complete blood cell counts), 955,
        1330
    cerebral arteriography, 464, 1341
    cerebrospinal fluid analyses, 1345-46
    coagulation tests, 1331
    colposcopy, 1346
    CT scanning, 494, 1334
    cystoscopy, 849, 1347
    ECG, 654, 655-57, 671, 1251, 1343-44
    echocardiography, 634, 683, 1342
    EEG, 1344
    electrical, 654, 655-57, 671, 1251, 1343-44
    EMG, 1344
    endoscopic, 817, 1333-34
    for enzymes, 1331
    ESRs (erythrocyte sedimentation rates),
        1331
    exercise tolerance, 655, 1344
    fluorescein angiography, 1342
    gallium scanning, 1338
    heart catheterization, 1340-41
    heart scans, 1339-40
    hysterosalpingography, 1346
    impedance plethysmography, 1342-43
    indium-labeled white blood cell scan-
        ning, 1338-39
    kidney X-rays, 829, 1341
    laparoscopy, 174, 1346-47
    laryngoscopy, 1333-34
    for lipids, 1250-51, 1331
    liver biopsies, 807, 1333
    liver scans, 1336-37
    lung scans, 1336
    microbiologic, 1345-46
    MRI, 494, 1334
    myelography, 510, 1341
    myocardial perfusion imaging, 1339
    ophthalmoscopy, 1342
    pancreatic duct X-rays, 816, 1341
    perspectives on radiologic examina-
        tions, 1335
    for pregnancy, 198
    in pregnancy, *see* prenatal tests
    for presence of drugs, 1331
    radionuclide angiography, 656, 1339-40
    radionuclide scans, 1336-40
    RAIU (radioactive iodine uptake), 1337
    reproductive tests, 1346-48
    scanning for infections, 1338-39
    synovial fluid analyses, 1345
    throat cultures, 678, 1345
    thyroid scans, 1337
    thyroid studies, 1331
    tumor imaging, 1337-38

ultrasonography, 180, 683, 1335
urine tests, 1347-48
venography, 1342-43
X-rays, *see* X-rays
see also blood tests
Medicare, 1264, 1265
home care and, 1321
medications, *see* drugs, therapeutic
medicine calendars, 1278
medicine chests, 1276
medullary sponge kidney, 830
medullary thyroid cancer, 946
megacolon, 791-92
congenital, 57
melanomas:
acral lentiginous, 1006, C-6
of eyes, 546, C-11
lentigo maligna, 1006, C-6
malignant, 1005-6, C-6
nodular, C-6
superficial spreading, C-6
membranes, premature rupture of, 205
membranous glomerulonephritis, 838
memory, in elderly, 237-38
men:
birth control pills for, 166
coitus interruptus and, 165-66
condoms for, 165
contraception for, 165-67
genital organs of, 163-67, 1196, A-13
hygiene for, 1205
in preventing pregnancy, 165-67
sexual function of, 164-66, 229-30, 242,
1225-29
testing fertility of, 1216
vasectomies for, 166-67
young-adult, 163-67
men, health problems of, 1196-1212
acute prostatitis, 1210-11
balanitis, 1205-6
bladder disorders, 1203-4, 1207-8
blood in semen, 1228
BPH (benign prostatic hyperplasia),
1209, B-5
cancer of penis, 1206-7
cancer of prostate, 1211-12, 1295, B-5
cancer of testicles, 1202-3, 1295
chronic prostatitis, 1211
curvature of penis, 1206, 1227-28
cystitis, 1203-4
enlarged prostate, 1209-10
epididymitis, 1198-99
erection abnormalities, 1227-28
hydrocele, 49, 1200
impotence, 229, 230, 1225-27
injuries to testicles, 1198
loss of sexual desire, 1229
noninfectious urethral discharge, 1205
orchitis, 1201-2
paraphimosis, 47, 1206
penile disorders, 1206-7
penile warts, 1204
premature ejaculation, 1228-29
priapism, 1206, 1228
prostate gland disorders, 1208, 1209-12,
B-5
retrograde ejaculation, 1229
scrotal masses, 1199
scrotal problems, 1199-1202
self-examination of testicles for, 1200
STDs (sexually transmitted diseases),
1206

testicular disorders, 1197-1203
testicular failure, 1198
testicular torsion, 1197-98
undescended testicles, 1202
urethral disorders, 1204-5
urethral stricture, 1205
urethritis, 1204-5
urinary incontinence, 1207-8
urinary tract infections, 1208
varicocele, 1201
see also sexual partners, health issues of
menarche, puberty and, 1143-44
Ménétrier's disease, 764
Meniere, Prosper, 583
Meniere's disease, 582-83
meningitis, 382, 481-82
head pain in, 433
meningococcal meningitis vaccination, 382
menopause, 1153-55
depression during, 228-29, 1153
exercise and, 1154-55
in middle years, 228
nutrition and, 1154-55
sex and, 228, 1153
treatment of, 1154-55, 1294
menorrhagia (heavy periods), 1150-52
menses and menstrual disorders, 1143-57
absence of periods, 1148-49
adrenal gland abnormalities, 1156-57
anovulation, 1217
D and C for, 1151
dysfunctional uterine bleeding, 1152
estrogen in, 1144, 1150
heavy periods, 1150-52
hypothalamus abnormalities, 1156-57
infrequent periods, 1149-50
menopause, 228, 1153-55, 1294
mittelschmerz, 1148
ovary abnormalities, 1156-57
painful menses, 159, 1148
pituitary abnormalities, 1156-57
PMS (premenstrual syndrome), 1147
postmenopausal bleeding, 1155
primary ovarian failure, 1155-56
sports and, 1150
thyroid abnormalities, 1156-57
TSS (toxic shock syndrome), 1145-47
menstrual care, 1145
menstrual cycle, normal, 1144-45
mental health, definition of, 1095-96
mental health facilities, 1256
mental problems, 1096-1137
absent grief reaction, 1110
addictive behavior, 1129-31
in adjusting to adolescence, 1096-97
in adjusting to adulthood, 1097
in adjusting to aging, 1097
in adolescence, 1101-3
adolescent depression, 154-55, 1101
alcohol abuse, 1102-3
alcohol dependence, 1129-30
alcohol-induced psychosis, 1129
anorexia nervosa, 152, 1102
antianxiety medications for, 1120, 1279
antisocial personality disorder, 1106
anxiety reactions, 1118-19
avoidant personality disorder, 1108
biofeedback for, 1121
borderline personality disorder, 1106-7
brief reactive psychosis, 1128
bruxism, 1117
bulimia nervosa, 152, 1102-3

caffeine addiction, 1131
in childhood, 1097-1100
chronic pain disorders, 1136-37
compulsive gambling, 1130
conversion disorder, 1135
dependence on barbiturates, 1131-32
dependence on benzodiazepines, 1132
dependence on cannabis compounds,
1134
dependence on central nervous system
depressants, 1131-32
dependence on central nervous system
stimulants, 1132-33
dependence on glue, 1131
dependence on hallucinogens, 1134
dependence on marijuana, 342-43, 1134
dependence on opioids, 1133
dependent personality disorder, 1108
depression and mood disorders, 1122-27
depression in elderly, 243-44, 1103-4
developmental, 1096-1137
drug abuse, 1102-3
drug dependence, 1131-34
drug-induced psychosis, 1129
in elderly, 243-44, 1103-5
encopresis, 89, 1098-99
enuresis, 89, 1098
grieving, 1109-11
histrionic personality disorder, 1107
hyperventilation in, 1119
hypochondriasis, 1135-36
infantile autism, 1100
insomnia, 1112-14
knot in stomach, 1118
major depressive disorder, 1123-25
manic-depressive illness, 1125-26
MMPI (Minnesota Multiphasic
Personality Inventory) in, 1137
narcissistic personality disorder, 1107-8
narcolepsy, 1114-15
night terrors, 1116
nightmares, 1116
obesity as, 1099
obsessive-compulsive disorders,
1108-9, 1121
panic attacks, 151, 1119
paranoid personality disorder, 1105
paranoid reactions in elderly, 1104
passive-aggressive personality disorder,
1109
personality-related, 1105-9
phobias, 91-92, 133-34, 1119-20
post-traumatic stress disorder, 1121-22
Prozac and, 1123
psychosomatic illness, 1135-37
psychotherapy for, 334, 1096, 1107,
1124, 1227
restless legs, 1115-16
retardation, 108-9, 1099-1100, 1328
schizoid personality disorder, 1105-6
schizophrenia, 1127-28
schizotypal personality disorder, 1106
seasonal affective disorder, 1126-27
situational depression, 1122-23
sleep apnea, 1114
sleep clinics for, 1115
sleepwalking, 1116-17
somatization disorder, 1135
teenage pregnancy, 147-48
teenage suicide, 154-55, 1101
thought disorders, 1127-29
victims of violence, 1103

warning signs of potential suicide in, 1125

see also anxiety, anxiety disorders; learning problems; sleep disorders

mental retardation, 1099-1100
group homes and, 1328
in preschool children, 108-9

mental status, 460

mentally ill, group homes for, 1328

mesangial proliferative glomerulonephritis, 838

metabolic disorders in newborns, 8-9, 13

metabolism, nutrition and, 257-58

metatarsalgia, 889

metered-dose inhalers (MDIs), 1046

methyl mercury, 270

methyltestosterone, 186

Metropolitan Life Insurance Company, 258

Michigan Alcoholism Screening Test, 330

microbiologic tests, 1345-46
cerebrospinal fluid analyses, 1345-46
synovial fluid analyses, 1345
throat cultures, 678, 1345

microphthalmia, 35

microwave ovens, safety of, 354

midcycle pelvic pain, 1188

middle years, 219-30
arthritis in, 226-27
baldness in, 227
bones in, 226
cardiovascular system in, 225
depression in, 223-24
digestive system in, 225-26
divorce in, 221
drug and alcohol abuse in, 221
family life in, 220-22
hair in, 227
joints in, 226-27
life in, 220-24
loss of parents in, 221
loss of spouse in, 221-22
meaning of, 220
menopause in, 228
midlife crisis in, 224
night jobs in, 222
osteoporosis in, 226
parenting in, 220-21
physical aging in, 224-30
planning for retirement in, 222-23
sexual changes in, 228-30
skin in, 227-28
suicides in, 223
women in, 228-30
work in, 222

migraine headaches, 120, 432-33, 502-4
acute, 503-4
in teenagers, 159

milia, 15, 69, C-2

milk and milk products, 262, 266
examples of servings of, 262
for preschool children, 113
for school-age children, 122

milk ducts, blocked, 216

mind-altering drugs, 430-31

minerals, 255, 284-85
for infants, 80
for newborns, 39
for nutrition and weight control in pregnancy, 183-84
organic vs. synthetic, 284-85

Minnesota Multiphasic Personality Inventory (MMPI), 1137

miscarriages, 197-98

mitral balloon valvuloplasty, 681

mitral valve problems, 680-82
complications from, 681
regurgitation, 680
stenosis, 680

mitral valve prolapse, 682

mittelschmerz, 1148

MMPI (Minnesota Multiphasic Personality Inventory), 1137

mobility, impairment of, 239-40

modified radical mastectomies, 1166, B-4

mold, respiratory allergies to, 1042-44

moldy food, proper handling of, 273

moles, 1003, C-5

molluscum contagiosum, 1012, C-13

Monday fever, 731-33

monoclonal antibodies, 1299, 1337-38

monoclonal gammopathy of undetermined significance, 973

monocytic leukemia, 965-66

mononucleosis, infectious, 158-59, 1064-65

monosodium glutamate (MSG), 1049

mons pubis, 1140

mood disorders, 1122-27
major depressive, 1123-25
manic-depressive illness, 1125-26
Prozac and, 1123
seasonal affective, 1126-27
situational, 1122-23
see also depression

morning sickness, 187, 197

Moro reflex, 33

morphine, 1133

Morton's neuroma, 890

motility agents, 1280

motility studies, esophageal, 746

motor development:
in infants, 7-8, 61-62
in newborns, 7-8

motor vehicle exhaust, air pollution from, 373

Motor Vehicle Safety Standards, Federal, 24

mountain bicycles, 299

mountain sickness, 417-18

mouth, infections and diseases of, 617-22, C-10
acute glossitis, 619
canker sores, 617, 1010-11, C-10
developmental, 614-17
discolored tongue, 621
geographic tongue, 620
gingivostomatitis, 618
hairy tongue, 620-21, C-10
halitosis, 620
leukoplakia, 618-19, C-10
oral cancer, 621-22, 1295
oral lichen planus, 619, C-10
oral thrush, 618, C-10
tongue disorders, 619-21

mouth-to-mouth resuscitation, obstructed airways in, 408

MRI (magnetic resonance imaging), 1334
of head, 494

MS (multiple sclerosis), 475-77

MSG (monosodium glutamate), 1049

mucothermal method of contraception, 171

MUGA scans, 1339-40

mullerian agenesis, 1169

multicystic dysplasia, 829

multifactorial inheritance, 43

multiple drug use, 245
abuse in, 340
hazards of, 1277

multiple myeloma, 973-74

multiple pregnancies, 213

multiple sclerosis (MS), 475-77

mumps, 1077-78, C-1
vaccination against, 1079

murmurs, 16, 634

muscle relaxants, 1280

muscle relaxation techniques, 504

muscles, 862-63, A-2-3

muscles, disorders of:
in back strains and spasms, 900-4
baseball finger, 874
cancer, 888
cramps, 871-72
fibromyalgia, 883
muscle spasms, 871-72
muscular dystrophy, 888
neck pain, 871
pulls, 868-69
strains, 868-69, 900-4
thigh bruises, 872
tumors, 888

muscles, tone of, 460

muscular dystrophy, Duchenne's, 888

musculoskeletal system, 861-63

musculoskeletal system, disorders of:
absence or loss of limbs, 450-51, 879-80
Achilles tendinitis, 874
acute painful shoulder, 917
allergic angiitis, 921
ankylosing spondylitis, 913, 914
arthritis at base of thumb, 885-86
arthritis of inflammatory bowel disease, 913
arthroscopy for, 878
back muscle strains and spasms, 900-4
Baker's cyst, 909
baseball finger, 874
bone disorders, *see* bones, disorders of
bone tumors, 899
bunions, 891-92
burning feet, 890
bursitis, 917-18
calluses, 890-91
carpal tunnel syndrome, 884-85
of childhood, 912
chondromalacia, 876
clubfoot, 46, 912
common problems, 863-79
congenital, 46
congenital dislocation of hip, 46, 912
corns, 890-91
corticosteroid drugs for, 919
costochondritis, 434, 883-84
cranial arteritis, 565-66, 921
dermatomyositis, 920-21
Dupuytren's contracture, 886-87
dwarfism, 46
fibromyalgia, 883
fibrous dysplasia, 898
flatfeet, 95-96, 892
foot ulcers, 893-94
ganglion, 886
gigantism and, 898
gonococcal arthritis, 915
gout, 437, 916, 1280
granulomatosis, 921
hammer toe, 892-93
heel pain, 874-76

hyperparathyroidism and, 898
hypersensitivity vasculitis, 921
hypopituitarism and, 898
immunologic, *see* immunologic
    rheumatic disorders
infectious arthritis, 915
inflammatory arthritis, 913-14
ingrown toenails, 893, 1022
joint replacement in, 911
juvenile rheumatoid arthritis, 911-13
knee injuries, 876-77
knee pain, 876
knee swelling, 877
Legg-Calvé-Perthes disease, 912
loose bodies in knees, 877
lumbar stenosis, 906
Lyme disease, 396, 915, 1067, C-14
mallet toe, 892-93
meniscal tears in knees, 876
metatarsalgia, 889
Morton's neuroma, 890
muscle cramps, 871-72
muscle strains, 868-69, 900-4
muscle tumors, 888
muscular dystrophy, 888
myelomeningocele, 514
neck pain, 871
nursemaid's dislocation, 866
Osgood-Schlatter disease, 159, 912
osteoarthritis, 509, 906, 907-9, B-1
osteomalacia, 896-97
osteomyelitis, 899
osteoporosis, *see* osteoporosis
Paget's disease of bone, 897-98
polyarteritis, 921
polymyalgia rheumatica, 922
polymyositis, 920-21
problems of feet, 889-94
prolapsed discs, 904-6
psoriatic arthritis, 913
pulled muscles, 868-69
reflex sympathetic dystrophy syn-
    drome, 887
Reiter's syndrome, 913-14
rheumatic fever arthritis, 915
rheumatoid arthritis, 909-11
rickets, 833, 896-97
runner's knee, 873
sciatica, 905, B-1
scleroderma, 771, 919-20
scoliosis, 159, 906-7
severed tendons, 867-68
shin splints, 870-71
Sjögren's syndrome, 920
slipped capital femoral epiphysis, 912
spinal cord disorders, *see* spinal cord,
    disorders of
spondylosis, 906
sports injuries, 160, 302-4, 867, 870
sprains, 449, 869-70
staphylococcal arthritis, 915
syringomyelia, 514
systemic lupus erythematosus, 918-19
tendinitis, 882-83
tennis elbow, 872-73
tenosynovitis, 881-82
thigh bruises, 872
tired feet, 892
tuberculous arthritis, 915
tumors, 899
vasculitis, 921
viral arthritis, 915

see also dislocations; fractures; joints,
    disorders of
mushroom picker's disease, 731
myalgias, tension, 883
myasthenia gravis, 479-81
myelocytic leukemia, 965-66
myelofibrosis, idiopathic, 972-73
myelogenic leukemia, 965-66
myelogenous leukemia:
    acute, 965-66
    chronic, 964-65
myelography, 510, 1341
myelomeningocele, 514
myocardial infarctions, *see* heart attacks
myocardial perfusion imaging, 1339
myocarditis, 687
myomas, 1182
myopia (nearsightedness), 523-25
    corrective lenses for, 525
myxedema coma, 948, 949

N

nabothian cysts, 1179
nails, 1021-23, C-7
    healthy, 985
    proper care of, 1023
    trimming of, 25
nails, disorders of, 1021-23
    deformation, 1023
    discoloration, 1023
    fungal infections, 1022-23
    ingrown toenails, 893, 1022
    leukonychia, C-7
    paronychia, 1021-22, C-7
naps, 1116
narcissistic personality disorder, 1107-8
narcolepsy, 1114-15
narcotics, 1278
    abuse of, 346
    intoxication from, 431
    in labor and delivery, 211
nasal obstruction, 588
nasal polyps, 1041-42
nasal septum, dislocation of, 22
nasolacrimal duct, congenital obstruction
    of, 50-51
National Cancer Institute (NCI), 280-81,
    1301-3
National Cholesterol Program, 284, 639
National Hospice Organization, 1307
National Institute of Drug Abuse, 340
National Institutes of Health, 933
NCI (National Cancer Institute), 280-81,
    1301-3
nearsightedness (myopia), 523-25
    corrective lenses for, 525
neck pain, 871
necrotizing subcutaneous infection, 1016
necrotizing ulcerative gingivitis, 612-13
neonatal genetic disorders, *see* genetic
    disorders
neonatal jaundice, 13-14
nephritis, acute interstitial, 836
nephropathy:
    acute uric acid, 835
    analgesic, 835
    diabetic, 838-39, 930
    IgA, 838
    lead, 835
    from solvents and fuels, 835
nephrotic syndrome, 840-41

congenital, 833
nephrotoxic agents, 853
nervous breakdowns, 1096
nervous system, *see* brain and nervous sys-
    tem
neuralgias, 514-15
    trigeminal, 515-16
neuritis, optic, 560
neuroblastomas, 493
neurodermatitis, 988-89, C-3
neurologic examinations, 460
neurologists, 460
neuromas:
    acoustic, 584
    Morton's, 890
neurons, 458
neuropathies:
    diabetic, 930
    optic, 560
    peripheral, 509-11
neurosis, hysterical, 1135
neurosurgeons, 460
neutropenia, 974
nevi, pigmented (moles), 1003, C-5
newborn intensive care units, for premature
    babies, 18
newborns, 4-58
    abnormal feet in, 45-46
    ambiguous genitals in, 49
    aortic stenosis in, 53
    Apgar score of, 6
    appetite of, 10, 14
    atonic cerebral palsy in, 55
    atrial septal defect in, 52
    bathing of, 27-28
    behavior in, 36-37
    biliary atresia in, 56
    birth injuries to, 21-22
    birthmarks in, 15-16
    blindness in, 35-36
    blink reflex in, 4, 34
    bonding in, 6, 31-32
    bottle-feeding for, 39-40
    bowel movements of, 7-8
    breastfeeding of, 6, 39-41
    breathing difficulties in, 5, 6, 9, 19-21
    bronchopulmonary dysplasia in, 20
    calories for, 38
    campylodactyly in, 45
    caput succedaneum in, 21
    car seats for, 23-24
    cataracts in, 35
    central nervous system disorders in,
        53-55
    cephalhematomas in, 21
    cerebral palsy in, 54-55
    circumcision of, 7
    cleft lip and cleft palate in, 51
    clitoral enlargement in, 49
    clothing for, 23
    clubfoot in, 46, 912
    clubhand in, 45
    coarctation of aorta in, 52
    colic in, 11-12
    common concerns about, 9-17
    congenital adrenal hyperplasia in, 9,
        941, 1169
    congenital dislocation of hip in, 46
    congenital disorders of skeleton in, 46
    congenital gastrointestinal tract dis-
        orders in, 55-58
    congenital heart disorders in, 51-53

congenital lobar emphysema in, 58
congenital obstruction of nasolacrimal
    duct in, 50-51
constipation in, 13
cradle cap in, 14, 68
cribs for, 28
crying of, 5, 7, 8, 9, 11-12
    after delivery, 5-6
    of diabetic mothers, 21
diaper rash in, 14
diapers for, 28-29
diaphragmatic hernias in, 57-58
diarrhea in, 10, 13
dislocation of nasal septum in, 21
Down syndrome in, 44
drinking water for, 38-39
drug withdrawal in, 22
dwarfism in, 46
emotional needs of, 36
enlarged breasts in, 50
Epstein pearls in, 50
erythema toxicum in, 16
esophageal atresia in, 56
excessive crying by, 9, 11-12
exposure of, to sun and wind, 24-25
extrapyramidal cerebral palsy in, 55
extra toes in, 46
extremities of, 10
eyes and ears of, 5, 25
facial nerve palsies in, 22
feeding of, 7, 39-42
fevers in, 9, 10-11, 424
fingernails of, 25
in first month of life, 4-5
fontanelles of, 26
fractured collarbones in, 22
gag reflex in, 34
galactosemia in, 8
gastroschisis in, 58
general care of, 22-30
genetic disorders in, 42-51
growth and development of, 7-8
hair of, 5
head of, 5, 7, 26
healthy, 5-9
hearing in, 7, 34-35
heart murmurs in, 16
hemangiomas in, 15-16
Hirschsprung's disease in, 57
hydrocele in, 49
hydrocephalus in, 54
hypospadias in, 48-49
hypothyroidism in, 9
imperforate anus in, 57
infant carriers for, 24
infantile eczema in, 14-15, 989, 1038, C-2
innocent heart murmurs in, 16
intensive care units for, 18
intestinal atresia in, 57
in-toeing in, 45
jaundice in, 10, 13-14
language of, 7
lethargy in, 10
limited abilities of, 4
loose stools in, 13
metabolic disorders in, 8-9, 13
milia in, 15
Moro reflex in, 33
nutrition in, 38-42
omphalocele in, 58
orienting response in, 34
out-toeing in, 45

pacifiers for, 24
palmar grasp in, 33
paraphimosis in, 47
patent ductus arteriosus in, 52
pectus excavatum in, 46-47
personality and behavior in, 30-37
phenylketonuria in, 8
phimosis in, 47
physical appearance of, 5
PKU screening of, 8
plantar reflex in, 33
pneumothorax in, 20-21
polydactyly in, 45
posture and motor capabilities of, 7-8
premature, 17-19
preventing disease in, 29-30
pulmonary stenosis in, 53
pyloric stenosis in, 55-56
reflexes of, 4, 19, 32-34
required screening for, 8-9
respiratory distress syndrome in, 19-20
responses in, 32-34
rooting reflex in, 33
salmon patches (stork bites) in, 15
sexual organs of, 47-49
signs and symptoms of illness in, 8,
    9-17
size of, 5
skin of, 5, 25
sleeping of, 8
sleeping problems in, 36, 37
spastic cerebral palsy in, 55
special concerns about, 17-22
spina bifida occulta in, 53-54
spitting up by, 12-13
spoiling of, 36
sucking reflex of, 33
supernumerary nipples in, 49-50
supernumerary teeth in, 50
syndactyly of fingers in, 45
syndactyly of toes in, 45-46
taking rectal temperature of, 10
tetralogy of Fallot in, 53
thrush in, 16
tonic neck reflex in, 33
toys for, 26-27
transient tachypnea in, 20
transposition of great vessels in, 53
trimming nails of, 25
twinship in, 33
umbilical hernias in, 17
umbilicus of, 30
undescended testes in, 47-48
vaginal bleeding in, 49
vaginal discharge in, 49
ventricular septal defect in, 52
vernix on, 5, 178
vision of, 7, 35-36
vomiting by, 10, 12-13
weights of, 5, 6, 14
    see also babies, healthy; infants
newspapers, health in, 1270
nickel dermatitis, C-3
Nicorette, 323
nicotine, addiction to, 316
    see also smoking
nicotine gum, 323
nicotine polacrilex, 323
nicotinic acid, 642
NIDDM (non-insulin-dependent diabetes
    mellitus), 926-27
night blindness, 561-62

night jobs, 222
night terrors, 1116
night vision, problems in, 239
nightmares, 1116
nipple problems, 1161-62
    cracking, 216
    soreness, 39
    supernumerary, 49-50
    yeast infections, 1161
nitrates, 1280
    in drinking water, 372
    in treating heart attacks, 664
nodular melanomas, C-6
nodules, singer's, 596
noise:
    ear disorders and, 573
    protection from, 358
nonfunctioning pituitary tumors, 943
non-Hodgkin's lymphomas, 970-71
nonlymphocytic leukemia, acute, 965-66
nonspecific urethritis, 1174-75
nonspecific vaginitis, 1173-74
nontropical sprue, 770-71
Norwalk virus, 767
nose:
    anatomy of, 569
    foreign bodies in, 427
    fractures of, 427
nose drops:
    addiction to, 587
    administration of, 1275
nose and sinuses, disorders of, 403, 586-92
    juvenile angiofibromas, 589
    loss of sense of smell, 589-90
    nasal obstruction, 588
    postnasal drip, 590
    rhinophyma, 589
    running nose, 589
    sick sinus syndrome, 670
    sinusitis, 590-91
nosebleeds, 403, 586-87
    cautery for, 587
    emergency treatment of, 403
nuclear scans, see radionuclide scans
nuclear sclerosis, 554
nummular dermatitis, C-15
nursemaid's dislocation, 866
nurses, 1243-44
    licensed practical, 1243
    pediatric, 5
    registered, 1243-44
nursing, see breastfeeding
nursing homes, 1255
    cost of, 248
    selection of, 247-48
nutrition:
    for acute kidney failure, 854
    Addison's disease and, 939
    alcoholism and, 286
    amyloidosis and, 975
    antioxidants and, 265-66
    balanced diet in, 113
    basic components of food in, 253-56
    body composition and, 256-57
    in bottle-feeding, 39-40
    in breastfeeding, 39-41
    calories in, see calories
    cancer and, 280-83, 373, 1294, 1303
    carbohydrates in, see carbohydrates
    and changing body composition, 257
    chronic kidney failure and, 854-55
    Crohn's disease and, 776

for diabetes insipidus, 945
diabetes mellitus and, 284-85, 932
drinking water in, 274-75
for elderly, 241
fats in, *see* fats
feeding problems and, *see* feeding
problems
feeding recommendations for, 78-79
folic acid anemia and, 960
Food Guide Pyramid in, 183, 261-62
fruits and vegetables in, 113, 122, 261,
262
gout and, 916
grains in, 113, 261, 262, 288
growth disorders related to, 83
health and, 251-88
hyperthyroidism and, 948
hypothyroidism and, 949-50
in infants, 78-80
for kidney stones, 845
lactation and, 215-16
lumps in breasts and, 1159
meats in, 113, 122, 262, 272
menopause and, 1154-55
metabolism and, 257-58
milk and dairy products in, 113, 122,
262, 266
minerals in, *see* minerals
in newborns, 38-42
non-Hodgkin's lymphomas and, 971
obesity and, *see* obesity
peptic ulcers and, 756
for PMS (premenstrual syndrome), 1147
in pregnancy, 182-85
in preschool children, 83, 112-14
protein in, *see* protein
in school-age children, 121-24
in school lunches, 123
sports and, 274-76
in teenagers, 140-41
ulcerative colitis and, 779
U.S. government guidelines for, 258-62
vitamins in, *see* vitamins
see also diets; food
nutrition services, 247
nystagmus, 36

O

obesity, 83, 1099
contributors to, 123-24
exercise programs for, 296
in heart and blood vessel disorders, 643
Heimlich maneuver and, 407
heredity as cause of, 124, 288
physical inactivity as cause of, 123-24
in preschool children, 113-14
in school-age children, 123-24
obsessive-compulsive personality disorder, 1108-9, 1121, 1123
obstructed airways:
in choking children, 408
clearing of, 406-8
finger sweep for, 407
mouth-to-mouth resuscitation and, 408
recognition of, 406
in unconscious victims, 408
obstructive pulmonary disease, chronic
(COPD), 714, 715-20
occiput anterior, 209
occiput posterior, 210
occupational asthma, 731

occupational hearing loss, 572-74
occupationally related lung disease, 728-34
allergic alveolitis, 731
asbestosis, 728-30
byssinosis, 731-33
farmer's lung, 733
from fumes, smoke, and gases, 732
industrial bronchitis, 733
occupational asthma, 731
pneumoconiosis, 730-31
silicosis, 730-31
silo-filler's disease, 733-34
Occupational Safety and Health
Administration (OSHA), 375
occupational therapists, 1326-27
office-based practices, 1254
oils, 122
oligomenorrhea (infrequent periods), 1149-
50
Olympic Committee, U.S., 347
omphalocele, 58
onychomycosis, C-8
open-angle glaucoma, 551
open-heart surgery, 684
ophthalmologists, 522
ophthalmopathy, Graves', 563-64
ophthalmoscopes, 524
ophthalmoscopy, 1342
opiates:
abuse of, 344-45
dependence on, 1133
optic neuritis, 560
optic neuropathy, 560
opticians, 522
optometrists, 522
oral and maxillofacial surgeons, 604
oral cancer, 621-22
screening for, 1295
oral contraceptives, 166, 171-72, 1146
drug interactions with, 1146
side effects of, 1146
oral disorders, *see* dental and oral
disorders
oral hygiene, 617
oral hypoglycemic agents, 934-35
oral lichen planus, 619, C-10
oral surgery, heart valve disorders and,
679
oral thermometers, 424
oral thrush, 618, C-10
orbital cellulitis, 452-53, 545, C-11
orbital tumors, laser therapy for, 558
orchitis, 1201-2
organ donation, 688, 1315
organs, A-6
see also specific organs
orgasm, orgasm disorders, 1223-25,
1228-29
in men, 229, 1228-29
in women, 170, 228-29, 1223-25
orienting response, 34
orthodontic treatment, 615-17
making changes in, 616-17
oral hygiene after, 617
problem identification in, 615-16
orthodontists, 604
orthopedic disorders:
bowlegs, 97
flatfeet, 95-96, 892
knock-knees, 96-97
pigeon toe, 96
in preschool children, 95-97

Osgood-Schlatter disease, 159, 912
OSHA (Occupational Safety and Health
Administration), 375
osseointegration, 628
osteitis deformans, 897-98
osteoarthritis, 907-9, B-1, B-6
cervical, 509
of the spine, 906
osteomalacia, 896-97
osteomyelitis, 899
osteoporosis, 290, 894-96, B-1
calcium and, 266-67
exercise and, 895
during menopause, 1153-55
in middle years, 226
OTC (over-the-counter) drugs, prescription drugs vs., 1274
otitis, external, 570-71
otitis media:
acute, 574-75
chronic, 575-76
otosclerosis, 578-79
hearing aids and, 579
outpatient departments, 1254
outpatient surgery, 1262-63
out-toeing, 45
ovarian cancer, 1190-91
chemotherapy for, 1191
radiation therapy for, 1191
ovarian disorders, 1189-91
benign tumors, 1189-90
cysts, 436, 1189-90
menses and menstrual disorders
related to, 1156-57
polycystic ovarian syndrome, 1191
primary ovarian failure, 1155-56
ovaries, 167, 1140, 1143, 1215
overfeeding, 41, 80
Overseas Citizens' Emergency Center, 380
over-the-counter (OTC) drugs, prescription
drugs vs., 1274
ovulation, 167
oxygen supplies, 718
oxytocin, 941, 1162

P

pacemakers, 675
pacifiers, 24
Paget's disease of bone, 897-98
pain:
abrupt onset of, 432
anal, 798
in cancer, 1303-4
growing, 119-20
in heels, 874-76
in minor illnesses, 393
psychosomatic, 1135-37
recurrent abdominal, 120
vaginal, 1175
pain centers, chronic, 1136
pain disorders, chronic, 1136-37
pain emergencies, 432-37
abdominal pain, 120, 435-36
acute arterial occlusion, 437
acute ear pain, 433
appendicitis, 436
bowel obstruction, 436
chest pains, 433-35
cystitis, 436
dental abscesses, 433

diverticulitis, 436
in extremities, 436-37
gallstones, 435
gastroenteritis, 435
head pain, 432-33
heart attacks, 434
in joints, 437
kidney stones, 436
meningitis, 433
migraine headaches, 432-33
ovarian cysts, 436
pancreatitis, 435
in pelvis, *see* pelvic pain
perforated peptic ulcers, 435
pneumonia with pleurisy, 434-35
pulmonary embolisms, 434
pyelonephritis, 436
ruptured ectopic pregnancy, 436
from thrombophlebitis, 437
ureteral stones, 436
pain relief:
in labor and delivery, 211-12
see also analgesics
painful heel syndrome, 874-76
painful intercourse (dyspareunia), 170, 1188
painful menses (dysmenorrhea):
primary, 1148
secondary, 1148
in teenagers, 159
painful shoulder, acute, 917
painkillers, *see* analgesics
palmar grasp, 33
palsies:
Bell's, 493-95
cerebral, *see* cerebral palsy
of facial nerves, 22, 493-95
shaking, 472
third nerve, 563
pancreas, 741
pancreas divisum, 822
pancreatic diseases, 818-22, 925-36
acute pancreatitis, 818-19
annular pancreas, 822
arteriosclerosis in, 929-30
cancer, 820-21, 936
chronic pancreatitis, 819-20
congenital, 822
coronary artery disease in, 929-30
diabetes mellitus, *see* diabetes mellitus
gastrinomas, 757-58, 936
glucagonomas, 936
hyperosmolar coma, 423, 926, 929-30
hypertension in, 929-30
hypoglycemic coma, 926, 927-28
insulin reaction in, 927-28
insulinomas, 936
islet cell tumors, 757-58, 936
ketoacidosis, 423, 926, 928-29
pancreas divisum, 822
reactive hypoglycemia and, 929
tumors, 820-21, 936
vision problems in, 930
pancreatic ducts, X-rays of, 816, 1341
pancreatitis:
abdominal pain from, 435
acute, 818-19
chronic, 819-20
panic attacks, 1119
in teenagers, 151
Pap smears, 168, 1141, 1181, 1204, 1250
Papanicolaou, G. N., 1181
papillomas:

intraductal, 1163
juvenile, 597
in pregnancy, 193
on vocal cords, 597
paracervical block, 211
paralysis, pharyngeal, 747-48
paralysis agitans, 472
paranoid personality disorder, 1105
paranoid reactions, 1104
paraphimosis, 47, 1206
paraplegia, rehabilitation for, 508
parasitic agents, 1059-60
parasitic digestive system disorders, 768-69
parasitic infestations, 1080-84
ascariasis, 1083-84
hookworm, 1084
malaria, 382-83, 1080-81
pinworms, 1082-83
strongyloidosis, 1083
tapeworm, 1081-82
trichinosis, 1082
parathyroid disorders, 950-52
hyperparathyroidism, 898, 950-51
hypoparathyroidism, 951-52
parathyroid hormone, 950, 951
parents:
in bonding with newborns, 6, 31-32
of children with cancer, 1307-8
death of, 221, 1318
in managing behavior of newborns,
36-37
in middle years, 220-21
of teenage alcohol abusers, 332
and teenage sexuality, 146
young adults as, 162-63
Parents Anonymous, 110
Parkinson, James, 472
Parkinson's disease, 472-74
paronychia, 1021-22, C-7
parotitis, epidemic, *see* mumps
paroxysmal atrial tachycardia, 671-72
partners, sexual, *see* sexual partners, health
issues of
passive-aggressive personality disorder,
1109
patent ductus arteriosus, 52
pathologic fractures, 446
patients:
communication between physicians
and, 1247-49, 1258, 1272
expectations and responsibilities of,
1247-48
and families in hospice system, 1306
medications and, 1272-73
visits to hospital, 1259
pauciarticular juvenile rheumatoid arthritis,
911
PCBs (polychlorinated biphenyls), 269-70
PCP (phencyclidine), 344, 1129, 1134
peak flowmeters, 1045
pectus excavatum, 46-47
pediatric dentists, 604
pediatric nurse practitioners, 5
pediculosis pubis, 1173
peer relationships, 126
pelvic examinations, 168, 1141-42, 1250
pelvic fractures, 448-49
pelvic inflammatory disease (PID), 168-69,
1187-89
pelvic organs, support of:
in elderly women, 244
loss of, 1175-76

pelvic pain, 436
acute, 1187-88
in adenomyosis, 1188
chronic, 1188
in chronic salpingitis, 1188
in cystitis, 436
in dyspareunia, 1188
in early pregnancy, 1187
in ectopic pregnancy, 436, 1187
in endometriosis, 1188
episodic, 1188
from kidney stones, 436
midcycle, 1188
nongynecologic causes of, 1187-88
from ovarian cysts, 436
from pyelonephritis, 436
from ruptured ectopic pregnancy, 436
from ureteral stones, 436
pelvic pain syndrome, 1188
penicillin, 1279
penis, 164, 1196
penis, disorders of, 1206-7
balanitis, 1205-6
cancer, 1206-7
curvature, 1206, 1227-28
erection abnormalities, 1227-28
impotence, 229, 230, 1225-27
paraphimosis, 47, 1206
phimosis, 47
priapism, 1206, 1228
warts, 1204
peptic ulcers, 753-57
hyperparathyroidism and, 951
nutrition and, 756
perforated, 435
upper gastrointestinal endoscopy for,
760-61
peptides, 1337
Perceived Exertion Scale, 295, 646
percutaneous transhepatic cholangiography
(PTHC), 815
percutaneous transluminal coronary
angioplasty (PTCA), 666
percutaneous umbilical cord sampling, 181
periarthritis of the shoulder, 917
pericarditis, 687-89
acute, 689
constrictive, 689
pericardium, diseases of, 686, 687-89
acute pericarditis, 689
cardiac tamponade, 689
constrictive pericarditis, 689
periodontal disease, 364-65, 609-13
gingivitis, 364-65, 610-11, 612-13
periodontitis, 611-12
prevention of, 613
trench mouth, 612-13
periodontists, 604
periods, *see* menses and menstrual disorders
perioral dermatitis, C-15
peripheral nervous system, 459
peripheral nervous system, disorders of,
506, 509-16
Charcot-Marie-Tooth disease, 513-14
Guillain-Barré syndrome, 513
neuralgias, 514-15
peripheral neuropathies, 509-11
peritoneal dialysis, 857
peritonitis, 792
spontaneous bacterial, 808
peritonsillar abscesses, 595

pernicious anemia, 958-59
personality, 1095
    sudden changes in, 430
    suicide potential in, 1125
    see also psychosocial development of
        personality and behavior
personality disorders, 1105-9
    antisocial, 1106
    avoidant, 1108
    borderline, 1106-7
    dependent, 1108
    histrionic, 1107
    narcissistic, 1107-8
    obsessive-compulsive, 1108-9, 1121
    paranoid, 1105
    passive-aggressive, 1109
    schizoid, 1105-6
    schizotypal, 1106
Perthes' disease, 912
pertussis (whooping cough), 1075
    vaccination against, 382, 1079
pervasive developmental disorder, 108, 1100
pesticides:
    farm safety and, 360
    food contaminated with, 268
petit mal seizures, 497
pets, allergies to, 1035, 1042-44
PET (positron emission tomography) scans,
    1338
Peyronie's disease, 1206, 1227-28
pharyngeal diverticula, 746-47
pharyngeal paralysis, 747-48
pharyngitis, 592-94
phencyclidine (PCP), 344, 1129, 1134
phenothiazines, 1280
phenylketonuria (PKU), 8
pheochromocytomas, 939
phimosis, 47
phlebitis, 694-95
phobias, 1119-20
    in preschool children, 91-92
    school, 133-34
photosensitivity, 998
phototherapy:
    for neonatal jaundice, 13
    for psoriasis, 993
physical abuse, 1231-33
physical examinations, see checkups
physical inactivity, obesity due to, 123-24
physical therapy:
    for backaches, 904
    getting most from visit to, 1246
    in rehabilitation for chronic neurologic
        problems, 480
    for spinal stenosis, 517
    see also exercise
physicians, 1245-47
    in cancer treatment, 1299-1300
    changing, 1249
    communication between patients and,
        1247-49, 1258, 1272
    and expectations and responsibilities of
        patients, 1247-48
    medical examinations by, see checkups
    medications and, 1272-73
    personal, 1245-47, 1299-1300
    prenatal care and, 178-79
    second opinions from, 1247
    selection of, 1246, 1299-1300
    ten questions for, 1258
    training of, 1241-43
    travel and, 280

in treating allergies, 1032-34
pica, 90
picnics, food safety at, 269
PID (pelvic inflammatory disease), 168-69,
    1187-89
pigeon toe, 96
pigmentary changes, 190, 994-95, C-7
pigmented nevi (moles), 1003, C-5
piles, see hemorrhoids
pill-box strategy, 244-45
pill-induced esophagitis, 745
pills, administration of, 1274-75
pimples, see acne
pinkeye, see conjunctivitis
pinworms, 1082-83
pipe smoke:
    emphysema and, 719
    see also smoking
pituitary adenomas, 943
pituitary gland disorders, 941-45
    diabetes insipidus, 944-45
    hypopituitarism, 898, 943-44
    menses and menstrual disorders
        related to, 1156-57
pituitary gland tumors, 942-44
    acromegaly caused by, 898, 942
    gigantism caused by, 898, 942
    nonfunctioning pituitary tumors, 943
    prolactinomas, 942-43, 1163
pityriasis rosea, 993, C-15
PKU (phenylketonuria), 8
placenta, retained, 214
placenta previa, 205-6
plague vaccination, 383
plantar reflex, 33
plantar warts, 1004
plants, poisonous, 440
plaque formation:
    in blood vessels, 467
    on teeth, 367
plasma, 955
    fresh-frozen, 980
plastic surgery, see cosmetic surgery
platelets (thrombocytes), 955
    aspirin and, 663
    transfusions of, 981
play, safety for children at, 99-100, 353
plethysmography, impedance, 1342-43
pleurisy, pneumonia with, 434-35, 711
Plummer's disease, 947
PMS (premenstrual syndrome), 1147
    exercise for, 1147
    nutrition for, 1147
pneumococcal pneumonia vaccination,
    226, 382
pneumoconiosis, 730-31
pneumonia, 704-5
    aspiration, 704
    community-acquired, 704
    hospital-acquired, 704
    with pleurisy, 434-35, 711
    vaccination against, 382, 1080
pneumothorax, 723-24
    in newborns, 20-21
Poison Control Centers, 438
poisoning, 437-41
    from acids and alkalis, 439
    botulism, 268-69, 441, 488-89
    from Clostridium perfringens, 268
    from CO (carbon monoxide), 376, 419
    from contaminated fish, 269-70
    emergency treatment of, 437-41

from food, 267-70, 440-41, 488-89, 769
gastroenteritis in, 440-41
hepatitis A from, 269
labels for, 352
lead, 71
from medications, 439-40
from plants, 440
in preschool children, 99-100
prevention of, 351-52
recognition of, 438
from Salmonella, 268, 767-68
from Staphylococcus aureus, 268
traveler's diarrhea and, 269
poison ivy, 987, 1035, 1036, C-3
poison oak, 1035, 1036
poison sumac, 1035, 1036
poisonous stings, first aid for, 397-98
poliomyelitis, 485-86
    post-polio syndrome after, 487
    vaccination against, 382, 1079
pollen, respiratory allergies to, 1042
pollution:
    of air, 373-75, 726, 732
    from chlorofluorocarbons, 373-74
    from cigarette smoke, 374
    from formaldehyde, 374
    from household products, 374
    indoor, 374-75
    from industrial and power plants, 373
    from lawn chemicals, 375
    from motor vehicle exhaust, 373
    taking action on, 375
    of water, 372
polyarteritis, 921
polyarticular juvenile rheumatoid arthritis,
    911
polychlorinated biphenyls (PCBs), 269-70
polycystic kidney disease, 831-32
polycystic ovarian syndrome, 1191
polycythemia vera, 971-72
polydactyly, 45
polymyalgia rheumatica, 922
polymyositis, 920-21
polyps:
    cervical, 1178-79
    in colon, 786-89, 797
    endometrial, 1182
    nasal, 1041-42
    in rectum, 797
    on vocal cords, 596
popliteal bursitis, 909
popliteal cysts, 876
pork, proper handling of, 272
porphyrias, 961
portal hypertension, 807
Portuguese man-of-war stings, 398-99,
    1015-16, C-13
port-wine stains, 16, C-2
positron emission tomography (PET)
    scans, 1338
postmaturity (prolonged pregnancy), 206
postmenopausal bleeding, 1155
postnasal drip, 590
postoperative recovery, 1262
postpartum bleeding, 214
postpartum depression, 216-18
postpartum psychosis, 217-18
post-polio syndrome, 487
post-traumatic stress disorder, 218, 1121-22
postural drainage, 709
postural hypotension, 650
posture:

in exercise, 303
of healthy babies, 7, 61-62
importance of, 902-3
of newborns, 7
poor, 902
proper, 902
poultry, proper handling of, 272
power plants, air pollution from, 373-74
powers of attorney for health care, durable, 1249, 1383, 1385-86
PPOs (preferred provider organizations), 1267
pravastatin, 642
precocity, sexual, 135
prednisone, 944
preeclampsia, 204-5
preferred provider organizations (PPOs), 1267
pregnancy:
    abnormal fetal positions in, 209-10
    age as risk factor in, 194
    AIDS in, 193
    alcohol as risk factor in, 195
    alcohol consumption in, 195, 328
    alpha-fetoprotein analysis in, 180-81
    anemia in, 188
    antepartum hemorrhage in, 205
    asthma in, 190
    baby blues after, 216-17
    backaches in, 187-88
    bleeding in, 178
    breast problems after, 216
    breastfeeding after, 215-16
    breastfeeding to prevent, 1156, 1162
    caffeine and, 185, 186, 194
    cesarean sections and, 212-13
    chickenpox in, 191
    chlamydial infections in, 193
    chorionic villus sampling in, 181
    common discomforts in, 186-89
    concerns after, 214-18
    concerns in, 175-96
    constipation in, 187
    contraception after, 218
    cytomegalovirus in, 193
    diabetes in, 21, 189
    diet as risk factor in, 194
    drug abuse in, 336
    eclampsia in, 204-5
    ectopic, 199-200, 436, 1187
    edema in, 189
    endometriosis in, 1186
    epilepsy in, 190
    exercise and, 195-96, 296
    false labor in, 208
    fertilization in, 176
    first trimester of, 177, 196-200
    genetic amniocentesis in, 181
    genital herpes in, 191
    German measles in, 191
    gonorrhea in, 193
    group B streptococci in, 193
    heart disorders in, 190
    heartburn in, 187
    Heimlich maneuver in, 407
    hemorrhoids in, 188
    hepatitis B in, 192-93
    hot tubs and, 195
    hydramnios in, 202-3
    hypertension in, 189-90
    illegal drugs in, 195
    incompetent cervix in, 203

infectious diseases in, 191-93
    intrauterine death in, 206
    intrauterine growth retardation in, 179
    labor and delivery in, 207-14
    medical problems of, 189-90
    medications in, 185-86
    morning sickness in, 187, 197
    with multiple fetuses, 213
    nutrition and weight control in, 182-85
    office Doppler and, 179-80
    papillomas in, 193
    pelvic pain early in, 1187
    percutaneous umbilical cord sampling in, 181
    pigmentation changes in, 190
    placenta previa in, 205-6
    postmaturity in, 206
    postpartum depression after, 216-18
    postpartum hemorrhage and, 214
    postpartum psychosis after, 217-18
    post-traumatic stress disorder after, 218
    preeclampsia in, 204-5
    premature labor in, 201-2
    premature rupture of membranes in, 205
    prenatal care for, 178-79
    prenatal development in, 177-78
    prenatal testing in, 179-82
    preparation for, 175
    prevention of, see contraception
    prolonged, 206
    prolonged labor and, 208
    pruritus in, 190
    radiation as risk factor in, 194
    retained placenta and, 214
    Rh incompatibility as risk factor in, 192
    risk factors and, 194-95
    second trimester of, 177-78, 200-203
    seizure disorders in, 190
    sex after, 217
    skin problems in, 190
    sleeping problems in, 188
    smoking in, 194-95, 320
    STDs (sexually transmitted diseases) in, 193
    syphilis in, 193
    of teenagers, 147-48, 194
    termination of, 199
    tests for, 198
    third trimester of, 178, 203-6
    toxoplasmosis in, 191
    travel in, 196
    with twins, 213
    ultrasonography in, 180, 1335
    varicose veins in, 188
premature babies, 17-19
    gestational ages of, 17-19
    newborn intensive-care units for, 18
    respiratory distress syndrome in, 19-20
    retinopathy in, 35
    size of, 19
premature ejaculation, 1228-29
premature labor, 201-2
premature puberty, 135
premature rupture of membranes, 205
premenstrual syndrome (PMS), 1147
    exercise for, 1147
    nutrition for, 1147
prenatal care, 178-79
prenatal development, 177-78
    in first trimester, 177
    in second trimester, 177-78

in third trimester, 178
prenatal tests, 179-82
    alpha-fetoprotein analysis, 180-81
    chorionic villus sampling, 181
    electronic fetal nonstress and stress, 182
    genetic amniocentesis, 181
    office Doppler, 179-80
    percutaneous umbilical cord sampling, 181
    ultrasound, 180, 1335
presbycusis, 579-81
presbyopia, 526-27
preschool children, 81-114
    abuse of, 110
    amblyopia in, 90
    balanced diet for, 113
    behavioral development in, 103-4
    bowlegs in, 97
    breathing changes in, 85
    brushing teeth of, 101
    burns and, 99
    car safety for, 100
    caring for teeth of, 101
    central auditory disorders in, 107
    choking by, 100
    chronic diseases in, 83
    common concerns about, 84-87
    common and recurrent colds in, 86-87
    conductive hearing loss in, 107
    constipation in, 87
    day-care centers for, 101-2
    decreased appetite of, 85
    delayed psychomotor development in, 106
    dentists for, 101
    diaper care for, 98
    diarrhea in, 85, 87-88
    diet for teeth of, 101
    drowning and, 99
    encopresis in, 89
    enuresis in, 89
    falls by, 92, 100
    fears and phobias of, 91-92
    fevers of, 85
    fighting by, 105
    finger sucking by, 106
    flatfeet of, 95-96
    fluoride for teeth of, 101
    general care for, 97-102
    growth disorders in, 83
    handicapped, 110-12
    hearing disorders in, 106-7
    hormonal disorders in, 83
    imagination of, 105
    knock-knees of, 96-97
    learning problems in, 106-8
    lethargy in, 85
    mental retardation in, 108-9
    mixed hearing loss in, 107
    negativism in, 104-5
    normal growth and development of, 82-84
    nutrition in, 83, 112-14
    nutritional deficiencies in, 83
    obesity of, 113-14
    orthopedic concerns and, 95-97
    personality and behavior in, 102-10
    pigeon toe in, 96
    poisoning in, 99-100
    preventing spread of disease to, 98
    quarrels of, 105
    rapid changes in, 82

safety at home and play for, 99-100
sensorineural hearing loss in, 107
sexual abuse of, 109-10
sexuality of, 109
sibling problems of, 105-6
signs of illness in, 84-86
sleep problems of, 90-91
speech and language development in, 92-94
speech and language disorders of, 107
strabismus in, 90
stuttering in, 93
tantrum throwing and breath holding by, 92
teething problems of, 89-90
thumb sucking by, 106
toilet training for, 88-89
toys shared by, 105-6
urinary tract infections in, 94-95
vision problems of, 90, 107-8
vomiting by, 85-86
walking by, 92
prescription drugs, OTC drugs vs., 1274
presurgical evaluations, 1260
priapism, 1206, 1228
prickly heat rash, 988, C-3
primary dysmenorrhea, 1148
primary health-care centers, 1255
primary sclerosing cholangitis (PSC), 814-15
probucol, 642
proctitis, 797, 798-99
proctosigmoidoscopy, 1250
   in colon cancer screening, 791
professional cramps, 871
professionals, health care, 1241-44
   M.D.s, see physicians
   nurses, 5, 1243-44
   specialties of, 1242, 1252-53
progesterone, 1152, 1156, 1157, 1189
progestin:
   in birth control pills, 171, 1146
   in birth control shots, 173
   in estrogen replacement therapy, 1154
progressive systemic sclerosis, 919-20
prolactin, 943, 1156, 1157, 1162, 1218
prolactinomas, 942-43, 1163
prolapsed (herniated) discs, 904-6, B-1
prostate, 164, 229, 1196
prostate cancer, 1211-12, 1295, B-5
prostate gland, disorders of, 1208, 1209-12, B-5
   acute prostatitis, 1210-11
   chronic prostatitis, 1211
   enlarged prostate (benign prostatic hyperplasia; BPH), 1209-10, B-5
   transurethral resections for, 1210
prostate-specific antigen (PSA) test, B-5
prostatitis:
   acute, 1210-11
   chronic, 1211
prosthesis, 598, 879
prosthetic silicone implants, 1167
prosthodontic treatment, 626-29
   dentures in, 626-29
   osseointegration of teeth in, 628
   partial dentures in, 626
prosthodontists, 604
protein, 253
   for newborns, 38
   for nutrition and weight control in pregnancy, 184
protein-losing enteropathy, 774

protozoa, 1060
protruding ears, 585
Prozac, 1123
pruritus, see itching
pruritus ani, 796
pruritus vulvae, 1170-71
PSC (primary sclerosing cholangitis), 814-15
pseudofolliculitis barbae, 1007
pseudogout, 916
pseudohemophilia, 977
pseudohermaphroditism:
   female, 49
   male, 49
pseudohypertrophic muscular dystrophy, 888
psoriasis, 992-93, C-16
psoriatic arthritis, 913
psychiatrists, 1096
psychoactive substance-induced organic mental disorder, 1129
psychoanalysis, see psychotherapy
psychogenic megacolon, 792
psychological changes, 144
psychological dependence:
   on analgesics, 341, 346
   on marijuana, 342-43, 1134
   on tranquilizers, 340-41
psychological support, 334
psychologists, 1096
psychomotor development, delayed, 106
psychomotor stimulant drugs, 346
psychoses, 1095
   alcohol-induced, 1129
   brief reactive, 1128
   drug-induced, 1129
   postpartum, 217-18
psychosocial development of personality and behavior:
   alcohol use and, 152, 153
   anxiety and, 151
   bizarre behavior and, 150-51
   bonding in, 6, 31-32
   dealing with physical illness and hospitalization, 128-29
   delayed psychomotor development and, 106
   depression and, 154-55
   developmental milestones in, 75-76
   and development of standards, 144-45
   and drug abuse and addiction, 152-53
   eating disorders and, 152
   fighting and, 105
   finger sucking and, 106
   healthy, 30-31, 103-4, 124-26
   hearing disorders and, 106-7
   imagination and, 105
   in infants, 36-37, 75-78
   learning problems and, 106-8
   mental retardation and, 108-9
   negativism and, 104-5
   newborn hearing and, 34-35
   in newborns, 30-37
   panic attacks and, 151
   peer relationships and, 126
   of preschool children, 102-10
   psychological changes, 144
   quarrels and, 105
   reflexes in, see reflexes
   refusal to share toys and, 105-6
   in school-age children, 124-29
   school problems and, 151

sexual abuse and, see sexual abuse
sexuality and, 109, 126-28
sibling relationships and, 77-78, 105-6, 126
sleeping problems and, 36, 37, 77
smoking and, 152
speech and language disorders and, 107
suicide and, 154-55
teenage rebellion and, 150
in teenagers, 143-45, 149-55
thumb sucking in, 106
of twins, 33
in typical 1-year-olds, 103
in typical 2-year-olds, 103
in typical 3-year-olds, 103-4
in typical 4-year-olds, 104
in typical 5-year-olds, 104
vision and, 35-36, 107-8
psychosomatic allergies, 1034-35
psychosomatic illness, 1135-37
   chronic pain disorders, 1136-37
   conversion disorder, 1135
   hypochondriasis, 1135-36
   somatization disorder, 1135
psychotherapy, 1096, 1107, 1124, 1227
   for alcoholism, 334
   for impotence, 1227
   for major depressive disorder, 1124
PTCA (percutaneous transluminal coronary angioplasty), 666
PTHC (percutaneous transhepatic cholangiography), 815
ptosis, 540
puberty:
   menarche and, 1143-44
   premature, 135
   see also teenagers
pubic lice, 1173
pudendal block, 211
pulmonary alveolar proteinosis, 722
pulmonary edema, 660-61
pulmonary embolism, 434, 734-35
pulmonary fibrosis, idiopathic, 722
pulmonary stenosis, 53
pulmonary valve problems, 685
pulse, measurement of, 645
punctures, first aid for, 401
purpura, senile, 244
pursed-lip breathing, 717
pyelonephritis:
   acute, 841-42
   pelvic pain from, 436
pyloric stenosis, 55-56
pyorrhea, 611-12

Q

quackery, 1268-70
   dangers of, 1269
   identification of, 1269-70
   thwarting of, 1270
quadriplegia:
   rehabilitation for, 508
   spastic, 55
quality assurance, autopsies for, 1316
quarrels, 105
quinsy, 595

R

rabies, 382, 395, 1070-71
   vaccination against, 382, 1079

radial keratotomy, 525
radiation:
  cancer from, 1294
  from dental X-rays, 369
  health risks associated with, 376-78
  as pregnancy risk factor, 194
  from radon, 378
  from X-rays, 369, 376-77
radiation esophagitis, 744
radiation therapy, 1297
  for breast cancer, 1165-68
  for cervical cancer, 1181
  for Hodgkin's disease, 970
  for ovarian cancer, 1191
  for uterine cancer, 1184-85
radical mastectomies, 1166
radical prostatectomies, B-5
radioactive iodine, 948
radioactive iodine uptake (RAIU) tests, 1337
radioallergosorbent test (RAST), 1032
radioisotopes, tumor-specific, 1338
radiologic examinations, see X-rays
radionuclide (nuclear) scans, 1336-40
  angiography, 656, 1339-40
  of bones, 1336
  gallium, 1338
  of heart, 656, 1339-40
  indium-labeled white blood cell,
    1338-39
  for infections, 1338-39
  of liver, 1336-37
  of lungs, 1336
  myocardial perfusion imaging, 1339
  RAIU (radioactive iodine uptake) tests,
    1337
  of thyroid, 1337
  tumor imaging, 1337-38
radiotherapy, see radiation therapy
radon, 378
RAIU (radioactive iodine uptake) tests,
  1337
rape, 1230-31
  see also sexual abuse
rashes:
  cradle cap, 14, 68, C-2
  diaper, 14, 29, 68, C-2
  from drool, 69
  from drugs, 996, C-15
  from heat, 69
  infant acne, 69
  in infants, 68-69
  milia, 15, 69, C-2
  prickly heat, 988, C-3
RAST (radioallergosorbent test), 1032
Raynaud's disease, 697-98, C-16
Raynaud's phenomenon, 697
R.D. (registered dietitian), 252
RDS (respiratory distress syndrome), 19-20
reactive hypoglycemia, 929
rebellion, 150
recessive genes, 42-43
rectal bleeding, 797
  first aid for, 403
rectal prolapse, 797
rectal thermometers, 424
  for newborns, 10
rectum:
  cancer of, 789-91
  digital examination of, 1250
  polyps in, 797
  sexually transmitted infection of, 799
  see also anorectal disorders

red blood cells, transfusions of, 980
red bugs (chiggers), 1086-87, C-14
reflexes:
  Babinski, 460
  blink, 4, 34
  gag, 4, 34
  grasp, 33
  of infants, 32-34
  Moro, 33
  of newborns, 4, 19, 32-34
  plantar, 33
  rooting, 33
  sucking, 19, 33
  tendon, 460
  tonic neck, 33
reflex sympathetic dystrophy syndrome,
  887
reflux:
  esophageal (heartburn), 187, 435,
    742-44
  vesicoureteral, 95, 830-31
reflux (spitting up):
  feeding problems due to, 41
  vomiting compared with, 12
refraction problems, 522-28
  astigmatism, 527-28
  blood sugar concentration as cause of,
    527
  farsightedness, 525-26
  nearsightedness, 523-25
  presbyopia, 526-27
  radial keratotomy for, 525
registered dietitian (R.D.), 252
registered nurse (R.N.), 1243-44
regurgitation:
  aortic, 685
  by infants, 63, 67-68, 80
  mitral valve, 680
rehabilitation:
  in cancer treatment, 1304-7
  cardiac, 668
  after coronary angioplasties, 666
  for dislocations, 866
  for fractures, 865
  in home care, 1326-27
  hospices in, 1305-7
  for knee injuries, 877
  for loss of limbs, 880
  for paraplegia, 508
  physical therapy in, 480
  for quadriplegia, 508
  for severed tendons, 868
  after sports injuries, 870
  after strokes, 469
rehabilitation centers, 1257-58
  services provided by, 1257
  settings of, 1257-58
Reiter's syndrome, 913-14
relaxation techniques, 312
renal adenocarcinomas, 847
renal artery stenosis, 851
renal cell carcinomas, 847
renal failure, see kidney failure
renal ischemia, 853
renal lithiasis, see kidney stones
renal tubular acidosis, 833
renal tubule defects, 833
renal vein thrombosis, 852
reproduction, normal, 1214-15
reproductive organs, see sexual organs
reproductive technology, assisted (ART),
  1219-21

reproductive tests, 1346-48
  colposcopy, 1346
  hysterosalpingography, 1346
  laparoscopy, 1346-47
respiratory allergies, 1029-37
  to animals, 1035, 1042-44
  asthma, see asthma
  hay fever, 1029, 1040-41
  to mold, dander, and dust, 1035, 1042-44
  nasal polyps, 1041-42
  to pollen, 1042
respiratory distress syndrome (RDS), 19-20
respiratory system, 700-1
respiratory system, disorders of, 701-36
  acute bronchitis, 702
  allergic alveolitis, 731
  asbestosis, 728-30
  aspergillosis, 712
  aspiration pneumonia, 704
  asthma, see asthma
  atelectasis, 723
  bronchiectasis, 708, 709
  bronchiolitis, 701-2
  bronchitis, 413, 702, 714-15, 733
  bronchoscopy for, 726
  byssinosis, 731-33
  cardiovascular system and, 734-36
  chest percussion for, 709
  chronic bronchitis, 714-15
  chronic lung conditions, 714-27
  coccidioidomycosis, 713
  community-acquired pneumonia, 704
  cor pulmonale and, 735
  cryptococcosis, 712-13
  cystic fibrosis, 709, 720-21
  emphysema, 58, 715-20
  empyema, 710-11
  farmer's lung, 733
  fungal diseases of lungs, 711-13
  Goodpasture's syndrome, 722-23
  heart-lung transplantation in, 736
  heart valve disorders and, 679
  histoplasmosis, 711-12
  hospital-acquired pneumonia, 704
  idiopathic pulmonary fibrosis, 722
  industrial bronchitis, 733
  infections, 701-11, 720-21
  interstitial lung disease, 721-23
  legionnaires' disease, 707
  lung abscesses, 708-10
  lung cancer, 723-27, 1295
  occupational asthma, 731
  occupationally related lung disease,
    728-34
  pleurisy and pleural effusions, 434-35,
    711
  pneumoconiosis, 730-31
  pneumonia, see pneumonia
  pneumothorax, 20-21, 723-24
  postural drainage for, 709
  in premature babies, 19-20
  pulmonary alveolar proteinosis, 722
  pulmonary embolisms and, 434, 734-35
  sarcoidosis, 721
  silicosis, 730-31
  silo-filler's disease, 733-34
  TB (tuberculosis), 705-7
respiratory tract surgery, heart valve disorders and, 679
respite care programs:
  day, 246
  for elderly, 246

restless legs (nocturnal jerking movements), 1115-16
restrictive cardiomyopathy, 686
resuscitation, 406-14
    cardiopulmonary, *see* cardiopulmonary resuscitation
retardation:
    of intrauterine growth, 179
    mental, 108-9, 1099-1100, 1328
    in preschool children, 108-9
retin-A, 999
retinal detachment, 452, 557-59
retinal reattachment, laser therapy in, 558
retinal vessel occlusion, 559-60
retinitis pigmentosa, 561-62
retinoblastomas, 545-46
retinopathy:
    diabetic, 558, 562-63, 930
    in premature babies, 35
retirement, planning for, 222-23
retirement communities, 246
retrograde ejaculation, 1229
retrolental fibroplasia, 35
Reye's syndrome, 484
rhabdomyosarcoma, 888
rhesus (Rh) incompatibility, 192
rheumatic disorders, *see* immunologic rheumatic disorders
rheumatic fever, 677-78
rheumatic fever arthritis, 915
rheumatica, 922
rheumatoid arthritis, 909-11
Rh (rhesus) incompatibility, 192
rhinophyma, 589
rickets, 896-97
    vitamin D-resistant hypophosphatemic, 833
ringworm, B-8
R.N. (registered nurse), 1243-44
Rocky Mountain spotted fever, 1068
rollerskating, 160
Röntgen, Wilhelm Conrad, 377
root canal, 607
rooting reflex, 33
rosacea, 991-92
roseola, 1074-75, C-1
rotational burr angioplasty, B-3
rotavirus, 766-67
rowing machines, 299
royal disease, 976
rubella (German measles), 1074, C-1
    in pregnancy, 52, 191
    vaccination against, 1079
rubeola, *see* measles
runner's knee, 873
running nose, simple remedy for, 589
ruptured eardrums, 572
ruptured ectopic pregnancy, pelvic pain from, 436

S

SAAST (Self-Administered Alcoholism Screening Test), 330
Safe Drinking Water Act (1974), 270
safe sex, 1091
safety, 350-62
    in basement, garage, and utility room, 355
    in bathroom, 240, 354
    in bedroom, 240, 354
    in bicycling, 357

on boats, 361
in car, *see* car safety
for children at play, 99-100, 353
for children on farms, 360
elements (weather) and, 357, 361-62
in entrances and stairways, 240, 354-55
for food, 267-71
with fumes, smoke, dust, and gas hazards, 358-59
with guns in home, 356
of herbal supplements, 355
in hiking and camping, 360-61
in home, 350-56
at home and play for preschool children, 99-100
in hotels, 357-58
for infants, 26-28, 71-72, 352-53
in intense cold, 362
in kitchen, 353-54
with lawn chemicals, 375
lightning and, 361-62
in living room, 354
in medication, drug, and alcohol use, 359
for microwave ovens, 354
in operating farm machinery, 359-60
outside of home, 356-62
poisonings and, 351-52
and protection from noise, 358
and protection from sun, 362
protective eye wear for, 358, 532
seat belts for, 356
in swimming, 361
for toys, 73
for VDT (video display terminal) use, 359
weather conditions and, 357, 361-62
in workplace, 358-59
salicylate sensitivity, 1049
salivary gland disorders, 622-23
    in marijuana, 342
    infections, 622
    salivary duct stones, 623
    salivary duct tumors, 623
Salmonella, 268, 767-68
salmon patches (stork bites), 15
salpingitis, chronic, 1188
salt, sodium, 123, 283-84
    in drinking water, 283
    hypertension and, 283-84, 653
    in pregnancy, 184
    restricting intake of, 653
same-day surgery, 1262-63
saphenous vein bypass, B-3
sarcoidosis, 721, 951
sarcoma, Kaposi's, 1006, C-6
scabies, 1085, C-14
scarlet fever, 1080, C-1
scarring, hypertrophic, 1003
schizoid personality disorder, 1105-6
schizophrenia, 1127-28
schizotypal personality disorder, 1106
school:
    phobia, 133-34
    teenage drug abuse and, 338
    teenagers' problems with, 151
school-age children, 115-36
    accidents and injuries of, 119
    adrenarche in, 135
    attention deficit disorder in, 132-33
    breast abnormalities in, 134
    common concerns about, 118-24
    controlling weight of, 124

in dealing with physical illness and hospitalization, 128-29
dental care for, 118-19
dyslexia in, 131-32
fevers in, 120-21
general care for, 118-19
genital infections in, 136
growing pains in, 119-20
hygiene in, 118
hyperactivity in, 133
immunizations for, 118
infectious diseases in, 118
learning problems in, 129-34
lifestyles of, 119
normal growth and development of, 116-17
nutrition in, 121-24
obesity in, 123-24
premature puberty in, 135
psychosocial development of personality and behavior in, 124-29
recurrent abdominal aches in, 120
recurrent headaches in, 120
regular checkups for, 118
school lunches for, 123
school phobia in, 133-34
sexual abuse of, 127
sexual development and gynecologic disorders in, 134-36
sexual precocity in, 135
sexuality in, 126-28
sibling and peer relationships of, 126
sick, caring for, 120-21
sleep requirements of, 118
speech disorders in, 132
vaginal bleeding in, 134-35
school lunches, 123
sciatica, 905, B-1
scleritis, 543-44
scleroderma, 771, 919-20, C-16
    of esophagus, 744
sclerosis, progressive systemic, 919-20
sclerotherapy, 1001
scoliosis, 906-7
    in teenagers, 159
scorpion bites, 396
scrotum, 164, 1196
scrotum, problems related to, 1199-1202
    hydrocele, 49, 1200
    orchitis, 1201-2
    scrotal masses, 1199
    varicocele, 1201
seamstress's cramp, 871
seasonal affective disorder, 1126-27
seat belts, 356
sebaceous cysts, 990, 1172
seborrheic dermatitis, 989, 990, C-3
seborrheic eczema, 14, 68, C-2
seborrheic keratoses, 1002, C-4
second-degree burns, 404
second-hand smoke, 320-21
second opinions, 1247
second sight, 554
secondary dysmenorrhea, 1148
sedimentation rate tests, 1331
seizure disorders, in pregnancy, 190
seizures, 204-5, 421, 495-99
    emergency treatment of, 421
    febrile, 69, 70, 120-21, 497-98
    without fever, 70
    grand mal, 496-97
    in infants, 69

petit mal, 497
temporal lobe, 498-99
selective serotonin re-uptake inhibitors (SSRIs), 1123
Self-Administered Alcoholism Screening Test (SAAST), 330
self-esteem, lack of, 1095
semen, 164
blood in, 1228
seminal vesicles, 164, 1196, 1216
senile lentigines, 1003, C-4
senile purpura, 244
senile skin, 1000
sensation disorders, 1222-23
senses, A-14, A-15
see also specific senses
sensorineural hearing loss, 573
in infants, 64
in newborns, 35
in preschool children, 107
sensory function, 460
septic shock, 444
emergency treatment of, 444
septum, dislocation of, 21
sequoiosis, 731
serotonin, 1123
severed tendons, 867-68
sexual abuse, 428, 1233-34
of adolescents, 153-54, 1233-34
of preschool children, 109-10
of school-age children, 127
signs and symptoms of, 109-10, 127
susceptibility to, 110, 127
of teenagers, 153-54, 1233-34
sexual assault, 428
sexual changes:
in elderly, 242
in middle years, 228-30
in teenage boys, 139-40
in teenage girls, 140
sexual crises, 1230-34
information on, 1233
physical abuse, 1231-33
rape, 1230-31
sexual abuse of adolescents, 153-54, 1233-34
sexual desire:
in elderly, 242
loss of, 1229
in men, 1229
short- and long-term effects of alcohol on, 329
sexual development and gynecologic disorders, 134-36
adrenarche, 135
breast abnormalities, 134
genital infections in young girls, 136
premature puberty, 135
sexual precocity, 135
vaginal bleeding, 134-35
sexual dysfunction:
arthritis and, 230
atherosclerosis and, 230
blood in semen, 1228
cancer and, 230
desire disorders in women, 1222, 1225
diabetes and, 230
erection abnormalities, 1227-28
heart disease and, 230
impotence, 229, 230, 1225-27
loss of sexual desire in men, 1229
medications and, 230

menopause and, 228, 1153
orgasm disorders in women, 170, 228-29, 1223-25
premature ejaculation, 1228-29
retrograde ejaculation, 1229
sensation disorders in women, 1222-23
in women, 169-70, 1222-25
sexual fantasies, 149
sexual intercourse:
after colostomies, 778
after heart attack, 229, 667
after hysterectomies, 229-30
after ileostomies, 778
pain in, 170, 1188
after pregnancy, 217
after prostate surgery, 229
safe sex in, 1091
sexual organs, A-12, A-13
ambiguous, 49
anabolic steroids and, 345-46
infections of, 136
of men, 163-67, 1196, A-13
of newborns, 47-49
trauma to, 428-29
well-being of, 168-69
of women, 167-68, 1140-43, A-12
sexual partners, health issues of, 1213-34
blood in semen, 1228
erection abnormalities, 1227-28
impotence, 229, 230, 1225-27
infertility, 1215-21
loss of sexual desire in men, 1229
loss of sexual desire in women, 1222, 1225
orgasm disorders in women, 170, 228-29, 1223-25
physical abuse, 1231-33
premature ejaculation, 1228-29
rape, 1230-31
retrograde ejaculation, 1229
sensation disorders in women, 1222-23
sexual precocity, 135
sexuality:
of preschool children, 109
of school-age children, 126-28
sexuality, teenage, 145-49
activity in, 147
contraception in, 148-49
fantasies in, 149
homosexuality in, 149
initiation of, 146-47
masturbation in, 149
parents and, 146
pregnancy in, 147-48, 194
sexuality and sexual dysfunction, 169-70, 1221-29
sexually transmitted diseases (STDs), 1087-92
chlamydial infections, 193, 1088-89
genital herpes, 191, 1090-92, C-13
genital warts, 1092, 1171-72
gonorrhea, 193, 1087-88
medication for, 158, 1088, 1089, 1090, 1092
in men, 1206
in pregnancy, 193
of rectum, 799
safe sex and, 1091
syphilis, 193, 1089-90
in teenagers, 146, 157-58
see also AIDS
shaking palsy, 472

shallow breathing, 20
shift disorders, 1117
Shigella, 768
shin splints, 870-71
shingles, 1011-12, C-13
shock, 441-45
in Addisonian crises, 443
anaphylactic, 444-45, 1029, 1033-34, 1053, 1277
bleeding and, 441-43
cardiogenic, 443-44
in cholera, 443
dehydration and, 443
in electrical injuries, 418
in excessive use of diuretics, 443
first aid for, 418, 441-45
in fractures, 447
in gastroenteritis, 443
heart-related, 443-44
hypovolemic, 441-43
kinds of, 441
recognition of, 442
septic, 444
in traumatic amputations, 450
TSS (toxic shock syndrome), 445
vasogenic, 441
shock (electroconvulsive) therapy, 1124-25
shoes, shopping for, 890
short-bowel syndrome, 772
shots, birth control, 173-74
shoulder:
acute painful, 917
periarthritis of the, 917
sibling relationships:
of infants, 77-78
of preschool children, 105-6
of school-age children, 126
sick sinus syndrome, 670
sickle cell disease, 833-34, 960-62
sideroblastic anemia, 963
SIDS (sudden infant death syndrome), 69-71
sight, sense of, A-14
mechanism of, 522
see also eyes
silicosis, 730-31
silo-filler's disease, 733-34
simvastatin, 642
singer's nodules, 596
sinuses, disorders of, *see* nose and sinuses, disorders of
sinusitis, 590-91
situational depression, 1122-23
Sjögren's syndrome, 920
skateboarding, 160
skating, in-line, 160
ski machines, cross-country, 299
skin, A-1
balanced, 986
bathing basic for, 994
combination, 986
damaged, 999, 1000, C-4
dry, 986, 994, C-15
healthy, 984-85
in middle years, 227-28
of newborns, 5, 25
oily, 986
proper care of, 986
wrinkled, 318, 1000
skin allergies, 1029, 1035-39
angioedema in, 415, 1038-39
atopic dermatitis, 14-15, 989, 1038, C-2

contact dermatitis, *see* contact dermatitis
to heat and cold, 1039
hives in, 415, 994, 1038-39, C-9
skin cancers, 1004-6, C-6
basal cell, 1005, C-6
in elderly, 244
Kaposi's sarcoma, 1006, C-6
screening for, 1295
squamous cell cancer, 1005, C-6
skin disorders, 987-1016, C-1-16
acne, 69, 158, 990-91, C-9
acne rosacea, C-9
actinic keratoses, 1002, C-4
angioedema, 415, 1038-39, C-9
from animal bites, 394-95, 1016
asteatosis, 244, 994, C-15
athlete's foot, 1013-14, C-8
atopic dermatitis, 14-15, 989, 1038, C-2
benign skin tumors, *see* skin tumors, benign
birthmarks, *see* birthmarks
blisters, 360, 1010
boils, 1009
candidiasis, C-2, C-10
canker sores, 617, 1010-11, C-10
carbuncles, 1009, C-12
cellulitis, 1009-10, C-12
chemical peels for, 999
cherry angiomas, 1002, C-4
chloasma patches, 995, C-7
cold sores, 1010-11, C-10
collagen injections for, 999
contact dermatitis, *see* contact dermatitis
cutaneous abscesses, 1016
damaged skin, 999, 1000, C-4
dandruff, 990
dermabrasion for, 999
dermographism, C-9
diaper rash, C-2
dishpan hands, C-3
drug rashes, 996, C-15
dry skin, 986, 994, C-15
in elderly, 244
erysipelas, 1009-10
folliculitis, 1007, C-12
fungal infections, 1012-14, B-2, B-8, C-2, C-8
from gas gangrene, 1016
heart valve disorders and, 679
hives, 415, 994, 1038-39, C-9
from human bites, 1015
ichthyosis, 994, C-15
impetigo, 1007, C-12
infections, *see* infections of the skin
from insect bites, 395-96, 1014-15, 1087, C-14
intertrigo, C-8
itching, *see* itching
jock itch, 1013-14, C-8
keloids, 1003, C-5
lasers for, 1004
lichen planus, 993
liver spots, 227-28, 244, 1003, C-4
lymphadenitis, 1010
lymphangitis, 1010
malignant melanomas, 1005-6, C-6
moles, 1003, C-5
molluscum contagiosum, 1012, C-13
necrotizing subcutaneous infection, 1016
neurodermatitis, 988-89, C-3

nickel dermatitis, C-3
nummular dermatitis, C-15
onychomycosis, C-8
overtreatment dermatitis, 990
perioral dermatitis, C-15
photosensitivity, 998
pigmentary changes, 190, 994-95, C-7
pityriasis rosea, 993, C-15
from poisonous plants, 440
from Portuguese man-of-war stings, 398-99, 1015-16, C-13
in pregnancy, 190
prickly heat rash, 988, C-3
psoriasis, 992-93, C-16
retin-A for, 999
ringworm, C-8
rosacea, 991-92
scleroderma, 919-20, C-16
sclerotherapy for, 1001
seborrheic dermatitis, 989, 990, C-3
seborrheic keratoses, 1002, C-4
senile skin, 1000
shingles, 1011-12, C-13
skin tags, 1002, C-4
solar elastosis, 998-1000
spider veins, 1001, C-15
stasis dermatitis, 989, C-3
sunburn, 414, 996-98
tinea versicolor, C-8
vitiligo, 995-96, C-7
warts, 1003-4, 1092, 1171-72, 1204, C-5
wound infections, 1016
xanthelasmas, 1001, C-11
xanthomas, 1001
skin emergencies:
hives and angioedema, 415
severe contact dermatitis, 415
skin tags, 1002, C-4
skin tests, 1031-32
skin tumors, benign, 1001-4
actinic keratoses, 1002, C-4
birthmarks, 15-16, 1002
cherry angiomas, 1002, C-4
keloids, 1003, C-5
liver spots, 227-28, 244, 1003, C-4
moles, 1003, C-5
seborrheic keratoses, 1002, C-4
skin tags, 1002, C-4
warts, 1003-4, 1092, 1171-72, 1204, C-5
skull, A-5
fractures of, 451
of infants, 63
of newborns, 5, 7, 26
see also head
sleep, dreams in, 1117
sleep disorders, 1112-17
alcohol and, 328
bruxism, 1117
in elderly, 1104-5
feeding problems due to, 41
in infants, 61, 77
insomnia, 1112-14
naps and, 1116
narcolepsy, 1114-15
in newborns, 36, 37
night terrors, 1116
nightmares, 1116
in pregnancy, 188
in preschool children, 90-91
restless legs, 1115-16
shift disorders, 1117
sleep apnea, 1114

sleep clinics for, 1115
sleepwalking, 1116-17
snoring, 1114
sleep patterns:
of elderly, 233
infant behavior and, 37
of newborns, 8
normal, 61, 1112
of preschool children, 85
of school-age children, 118
sleep position, SIDS and, 70
slipped capital femoral epiphysis, 912
slipped discs, 904-6, B-1
small intestine, 740
barium X-rays of, 762-63
disorders of, *see* intestines, disorders of
tumors of, 779-81
smallpox, 1077
vaccination against, 383
smell, sense of, A-15
loss of, 589-90
smoke, 358-59
inhalation of, 419
occupationally related lung disease from, 726, 732
smoker's keratosis, C-10
smoking, 315-24
advertising for, 317
in arteriosclerosis, 691
in bed, 351
cancer and, 1294
chewing tobacco and, 319-20
common health effects of, 317-20
emphysema and, 715-16, 718, 719
hazards of, 317-21
in heart and blood vessel disorders, 639
after heart attack, 668
indoor pollution from, 374-75
lesser-known health effects of, 318
lung cancer and, 723-27
passive, 320-21, 373
in pregnancy, 194-95, 320
reasons for, 316
secondhand, SIDS and, 70
skin wrinkles from, 318
stopping of, 321-23, 719
by teenagers, 152, 320
snacks, in pregnancy, 184
snake bites, emergency treatment of, 398
Snellen charts, 524
snoring, 1114
snuff, 319
snuff keratosis, C-10
sociopaths, 1106
sodium, *see* salt, sodium
soft spots (fontanelles):
in infants, 63
in newborns, 26
soft tissue, disorders of:
carpal tunnel syndrome, 884-85
costochondritis, 434, 883-84
Dupuytren's contracture, 886-87
fibromyalgia, 883
reflex sympathetic dystrophy syndrome, 887
soft tissue injuries, first aid for, 401
solar elastoses, 998-1000
solar keratoses, 1002, C-4
solvents, nephropathy from, 835
somatization disorder, 1135
somatoform pain disorder, 1136-37
somatostatin, 925

sonography (ultrasonography), 180, 683, 1335
sound levels, 573
spasms:
    in back muscles, 900-4
    diffuse, 746
    muscle, 871-72
spastic colon, 782
    minimizing symptoms of, 782
spastic quadriplegia, 55
specific reading disability (dyslexia), 131-32
speech:
    esophageal, 598
    after laryngectomies, 598
    see also communicating; language
speech pathologists, 93
sperm, 164
spermatic cysts, 1199
spermatoceles, 1199
spherocytosis, 962
sphygmomanometers, 649
spider bites, 396, 1014, C-14
spider veins, 1001, C-15
spina bifida:
    occulta, 53-54
    open, 514
spinach, 288
spinal anesthesia, 211-12
spinal cord, 459, A-5
spinal cord, disorders of, 506-9, 514
    cancer, 508-9
    cervical spondylosis, 509
    injuries, 448
    lumbar stenosis, 906
    myelomeningocele, 514
    prolapsed disc, 904-6
    scoliosis, 159, 906-7
    spinal stenosis, 516-17
    spondylosis, 906
    syringomyelia, 514
    from trauma, 448, 506-8
    tumors, 508-9
    see also backaches
spinal stenosis, 516-17
spinal tap (lumbar puncture), 485, 510
spine, osteoarthritis of, 906
spitting up (reflux):
    feeding problems due to, 41
    vomiting compared with, 12
spleen, enlarged, 954
splints, 865
spondylitis, ankylosing, 913, 914
spondylosis, 906
    cervical, 509
sponge baths, 27
sports:
    drug abuse and, 345-47
    menses and, 1150
    protecting eyes in, 532
    see also athletes
sports injuries, 302-4, 867
    rehabilitation after, 870
    teenagers and, 160
sprains, 449, 869-70
    degrees of, 869
    first aid for, 449
    heat vs. cold treatment for, 869
sprue:
    celiac, 285, 770-71
    nontropical, 770-71
    tropical, 771

squamous cell cancer, 1005, C-6
SSRIs (selective serotonin re-uptake inhibitors), 1123
stair-climbers, 299
stairways, safety and, 240, 354-55
standards, development of, 144-45
staphylococcal arthritis, 915
Staphylococcus aureus, food poisoning from, 268
stasis dermatitis, 989, C-3
statins, 642
stationary bicycles, 299
STDs, see sexually transmitted diseases
Stein-Leventhal syndrome, 1191
stenosis, spinal, 516-17
stent, B-3
stereotaxic breast biopsy, 1164
sterilization, of women, 174-75
steroids, anabolic, 345-46, 1278
stethoscopes, 634
sties, 536-37, C-11
stiff neck, fevers accompanied by, 424
stiffness, of back, 902
stings, see bites and stings
stomach, 739-40
    barium X-rays of, 762-63
    knot in, 1118
stomach problems, 751-64
    dilation, 764
    drug-induced, 758-59
    duodenal ulcers, 753-54
    eosinophilic gastroenteritis, 764
    gastric ulcers, 754-55
    gastritis, 758
    gastrostomies in, 747
    indigestion, 752-53
    Ménétrier's disease, 764
    peptic ulcers, 435, 753-57, 760-61
    Zollinger-Ellison syndrome, 757-58, 936
stomach tumors, 761-64
stools, loose, in newborns, 13
stork bites (salmon patches), 15
strabismus, 534-36
    corrective measures for, 535-36
    early recognition of, 534-35
    in infants, 65-66
    optical approaches to, 536
    in preschool children, 90
strains, 868-69, 900-904
strawberry hemangiomas, 15-16, C-2
street drugs, see drugs, illegal
strep throat, contagiousness of, 102
streptococci, group B, 193
streptomycin, 186
stress:
    anal itch due to, 796
    control of, 307-14
    coping with, 311-14
    dealing with, 309-11
    in family conflicts, 310
    fight-or-flight response and, 308
    after heart disease, 668
    in interpersonal conflicts, 310
    in job conflicts, 310
    in marital conflicts, 310
    medical problems affected by, 312
    physical fitness in coping with, 313-14
    post-traumatic, 1121-22
    recognition of, 309
    relaxation techniques for, 312
    relaxed breathing for, 313
stretches, 292, 293

calf, 293
hamstring, 293
thigh, 293
strokes and vascular disorders, 421-22, 461-69, B-2
    aspirin and, 663
    brain attack, 461
    diagnosis of, 564-65
    emergency treatment of, 422
    extradural hemorrhages, 468-69
    eye disorders as warning signs of, 564-65
    hemorrhagic, 462
    hypertension as cause of, 650
    ischemic, 564
    medication for, 463, 565, 663
    rehabilitation after, 469
    signs and symptoms of, 564-65
    subdural hemorrhages, 466-68
    surgery for, 463, 565
    TIA (transient ischemic attack), 463-66
    treatment of, 421-22, 565
    see also vascular problems of bowel
strongyloidosis, 1083
struvite kidney stones, 844
stuttering, 93
suberosis, 731
substance abuse, see alcohol abuse; drug abuse
substance-induced organic mental disorder, psychoactive, 1129
sucking reflex, 19, 33
sudden cardiac death, 674-76
sudden infant death syndrome (SIDS), 69-71
sugar:
    in school lunches, 123
    tooth decay related to intake of, 608
suicides:
    in middle years, 223
    Prozac and, 1123
    of teenagers, 154-55, 1101
    warning signs of, 431, 1125
sulfite sensitivity, 1049
sun exposure:
    cancer and, 373, 1294
    for newborns, 24-25
    safety and, 362
    skin damage from, 1000, C-4
sunburn, 414, 996-98
    emergency symptoms of, 996
    first aid for, 414
    mild, 414
    severe, 414
sunglasses, 532
supernumerary nipples, 49-50
supernumerary teeth, 50
support braces, 879
support stockings, value of, 696
suppositories, administration of, 1275
surgery, 1260-63
    for acne, 991
    for acute appendicitis, 773
    for acute ear infection, 575
    for acute pancreatitis, 819
    ambulatory, 1262-63
    anesthesia for, 1260-62
    for angina pectoris, 659
    for anorectal abscesses, 798
    for aortic aneurysms, 694
    for aortic valve problems, 685
    for arterial embolisms, 694

for arteriosclerosis of extremities, 691-92
for backaches, 904
for bile duct obstructions, 817
for breast cancer, 1166-67
for breast infections, 1161
for bronchiectasis, 708
for cancer, 1297
for carpal tunnel syndrome, 884-85
for cataracts, 554-56, 558
for cervical cancer, 1180-81
for cervical dysplasia, 1179-80
for cervical polyps, 1179
for cervical spondylosis, 509
for chronic ear infection, 575-76
for chronic glaucoma, 551
for chronic lymphocytic leukemia, 966
for chronic myelogenous leukemia, 966
for chronic pancreatitis, 820
for coccidioidomycosis, 713
for colon cancer, 791
for congestive heart failure, 660
coronary artery bypass, 665, B-3
for Crohn's disease, 776-77
for Cushing's syndrome, 938
for developmental disorders of cervix,
   1178
for developmental disorders of teeth,
   617
for developmental disorders of uterus,
   1178
for developmental disorders of vagina
   and vulva, 1169-70
for diabetes insipidus, 945
for Dupuytren's contracture, 887
for dysfunctional uterine bleeding, 1152
for empyema, 710-11
for endometrial polyps, 1182
for endometriosis, 1186
for enlarged prostate, 1210
for epidural abscess, 488
for esophageal tumors, 750
for extradural hemorrhages, 469
for foot ulcers, 894
for fractures, 865
for galactorrhea, 1163
for gallbladder removal, 817
for gallstones, 813
for ganglion, 886
general anesthesia for, 1261-62
for grand mal seizures, 497
for hair replacement, 1018
for hearing loss, 243
on heart valves, 681-82, 684
for heartburn, 744
for hemolytic anemia, 962
for hemophilia, 977
for hernias, 823
for herniated (slipped) discs, 905
for Hodgkin's disease, 970
for hydatidiform moles, 1185
for hydrocele, 1200
for hydrocephalus, 490
for hyperthyroidism, 948
for impotence, 1227
for infective endocarditis, 680
for iron-deficiency anemia, 958
for kidney injuries, 834
for kidney stones, 845
laparoscopic, 817, B-7
local anesthesia for, 1261
for loss of pelvic support, 1176
for lumps in breasts, 1159

for Meniere's disease, 583
for menorrhagia, 1152
for mitral valve problems, 681-82
for multiple myeloma, 973-74
for myasthenia gravis, 481
for nabothian cyst, 1179
for nearsightedness, 525
for non-Hodgkin's lymphomas, 970
for nosebleeds, 587
open-heart, 684
for osteoarthritis, 909
for osteoporosis, 896
for otosclerosis, 578-79
outpatient, 1262-63
for ovarian cancer, 1191
for ovarian cysts and benign tumors,
   1190
own blood used in, 982
for Paget's disease of bone, 898
for pancreatic cancer, 821
for Parkinson's disease, 474
for penile cancer, 1207
for peptic ulcers, 755-56
for pericarditis, 689
for periodontitis, 612
for PID (pelvic inflammatory disease),
   1189
for polycystic ovarian syndrome, 1191
for polycythemia vera, 972
postoperative recovery from, 1262
presurgical evaluation for, 1260
for primary ovarian failure, 1156
for prolapsed discs, 905
for prostate cancer, 1212
for protruding ears, 585
for pruritus vulvae, 1171
for pulled muscles, 869
for pulmonary embolisms, 735
for reattaching severed limbs, 880
regional anesthesia for, 1261
for rheumatoid arthritis, 912
for rickets, 897
same-day, 1262-63
for scrotal masses, 1199
for severed tendons, 868
for sinusitis, 591-92
for slipped (herniated) discs, 905
for spinal cord trauma, 507
for spinal stenosis, 517
for sprains, 870
for stomach tumors, 764
for strabismus, 536
for strokes, 463, 565
for subdural hemorrhages, 468
for temporal lobe seizures, 499
for tendinitis, 882
for tenosynovitis, 882
for testicular cancer, 1203
for testicular torsion, 1198
for thrombocytopenia, 979
for thrombophlebitis, 695
for TIA, 466
for traumatic injury to bladder and
   urethra, 836
for ulcerative colitis, 780
for undescended testicles, 1202
for urine loss problems, 1193, 1208
for uterine cancer, 1183-85
for vaginal cancer, 1177
for vaginal cysts, 1174
for varicocele, 1201
for varicose veins, 697

for vesicoureteral reflux, 830-31
   see also specific procedures
swallowed foreign objects, 90, 427
swallowing problems, 745-48
   achalasia, 745-46
   diffuse spasm, 746
   emergency symptoms of, 745
   pharyngeal diverticula, 746-47
   pharyngeal paralysis, 747-48
   upper gastrointestinal endoscopy for,
      760-61
sweeteners, artificial, in pregnancy, 184
sweets, 122
swelling (edema):
   in pregnancy, 189
   pulmonary, 660-61
swimmer's ear, 570-71
swimming, safety in, 361
swings, 73
sympathomimetic amines, 346
synapses, 458
syncope (fainting spells), 420, 674
   first aid for, 420
   while lying down, 420
   other symptoms in, 420
   while seated, 420
   taking it easy after, 420
syndactyly (webbing):
   of fingers, 45
   of toes, 45-46
syngeneic bone marrow transplants, 967
synovial cyst of the popliteal space, 909
synovial fluid analyses, 1345
syphilis, 1089-90
   in pregnancy, 193
syringomyelia, 514
systemic diseases, eyes in, 562-66
systemic lupus erythematosus, 918-19

T

tachypnea, transient, 20
tags, skin, 1002, C-4
talipes equinovarus, 912
tamoxifen, 1168
tantrums, 92
tapeworm, 1081-82
tartar, 365
   control of, 367-68
taste, sense of, A-15
TB (tuberculosis), 705-7
T cells, 1026-28, 1057, 1299
tear ducts, infections of, 539
tearing problems, 537-39
   dry eyes, 538
   eyedrops for, 538
   infections of tear ducts, 539
   watering eyes, 538-39
teenagers, 137-60, 1101-3
   acne in, 158
   alcohol use by, 152, 153, 332, 1102-3
   anorexia nervosa in, 1102
   anxiety attacks in, 151
   in automobile accidents, 160
   in bicycle accidents, 160
   bizarre behavior in, 150-51
   bulimia nervosa in, 1102
   causes of death in, 154-55
   checkups for, 156-57
   common concerns about, 155-60
   complications in pregnancies of, 194
   contraception used by, 148-49

depression in, 154-55, 1101
development of standards in, 144-45
developmental problems of, 1096-97
drug abuse and addiction in, 152-53,
    338, 1102-3
dysmenorrhea in, 159
eating disorders in, 152
epiphysitis in, 159
hearing disorders in, 160
homosexuality in, 149
infectious mononucleosis in, 158-59
initial sexuality in, 146-47
intellectual growth and development
    of, 142
iron-deficiency anemia in, 159
masturbation by, 149
migraine headaches in, 159
normal growth and development of,
    139
nutrition in, 140-41
panic attacks in, 151
parents and sexuality of, 146
physical growth of, 138-40
pregnancy of, 147-48, 194
psychological and behavioral concerns
    about, 149-55
psychological changes in, 144
psychosocial development of personal-
    ity and behavior in, 143-45, 149-55
rebellion in, 150
school problems in, 151
scoliosis in, 159
sexual abuse of, 153-54, 1233-34
sexual changes in, 139-40
sexuality of, 145-49
smoking by, 152, 320
sports injuries in, 160
STDs (sexually transmitted diseases)
    in, 146, 157-58
suicides of, 154-55, 1101
urinary tract infections in, 159
as victims of violence, 1103
vision problems in, 160
teeth:
    brushing of, 101, 366-67
    deformation of, 614-15
    development of, 602
    developmental disorders of, 614-17
    discolored, 614-15
    grinding of (bruxism), 1117
    impacted, 614
    loss of (avulsions), 624
    misshapen, 614-15
    orthodontic treatment of, 615-17
    osseointegration of, 628
    parts of, 602-3
    of preschool children, 101
    of school-age children, 118-19
    sensitive, 365
    supernumerary, 50
    see also tooth care; tooth decay
teething problems, 89-90
telescopes, 239
television, health news on, 1270
temperature, room, SIDS and, 70
temporal arteritis, 565-66
temporal lobe seizures, 498-99
temporomandibular joint problems,
    624-25
tendinitis, bicipital, 917
tendon reflexes, 460
tendons, disorders of:

Achilles tendinitis, 874
ganglion, 886
severed tendons, 867-68
sprains, 449, 869-70
tendinitis, 874, 882-83
tennis elbow, 872-73
tenosynovitis, 881-82
tennis elbow, 872-73
tenosynovitis, 881-82
tension myalgias, 883
TEP (tracheoesophageal puncture), 598
terminal illnesses, 1310-14
testicles, 163-64, 1196
testicles, problems related to, 1197-1203
    cancer, 1202-3, 1295
    epididymitis, 1198-99
    injuries, 1198
    orchitis, 1201-2
    self-examination for, 1200
    testicular failure, 1198
    undescended testicles, 47-48, 1202
testicular feminization, 1155-56, 1169
testicular torsion, 428, 1197-98
testosterone, 164, 1196, 1197
tetanus, 1070
    vaccination against, 226, 382, 393, 1079
tetracycline, 5, 186
tetralogy of Fallot, 53
thalamus, 458-59
thalassemia, 962-63
thallium exercise scans, 656
thelarche, 134
therapeutic abortions, 199
thermometers:
    oral, 424
    reading of, 1072
    rectal, 10, 424
thigh bruises, 872
thigh stretches, 293
third-degree burns, 404
third nerve palsy, 563
thought disorders, 1127-29
    alcohol-induced psychosis, 1129
    brief reactive psychosis, 1128
    drug-induced psychosis, 1129
    schizophrenia, 1127-28
threadworm, 1083
throat, anatomy of, 569
throat, disorders of, 592-600
    adenoidectomies in, 593
    contact ulcers, 596-97
    epiglottitis, 413, 594-95
    laryngectomies in, 598
    laryngitis, 595-99
    leukoplakia, 597
    lump in throat, 593
    peritonsillar abscesses, 595
    pharyngitis, 592-94
    singer's nodules, 596
    tonsillectomies in, 593
    tonsillitis, 594
    vocal cord polyps, 596
    vocal cord problems, 596-97
throat, swelling of, fevers accompanied by,
    424
throat cancers, 599-600, 1295-96
throat cultures, 1345
    rheumatic fever and, 678
thrombocytes (platelets), 955
    aspirin and, 663
    transfusions of, 981
thrombocytopenia, 978-79

isolated secondary, 978
thrombocytopenic purpura, idiopathic,
    978-79
thrombophlebitis, 694-95
    pain in, 437
    superficial, 694
thrombosis, 463
    deep-vein, 695
    renal vein, 852
thrombus, 461
thrush:
    in newborns, 16
    oral, 618, C-10
thumb:
    arthritis at base of, 885-86
    sucking of, 106
thymine, B-8
thyroid disorders, 945-50
    adenomatous goiters, 946
    cancer, 946
    goiters, 946
    Graves' disease, 563-64, 946, 947
    hyperfunctioning thyroid nodules, 947
    hyperthyroidism, 947-48
    hypothyroidism, 9, 948-50
    lymphocytic thyroiditis, 946
    medullary cancer, 946
    menses and menstrual disorders
        related to, 1156-57
    simple goiters, 946
    subacute thyroiditis, 946
thyroid scans, 1337
thyroid-stimulating hormone (TSH), 947,
    948
thyroid studies, 1331
thyroxine, 945, 947
TIA (transient ischemic attack), 463-66
tic disorders, 475
tic douloureux, 515
tick bites, 396, 398, 1087, C-14
Tietze's syndrome, 434, 883-84
tinea corporis, B-8
tinea cruris (jock itch), 1013-14, C-8
tinea pedis (athlete's foot), 1013-14, C-8
tinea versicolor, C-8
tinnitus, 582
tired feet, 892
tobacco:
    smokeless, 152
    see also smoking
toddler's diarrhea, 87-88
toenails, 1021-23
    disorders of, 893, 1021-23
    healthy, 985
    of newborns, 25
    proper care of, 1023
toes:
    extra, 46
    syndactyly of, 45-46
toilet training, 88-89
tongue disorders, 619-21
    acute glossitis, 619
    discolored tongue, 621
    geographic tongue, 620
    hairy tongue, 620-21, C-10
tonic-clonic seizures, 496
tonic neck reflex, 33
tonometers:
    air-puff, 553
    applanation, 553
tonometry, 553
tonsillectomies, 593

tonsillitis, 594
tooth abscesses, 607-8
tooth avulsion, 453
tooth care, 101, 118-19, 363-70
tooth decay, 370, 605-9
    abscesses in, 607-8
    checkups in prevention of, 603-4
    development of, 605-6
    fillings in, 606-7
    fluoride and, 101, 370, 608-9
    prevention of, 608-9
    root canal in, 607
    sugar and carbohydrate intake related
        to, 608
    tooth sealants in prevention of, 609
    treatments of, 606-7
toothbrushes, selection of, 365
toothpaste, selection of, 367-68
torticollis, 479
total allergy syndrome, 374, 1033
toupees, 227
Tourette's syndrome, 475
touring bicycles, 299
tourniquets, 450
toxic hepatitis, 803
toxic shock syndrome (TSS), 445, 1145-47
toxoplasmosis, 191
toys:
    for infants, 73
    for newborns, 26-27
    refusal to share, 105-6
tracheoesophageal puncture (TEP), 598
traction, 865
tranquilizers, 186
    addictiveness of, 341
    alcohol interactions with, 340
    dependence on, 340-41
    mixing other drugs with, 341
transfusions, blood, 979-82
transient ischemic attack (TIA), 463-66
transitional cell cancer, 847
transplantation:
    of bone marrow, 967-68
    of corneas, 548
    of heart, 688
    of heart-lung, 736
    of kidneys, 857-58
    of liver, 811
transposition of great vessels, 53
transurethral resections, 1210, B-5
transverse presentation, 209
trauma, 445-53
    acoustic, 582
    acute conjunctivitis, 453
    acute glaucoma, 452, 550-51
    acute iritis, 453
    after amputations, 450-51
    arm fractures, 447-48
    bile duct obstruction due to, 814
    to bladder, 835-36
    blood in eye, 452, 544
    central retinal artery occlusion, 452
    from concussions, 451, 490-91
    dislocations, 449
    emergency treatment of, 428-29, 445-53
    to external genitals, 428-29
    eyelid laceration, 452
    to eyes, 452-53, 531-33
    facial, 623-25
    fractures, 445-49
    to head, 451-52, 490-91
    hip fractures, 448-49

    in intracranial hematomas, 451
    leg fractures, 448
    limb fractures, 445-48
    mandibular, 623-25
    orbital cellulitis, 452-53
    pelvic fractures, 448-49
    retinal detachment, 452, 557-59
    from skull fractures, 451
    to spinal cord, 448, 506-8
    sprains, 449, 869-70
    tooth avulsion, 453
    to urethra, 835-36
travel, 379-86
    cholera vaccination for, 383
    diphtheria vaccination for, 382
    hepatitis A vaccination for, 382
    hepatitis B vaccination for, 382
    immunizations for, 380-83
    influenza vaccination for, 382
    jet lag in, 385-86
    malaria vaccination for, 382-83
    medical records for, 381
    medications for, 381
    meningococcal meningitis vaccination
        for, 382
    pertussis vaccination for, 382
    plague vaccination for, 383
    planning for, 380
    pneumococcal pneumonia vaccination
        for, 382
    polio vaccination for, 382
    pregnancy and, 196
    rabies vaccination for, 382
    smallpox vaccination for, 383
    tetanus vaccination for, 382
    typhoid vaccination for, 383
    yellow fever vaccination for, 383
traveler's diarrhea, 383-85
    food poisoning and, 269
    replacing fluids lost in, 384
treadmills, 299
treatment, discontinuing, withholding, or
        limiting of, 1312-13
trench mouth, 612-13
trichinosis, 1082
trichomoniasis, 1173
tricuspid valve problems, 685
trigeminal neuralgia, 515-16
trihalomethanes, 372
tropical sprue, 771
TSS (toxic shock syndrome), 445, 1145-47
tubal ligation, 174-75
    reversal of, 174
tubal pregnancy, 199-200, 436, 1187
tuberculosis (TB), 705-7
tuberculous arthritis, 915
tumor imaging, 1337-38
tumor necrosis factors, 1299
tumor-specific radioisotopes, 1338
tumors, benign:
    angle, 584
    in ears, 571
    of muscles, 888
    ovarian, 1189-90
    of skin, see skin tumors, benign
tumors, malignant, see cancer
Turner's syndrome, 1155
20th century syndrome, 374, 1033
twins, 213
    caring for, 33
2,4-D (lawn chemical), 375
typhoid fever, 383, 1068-70

U

ulcerative colitis, 777-79
ulcerative gingivitis, necrotizing, 612-13
ulcers:
    antibiotics for, 754
    aphthous, 617, C-10
    contact, 596-97
    corneal, 547
    duodenal, 753-54
    on feet, 893-94
    gastric, 754-55
    peptic, 435, 753-57, 760-61
    on vocal cords, 596-97
ultrasonography (sonography), 180, 683,
        1335
umbilical cord:
    clamping of, 5
    percutaneous sampling of, 181
umbilical granulomas, 30
umbilical hernias, 17
umbilicus, care of, 30
unconscious victims, obstructed airways
        in, 408
undereating, 41
underfeeding, 41, 80
undescended testicles, 47-48, 1202
UPJ (ureteral pelvic junction) obstruction,
        828
upper gastrointestinal endoscopy, 760-61
    for cancer, 761
    for esophagitis, 760
    for gastrointestinal tract bleeding, 761
    for peptic ulcers, 760-61
    for swallowing problems, 760
ureteral pelvic junction (UPJ) obstruction,
        828
ureteral stones, pelvic pain from, 436
ureters:
    cancer of, 847-48
    injury to, 834-35
urethra:
    in men, 1196
    in women, 1040-41
urethral disorders, 1192-94
    irritable bladder, 1193-94
    in men, 1204-5, 1208
    noninfectious urethral discharge, 1205
    traumatic injury, 835-36
    urethral stricture, 1205
    urine loss problems, 1193
urethritis, 842-43
    chronic, 1192-93
    in men, 1204-5
    nonspecific, 1174-75
uric acid kidney stones, 844
uric acid nephropathy, acute, 835
urinary incontinence, see incontinence,
        urinary
urinary tract, A-12, A-13
    workings of, 826-27
urinary tract, disorders of:
    acute pyelonephritis, 841-42
    bladder stones, 845-47
    cancer, screening for, 1296
    cancer of bladder, 848-50, 1296
    cancer of ureter, 847-48
    cystitis, 94-95, 159, 436, 842, 1192,
        1203-4
    cystoscopy in evaluation of, 849, 1347
    hematuria in, 403, 832

injury to ureters, 834-35
interstitial cystitis, 842, 1193
traumatic injury to bladder and urethra, 835-36
urethritis, 842-43, 1174-75, 1192-93, 1204-5
urinary tract infections (UTIs), 841-43
in men, 1208
in preschool children, 94-95
in teenagers, 159
urination, frequent, 197
urine, blood in, 403, 832
urine tests, 1347-48
urography, excretory, 829, 1341
urologic surgery, heart valve disorders and, 679
urologic tests:
cystoscopy, 849, 1347
urine tests, 1347-48
urticaria (hives), 415, 994, 1038-39, C-9
urushiol, 1036
uterine bleeding, dysfunctional, 1152
uterine cancer, 1183-85
uterus, 168, 1140-41
uterus, disorders of, 1182-86
adenomyosis, 1186, 1188
developmental, 1178
endometrial hyperplasia, 1183
endometrial polyps, 1182
endometriosis, 1185-86, 1188
fibroids, 1182
hydatidiform moles, 1185
utility room, safety in, 355
utilization review boards, 1267
UTIs, see urinary tract infections
uveitis, 544

V

vaccinations, see immunizations
vacuum extraction deliveries, 211
vagina, 1140-41
developmental disorders of, 49, 1169-70
hygiene for, 1171
middle years changes in, 228
vaginal bleeding, 49
first aid for, 403
in school-age children, 134-35
vaginal cancer, 1176-77
vaginal discharge, 49
vaginal disorders, 1168-77
atrophic vaginitis, 1174
Bartholin's gland abscess, 1172
cysts, 1174
developmental, 1169-70
loss of pelvic support, 1175-76
nonspecific urethritis, 1174-75
nonspecific vaginitis, 1173-74
pain, 1175
pubic lice, 1173
sebaceous cysts, 990, 1172
trichomoniasis, 1173
vaginitis, 1173-74
warts, 1171-72
yeast infections, 1173
vaginal sponges, 173
vaginismus, pain in, 170
vaginitis, 1172-73
Valium, 186
valve repairs, 684

valve replacements, 684
valvuloplasty, heart valve, 681
varicella (chickenpox), 1076-77, 1080, C-1
contagiousness of, 102
in pregnancy, 191
varicocele, 1201
varicose veins, 695-97
in pregnancy, 188
support stockings for, 696
vascular disorders, see heart and blood vessels, disorders of; strokes and vascular disorders
vascular hemophilia, 977
vascular problems of bowel, 794
angiodysplasia of colon, 794
ischemic colitis, 794
mesenteric ischemia, 794
vascular system, 634-35
vasculitis, 921
hypersensitivity, 921
vas deferens, 164, 1196, 1197
vasectomies, 166-67
reversing of, 166
vasoconstrictors, 538
vasodilators, 1280
vasogenic shock, 441
vasovasectomy, 166
VDTs (video display terminals), safety and, 359
vegetables, 261
examples of servings of, 262
intolerance to, 1049
for preschool children, 113
for school-age children, 122
vegetarian diets, 276-77
in pregnancy, 184
veins:
bleeding from, 399
spider, 1001, C-15
varicose, 188, 695-97
venereal disease, see sexually transmitted diseases
venereal (genital) warts, 1092, 1171-72
venography, 1342-43
venous obstruction, acute, 437
ventricles, clicks of, 634
ventricular premature complexes (VPCs), 672
ventricular septal defect (VSD), 52
ventricular tachycardia and fibrillation, 672
vernix, 5, 178
verruca vulgaris, 1003-4, C-5
vertebrae, see spinal cord
vertigo, benign paroxysmal positional (BPPV), 584-85
vesicoureteral reflux, 95, 830-31
Victoria, queen of England, 976
video display terminals (VDTs), safety and, 359
video systems, 239
Vincent's infection, 612-13
violence, adolescents as victims of, 1103
viral arthritis, 915
viral gastroenteritis, acute, 766-67
viral hepatitis, acute, 801-8
viruses, 1059
vision:
of newborns, 7, 35-36
see also eyes
vision disorders, 548-62
acute glaucoma, 452, 550-51

cataracts, 35, 266, 553-56, 558
choroiditis, 560-61
chronic glaucoma, 551-53
colobomas, 560
color blindness, 548-50
double vision, 535
farsightedness (hyperopia), 525
in elderly, 238-39
in endocrine disorders, 562-63, 930
floaters, 561
glaucoma, 452, 550-53, 558, 1250
in infants, 65-66
laser therapy for, 558
macular degeneration, 556-57
nearsightedness (myopia), 523
at night, 239
optic neuritis, 560
optic neuropathy, 560
in preschool children, 90, 107-8
retinal detachment, 452, 557-59
retinal vessel occlusion, 559-60
retinitis pigmentosa, 561-62
spots, 561
in teenagers, 160
see also blindness; eyes, disorders of
vitamin A, deficiency in, 547
vitamin B complex, 642
vitamin B_{12}, deficiency in, 959
vitamin D, 255
vitamin D-resistant hypophosphatemic rickets, 833
vitamin K, 6
vitamins, 254-55
brand name vs. generic name, 285
for infants, 80
myths about, 288
for newborns, 39
for nutrition and weight control in pregnancy, 183-84
organic vs. synthetic, 285
vitiligo patches, 995-96, C-7
vitreous, changes in, 561
vitreous collapse, 561
vocal cord problems, 596-97
voice:
in elderly, 243
proper use of, 597
voice aids:
artificial, 598
after laryngectomies, 598
voice prosthesis, 598
vomiting:
of blood, 12, 402
causes of, 12
feeding problems and, 41, 80
of green bile, 13
home care and, 1325
by infants, 63, 67-68, 80
in minor illnesses, 394
by newborns, 10, 12-13
by preschool children, 85-86
shock and, 442
spitting up compared with, 13
von Willebrand's disease, 977
VPCs (ventricular premature complexes), 672
VQ (lung) scanning, 1336
VSD (ventricular septal defect), 52
vulva, 1140
cancer of, 1172-73
disorders of, 49, 1168-93
vulvovaginitis, 136

W

walkers, 73
walking:
    for cardiovascular fitness, 297-98, 647
    for exercise, 297-98, 647
    by preschool children, 92
warm-ups, 292, 647, 867
warts, 1003-4, C-5
    genital, 1092, 1171-72
    penile, 1204
wasp stings, 396
watchmaker's cramp, 871
water, drinking, 274-75
    asbestos and heavy metals in, 372
    camping and, 360-61
    in ideal diet, 253
    for newborns, 38-39
    nitrates in, 372
    in nutrition, 274-75
    safety of, 270-71
    salt in, 283
    solutions for contamination of, 372
    traveler's diarrhea and, 384
    trihalomethanes in, 372
water safety, 361
wax blockage, 585-86
weaning, 216
wear-and-tear arthritis, 908
weather, safety and, 357, 361-62
webbing (syndactyly):
    of fingers, 45
    of toes, 45-46
weight control:
    curbing appetite in, 278
    daily calorie deficit in, 277
    exercise and, 278-80
    "healthy" weight and, 258-59
    after heart attack, 668
    myths about, 288
    in pregnancy, 182-85
    for school-age children, 124
    setbacks in, 278
    setting pace for, 277-78
    weight loss and, 277-78
weight gain:
    feeding problems and, 42
    by infants, 63-64
    by newborns, 6, 14
    and stopping smoking, 323-24
weight loss:
    backaches and, 304, 902
    myths about, 288
    rates of, 277-78
weight tables, 259
weight training:
    cautions for, 302
    designing program for, 300-301
    establishing routines in, 302
    for fitness, 300-302
    free weights in, 301
    machines in, 301-2
    types of, 300
    weights in, 300-302
weights and measures, 1351-54
Wernicke-Korsakoff's syndrome, 328
wheat intolerance, 1049
Whipple's disease, 771
white blood cells (leukocytes), 955
whiteheads, 990
WHO (World Health Organization), 272,
    1077

whooping cough (pertussis), 1075
    vaccination against, 382, 1079
wills, living, 1248-49, 1312, 1384, 1387-89
Wilms' tumor, 847-48
Wilson's disease, 807
wind, newborn exposure to, 24-25
winter blahs, 1127
winter itch, 994
winter vomiting disease, 767
withdrawal:
    from acute drug intoxication, 431
    from alcohol intoxication, 330, 333,
        429-30
    from drugs in newborns, 22
    from nicotine, 323
    in treating alcoholism, 333
withholding treatment, 1312-13
women:
    in abusive relationships, 1223
    antepartum hemorrhage in, 205
    barrier methods of contraception for,
        172-73
    birth control pills for, 171-72, 1146
    birth control shots for, 173-74
    bleeding in pregnancy of, 178
    breast disorders in, see breast problems
    calendar method of contraception for,
        171
    cervical caps for, 173
    childbearing, 167-75
    common discomforts in pregnancy of,
        186-89
    contraceptive implants in, 173
    diaphragms for, 172-73
    ectopic pregnancy of, 199-200, 436, 1187
    elderly, support of pelvic organs in, 244
    exercise in pregnancy of, 195-96, 296
    failure to reach orgasm in, 170, 228-29,
        1223-25
    false labor of, 208
    family planning for, 170-74
    fertilization of, 176
    genitals of, 167-68, 1140-43, A-12
    gynecologists and, 1142
    hydramnios in, 202-3
    incompetent cervix in, 203
    infectious diseases in pregnancy of,
        191-93
    intrauterine growth retardation in, 179
    IUDs (intrauterine devices) for, 172
    in labor and delivery, 207-14
    laparoscopy in, 1346-47
    medical problems in pregnancy of,
        189-90
    in middle years, 228-30
    mucothermal method of contraception
        for, 171
    mucus inspection method of contra-
        ception for, 171
    natural family planning for, 171
    nutrition and weight control in preg-
        nancy of, 182-85
    painful intercourse in, 170
    pelvic examinations of, 168, 1141-42,
        1250
    placenta previa in, 205-6
    postmaturity in, 206
    preeclampsia and eclampsia in, 204-5
    pregnancy concerns of, 175-96
    pregnancy prevention for, 170-74, 218
    pregnancy tests for, 198
    premature labor in, 201-2

    premature rupture of membranes in, 205
    prenatal care for, 178-79
    prenatal development in, 177-78
    in preparing for pregnancy, 175
    preventing rape of, 1231
    sexual and reproductive health of,
        168-69, 228, 242
    sexual dysfunction in, 169-70, 1222-25
    sterilization operations for, 174-75
    temperature method of contraception
        for, 171
    testing fertility of, 1216-17
    therapeutic drugs in pregnancy of,
        185-86
    travel in pregnancy of, 196
    vaginal sponges for, 173
    young-adult, 167-218
women, health problems of, 1139-94
    absence of periods, 1148-49
    adenomyosis, 1186, 1188
    adrenal gland abnormalities, 1156-57
    atrophic vaginitis, 1174
    atrophic vulvar dystrophy, 1170
    Bartholin's gland abscess, 1172
    bladder disorders, 1192-94
    breast infections, 1160-61
    cancer of the breast, 169, 1163-68, 1250,
        1294, B-4
    cancer of cervix, 1180-81, 1294
    cancer of endometrium, 1295
    cancer of ovaries, 1190-91
    cancer of uterus, 1183-85
    cancer of vagina, 1176-77
    cancer of vulva, 1172-73
    cervical dysplasia, 1179-80
    cervical polyps, 1178-79
    cervicitis, 1179
    cervix disorders, 1177-81
    chronic urethritis, 1192-93
    D and C for, 1151
    developmental disorders of cervix,
        uterus, and fallopian tubes, 1178
    developmental disorders of vagina and
        vulva, 1169-70
    dysfunctional uterine bleeding, 1152
    endometrial hyperplasia, 1183
    endometrial polyps, 1182
    endometriosis, 1185-86, 1188
    fallopian tube disorders, 168-69, 1178,
        1187-89
    fibroids, 1182
    galactorrhea, 1162-63
    genital warts, 1171-72
    heavy periods, 1150-52
    hydatidiform mole, 1185
    hypothalamus abnormalities, 1156-57
    hysterectomies for, 229-30, 1184
    infrequent periods, 1149-50
    intraductal papillomas, 1163
    irritable bladder, 1193-94
    loss of pelvic support, 1175-76
    lumps in breasts, 1158-59, B-4
    menopause, 228, 1153-55, 1294
    menstrual disorders, see menses and
        menstrual disorders
    mittelschmerz, 1148
    nabothian cysts, 1179
    nipple problems, 39, 49-50, 216, 1161-62
    nonspecific urethritis, 1174-75
    nonspecific vaginitis, 1173-74
    orgasm disorders, 170, 228-29, 1223-25
    ovarian abnormalities, 1156-57

ovarian benign tumors, 1189-90
ovarian cysts, 436, 1189-90
ovarian disorders, *see* ovarian disorders
painful menses, 159, 1148
Pap smears in detection of, 168, 1181, 1250
pelvic pain, *see* pelvic pain
PID (pelvic inflammatory disease), 168-69, 1187-89
pituitary abnormalities, 1156-57
PMS (premenstrual syndrome), 1147
polycystic ovarian syndrome, 1191
postmenopausal bleeding, 1155
premenstrual tenderness and swelling of breasts, 1158
primary ovarian failure, 1155-56
pruritus vulvae, 1170-71
pubic lice, 1173
sebaceous cysts, 990, 1172
sensation disorders, 1222-23
sexual desire disorders, 1222, 1225
sexual dysfunction, 169-70, 1222-25
thyroid abnormalities, 1156-57
trichomoniasis, 1173
TSS (toxic shock syndrome), 1145-47
urethral disorders, 1192-94
urine loss problems, 1193
uterine disorders, 1178, 1182-86
vaginal and vulvar disorders, 1168-77
vaginal cysts, 1174
vaginal pain, 1175
vaginitis, 1173-74
vulvitis, 1170
yeast infections, 1161, 1173
see also breast problems; sexual partners, health issues of
workplace:
cancer prevention in, 373
fumes, smoke, dust, and gas hazards in, 358-59, 728-34
medication, drug, and alcohol use in, 358-59
in middle years, 222
noise in, 358, 573
planning retirement and, 222-23
protecting eyes at, 358, 532
safety in, 358-59
shifts in, 222, 359
stress in, 310
VDTs (video display terminals) in, 359
World Health Organization (WHO), 272, 1077
wounds:
to abdomen, 401
first aid for bleeding from, 399-403
infections from, 1016

minor, 392
tetanus immunization for, 393
wrinkles, skin, 318, 1000
writer's cramp, 871

X

xanthelasmas, 1001, C-11
xanthines, 1280
xanthomas, 1001
xenotransplantation, 689
X-linked disorders, 43
X-ray therapy, *see* radiation therapy
X-rays, 1341
arthrography, 1341
barium, 762-63
of bile duct, 815, 816, 1341
cerebral arteriography, 464, 1341
of chest, 657, 1251
dental, 369
in diagnosing coronary artery disease, 657
of esophagus, 762-63
of kidneys, 829, 1341
myelography, 510, 1341
of pancreatic duct, 816, 1341
perspectives on safety of, 1335
radiation from, 369, 376-77

Y

yeast hypersensitivity treatment, 1031
yeast infections, 1161, 1173
yellow fever vaccination, 383
yellow jacket stings, 396
YMCA, 391
yohimbine, 355
young adults, 161-218
antepartum hemorrhage in, 205
barrier methods of contraception for, 172-73
birth control pills for, 166, 171-72, 1146
birth control shots for, 173-74
bleeding in pregnancy of, 178
breast disorders in, 169
calendar method of contraception for, 171
cervical caps for, 173
childbearing of, 167-75
coitus interruptus and, 165-66
condoms for, 165
contraceptive implants for, 173
diaphragms for, 172-73
ectopic pregnancy of, 199-200
exercise in pregnancy for, 195-96
failure to reach orgasm in, 170, 1223-25

false labor of, 208
family planning for, 170-74
female reproductive system of, 167-68
fertilization of, 176
hydramnios in, 202-3
incompetent cervix in, 203
infectious diseases in pregnancy in, 191-93
intrauterine death in, 206
intrauterine growth retardation in, 179
IUDs (intrauterine devices) for, 172
in labor and delivery, 207-14
male reproductive organs in, 163-67
medical problems of pregnancy in, 189-90
mucothermal method of contraception for, 171
mucus inspection method of contraception for, 171
natural family planning for, 171
nutrition and weight control in pregnancy for, 182-85
painful intercourse in, 170
parenthood for, 162-63
placenta previa in, 205-6
postmaturity in, 206
preeclampsia and eclampsia in, 204-5
pregnancy concerns of, 175-96
pregnancy prevention in, 165-67, 170-74, 218
pregnancy tests for, 198
premature labor in, 201-2
premature rupture of membranes in, 205
prenatal care for, 178-79
prenatal development in, 177-78
in preparing for pregnancy, 175
sexual and reproductive health of, 168-69
sexual dysfunction in, 169-70, 1222-25
sexual function of, 164-65
sterilization operations for, 174-75
temperature method of contraception for, 171
therapeutic drugs in pregnancy for, 185-86
travel in pregnancy for, 196
vaginal sponges for, 173
vasectomies for, 166
in years of transition, 162

Z

Zollinger-Ellison syndrome (gastrinomas), 757-58, 936